CUTANEOUS MEDICINE AND SURGERY

An Integrated Program in Dermatology

CUTANEOUS MEDICINE AND SURGERY

An Integrated Program in Dermatology

Volume 2

KENNETH A. ARNDT, MD
Dermatologist-in-Chief
Beth Israel Hospital
Professor of Dermatology
Harvard Medical School
Boston, Massachussetts

PHILIP E. LeBOIT, MD
Associate Professor of Pathology
  and Dermatology
University of California, San Francisco
San Francisco, California

JUNE K. ROBINSON, MD
Professor of Dermatology and Surgery
Departments of Dermatology and Surgery
Northwestern University Medical School
Chicago, Illinois

BRUCE U. WINTROUB, MD
Professor and Chairman
Department of Dermatology
Associate Dean
School of Medicine
University of California, San Francisco
San Francisco, California

W.B. SAUNDERS COMPANY
A Division of Harcourt Brace & Company
Philadelphia • London • Toronto • Montreal • Sydney • Tokyo

W.B. SAUNDERS COMPANY
A Division of Harcourt Brace & Company

The Curtis Center
Independence Square West
Philadelphia, Pennsylvania 19106

Library of Congress Cataloging-in-Publication Data

Cutaneous medicine and surgery: an integrated program in dermatology / [edited by] Kenneth A. Arndt . . . [et al.].

    p.   cm.

  ISBN 0-7216-4852-5

  1. Dermatology. 2. Skin—Surgery. I. Arndt, Kenneth A.
  [DNLM: 1. Skin Diseases—physiopathology. 2. Skin Diseases—therapy. 3. Skin—surgery.
WR 140 C9885 1996]
  RL71.C96 1996
  616.5—dc20

  DNLM/DLC   94-6429

Cutaneous Medicine and Surgery: An Integrated Program in Dermatology   ISBN 0-7216-4852-5
                                                     Volume 1: 0-7216-4853-3
                                                     Volume 2: 0-7216-4854-1

Copyright © 1996 by W.B. Saunders Company.

All rights reserved. No part of this publication may be reproduced or transmitted in any form or by any means, electronic or mechanical, including photocopy, recording, or any information storage and retrieval system, without permission in writing from the publisher.

Printed in the United States of America.

Last digit is the print number: 9   8   7   6   5   4   3   2   1

***Dedicated to the One(s) We Love**

Anne, David, Jennifer, and Pablo; Joseph, Mollie, Marian, Glenn,
Erik, Karen, Jonah, and Tory; William; Marya, Anne, Ben, Molly,
and Max; and to our parents.*

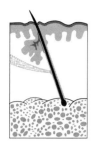

Contributors

DONALD C. ABELE, M.D.
Professor of Dermatology, Medical College of Georgia, Augusta, Georgia.
Lyme Borreliosis

MOHAMED AMER, M.D.
Professor and Chairman, Department of Dermatology and Venereology, Zagazig University, (Dokki) Cairo, Egypt; Professor of Dermatology, Thomas Jefferson University, Philadelphia, Pennsylvania
Parasitic Diseases

HONNAVARA N. ANANTHASWAMY, PH.D.
Associate Professor, The University of Texas M.D. Anderson Cancer Center, Houston, Texas
Molecular Mechanisms of Photocarcinogenesis: The Role of ras and p53 Alterations

ELLIOT J. ANDROPHY, M.D.
Associate Professor of Dermatology, Molecular Biology and Microbiology, Tufts University School of Medicine; New England Medical Center, Boston, Massachusetts
Human Papillomavirus Infection

GRANT J. ANHALT, M.D.
Professor, Johns Hopkins School of Medicine; Johns Hopkins Hospital, Baltimore, Maryland
Pemphigus Vulgaris and the Pemphigus Disease Spectrum

OSCAR E. ARAUJO, PH.D.
Professor of Pharmacy Practice and Dermatology, College of Pharmacy, University of Florida, Gainesville, Florida
Topical Corticosteroid Therapy

JACK L. ARBISER, M.D., PH.D.
Fellow in Dermatology, Howard Hughes Medical Institute, Harvard Medical School; Childrens Hospital, Division of Surgical Research, Harvard Medical School, Boston, Massachusetts
Congenital Alopecias and Disorders of Melanosome Transfer to Hair Follicles

ZSOLT B. ARGENYI, M.D.
Associate Professor of Dermatology and Pathology, Director of Dermatopathology, University of Iowa Hospitals and Clinics, Iowa City, Iowa
Neural Tumors (Other than Tuberous Sclerosis and Neurofibromatosis)

RAYMOND L. BARNHILL, M.D.
Associate Professor of Pathology, Harvard Medical School; Director, Dermatopathology Division, Department of Pathology, Brigham and Women's Hospital, Children's Hospital, Harvard Community Health Plan, Boston, Massachusetts
Melanoma

DONALD V. BELSITO, M.D.
Associate Professor, Dermatology and Pathology, New York University Medical Center; Attending Physician, Tisch Hospital, Bellevue Medical Center, Manhattan VA Medical Center, New York, New York
Basic Photobiology, Phototoxicity, and Photoallergy

TIMOTHY G. BERGER, M.D.
Associate Clinical Professor, University of California, San Francisco; Chief, Dermatology Service, San Francisco General Hospital, San Francisco, California
Syphilis and the Treponematoses; Human Immunodeficiency Virus Infection and the Cutaneous Complications of Immunosuppression

JEFFREY D. BERNHARD, M.D.
Professor of Medicine, Director, Division of Dermatology, University of Massachusetts Medical School, Worcester, Massachusetts
Lichen Simplex Chronicus, Prurigo Nodularis, and Notalgia Paresthetica

ERIC F. BERNSTEIN, M.D.
Assistant Professor, Department of Dermatology, Jefferson Medical College; Director, Jefferson Cutaneous Laser Center, Department of Dermatology, Thomas Jefferson University, Philadelphia, Pennsylvania
The Dermis

KARL BEUTNER, M.D., PH.D.
Associate Clinical Professor of Dermatology, University of California, San Francisco, San Francisco, California; Department of Medicine, Sutter Solano Medical Center, Vallejo, California
Human Papillomavirus Infection

JAG BHAWAN, M.D.
Professor of Dermatology and Pathology, Head, Dermatopathology Section, Boston University School of Medicine, Boston, Massachusetts
Cysts of Epithelial Adnexal Origin

MICHAEL BIGBY, M.D.
Assistant Professor of Dermatology, Harvard Medical School; Assistant in Dermatology and Immunology, Massachusetts General Hospital and Associate in Dermatology, Beth Israel Hospital, Boston, Massachusetts
What Is Normal Skin? Lichenoid Dermatitides (Lichen Planus, Lichen Nitidus, Keratosis Lichenoides Chronica, and Erythema Dyschromicum Perstans)

MIROSLAV BLUMENBERG, PH.D.
Associate Professor of Dermatology and Biochemistry, New York University Medical Center, New York, New York
Keratinocytes: Biology and Differentiation

RAYMOND E. BOISSY, PH.D.
Associate Professor of Dermatology and Cell Biology/Anatomy, University of Cincinnati College of Medicine, Cincinnati, Ohio
Biology of Melanocytes; Vitiligo

JEAN L. BOLOGNIA, M.D.
Associate Professor, Dermatology, Yale University School of Medicine; Attending Physician, Yale–New Haven Hospital, New Haven, Connecticut
Albinism and Other Disorders of Hypopigmentation

KATHRYN E. BOWERS, M.D.
Clinical Instructor in Dermatology, Harvard Medical School; Dermatologist, Beth Israel Hospital, Boston, Massachusetts
Pigmented Purpuric Dermatoses

DOMINIC A. BRANDY, B.S., M.D.
Clinical Instructor, Department of Dermatology, University of Pittsburgh Medical Center; Faculty, St. Francis Central Hospital, Pittsburgh, Pennsylvania
Biochemistry and Control of Hair Growth

KATHRYN L. BRANDY, R.N., C.N.O.R.
Nursing Administrator, Cosmetic Surgery Center, Pittsburgh, Pennsylvania
Biochemistry and Control of Hair Growth

ERIC BREISCH, PH.D.
Assistant Clinical Professor of Pathology, University of California at San Diego, School of Medicine, Department of Pathology, La Jolla, California; Clinical Anatomist, Children's Hospital and Health Center, Department of Pathology, San Diego, California
What Basic Surgical Concepts and Procedures Are Required for the Practice of Cutaneous Medicine and Surgery?

DARRYL M. BRONSON, M.D., M.P.H.
Clinical Professor of Dermatology, University of Illinois, Chairman, Division of Dermatology, Cook County Hospital, Chicago, Illinois
Acrodermatitis Enteropathica

STANISLAW A. BUECHNER, M.D.
Professor of Dermatology, Department of Dermatology, University of Basel, Basel, Switzerland; Former Visiting Clinician at Department of Dermatology, Mayo Clinic and Mayo Foundation, Rochester, Minnesota
Leukemia Cutis

CHRISTOPHER B. BUNKER, M.D., M.R.C.P.
Consultant Dermatologist, Charing Cross and Westminster Medical School, University of London; Chelsea and Westminster Hospital, London, England
Raynaud's Phenomenon

GÜNTER BURG, M.D.
Professor and Doctor of Medicine, Klinikdirektor, University Hospital of Zürich, Clinic of Dermatology, Zürich, Switzerland
Other Cutaneous Lymphomas: B-Cell Lymphoma, Non–Mycosis Fungoides T-Cell Lymphoma, and Adult T-Cell Lymphoma/Leukemia

WALTER H. C. BURGDORF, M.D.
Clinical Lecturer, Department of Dermatology, Ludwig-Maximilian University, Munich, Germany
Cutaneous Reactions to Chemotherapeutic Agents

JEFFREY P. CALLEN, M.D.
Professor of Medicine (Dermatology), Chief, Division of Dermatology, University of Louisville School of Medicine, Louisville, Kentucky
Dermatologic Manifestations of Internal Disease

CHARLES CAMISA, M.D.
Head, Section of Clinical Dermatology, Department of Dermatology, Cleveland Clinic Foundation, Cleveland, Ohio; Associate Professor of Medicine, Ohio State University College of Medicine, Columbus, Ohio
Lichenoid Dermatitides (Lichen Planus, Lichen Nitidus, Keratosis Lichenoides Chronica, and Erythema Dyschromicum Perstans)

S. WRIGHT CAUGHMAN, M.D.
Associate Professor and Director of Research, Department of Dermatology, Emory University School of Medicine, Atlanta, Georgia
Pathways of Inflammation

RINO CERIO, B.S., F.R.C.P., D.P.R.C.PATH.
Consultant and Director of Dermatology, Senior Lecturer in Dermatopathology, The Royal London Hospital and London Hospital Medical School; London Hospital Medical College (University of London), London, England
Tuberculous Mycobacterial Infections of the Skin

MARC D. CHALET, M.D.
Clinical Professor of Medicine/Dermatology, University of California at Los Angeles; Assistant Chief, Dermatology Service, West Los Angeles VA Medical Center; Chief, Dermatology Outpatient Clinic, West Los Angeles, VA Medical Center, Los Angeles, California
Transient Acantholytic Dermatosis

LAWRENCE S. CHAN, M.D.
Assistant Professor of Dermatology and Director of Immunodermatology Unit, Northwestern University Medical School; Staff Physician, Northwestern Memorial Hospital; Staff Physician, VA Lakeside Medical Center, Chicago, Illinois
Epidermolysis Bullosa Acquisita

LIZA W. CHANG, M.D.
Department of Dermatology, Cleveland Clinic Foundation, Cleveland, Ohio
Deep Fungal and Opportunistic Mycoses

PAUL CHU, M.D.
Assistant Clinical Professor of Medicine, Albert Einstein College of Medicine of Yeshiva University, Bronx, New York; Clinical Assistant Professor of Dermatology, State University of New York at Stony Brook, School of Medicine, Stony Brook, New York
Multicentric Reticulohistiocytosis and Sinus Histiocytosis

RICHARD A. F. CLARK, M.D.
Professor and Chairman, Department of Dermatology, SUNY Stony Brook; Chief of Service, University Hospital, SUNY at Stony Brook, Stony Brook, New York
Atopic Dermatitis

JAMES E. CLEAVER, PH.D.
Professor, Laboratory of Radiobiology and Environmental Health, University of California, San Francisco, San Francisco, California
Xeroderma Pigmentosum

CLAY J. COCKERELL, M.D.
Associate Professor—Dermatology and Pathology; University of Texas Southwestern Medical Center; Director HIV-Related Skin Disease Clinic, Parkland Hospital, Dallas, Texas
How Are Abnormalities of the Skin Described? Melanocytic Nevi

BERNARD A. COHEN, M.D.
Associate Professor of Pediatrics and Dermatology, Director of Pediatric Dermatology, Johns Hopkins Children's Center, Johns Hopkins University, School of Medicine, Baltimore, Maryland
Pediatric Dermatology

PHILIP R. COHEN, M.D.
Assistant Professor, Department of Dermatology and Pathology, University of Texas–Houston Medical School; Department of Medical Specialties (Section of Dermatology), University of Texas M. D. Anderson Cancer Center, Houston, Texas
Pityriasis Rubra Pilaris

BRETT COLDIRON, M.D., F.A.C.P.
Clinical Assistant Professor of Dermatology and Otolaryngology, University of Cincinnati; Clinical Assistant Professor of Dermatology, University of Illinois at Chicago, Chicago, Illinois; Clinical Assistant Professor, University of Cincinnati, University Hospital, Cincinnati, Ohio
Neoplasms of the Pilosebaceous Unit; Neoplasms with Eccrine or Apocrine Differentiation

GARY W. COLE, M.D.
Adjunct Professor, University of California, Irvine; Chief, Dermatology Service, Veterans Affairs Medical Center, Long Beach, California
Cutaneous Candidiasis

WILLIAM P. COLEMAN, III, M.D.
Clinical Professor of Dermatology, Tulane University School of Medicine, New Orleans, Louisiana; Chief of Dermatology, East Jefferson Hospital, Metairie, Louisiana
Acne; Hidradenitis Suppurativa; Biology and Disorders of Sweat Glands; Neoplasms of Muscle and Fat, Liposuction Surgery of Fat Hypertrophy

KARI CONNOLLY, M.D.
Assistant Professor of Dermatology and Medicine, University of California, San Francisco, San Francisco, California
Lupus Erythematosus; Chemically Induced Scleroderma

SERGE A. COOPMAN, M.D.
Clinical Consultant, University Hospital of Leuven, Leuven, Belgium; Head, Department of Dermatology, Eeuwfeest Clinic, Antwerpen, Belgium
Photodamage and Photoaging

THOMAS G. CROPLEY, M.D.
Assistant Professor, Division of Dermatology, Department of Medicine, University of Massachusetts Medical Center, Worcester, Massachusetts
Seborrheic Dermatitis

PONCIANO D. CRUZ, JR., M.D.
Associate Professor and Director of Residency Training Program, University of Texas Southwestern Medical Center, Dallas, Texas
Contact Dermatitis

WILLIAM CUNLIFFE, M.D., F.R.C.P.
Professor of Dermatology, Leeds General Infirmary, Leeds, England
Acne

CHRISTOPHER J. DANNAKER, D.O., M.P.H.
Assistant Professor, University of California, San Francisco, Department of Dermatology, San Francisco, California
Responses to Friction and Hydration

ANIR DHIR, M.D.
Resident, Baylor College of Medicine, Houston, Texas
Chancroid, Granuloma Inguinale, and Lymphogranuloma Venereum

STEFAN DOMMANN, M.D.
Doctor of Medicine (Assistenzarzt), University Hospital of Zürich, Clinic of Dermatology, Zürich, Switzerland
Other Cutaneous Lymphomas: B-Cell Lymphoma, Non–Mycosis Fungoides T-Cell Lymphoma, and Adult T-Cell Lymphoma/Leukemia

JEFFREY S. DOVER, M.D., F.R.C.P.C.
Assistant Professor of Dermatology, Harvard Medical School; Chief of Dermatology, New England Deaconess Hospital, Boston, Massachusetts
The Idiopathic Photodermatoses; Cutaneous Effects of Heat and Cold; Sports-Related Skin Disease

PAULINE M. DOWD, M.D., F.R.C.P.
Reader in Dermatology, University College London Medical School; Consultant Dermatologist, University College London Hospitals, London, England
Mechanisms of Pruritus; Raynaud's Phenomenon; Cutaneous Effects of Heat and Cold

JEFFREY C. DRALUCK, M.D.
Consultant, Cook County Hospital, Division of Dermatology, Chicago, Illinois
Acrodermatitis Enteropathica

REINHARD DUMMER, M.D.
Doctor of Medicine (Oberarzt), University Hospital of Zürich, Clinic of Dermatology, Zürich, Switzerland
Other Cutaneous Lymphomas: B-Cell Lymphoma, Non–Mycosis Fungoides T-Cell Lymphoma, and Adult T-Cell Lymphoma/Leukemia

RICHARD L. EDELSON, M.D.
Professor and Chairman, Department of Dermatology, Yale University, New Haven, Connecticut
Cutaneous T-Cell Lymphoma

DRORE EISEN, M.D., D.D.S.
Staff, Mercy Hospitals of Cincinnati, Children's Hospital Medical Center, Cincinnati, Ohio
Disorders of Oral Mucous Membranes

ROKEA A. EL-AZHARY, M.D., PH.D.
Assistant Professor of Dermatology, Mayo Medical School, Rochester, Minnesota; Consultant in Dermatology, Mayo Clinic; St. Luke's Hospital, Jacksonville, Florida
Erythema Elevatum Diutinum and Granuloma Faciale

BONI E. ELEWSKI, M.D.
Associate Professor of Dermatology, University Hospitals, Case Western Reserve University, Cleveland, Ohio
Common Superficial Mycoses; The Dermatophytoses

MERVYN L. ELGART, M.D.
Professor of Pediatrics, Professor of Medicine, and Professor and Chairman, Department of Dermatology, The George Washington University School of Medicine; Chief of Dermatology Service, The George Washington University Hospital; Consultant Dermatologist, Children's Hospital National Medical Center, Washington Hospital Center, Washington, D.C.
Insect Bites and Stings; Myiasis and Tungiasis

PETER M. ELIAS, M.D.
Professor of Dermatology and Vice-Chairman, Department of Dermatology, University of California, San Francisco; Chief, Dermatology Service, Veterans Affairs Medical Center, San Francisco, California
What Does Normal Skin Do?; Staphylococcal Toxin–Mediated Syndromes

ERVIN EPSTEIN, JR., A.B., M.D.
Research Dermatologist, Clinical Professor, Dermatology, University of California, San Francisco, San Francisco, California
Basal Cell Nevus Syndrome

JOHN EPSTEIN, M.D., M.S.
Clinical Professor, Department of Dermatology, University of California, San Francisco, San Francisco, California
Xeroderma Pigmentosum

RONALD J. FALK, M.D.
Associate Professor of Medicine, School of Medicine, University of North Carolina at Chapel Hill; Director, Division of Nephrology and Hypertension, Department of Medicine, University of North Carolina Hospitals, Chapel Hill, North Carolina
Microscopic Polyarteritis, Wegener's Granulomatosis, and Churg-Strauss Syndrome

DAVID S. FEINGOLD, M.D.
Professor and Chairman, Department of Dermatology, Tufts University School of Medicine; Dermatologist-in-Chief, New England Medical Center, Boston, Massachusetts
Skin Infections Caused by Unusual Bacterial Pathogens

JAMES FERGUSON, M.D.
Honorary Senior Lecturer, University of Dundee, Ninewells Hospital and Medical School; Consultant Dermatologist, Ninewells Hospital and Medical School, Dundee, Scotland
The Idiopathic Photodermatoses

JESSICA L. FEWKES, M.D.
Assistant Professor, Harvard University; Associate Dermatologist, Massachusetts General Hospital, Boston, Massachusetts
What Basic Surgical Concepts and Procedures Are Required for the Practice of Cutaneous Medicine and Surgery?

VIRGINIA C. FIEDLER, M.D.
Professor of Dermatology, University of Illinois at Chicago, Chicago, Illinois
Alopecia Areata and Other Nonscarring Alopecias

JO-DAVID FINE, M.D., M.P.H.
Professor of Dermatology, Adjunct Professor of Epidemiology, Schools of Medicine and Public Health, University of North Carolina at Chapel Hill; Principal Investigator, National Epidermolysis Bullosa Registry; Attending Physician, North Carolina Memorial Hospital, Chapel Hill, North Carolina
The Dermoepidermal Junction: Structure, Biochemistry, Antigenicity, and Recent Molecular Biologic Studies; Epidermolysis Bullosa; The Ectodermal Dysplasias

GAYLE FISCHER, M.B., B.S., F.A.C.D.
Lecturer in Dermatology, University of Sydney; Visiting Dermatologist, Royal Alexandra Hospital for Children, Sydney, Australia
Nevoid Conditions of Epidermis, Dermis, and Subcutaneous Tissue

FREDERICK S. FISH, M.D., F.A.C.P.
Assistant Clinical Professor of Dermatology, University of Minnesota, Minneapolis, Minnesota
Fibrous Neoplasms

JAMES E. FITZPATRICK, M.D.
Chief, Dermatology Service, Fitzsimmons Army Medical Center, Aurora, Colorado; Associate Clinical Professor, Department of Dermatology, University of Colorado School of Medicine, Denver, Colorado
Neoplasms of Muscle and Fat, Liposuction Surgery of Fat Hypertrophy

NICHOLAS FIUMARA, A.B., M.D., M.P.H.
Clinical Professor of Dermatology, Adjunct Professor of Dermatology, Boston University School of Medicine; Chief of STD Clinic, New England Medical Center, Boston, Massachusetts
Syphilis and the Treponematoses

FRANKLIN P. FLOWERS, M.D.
Professor, University of Florida College of Medicine, Department of Medicine, Division of Dermatology; Shands Hospital, University of Florida, Gainesville VA Medical Center, Gainesville, Florida
Topical Corticosteroid Therapy

DAVID F. FRETZIN, M.D.
Professor of Pathology, University of Illinois; Attending, Department of Pathology; Michael Reese Hospital and Medical Center, Chicago, Illinois
Sclerema Neonatorum and Subcutaneous Fat Necrosis of the Newborn

BRUCE FREUNDLICH, M.D.
Associate Professor of Medicine, University of Pennsylvania; Chief of Rheumatology, The Graduate Hospital, Philadelphia, Pennsylvania
Scleroderma

ILONA J. FRIEDEN, M.D.
Associate Clinical Professor, Dermatology and Pediatrics, University of California, School of Medicine; Chief, Pediatric Dermatology Clinics, University of California, School of Medicine, San Francisco, California
Blistering and Pustular Disorders of the Neonate; Viral Exanthems; Angiogenesis, Vascular Malformations and Proliferations; Focal Dermal Hypoplasia and Aplasia Cutis Congenita

JOSIAH FRIEDLANDER, M.D.
Research Fellow, Skin Research Foundation of California, Santa Monica, California
Sunscreens

ELAINE V. FUCHS, PH.D.
Amgen Professor of Basic Sciences, University of Chicago; Investigator, Howard Hughes Medical Institute, Chicago, Illinois
The Dermoepidermal Junction: Structure, Biochemistry, Antigenicity, and Recent Molecular Biologic Studies

ANNE-SOPHIE GADENNE, M.D.
Resident in Dermatology, Harvard Medical School, Boston, Massachusetts
Lichenoid Dermatitides (Lichen Planus, Lichen Nitidus, Keratosis Lichenoides Chronica, and Erythema Dyschromicum Perstans)

J. MICHAEL GAGNIER, M.D.
Pathologist/Dermatopathologist, National Health Labs, Inc., Herndon, Virginia
Cutaneous Metastases

EDITH GARCIA, M.D.
Coordinator of Dermatology, Instituto Nacional de Perinatologia (National Institute of Perinatology), Mexico City, Mexico
Parasitic Diseases

MARJAN GARMYN, M.D., PH.D.
Assistant Professor of Medicine, University of Leuven; Supervisor in Dermatology, Department of Dermatology, University Hospital, Leuven, Leuven, Belgium
Photodamage and Photoaging

JOHN K. GEISSE, M.D.
Assistant Clinical Professor, Departments of Dermatology and Pathology, University of California, San Francisco, San Francisco, California
Malignant Neoplasms of Keratinocytes

ROBERT H. GELBER, M.D.
Clinical Professor, University of California, San Francisco; Attending Physician, University of California, San Francisco, Mount Zion Campus, San Francisco, California
Leprosy

ROY G. GERONEMUS, M.D.
Clinical Associate Professor of Dermatology, New York University Medical Center; Director, Laser and Skin Surgery Center of New York, New York, New York
Angiogenesis, Vascular Malformations and Proliferations

RUBY GHADIALLY, M.D.
Assistant Professor in Residence, University of California at San Francisco, San Francisco, California
Granuloma Annulare and Actinic Granuloma

LAWRENCE E. GIBSON, M.D.
Associate Professor of Dermatology, Mayo Medical School; Consultant in Dermatology, Mayo Clinic, Rochester, Minnesota
Erythema Elevatum Diutinum and Granuloma Faciale

RICHARD G. GLOGAU, M.D.
Clinical Professor of Dermatology, University of California, San Francisco, San Francisco, California
Photodamage and Photoaging

NEIL S. GOLDBERG, M.D.
Associate Professor of Dermatology, New York Medical College, Valhalla, New York; Attending Physician, Westchester County Medical Center, Valhalla, New York; Lawrence Hospital, Bronxville, New York; St. Agnes Hospital, White Plains, New York
Neurofibromatosis, Tuberous Sclerosis, and Other Neurocutaneous Disorders

HERBERT GOLDSCHMIDT, M.D.
Clinical Professor of Dermatology, University of Pennsylvania School of Medicine; Hospital of the University of Pennsylvania, Philadelphia, Pennsylvania
Radiation Dermatitis

SANFORD M. GOLDSTEIN, M.D.
Associate Clinical Professor, University of California, San Francisco; Physician, Department of Dermatology, The Permanente Medical Group, San Francisco, California
Urticaria

LOREN E. GOLITZ, M.D.
Professor of Dermatology and Pathology, University of Colorado School of Medicine; Chief of Dermatology, Clinical Director, Ambulatory Care Center, Denver General Hospital, Denver, Colorado
Incontinentia Pigmenti

HARALD GOLLNICK, M.D.
Chairman and Head, Professor, Department of Dermatology and Venereology, Medical Faculty, Otto von Guericke University, Magdeburg, Germany
Acne

ERNESTO GONZALEZ, M.D.
Associate Professor of Dermatology, Harvard Medical School; Dermatologist, Massachusetts General Hospital, Boston, Massachusetts
Pityriasis Rosea

ALDO GONZÁLEZ-SERVA, M.D.
Assistant Professor of Dermatology, Tufts University; Assistant Professor of Pathology, Boston University; Lecturer in Pathology, Harvard University, Boston, Massachusetts; Dermatopathologist, Pathology Services, Inc., Cambridge, Massachusetts
Photodamage and Photoaging

GLORIA GRAHAM, M.D.
Clinical Professor of Dermatology, University of North Carolina, Chapel Hill, North Carolina; Private Practice, Morehead City, North Carolina
Benign Neoplasms of the Epidermis

HUBERT T. GREENWAY, JR., M.D.
Clinical Instructor of Medicine, School of Medicine, University of California, San Diego; Head, Mohs Surgery and Cutaneous Laser Unit, Division of Dermatology and Cutaneous Surgery, Department of Medicine; Director, Cutaneous Oncology, Green Cancer Center, Scripps Clinic and Research Foundation, La Jolla, California
What Basic Surgical Concepts and Procedures Are Required for the Practice of Cutaneous Medicine and Surgery?

ROY C. GREKIN, M.D.
Associate Clinical Professor, Department of Dermatology, University of California, San Francisco, California
Malignant Neoplasms of Keratinocytes

SUZANNE A. GREVELINK, M.D.
Resident in Dermatology, Harvard Medical School, Boston, Massachusetts
Leishmaniasis

RICHARD W. GROVES, M.B., B.S., M.R.C.P.
Instructor in Dermatology, Harvard Medical School; Associate Dermatologist, Brigham and Women's Hospital, Boston, Massachusetts
Poxviruses

ROY GULICK, M.D., M.P.H.
Instructor, New York University School of Medicine;
Director, HIV Research Clinic, Bellevue Hospital,
New York, New York
Herpesvirus Infections

ARNOLD W. GUREVITCH, M.D.
Professor of Clinical Medicine, UCLA School of Medi-
cine; Chief, Division of Dermatology, Harbor-UCLA
Medical Center, Torrance, California
Nummular Dermatitis

SUSAN HADLEY, M.D.
Assistant Professor of Internal Medicine, The Ohio
State University, College of Medicine; The Ohio State
University Medical Center, Columbus, Ohio
*Rocky Mountain Spotted Fever and Other Rickettsial
Diseases*

RUSSELL P. HALL, III, M.D.
Associate Professor, Duke University Medical Center,
Durham VA Hospital, Durham, North Carolina
Dermatitis Herpetiformis

SCOTT M. HAMMER, M.D.
Associate Professor of Medicine, Harvard Medical
School; Director, Research Virology Laboratory, New
England Deaconess Hospital, Boston, Massachusetts
*Rocky Mountain Spotted Fever and Other Rickettsial
Diseases*

JAMES A. HARKER, M.D., M.B.A.
Associate Clinical Professor, University of Illinois Col-
lege of Medicine; Staff Pathologist, Methodist Medical
Center, Peoria, Illinois
*Sclerema Neonatorum and Subcutaneous Fat Necrosis
of the Newborn*

GERALD D. HARRIS, M.D.
Associate Clinical Professor, Department of Surgery,
Northwestern University; Northwestern Memorial-
Chief, Hand Surgery; Children's Memorial, Lutheran
General, Evanston Hospital, Glenbrook Hospital, Co-
lumbus Hospital, Shriner's Hospital, V.A. Lakeside,
Chicago, Illinois
Dupuytren's Disease

DAVID T. HARVEY, M.D.
Resident in Dermatology, Department of Dermatology and Cutaneous Surgery, University of South Florida College of Medicine, Tampa, Florida
Lymphedema

KEN HASHIMOTO, M.D.
Professor and Chairman, Department of Dermatology,
Wayne State University School of Medicine, Detroit,
Michigan
Amyloidosis

JOHN L. M. HAWK, B.SC., M.D., F.R.C.P.
Consultant Dermatologist and Head of Photobiology
Department, St. John's Institute of Dermatology, St.
Thomas' Hospital, London, England
Chronic Actinic Dermatitis

PETER W. HEALD, M.D.
Associate Professor, Yale School of Medicine, Yale-
New Haven Hospital, New Haven, Connecticut
Cutaneous T-Cell Lymphoma

ADELAIDE A. HEBERT, M.D.
Associate Professor of Dermatology and Pediatrics,
University of Texas Medical School, Houston, Texas
Inherited Enzyme Diseases

CAROLINE HIGGINS, M.B., B.S., M.R.C.P.
Registrar (Semi-resident)—Dermatology, Royal Lon-
don Hospital, London, England
Tuberculous Mycobacterial Infections of the Skin

JAN V. HIRSCHMANN, M.D.
Professor of Medicine, University of Washington
School of Medicine; Assistant Chief, Medical Service,
VA Medical Center, Seattle, Washington
*Skin Infections Caused by Staphylococci, Streptococci,
and the Resident Cutaneous Flora*

PETER HOGAN, M.B., B.S., BSCMED., F.A.C.D.
Lecturer in Dermatology, University of Sydney; Visiting Dermatologist, Royal Alexandra Hospital for Children, Sydney, Australia
*Nevoid Conditions of Epidermis, Dermis, and Subcu-
taneous Tissue*

MARIA K. HORDINSKY, M.D.
Associate Professor, Department of Dermatology,
University of Minnesota; University of Minnesota
Hospital and Clinics, Minneapolis, Minnesota
Biochemistry and Control of Hair Growth

THOMAS D. HORN, M.D.
Associate Professor of Dermatology and Pathology,
The Johns Hopkins University School of Medicine;
Associate Professor of Dermatology and Pathology,
Director, Division of Dermatopathology, The Johns
Hopkins Medical Institutions, Baltimore, Maryland
Graft-versus-Host Disease

RENÉE HOWARD, M.D.
Chief Resident, Department of Dermatology, Univer-
sity of California, San Francisco, San Francisco,
California
Viral Exanthems

ARTHUR C. HUNTLEY, M.D.
Associate Professor of Dermatology, University of Cal-
ifornia, Davis, Davis, California
Hirsutism and Its Related Endocrine Disorders

SIMON M. JACKSON, PH.D.
Post-Doctoral Fellow, Department of Biological Chemistry, Center for Health Sciences, University of California at Los Angeles, Los Angeles, California
What Does Normal Skin Do?

J. CHARLES JENNETTE, M.D.
Professor of Pathology and Medicine, School of Medicine, University of North Carolina at Chapel Hill; Director, Nephropathology Laboratory, University of North Carolina Hospitals, Chapel Hill, North Carolina
Microscopic Polyarteritis, Wegener's Granulomatosis, and Churg-Strauss Syndrome

ANTHONY WILLIAM JOHNSON, B.SC. BIOCHEMISTRY, PH.D. BIOCHEMISTRY
Manager, Skin Biosciences, Vaseline Research, Chesebrough-Pond's Research Laboratories, Trumbull, Connecticut
The Care of Normal Skin

TIMOTHY M. JOHNSON, M.D.
Assistant Professor, Department of Dermatology, Otorhinolaryngology, and Surgery (Division of Plastic Surgery), University of Michigan Medical Center, Ann Arbor, Michigan
Melanocytic Nevi

JOSEPH L. JORIZZO, M.D.
Professor and Chairman, Department of Dermatology, Bowman Gray School of Medicine of Wake Forest University, Winston-Salem, North Carolina
Neutrophilic Dermatoses; Sclerosing Panniculitis and Protease Inhibitor Deficiency Panniculitis; Dermatologic Manifestations of Internal Disease

MARSHALL E. KADIN, M.D.
Associate Professor of Pathology, Harvard Medical School; Chief of Hematopathology, Senior Pathologist, Beth Israel Hospital, Boston, Massachusetts
Lymphomatoid Papulosis

DEBRA CHESTER KALTER, M.D.
Late Assistant Clinical Professor, Department of Dermatology, George Washington University, Washington, D.C.; Assistant Professor of Dermatology, Uniformed Services University of Health Sciences, Bethesda, Maryland; Consultant to Walter Reed Army Institute of Research (WRAIR), Washington, D.C.
Nocardiosis and Actinomycosis; Parasitic Diseases

HIDEKO KAMINO, M.D.
Associate Professor of Dermatology and Pathology, Director of Dermatopathology, New York University Medical Center, New York, New York
Fibrous Neoplasms

NEAL KANE, PH.D.
Research Assistant II, Department of Dermatology, University of Iowa College of Medicine, Iowa City, Iowa
Biology and Disorders of Sweat Glands

GWENDOLYN F. KANE-WANGER, M.D.
Research Fellow in Medicine, Harvard Medical School; Department of Rheumatology/Immunology, Brigham and Women's Hospital, Boston, Massachusetts
Reiter's Syndrome

SAGARIKA KANJILAL, PH.D.
Research Associate, The University of Texas M.D. Anderson Cancer Center, Houston, Texas
Molecular Mechanisms of Photocarcinogenesis: The Role of ras *and* p53 *Alterations*

L. MASAE KAWAMURA, M.D.
Clinical Instructor, University of California, San Francisco; Attending, Tuberculosis Clinic, San Francisco General Hospital; Medical Supervisor (TB Compliance Study), Urban Health Study, San Francisco, California
Leprosy

PAUL KECHIJIAN, M.D.
Chief of Nail Section and Clinical Associate Professor of Dermatology, New York University Medical School; New York, New York; Associate Attending Physician, Tisch Hospital and Bellam Hospital; Senior Assistant Attending Physician, North Shore University Hospital, Manhasset, New York
Biology and Disorders of Nails

A. PAUL KELLY, M.D.
Professor of Medicine (Dermatology), Charles R. Drew University of Medicine and Science; Staff Physician, King/Drew Medical Center, Chief, Division of Dermatology, Chairman, Department of Internal Medicine, Los Angeles, California
Pseudofolliculitis Barbae

MAUREEN KEOGH, M.D.
Duke University Medical Center, Durham, North Carolina
Dermatitis Herpetiformis

FRANCISCO A. KERDEL, B.SC., M.B.B.S.
Associate Professor of Dermatology, University of Miami School of Medicine; Attending Physician, Cedars Medical Center, Jackson Memorial Medical Center, Mt. Sinai Medical Center, Miami, Florida
Sarcoidosis

SUZANNE LINSMEIER KILMER, M.D.
Instructor in Dermatology, Harvard Medical School, Boston, Massachusetts; Assistant Clinical Professor, University of California, Davis, Medical School; UC Davis Medical Center, Mercy Hospitals of Sacramento, Sutter Hospitals, Sacramento, California
Tattoos, Foreign Body Granulomas, and Their Treatment

YULY KIPERVARG, M.D.
Resident in Dermatology, University of California, San Francisco, San Francisco, California
Chemically Induced Scleroderma

ROBERT S. KIRSNER, M.D.
Chief Resident in Dermatology, University of Miami School of Medicine, Department of Dermatology and Cutaneous Surgery, Miami, Florida
Sarcoidosis

SUSAN E. KOCH, M.D.
Assistant Professor of Dermatology, Johns Hopkins Medical Institutions, Department of Dermatology, Baltimore, Maryland
Cutis Laxa

JANE E. KOEHLER, M.D.
Assistant Professor of Medicine, University of California, San Francisco, San Francisco, California
Bacillary Angiomatosis, Cat-Scratch Disease, and Bartonellosis

HOWARD K. KOH, M.D., F.A.C.P.
Professor of Dermatology, Medicine and Public Health, Director of Cancer Prevention and Control, Boston University Schools of Medicine and Public Health; Attending Physician, Boston University Medical Center Hospital and Boston City Hospital, Boston, Massachusetts
Melanoma

JOHN Y. M. KOO, M.D.
Assistant Professor, Department of Dermatology, UCSF Medical Center; Director, Psoriasis Treatment Center and Phototherapy Unit, Clinical Research Unit, Psychodermatology Clinic; Vice Chairman, Department of Dermatology, University of California, San Francisco, Medical School, San Francisco, California
Psychocutaneous Disorders

NEIL J. KORMAN, PH.D., M.D.
Assistant Professor, Department of Dermatology, Case Western Reserve University School of Medicine; Dermatologist, University Hospitals of Cleveland, Cleveland, Ohio
Bullous Pemphigoid

LEONARD KRISTAL, M.D.
Assistant Professor, Department of Dermatology, SUNY at Stony Brook; Staff Physician, University Hospital, SUNY at Stony Brook, Stony Brook, New York
Atopic Dermatitis

JOSEPH C. KVEDAR, M.D.
Assistant Professor in Dermatology at Harvard Medical School; Assistant in Dermatology at Massachusetts General Hospital, Boston, Massachusetts
Disorders of Follicular Keratinization

ALFRED T. LANE, M.D.
Associate Professor of Dermatology and Pediatrics, Director of Pediatric Dermatology, Lucile Packard Children's Hospital, Stanford University Hospital, Palo Alto, California
Diaper Dermatitis

JEAN CHRISTOPHE LAPIERE, M.D.
Research Associate, Northwestern University Medical School, Chicago, Illinois
Epidermolysis Bullosa Acquisita

CLIFFORD M. LAWRENCE, M.D., F.R.C.P.
Clinical Lecturer, Newcastle University Medical School; Consultant Dermatologist, Royal Victoria Infirmary, Newcastle, England
Chondrodermatitis Nodularis

ZELMIRA LAZAROVA, M.D.
Visiting Fellow, National Institutes of Health–National Cancer Institute, Dermatology Branch, Bethesda, Maryland
Dermatoses of Pregnancy

PHILIP E. LEBOIT, M.D.
Associate Professor of Pathology and Dermatology, University of California, San Francisco, San Francisco, California
What Basic Surgical Concepts and Procedures Are Required for the Practice of Cutaneous Medicine and Surgery?; Angiogenesis, Vascular Malformations and Proliferations; Cutaneous T-Cell Lymphoma; The Ichthyoses: Disorders of Cornification

KRISTIN M. LEIFERMAN, M.D.
Associate Professor of Dermatology, Mayo Medical School; Consultant, Department of Dermatology, Mayo Clinic and Mayo Foundation; Rochester, Minnesota
Hypereosinophilic Syndrome

ETHAN A. LERNER, M.D., PH.D.
Assistant Professor, Department of Dermatology, Harvard Medical School; Physician, Brigham and Women's Hospital, Boston, Massachusetts
Leishmaniasis

BARRY LESHIN, M.D.
Associate Professor of Dermatology and Otolaryngology, Bowman Gray School of Medicine of Wake Forest University, Winston-Salem, North Carolina
Malignant Neoplasms of Keratinocytes

MOISE L. LEVY, M.D.
Associate Professor of Dermatology and Pediatrics, Baylor College of Medicine; Chief, Dermatology Service, Texas Children's Hospital, Houston, Texas
Genodermatoses

HENRY W. LIM, M.D.
Professor of Dermatology, New York University School of Medicine; Chief of Staff, New York VA Medical Center, New York, New York
Basic Photobiology, Phototoxicity, and Photoallergy

JACK LONGLEY, M.D.
Associate Professor of Dermatology and Pathology, Yale University School of Medicine, Department of Dermatology, New Haven, Connecticut
Mastocytosis

NICHOLAS J. LOWE, M.D., F.R.C.P., F.A.C.P.
Clinical Professor of Dermatology, UCLA School of Medicine; Clinical Professor, UCLA; Consultant, VA Wadsworth-UCLA Medical Center; St. John's Hospital, Santa Monica, Santa Monica Hospital, Los Angeles/Santa Monica, California
Sunscreens

AÍDA LUGO-SOMOLINOS, M.D.
Assistant Professor, University of Puerto Rico School of Medicine, San Juan, Puerto Rico
Small Plaque Parapsoriasis

HARVEY LUI, M.D., F.R.C.P.C.
Assistant Professor, Division of Dermatology, University of British Columbia, Division of Dermatology; Director, Lions Laser Skin Centre; Active Staff, Vancouver Hospital and Health Sciences Centre, Vancouver, British Columbia, Canada
Paraneoplastic Syndromes

GEORGE P. LUPTON, B.S., M.D.
Chairman, Department of Dermatopathology, Armed Forces Institute of Pathology, Washington, D.C.
Cutaneous Metastases

JACKSON MACHADO-PINTO, M.D., M.SC.
Professor of Dermatology, Faculdade de Ciencias Medicas de Minas Gerais; Head, Department of Dermatology, Hospital de Santa Casa de Miserif Cordia, Belo Horizonte, Brazil
Incontinentia Pigmenti

JENNIFER F. MADISON, M.D.
Assistant Professor, Yale University, New Haven, Connecticut
Cutaneous T-Cell Lymphoma

ANTHONY J. MANCINI, M.D.
Resident (PGY-2), Dermatology, Stanford University School of Medicine, Palo Alto, California
Diaper Dermatitis

LAWRENCE W. MARGOLIS, M.D.
Clinical Professor and Vice Chairman, University of California, San Francisco (UCSF), UCSF/Mt. Zion Cancer Center; University of California, San Francisco (UCSF), UCSF/Mt. Zion Cancer Center; University of California, Davis (UCD); Kaiser San Francisco as Consultant, San Francisco, California
Malignant Neoplasms of Keratinocytes

TIMOTHY H. MCCALMONT, M.D.
Assistant Clinical Professor, Departments of Pathology and Dermatology, University of California Medical Center, San Francisco, California
Behçet's Disease; Noninflammatory Small Vessel Occlusive Diseases

S. TERI MCGILLIS, M.D.
Staff Physician, Section of Dermatologic Surgery, Cleveland Clinic Foundation, Cleveland, Ohio
Cysts of Epithelial Adnexal Origin

JOHN A. MCGRATH, M.D., M.R.C.P. (UK)
Post-Doctoral Research Fellow, Department of Dermatology, Jefferson Medical College, Philadelphia, Pennsylvania; Senior Registrar, St. John's Institute of Dermatology; St. Thomas' Hospital, London, England
The Dermis

KEVIN E. MCKENNA, M.R.C.P., M.D.
Clinical Research Fellow (Phototherapy), Department of Dermatology, Beth Israel Hospital, Harvard Medical School, Boston, Massachusetts
Hand and Foot Dermatitis

DAVID I. MCLEAN, M.D., F.R.C.P.C.
Assistant Dean of Research, Head, Division of Dermatology, University of British Columbia; Director of Research, Vancouver Hospital and Health Sciences Center, Vancouver, British Columbia, Canada
Paraneoplastic Syndromes

N. SCOTT MCNUTT, M.D.
Professor of Pathology, Cornell University Medical Center; Chief, Dermatopathology Division, Department of Pathology and Dermatology, New York Hospital, New York, New York
Langerhans Cell Histiocytosis

TERRI LYNN MEINKING, B.A.
Research Assistant Professor, Department of Dermatology and Cutaneous Surgery, University of Miami School of Medicine, Miami, Florida
Parasitic Diseases

JOHN W. MELSKI, M.D.
Associate Professor of Medicine, University of Wisconsin, Madison, Wisconsin; Saint Joseph's Hospital, Marshfield, Wisconsin
Wells' Syndrome

HÉLÈNE DU P. MENAGÉ, B.SC., M.R.C.P.
Senior Registrar, St. John's Institute of Dermatology, St. Thomas' Hospital, London, England
Chronic Actinic Dermatitis

O. FRED MILLER, III, M.D.
Director, Department of Dermatology, Geisinger Medical Center, Danville, Pennsylvania
Dermatomyositis and Polymyositis

LYNNE H. MORRISON, M.D.
Assistant Professor of Dermatology and Active Staff, Oregon Health Sciences University, Portland, Oregon
Cicatricial Pemphigoid

JANET A. MOY, M.D.
Assistant Professor, New York University School of Medicine; NYU Department of Dermatology—Tisch Hospital, Bellevue Hospital Medical Center, Manhattan VA Medical Center, New York, New York
Physical Trauma to the Skin and Emergency Department Dermatology

DANIEL J. NAGLE, M.D.
Assistant Professor of Clinical Orthopaedic Surgery, Northwestern University Medical School; Attending Staff, Northwestern Memorial Hospital; Courtesy Attending Staff, Children's Memorial Hospital; Associate Staff, Shriners Hospital for Crippled Children; WOC Physician, Lakeside Veteran's Administration; Attending Staff, Lutheran General Hospital; Associate Staff, Columbus Hospital, Chicago, Illinois
Dupuytren's Disease

KENNETH H. NELDNER, M.D., M.S. (DERMATOLOGY)
Professor of Dermatology, Texas Tech University Health Sciences Center; University Medical Center, Lubbock, Texas
Inherited Elastic Tissue Malformations

ALBERT J. NEMETH, M.D.
Clinical Assistant Professor, Department of Dermatology and Cutaneous Surgery, University of South Florida College of Medicine, Tampa, Florida
Lymphedema

JAMES R. NETHERCOTT, M.D.
Professor, Departments of Dermatology and Epidemiology, University of Maryland; Attending Physician, Department of Dermatology, University of Maryland Medical Center, Johns Hopkins Hospital, Baltimore, Maryland
Contact Dermatitis

SUSAN NETTESHEIM, B.S. PHARMACY
Manager of Skincare Product Development, The Pond's Institute, Trumbull, Connecticut
The Care of Normal Skin

ERIC D. NEWMAN, M.D., F.A.C.P.
Clinical Assistant Professor, Jefferson Medical College, Philadelphia, Pennsylvania; Associate, Department of Rheumatology, Geisinger Medical Center, Danville, Pennsylvania
Dermatomyositis and Polymyositis

JAMES NIGRO, M.D.
Resident, Department of Dermatology, Medical College of Wisconsin, Milwaukee, Wisconsin
Angiogenesis, Vascular Malformations and Proliferations

JAMES J. NORDLUND, M.D.
Professor and Chairman, University of Cincinnati College of Medicine, Department of Dermatology; Attending, University of Cincinnati Medical Center, Children's Hospital Medical Center, Cincinnati, Ohio
Biology of Melanocytes; Vitiligo

HOPE NORTHRUP, M.D.
Associate Professor, Division of Medical Genetics, Department of Pediatrics, University of Texas Medical School–Houston, Houston, Texas
Inherited Enzyme Diseases

MARIANNE NELSON O'DONOGHUE, M.D.
Associate Professor of Dermatology, Rush–Presbyterian–St. Luke's Medical Center and School; Staff, Rush–Presbyterian–St. Luke's Medical Center, West Suburban Hospital, Oak Park Hospital, Chicago, Illinois
Perioral Dermatitis

SUZANNE OLBRICHT, M.D.
Instructor in Dermatology, Harvard Medical School; Director, Dermatologic Surgery, Beth Israel Hospital, Boston, Massachusetts
Human Papillomavirus Infection

KATIA C. ONGENAE, M.D.
Dermatology Fellow, Boston University School of Medicine, Boston, Massachusetts
Leg Ulcers and Wound Healing

FRANK PARKER, M.D.
Professor of Dermatology, Oregon Health Sciences University, Portland, Oregon
Xanthomas

JAMES W. PATTERSON, M.D., F.A.C.P.
Clinical Professor of Pathology and Dermatology, Medical College of Virginia; Consulting Dermatologist, Johnston-Willis Hospital, Chippenham Medical Center, Retreat Hospital, Stuart Circle Hospital, Henrico Doctor's Hospital, St. Mary's Hospital, Richmond, Virginia
Rheumatoid Nodule, Necrobiosis Lipoidica, and Necrobiotic Xanthogranuloma; Other Forms of Panniculitis

RAFFAELE PENNELLA, M.D.
Resident, Dermatology, University of California, San Francisco, San Francisco, California
Noninflammatory Small Vessel Occlusive Diseases

TANIA J. PHILLIPS, M.D., M.R.C.P.C.
Associate Professor, Boston University School of Medicine; Attending Physician, BUMC–University Hospital, Boston City Hospital, Boston, Massachusetts
Leg Ulcers and Wound Healing

MAUREEN B. POH-FITZPATRICK, M.D.
Professor of Dermatology, College of Physicians and Surgeons of Columbia University, New York, New York
The Porphyrias

SHELDON V. POLLACK, M.D., F.R.C.P.C., F.A.C.P.
Associate Professor of Medicine (Dermatology); Director of Dermatologic Surgery Training, Faculty of Medicine, University of Toronto, Toronto, Ontario, Canada
Rosacea (With Discussion of Electrosurgery)

JEROME POTOZKIN, M.D.
Clinical Instructor, University of California, San Francisco, School of Medicine, San Francisco, California
Malignant Neoplasms of Keratinocytes

FRANK C. POWELL, F.R.C.P.I.
Consultant Dermatologist, Regional Centre of Dermatology, Mater Hospital, Dublin, Ireland
Morphea and Morphea Profunda

JANET H. PRYSTOWSKY, M.D., PH.D.
Irving Assistant Professor of Dermatology, Columbia University, College of Physicians and Surgeons; Assistant Attending, The Presbyterian Hospital in the City of New York, New York, New York
Pityriasis Rubra Pilaris

SHARON S. RAIMER, M.D.
Professor of Dermatology and Pediatrics, University of Texas Medical Branch, Galveston, Texas
Other Histiocytoses of Childhood

RONALD P. RAPINI, M.D.
Professor and Chairman, Department of Dermatology, Professor, Department of Pathology, Texas Tech University, Lubbock, Texas
Perforating Disorders

JAMES E. RASMUSSEN, M.D.
Professor of Dermatology, Professor of Pediatrics, University of Michigan Medical Center; Mott Children's Hospital, University of Michigan Medical Center, Ann Arbor VA Hospital, Ann Arbor, Michigan
Body Lice, Head Lice, Pubic Lice, and Scabies

ALFREDO REBORA, M.D.
Full Professor of Dermatology, University of Genoa, Medical School; Chairman, Department of Dermatology, University of Genoa, Genoa, Italy
The Cutaneous Mucinoses

LUIS REQUENA, M.D.
Associate Professor, School of Medicine, Universidad Autonoma; Associate Chief, Fundacion Jimenez Diaz, Madrid, Spain
Erythema Nodosum and Nodular Vasculitis

STEVEN D. RESNICK, M.D.
Associate Professor of Dermatology and Pediatrics, The University of North Carolina at Chapel Hill; Attending Physician, UNC Hospitals and Clinics (North Carolina Memorial Hospital; North Carolina Children's Hospital), Chapel Hill, North Carolina
Staphylococcal Toxin–Mediated Syndromes

JEAN-EDOUARD REVUZ, M.B.
Professor of Dermatology, Univerité Paris-Val de Marne; Chairman, Department of Dermatology, Hôpital Henri Mondor, Creteil, France
Toxic Epidermal Necrolysis

JUNE K. ROBINSON, M.D.
Professor of Dermatology and Surgery, Departments of Dermatology and Surgery, Northwestern University Medical School, Chicago, Illinois
What Basic Surgical Concepts and Procedures Are Required for the Practice of Cutaneous Medicine and Surgery? Merkel Cell Carcinoma

RANDALL K. ROENIGK, M.D.
Professor in Dermatology; Consultant, Department of Dermatology, Mayo Clinic/Foundation, Rochester, Minnesota
Neurofibromatosis, Tuberous Sclerosis, and Other Neurocutaneous Disorders

GARY S. ROGERS, M.D.
Associate Professor, Boston University School of Medicine; Associate Professor, Departments of Dermatology and Surgery; Director of Dermatologic Surgery, The University Hospital, Co-Director, The Skin Oncology Program, Boston University Medical Center, Boston University, Medical Center Hospital, Boston, Massachusetts
Melanoma

MAUREEN ROGERS, M.B., B.S., F.A.C.D.
Lecturer in Dermatology, University of Sydney; Visiting Dermatologist, Head of Department of Dermatology, Royal Alexandra Hospital for Children, Sydney, Australia
Nevoid Conditions of Epidermis, Dermis, and Subcutaneous Tissue

FRANCO RONGIOLETTI, M.D.
Assistant Professor of Dermatology, University of Genoa School of Medicine, Genoa, Italy
The Cutaneous Mucinoses

THEODORE ROSEN, M.D.
Professor of Dermatology, Baylor College of Medicine; Chief, Dermatology Service, VA Medical Center–Houston, Houston, Texas
Chancroid, Granuloma Inguinale, and Lymphogranuloma Venereum

JEAN-CLAUDE ROUJEAU, M.D.
Professor of Dermatology, Université Paris XII; Service de Dermatologie, Hôpital Henri Mondor Creteil, France
Toxic Epidermal Necrolysis

STUART J. SALASCHE, M.D.
Associate Professor, University of Arizona; University of Arizona Health Science Center, Tucson, Arizona
Biology and Disorders of Nails

JORGE L. SÁNCHEZ, M.D.
Professor and Chairman, Department of Dermatology, University of Puerto Rico School of Medicine, San Juan, Puerto Rico
Small Plaque Parapsoriasis; Melasma and Other Disorders of Hyperpigmentation

MIGUEL R. SANCHEZ, M.D.
Assistant Professor, New York University School of Medicine; Department of Dermatology, New York University, Bellevue Hospital, Manhattan VA Medical Center, Tisch Hospital, New York, New York
Physical Trauma to the Skin and Emergency Department Dermatology

RAMON L. SANCHEZ, M.D.
Associate Professor, Dermatology and Pathology, Department of Dermatology, University of Texas Medical Branch, Galveston, Texas
Other Histiocytoses of Childhood

OMAR P. SANGÜEZA, M.D.
Associate Professor of Pathology, Medical College of Georgia; Staff Dermatopathologist and Pathologist, Medical College of Georgia Hospitals, Augusta, Georgia
What Is Normal Skin?

FUSAKO SATO, M.S.
Research Assistant III, Department of Dermatology, University of Iowa College of Medicine, Iowa City, Iowa
Biology and Disorders of Sweat Glands

KENZO SATO, M.D., PH.D.
Professor of Dermatology, Department of Dermatology, University of Iowa College of Medicine, Iowa City, Iowa
Biology and Disorders of Sweat Glands

DANIEL N. SAUDER, M.D., F.R.C.P.(C).
Professor and Chief of Dermatology, University of Toronto, Sunnybrook Health Science Centre; Director of Dermatology, Sunnybrook Health Science Centre, Toronto, Ontario, Canada
Pathways of Inflammation

MARTY E. SAWAYA, M.D., PH.D.
Assistant Professor of Medicine and Dermatology, University of Florida College of Medicine, Gainesville, Florida
Biochemistry and Control of Hair Growth

MARK JORDAN SCHARF, M.D.
Assistant Professor, Department of Medicine, Division of Dermatology, University of Massachusetts Medical School, Worcester, Massachusetts
Aquatic Dermatology

NORBERT T. SEPP, M.D.
Assistant Professor, Department of Dermatology, University of Innsbruck, Innsbruck, Austria
Angiogenesis, Vascular Malformations and Proliferations

JOHN SEXTON, D.M.D., M.S.D.
Clinical Instructor, Department of Oral and Maxillofacial Surgery, Harvard University; Chief, Oral and Maxillofacial Surgery; Director, Maxillofacial Trauma Service, Beth Israel Hospital, Boston, Massachusetts
Disorders of Oral Mucous Membranes

PHILIP E. SHAPIRO, M.D.
Assistant Professor of Dermatology and Pathology, Yale University School of Medicine; Attending Physician, Yale–New Haven Hospital, New Haven, Connecticut
Albinism and Other Disorders of Hypopigmentation; Cutaneous T-Cell Lymphoma

CHRISTOPHER R. SHEA, M.D.
Assistant Professor of Dermatology and Pathology, Cornell University Medical College; Assistant Attending Dermatologist and Pathologist, Assistant Director, Laboratory of Dermatopathology, New York Hospital–Cornell Medical Center, New York, New York
Langerhans Cell Histiocytosis

NEIL H. SHEAR, M.D., F.R.C.P.C.
Deputy Director, Dermatology, and Director, Clinical Pharmacology, University of Toronto Medical School; Director, Adverse Reaction Clinic, Sunnybrook Health Science Centre, Toronto, Ontario, Canada
Cutaneous Reactions to Drugs and Biologic Response Modifiers

ELIZABETH F. SHERERTZ, M.D.
Professor and Vice Chairman, Department of Dermatology, Bowman Gray School of Medicine of Wake Forest University, Winston-Salem, North Carolina
Inherited Abnormalities of Amino Acid Metabolism

WILLIAM K. SHERWIN, M.D., PH.D.
Clinical Assistant Professor of Dermatology, University of Pennsylvania School of Medicine; Full Active Staff, The Lankenau Hospital, Hospital of the University of Pennsylvania; Philadelphia, Pennsylvania
Radiation Dermatitis

ROBERT H. SHMERLING, M.D.
Assistant Professor in Medicine, Harvard Medical School; Associate Physician, Beth Israel Hospital, Boston, Massachusetts
Temporal Arteritis

JEFFREY K. SHORNICK, M.D.
Affiliate Position, University of Washington; Full Time Staff, Group Health Cooperative of Puget Sound, Seattle, Washington
Herpes Gestationis

JAMES E. SLIGH, JR., PH.D.
Student, Medical Scientist Training Program, Baylor College of Medicine, Houston, Texas
Genodermatoses

KENNETH B. SLOAN, PH.D.
Associate Professor, Department of Medicinal Chemistry, University of Florida, Gainesville, Florida
Topical Corticosteroid Therapy

EILEEN PAZDERKA SMITH, M.D.
Resident, Division of Dermatology, University of Utah Health Sciences Center, Division of Dermatology, Department of Internal Medicine, Salt Lake City, Utah
Linear IgA Bullous Dermatosis

BRUCE R. SMOLLER, M.D.
Associate Professor of Pathology and Dermatology, Director, Dermatopathology, Stanford University Medical School, Stanford, California
Polyarteritis Nodosa; Benign Neoplasms of the Epidermis; Neoplasms of the Pilosebaceous Unit; Neoplasms with Eccrine or Apocrine Differentiation

ALVIN R. SOLOMON, M.D.
Associate Professor of Dermatology and Pathology, Emory University School of Medicine, Atlanta, Georgia
Neutrophilic Dermatoses; Sclerosing Panniculitis and Protease Inhibitor Deficiency Panniculitis; Scarring Alopecia

GYULA SOOS, M.D.
Postdoctoral Associate, Department of Dermatology, University of Iowa College of Medicine, Iowa City, Iowa
Biology and Disorders of Sweat Glands

NICHOLAS A. SOTER, M.D.
Professor of Dermatology, New York University School of Medicine; Medical Director, Charles C. Harris Skin and Cancer Pavilion; Attending Physician, Tisch Hospital–The University Hospital of New York University, New York, New York
Cutaneous Venulitis (Necrotizing Vasculitis, Leukocytoclastic Vasculitis)

OLIVER STANTON, M.D.
Former Fellow, Dermatopathology, University of California, San Francisco, San Francisco, California
Anetoderma

ROBERT S. STERN, M.D.
Associate Professor of Dermatology, Harvard Medical School; Dermatologist, Beth Israel Hospital, Boston, Massachusetts
Psoriasis; Cutaneous Reactions to Drugs and Biologic Response Modifiers

W. P. DANIEL SU, M.D.
Consultant, Department of Dermatology, Mayo Clinic and Mayo Foundation; Professor of Dermatology, Mayo Medical School, Rochester, Minnesota
Morphea and Morphea Profunda; Leukemia Cutis

NEIL A. SWANSON, M.D.
Professor and Interim Chair, Department of Dermatology, Professor, Department of Otolaryngology, Oregon Health Sciences University; University Hospitals and Clinics, Portland VA Medical Center, St. Vincent Hospital, Legacy Hospitals, Portland, Oregon
Melanocytic Nevi

ROBERT A. SWERLICK, M.D.
Associate Professor, Emory University School of Medicine; Emory University Hospital, Grady Memorial Hospital, Veterans Affairs Medical Center, Atlanta, Georgia
Angiogenesis, Vascular Malformations and Proliferations

JORDAN W. TAPPERO, M.D., M.P.H.
Medical Epidemiologist, Centers for Disease Control and Prevention, Atlanta, Georgia
Bacillary Angiomatosis, Cat-Scratch Disease, and Bartonellosis; Human Immunodeficiency Virus Infection, and The Cutaneous Complications of Immunosuppression

STEPHEN F. TEMPLETON, M.D.
Assistant Professor of Dermatology and Pathology, Emory University School of Medicine; Faculty at Emory University Hospital, Atlanta, Georgia
Neutrophilic Dermatoses; Sclerosing Panniculitis and Protease Inhibitor Deficiency Panniculitis; Scarring Alopecia

MICHAEL D. THARP, M.D.
Professor and Vice Chairman, Department of Dermatology, University of Pittsburgh, Pittsburgh, Pennsylvania
Urticaria

KRISTIAN THESTRUP-PEDERSEN, M.D., PH.D.
Professor and Chairman, Department of Dermatology, Marselisborg Hospital, Aarhus University, Aarhus, Denmark
Erythroderma

BRUCE H. THIERS, M.D.
Professor, Department of Dermatology, Medical University of South Carolina; Attending Physician, Medical University Hospital; Chief, Dermatology Service, Veterans Administration Medical Center, Charleston, South Carolina
Pyoderma Gangrenosum

KENNETH J. TOMECKI, M.D.
Department of Dermatology, Cleveland Clinic Foundation, Cleveland, Ohio
Deep Fungal and Opportunistic Mycoses

MARCIA G. TONNESEN, M.D.
Associate Professor of Medicine and Dermatology, State University of New York at Stony Brook School of Medicine; Dermatologist and Director of Phototherapy, University Hospital, Stony Brook, New York; Chief of Dermatology, VA Medical Center, Northport, New York
Erythema Multiforme; Cutaneous Effects of Heat and Cold

JOHAN TOONSTRA, M.D.
Staff Member, Department of Dermatology, Utrecht University, Utrecht, The Netherlands
Jessner's Lymphocytic Infiltrate

JORGE E. TORRES, M.D.
Assistant Professor of Dermatology, University of Puerto Rico School of Medicine, Department of Dermatology, San Juan, Puerto Rico
Melasma and Other Disorders of Hyperpigmentation

TAKASHI TOYOMOTO, M.D.
Postdoctoral Associate, Department of Dermatology, University of Iowa College of Medicine, Iowa City, Iowa
Biology and Disorders of Sweat Glands

DAVID E. TRENTHAM, M.D.
Associate Professor of Medicine, Harvard Medical School; Chief, Division of Rheumatology, Beth Israel Hospital, Boston, Massachusetts
Relapsing Polychondritis

JAIME A. TSCHEN, M.D.
Clinical Associate Professor, Baylor College of Medicine; St. Joseph Hospital, Houston, Texas
Figurate Erythemas

MARIA L. CHANCO TURNER, M.D.
Clinical Professor, George Washington University Medical School, Washington, D.C.; Medical Officer, Dermatology Branch, National Institutes of Health, Bethesda, Maryland
Genital Disorders

JOUNI UITTO M.D., PH.D.
Professor of Dermatology, and Biochemistry and Molecular Biology, Jefferson Medical College; Chairman, Department of Dermatology, Thomas Jefferson University, Philadelphia, Pennsylvania
The Dermis

MARIE-DOMINIQUE VIGNON-PENNAMEN, M.D.
Ancien Chef de Clinique, Paris University; Attachée, Dermatology Department, Hôpital Saint Louis, Paris, France
Subcorneal Pustular Dermatosis

DANIEL WALLACH, M.D.
Maître de Conférences, Paris University; Hôpital Cochin-Tarnier, Paris, France
Subcorneal Pustular Dermatosis

KALMAN L. WATSKY, M.D.
Assistant Clinical Professor, Yale University School of Medicine; Section Chief of Dermatology, Hospital of Saint Raphael, New Haven, Connecticut
Cutaneous Ossification and Calcification

ROBERT A. WEISS, M.D.
Assistant Professor, Department of Dermatology, Johns Hopkins University School of Medicine, Baltimore, Maryland
Phlebology and Sclerotherapy

DALE R. WESTROM, M.D., PH.D.
Assistant Clinical Professor, University of California, San Francisco; Moffit Hospital, San Francisco, California; Memorial Hospital Santa Rosa, California; Yountville Veterans Hospital, Yountville, California; Warrack Hospital, Santa Rosa, California
The Zoonoses

RONALD G. WHEELAND, M.D.
Professor and Chairman, Department of Dermatology, University of New Mexico; University of New Mexico Health Sciences Center, Albuquerque, New Mexico
Keloids and Hypertrophic Scars

CLIFTON R. WHITE, JR., M.D.
Professor of Dermatology and Pathology, Oregon Health Sciences University; Associate Chairman, Department of Dermatology, Oregon Health Sciences University; Chief, Dermatology Service, Portland Veterans Affairs Hospital, Portland, Oregon
What Is Normal Skin?

WAIN L. WHITE, M.D.
Associate Professor of Pathology and Dermatology, Bowman Gray School of Medicine, Wake Forest University, Winston-Salem, North Carolina
Malignant Neoplasms of Keratinocytes

MARGOT WHITFELD, M.B., B.S., D.T.M.&H., F.A.C.D.
Fellow in Dermatology, University of California, San Francisco, San Francisco, California
Syphilis and the Treponematoses

THOMAS A. WIEDRICH, M.D.
Assistant Professor of Clinical Surgery, Northwestern University Medical School; Attending Physician, Northwestern Memorial Hospital; Attending Physician, Children's Memorial Hospital; Consultant, Shriners Hospital for Crippled Children, Chicago Unit, Chicago, Illinois
Dupuytren's Disease

JONATHAN K. WILKIN, M.D.
Professor, Departments of Pharmacology and Medicine; Director, Division of Dermatology, Ohio State University; Ohio State University Medical Center, Columbus, Ohio
Erythromelalgia, Erythermalgia, and Flushing

MARY L. WILLIAMS, M.D.
Adjunct Professor of Dermatology and Pediatrics, University of California, San Francisco; Chief, Pediatric Dermatology Service, University of California, San Francisco, San Francisco, California
The Ichthyoses: Disorders of Cornification

KAREN WISS, M.D.
Assistant Professor of Medicine and Pediatrics, University of Massachusetts Medical School; Director of Pediatric Dermatology, University of Massachusetts Medical Center, Worcester, Massachusetts
Lichen Striatus

GARY S. WOOD, M.D.
Associate Professor of Dermatology and Pathology, Case Western Reserve University; Chief, Dermatology Service, Veterans Affairs Medical Center, Cleveland, Ohio
Pityriasis Lichenoides; Cutaneous Lymphoid Hyperplasia

DAVID T. WOODLEY, M.D.
Professor and Chairman, Department of Dermatology, Northwestern University; Dermatologist-in-Chief, Northwestern Memorial Hospital, Chicago, Illinois
Epidermolysis Bullosa Acquisita

JOHN T. WOOSLEY, M.D., PH.D.
Assistant Professor of Pathology and Dermatology, School of Medicine, University of North Carolina at Chapel Hill; Associate Director, Surgical Pathology, Director, Dermatopathology, University of North Carolina Hospitals, Chapel Hill, North Carolina
Microscopic Polyarteritis, Wegener's Granulomatosis, and Churg-Strauss Syndrome

PAUL D. WORTMAN, M.D.
Assistant Professor, Department of Dermatology, Bowman Gray School of Medicine, Wake Forest University Medical Center, Winston-Salem, North Carolina
Nocardiosis and Actinomycosis

J. TIMOTHY WRIGHT, D.D.S., M.S.
Associate Professor, Department of Pediatric Dentistry, School of Dentistry, University of North Carolina at Chapel Hill, Chapel Hill, North Carolina
The Ectodermal Dysplasias

JESSICA P. WU, M.D.
Resident Instructor, University of Southern California School of Medicine; Resident, Los Angeles County–University of Southern California Medical Center, Los Angeles, California
Psoriasis

KIM B. YANCEY, M.D.
Adjunct Associate Professor, Department of Dermatology, Uniformed Services University of the Health Sciences; Senior Investigator, Dermatology Branch, National Cancer Institute, National Institutes of Health, Bethesda, Maryland
Dermatoses of Pregnancy

JOHN M. YARBOROUGH, M.D.
Clinical Professor of Dermatology, Tulane University School of Medicine, New Orleans, Louisiana
Acne

EVARISTO SÁNCHEZ YUS, M.D.
Professor of Dermatology, School of Medicine, Universidad Complutense; Associate Chief, Hospital Universitario San Carlos, Madrid, Spain
Erythema Nodosum and Nodular Vasculitis

JOHN J. ZONE, M.D.
Chief, Dermatology Section, Veterans Administration Medical Center, Salt Lake City, Utah
Linear IgA Bullous Dermatosis

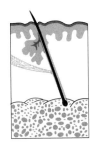

Preface

The last decade has witnessed an explosion in biologic sciences unequaled in human history. These events have revolutionized our understanding of cutaneous biology and disease. Dermatologists have applied this knowledge to the treatment of cutaneous diseases, expanding the range of therapeutic choices to include new medical and surgical techniques. Just as there have been extraordinary advances in knowledge, so should there be an imaginative educational program that synthesizes and updates this information for the clinician.

The background and experiences of each of the four editors represent the broad scope of dermatology. The purpose of this program is to present cutaneous medicine and surgery as an integration of clinical dermatology, dermatopathology, mechanisms of disease, and medical and surgical therapies. In an effort to do this, we have organized dermatology into practical categories, then translated each into a question that will help guide the reader to a rational diagnosis and management. Additional tables of contents will help guide the reader who has a special interest in medical and surgical therapies or basic sciences to pertinent information. The organization not only summarizes current understanding of the etiology and presentation of dermatologic diseases, but also reflects the editors' vision of the evolution of the field.

The main text in this program is composed of contributions from numerous emerging and established leaders in the field. In many cases, clinical dermatologists, dermatopathologists, and dermatologic surgeons collaborated on single chapters in order to bring their combined expertise to the subject matter. In clinical areas where biologic sciences have had the greatest impact, several authors have been invited in order to integrate their knowledge and develop a comprehensive and balanced presentation for the reader. The sections on pathology have been written either by a dermatopathologist or in collaboration with one of the editors, who is a dermatopathologist. Photos and illustrations have been carefully selected by the contributors and editors. Though this book contains an abundance of illustrative material, the reader will note that only when necessary do photos appear in color. This has been done purposely, in an effort to maintain an attractive price on the book and to reach as many health care providers as possible with this program. Should the reader be interested in color figures, there are, of course, several excellent atlases—some of them electronic—currently available.

This text is the "flagship" for an entire educational program. Each component is intended to enhance the clinician's understanding and practical application of cutaneous medicine and surgery. Along with the flagship text, the program consists of a series of related books. Publishing simultaneously with the main text are the following books, with additional projects underway:

Atlas of Cutaneous Surgery. This text/atlas will enable clinicians to fully explore the range of cutaneous surgical techniques, including excisional surgery and aesthetic reconstructive surgery. These surgical procedures are illustrated in color and described in detail. Case studies are provided, many including long-term results. Readers of the flagship text are referred to the atlas whenever possible for expanded coverage of these surgical methods.

Cutaneous Medicine and Surgery: Self-Assessment and Review. A workbook to test your comprehension of the scope of dermatology, this book may be used by clinicians and residents for board review, recertification, and self-assessment. It contains more than 2000 board-style questions, along with rationales for determining each answer and a detailed discussion of the topic in question. Each chapter is keyed to the relevant section in *Cutaneous Medicine and Surgery* for further information.

Cutaneous Medicine and Surgery: Pocket Guide. Designed to contain key elements of the flagship text that are pertinent to clinical practice, such as differential diagnosis and therapy, this pocket-size book will be an excellent resource for postgraduate trainees, medical students, and other health care professionals.

We are delighted to have been able to participate in the growth and evolution of cutaneous medicine and surgery. We have certainly learned a great deal while editing this program, and we hope that patient care will be improved by those health care providers who gain knowledge through the use of it. The completion of this project would not have been possible without the expertise and tireless devotion to excellence of the editors, Judith Fletcher and Dolores Meloni. We also wish to thank the production staff of WB Saunders for their help and guidance throughout the production process.

KENNETH A. ARNDT
PHILIP E. LEBOIT
JUNE K. ROBINSON
BRUCE U. WINTROUB

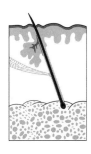

Contents

Color plates follow page xl.

VOLUME 1

section one

What Fundamental Information Is Necessary to Understand Cutaneous Medicine and Surgery? 1

chapter 1
What Is Normal Skin?. 3
CLIFTON R. WHITE, JR., MICHAEL BIGBY, and
OMAR P. SANGÜEZA

chapter 2
What Does Normal Skin Do? 46
PETER M. ELIAS and SIMON M. JACKSON

chapter 3
Keratinocytes: Biology and
Differentiation 58
MIROSLAV BLUMENBERG

chapter 4
The Care of Normal Skin 75
ANTHONY WILLIAM JOHNSON and
SUSAN NETTESHEIM

chapter 5
How Are Abnormalities of the Skin
Described? 84
CLAY J. COCKERELL

chapter 6
What Basic Surgical Concepts and
Procedures Are Required for the
Practice of Cutaneous Medicine and
Surgery?. 111
  Fundamental Anatomy, 111
    Eric Breisch and Hubert T. Greenway, Jr.

  Biopsy Techniques: Description and Proper
  Use, 120
    June K. Robinson and Philip E. LeBoit

  Antisepsis, Anesthesia, Hemostasis, and
  Suture Placement, 128
    Jessica L. Fewkes

section two

What Disorders Present with Inflamed Skin?. 139

*Mechanisms, Symptoms, and Treatment of
Inflammation* 141

chapter 7
Pathways of Inflammation 141
S. WRIGHT CAUGHMAN and DANIEL N. SAUDER

chapter 8
Mechanisms of Pruritus. 154
PAULINE M. DOWD

chapter 9
Topical Corticosteroid Therapy 160
KENNETH B. SLOAN, OSCAR E. ARAUJO, and
FRANKLIN P. FLOWERS

*Inflammatory Diseases that Principally
Affect the Epidermis and Dermis* 167

chapter 10
Contact Dermatitis. 167
  Allergic Contact Dermatitis: Cell-Mediated
  Immunity and Langerhans Cell Biology, 167
    Ponciano D. Cruz, Jr.

  Contact Dermatitis and Occupational
  Dermatology, 173
    James R. Nethercott

chapter 11
Diaper Dermatitis. 184
ANTHONY J. MANCINI and ALFRED T. LANE

chapter 12
Hand and Foot Dermatitis 188
KEVIN E. McKENNA

chapter 13
Atopic Dermatitis. 193
LEONARD KRISTAL and RICHARD A. F. CLARK

chapter 14
Lichen Simplex Chronicus,
Prurigo Nodularis, and Notalgia
Paresthetica 205
JEFFREY D. BERNHARD

chapter 15
Nummular Dermatitis 211
ARNOLD W. GUREVITCH

chapter 16
Seborrheic Dermatitis. 214
THOMAS G. CROPLEY

chapter 17
Pityriasis Rosea. 218
ERNESTO GONZALEZ

chapter 18
Small Plaque Parapsoriasis. 222
JORGE L. SÁNCHEZ and AÍDA LUGO-SOMOLINOS

chapter 19
Graft-versus-Host Disease 225
THOMAS D. HORN

chapter 20
Lichenoid Dermatitides (Lichen Planus,
Lichen Nitidus, Keratosis Lichenoides
Chronica, and Erythema Dyschromicum
Perstans). 235
ANNE-SOPHIE GADENNE, MICHAEL BIGBY, and
CHARLES CAMISA

chapter 21
Lichen Striatus. 244
KAREN WISS

chapter 22
Erythema Multiforme. 247
MARCIA G. TONNESEN

chapter 23
Pityriasis Lichenoides 256
GARY S. WOOD

chapter 24
Lupus Erythematosus. 260
KARI CONNOLLY

chapter 25
Dermatomyositis and Polymyositis. 283
O. FRED MILLER, III, and ERIC D. NEWMAN

chapter 26
Pigmented Purpuric Dermatoses 291
KATHRYN E. BOWERS

chapter 27
Psoriasis 295
ROBERT S. STERN and JESSICA WU

chapter 28
Reiter's Syndrome 322
GWENDOLYN F. KANE-WANGER

chapter 29
Subcorneal Pustular Dermatosis. 327
DANIEL WALLACH and
MARIE-DOMINIQUE VIGNON-PENNAMEN

chapter 30
Pityriasis Rubra Pilaris 331
PHILIP R. COHEN and JANET H. PRYSTOWSKY

chapter 31
Erythroderma 336
KRISTIAN THESTRUP-PEDERSEN

chapter 32
Transient Acantholytic Dermatosis 341
MARC D. CHALET

chapter 33
Jessner's Lymphocytic Infiltrate 344
JOHAN TOONSTRA

chapter 34
Figurate Erythemas 348
JAIME A. TSCHEN

chapter 35
Hypereosinophilic Syndrome 352
KRISTIN M. LEIFERMAN

chapter 36
Wells' Syndrome. 360
JOHN W. MELSKI

chapter 37
Dermatoses of Pregnancy 365
KIM B. YANCEY and ZELMIRA LAZAROVA

chapter 38
Neutrophilic Dermatoses 372
STEPHEN F. TEMPLETON, JOSEPH L. JORIZZO, and
ALVIN R. SOLOMON

chapter 39
Pyoderma Gangrenosum. 379
BRUCE H. THIERS

chapter 40
Behçet's Disease 385
TIMOTHY H. MCCALMONT

chapter 41
Urticaria. 392
SANFORD M. GOLDSTEIN and
MICHAEL D. THARP

chapter 42
Perforating Disorders 407
RONALD P. RAPINI

chapter 43
Cutaneous Reactions to Drugs and
Biologic Response Modifiers 412
ROBERT S. STERN and NEIL H. SHEAR

chapter 44
Cutaneous Reactions to
Chemotherapeutic Agents 426
WALTER H. C. BURGDORF

Granulomatous Inflammation 433

chapter 45
Sarcoidosis 433
ROBERT S. KIRSNER and FRANCISCO A. KERDEL

chapter 46
Granuloma Annulare and
Actinic Granuloma 438
RUBY GHADIALLY

chapter 47
Rheumatoid Nodule, Necrobiosis
Lipoidica, and Necrobiotic
Xanthogranuloma 444
JAMES W. PATTERSON

chapter 48
Tattoos, Foreign Body Granulomas, and
Their Treatment 452
SUZANNE LINSMEIER KILMER

Follicular Inflammation 461

chapter 49
Acne 461
Sebaceous Gland Science, Clinical
Description, and Therapies, 461
William Cunliffe and Harald Gollnick

Surgical Treatment of Scars, 473
John M. Yarborough and William P. Coleman, III

chapter 50
Hidradenitis Suppurativa 481
WILLIAM P. COLEMAN, III

chapter 51
Rosacea (With Discussion of
Electrosurgery) 485
SHELDON V. POLLACK

chapter 52
Perioral Dermatitis 497
MARIANNE NELSON O'DONOGHUE

chapter 53
Pseudofolliculitis Barbae 499
A. PAUL KELLY

chapter 54
Disorders of Follicular Keratinization 503
JOSEPH C. KVEDAR
Chondritis, 503

chapter 55
Chondrodermatitis Nodularis 507
CLIFFORD M. LAWRENCE

chapter 56
Relapsing Polychondritis 512
DAVID E. TRENTHAM

Vasculitis and Disorders of Vascular
Reactivity 515

chapter 57
Temporal Arteritis 515
ROBERT H. SHMERLING

chapter 58
Polyarteritis Nodosa 519
BRUCE R. SMOLLER

chapter 59
Microscopic Polyarteritis,
Wegener's Granulomatosis, and
Churg-Strauss Syndrome 522
J. CHARLES JENNETTE, JOHN T. WOOSLEY, and
RONALD J. FALK

chapter 60
Erythema Elevatum Diutinum and
Granuloma Faciale 528
ROKEA A. EL-AZHARY and LAWRENCE E. GIBSON

chapter 61
Erythromelalgia, Erythermalgia, and
Flushing 533
JONATHAN K. WILKIN

chapter 62
Raynaud's Phenomenon 537
CHRISTOPHER B. BUNKER and PAULINE M. DOWD

chapter 63
Noninflammatory Small Vessel
Occlusive Diseases 543
TIMOTHY H. McCALMONT and RAFFAELE PENNELLA

chapter 64
Lymphedema 554
DAVID T. HARVEY and ALBERT J. NEMETH

chapter 65
Leg Ulcers and Wound Healing 558
KATIA C. ONGENAE and TANIA J. PHILLIPS

chapter 66
Phlebology and Sclerotherapy 574
ROBERT A. WEISS

chapter 67
Cutaneous Venulitis
(Necrotizing Vasculitis,
Leukocytoclastic Vasculitis) 584
NICHOLAS A. SOTER

Panniculitis 591

chapter 68
Erythema Nodosum and
Nodular Vasculitis 591
EVARISTO SÁNCHEZ YUS and LUIS REQUENA

chapter 69
Sclerema Neonatorum and
Subcutaneous Fat Necrosis
of the Newborn 599
JAMES A. HARKER and DAVID F. FRETZIN

chapter 70
Sclerosing Panniculitis and Protease
Inhibitor Deficiency Panniculitis 603
STEPHEN F. TEMPLETON, JOSEPH L. JORIZZO, and
ALVIN R. SOLOMON

chapter 71
Other Forms of Panniculitis 608
JAMES W. PATTERSON

section three

**What Diseases Cause Blistering of
the Skin?** 615

chapter 72
The Dermoepidermal Junction:
Structure, Biochemistry, Antigenicity,
and Recent Molecular
Biologic Studies 617
JO-DAVID FINE and ELAINE V. FUCHS

chapter 73
Epidermolysis Bullosa 635
JO-DAVID FINE

chapter 74
Pemphigus Vulgaris and the Pemphigus
Disease Spectrum 651
GRANT J. ANHALT

chapter 75
Bullous Pemphigoid.................. 664
NEIL J. KORMAN

chapter 76
Cicatricial Pemphigoid............... 674
LYNNE H. MORRISON

chapter 77
Herpes Gestationis.................. 679
JEFFREY K. SHORNICK

chapter 78
Epidermolysis Bullosa Acquisita 685
JEAN CHRISTOPHE LAPIERE, LAWRENCE S. CHAN,
and DAVID T. WOODLEY

chapter 79
Dermatitis Herpetiformis.............. 691
MAUREEN KEOGH and RUSSELL P. HALL, III

chapter 80
Linear IgA Bullous Dermatosis.......... 698
EILEEN PAZDERKA SMITH and JOHN J. ZONE

chapter 81
Toxic Epidermal Necrolysis 704
JEAN-EDOUARD REVUZ and
JEAN-CLAUDE ROUJEAU

chapter 82
Blistering and Pustular Disorders
of the Neonate....................... 712
ILONA J. FRIEDEN

section four

**What Diseases Are Caused by
Environmental Exposure or
Physical Trauma?**................... 723

chapter 83
Basic Photobiology, Phototoxicity, and
Photoallergy 725
HENRY W. LIM and DONALD V. BELSITO

chapter 84
Photodamage and Photoaging 732
SERGE A. COOPMAN, MARJAN GARMYN,
ALDO GONZÁLEZ-SERVA, and
RICHARD G. GLOGAU

chapter 85
Sunscreens 751
JOSIAH FRIEDLANDER and NICHOLAS J. LOWE

chapter 86
The Idiopathic Photodermatoses 758
JAMES FERGUSON and JEFFREY S. DOVER

chapter 87
Chronic Actinic Dermatitis............. 768
HÉLÈNE DU P. MENAGÉ and JOHN L. M. HAWK

chapter 88
Responses to Friction and Hydration.... 772
CHRISTOPHER J. DANNAKER

chapter 89
Psychocutaneous Disorders............ 779
JOHN Y. M. KOO

chapter 90
Aquatic Dermatology................. 787
MARK JORDAN SCHARF

chapter 91
Insect Bites and Stings 804
MERVYN L. ELGART

chapter 92
Myiasis and Tungiasis 818
MERVYN L. ELGART

chapter 93
Cutaneous Effects of Heat and Cold 823
JEFFREY S. DOVER, PAULINE M. DOWD, and
MARCIA G. TONNESEN

chapter 94
Radiation Dermatitis 836
WILLIAM K. SHERWIN and HERBERT GOLDSCHMIDT

chapter 95
Physical Trauma to the Skin and
Emergency Department
Dermatology 839
JANET A. MOY and MIGUEL R. SANCHEZ

chapter 96
Sports-Related Skin Disease 849
JEFFREY S. DOVER

section five

What Disorders Change the Structure of the Dermis?

What Disorders Change the Structure
of the Dermis? 855

chapter 97
The Dermis 857
JOUNI UITTO, ERIC F. BERNSTEIN, and
JOHN A. MCGRATH

chapter 98
Scleroderma 882
BRUCE FREUNDLICH

chapter 99
Chemically Induced Scleroderma 891
YULY KIPERVARG and KARI CONNOLLY

chapter 100
Morphea and Morphea Profunda 895
W. P. DANIEL SU and FRANK C. POWELL

chapter 101
Keloids and Hypertrophic Scars 900
RONALD G. WHEELAND

chapter 102
Dupuytren's Disease 908
GERALD D. HARRIS, DANIEL J. NAGLE, and
THOMAS A. WIEDRICH

chapter 103
Anetoderma 910
OLIVER STANTON

chapter 104
Cutis Laxa 913
SUSAN E. KOCH

VOLUME 2

section six

What Infections and Infestations Affect the Skin?

What Infections and Infestations
Affect the Skin? 917

chapter 105
Skin Infections Caused by
Staphylococci, Streptococci, and the
Resident Cutaneous Flora 919
JAN V. HIRSCHMANN

chapter 106
Staphylococcal Toxin–Mediated
Syndromes 931
STEVEN D. RESNICK and PETER M. ELIAS

chapter 107
Skin Infections Caused by Unusual
Bacterial Pathogens 939
DAVID S. FEINGOLD

chapter 108
Syphilis and the Treponematoses 949
TIMOTHY G. BERGER, NICHOLAS FIUMARA, and
MARGOT WHITFELD

chapter 109
Lyme Borreliosis 965
DONALD C. ABELE

chapter 110
Chancroid, Granuloma Inguinale, and
Lymphogranuloma Venereum 973
THEODORE ROSEN and ANIR DHIR

chapter 111
Tuberculous Mycobacterial Infections
of the Skin 983
CAROLINE HIGGINS and RINO CERIO

chapter 112
Leprosy 993
L. MASAE KAWAMURA and ROBERT H. GELBER

chapter 113
Nocardiosis and Actinomycosis 1006
PAUL D. WORTMAN and DEBRA CHESTER KALTER

chapter 114
Rocky Mountain Spotted Fever and
Other Rickettsial Diseases 1011
SUSAN HADLEY and SCOTT M. HAMMER

chapter 115
Bacillary Angiomatosis, Cat-Scratch
Disease, and Bartonellosis............ 1023
JORDAN W. TAPPERO and JANE E. KOEHLER

chapter 116
The Zoonoses 1030
DALE R. WESTROM

chapter 117
Common Superficial Mycoses......... 1037
BONI E. ELEWSKI

chapter 118
The Dermatophytoses................ 1043
BONI E. ELEWSKI

chapter 119
Cutaneous Candidiasis 1056
GARY W. COLE

chapter 120
Deep Fungal and Opportunistic
Mycoses........................... 1060
LIZA W. CHANG and KENNETH J. TOMECKI

chapter 121
Herpesvirus Infections.............. 1074
ROY GULICK

chapter 122
Poxviruses 1093
RICHARD W. GROVES

chapter 123
Human Papillomavirus Infection....... 1100
ELLIOT J. ANDROPHY, KARL BEUTNER, and
SUZANNE OLBRICHT

chapter 124
Viral Exanthems 1123
RENÉE HOWARD and ILONA J. FRIEDEN

chapter 125
Human Immunodeficiency
Virus Infection and the
Cutaneous Complications of
Immunosuppression 1137
TIMOTHY G. BERGER and JORDAN W. TAPPERO

chapter 126
Leishmaniasis 1163
ETHAN A. LERNER and SUZANNE A. GREVELINK

chapter 127
Parasitic Diseases 1172
DEBRA CHESTER KALTER, TERRI LYNN MEINKING,
EDITH GARCIA, and MOHAMED AMER

chapter 128
Body Lice, Head Lice, Pubic Lice, and
Scabies 1190
JAMES E. RASMUSSEN

section seven

What Diseases Alter Skin Color? 1201

chapter 129
Biology of Melanocytes.............. 1203
RAYMOND E. BOISSY and JAMES J. NORDLUND

chapter 130
Vitiligo 1210
RAYMOND E. BOISSY and JAMES J. NORDLUND

chapter 131
Albinism and Other Disorders of
Hypopigmentation.................. 1219
JEAN L. BOLOGNIA and PHILIP E. SHAPIRO

chapter 132
Melasma and Other Disorders of
Hyperpigmentation 1233
JORGE E. TORRES and JORGE L. SÁNCHEZ

section eight

What Diseases Alter Hair, Nails, and Sweat Glands? 1243

chapter 133
Biochemistry and Control of
Hair Growth 1245
    Anatomy, 1245
        Marty E. Sawaya
    Androgenetic Disorders, 1250
        Maria K. Hordinsky
    Hair Replacement Surgery, 1258
        Dominic A. Brandy and Kathryn L. Brandy

chapter 134
Alopecia Areata and Other
Nonscarring Alopecias............... 1269
VIRGINIA C. FIEDLER

chapter 135
Scarring Alopecia 1280
STEPHEN F. TEMPLETON and ALVIN R. SOLOMON

chapter 136
Biology and Disorders of Nails 1295
PAUL KECHIJIAN and STUART SALASCHE

chapter 137
Biology and Disorders of
Sweat Glands 1307
    Sweat Gland Science, 1307
        Kenzo Sato, Neal, Kane, Gyula Soos,
        Takashi Toyomoto, and Fusako Sato
    Pathology and Surgery, 1311
        William P. Coleman, III, Kenzo Sato, Neal Kane,
        Gyula Soos, Takashi Toyomoto, and
        Fusako Sato

section nine

What Diseases Alter Mucous Membranes? 1321

chapter 138
Disorders of Oral Mucous Membranes .. 1323
DRORE EISEN and JOHN SEXTON

chapter 139
Genital Disorders 1340
MARIA L. CHANCO TURNER

section ten

What Benign and Malignant Proliferations of Cells Affect the Skin, and How Are They Treated? 1361

chapter 140
Molecular Mechanisms of Photocarcinogenesis: The Role of *ras* and *p53* Alterations................... 1363
SAGARIKA KANJILAL and HONNAVARA N. ANANTHASWAMY

chapter 141
Malignant Neoplasms of Keratinocytes 1378

Disease Description: Actinic (Solar) Keratosis, Bowen's Disease, Keratoacanthoma, Squamous Cell Carcinoma, Basal Cell Carcinoma, and Merkel Cell Carcinoma, 1378
Barry Leshin and Wain L. White

Treatment, 1393
Roy C. Grekin, John K. Geisse, Lawrence W. Margolis, and Jerome Potozkin

chapter 142
Benign Neoplasms of the Epidermis 1441
BRUCE R. SMOLLER and GLORIA GRAHAM

chapter 143
Cysts of Epithelial Adnexal Origin 1450
JAG BHAWAN and S. TERI MCGILLIS

chapter 144
Neoplasms of the Pilosebaceous Unit 1464
BRETT COLDIRON and BRUCE R. SMOLLER

chapter 145
Neoplasms with Eccrine or Apocrine Differentiation 1476
BRUCE R. SMOLLER and BRETT COLDIRON

chapter 146
Angiogenesis, Vascular Malformations and Proliferations................... 1492
JAMES NIGRO, ROBERT A. SWERLICK, NORBERT T. SEPP, ROY G. GERONEMUS, PHILIP E. LEBOIT, and ILONA J. FRIEDEN

chapter 147
Neoplasms of Muscle and Fat, Liposuction Surgery of Fat Hypertrophy 1522
JAMES E. FITZPATRICK and WILLIAM P. COLEMAN, III

chapter 148
Neural Tumors (Other than Tuberous Sclerosis and Neurofibromatosis) 1536
ZSOLT B. ARGENYI

chapter 149
Fibrous Neoplasms................... 1552
FREDERICK S. FISH and HIDEKO KAMINO

chapter 150
Melanocytic Nevi.................... 1561

Benign Melanocytic Neoplasms: Congenital and Acquired Nevi, 1561
Clay J. Cockerell, Timothy M. Johnson, and Neil A. Swanson

Atypical Melanocytic Nevi, 1571
Clay J. Cockerell

chapter 151
Melanoma.......................... 1576
HOWARD K. KOH, RAYMOND L. BARNHILL, and GARY S. ROGERS

chapter 152
Mastocytosis 1602
JACK LONGLEY

chapter 153
Langerhans Cell Histiocytosis 1610
CHRISTOPHER R. SHEA and N. SCOTT MCNUTT

chapter 154
Multicentric Reticulohistiocytosis and Sinus Histiocytosis 1616
PAUL CHU

chapter 155
Other Histiocytoses of Childhood 1620
SHARON S. RAIMER and RAMON L. SANCHEZ

chapter 156
Cutaneous Lymphoid Hyperplasia...... 1626
GARY S. WOOD

chapter 157
Lymphomatoid Papulosis 1631
MARSHALL E. KADIN

chapter 158
Cutaneous T-Cell Lymphoma 1639
PETER W. HEALD, PHILIP E. SHAPIRO, JENNIFER F. MADISON, PHILIP E. LEBOIT, and RICHARD L. EDELSON

chapter 159
Other Cutaneous Lymphomas: B-Cell
Lymphoma, Non–Mycosis Fungoides
T-Cell Lymphoma, and Adult T-Cell
Lymphoma/Leukemia 1660
GÜNTER BURG, REINHARD DUMMER, and STEFAN
DOMMANN

chapter 160
Leukemia Cutis..................... 1670
STANISLAW A. BUECHNER and W. P. DANIEL SU

chapter 161
Cutaneous Metastases............... 1674
GEORGE P. LUPTON and J. MICHAEL GAGNIER

section eleven

What Diseases of the Skin Are
Malformations or Are Predominantly
Inherited?......................... 1679

chapter 162
The Ichthyoses: Disorders of
Cornification 1681
MARY L. WILLIAMS and PHILIP E. LeBOIT

chapter 163
Congenital Alopecias and
Disorders of Melanosome Transfer to
Hair Follicies 1712
JACK L. ARBISER

chapter 164
The Ectodermal Dysplasias 1721
J. TIMOTHY WRIGHT and JO-DAVID FINE

chapter 165
Incontinentia Pigmenti 1725
JACKSON MACHADO-PINTO and LOREN E. GOLITZ

chapter 166
Neurofibromatosis, Tuberous
Sclerosis, and Other Neurocutaneous
Disorders 1729
NEIL S. GOLDBERG and RANDALL K. ROENIGK

chapter 167
Basal Cell Nevus Syndrome........... 1742
ERVIN EPSTEIN, JR.

chapter 168
Xeroderma Pigmentosum 1747
JAMES E. CLEAVER and JOHN EPSTEIN

chapter 169
The Porphyrias 1753
MAUREEN B. POH-FITZPATRICK

chapter 170
Acrodermatitis Enteropathica 1763
JEFFREY C. DRALUCK and DARRYL M. BRONSON

chapter 171
Inherited Enzyme Diseases 1766
Gaucher's Disease, 1766
Adelaide A. Hebert and Hope Northrup
Hartnup's Disorder, 1768
Hope Northrup and Adelaide A. Hebert

chapter 172
Inherited Elastic Tissue
Malformations..................... 1770
KENNETH H. NELDNER

chapter 173
Focal Dermal Hypoplasia and Aplasia
Cutis Congenita.................... 1780
ILONA J. FRIEDEN

chapter 174
Nevoid Conditions of Epidermis, Dermis,
and Subcutaneous Tissue 1787
MAUREEN ROGERS, GAYLE FISCHER, and
PETER HOGAN

chapter 175
Genodermatoses.................... 1796
JAMES E. SLIGH, JR., and MOISE L. LEVY

section twelve

What Are the Disorders of Deposition
and Cellular Secretion? 1807

chapter 176
Xanthomas 1809
FRANK PARKER

chapter 177
Amyloidosis........................ 1818
KEN HASHIMOTO

chapter 178
Cutaneous Ossification and
Calcification 1828
KALMAN L. WATSKY

chapter 179
The Cutaneous Mucinoses............ 1832
ALFREDO REBORA and FRANCO RONGIOLETTI

section thirteen

What Are the Dermatologic
Manifestations of Internal Disease?
What Are the Dermatologic
Disorders Commonly Found in
Pediatrics?........................ 1841

chapter 180
Paraneoplastic Syndromes 1843
DAVID I. MCLEAN and HARVEY LUI

chapter 181
Hirsutism and Its Related Endocrine
Disorders 1853
ARTHUR C. HUNTLEY

chapter 182
Inherited Abnormalities of Amino Acid
Metabolism 1858
ELIZABETH F. SHERERTZ

chapter 183
Dermatologic Manifestations of Internal
Disease 1863
JOSEPH L. JORIZZO and JEFFREY P. CALLEN

chapter 184
Pediatric Dermatology 1889
BERNARD A. COHEN

Index i

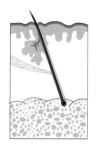

Contents Medical and Surgical Therapies

Antihistamines (Chapter 41, pp. 401–402; Chapter 152, p. 1607)

Antisepsis, Anesthesia, Hemostasis, Suture Placement, and Techniques for Skin Biopsy (Chapter 6, p. 128)

Biopsy Techniques: Description and Proper Use (Chapter 6, p. 120)

Care of Normal Skin: Everyday Skin Care (Chapter 4, p. 79)

Cartilage Excision in Chondrodermatitis Nodularis (Chapter 55, pp. 507–510)

Chemical Peels for Photodamage (Chapter 84, pp. 741–746)

CO_2 Laser Treatment for Cutaneous Disorders (Chapter 123, pp. 1114–1117)

Cryosurgery (Chapter 123, p. 1113; Chapter 142, pp. 1443, 1446–1448)

Cyclosporine Use in Psoriasis and Other Diseases (Chapter 27, p. 310)

Cysts: Incision, Excision, and Drainage (Chapter 143, pp. 1454–1462)

Dapsone (Chapter 65, p. 79)

Dermabrasion Technique (Chapter 49, pp. 473–479)

Electron Beam Radiotherapy for Cutaneous T-Cell Lymphoma (Chapter 158, p. 1639)

Electrosurgery: Principles and Use (Chapter 51, pp. 489–495)

Excisional Biopsy of Suspicious Pigmented Lesions (Chapter 6, p. 127; Chapter 151, p. 1576)

Extracorporeal Photochemotherapy for Cutaneous T-Cell Lymphoma (Chapter 158)

Flaps and Grafts in Dermatology (Chapter 141, pp. 1408–1417)

Hair Replacement Surgery (Chapter 133, pp. 1258–1263)

Interferons in the Treatment of Cutaneous Malignancies (Chapter 141, pp. 1427–1429)

Iontophoresis for Hyperhidrosis (Chapter 137, pp. 1314–1315)

Keloid Surgery (Chapter 101, p. 905)

Keratinocyte Grafts and Autografts (Chapter 65, p. 569)

Laser Treatment of Cutaneous Vascular Lesions (Chapter 146, pp. 1499–1500, 1502)

Liposuction
- General Principles: Treatment of Benign Tumors and Hypertrophy of Fat (Chapter 147, pp. 1530–1534)
- of the Axilla in Hidradenitis Suppurativa (Chapter 50, pp. 482–483)
- for the Treatment of Axillary Hyperhidrosis (Chapter 137, pp. 1316–1317)

Methotrexate Use for Psoriasis and Other Diseases (Chapter 27, p. 307)

Mohs Micrographic Surgery (Chapter 141, pp. 1393–1394, 1403–1408)

Nail Biopsy (Chapter 136, p. 1295)

Photodynamic Therapy: Mechanism of Action, Technique, and Application in the Treatment of Cutaneous Malignancy (Chapter 141, pp. 1423–1427)

Phototherapy and Photochemotherapy (Chapter 27, p. 312)
- For the Treatment of Vitiligo (Chapter 130, p. 1214)
- Topical Photochemotherapy (including Table 12–3) (Chapter 12, p. 192)

Q-Switched Laser Treatment for Pigmented Lesions: Principles of Use (Chapter 48, p. 453)

Retinoids
- Use of Systemic Retinoids in Psoriasis (Chapter 27, pp. 309–310)
- Isotretinoin in the Treatment of Acne (Chapter 49, pp. 468, 470, 472–473)
- Topical Retinoids for the Treatment of Photodamaged Skin (Chapter 84, pp. 740–741)
- Retinoids in the Treatment of Cutaneous Malignancies (Chapter 141, pp. 1429, 1431)

Sclerotherapy (Chapter 66, pp. 574–575, 580, 581)

Sunscreens in the Prevention of Photodamage and Photoaging (Chapters 84 and 85, pp. 739, 752–757)

Surgical Excision of the Axilla for Hyperhidrosis (Chapter 137, pp. 1314–1317)

Surgical Treatment of Vitiligo (Chapter 130, pp. 1214–1216)

Tattooing for Depigmentation in the Treatment of Vitiligo (Chapter 130, pp. 1214–1216)

Topical Corticosteroid Therapy
• Types of Formulations (Chapter 9, p. 161)
• Table Ranking of Some Commonly Used Topical Steroids by Potency (Chapter 9, p. 162)
• Clinical Considerations in the Use of Topical Corticosteroids (Chapter 9, p. 163)
• Side Effects (Chapter 9, p. 165)

Topical Nitrogen Mustard Therapy for Cutaneous T-Cell Lymphoma (Chapter 158, pp. 1651–1652)

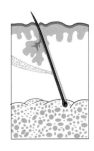

Contents Biology of the Skin

Angiogenesis (Chapter 146, pp. 1492–1521)

Dermis: Structure, Biochemistry, and Molecular Biology (Chapter 97, p. 857)

Dermoepidermal Junction: Structure, Biochemistry, Antigenicity, and Molecular Biology (Chapter 72, p. 617)

Hair: Biochemistry and Control of Growth (Chapter 133, pp. 1245–1268)

Inflammation, Immunity, and the Skin
- Adhesion Molecules (pp. 146–151)
- Biochemistry of Inflammation (pp. 140–153)
- Cell-Mediated Immunity (pp. 167–173)
- Cytokines (pp. 143–146)
- Langerhans Cells: Morphology and Function (pp. 170–172)
- Major Histocompatibility Complex (p. 226)
- Mast Cells: Biochemistry and Biology (Chapter 41, pp. 396–399)
- Pruritus: Mechanisms (pp. 154–159)

Keratinocyte Biology and Differentiation (pp. 58–74)

Melanocyte Biology (Chapter 129, pp. 1206–1207)

Nail: Anatomy, Biology, and Growth (Chapter 136, pp. 1295–1306)

Normal Skin
- Anatomy (pp. 111–119)
- Structure, Development, and Function (pp. 3–57)

Photobiology (Chapter 83, pp. 725–727)

Photocarcinogenesis (Chapter 140, p. 1367)

Sebaceous Gland Biology (Chapter 49, pp. 461–480)

Sweat Glands: Anatomy and Biology (Chapter 137, pp. 1307–1319)

Wound Healing (Chapter 65, pp. 558–573)

Color Plates

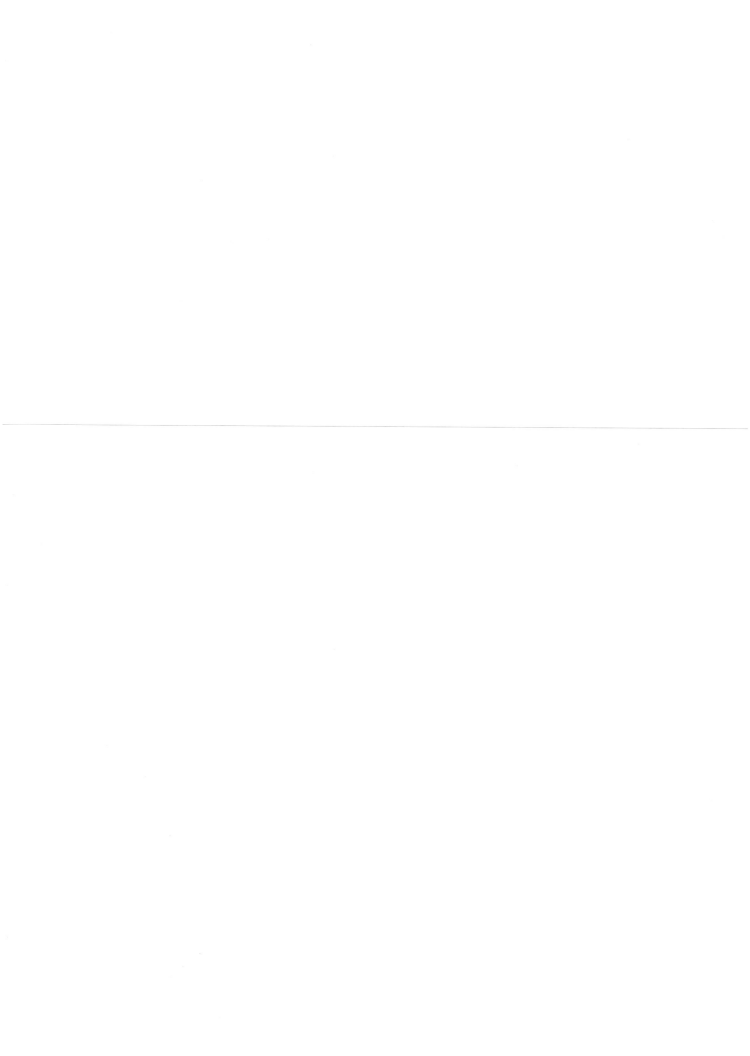

PLATE 6

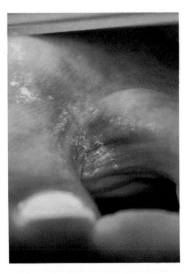

FIGURE 105-7. Erythrasma. The lesion shown in Figure 105-6 (see p. 927) fluoresces a coral-pink color with Wood's lamp, confirming the diagnosis.

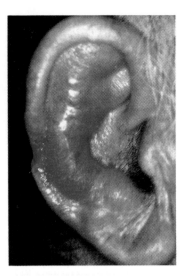

FIGURE 107-1. External otitis due to *Pseudomonas aeruginosa.*

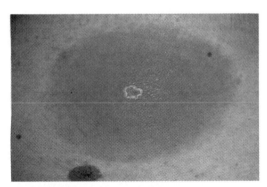

FIGURE 109-1. Primary erythema migrans: solid erythema with early collarette of scale. (From Melski JW. Lyme borreliosis in Wisconsin: Lessons in diagnosing and treating erythema migrans. Fitzpatrick's J Clin Dermatol 1994;May/June:14-25. Photograph by John W. Melski, M.D.)

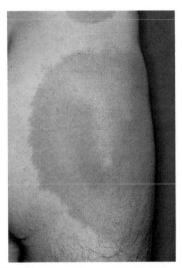

FIGURE 109-2. Secondary erythema migrans: large annular lesion. (From Melski JW. Lyme borreliosis in Wisconsin: Lessons in diagnosing and treating erythema migrans. Fitzpatrick's J Clin Dermatol 1994; May/June:14-25. Photograph by John W. Melski, M.D.)

PLATE 7

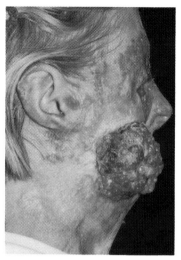

FIGURE 111–2. Long-standing lupus vulgaris with squamous cell carcinoma arising from cheek.

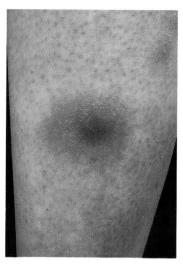

FIGURE 111–5. Erythema induratum of Bazin on the calf.

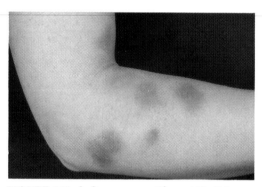

FIGURE 111–8. Same case as Figure 111–7 (see p. 990), showing sporotrichoid spread along the forearm.

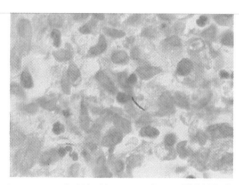

FIGURE 111–9. Skin biopsy specimen. Ziehl-Neelsen stain reveals an isolated acid-fast bacillus.

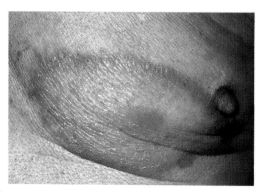

FIGURE 112–2. A hypopigmented macule of tuberculoid leprosy shows a defined border.

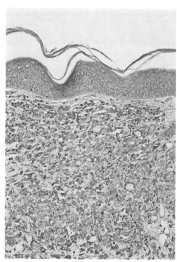

FIGURE 112–5. A Fite-Faracco stain of the dermis in untreated lepromatous leprosy shows the numerous clustered bacilli, or globi.

PLATE 8

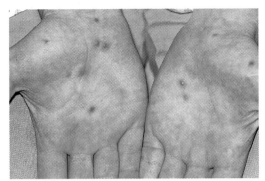

FIGURE 115–1. Small vascular papules of bacillary angiomatosis on the palms.

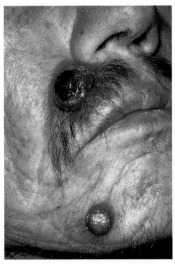

FIGURE 115–2. Characteristic exophytic angiomatous nodules of bacillary angiomatosis with and without surrounding cellulitic erythema.

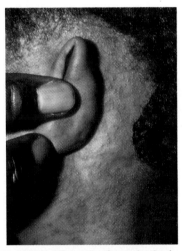

FIGURE 124–1. The rash of measles begins behind the ears. (From Frieden IJ, Penneys N. In: Schachner L, Hansen R, eds. Pediatric Dermatology. New York: Churchill Livingstone, 1988.)

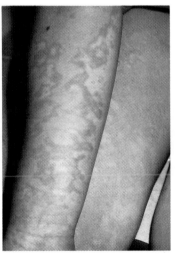

FIGURE 124–2. Erythema infectiosum: Characteristic reticulate pattern on the arm (From Frieden IJ. Viral exanthems. In: Sams W, Lynch P, eds. Principles and Practice of Dermatology. New York: Churchill Livingstone, 1990.)

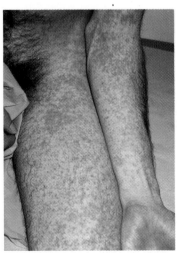

FIGURE 124–4. Exanthem of primary HIV infection.

PLATE 9

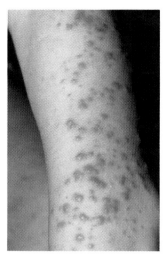

FIGURE 124–6. Gianotti-Crosti syndrome due to Epstein-Barr virus infection.

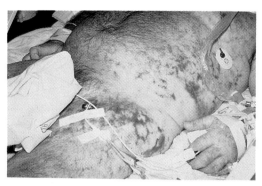

FIGURE 127–9. Premorbid strongyloidiasis in a case of superinfection. (Courtesy of the Armed Forces Institute of Pathology.)

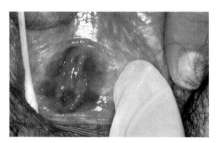

FIGURE 139–12. In vulvar vestibulitis syndrome, there is marked erythema in the vulvar vestibule around the openings of Bartholin's ducts and Skene's ducts. Application of light pressure on these areas by an applicator tip elicits exquisite tenderness.

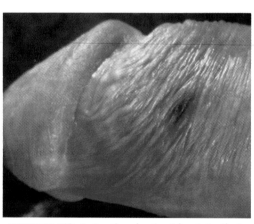

FIGURE 150–1. Lentigo simplex (simple lentigo).

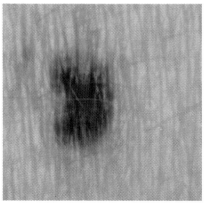

FIGURE 150–3. Junctional nevus.

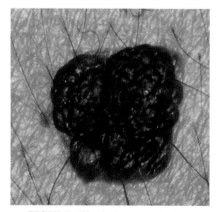

FIGURE 150–4. Compound nevus.

PLATE 10

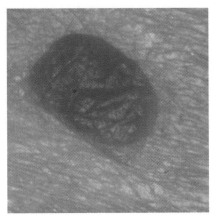

FIGURE 150-5. Intradermal nevus.

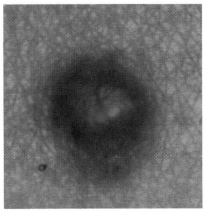

FIGURE 150-9. Spitz nevus (spindle and epithelioid nevus).

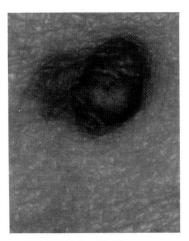

FIGURE 150-13. Blue nevus.

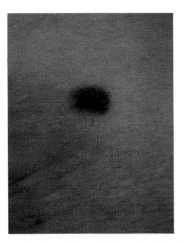

FIGURE 150-18. Compound type of atypical melanocytic nevus. Note the peripheral spread of pigment. Lesion is located at the junction of the areola in a young woman. (Courtesy of June K. Robinson, M.D.)

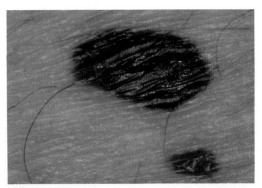

FIGURE 150-19. Junctional type of atypical melanocytic nevus. Two lesions are located very close to each other.

PLATE 11

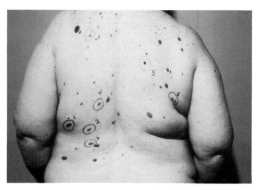

FIGURE 150-21. Patient with familial multiple atypical nevi and melanoma. Lesion 1 was shown to represent melanoma following excision.

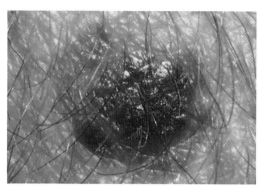

FIGURE 151-3. Melanoma in situ.

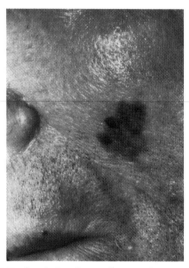

FIGURE 151-4. Lentigo maligna melanoma on the face.

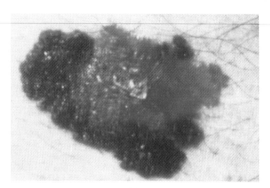

FIGURE 151-5. Superficial spreading melanoma.

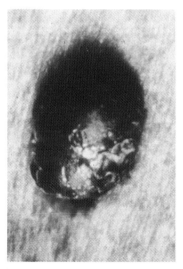

FIGURE 151-6. Nodular melanoma.

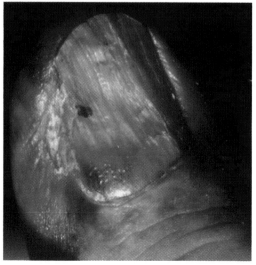

FIGURE 151-7. Acral lentiginous melanoma demonstrates Hutchinson's sign, the spreading of pigmentation onto the proximal nail fold. (Reprinted with permission from the New England Journal of Medicine, 1991;325:171-182.)

PLATE 12

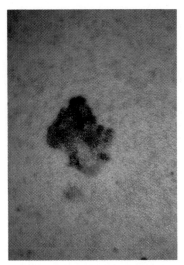

FIGURE 151–8. Regression of melanoma results in flat white or gray areas within a melanoma. (Courtesy of June K. Robinson, M.D.)

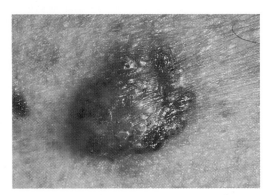

FIGURE 151–15. Pigmented basal cell carcinoma.

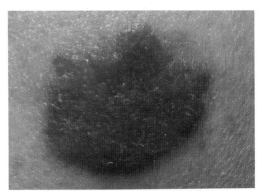

FIGURE 151–16. Kaposi's sarcoma.

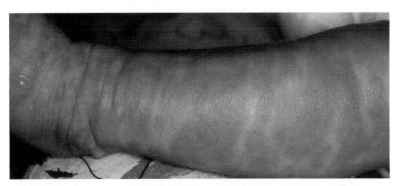

FIGURE 152–3. Hyperpigmented and thickened skin in an infant with diffuse cutaneous mastocytosis. Subepidermal bulla (*far left, dorsal ankle*) is caused by edema of the superficial dermis, secondary to mast cell mediator release.

PLATE 13

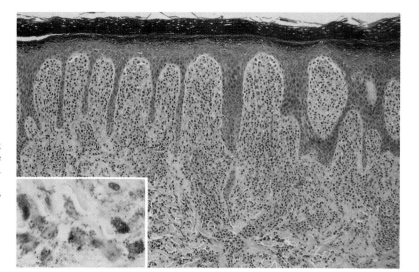

FIGURE 152–4. Infiltrating mast cells in cutaneous mastocytosis are larger than normal mast cells and resemble fried eggs. Highly charged, sulfated acid mucopolysaccharides cause metachromatic (purple) staining of mast cell granules in Giemsa-stained sections (*inset*), in contrast to the eosinophilic (pink) granules of eosinophils recruited by mast cell degranulation.

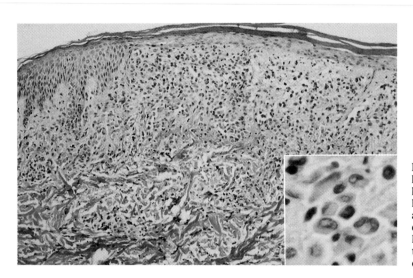

FIGURE 153–3. Biopsy specimen has a nodular infiltrate of Langerhans cells in the dermis, with focal hemorrhage, epidermal atrophy, and parakeratosis (hematoxylin-eosin, × 200). *Inset,* Demonstrates lobular nuclei and eosinophilic cytoplasm of the dermal Langerhans cell infiltrate (× 1300).

PLATE 14

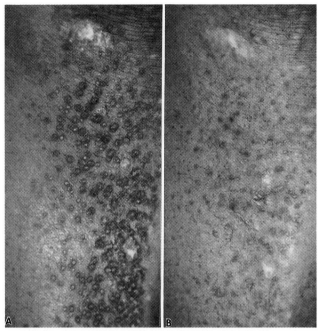

FIGURE 177–3. Lichen amyloidosus. In *A*, hyperkeratotic papulonodules become confluent in lower part of this picture. In *B*, after the treatment with mercaptoethanol-urea solution (see p. 1827, reference 36), most papules have subsided but hyperpigmentation remains; this is the picture of biphasic amyloidosis.

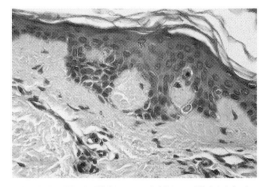

FIGURE 177–6. Lichen amyloidosus. Pink globular materials accumulated in dilated papillary dermis. An apoptotic basal cell with a pyknotic nucleus is seen in acanthotic epidermis (hematoxylin-eosin, × 130).

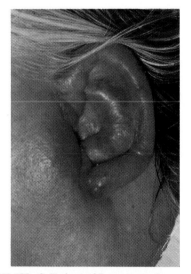

FIGURE 180–3. Patient with acute myelogenous leukemia and Sweet's syndrome.

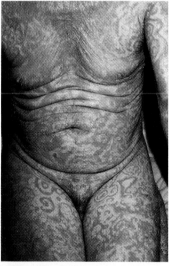

FIGURE 180–4. Erythema gyratum repens secondary to internal cancer. (Courtesy of D. Lookingbill, M.D., Hershey, PA.)

PLATE 15

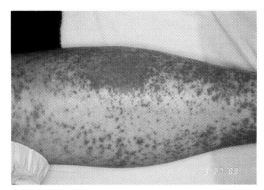

FIGURE 183-3. Small vessel vasculitis in Sjögren's syndrome.

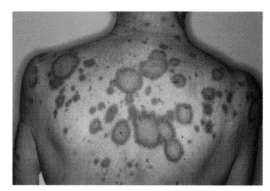

FIGURE 183-4. Subacute cutaneous lupus erythematosus in a patient with Sjögren's syndrome.

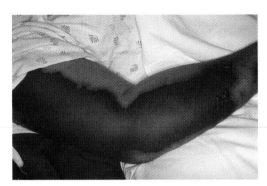

FIGURE 183-9. Disseminated intravascular coagulation.

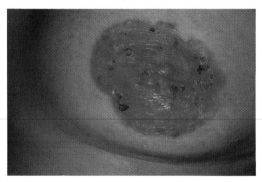

FIGURE 183-16. Paget's disease. (From Callen JP. Skin signs of internal malignancy. In: Callen JP, Jorizzo JL, et al., eds. Dermatological Signs of Internal Disease, 2nd edition. Philadelphia: WB Saunders Co., 1995:111-121.)

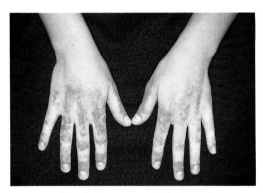

FIGURE 183-19. Dermatomyositis (KAA interpretation).

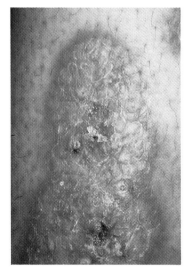

FIGURE 183-22. Necrobiosis lipoidica diabeticorum.

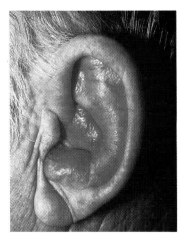

FIGURE 183-45. Relapsing polychondritis.

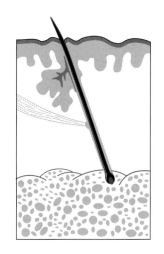

What Infections and Infestations Affect the Skin?

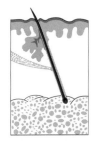

Skin Infections Caused by Staphylococci, Streptococci, and the Resident Cutaneous Flora

JAN V. HIRSCHMANN

Several characteristics of skin help protect it from infection by pathogens.[1] The dry, tough stratum corneum is largely impenetrable to invasion by organisms and is inhospitable to the growth of many types, especially those requiring substantial moisture. Beneath the stratum corneum, the cells of the granular and spinous layers are tightly joined together by a "cement," a complex mixture of lipids that also protects the skin by sealing the entry to hair follicles and inhibiting the proliferation of many organisms. In addition, the constant shedding of cutaneous cells as epidermal production continues may help eliminate any pathogens attached to them. Other factors potentially subduing invaders include an acidic pH, the presence of immunoglobulins in sweat, and the various kinds of resident skin flora that compete for nutrients and can produce antimicrobial substances harmful to other microbes.

Cutaneous infections usually occur when trauma, inflammatory skin diseases, excessive hydration, or other processes disrupt these protective mechanisms. The organisms causing these infections may be part of the resident flora on adjacent skin or contiguous mucous membranes, or they may originate from sources external to the host, such as other persons, the environment, or contaminated inanimate objects. Many pyogenic infections in humans occur from *Staphylococcus aureus* and *Streptococcus pyogenes*, which normally reside on the skin or mucous membranes of some persons.

The main location for *Staphylococcus aureus* is the anterior nares, which it colonizes in about 30% of the normal population.[2] A majority of these hosts also carry this organism on the turbinates and the posterior nasal surfaces. Long-term studies indicate that some persons are chronic carriers, others are intermittent or transient carriers, and many are never colonized. Hereditary factors, alterations in nasal anatomy (such as septal deviation), and certain other host characteristics influence the carriage rate; it may be higher in diabetics, users of illicit intravenous drugs, persons with acquired immunodeficiency syndrome, and renal dialysis patients, but the evidence has often been conflicting. About 2% of the population are chronic axillary carriers, and about 7% are transient carriers; the corresponding numbers for permanent and temporary perineal carriage are about 6% and 7%, respectively. The organism is found in the toe webs in about 5%. *Staphylococcus aureus* is unusual elsewhere on normal skin; generally, it is present in less than 5% of the healthy population, but its prevalence markedly increases in those patients with diabetes mellitus and certain dermatologic diseases, especially atopic eczema, where skin cultures are positive in nearly all patients. From these locations the bacteria may cause cutaneous infections in the host, spread to colonize or infect other persons, or contaminate objects, such as medical instruments, which can then become sources of infection.

Streptococcus pyogenes often inhabits the nasopharynx of healthy persons.[3] From this site the organism can disperse to contaminate the skin, but epidemiologic studies of outbreaks of streptococcal skin infections suggest that a skin source is more frequently the predisposing factor than one in the respiratory tract. In fact, the presence of *Streptococcus pyogenes* in the nasopharynx in those with it also present on the skin surface is usually a consequence of the cutaneous colonization rather than the cause. The skin, however, is ordinarily an inhospitable location for this organism; experimental inoculation onto normal skin typically fails to initiate colonization, probably because of the inhibitory effects of unsaturated fatty acids. Streptococci, however, will sometimes inhabit areas of abnormal skin, and the source of most streptococci causing skin infections is probably organisms present on the cutaneous surface of the host before the initiating injury. Other possible mechanisms of streptococcal skin infections besides autoinoculation include direct transmission of the bacteria from other persons colonized or infected with them, contaminated objects in the environment, pets, or, rarely, contaminated insects.

IMPETIGO

The nature of the cutaneous infections caused by *Staphylococcus aureus* and *Streptococcus pyogenes* depends on the location of the bacteria in the skin. The most superficial of these is impetigo. Once regarded as primarily of streptococcal origin, nonbullous impetigo is now recognized as a manifestation of infection with either or both of these organisms. In fact, studies have revealed that most cases of impetigo are due solely to *Staphylococcus aureus*, some to a combination of both organisms, and few to *Streptococcus pyogenes* alone.[4, 5] Impetigo, which is considerably more common in children than adults, usually develops on exposed areas of the skin, especially the face and distal extremities, and typically follows trauma, such as abrasions, insect bites, excoriations from scratching pruritic areas, and cuts. It is more common in hot, humid climates than more temperate ones, perhaps because overhydrated skin is more easily injured, heals more slowly, or is more readily colonized with these pyogenic bacteria. Poor hygiene is also a predisposing factor, as are crowded living conditions, which allow easy interpersonal spread of the pathogens.

Impetigo usually starts as red papules that transform into vesicles and pustules, which, because they are located in the superficial epidermis, rupture readily to create thick, adherent, honey-colored crusts surmounting an enlarging, erythematous base (Fig. 105–1). The lesions, which are often numerous, may be pruritic but are not usually painful and are sometimes associated with tender regional lymph node enlargement. On the face impetigo is commonly periorificial, and in any location the lesions may coalesce to form large areas of exudation and crusting. Cultures of impetigo will usually yield the responsible pathogens but are often unnecessary in clinically obvious cases.

On skin biopsy specimens, which are rarely required for the diagnosis, vesicopustules containing neutrophils, gram-positive cocci, and, sometimes, acantholytic cells are present above, within, or below the granular layer. The epidermis beneath displays spongiosis and neutrophils migrating through it from the underlying inflamed dermis, which contains a mixed population of neutrophils and lymphocytes.

Impetigo may complicate various eczemas, but the distinction between superinfection and noninfectious in-

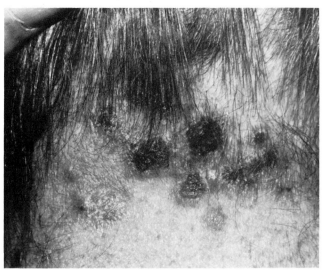

FIGURE 105–1. Impetigo. Several erythematous, crusted lesions are present on the posterior neck. Culture of the lesions yielded a pure growth of *Staphylococcus aureus.*

flammation can be difficult, since exudation, erythema, and crusting may be present with either. Furthermore, the common isolation of *Staphylococcus aureus* from eczematous lesions of all grades of severity suggests that it is often a harmless, colonizing organism rather than a pathogen. Some have argued that these bacteria cause eczema to worsen when they exceed a certain concentration,[6] but the validity of this claim is uncertain; and, furthermore, quantitative cultures are not routinely done. The most convincing clinical manifestations of superinfection are pustules,[7] substantial surrounding cellulitis, fever, lymphangitis (i.e., red streaks coursing proximally from the site), and regional lymphadenitis. Many clinicians treat severe eczema with topical or systemic antistaphylococcal antibiotics even in the absence of these features. The evidence to support this practice is conflicting,[8, 9] and therapy for eczema with topical corticosteroids alone substantially reduces the concentration of staphylococci as the underlying inflammation improves.[10]

Sometimes, impetigo is self-limited, but treatment will relieve symptoms more rapidly, halt the formation of new lesions, and promote more prompt resolution for those already present (Table 105–1). Healing occurs without scarring since the pathologic process does not reach the dermis. Systemic antimicrobial therapy is very effective. Although agents active only against *Streptococcus pyogenes*, such as penicillin, are often satisfactory, a better overall response occurs with treatment directed against both *Staphylococcus aureus* and *Streptococcus pyogenes*, confirming the importance of staphylococci in the pathogenesis of nonbullous impetigo.[11, 12] In most locales oral erythromycin remains effective, but resistant staphylococci may be frequent, and alternatives include dicloxacillin or an oral first-generation cephalosporin such as cephalexin or cephradine. Many topical antibiotics such as bacitracin or the neomycin-bacitracin combinations provide some benefit, but the best topical agent

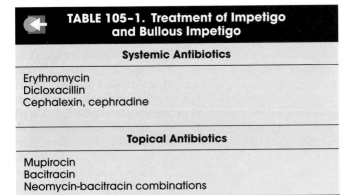

TABLE 105-1. Treatment of Impetigo and Bullous Impetigo

Systemic Antibiotics
Erythromycin
Dicloxacillin
Cephalexin, cephradine

Topical Antibiotics
Mupirocin
Bacitracin
Neomycin-bacitracin combinations

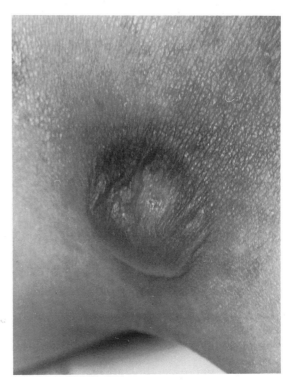

FIGURE 105-2. Bullous impetigo. A flaccid bulla on an erythematous base appears on the knee of a child. Culture of the blister fluid yielded *Staphylococcus aureus.*

is mupirocin, which, when applied three times a day for 7 to 8 days, is equivalent in efficacy to oral erythromycin.[5, 13-15] The presence of widespread lesions or the involvement of several family members may make topical therapy inconvenient, and it has the disadvantage of not eradicating streptococci from the respiratory tract, which may sometimes be a reservoir for reinfection or spread of the organism to others. This limitation of topical therapy is especially of concern in epidemic situations or when the streptococci are "nephritogenic strains," those uncommon isolates of *Streptococcus pyogenes* capable of initiating poststreptococcal glomerulonephritis. Whether antimicrobial therapy of any sort decreases the rare risk of this renal disease is uncertain; often the kidney abnormality is already present when the patient seeks medical attention for the skin infection.[16] The benefit of systemic antimicrobial therapy in that setting is more clearly to prevent spread of these dangerous bacteria to uninfected contacts. Fortunately, cutaneous infections caused by *Streptococcus pyogenes* do not lead to another nonsuppurative complication, acute rheumatic fever, which occurs only after respiratory infections with the organism.

Unlike the nonbullous form, bullous impetigo is strictly due to certain strains of *Staphylococcus aureus*, primarily phage II, group 71, which produce a toxin, exfoliatin, that causes cleavage in the granular layer of the epidermis. When absorbed in large quantities into the bloodstream this toxin is responsible for the staphylococcal scalded skin syndrome. When produced in the localized skin infection of bullous impetigo it causes vesicles and bullae to form on an erythematous base (Fig. 105-2). Because the skin separation produced is so high in the epidermis, the blisters are fragile and disrupt easily to spill their fluid contents onto the skin surface, where the liquid dries to produce a thin, brownish, lacquer-like covering. Although intact bullae may be present, often only erosions are apparent, which may coalesce to form large, clearly demarcated areas surrounded by erythema. Bullae, which form in the granular layer or beneath the stratum corneum, contain neutrophils and clusters of cocci. The upper dermis may disclose inflammation from a mixture of neutrophils and lymphocytes.

Appropriate therapy for bullous impetigo is an oral agent active against *Staphylococcus aureus*, such as erythromycin, a first-generation cephalosporin, or dicloxacillin. Topical mupirocin is an alternative. In hot, humid climates where the risk of impetigo is high, its frequency can be reduced in children by applying topical neomycin-bacitracin prophylactically to areas of minor trauma, such as scratches, abrasions, and insect bites.[17]

ECTHYMA

Ecthyma, a Greek term for pustule derived from a word meaning "breaking out," refers to an infection resembling impetigo but located deeper in the skin. Like impetigo, it may be caused by *Streptococcus pyogenes*, *Staphylococcus aureus*, or a combination of the two, but it produces ulceration that reaches the dermis and, unlike impetigo, heals with scarring. It usually occurs in patients with preceding trauma, frequently in the setting of poor hygiene, and commonly affects the lower extremities, often with several lesions. It begins with pustules and vesicles, but the infection penetrates beneath the skin surface to create ulcerations with surrounding erythema. The lesions are typically covered with thick, adherent crusts (Fig. 105-3). Biopsy of the lesion demonstrates a nonspecific ulcer with abundant neutrophils present in the dermis and the overlying serous exudate. Treatment should be an oral antimicrobial agent with activity against both *Staphylococcus aureus* and *Streptococcus pyogenes*, such as dicloxacillin.

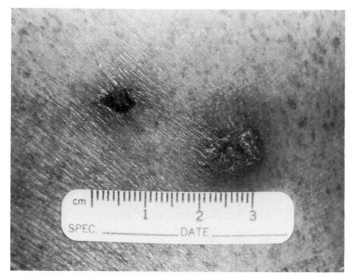

FIGURE 105-3. Ecthyma. Two erythematous lesions appear on the leg. The left lesion has an adherent crust, and the right lesion has a small ulcer in the center. Culture of the ulcer grew 100% *Staphylococcus aureus*.

BLISTERING DISTAL DACTYLITIS

Blistering distal dactylitis is usually caused by *Streptococcus pyogenes*, but *Staphylococcus aureus* is occasionally responsible. Most reported cases have occurred in children.[18] A tender, superficial bulla on an erythematous base develops on the volar fat pad of a finger, thumb, or, rarely, a toe[19] and may extend to involve the hyponychial area. Several digits may be affected, and the contents of the blister vary from thin and watery to purulent. Gram stains of aspirated fluid typically demonstrate neutrophils and gram-positive cocci in chains, and cultures usually yield *Streptococcus pyogenes*. Gram-positive cocci in clusters on Gram stain should suggest *Staphylococcus aureus*. When combined with incision and drainage for tense, painful blisters, systemic penicillin is satisfactory therapy except for the rare staphylococcal lesion, which should be treated with an agent such as dicloxacillin.

FOLLICULITIS

Folliculitis, inflammation of the epithelium of the hair follicle, is a common dermatologic problem with several different causes. One element in its pathogenesis is occlusion of the follicular orifice by keratinaceous material, excessive hydration of the surrounding skin, or adjacent cutaneous inflammation of microbial, chemical, mechanical, or immunologic origin. Organisms beneath the obstructed ostium can then proliferate, causing follicular inflammation and purulence. Sometimes, *Staphylococcus aureus* is isolated from the pus, but often the cultures yield a mixture of normal cutaneous flora or are sterile. The yeast *Pityrosporum orbiculare* is another cause. Staphylococcal folliculitis has been most common in children, appearing usually on the scalp or extremities. Erythematous papules or pustules surrounding hairs may

occur singly or in crops; this disorder responds promptly to systemic antistaphylococcal antimicrobial therapy.

FURUNCLES AND CARBUNCLES

When staphylococci infect the hair follicle at a deeper level than in folliculitis, the inflammation extends to the dermis, causing furuncles or carbuncles. An inflammatory nodule develops, topped by a pustule through which a hair emerges. Individual lesions are called furuncles or boils and can appear anywhere on the hairy skin but are most common on the legs and face. When the infection involves several adjacent follicles to create an inflammatory mass from which pus discharges through several follicular orifices, the lesion is called a carbuncle. Carbuncles typically occur on the back of the neck and appear to be more common in diabetics than in the general population. Moist heat, which may promote drainage, is often satisfactory therapy for small furuncles; incision and drainage are required for larger furuncles and for carbuncles. Unless substantial surrounding cellulitis or fever is present, systemic antistaphylococcal antibiotics are usually unnecessary.

RECURRENT STAPHYLOCOCCAL SKIN INFECTIONS

Some patients are afflicted by recurrent episodes of staphylococcal skin infections. Diabetes mellitus, chronic renal dialysis, intravenous drug abuse, and certain granulocytic or immunologic diseases are predisposing factors, but most patients have no obvious underlying disorder. They are probably chronic staphylococcal nasal carriers who disperse the organisms onto the skin, where trauma, often mild and inapparent, allows the staphylococci to invade the skin and cause infections.

Approaches to preventing these recurrent pyodermas have included bathing with various antiseptics, sterilizing the patient's laundry, treating other family members with antistaphylococcal antibiotics, inoculating the patient's anterior nares with nonpathogenic staphylococci, and protracted therapy with topical or systemic antimicrobial agents in an attempt to eliminate staphylococcal carriage. These techniques are usually impractical and ineffectual. Many topical antibiotics applied to the anterior nares eradicate the organisms (Table 105-2), but the bacteria quickly reappear once the agent is discontinued, in many cases probably because staphylococci also reside more posteriorly in the nose. The most effective topical medication is mupirocin, which often eliminates *Staphylococcus aureus* for long periods even after the course of application has ended. Unfortunately, widespread or protracted use has led to the emergence of resistance to the drug. Most oral antibiotics are ineffective, probably because they achieve poor concentrations in the nasal secretions. Exceptions include rifampin and the fluoroquinolones, such as ciprofloxacin, but resistance to these agents is a major concern when they are used alone. Clindamycin is probably the best antimicrobial agent for this purpose. When given as a single 150-mg tablet daily

TABLE 105-2. Medications for Treating Staphylococcal
and Streptococcal Skin Infections

Medication	Adult Dosage	Duration of Therapy	Comments
Cefazolin	500 mg bid–tid IM or IV	7–10 days	For severe infections requiring parenteral therapy; with clinical improvement, treatment can be changed to oral cephalexin or cephradine.
Cephalexin Cephradine	250 mg qid PO	7–10 days	
Clindamycin	150 mg qid PO or IV	7–10 days	*Staphylococcus aureus* occasionally resistant; one tablet daily for several months is effective prophylaxis against recurrent staphylococcal skin infections; *Clostridium difficile* colitis is a very rare complication with outpatient therapy.
Dicloxacillin	250 mg qid PO	7–10 days	
Erythromycin base or stearate	250 mg qid PO	7–10 days	Variable resistance of *S. aureus* depending on community.
Mupirocin	Apply topically tid	7–10 days	Good for impetigo; mupirocin is active against streptococci and *S. aureus*, both methicillin sensitive and resistant strains; prolonged treatment (months) may lead to development of resistance in *S. aureus*.
Nafcillin Oxacillin	500 mg qid IV	7–10 days	For severe infections requiring parenteral therapy; with clinical improvement, treatment can be changed to oral dicloxacillin.
Penicillin G Benzathine	1.2 million units IM	Single dose	Single dose provides adequate tissue and blood levels for about 4 weeks against streptococci and penicillin-sensitive staphylococci; can be given monthly to prevent recurrent cellulitis.
Penicillin V	250 mg qid PO	7–10 days	For infections due to streptococci and penicillin-sensitive staphylococci; good for mild to moderately severe erysipelas.
Vancomycin	1 g bid IV	7–10 days	For severe infections requiring parenteral therapy; parenteral drug of choice for methicillin-resistant *S. aureus*.

for 3 months, it eradicated recurrent staphylococcal skin infections in 82% of patients with a preceding history of them, compared with patients receiving placebo, 64% of whom continued to develop them. After discontinuing the clindamycin, most patients remained free of infections for at least 9 months, suggesting that staphylococcal carriage was eliminated, although nasal cultures were not done.[20]

ERYSIPELAS AND CELLULITIS

Erysipelas and cellulitis are acute, rapidly spreading, nonsuppurative infections of the skin and underlying soft tissues but not including the muscle. Erysipelas is more superficial than cellulitis and involves the dermis, predominantly the upper part. Cellulitis affects the deep dermis and subcutaneous fat. The clinical distinction between the two supposedly rests on the demarcation of the cutaneous erythema and edema from the surrounding tissue: there is sharp delineation in erysipelas but less clear differentiation in cellulitis, in which these abnormalities more gradually merge with the adjacent skin and soft tissues. The diagnostic difference is frequently difficult to appreciate, and, for many, the term *erysipelas* applies only to facial involvement. Erysipelas so defined is most common in the elderly, may occur after obvious facial injury or without any apparent cause, and typically affects the cheeks, often spreading across the nasal bridge to form a butterfly pattern. From this area and other common sites such as the forehead and ears, the process may spread to the eyelids (Fig. 105–4). It is usually a painful, sometimes pruritic, bright-red, spreading edema on which vesicles, bullae, and exudation may develop. It

is hot and tender to the touch. Fever and chills are common, but not invariable, accompaniments; occasionally, they precede any cutaneous findings by several hours. Some patients become confused or delirious from the toxicity of the infection, and many patients have leukocytosis. Erysipelas is considered to be a streptococcal infection, usually due to group A (*Streptococcus pyogenes*) but sometimes to other groups, such as G and C.[21]

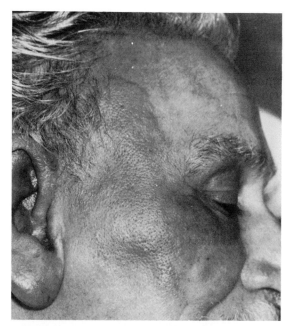

FIGURE 105–4. Erysipelas. Swelling and erythema involve the ear, temporal area, cheek, and right lower eyelid. Fluid oozing from the surface of the ear grew group C streptococci.

Cellulitis commonly involves the extremities, particularly the calf area. Often there is preceding trauma, an ulcer, or other damaged skin from which the infection emanates. Lymphedema is a predisposing factor, as is saphenous vein removal for vascular procedures. Sometimes, the site of cutaneous damage is subtle, such as a small fissure in the skin, particularly in the toe webs from tinea pedis, but frequently no obvious abnormality is present to explain why cellulitis has occurred. As in erysipelas, fever and chills may accompany, or even precede, the cutaneous findings, but many patients are afebrile and do not appear seriously ill. The skin is red, hot, and edematous; the margin of the inflammation is irregular; and, as in erysipelas, vesicles, bullae, and exudation of fluid from the surface of the lesion may occur. Especially on the lower extremities, because of the high vascular hydrostatic pressure, petechiae, purpura, or hemorrhagic bullae sometimes develop (Fig. 105–5). Lymphangitis and regional lymphadenitis can also occur but are commonly absent.

The clinical diagnosis of cellulitis is usually simple, although some clinicians find the distinction between it and venous thrombosis difficult (Table 105–3). In superficial thrombophlebitis the erythema and edema are linear and clearly overlie a tender, easily palpable vascular structure, making the diagnosis easy. In deep venous thrombosis of the leg, the occluded, possibly inflamed vein lies very deep; between it and the skin are large muscle groups, fascia, and substantial subcutaneous tissue. Accordingly, inflammation arising from the vein cannot spread through all those structures to involve the cutaneous surface, and, therefore, the skin is not red or hot. An exception is thrombosis of the ileofemoral vein, which lies close to the skin surface as it enters the groin area. Even in that circumstance, although erythema and heat may occur on the overlying skin, they typically have a linear distribution along the course of the underlying vein.

A more difficult differentiation is between acute gout and cellulitis of the foot and ankle. In gout, soft tissue inflammation can spread from the involved joint to cause heat and erythema in the surrounding skin. Fur-

TABLE 105–3. Differential Diagnosis of Cellulitis

Superficial thrombophlebitis
Deep venous thrombosis
Acute gout

thermore, some patients have fever. Helpful clues suggesting gout are marked pain with movement of the involved joint and a history of previous attacks. In some cases, aspiration of the joint is prudent to confirm the suspicion of gout. The presence of lymphangitis, lymphadenitis, bullae, or vesicles, on the other hand, indicates cellulitis.

A definitive bacteriologic diagnosis of erysipelas and cellulitis is difficult to obtain. Needle aspiration of the affected skin has a 5% to 10% yield on culture,[22] although the return may be higher in those with diabetes or malignancy.[23] Cultures of skin biopsy specimens were positive in about 20% in one study.[22] Blood cultures, positive in about 5%, have usually grown *Streptococcus pyogenes*, but streptococci of other serogroups such as G, C, or F are occasional isolates. The meager frequency of positive cultures suggests that the number of organisms present in the tissues is small, and most of the inflammatory reaction may be an immune response to bacterial antigens or toxins rather than the effects of intact, live bacteria.[24] Immunofluorescent microscopic evaluation of skin biopsy specimens indicates that most cases of erysipelas and cellulitis are due to various streptococci.[25] Serologic evidence of recent streptococcal infection may confirm the etiology, but these techniques have not been widely employed in studies of cutaneous infections. Testing for Anti–streptolysin O is not helpful because streptococcal skin infections do not commonly elicit this antibody. Anti–DNAse B is sensitive and specific for *Streptococcus pyogenes* but will not detect infections with other streptococcal serogroups.

The histologic features of erysipelas and cellulitis are edema, dilated lymphatics, and diffuse neutrophilic infil-

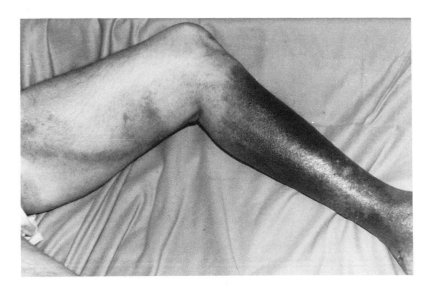

FIGURE 105–5. Cellulitis with lymphangitis. Erythema and purpura on the calf. Linear erythema extends along the inner thigh, indicating proximal lymphangitis.

tration throughout the dermis. The inflammation, often more pronounced around blood vessels, may elicit red blood cell extravasation and may extend into the subcutaneous fat. Severe papillary edema may be associated with subepidermal vesiculation. Brown-Brenn or Giemsa stains may reveal gram-positive cocci in the tissues.

Staphylococcus aureus can sometimes cause cellulitis, but it is usually associated with a cutaneous abscess or an ulcer, and the erythema and edema are typically circumscribed to a small area around the site of origin. Unusual forms of cellulitis, such as those associated with severe neutropenia, immersion injuries, or animal bites are discussed in Chapter 106.

Treatment of erysipelas and cellulitis includes local measures and antimicrobial agents (Table 105–4). The affected inflamed area should be elevated to help promote resolution of the edema and drainage of the inflammatory products. Patients with erysipelas should keep their heads upright throughout the day and night, sleeping with several pillows or with the head of the bed raised. Patients with leg cellulitis should remain recumbent as much as possible with the affected lower extremity elevated to a position above the level of the heart. Cool, moist dressings may help relieve discomfort but are usually unnecessary and do not hasten recovery.

Because erysipelas is nearly always streptococcal, the treatment of choice remains penicillin, given by mouth or parenterally, depending on the severity of the infection and the ability of the patient to take oral medications. Benzathine penicillin, 1.2 million units intramuscularly, is very effective for outpatient management, since a single dose provides therapeutic levels for several weeks and ensures adequate treatment for those who may be unreliable in taking oral medication. In severely ill patients requiring hospitalization, intravenous aqueous penicillin G is the drug of choice; a first-generation cephalosporin (e.g., cefazolin), clindamycin, and vancomycin are alternatives.

Some clinicians believe that most cases of cellulitis are also due to streptococci and treat this disorder with penicillin as well. Others are concerned about the possible role of *Staphylococcus aureus* and employ an agent active against both pathogens. For oral therapy, erythromycin, dicloxacillin, clindamycin, and a first-generation cephalosporin such as cephradine or cephalexin are reasonable choices. Parenteral therapy for hospitalized patients could include an antistaphylococcal penicillin such as nafcillin or oxacillin or a first-generation cepha-

losporin such as cefazolin. Because many of the features of erysipelas and cellulitis arise from inflammation, the addition of systemic corticosteroids (e.g., prednisone, 40 mg daily, for a few days) to antimicrobial therapy is a theoretically attractive, but untested, approach to hasten the resolution of the clinical findings and diminish lymphatic damage.

Patients treated for erysipelas or cellulitis often appear to worsen in the first 1 or 2 days of antimicrobial therapy. The erythema may extend, the fever increase, and the patient's toxic appearance intensify. These apparently worrisome features are probably due to the dying organisms suddenly releasing enzymes, such as streptokinase, hyaluronidase, and DNAse, that provoke a potent inflammatory response and are probably responsible for most of the cutaneous and systemic findings in these infections. No change in antimicrobial therapy is necessary, and improvement is usually evident within a day or so.

Some patients have recurrent episodes of erysipelas or cellulitis. Each attack probably causes some lymphatic damage from inflammation and scarring; the resulting cutaneous edema and impaired drainage of lymph may increase the likelihood of further episodes. Lymphatic injury from other causes, such as surgery[26] or radiation therapy, imposes a similar risk. Any long-standing or permanent cutaneous injury can also predispose to such recurrent infections. An example is a preceding saphenous venectomy performed for vascular disease or coronary artery surgery. In many of these patients there has been an associated tinea pedis, the treatment of which has ended the repeated episodes.[27] Perhaps the area of fungal infection has provided a portal of entry for the infecting streptococci. An alternative, but unconfirmed, explanation is that the responsible streptococci, which ordinarily do not survive on normal skin, colonize the area of fungal infection, from where they can easily disperse to reach and invade the scarred skin at the site of vein removal.

When patients have recurrent cellulitis in the same location, the clinician should treat any remediable predisposing skin condition, such as tinea pedis, eczema, or dry skin. If recurrences continue, an effective prophylactic program is monthly intramuscular injections of benzathine penicillin. An alternative approach is oral penicillin or erythromycin given daily or for 1 week once a month.[28]

UNCOMMON STREPTOCOCCAL AND STAPHYLOCOCCAL INFECTIONS

Perianal Cellulitis[29, 30]

Streptococcus pyogenes can cause a painful or itchy perianal eruption, usually in young children, that may be present for weeks to months. It typically consists of a bright, moist, and tender erythema, sometimes with painful fissures and a purulent or mucoid discharge that may stain the underclothes. Pustules are occasionally present. The origin of the bacteria is uncertain; streptococci from the upper respiratory tract may be swallowed

TABLE 105–4. Treatment of Cellulitis and Erysipelas

Elevate inflamed area.
Apply cold compresses.
Administer antibiotics.
Use intravenous penicillin for very ill patients.
  Alternates: cefazolin, clindamycin, vancomycin
Use oral antibiotics for mild-moderate infections.
  Erythromycin
  Dicloxacillin
  Clindamycin
  Cephalexin or cephradine

or transferred by contaminated hands to the anal area. Therapy with penicillin is effective.

Botryomycosis[31, 32]

Botryomycosis is a rare, chronic suppurative disease characterized histologically by the presence of granules formed by clumps of bacteria within foci of chronic granulomatous and suppurative inflammation. The usual location is on the extremities, but lesions can occur on the trunk, face, and perianal area. They are typically chronic, slowly enlarging plaques or masses with a verrucous surface within which may be nodules, crusting, and sinuses that drain pus and firm granules. *Staphylococcus aureus* has been a common isolate, often in pure culture, but many other bacteria, alone or in combination, have been implicated, including *Pseudomonas aeruginosa*, *Escherichia coli*, and species of *Proteus*, *Peptostreptococcus*, and *Bacillus*. Possible predisposing factors include trauma, diabetes mellitus, and immune deficiencies, but the pathogenesis of botryomycosis is unknown. Protracted treatment with an appropriate antibiotic is usually successful in eradicating the infection.

Necrotizing Fasciitis and Streptococcal Toxic Shock Syndrome

These unusual streptococcal soft tissue infections are discussed in Chapters 106 and 108.

THE NORMAL CUTANEOUS FLORA[1]

The introduction to this chapter mentioned some of the characteristics affecting the growth of organisms on the cutaneous surface. A few kinds of bacteria, "residents," can complete their life cycle on the skin; their ability to do so relates partly to their capacity to attach to cutaneous cells. In contrast, "transients," which reach the skin surface from the environment or contiguous body areas, such as mucous membranes, do not adhere well to squames and cannot flourish on the skin for protracted periods. The normal resident flora lives as mixed microcolonies, predominantly between the layers of the outer stratum corneum but also in the hair follicles. The density of the bacteria ranges from $10^2/cm^2$ on dry skin to $10^7/cm^2$ in moist areas such as the toe webs or axillae. Anaerobes are infrequent in most sites but reach densities of 10^4 to $10^6/cm^2$ in locations with abundant sebaceous glands, such as the face and scalp, and populate the deeper parts of the hair follicles and sebaceous glands.

Coagulase-negative staphylococci are the most numerous bacteria on the skin. *Staphylococcus epidermidis* predominates on most of the cutaneous surface, especially the upper body, but *S. hominis* is also frequently present. *S. capitis* is common on the scalp and face, and other isolates include *S. cohnii*, *S. warneri*, *S. simulans*, *S. xylosus*, and *S. saprophyticus*. The related gram-positive cocci, *Micrococcus* species (primarily *M. luteus* and *M. varians*) are also common skin organisms.

Coryneform bacteria are aerobic or anaerobic gram-positive bacilli that do not form spores, do not branch, and are not acid fast.[33] Some of those on the skin require lipids for growth and are designated "lipophilic" or "lipid dependent." These bacteria are major elements of the cutaneous flora, especially in moist areas such as the nose, axilla, perineum, and toe interspaces. Aerobic non–lipid-dependent coryneforms commonly present on the skin include *Corynebacterium minutissimum*, *C. xerosis*, and *Brevibacterium epidermidis*, all of which are prevalent primarily in the perineum and toe interspaces. Anaerobic coryneforms are *Propionibacterium* species. *P. acnes*, the most common, is present mostly in areas with abundant sebaceous glands such as the face and scalp, as is *P. granulosum*. *P. avidum* is usually found in moist areas, such as the nose, axilla, perineum, and anal regions.

Gram-negative bacilli are uncommon on the skin, except for *Acinetobacter* species, which are carried by about 25% of adults in moist areas, including the axillae, groin, toe webs, and antecubital fossae. Carriage is more common in the summer months, presumably because of increased sweating.

RESIDENT FLORA AS CUTANEOUS PATHOGENS

Cutaneous Abscesses[34, 35]

Most clinicians associate cutaneous abscesses with *Staphylococcus aureus*. This organism, however, is isolated in only about 25% of cases, usually in pure culture. The location of the abscess determines the identity of the infecting flora. *S. aureus* is present in more than 50% of finger paronychiae, breast abscesses in puerperal women, and axillary abscesses. It is isolated in 20% to 40% of breast abscesses in nonpuerperal women, toe paronychiae, and abscesses of the hands, buttocks, extremities, trunk, and inguinal areas.

When *S. aureus* is not the cause, the bacteriology is usually anaerobes alone or a mixture of aerobic and anaerobic organisms, typically members of the resident regional flora or transients from contiguous mucous membranes. Abscesses of the perineal area, including those of the vulvovaginal, scrotal, inguinal, perianal, and buttocks regions, commonly grow fecal flora, such as anaerobic gram-positive cocci, streptococci, and *Bacteroides* species. Abscesses of the head and neck typically yield *Staphylococcus epidermidis*, *Propionibacterium* species, and anaerobic gram-positive cocci.

Cutaneous abscesses are usually tender, erythematous, fluctuant masses, sometimes with a purulent top. Removal of the pus by incision and drainage is the appropriate therapy; leaving the resultant cavity open, packing it with gauze, or suturing the incision are therapeutic alternatives with different proponents. Gram stain and culture of the pus are usually unnecessary, as is antibiotic therapy,[34] which should be reserved for those patients with extensive surrounding cellulitis, seriously impaired host defenses, cutaneous gangrene, or systemic manifestations of infection.

Erythrasma

Erythrasma is characterized by red to brown scaling patches. It is apparently caused by *Corynebacterium minutissimum*,[36] although the evidence implicating this specific organism, as opposed to other coryneforms, is not entirely convincing. Usually producing no symptoms, erythrasma tends to affect intertriginous areas such as the groin, submammary regions, axillae, and toe webs, probably because the high moisture content, friction, and maceration damage the stratum corneum, allowing this organism to proliferate. Diabetes mellitus, increasing age, obesity, and residence in tropical climates (where the lesions are often more extensive than in temperate locations) are predisposing factors. The most common form of erythrasma, which may occur in 20% or more of the population, affects the toe webs, especially the fourth interspace, producing scaling, fissuring, and maceration (Figs. 105–6 and 105–7; see color plate). Elsewhere, the typical lesions are irregular, scaly, slightly brown or erythematous patches with well-demarcated borders.

Because these infecting organisms produce porphyrins, the involved areas fluoresce coral-pink to orange-red with ultraviolet light from Wood's lamp. This test confirms the diagnosis; cultures are not rewarding. Lesions are sometimes biopsied to rule out other conditions. Erythrasma is a noninflammatory condition, and the only diagnostic finding is the presence of fine linear arrays of coccobacilli within compact hyperkeratosis. The diagnosis can be confirmed by Brown-Brenn or Gomori's methenamine silver stain.

Vigorous washing with soap sometimes suffices as treatment. Another approach is topical therapy with azoles, such as miconazole, clotrimazole, or econazole (but not ketoconazole), which have activity against some

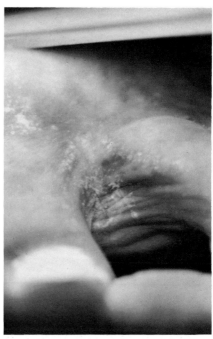

FIGURE 105–7. Erythrasma. The lesion shown in Figure 105–6 fluoresces a coral-pink color with Wood's lamp, confirming the diagnosis. (See color plate.)

gram-positive bacteria as well as fungi.[37] Topical erythromycin, clindamycin, and Whitfield's ointment are also effective, as is oral erythromycin.[38, 39]

Trichomycosis Axillaris

Yellow, red, or black waxy nodules forming on axillary hair characterize trichomycosis axillaris (Fig. 105–8).[40] They may fluoresce various colors under Wood's light. Similar lesions occasionally occur on pubic or facial hair. This process is produced by large colonies of coryneform bacteria coating the cuticular layers of the hair and perhaps elaborating enzymes that partly destroy the superficial hair keratins.[41, 42] The disorder occurs primarily in patients who have poor personal hygiene, sweat excessively, and do not use deodorants. Shaving the hair and using axillary deodorants are usually successful in treating the disease. Topical clindamycin or erythromycin may also be effective.

Axillary Odor

Studies on axillary flora indicate that common isolates are gram-positive cocci (including *Staphylococcus* and *Micrococcus* species), lipophilic coryneforms, and large-colony coryneforms.[43, 44] About 65% of females and 25% of males have a cocci-dominant flora, defined as constituting more than 75% of the aerobes. The density of organisms in these persons is relatively low, less than $1 \times 10^6/cm^2$. In about 65% of males and 25% of females coryneforms dominate and are present in high concentrations, about $2 \times 10^6/cm^2$. Persons with a coryneform-

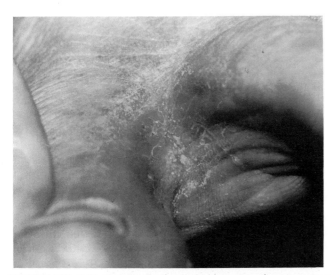

FIGURE 105–6. Erythrasma. Scaling and white maceration are present between the first and second toes.

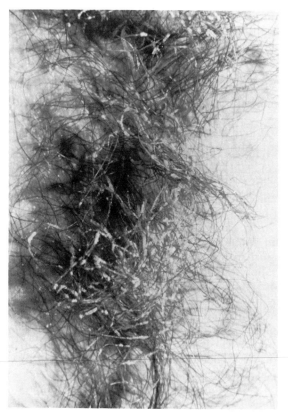

FIGURE 105–8. Trichomycosis axillaris. Nodular thickening appears along the axillary hairs.

dominant flora have a more intense axillary odor. Sterile apocrine sweat has no smell, but when incubated with lipophilic or large-colony coryneforms on the forearm, axillary odor is reproduced. Incubation of the sweat with staphylococci or *Escherichia coli* does not reproduce the aroma.[44] Further evidence for the role of bacteria is the effectiveness of topical neomycin in reducing the gram-positive flora and eliminating axillary odor.[45] In fact, a principal action of many axillary deodorants lies in their antibacterial properties. The odor probably derives from a mixture of volatile substances, including fatty acids, androstenedione, and, perhaps most importantly, 3-methyl-2-hexanoic acid, a product of bacterial action on axillary sweat.[46]

Pitted Keratolysis

Pitted keratolysis is the presence of pits 1 to 7 mm in diameter on the soles or, less commonly, collarettes on the palms.[47] Patients are usually asymptomatic, but pruritus, burning, pain, and tenderness may be present, as may a cheesy malodor. Scaling, erythema, and fissuring may occur, and sometimes the pitted areas coalesce to form larger erosions and erythematous plaques (Fig. 105–9). The lesions become more prominent when soaked in water for 10 to 15 minutes. Pitted keratolysis seems to occur in association with increased moisture from occlusive footwear, frequent contact with water, or excessive sweating. Bacteria appear responsible for this

disorder and may produce enzymes that digest keratin to create the pits or erosions in the stratum corneum. Some evidence suggests that coryneforms are the cause, and inoculating *Corynebacterium* strains onto the skin of human volunteers reproduced the disease. Another investigation found both *C. minutissimum* and *Micrococcus sedentarius* in all cases of pitted keratolysis and produced the disorder by applying a pure culture of *M. sedentarius* under occlusion on a volunteer's heel.[48] Perhaps, both coryneforms and *M. sedentarius* alone or together can cause the disease. *M. sedentarius* elaborates volatile, malodorous thiols and thiol esters that may explain the foot odor. Biopsy specimens show pits within the cornified layer of affected acral skin, lined by filamentous arrays of minute cocci. Several therapies seem to be effective, including topical azoles such as miconazole and clotrimazole (which are active against many gram-positive bacteria); topical erythromycin or clindamycin; antiseptics, such as glutaraldehyde and formaldehyde; and oral erythromycin.[47]

Interdigital Toe Space Infections

The normal flora of the toe spaces includes coagulase-negative staphylococci, lipophilic coryneforms, large-colony coryneforms, and, to a lesser extent, gram-negative bacilli (predominantly *Acinetobacter* species) and yeasts.[49, 50] Interdigital toe space infections or "athlete's foot" usually begins as scaling and fissuring.[51] Although some of the infections are erythrasma, dermatophytes are present in about 85% of cases and the normal flora is increased in density. As the infection becomes more severe and maceration develops, the normal flora, especially large-colony coryneforms including *Brevibacterium epidermidis* and *Corynebacterium minutissimum*, continues to proliferate, and other bacteria become more prevalent, including gram-negative bacilli and *Staphylococcus aureus*. Cultures for dermatophytes are positive in about 60%. In severe "athlete's foot," characterized by

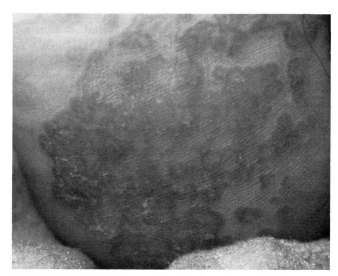

FIGURE 105–9. Pitted keratolysis. Erosions, pits, and collarettes are present on the heel. The foot was also malodorous.

redness, maceration, itching, and malodor, cultures yield dermatophytes in about 35%, more numerous normal flora, and a marked increase in gram-negative bacilli and large-colony coryneforms. The worst stage of interdigital toe infections involves erosions and pus. *Pseudomonas aeruginosa* predominates, and dermatophytes grow in about 33% of cases.

The proposed sequence of interdigital toe space infections begins with damage to the stratum corneum by dermatophytes and is known as dermatophytosis simplex.[50] These fungi produce penicillin, which decreases the sensitive lipophilic coryneforms and encourages the growth of penicillin-resistant organisms, including large-colony coryneforms, *Staphylococcus aureus*, gram-negative bacilli, and *Micrococcus sedentarius*. These "pathogens" may provoke inflammation and maceration, and *Brevibacterium epidermidis*, in particular, produces proteolytic enzymes that further damage the stratum corneum. Moreover, it elaborates several sulfur compounds, such as methanethiol, which discourage the growth of fungi and cause malodor. This condition is called dermatophytosis complex, because it appears to represent the effects not only of the fungi but also of the overgrowth of bacteria. The dermatophytes, inhibited by the bacteria and forced lower in the stratum corneum, are more difficult to isolate from superficial scrapings, but biopsy specimens from the interdigital skin typically show sparse fungal filaments in the deep stratum corneum.

In mild interdigital infections dermatophytes are the main cause, and antifungal agents should suffice in most cases. In studies of moderately severe infections a purely antibacterial substance (i.e., framycetin) produced modest improvement, a purely antifungal agent (i.e., tolfanate) was also fairly effective,[52] but azoles (e.g., clotrimazole, econazole, or miconazole but not ketoconazole), which are active against both fungi and the bacteria, were better than the other medications.[52, 53] Experiments on volunteers confirm the pathogenic significance of both fungi and bacteria.[51] Interspace occlusion in those without dermatophyte infection caused an increase in the population of large-colony coryneforms but only mild clinical changes. When dermatophyte infection was already present, occlusion caused a marked increase in large-colony coryneforms and the interspace became soggy, white, and macerated, with malodor and pruritus. Treatment of the interspace with antibacterial agents (povidone-iodine and topical chloramphenicol) during the period of occlusion in those patients with dermatophyte infection prevented the bacterial overgrowth, and the interspace remained nearly normal. In moderately severe and severe interdigital infections, therefore, both dermatophytes and bacteria, especially gram-positive organisms, seem important, and azoles, with their activity against both types of organisms, are probably the best topical agents. When "gram-negative" interdigital infection occurs, characterized by erosions and pus, an azole may still be effective,[53] even though it is inactive against gram-negative bacilli, perhaps because decreasing the other flora may remove the conditions that allow gram-negative bacilli to thrive. Drying the interspaces by removal of footwear, separation of the toes, and application of astringents such as aluminum chloride may also be helpful in severe cases.

References

1. Roth RR, James WE. Microbiology of the skin: Resident flora, ecology, infection. J Am Acad Dermatol 1980;20:367–390.
2. Noble WC. Staphylococci on the skin. In: Noble WC, ed. The Skin Microflora and Microbial Skin Disease. Cambridge, England: Cambridge University Press, 1992:135–152.
3. Barnham M. Streptococci and the skin. In: Noble WC, ed. The Skin Microflora and Microbial Skin Disease. Cambridge, England: Cambridge University Press, 1992:173–209.
4. Barton LL, Friedman AD. Impetigo: A reassessment of etiology and therapy. Pediatr Dermatol 1987;4:185–188.
5. Barton LL, Friedman AD, Sharkey AM, et al. Impetigo contagiosa: III. Comparative efficacy of oral erythromycin and topical mupirocin. Pediatr Dermatol 1989;6:134–138.
6. Leyden JJ, Marples RR, Kligman AM. *Staphylococcus aureus* in the lesions of atopic dermatitis. Br J Dermatol 1974;90:525–530.
7. Hanifin JM, Rogge JL. Staphylococcal infections in patients with atopic dermatitis. Arch Dermatol 1977;113:1383–1386.
8. Wachs GN, Maibach HI. Co-operative double-blind trial of an antibiotic corticoid combination in impetiginized atopic dermatitis. Br J Dermatol 1976;95:323–328.
9. Lever R, Hadley K, Downey D, et al. Staphylococcal colonization in atopic dermatitis and the effect of topical mupirocin therapy. Br J Dermatol 1988;119:189–198.
10. Nilsson EJ, Henning CG, Magnusson J. Topical corticosteroids and *Staphylococcus aureus* in atopic dermatitis. J Am Acad Dermatol 1992;27:29–34.
11. Dagan R, Bar-David Y. Comparison of amoxicillin and clavulanic acid (Augmentin) for the treatment of nonbullous impetigo. Am J Dis Child 1989;143:916–918.
12. Demidovich CW, Wittler RR, Ruff ME, et al. Impetigo: Current etiology and comparison of penicillin, erythromycin, and cephalexin therapies. Am J Dis Child 1990;144:1313–1315.
13. McLinn S. Topical mupirocin vs. systemic erythromycin treatment of pyoderma. Pediatr Infect Dis J 1988;7:785–790.
14. Goldfarb J, Crenshaw D, O'Horo J, et al. Randomized clinical trial of topical mupirocin versus oral erythromycin for impetigo. Antimicrob Agents Chemother 1988;32:1780–1783.
15. Mertz PM, Marshall DA, Eaglstein WH, et al. Topical mupirocin treatment of impetigo is equal to oral erythromycin therapy. Arch Dermatol 1989;125:1069–1073.
16. Dillon HC. The treatment of streptococcal skin infections. J Pediatr 1970;76:676–684.
17. Maddox JS, Ware JC, Dillon HC. The natural history of streptococcal skin infection: Prevention with topical antibiotics. J Am Acad Dermatol 1985;13:207–212.
18. McCray MK, Esterly NB. Blistering distal dactylitis. J Am Acad Dermatol 1981;5:592–594.
19. Telfer NR, Barth JH, Dawber RPR. Recurrent blistering distal dactylitis of the great toe associated with an ingrowing toenail. Clin Exp Dermatol 1989;14:380–381.
20. Klempner MS, Styrt B. Prevention of recurrent staphylococcal skin infections with low-dose oral clindamycin therapy. JAMA 1988;260:2682–2685.
21. Chartier C, Grosshans E. Erysipelas. Int J Dermatol 1990;29:459–467.
22. Hook EW, Hooten TM, Horton CA, et al. Microbiologic evaluation of cutaneous cellulitis in adults. Arch Intern Med 1986;146:295–297.
23. Kielhofner MA, Brown B, Dall L. Influence of underlying disease process on the utility of cellulitis needle aspirates. Arch Intern Med 1988;148:1451–2452.
24. Sachs MK. Cutaneous cellulitis. Arch Dermatol 1991;127:493–496.
25. Bernard P, Bedane C, Mounier M, et al. Streptococcal cause of erysipelas and cellulitis in adults. Arch Dermatol 1989;125:779–782.
26. Simon MS, Cody RL. Cellulitis after axillary lymph node dissection for carcinoma of the breast. Am J Med 1992;93:543–548.
27. Baddour LM, Bisno AL. Recurrent cellulitis after coronary artery

surgery: Association with superficial fungal infection in saphenous venectomy limbs. JAMA 1984:251:1049–1052.

28. Babb RR, Spittell JA, Martin WJ, Schirger A. Prophylaxis of recurrent lymphangitis complicating lymphedema. JAMA 1966; 195:871–873.
29. Rehder PA, Eliezer ET, Lane AT. Perianal cellulitis: Cutaneous group A streptococcal disease. Arch Dermatol 1988;124:702–704.
30. Krol AL. Perianal streptococcal dermatitis. Pediatr Dermatol 1990;7:97–100.
31. Picou K, Batres E, Jarratt M. Botryomycosis: A bacterial cause of mycetoma. Arch Dermatol 1979;115:609–610.
32. Mehregan DA, Su WPD, Anhalt JP. Cutaneous botryomycosis. J Am Acad Dermatol 1991;24:393–396.
33. Leyden JJ, McGinley KJ. Coryneform bacteria. In: Noble WC, ed. The Skin Microflora and Microbial Skin Disease. Cambridge, England: Cambridge University Press, 1992;102–117.
34. Meislin HW, Lerner SA, Graves MH, et al. Cutaneous abscesses: Anaerobic and aerobic bacteriology and outpatient management. Ann Intern Med 1977;87:145–149.
35. Brook I, Frazier RH. Aerobic and anaerobic bacteriology of wounds and cutaneous abscesses. Arch Surg 1990;125:1445–1451.
36. Sarkany I, Taplin D, Blank H. The etiology and treatment of erythrasma. J Invest Dermatol 1961;37:283–290.
37. Pitcher DG, Noble WC, Seville RH. The treatment of erythrasma with miconazole. Clin Exp Dermatol 1979;4:453–456.
38. Seville RH, Somerville DA. The treatment of erythrasma in a hospital for the mentally subnormal. Br J Dermatol 1970;83:502–506.
39. Cochran RJ, Rosen T, Landers T. Topical treatment for erythrasma. Int J Dermatol 1981;20:562–564.
40. Savin JA, Somerville DA, Noble WC. The bacterial flora of trichomycosis axillaris. J Med Microbiol 1970;3:352–356.
41. McBride ME, Freeman RG, Knox JM. The bacteriology of trichomycosis axillaris. Br J Dermatol 1968;80:509–513.
42. Orfanos CE, Schloesser E, Mahrle G. Hair-destroying growth of *Corynebacterium tenuis* in the so-called trichomycosis axillaris. Arch Dermatol 1971;103:632–639.
43. Jackman PJH, Noble WC. Normal axillary skin microflora in various populations. Clin Exp Dermatol 1983;8:259–268.
44. Leyden JJ, McGinley KJ, Holzle E, et al. The microbiology of the human axilla and its relationship to axillary odor. J Invest Dermatol 1981;77:413–416.
45. Shelley WB, Cahn MM. Effect of topically applied antibiotic agents on axillary odor. JAMA 1955;159:1736–1738.
46. Leyden JJ, Zeng XN, McGinley KJ, et al. Characterization of pungent axillary odors. J Invest Dermatol 1990;94:549.
47. Zaias N. Pitted and ringed keratolysis: A review and update. J Am Acad Dermatol 1982;7:787–791.
48. Nordstrom KM, McGinley KJ, Capiello L, et al. Pitted keratolysis: The role of *Micrococcus sedentarius*. Arch Dermatol 1987; 123:1320–1325.
49. Marshall J, Leeming JP, Holland KT. The cutaneous microbiology of normal human feet. J Appl Bacteriol 1987;62:139–146.
50. Kates SG, Nordstrom KM, McGinley KJ, et al. Microbial etiology of interdigital infections of the toe web spaces. J Am Acad Dermatol 1990;22:578–582.
51. Leyden JJ, Kligman AM: Interdigital athlete's foot. Arch Dermatol 1978;114:1466–1472.
52. Talwar P, Kumar B, Ayyagirl A, Kaur S. Prevalence of bacteria and fungi in athlete's foot of varying severity and response to antibacterial and antifungal therapies. Sabouraudia 1985;23:303–312.
53. Kates SG, Myung KB, McGinley KJ, et al. The antibacterial efficacy of econazole nitrate in interdigital toe web infections. J Am Acad Dermatol 1990;22:583–586.

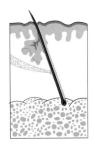

chapter 106

Staphylococcal Toxin-Mediated Syndromes

STEVEN D. RESNICK and PETER M. ELIAS

Toxic exanthems in children and adults represent a common clinical problem. Two distinct staphylococcal toxin–mediated syndromes are included among the numerous infectious etiologies of such exanthems. Toxic shock syndrome (TSS) and the staphylococcal scalded skin syndrome (SSSS) are uncommon but important clinical problems in which early diagnosis of the exanthem can impact significantly in reducing both morbidity and mortality. These syndromes are important as models for understanding the pathogenesis of bacterial toxin–mediated diseases.

Toxic Shock Syndrome

CLINICAL DESCRIPTION

Staphylococcal TSS is characterized by sudden onset of high fever associated with vomiting, diarrhea, headache, pharyngitis, profound myalgia, and significant hypotension.[1] Multisystem organ involvement is an additional characteristic feature that results from both poor tissue perfusion and direct damage from mediators. Potentially fatal complications include refractory shock, oliguric renal failure, ventricular arrhythmia, disseminated intravascular coagulation, and adult respiratory distress syndrome.

Both cutaneous and mucocutaneous findings are prominent in TSS. A diffuse, flexurally accentuated,

scarlatiniform exanthem appears early in the illness. The eruption initially may appear over the trunk, but inevitably it spreads to the arms and legs. Petechiae, vesicles, and bullae are uncommon. Erythema and edema of the palms and soles occur frequently. "Strawberry tongue" may occur along with intense erythema of the mucous membranes and conjunctivae.

Generalized desquamation with prominent sheet-like peeling of the hands and feet usually occurs between 10 and 21 days after presentation. A late-onset, pruritic, generalized macular and papular skin eruption, appearing 9 to 13 days after initial onset of symptoms was seen in 12 of a series of 33 patients,[2] and has been described in other studies. Reversible patchy alopecia and shedding of fingernails has been described in 25% of patients in one series of patients with TSS.[3] Although the hair loss has been characterized as a typical telogen effluvium, the rapid onset of hair loss might be better explained as a toxin-induced anagen effluvium.

Epidemiology

The staphylococcal toxic shock syndrome was defined formally in 1978 with an initial report of seven children.[4] Subsequently, attention has focused on the association of TSS with tampon use in menstruating women.[5] This acute onset and multiorgan illness, however, can affect patients of both sexes, of all ages, and within various settings of occult, trivial, or severe staphylococcal infection. The diagnosis requires the identification of clinical criteria, as delineated by the case definition (Table 106–1).

Menstruating women, especially adolescents, continue to be the group at highest risk for the development of TSS.[6] But nonmenstrual TSS has been increasing in importance since the dramatic cluster of menstrual TSS cases in the early 1980s. In 1986, 45% of the cases identi-

Portions of this chapter taken from Resnick SD. Staphylococcal toxin–mediated syndromes in childhood. Semin Dermatol 1992; 11:11–19.

**TABLE 106-1. Clinical Features of
Toxic Shock Syndrome***

Fever, with temperature greater than 38.9°C (102°F)
Diffuse macular or scarlatiniform skin eruption
Desquamation, 1 to 2 weeks after onset of illness[†]
Hypotension
Involvement of three or more organ systems:
  Gastrointestinal (usually vomiting and diarrhea)
  Muscular
  Mucous membrane erythema
  Renal
  Hepatic
  Hematologic (platelet count less than 100,000/mm³)
  Central nervous system
  Efforts should be made to rule out other treatable causes of
    illness (i.e., Rocky Mountain spotted fever, leptospirosis)

*Probable toxic shock syndrome is considered the same illness except one major criterion is absent.
[†]Desquamation is not necessary in fatal cases.

fied by active case finding were nonmenstrual.[6] Although nonmenstrual cases account for only about 11% of all reported cases of TSS, the true extent of the problem probably has been obscured by failure to recognize nonmenstrual TSS. A growing list of clinical settings for the development of TSS emphasizes the point that TSS is not exclusively a "tampon disease." The associated spectrum of localized staphylococcal infections includes postpartum infection and septic abortion, as well as infections complicating the use of the contraceptive sponge and the contraceptive diaphragm. Additional, less commonly reported settings for TSS include empyema, fasciitis, osteomyelitis, peritonsillar abscess, cutaneous abscess, surgical wound infection, bacteremia,[7] infection at insulin pump infusion sites in diabetics,[8] and following ear piercing.[9]

Nonmenstrual Pediatric Toxic Shock Syndrome

There are approximately 60 reports of nonmenstrual TSS in children.[4, 10] Many of the associated infections have been minor or occurred in commonplace clinical settings, including the previously mentioned case occurring after ear piercing, a case associated with poison oak dermatitis,[11] and two recent cases in children involving secondarily infected abrasions caused by orthopedic casts.[12] Although any infection with toxigenic *Staphylococcus aureus* may result in pediatric TSS, certain clinical settings have been reported more frequently.[10] Fourteen of the 60 reported cases of nonmenstrual TSS in children have occurred in a setting of upper airway infections, including bacterial tracheitis,[13-16] bacterial tracheobronchitis after influenza B,[17] and sinusitis.[18] Children with burn injuries may also represent a group at relatively high risk, based on the development of TSS in 14 children after secondary wound infections in two British burn units. Both the clinical features and the course of nonmenstrual pediatric TSS is similar to the syndrome in adults except that there may be a higher incidence of respiratory failure requiring mechanical ventilation.

PATHOLOGY

Although the diagnosis of TSS is usually made on clinical grounds, there are characteristic histopathologic findings.[19] These include sparse infiltrates of lymphocytes, neutrophils, and sometimes eosinophils around vessels of the superficial plexus and small foci of spongiosis, some of which have clusters of necrotic keratinocytes accompanied by neutrophils. The lesions, in their desquamative phase, resolve with parakeratosis.

PATHOGENESIS AND ETIOLOGY

TSS is caused by infection with certain toxin-producing strains of *S. aureus* in persons lacking protective antibodies at the time of infection. The full expression of the clinical syndrome is dependent on the interaction of both bacterial and host factors. Toxic shock syndrome toxin-1 (TSST-1), a 22,049-dalton protein with a known nucleotide sequence, is one of the significant mediators of pathogenicity in TSS. TSST-1 is generated by strains from virtually all menstrual and many nonmenstrual cases of TSS. However, TSST-1 is not the exclusive agent responsible for the pathogenesis of TSS. Indeed, nonmenstrual cases of TSS are more likely to be due to strains of *S. aureus* that do not produce TSST-1; 40% to 64% of nonmenstrual isolates produce the toxin, compared with 91% to 100% of menstrual isolates. Staphylococcal enterotoxins (A through E), well-known for their role in staphylococcal food poisoning, may also cause TSS under certain conditions, or they could worsen disease caused by TSST-1 in others.[20] Enterotoxin B is the most common TSS toxin among TSST-1–negative strains from cases of nonmenstrual TSS.

Host factors play a major role in the development of TSS. Susceptibility to disease correlates with the absence of a protective level of antibody to TSST-1 in menstrual TSS, and presumably a similar susceptibility exists for those lacking antibodies to enterotoxin B (and probably C). Neonates have passively acquired immunity, unless the mother lacks immunity. Beyond infancy, the likelihood of protective immunity to TSST-1 and enterotoxins changes with age. Approximately half of all children have antibody to TSST-1 by age 10, and it appears that either colonization or subclinical infection with TSST-1–producing staphylococci is adequate to induce the immune response.[21]

In the absence of protective immunity, several biologic activities of TSST-1 and TSS-causing staphylococcal enterotoxins figure prominently in the pathogenesis of TSS. First, the toxins produce marked T-lymphocyte activation and proliferation as a function of their activity as "superantigens."[22, 23] Conventional antigens are processed by antigen-presenting cells (APC) and presented to T lymphocytes in the "binding groove" of the class II major histocompatibility (MHC) molecule on the surface of APC. The complex of antigen bound to the class II MHC then is recognized by a specific T-cell receptor, and the interaction is restricted by T-cell receptor recognition of MHC elements as well as the antigen, resulting in limited recruitment of T lymphocytes. In contrast, superantigens such as TSST-1 and enterotoxin B bind directly to class II MHC, and since binding occurs outside the conventional "binding groove," recognition and processing by APC are not required. The complex of superantigen and class II MHC on APC can then interact with a relatively large number of T lymphocytes because binding to the T-cell receptor is restricted only by the specificity of one region of the T-cell receptor—the V beta region. This relatively unrestricted binding can lead to activation of up to 10% of circulating T lymphocytes, an order of magnitude greater than conventional antigens.[22, 23] Superantigenic T-cell activation leads in turn to massive production of cytokines, including tumor necrosis factor. Many of the signs and symptoms of TSS can be explained by the known effects of cytokines, including fever, shock, and multiple organ system dysfunction.

TSST-1 and enterotoxin B also directly induce monocyte production of interleukin-1 and tumor necrosis factor.[24] Although the superantigenic properties of the toxins have received much attention in the literature, the direct stimulation of cytokine production in monocytes by toxins may be as important or more important than production of cytokines by superantigen-activated lymphocytes. Additional details of investigations into the pathogenesis of TSS can be found in two recent reviews.[10, 20]

DIFFERENTIAL DIAGNOSIS

Intense conjunctival hyperemia is a very frequent and characteristic finding in TSS, but it also occurs in Kawasaki disease, erythema multiforme, Rocky Mountain spotted fever, rubeola, leptospirosis, and enteroviral infections. These diseases, along with early SSSS, make up the important differential diagnosis of TSS (Table 106–2). In children, the distinction between Kawasaki disease and TSS can be very difficult, especially early in the course of illness. The characteristic thrombocytosis and lymphadenopathy of Kawasaki disease are the most helpful distinguishing features, but these features may not always be present.

Also, in recent years, cases of a severe TSS-like streptococcal disease have appeared, associated with reemergence of type A (and type B) pyrogenic exotoxin-producing streptococci.[25–27] The illness is distinct from classic scarlet fever and may not be accompanied by any exanthem. Other features may be indistinguishable clinically from staphylococcal TSS, including multiorgan involvement, toxicity, conjunctival hyperemia and profound hypotension. Typical patients with streptococcal TSS-like syndrome have been previously healthy adults with bacteremia and extensive necrotizing streptococcal soft tissue infections. In contrast, staphylococcal TSS is typically associated with occult or minor focal infections. In Pima County, Arizona, 128 patients with invasive streptococcal infections were retrospectively identified, and streptococcal TSS-like syndrome occurred in 8% of the cases identified since 1988 but none of the cases identified between 1985 and 1987.[28] The first reported case of streptococcal TSS-like syndrome in a child in recent decades was reported in January 1991.[29] Unlike the adult cases of streptococcal TSS-like syndrome, the associated illness in this otherwise normal child was mild primary varicella infection complicated by a secondary skin infection leading to streptococcal bacteremia, but there was no necrotizing soft tissue infection.

It appears that streptococcal pyrogenic exotoxin A shares many biologic properties with TSST-1[30] and possesses structural homology to staphylococcal enterotoxin B.[31] Indeed, the staphylococcal enterotoxins as a group, along with TSST-1 and the streptococcal pyrogenic exotoxins, represent a related family of toxins with strong structural and functional commonalities. The biologic similarities (including superantigen activity) of streptococcal pyrogenic exotoxin A to the TSS-associated staphylococcal toxins help to explain the clinical similarity of streptococcal TSS-like syndrome to TSS.

TREATMENT

Prompt intervention is the key to the successful management of the shock and the resulting multiorgan involvement in TSS. Removal of infected foreign bodies, drainage of infected sites, and institution of penicillinase-resistant antistaphylococcal antibiotics are essential to eradicate the focus of toxin-producing organisms. Massive volume replacement may be needed in the setting of severe intravascular volume depletion accompanied by both a decrease in vasomotor tone and capillary leakage. Cardiovascular support may be necessary, including both inotropic and antiarrhythmic measures. Pediatric patients may require ventilatory support for respiratory distress more often than adult patients. Metabolic acidosis, hypomagnesemia, hypocalcemia, and hypophosphatemia may accompany renal disease, requiring aggressive monitoring and management.

In addition, two somewhat controversial therapies merit consideration in the sickest patients with TSS. First, systemic corticosteroids have been used in the management of severely affected patients. A retrospective study of 25 patients with TSS treated within 3 to 4 days of disease onset with corticosteroids showed reduced severity of illness and duration of fever when compared with 20 patients with TSS who did not receive such therapy.[32] However, other studies have noted no favorable correlation between outcome and the use of corticosteroids.[1] Unless there is evidence of adrenal insufficiency, steroids should probably be considered only when a patient's hypotension is not responsive to removal or drainage of the focus of infection and several hours of fluid administration. Second, administration of immune globulin (400 mg/kg as single dose infused over 2 to 3 hours) is a rational approach to providing specific neutralizing antibody to patients with TSS who typically lack immunity to TSST-1 (or enterotoxins). All commercial preparations of immunoglobulin contain high levels of antibody to TSST-1.[21] This costly therapy, however, has not been critically evaluated and should be reserved for severely ill patients with undrainable or nonresectable foci of infection, such as pneumonia or endometritis (in

TABLE 106-2. Differential Diagnosis of Toxic Shock Syndrome and Staphylococcal Scalded Skin Syndrome

Toxic Shock Syndrome

Most common in young women; associated with menstruation, but nonmenstrual disease occurs in association with focal staphylococcal infections
Hypotension, multiorgan involvement, thrombocytopenia, fever, scarlatiniform rash with flexural accentuation, palmar erythema, mucous membrane erythema, "strawberry tongue" and conjunctival hyperemia, delayed desquamation (especially hands and fingers), alopecia, and nail shedding

Streptococcal Toxic Shock-like Syndrome

Most cases have occurred in adults 20 to 50 years old, without underlying illness; often associated with minor nonpenetrating trauma leading to deep bruising and subsequent deep soft tissue infection; childhood cases have occurred after secondary infection of cutaneous lesions of varicella
Similar to toxic shock syndrome in terms of sudden hypotension, multiorgan involvement, fever, and edema; distinct from toxic shock syndrome because of severe pain of abrupt onset (often in an extremity) and lack of an exanthem

Staphylococcal Scalded Skin Syndrome

Primarily occurs in children younger than 5 years old but seen in older children and adults; caused by epidermolytic toxins A and B produced by strains of phage group II S. aureus
Flexural or generalized erythema, fragile bullae and extensive superficial desquamation, purulent conjunctivitis, rare oral and genital findings, characteristic cutaneous histopathology with separation seen in the granular layer

Kawasaki Disease

Primarily occurs in children younger than 5 years old; reported in some adults
Nonpurulent cervical lymphadenopathy, thrombocytosis, fever, polymorphic maculopapular erythema, mucous membrane erythema, "strawberry tongue" and conjunctival hyperemia, delayed desquamation of fingertips, cardiac sequelae

Scarlet Fever

Occurs in children 2 to 8 years old, resulting from infection with group A β-hemolytic streptococci
Fever, characteristic macular erythema, flexural accentuation (Pastia's lines), sandpaper-like texture, circumoral pallor, pharyngitis, postexanthematous desquamation of fingertips, positive ASO titer

Rocky Mountain Spotted Fever

Caused by Rickettsia rickettsiae, acquired through exposure to ticks
Fever, frontal headache, followed by a characteristic eruption that begins on the wrists and ankles, and spreads centripetally with macular, papular, and characteristically petechial/purpuric components; conjunctival hyperemia may be prominent

Leptospirosis

Infecting organisms acquired through exposure to rats or their urine
Fever, myalgia.petechial/purpuric skin lesions are characteristic but not invariably present; conjunctival hyperemia

Erythema Multiforme Major (Stevens-Johnson Syndrome)

Associated most often with recurrent herpes simplex and drug reactions
Target (iris) lesions, palmar/plantar lesions, crusted and/or inflammatory conjunctival lesions, severe oral inflammation, crusted lips

Adapted from Resnick SD. Staphylococcal toxin–mediated syndromes in childhood. Semin Dermatol 1992;11:11-18.

whom toxemia might persist for some time beyond initiation of antibiotic therapy).

Staphylococcal Scalded Skin Syndrome

SSSS is a potentially life-threatening but treatable, toxin–mediated manifestation of localized infection with certain strains of staphylococci. The syndrome includes a range of limited to extensive cutaneous and systemic disease characterized by tenderness, blistering, and superficial denudation of the skin. SSSS results from the effects of one of the two epidermolytic toxins: ET-A and ET-B. First described in 1878 by Ritter von Rittershain,[33] SSSS is now clearly distinguished from other diseases of generalized epidermal necrolysis such as toxic epidermal necrolysis.

CLINICAL DESCRIPTION

Bullous impetigo, the most common expression of the SSSS spectrum, is caused by a localized skin infection with epidermolytic toxin–producing staphylococci (Fig. 106–1). Bullous impetigo is rarely associated with systemic illness, occurs predominantly in children, but is also seen in adults.[34, 35] The lesions of bullous impetigo contain staphylococci.

Systemic findings and generalized involvement leading to the clinical appearance of scalded skin are the hallmarks of the Ritter disease presentation that most clinicians associate with SSSS. Infections leading to SSSS typically originate in the nasopharynx and frequently go unrecognized. Other primary foci of infection leading to SSSS have included the umbilicus, urinary tract, conjunctivae, and blood. Sudden onset of fever, irritability, cutaneous tenderness, and scarlatiniform erythema heralds the syndrome. The erythema is often accentuated in

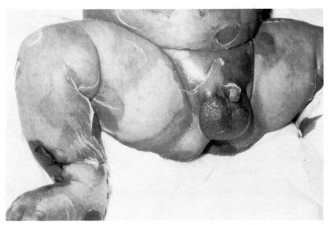

FIGURE 106–2. Generalized epidermolysis and erythema in the Ritter variant of staphylococcal scalded skin syndrome.

flexural and periorificial areas. Flaccid blisters and erosions develop within 24 to 48 hours in the Ritter disease form of SSSS (Fig. 106–2). The blisters and erosions yield no organisms when sampled for bacterial culture. Important clinical clues to diagnosis include prominent denudation in areas of mechanical stress, easy disruption of skin with firm rubbing (Nikolsky's sign), and skin tenderness. A facies with conjunctival inflammation and circumoral erythema evolving to prominent crusting is characteristically seen a few days into the course of the skin disease (Fig. 106–3). Although lip involvement with

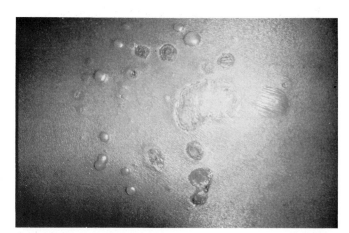

FIGURE 106–1. Localized lesions of bullous impetigo, demonstrating various stages, including tense bullae, denuded blisters, and dried, annular crusted sites of older lesions.

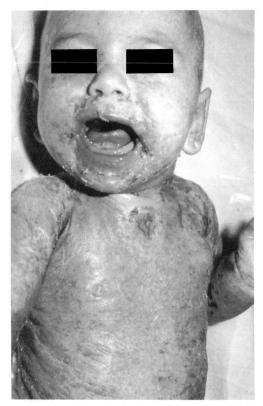

FIGURE 106–3. Prominent perioral crusting, a characteristic clinical feature of the staphylococcal scalded skin syndrome.

fissures is characteristic of this exfoliative phase, intraoral mucosal lesions are distinctly unusual. Recovery from SSSS is common, but sepsis as well as serious fluid and electrolyte disturbances can lead to morbidity and mortality (1% to 10% in the antibiotic era).[36]

An abortive form of SSSS, known as the scarlatiniform variant, shows the early erythrodermic and final desquamative stages seen in Ritter's disease, but the bullous stage does not occur. Such cases may be confused with other toxic exanthems, including TSS. Other intermediate forms of SSSS may be seen that begin as localized bullous impetigo but may evolve to produce regionally limited bullae and denuded areas that may or may not harbor staphylococci.

Epidemiology

SSSS is predominantly a disease of infancy and early childhood with most cases seen before the age of 5. Factors responsible for the age distribution include renal immaturity leading to decreased toxin clearance in neonates and lack of immunity to the toxins.[37] Not surprisingly, neonatal nurseries have been important, high-risk areas for outbreaks of SSSS.[38] Nursery or maternity staff who are infected or colonized with epidermolytic toxin–producing S. aureus are typically the source of such outbreaks. Standard infection control measures such as the use of chlorhexidine hand washing may not be sufficient for control, and asymptomatic nasal carriage by an adult can be a point source for infection.[39] The importance of follow-up surveillance of nursery personnel with documented nasal carriage has been emphasized, along with the utility of mupirocin ointment for eradication of persistent nasal carriage. As mentioned previously, adult SSSS also occurs, but it is uncommon and usually is found in the setting of renal or immunologic compromise.[34, 35, 40] There has been a single case report of congenital SSSS in a neonate with sepsis born to a mother with staphylococcal chorioamnionitis.[41]

PATHOLOGY

Bullous impetigo is characterized by a blister whose roof is composed by the granular and cornified layers and whose cavity contains neutrophils. As in any process in which neutrophils and keratinocytes come into proximity, acantholysis can occur as a result of neutrophilic enzymes and single acantholytic keratinocytes are often evident in blister cavities as well. Modified Gram stains for use in tissue sections, such as the Brown-Brenn method, will often show cocci in the blister cavity, but early lesions will sometimes appear to be devoid of cocci, since the number of organisms is initially low.

SSSS is an acantholytic intraepidermal blistering process, in which clefts appear in the granular layer or just beneath the stratum corneum (Fig. 106–4). In fresh lesions, the clefts contain neither plasma, cocci, nor inflammatory cells and inflammatory cells are uncommon in the dermis. Older lesions can become superinfected, obscuring the diagnosis of SSSS. In bullous impetigo, the

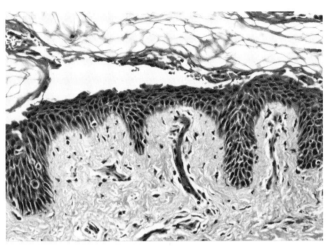

FIGURE 106–4. Subgranular epidermolysis, a characteristic histopathologic feature of the staphylococcal scalded skin syndrome, as well as bullous impetigo (hematoxylin-eosin, × 40).

superficial blisters contain neutrophils and cocci, although very early lesions will sometimes fail to demonstrate organisms. The histopathologic distinction between blisters caused by the superficial forms of pemphigus, bullous impetigo, SSSS, and subcorneal pustular dermatosis can be problematic on occasion.

PATHOGENESIS AND ETIOLOGY

Two distinct epidermolytic toxins are responsible for the blistering in SSSS. In bullous impetigo, toxin is produced and has its effect locally. In generalized forms of SSSS, toxin diffuses from an infected focus and, in the absence of specific antitoxin antibody, spreads hematogenously to produce its widespread effects. Although most toxigenic strains of S. aureus are identified by group II phage (types 71 and 55), toxin producers also have been identified among phage group I and III staphylococci.[42]

It has been generally accepted that ET-A is genetically encoded on a bacterial chromosome, while ET-B is plasmid encoded, but recently this view has been challenged.[43] Both of the epidermolytic toxins produce blistering and denudation by disruption of the epidermal granular cell layer through interdesmosomal splitting.[37] The histologic correlate of this is the formation of intraepidermal blisters at the granular cell layer (see Fig. 106–4). The mechanism of action of epidermolytic toxin in the epidermis is not completely understood and is an area of ongoing investigation. The role of ionic calcium appears to be important but uncertain, with earlier reports of calcium-induced inhibition of epidermolytic toxin[44] contradicted by recent evidence of calcium dependence.[45] The notion that epidermolytic toxin directly affects desmosomes is supported by the finding that it appears to bind desmoglein I.[46]

The epidermolytic toxins display limited homology to the staphylococcal enterotoxins and TSST-1, and there are reports of documented in vitro superantigenic activity of epidermolytic toxins. However, toxic shock–like presentations have not yet been described in patients infected with epidermolytic toxin–producing staphylococci. Recombinant ET-A has been shown to possess no superantigenic activity, and it was proposed that previous reports of superantigenic activity of epidermolytic toxins resulted from the use of preparations contaminated by minute quantities of other staphylococcal exotoxins (i.e., enterotoxin or TSST-1).[47]

DIAGNOSIS AND DIFFERENTIAL DIAGNOSIS

The diagnosis of SSSS can be made rapidly on frozen sections of skin biopsy specimens or from exfoliated skin samples prepared for frozen section. In both cases, the characteristic intraepidermal level of blistering should be easily recognized. Alternatively, a cytologic examination prepared as a Tzanck smear will reveal acantholytic, squamous nucleated cells, but correct interpretation requires an experienced observer. The major entity in the differential diagnosis is toxic epidermal necrolysis, a life-threatening, but rare disease in infancy. In contrast to SSSS, toxic epidermal necrolysis produces full-thickness epidermal necrosis and histologically demonstrates dermoepidermal separation, rather than the granular layer split in the epidermis characteristic of SSSS. The scarlatiniform variant of SSSS may be confused with TSS or other toxic exanthems, as previously mentioned. The distinguishing features of toxic exanthems are summarized in Table 106–2.

TREATMENT

Therapy for SSSS in affected patients should be directed toward eradication of staphylococci from the focus of infection, which generally requires intravenous penicillinase-resistant antistaphylococcal antibiotics. Usually, oral antibiotic therapy can be substituted within several days or sooner. Antibiotics, supportive skin care, and appropritae attention to fluid and electrolyte management in the presence of disrupted barrier function will usually ensure rapid recovery. The superficial nature of the erosions in SSSS makes rapid re-epithelialization with minimal or no scarring a predictable result after appropriate therapy.

As noted earlier, it is vital to recognize the potential for epidemic SSSS in neonatal nurseries,[38] and identification of health care workers colonized or infected with toxigenic *S. aureus* is an integral part of managing the problem. Control measures should be applied, including strict enforcement of chlorhexidine hand washing, oral antibiotic therapy for infected workers, and mupirocin ointment for eradication of persistent nasal carriage.[39]

References

1. Chesney PJ, Davis JP, Purdy WK, et al. Clinical manifestations of the toxic shock syndrome. JAMA 1981;246:741–748.
2. Chesney PJ, Crass BA, Polyak MB, et al. Toxic shock syndrome: Management and long-term sequelae. Ann Intern Med 1982; 96:847–851.
3. Tofte R, Williams DN. Toxic shock syndrome: Clinical and laboratory features in 15 patients. Ann Intern Med 1981;94:149–156.
4. Todd J, Fishaut M, Kapral F, et al. Toxic shock syndrome associated with phage-group I staphylococci. Lancet 1978;2:1116–1118.
5. Shands KN, Schmid BP, Dan BB, et al. Toxic shock syndrome in menstruating women: Its association with tampon use and *Staphylococcus aureus* and the clinical features in 52 cases. N Engl J Med 1980;303:1436–1442.
6. Gaventa S, Reingold AL, Hightower AW, et al. Active surveillance for toxic shock syndrome in the United States, 1986. Rev Infect Dis 1989;2(Suppl 1):S28–S34.
7. Reingold AL, Hargrett NT, Dan BB, et al. Nonmenstrual toxic shock syndrome: A review of 130 cases. Ann Intern Med 1982; 96:871–874.
8. Tanner MH, Liljenquist JE. Toxic shock syndrome from *Staphylococcus aureus* infection at insulin pump infusion sites. JAMA 1988;259:394–395.
9. McCarthy VP, Peoples WM. Toxic shock syndrome after ear piercing. Pediatr Infect Dis J 1988;7:741–742.
10. Resnick SD. Toxic shock syndrome: Recent developments in pathogenesis. J Pediatr 1990;116:321–328.
11. Kishaba RG, Losek JD. Toxic shock syndrome associated with poison oak dermatitis. Pediatr Emerg Care 1989;5:40–42.
12. Spearman PW, Barson WJ. Toxic shock syndrome occurring in children with abrasive injuries beneath casts. J Pediatr Orthop 1992;12:169–172.
13. Solomon R, Truman T, Murray DL. Toxic shock syndrome as a complication of bacterial tracheitis. Pediatr Infect Dis J 1983; 4:298–299.
14. Surh L, Read SE. Staphylococcal tracheitis and toxic shock syndrome in a young child. J Pediatr 1984;105:585–587.
15. Cheneaud M, Leclerc F, Martinot A. Bacterial croup and toxic shock syndrome. Eur J Pediatr 1986;145:306–330.
16. Donaldson JD, Maltby CC. Bacterial tracheitis in children. J Otolaryngol 1989;18:101–104.
17. MacDonald KL, Osterholm MT, Hedberg CW, et al. Toxic shock syndrome: A newly recognized complication of influenza and influenzalike illness. JAMA 1987;257:1053–1058.
18. Ferguson MA, Todd J. Toxic shock syndrome associated with *Staphylococcus aureus* sinusitis. J Infect Dis 1990;161:953.
19. Hurwitz RM, Ackerman AB. Cutaneous pathology of the toxic shock syndrome. Am J Dermatopathol 1985;7:563–578.
20. Parsonnet J. Mediators in the pathogenesis of toxic shock syndrome: Overview. Rev Infect Dis 1989;2(Suppl 1):S263–S269.
21. Parsonnet J. Toxic shock syndrome. In: Kass EH, Platt R, eds. Current Therapy of Infectious Diseases. St. Louis: BC Decker, 1990:73–78.
22. Marrack P, Kappler J. The staphylococcal enterotoxins and their relatives. Science 1990;248:710–711.
23. Johnson HM, Russell JK, Pontzer CH. Staphylococcal enterotoxin microbial superantigens. FASEB J 1991;5:2706–2712.
24. Fast DJ, Schlievert PM, Nelson RD: Toxic shock syndrome-associated staphylococcal and streptococcal pyrogenic toxins are potent inducers of tumor necrosis factor production. Infect Immun 1989;57:291–294.
25. Cone LA, Woodard DR, Schlievert PM, et al. Clinical and bacteriologic observations of a toxic shock–like syndrome due to *Streptococcus pyogenes*. N Engl J Med 1987;317:146–149.
26. Klein JO. Group A streptococcal infections: An era of growing concern. Pediatr Infect Dis J 1991;10(Suppl):s3–s78.
27. Breiman RF, and the Working Group on severe streptococcal diseases: Defining the group A streptococcal toxic shock syndrome. JAMA 1993;269:390–391.
28. Hoge CW, Schwartz B, Talkington DF, et al. The changing epidemiology of invasive group A streptococcal infection and the emergence of streptococcal toxic shock-like syndrome. JAMA 1993;269:384–389.
29. Bradley JS, Schlievert PM, Sample TG Jr. Streptococcal toxic shock–like syndrome as a complication of varicella. Pediatr Infect Dis J 1991;10:77–79.
30. Stevens DL. Invasive group A streptococcal infections. Clin Infect Dis 1992;14:2–13.
31. Johnson LP, L'Italien JJ, Schlievert PM. Streptococcal pyrogenic exotoxin type A (scarlet fever toxin) is related to *Staphylococcus aureus* enterotoxin B. Mol Gen Genet 1986;203:354–356.

32. Todd TK, Rossman M, Castor SA, et al. Corticosteroid therapy for patients with toxic shock syndrome. JAMA 1984;252:3399–3402.

33. Ritter von Rittershain G: Die exfoliativa dermatitis jungerer sauglinge. Zentralzeit Kinderheilkd 1878;2:3–23.

34. Elias PM, Levy SW. Bullous impetigo: Occurrence of localized scalded skin syndrome in an adult. Arch Dermatol 1976;112:856–858.

35. Beers B, Wilson B. Adult staphylococcal scalded skin syndrome. Int J Dermatol 1990;29:428–429.

36. Elias PM, Fritsch P, Epstein EE Jr. Staphylococcal scalded skin syndrome. Arch Dermatol 1977;113:207–219.

37. Resnick SD, Fritsch P, Elias PM. The staphylococcal scalded skin and toxic shock syndromes. In: Goldsmith LA, ed. Physiology, Biochemistry, and Molecular Biology of the Skin, 2nd ed. New York: Oxford University Press, 1991.

38. Dancer SJ, Simmons NA, Poston SM, et al. Outbreak of staphylococcal scalded skin syndrome among neonates. J Infect 1988;16:87–103.

39. Hoeger PH, Elsner P. Staphylococcal scalded skin syndrome: Transmission of exfoliatin-producing *S. aureus* by an asymptomatic carrier. Pediatr Infect Dis J 1988;7:340–342.

40. Goldberg NS, Ahmed T, Robinson B, et al. Staphylococcal scalded skin syndrome mimicking acute graft versus host disease in a bone marrow recipient. Arch Dermatol 1989;125:85–87.

41. Loughead JL. Congenital staphylococcal scalded skin syndrome: Report of a case. Pediatr Infect Dis J 1992;11:413–414.

42. Florman A, Holzman RS. Nosocomial scalded skin syndrome. Am J Dis Child 1980;134:1043–1047.

43. Murono K, Fujita K, Yoshioka H. Microbiologic characteristics of exfoliative toxin-producing *Staphylococcus aureus*. Pediatr Infect Dis J 1988;7:313–315.

44. Dimond RL, Erickson KC, Wuepper KD. The role of divalent cations in epidermolysis. Br J Dermatol 1976;95:25–34.

45. Taniguchi S, Makoto I. Effects of proteinase inhibitors and calcium antagonist on experimental epidermolysis caused by recombinant epidermolytic toxin A. J Invest Dermatol 1990;94:584a.

46. Takagi Y, Futamura S, Asada Y. Action site of exfoliative toxin on keratinocytes. J Invest Dermatol 1990;94:52a.

47. Fleischer B, Bailey CJ. Recombinant epidermolytic toxin A of *Staphylococcus aureus* is not a superantigen. Med Microbiol Immunol 1992;180:273–278.

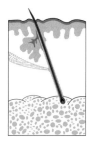

Skin Infections Caused by Unusual Bacterial Pathogens

DAVID S. FEINGOLD

Staphylococcus aureus, Streptococcus pyogenes, and the organisms of the resident cutaneous flora cause the large majority of skin infections. These infections are discussed in Chapter 105. Other bacteria may infect the skin, especially in hosts with impaired cellular or humoral defenses against infection or in particular epidemiologic situations. Because proper antibiotic treatment varies with the infecting organism and aggressive treatment is required in infected impaired hosts, it is especially important to identify the etiologic bacteria causing these unusual infections of the skin. Here, unusual skin infections are defined as those bacterial infections caused by organisms other than *Staphylococcus aureus, Streptococcus pyogenes,* or the resident cutaneous flora.

Mycobacterial infections of the skin (see Chapters 111 and 112), Lyme borreliosis (see Chapter 109), and cat-scratch disease or bacillary angiomatosis (see Chapter 115) are only mentioned here in the context of differential diagnosis. Some of the very rare cutaneous infections such as anthrax and cutaneous diphtheria are not discussed.

Table 107–1 is a list of bacteria that cause skin infections. The type of infection depends on the depth of involvement and the characteristics of the pathogen, as described in Chapter 105. For example, streptococcal cellulitis is spreading infection of the dermis and/or subcutaneous tissue and staphylococcal folliculitis is loculated infection originating in hair follicles. Some organisms, such as *Clostridium perfringens,* cause a rapidly spreading cellulitis, while others, such as *Erysipelothrix rhusiopathiae,* cause a slow-paced infection.

For the purposes of this discussion the infections are classified as endogenous or exogenous. The former are infections caused by organisms that are frequently present in body flora. The latter are infections caused by environmental bacteria. Septic bacterial skin lesions, those that are metastatic to the skin during sepsis or spread from internal foci of infection, may be very helpful for diagnosing the underlying infection and are discussed as a separate category. Several noninfectious cutaneous lesions occur as complications of generalized infections (*e.g.,* vasculitis, erythema nodosum, and erythema multiforme). These infection-associated but noninfected lesions may also help in the diagnosis of systemic infections.

ENDOGENOUS SKIN INFECTIONS

Haemophilus influenzae Infections

Haemophilus influenzae are pleomorphic, gram-negative, coccobacillary organisms. They are primarily respiratory tract pathogens. Most severe infections with *H. influenzae,* including meningitis, pneumonia, epiglottitis, and cellulitis, are caused by encapsulated type b strains. The ribosylribitol polymer capsule inhibits phagocytosis in the nonimmune individual. Greatest susceptibility to *H. influenzae* type b infection occurs at 3 months to about 3 years of age.

In healthy young children, *H. influenzae* is frequently part of the upper respiratory tract flora. Cellulitis caused by *H. influenzae* type b usually accompanies an upper respiratory tract infection or otitis media. Typically in a young child with an upper respiratory tract infection an edematous and erythematous area develops on the face or upper body accompanied by high fever. The margins of the skin infection are usually indistinct. In infants, a

**TABLE 107-1. Organisms Causing
Less Common Skin Infections**

Organisms Present in Some Body Flora

Haemophilus influenzae
Streptococcus pneumoniae
Pseudomonas aeruginosa
Gram-negative bacilli
Clostridium perfringens

Environmental Bacteria

Vibrio vulnificus
Aeromonas hydrophila
Erysipelothrix rhusiopathiae
Mycobacterium species
Pasteurella multocida
Francisella tularensis
Borrelia burgdorferi

characteristic purplish colored cellulitis has been described. Marked tenderness and swelling may develop. The presence of buccal cellulitis is frequently accompanied by otitis media; the mechanism of this association is unclear.[1] The patients are often acutely ill with a high fever, leukocytosis, and lethargy. Bacteremia is present about one half of the time. During the illness one must be on the lookout for complications of H. influenzae sepsis, including meningitis.

H. influenzae type b cellulitis is unusual in adults, but several cases have been described.[2, 3] It usually begins with pharyngitis and may progress rapidly to dysphagia, neck swelling, and erythema. Although the purplish hue of the cellulitis has also been reported in adults, most cases are indistinguishable morphologically from the common streptococcal cellulitis described in Chapter 105.

Two separate large-scale studies in the United States have demonstrated that immunization against H. influenzae type b with conjugated ribosylribitol phosphate polymers, the capsular antigen of the organism, has decreased the incidence of infections with the organisms, including cellulitis.[4, 5]

Streptococcus pneumoniae Infections

Streptococcus pneumoniae, or the pneumococcus, is the most common cause of bacterial pneumonia and frequently a part of the respiratory flora in healthy adults. Although it is an aggressive pathogen, it is noteworthy how infrequently it infects the skin. Only 13 cases of pneumococcal cellulitis of adults were found in a recent review of the literature.[6] Most of the cases occurred in chronically ill or immunocompromised patients. In one series of 12 pneumococcal soft tissue infections including cellulitis, an association with connective tissue diseases was noted.[7] Characteristics of pneumococcal cellulitis included face or upper body involvement, brawny erythema, bullae, a purplish color, and pneumococcal bacteremia in about 50% of the patients. Of the bacteria commonly found in the flora of the upper

respiratory tract only H. influenzae, Streptococcus pneumoniae, S. pyogenes, and Staphylococcus aureus are well-described cutaneous pathogens.

Pseudomonas aeruginosa Infections

Pseudomonas aeruginosa is a ubiquitous, gram-negative, aerobic bacillus responsible for frequent and often distinctive skin infections. It is found widely in wet areas in the environment. In healthy persons the organism colonizes moist parts of the body such as web spaces or the external auditory canal about 5% of the time and the bowel flora up to 20% of the time. Even a larger percentage of hospitalized patients are colonized. P. aeruginosa becomes pathogenic when local tissue conditions foster overgrowth or when altered host defenses become permissive. The infections vary from life-threatening septicemia to serious localized infections such as otitis to the more common manifestations of bacterial overgrowth in moist cutaneous areas. Skin lesions secondary to P. aeruginosa septicemia may be diagnostic. They are discussed later in the chapter together with other skin lesions seen in bacterial sepsis.

Paronychiae typically occur in those persons with occupational chronic water immersion of the hands, such as bartenders or nurses. Acute paronychiae are often caused by S. aureus and characterized by pain, swelling, erythema, and purulence. In chronic infection, P. aeruginosa and Candida albicans are usually etiologic. These two organisms are also the ones that most often colonize and may overgrow in other moist body loci. Chronic paronychiae are characterized by intermittent tenderness and erythema, resulting in often extensive nail dystrophy. In the case of Pseudomonas, green to blue discoloration of the nail may be seen either diffusely or in bands reflecting intermittent infectious activity.

Pseudomonas overgrowth in moist, intertriginous areas such as toe web spaces is usually characterized by superficial erosions with exudation. The typical fruity smell of P. aeruginosa or the pigment production may be evident. In the moist external auditory canal, Pseudomonas organisms often overgrow, causing inflammation with swelling, discomfort, and discharge. This "swimmer's ear" or external otitis is common. A variety of organisms can be cultured from the site, but P. aeruginosa is the most frequent isolate,[8] and it usually results in a self-limited infectious process.

When external otitis becomes invasive it may involve the cartilage of the pinna, causing intense swelling (Fig. 107-1; see color plate) and pain. In its most severe form the infection spreads to the soft tissues at the base of the skull, often causing multiple cranial neuropathies and osteomyelitis of the base of the skull. Although this scenario is usually seen in diabetics, normal elderly patients may also be afflicted.[9] Minor trauma or a surgical procedure can trigger conversion of a pesky external otitis to an invasive, life-threatening infection, sometimes called malignant external otitis. Early treatment can be life saving.

Pseudomonas folliculitis is a common infection occurring in persons exposed to closed-cycle recreational water

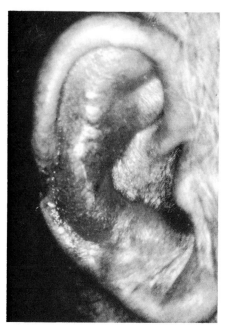

FIGURE 107-1. External otitis due to *Pseudomonas aeruginosa*. (See color plate.)

sources such as hot tubs or pools in which contamination with *P. aeruginosa* is frequent. The organisms are able to resist relatively high temperatures and chlorine levels, making them very difficult to eradicate. Dozens of epidemics of folliculitis in those exposed to such water sources have been reported.[10, 11] The clinical picture (Fig. 107-2) is characterized by erythematous papulopustular lesions on the trunk and proximal extremities 2 to 4 days after exposure. Prolonged exposure with maceration of the skin is a risk factor. *Pseudomonas* colonization of the skin does not result in folliculitis unless there is concomitant superhydration of the skin from occlusion.[12, 13] External otitis or intertriginous infection may be seen along

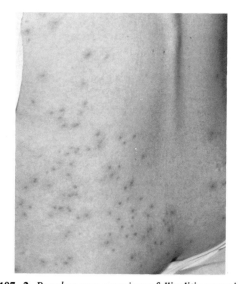

FIGURE 107-2. *Pseudomonas aeruginosa* folliculitis occurring after immersion in a hot tub.

with folliculitis. Malaise and low-grade fever have been reported.

When a patient with folliculitis reports exposure to potentially contaminated sources the diagnosis is clear cut. The diagnosis is more difficult without a relevant epidemiologic history. A case associated with use of a contaminated loofah sponge has been reported.[14] The wet sponge was overgrown with large numbers of *P. aeruginosa*. These widely used sponges can be hazardous when left continually wet in the shower or tub. Drying the sponge after each use restricts *Pseudomonas* contamination. Recently two cases of *Pseudomonas* folliculitis without any obvious source of the organisms were reported.[15] In one of the cases folliculitis of the legs after epilation occurred in a young woman; in the other case *Pseudomonas* folliculitis was widespread without any discernible predisposing cause.

In the normal host, *Pseudomonas* folliculitis is usually self-limited. The situation was quite different in a small series reported from a cancer center of immunosuppressed patients.[16] These patients with *Pseudomonas* folliculitis rapidly developed progressive infection and required aggressive treatment. The organism was contaminating the water sources in the patients' hospital rooms.

Gram-Negative Folliculitis

Gram-negative folliculitis is the term used to describe the infection of facial lesions of acne vulgaris with various gram-negative bacilli. It is usually seen in patients on long-term oral antibiotic treatment for acne. Two varieties of infection are described.[17] Lactose-fermenting Enterobacteriaceae such as *Escherichia coli* or *Klebsiella aerogenes* are responsible for superficial pustules in 80% of the patients. *Proteus* species cause deep nodular lesions in about 20% of patients. *P. aeruginosa* may also cause gram-negative folliculitis; often this is associated with *Pseudomonas* external otitis. Usually, discontinuation of the long-term antibiotic therapy and specific systemic antibiotic treatment for the offending gram-negative bacillus is curative.[18]

A unique outbreak of gram-negative folliculitis has been described.[19] Dermatitis palaestrae limosae, or mud wrestling–induced pustular dermatitis, has occurred in college students participating in this activity. Various members of the Enterobacteriaceae were the offending organisms. Increased immersion time during wrestling increased the risk of infections. The authors likened this infection to recreational *Pseudomonas* folliculitis with cutaneous superhydration and concomitant exposure to large numbers of gram-negative bacilli.

Wound Infections

Organisms of the gastrointestinal flora rarely cause cellulitis, except in the instance of bowel-associated wound infections. *Clostridium perfringens* and other clostridial species cause a characteristic wound infection — anaerobic cellulitis. The rapidly spreading infection occurs postoperatively, after dirty surgery or a wound resulting in devitalized tissue. The infection usually results in the accumulation of large amounts of tissue gas, causing crepitus, swelling, and often very little other cutaneous change. This type of clostridial cellulitis is readily cured with minor debridement and antibiotics. If muscle becomes involved, the clinical picture is dramatically altered and a pesky cellulitis becomes a life-threatening infection, clostridial myonecrosis, or gas gangrene. The transition is usually marked by the development of severe pain. The patient with clostridial myonecrosis is acutely ill and may require extensive debridement to remove all involved muscle.

Necrotizing fasciitis is an aggressive cellulitis centered in the superficial fascia and subcutaneous tissue. The outstanding characteristic of necrotizing fasciitis is the extensive undermining of the tissue caused by the necrosis in the superficial fascia. Because nerves and blood vessels that penetrate the fascia are often damaged, clinically one sees patchy necrosis and anesthesia of the overlying skin. Necrotizing fasciitis must be considered when the cellulitis is atypical or does not respond to appropriate treatment for the usual streptococcal cellulitis.

Type 1 and type 2 necrotizing fasciitis are caused by different organisms and hence have different signs and symptoms. These are listed in Table 107–2. The type 1 or bowel-associated infections often grow mixtures of Enterobacteriaceae, an enterococcus, and an anaerobe, such as *Bacteroides fragilis*. The type 2 infection is caused by a single organism, usually *Streptococcus pyogenes* but rarely other organisms such as *Vibrio vulnificus*.[20]

Fournier's gangrene is a unique necrotizing fasciitis that usually involves the genitalia of middle-aged men, but any age male can be infected.[21, 22] The illness, which often occurs in diabetics, may be explosive in onset and progression. More often it is moderately paced in its progression, resulting in erythema, often dramatic swelling, and crepitus. The infection can spread anteriorly up the abdominal wall or posteriorly through the perineum. Most of the patients have predisposing trauma, which may be perianal suppuration, local trauma, or perineal surgery. Usually, mixed bowel organisms are etiologic in Fournier's gangrene. Rarely, type 2 necrotizing fasciitis due to *Streptococcus pyogenes* can cause the clinical picture of Fournier's gangrene, at times without a recognized antecedent trauma.

EXOGENOUS SKIN INFECTIONS

Skin infections from organisms not usually found in the human microbial flora are most often seen in two situations: skin injury in a marine environment or bites from animals or insect vectors. Infections resulting from skin injury in a marine environment include infections with *Vibrio vulnificus, Aeromonas hydrophilia, Erysipelothrix rhusiopathiae,* and *Mycobacterium marinum.* Cutaneous involvement with *M. marinum* and other mycobacteria are discussed in Chapter 111. The patient's history and especially recent travel history usually trigger consideration of these exogenous skin infections.

Vibrio vulnificus Infections

V. vulnificus is a noncholera vibrio, first described in 1979,[23] that prefers to grow in water warmer than 20°C and with a salt concentration of 0.7% to 1.6%. The organism is found widely in warmer coastal waters and infects up to 10% of raw shellfish on the market in the United States.[24] The per cent is highest in warm water areas. Unique among the vibrios, *V. vulnificus* is virulent in normal as well as compromised hosts. This virulence may reflect a polysaccharide capsule that resists phagocytosis or the production of an extracellular cytolytic toxin.[25]

Two distinct clinical syndromes caused by *V. vulnificus* predominate. The first is a bacteremia following ingestion of the organism, almost always related to consumption of raw oysters. Seeding of the soft tissues regularly occurs during *V. vulnificus* bacteremia with resultant, chacteristically bullous cellulitis. The skin lesions occur early in the course of the illness and are an important clue to the proper diagnosis. Fasciitis, myositis, and necrotic skin ulcers are also reported during bacteremia. As with other causes of gram-negative septicemia, shock is common and, when it occurs, the end result is usually fatal. Most of the patients with primary *V. vulnificus* bacteremia have liver disease (usually cirrhosis). In a 1992 literature review of all reported cases of primary *V. vulnificus* bacteremia, 95% of patients had underlying diseases.[26]

Gastroenteritis without bacteremia is seen with *V. vulnificus* ingestion, as well as with other vibrios such as *V. parahaemolyticus, V. damsela,* and non-01 *V. cholerae.* It is likely that *V. vulnificus* gastroenteritis without bacteremia and related to consumption of raw oysters is common, especially in the regions bordering the Gulf of Mexico. Consequent bacteremia and its sequelae are essentially limited to impaired hosts. Rarely, the other vibrios may also cause bacteremia.

The second clinical syndrome of *V. vulnificus* infection occurs when wounds are contaminated by sea water, often related to trauma during water sports or fishing. The severity of infection varies from a mild cellulitis to cellulitis with bullae and gangrenous areas to necrotizing fasciitis. Bacteremia with its severe sequelae may also occur when wound infection is primary.[27] Although many of the reported patients with this type of *V. vulnificus* cellulitis are also impaired hosts, clearly the infection occurs frequently in normal persons with contaminated wounds.

TABLE 107–2. Clinical Features of Necrotizing Fasciitis

Clinical Feature	Type 1 Infection	Type 2 Infection
Pain	Painful	Painful
Tissue gas	Often present	Absent
Odor of exudate	Foul	Little
Skin changes	Redness, patchy necrosis, and anesthesia with extensive undermining by necrotic fascia	
Systemic toxicity	Prominent	Prominent
Progression	Rapid	Rapid
Predisposing factors	Follows abdominal or perineal surgery, skin popping	Spontaneous or follows minor trauma

Aeromonas hydrophila Infections

Aeromonas hydrophila is a facultative anaerobic gram-negative rod that, unlike *V. vulnificus,* does not require salt to grow. It is widespread in fresh and brackish water sources. The organism is pathogenic for fish and amphibians as well as humans. Various extracellular toxins and enzymes are probably responsible for the virulence of the organism.

In humans, infections include acute gastroenteritis; sepsis usually in patients with cancer or cirrhosis; various focal infections including pneumonia, endocarditis, and osteomyelitis; and skin and soft tissue infections following trauma, usually with water exposure. Gastroenteritis caused by *Aeromonas hydrophila* is the most common infection with this organism, followed by infection of the skin and soft tissues. The spectrum of infection is very similar to that seen with *V. vulnificus* except for the lack of skin tropism during bacteremia, which is such a prominent part of the clinical picture of *V. vulnificus* infection.

Although sepsis is usually seen in patients with malignancy or cirrhosis, soft tissue infections usually occur in immunocompetent hosts. As with *V. vulnificus* infection, skin infection with *A. hydrophila* usually occurs in the setting of soft tissue trauma with water exposure. Both organisms must be considered when infection follows injury in salt or brackish water. Cases are most often sporadic, but a few small nosocomial outbreaks have been reported. In California, clinical isolates of *Aeromonas* species are reportable. From May 1988 through April 1989 the incidence of reported wound infections with *Aeromonas* was only 0.7 per 1 million population.[28] Thus soft tissue infections with *A. hydrophila* or related *Aeromonas* species are either very rare or rarely diagnosed.

A. hydrophila wound infections after trauma may be indistinguishable from group A β-hemolytic streptococcal cellulitis. Subcutaneous abscess formation is common, occurring in 9 of 11 patients reported by Gold and Salit.[29] When present, this distinguishes *A. hydrophila* infection from streptococcal cellulitis. Abscesses may spread rapidly along fascial planes. Because *A. hydrophila* produces gas, it is not surprising that crepitant cellulitis with the organism has been reported. *A. hydrophila* may involve muscle and produce a clinical picture similar to clostridial gas gangrene. Over 80% of the time culture yields more than one pathogen. The discharge in infection is frequently described as a foul or fishy odor. *Edwardsiella tarda,* one of the Enterobacteriaceae, has been reported to cause the same spectrum of clinical syndromes as *A. hydrophila.*[30]

Erysipelothrix rhusiopathiae Infections

Erysipelothrix rhusiopathiae, a pleomorphic gram-positive rod, is another organism responsible for skin infection following trauma in a marine environment, as well as occupational infections. It is a commensal of many animals and fish and causes an economically important infection in swine. From animals the organisms contaminate the environment. There the organisms can persist in water (including sea water) for weeks. Infection following trauma is seen in fish, meat, and poultry handlers as well as farmers.[31]

Skin infection is the usual manifestation of infection with *E. rhusiopathiae,* although rarely systemic disease is reported. The usual manifestation is Rosenbach's erysipeloid, a distinctive cellulitis. Lesions usually begin on the fingers or hands at sites of trauma. Purplish red indurated plaques develop and extend peripherally, often with central clearing. Hemorrhagic vesicles may occur in the involved area. There may be stiffness of joints in the area and local pain. The infection spreads slowly and usually runs a self-limited course over about 3 weeks. The pace of the infection is slow compared with erysipelas, from which the name erysipeloid was derived. Occasionally there is associated fever, malaise, regional lymphadenopathy, and diffuse arthralgias. Other names for erysipeloid include whale or seal finger, blubber finger, and fish-handler's disease. The rarely occurring systemic disease is associated with endocarditis about 90% of the time.[32] In about one third of the patients with endocarditis, concurrent lesions of erysipeloid are present. The organisms may cause other focal lesions, such as brain abscess, pericarditis, or septic arthritis.

Bite-Associated Infections

Soft tissue infections frequently follow animal or insect bites. When secondary wound infections occur, the usual etiologic agents of pyodermas, namely, *Staphylococcus aureus* and *Streptococcus pyogenes,* are the cause. There are, however, a few exogenous bacteria that cause characteristic infections following bites. *Pasteurella multocida* and *Francisella tularensis* infections are discussed here. Lyme borreliosis and the skin lesions of erythema migrans that may result from the bite of an infected deer tick are discussed in Chapter 109. *Yersinia pestis* infection, or plague, is secondary to rat flea bites; usually no skin lesions are seen in plague.

The salivary flora of dogs and cats is complex, and bite wound infections are frequently polymicrobial.[33] *Pasteurella multocida,* a gram-negative coccobaccillus, is present in the mouth of the majority of cats and is frequently present in dog saliva. It may cause serious epizootic infection in a variety of animals. In as many as 50% of infected human bite wounds from these animals *Pasteurella multocida* is etiologic. A definitive review of 34 cases from the Massachusetts General Hospital was reported in 1984.[34] Often within hours after a bite pain, swelling, erythema, and purulent or serosanguineous drainage result from infection with the organism. The hand is frequently infected because it is the most common bite site, and local complications of osteomyelitis, tenosynovitis, or arthritis may occur. Low-grade fever, lymphadenopathy, and, rarely, bacteremia are seen.

Tularemia (rabbit fever or deerfly fever) is caused by infection with *Francisella tularensis,* a small gram-negative coccobaccillus that is widely distributed in animals and insects. It is spread by contact with infected animal fluids, usually those of rabbits. Humans become infected by the cutaneous route, probably though inapparent breaks in the skin rather than by penetration through intact skin. Less commonly, the organism enters through

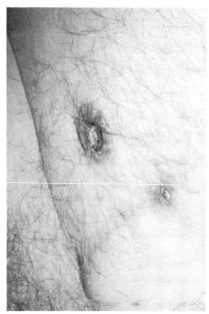

FIGURE 107–3. Abdominal skin lesions occurring at the sites of tick bites in a patient with ulceroglandular tularemia.

pulmonary or ocular mucous membranes. Vector-borne tularemia is becoming increasingly important. Bites of insect vectors, usually the tick or deerfly and, rarely, bites from other animals are responsible. In 75% to 85% of the patients, cutaneous inoculation yields an inflammatory papule or an area of cellulitis that ulcerates and crusts. A typical skin lesion of tularemia is shown in Figure 107–3. Among 53 tularemic cutaneous ulcers reported by Evans and associates,[35] the size varied from 0.4 cm to 3.0 cm in diameter; the ulcers were on the upper extremity 79% of the time. Fever, chills, headache, and painful regional lymphadenopathy complete the usual clinical presentation. Several other clinical syndromes of tularemia are seen in the absence of cutaneous lesions, including glandular, typhoidal, oculoglandular, and oropharyngeal tularemia. Fifteen cases of tularemia related to cat bites have been reported recently.[36]

DISSEMINATED SKIN INFECTIONS

Table 107–3 is a list of some of the systemic infections that involve the skin in a characteristic way. In many instances the skin infection component, either morphologically or by Gram stain or culture, can lead to diag-

TABLE 107–3. Some Disseminated Skin Infections (Excluding Mycobacterial Infections)

Bacterial endocarditis (acute)
Meningococcemia
Disseminated gonococcal infection
Pseudomonas aeruginosa sepsis
Salmonellosis
Syphilis
Vibrio vulnificus infection

nosis of the primary infection. Good examples are the cutaneous abscesses or the purulent petechiae that may occur secondary to high-grade bacteremia in staphylococcal endocarditis. Skin lesions are commonly seen during episodes of endocarditis of various causes. Most often the skin lesions reflect vasculitis rather than metastatic infection. Although there has been lively controversy about the etiology of Osler's nodes, Janeway's lesions, and the petechiae seen in endocarditis, the consensus is that all are secondary to manifestations of a vasculitis.[37]

In acute meningococcemia three types of skin lesions are seen:[38, 39] (1) early on a transient urticarial or macular eruption may occur; (2) later, one may see the purpura of disseminated intravascular coagulation; and (3) the most characteristic skin lesions in meningococcemia are purulent petechiae. These are manifestations of a septic vasculitis with fibrin thrombi in the luminia of venules, organisms, and polymorphonuclear leukocytes in vessel walls and sparse perivascular infiltrates of neutrophils without leukocytoclasis. Extravasation of red blood cells yields petechiae that develop gray to yellow centers as the organism multiplies and more white blood cells accumulate.

The clinical picture in disseminated gonococcal infection is characteristic and often the only way to make the diagnosis. In 1% to 3% of patients with gonorrhea (usually women), disseminated gonococcal infection occurs. It is manifested by the abrupt onset of fever, chills, and joint pain, usually at the time of menses. An acral eruption occurs, characterized by a small number of lesions that tend to be concentrated near joints; it consists of erythematous papules that evolve into hemorrhagic vesicles. A typical hemorrhagic vesicle is shown in Figure 107–4. Migratory tenosynovitis completes the usual clinical picture. Since blood cultures and cultures of the skin lesions may be negative, it is essential to recognize and think of this clinical picture. Cultures of the uterine cervix, if done during the episode of disseminated gonococcal infection, will often be positive for *Neisseria gonorrhoeae.* Biopsy of a papulopustule in a patient with gonococcemia reveals thrombi in small vessels and dense dermal infiltrates of neutrophils, which accumulate in an

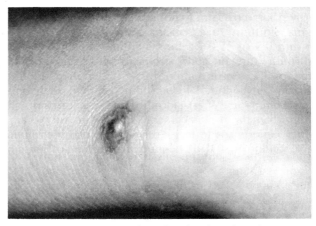

FIGURE 107–4. Typical skin lesion in disseminated gonococcal infection.

edematous papillary dermis. Organisms are exceedingly rare, and tissue staining with Gram stain is almost always negative. Immunofluorescent examination has shown gonococcal antigens in pustular lesions, however.

Several types of skin lesions may occur during the course of *Pseudomonas* septicemia.[40] The organism has a predilection to settle and multiply in the walls of small vessels, especially veins, in the skin, causing a necrotizing vasculitis, usually with sparing of the intima. The overgrowth of organisms in *Pseudomonas* septicemia can be so dramatic that they are visible as basophilic encrustations that obscure the walls of blood vessels in biopsy specimens. In some immunosuppressed hosts, this picture is seen in the absence of inflammatory cells (Fig. 107–5). There is extravasation of red blood cells and often extensive perivascular edema and necrosis with consequent interference with blood supply. Organisms spread through the vessels and invade the skin. This process results in the several different morphologic types of skin lesions that have been described:

1. Vesicles and bullae may occur in crops or singly anywhere on the body.
2. Ecthyma gangrenosum, which is a sharply demarcated, painless, indurated, necrotic ulcer or eschar with surrounding erythema (Fig. 107–6), is often present in the anogenital area or other apocrine gland areas. Although characteristic for *P. aeruginosa* septicemia, similar lesions may rarely be seen during the course of other gram-negative septicemias. A nonsepticemic form of ecthyma gangrenosum has also been described. In apocrine gland areas, usually in immunocompromised hosts, a primary cutaneous infection with the organism yields lesions similar in morphology to bacteremic ecthyma gangrenosum.[41, 42]
3. Small, erythematous, blanchable macular or papular lesions that resemble the rose spots of typhoid fever
4. Focal gangrenous cellulitis

Since the lesions all reflect a necrotizing vasculitis or colonization of vessel walls without inflammation,[43] it is not surprising that one morphologic form may evolve into another and that several different types of skin lesions may be present at any one time during the course of

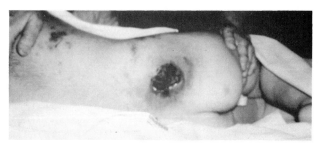

FIGURE 107–6. Ecthyma gangrenosum in a 5-year-old boy with *Pseudomonas* sepsis.

Pseudomonas septicemia. Similar focal lesions may occur in other parenchymatous organs.

In typhoid fever due to *Salmonella typhi*, rose spots are regularly seen. It is unusual to see rose spots in other enteric fevers. They occur early in the course during the acute febrile period. They are raised, pink, blanchable, nontender papules a few millimeters in size. Crops of 10 to 20 lesions occur, usually on the trunk, and fade gradually over several days. Biopsy reveals a dilated dermal vessel infiltrated with macrophages that may contain intracellular organisms.[44]

One does not usually think of syphilitic skin lesions as due to bacteremic spread to the skin, but indeed secondary lesions are just that. After the primary lesion or chancre there is a spirochetemia and organisms are deposited in the dermal vessels. The various skin manifestation of secondary syphilis reflect multiplication of the organisms in the skin and the subsequent tissue response.

Bacteremic spread of *V. vulnificus* to the skin causing often multiple areas of cellulitis has been referred to earlier.

DIAGNOSIS

The staphylococcal and streptococcal pyodermas discussed in Chapter 105 constitute the majority of bacterial skin infections. One should be concerned about a different infectious process in three clinical situations: (1) when the infection does not fit the clinical picture of the typical pyoderma, or the infection does not respond promptly to standard therapy for staphylococcal or streptococcal cutaneous infections; (2) when the host is impaired in his or her ability to combat infections; and (3) when there is an epidemiologic history of potential exposure to an unusual cutaneous pathogen.

The diagnosis of streptococcal cellulitis must be suggested if areas of necrosis, bullae, or anesthesia complicate the clinical picture. Streptococcal cellulitis should begin to respond to antibiotic treatment within 24 hours. If the response is delayed, the diagnosis must be questioned. Both of these clinical instances suggest the possibility of necrotizing fasciitis, a diagnosis that must be made promptly so that required debridement can be done. The diagnosis of necrotizing fasciitis rests on proving that the superficial fascia is extensively involved in the infection either on incision when a blunt instrument falls into the fascial space or on biopsy, showing infection histologically.[45] Soft tissue radiographs may be helpful in

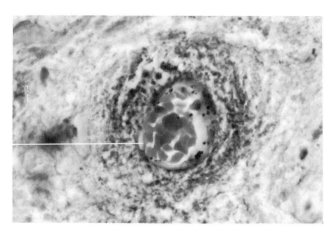

FIGURE 107–5. In ecthyma gangrenosum, pseudomonads colonize the walls of vessels in such numbers that they are visible even without special stains.

detecting gas in tissues or tissue necrosis. Impaired hosts are much more likely to have unusual and more aggressive skin infections than normal persons. If a primary lesion is present, it should be Gram stained and cultured. Biopsy for histology and culture should be done early if there is not prompt response to treatment.

The diagnosis of infection by one of the exogenous or environmental pathogens depends first on the history eliciting the possibility. For example, Lyme borreliosis must be considered when a patient with a skin lesion that fits the erythema migrans spectrum has been in an endemic area. *Vibrio vulnificus, Aeromonas hydrophila,* or *Erysipelothrix rhusiopathiae* must be considered when wounding occurs during water sports or water exposure. Wound culture is diagnostic in the first two instances, but rarely are cultures positive in erysipeloid. Erysipeloid is a clinical diagnosis based on morphology and history. Rarely, blood cultures are positive. The microbiology laboratory should be warned that *Erysipelothrix rhusiopathiae* is being considered to avoid mistaking a positive blood culture for "diphtheroids."

The diagnosis of skin infection is usually straightforward, based on the epidemiology and the clinical picture. In a few clinical situations one must be aggressive in trying to make specific diagnoses. The main diagnostic tools include Gram stain and culture of exudate or aspirant, incision for tissue examination, and biopsy. Serologic tests are not helpful. Immunofluorescent examination of biopsy material may identify organisms that are difficult to culture, but this is a research tool rather than a widely available clinical tool.[46] Finally, the polymerase chain reaction holds great promise for the rapid identification of hard-to-grow organisms once the problem of false-positive reactions is minimized and understood. Several studies of diagnoses of skin infections by polymerase chain reaction have been reported,[47-50] and many more are in progress. Clearly this will be a helpful clinical test; how helpful is yet to be determined.

TREATMENT

The principles of treating cutaneous bacterial infections are the same as those that apply to all bacterial infections: (1) accumulations of pus must be drained; (2) necrotic tissue must be debrided; and (3) antibiotic treatment must be guided ultimately by sensitivity determinations but initially by an educated guess. In Table 107–4 treatment recommendations for many of the infections discussed in the chapter are presented. The following are expanded treatment recommendations for the various infections organized in the order they are discussed in the text.

Since *H. influenzae* cellulitis is a fascial cellulitis of young children that is usually indistinguishable from classic streptococcal cellulitis, therapy for fascial cellulitis should be chosen to be effective against this organism also. Ampicillin resistance is now common in *H. influenzae;* thus a second-generation cephalosporin, such as cefaclor at 20 mg/kg per day in three divided doses, or a combination drug containing a penicillin and a penicil-

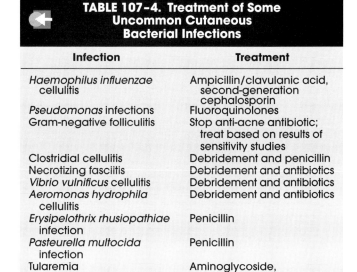

TABLE 107–4. Treatment of Some Uncommon Cutaneous Bacterial Infections	
Infection	**Treatment**
Haemophilus influenzae cellulitis	Ampicillin/clavulanic acid, second-generation cephalosporin
Pseudomonas infections	Fluoroquinolones
Gram-negative folliculitis	Stop anti-acne antibiotic; treat based on results of sensitivity studies
Clostridial cellulitis	Debridement and penicillin
Necrotizing fasciitis	Debridement and antibiotics
Vibrio vulnificus cellulitis	Debridement and antibiotics
Aeromonas hydrophila cellulitis	Debridement and antibiotics
Erysipelothrix rhusiopathiae infection	Penicillin
Pasteurella multocida infection	Penicillin
Tularemia	Aminoglycoside, doxycycline

linase-inhibitor, such as amoxacillin/calvulanic acid, is indicated. Penicillin resistance in treatment of pneumococcal infection is still relatively rare; thus, penicillin remains the treatment of choice for pneumococcal cellulitis. Since this infection generally occurs in compromised hosts, parenteral treatment is preferred.

Reliable oral antibiotic treatment for the various *Pseudomonas* cutaneous infection syndromes has finally been achieved with the development of the fluoroquinolones. Ciprofloxacin, 750 mg twice daily, is recommended for *Pseudomonas* paronychia, *Pseudomonas* erosive intertriginous infection, *Pseudomonas* folliculitis, and *Pseudomonas* external otitis. Recreational *Pseudomonas* folliculitis may be cleared without antibiotics by withdrawing the patient from the reservoir of *P. aeruginosa. Pseudomonas* malignant external otitis may require adjunctive surgical management, including canal debridement and mastoidectomy.

The acne-associated, gram-negative folliculitis may be caused by a variety of bacilli. Discontinuance of the antibiotic treatment of the acne may cause regression of the superinfection; however, antibiotic therapy based on the determined sensitivity is usually required. Development of the oral second- and third-generation cephalosporins and the fluoroquinolones has improved therapy, obviating the need for parenteral antibiotic treatment. Patients with gram-negative folliculitis complicating acne are excellent candidates for isotretinoin therapy.

Necrotizing fasciitis, regardless of the bacterial etiology, cannot be cured unless the necrotic fascia is debrided. Type 1 infection due to mixed bowel flora also requires aggressive antibiotic treatment with a combination such as clindamycin and an aminoglycoside. In type 2 infection with *Streptococcus pyogenes,* penicillin is the drug of choice. Similarly, incision and drainage is mandatory in the genital area to cure Fournier's gangrene. Plastic reconstruction to repair the necrotic and debrided areas is often a difficult task after recovery from Fournier's gangrene.

Vibrio vulnificus and *Aeromonas hydrophila* wound infection and cellulitis often require surgical debridement as well as antibiotics. When an oral drug is indicated, fluoroquinolones or a cephalosporin is usually the first choice for antibiotic treatment, although results of sensitivity studies should be the guide. One of the penicillin preparations remains the antibiotic of choice for therapy for skin infections with *Erysipelothrix rhusiopathiae* and *Pasteurella multocida*. The aminoglycosides streptomycin (20 mg/kg per day in two divided doses) or gentamicin (5 mg/kg per day) probably remain the most effective drugs to treat tularemia, but they must be given parenterally. Chloramphenicol, 2 to 4 g per day given orally in four divided doses, is often effective but is associated with more relapses than the aminoglycosides.

References

1. Nelson JD, Ginsburg CM. An hypothesis on the pathogenesis of *Hemophilus influenzae* buccal cellulitis. J Pediatr 1976;88:709–710.
2. Drapkin MS, Wilson ME, Shrager SM, Rubin RH. Bacteremic *Hemophilus influenzae* type B cellulitis in the adult. Am J Med 1977;63:449–452.
3. McDonnell WM, Roth MS, Sheagren JN. *Hemophilus influenzae* type B cellulitis in adults. Am J Med 1986;81:709–712.
4. Adams WG, Deaver KA, Cochi SL, et al. Decline of childhood *Haemophilus influenzae* type B (Hib) disease in the Hib vaccine era. JAMA 1993;269:221–226.
5. Broadhurst LE, Erickson RL, Kelley PW. Decreases in invasive *Haemophilus influenzae* diseases in US Army children, 1984 through 1991. JAMA 1993:269:227–231.
6. Lawlor MT, Crowe HM, Quintiliani R. Cellulitis due to *Streptococcus pneumoniae*: Case report and review. Clin Infect Dis 1992;13:237–250.
7. DiNubile MJ, Albornoz MA, Stumacher RJ, et al. Pneumococcal soft tissue infections: Possible association with connective tissue diseases. J Infect Dis 1991;163:897–900.
8. Brook I, Frazier EH, Thompson DH. Aerobic and anaerobic microbiology of external otitis. Clin Infect Dis 1991;15:955–958.
9. Doroghazi RM, Nadol JB, Hyslop NE, et al. Invasive external otitis. Am J Med 1991;71:603–614.
10. Gustafson TL, Band JD, Hutcheson RH, et al. *Pseudomonas* folliculitis: An outbreak and review. Rev Infect Dis 1983;5:1–8.
11. Ratnam S, Hogan K, March SB, et al. Whirlpool associated folliculitis caused by *Pseudomonas aeruginosa*: Report of an outbreak and review. J Clin Microbiol 1986;23:655–659.
12. Hojyo-Tomoka MT, Marples RR, Kligman AM. *Pseudomonas* infection in superhydrated skin. Arch Dermatol 1973;107:723–727.
13. Leyden JJ, Stewart R, Kligman AM. Experimental infection of *Pseudomonas aeruginosa* and *Pseudomonas cepacia* on human skin. J Cosmet Chem 1990;31:19–28.
14. Bottone EJ, Perez AA. *Pseudomonas aeruginosa* folliculitis acquired through use of a contaminated loofah sponge: An unrecognized potential public health problem. J Clin Microbiol 1993;31:480–483.
15. Trueb RM, Panizzon RG, Burg G. Non-recreational *Pseudomonas aeruginosa* folliculitis: Report of two cases and review of the literature. Eur J Dermatol 1993;3:269–272.
16. Blaze PE, Thyss A, Caldani C, et al. *Pseudomonas aeruginosa* 0-11 folliculitis. Arch Dermatol 1985;121:873–876.
17. Leyden JJ, Marples RR, Mills OH, et al. Gram-negative folliculitis: A complication of antibiotic therapy in acne vulgaris. Br J Dermatol 1973;88:533–538.
18. Blankenship ML. Gram-negative folliculitis. Arch Dermatol 1984;120:1301–1303.
19. Adler AI, Altman J. An outbreak of mud wrestling–induced pustular dermatitis in college students: Dermatitis palaestrae limosae. JAMA 1993;269:502–504.
20. Guiliano A, Lewis F Jr, Hadley K, et al. Bacteriology of necrotizing fasciitis. Am J Surg 1977;134:52–57.
21. Jones BB, Hirschmann JV, Brown GS, et al. Fournier's syndrome: Necrotizing subcutaneous infection of the male genitalia. J Urol 1979;122:279–282.
22. Clayton MD, Fowler JE Jr, Sharifi R, et al. Causes, presentation and survival of fifty-seven patients with necrotizing fasciitis of the male genitalia. Surg Gynecol Obstet 1990;170:49–55.
23. Blake PA, Merson MH, Weaver RE, et al. Disease caused by a marine vibrio: Clinical characteristics and epidemiology. N Engl J Med 1979;300:1–5.
24. Centers for Disease Control and Prevention. *Vibrio vulnificus* infections associated with raw oyster consumption—Florida, 1981–1992. MMWR 1993;42:405–407.
25. Gray LD, Kreger AS. Mouse skin damage caused by cytolysin from *Vibrio vulnificus* and by *V. vulnificus* infection. J Infect Dis 1987;155:236–241.
26. Chuang YC, Yuan CY, Liu CY, et al. *Vibrio vulnificus* infection in Taiwan: Report of 28 cases and review of clinical manifestations and treatment. Clin Infect Dis 1992;15:271–276.
27. Case Records of the Massachusetts General Hospital. N Engl J Med 1989;321:1029–1038.
28. *Aeromonas* wound infections associated with outdoor activities—California. MMWR 1990;39:334–341.
29. Gold WL, Salit IE. *Aeromonas hydrophila* infections of skin and soft tissue: Report of 11 cases and review. Clin Infect Dis 1993;16:69–74.
30. Janda JM, Abbott SL. Infections associated with the genus *Edwardsiella*: The role of *Edwardsiella tarda* in human disease. Clin Infect Dis 1993;17:742–748.
31. Barnett JH, Estes SA, Wirman JA, et al. Erysipeloid. J Am Acad Dermatol 1983;9:116–123.
32. Gorby GI, Peacock JE. *Erysipelothrix rhusiopathiae* endocarditis: Microbiologic, epidemiologic, and clinical features of an occupational disease. Rev Infect Dis 1988;10:317–325.
33. Kizer KW. Animal bites. In: Gorbach SL, Bartlett JG, Blacklow NR, eds. Infectious Diseases. Philadelphia: WB Saunders Co., 1992:1277–1281.
34. Weber DJ, Wolfson JS, Swartz MN, et al. *Pasteurella multocida* infections: Report of 34 cases and review of the literature. Medicine 1984;63:133–154.
35. Evans ME, Gregory DW, Schaffner W, et al. Tularemia: A 30-year experience with 88 cases. Medicine 1985;64:251–269.
36. Capellan J, Fong IW. Tularemia from a cat bite: Case report and review of feline-associated tularemia. Clin Infect Dis 1993;15:472–475.
37. Kingston ME, Mackey D. Skin clues in the diagnosis of life threatening infections. Rev Infect Dis 1986;8:1–11.
38. Sotto MN, Langer B, Hoshino-Shimizu S, et al: Pathogenesis of cutaneous lesions in acute meningococcemia in humans: Light, immunofluorescent and electron microscopic studies of skin biopsy specimens. J Infect Dis 1976;133:506–514.
39. Weinberg AN, Swartz MN. Gram-negative coccal and bacillary infections. In: Fitzpatrick TB, Eisen AZ, Wolff K, et al., eds. Dermatology in General Medicine, 4th ed. New York: McGraw-Hill, 1993;2334–2335.
40. Weinberg AN, Swartz MN. Gram-negative coccal and bacillary infections. In: Fitzpatrick TB, Eisen AZ, Wolff K, et al., eds. Dermatology in General Medicine, 4th ed. New York: McGraw-Hill, 1993;2341.
41. Boissoau AM, Sarlangue J, Perel Y. Perineal ecthyma gangrenosum in infancy and early childhood: Septicemic and nonsepticemic forms. J Am Acad Dermatol 1992;27:415–418.
42. Blaze P, Thyss A, Vinti H, et al. A study of nineteen immunocompromised patients with extensive skin lesions caused by *Pseudomonas aeruginosa* with and without bacteremia. Acta Derm Venereol 1991;71:411–415.
43. Teplitz C. Pathogenesis of *Pseudonomas* vasculitis in septic lesions. Arch Pathol 1965;80:297–307.
44. Litwack KD, Hoke AW, Borchardt KA. Rose spots in typhoid fever. Arch Dermatol 1972;105:252–255.

45. Stamenkovic I, Lew PD. Early recognition of potentially fatal necrotizing fasciitis. N Engl J Med 1984;210:1689–1693.
46. Bernard P, Bedane C, Mounier M, et al. Streptococcal cause of erysipelas and cellulitis in adults. Arch Dermatol 1989;125:779–782.
47. Engleberg NC, Eisenstein BI. Detection of microbial nucleic acids for diagnostic purposes. Annu Rev Med 1992;43:147–155.
48. Koehler JE, Quinn FD, Berger TG, et al. Isolation of *Rochalimaea* species from cutaneous and osseous lesions of bacillary angiomatosis. N Engl J Med 1992;237:1625–1631.
49. Beard JS, Benson PM, Skillman L. Rapid diagnosis of coccidioidomycosis with a DNA probe to ribosomal RNA. Arch Dermatol 1993;129:1589–1593.
50. Penneys NS, Leonardi CL, Cook S, et al. Identification of *Mycobacterium tuberculosis* DNA in five different types of cutaneous lesions by the polymerase chain reaction. Arch Dermatol 1993;129:1594–1598.

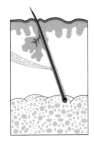

chapter 108

Syphilis and the Treponematoses

TIMOTHY G. BERGER, NICHOLAS FIUMARA,
and MARGOT WHITFELD

DEFINITION

Syphilis is an acute or chronic infectious disease caused by the spirochete *Treponema pallidum*. It is usually sexually transmitted during infectious stages of the disease, except in the case of congenital syphilis, which is spread from mother to fetus. Classically, the disease passes through four stages. The primary stage is characterized by a chancre, an ulceration at the site of inoculation. The secondary stage may have a host of systemic symptoms, usually including adenopathy and rash. The latent stage is an asymptomatic period of variable duration with reactive serologic tests. In tertiary syphilis mucocutaneous, osseous, visceral, cardiovascular, and neural involvement may be seen. Infectious syphilis consists of the primary, secondary, and early latent phase. It is during these stages that syphilis may be spread sexually. [1] During pregnancy, however, syphilis in all stages is potentially infectious to the developing fetus.[2]

CLINICAL MANIFESTATIONS

Primary Syphilis

After an incubation period of 9 to 90 days, with an average of 3 weeks, the primary stage appears. It is characterized by the chancre, which emerges at the point of inoculation. Inasmuch as 90% of all syphilis is transmitted sexually, most chancres appear on the genitalia either as single or multiple lesions. The chancre begins as a papule and soon erodes and becomes ulcerative. It is characteristically painless, indolent, punched out and clean, with a scanty, yellow, serous discharge (Fig. 108–1). The borders of the ulcer are raised, smooth, and sharply defined; the base is finely granular and hard; and the entire lesion is indurated or rubbery to palpation (Fig. 108–2). The neighboring lymph nodes are discretely enlarged and firm but do not suppurate. Most chancres of the penis occur on the prepuce, coronal sulcus, glans, or frenulum. Anorectal chancres often occur in the posterior midline of the anal ring and superficially resemble an anal fissure. The patient complains of pain and bleeding on defecation; however, in contrast to an anal fissure, the ulcer is indurated and there is usually bilateral inguinal adenopathy. Any anal fissure not occurring in the midline must be considered a chancre until proven otherwise. Chancres of the rectum are less common and appear as an indurated, ulcerated area that superficially resembles a carcinoma. In women, the labia are the most common sites, but chancres may appear on the fourchette, urethra, perineum and cervix.

The lips are the commonest site for chancres of the oral cavity.[3] Chancres of the tongue, next in frequency, take the form of painless ulcers. Tonsillar chancres are unilateral and for some still unknown reason, are more common on the left. The uvula is erythematous and pulled over to the left, "looking at the chancre." The gag reflex is diminished to absent. The foliate papillae are enlarged, the left anterior tonsillar pillar is red, and the tonsil is ulcerated, hard, and nontender. The anterior cervical node is enlarged.

The diagnosis of primary syphilis is established by the finding of *T. pallidum* on darkfield examination (except in the mouth), and by the reagin and treponemal blood tests. Early in primary syphilis the reaginic test may not be reactive. The Rapid Reagin Plasma test becomes positive sooner than the Venereal Disease Research Laboratory test. The specific treponemal tests (especially the fluorescent treponemal antibody absorption test [FTA-ABS]) will often be positive. In the patient with a suspicious mucocutaneous lesion, no prior history of syphilis,

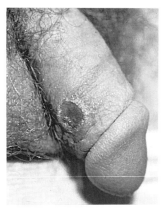

FIGURE 108-1. In primary syphilis, the chancre is a hard, indurated, non-tender ulceration of the penis with hard discrete non-tender inguinal nodes. Sixty per cent of chancres are singular lesions; 40% are multiple.

and a negative reaginic test, a specific treponemal test may be useful in diagnosing primary syphilis.

Secondary Syphilis

The secondary stage follows the onset of the chancre by 3 to 6 weeks, or about 6 to 8 weeks following infection. The chancre is present in about 25% of cases of secondary syphilis but usually is healing. The signs and symptoms of secondary syphilis are protean.[4, 5]

Early in this stage, the patient complains of an influenza or flu-like syndrome consisting of headaches, lacrimation, nasal discharge, sore throat, and generalized arthralgia. With these constitutional symptoms, the patient will have enlargement of the lymph nodes. The lymph nodes are not painful, and have a rubbery character. Adenopathy usually precedes the cutaneous eruption. Palpation of the abdomen may reveal an enlarged spleen and, less commonly, an enlarged liver as well.

The generalized eruption completes the picture of secondary syphilis. The eruption is painless and often non-

pruritic. Mucous membrane lesions (mucous patches) and alopecia may be found. Skin lesions tend to follow to some extent the skin tension lines, especially on the trunk. Secondary syphilis has a special predilection for the palms and soles. These lesions are discrete and sharply demarcated rather than confluent and have a coppery hue. The color becomes more intensified as one proceeds from the periphery to the center. The eruption of early secondary syphilis is usually not particularly scaly, with the exception of the hard, indurated papules on the palms and soles. The eruption is bilateral and symmetrical, tending to be more profuse on the upper extremities and upper trunk than on the abdomen and lower extremities.

The eruption is most commonly macular, papular, pustular, or some combination, but may show any morphology except a vesicular or bullous eruption. The eruption may last a few weeks to as long as 12 months. This is followed by a period of latency, which, in at least 25% of untreated cases, is interrupted by signs and symptoms of clinical secondary relapse.

The pattern of eruption is related to the duration of infection. The earliest cutaneous expression of secondary syphilis is the macular or erythematous eruption, which appears about 6 to 8 weeks after the infectious exposure. It begins on the sides of the trunk, shoulders, upper extremities, and the flexors of the arms and forearms, and tends to spare the face, palms, and soles. Individual lesions are oval 1- to 2-cm patches that may coalesce. The eruption is not indurated and the lesions will blanch with pressure. The rash is transient and fades within 2 weeks.

The macular stage is the forerunner of the maculo-papular eruption, which is the usual textbook description of the rash of secondary syphilis. This eruption is generalized, involving the middle of the face, chest, back, abdomen, the flexors of the forearms and arms, and, to a lesser extent, the lower extremities. During this stage, there are lesions on the palms and soles (Fig. 108-3). The eruption is coppery red. Lesions involving the mucous membranes are called mucous patches. These lesions may also appear on the moist surfaces of the

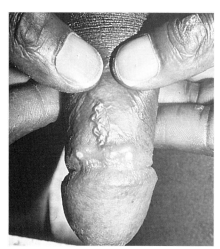

FIGURE 108-2. An atypical chancre is indurated and non-tender. Half of chancres are atypical.

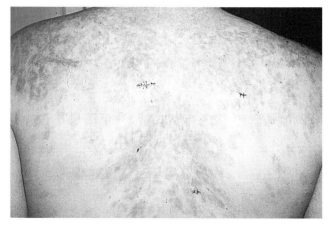

FIGURE 108-3. In secondary syphilis, macules and papules appear on the palms and soles, chest, and back. Mucous patches appear in the mouth. Lesions are oval in skin tension lines and are approximately the same size. This patient presented with uveitis.

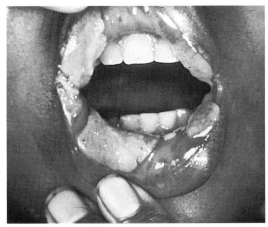

FIGURE 108–4. Mucous patches of lips in secondary syphilis. They may appear in the oral cavity on buccal mucous membrane, tongue, and pharyngeal mucosa. On moist surface of glans penis, foreskin, or labia, they are shallow erosions covered by a grayish-white membrane.

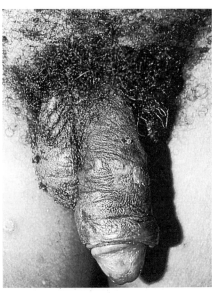

FIGURE 108–6. Papulosquamous secondary syphilis. Lesions may be concentrated on the penis and scrotum and resemble psoriasis.

genitalia, particularly on the glans and foreskin or the labia. The typical mucous patch is an oval lesion with a slightly raised border within which is a shallow ulcer or erosion covered by a grayish-white membrane (Fig. 108–4). On the tip and sides of the tongue, mucous patches show more ulceration than elsewhere in the mouth.

Papular lesions of secondary syphilis appear next. They are fewer in number and larger. They may be *follicular*, and associated with a nonscarring, nonerythematous alopecia of the scalp and beard, and patchy alopecia of the eyebrows (Fig. 108–5). The *lenticular*, or flat-topped, small papules superficially resemble lichen planus and are generalized. The *papulosquamous* lesions are also generalized and resemble psoriasis (Fig. 108–6). *Corymbose* lesions consist of a central larger papule surrounded by smaller papules. The number of lesion groups is small and lesions are asymmetrical. This is a sign of later secondary syphilis. *Nodular* syphilis presents as large asymmetrical lesion(s) (Fig. 108–7).

In contrast to the coppery-red hue of maculopapular syphilis, papular lesions tend to be of a darker red to reddish-brown color. The induration of the individual

lesions is more pronounced, and there is greater tendency toward postinflammatory hyperpigmentation as the lesions heal. The regression of papular lesions is slower than that of either macular or maculopapular lesions. Papular lesions are almost invariably found on the palms and soles where they are seen as deep-seated, flat-topped papules or scaly papulosquamous lesions (Fig. 108–8). After treatment, the papules disappear last from the palms and soles, respectively. The papular lesions of secondary syphilis that occur on the moist areas of the body are called condylomata lata (Fig. 108–9). They are elevated, reddish-brown or gray, flat topped, and moist. These lesions teem with spirochetes.

Pustular lesions follow and are less common than either maculopapular or papular lesions. Pustular lesions begin as papules that soften, ulcerate, and then crust. They may be generalized. Pustular syphilis may resemble chickenpox or generalized impetigo and, as in chickenpox in the adult, the patient is sicker, with fever, head-

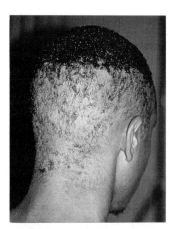

FIGURE 108–5. Syphilitic alopecia is a patchy non-scarring alopecia of scalp. On the eyebrows, the alopecia is usually lateral. The hair grows back after treatment.

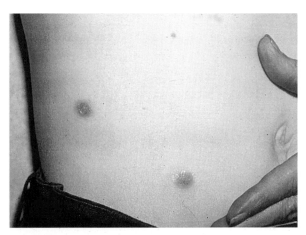

FIGURE 108–7. Nodular secondary syphilis. Fewer lesions, larger in size, but still with characteristic red-brown color.

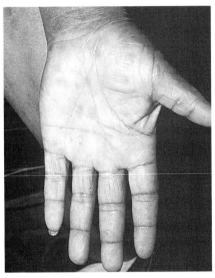

FIGURE 108-8. Secondary syphilis of the palms. The lesions may be maculopapular, papular, papulopustular, or pustular.

aches, and arthralgia. The lesions are frequently seen around the fingernails and toenails, as well as on the palms and soles. The lesions teem with treponemes, and darkfield examination is usually positive.

Annular syphilis tends to be papular, and during the protracted course of untreated secondary syphilis, the lesions may appear and disappear, with various intervals of quiescence. The lesions of recurrent secondary syphilis tend to be larger, more discrete, and darker in color than the earlier manifestations. Annular lesions are more frequently seen in dark-skinned persons. Recurrent annular secondary syphilis may also appear with condylomata lata of the anogenital areas.

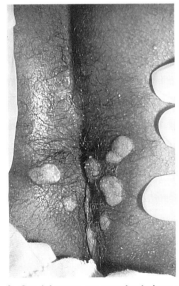

FIGURE 108-9. Condylomata are papular lesions coalescing in the flexural creases in the moist areas of the body—nasolabial, axillary, genitocrural, perianal, and webs of fingers and toes.

Secondary syphilis may involve virtually any other organ system, but certain patterns are characteristic.[6] Syphilitic *hepatitis* occurs in up to 10% of patients with early syphilis, is most commonly asymptomatic, and the alkaline phosphatase level is usually more elevated than the level of transaminases. *Gastritis* presents similarly to peptic ulcer disease. Syphilitic *renal* disease is an immune complex glomerulonephritis, usually presenting as nephrotic syndrome. As many as one third of patients develop *musculoskeletal* symptoms manifested by tenosynovitis, symmetrical polyarthritis, periostitis, or, rarely, syphilitic osteomyelitis.

Both the reaginic and treponemal tests are always reactive in secondary syphilis. The titer of nontreponemal tests is usually higher than that seen in primary syphilis. Very high titer antibody may lead to a false-negative result, called the *prozone* phenomenon.[7] In such instances, the quantitative reagin will be nonreactive in undiluted or low-titer sera (1:1 and 1:2), but as the serum is diluted, a positive reaction is found. Agglutination reactions occur only within fixed limits of antibody and antigen. In the prozone reaction, the patient has a surplus amount of antibody for the amount of antigen used; thus, no agglutination occurs. The specific treponemal tests are not affected by the prozone reaction, and will be reactive.

Latent Syphilis

Latency is defined as acquired or congenital syphilis that is without signs or symptoms (of early or late symptomatic syphilis) and characterized by repeated reactive reagin and treponemal tests, and a nonreactive spinal fluid. Latent syphilis is divided into early or late latent syphilis. The Centers for Disease Control and Prevention considers early latent syphilis as syphilis under 1 year's duration, if there is a history of untreated primary or secondary syphilis, or of lesions consistent with primary or secondary syphilis within the past year, or if the patient has had a nonreactive reagin test within the past year. Within this constellation, there will be patients with incubating syphilis, patients who are between the primary and secondary stages, and others who have already had secondary syphilis. Early latent syphilis is potentially infectious. The World Health Organization considers early latency to encompass the first 2 years of infection. About 25% of patients with untreated latent syphilis will have the reappearance of mucocutaneous lesions, usually within the first year of infection.

Late Mucocutaneous Syphilis

Late syphilis of the skin may appear from 5 to 10 years or as long as 20 years after the primary infection. The lesions may be nodular, noduloulcerative, or gummatous. Characteristically, the lesions are chronic, painless, asymptomatic, asymmetric, indolent, slow-growing, and progressively destructive. They are hard and indurated, with sharply demarcated borders.

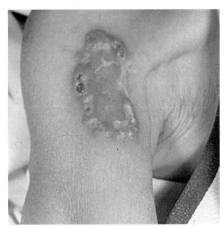

FIGURE 108-10. Late (tertiary) mucocutaneous syphilis with noduloulcerative lesion—chronic, deep-seated ulceration that is hard, nontender, and scarring.

Nodular Lesions

These lesions may vary in size from a few millimeters to several centimeters. The color is generally reddish brown. The lesions appear asymmetrically in clusters or large plaques. Lesions progress centrifugally, forming annular or arciform lesions with central scarring. They may involve any area of the skin, including the scalp, palms, and soles.

Noduloulcerative Lesions

These lesions are often seen with nodular tertiary syphilis and represent lesions that have ulcerated. The ulcerations are multiple and usually deep (Fig. 108-10).

Gummas

In contrast to the multiple lesions of the nodular and noduloulcerative stages, gummas tend to be solitary lesions. They usually develop at sites of trauma. A gumma arises deep in the dermis, appearing first as a soft tissue tumor-like swelling. Ulceration may occur. Lesions may progress, remain stable, or spontaneously heal. Gummas may be seen in many other organ systems, most commonly the bones, upper respiratory tract, and mucous membrane of the mouth. Involvement of the nasal bones/cartilage may lead to a saddle-nose deformity, and involvement of the palate may lead to perforation. The long bones are more likely to be attacked by syphilis. Of the long bones, the tibia is involved most frequently. The skull and the clavicle, particularly at its sternal end, are also involved.

EPIDEMIOLOGY

In the United States, there was a slow but steady increase in the incidence of syphilis—primary and secondary stages—from 1920 to 1935. Then in 1936, reported cases of syphilis rose sharply and continued during World War II, reaching a peak of nearly 100,000 cases in

1946. After the war, with peace and penicillin, there was a dramatic drop in reported primary and secondary syphilis until the mid 1950s, with about only 6500 cases yearly. In the late 1950s and 1960s this trend reversed, averaging between 19,000 and 26,000 cases annually. Rates increased through the 1970s, with many cases among homosexual men. Rates fell in the early 1980s due to changes in sexual behavior among gay men with the onset of the acquired immunodeficiency syndrome epidemic. In 1985 syphilis began to increase dramatically among heterosexual men and women, with an associated increase in congenital syphilis. By 1990 with 50,223 cases, syphilis had increased 75% in just 5 years. This increase reflected even more dramatic increases among black men (126%) and black women (231%), while rates in other segments of the population remained stable, or even declined. Much of this increase is linked to the urban "crack" cocaine epidemic, and trading sex for drugs. Outreach programs to this segment of the inner-city population has led to a decrease in cases—34,547 in 1992.[9]

TRANSMISSION

Syphilis may be contracted in one of five ways:

1. Sexual exposure: About 90% of all syphilis is transmitted sexually. Today, it is known that a patient is most infectious sexually during the first year of infection and becomes less so with each succeeding year, until, by the end of the second year, for all practical purposes, the patient cannot spread syphilis by this means.

2. Kissing: Kissing a person who has lesions of primary or secondary syphilis on the lips or in the oral cavity can transmit the disease.

3. Prenatal transmission: The mother infects the fetus in utero.

4. Transfusion: This is rarely seen today because all blood donors must have a nonreactive blood test before their blood can be used. However, needle sharing by intravenous drug users may transmit syphilis.

5. Accidental direct inoculation: Laboratory workers handling live spirochetes may be infected.

PATHOLOGY

The pathologic findings of syphilis depend on the stage of the disease and the type of lesion sampled. Infiltrates containing plasma cells and spirochetes are common to all three stages, although either can be scant. Swollen endothelial cells are frequently touted as a hallmark of syphilis, but are present in many other conditions.

Chancres of primary syphilis are ulcers whose beds are covered by neutrophils and fibrin that are often flanked by epithelial hyperplasia. There are often dense infiltrates of lymphocytes and plasma cells at the base of the ulcer, and thrombi can be present in the lumina of vessels just beneath the ulcer. Spirochetes tend to be numerous in chancres of primary syphilis, and can be demonstrated with an appropriate silver stain, such as the Warthin-Starry, Levaditi, or Steiner methods, or by immunoperoxidase staining. The direct fluorescent antibody tissue test for *T. pallidum* may be used in combination with histological stains to demonstrate pathogenic treponemes in formalin-fixed tissues. The spirochetes of syphilis are visible in specially stained preparations as spiral organisms that range from 7 to 15 μ in length and are 0.25 μ in diameter (Fig. 108–11).

Macules of secondary syphilis feature superficial and deep perivascular infiltrates of lymphocytes, macrophages, and plasma cells without epidermal change, or accompanied by slight vacuolar change at the dermoepidermal interface.

Papules and plaques of secondary syphilis most often show dense superficial and deep infiltrates of lymphocytes, macrophages, and plasma cells. These cells are usually distributed in a band-like pattern in the papillary dermis, accompanied by psoriasiform epidermal hyperplasia and hyperkeratosis.[10] The presence of numerous macrophages often gives the infiltrates a pallid appearance at scanning magnification (Fig. 108–12). Spirochetes can be found either within the epidermis around superficial capillaries and venules. Plasma cells are said to be absent in 10% of cases, and scant in 15%.[11] As lesions age, macrophages become more numerous, so

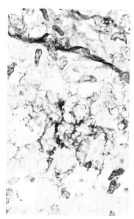

FIGURE 108–12. A Warthin-Starry stain of a lesion of secondary syphilis demonstrates spiral-shaped organisms just beneath the silver-positive basement membrane.

that in late secondary lues, granulomatous foci are often present. In pustular lesions, there is pallor of epidermal or follicular keratinocytes, with spongiform neutrophilic pustules. Spirochetes are more plentiful in such areas than in any other form of secondary lues. Follicular pustules feature infiltrates of plasma cells and macrophages in the adventitial dermis around infundibula, and neutrophils both within infundibular epithelium and in the follicular ostium. Condylomata have spongiform pustules within areas of papillated epithelial hyperplasia that teem with spirochetes. In the "moth-eaten" alopecia of secondary syphilis there are superficial and deep infiltrates of lymphocytes and plasma cells, focally obscuring the dermoepidermal junction, and increased numbers of follicles in devolutional stages. In a vasculitic form of secondary syphilis known as lues maligna, fibrin thrombi are present in some superficial venules, and neutrophils can be found within and around vessels. Ulceration can be present, and resolves with fibrosis.[12]

Nodular lesions of late syphilis usually have changes that resemble those of secondary lesions, with the addition of tuberculoid granulomas. The epidermis in such lesions can be atrophic rather than hyperplastic. In gummas, there is necrosis of cells within granulomas. Spirochetes are scant, even in necrotic foci.

LABORATORY TESTS

The diagnosis of syphilis is usually confirmed by one of four methods.[13, 14]

The Darkfield Examination

The darkfield examination may be performed on any exudate from a suspicious genital ulceration, wet lesion of secondary syphilis (or if dry, scraped until oozing), umbilical cord in congenital syphilis, or the aspirate of an enlarged lymph node in primary or secondary syphilis (Fig. 108–13). *T. pallidum* is a slender, motile, spiral organism 7 to 15 μ long and 0.25 μ thick. The spirals are evenly spaced and are about 1 μ apart.

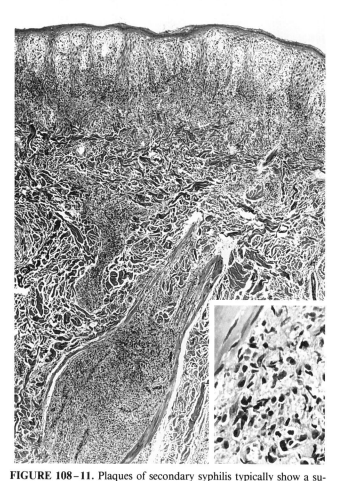

FIGURE 108–11. Plaques of secondary syphilis typically show a superficial and deep lichenoid infiltrate coupled with psoriasiform epidermal hyperplasia. There is a dense infiltrate of plasma cells and macrophages adjacent to an arrector pili muscle (inset, lower right).

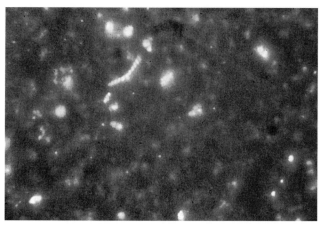

FIGURE 108–13. Positive darkfield examination reveals a motile spirochete 7 to 15 μ long, about the diameter of a red blood cell. It has four movements—rotation, opening and closing of coils, flexion and extension, and true motion or progression.

In lesions in the mouth, a darkfield examination is unreliable because the normal commensal *T. microdentium* cannot be distinguished with certainty from *T. pallidum*. If a darkfield microscope is not available, the exudate may be allowed to dry on the slide and be sent to a laboratory for direct fluorescent antibody examination for *T. pallidum*.

Nontreponemal Tests (The Reagin Blood Test)

The Venereal Disease Research Laboratory test and the Rapid Plasma Reagin (RPR) tests are currently performed in the United States, the latter gradually replacing the former.[15] These tests measure antilipid antibodies formed by the host against the lipid on the treponemal cell surface.[16] They are less sensitive and less specific than the treponemal tests (see below), but are used as screening tests owing to their ease and low cost. A positive result of a nontreponemal test should always be confirmed by a specific treponemal test. The reagin tests, in addition to their usefulness in diagnosing syphilis, are also essential in assessing the effectiveness of treatment and the detection of possible relapse or reinfection.

Treponemal Tests

These tests use *T. pallidum* or a portion of it as the antigen. The *Treponema pallidum* immobilization test, when positive, is specific for syphilis or a treponematosis (yaws, pinta, bejel). The test measures the ability of the patient's serum to immobilize and kill live *T. pallidum* in the presence of complement. Except for research, it is no longer used in the United States. The FTA-ABS is an indirect fluorescent antibody test in which the patient's serum is placed on a slide to which a suspension of *T. pallidum* has been fixed. Then a fluorescein-labeled antihuman globulin is added that binds specifically to the patient's serum antibodies adhering to the *T. pallidum*, resulting in a visible reaction under fluorescent micros-

copy. The microhemagglutination assay for *T. pallidum* is gradually replacing the FTA-ABS because it is easier to perform, less expensive, and has about the same sensitivity and specificity. Treponemal tests usually remain positive for life and are therefore not useful in diagnosing other than the initial episode of syphilis. Recent studies, however, have demonstrated loss of positivity of both the FTA-ABS and the microhemagglutination assay for *T. pallidum* in between 13% and 24% of patients, respectively. This was independent of stage of syphilis and human immunodeficiency virus (HIV) serologic status.[17, 18]

The biologic false-positive (BFP) reaction is a positive RPR or other reaginic serologic test with a negative treponemal test in a patient without a history of syphilis. Ninety per cent of BFP tests are of low titer (<1:8).[19] There are two types of BFP reactions, acute and chronic. The acute reaction occurs in those patients whose reagin blood tests are reactive for less than 3 to 6 months. Many infectious diseases, immunizations, and pregnancy may cause this reaction (Table 108–1). Chronic BFP reactions occur in patients whose reagin tests are reactive for more than 3 to 6 months. Connective tissue diseases, especially systemic lupus erythematosus, chronic liver disease, multiple blood transfusions/intravenous drug usage, and advancing age are the most common causes. Treponemal tests less frequently can be falsely positive, but because they are used only to confirm positive reaginic tests, this is rarely a clinical problem. Lyme disease may cause a positive FTA-ABS, but is not a common cause of BFP reaginic tests.[8]

Histopathology

Biopsy specimens from affected organs contain spirochetes in all stages of disease. Organisms are most abundant in early syphilis, and much fewer in late disease. Silver stains are used most commonly, and in the skin identify spirochetes in the epidermis and around blood vessels in the dermis. Immunofluorescent techniques using specific antitreponemal antibodies may also be performed on paraffin-fixed material, and greatly enhance the detection of organisms.

DIFFERENTIAL DIAGNOSIS (Table 108–2)

Primary Syphilis

The differential diagnosis is that of a patient with a genital ulcer.[20] About 5% of patients with genital ulcer disease have multiple pathogens simultaneously.

Herpes Simplex. Primary or recurrent herpes simplex can produce genital ulcerations. In primary herpes the incubation period is generally shorter (less than 1 week). Herpetic lesions begin as grouped blisters that erode, forming shallow, nonindurated ulcerations. They are usually exquisitely tender and often painful. Inguinal lymph nodes may be enlarged and tender. The Tzanck test smear is positive, revealing multinucleated giant cells; viral culture is usually positive.

TABLE 108-1. Potential Causes of False-Positive Serologic Tests for Syphilis

Tests	Infectious Causes	Noninfectious Causes
Reaginic or nontreponemal tests (RPR, VDRL) Bacterial	Pneumococcal pneumonia Scarlet fever Leprosy Lymphogranuloma venereum Relapsing fever Bacterial endocarditis Malaria Rickettsial disease Psittacosis Leptospirosis Chancroid Tuberculosis Mycoplasmal pneumonia Trypanosomiasis	Pregnancy Chronic liver disease Advanced cancer Intravenous drug use Multiple myeloma Advancing age Connective-tissue disease Multiple blood transfusions
Viral	Vaccinia (vaccination) Chickenpox HIV Measles Infectious mononucleosis Mumps Viral hepatitis	
Treponemal tests (FTA-ABS, MHA-TP)	Lyme disease Leprosy Malaria Infectious mononucleosis Relapsing fever Leptospirosis	Systemic lupus erythematosus

Reprinted by permission of *The New England Journal of Medicine*, Hook EW, Marra CM. Acquired syphilis in adults. N Engl J Med 1992;326:1060–1067. Copyright 1992, Massachusetts Medical Society.

RPR, Rapid Plasma Reagin; VDRL, Venereal Disease Research Laboratory; HIV, human immunodeficiency virus; FTA-ABS, fluorescent treponemal, antibody absorption; MHA-TP, microhemagglutination assay for *Treponema pallidum*.

Traumatic Erosions and Ulcerations. Lesions and pain appear almost immediately following sexual activity.

Allergic Contact Dermatitis. The most common allergens are contraceptive vaginal creams or foam, condoms, or topical medication.

Fixed Drug Eruption. These lesions are most frequently due to sulfamethoxazole/trimethoprim, nonster-

TABLE 108-2. Differential Diagnosis of Primary and Secondary Syphilis

Primary Syphilis

Herpes simplex
Traumatic lesions
Contact dermatitis
Fixed drug eruption
Chancroid
Granuloma inguinale
Lymphogranuloma venereum

Secondary Syphilis

Pityriasis rosea
Lichen planus
Psoriasis
Drug eruption
Viral exanthems
Rubella
Dermatophytoses

oidal anti-inflammatory agents, or tetracycline. Lesions are larger than chancres, nonindurated, more superficial, and tender.

Chancroid.[21, 22] The incubation period is 3 to 5 days. The primary lesion is a painful erythematous papule that rapidly ulcerates with an erythematous halo. The ulceration is deep, not shallow as in herpes. The edges are ragged and the ulcer spreads laterally, burrowing under the skin and giving the lesion the characteristically undermined edges. The ulcers are soft and tender. The contiguous areas of the skin become infected (autoinoculation) and ulcerate. Diagnosis is confirmed by Gram's stain and culture on special media.

Granuloma Inguinale. Granuloma inguinale is a relatively rare disease in the United States, with fewer than 50 cases annually. The incubation period is 8 days to 3 months. Lesions begin as a beefy-red, moist papule that appears often on the corona or shaft of penis. Ulcerations typically have an elevated and rolled border, and the base has a rough cobblestone appearance. Lesions may expand, become granulomatous, and coalesce. Long-standing untreated lesions may give rise to a squamous carcinoma. Diagnosis is confirmed by biopsy or a touch preparation stained with Wright's or Giemsa stain.

Lymphogranuloma Venereum. Lymphogranuloma venereum is also a rare disease in the United States, with fewer than 500 cases a year reported. It is more common in Central and South America, Southern Asia, and Africa. The incubation period varies from 3 to 30 days.

The primary lesion is a painless papule or small papulo-vesicle that heals without scarring in 2 to 3 days. The site of the primary lesion determines which group of lymph nodes will be involved. If the lesion is on the penis, labia, or perianal area, the inguinal nodes will be affected. If the primary lesion appears on the cervix or in the rectum, the perirectal and deep iliac nodes will enlarge.

Secondary Syphilis

The rash of secondary syphilis may be macular, maculopapular, papular, papulopustular, pustular, or relapsing with annular macular or papular rings. The differential diagnosis is principally that of the papulosquamous eruptions.

Pityriasis Rosea. In pityriasis rosea there may be a herald patch. The eruption is generalized from the neck to the elbows, and on the trunk down to the thighs. It tends to spare the face, forearms, palms, legs, and soles of feet, and may be very pruritic. In pityriasis rosea, the lesions are oblong, of varying sizes, and follow the lines of cleavage. The lesions of pityriasis rosea are lighter, especially in their centers, whereas in syphilis the lesions are darker in the center. There is no generalized adenopathy in pityriasis rosea.

Lichen Planus. In lichen planus, lesions are usually violaceous, flat-topped polygonal papules with white lines on their surface. Pruritus is common and may be severe. Mucosal lesions are reticulate and favor the buccal surfaces. There is no adenopathy.

Psoriasis. Psoriatic lesions are papular with silvery scales that when scraped result in minute bleeding points (Auspitz sign). Papules may coalesce to form plaques. There is no adenopathy.

Drug Eruptions. Lesions are generalized, erythematous, and morbilliform. Pruritus is common, and adenopathy is unusual except in eruptions due to anticonvulsants.

Late Mucocutaneous Syphilis

The differential diagnosis of late mucocutaneous syphilis is listed in Table 108–3.

TABLE 108-3. Differential Diagnosis of Late Mucocutaneous Syphilis

Cutaneous tuberculosis
    Lupus vulgaris
    Erythema induratum
    Papulonecrotic tuberculid
    Scrofuloderma
Sarcoidosis
    Nonmelanoma skin cancer
    Psoriasis
    Granuloma annulare
    Stasis ulcer
    Bromoderma
    Hansen's disease
    Sporotrichosis
    Blastomycosis

TABLE 108-4. Treatment Recommendations for Syphilis

Early Syphilis (Primary, Secondary and Early Latent)

Benzathine Penicillin G, 2.4 million units intramuscularly weekly for 2 weeks; a total of 4.8 million units.
Penicillin allergy: doxycycline, 100 mg orally every 12 hours, or tetracycline, 500 mg every 6 hours for 14 days.

Late Syphilis (Excluding Neurosyphilis), Late Latent Syphilis, or Syphilis of Unknown Duration

Benzathine penicillin G, 2.4 million units weekly for 3 weeks; a total of 7.2 million units.
Penicillin allergy: doxycycline, 100 mg orally every 12 hours, or tetracycline, 500 mg every 6 hours for 28 days.*

Neurosyphilis

Aqueous crystalline penicillin G, 12–24 million units daily administered as 2–4 million units intravenously every 4 hours for 10–14 days.
Alternatively, 2.4 million units procaine penicillin intramuscularly daily, plus probenicid, 500 mg orally four times a day, both for 10–14 days.

Congenital Syphilis

Aqueous crystalline penicillin G, 100,000–150,000 units/kg/day (administered as 50,000 units/kg every 12 hours during the first 7 days of life and every 8 hours thereafter) for 10–14 days.
Alternatively, procaine penicillin G, 50,000 units/kg intramuscularly in a single dose for 10–14 days.†

*Patients treated with regimens not including penicillin should have a lumbar puncture prior to therapy (to exclude asymptomatic neurosyphilis).
†If more than 1 day of therapy is missed, the entire course is restarted. An infant with a completely normal evaluation, whose mother was treated with erythromycin, treated less than 1 month before delivery, or treated with an appropriate regimen before pregnancy but did not have an adequate response documented may be treated with benzathine penicillin G, 50,000 units/kg in a single dose.
Data from references 8 and 34.

TREATMENT

The drug of choice for the treatment of syphilis is penicillin, and the depot preparations of penicillin are preferred because they are inexpensive, are easy to administer, provide sustained blood levels of active drug, and do not require frequent patient visits (Table 108–4). Erythromycin is not recommended because it is poorly tolerated and has a high failure rate. All syphilis patients should be tested for HIV disease, as the presence of coexistent HIV infection may increase the risk of treatment failure or early central nervous system relapse.[23] Therapeutic alternatives to penicillin are recommended for early syphilis, late and late latent syphilis if the central nervous system is not involved. Only 10% of persons with a history of penicillin allergy have positive skin tests. Skin testing followed by desensitization if tests are positive and treatment with penicillin are recommended in neurosyphilis, all stages of syphilis in pregnancy, and in HIV-infected persons with syphilis.[24]

The objective of treatment in early syphilis is not only clinical cure but also a serologic cure, with the reagin test reverting to seronegativity (seroreversion). Patients should be seen every 3 months for the first year, every 6 months in the second year, and yearly thereafter. Because different treatment regimens have been used in different studies, the expected outcomes reported are somewhat different.[25, 26] Brown and associates found that the quantitative RPR titer declined fourfold by the third month, and eightfold by the sixth month in patients with their first episode of syphilis.[27] All patients with primary syphilis were nonreactive at 12 months, and those with secondary syphilis in 24 months. About 95% of patients with early latent syphilis were RPR nonreactive in 2 years and the remaining 5% within 4 years. If the patient had previously treated syphilis and was reinfected, the reagin titers are slower to decline after treatment and some patients do not achieve seronegativity.[18, 28] Romanowski and colleagues found that 72% of patients with first episode primary or secondary syphilis were RPR negative by 36 months.[18] A fourfold reduction in titer was seen at 6 months and an eightfold reduction by 12 months. Early latent syphilis had only a fourfold reduction in titer by 12 months. In this study, seroreversion of specific treponemal tests also occurred, so that by 36 months 24% of patients had a negative FTA-ABS and 13% had a negative microhemagglutination assay for *T. pallidum.*

Patients treated for late latent or late symptomatic syphilis should be examined every 3 months the first year, every 6 months during the second year, and yearly thereafter. The reagin titer will decline slowly, with about 45% becoming seronegative in 5 years, and the rest becoming reagin fast.[29]

The treatment of syphilis in pregnancy is appropriate treatment for that patient's stage of disease, i.e. for early syphilis a minimum of benzathine penicillin G 2.4 million units I.M. weekly for two consecutive weeks for a total of 4.8 million units.[30, 31] The pregnant patient who is allergic to penicillin presents a therapeutic dilemma. Tetracyclines are contraindicated and erythromycin therapy lacks efficacy in curing the mother and fetus and is not recommended.[32, 33] Desensitization and treatment with penicillin is recommended.[24, 34-36]

The deciduous teeth are fully formed by the eighteenth week of pregnancy, and treatment prior to this time will prevent the formation of the hypoplastic and malformed deciduous teeth. Treatment of the infected mother during the second and third trimester will cure the fetus if infected. If the mother is treated with the two doses of benzathine penicillin G within 14 days of delivery, the fetus is considered effectively treated and should not develop the early signs of neonatal syphilis. Babies will escape the development of the Hutchinson's incisors and the mulberry molars of the permanent dentition if the mother has been treated during pregnancy, or if the infant is treated within 3 months of delivery.

The Jarisch-Herxheimer Reaction

The Jarisch-Herxheimer reaction is a brief, self-limited flu-like syndrome following penicillin treatment of some cases of primary, many cases of secondary, and some cases of early latent syphilis. Symptoms include chills, fever, headache, and myalgias that appear 2 to 6 hours after treatment. Doxycycline or tetracycline treatment causes this reaction only rarely. The chancre or rash may be exacerbated. This reaction lasts for several hours, and is also seen following treatment of neonatal syphilis. The reaction is believed to be to the breakdown of the spirochetes.

NEUROSYPHILIS

Involvement of the central nervous system in syphilis occurs early in the disease. Forty per cent of patients with untreated primary or secondary syphilis have cerebrospinal fluid (CSF) pleocytosis.[24] Twenty-four per cent of patients with secondary syphilis have a reactive CSF Venereal Disease Research Laboratory test, and *T. pallidum* can be recovered from the CSF of 30% of patients with early syphilis, in one third of whom the CSF is otherwise normal. The importance of this latter finding is unknown.[8]

In two thirds of patients, CSF abnormalities resolve by the end of the secondary stage.[20] Patients with more abnormalities of their CSF are more likely to develop symptomatic neurosyphilis. Patients with normal CSF examinations do not develop symptomatic neurosyphilis. It is therefore important to identify those persons with no neurologic findings but abnormal CSF findings (asymptomatic neurosyphilis) because they are at risk for the development of neurosyphilis. Ten per cent of males and 5% of females with untreated syphilis develop neurosyphilis.

Neurosyphilis can occur at any stage of syphilis after the primary stage. Neurosyphilis is not just a finding of tertiary syphilis. Several characteristic patterns of central nervous system involvement occur, and they tend to occur at certain times following infection, with some overlap (Fig. 108–14).

Meningeal syphilis (syphilitic meningitis) usually occurs in the first year of infection and is characterized by headache, fever, stiff neck, cranial nerve findings (es-

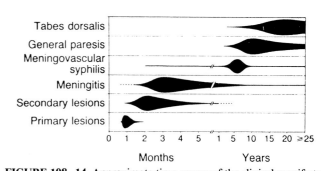

FIGURE 108–14. Approximate time course of the clinical manifestations of early syphilis and neurosyphilis. Shaded areas corresponding to each syndrome represent the approximate proportion of patients with the syndrome specified and do not indicate the proportion of all patients with syphilis who have that syndrome. (Reprinted by permission of *The New England Journal of Medicine*, Hook EW, Marra CM. Acquired syphilis in adults. N Engl J Med 1992;326:1059–1068. Copyright 1992, Massachusetts Medical Society.)

pecially hearing loss), facial palsies, and ophthalmic findings (photophobia, uveitis, retinitis, and optic neuritis). Meningovascular syphilis occurs 5 to 12 years after infection and is characterized by focal central nervous system findings of ischemia or stroke, such as hemiplegia, hemiparesis, aphasia, or seizures. Premonitory signs of headache, dizziness, insomnia, memory loss, and psychiatric symptoms occur in about half of cases.[37] Ten per cent of patients with meningovascular syphilis have Argyll Robertson pupils (react to accommodation but not light). In these early forms of neurosyphilis, both blood and CSF nontreponemal tests are positive, as well as the CSF exhibiting pleocytosis. Meningeal syndromes in Lyme disease are distinguished by the clinical features and negative nontreponemal tests in serum and CSF. Syphilis may be a cause of false positive Lyme serologies by enzyme-linked immunosorbent assay and by immunofluorescent assay.[38, 39]

Parenchymatous neurosyphilis is divided into two classic forms, general paresis and tabes dorsalis. General paresis is syphilitic meningoencephalitis caused by direct invasion of the cerebrum by spirochetes.[40] It appears 15 to 20 years after initial infection. The clinical manifestations are numerous but are typically psychiatric early and dementia-like later in the course.

Tabes dorsalis occurs 20 to 25 years after infection, and is manifested early by lightning pains of the legs or viscera (visceral crises). Ataxia, paresthesias, bowel and bladder disturbances, and visual loss (optic atrophy) may occur. Multiple neurologic abnormalities may be found on examination, but pupillary abnormalities and abnormalities of the reflexes of the lower extremities are virtually always found. As the disease progresses, the joints of the neurologically impaired lower extremities may be destroyed by trauma (Charcot's joints), and nonhealing trophic ulcers of the soles may occur.

A positive nontreponemal test in the CSF is very specific for neurosyphilis, and sufficient for the diagnosis of neurosyphilis even if the serum test is of very high titer. The diagnosis of late neurosyphilis is complicated by the fact that only 50% to 70% of patients with late syphilis have a positive serum nontreponemal test. A persistently positive serum treponemal test is not indicative of active infection, and the meaning of a positive CSF treponemal test is unclear, and cannot be used to make the diagnosis of neurosyphilis. A negative CSF FTA-ABS appears to exclude the diagnosis of neurosyphilis, however.[20] A combination of serum and CSF serologic tests (and their ratios), the clinical findings, and computed tomography may be required to establish a diagnosis.

CONGENITAL SYPHILIS

Congenital syphilis occurs when spirochetes from an infected, untreated mother enter the placenta and the fetal circulation.[41] Congenital syphilis is divided into two stages—early and late. It is early congenital syphilis if the disease is found within the first 2 years of life, and late congenital after this time.

Spontaneous abortion is the most common outcome of syphilis in the second and early third trimester.[42, 43] Stillbirths and perinatal death occur in about 40% of pregnancies of mothers with untreated early syphilis and over 20% of births of mothers with untreated late syphilis.[44]

Infants of women who meet any of the following criteria should be evaluated for congenital syphilis: (a) untreated syphilis, inadequate treatment, or no documentation of adequate treatment; (b) treatment of syphilis with erythromycin; (c) treatment less than 1 month before delivery; (d) inadequate response to treatment; (e) appropriate treatment before pregnancy, but insufficient serologic follow-up to document adequacy of therapy. The results of serologic tests for syphilis for every woman delivering a baby must be known prior to the discharge of that baby from the hospital. Serologic testing of the mother and child at delivery are recommended. Evaluation of children of women noted above should include: (a) a complete physical examination for findings of congenital syphilis; (b) nontreponemal serology of the infant's sera (not cord blood); (c) CSF evaluation; (d) long bone radiographs; and (e) pathologic evaluation of the placenta using specific antitreponemal antibody staining. For infants with no evidence of congenital syphilis on the above evaluations, determination of specific antitreponemal IgM should be considered.[34]

Early Congenital Syphilis

Inasmuch as the inoculation is directly into the fetal circulation, not focal (as in acquired syphilis), the manifestations of early congenital syphilis resemble those of acquired secondary syphilis. Chancres do not occur in early congenital syphilis. Most infants appear healthy at birth. In two thirds of cases the early signs appear in the third to eighth week, and in nearly all cases by the third month. Neonates who are symptomatic at birth are apt to be premature, potbellied, and emaciated. The prognosis is poor. The findings of early congenital syphilis are noted in Table 108–5.[45–49]

Late Congenital Syphilis

This stage occurs in children age 2 years or older. Eighty per cent of children eventually diagnosed with congenital syphilis are undetected in the early stage.[50] Usually, these patients are referred to the physician because the screening reagin blood test, taken during the evaluation of a totally unrelated disease, is found to be reactive.[49] The findings of late congenital syphilis are either malformations of tissues affected at critical growth periods earlier in life, or persistent inflammatory foci (Table 108–6; Fig. 108–15).[51]

Congenital neurosyphilis presents in a pattern similar to acquired syphilis. Meningitis appears in the first year, meningovascular syphilis in the first two years, and general paresis or tabes dorsalis between age 6 and 21, usually in adolescence.

SYPHILIS AND HUMAN IMMUNODEFICIENCY VIRUS

Most HIV-infected patients with syphilis exhibit the classic clinical manifestations with appropriate serologic

TABLE 108-5. Early Congenital Syphilis

1. *Snuffles*, the earliest sign—thick, tenacious, mucoid nasal discharge, often blood tinged. The discharge is teeming with spirochetes, an easy way to confirm the diagnosis.
2. *Central nervous system involvement*—Abnormal spinal fluid to frank stiff neck, bulging fontanelle, convulsions, positive Kernig's sign; chronic meningovascular syphilis with cranial nerve palsies, hydrocephalus.
3. *Iritis, chorioretinitis.*[45]
4. *Hoarse cry*, cracked cry and finally aphonic.
5. *Pseudoparalysis of Parrot*, osteochondritis by radiograph—spontaneous fractures.[46]
6. *Generalized lymphadenopathy*—hard, discrete, nontender nodes—anterior and posterior cervical, epitrochlear, inguinal, less often axillary—least often popliteal.
7. *Hepatosplenomegaly.*
8. *Potbelly.*
9. *Anemia*, hypochromic normocytic.[47]
10. *Thrombocytopenia*—purpura.
11. *Low serum protein*—marked reduction in albumin.
12. *Generalized edema.*
13. *Jaundice.*
14. *Ascites.*
15. *Skin lesions*: Skin lesions occur in 30%—60% of infants.[48]
    a. Maculopapular—as in acquired secondary syphilis with mucous patches in mouth, nares, pharynx, or trachea.[49]
    b. Papular—with condyloma lata—nasolabial, axillary, genito-crural.
    c. Bullous—on areas of pressure, palms and soles, "syphilitic pemphigoid," a sign of severe disease.
    d. Pustules frequently periungual.
    e. Rhagades—moist deep fissures around the mouth. They scar in a radiating linear fashion.
    f. Alopecia.
    g. Desquamation—often periungual, but may be generalized.

TABLE 108-6. Characteristic Findings of Late Congenital Syphilis

1. *Frontal bossing* of Parrot represents a localized periostitis of the frontal and parietal bones.
2. *Short maxilla, protuberant mandible, high palatal arch, and saddle nose.* Syphilitic nasal chondritis causes a collapsed "saddle nose." If this process affects the maxilla and palate, a concave or shallow-dish configuration in the middle section of the face and a high arched palate may result. The mandible appears prominent due to the shortened maxilla.
3. *Periostitis* of the long bones most commonly affects the tibia, clavicle, and scapula. *Saber shin* is bowing of the tibia. *Higoumenakis' sign* is an irregular thickening or enlargement of the sternoclavicular portion of the clavicle. *Scaphoid scapula*, a concavity of the vertebral border of the scapula, is a stigma, but not diagnostic of congenital syphilis.
4. *Hutchinson's teeth.* This abnormality of the upper central incisors of the permanent dentition does not appear until age 6 years or older. The incisors and canines are small, tapered toward the apex, widely spaced, and the biting edge is notched (Fig. 108-15).
5. *Mulberry molars.* Although all the molars may be affected in congenital syphilis, the tooth that is diagnostic is the lower first molar. This sixth-year molar of the permanent dentition develops at the same time as the upper central incisors. It is characterized by multiple small cusps in a circle.
6. *Eighth nerve deafness.*
7. *Interstitial keratitis.*
8. *Rhagades* are linear scars like spokes of a wheel, radiating from the angles of the eyes, nose, mouth, chin, and anus. Although they appear in the newborn period, they persist throughout life.
9. *Clutton's joint.* This is a rare manifestation of congenital syphilis that appears at about the age of puberty. The knee joint is the primary target, although the other joints can be involved. It is a painless synovitis with a doughy swelling of the joint.

titers for that stage of disease. Response to treatment, both clinical and serologic in HIV-infected patients with syphilis, generally follows the clinical and serologic patterns seen in patients without coexisting HIV infection.[17, 52-55] In a large study that compared HIV-positive to HIV-negative syphilis patients, patients with HIV were more likely to present with secondary syphilis (53% vs. 33%) and were more likely to have a chancre persisting when they had secondary syphilis (43% vs. 15%).[6] Unusual clinical manifestations of syphilis in HIV include florid skin lesions to few atypical ones, but these are exceptions, not the rule.[53, 54, 57, 58]

In general the nontreponemal tests are of higher titer in HIV-infected persons as a result of their enhanced B-cell activity.[17, 55] Rarely, the serologic response to infection may be impaired or delayed, and seronegative secondary syphilis has been reported.[59-61] Biopsy of the skin lesions and histopathologic evaluation with silver stains will confirm the diagnosis of syphilis in such cases. This approach, as well as darkfield examination of appropriate lesions, should be considered if the clinical eruption is characteristic of syphilis and the serologic tests are negative.

Neurosyphilis has been frequently reported in HIV-infected persons, even after appropriate therapy for early syphilis.[62, 63] Manifestations have been those of early neurosyphilis—meningeal or meningovascular syphilis.

These have included headache, fever, hemiplegia, and cranial nerve deficits, especially deafness (CN VIII), decreased vision (CN II), and ocular palsies (CN III and VI). Whether HIV-infected persons are at increased risk for these complications or whether they occur more quickly is unknown. It is known that spirochetes are no

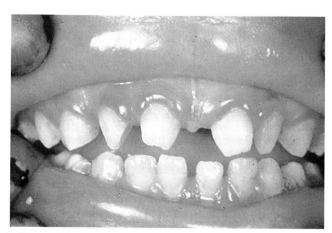

FIGURE 108-15. Congenital syphilis—Hutchinson's teeth, upper central incisors of the permanent dentition. The incisors are widely spaced, shorter than the lateral incisors, barrel shaped or peg shaped, and the width of the biting surface is less than the gingival margin. There is notching at the biting surface.

more likely to remain in the CSF after treatment in HIV-infected persons than in HIV-uninfected persons. Whether the impaired host immunity allows these residual spirochetes to more frequently or more quickly cause clinical relapse in the setting of HIV is unknown.

HIV-infected patients who have primary or secondary syphilis, are not allergic to penicillin, and are without any neurologic or psychiatric findings should be treated with benzathine penicillin G 2.4 million units intramuscularly weekly for a minimum of two doses and preferably three.[64] The third dose, although it may be unnecessary, will not harm the patient and reassures the physician that the patient's treatment was adequate. Patients allergic to penicillin should be desensitized and treated with penicillin. Following treatment, the patient should have monthly serologic follow-up with quantitative nontreponemal tests for the first 6 months. Failure of the titer to fall is an indication for reevaluation, including lumbar puncture.

As a result of the concerns about neurologic relapse in the setting of HIV disease, careful evaluation of the central nervous system is recommended.[65] Lumbar puncture is recommended in HIV-infected persons with latent syphilis (of any duration), late syphilis (even with a normal neurologic examination), and HIV-infected persons with any neurologic or psychiatric signs or symptoms. Treatment in these patients will be determined by the result of their CSF evaluation. HIV-infected persons with primary and secondary syphilis should be counseled about their possible increased risk of central nervous system relapse, and offered lumbar puncture.

ENDEMIC TREPONEMATOSES (ENDEMIC SYPHILIS, PINTA, AND YAWS)

These three diseases are caused by spirochetes morphologically identical to *T. pallidum*. They are spread nonsexually, affecting primarily children. They are endemic to certain geographic regions, especially rural regions where malnutrition and poor hygiene are common.

Endemic Syphilis

Endemic syphilis is caused by a spirochete identical to or closely related to *T. pallidum*, *T. pallidum* subspecies *endemicum*.[66, 67] It is found primarily among nomadic tribes in Southwest Asia, especially Saudi Arabia, and sub-Saharan Africa. In these regions seropositivity reaches as high as 40% and early lesions occur in 2% to 20% of children. Children ages 2 to 15 years represent the main reservoir, and both sexes are affected equally. It is spread from a lesion or saliva to the skin or mouth via contaminated drinking vessels or infected saliva, or by contaminated fingers. Early and late stages of disease occur. Early lesions are primary and secondary lesions very similar to venereal syphilis. Late disease consists of late latent disease and tertiary lesions. Primary lesions are often in the oropharynx and usually undiagnosed. Presentation is usually in the secondary stage with

mucous patches, shallow relatively painless oral ulcerations, angular stomatitis, condylomata, nonpruritic skin eruptions, and generalized adenopathy. Osteoperiostitis of the long bones may cause leg pains. Late disease is usually latent, but may present as gummas of the skin, bones, or cartilage. Destruction of the nose and palate may occur. Bone pain (especially tibial) with subtle radiologic findings of the tibia, fibula, radius, or ulna may be more common than previously reported.[67] Neurologic and cardiac involvement are rarely seen, but ocular complications, especially uveitis, occur.[68] An attenuated form of endemic syphilis has been described in Saudi Arabia, with less severe disease, leg pain being the most common manifestation.

Diagnosis

The diagnosis of endemic syphilis must be considered in persons from endemic regions. Serologic tests for syphilis are positive, and biopsy specimens or smears of active lesions demonstrate spirochetes. Distinction of early lesions from venereal syphilis is largely clinical. Late lesions must be differentiated from yaws, leishmaniasis, histoplasmosis, rhinoscleroma, rhinosporidiosis, tuberculosis, leprosy, and Wegener's/lethal midline granuloma.

Pinta

Pinta, caused by *T. carateum*, is prevalent in remote tropical regions of Central and South America.[66-68] In highly endemic areas, seroprevalence may reach 20%, and 2% to 3% of children have skin lesions. Both sexes and all races are equally affected. Transmission is through injured skin or mucous membranes. Pinta is the most benign of the endemic treponematoses, affecting the skin only.

Early pinta is characterized by primary and secondary lesions. The primary lesion appears 1 week to 2 months after inoculation (average 10 days), as a small scaling papule on the lower legs, face, arms, or trunk. It expands over several months to a plaque of about 10 cm. It may then resolve or continue to persist into the secondary stage. Secondary lesions (pintids), appearing 2 to 6 months or even longer after the primary stage, are identical to the primary lesion, but usually smaller. Secondary lesions are frequently hyper- or hypopigmented and hyperkeratotic (psoriasiform), and tend to be asymmetrical. Lesions tend to fade, intermix, and relapse, forming polycyclic plaques. There is generalized lymphadenopathy.

Late (tertiary) pinta develops 2 to 5 or more years after the early lesions, and tends to be generalized and symmetrical. Tertiary lesions are less erythematous and hyperkeratotic, may be atrophic, and are more dyspigmented. Increased, decreased, or absent pigmentation may be seen. Depigmented areas are permanent, even after effective treatment.

Biopsy specimens of pinta are said to show superficial and deep infiltrates of lymphocytes, plasma cells, and neutrophils, coupled with epidermal hyperplasia, spongiosis, and parakeratosis. The organisms of pinta are visible in sections stained with silver methods appropriate for syphilis. The depigmented areas are due to loss of melanin (and presumably melanocytes) from the basal layer.[65]

The diagnosis must be suspected in persons from endemic areas. Skin biopsies, darkfield examinations, and serologic tests for syphilis are all useful in confirming the diagnosis. Serologic tests become positive 2 to 4 months after the appearance of the primary lesion.[68, 69] Early pinta must be distinguished from tinea, psoriasis, pellagra, and eczematous eruptions. Dyspigmented lesions must be distinguished from vitiligo, tinea versicolor, leprosy, lupus erythematosus, pityriasis alba, and lichen planus actinicus/erythema dyschromicum perstans.

Yaws

Yaws, caused by *T. pallidum* subspecies *pertenue*, is found in Africa, Southeast Asia, South and Central America, and areas of the Pacific.[67, 70] Although a widespread eradication program sponsored by the World Health Organization and UNICEF in the 1950s and 1960s produced a dramatic reduction in the prevalence of yaws, there has been a slow resurgence in many areas.[71]

Yaws is spread by direct contact with broken skin, so exposed areas, mainly the legs, are the most common sites of involvement. Children under 15 remain the principal reservoir and the most commonly affected.

Skin lesions occur both early (primary and secondary stages) and late (tertiary stage). The primary stage consists of the primary lesion or "mother yaw" occurring between 9 and 90 days (average 21) after inoculation (Fig. 108–16). The primary yaw begins as a red papule

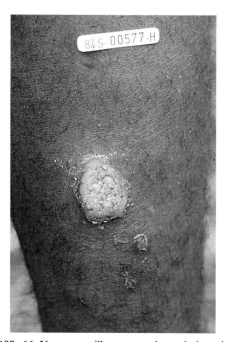

FIGURE 108–16. Yaws—papillomatous primary lesion with a small satellite lesion.

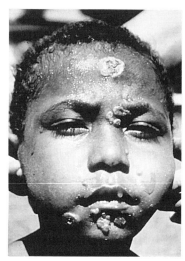

FIGURE 108–17. Yaws—multiple ulcerating and papillomatous lesions. (Courtesy of B. J. Hudson, M. D., Sydney, Australia.)

that enlarges, develops a crust, then ulcerates. The surface may resemble a raspberry, thus accounting for the name *framboesia* given to this disease by early workers. They are usually painless unless secondarily infected, and heal spontaneously after a few weeks to months. Associated features include fever, joint pain, and lymphadenopathy.[67, 70]

The secondary lesions or "daughter yaws" may arise before the primary lesion has resolved. They are often multiple papules and ulcers that, although widespread, often develop periorificially and in the axillae and groin. Secondary lesions may also be clustered around the site of the primary lesion (Fig. 108–17). Other morphologies include micropapular, annular, and hyperkeratotic forms.[72, 73] The last form occurs particularly on the soles, where lesions may be painful, resulting in a crab-like gait known as *crab yaws*. The duration of the papillomatous (secondary) stage averages 6 months for the first crop of papillomas, and subsequent outbreaks may last another 6 months[74] or longer, up to 5 years. The early lesions vary somewhat with disease prevalence, and an "attenuated" form of yaws has been described with fewer, drier, flatter lesions in areas of low endemicity and high altitude.[74] These atypical lesions are less infectious and easily misdiagnosed. Secondary yaws is followed by a latent period. Tertiary yaws develops in about 10% of untreated patients,[74] and is characterized by nodular, hyperkeratotic, and plaque-like cutaneous lesions, juxta-articular nodules, as well as gummatous lesions. Bony involvement includes gangosa (a deforming rhinopharyngitis), goundou (production of exostoses of the maxilla), and a deforming osteoperiostitis mainly of the long bones but also of the metatarsals and metacarpals. Extensive tibial involvement can produce a sabre shin.[67, 72] Although it is widely believed that the neurologic and cardiovascular abnormalities seen in syphilis do not occur in yaws, the opposite has been proposed by some authors.[75, 76]

Both primary and early secondary lesions of yaws are said to show dense diffuse dermal infiltrates of lymphocytes, plasma cells, macrophages, and eosinophils, coupled with irregular or psoriasiform papillated epidermal hyperplasia and intraepidermal spongiotic vesiculation and spongiform pustules. Late secondary lesions reportedly resemble those of late secondary syphilis. The same silver stains that demonstrate *T. pallidum* also stain *T. p. pertenue.*[77] The diagnosis must be considered in persons who have lived in or visited endemic areas. Darkfield examinations with serologic confirmatory tests for syphilis are appropriate for early lesions, and biopsy with serology is appropriate for atypical lesions or if the darkfield examination is negative.[76]

Differential Diagnosis

Early yaws must be distinguished from topical ulceration, venereal syphilis, leishmaniasis, ecthyma, scabies, eczema, psoriasis, and keratodermas. The bony lesions may mimic venereal and endemic syphilis, tuberculosis, and osteomyelitis, whereas the nasopharyngeal lesions may resemble leprosy, leishmaniasis, deep fungal infections, and tuberculosis.

Treatment of the Endemic Treponematoses

A single intramuscular injection of benzathine penicillin is the recommended treatment for yaws, pinta, and endemic syphilis. Adults are given 1.2 to 2.4 million units and children under 10, 0.6 to 1.2 million units. Depending on how endemic the disease is in a given region, everyone, children only, or just all active cases and their families are treated. In penicillin-allergic persons oral tetracycline or erythromycin may be used, in doses used to treat early venereal syphilis.

References

1. Fiumara NJ. Infectious syphilis. Dermatol Clin North Am 1983;1:3–21.
2. Fiumara NJ. A legacy of syphilis. Arch Dermatol 1965; 92:676–678.
3. Allison SD. Extragenital syphilitic chancres. J Am Acad Dermatol 1986;14:1094–1095.
4. Felman M, Nikitas JA. Secondary syphilis. Cutis 1982; 29:322–329.
5. Hira SK. Clinical manifestation of secondary syphilis. Int J Dermatol 1987;26:103–107.
6. McPhee SJ. Secondary syphilis: Uncommon manifestations of a common disease. West J Med 1984;140:35–42.
7. Jurado RL, Campbell J, Martin PD. Prozone phenomenon in secondary syphilis. Arch Intern Med 1993;153:2496–2498.
8. Hook EW, Marra CM. Acquired syphilis in adults. N Engl J Med 1992;326:1060–1067.
9. Sexually transmitted disease surveillance 1992. US Dept Health & Welfare, Public Health Services, 1992.
10. Jeerapaet P, Ackerman AB. Histologic patterns of secondary syphilis. Arch Dermatol 1973;107:373–377.
11. Abell E, Marks R, Wilson JE. Secondary syphilis. A clinicopathologic review. Br J Dermatol 1975;93:53–61.
12. Fisher DA, Chang LW, Tuffanelli DL. Lues maligna. Arch Dermatol 1969;99:70–73.
13. Larsen SA, Hunter EF, Kraus SJ, eds. A Manual of Tests for Syphilis. Washington, DC: American Public Health Association, 1990:1–167.
14. Wentworth RB, Judson FW, Gilchrist M Jr, eds. Laboratory Methods for the Diagnosis of Sexually Transmitted Diseases, 2nd edition. Washington, DC: American Public Health Association, 1991:1–52.
15. Portnoy J, Brewer JH, Harris A. Rapid plasma reagin card test for syphilis. Public Health Reports 1962;645–652.
16. Larsen SA, Hunter EF, Creighton ET. Syphilis. In: Holmes KK, Mardh P-A, Sparling PJ, et al., eds. Sexually Transmitted Diseases, 2nd edition. New York: McGraw-Hill, 1990:928–929.
17. Gourevitch MN, Selwyn Pa, Davenny K, et al. Effects of HIV infection on the serologic manifestations and response to treatment of syphilis in intravenous drug users. Ann Intern Med 1993; 118:350–355.
18. Romanowski B, Sutherland R, Fick GH, et al. Serologic response to treatment of infectious syphilis. Ann Intern Med 1991;114: 1005–1009.
19. Larsen SA, Hunter EF, Creighton ET. Syphilis. In: Holmes, Mardh, Sparling, et al., eds. Sexually Transmitted Diseases, 2nd edition. 1990:929–930.
20. Schmid GP. Approach to the patient with genital ulcer disease. Med Clin North Am 1990;74(6):1559–1572.
21. Fiumara NJ, Rachman K, Tang S. The diagnosis and treatment of chancroid. J Am Acad Dermatol 1986;15:939.
22. Schmid GP, Sanders LL, Blount J, et al. Chancroid in the United States. JAMA 1987;258:3265.
23. Lukehart SA, Hook EW III, Baker-Zander SA, et al. Invasion of the central nervous system by *Treponema pallidum*: Implication for diagnosis and treatment. Ann Intern Med 1988;109:855–862.
24. Beall GN. Immediate hypersensitivity reactions to beta lactone antibiotics. Ann Intern Med 1987;107:204–215.
25. Fiumara NJ. Treatment of primary and secondary syphilis: Serologic response. J Am Acad Dermatol 1986;14:487–491.
26. Fiumara NJ. The treatment of early latent syphilis under one year—an evaluation of 275 patients. Sex Transm Dis 1978;5: 85–88.
27. Brown ST, Zaidi A, Larsen SA, et al. Serologic response to syphilis treatment: A new analysis of old data. JAMA 1985;253: 1296–1299.
28. Fiumara NJ. Reinfection primary, secondary and latent syphilis. Sex Transm Dis 1980;7:111–115.
29. Fiumara NJ. Serologic response to treatment of 128 patients with late latent syphilis. Sex Transm Dis 1979;6:243–246.
30. Miesher DM. How much penicillin cures early syphilis. Ann Intern Med 1988;109:849–851.
31. Markovitz DM, Benter KR, Maggio RP, et al. Failure of recommended treatment for secondary syphilis. JAMA 1986; 255:1767–1768.
32. Kline AH, Blottner RJ, Lunin M. Transplacental effect of tetracycline on teeth. JAMA 1964;188;178–180.
33. Hashisaki P, Wertzberger GC, Conrad GL, et al. Erythromycin failure in the treatment of syphilis in pregnancy. Sex Transm Dis 1983;10:36–38.
34. Centers for Disease Control. 1993 Sexually Transmitted Diseases Treatment Guidelines; 27–46.
35. Wendel GD, Stark BJ, Jamison RB, et al. Penicillin allergy and desensitization in serious infections during pregnancy. N Engl J Med 1985;312:1229–1232.
36. Ziaya PR, Hankins G, Gilstrap L, et al. Intravenous penicillin desensitization and treatment during pregnancy. JAMA 1986; 2561–2562.
37. Swartz MN. Neurosyphilis. In: Holmes KK, Mardh P-A, Sparling PJ, et al., eds. Sexually Transmitted Diseases, 2nd edition. New York: McGraw-Hill, 1990:234.
38. Russell H, et al. Enzyme-linked immunosorbent assay and indirect immunofluorescence assay for Lyme disease. J Infect Dis 1984; 249:465.
39. Marnarelli LA, et al. Cross-reactivity in serological tests for Lyme disease and other spirochetal infections. J Infect Dis 1987;156:183.
40. Swartz MN. Neurosyphilis. In: Holmes KK, Mardh P-A, Sparling PJ, et al, eds. Sexually Transmitted Diseases, 2nd edition. New York: McGraw-Hill, 1990:236.
41. Hater WD. Transplacental transmission of spirochetes in congenital syphilis. Sex Transm Dis 1986;5:122.
42. Harter, Benirschke K. Fetal syphilis in the first trimester. Am J Obstet Gynecol 1976;124:705.
43. Dippel AL. The relationship of congenital syphilis to abortion and miscarriage, and the mechanism of uterine protection. Am J Obstet Gynecol 1944;47:369.
44. Schulz KF, Murphy FK, Patamasucon P, et al. Congenital syphilis.

In: Holmes KK, Mardh P-A, Sparling PF, et al., eds. Sexually Transmitted Diseases, 2nd edition. New York: McGraw-Hill, 1990:825.

45. Contreras R, Pereda J. Congenital syphilis of the eye with liver involvement. Arch Ophthalmol 1978;96:1052.

46. Solomon A, Rosen E. Focal osseous lesions in congenital lues. Pediatr Radiol 1978;7:36.

47. Whitaker TA. Hematological aspects of congenital syphilis. J Pediatr 1965;66:629.

48. Schulz KF, Murphy FK, Patamasucon P, et al. Congenital syphilis. In: Holmes KK, Mardh P-A, Sparling PF, et al., eds. Sexually Transmitted Diseases, 2nd edition. New York: McGraw-Hill, 1990:829.

49. Dorfman DH, Glasen JH. Congenital syphilis presenting in infants after the newborn period. N Engl J Med 1990;323:1299.

50. Schulz KF, Murphy FK, Patamasucon P, et al. Congenital syphilis. In: Holmes KK, Mardh P-A, Sparling PF, et al., eds. Sexually Transmitted Diseases, 2nd edition. New York: McGraw-Hill, 1990:832.

51. Fiumara JN, Lessell S. The stigmata of late congenital syphilis—an analysis of 100 patients. Sex Transm Dis 1983;10:26–129.

52. Fiumara NJ. Human immunodeficiency virus infection and syphilis. J Am Acad Dermatol 1989;21:141–142.

53. Glover RA, Praquadio DJ, Kern S, et al. An unusual presentation of secondary syphilis in a patient with human immunodeficiency virus infection. Arch Dermatol 1992;128:530–534.

54. Gregory N, Sanchez M, Buchness MR. The spectrum of syphilis in patients with human immunodeficiency virus infeciton. J Am Acad Dermatol 1990;22:1061–1067.

55. Hutchinson CM, Rompalo AM, Reichart CA, et al. Characteristics of patients with syphilis attending Baltimore STD clinics. Arch Intern Med 1991;151:511–516.

56. Hutchinson CM, Hook EW, Shepherd M, et al. Altered clinical presentation of early syphilis in patients with human immunodeficiency virus infeciton. Ann Intern Med 1994;121:94–99.

57. Shulkin D, Tripoli L, Abell E. Lues maligna in a patient with human immunodeficiency virus infection. Am J Med 1988;85:425–427.

58. Radolf JD, Kaplan RP. Unusual manifestations of secondary syphilis and abnormal humoral immune response to *Treponema pallidum* antigens in a homosexual man with asymptomatic human immunodeficiency virus infection. J Am Acad Dermatol 1988;18:423–428.

59. Hicks CB, Benson PM, Lupton GP, et al. Seronegative secondary syphilis in a patient infected with the human immunodeficiency virus (HIV) with Kaposi sarcoma. Ann Intern Med 1987;107:491–495.

60. Tikjob G, Russel M, Petersen CS, et al. Seronegative secondary syphilis in a patient with AIDS: Identification of *Treponema pallidum* in biopsy specimen. J Am Acad Dermatol 1991;24:506–508.

61. Zalka A, Grossman ME. "Seronegative" syphilis in AIDS. Ann Intern Med 1991;114:521–522.

62. Johns DR, Tierney M, Felsenstein D. Alteration in the natural history of neurosyphilis by concurrent infection with the human immunodeficiency virus. N Engl J Med 1987;316:1569–1572.

63. Berry CD, Hooton TM, Collier AC, et al. Neurologic relapse after benzathine penicillin therapy for secondary syphilis in a patient with HIV infection. N Engl J Med 1987;316:1587–1589.

64. Manganoni AM, Graifemberghi S, Facchetti F, et al. Effectiveness of penicillin G benzathine therapy for primary and secondary syphilis. J Am Acad Dermatol 1990;23:1185–1186.

65. Bolan G. Management of syphilis in HIV-infected persons. In: Sande MA, Volberding PA, eds. The Medical Management of AIDS, 4th edition. Philadelphia: WB Saunders Co., 1995: 537–554.

66. Engelkens HJH, Niemel PLA, van der Sluis JP, et al. Endemic treponematoses. Part II. Pinta and endemic syphilis. Int J Dermatol 1991;30:231–238.

67. Koff AB, Rosen T. Nonvenereal treponematoses: Yaws, endemic syphilis, and pinta. J Am Acad Dermatol 1993;29:519–535.

68. Tabbara KF, Al Kaff AS, Fadel T. Ocular manifestations of endemic syphilis (bejel). Ophthalmology 1989;96:1087–1091.

69. Fuchs J, Milbradt R, Pecher SA. Tertiary pinta: Case reports and overview. Cutis 1993;51:425–430.

70. Engelkens HJH, Judanarso J, Oranje AP, et al. Endemic treponematoses. Part 1. Yaws. Int J Dermatol 1991;30:77–83.

71. Engelkens HJH, Niemal PLA, van der Sluis JJ, et al. The resurgence of yaws. World-wide consequences. Int J Dermatol 1991;30:99–101.

72. Perine PL, Hopkins DR, Niemel PLA, et al. Yaws, endemic syphilis and pinta. In: Handbook of endemic treponematoses. Geneva: World Health Organization, 1984:1–53.

73. Hackett CJ. An international nomenclature of yaws lesions. WHO monograph series number 36. Geneva: World Health Organization, 1957.

74. Vorst FA. Clinical diagnosis and the changing manifestations of treponemal infection. Rev Infect Dis 1986;7:S327–S331.

75. Roman GC, Roman LN. Occurrence of congenital, cardiovascular, visceral, neurologic, and neuro-ophthalmologic complications in late yaws: A theme for future research. Rev Infect Dis 1986;8:760–770.

76. Smith JL, David NJ, Indgin S, et al. Neuro-ophthalmological study of late yaws and pinta II. The Caracas project. Br J Vener Dis 1971;47:226–227.

77. Hasselman CM. Comparative studies on the histopathology of syphilis, yaws and pinta. Br J Vener Dis 1957;33:5–23.

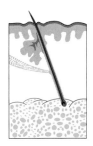

chapter 109

Lyme Borreliosis

DONALD C. ABELE

DEFINITION

Lyme borreliosis is a complex, multisystemic disorder caused by infection with the spirochete *Borrelia burgdorferi*. It has protean manifestations that are acute or chronic. The most striking signs and symptoms involve the joints, central and peripheral nervous systems, heart, and skin.

The disease was first recognized in Europe by Afzelius as a purely cutaneous disorder, erythema chronicum migrans which he believed was a reaction to tick bites.[1, 2] Subsequently an association was made with meningitis.[3] The demonstration of spirochetes in lesions of erythema chronicum migrans by Lennhoff,[4] successful treatment by antibiotics,[5] human to human transmission,[6] and isolation of a spirochete in rabbit testes injected with tissue from patients with erythema chronicum migrans,[7] reinforced the concept that the disease was infectious and most likely caused by a spirochete.

In the United States, epidemics in New England of what was thought to be juvenile rheumatoid arthritis led to an investigation by Steere and coworkers[8] and the recognition of the disorder now called Lyme disease or Lyme borreliosis. The eruption in many of these patients was recognized as erythema chronicum migrans, leading to studies that suggested Lyme disease was caused by an agent transmitted by *Ixodes* ticks.[9, 10] In 1982, Burgdorfer and coworkers isolated a spirochete from *I. dammini* that was subsequently recognized as the cause of Lyme disease.[11] Similar organisms were later isolated from ticks in Europe[12] and from blood,[13, 14] skin,[13] and cerebrospinal fluid[13] of patients with Lyme disease. In 1984, the spirochete transmitted by *I. dammini* was shown to be a new species, *Borrelia burgdorferi*.[15, 16] It has amino acid sequences related to the variant antigens of the borrelial species that cause relapsing fever.[15, 16] *Borrelia* have the ability to vary their major surface antigens, thereby evading the host's immune defenses; as one antigenic type is cleared by the immune system, it may be replaced by other serotypes to which the host mounts

a new antibody response. This may account for the chronic, recurrent nature of some manifestations of Lyme disease.[17] Differences among *B. burgdorferi* isolates[18] from the United States and Europe may account for variations in the clinical manifestations described from these areas.

CLINICAL DESCRIPTION

Epidemiology

Ixodes ticks are the primary vectors for Lyme borreliosis, and the disease occurs in areas where these ticks are endemic. *I. scapularis (dammini)*[19] is the major vector in the eastern United States and *I. pacificus* is the vector in the western part of the country.[10] *I. ricinus* is the major vector in Europe. Lyme disease is the most commonly reported tick-borne disease in the United States.[20] Reported in nearly all states, the disease is most common in the Northeast, upper midwest, California, and Oregon. It occurs in all continents except Antarctica.

The life cycle of the ticks lasts 2 years.[21] The adult female deposits ova in the spring and its larvae feed on small mammals, especially the white-footed mouse (*Peromyscus leucopus*), which is the main reservoir for *B. burgdorferi*. A larva feeds once and may acquire the organism from an infected mouse. The larva then molts, rests through winter, and emerges in spring as a nymph, which is the most infectious form of the vector. The nymph feeds once and develops into an adult that overwinters on the white-tailed deer (*Odocoileus virginianus*). The female, after mating, drops to the ground where she deposits eggs in the spring to complete the cycle.

Ticks are most commonly found attached to plants in grassy, wooded, or bushy areas and are transferred on contact to animals or humans, who are incidental hosts. In endemic areas, even parks[22] and lawns[23] may harbor many infected ticks. The risk of contracting disease depends on the population density of ticks, their degree of parasitism, and the duration of attachment to an animal or human. In some parts of the eastern United States, up to 60% of *I. dammini* may be parasitized by *B. burgdorferi*, compared with only 1% to 2% of *I. pacificus* in the west.[24]

The bite of an infected tick is painless and often unnoticed. Spirochetes are transmitted to the host after 1 to 3 days of attachment.[24] If the tick is removed promptly, transmission of infection may be avoided.[25] Because of its very small size, the nymph may not be noticed and removed in time to prevent infection.

Stages of Lyme Disease

The manifestations of infection with *B. burgdorferi* vary from early to late in the course. Because of some similarities to syphilis, another spirochetal disorder, early attempts were made relating the manifestations to the classic major stages of syphilis: primary, secondary, and late.[13, 26]

Stage 1 disease begins 3 to 30 days after a tick bite, which is recalled by fewer than one half of patients. The disease is characterized by flu-like symptoms, including fever, chills, fatigue, headache, and arthralgias. Early joint complaints are vague and migratory, often without objective findings. Erythema chronicum migrans, which is a diagnostic manifestation, is present in up to 75% of patients. Classic erythema chronicum migrans starts as an erythematous papule at the bite site and then evolves into an annular, erythematous ring (Fig. 109-1; see color plate). There are few symptoms associated with erythema chronicum migrans, although some patients complain of mild pruritus or tenderness. Erythema chronicum migrans clears spontaneously within weeks or months in most cases. Although the lesions are usually annular with central clearing, they may remain as an enlarging, bluish-red plaque or develop central vesiculation, necrosis, or both. Less characteristic skin manifestations may include malar erythema, urticaria, periorbital edema, and erythema nodosum.[27] Other findings include temporomandibular joint pain,[28] conjunctivitis,[29] and testicular swelling.[29]

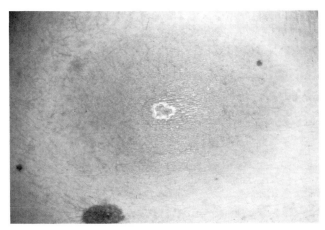

FIGURE 109-1. Primary erythema chronicum migrans: solid erythema with early collarette of scale. (See color plate.) (From Melski JW. Lyme borreliosis in Wisconsin: Lessons in diagnosing and treating erythema migrans. Fitzpatrick's J Clin Dermatol 1994;May/June:14–25. Photograph by John W. Melski, M.D.)

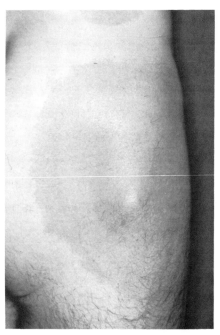

FIGURE 109-2. Secondary erythema chronicum migrans: large annular lesion. (See color plate.) (From Melski JW. Lyme borreliosis in Wisconsin: Lessons in diagnosing and treating erythema migrans. Fitzpatrick's J Clin Dermatol 1994;May/June:14–25. Photograph by John W. Melski, M.D.)

Stage 2 begins after weeks or months and primarily involves the nervous and cardiovascular systems. Regional or generalized lymphadenopathy may be present. Cutaneous findings may include multiple annular, erythematous lesions (Fig. 109-2; see color plate), which may simulate secondary syphilis,[30] and lymphadenosis benigna cutis.

Stage 3 disease develops weeks or months after primary infection and chiefly involves the musculoskeletal, nervous system, and eye. A late cutaneous manifestation is acrodermatitis chronica atrophicans.

Another classification of Lyme disease considers the disorder as either "early" or "late" disease.[31, 32] "Late" disease is considered as occurring more than 1 year after infection; thus "early" disease essentially combines stage 1 and 2 as described earlier.

Although these classifications have some utility in thinking about pathogenesis and treatment, neither is entirely satisfactory because orderly progression from one stage or another is not often found. Some patients appear to recover spontaneously from "early" infection and never progress to later stages, and some patients present initially with "late" manifestations. Others may have symptoms or findings of several stages simultaneously. Because of these discrepancies, the various manifestations of Lyme disease are categorized here by their effects on each organ system.

Musculoskeletal System

The musculoskeletal manifestations of early Lyme disease have already been mentioned. In about 60% of untreated cases the patient may develop arthritis later in the course of the disease.[8, 28] Large joints, especially the knees, are usually involved. The arthritis tends to be intermittent, and many cases may resolve; however, 10% of patients may develop chronic, erosive arthritis. The chronic arthritis associated with Lyme disease differs from rheumatoid arthritis by its tendency to be oligoarthritic, while rheumatoid disease is symmetrical and associated with rheumatoid nodules and rheumatoid factor. Radiographic findings of joints range from normal to joint space narrowing to erosive, osteophytic changes. The features are similar to other inflammatory arthritides and are not diagnostic for Lyme disease.[33] Children may have a higher incidence of arthritis than adults.[34, 35] An association of chronic Lyme arthritis has been made with the presence of HLA-DR4 combined with HLA-DR3 or DR2 antigens.[36, 37] Although there has seemed to be a lower incidence of arthritides in Europe than in the United States, such may not be the case.[38]

Cardiovascular System

Cardiac manifestations occur in about 8% of patients with Lyme disease,[39] with the most common finding being fluctuating degrees of atrioventricular block. The involvement is usually transient with spontaneous resolution but high-grade block may require a temporary transvenous pacemaker; occasionally a permanent pacemaker may be required.[40, 41] Some patients may have myopericarditis or mild left ventricular dysfunction. Pancarditis and cardiomyopathy may occur. Spirochetes have been demonstrated in cardiac tissue at autopsy and by myocardial biopsy cultures.[42, 43]

Nervous System

Neurologic disorders may occur in 15% of untreated patients with Lyme disease.[29] Numerous manifestations have been reported, many of which are on tenuous grounds. Several excellent reviews should be consulted for detailed information.[44-46] The disease may involve the peripheral or central nervous system. Patients in early stage disease may have aseptic meningitis, cranial nerve palsies (especially Bell's palsy), radiculitis, and encephalitis. The cerebrospinal fluid typically reveals a lymphocytic pleocytosis, and spirochetes may be cultured.[47] The triad of meningitis, cranial neuritis, and radiculoneuritis is virtually unique to Lyme disease and is almost diagnostic in a patient from an endemic area.[48] Patients with late or chronic Lyme disease may have encephalitis, encephalopathy, chronic neuropathy, and entrapment neuropathies such as carpal tunnel syndrome. There appears to be no relationship of chronic neuroborreliosis to chronic fatigue syndromes or multiple sclerosis.[49]

Ophthalmologic Manifestations

A variety of ophthalmologic manifestations can occur at any stage of the disease. The most common finding is conjunctivitis seen early in the course of the disease.[50]

Other manifestations, some anecdotal, include iritis, iridocyclitis, optic neuritis, exudative retinal detachments, panophthalmitis with blindness, papilledema with and without pseudotumor cerebri, diplopia due to cranial nerve palsies, and Argyll Robertson pupils. Many of the changes are similar to those seen in syphilis.[51]

Specific Cutaneous Manifestations

There are several cutaneous manifestations of Lyme disease that seem unquestioned: erythema migrans chronicum,[7, 9] acrodermatitis chronica atrophicans,[52, 53] and lymphadenosis benigna cutis.[54] These have been reviewed in detail.[55, 56]

Acrodermatitis Chronica Atrophicans

Acrodermatitis chronica atrophicans has been reported in Europe for many years but is not commonly recognized in the United States.[57, 58] It is characterized by two stages: early inflammatory and late atrophic. Early lesions are erythematous nodules or plaques, that may have central clearing. These lesions progress slowly over months or years. Eventually atrophic, poikilodermatous areas develop with subcutaneous nodules, sclerosis, and fibrous bands that may result in joint immobility. Erythema chronicum migrans may precede the appearance of acrodermatitis chronica atrophicans in some patients.[59]

Many systemic complaints have been associated with acrodermatitis chronica atrophicans, especially a peripheral polyneuropathy.[60, 61] Asbrink[52] reported that patients had dysesthesias, cramps, and pain in the affected extremities, and some had weight-loss arthralgias, deforming arthritis, periosteal changes, as well as scleroderma-like or lichen sclerosus et atrophicus–like changes.

Lymphadenosis Benigna Cutis

Lymphadenosis benigna cutis is the term used for lesions of cutaneous lymphoid hyperplasia in which lymphoid follicles are present. It occurs in Lyme disease, most commonly in European patients. It is identical to sporadic cutaneous lymphoid hyperplasia in its clinical presentation (see Chapter 150), namely reddish violaceous nodules and plaques.[61a-61c]

Many reports suggested an infectious etiology for some cases of this disorder.[54, 56]

Other Possible Cutaneous Manifestations

There are conflicting reports concerning whether *B. burgdorferi* may be the cause of some forms of morphea and lichen sclerosus et atrophicus.[56] Most reports of an association come from Europe and are based primarily on positive serologic tests associated with compatible clinical lesions, although spirochetes have been demonstrated histologically and by culture in some instances. Reports from the United States appear to refute an association. Perhaps the controversy will be resolved by more specific and sensitive methods for detection of the organism in skin lesions.[62]

Among other cutaneous disorders reported to be associated with *B. burgdorferi* infections are benign lymphocytic infiltration of the skin (Jessner-Kanof,[63, 64] progressive facial hemiatrophy (Parry-Romberg),[65] eosinophilic fasciitis,[56] granuloma annulare, erythema nodosum, urticaria[66] urticarial vasculitis,[67] and periarticular fibrous nodules.[68] B-cell lymphoma of the skin (usually low grade) has been reported in European patients with borreliosis.[69]

PATHOLOGY

Erythema Chronicum Migrans. Several patterns of histologic changes may be found.[70] Most commonly there are superficial and deep perivascular and interstitial infiltrations of primarily lymphocytes with some plasma cells. Specimens from the centers of lesions show superficial and deep perivascular and interstitial lymphocytic infiltration with eosinophils but no plasma cells, similar to an arthropod bite reaction. A third pattern may have only lymphocytes. Spirochetes may be demonstrated with silver stains but not consistently.[71]

Acrodermatitis Chronica Atrophicans. In the early inflammatory stage, dermal edema and telangiectasia with perivascular lymphocytes and plasma cells are present. In later stages there is epidermal atrophy, loss of appendages and a sclerosis resembling morphea. The papillary dermis can be edematous, resembling the changes of lichen sclerosus et atrophicus.[53]

Lymphadenosis Benigna Cutis. The changes are identical to those seen in the follicular pattern of cutaneous lymphoid hyperplasia,[72] except that in some cases spirochetes can be demonstrated in tissue sections using silver stains.

Other Organ Systems. The findings in the musculoskeletal,[73, 74] cardiovascular,[73, 74] and nervous system,[44, 46, 73, 74] and the eyes[73, 74] are reviewed in detail elsewhere.

PATHOGENESIS

The pathogenesis of the various manifestations of Lyme borreliosis is not well understood. Some manifestations are due to the host inflammatory response to the organism, while others may be due to the triggering of autoimmune reactions.[74–78]

Several days to weeks after the bite of an infected tick the organism migrates in the skin, causing erythema chronicum migrans. This is then followed by dissemination to regional lymph nodes or throughout the bloodstream to other organs of the body or other areas of skin, resulting in secondary annular lesions. During this period of dissemination circulating antigen–antibody complexes are present that may cause arthritis and other symptoms.[79]

More chronic manifestations of the diseases may be due to long-term persistence of the organism, which may occur even after antibiotic therapy and the development of host immune response, as evidenced by demonstration of organisms in tissues as well as an expanding antibody response over time shown by Western blotting studies.[80] Some manifestations such as chronic arthritis and acrodermatitis chronica atrophicans seem to occur more frequently in persons with certain immunogenetic backgrounds (e.g., DR2, DR3, DR4 alloantigens).[35, 36, 81] Autoimmune reactions may be another pathogenetic mechanism due to the elicitation of host immune response to cross-reacting epitopes of the organism and human tissues (molecular mimicry).[82] Chronic immune stimulation could account for the occurrence of B-cell lymphomas in patients with borreliosis.

DIAGNOSIS AND DIFFERENTIAL DIAGNOSIS

Acute early Lyme disease presents as a "flu-like" syndrome that may be indistinguishable from many viral illnesses or various connective tissue disorders. The diagnosis may be suspected and confirmed by the characteristic eruption, erythema chronicum migrans, which occurs in 50% to 70% of patients. At this stage the diagnosis is primarily based on clinical grounds since serologic tests may not become positive for a number of weeks. An acute reaction may occur at the site of a tick bite and must be distinguished from erythema chronicum migrans; this reaction occurs within a day, is usually less than 2.0 cm in diameter, and regresses within several days rather than expanding. Conditions to consider in the differential diagnosis of various cutaneous manifestations are summarized in Table 109–1. The differential diagnosis of other manifestations (cardiac, neurologic, musculoskeletal, ophthalmologic) are beyond the scope of this text but may be found in the references cited for the various organ systems.

As with any infection, the diagnosis is best made by the identification of organisms. Spirochetes have been cultured from lesions of erythema chronicum migrans,[83] but as yet this test is not routinely available. Organisms may also be cultured from blood, spinal fluid, and other tissues during acute phases, but again this is not a routinely available or reliable procedure.[13, 14] Occasional cultures have been reported from other cutaneous and internal sites.[73, 74] Spirochetes may also be demonstrated by silver stains and immunofluorescent techniques in a variety of tissues.[74] Interpretation is difficult, and the sensitivity is too low to make these techniques routinely useful or reliable for diagnosis.

Serum antibodies to *B. burgdorferi* develop within weeks of infection. The two most common methods used for detection are the indirect immunofluorescent (IFA) or the enzyme-linked immunosorbent assay (ELISA). The ELISA tests are believed to be more sensitive and reproducible,[85, 86] but the IFA tests are useful in determining titers of antibody. IgM antibody appears first and usually declines in 4 to 6 months; persistence of IgM antibody or reappearance at a later time may predict

TABLE 109-1. Major Cutaneous Manifestations of
Lyme Disease (Differential Diagnosis)

Erythema Chronicum Migrans		Acrodermatitis Chronica Atrophicans		Lymphadenosis Benigna Cutis
Primary	*Secondary (Multiple)*	*Early*	*Late*	
Bacterial cellulitis	Erythema multiforme	Cellulitis	Linear morphea	Granuloma faciale
Contact dermatitis	Secondary syphilis	Stasis dermatitis	Atrophodermas	Discoid lupus erythematosus
Fixed drug eruption	Pityriasis rosea		Lichen sclerosus et	Rosacea (granulomatous)
Tinea corporis	Erythema annulare		atrophicus	Polymorphic light eruption
Spider bite	centrifugum		Necrobiosis lipoidica	Sarcoid
	Annular urticaria		diabeticorum	Lymphoma cutis
				Benign lymphocytic infiltrate (Jessner-Kanof)

continued infection and a greater risk of complications. IgG antibodies appear later and remain elevated in patients with long-term infection.[85] Antibodies in the cerebrospinal fluid may be a sensitive and reliable indicator of neuroborreliosis.[87]

Unfortunately there is no standardization of these serologic tests, and thus interpretation is difficult.[88-90] Failure to correlate test results with clinical findings may lead to misdiagnosis.[91] There also may be cross-reacting antibodies in patients with other treponemal diseases, leprosy, venereal diseases, and connective tissue disorders that complicate interpretation.[92, 93]

Western blotting techniques may be useful to clarify results of ELISA testing, particularly in cases of long-standing infection.[88, 94, 95] A test using the polymerase chain reaction has been developed and may prove to be a more reliable and specific means of diagnosis.[96-98]

TREATMENT

The best antibiotic treatment for the various manifestations of Lyme disease is as yet unsettled. Efficacy, dosage, and duration of therapy are still under study. Few controlled studies have been reported.[99-102] Recommendations for therapy are continually changing, and the current literature should be consulted for up-to-date therapeutic recommendations.

In general, early manifestations of Lyme disease are satisfactorily treated with oral regimens of doxycycline or amoxicillin. Erythromycin may be satisfactory therapy in children who cannot be given tetracyclines or in children and adults who are allergic to penicillin; however, erythromycin is thought to be less effective. Late manifestations of the disease and meningitis more likely require parenteral therapy. Table 109-2 is a

TABLE 109-2. Treatment of Lyme Disease

	Doxycycline	Amoxicillin	Erythromycin	Penicillin G	Ceftriaxone
Early Lyme disease					
Erythema chronicum migrans (solitary or multiple) Isolated facial nerve palsy Carditis (mild)	100 mg PO bid × 3 wk	500 mg tid PO × 3 wk	1.0 g daily PO × 3 wk		
Lymphadenosis benigna cutis	100 mg PO bid × 4-6 wk	500 mg qid PO × 4-6 wk			
Acrodermatitis chronica atrophicans	100 mg PO bid* × 4-6 wk	500 mg qid* PO × 4-6 wk			
Neurologic disease (other than isolated facial nerve palsy)				20 million units IV daily for 2-3 wk	2 gm daily IV × 2-3 wk
Carditis (other than mild)				20 million units IV daily × 2 wk	2 gm daily IV × 2 wk
Arthritis	100 mg PO bid × 3-4 wk	500 mg PO† qid × 4 wk		20 million units IV daily × 2-3 wk	2 gm daily IV × 2-3 wk
During pregnancy					
Early disease		500 mg tid PO × 3 wk			
Disseminated early or late disease				20 million units IV daily × 2-3 wk	

*May require longer therapy or use of IV penicillin or ceftriaxone.
†Plus probenecid, 500 mg qid.

list of some guidelines for therapy based on a number of sources.[103-105] For more serious or chronic infections these and other sources should be consulted. It is important to keep in mind that Lyme disease during pregnancy may result in fetal malformations and therapy should generally be undertaken with appropriate drugs.[105, 106] It also should be understood that while antibiotic therapy of early Lyme disease may decrease the incidence of complications, a permanent cure may not result.[107]

Prevention

Attempts have been made to reduce the prevalence of Lyme disease by reducing the tick populations in endemic areas. Methods involving biologic control, environmental modification, and chemical control have been attempted but with little success.[104] Personal protection remains the most effective means of reducing infections and involves the use of permethrin-based repellents, the wearing of appropriate clothing, and a careful search for and prompt removal of ticks. As yet there is no firm recommendation for prophylactic antibiotic treatment of all tick bites, even in endemic areas.[105, 109]

References

1. Afzelius A. Verhandlungen der Dermatologischen. Gesellsch Stockholm 1909;101:404.
2. Afzelius A. Erythema chronicum migrans. Acta Derm Venereol 1921;2:120–125.
3. Hellerstrom S. Erythema chronicum migrans Afzelius with meningitis. Acta Derm Venereol 1951;31:227–234.
4. Lennhoff C. Spirochetes in aetiologically obscure diseases. Acta Derm Venereol 1948;28:295–324.
5. Hollstrom E. Successful treatment of erythema chronicum migrans Afzelius. Acta Derm Venereol 1951;31:235–243.
6. Binder E, Doepfmer R, Hornstein O. Experimentelle Übertragung des Erythema chronicum migrans von Mensch zu Mensch. Hautarzt 1955;6:494–496.
7. Asbrink E, Hederstedt B, Hovmark A. The spirochetal etiology of erythema chronicum migrans Afzelius. Acta Derm Venereol 1984;64:291–295.
8. Steere AC, Malawista SE, Snydman DR, et al. Lyme arthritis: An epidemic of oligoarticular arthritis in children and adults in three Connecticut communities. Arthritis Rheum 1977;20:7–17.
9. Steere AC, Broderick TF, Malawista SE. Erythema chronicum migrans and Lyme arthritis: Epidemiologic evidence for a tick vector. Am J Epidemiol 1978;108:312–321.
10. Steere AC, Malawista SE. Cases of Lyme disease in the United States: Locations correlated with the distribution of *Ixodes dammini*. Ann Intern Med 1979;91:730–733.
11. Burgdorfer W. Discovery of the Lyme disease spirochete and its relation to tick vectors. Yale J Biol Med 1984;57:515–520.
12. Barbour AG, Burgdorfer W, Hayes SE, et al. Isolation of a cultivable spirochete from *Ixodes ricinus* ticks of Switzerland. Curr Microbiol 1983;8:123–126.
13. Steere AC, Grodzicki MS, Kornblatt AN, et al. The spirochetal etiology of Lyme disease. N Engl J Med 1983;308:722–740.
14. Benach JL, Bosler EM, Hanrahan JP, et al. Spirochetes isolated from the blood of two patients with Lyme disease. N Engl J Med 1983;308:740–742.
15. Schmid GP, Steigerwalt AG, Johnson SE, et al. DNA characterization of the spirochete that causes Lyme disease. J Clin Microbiol 1984;20:155–158.
16. Schmid GP, Steigerwalt AG, Johnson S, et al. DNA characterization of Lyme disease spirochetes. Yale J Biol Med 1984; 57:539–542.
17. Hayes L, Wright DJM, Archard LC. A short amino acid sequence is shared by surface antigens of *Borrelia duttonii, Borrelia herm-*
sii, and *Borrelia burgdorferi.* Ann NY Acad Sci 1988; 539:381–382.
18. Wilske B, Preac-Mursic V, Schierz G, et al. Antigenic variability of *Borrelia burgdorferi.* Ann NY Acad Sci 1988;534:126–143.
19. Oliver JH, Owsley MR, Hutcheson HJ, et al. Conspecificity of the ticks *Ixodes scapularis* and *I. dammini* (Acari: Ixodidae). J Med Entomol 1993;30:54–63.
20. Ciesielski CA, Markowitz LE, Hensley R, et al. The geographic distribution of Lyme disease in the United States. Ann NY Acad Sci 1988;539:283–288.
21. Dammini GJ. Lyme disease: Its transmission and diagnostic features. Lab Manage 1986;24:33–38.
22. Falco RC, Fish D. Potential for exposure to tick bites in recreational parks in a Lyme disease endemic area. Am J Public Health 1989;79:12–15.
23. Falco RC, Fish D. Prevalence of *Ixodes dammini* near the homes of Lyme disease patients in Westchester County, New York. Am J Epidemiol 1988;127:826–830.
24. Riberio JMC, Mathier TN, Piesman J, et al. Dissemination and salivary delivery of Lyme disease spirochetes in vector ticks (Acari: Ixodae). J Med Entomol 1987;24:201–205.
25. Piesman J, Mathier TN, Sinsky RJ, et al. Duration of tick attachment and *Borrelia burgdorferi* transmission. J Clin Microbiol 1987;25:557–558.
26. Andiman WA. Lyme disease: Epidemiology, etiology, clinical spectrum, diagnosis, and treatment. Adv Pediatr Infect Dis 1987;1:163–186.
27. Hurwitz S. Erythema chronicum migrans and Lyme disease. Pediatr Dermatol 1985;2:266–274.
28. Steere AC, Schoen RT, Taylor E. The clinical evolution of Lyme arthritis. Ann Intern Med 1987;107:725–731.
29. Steere AC, Bartenhagen NH, Croft JE, et al. Clinical manifestations of Lyme disease. Zentralbl Bakt Hyg [A] 1986;263: 201–205.
30. Burke WA, Steinbaugh JR, O'Keefe EJ. Lyme disease mimicking secondary syphilis. J Am Acad Dermatol 1987;14:137–139.
31. Asbrink E, Hovmark A. Early and late cutaneous manifestations in *Ixodes*-borne borreliosis (erythema migrans borreliosis, Lyme borreliosis). Ann NY Acad Sci 1988;539:4–15.
32. Steere AC. Lyme disease. N Engl J Med 1989;321:586–596.
33. Lawson JP, Steere AC. Lyme arthritis: Radiologic findings. Radiology 1985;154:37–43.
34. Petersen LR, Sweeney AH, Checko PJ, et al. Epidemiological and clinical features of 1,149 persons with Lyme disease identified by laboratory-based surveillance in Connecticut. Yale J Biol Med 1989;62:253–263.
35. Davidson RS. Orthopaedic complications of Lyme disease in children. Biomed Pharmacother 1989;43:405–408.
36. Steere AC, Gibofsky A, Patarroyo ME, et al. Chronic Lyme arthritis: Clinical and immunogenetic differentiation from rheumatoid arthritis. Ann Intern Med 1979;90:896–901.
37. Steere AC, Feld J, Winchester R. Association of chronic Lyme arthritis with increased frequency of DR4 and 3 (abstract). Arthritis Rheum 1988;31:598.
38. Kryger P, Hansen K, Vinterberg H, et al. Lyme borreliosis among Danish patients with arthritis. Scand J Rheumatol 1990; 19:77–81.
39. Steere AC, Batsford WP, Weinberg M, et al. Lyme carditis: Cardiac abnormalities of Lyme disease. Ann Intern Med 1980; 93:8–16.
40. Van der Linde MR, Crijns HJGM, de Koning J, et al. Range of atrioventricular condition disturbances in Lyme borreliosis: A report of four cases and review of other published reports. Br Heart J 1990;63:162–168.
41. Mayer N, Kleber FX, Welske B, et al. Persistent atrioventricular block in Lyme borreliosis. Klin Wochenschr 1990;68:431–435.
42. Marcus LC, Steere AC, Duray PH, et al. Fatal pancarditis in a patient with coexistent Lyme disease and babesiosis: Demonstration of spirochetes in the myocardium. Ann Intern Med 1985;103:374–376.
43. Stanek G, Klein J, Bittner R, et al. Isolation of *Borrelia burgdorferi* from the myocardium of a patient with longstanding cardiomyopathy. N Engl J Med 1990;322:249–252.
44. Halperin JJ. Nervous system manifestations of Lyme disease. Rheumatol Dis Clin North Am 1989;15:635–647.

45. Kristoferitsch W. Lyme borreliosis in Europe: Neurologic disorders. Rheumatol Dis Clin North Am 1989;15:767–774.

46. Halperin JJ, Luft BJ, Volkman DJ, et al. Lyme neuroborreliosis: Peripheral nervous system manifestations. Brain 1990;113:1207–1221.

47. Karlsson M, Hovind-Hougen K, Svenungsson B, et al. Cultivation and characterization of spirochetes from cerebrospinal fluid of patients with Lyme borreliosis. J Clin Microbiol 1990;28:473–479.

48. Pachner AR, Steere AC. The triad of neurologic manifestations of Lyme disease: Meningitis, cranial neuritis and radiculoneuritis. Neurology 1985;35:47–53.

49. Schmutzhard E. Lyme borreliosis and multiple sclerosis. Biomed Pharmacother 1989;43:415–419.

50. Steere AC, Bartenhagen NH, Croft JE, et al. The early clinical manifestations of Lyme disease. Ann Intern Med 1983;99:76–82.

51. Kauffmann DJH, Wormser GP. Ocular Lyme disease: Case report and review of the literature. Br J Ophthalmol 1990;74:325–327.

52. Asbrink E. Erythema chronicum migrans Afzelius and acrodermatitis chronica atrophicans. Acta Derm Venereol 1985;118:1–63.

53. Asbrink E, Brehmer-Andersson E, Hovermark A. Acrodermatitis chronica atrophicans: A spirochetosis. Am J Dermatopathol 1986;8:209–219.

54. Hovmark A, Asbrink E, Olsson L. The spirochetal etiology of lymphadenosis benigna cutis solitaria. Acta Derm Venereol 1986;66:479–484.

55. Abele DC, Anders KH. The many faces and phases of borreliosis: I. Lyme disease. J Am Acad Dermatol 1990;23:167–186.

56. Abele DC, Anders KH. The many faces and phases of borreliosis: II. J Am Acad Dermatol 1990;23:401–410.

57. Lavoie PE, Wilson AJ, Tuffanelli DL. Acrodermatitis chronica atrophicans with antecedent Lyme disease in a Californian. Zentralbl Bakteriol Hyg [A] 1986;263:265.

58. Kaufman LD, Gruber BL, Phillips ME, et al. Late cutaneous Lyme disease: Acrodermatitis chronica atrophicans. Am J Med 1989;86:828–830.

59. Asbrink E, Hovmark A, Hederstedt B. The spirochetal etiology of acrodermatitis chronica atrophicans Herxheimer. Acta Derm Venereol 1984;64:506–512.

60. Hopf HCH. Peripheral neuropathy in acrodermatitis chronica atrophicans (Herxheimer). J Neurol Neurosurg Psychiatry 1975;28:452–458.

61. Kristoferitsch W, Sluga E, Grof M, et al. Neuropathy associated with acrodermatitis chronica atrophicans: Clinical and morphological features. Ann NY Acad Sci 1988;539:35–45.

61a. Spiegler E. Uber die sogenennte sarcomatosis cutis. Arch Derm Syph 1894;27:163.

61b. Fendt H. Beitrage zur kenntnis der sogenannten sarcoiden geschwaltze der haut. Arch Derm Syph 1900;53:213.

61c. Baverstadt B. Uber lymphadenosis benigna cutis, eine klinische und pathologich-anatomische studie. Stockholm: P.A. Nordstedt und Soner, 1943.

62. Schempp C, Bocklage H, Lange R, et al. Further evidence for *Borrelia burgdorferi* infection in morphea and lichen sclerosus et atrophicus confirmed by DNA amplification. J Invest Dermatol 1993;100:717–720.

63. Abele DC, Anders KH, Chandler FW. Benign lymphocytic infiltration (Jessner-Kanof): Another manifestation of borreliosis? J Am Acad Dermatol 1989;21:795–797.

64. Rabb DC, Lesher JL, Chandler FW. Polymerase chain reaction confirmation of *Borrelia burgdorferi* in benign lymphocytic infiltrate of dermis. J Am Acad Dermatol 1992;26:267–268.

65. Abele DC, Bedingfield RB, Chandler FW, et al. Progressive facial hemiatrophy (Parry-Romberg syndrome) and borreliosis. J Am Acad Dermatol 1990;22:531–533.

66. Berger BW. Cutaneous manifestations of Lyme borreliosis. Rheumatol Dis Clin North Am 1989;15:627–634.

67. Olsson JC, Esterly NB. Urticarial vasculitis and Lyme disease. J Am Acad Dermatol 1990;22:1114–1116.

68. Espana A, Torrelo A, Guerrero A, et al. Periarticular fibrous nodules in Lyme borreliosis. Br J Dermatol 1991;125:68–70.

69. Garbe C, Stein H, Dienemann D, et al. *Borrelia burgdorferi*-associated cutaneous B-cell lymphoma: Clinical and immunohistochemical characterization of four cases. J Am Acad Dermatol 1991;24:584–590.

70. Berger BW, Clemmensen OJ, Ackerman AB. Lyme disease is a spirochetosis. Am J Dermatopathol 1983;5:111–124.

71. Duray PH, Steere AC. The spectrum of organ and system pathology in human Lyme disease. Zentralbl Bakteriol Hyg [A] 1986;263:169–178.

72. Lever WF, Schaumburg-Lever G. Histopathology of the Skin. Philadelphia: JB Lippincott, 1983:753–756.

73. Duray PH. Histopathology of clinical phases of human Lyme disease. Rheumatol Dis Clin North Am 1989;15:691–710.

74. Duray PH. Clinical pathologic correlations of Lyme disease. Rev Infect Dis 1989; 2(Suppl 6):S1487–S1493.

75. Garcia-Monco JC, Benach JL. The pathogenesis of Lyme disease. Rheumatol Dis Clin North Am 1989;15:711–726.

76. Malawista SE. Pathogenesis of Lyme disease. Rheumatol Int 1989;9:233–235.

77. Aberer E, Brunner C, Suchanek G, et al. Molecular mimicry and Lyme borreliosis: A shared antigenic determinant between *Borrelia burgdorferi* and human tissue. Ann Neurol 1989;26:732–737.

78. Schoen RT. Pathogenesis, diagnosis, manifestations and treatment of Lyme disease. Curr Opin Rheumatol 1991;3:610–616.

79. Hardin JA, Steere AC, Malawista SE. Immune complexes and evaluation of Lyme arthritis: Dissemination and localization of abnormal C1q binding activity. N Engl J Med 1979;301:1358–1363.

80. Craft JE, Fischer DK, Shimamoto GT, et al. Antigens of *Borrelia burgdorferi* recognized during Lyme disease: Appearance of a new immunoglobulin M response and expansion of the immunoglobulin G response late in the illness. J Clin Invest 1986;78:934–939.

81. Kristoferistch W, Mayr WR, Partsch H, et al. HLA-DR in Lyme borreliosis (letter). Lancet 1986;2:278.

82. Aberer E, Brunner C, Suchanek G, et al. Molecular mimicry and Lyme borreliosis: A shared antigenic determinant between *Borrelia burgdorferi* and human tissue. Ann Neurol 1989;26:732–737.

83. Berger BW, Johnson RC, Kodner C, et al. Cultivation of *Borrelia burgdorferi* from erythema migrans lesions and perilesional skin. J Clin Microbiol 1992;30:359–361.

84. Duray PH, Asbrink E, Weber K. The cutaneous manifestations of human Lyme disease: A widening spectrum. Adv Dermatol 1989;4:255–276.

85. Craft JE, Grodzicki RL, Kornblatt AN, et al. Antibody response in Lyme disease: Evaluation of diagnostic tests. J Infect Dis 1984;149:789–795.

86. Dattwyler RJ, Luft BJ. Immunodiagnosis of Lyme borreliosis. Rheumatol Dis Clin North Am 1989;15:727–734.

87. Hansen K, Cruz M, Link H. Oligoclonal *Borrelia burgdorferi*-specific IgG antibodies in cerebrospinal fluid in Lyme neuroborreliosis. J Infect Dis 1990;161:1194–1202.

88. Schwartz BS, Goldstein MD, Ribeiro JMC, et al. Antibody testing in Lyme disease: A comparison of results in four laboratories. JAMA 1989;262:3341–3434.

89. Cristenson VD, White DH. Evaluation of four commercially available ELISA assays for the serologic diagnosis of Lyme disease. J Clin Lab Anal 1991;5:340–343.

90. Bakken LL, Case KL, Callister SM, et al. Performance of 45 laboratories participating in a proficiency testing program for Lyme disease serology. JAMA 1992;268:891–895.

91. Steere AC, Taylor E, McHugh GL, et al. The overdiagnosis of Lyme disease. JAMA 1993;269:1812–1816.

92. Magnarelli LA, Miller JN, Anderson JF, et al. Cross-reactivity of nonspecific treponemal antibody in serologic tests for Lyme disease. J Clin Microbiol 1990;28:1276–1279.

93. Mackworth-Young CG. Cross-reactive idiotypes in sera from patients with leprosy, lupus, and Lyme disease and from healthy individuals. Clin Exp Immunol 1990;79:78–82.

94. Karlsson M, Mollegard I, Stiernstedt G, et al. Comparison of Western blot and enzyme-linked immunosorbent assay for diagnosis of Lyme borreliosis. Eur J Clin Microbiol Infect Dis 1989;8:871–877.

95. Nelson JA, Bankowski MJ, Newton BJ, et al. Detection of antibodies in late Lyme disease. J Infect Dis 1990;161:1034–1035.

96. Malloy DC, Nauman RK, Paxton H. Detection of *Borrelia burgdorferi* using the polymerase chain reaction. J Clin Microbiol 1990;28:1089–1093.

97. Nielsen SL, Young KKY, Barbour AG. Detection of *Borrelia burgdorferi* DNA by the polymerase chain reaction. Mol Cell Probes 1990;4:73–79.

98. Picken RN. Polymerase chain reaction primers and probes derived from flagellin gene sequences for specific detection of the agents of Lyme disease and North American relapsing fever. J Clin Microbiol 1992;30:99–114.

99. Neu HC. A perspective on therapy of Lyme infection. Ann NY Acad Sci 1988;539:314–316.

100. Kohlhepp W, Oschmann P, Mertens HG. Treatment of Lyme borreliosis: Randomized comparison of doxycycline and penicillin G. J Neurol 1989;236:464–469.

101. Weber K, Preac-Mursic V, Wilske B, et al. A randomized trial of ceftriaxone versus oral penicillin for the treatment of early European Lyme borreliosis. Infection 1990;18:91–96.

102. Hassler D, Zöller L, Haude M, et al. Cefotaxime versus penicillin in the late state of Lyme disease: Prospective randomized therapeutic study. Infection 1990;18:16–20.

103. Luft BJ, Dattwyler RJ. Treatment of Lyme borreliosis. Rheumatol Dis Clin North Am 1989;15:747–755.

104. Luft BJ, Gorevic PD, Halperin JJ, et al. A perspective on the treatment of Lyme borreliosis. Rev Infect Dis 1989;2(Suppl 6):S1518–S1525.

105. Rahn DW, Malawista SE. Lyme disease: Recommendations for diagnosis and treatment. Ann Intern Med 1991;114:472–481.

106. MacDonald AB. Gestational Lyme disease: Implications for the fetus. Rheumatol Dis Clin North Am 1989;15:657–677.

107. Preac-Mursic V, Weber K, Pfister HW, et al. Survival of *Borrelia burgdorferi* in antibiotically treated patients with Lyme borreliosis. Infection 1989;17:355–359.

108. Anderson JF. Preventing Lyme disease. Rheumatol Dis Clin North Am 1989;15:757–766.

109. Centers for Disease Control, Bacterial Zoonoses Branch, Division of Vector-Borne Infectious Diseases, National Centers for Infectious Diseases, vol 2, No. 6, August 1991.

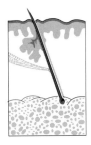

chapter 110

Chancroid, Granuloma Inguinale, and Lymphogranuloma Venereum

THEODORE ROSEN and ANIR DHIR

Sexually transmitted diseases (STDs) are often associated with cutaneous manifestations, such as pain or ulceration, that bring them to the attention of dermatologists. In the United States, genital ulcerative disease most commonly results from syphilis or herpes progenitalis. Other infectious causes of genital lesions such as chancroid, granuloma inguinale, and lymphogranuloma venereum are prevalent in developing Third World countries, but they are historically rare in Europe and North America. However, the incidence of chancroid has risen sharply in recent years, and the disease may now be endemic in some large urban centers in the United States. The rising number of cases, coupled with the recognition that genital ulcerative disease may facilitate transmission of human immunodeficiency virus (HIV), has led to renewed interest in these "minor" STDs.

Chancroid

DEFINITION

Chancroid, or soft chancre (ulcer molle), is a painful ulcerative genital disease caused by sexual transmission of *Haemophilus ducreyi*. Genital lesions are often associated with tender inguinal lymphadenopathy, which may progress to suppuration and bubo formation.

CLINICAL DESCRIPTION

Epidemiology

Chancroid is endemic in many tropical and subtropical countries, particularly in Africa and southeast Asia.[1] It is the most common cause of ulcerative genital disease in Kenya, Zimbabwe, and Gambia.[2] In fact, chancroid's worldwide incidence may exceed that of syphilis.[3] However, chancroid has historically been a relatively rare STD in the United States. The number of reported cases peaked in 1947, with a total of 9515 cases.[4] After World War II, the annual incidence steadily declined, with the exception of a brief rise during the Vietnam War. From 1971 to 1980, a mean of only 878 cases was reported annually.[1] This downward trend was reversed in the early 1980s, when an increased flow of immigrants from southeast Asia, Mexico, and the Caribbean contributed to a resurgence of chancroid in the United States.[2]

Since 1981, several large outbreaks have occurred in urban centers, including New York City, Boston, Atlanta, Palm Beach, Jacksonville, Orlando, Dallas, Houston, Orange County, and Los Angeles.[1-3] The disease may now be endemic in New York City and southern Florida.[5] In 1988 and 1989, 4891 and 4697 cases were reported, respectively. In 1990, 4223 cases were reported, with 88% of these clustered in New York, Georgia, Florida, Texas, and California.[6] Since 1979, the overall incidence of chancroid in the United States has increased 10-fold, from 0.2 to 2.1 per 100,000 population.[1] The actual incidence may be significantly higher since the disease has probably been underreported owing to difficulties in establishing unequivocal diagnosis.[6]

In the United States, unprotected sex with infected prostitutes plays a major role in transmission. Military personnel and merchant seamen are commonly affected, and recent outbreaks have primarily involved young black and Latino heterosexual men. Patients are often members of lower socioeconomic groups, and the male-to-female ratio is reportedly between 3:1 and 25:1.[3] It is unclear whether a significant asymptomatic female carrier state exists.[4] Studies have demonstrated a higher incidence of HIV seropositivity in patients with chancroid. In Kenya, chancroid is believed to play a major role in the transmission of HIV among heterosexuals. Similar studies have not shown an increased incidence of HIV antibodies among patients with nonulcerative STDs. Presumably, ulcerative genital disease facilitates entry of the virus into the body by circumventing the natural barrier function of the skin.[7]

Clinical Manifestations

Initial entry of *H. ducreyi* into the skin occurs through minor abrasions that disrupt epithelial integrity. The incubation period ranges from 3 to 14 days, although 4 to 7 days is most common.[1] There is no prodrome, and systemic symptoms are rare. The first manifestation of infection is a small, inflammatory papule, which progresses within 2 or 3 days to a pustule that rapidly ulcerates. Many patients do not notice the lesion until ulceration has occurred. The classic chancroidal lesion consists of one or more well-demarcated, nonindurated, tender ulcerations with ragged, undermined edges and surrounding erythema (Fig. 110–1). Autoinoculation of adjacent skin results in characteristic "kissing lesions." A gray or yellow, necrotic, often foul-smelling exudate usually overlies the friable, granulomatous base, which bleeds easily when scraped.[8]

Several morphologic variants of chancroid have been described. *Dwarf chancroid* is characterized by one or more small, rounded, shallow herpetiform ulcers with irregular bases and sharp hemorrhagic borders. *Giant chancroid* results when several smaller ulcers coalesce to form a large, sometimes serpiginous solitary lesion. In *transient chancroid*, the initial ulceration resolves rapidly within 4 to 6 days but is followed by acute inguinal lymphadenopathy with suppuration in 10 to 20 days; this form may be difficult to distinguish from lymphogranuloma venereum. Origination of the infection within the pilar apparatus may result in *follicular chancroid* that clinically mimics a folliculitis. Extensive ulceration that is unusually deep and destructive characterizes *phagedenic chancroid*. Finally, *pseudogranuloma inguinale* is a variant of chancroid that closely resembles granuloma inguinale.[9]

In males, the disease most commonly involves the distal prepuce, frenulum, and coronal sulcus; the glans, penis shaft, and anus are affected less frequently. Local extension may result in lesions involving the scrotum or inguinal creases. In females, ulcers are most often located on the labia, fourchette, vestibule, and clitoris and in the

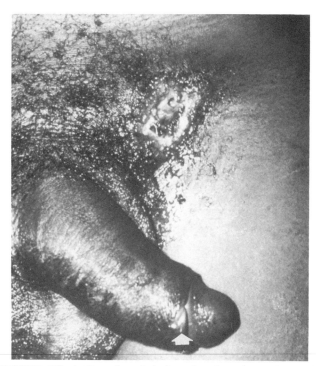

FIGURE 110–1. Ragged genital ulceration *(arrow)* associated with draining suppuration of a lymph node characteristic of chancroid.

perianal area.[4] Lesions in females may be more superficial and less tender and may heal more rapidly.[2] Painless cervical and vaginal lesions are also possible.[4] Potential complications of genital ulceration include paraphimosis, labial adhesions, and strictures.[2]

In approximately 50% of patients, chancroid is associated with painful inguinal, usually unilateral lymphadenopathy. Suppuration with bubo formation occurs in about 25% of cases. The skin overlying the bubo may become tense and erythematous, with rupture resulting in a deep, inguinal ulcer. Potential complications include scarring and lymphedema.[8]

PATHOLOGY

Microscopic examination of the base of the chancroidal ulcer reveals three distinct zones. The superficial zone contains necrotic tissue, fibrin, erythrocytes, neutrophils, and the causative bacteria. The middle zone is an area of neovascularization and thrombosed vessels. Finally, the deepest zone consists of a dense infiltrate of lymphocytes and plasma cells. Bacteria can be demonstrated by either Giemsa or silver stains.[10]

PATHOGENESIS AND ETIOLOGY

Chancroid, or soft chancre, was first differentiated from the indurated chancre of syphilis by Bassereau in France in 1852. He noted that new lesions could be formed in patients with soft chancre, but not syphilis, by autoinoculation of ulcer exudate into other skin sites. In 1889, Ducrey first identified *H. ducreyi* as the causative agent of chancroid by using autoinoculation to maintain 15 successive generations of ulcers on the forearms of three patients. After the sixth reinoculation, Ducrey discovered a single microorganism in each of the patients. He was also able to isolate this same organism from associated buboes.[4]

H. ducreyi is a short, compact gram-negative bacillus (1.5×0.5 μm) with rounded ends that often grows in chains. It is a facultative aerobe located both extracellularly and within neutrophils.[4] Istamanoff and Akspianz are credited with the first culture of *H. ducreyi* on a medium of agar and human skin. Modern cultural methods evolved from techniques developed by Teague and Deibert in 1920 and improved by Heyman and colleagues in 1945.[11] Inoculation of the chancroid bacillus into apes, chimpanzees, humans, and rabbits has resulted in experimental disease.[4] In addition, a mouse model of *H. ducreyi* has been developed that more closely resembles human disease and may be helpful in future study of chancroid pathogenesis.[12]

DIAGNOSIS AND DIFFERENTIAL DIAGNOSIS

Diagnosis of chancroid based solely on ulcer appearance is accurate in only 33% to 53% of cases.[13, 14] As discussed earlier, several morphologic variants exist. In addition, STDs such as herpes simplex, syphilis, lymphogranuloma venereum, and granuloma inguinale may mimic chancroid. The differential diagnosis also includes non-STDs such as Behçet's disease, extraintestinal Crohn's disease, and fixed drug eruption (Table 110–1).[15] Therefore, laboratory correlation is mandatory for accurate diagnosis.

Gram staining of an ulcer specimen may reveal gram-negative coccobacilli singly or in a "school of fish" formation, in which the bacilli are arranged in long parallel columns between cells or shreds of mucus. However, studies have shown that this "typical" Gram stain is seen in only 5% to 36% of culture-proven cases of chancroid.[14, 16] Accurate interpretation of the Gram stain is further hampered by frequent polymicrobial contamination of genital ulcers. Therefore, the Gram stain may be useful as an ancillary study, but its poor sensitivity

and specificity make it inadequate for definitive diagnosis.[8, 11, 17]

Biopsy of a suspected chancroidal ulcer is rarely performed because the histology may not be diagnostic, and biopsies are both painful and not readily performed in many STD clinics. The autoinoculation technique is no longer considered ethical, and earlier diagnostic methods such as the Ito-Reenstierna skin test and the complement fixation test are no longer used because of low sensitivity and lack of specificity.[8]

Definitive diagnosis of chancroid requires cultural isolation of *H. ducreyi*.[4, 8, 17] Unfortunately, isolation has proven difficult in the past because of the fastidious nature of this organism. The development of various selective solid media within the past 20 years has improved the situation, but cultural diagnosis remains problematic. The most promising results have been obtained through the use of Nairobi medium.[8, 18] Ideally, this medium consists of a biplate of (1) gonococcal agar base with 2% bovine hemoglobin, 5% fetal calf serum, and 3 mg/L of vancomycin and (2) Mueller-Hinton agar with 5% chocolatized horse blood and vancomycin. Studies in Kenya using this media yielded sensitivities of 75% to 81%,[17, 19] with an increase in sensitivity of 8% if a second culture was performed 48 hours later.[19] If Nairobi medium is unavailable, isolation may be attempted on chocolate Mueller-Hinton or BBL chocolate II with vancomycin.[8, 9] Most *H. ducreyi* strains are resistant to vancomycin, with minimum inhibitory concentrations of 32 to 128 mg/L. Therefore, this antibiotic is routinely incorporated into culture media to prevent the overgrowth of contaminants. However, strains of *H. ducreyi* with a minimum inhibitory concentration of 4 mg/mL have been reported, and repeated negative cultures in cases of strongly suspected chancroid should prompt screening for vancomycin-sensitive organisms.[8, 9]

Ulcers are cleaned with sterile, nonbacteriostatic saline and gauze, and specimens are obtained from the base and undermined margins using a cotton swab.[1, 9] Isolation of *H. ducreyi* from inguinal bubo aspirate may be attempted, but it is generally less successful than isolation of the organism from genital ulcers. Chancre exudate may be transported in Amies' or Stuart's medium if needed.[9] However, whenever possible, specimens should

	Duration	Recurrence	Pain	Size/Destruction	Induration	Enlarged Nodes
TABLE 110-1. Differential Diagnosis of Genital Ulcerations						
Sexually Transmitted						
Herpes simplex	Short	Yes	Yes	Small/no	No	Yes
Syphilis	Short	No	No	Small/rarely	Yes	Yes
Chancroid	Short	No	Yes	Small/no	No	Yes
Granuloma inguinale	Moderate	No	No	Large/yes	Slight	No
Lymphogranuloma venereum	Short	No	No	Small/no	No	Yes
Scabies	Short	No	No	Small/no	Slight	No
GC boil	Short	No	Yes	Small/no	Yes	No/rarely
Non-Sexually Transmitted						
Fixed drug eruption	Short	Maybe	Maybe	Small/no	No	No
Behçet's disease	Variable	Yes	Yes	Variable/maybe	Slight	If metastatic
Tumor	Long	No	No	Variable/yes	Yes	No
Crohn's disease	Variable	No	Maybe	Variable/no	Slight	No
Factitial disease	Variable	No	Maybe	Variable/maybe	If infected	If infected

be directly inoculated onto selective media for at least two reasons. First, survival of this fastidious organism in transport media has not been verified.[1] Second, dilution of the specimen in transport media may lead to false-negative cultures. Inoculation onto selective solid media should be done within 2 hours, and preferably within 1 hour.[8, 9, 20] A candle extinction jar containing six moist paper towels incubated at 33°C to 35°C will provide the humid, carbon dioxide–enriched (5%–10%) environment required by this bacterium.[1]

Colonies are characteristically yellow-gray, nonmucoid, raised, compact, and granular. They are generally pinpoint size at 24 hours and increase to 1 to 2 mm in 48 to 72 hours. Because of significant intercellular adhesion (demonstrated by electron microscopy), individual colonies remain intact when pushed across the agar surface with an inoculating loop. Size and opacity may vary between individual colonies, resulting in the appearance of a mixed culture.[4, 11]

H. ducreyi possesses very limited biochemical activity, but tests for nitrate reductase, alkaline phosphatase, cytochrome oxidase, and β-lactamase are characteristically positive. The organism is usually catalase negative. However, strains with exceptions to the aforementioned activities have been reported. Most strains of *H. ducreyi* require factor V (nicotinamide adenine dinucleotide) and factor X (hemin) for optimal growth.[8] The bacterium's identification profile in a standard biochemical screening panel (RapID-ANA) is 110500.[21]

Many suspected cases of chancroid are actually due to herpes simplex or syphilis that is negative on darkfield microscopy. Inadequate screening for other diseases in the past may have led investigators to overestimate the number of "culture negative" chancroid cases. Therefore, routine screening should include herpes simplex culture, Tzanck smear, darkfield examination for *Treponema pallidum*, and serologic testing for syphilis.[9]

Although culture is the diagnostic standard, efforts are underway to design a serologic test or DNA probe that will allow more rapid and sensitive diagnosis. Unfortunately, incomplete knowledge about the antigenic composition of the organism, as well as geographic variation in outer membrane profiles, has hindered the development of a diagnostic serologic test.[4] An indirect immunofluorescence test using monoclonal antibodies against outer membrane proteins has been described, but it lacks enough sensitivity for clinical use.[22] Other hybridoma-produced monoclonal antibodies have been used in an experimental immunofluorescence reagent with up to 93% sensitivity.[23] Parsons and colleagues[24] have developed a DNA probe labeled with ^{32}P that is both highly sensitive and specific for *H. ducreyi* grown in culture and in rabbit skin. Application of this probe in conjunction with the polymerase chain reaction may eventually simplify laboratory diagnosis.

TREATMENT

Untreated chancroidal ulcers may persist for 1 to 3 months, whereas appropriate antimicrobial therapy results in resolution within 7 to 14 days.[2] In the past, tetracycline was considered the drug of choice for chancroid. However, widespread plasmid-mediated resistance now exists to tetracyclines, as well as to sulfonamides, chloramphenicol, and kanamycin. Penicillin and ampicillin are also ineffective owing to β-lactamase production in the majority of clinical isolates. Therefore, these agents are no longer recommended.[1, 2, 17]

The current recommendations of the Centers for Disease Control and Prevention are ceftriaxone sodium, 250 mg intramuscularly in a single dose, or oral erythromycin, 500 mg four times daily for 1 week (Table 110–2).[25, 26] An alternative regimen is ciprofloxacin, 500 mg twice daily for 1 to 3 days,[25] which has resulted in 90% to 100% cure rates in both Africa and Asia.[27, 28] Chancroid also usually responds to oral amoxicillin/clavulanate, 500 mg/125 mg three times a day for 1 week. Trimethoprim-sulfamethoxazole, 160 mg/800 mg orally twice daily for 1 week has proven effective in most geographic areas except Thailand.[29] However, strains with minimal inhibitory concentrations of trimethoprim greater than 32 mg/mL have been reported in both Asia and Africa.[29, 30] Whenever possible, all sexual contacts of the index patient should be examined and should receive appropriate antibiotic therapy.

Treatment also includes prophylactic aspiration of buboes, particularly if they are fluctuant. A superior approach is preferred to avoid creating a fistulous tract. Warm, moist compresses should be applied both to ulcers and to enlarged lymph nodes. The healing of buboes tends to parallel the healing of ulcers if the bubo is no larger than 5 cm in diameter. Buboes exceeding this diameter usually heal more slowly than ulcers.[2]

As is true in all instances of genital ulcer disease, the patient should receive appropriate pretest counseling and HIV serologic evaluation.

	Drugs of Choice	**Alternatives**
TABLE 110-2. Treatment of Chancroid, Granuloma Inguinale, and Lymphogranuloma Venereum		
Chancroid	Ceftriaxone, 250 mg IM in a single dose Erythromycin, 500 mg PO qid for 7 days	Ciprofloxacin, 500 mg PO bid for 1–3 days
Granuloma inguinale	Tetracycline, 500 mg PO qid for 2–3 weeks	Trimethoprim-sulfamethoxazole, 160 mg/800 mg PO bid for 2–3 weeks
	Doxycycline, 100 mg PO bid for 2–3 weeks	Erythromycin, 500 mg PO qid for 2–3 weeks
Lymphogranuloma venereum	Doxycycline, 100 mg PO bid for 3 weeks	Erythromycin, 500 mg PO qid for 3 weeks
	Tetracycline, 500 mg PO qid for 3 weeks	Sulfisoxazole, 500 mg PO qid for 3 weeks

Granuloma Inguinale

DEFINITION

Granuloma inguinale (donovanosis, granuloma venereum) is a rare, chronic, indolent disease characterized by anogenital and inguinal ulcerogranulomatous lesions. It is generally considered to be caused by sexual transmission of *Calymmatobacterium granulomatis*.

CLINICAL DESCRIPTION

Epidemiology

Granuloma inguinale primarily occurs in small endemic foci located in tropical and subtropical areas of the world. The major regions from which the disease is usually reported include southeast India, New Guinea, the Caribbean (particularly Grenada), and the eastern half of South America.[31] Significant foci are also located in South Africa, Zambia, Vietnam, Japan, and Australia (among the aborigines). In some endemic areas, this disease represents 20% of all STD diagnoses in male patients.[32] Since granuloma inguinale was first noted in the United States in 1913, most cases have been reported from southern and southeastern states.[33] The incidence rate has been steadily decreasing in the United States, and fewer than 100 cases are now reported annually.[1] The disease is more common among individuals of low socioeconomic status, and males are affected about twice as often as females.[33]

Interestingly, the role of sexual transmission in granuloma inguinale remains controversial. Several epidemiologic studies done 20 years ago suggested a nonvenereal etiology.[34, 35] As supporting evidence, these researchers cited the occurrence of disease in very young and elderly sexually inactive patients, the low incidence among prostitutes, and the presence of only extragenital lesions in some cases. However, more recent epidemiologic data support the classification of granuloma inguinale as a venereal disease. Lal and Nicholas[36] cite the presence of genital lesions in 93% of cases, other concomitant STDs in 45% of cases, and disease in 52% of sexual partners. Further evidence of sexual transmission is seen in an outbreak of 20 cases in Houston in 1982–1983: one cluster of 5 cases involved a female prostitute, her husband, and 3 "customers."[38] In homosexual men, lesions are commonly located perianally.[31, 33] Finally, individuals are most often affected in the second to third decades of life, an age-specific incidence that closely parallels that of other STDs.[37] Studies have associated HIV seropositivity with granuloma inguinale in South Africa.[38]

Another unresolved issue is the relationship between granuloma inguinale and penile carcinoma. Reports suggest that squamous cell carcinoma may arise in ulcers of granuloma inguinale. One study found complement-fixing antibody to *C. granulomatis* in 15% of patients with penile carcinoma but not in control sera.[39] Histolog-ically and clinically, granuloma inguinale may resemble carcinoma.[40] Therefore, some cases of diagnosed penile carcinoma may actually represent long-standing granuloma inguinale. Clinicians should maintain a high index of suspicion for granuloma inguinale when finding morphology or histology suggestive of penile carcinoma in a younger individual.

Clinical Manifestation

Four morphologic variants of granuloma inguinale have been described: ulcerovegetative, nodular, hypertrophic, and cicatricial. In *ulcerovegetative* disease (the most common), papules or small nodules appear at the site of initial infection after an incubation period ranging from less than 2 weeks to 3 months. These nodules rapidly erode to form one or more painless ulcerations with a raised, rolled, sharp border and a clean, "beefy red" base containing exuberant, friable granulation tissue (Fig. 110–2). Ulcers slowly spread by direct extension and by autoinoculation of adjacent skin that results in "kissing lesions." In the *nodular* variant, lesions are soft, erythematous papules with a granulation tissue–like surface. *Hypertrophic* granuloma inguinale consists of large, vegetating masses that may closely resemble condyloma acuminatum or latum. Finally, the rare *cictaricial* form is characterized by expanding scarring plaques.[33]

Lesions in men occur most commonly on the prepuce, coronal sulcus, or perianally (in homosexuals); women usually present with labial lesions, although the vagina and cervix may also be involved.[33] Infection may spread to the inguinal lymph nodes, but true inguinal lymphadenopathy does not occur. Nevertheless, swelling and ulceration of the inguinal area are commonly seen. These seemingly contradictory events are reconciled by Richens,[31] who explains that infection tends to escape from the lymph nodes into surrounding tissues, causing a periadenitis. This may result in abscess (pseudobubo)

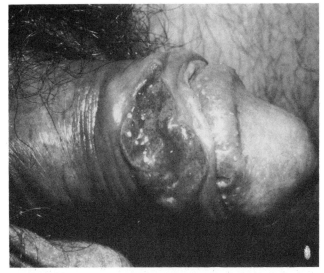

FIGURE 110–2. Large, friable genital ulceration typical of granuloma inguinale.

formation or ulceration of overlying skin. Anaerobic bacterial superinfection of genital ulcers may result in a foul-smelling exudate and pain, as well as true inguinal lymphadenopathy.

Granuloma inguinale can be mutilating if left untreated. Scarring and fibrosis may be prominent, and infrequent complications include phimosis, destruction of the penis, lymphedema, and an elephantiasis-like swelling of the external genitalia in women. Intrapelvic disease is associated with case–fatality rates from 5.2% to 14.3% in some series.[41, 42] Extragenital mucocutaneous lesions involving the face, mouth, neck, and other sites occur in less than 10% of patients.[33] In very rare cases, the infection may disseminate hematogenously, resulting in lesions affecting the bones, liver, spleen, or lung.[1, 31] Hematogenous disease is a life-threatening complication that usually occurs after several years of chronic genital infection. It is strongly associated with pregnancy.[31] Constitutional symptoms do not typically occur in granuloma inguinale unless intrapelvic spread, secondary infection, or hematogenous dissemination has occurred.

PATHOLOGY

Histopathology reveals endothelial proliferation and dilatation of dermal blood vessels as well as infiltration of the dermis by histiocytes containing 1- to 2-μm intracytoplasmic bacilli known as Donovan bodies. Donovan bodies are hard to see in hematoxylin and eosin–stained sections but can be demonstrated in sections stained with Warthin-Starry or Giemsa, in which their two polar bodies give them a safety pin–like appearance. Plasma cells are common, and the infiltrate also includes scattered microabscesses composed of neutrophils. Lymphocytes are notably scarce.[43]

PATHOGENESIS AND ETIOLOGY

McLeod[44] first recognized granuloma inguinale as a distinct disease in 1882 in southeast India. In 1905, Donovan described the intracellular inclusions (Donovan bodies) that represent the presumed causative organism within histiocytes.[45] C. granulomatis is a small (1 to 1.5 mm $\times$ 0.5 to 0.7 mm) gram-negative pleomorphic bacillus with a characteristic safety-pin appearance due to bipolar condensations of chromatin.[33] The organism was first isolated by Anderson in 1942 in the yolk sacs of chick embryos.[31] Fourteen isolates were subsequently reported, the last in 1962.

C. granulomatis has not been successfully grown on conventional solid media; thus, culture is rarely performed. As a result, this organism has been poorly characterized. It shares some antigenic specificity with both Klebsiella rhinoscleromatis and certain Enterobacteriaceae. Disease has reportedly been reproduced in humans by direct intradermal inoculation of lesional exudate or tissue, but inoculation of culture material has failed to produce experimental infection in both animals and humans.[33] Therefore, Koch's postulates have not been entirely satisfied.

DIAGNOSIS AND DIFFERENTIAL DIAGNOSIS

Morphologic diagnosis of genital ulcerative disease, including granuloma inguinale, is often inaccurate. The differential diagnosis includes primary and secondary syphilis, penile carcinoma, and chancroid (see Table 110–1). Condyloma acuminatum and anogenital amebiasis may also mimic granuloma inguinale. The pitfalls associated with morphologic diagnosis are highlighted by the fact that 30% to 45% of patients with granuloma inguinale also have positive syphilis serology.[38, 46] The existence of several variants of granuloma inguinale further complicates matters.

As a result, diagnosis is based on characteristic clinical appearance in conjunction with supportive laboratory findings. Since cultural isolation is not practical, the definitive diagnosis is established by direct visualization of the causative bacteria (Donovan bodies) within histiocytes in either crush preparations or biopsy specimens stained with Giemsa, Wright, Leishman, or Warthin-Starry silver stain. Hematoxylin-eosin is not recommended because it does not demonstrate the organisms well.[17]

Crush preparations are most often used. After cleaning the lesion with saline, tissue is removed from the leading edge of the ulcer using a scalpel, forceps, scissor, or punch biopsy. The deep portion of the moist specimen should be crushed between two slides immediately to avoid desiccation, which may lower yield owing to rupture of histiocytes.[31] The impression is then air dried and stained. O'Farrell and associates[47] have described a simpler, more rapid diagnostic stain that may be effective.[47] Specimens are obtained using cotton swabs and processed by a 1-minute rapid differentiation staining technique using eosin and thiasine dyes.

Routinely processed biopsy specimens stained with Giemsa or Warthin-Starry stains are also diagnostic in over 95% of cases.[48] Biopsy is preferred to crush preparation when the number of C. granulomatis organisms is likely to be low, as in very early, very sclerotic, or superinfected lesions.[31] Semi-thin sections cut from plastic-embedded tissue blocks and stained with toluidine blue provide the best results, and the added expense and time may be justified in diagnostically difficult cases.[49] Several complement fixation studies and skin tests with promising sensitivities and specificities have been reported, but none have yet become established diagnostic tools.[50-53] The frequent coexistence of syphilis with granuloma inguinale mandates screening for the former with darkfield examination and serologic testing.

TREATMENT

Treatment recommendations are based on empiric observations since in vitro antibiotic sensitivity testing of C. granulomatis has not been done. Granuloma inguinale apparently responds best to lipid-soluble antibiotics that achieve a high intracellular concentration and are effective against gram-negative bacilli.[31] Therapy is typically continued for 2 to 3 weeks or until healing is complete.[1]

The antibiotic of choice is tetracycline, 500 mg orally four times a day (see Table 110–2).[25, 26] This agent is generally quite effective, but resistance has been reported both in the United States and overseas.[37] However, this drug is still considered first-line therapy because it is inexpensive, relatively safe, and convenient. Minocycline has been successfully used to treat small numbers of patients, but it does not seem to offer any therapeutic advantage over tetracycline and is more expensive.[33]

Streptomycin, 20 to 30 g intramuscularly over 5 to 10 days, has been extensively employed in the past. However, it is now rarely used in the United States because of its association with multiple injections, potential ototoxicity, and a 9% failure rate.[25, 33] Chloramphenicol, 500 mg orally every 8 hours, has proven efficacy with a failure rate of only 2%, but it is also unpopular because of the potential for fatal blood dyscrasias, including aplastic anemia.[33]

A promising alternative regimen is oral trimethoprim-sulfamethoxazole, 160 mg/800 mg twice daily.[25] This agent was first used to treat granuloma inguinale in India in 1962, and both short- and long-term cure rates were confirmed in later studies.[54, 55] In an outbreak of disease in Houston in 1982–1983, this drug resulted in cure within 2 to 4 weeks in 19 of 19 patients, including 6 who had failed to respond to tetracycline. Side effects were limited to mild nausea, and no relapse occurred in up to 4 months of follow-up.[37]

Second-line antibiotics include erythromycin, lincomycin, and sodium methicillin.[1, 25, 33] Each has been successfully used in small numbers of patients. Erythromycin or other macrolides should be used to treat disease in pregnant patients, in whom tetracycline, chloramphenicol, and streptomycin are contraindicated and sulfonamides relatively prohibited.[33] Lesions may be less responsive to therapy in pregnancy. Norfloxacin has been used in India to successfully treat granuloma inguinale,[56] and it is likely that other quinolone antibiotics (ciprofloxacin, ofloxacin) would be efficacious.

Surgery may be necessary in the presence of complications such as strictures, fistulae, pelvic abscess, or elephantiasis. Granuloma inguinale is reportedly less responsive to therapy in patients co-infected with HIV.[57] HIV testing should be done on all patients with granuloma inguinale.

Lymphogranuloma Venereum

DEFINITION

Lymphogranuloma venereum is a systemic disease caused by the sexual transmission of specific serotypes of *Chlamydia trachomatis.* It is characterized by prominent lymphatic involvement, and three stages of disease are recognized.

CLINICAL DESCRIPTION

Epidemiology

Lymphogranuloma venereum is a worldwide disease that occurs more commonly in tropical and subtropical climates. It may be endemic in portions of Africa, southeast Asia, India, the Caribbean, and South America. A lack of reliable epidemiologic data makes accurate determination of prevalence and incidence difficult, but lymphogranuloma venereum represented 6% of all STDs reported in Madras, India, from 1968 to 1977.[58] The prevalence in Nigeria was 2% in another study,[59] and Piot and colleagues[60] diagnosed lymphogranuloma venereum in 3% to 10% of males with genital ulcerative disease in South Africa. In the United States, lymphogranuloma venereum is not an officially reportable disease, but the current incidence is estimated to be approximately 600 cases annually.[61] The incidence has been dropping steadily since a peak of 1300 to 2600 cases reported per year from 1941 to 1947.[62]

Clinical Manifestations

Lymphogranuloma venereum is classically divided into three clinical stages. The primary stage is characterized by the appearance of a small (5 to 6 mm), painless genital lesion after an incubation period of 3 to 30 days.[63] This lesion may be a shallow papule, erosion, ulcer, or herpetiform lesion. It may even present as nonspecific urethritis or cervicitis if internally located. Regardless of its form, the primary lesion is transient and goes unnoticed by more than 60% of patients.[58] In men, it is most commonly located on the glans, coronal sulcus, or scrotum or in the urethra. The typical locations in females are the labia, posterior vaginal wall, and cervix. In rare cases, the primary lesion may arise in extragenital areas such as the fingers or tongue. Primary anorectal infection characterized by purulent or bloody diarrhea and tenesmus may occur in men or women who practice receptive anal intercourse.[1] After a few days, the primary lesion typically heals without scarring. On occasion, however, the primary lesion may persist for 2 to 4 weeks.

The second stage, termed the *inguinal syndrome,* usually develops within 2 to 6 weeks of the appearance of the primary lesion, although a range of 10 days to 6 months is reported. This stage is characterized by painful, inflammatory inguinal and femoral lymphadenopathy and bubo formation (Fig. 110–3). The pathognomonic "groove sign" occurs in 15% to 20% of patients as the result of nodal enlargement above and below the inguinal ligament.[58] Constitutional symptoms such as fever, malaise, arthralgias, myalgias, and anorexia are common.[64] Erythema nodosum accompanies lymphogranuloma venereum in 2% to 10% of cases, usually appearing during the second stage.

Necrotic abscesses may develop and rupture, resulting in fistulae. Inflammation can lead to matting of nodes, fibrosis, lymphedema, and eventual elephantiasis. Although most men present with classic second stage disease, only one third of women develop inguinal adenop-

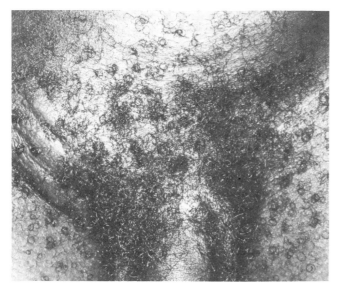

FIGURE 110–3. Massive inguinal lymphadenopathy, outlining the inguinal ligament, is typical of lymphogranuloma venereum.

athy, which is caused by frequent lymphatic drainage to deep iliac and perirectal nodes. Enlargement of these nodes in females may result in lower abdominal or back pain. In the rare cases of initial infection at an extragenital site, lymphadenopathy may present in axillary, supraclavicular, cervical, or submaxillary locations.[63]

The destructive tertiary stage, known as the *genitoanorectal syndrome*, occurs more commonly in females, probably owing to unrecognized and thus untreated second stage disease. Proctocolitis results in fever, pain, tenesmus, and "lymphorrhoids" (due to hyperplasia of perirectal lymphatic tissue). Eventually, perirectal abscesses, ulcerations, fistulae, and rectal strictures may occur. Chronic fibrosis of lymphatics and resultant lymphedema contribute to the development of elephantiasis and esthiomene, which is a hypertrophic enlargement of the labia. Lymphogranuloma venereum can become a chronic, disfiguring disease since increased ulceration and scarring lead to further ischemia and tissue necrosis.[1] Rare systemic complications include aseptic meningitis, conjunctivitis, pneumonia, pericarditis, and arthritis.[65]

Men usually have acute, classic bubonic lymphogranuloma venereum, while women tend to present later in the course of the disease.[63] As a result, later complications such as the anorectal syndrome are reported more frequently in women,[61] and these sequelae may cause women to visit gastroenterology or general medicine clinics rather than STD clinics. In homosexuals, lymphogranuloma venereum is often associated with proctocolitis.[64]

PATHOLOGY

The histopathology of the initial papule is nonspecific. However, microscopic examination of infected lymph nodes may reveal stellate microabscesses that are highly suggestive of lymphogranuloma venereum. The center of

the microabscess is composed primarily of neutrophils and occasional macrophages; epithelioid cells surround the center in a palisade formation. The causative chlamydial organisms are not visualized even by conventional special stains but can be shown by direct immunofluorescence with an antichlamydial antibody.[49]

PATHOGENESIS AND ETIOLOGY

Lymphogranuloma venereum was first described as a distinct clinical entity by Durand, Nicolas, and Favre in 1913.[66] This STD is caused by the L1, L2, and L3 serovars of *C. trachomatis.*[64] These serotypes tend to be much more virulent and invasive than the other 12 *C. trachomatis* immunotypes, which are associated with oculogenital infections limited to mucous membranes. Also, the lymphogranuloma venereum strains infect macrophages instead of the squamocolumnar cells selected by other serotypes.[1] *C. trachomatis* that causes lymphogranuloma venereum may exhibit a greater propensity for lymph node and systemic involvement owing to less specialized host cell receptor requirements.[63]

DIAGNOSIS AND DIFFERENTIAL DIAGNOSIS

Diagnosis is based on characteristic clinical features and appropriate laboratory confirmation. Frei[67] developed a diagnostic skin test in 1925 that was commercially available until 1974. The Frei test typically became positive 2 to 8 weeks after the onset of infection.[1] This test is no longer used because sensitivity was inadequate in early disease and specificity was low because of positive reactions in any chlamydial infection.[68]

Today, laboratory diagnosis most commonly involves serologic testing. The two major assays are the complement fixation (CF) test and the microimmunofluorescence (MIF) test. Of these, the CF test is the recommended assay for general clinical diagnosis of lymphogranuloma venereum.[68] Positive results usually develop within 2 weeks of the onset of infection. In the appropriate clinical setting, a single CF titer of greater than or equal to 1:64 is believed to be diagnostic of lymphogranuloma venereum. As many as 80% of infected patients will have titers greater than or equal to 1:128.[69] Lymphogranuloma venereum may also be diagnosed on the basis of a fourfold increase in titers, but this is generally less useful because most patients are seen after the acute stage. Like the Frei test, the CF test is only genus specific and antibodies to various chlamydial species and serotypes may cross-react. However, CF titers are rarely higher than 1:16 in association with routine chlamydial urethritis, cervicitis, or conjunctivitis.[61, 69]

The MIF test is the most accurate serologic assay because it measures antibodies produced against specific chlamydial serovars. It is also more sensitive than the CF test. However, the MIF test is used only by specialized research laboratories owing to a lack of commercially available reagents.[17]

The "gold standard" of diagnosis is cultural isolation and typing of lymphogranuloma venereum–related *C.*

trachomatis from a fluctuant lymph node.[68] However, culture remains technically difficult and expensive, and the recovery rate from cycloheximide-treated McCoy cells or diethylaminoethyl-treated HeLa cells is less than 50%.[17] Thus, isolation is rarely performed other than in research settings.

Staining with Giemsa, fluorescent antibody, and the immunoperoxidase reaction can be used in an attempt to demonstrate chlamydial organisms. However, specificity is again poor, owing to frequent polymicrobial contamination and an inability to distinguish specific *C. trachomatis* serotypes.[68]

Klotz and coworkers[70] have developed a promising fluorescent monoclonal antibody stain directed at the chlamydial group antigen and the L2 serotype antigen, but this test is not widely available. More recently, investigators have discovered sequence diversity in outer membrane proteins between the trachoma and lymphogranuloma venereum biovars of *C. trachomatis*.[71] Application of this research to the development of monoclonal antibody stains or nucleic acid probes may lead to more specific diagnostic tools.

The differential diagnosis of lymphogranuloma venereum includes other causes of lymphadenopathy and genital ulceration, such as syphilis, herpes simplex, chancroid, and tumor (see Table 110–1). Also, in diagnosing lymphogranuloma venereum, it is important to exclude other concomitant STDs. One study reported the presence of syphilis in as many as one third of patients with lymphogranuloma venereum.[58] Thus, patients should be screened for both syphilis and gonorrhea, as well as encouraged to be screened for HIV infection.

TREATMENT

The current drug of choice for treatment of lymphogranuloma venereum is oral doxycycline, 100 mg twice daily for 21 days (see Table 110–2). A 3-week course of tetracycline, 500 mg four times a day, is also acceptable first-line therapy. Alternatively, erythromycin or sulfisoxazole, both in a dosage of 500 mg four times daily, may be used.[25, 26] Appropriate antimicrobial treatment usually results in rapid resolution of constitutional symptoms.

Buboes typically require several weeks to heal. Fluctuant lymph nodes should be aspirated, and incision and drainage may be needed for abscesses. Disease in patients with HIV infection may be less amenable to therapy.[17] After adequate antimicrobial therapy, late sequelae of lymphogranuloma venereum may require surgery,[72] but results are often less than optimal owing to the extensive fibrosis and compromised local blood supply.[58]

References

1. Buntin DM, Rosen T, Lesher, JL, et al. Sexually transmitted diseases: Bacterial infections. J Am Acad Dermatol 1991;25: 287–299.
2. Boyd AS. Clinical efficacy of antimicrobial therapy in *Haemophilus ducreyi* infections. Arch Dermatol 1989;125:1399–1405.
3. Schmid GP, Sanders LL, Blount JH, et al. Chancroid in the United States: Reestablishment of an old disease. JAMA 1987;258: 3265–3268.
4. Morse SA. Chancroid and *Haemophilus ducreyi*. Clin Microbiol Rev 1989;2:137–157.
5. Ronald T, Plummer FA. Chancroid and granuloma inguinale. Sex Transm Dis 1989;9:535–543.
6. Schulte JM, Martich FA, Schmid GP. Chancroid in the United States, 1981–1990: Evidence for underreporting of cases. MMWR 1992;41:57–61.
7. Piot P, Laga M. Genital ulcers, other sexually transmitted diseases, and the sexual transmission of HIV. Br Med J 1989;298:623–624.
8. Jones CC, Rosen T. Cultural diagnosis of chancroid. Arch Dermatol 1991;127:1823–1827.
9. Jones CC, Rosen T, Clarridge, J, et al. Chancroid: Results from an outbreak in Houston, Texas. South Med J 1990;83:1384–1389.
10. Margolis RJ, Hood AF. Chancroid: Diagnosis and treatment. J Am Acad Dermatol 1982;6:493–499.
11. Albritton WL. Biology of *Haemophilus ducreyi*. Microbiol Rev 1989;53:377–389.
12. Tuffrey M, Abeck D, Alexander F, et al. A mouse model of *Haemophilus ducreyi* infection (chancroid). FEMS Microbiol Lett 1988;50:207–209.
13. Chapel TA, Brown WJ, Jeffries C, et al. How reliable is the morphological diagnosis of penile ulcerations? Sex Transm Dis 1977;4:150–152.
14. Sturm AW, Stolting GJ, Cormane RH, et al. Clinical and microbiological evaluation of 46 episodes of genital ulceration. Genitourin Med 1987;63:98–101.
15. Rosen T. Ulceration of the genitalia. In: Greer KE, eds. Common Problems in Dermatology. Chicago: Year Book Medical Publishers, 1988;384–392.
16. Choudhary BP, Kumari S, Bhati R, et al. Bacteriological study of chancroid. Indian J Med Res 1982;76:379–385.
17. Van Dyck E, Piot P. Laboratory techniques in the investigation of chancroid, lymphogranuloma venereum, and donovanosis. Genitourin Med 1992;68:130–133.
18. Nsanze H, Plummer FA, Maggwa AB, et al. Comparison of media for the primary isolation of *Haemophilus ducreyi*. Sex Transm Dis 1984;11:6–9.
19. Dylewski J, Nsanze H, Maitha G, et al. Laboratory diagnosis of *Haemophilus ducreyi*: Sensitivity of culture media. Diagn Microbiol Infect Dis 1986;4:241–245.
20. Lubwama SW, Plummer FA, Ndinya-Achola J, et al. Isolation and identification of *Haemophilus ducreyi* in a clinical laboratory. J Med Microbiol 1986;22:175–178.
21. Shawer R, Sepulveda J, Clarridge JE. Use of the RapID-ANA system and sodium polyanetholesulfonate disk susceptibility testing in identifying *Haemophilus ducreyi*. J Clin Microbiol 1990;28:108–111.
22. Schalla WO, Sanders LL, Schmid GP, et al. Use of dot-immunobinding and immunofluorescence assays to investigate clinically suspected cases of chancroid. J Infect Dis 1986;153:879–887.
23. Karim QN, Finn GY, Easmon CSF, et al. Rapid detection of *Haemophilus ducreyi* in clinical and experimental infections using monoclonal antibody. Genitourin Med 1989;65:361–365.
24. Parsons LM, Shayegani M, Waring AL, et al. DNA probes for the identification of *Haemophilus ducreyi*. J Clin Microbiol 1989; 27:1441–1445.
25. Abramowicz M, ed. The choice of antibacterial drugs. Med Lett Drugs Ther 1992;34:49–56.
26. Centers for Disease Control. 1989 sexually transmitted disease treatment guidelines. MMWR 1989;33:433–434.
27. Naamara W, Plummer FA, Greenblatt RM, et al. Treatment of chancroid with ciprofloxacin. Am J Med 1987;82(suppl 4):317–320.
28. Bodhidatta L, Taylor DN, Chitwarakorn A, et al. Evaluation of 500- and 1000-mg doses of ciprofloxacin for the treatment of chancroid. Antimicrobiol Agents Chemother 1988;32:723–725.
29. Taylor DN, Pitarangsi C, Echeverria P, et al. Comparative study of ceftriaxone and trimethoprim-sulfamethoxazole for the treatment of chancroid in Thailand. J Infect Dis 1985;152:1002–1006.
30. Plummer FA, Nsanze H, D'Costa LJ, et al. Short-course and single-dose antimicrobial therapy for chancroid in Kenya: Studies with rifampin alone and in combination with trimethoprim. Rev Infect Dis 1983;5(suppl):565–572.

31. Richens J. The diagnosis and treatment of donovanosis (granuloma inguinale). Genitourin Med 1991;67:441–452.
32. Hart G. Donovanosis. In: Holmes KK, Mardh P-A, Sparling PF, et al., eds. Sexually Transmitted Diseases, 2nd ed. New York: McGraw-Hill, 1990:273.
33. Rosen T, Tschen JA. Granuloma inguinale. In: Felman YM, ed. Sexually Transmitted Diseases. New York: Churchill Livingstone, 1986:113–120.
34. Goldberg J. Studies on granuloma inguinale: VII. Some epidemiological considerations of the disease. Br J Vener Dis 1964;40:140.
35. Peck S. Granuloma inguinale. Arch Dermatol 1968;98:555.
36. Lal S, Nicholas C. Epidemiological and clinical features in 165 cases of granuloma inguinale. Br J Vener Dis 1970;46:461.
37. Rosen T, Tschen JA, Ramsdell W, et al. Granuloma inguinale. J Am Acad Dermatol 1984;11:433–437.
38. O'Farrell N, Windsor I, Becker P. Risk factors for HIV-1 amongst STD clinic attenders in Durban, South Africa. Poster presented at the 6th International Conference on AIDS, San Francisco, 20–24 June 1990 (abstract F.C. 604).
39. Goldberg J, Annamunthodo, H. Studies on granuloma inguinale: VIII. Serological reactivity in sera from patients with carcinoma of the penis when tested with Donovania antigens. Br J Vener Dis 1966;42:205.
40. Jofre ME, Webling DD'A, James ST. Granuloma inguinale simulating advanced pelvic cancer. Med J Aust 1976;2:869–873.
41. Pund ER, McInnes GF. Granuloma venereum: A cause of death: Report of six fatal cases. Clinics 1944;3:221–234.
42. Arnell RE, Potekin JS. Granuloma inguinale of the cervix: An analysis of thirty-eight cases. Am J Obstet Gynecol 1940; 39:626–635.
43. Lever WF, Schaumburg-Lever G. Granuloma inguinale (donovanosis). In: Histopathology of the Skin, 7th ed. Philadelphia: JB Lippincott, 1990:341–342.
44. McLeod K. Precis of operations performed on the wards of the first surgeon Medical College Hospital during the year 1881. Indian Med Gaz 1882;17:121.
45. Donovan C. Medical cases from Madras General Hospital. Indian Med Gaz 1905;40:411.
46. Vacca A, MacMillan LL. Anogenital lesions in women in Papua New Guinea. P N G Med J 1982;23:70–73.
47. O'Farrell N, Hoosen AA, Coetzee K, et al. A rapid stain for the diagnosis of granuloma inguinale. Genitourin Med 1990; 66:200–201.
48. Sehgal VN, Shyamprasad AL, Beohart PC. The histopathological diagnosis of donovanosis. Br J Vener Dis 1984;60:45–47.
49. Alacoque B, Cloppe H, Dulmontel C, Moulin G. Histological, immunofluorescent, and ultrastructural features of lymphogranuloma venereum: A case report. Br J Vener Dis 1984;60:390–305.
50. Dunham W, Rake G. Cultural and serologic studies on granuloma inguinale. Am J Syphilis 1948;32:145–149.
51. Goldberg J, Weaver RH, Packer H, et al. Studies on granuloma inguinale: II. The complement fixation test in the diagnosis of granuloma inguinale. Am J Syphilis 1953;37:71–76.
52. Kornblith BA. An intradermal reaction as an aid in the diagnosis of granuloma inguinale. NY State J Med 1944;44:2476–2478.
53. Chen CH, Dienst RB, Greenblatt RB. Skin reaction of patients to Donovania granulomatis. Am J Syphilis 1949;33:60–64.
54. Garg BR, Lal S, Sivamani S. Efficacy of co-trimoxazole in donovanosis: A preliminary report. Br J Vener Dis 1978;54:348.
55. Lal S, Garg BR. Further evidence of the efficacy of co-trimoxazole in granuloma venereum. Br J Vener Dis 1980;56:412.
56. Ramanan C, Sarma PSA, Ghorpade A, et al. Treatment of donovanosis with norfloxacin. Int J Dermatol 1990;29:298–299.
57. Jardim ML, Barros ER, Silveira M. Donovanose em pacientes portadores de AIDS: Relato de dois casos. Anais Brasileiros Dermatol Sifil 1990;65:175–177.
58. Schachter J, Osoba AO. Lymphogranuloma venereum. Br Med Bull 1983;39:151.
59. Osoba AO. Lymphogranuloma venereum. In: Holmes KK, Mardh P-A. International Perspectives on Neglected Sexually Transmitted Diseases. New York: McGraw-Hill, 1983:193.
60. Piot P, Ballard RC, Fehler HG, et al. Isolation of Chlamydia trachomatis from genital ulceration in southern Africa. In: Mardh P-A, Holmes KK, Oriel SD, eds. Chlamydial Infections. Amsterdam: Elsevier Biomedical Press, 1982:115.
61. Perine PL, Osoba AO. Lymphogranuloma venereum. In: Holmes KK, Mardh P-A, Sparling PF, et al., eds. Sexually Transmitted Diseases, 2nd ed. New York: McGraw-Hill, 1990:195–204.
62. Centers for Disease Control: STD Fact Sheet, 35th ed. Atlanta: U.S. Department of Health and Human Services, 1981.
63. Hammerschlag MR. Lymphogranuloma venereum. In: Felman Y, ed. Sexually Transmitted Diseases. New York: Churchill Livingstone, 1986:93–104.
64. Burgoyne RA. Lymphogranuloma venereum. Primary Care 1990;17:153–157.
65. Myhre EB, Mardh P-A. Unusual manifestations of Chlamydia trachomatis infections. Scand J Infect Dis Suppl 1982;32:122–126.
66. Durand M, Nicolas J, Favre M. Lymphogranuomatose inguinale subaigue d'origine genital probable, peut-être vénérienée. Bull Mem Soc Med Hosp 1913;35:274.
67. Frei W. On the skin test in lymphogranuloma inguinale. J Invest Dermatol 1938:1:367.
68. Barnes RC. Laboratory diagnosis of human chlamydial infections. Clin Microbiol Rev 1989;2:119–136.
69. Treharne JD, Forsey T, Thomas BJ. Chlamydial serology. Br Med Bull 1983;39:194–200.
70. Klotz SA, Drutz DJ, Tam MR, et al. Hemorrhagic proctitis due to lymphogranuloma venereum serogroup L2: Diagnosis by fluorescent monoclonal antibody. N Engl J Med 1983;308:1563–1565.
71. de la Maza LM, Fielder TJ, Carlson EJ, et al. Sequence diversity of the 60-kilodalton protein and of a putative 15-kilodalton protein between the trachoma and lymphogranuloma venereum biovars of Chlamydia trachomatis. Infect Immun 1991;59:1196–1201.
72. Parkash S, Radhakrishna K. Problematic ulcerative lesions in sexually transmitted diseases: Surgical management. Sex Transm Dis 1986;13:127–133.

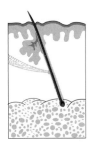

chapter 111

Tuberculous Mycobacterial Infections of the Skin

CAROLINE HIGGINS and RINO CERIO

DEFINITION

The genus *Mycobacterium* contains many members, perhaps its most famous being *M. tuberculosis* and *M. leprae.* The latter is discussed in Chapter 112. Besides these two important human pathogens, the genus also contains a number of nontuberculous mycobacteria (or atypical mycobacteria) that can be pathogenic to humans, as well as a number of harmless commensal organisms.

Mycobacteria are acid-fast, nonmotile, non–spore-forming anaerobic rods. They are usually stained by the Ziehl-Neelsen method. Acid-fastness is a distinguishing feature of this genus not found in any other bacteria of medical significance.

Mycobacterium tuberculosis and *Mycobacterium bovis*

Although five types of tubercle bacilli exist, each is adapted to a different animal host—human, bovine, murine, avian, and cold-blooded. The human type (*M. tuberculosis*) and the bovine type (*M. bovis*) have emerged as being the most important in human disease. These two mycobacteria grow poorly or not at all on ordinary laboratory media and are usually cultured on Löwenstein-Jensen medium, where colonies may take 6 to 8 weeks to grow. *M. tuberculosis* is responsible for most cases of human tuberculosis worldwide, the organism being spread by droplets. In primary tuberculosis there is a single focus of infection in the lung with hilar gland involvement. The infection usually resolves spontaneously and causes no symptoms, although in a few cases the infection can spread to bones, joints, kidneys, or meninges. In postprimary tuberculosis, reinfection by bacilli is usually from an exogenous source, although in some cases reactivation of bacilli present in primary lesions can occur. In postprimary tuberculosis, involvement of the apices of the lungs and regional lymph nodes is common. *M. bovis* is usually conveyed to humans by infected cow's milk and commonly involves the cervical glands, infected through the pharynx, and the abdominal glands, infected from the intestines. Pasteurization of milk has made infection with this organism rare.

Cutaneous Tuberculosis

Tuberculosis of the skin is caused by *M. tuberculosis, M. bovis,* and occasionally the bacillus Calmette-Guérin (BCG), which is an attenuated strain of *M. bovis.* The falling incidence in tuberculosis of the skin in the Western hemisphere over the past 40 years has left a generation of dermatologists unfamiliar with this treatable condition. Although developing countries have also seen a fall in the incidence of cutaneous tuberculosis, a survey from India in 1987 revealed that only 0.15% of all outpatient visits for skin disease were due to cutaneous tuberculosis.[1] Widespread immigration and an increasing incidence of tuberculosis among immunosuppressed persons has led to a resurgence of interest in this important condition.

CLINICAL DESCRIPTION

The clinical manifestations of cutaneous tuberculosis are legion, with the clinical presentation being dependent on the source of infection and the immune response of the host. Attempts to systematize the diverse clinical types of cutaneous tuberculosis over the years has led to a number of classifications based on (1) differentiating localized from hematogenous disease,[2] (2) describing the histopathologic forms of the disease and the immunologic state of the patient,[3] and (3) contrasting chronic and labile disease.[4] However, in 1980, Beyt and coworkers[5] devised a straightforward, clinically relevant classification based on the source of the tubercle bacilli. They identified three broad categories of infection: (1) Inoculation of cutaneous mycobacteriosis from an exogenous source, (2) cutaneous mycobacteriosis from an endogenous source, and (3) cutaneous mycobacteriosis from hematogenous spread.

Many would now add a fourth category to this list—the tuberculids.[6] Our modified form of this classification is illustrated in Table 111–1.

Inoculation Tuberculosis — Exogenous Source

Included in this category are tuberculous chancre, tuberculosis verrucosa cutis (warty tuberculosis), and some cases of lupus vulgaris.

Tuberculous Chancre

A chancre occurs after the inoculation of *M. tuberculosis* into the skin of a patient with no previous exposure to mycobacteria and is now a very rare form of primary tuberculosis, with most reported cases occurring in children.[5] The skin presents a formidable barrier to *M. tuberculosis* and normally requires injury before inoculation can take place. The type of injury reported is variable, and tuberculous chancres have followed circumcision,[5] tattooing,[7] and mouth-to-mouth resuscitation.[8] Clinically, multiplication of the organism at the site of inoculation leads to a brown papule or ulcer[6] with a hemorrhagic base. Lymphadenopathy usually occurs 3 to 6 weeks after inoculation. Most ulcers heal spontaneously, albeit slowly. Rarely the chancre may proceed to lupus vulgaris[6] or miliary tuberculosis.[5] The adenopathy eventually resolves, although it is not uncommon for nodes to calcify 2 to 3 years later.[9]

Warty Tuberculosis (Tuberculosis Verrucosa Cutis)

This is a form of cutaneous tuberculosis that results from the inoculation of *M. tuberculosis* in a person who has been previously sensitized to the organism. Like primary inoculation, a minor wound is often the site of entry. In most cases, the source of the tubercle bacilli is exogenous and many of the reported cases occur in pathologists and postmortem attendants—hence the expression "prosecutor's warts." Inoculation can, however, occur from a patient's own sputum.[10] Clinically, there is usually a single, slow-growing hyperkeratotic plaque (Fig. 111–1), although larger tumor-like lesions have been reported.[11] These lesions tend to occur on the hands of European adults but are more common on the lower extremities of Asian children.[12] Lymphadenopathy is rare. There are scanty acid-fast bacilli in the lesions, and results of cultures are often negative. Histologic features include epidermal hyperkeratosis, pseudoepitheliomatous hyperplasia, and dermal epithelioid cell granulomas with some necrosis, neutrophils, lymphocytes, and occasional giant cells. The course is usually slowly progressive,[13] although lesions may remain static for years and spontaneous remission can occur.

Cutaneous Tuberculosis from an Endogenous Source

Scrofuloderma

Scrofuloderma occurs when there is contiguous spread from an endogenous source, with breakdown of the overlying skin. Although the endogenous source is usually a lymph node (commonly cervical), tuberculosis of bones and joints and tuberculous epididymitis may produce the same effect. All age groups may be affected, but

TABLE 111–1. Classification of Cutaneous Tuberculosis

Inoculation tuberculosis

Tuberculous chancre
Warty tuberculosis
Lupus vulgaris

Tuberculosis from endogenous source

Scrofuloderma
Orificial tuberculosis

Hematogenous tuberculosis

Acute miliary tuberculosis
Lupus vulgaris
Metastatic tuberculous abscess and ulcer

Tuberculids

Lichen scrofulosorum
Papulonecrotic tuberculid
Erythema induratum

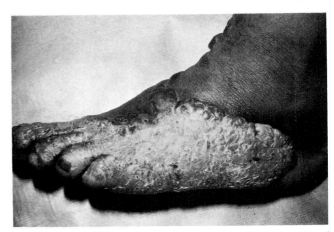

FIGURE 111–1. Warty tuberculosis on the foot. (Courtesy of Prof. E. Wilson-Jones.)

scrofuloderma is more common in children. Lesions develop as subcutaneous bluish-red nodules overlying the infected focus. These nodules then break down and perforate, leaving undermined ulcers and discharging sinuses.[13] Eventually, scarring occurs, which may be extensive, with fibrous masses coexisting with boggy discharging nodules.[6] Histologically, the peripheral areas of the abscesses or sinuses contain caseating granulomas and *M. tuberculosis* can be identified in these sections.[13] Tuberculin sensitivity is high.

Orificial Tuberculosis

Orificial tuberculosis is a rare condition that describes tuberculosis of the mucous membranes and skin surrounding orifices in patients with tuberculosis of internal organs (usually of the gastrointestinal tract, lungs, or occasionally the genitourinary tract). The disease is usually caused by autoinoculation, with mycobacteria being shed in large numbers from internal organs and subsequently being inoculated into the mucous membranes and the skin surrounding orifices. Lymphatic and hematogenous spread around orifices may also occur, and rarely exogenous sources of mycobacteria can cause this clinical picture.[14] Histopathology is variable and often shows a nonspecific inflammatory mixed mononuclear infiltrate, but caseation necrosis can be seen deep in the dermis and tubercle bacilli are easily demonstrated. The mouth is the most commonly affected site, particularly the tongue and both soft and hard palates. Anal and vulvar lesions can also occur. Lesions characteristically develop as a painful red nodule that subsequently ulcerates to form a punched-out ulcer. Most patients show a positive tuberculin reaction, although anergy may develop at a later stage. Since many of these patients have advanced internal disease, the prognosis is poor and these lesions tend to progress.

Hematogenous Tuberculosis

Cutaneous tuberculosis from hematogenous spread includes miliary tuberculosis, lupus vulgaris, and metastatic tuberculous ulcers.

Acute Miliary Tuberculosis of the Skin

This rare skin condition is caused by hematogenous dissemination of mycobacteria and is traditionally described in infants and young children. The mean age of affected patients does seem to be rising, however,[15] and this type of tuberculosis may emerge as a problem in immunosuppressed patients. The focus of infection is usually meningeal or pulmonary,[13] although in some cases a focus is not found.[15] The clinical features are variable, with crops of nodules,[15, 16] papules, vesicles, and pustules being described, usually in severely ill patients. Tuberculin test is usually negative. Mycobacteria are usually present in large numbers in the skin biopsy specimen. The outlook is usually poor in children, although a good response to chemotherapy has been reported in some adult patients.[15]

Lupus Vulgaris

Lupus vulgaris is a chronic, progressive form of cutaneous tuberculosis occurring in previously sensitized individuals. The most common form of cutaneous tuberculosis, it occurs almost exclusively on the head and neck and is reported as being more common in females (female-to-male ratio ranging from 2:1 to 3:1).[17] Immunity is thought to be only moderate in patients with lupus vulgaris, since lesions progress steadily and healing without therapy is rare.[13] The pathogenesis of lupus vulgaris is multifactorial. It originates from a tuberculous focus elsewhere and can arise by direct extension from underlying glands (often cervical), by lymphatic spread from the mucous membranes of the nose or throat,[18] by hematogenous dissemination, or rarely by direct inoculation or BCG vaccination.[19] Pulmonary tuberculosis and cervical adenitis are the most common underlying foci of infection.[13] Isolation of tubercle bacilli from the lesions is usually difficult. Clinically, the typical soft, brown plaque-like lesions usually start on the nose or cheek and gradually spread. Involvement of the limbs and trunk is much less common. Lesions are usually solitary. On diascopy, the characteristic "apple jelly" nodules are seen. Variations in this typical appearance include ulcerating, vegetating, tumor-like, papular and nodular forms. Mucous membrane involvement of the mouth, nose, and conjunctiva may occur and destruction of the nasal septum has been reported. Although lupus vulgaris is a slowly extending, chronic condition, progression is inevitable and relentless, and marked disfiguration may occur. Perhaps the most serious complication is the development of malignancy, with squamous cell carcinomas being far more common than basal cell carcinomas in this respect (Fig. 111–2; see color plate). Standard antituberculous chemotherapy should be given.

Metastatic Tuberculous Ulcer

Hematogenous dissemination from a primary focus may occur, leading to a distant subcutaneous abscess that may ulcerate. Tubercle bacilli may sometimes be isolated from these lesions (Fig. 111–3).

The Tuberculids

This category includes lichen scrofulosorum, papulonecrotic tuberculid, and erythema induratum of Bazin. Over the years the association of these clinical entities with *M. tuberculosis* infection has been the subject of much debate. It is now agreed that the tuberculids occur as the result of hematogenous dissemination of the tubercle bacilli in patients with a high degree of immunity. The presence of mycobacterial DNA in lesional skin has actually been demonstrated in papulonecrotic tuberculid[20] and erythema induratum of Bazin[21] using the polymerase chain reaction. The underlying focus of infection is, however, not always apparent clinically, and some patients are not aware that they have been previously infected with the bacterium. Changes in the immunologic status of the patient, stasis, skin temperature, and

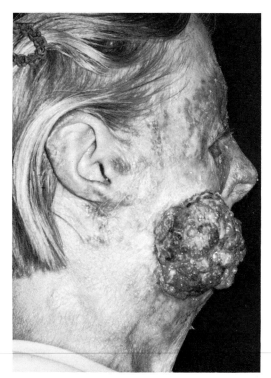

FIGURE 111-2. Long-standing lupus vulgaris with squamous cell carcinoma arising from cheek. (See color plate.)

blood supply seen to affect the development of the eruptions.[6] The tuberculids are united in having a rapid response to antituberculous chemotherapy, a strongly positive tuberculin test, and a striking absence of tubercle bacilli in biopsy specimens, taken from affected areas of skin.

Lichen Scrofulosorum

Lichen scrofulosorum is a rare eruption of asymptomatic, flat-topped, yellow to pink papules occurring most often on the skin of the trunk of patients with tuberculosis in lymph nodes and or bone.[22, 23] These lesions can develop into discoid plaques that may last for months but eventually resolve slowly. Treatment with chemotherapy causes rapid resolution.[24]

Papulonecrotic Tuberculid

Papulonecrotic tuberculid is characterized by symmetrical, necrotic papules that occur in showers over the extremities (Fig. 111-4). Occasionally, they may form chronic, ulcerating lesions that may persist for several months.[25] The lesions are usually asymptomatic and are generally more common in young adults.[26] As with all tuberculids, tubercle bacilli are not found in skin biopsy specimens, tuberculin sensitivity is high, and a good response to antituberculous chemotherapy is noted. The extracutaneous source of the tubercle bacilli is not always found.[25]

Erythema Induratum of Bazin

The typical clinical features of this tuberculid include dusky-red tender nodules, usually occurring on the lower legs in middle-aged women (Fig. 111-5; see color plate). These nodules tend to be persistent or recurrent and heal with scarring. Ulceration is not uncommon. In one large

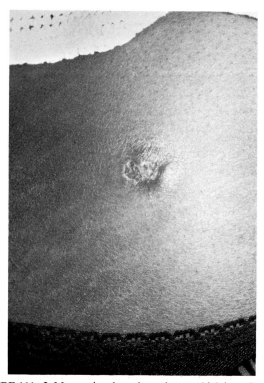

FIGURE 111-3. Metastatic tuberculous ulcer on thigh in patient with hematogenous spread of tubercle bacilli.

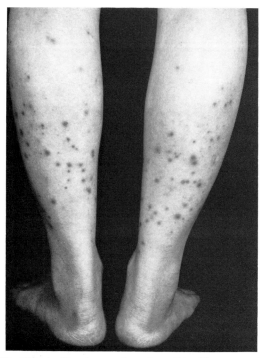

FIGURE 111-4. Papulonecrotic tuberculid. (Courtesy of Prof. E. Wilson-Jones.)

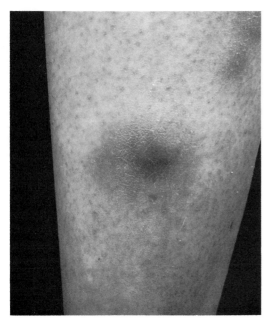

FIGURE 111–5. Erythema induratum of Bazin on the calf. (See color plate.)

series of 26 patients with erythema induratum,[27] only two fifths of the patients had a personal or family history of active tuberculosis, but all of the patients in this series had a strongly positive tuberculin test and clearing of lesions after antituberculous therapy, suggesting a latent tuberculous focus as the cause of these skin lesions. Tubercle bacilli are never found in skin lesions, but in one study[28] it was found that the infiltrating cells in skin biopsy specimens from patients with this disease were predominantly T lymphocytes, suggesting that erythema induratum may be due to a T-cell–mediated immune response to a tuberculous antigen. Erythema nodosum is also a nodular eruption occurring on the lower legs. However, ulceration and scarring do not occur. Primary tuberculosis can rarely produce this reaction, which is thought to be immune complex mediated.

There are a large number of conditions that were previously thought to be tuberculous in origin, based mainly on a granulomatous picture on histology. These include Lewandowsky's rosacea-like eruption and acne agminata (previously called lupus miliaris disseminatus faciei or acnitis). In Lewandowsky's rosacea-like eruption, small red-blue papules occur on the cheeks and forehead with an erythematous background. This is now accepted as representing a micropapular form of rosacea, with a tuberculoid pathology but no response to antituberculous chemotherapy. Similarly, the link of acne agminata with tuberculosis is purely historical. Clinically, this presents in young adults of both sexes as brown papules involving the central portion of the face. Although tuberculoid follicles with central caseation may be seen in the dermis,[6] mycobacteria are never isolated and there is no response to antituberculous chemotherapy. This condition tends to resolve spontaneously.

DIAGNOSIS AND DIFFERENTIAL DIAGNOSIS

Perhaps the most important facet to making a diagnosis of cutaneous tuberculosis is a high index of clinical suspicion. This can be particularly important with the tuberculids, where active tuberculosis elsewhere may not be obvious.

The tuberculin test is used to detect those persons previously infected with tubercle bacilli either by inoculation or invasion. The basis of the tuberculin reaction is a delayed hypersensitivity to tuberculous proteins. Purified protein derivative (PPD) of *M. tuberculosis* is injected intradermally using one of two techniques, either the Mantoux test or the Heaf test. The Mantoux test has the advantage of being able to inoculate various strengths of PPD from 1 to 100 tuberculin units. The test is read 48 hours later, and the degree of induration is noted. Induratum of more than 10 mm suggests previous exposure to tuberculosis. The Heaf test is more useful for mass screening; multiple (six) punctures of PPD are inoculated into the forearm in a circular distribution, and the reaction to this noted after 48 hours. The following grading system is used for Heaf testing:

Grade I: four to six papules
Grade II: complete circle of induration
Grade III: plaque of 12-mm induration
Grade IV: presence of vesiculation or ulceration

Although grade I and II reactions may indicate previous vaccination, grade III and IV reactions indicate past or present tuberculosis.

The tuberculin test, however, is not entirely specific for *M. tuberculosis*. Small, nonspecific reactions may occur, probably due to infection with nontuberculous mycobacteria.

Demonstration of acid-fast bacilli in the lesion remains the only available way to confirm the diagnosis with certainty. This can be achieved by the following:

1. Microscopy. Skin sections can be stained by the Ziehl-Neelsen or auramine methods and examined for acid-fast bacilli. This can provide a rapid diagnosis, allowing early treatment.
2. Culture. Skin biopsy specimens should always be submitted for culture since this provides a definitive diagnosis if they are positive. Culture may take up to 8 weeks but it has the advantage over microscopy of allowing identification of bacterial species and can determine what drug will be effective.
3. Polymerase chain reaction (PCR). This technique may be useful in amplifying mycobacterial DNA sequences and act as an aid to diagnosis.[29] PCR has been used to identify *M. tuberculosis* DNA in skin biopsy specimens in a patient with long-standing lupus vulgaris[30] and scrofuloderma,[31] as well as papulonecrotic tuberculid[20] and erythema induratum of Bazin.[21]

The histopathology of cutaneous tuberculosis varies depending on the classification and the balance between infection and immunologic response. In the tuberculous chancre an acute necrotic neutrophilic reaction changes to a mononuclear infiltrate and, after 4 to 6 weeks, into typical tubercles in which bacilli can no longer be identi-

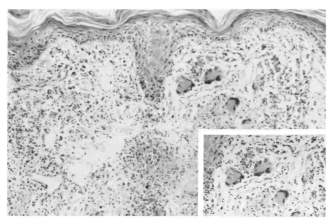

FIGURE 111-6. Lupus vulgaris. There is a mixed chronic inflammatory cell infiltrate with prominent Langhans' giant cells (hematoxylin-eosin, ×250).

TABLE 111-3. Differential Diagnosis of Tuberculosis

Type of Tuberculosis	Important Differential Diagnoses
Tuberculous chancre	Primary chancre Cat-scratch fever Tularemia Sporotrichosis Actinomycosis
Warty tuberculosis	Warts or keratoses Hypertrophic lichen planus Blastomycosis Chromoblastomycosis
Lupus vulgaris	Discoid lupus erythematosus Sarcoidosis Lymphocytoma Tertiary syphilis Deep mycoses
Scrofuloderma	Syphilitic gumma Sporotrichosis Actinomycosis Severe acne conglobata
Orificial tuberculosis	Syphilis Aphthous ulcers Squamous cell carcinoma
Metastatic tuberculous ulcer	Sporotrichosis
Lichen scrofuloderma	Lichen planus Lichen nitidus Micropapular sarcoidosis Eczema
Papulonecrotic tuberculid	Pityriasis lichenoides et varioliformis acuta
Erythema induratum	Nodular vasculitis

fied. A typical mature tubercle consists of epithelioid cells surrounded by a wall of mononuclear cells. A few Langhans' giant cells may be present among the epithelioid cells (Fig. 111-6). The center of the tubercle undergoes caseation necrosis and may calcify. These typical tubercles do not always form, however, and sparse collections of epithelioid cells within an inflammatory infiltrate without necrosis or giant cells can occur. In miliary and orificial forms the characteristic tubercle does not form or is imperfect. Bacilli are numerous. In scrofuloderma the skin is destroyed by nonspecific abscess formation and ulceration. Typical tubercle formation at the periphery can occur. In verrucous tuberculosis, typical dermal changes are missing but there is verrucous epidermal hyperplasia and hyperkeratosis. The histopathologic features of lupus vulgaris can be variable. Although typical tubercles are often present in the dermis, the extent of the mononuclear infiltrate varies and when extensive can cause diagnostic difficulties. Healing with intense fibrosis may also cause diagnostic difficulties. Squamous cell carcinoma may arise in long-standing lesions. These histologic changes are classified in Table 111-2.

Response to antituberculous chemotherapy may also aid in making the diagnosis.

New approaches to allow the rapid and accurate diagnosis of tuberculosis include the measurement in serum of the humoral response to mycobacterial antigens.[32] Although no widespread test is yet available, one study using monoclonal antibodies to an *M. tuberculosis*-specific antigen gave positive results in 70% to 80% of cases of extrapulmonary tuberculosis.[33]

The differential diagnosis of cutaneous tuberculosis is very wide for all types of cutaneous tuberculosis and is summarized in Table 111-3.

TREATMENT

The standard chemotherapy regimen for tuberculosis, as recommended by the Joint Tuberculosis Committee

TABLE 111-2. Histopathology of Cutaneous Tuberculosis

	Primary Inoculation Tuberculosis, Miliary Tuberculosis, Scrofuloderma	Verrucosa Cutis	Lupus Vulgaris
Epidermis	Variable epidermal ulceration	Hyperkeratosis, acanthosis, and papillomatosis (which may be pseudoepitheliomatous)	Atrophy, hyperplasia, or ulceration
Dermal	Diffuse and mixed with many neutrophils and variable granulomatous component later	Neutrophilic microabscesses in epidermis; diffuse polymorphonuclear lymphocytes in upper dermis	Tuberculoid granuloma often at periphery and upper dermis with caseation necrosis and Langhans'-type giant cells
Acid-Fast	+++ seen on Ziehl-Neelsen stain	+ sometimes present	Cannot be demonstrated

of the British Thoracic Society,[34] is a 2-month regimen of four drugs: isoniazid, rifampicin, pyrazinamide, and ethambutol. This is followed by rifampicin and isoniazid for an additional 4 months. The American Thoracic Society recommends the same regimen.

1. Isoniazid. This is the most effective bactericidal drug, the usual dose being 300 mg daily. Its main side effect is peripheral neuropathy, which can be prevented by taking pyridoxine, 10 mg daily. This regimen is recommended in those at risk of neuropathy (i.e., patients with alcoholism, diabetes, or renal failure). Hepatitis can also occur.

2. Rifampicin. This drug is particularly important in preventing the emergence of resistance to other drugs. Recommended daily doses are 450 mg if the patient weighs less than 50 kg and 600 mg if the patient weighs more than 50 kg. It is not uncommon for the serum transaminase levels to be elevated during treatment. This is not in itself an indication to stop treatment unless further liver damage ensues. Gastrointestinal upsets may also occur, and patients must be warned that urine, sweat, and tears may be colored orange.

3. Pyrazinamide. Dosage depends on the patient's weight: 1.5 g daily if weighing less than 50 kg, 2.0 g daily if weighing between 50 and 74 kg, and 2.5 kg daily if weighing more than 75 kg. Side effects include rash, nausea, anorexia, vomiting, and raised serum uric acid levels. This last effect may be overcome by intermittent dosing.

4. Ethambutol. Recommended dose is 15 mg/kg daily. This drug can be complicated by a dose-related optic neuropathy. Patients should be warned to stop the drug immediately if any visual symptoms occur. This drug should be avoided in patients in renal failure.

It is now generally accepted that this regimen should be employed for all cases of cutaneous tuberculosis, and in drug-susceptible tuberculosis a cure rate of more than 95% can be expected. Other methods that can also be used include surgery. Small lesions of lupus vulgaris and warty tuberculosis can be excised, and reconstructive surgery can be helpful in the disfigurement caused by lupus vulgaris.[6] The therapy for all types of cutaneous mycobacteriosis is summarized in Table 111–4.

Drug-Resistant Tuberculosis

Strains of *M. tuberculosis* that are resistant to standard antituberculous chemotherapy are emerging. This resistance is promoted by poor compliance with therapy and the incorrect use of single antituberculous agents. Drug-resistant tuberculosis seems to particularly occur in patients affected with the human immunodeficiency virus[35, 36] and has the ability to spread by nosocomial transmission.[37]

Atypical Mycobacteria

These mycobacteria form a heterogeneous group, and the epidemiology of infections caused by these pathogens

◀ TABLE 111–4. Treatment of Common Cutaneous Mycobacterial Infections

Type of Mycobacteria	Treatment
Mycobacterium tuberculosis	Two months of 4 drugs: isoniazid, rifampicin, pyrazinamide and ethambutol; followed by rifampicin and ethambutol for 4 months
Mycobacterium marinum	Combinations of rifampicin and ethambutol or sulfamethoxazole plus trimethoprim have proved successful; minocycline as a single agent also suggested
Mycobacterium ulcerans	Surgery is treatment of choice; drug therapy disappointing
Mycobacterium kansasii	Standard tuberculous chemotherapy: isoniazid, rifampicin, streptomycin, and ethambutol; minocycline may also be helpful
Mycobacterium avium complex	Not very responsive to standard chemotherapy; surgical treatment most effective for localized disease
Mycobacterium fortuitum complex (including *M. chelonei*)	Amikacin or doxycycline in either infection; erythromycin and tobramycin in *M. chelonei* infections, ciprofloxacin or sulfamethoxazole in *M. fortuitum*

Ultimately, in all of these infections, one needs to be guided by in vitro antibiotic sensitivity studies.

is different from that of tuberculosis. Between 1954 and 1959 Runyon classified these atypical mycobacteria, dividing them into slow-growing and fast-growing groups.[38] The slow growers were further subdivided according to their ability to form pigment on exposure to light, giving the groups listed in Table 111–5. Cutaneous lesions are usually caused by *M. marinum* and *M. ulcerans*.

TABLE 111–5. Atypical Mycobacteria

Group I Photochromogens, able to form pigment on exposure to light:
    M. marinum
    M. kansasii
    M. simiae
Group II Scotochromogens, able to form pigment without exposure to light:
    M. scrofulaceum
    M. szulgai
Group III Normochromogens:
    M. ulcerans
    M. xenopi
    M. avium-intracellulare
Group IV Rapid growers:
    M. fortuitum complex

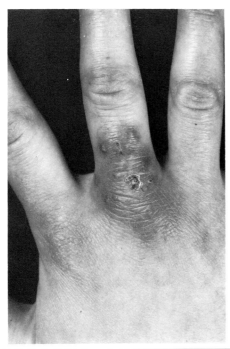

FIGURE 111–7. *Mycobacterium marinum* infection in a tropical fish breeder.

Mycobacterium marinum Infection

This atypical mycobacterium grows mainly in water that is not often replenished, and therefore human infection usually occurs from swimming pools and fish tanks, hence the often used terms *swimming pool granuloma* or *fish tank granuloma* to describe these lesions. Clinically, the usual presentation is of a single nodule or pustule, usually on the hands in fish-keepers and at the sites of trauma in other cases. These nodules may ulcerate and suppurate.[39] In many cases these nodules can spread along the line of lymphatic vessels, called sporotrichoid spread (Figs. 111–7 and 111–8; see color plates). The diagnosis may be missed, since acid-fast bacilli are often

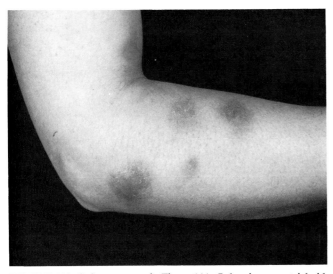

FIGURE 111–8. Same case as in Figure 111–7 showing sporotrichoid spread along the forearm. (See color plate.)

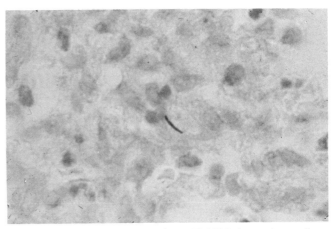

FIGURE 111–9. Skin biopsy specimen. Ziehl-Neelsen stain reveals an isolated acid-fast bacillus. (See color plate.)

scanty (Fig. 111–9; see color plate) and may not be seen on microscopy of affected skin. Also, *M. marinum* grows best on culture media at low temperatures (25°C to 32°C). Therefore, samples cultured at 37°C, the usual temperature used for culturing mycobacteria, may yield no growth and lead to a delay in diagnosis. Lesions may spontaneously resolve, but this can take months.[40] Three drug regimens have proved successful in treatment: (1) rifampicin and ethambutol, (2) tetracyclines, and (3) sulfamethoxazole plus trimethoprim. Many clinicians now recommend minocycline (or doxycycline) 200 mg daily, as the drug of choice.[41] Treatment may be necessary for several weeks.[42]

Mycobacterium ulcerans Infection

M. ulcerans generally occurs in subequatorial regions, with cases clustered in the Nile bed areas of Uganda. Like *M. marinum*, it grows best below body temperature at 32°C to 33°C. This property of growth at low temperatures probably accounts for the fact that both of these mycobacteria only affect the skin of humans; they are unable to survive warmer, core temperatures. Most cases in Africa are in children, in the 5- to 15-year-old age group.[43] Most patients present with a solitary nodule that will ulcerate in many cases to form a crater with typical undermined edges. Lesions are usually on the arms and legs. Healing may occur after 6 to 9 months,[6] but some cases may extend widely to involve an entire limb.[43] Histology shows acute necrosis of dermis and fat; a septate panniculitis is typical.[6] Mycobacteria can be seen in clumps in the fatty septa.

M. ulcerans is sensitive to a number of drugs, including rifampicin in vitro.[43] Drug therapy, however, remains disappointing, and surgery to excise the diseased tissue is the treatment of choice.

Other Mycobacteria in Skin Disease

Mycobacterium kansasii

This unusual skin pathogen is more commonly associated with pulmonary disease in middle-aged men. The clinical features of *M. kansasii* skin lesions are variable, verrucous nodules with sporotrichoid spread, papulopustules, and crusted ulcerations.[43] In the same study it was noted that three of the eight patients reported were immunosuppressed. Standard antituberculous chemotherapy (including isoniazid, rifampicin, streptomycin, and ethambutol) has been used with success.[44] Minocycline has also been reported as healing lesions,[40] although ultimately one has to be guided by in vitro sensitivity test results.

Mycobacterium scrofulaceum

This slow-growing mycobacterium can occasionally cause skin abscesses.[46]

Mycobacterium avium Complex

This organism commonly infects the lungs and lymph nodes. A variety of cutaneous lesions, including papules and ulcers, can occur secondary to hematogenous dissemination.[47] This picture is particularly common in patients with the acquired immunodeficiency syndrome. Skin lesions following direct inoculation can occur but are rare.[6] If possible, surgical treatment is the most effective, since the organism is not very responsive to chemotherapy.[13] Obviously, with disseminated disease surgery is not possible and a combination of antituberculous chemotherapy will need to be tried.

Mycobacterium fortuitum Complex

This complex includes *M. chelonei*. Organisms are both widely distributed and rapid growers, which most commonly causes abscesses after injections or surgical procedures. Typical lesions show a red, painful node at the site of injection, with subsequent abscess formation. Standard antituberculous chemotherapy is not helpful with these organisms. Amikacin or doxycycline may be used in either infections; and while erythromycin and tobramycin are more useful in *M. chelonei* infections, *M. fortuitum* responds better to ciprofloxacin or sulfamethoxazole.[47] Ultimately, the best approach to treatment is to identify the organism and be guided by in vitro antibiotic sensitivity studies.

Acquired Immunodeficiency Syndrome and Mycobacterial Infections

Patients with the acquired immunodeficiency syndrome have a high incidence of mycobacterial infections, and this has led to a resurgence of cases in inner city areas where these patients are clustered.[45] Most of these infections are due to *M. avium* complex, about 10% are due to *M. tuberculosis,* with *M. kansasii* and *M. scrofulosorum* commonly seen.[6] Many of these patients have disseminated disease and can develop cutaneous macules, papules, ulcers, and abscesses in which acid-fast bacilli can be identified.[49] Bacilli are generally abundant. "Histoid" reactions to *M. kansasii*, in which there are dermal nodules of spindled macrophages that are parasitized by bacilli, can be mistaken for spindle cell neoplasms.

References

1. Sehgal VN, Srivastava MD, Khurana VK, et al. An appraisal of epidemiologic, clinical, bacteriological, histopathologic and immunologic parameters in cutaneous tuberculosis. Int J Dermatol 1987;26:521–526.
2. Montgomery H. Histopathology of various types of cutaneous tuberculosis. Arch Dermatol 1937;35:1937.
3. Pinkus H, Mehregan AH. A Guide to Dermatohistopathology, 2nd ed. New York: Appleton-Century-Crofts, 1976:289.
4. Michelson HE, Laymon CW. Classification of tuberculosis of the skin. Arch Dermatol 1945;52:108.
5. Beyt BE, Ortbals DW, Santa Cruz DJ, et al. Cutaneous tuberculosis: Analysis of 34 cases with a new classification of the disease. Medicine 1980;69:95–109.
6. Savin JA. Mycobacterial infections. In: Rook A, Wilkinson DS, Ebling FJG, Champion RH, Burton JL, eds. Textbook of Dermatology, 5th ed, vol II. Oxford: Blackwell Scientific Publications, 1991:1033–1063.
7. Horney DA, Gaither JM, Caurer R, et al. Cutaneous inoculation tuberculosis secondary to jail-house tattooing. Arch Dermatol 1985;121:648–650.
8. Heilman KM, Muschenheim C. Primary cutaneous tuberculosis resulting from mouth to mouth respiration. N Engl J Med 1965;273:1035–1036.
9. Miller FJW, Cashman JM. The natural history of peripheral tuberculosis lymphadenitis associated with a visible primary focus. Lancet 1955;1:1286.
10. Wortman PD. Pulmonary and cutaneous tuberculosis. J Am Acad Dermatol 1992;27:457–460.
11. Iizawa O, Alba S, Tagami H. Tuberculosis verrucosa cutis in a tumour-like form. Br J Dermatol 1991;125:79–80.
12. Wong KO, Lee KP, Chin SF. Tuberculosis of the skin in Hong Kong: A review of 160 cases. Br J Dermatol 1968;80:424–429.
13. Wolff K, Tappeiner G. Mycobacterial diseases: Tuberculosis and atypical mycobacterial infections. In: Fitzpatrick TB, Eisen AZ, Wolff K, Freedburg IM, Austen KF, eds. Dermatology in General Medicine, 3rd ed, vol II. New York: McGraw-Hill, 1987: 2152–2180.
14. Ratcliff DP. Tuberculosis of the mandible. Br Dent J 1973;135: 122–124.
15. Kennedy C, Knowles GK. Miliary tuberculosis presenting with skin lesions. Br Med J 1975;9:356.
16. Kounis NG, Constantinidis K. Unusual tuberculous skin manifestations. Practitioner 1979;222:390–393.
17. Werschler WP, Elgart ML, Williams CM. Progressive asymptomatic annular facial skin lesions. Arch Dermatol 1990;126: 1225–1230.
18. Morrison JGL, Foyrce ED. The papulonecrotic tuberculide. Br J Dermatol 1974;91:263–270.
19. Marcussen PV. Lupus vulgaris following BCG vaccination. Br J Dermatol 1954;66:121.
20. Victor T, Jordann HF, Van Niekerk DJT, et al. Papulonecrotic tuberculid: Identification of *Mycobacterium tuberculosis* DNA by polymerase chain reaction. Am J Dermatopathol 1992;14: 491–495.
21. Degitz K, Messer G, Schirren H, et al. Successful treatment of erythema induratum of Bazin following rapid detection of mycobacterial DNA by polymerase chain reaction. Arch Dermatol 1993;129:1619–1620.
22. Graham-Brown RAC, Sarkany I. Lichen scrofulosorum with tuberculous dactylitis. Br J Dermatol 1980;103:561–564.
23. Hudson PM. Tuberculide (lichen scrofulosorum) secondary to osseous tuberculosis. Clin Exp Dermatol 1976;1:391–394.
24. Smith NP, Ryan TJ, Sanderson KV, et al. Lichen scrofulosorum: A report of four cases. Br J Dermatol 1976;94:319.
25. Wilson-Jones E, Winklemann RW. Papulonecrotic tuberculid: A neglected disease in Western countries. J Am Acad Dermatol 1986;14:815–826.
26. Morrison JGL, Fourie ED. The papulonecrotic tuberculid: From Arthus reaction to lupus vulgaris. Br J Dermatol 1974;91: 263–270.
27. Rademaker M, Lowe DG, Munro DD. Erythema induratum (Bazin's disease). J Am Acad Dermatol 1989;21:740–745.
28. Kuramoto Y, Aiba S, Tagami H. Erythema induratum of Bazin as a type of tuberculid. J Am Acad Dermatol 1990;22:612–616.

29. Penneys NS, Leonardi CL, Cook S, et al. Identification of *Mycobacterium tuberculosis* DNA in five different types of cutaneous lesions by the polymerase chain reaction. Arch Dermatol 1993;129:1594,1618–1620.

30. Sefling U, Pennys N, Leonardi CL. Identification of *Mycobacterium tuberculosis* DNA in a case of lupus vulgaris. J Am Acad Dermatol 1993;28:318–322.

31. Taniguchi S, Chanoki M, Hamada T. Scrofuloderma: The DNA analysis of mycobacteria by the polymerase chain reaction. Arch Dermatol 1993;129:1618–1619.

32. Woodhead M. New approaches to the rapid diagnosis of tuberculosis. Thorax 1992;47:264.

33. Wilkins EGL, Ivanyi J. Potential value of serology for the diagnosis of extrapulmonary tuberculosis. Lancet 1990;336:641–644.

34. Ormerod LP, for a subcommittee of the Joint Tuberculosis Committee. Chemotherapy and management of tuberculosis in the United Kingdom: Recommendations of the Joint Tuberculosis Committee of the British Thoracic Society. Thorax 1990;45:403–408.

35. Edlin BR, Tokars JL, Grieco MH, et al. An outbreak of multidrug-resistant tuberculosis among hospitalised patients with the acquired immunodeficiency syndrome. N Engl J Med 1992;326:1514–1521.

36. Fischl MA, Daikos GL, Uttamchandani RB, et al. Clinical presentation and outcome of patients with HIV infection and tuberculosis caused by multiple-drug–resistant bacilli. Ann Intern Med 1992;117:184–190.

37. Barnes PF, Barrows SA. Tuberculosis in the 1990s. Ann Intern Med 1993;119:400–410.

38. Runyon EH: Pathogenic mycobacteria. Adv Tuberc Res 1965;14:235.

39. Gray SF, Stanwell Smith R, Reynolds NJ, et al. Fish tank granuloma. Br Med J 1990;300:1069–1070.

40. Black MM, Eykyn SJ. The successful treatment of tropical fish tank granuloma (*Mycobacterium marinum*) with co-trimoxazole. Br J Dermatol 1977;97:689–692.

41. Brown JW, Sanders CV. *Mycobacterium marinum* infections: A problem of recognition not therapy (editorial)? Arch Intern Med 1987;147:817–818.

42. Huminer D, Pitlik SD, Block C, et al. Aquarium-borne *Mycobacterium marinum* skin infection. Arch Dermatol 1986;122:698–703.

43. Barker DJP. Mycobacterial skin ulcers. Br J Dermatol 1974;91:473–474.

44. Hanke CW, Temofeew RK, Slama SL. *Mycobacterium kansasii* infection with multiple cutaneous lesions. J Am Acad Dermatol 1987;16:1122–1128.

45. Dore N, Collins JP, Mankiewicz E. A sporotrichoid-like *M. kansasii* infection of the skin treated with minocycline hydrochloride. Br J Dermatol 1979;101:75–79.

46. Murray-Leisure KA, Egan N, Weitecamp MR. Skin lesions caused by *M. scrofulosorum.* Arch Dermatol 1987;123:369–370.

47. Freed JA, Pervez NK, Chen V, et al. Cutaneous mycobacteriosis: Occurrence and significance in two patients with the acquired immunodeficiency syndrome. Arch Dermatol 1987;123:1601–1603.

48. Wallace RJ. The clinical presentation, diagnosis and therapy of cutaneous and pulmonary infections due to the rapidly growing mycobacteria *M. fortuitum* and *M. chelonei.* Clin Chest Med 1989;10:419–429.

49. Reider HL, Canthen GM, Kelly GD, et al. Tuberculosis in the United States. JAMA 1989;262:385–389.

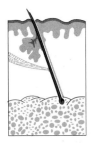

chapter 112

Leprosy

L. MASAE KAWAMURA and ROBERT H. GELBER

DEFINITION

Leprosy, or Hansen's disease, which dates to man's earliest historical records, remains one of the world's major unresolved infectious diseases. This chronic infection of slow onset is caused by the acid-fast bacillus *Mycobacterium leprae*, whose medical sequelae are primarily determined by the unique tropism of the causative organism, among bacteria, for invasion and consequent pathology of the peripheral nervous system and the host's specific immunologic response. *M. leprae* invades the cooler tissues of the body, namely, the skin, peripheral nerves, upper respiratory tract, anterior chamber of the eyes, and testes, resulting in clinical signs and symptoms that are largely confined to these cooler tissues. Depending on host cellular immunity, the disease may be benign or malignant, with its course further being complicated by intercurrent immune-mediated reactional states. If leprosy is severe and left untreated, its aggressive course can cause severe debilitating deformity, which until this day unfortunately results in unreasonable stigma and social ostracism. Although *M. leprae* was identified in 1873 by a Norwegian physician, G. Armauer Hansen,[1] the first effective treatment, the sulfones, was not introduced until 1943.[2] Because antimicrobial therapy can arrest and even at times cure disease, early diagnosis and therapy are critical in preventing deformity and resulting in a salutary outcome.

CLINICAL DESCRIPTION

Epidemiology

The prevalence of leprosy worldwide is estimated at about 5.5 million people.[3] Among these, approximately 6000 patients reside in the United States, with 95% or more acquiring their disease in developing countries. Over the past 2 decades, the number of reported cases in the United States (200 to 300 per year) has risen dramati-

cally, resulting almost exclusively from immigration, primarily from the Philippines, Southeast Asia, and Mexico. States with large immigrant populations (e.g., California, Texas, Hawaii, and New York) have the largest proportion of new cases.

The majority of affected persons reside in the tropics and subtropics, with prevalence being generally inversely proportional to a nation's per capita income. Unlike tuberculosis, leprosy is more a rural than an urban disease. Leprosy is endemic in Asia, Africa, the Pacific Basin, and Latin America (excluding Chile). Eighty per cent of worldwide cases are found in five countries: India (accounting for 60% of cases worldwide), Myanmar, Indonesia, Brazil, and Nigeria. Within the United States, Hawaii, Louisiana, and Texas still report rare cases in individuals without a history of previous Third World travel or residence.

Leprosy affects all races and age groups, with a peak incidence of onset in the second and third decades of life. It is rarely seen in children younger than the age of 2 and can present in the seventh and eighth decades. In children, the tuberculoid form predominates and is without gender preference. In adults, lepromatous leprosy is more common in men than in women (2:1).[4] In highly endemic areas such as India and Africa, tuberculoid leprosy predominates, whereas among Mexicans the majority of cases are lepromatous and among the Chinese there are equal numbers of lepromatous and tuberculoid cases. Genetic predisposition may account for this difference, as suggested by studies linking specific class II major histocompatibility complex loci to the predilection of both tuberculoid and lepromatous leprosy.[5, 6]

Most persons are immune to leprosy, with subclinical infection being believed to be common in endemic areas and only a minority of exposed individuals progressing to actual disease.[7, 8] Owing to *M. leprae*'s uniquely long generation time, the incubation period of leprosy can be measured in years, with a range of 2 to 30 or more years and an average of 5 years. Children appear more susceptible to disease, and adults are relatively resistant, as suggested by only a 5% incidence of conjugal leprosy (leprosy acquired from a marriage partner).[9] Because the initial pathophysiologic process is unknown, it is unclear whether the disease arises from primary infection or reactivation.

Transmission of leprosy is not completely understood. Only lepromatous leprosy (multibacillary disease) is considered infectious. Tuberculoid leprosy (paucibacillary disease—no bacilli demonstrable in the dermis) is noninfectious. Although it was long held that close prolonged contact with a highly bacilliferous lepromatous case is the primary mode of transmission, more than 50% of patients with leprosy have no known history of contact with another known patient with leprosy.[10] Intact skin-to-skin transmission has been generally discounted, since *M. leprae* is found only in deeper dermal tissue and transepidermal shedding of the bacillus appears to be negligible.[11] However, ulcerated lesions or denuded skin may serve as a potential source of infection. Most authorities favor respiratory transmission from heavily infected nasal droplets as the primary mode of transmission.[12, 13] The number of acid-fast bacilli in a sneeze from an untreated lepromatous patient is similar to that found in a cough from untreated patients with cavitary tuberculosis,[14] and immunosuppressed mice placed in an aerosol of *M. leprae* become diseased.[15] Other possible modes of transmission include environmental factors such as insect vectors and infected soil. Blood-sucking insects have long been suspected as vectors of leprosy. Bedbugs and mosquitos found in the vicinity of leprosaria regularly harbor *M. leprae*,[16] and Narayanan and colleagues[17] demonstrated that mosquitos are capable of infecting mice from lepromatous volunteers as long as 48 hours after the blood meal. *M. leprae* has also been found in soil.[10, 18, 19] Although rare, direct dermal inoculation through tattoo[20] and hypodermic needles has resulted in infection. Therefore, it is possible that the preponderantly rural prevalence of leprosy may be the result of contact with infected soil and transcutaneous inoculation, possibly, at least in part, from walking barefoot.

For unclear reasons, in nonendemic locales, household spread is significantly decreased, such that some clinicians report no disease at all in household contacts.[21, 22] The household risk of developing disease in endemic areas from a lepromatous patient is about 10%,[23] and in nonendemic areas it is estimated at 1%. In the United States, affected immigrants with the disease pose no threat to nonhousehold contacts. Casual contacts and medical caregivers are not at risk. Isolation procedures in the hospital setting are unnecessary even for the untreated patient with leprosy.

Clinical and Immunologic Features

Classification and Skin Testing (Lepromin)

Based on clinical findings and dermatopathology, Ridley and Jopling[24] devised a classification scheme that is widely accepted, places patients accurately on the immunologically determined disease spectrum, and can be extremely useful to clinicians in predicting outcome, likely complications, and possible reactional states. The clinical pathologic features of the Ridley-Jopling classification are summarized in Table 112–1.

Lepromin is a homogenate of heat-killed *M. leprae* that, injected intradermally, is useful in determining whether cellular immunity to *M. leprae* is intact, with skin test site induration at 3 to 4 weeks (the Mitsuda reaction) being the preferred method for evaluation. The Mitsuda reaction is positive if the induration is 5 mm or more, intermediate if 3 to 5 mm, and negative if less than 3 mm. The lepromin test is positive in tuberculoid patients and invariably negative in multibacillary disease.

Tuberculoid Leprosy. The tuberculoid lesion first appears as an erythematous, anesthetic macule that tends to heal centrally, leaving a hypopigmented, slightly atrophic, and depressed center (Fig. 112–2; see color plate). In tuberculoid leprosy, lesions are either singular or few. The borders are always sharply demarcated and, with increased immune activity, can be raised and erythematous. An enlarged nerve is typically palpated in the vicinity of the lesion.

In polar tuberculoid disease, intact cell-mediated immunity to *M. leprae* results in containment of infection and acid-fast bacilli are absent. Well-organized granulomatous inflammation results, causing early nerve destruction and its consequent anesthesia or muscle weakness. With the organism's predilection for cooler sites of the body, thickened nerve trunks occur especially where they are most superficial and susceptible to trauma, particularly the ulnar nerve at the elbow. The end result is a self-limited, well-demarcated anesthetic lesion, limited in number and at times associated with an enlarged nerve. Neural involvement in the absence of cutaneous lesions occurs and is called pure "neural leprosy."

Lepromatous Leprosy. The skin lesions of polar lepromatous disease are not particularly anesthetic but are numerous, diffuse, infiltrated lesions with a smooth and often shiny appearance, sparing only the warmer parts of the body (the axilla, groin, hair-bearing scalp, and midline of the back) (Fig. 112–4). They are usually nodular with indefinite borders, but sharply demarcated papules resembling dermatofibromas can occur. This phenomenon has been termed *histoid leprosy* and is more common in relapse than on initial presentation. Polar lepromatous lesions may coalesce, appearing more plaque-like, and may eventually lead to diffuse thickening of the skin, giving it a "doughy" texture and appearance. Mexican patients particularly have a form of leprosy without visible skin lesions but a thickened dermis and loss of body hair termed *diffuse lepromatosis*. As the skin gets progressively infiltrated, loss of body hair occurs, especially affecting the eyebrows and eyelashes. The earlobes become swollen and "succulent." The "leonine" face of leprosy results from deepened facial lines from diffuse infiltration. Because of early bacillary invasion of the nasal mucosa and at times cartilage, patients commonly present with chronic nasal congestion and occasionally septal perforation and saddle-nose deformity. Other findings include edema of the eyelids, lips, and distal extremities and fusiform swelling of the fingers resembling that of scleroderma. "Stocking-and-glove" anesthesia occurs late in the disease with uni-

TABLE 112–1. Some Clinical and Histologic Features of the Ridley-Jopling Classification of Leprosy

Clinical and Histologic Features	Tuberculoid (TT)	Borderline Tuberculoid (BT)	Borderline (BB)	Borderline Lepromatous (BL)	Lepromatous (LL)
Skin lesions	Up to three; sharply defined asymmetrical plaques with tendency for central clearing and elevated borders	Smaller or larger than TT; potentially more numerous than lesions of TT; usually annular lesions with sharp margination on exterior and interior borders. Borders not as elevated as in TT.	Dimorphic lesions intermediate between BT and BL	Few or many LL-type lesions; ill-defined plaques with an occasional sharp margin; shiny appearance	Symmetrical; poorly marginated, multiple infiltrated nodules and plaques or diffuse infiltration; xanthoma-like or dermatofibroma papules; leonine facies and eyebrow alopecia
Nerve lesions	Skin lesions anesthetic early; nerve near lesion may be enlarged	Skin lesions anesthetic early. Nerve trunk palsies asymmetrical. Nerve abscesses most common in BT.	Anesthetic skin lesions and nerve trunk palsies	Skin lesions usually hypesthetic; may be anesthetic; nerve trunk palsies common and frequently symmetrical	Hyperesthesia a *late* sign; nerve palsies variable; acral, distal, symmetrical anesthesia common
Lepromin skin test	Positive	Usually positive (80% to 90%)	Negative	Negative	Negative
Lymphocytes	Dense peripheral infiltration about epithelioid tubercle; infiltration into epidermis well developed	Less numerous than TT; peripheral infiltration about granuloma; variable epidermal infiltration usually focal	Lymphopenic	Moderately dense and in the same distribution as macrophages	Scant; diffuse or focal in distribution
Macrophage differentiation	Epithelioid	Epithelioid	Epithelioid	Usually undifferentiated; epithelioid foci may be present; may show foamy change	Foamy change the rule; may be undifferentiated in early lesions
Langhans' giant cells	Present, well developed	May be present; usually few in number	Absent	Absent	Absent
Acid-fast bacilli	Rare, less than 1 per 100 oil immersion fields (i.e., bacteriologic index [BI] of zero (paucibacillary)	Rare, usually BI of zero (paucibacillary). If acid-fast bacilli present, consider a reversal reaction	1–10 per oil immersion field or BI of 3 to 4.	10–100 per oil immersion field or BI of 4 to 5.	100–1000 per oil immersion field or BI of 4 to 6; globi

From Rea TH, Modlin RL. Leprosy. In: Demis DJ, ed. Clinical Dermatology, 19th revision, vol 3, unit 16–29. Philadelphia: JB Lippincott, 1992.

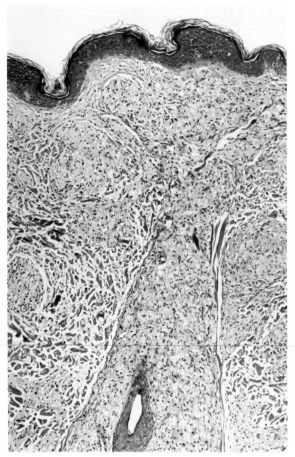

FIGURE 112-1. The dermis in lepromatous leprosy contains nodules of foam cells.

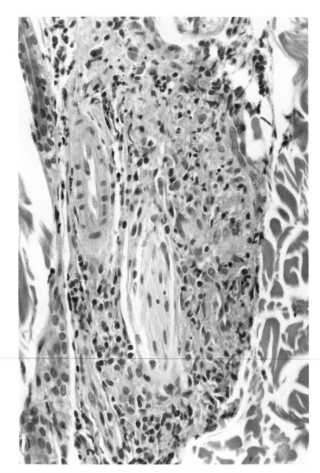

FIGURE 112-3. A compact granuloma surrounds a nerve in tuberculoid leprosy.

formly enlarged nerve trunks and corresponding sensory and motor dysfunction.

Specific cell-mediated anergy to *M. leprae* in lepromatous leprosy leads to widespread, primarily lymphohematogenous, dissemination. With the exception of the central nervous system, the gastrointestinal tract, and the lungs, bacilli can be found in virtually every organ system, including the skin, peripheral nerves, eyes, upper

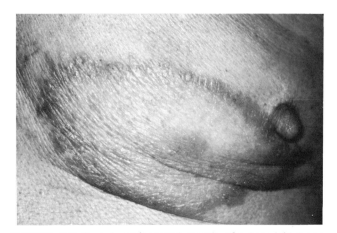

FIGURE 112-2. A hypopigmented macule of tuberculoid leprosy shows a defined border. (See color plate.)

respiratory tract (especially the nose), and reticuloendothelial system. A continuous, asymptomatic bacteremia occurs. Paradoxically, this diffuse dissemination greatly predates any skin lesions and, despite the tremendous bacillary load, the patient usually feels remarkably well.

The mechanism of nerve damage in lepromatous disease differs from that in tuberculoid disease in that damage results from the massive bacillary infiltration, compression, and eventual fibrosis of the dermal nerves and not from the inflammatory response of an intact cell-mediated response. As a result, in lepromatous leprosy the onset of anesthesia occurs late and is bilateral and symmetrical.

Patients with lepromatous leprosy have an *M. leprae*-specific anergy[25, 26] and are not subject to opportunistic infections such as are patients with the acquired immunodeficiency syndrome. The immune defect in lepromatous leprosy has been found to be associated with both a loss of *M. leprae*-responsive T-cell precursors[27] and enhanced suppressor T-cell activity.[28, 29] On the other hand, patients with lepromatous leprosy have a polyclonal hyperglobulinemia, resulting commonly in false-positive serologic tests for syphilis, rheumatoid arthritis, lupus erythematosus, and so on. Although phagocytosis and microbicidal activity of lepromatous macrophages for other organisms have been demonstrated to be unim-

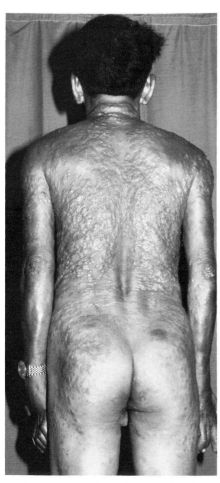

FIGURE 112–4. Infiltrated lesions of lepromatous leprosy. Note the sparing of the midline of the back, the dermis therein being 5°C warmer than at the posterior axillary line. Other warm areas—scalp, axilla, and groin—are also generally spared in lepromatous leprosy.

paired, lepromatous macrophages have been found to be impaired in their ability to kill *M. leprae*.[30, 31] There is an abundant literature demonstrating that certain *M. leprae* products, particularly phenolic glycolipid-1 and lipoarabinomannan, impair both lymphocyte and macrophage function in vitro.[32–34] As compared with tuberculoid patients, lepromatous patients have reduced amounts of protective cytokines, interleukin-2,[35] and interferon gamma within the dermis,[36] as well as increased amounts of suppressive antibody-inducing cytokines, interleukin-4, interleukin-5, and interleukin-10.[37] Local injection of interleukin-2[38] and interferon gamma[39] into leprous nodules has resulted in decreased numbers of acid-fast bacilli and conversion of immunohistologic features toward the tuberculoid end of the spectrum, once again suggesting that cytokine expression is critical to protective immunity in leprosy.

Borderline Leprosy. Most patients diagnosed with leprosy are intermediate between the two polar forms, clinically and histologically manifesting characteristics of both polar extremes. The degree of similarity to the polar extremes is determined by their precise degree of immunocompetence. These patients with borderline leprosy frequently develop reactional states manifested pri-

marily by skin and neural inflammation (lepra type 1 reactions), which complicate their course.

BORDERLINE TUBERCULOID LEPROSY. In borderline tuberculoid leprosy immunity to *M. leprae*, as in polar tuberculoid patients, is intact. The lesions of borderline tuberculoid disease resemble those of polar tuberculoid leprosy except that they may be more in number, often presenting as coalescing satellite lesions, and can have a more symmetrical distribution. They frequently upgrade immunologically, turning the lesion into an erythematous plaque with serpiginous borders.

MID-BORDERLINE LEPROSY. This form of leprosy is exceedingly rare. The skin lesions are more numerous and are classically dimorphic, having features of both polar forms, giving a "punched out" or "Swiss cheese" appearance. These annular lesions have poorly defined outer borders, resembling those of lepromatous leprosy, and sharp well-defined inner borders, resembling those of tuberculoid leprosy with central normal-appearing but anesthetic skin.

Patients with mid-borderline leprosy may have a weakly positive lepromin test and acid-fast bacilli may be seen on biopsy.

BORDERLINE LEPROMATOUS LEPROSY. As the host loses its last vestiges of cellular immunity, borderline lepromatous disease is seen (lepromin-negative). The skin lesions are more numerous than in mid-borderline disease, tend to be smaller, and have appearances of lesions representative of the whole spectrum of leprosy: hypopigmented macules, annular lesions, plaques, nodules, sometimes papules, and variable combinations of these are seen. Nerve palsies vary from few to multiple and tend to be symmetrical. Acid-fast bacilli are always present in biopsy samples but the patient is less bacilliferous than in lepromatous leprosy, and nasal skin smears are usually negative.

Indeterminate Leprosy. Indeterminant leprosy is a form of early leprosy, usually found in a child, who has theoretically not yet declared his or her immunologic status to the disease. It is thought to be leprosy at its earliest stage and usually presents as a hypopigmented or slightly erythematous macule that is mildly hypesthetic.

Complications

Reactional States. The reactional states complicating leprosy occur in as many as 50% of patients after the initiation of therapy. They may cause considerable morbidity and be a source of confusion to the patient, whose expectation is improvement and not the appearance of new skin lesions, painful neuropathy, and so on. Two major types of reaction occur and are different clinically and immunologically.

REVERSAL AND DOWNGRADING REACTIONS (LEPRA TYPE 1). Lepra type 1 reactions affect individuals with borderline disease. When they occur before the initiation of therapy they are called "downgrading" reactions and represent a shift toward the lepromatous pole. Reactions that occur after the initiation of therapy are clinically indistinguishable. These "reversal" reactions signify a shift toward tuberculoid disease. Reactions are confined only to lesional skin or inapparent foci and nerves where leprosy antigen is present. Therefore, lepra type 1 reactions are not associated with systemic symptoms such as fever (except low grade) or arthralgias. Lepra type 1 reactions are worse, more prolonged, and most common in borderline lepromatous disease, where more antigen is present. Existing lesions become inflamed and tender. New inflammatory "satellite" lesions may appear for the first time. Although reversal reactions frequently occur only in the skin, they can dramatically present as acute painful nerve-trunk palsies within 24 to 36 hours, making these events one of the few emergencies in leprosy.[40] On examination, involved nerves are typically enlarged and tender. Many patients also experience "silent" neuritides that occur slowly and painlessly, often presenting as peripheral dysfunction only when there is little hope of reversal from treatment.

Reversal reactions result in both clinical and dermatopathologic shifts toward the tuberculoid end of the spectrum. During these reactions the dermis has been demonstrated to contain increased numbers of CD4-positive helper cells and increased levels of interferon gamma, interleukin-2, and gamma/delta T cells.[41]

ERYTHEMA NODOSUM LEPROSUM (LEPRA TYPE 2). Erythema nodosum leprosum occurs in half of patients with borderline lepromatous and lepromatous leprosy. Although erythema nodosum leprosum may be seen on initial presentation and be a precipitating cause for a patient to seek medical attention, it more commonly (90% of the time) develops within the first few years after therapy has begun, and episodes of the disease resolve spontaneously generally after about 5 years of treatment. The most common clinical manifestation is crops of erythematous, painful nodules of the skin and subcutaneous tissues. If the disease is severe, pustules develop, which can ulcerate and result in suppurative wounds and subsequent scarring. Unlike erythema nodosum, erythema nodosum leprosum is not limited to the lower extremities, being found virtually anywhere, but most often on the extensor surface of the forearms, medial thighs, and occasionally the face. Unlike erythema nodosum, individual lesions of erythema nodosum leprosum last only a few days. Like certain other rheumatologic diseases, erythema nodosum leprosum is a systemic disorder at times associated with fever, malaise, anorexia, leukocytosis, and anemia. Erythema nodosum leprosum may also result in synovitis, nephritis, neuritis, iritis, lymphadenitis, and epididymo-orchitis.

Histologically erythema nodosum leprosum shows infiltrates of lymphocytes, macrophages, and particularly neutrophils, sometimes accompanied by a leukocytoclastic vasculitis that can involve both the dermis and subcutis. It appears to be caused by circulating immune complexes, and C3 and IgG can be present in the walls of venules.[42] Erythema nodosum leprosum has been demonstrated to be associated with elevated levels of tumor necrosis factor.[43] It is also associated with a local increase in cell-mediated immunity (i.e., increased numbers of T-helper cells, interleukin-2, and interferon gamma, and loss of suppressor T-cell activity).[21]

LUCIO'S PHENOMENON. Rarely encountered is Lucio's phenomenon, which occurs almost exclusively in Latin Americans, particularly in patients from certain states of western Mexico. These patients have a form of lepromatous leprosy referred to earlier as diffuse lepromatosis. The Lucio reaction results in large bullous lesions that ulcerate, especially below the knees. The lesions are a consequence of dermal ischemic infarction, resulting, in turn, from leukocytoclastic vasculitis of small vessels in some cases and thrombi in superficial vessels in others. Bacilli are often present within endothelial cells. Secondary infection of widespread Lucio's ulcers can lead to sepsis and commonly death. Unlike erythema nodosum leprosum, which tends to occur after the initiation of treatment, Lucio's phenomenon is frequently present at the time of initial diagnosis.

Specially Affected Organs

Nerves. The peripheral nerve pathology in leprosy results from bacillary invasion, particularly of Schwann cells (in lepromatous leprosy), the host's granulomatous response to the intradermal bacilli (in tuberculoid leprosy), or because of various reactional states. Patients lose fine touch and hot, cold, and pain sensations, while generally maintaining position and vibration sense. The most common nerve trunk involved is the ulnar nerve at the elbow, which results in clawing of the fourth and fifth digits and the wasting of the dorsal interosseous muscles of the hand. Other nerve trunks involved less often include the peroneal, median, posterior tibial, and posterior auricular nerves and the zygomatic branch of the facial nerve. The late acral distal numbness of lepromatous leprosy commonly leads to repeated burns and trauma of the distal extremities. The insensitive plantar surface of the feet often results in trophic ulceration, a major cause of disease morbidity: treatment includes therapy for secondary infection, avoidance of weight bearing (which can be accomplished with a total-contact cast with a heel pad for walking), aggressive callus care of healed tissues to prevent recurrence (which may be frequent), and extra-depth or specially molded shoes. Tendon transfers may ameliorate lost function, particularly that resulting from ulnar, medial, and peroneal nerve involvement.

Eye and Nose. In lepromatous leprosy, involvement of the anterior chamber of the eye is caused by several mechanisms of injury. Direct invasion by *M. leprae* of the anterior chamber causes characteristic beaded corneal nerves and iris pearls on slit lamp examination. Such involvement of the anterior chamber and erythema nodosum leprosum–induced iritis may result in secondary glaucoma. Lagophthalmos (inability to close the eye) and corneal and conjunctival insensitivity from seventh and fifth cranial nerve involvement may lead to corneal trauma, infection, scarring, and eventual blindness. Lepromatous leprosy is also associated with the loss of eyebrows and eyelashes, which may be of considerable cosmetic concern to patients. To prevent corneal trauma in patients with lagophthalmos, corneal eye drops during the day and ointments at night are useful. Corrective surgery for lagophthalmos is often required.

Frequently, epistaxis occurs in patients with lepromatous leprosy and may be ameliorated by hydration and products such as Cortisporin (hydrocortisone-neomycin-bacitracin-polymyxin B) ointment. When nasal collapse occurs in lepromatous patients, reconstructive surgery may successfully reverse this cosmetic defect.

Testes. The testes are commonly involved in the lepromatous male patient and can cause infertility from hypospermia and decreased levels of testosterone with increased levels of follicle-stimulating hormone and luteinizing hormone.[44, 45] Testicular atrophy, gynecomastia, and impotence may result, a process far more common in patients with polar lepromatous leprosy than borderline lepromatous leprosy. Monthly intramuscular injections of testosterone enanthate, 200 mg, may ameliorate sexual dysfunction.

Kidneys. Once common in autopsies of untreated patients with lepromatous leprosy,[46, 47] secondary amyloidosis and renal failure are rarely seen today, probably owing to effective chemotherapy and treatment for erythema nodosum leprosum.

PATHOLOGY

Tuberculoid Leprosy. Specimens for histologic evaluation must be obtained from involved tissue, preferably the advancing edge of skin lesions. Histologically, in tuberculoid leprosy, well-developed epithelioid granulomas typically form, sometimes around neurovascular structures, collared by abundant lymphocytic infiltrates that extend into the epidermis. Langhans' giant cells are common, and dermal nerves are either completely destroyed or greatly swollen from intraneural granuloma, rarely with central caseating necrosis (see Fig. 112–3).

Lepromatous Leprosy. The random skin biopsy of a lepromatous patient from virtually any site (except the hair-bearing scalp) shows poorly organized collections of foamy macrophages (Virchow's or foam cells) with a clear subepidermal free zone (see Fig. 112–1). Fite-Faracco staining reveals bundles of acid-fast bacilli and spheroidal masses of intracellular bacilli known as "globi" (Fig. 112–5; see color plate). Lymphocytes are generally scanty, and giant cells are typically absent. Schwann cells and perineural cells of nerve bundles are laden with bacilli yet are structurally more preserved than in tuberculoid disease.

Borderline Tuberculoid Leprosy. Histologically, well-developed epithelioid granulomas are present but with few-to-absent Langhans' giant cells. Unlike in tuberculoid leprosy, few lymphocytes are present in the epidermis. Acid-fast bacilli are absent to rare and more likely to be found in dermal nerves.

Mid-Borderline Leprosy. The epithelioid granulomas are more diffuse, and giant cells are typically absent. There is a clear subepidermal zone resembling polar lepromatous histology.

Borderline Lepromatous Leprosy. Skin biopsy shows granulomas with slight foamy changes and numerous lymphocytes. Nerves often take on a multilaminated appearance or classic "onion skin" change from the infiltration of the perineurium with plasma cells and lymphocytes. Foci of epithelioid macrophages may be seen, representing minimal cell-mediated immunity.

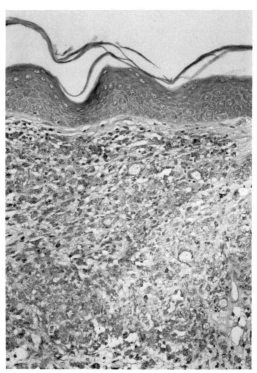

FIGURE 112–5. A Fite-Faracco stain of the dermis in untreated lepromatous leprosy shows the numerous clustered bacilli, or globi. (See color plate.)

Indeterminate Leprosy. On biopsy, nonspecific findings are typical, with scattered histiocytes and lymphocytes around dermal appendages and nerves in the deeper dermis. Acid-fast bacilli are at times present and the only certain means generally to confirm this diagnosis.

PATHOGENESIS AND ETIOLOGY

Mycobacterium leprae is an obligate intracellular acid-fast bacillus that is preferentially stained with the Fite-Faracco method. The leprosy bacillus is inert, is nonmotile, and is incapable of producing toxin; yet it has a unique capacity to enter nerves, which causes most of its medical sequelae. All attempts to grow *M. leprae* on artificial media or tissue culture have failed. However, *M. leprae* can be grown in the footpads of mice with a unique 14-day doubling time and in which antimicrobial susceptibility can be evaluated. Humans were once believed to be the only reservoir or host of *M. leprae* until natural infection was discovered in the nine-banded armadillo.

M. leprae shares morphologic, biochemical, antigenic, and genetic similarities with other mycobacteria. However, the acid-fast nature of its staining can be abrogated: pyridine extraction results in loss of its acid-fast nature, and decolorization can be used to separate *M. leprae* from other mycobacteria. Also, *M. leprae* is unique among the mycobacteria in having dopa oxidase activity.

The cell wall of *M. leprae* is indigestable, waxy, and primarily lipid, composed largely of a unique *M. leprae* antigen, phenolic glycolipid-1. IgM antibody to phenolic glycolipid-1 can be detected serologically and its presence and titer appear to directly correlate with bacillary load. It is detected only 50% to 70% of the time in patients with tuberculoid leprosy (paucibacillary) but is virtually always positive in multibacillary patients, wherein titers fall with effective therapy.[48-52]

DIAGNOSIS AND DIFFERENTIAL DIAGNOSIS

Although the variable skin lesions of leprosy may mimic innumerable other dermatologic diseases (Table 112–2), the combination of skin and nerve involvement in a patient from a known leprosy-endemic area should clearly raise suspicion for leprosy, and its diagnosis should be pursued until proven otherwise. The finding of acid-fast bacilli or granuloma within a nerve is seen only in leprosy. No other disease will result in an anesthetic skin lesion or a unilaterally enlarged nerve associated with palsy and/or anesthesia. A few rare genetic diseases also cause enlarged nerves and associated palsies but are always bilateral and not associated with skin lesions (e.g., Charcot-Marie-Tooth disease).

In multibacillary disease, despite the occasional lack of neurologic findings (a late sign), diagnosis is easily made by the presence of acid-fast bacilli in the biopsy of skin lesions and even normal skin (in the case of lepromatous leprosy). For skin biopsy specimens a Fite-Faracco stain should be employed since the classic Ziehl-Neelsen stain may not at times reveal acid-fast bacilli.

The biopsy of the tuberculoid or borderline tuberculoid lesion is less useful, since the usual lack of acid-fast bacilli can mimic other cutaneous granulomatous diseases (especially cutaneous sarcoidosis). However, granuloma within nerves is pathognomonic of leprosy. In pure neural leprosy, where there is an absence of skin lesions and the presence of an enlarged nerve trunk, nerve biopsy may reveal typical granulomatous pathology and

TABLE 112-2. Differential Diagnosis of Leprosy
Sarcoidosis
Pityriasis alba
Tinea versicolor
Hypopigmented birthmarks
Contact dermatitis
Vitiligo
Avitaminosis B
Psoriasis
Granuloma annulare
Lupus vulgaris
Tuberculosis verrucosa cutis
Tinea circinata
Neurofibromatosis
Leukemia cutis
Xanthomatosis
Dermal leishmaniasis
Lymphoma
Syphilis
Yaws

acid-fast bacilli. Because nerve biopsy can result in dysfunction, only lateral fascicles should be taken and motor nerve trunks optimally avoided.

Because of the absence of demonstrable acid-fast bacilli, tuberculoid leprosy may be confused with a number of granulomatous dermatitides, which include lupus vulgaris, sarcoidosis, dermal leishmaniasis, lymphoma, syphilis, yaws, and granuloma annulare. Sputum smears from lepromatous patients will contain noncultivable acid-fast bacilli that are morphologically indistinguishable from *M. tuberculosis*. In sarcoidosis there may be evidence of peripheral neuropathy, with granulomas surrounding dermal nerves and pathology of the perineurium but no actual granuloma within nerves as in leprosy.

The lepromin test unfortunately cannot be used to diagnose infection because it is negative in patients with lepromatous leprosy and often positive in individuals without leprosy and even with no prior history of exposure.[53-55] Unfortunately, serology for leprosy is also of little diagnostic value: in paucibacillary leprosy, when the absence of acid-fast bacilli at times renders the diagnosis of leprosy difficult, there commonly (50%–70% of the time) are not demonstrable circulating antibodies to PGL-1,[50, 52] while many individuals, particularly in endemic countries, have antibody to *M. leprae* but no disease.[7]

TREATMENT

Antimicrobial Therapy

Antimicrobials to Treat Leprosy

Dapsone. Dapsone (4,4'-diaminodiphenylsulfone or DDS) is the drug of choice for treating all forms of leprosy but is principally only bacteriostatic for *M. leprae*. It is inexpensive ($1 per year per patient) and very well tolerated on long-term administration. Other virtues include high serum concentrations (500 times higher than dapsone's minimum inhibitory concentration against *M. leprae*), allowing for a very large therapeutic index, and a prolonged half-life, which allows for some minor lapses in compliance. The usual adult dose is 100 mg per day. Although a dose-related hemolysis is common,[56] severe anemia is rare except in the setting of glucose-6-phosphate dehydrogenase deficiency. Also, dapsone may rarely cause bone marrow aplasia and a mononucleosis-type blood picture, associated with fever and exfoliative dermatitis, termed the *dapsone syndrome*. The dapsone syndrome generally responds to drug discontinuation and systemic corticosteroid therapy. Other infrequent side effects include cutaneous drug reactions (occasionally erythema multiforme), dose-related methemoglobinemia, and sulfhemoglobinemia.

Rifampin. Rifampin is rapidly bactericidal for *M. leprae* with a daily adult dose of 600 mg and acts to selectively inhibit bacterial and not mammalian DNA-dependent RNA polymerase.[57, 58] It is quickly and easily absorbed through the gastrointestinal tract, is widely distributed, and penetrates well into both tissues and cells. Rifampin discolors urine and body secretions orange and is often worrisome to the patient who is not informed of this banal side effect. Since the drug is a potent inducer of hepatic microsomal enzymes, accelerated metabolism of other drugs concurrently taken can occur. Notable drug interactions that may cause increased dose requirements occur with oral contraceptives, steroids (i.e., prednisone), warfarin, oral hypoglycemic agents, and certain antiseizure medications. Although fairly nontoxic, side effects include hepatotoxicity (especially in those with underlying liver disease), allergic skin eruptions, and febrile or flu-like episodes. With intermittent therapy, rare thrombocytopenia, severe hemolytic anemia, and renal failure are known to occur.

Unfortunately, rifampin is not affordable on a daily basis in poor, developing countries, where the prevalence of leprosy is highest. For this reason, the World Health Organization (WHO) multidrug regimens advocate intermittent, single-dose rifampin once monthly. Whether such long-term, intermittent usage will lead to rifampin resistance is of some concern.

Clofazimine. Clofazimine is a riminophenazine dye that is bacteriostatic against *M. leprae* in adult doses of 50 mg daily to 100 mg three times weekly. The drug accumulates in fatty tissues and cells of the reticular endothelial system. At higher doses of 200 to 300 mg per day it has a moderate anti-inflammatory effect against erythema nodosum leprosum. Unfortunately, clofazimine results in a red-black skin discoloration that tends to accentuate the appearance of leprous lesions. This is often unacceptable to patients, especially those of lighter skin, who believe the medication draws even more attention to the lesions they are trying to conceal and forget. Hence, if compliance is of issue, clofazimine is best avoided. Additionally, clofazimine may cause a variety of gastrointestinal side effects.

Ethionamide. Ethionamide is bactericidal against *M. leprae* and kills the bacilli faster than dapsone. However, its frequent gastrointestinal side effects and hepatotoxicity (especially when used with rifampin) limit its usefulness. The usual dose is 250 to 500 mg per day. Dividing this daily dose and administering it with large meals has been found useful in diminishing this drug's gastrointestinal toxicity.

Newer Antimicrobials. Promising new antimicrobial agents are under investigation. Minocycline hydrochloride,[59, 60] clarithromycin,[60-62] and a number of fluoroquinolones[63-65] have been found to be bactericidal against *M. leprae* in mice. Furthermore, minocycline,[66, 67] clarithromycin,[67] and two fluoroquinolones (pefloxacin and ofloxacin)[68] have been found to be more rapidly effective than either dapsone or clofazimine in clinical trials. In addition, preliminary observations suggest that minocycline may have an anti-inflammatory effect that decreases the incidence of erythema nodosum leprosum. Since its long-term side effects have proved to be minimal as a result of our considerable experience in the treatment of acne, minocycline appears the most promising of these three new classes of antimicrobial agents.

Regimens to Treat Leprosy

There are two important issues affecting the appropriate selection of treatment regimens for the different polar ends of the leprosy spectrum: the number of bacilli and the presence or absence of specific cellular immunity. It naturally follows that in multibacillary disease (lepromatous, borderline, and mid-borderline), more intensive drug regimens for a greater duration are required. Lifelong therapy for lepromatous leprosy, usually monotherapy with dapsone, had become standard from 1943 to 1970. With the advent of rifampin, which is far more bactericidal, shorter courses of multidrug therapy are advised.

Chemotherapy in leprosy rapidly renders the patient noninfectious to others, probably within the first few weeks of therapy. However, viable drug-sensitive bacterial persistence,[57, 69, 70] despite prolonged multidrug regimens including rifampin treatment, presents vital concerns as to our ability to cure lepromatous leprosy. Nevertheless, in 1982, the WHO[71] proposed and advocated multidrug regimens of limited duration after the model of chemotherapy for tuberculosis (Table 112-3). For multibacillary leprosy the WHO[71] recommends dapsone, 100 mg daily, plus clofazimine, 50 mg, and monthly (supervised) rifampin, 600 mg, plus clofazimine, 300 mg, for at least 2 years or until smear-negativity. For paucibacillary leprosy the WHO[71] recommends

	Type of Treatment	
Source	*Paucibacillary*	*Multibacillary*
World Health Organization	Dapsone, 100 mg per day, and supervised rifampin, 600 mg per month for 6 months	Dapsone, 100 mg per day, with clofazimine, 50 mg per day, and supervised rifampin, 600 mg plus clofazimine, 300 mg per month; therapy continued at least 2 years or until skin smears are negative (generally 5 years)
Authors	Dapsone, 100 mg per day for 5 years	Dapsone, 100 mg per day for life, and rifampin, 600 mg per day for 3 years or until acid-fast bacilli skin smear is negative

TABLE 112-3. Treatment of Leprosy*

*These recommendations are for adult patients.

dapsone, 100 mg daily, plus monthly (supervised) rifampin, 600 mg, for a total duration of 6 months. The rationale behind their use was that multidrug chemotherapy rapidly eradicates contagion, can be inexpensive (hence monthly and not daily rifampin), and prevents drug resistance, and that a limited or short course will improve compliance and is operationally more feasible. Unfortunately, these recommendations antedated supportive clinical trials, and, furthermore, the tremendous bacillary load of lepromatous leprosy in these *M. leprae*-anergic hosts, the long time to relapse after discontinuation of rifampin-containing regimens (averaging 7 years), and the affordability of available chemotherapy (as in the United States) caused some leprologists to resist these recommendations. Although initially relapse rates in multibacillary patients were reportedly low, by 8 years or more after the discontinuation of therapy relapse rates have been at the unacceptably high rate of 10% to 20%.[72]

Hence, the authors and many American leprologists have opted to use more conservative regimens until firm scientific evidence of the efficacy of limited short-course regimens has been proven (see Table 112–3). We treat multibacillary leprosy with dapsone, 100 mg, daily for a lifetime and rifampin, 600 mg, daily for the initial 3 years or until skin smears for acid-fast bacilli are negative. For paucibacillary leprosy we recommend dapsone, 100 mg daily, alone for a total of 5 years.

In the United States, clinically relevant primary dapsone resistance does not occur.[73] Therefore, dapsone's efficacy as effective monotherapy for paucibacillary or as a part of multidrug therapy for multibacillary leprosy can be relied on in the United States. This abrogates the need for rifampin additionally for paucibacillary leprosy and the requirement for clofazimine, in addition to dapsone and rifampin, for multibacillary disease. Furthermore, in multibacillary leprosy daily rifampin therapy has proved to be more effective than various intermittent rifampin schedules,[72] and, because in the United States daily rifampin is certainly affordable, we recommend that rifampin be administered daily.

Monitoring Therapy

Slit-skin smears obtained by scraping the dermis with a scalpel or razor blade are useful in determining the efficacy of treatment as well as in establishing an initial baseline of disease severity. The skin smears are examined microscopically for (1) density of organisms (bacteriologic index) and (2) percentage of bacilli that stain uniformly and correlate with actual *M. leprae* viability (morphologic index). The smears are traditionally taken from six different skin sites: the earlobes, posterior elbows, and anterior knees (although other lesional sites can be substituted). In lepromatous leprosy, initial skin smears typically have a bacteriologic index of 4 to 6+, which falls by 1+ per year with effective therapy, becoming 0 usually at about 5 years. The morphologic index falls to 0 rapidly within days to weeks with rifampin use and within a few months with dapsone monotherapy.

Although antibody titers to *M. leprae*-specific phenolic glycolipid-1 fall with therapy, they are often still present at low titer long after smear negativity, and their rate of fall is so variable as to be of limited value to clinicians.[52]

Treatment of Complications

Reactional States

Because of the common propensity of reactional states for morbidity, particularly neuritis and its resultant permanent neurologic sequelae, their recognition and treatment are as important as antimicrobial therapy.

Erythema Nodosum Leprosum. If mild, skin lesions of erythema nodosum leprosum can be treated symptomatically with aspirin or other nonsteroidal anti-inflammatory agents. However, if episodes are severe with multiple erythema nodosum leprosum skin lesions, are generalized with symptoms of fever and malaise, or are associated with neuritis, orchitis, lymphadenitis, arthritis, or other similar condition, initiation of treatment with prednisone is indicated. Initial doses of 40 to 60 mg daily usually rapidly improve symptoms within 24 to 48 hours, and corticosteroids can be discontinued abruptly in 1 week. If erythema nodosum leprosum occurs repeatedly, then thalidomide can be used in patients of non–child-bearing potential for long-term control. Thalidomide in doses of 100 to 300 mg per night is as effective as prednisone in treating erythema nodosum leprosum but has a more delayed onset of action, generally several days to a week. Its effectiveness is probably due to thalidomide-induced impairment of IgM synthesis, polymorphonuclear leukocyte migration, and reduction of level of circulating tumor necrosis factor.[43, 74] Thalidomide, a sedative-hypnotic drug, is relatively free of other side effects except for constipation and mild leukopenia. However, if it is given during pregnancy, especially in the first trimester, severe birth deformities result. Consequently, thalidomide is now under an investigational license held by the G. W. Long Hansen's Disease Center with co-investigators at its regional centers and is available for the treatment of erythema nodosum leprosum in men and strictly in women of non–child-bearing potential. Unfortunately, refractory erythema nodosum leprosum occasionally occurs in young females, requiring chronic high doses of steroids. It is most tragic that, short of a tubal ligation, thalidomide cannot be used when secondary steroid side effects of cushingoid appearance, steroid acne, premature osteoporosis, and cataract formation develop. Unfortunately, although clofazimine (200–300 mg daily) may reduce the steroid requirement of erythema nodosum leprosum, it is not particularly effective and is often not accepted by the young female patient because of its red-black discoloration. Implanted contraceptives, such as levonorgestrel (Norplant), when compliance is not an issue, may in the future hold some hope for young women with refractory erythema nodosum leprosum if approved to be used concurrently with thalidomide.

Reversal Reactions. Unlike the case with erythema nodosum leprosum, corticosteroids for a few months are the only reliably effective treatment for reversal reactions (shorter courses are unfortunately associated with relapse). Hence, minor skin inflammation should be tolerated. Therapy is required for neuritis, lesions that threaten to ulcerate, and those at cosmetically important places such as the face. Although irreversible nerve damage may result if steroids are not initiated within 24 hours of the onset of reversal reaction-associated neuritis, corticosteroids may reverse such established neurologic damage of even a few months' duration. An initial dose of 40 to 60 mg of prednisone per day is usually adequate. Slow tapers over 2 to 3 months after control has been achieved are required to prevent these frustrating recurrences. Usually the prednisone dose may be decreased by 5 to 10 mg per week to 20 mg daily. Thereafter, maintenance at that dose or slower taper of 5 mg per week is recommended. The duration of steroid treatment required varies but generally tends to be longer as one approaches the lepromatous end of the spectrum, with patients with borderline tuberculoid disease requiring treatment for 4 to 9 months; those with mid-borderline disease, 6 to 12 months; and those with borderline lepromatous disease, 6 to 24 months.[40]

Other Reactions

LUCIO'S PHENOMENON. In Lucio's phenomenon, neither corticosteroids nor thalidomide is reliably effective. New Lucio lesions usually do not occur after 1 week of rifampin therapy[21]; hence chemotherapy is the mainstay of treatment of Lucio's phenomenon. Appropriate antimicrobial treatment of secondary infection and particularly bacteremia is indicated, and plasmapheresis has been successful in refractory cases, especially those with very high levels of circulating cold agglutinins.[75]

NERVE ABSCESSES. Profound nerve inflammation in patients with leprosy, particularly those with borderline disease, may present as an abscess with rapid loss of nerve function secondary to compression. Surgical drainage can result in return of nerve function and should be advised early whenever this diagnosis is made.

PROPHYLAXIS

It is advised that all household contacts of lepromatous patients, especially children, should be examined annually by experienced personnel for a period of 5 years after the diagnosis of the index case. Dapsone prophylaxis of household contacts of lepromatous patients is no longer advocated since it does not prevent the development of lepromatous leprosy and only partially reduces the subsequent prevalence of tuberculoid leprosy.[76]

Trials of vaccine prophylaxis with bacille Calmette-Guérin (BCG) have proven to be only moderately to minimally effective against M. leprae.[77-81] In lepromatous patients, the combination of BCG and heat-killed M. leprae is known to boost cell-mediated immunity and clear acid-fast bacilli,[82, 83] and yet clinical trials with this vaccine have not proved to be more effective than BCG alone.[84] Perhaps the lack of efficacy of such vaccines is because whole mycobacterial vaccines contain immunosuppressive mycobacterial products, especially phenolic glycolipid-1 and lipoarabinomannan.[32-34] Vaccination of mice with subunits of M. leprae that are largely protein and devoid of these immunosuppressant lipids and carbohydrates are more effective than whole killed M. leprae and offer potential for future application to disease control.[85, 86] Furthermore, specific proteins of M. leprae have been identified, cloned in Escherichia coli, and expressed in BCG, some of which have proved protective vaccines in mice.[87]

References

1. Hansen GA. Undwersogelser angaend spedalskhedens arsager. Norsk Mag Laegevid 1874;4:1–88.
2. Faget GH, Pogge RC, Johansen FA, et al. The promin treatment of leprosy: A progress report. Public Health Rep 1943;58:1729–1741.
3. Noordeen SK, Lopez-Bravo L, Sundaresan TK. Estimated number of leprosy cases in the world. Bull WHO 1992;70:7–10.
4. Newell KW. An epidemiologist's view of leprosy. Bull WHO 1966;34:827–857.
5. Xu K, de Vries RRP, van Leeuwen A, et al. HLA-linked control of predisposition of lepromatous leprosy. Int J Lepr 1985;53:56–63.
6. Ottenhoff THM, de Vries RRP. HLA class II immune response and suppression genes in leprosy. Int J Lepr 1987;55:521–534.
7. Abe M, Minagawa F, Yoshi Y, et al. Fluorescent leprosy antibody absorption (FLA-ABS) test for detecting subclinical infection with *Mycobacterium leprae*. Int J Lepr 1980;48:109–119.
8. Godal T, Negassi K. Subclinical infection in leprosy. Br Med J 1973;3:557–559.
9. Jopling WH. Handbook of Leprosy, 3rd ed. London: William Heinemann Books, 1984.
10. Blake LA, West BC, Lary CH, et al. Environmental nonhuman sources of leprosy. Rev Infect Dis 1987;9:3;562–577.
11. Pedley JC. Composite skin contact smears: A method of demonstrating nonemergence of *Mycobacterium leprae* from intact lepromatous skin. Lepr Rev 1970;41:31–43.
12. Rees RJW, McDougall AC, Weddell AG. The nose in mice with experimental human leprosy. Lepr Rev 1974;45:112–120.
13. Shepard CC. Acid-fast bacilli in nasal secretions in leprosy and results of inoculation of mice. Am J Hyg 1960;71:147–157.
14. Davey TF, Rees RJW. The nasal discharge in leprosy: Clinical and bacteriological aspects. Lepr Rev 1974;45:121–134.
15. Rees RJW. Airborne infection with *Mycobacterium leprae* in mice. Int J Lepr 1976;44:99–103.
16. Narayanan E, Manja KS, Bedi BMS, et al. Arthropod feeding experiments in lepromatous leprosy. Lepr Rev 1972;43:188–193.
17. Narayanan E, Sreevatsa Raj AD, Kirchheimer WF, Bedi BM. Transfer of leprosy bacilli from patients to mouse footpads by *Aedes aegypti*. Lepr India 1977;49:181–186.
18. Truman RW, Franzblau SG, Job CK. The nine-banded armadillo, *Dasypus novemcinctus*, as an animal model to study the transmission of leprosy. In: Abstracts of the 86th annual meeting of the American Society for Microbiology (abstract U-23). Washington, DC: American Society for Microbiology, 1986.
19. Kazda J, Irgens LM, Kolk AHJ. Acid-fast bacilli found in sphagnum vegetation of coastal Norway containing *Mycobacterium leprae*-specific phenolic glycolipid-1. Int J Lepr 1990;58:353–357.
20. Porritt RJ, Olsen RS. Two simultaneous cases of leprosy developing in tattoos. Am J Pathol 1947;23:805–817.
21. Rea TH, Modlin RL. Leprosy. In: Demis DJ, ed. Clinical Dermatology, 19th revision, vol 3, unit 16–29. Philadelphia: JB Lippincott, 1992.
22. Brown SG. The epidemiological situation of leprosy in Great Britain. Quad Coop Sani 1978;1:34–35.
23. Worth RM, Wong TO. Further notes on the prevalence of leprosy in Hong Kong Chinese living with 9 lepromatous patients. Int J Lepr 1971;39:744–748.
24. Ridley DS, Jopling WH. Classification of leprosy according to immunity: A five group system. Int J Lepr 1966;34:255–273.
25. Myrvang B, Godal T, Ridley DS, et al. Immune responsiveness to *Mycobacterium leprae* and other mycobacterial antigens throughout the clinical and histopathological spectrum of leprosy. Clin Exp Immunol 1973;14:541–543.
26. Rea TH, Quismorio FP, Harding B, et al. Immunologic responses in patients with lepromatous leprosy. Arch Dermatol 1976;112:791–800.

27. Mohagheghpour N, Gelber RH, Larrick JW, et al. Defective cell-mediated immunity in leprosy: Failure of T cells from lepromatous leprosy patients to respond to *Mycobacterium leprae* is associated with defective expression of interleukin 2 receptors and is not reconstituted by interleukin 2. J Immunol 1985;135:1443–1449.

28. Mehra V, Mason LH, Fields JP, et al. Lepromin-induced suppressor cells in patients with leprosy. J Immunol 1979;123:1813–1817.

29. Nath I, Singh R. The suppressive effect of *M. leprae* of the in vitro proliferative responses of lymphocytes from patients with leprosy. Clin Exp Immunol 1980;41:406–414.

30. Klebanoff SJ, Shepard CC. Toxic effect of the peroxidase–hydrogen peroxide–halide antimicrobial system on *Mycobacterium leprae*. Infect Immun 1984;44:534–536.

31. Horwitz MA, Levis WR, Cohn ZA. Defective production of monocyte-activating cytokines in lepromatous leprosy. J Exp Med 1984;159:666–678.

32. Mehra V, Brennan PJ, Rada E, et al. Lymphocyte suppression in leprae induced by unique *Mycobacterium leprae* glycolipid. Nature 1984;308:194–196.

33. Kaplan G, Gandhi RR, Weinstein DE, et al. *Mycobacterium leprae* antigen–induced suppression of T-cell proliferation in vitro. J Immunol 1987;138:3028–3034.

34. Sibley LD, Hunter SW, Brennan PJ, et al. Mycobacterial lipoarabinomannan inhibits gamma interferon–mediated activation of macrophages. Infect Immun 1988;56:1232–1236.

35. Modlin RL, Hofman FM, Horwitz DA, et al. In situ identification of cells in human leprosy granulomas with monoclonal antibodies to interleukin 2 and its receptor. J Immunol 1984;132:3085–3090.

36. Cooper CL, Mueller C, Sinchaisri T-A, et al. Analysis of naturally occurring delayed-type hypersensitivity reactions in leprosy by in situ hybridization. J Exp Med 1989;169:1565–1581.

37. Yamamura M, Uyemura K, Deans RJ, et al. Defining protective responses to pathogens: Cytokine profiles in leprosy lesions. Science 1991;254:277–279.

38. Kaplan G, Kiessling R, Teklemariam S, et al. The reconstitution of cell-mediated immunity in the cutaneous lesions of lepromatous leprosy by recombinant interleukin 2. J Exp Med 1989;169:893–907.

39. Nathan CF, Kaplan G, Levis WR, et al. Local and systemic effects of intradermal recombinant interferon-gamma in patients with lepromatous leprosy. N Engl J Med 1986;315:6–15.

40. Rose P, Waters MFR. Reversal reactions in leprosy and their management. Lepr Rev 1991;62:113–121.

41. Modlin RL, Pirmez C, Hofman FM, et al. Lymphocytes bearing antigen-specific gamma/delta T-cell receptors in human infectious disease lesions. Nature 1989;339:544–548.

42. Waters MFR, Turk JL, Wemambu SN. Mechanisms of reactions in leprosy. Int J Lepr 1971;39:417–428.

43. Sampaio EP, Sarno EN, Galilly R, et al. Thalidomide selectively inhibits tumor necrosis factor alpha production by stimulated human monocytes. J Exp Med 1991;173;699–703.

44. Rea TH. A comparative study of testicular involvement in lepromatous and borderline lepromatous leprosy. Int J Lepr 1988;56:383–388.

45. Job CK. Gynecomastia and leprous orchitis, a preliminary study. Int J Lepr 1961;29:423–441.

46. Mitsuda K, Ogawa M. A study of one hundred and fifty autopsies on cases of leprosy. Int J Lepr 1973;5:53–60.

47. Powell CS, Swan LL. Leprosy: Pathologic changes observed in fifty consecutive necropsies. Am J Pathol 1955;31:1131–1147.

48. Levis WR, Meeker HC, Schuller-Levis G, et al. IgM and IgG antibodies to phenolic glycolipid I from *Mycobacterium leprae* in leprosy: Insight into patient monitoring, erythema nodosum leprosum and bacillary persistance. Invest J Dermatol 1986;86:529–534.

49. Cho SN, Fujiwara T, Hunter SW, et al. Use of an artificial antigen containing the 3,6-di-O-methyl-beta-D-glucopyranosyl epitope for the serodiagnosis of leprosy. J Infect Dis 1984;150:311–322.

50. Cho SN, Yanagihara DL, Hunter WS, et al. Serological specificity of phenolic glycolipid I from *Mycobacterium leprae* and use in serodiagnosis of leprosy. Infect Immun 1983;41:1077–1083.

51. Young DB, Buchanan TM. A serological test for leprosy with a glycolipid specific for *Mycobacterium leprae*. Science 1983;221:1057–1059.

52. Gelber RH, Li F, Cho SN, et al. Serum antibodies to defined carbohydrate antigens during the course of treating leprosy. Int J Lepr 1989;57:744–751.

53. Rotberg A, Bechelli LM, Keil H. The Mitsuda reaction in a nonleprous area. Int J Lepr 1950;18:209–220.

54. Rees RJW. The significance of the lepromin reaction in man. Prog Allerg 1964;8:258–264.

55. Gill HK, Mustafa AS, Godal T. Vaccination of human volunteers with heat-killed *M. leprae*: Local responses in relation to the interpretation of the lepromin reaction. Int J Lepr 1988;56:36–44.

56. Byrd SR, Gelber RH. Effect of dapsone on haemoglobin concentration in patients with leprosy. Lepr Rev 1991;62:171–178.

57. Waters MF, Rees RJ, Pearson JM, et al. Rifampicin for lepromatous leprosy: Nine years' experience. Br Med J 1978;1:133–136.

58. Shepard CC, Levy L, Fasal P. Rapid bactericidal effect of rifampin on *Mycobacterium leprae*. Am J Trop Med Hyg 1972;21:446–449.

59. Gelber RH. Activity of minocycline in *Mycobacterium leprae*-infected mice. J Infect Dis 1987;156:236–239.

60. Ji BH, Perani EG, Grosset JH. Effectiveness of clarithromycin alone and in combination against experimental *Mycobacterium leprae* infection in mice. Antimicrob Agents Chemother 1991;35:579–581.

61. Franzblau SG, Hastings RC. In vitro and in vivo activities of macrolides against *Mycobacterium leprae*. Antimicrob Agents Chemother 1988;32:1758–1762.

62. Gelber RH. Activities of various macrolide antibiotics against *Mycobacterium leprae* infection in mice. Antimicrob Agents Chemother 1991;35:760–763.

63. Guelpa-Lauras C-C, Perani EG, Giroir A-M, et al. Activities of pefloxacin and ciprofloxacin against *Mycobacterium leprae* in the mouse. Int J Lepr 1987;55:70–77.

64. Grosset JH, Ji B, Guelpa-Lauras C-C, et al. Activity of ofloxacin against *Mycobacterium leprae* in the mouse. Int J Lepr 1988;56:259–264.

65. Gelber RH, Iranmanesh A, Murray L, et al. Activities of various quinolone antibiotics against *Mycobacterium leprae* in infected mice. Antimicrob Agents Chemother 1992;36:2544–2547.

66. Gelber RH. A clinical trial of minocycline in lepromatous leprosy. Br Med J 1992;304:91–92.

67. Ji B, Jamet P, Perani EG, et al. Powerful bactericidal activities of clarithromycin and minocycline against *Mycobacterium leprae* in lepromatous leprosy. J Infect Dis 1993;168:188–190.

68. Grosset JH, Ji BH, Guelpa-Lauras C-C, et al. Clinical trial of pefloxacin and ofloxacin in the treatment of lepromatous leprosy. Int J Lepr 1990;58:281–295.

69. Waters MF, Rees RJ, McDougall AC, et al. Ten years of dapsone in lepromatous leprosy: Clinical, bacteriological and histological assessment and the finding of viable leprosy bacilli. Lepr Rev 1974;45:288–298.

70. Subcommittee on Clinical Trials of THELEP and SWG of the UNDP/World Bank/WHO Special Program for Research and Training in Tropical Diseases. Int J Lepr 1987;55:864–871.

71. WHO Expert Committee on Leprosy. Geneva, Switzerland: World Health Organization; 1988. Technical Report Series 768.

72. Pattyn SR. Search for effective short-course regimens for the treatment of leprosy. Int J Lepr 1993;61:76–81.

73. Gelber RH, Rea TH, Murray LP, et al. Primary dapsone-resistant Hansen's disease in California: Experience with over 100 *Mycobacterium leprae* isolates. Arch Dermatol 1990;126:1584–1586.

74. Hastings RC, Morales MJ, Belk SE, et al. Thalidomide analogs with potential activity in erythema nodosum leprosum. Int J Lepr 1979;47:672–673.

75. Piepkorn M, Brown C, Zone J. Auricular chrondritis as a rheumatologic manifestation of Lucio's phenomenon: Clinical improvement after plasmapheresis. Ann Intern Med 1983;98:49–50.

76. Shepard CC, Fasal P, Worth RM, et al. Acedapsone in the prevention of leprosy: Field trial in three high prevalence villages in Micronesia. Am J Trop Med Hyg 1979;28:559–563.

77. Stanley SJ, Howland C, Stone MM, et al. BCG vaccination of children against leprosy in Uganda: Final results. J Hyg 1981;87:233–248.

78. Irwin KT, Sundaresan T, Gyi MM. BCG vaccination of children against leprosy: Fourteen-year findings of the trial in Burma. Bull WHO 1985;63:1069–1078.

79. Noordeen SK. Vaccination against leprosy: Recent advances and practical applications. Lepr Rev 1985;56:1–3.

80. Stanford JL. The BCG trials. Practitioner 1983;227:10–13.

81. Tripathy SP. The case for BCG. Ann Natl Acad Med Sci (India) 1983;19:11–21.

82. Convit J, Aranzazu N, Ulrich M, et al. Immunotherapy with a mixture of *Mycobacterium leprae* and BCG in different forms of leprosy and in Mitsuda-negative contacts. Int J Lepr 1982; 50:415–424.

83. Convit J, Aranzazu N, Pinardi M, et al. Immunological changes observed in indeterminate and lepromatous leprosy patients and Mitsuda-negative contacts after the inoculation of a mixture of *Mycobacterium leprae* and BCG. Clin Exp Immunol 1979; 36:214–220.

84. Convit J, Sampson C, Zuniga M, et al. Immunoprophylactic trial with combined *Mycobacterium leprae*/BCG vaccine against leprosy: Preliminary results. Lancet 1992;339:446–450.

85. Gelber RH, Brennan PJ, Hunter SW, et al. Effective vaccination of mice against leprosy bacilli with subunits of *Mycobacterium leprae*. Infect Immun 1990;58:711–718.

86. Gelber RH, Murray L, Siu P, et al. Vaccination of mice with a soluble protein fraction of *Mycobacterium leprae* provides consistent and long-term protection against *M. leprae* infection. Infect Immun 1992;60:1840–1844.

87. Gelber RH, Azouaou N, Abel K, et al. Protection of mice from *M. leprae* infection by T cells and protein vaccines. Int J Lepr 1992;60:715–716.

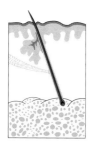

chapter 113

Nocardiosis and Actinomycosis

PAUL D. WORTMAN and DEBRA CHESTER KALTER*

Nocardiosis

DEFINITION

Nocardiosis refers to the spectrum of disease caused by filamentous bacteria of the genus *Nocardia*. In humans, nocardiosis is caused predominantly by *N. asteroides* and *N. brasiliensis* and less often by *N. caviae* and *N. transvalensis*. Infection may be initiated by inhalation or traumatic inoculation, with possible dissemination.[1-5] Cutaneous manifestations have been categorized as mycetoma and lymphocutaneous, cervicofacial, superficial, and disseminated infections.[4]

CLINICAL DESCRIPTION

N. asteroides is isolated from soil in temperate areas. *N. brasiliensis* is endemic in regions of Mexico and Central and South America; it is also occasionally found in the United States. Males are infected more often than females (3 : 1), and the incidence of infection is highest in the 20- to 50-year old age group, suggesting some occupational exposure.[1, 6] Approximately 85% of cases are pulmonary or systemic infections and 15% are localized to the skin and soft tissue.[3] *N. asteroides* accounts for the majority of pulmonary and systemic infections, often occurring opportunistically.[3] Rarely, *N. asteroides* causes primary cutaneous infection.[7] *N. brasiliensis* usually infects the skin and soft tissue in immunocompetent patients.[4, 8] Occasionally, *N. brasiliensis* produces primary

pulmonary infection or disseminated disease in immunocompromised and immunocompetent hosts.[3, 8]

Nocardial pulmonary infections may cause necrotizing pneumonia, cavitation, abscesses, pleural effusions, and penetration of sinus tracts through the chest wall.[1, 2, 8] Systemic dissemination occurs most frequently in patients with pulmonary infection; however, it may follow primary cutaneous infection.[7] The central nervous system is involved most often (occurring in up to one third of cases), with single or multiple brain abscesses.[1, 2] The skin and soft tissues are the second most common sites of dissemination (10%–15%). Nodules, pustules, and abscesses occur and may become ulcerated.[3, 4] Other reported sites of dissemination include the kidneys, liver, spleen, adrenals, pericardium, myocardium, and eyes.[1]

The most common manifestation worldwide of primary skin and soft tissue infection is mycetoma (Fig. 113–1).[8] A mycetoma is a chronic infection that usually occurs on the lower extremity as a painless, firm swelling with multiple sinus tracts draining purulent material. Underlying bone is often involved. Mycetomas may be caused by *Nocardia* and other actinomycetes (actinomycetoma) or by true fungi (eumycetoma).[9] Primary cutaneous infection alternatively may occur as pustules, abscesses, ulcers, or cellulitis, which may mimic infection caused by more common gram-positive bacteria.[4, 8] A sporotrichoid pattern of linear erythematous nodules, often suppurative or ulcerated, can also be seen along an extremity.[10] A cervicofacial variant has occurred in children, who have an erythematous papule or pustule on the face, submandibular lymphadenopathy, and fever.[11]

PATHOLOGY

Cutaneous lesions other than mycetomas reveal neutrophilic abscesses with rare fibrosis, Langhans' giant

---

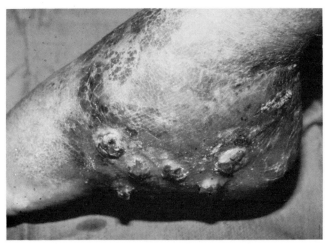

FIGURE 113-1. Mycetoma due to *Nocardia brasiliensis* frequently involves the lower extremity with induration and chronically draining sinus tracts. (From Wortman PD. Treatment of a *Nocardia brasiliensis* mycetoma with sulfamethoxazole and trimethoprim, amikacin, and amoxicillin and clavulanate. Arch Dermatol 1993;129:564–567. Copyright 1993, American Medical Association.)

cells, and caseation necrosis.[1] The organisms are not seen in hematoxylin and eosin–stained sections.[1] Grains or granules, which represent microbial colonies, can be seen in mycetomas, surrounded by an infiltrate of neutrophils with some plasma cells and macrophages.[12] Intact neutrophil function and cell-mediated immunity are necessary to control nocardial infection.[13]

DIAGNOSIS AND DIFFERENTIAL DIAGNOSIS

Gram and modified acid-fast stains and culture of clinical specimens (sputum, pus, tissue) establish the diagnosis.[1, 2] *Nocardia* species are aerobic, weakly gram-positive, variably acid-fast, filamentous bacteria. Growth of *Nocardia* organisms may take a week or more on Sabouraud's glucose agar and is impeded on media containing antimicrobial agents or by the presence of other bacteria.[1, 2] Serologic tests are unreliable because of cross-reactivity with other infections, particularly tuberculosis and leprosy.[14] Cross-reactivity results from shared antigens on the cell walls of *Nocardia* species and mycobacteria.[15] An enzyme immunoassay using a specific antigen from *N. asteroides* is more sensitive and specific than prior tests.[16]

Since the clinical presentation of nocardiosis is pleomorphic, so is the differential diagnosis (Table 113–1).

TABLE 113-1. Differential Diagnosis of Nocardiosis and Actinomycosis	
Nocardiosis	**Actinomycosis**
Tumors	Staphylococcal
Bacterial infections	botryomycosis
Foreign body granuloma	Deep fungal infections
Deep fungal infections—	Dental abscess
sporotrichosis	

Other infectious and granulomatous diseases, as well as tumors, must be excluded during evaluation.

TREATMENT

Antimicrobial chemotherapy is administered for prolonged periods, often in combination with surgery to drain abscesses, excise small mycetomas, or debulk larger mycetomas.[2, 12, 17] Sulfonamides, such as sulfadiazine and trimethoprim-sulfamethoxazole, have been considered the most effective antibiotic agents; however, primary resistance and late relapse are problematic.[2] Other antibiotics that may be effective, as suggested by in vitro or clinical studies, include minocycline, amikacin, amoxicillin-clavulanic acid, imipenem, cefotaxime, ceftriaxone, and cefuroxime (Table 113–2).[2, 18] Combinations of antibiotics may act synergistically.[2] In vitro sensitivity testing is helpful, if available, since individual isolate sensitivities are variable.[2]

Actinomycosis

DEFINITION

Actinomycosis is a chronic, suppurative, granulomatous, and fibrosing infection that most often involves the cervicofacial, thoracic, and abdominal areas. It is caused primarily by the endogenous oral bacterium *Actinomyces israelii*. Infection frequently spreads to adjacent tissues, forming cutaneous sinus tracts that discharge "sulfur granules," which are colonies of the causative organism. Less common causes of actinomycosis in humans include *A. naeslundii*, *A. viscosus*, *A. odontolyticus*, *A. meyeri*, and *Arachnia propionica*.[1, 19, 20]

CLINICAL DESCRIPTION

Actinomycosis occurs worldwide with a higher incidence in rural areas. It is seen most commonly in the 30- to 60-year age group and rarely in children and affects males more often than females.[20, 21] Cervicofacial infection occurs in 32% to 63% of cases, with thoracic infection in 13% to 34% and abdominal infection in 13% to 23%.[21–23] Actinomycosis is caused by normal flora in the human oral cavity. *A. israelii* is also found in the intestines and vagina.[1, 19]

Patients with actinomycosis, regardless of site, may complain of localized pain and can have a low-grade fever and a normal or mildly elevated white blood cell count.[22] Cervicofacial actinomycosis, or "lumpy jaw," is believed to begin as a periodontal abscess that forms in the mandible or maxilla after dental extraction, oral surgery, or other trauma in the setting of poor oral hygiene (Fig. 113–2).[20, 24] The infection then characteristically spreads (acutely or chronically) to adjacent tissues, form-

TABLE 113-2. Treatment of Nocardiosis and Actinomycosis				
	Norcardiosis		**Actinomycosis**	
	Drug	**Dosage***	**Drug**	**Dosage***
Preferred Therapy	Sulfadiazine or sulfisoxazole	1 g q4h PO	Penicillin G	10-20 million units per day IV
	Trimethoprim-sulfamethoxazole	6 tabs (80/400) q6h PO	Followed by penicillin V	2-4 g per day PO
	Surgery (may be required)		Surgery (may be required)	
Alternative Therapy	Minocycline	100 mg q12h PO	Tetracycline	500 mg q6h PO
	Amikacin	5 mg/kg q8h or 7.5 mg q12h IV	Erythromycin	500 mg q6h PO
			Clindamycin	300-450 mg q6h PO
	The optimal duration of treatment for nocardiosis is not known; prolonged therapy (often for many months after clinical cure) is required to prevent relapses.[2]		Duration of treatment for actinomyosis is intravenous penicillin X 4-6 weeks followed by oral penicillin for 6-12 months.*	

*Data from the Sanford Guide to Antimicrobial Therapy (1993), Antimicrobial Therapy, Inc., with permission.

ing sinuses to the skin or mouth that drain purulent material, sometimes containing granules. The skin overlying the indurated mass may exhibit a violaceous color. There is usually no regional lymphadenopathy.[23, 24] Bone involvement results from direct spread of infection and occurs as periostitis and osteomyelitis.[20, 24] Penetration into the central nervous system from foci in the jaw, ears, or sinuses may occur, with resultant brain abscesses or meningoencephalitis.[25]

Thoracic actinomycosis most frequently occurs after aspiration from the oral cavity.[19, 20, 23] The lung parenchyma (typically basilar), pleura, mediastinum, and chest wall may all be involved.[19, 23] Underlying lung diseases such as tuberculosis, bronchiectasis, and carcinoma predispose to infection.[20] Roentgenographic features that suggest the diagnosis are (1) penetration of a pulmonary focus of infection through the chest wall; (2) destruction of adjacent ribs; (3) spread of infection across interlobar fissures; and (4) erosion of the vertebral body and processes.[26]

Abdominal actinomycosis most often involves the ileocecal region. Infection tends to start at sites where the bowel mucosa has been injured by inflammatory disorders, ulcerations, perforations, surgery, or other trauma.[19, 27] Abscess formation, draining sinus tracts, induration, and strictures are typical.[19] Intrauterine contraceptive devices predispose to pelvic infection.[28]

Hematogenous dissemination occurs most often secondary to thoracic infection and may occur in 10% of all patients with actinomycosis.[21] Sites of dissemination include the central nervous system, kidney, liver, spleen, bowel, pericardium, thyroid, skin, and soft tissues.[19, 21, 29] Traumatic inoculation into the skin, usually of the extremities, may result in abscesses and sinus tract formation.[30] Unlike infection with *N. asteroides*, actinomycosis does not occur more frequently as an opportunistic infection.[19]

PATHOLOGY

Gross pathologic examination of infected tissue reveals suppurative and fibrotic masses with multiple sinus tracts.[1, 21] Yellow "sulfur granules," 0.25 to 2.0 mm in diameter, suggest the diagnosis when present within the purulent material.[29] Neutrophilic abscesses are surrounded by a mixed infiltrate of lymphocytes, plasma cells, macrophages, and fibroblasts. When stained with hematoxylin and eosin, the irregularly shaped sulfur granules are basophilic, with a rim of eosinophilic clubs radiating outward, surrounded by neutrophils (Fig. 113-3).[31]

DIAGNOSIS AND DIFFERENTIAL DIAGNOSIS

The presence of granules in tissue is not pathognomonic of actinomycosis. Similar granules can be seen in

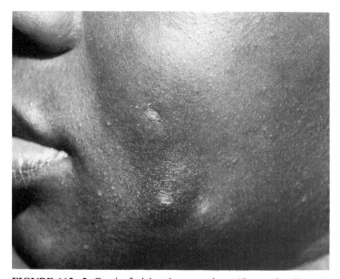

FIGURE 113-2. Cervicofacial actinomycosis, or "lumpy jaw," results in abscess formation with subsequent drainage through the skin. (Courtesy of Alan B. Fleischer, Jr., M.D.)

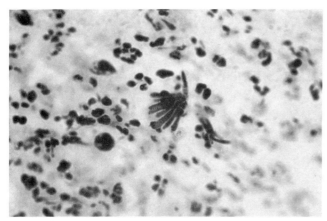

FIGURE 113-3. A clump of bacilli forming a small actinomycotic sulfur granule is seen within a field of polymorphonuclear cells (Gram stain, ×400). (From Katz BJ, Kalter DC, Bruce S. Subcutaneous nodules in a man diagnosed as having tuberculosis. Arch Dermatol 1988;124:121–122, 124–125. Copyright 1988, American Medical Association.)

mycetomas (caused by fungi, *Nocardia*, *Streptomyces*, or *Actinomadura*) and in staphylococcal botryomycosis.[1, 12, 19] Distinguishing features exist: the eosinophilic clubbed fringe typical of actinomycosis is usually absent in mycetomas and botryomycosis; the true fungi, which cause enmycetomas, exhibit wide septate hyphae, best seen with special stains; granules in nocardia mycetomas are more loosely aggregated than in actinomycosis; and the granules in staphylococcal botryomycosis are composed of cocci.[1, 12, 21] The composition of granules is sometimes more evident in Brown-Brenn–stained sections. *Actinomyces* species are gram-positive non–acid-fast, branching, long, slender filamentous bacteria.[1] Clinically, other infectious agents and tumors must be excluded (see Table 113–1).

The definitive diagnosis of actinomycosis is made by identifying the organism in culture. A granule (after careful washing in sterile nonbacteriostatic saline to remove bacterial contaminants) or homogenized tissue is plated onto a brain-heart infusion or blood agar, without antimicrobials, and incubated anaerobically at 37°C for 4 to 6 days.[23] Some species are microaerophilic or facultative aerobes.[1] *Actinobacillus actinomycetemcomitans* is frequently isolated in association with *Actinomyces* in cervicofacial and thoracic infections, while *Escherichia coli* and anaerobic bacteria may accompany abdominal disease.[19, 23]

TREATMENT

Actinomycosis is treated with a combination of long-term (weeks to months) high-dose penicillin and surgical debridement of abscesses and fibrotic tissue.[32] Other antimicrobial agents that may be effective, as suggested by in vitro susceptibility studies, include erythromycin, cephalothin, minocycline, tetracycline, clindamycin, and chloramphenicol (see Table 113–2).[33] High doses of antibiotics are required to penetrate fibrotic tissue and the microbial granules.[32]

References

1. Rippon JW. Medical Mycology: The Pathogenic Fungi and the Pathogenic Actinomycetes, 3rd ed. Philadelphia: WB Saunders Co., 1988:30–68.
2. Lerner PI. *Nocardia* species. In: Mandell GL, Douglas RG Jr, Bennett JE, eds. Principles and Practice of Infectious Diseases, 3rd ed. New York: Churchill Livingstone, 1990:1926–1932.
3. Beaman BL, Burnside J, Edwards B, et al. Nocardial infections in the United States, 1972–1974. J Infect Dis 1976;134:286–289.
4. Kalb RE, Kaplan MH, Grossman ME. Cutaneous nocardiosis: Case reports and review. J Am Acad Dermatol 1985;13:125–133.
5. Schiff TA, Goldman R, Sanchez M, et al. Primary lymphocutaneous nocardiosis caused by an unusual species of *Nocardia*: *Nocardia transvalensis*. J Am Acad Dermatol 1993;28:336–340.
6. Rippon JW. *Nocardia*: A geographic prevalence. (Letter). Arch Dermatol 1977;113:237.
7. Kahn FW, Gornick CG, Tofte RW. Primary cutaneous *Nocardia asteroides* infection with dissemination. Am J Med 1981;70:859–863.
8. Smego RA Jr, Gallis HA. The clinical spectrum of *Nocardia brasiliensis* infection in the United States. Rev Infect Dis 1984;6:164–180.
9. Magana M, Magana-Garcia M. Mycetoma. Dermatol Clin 1989;7:203–217.
10. Schwartz JG, McGough DA, Thorner RE, et al. Primary lymphocutaneous *Nocardia brasiliensis* infection: Three case reports and a review of the literature. Diagn Microbiol Infect Dis 1988;10:113–120.
11. Lampe RM, Baker CJ, Septimus EJ, et al. Cervicofacial nocardiosis in children. J Pediatr 1981;99:593–595.
12. Lavalle P. Mycetoma. In: Canizares O, Harman RRM, eds. Clinical Tropical Dermatology, 2nd ed. Boston: Blackwell Scientific Publications, 1992:41–60.
13. Filice GA, Niewoehner DE. Contribution of neutrophils and cell-mediated immunity to control of *Nocardia asteroides* in murine lungs. J Infect Dis 1987;156:113–121.
14. Shainhouse JZ, Pier AC, Stevens DA. Complement fixation antibody test for human nocardiosis. J Clin Microbiol 1978;8:516–519.
15. Boiron P, Stynen D. Immunodiagnosis of nocardiosis. Gene 1992;115:219–222.
16. Angeles AM, Sugar AM. Rapid diagnosis of nocardiosis with an enzyme immunoassay. J Infect Dis 1987;155:292–296.
17. Mahgoub ES. Agents of mycetoma. In: Mandell GL, Douglas RG, Jr, Bennett JE, eds. Principles and Practice of Infectious Diseases, 3rd ed. New York: Churchill Livingstone, 1990:1977–1980.
18. Gutmann L, Goldstein FW, Kitzis MD, et al. Susceptibility of *Nocardia asteroides* to 46 antibiotics, including 22 β-lactams. Antimicrob Agents Chemother 1983;23:248–251.
19. Lerner PI. *Actinomyces* and *Arachnia* Species. In: Mandell GL, Douglas RJ Jr, Bennett JE, eds. Principles and Practice of Infectious Diseases, 3rd ed. New York: Churchill Livingstone, 1990:1932–1942.
20. Hay RJ, Roberts SOB, MacKenzie DWR. Mycology: Actinomycosis. In: Champion RH, Burton JL, Ebling FJG, eds. Textbook of Dermatology, 5th ed. Oxford: Blackwell Scientific Publications, 1992:1213–1214.
21. Brown JR. Human actinomycosis: A study of 181 subjects. Hum Pathol 1973;4:319–330.
22. Weese WC, Smith IM. A study of 57 cases of actinomycosis over a 36-year period: A diagnostic "failure" with a good prognosis after treatment. Arch Intern Med 1975;135:1562–1568.
23. Bennhoff DF. Actinomycosis: Diagnostic and therapeutic considerations and a review of 32 cases. Laryngoscope 1984;94:1198–1217.
24. Lerner PI. The lumpy jaw: Cervicofacial actinomycosis. Infect Dis Clin North Am 1988;2:203–220.
25. Smego RA Jr. Actinomycosis of the central nervous system. Rev Infect Dis 1987;9:855–865.
26. Flynn MW, Felson B. The Roentgen manifestations of thoracic actinomycosis. AJR 1970;110:707–716.
27. Bernardi RS. Abdominal actinomycosis. Surg Gynecol Obstet 1979;149:257–266.
28. Burkman R, Schlesselman S, McCaffrey L, et al. The relationship

of genital tract actinomycetes and the development of pelvic inflammatory disease. Am J Obstet Gynecol 1982;145:585–589.

29. Katz BJ, Kalter DC, Bruce S. Subcutaneous nodules in a man diagnosed as having tuberculosis. Arch Dermatol 1988;124: 124–125.

30. Reiner SL, Harrelson JM, Miller SE, et al. Primary actinomycosis of an extremity: A case report and review. Rev Infect Dis 1987;9:581–589.

31. Lever WF, Schaumberg-Lever G. Histopathology of the Skin, 7th ed. Philadelphia: JB Lippincott, 1990:385–386.

32. Peabody JW, Jr, Seabury JH. Actinomycosis and nocardiosis: A review of basic differences in therapy. Am J Med 1960;28:99–115.

33. Lerner PI. Susceptibility of pathogenic actinomycetes to antimicrobial compounds. Antimicrob Agents Chemother 1974;5: 302–309.

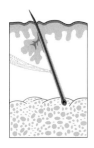

chapter 114

Rocky Mountain Spotted Fever and Other Rickettsial Diseases

SUSAN HADLEY and SCOTT M. HAMMER

Rocky Mountain spotted fever and other rickettsial infections are diseases that are caused by obligate intracellular bacterial organisms belonging to the family Rickettsiaceae. This family subsumes the genera *Rickettsia, Coxiella,* and *Ehrlichia,* which are responsible for the spotted fever/typhus illnesses, Q fever, and ehrlichiosis, respectively (Table 114–1). All have the capacity to produce febrile infectious syndromes, and the spotted fever/typhus group of illnesses have the most distinctive cutaneous manifestations. These diseases are zoonotic infections that are transmitted to humans by arthropod vectors or by aerosol (e.g., Q fever). Recognition of these illnesses requires a careful history in addition to a detailed examination in that an individual's activities, travels, and arthropod or animal exposures are often the key to suspecting the diagnosis. This is critical in the case of Rocky Mountain spotted fever, the most important disease in this category, as a delay in diagnosis may result in tragic consequences. Rickettsial infections should always be considered in the differential diagnosis of fever and rash, and thus a thorough knowledge of the cutaneous manifestations of these diseases is important in trying to make an early diagnosis and institute effective antimicrobial therapy.

Rocky Mountain Spotted Fever

CLINICAL DESCRIPTION

Rocky Mountain spotted fever is caused by the obligate intracellular parasite *Rickettsia rickettsii* and is transmitted to humans by the bite of a tick. In 1993, approximately 450 cases were reported in the United States, although this figure likely represents underreporting of the disease.[1] In the western United States, the primary vector is the wood tick, *Dermacentor andersoni*; the dog tick, *Dermacentor variabilis,* is the principal vector in the eastern and southern states.[2] The reservoirs of the organism are primarily small rodents, but ticks may infect their offspring transovarially, thus perpetuating generations of infected ticks. Adult ticks feed on humans; therefore, the peak incidence of disease is in the late spring and early summer when nymphs molt to become adults. Although the disease was first reported in the Rocky Mountain region, the highest incidence of disease now occurs in the South Atlantic states of North and South Carolina extending to the central middle states of Tennessee, Oklahoma, and Texas. Children have the highest incidence of disease, accounting for up to 50% of cases, likely reflecting the seasonal peak of the adult ticks and outdoor activities of children.[2–6]

After inoculation, the incubation period ranges from 2 to 14 days with an average of 7 days. The onset of symptoms is more often abrupt but may be insidious.[2, 5, 7, 8] Early symptoms are usually nonspecific and include fever (100 to 104° F), headache (often severe), myalgias, arthralgias, and malaise. The classic triad of fever, rash, and headache history of tick exposure may occur infrequently in the first 3 days of illness but is reported in 50% to 60% of confirmed cases.[8, 9]

Rash is the sign most helpful in making the correct diagnosis (Fig. 114–1). The mean time of onset is 3 or 4 days and ranges from 1 to 14 days.[2, 7, 10] It is important to note that at least 4% to 10% of patients may not develop a rash or may develop one so late in the course of illness

TABLE 114–1. Epidemiologic and Cutaneous Characteristics of Rickettsial Infections

Disease	Organism	Geographic Distribution	Hosts	Mode of Transmission	Rash Nature	Rash Spread	Eschar
Spotted fever group							
Rocky Mountain spotted fever	R. rickettsii	North America, Central and South America	Rodents, dogs	Tick bite	Maculopapular, petechial	Centripetal	No
Mediterranean spotted fever	R. conorii	Mediterranean basin, Asia	Rodents, dogs	Tick bite	Maculopapular	Centripetal	Yes (tache noir)
South African tick-bite fever	R. conorii	Africa					
Siberian tick typhus	R. sibirica	Russia, Mongolia	Rodents	Tick bite	Maculopapular	Centripetal	Yes
Queensland tick typhus	R. australis	Australia	Rodents, marsupials	Tick bite	Maculopapular	Centripetal	Yes
Oriental spotted fever	R. japonica	Japan	?	Tick bite			
Rickettsialpox	R. akari	North America, Ukraine, Korea	Mice	Mite bite	Papulovesicular	Centrifugal	Yes
Typhus group							
Epidemic typhus (louse-borne)	R. prowazekii	Africa, Central and South America, U.S., Asia	Humans (flying squirrels)	Louse feces	Maculopapular	Centrifugal	No
Brill-Zinsser (recrudescent louse-borne typhus)	R. prowazekii	Worldwide (immigration-dependent)	Humans	Latent infection	Maculopapular (may be absent)	Centrifugal	No
Murine typhus	R. typhi	Worldwide (southern U.S., Texas)	Rodents	Flea feces	Maculopapular	Centrifugal	No
Scrub typhus	R. tsutsugamushi	Southeast Asia, South Pacific	Rodents	Mite (chigger bite)	Maculopapular	Centrifugal	Yes
Q fever	Coxiella burnetii	Worldwide	Cattle, sheep, goats	Inhalation	Usually none	Centrifugal, if present	No
Ehrlichiosis	E. chaffeensis	Southeastern, South Central and Middle Atlantic states, Europe, Africa	?	Tick bite	Maculopapular (minority of cases)	No classic pattern	

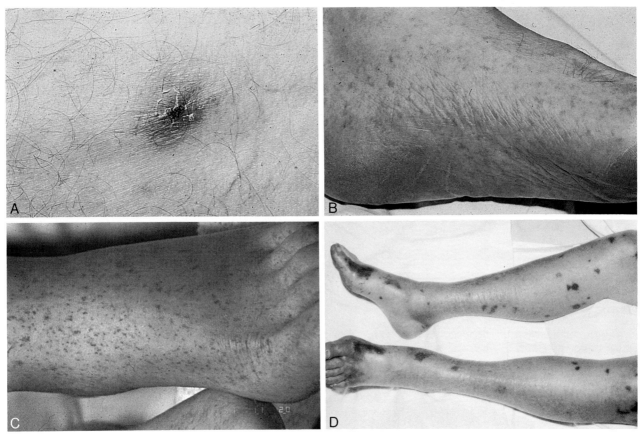

FIGURE 114-1. The rash of Rocky Mountain spotted fever. *A*, Site of the tick bite. *B*, Macular lesions of the early rash. *C*, Petechial component of the later rash. *D*, Confluent ecchymoses on extremity and gangrene of toes in a patient with severe illness. (Courtesy of Barney Graham, M.D., Vanderbilt University, Division of Infectious Diseases, Memphis, TN.)

that the delayed diagnosis and treatment may result in death.[3,4,7,8] The eruption is initially characterized by pink macules beginning on the wrists, ankles, palms, and soles that fade with pressure. Application of a warm compress to the extremity or a rise in body temperature in the early stages may accentuate the rash and assist in early diagnosis.[10] Centripetal spread to axillae, buttocks, trunk, and face is characteristic. The color of lesions deepens, and papules evolve 2 to 3 days after onset. In approximately 4 days, petechiae usually develop and may coalesce to form large ecchymotic lesions. Capillary fragility may be evidenced by the development of petechiae at a tourniquet or blood pressure cuff site (Rumpel-Leede phenomenon).[10] The rash generally fades into hyperpigmented spots at the site of previous lesions and may persist for several weeks during convalescence.[10] The severity of the eruption often correlates with the severity of the illness. Patients with prolonged hypotension with or without evidence of disseminated intravascular coagulation may develop confluent ecchymoses and gangrene of fingers, toes, penis, and/or scrotum requiring surgical debridement or amputation.[15-17]

R. rickettsii infection is a multisystem organ disease reflecting a widespread infectious vasculitic process. While a petechial eruption is the hallmark of the disease, a variety of symptoms at presentation or during the course of illness reflect systemic involvement. Gastrointestinal manifestations such as nausea, vomiting, diarrhea, and/or abdominal pain occur in 30% to 50%.[7,8,18-20] Pneumonitis occurs in approximately 12% to 20% and is more common (up to 36%) in fatal cases.[3,7,8] Capillary leakage resulting in noncardiogenic pulmonary edema occurs in cases with severe vasculitis.[21,22] Myocarditis with cardiac dysfunction may develop in 5% to 26% of patients. Skeletal muscle necrosis is manifested by severe myalgias and rises in creatine kinase and aldolase levels, and may occur in 17% to 46% of patients.[7,8] Azotemia secondary to volume depletion is not uncommon, and interstitial nephritis is the hallmark of renal pathology.[23] Neurologic manifestations are common. Headache is the most frequent complaint, and meningismus occurs in approximately 25%.[7,8] Seizures and coma occur in 8% to 9% of hospitalized patients, with focal deficits, hearing loss, papilledema, and ataxia occurring less often. Other manifestations of disease include conjunctivitis, retinitis, parotitis, and orchitis.[8]

PATHOLOGY

A widespread small vessel thrombotic vasculitis is the pathologic hallmark of many forms of rickettsial disease.[24-26] Infections with *R. rickettsii* produce the most severe vasculitis and the prototypical pathologic changes. After inoculation by the vector, local replication of the organism occurs followed by invasion of the blood stream and lymphatics and dissemination to multiple organs. Endothelial cells of small vessels and, in *R. rickettsii* infection, smooth muscle cells of the vessel wall are the initial targets of infection. Organisms enter cells by induced phagocytosis, escape from the phagosome, and readily multiply in the cytoplasm.[27] *R. rickettsii* replicates in the nucleus as well. Endothelial cell swelling and death occur, leading to thrombosis of the vessel and vascular and perivascular necrosis (Fig. 114–2).

Multiple organs may be involved, including the skin, heart, lungs, kidney, brain, skeletal muscle, and gastrointestinal tract.[19, 21-23, 28] Microscopic examination of cutaneous lesions shows perivascular infiltrates of lymphocytes and sometimes a few neutrophils around venules that have fibrin in their walls and often in their lumina. Eschars are due to necrosis of the epidermis. Extravasated erythrocytes are commonly present. Proliferation of endothelial and surrounding mononuclear cells results in formation of an identifiable histopathologic nodule in many organs.[24] Central nervous system infection is associated with "Fraenkel nodules" or infiltration of mononuclear inflammatory cells around central vessels.[24,25,28,29] In his extensive pathologic studies, Wolbach noted that the progression of the skin rash reflected the extensive endothelial cell damage, and Harrell emphasized the correlation of the pathologic lesions with the clinical course.[24, 30]

PATHOGENESIS

The pathogenesis of the vasculitis is not completely understood but appears to be mediated by direct toxic effects of the organism. Ultrastructural studies of cultured endothelial cells infected with *R. rickettsii* have shown early dilatation of endoplasmic reticulum and outer nuclear membranes with subsequent intracisternal swelling.[31, 32] The cytopathic changes in *R. rickettsii* infections do not seem to correlate with the intracellular organism burden as they do in *R. prowazekii* infections, where cell lysis occurs with increasing organism load.[33, 34] Beause of the demonstrated membrane abnormalities, free radical–induced lipid peroxidation has been hypothesized to be the physiologic cause of endothelial cell injury.[33] Alteration of anticoagulant functions of endothelial cells either via antibodies to endothelial cells and/or phospholipids or via rickettsial-induced release of von Willebrand's factor from Weibel-Palade bodies or via increased platelet adherence and activation may also be involved in the pathogenesis of the vasculitis and thrombosis.[35-39] Increased phospholipase A activity of *Rickettsia* species with subsequent release of soluble immune mediators such as prostaglandin I_2, prostaglandin E_2, and leukotriene B_4 from endothelial and macrophage cells noted in vitro may contribute to the increased vascular permeability accompanying Rocky Mountain spotted fever and severe typhus seen in vivo.[29, 40-45] There is little compelling evidence for a role of the host immune response in the pathogenesis of rickettsial diseases.

DIAGNOSIS AND DIFFERENTIAL DIAGNOSIS

Routine laboratory evaluation is of little help in distinguishing the disease process. Diagnosis is most commonly confirmed serologically or by direct visualization of organisms in tissue by immunofluorescence staining. The most sensitive and specific serologic diagnostic tests are the indirect hemagglutination (IHA) and indirect fluorescent antibody (IFA) tests.[46] Less sensitive tests include latex agglutination, complement fixation, and the Weil-Felix reaction (based on the cross-reactive agglutination of *Proteus* strains OX-19 and OX-2). No serologic test, however, can be used for acute diagnostic purposes. Early specific diagnosis can be achieved with identification of rickettsiae in skin tissue specimens by immunofluorescence staining of the organism in the blood vessel walls (Fig. 114–3).[47-51] More rapid techniques utilizing avidin-biotin immunoperoxidase demonstration of intracellular rickettsial organisms have been developed.[52] Polymerase chain reaction technology has been applied successfully to amplify a region of the *R. rickettsii* genome from the sera of several patients with known Rocky Mountain spotted fever and may prove to be the most sensitive early diagnostic tool for accurate detection of rickettsial infection, but it is available only in research settings at this time.[53, 54] Isolation of the organism is not performed outside of the research laboratory, and the diagnosis today is most often confirmed with acute and convalescent serologic titers with or without immunoflu-

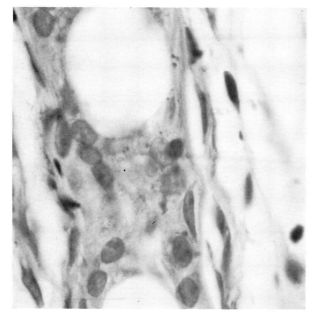

FIGURE 114–2. Histopathology of the vasculitis of Rocky Mountain spotted fever: Giemsa stain of skin biopsy showing organisms within endothelial cells. (Courtesy of Barney Graham, M.D., Vanderbilt University, Division of Infectious Diseases, Memphis, TN.)

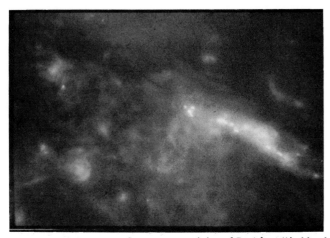

FIGURE 114-3. Immunofluorescence staining of *R. rickettsii* in blood vessel wall of skin tissue biopsy specimen. (Courtesy of David H. Walker, M.D., The University of Texas Medical Branch at Galveston, Department of Pathology, Galveston, TX.)

orescence staining of skin tissue specimens. Thus, most often the early diagnosis of Rocky Mountain spotted fever is a clinical one based on symptoms, signs, and supporting epidemiologic history.

The differential diagnosis for Rocky Mountain spotted fever is broad (Table 114-2). The most important potentially fatal disease to rule out is meningococcemia. Rash may be similar in distribution and character but usually occurs earlier in the course of illness in meningococcemia, and a Gram stain of an unroofed lesion may reveal the organism. Early in the course of Rocky Mountain spotted fever, especially if rash is not present, the diagnosis may be elusive, leading to delay in initiation of appropriate therapy. The nonspecific symptoms may suggest viral diseases such as enteroviral infection, measles or atypical measles, rubella, infectious mononucleosis, or hepatitis.[2, 55] Viral exanthems caused by the enteroviruses are much less often associated with petechiae. Other illnesses that may be confused with Rocky Mountain spotted fever include typhoid fever, leptospirosis, relapsing fever, secondary syphilis, gonococcemia, and noninfectious vasculitides such as immune thrombocytopenic purpura, thrombotic thrombocytopenic purpura, and immune complex vasculitis. Other rickettsial infections such as murine typhus, seen primarily in the southeastern United States and Texas, ehrlichiosis, and rickettsialpox are important considerations. Centrifugal spread and sparing of the palms and soles are most typical of the rash of murine typhus. Ehrlichiosis is less commonly associated with a petechial rash, and rickettsialpox is notable for a distinctive vesicular rash, an eschar at the site of the mite bite, and spread of the rash from the bite site to the torso and extremities.

TREATMENT

Without treatment, mortality from Rocky Mountain spotted fever approaches 70%.[56] Appropriate early antibiotic and supportive therapy has reduced mortality to 2% to 7%.[3, 4, 7, 8] The bacteriostatic agents tetracycline (and its analogues) and chloramphenicol are the mainstays of antibiotic therapy (Table 114-3). Newer fluoroquinolones such as ciprofloxacin and pefloxacin (not available in the United States) have been successfully used to treat other spotted fever rickettsioses and are effective in vitro against *R. rickettsii*, but proof of their clinical efficacy in Rocky Mountain spotted fever is lacking.[57]

The recommended treatment includes doxycycline, 200 mg per day orally in divided doses; or tetracycline hydrochloride, 25 to 30 mg/kg per day orally in four divided doses; or chloramphenicol sodium succinate, 50 mg/kg loading dose, followed by 50 mg/kg per day orally in divided doses. Patients severely ill or unable to take oral medication should be treated with intravenous medications in the following doses: doxycycline, 4.4 mg/kg per day up to 200 mg per day in divided doses every 12 hours; tetracycline, 15 mg/kg loading dose followed by 15 mg/kg per day in divided doses every 6 hours; or chloramphenicol, 15 to 20 mg/kg loading dose followed by 30 to 50 mg/kg per day in divided doses every 6 hours. Sulfonamides should not be used when Rocky Mountain spotted fever is suspected, as they are ineffective and have been reported to exacerbate the disease.[58] Defervescence is usually prompt within 24 to 72 hours, with improvement of general well-being. Treatment is continued until the patient has been afebrile for at least 2 to 3 days.

Supportive therapy with volume replacement including intravenous fluids or blood products may be necessary for the critically ill patient. Corticosteroids may have a role in the treatment of critically ill patients with diffuse vasculitis and shock secondary to increased capillary permeability,[9, 29, 59] but their efficacy is unknown.

Careful epidemiologic history, detailed physical examination, and a high index of suspicion are necessary for

TABLE 114-2. Differential Diagnosis of Rocky Mountain Spotted Fever		
Common	**Less Common**	**Rare**
Meningococcemia	Gonococcemia	Borreliosis (relapsing fever)
Other rickettsial diseases	Measles (if unvaccinated)	Immune thrombocytopenic purpura
Enteroviral infections	Rubella (if unvaccinated)	Thrombotic thrombocytopenic purpura
Typhoid fever	Infectious mononucleosis (Epstein-Barr virus,	Immune complex vasculitis
Secondary syphilis	cytomegalovirus)	
Scarlet fever	*Mycoplasma pneumoniae* infection	
Drug eruption	Atypical measles	
	Leptospirosis	

TABLE 114-3. Treatment of Rocky Mountain Spotted Fever

Agent	Dose	Comments
Doxycycline	100 mg PO bid or 4.4 mg/kg per day IV up to 200 mg per day in divided doses	Tetracyclines are contraindicated in children under 8 years old
Tetracycline hydrochloride	500 mg PO qid or 15 mg/kg IV loading dose, then 15 mg/kg per day in four divided doses	
Chloramphenicol	50 mg/kg loading dose, then 50 mg/kg per day in divided doses; or 15–20 mg/kg IV loading dose, then 30–15 mg/kg per day in four divided doses	Aplastic anemia is a rare complication
? Fluoroquinolones		Effective in vitro against *R. rickettsii* but clinical efficacy not proven and not recommended for use in children <12 years old

successful early intervention in this disease. Rocky Mountain spotted fever is a disease for which empiric therapy is indicated. When a rash is present, early biopsy and immunofluorescence staining may be crucial.

Other Rickettsial Diseases

TICK-BORNE SPOTTED FEVERS

Other tick-borne spotted fevers include Mediterranean spotted fever (boutonneuse fever), South African tick-bite fever, Siberian tick typhus, Oriental spotted fever, and Queensland tick typhus.

These diseases are caused by rickettsiae from varying geographic distributions. *R. conorii* is the cause of Mediterranean spotted fever (also known as boutonneuse fever) and South African tick-bite fever and is endemic to the Mediterranean basin and Africa. Siberian tick typhus is caused by *R. sibirica* and occurs in Asia. Newly reported Oriental spotted fever in Japan is caused by *R. japonica*, and *R. australis* is the cause of Queensland tick typhus in Australia. The vectors are predominantly dog ticks; the vector of Oriental spotted fever has not yet been identified.[60]

Mediterranean spotted fever, caused by *R. conorii,* is the prototype of the tick-borne spotted fevers in this group. After an incubation period of 6 to 10 days, a systemic illness of abrupt onset characterized by fever, myalgias, arthralgias, and headache is the usual presentation in a person with a history of dog exposure. A distinguishing lesion, the "tache noire" (Fig. 114–4), results at the site of the tick bite, appearing as a black eschar with or without ulceration and with a surrounding rim of erythema.[61] Lymphadenitis may occur near the site of the tache noire. Studies of the histopathology of the taches noires of Mediterranean spotted fever have shown necrosis of the epidermis, intense focal inflammation from the papillary and reticular dermis to the subcutaneous tissues involving small blood vessels, swollen endothelial cells and thrombosis of the microcirculation, and the presence of *R. conorii* in the eschar.[61, 62] A maculo-

papular rash erupts most often 3 days (range, 2 to 10 days) after the onset of symptoms in approximately 50% of patients and spreads in a centripetal fashion; typically, it may also involve the palms and soles.[60, 61] Petechiae develop rarely and usually signify severe disease. The histopathology of the maculopapular lesions reveals a dermal perivascular lymphohistiocytic infiltrate with diffuse vasculitis and swelling of endothelial cells.[61, 62] Atypical papulovesicular eruptions have been reported in *R. conorii* and *R. australis* infections.[63, 64] Disease without a rash has also been reported.[65]

The illness is generally milder than that of Rocky Mountain spotted fever but can be fatal as a result of multiorgan involvement. Diagnosis is established by serology or demonstration of organisms by immunofluorescence staining of tissue specimens.[66-68] The differential diagnosis is similar to that of Rocky Mountain spotted

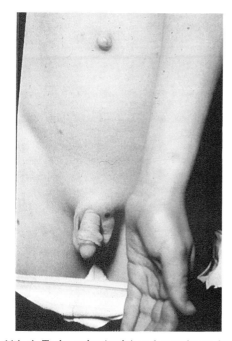

FIGURE 114–4. Tache noire (groin) and maculopapular rash in a patient with South African tick bite fever. (Courtesy of Arnold Weinberg, M.D., Harvard Medical School, Infectious Diseases Unit, Massachusetts General Hospital, Boston, MA.)

fever (see Table 114–2). Treatment with tetracycline or chloramphenicol is effective; a 1-day course of doxycycline may be as effective as a 10-day course.[69] Ciprofloxacin has been shown to be effective in vitro and in vivo.[57, 70] Sulfonamides may be contraindicated in patients with Mediterranean spotted fever.[71]

RICKETTSIALPOX

R. akari is the cause of rickettsialpox and is transmitted to humans by the bite of a mouse mite. The disease is most commonly seen in urban areas and has been reported in outbreaks in New York City, Ohio, Utah, Arizona, and Russia. This self-limited spotted fever illness is characterized by a primary lesion at the site of the mite bite commencing as an erythematous papule in which a central vesicle develops. The vesicle eventually dries, leaving a brown or black eschar on a large indurated base.[72–74] Nonspecific symptoms of fever, headache, myalgias, and malaise develop after an incubation period of 9 to 14 days. Regional lymphadenitis often develops near the site of the eschar, and the appearance of a generalized eruption of erythematous papules with central vesicles, sparing the palms and soles, occurs within 3 days (range, 1 to 4 days) of the onset of systemic symptoms. A vacuolar interface dermatitis with dense mixed perivascular infiltrates, swollen endothelial cells, and, sometimes, fibrin thrombi characterizes the histopathology of the papulovesicular lesions.[72] Diagnosis is made serologically by IFA; the Weil-Felix reaction is negative. The differential diagnosis of rickettsialpox includes other rickettsioses such as spotted fevers associated with tache noire lesions (Mediterranean spotted fever [boutonneuse fever], Siberian tick typhus, South African tick-bite fever, and Queensland tick typhus), which may be indistinguishable from the eschar of rickettsialpox, and scrub typhus. Nonrickettsial infections in the differential diagnosis include varicella, smallpox (now eradicated), enteroviruses, eczema herpeticum, and eczema vaccinatum; however, an eschar is evident only in rickettsialpox.[75] Tetracycline or chloramphenicol is an effective therapy, although untreated cases usually resolve without relapse. Either control of environmental contamination of mouse mites or underreporting is responsible for a decline in the reported incidence of this disease in the past 30 years.

TYPHUS FEVER GROUP

Epidemic (Louse-Borne) Typhus

Epidemic (louse-borne) typhus is caused by *R. prowazekii* and is transmitted to its human reservoir by the body louse, *Pediculus humanus corporis*. Epidemics of typhus have been reported since the early sixteenth century and are responsible for millions of deaths in times of war, famine, and human conditions promoting malnutrition, poor hygiene, and overcrowding. Seasonal occurrence in colder months is most common. During a blood meal, the infected louse defecates and deposits infected feces onto the skin of the human, inoculating the site of the bite. The organisms gain entry into the host and after replication at the site of entry disseminate and infect endothelial cells, causing their proliferation and infiltration of mononuclear cells resulting in diffuse vasculitis.[76, 77] Today, countries reporting cases of epidemic typhus include those in central Africa, and Central and South America.[78] Humans were thought to be the only reservoir for the organism, with body lice facilitating person-to-person transmission, until sporadic cases reported in the United States in the 1970s showed an epidemiologic association with flying squirrels or their ectoparasites.[79–85] Transmission to humans may occur via inhalation of aerosolized feces from infected squirrel lice, or directly by the bite of the squirrel flea.[86]

In epidemic (louse-borne) typhus, the incubation period averages 10 days.[75, 77, 87–89] Abrupt onset of fever, severe headache, myalgias, and arthralgias is the usual presentation. Fever and headache are unremitting, and the patient quickly becomes prostrate. Cutaneous eruption develops 4 to 7 days after the onset of systemic symptoms[75, 76] and is characterized by erythematous macules that fade with pressure, beginning in the axillary folds and spreading to the trunk and extremities. Palms and soles are spared, except in severe cases, where generalized petechiae and purpuric lesions may develop that may lead to necrosis, especially over bony prominences.[29, 76] Eschars do not occur. The rash is absent in 10% to 50% of patients.[78, 89] Neurologic complications such as abnormal mental status, focal cranial neuropathies, and, less often, coma may develop. Other signs and symptoms include conjunctival suffusion, relative bradycardia in the early stages, dry cough, constipation, and abdominal pain.[78] Disease severity correlates with age; indigenously acquired *R. prowazekii* infection may have a less severe course.[84] Severe vasculitis may predispose the patient to cerebral thrombosis or symmetrical gangrene of the distal digits. Both complications may resolve with treatment without long-term sequelae.[78]

The histopathology of the vasculitis is similar to that of Rocky Mountain spotted fever. Diagnosis is best made serologically with the more sensitive and specific IFA assay;[90] in cases in which the Weil-Felix reaction is employed, it is positive with cross-reactive antibodies to *Proteus* OX-19.[75, 78] Immunofluorescence staining of skin specimens has not been reported. Other illnesses presenting with fever and rash are usually distinguished from epidemic (louse-borne) typhus by the character and mode of spread of the rash and by the epidemiologic setting in which the illness occurs. If the illness suggests Rocky Mountain spotted fever but the season is autumn or winter, louse-borne or flying squirrel–borne typhus should be suspected.[91]

Prompt improvement of symptoms occurs with treatment. Tetracycline or chloramphenicol is the recommended treatment and is continued until 2 or 3 days after defervescence. A single dose of 100 mg or 200 mg of doxycycline may be effective.[92, 93] Early treatment may be associated with relapse as a result of an ineffective immune response and incomplete eradication of the organism. Mortality ranges from 10% to 40%; there were no deaths in one report of 60 cases.[75, 77, 78]

Brill-Zinsser Disease

Recrudescent typhus may occur years later in the form of Brill-Zinsser disease, an entity now rarely reported. Latent organisms are believed to reactivate under conditions of stress for the host and cause an illness similar to but less severe than classic epidemic typhus.[94] The disease was seen most commonly in the United States among immigrants from Eastern Europe or survivors of World War II concentration camps who had a history of a typhus-like illness and presented with the sudden onset of fever and severe headache.[95, 96] Rash is not always present but may develop by the fourth to seventh day and is initially characterized by faint erythematous discrete macules that fade with pressure in a similar distribution to those of louse-borne typhus, but may also involve the palms and soles.[89, 95] Petechiae are less common in this illness. A brisk acute-phase IgG anamnestic response is characteristic, and IFA serology is useful for the diagnosis.[90] Unlike louse-borne typhus, the Weil-Felix reaction is usually negative. Effective treatment is similar to that of classic epidemic typhus.

Endemic (Murine) Typhus

Endemic (murine) typhus is a worldwide disease caused by *R. typhi,* which is transmitted to humans from its unaffected rat host by the rat flea, *Xenopsylla cheopis.* Man is a dead-end host for the organism. In the United States, the southern Gulf states, particularly southern Texas, have the highest incidence of reported disease of approximately 100 cases per year.[97] Persons working in areas of food storage are at increased risk of infection. The organism is transmitted when the flea defecates after its blood meal and infected feces are rubbed into the abraded skin.

After an incubation period of 6 to 14 days, a prodrome of mild headache, malaise, nausea, cough, chest pain, coryza, and myalgias may develop, followed by abrupt onset of fever, chills, more severe headache, and intense myalgias. Rash occurs in 50% to 65% by the fifth or sixth day of symptoms.[98, 99] Pink, blanching macules, originating on the trunk and spreading to the extremities sparing palms and soles, are the characteristic early exanthemas of murine typhus.[98, 100] Papular lesions that may become petechial and, rarely, hemorrhagic develop as the rash ages.[98] Overall, the rash is less severe than that seen in classic epidemic typhus and usually fades in 2 to 9 days.[98] In severe cases, thrombosis of large vessels can occur with resultant gangrene of an extremity. Other common symptoms and signs include mental status changes, cranial neuropathies (especially neurosensory deafness), pulmonary infiltrates on chest x-ray, hypotension, vomiting, and prerenal azotemia.[98, 99]

Histologic examination of skin biopsy specimens reveals vascular injury, hemorrhage, and vesicle formation.[100] The Weil-Felix reaction is positive with *Proteus* OX-19 agglutination, but this does not distinguish between Rocky Mountain spotted fever and the typhus fever group. Specific diagnosis is confirmed with IFA. Immunohistologic demonstration of *R. typhi* in tissues

with fluorescein-conjugated antiserum reactive with typhus group rickettsiae has confirmed the diagnosis in a fatal case of murine typhus.[101] The differential diagnosis is similar to that of Rocky Mountain spotted fever (see Table 114–2).

Treatment with tetracycline, doxycycline, or chloramphenicol is usually successful; efficacy of ciprofloxacin has also been demonstrated.[102] Mortality is generally low, ranging from 1% to 4% in untreated cases.[98, 99] Sulfa drugs have been reported to exacerbate the disease.[99, 103]

Scrub Typhus

Scrub typhus is caused by *R. tsutsugamushi* and is transmitted to humans by the bite of the larval form (chigger) of a mite. The disease is endemic to the Far East in Japan, China, Southeast Asia, India, and Australia, but imported cases have been reported in the United States.[89] The name "scrub" reflects the low vegetation harboring chiggers that carry the organism. Transovarial transmission of the organism occurs in the mites, and because chiggers do not travel far and require only one blood meal, focal areas of high infection occur in endemic areas. *R. tsutsugamushi* is the one rickettsial organism with multiple serotypes; therefore, infection with one does not confer immunity against others.

Chiggers bite with a predilection for pressure points (boot tops, waist line), inoculating organisms into the skin. Local replication followed by dissemination occurs. At the site of the chigger bite, an erythematous papule develops that becomes a small bulla and sloughs to form a shallow ulcer.[104] Necrosis occurs and an eschar on a raised erythematous base forms, which is noted in 66% to 80% of cases[104, 105] (Fig. 114–5*A*). After an incubation period of 6 to 21 days,[89, 106] a prodrome of headache, chills, and anorexia develops.[104] Unremitting fever, headaches, and myalgias are the rule and may be accompanied by a dry cough.

The cutaneous eruption occurs in approximately 30% to 35% of cases by the fifth day (range, 3 to 8 days) and is characterized by a self-limited erythematous maculopapular rash beginning on the trunk, spreading centrifugally, and sparing palms and soles (Fig. 114–5*B*).[104, 105] Purpuric lesions are noted in a minority of patients, and larger vessel thrombosis rarely occurs.[75, 105]

The most common physical sign is generalized lymphadenopathy, and the diagnosis can be confused with infectious mononucleosis.[104] Splenomegaly may be present in 20% to 50%.[104, 105] Prominent ocular signs include conjunctivitis, retinal vein engorgement, and papilledema.[89, 105, 107] Diagnosis is most accurately made with IFA or indirect immunoperoxidase testing; the Weil-Felix OX-K test is less specific and may yield false-positive results with leptospirosis, malaria, and *Proteus* infections.[108] If an eschar is present, the differential diagnosis is limited in an epidemiologically exposed individual; otherwise, other systemic illnesses such as leptospirosis, brucellosis, typhoid fever, viral infectious mononucleosis syndromes, toxoplasmosis, and endemic viral diseases such as dengue fever must be considered.[106] Treatment with tetracycline or chloramphenicol reduces the length

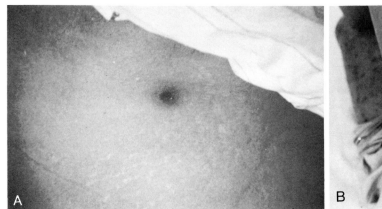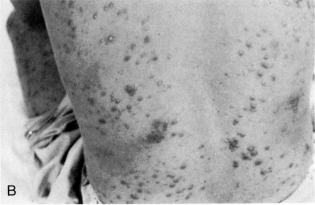

FIGURE 114–5. *A*, Eschar at the site of the chigger bite in scrub typhus. *B*, Truncal maculopapular rash of scrub typhus. (*A* and *B* Courtesy of Susumu Ito, Ph.D., Harvard Medical School, Department of Neurobiology, Boston, MA.)

of illness, but relapses can occur.[105] Ciprofloxacin has been shown to be effective in animal models.[109] Mortality is generally low in this disease; fatal complications are associated with the effects of severe vasculitis in untreated cases.[105]

Q FEVER

Q fever is the one rickettsial disease that is not usually transmitted by a vector, but rather is acquired through inhalation or rarely through ingestion. The illness is caused by *Coxiella burnetii,* which primarily infects cattle, sheep, and goats. Infection occurs when birth products are aerosolized. Acute onset of systemic symptoms of fever, headache, chills, and anorexia occurs. Pneumonitis is common, and hepatitis may develop.[110] Radiographic findings reveal diffuse patchy infiltrates and together with a nondiagnostic sputum examination suggest atypical pneumonia. Chronic infections in the form of endocarditis, osteomyelitis, meningoencephalitis, or granulomatous hepatitis may also occur.[111–115] A rash is unusual in this disease and occurs in 5% or less of cases. It appears as discrete erythematous macules that begin on the trunk and may spread centrifugally.[116] The histopathology is unique among rickettsial diseases. Granulomas with central clearing surrounded by inflammatory cells and a fibrin ring (doughnut lesion) are the distinguishing features.[110, 117, 118] Serologic diagnosis is made with complement-fixation antibody titers or with IFA.[119] Early in the illness, the differential diagnosis includes entities causing systemic illness such as salmonellosis, brucellosis, leptospirosis, viral mononucleosis syndromes, and viral hepatitis.[9] Treatment with tetracycline is effective; ciprofloxacin may also be successful.

EHRLICHIOSIS

Human ehrlichiosis is a rickettsial disease caused by the species *Ehrlichia chaffeensis,* which is probably transmitted to humans by a tick bite.[120–124] Unlike other rickettsial organisms, *Ehrlichia* species invade leukocytes

and replicate within intracytoplasmic membrane bound vacuoles until cell lysis occurs.[125] Distinct forms within the leukocytes, morulae, may be visualized by light microscopy and represent mature intraleukocytic inclusions of the organisms.

The endemic focus in the United States appears to be primarily in the south central and southeastern states, but whether this is an artifact of overdetection as a result of suspicion for Rocky Mountain spotted fever is not known. The peak incidence of disease is in the warmer months, particularly April to June. The clinical manifestations of the illness are similar to those of other rickettsial diseases. After an incubation period of 10 to 15 days, a prodrome of malaise and anorexia is followed by abrupt onset of fever, headache, chills, and myalgias.[125, 126] An erythematous maculopapular rash occurs in 20% to 47% without a typical distribution, and involvement of the palms and soles is rare.[125–127] Pulmonary and central nervous system complications (aseptic meningitis and encephalopathy) are not uncommon.[126, 127] In general, however, the disease is milder than Rocky Mountain spotted fever and may be subclinical in some patients.[126, 128] Laboratory findings are potentially more helpful in that a majority of patients may present with leukopenia and/or thrombocytopenia, and inclusion bodies may be seen in leukocytes on the peripheral smear. Diagnosis may now be made by IFA serology. Polymerase chain reaction has successfully amplified *E. chaffeensis* DNA from patients' sera, and immunohistology with labeled avidin-biotin immunoperoxidase may be useful for tissue identification of the organism.[124, 129] The differential diagnosis is similar to that of other rickettsial diseases and includes early Lyme disease, babesiosis, and Colorado tick fever as well.[9, 125, 130] Chloramphenicol and tetracycline appear to be equally effective treatments.[126, 131]

References

1. Centers for Disease Control and Prevention. Cases of selected notifiable disease, United States, weeks ending December 18, 1993, and December 12, 1992. MMWR Dec. 24, 1993;42:977.
2. Weber DJ, Walker DH. Rocky Mountain spotted fever. Infect Dis Clin North Am 1991;5:19–35.

3. Hattwick MAW, O'Brien RJ, Hanson BF. Rocky Mountain spotted fever: Epidemiology of an increasing problem. Ann Intern Med 1976;84:732–739.

4. Kirk JL, Fine DP, Sexton DJ, et al. Rocky Mountain spotted fever: A clinical review based on 48 confirmed cases, 1943–1986. Medicine 1990;69:35–45.

5. Wilfert CM, MacCormack JN, Kleeman K, et al. Epidemiology of Rocky Mountain spotted fever as determined by active surveillance. J Infect Dis 1984;150:469–479.

6. Fishbein DB, Kaplan JE, Bernard KW, et al. Surveillance of Rocky Mountain spotted fever in the United States, 1981–1983. J Infect Dis 1984;;150:609–611.

7. Kaplowitz LG, Fischer JJ, Sparling PF. Rocky Mountain spotted fever: A clinical dilemma. In: Remington JS, Swartz MN, eds. Current Clinical Topics in Infectious Disease 1980. New York: McGraw-Hill, 1981:89–108.

8. Helmick CV, Bernard KW, D'Angelo LJ. Rocky Mountain spotted fever: Clinical, laboratory, and epidemiological features of 262 cases. J Infect Dis 1984;150:480–488.

9. Relman DA, Swartz MN. Rickettsial diseases. In: Rubenstein E, Federman DD, eds. Scientific American Medicine. New York: Scientific American, 1993:1–14.

10. Woodward TE. Rocky Mountain spotted fever. Resident & Staff Physician May 1978:52–61.

11. Hattwick MA, Retailliau H, O'Brien RJ, et al. Fatal Rocky Mountain spotted fever. JAMA 1978;240:1499–1503.

12. Cohen JI, Corson AP, Corey GR. Late appearance of skin rash in Rocky Mountain spotted fever. South Med J 1983;76:1457–1458.

13. Sexton DJ, Banks PM, Weig S, et al. Late appearance of skin rash and abnormal serum enzymes in Rocky Mountain spotted fever: A case report. J Pediatr 1975;87:580–582.

14. Sexton DJ, Corey G. Rocky Mountain "spotless" and "almost spotless" fever: A wolf in sheep's clothing. Clin Infect Dis 1992;15:439–448.

15. Griffith GL, Luge EA. Massive skin necrosis in Rocky Mountain spotted fever. South Med J 1978;71:1338–1340.

16. Kirkland KB, Marcom PK, Sexton DJ, et al. Rocky Mountain spotted fever complicated by gangrene: Report of six cases and review. Clin Infect Dis 1993;16:629–634.

17. Weiser IB, Green CE. Dermal necrosis associated with Rocky Mountain spotted fever in four dogs. J Am Vet Med Assoc 1989;195:1756–1758.

18. Middleton DB. Rocky Mountain spotted fever: Gastrointestinal and laboratory manifestations. South Med J 1978;71:629–632.

19. Walker DH, Lesesne HR, Varma VA, et al. Rocky Mountain spotted fever mimicking acute cholecystitis. Arch Intern Med 1985;145:2194–2196.

20. Davis AE, Bradford WD. Abdominal pain resembling acute appendicitis in Rocky Mountain spotted fever. JAMA 1982;247:2811–2812.

21. Walker DH, Crawford CG, Cain BG. Rickettsial infection of the pulmonary microcirculation: The basis for interstitial pneumonitis in Rocky Mountain spotted fever. Hum Pathol 1979;II:263–272.

22. Donohue JF. Lower respiratory tract involvement in Rocky Mountain spotted fever. Arch Intern Med 1980;140:223–227.

23. Walker DH, Mattern WD. Acute renal failure in Rocky Mountain spotted fever. Arch Intern Med 1979;139:443–448.

24. Wolbach SB. Studies on Rocky Mountain spotted fever. J Med Res 1919;41:1–197.

25. Woodward TE, Walker DH, Dumler JS. The remarkable contributions of S. Burt Wolbach on rickettsial vasculitis updated. Trans Am Clin Climatol Assoc 1992;103:78–94.

26. Walker DH, Mattern WD. Rickettsial vasculitis. Am Heart J 1980;100:896–906.

27. Walker TS. Rickettsial interactions with human endothelial cells in vitro: Adherence and entry. Infect Immun 1984;44:205–210.

28. Katz DA, Sworzack DL, Horowitz EA, et al. Encephalitis associated with Rocky Mountain spotted fever. Arch Pathol Lab Med 1985;109:771–773.

29. Woodward TE. Commentary: Rocky Mountain spotted fever: A present-day perspective. Medicine 1992;71:240–255.

30. Harrell GT. Rocky Mountain spotted fever. Medicine 1949;28:333–370.

31. Silverman DJ, Bond SB. Infection of human vascular endothelial cells by Rickettsia rickettsii. J Infect Dis 1984;149:201–206.

32. Silverman DJ. Rickettsia rickettsii–induced cellular injury of human vascular endothelium in vitro. Infect Immun 1984;44:545–553.

33. Silverman DJ, Santucci LA. Potential for free radical–induced lipid peroxidation as a cause of endothelial cell injury in Rocky Mountain spotted fever. Infect Immun 1988;56:3110–3115.

34. Silverman DJ, Wisseman CL, Waddel A. In vitro studies of rickettsia-host interactions: Ultrastructural changes induced by Rickettsia prowazekii infections of chicken embryo fibroblasts. Infect Immun 1980;29:778–790.

35. Walker TS, Triplett DA. Serologic characterization of Rocky Mountain spotted fever: Appearance of antibodies reactive with endothelial cells and phospholipids, and factors that alter protein C activation and prostacyclin secretion. Am J Clin Pathol 1991;95:725–732.

36. Sporn LA, Shi R, Lawrence SO, et al. Rickettsia rickettsii infection of cultured endothelial cells induces release of large von Willebrand factor multimers from Weibel-Palade bodies. Blood 1991;78:2595–2602.

37. Silverman DJ. Adherence of platelets to human endothelial cells infected by Rickettsia rickettsii. J Infect Dis 1986;153:694–700.

38. Rao AK, Schapira M, Clements ML, et al. A prospective study of platelets and plasma proteolytic systems during the early stages of Rocky Mountain spotted fever. N Engl J Med 1988;318:1021–1028.

39. Walker TS, Mellott GE. Rickettsial stimulation of endothelial platelet-activating factor synthesis. Infect Immun 1993;61:2024–2029.

40. Winkler HH, Milller ET. Phospholipase A activity in the hemolysis of sheep and human erythrocytes by Rickettsia prowazekii. Infect Immun 1980;29:316–321.

41. Winkler HH, Miller ET. Phospholipase A and the interaction of Rickettsia prowazekii and mouse fibroblasts (L-929). Infect Immun 1982;38:109–113.

42. Winkler HH, Miller ET. Activated complex of L-cells and Rickettsia prowazekii with N-ethylmaleimide–insensitive phospholipase A. Infect Immun 1984;45:577–581.

43. Raoult D, Arnoux D, Drancourt M, et al. Enzyme secretion by human endothelial cells infected with Rickettsia conorii. Acta Virol 1987;31:352–356.

44. Walker TS, Brown JS, Hoover CX, et al. Endothelial prostaglandin secretion: Effects of typhus rickettsiae. J Infect Dis 1990;162:1136–1144.

45. Walker TS, Dersch MW, White WE. Effects of typhus rickettsiae on peritoneal and alveolar macrophages: Rickettsiae stimulate leukotriene and prostaglandin secretion. J Infect Dis 1991;163:569–573.

46. Kaplan JE, Schonberger LB. The sensitivity of various serologic tests in the diagnosis of Rocky Mountain spotted fever. Am J Trop Med Hyg 1986;35:840–844.

47. Woodward TE, Pedersen CE, Oster CN, et al. Prompt confirmation of Rocky Mountain spotted fever: Identification of rickettsiae in skin tissues. J Infect Dis 1976;134:297–301.

48. Walker DH, Cain BG. A method for specific diagnosis of Rocky Mountain spotted fever on fixed, paraffin-embedded tissue by immunofluorescence. J Infect Dis 1978;137:206–209.

49. Walker DH, Cain BG, Olmstead PM. Laboratory diagnosis of Rocky Mountain spotted fever by immunofluorescent demonstration of Rickettsia rickettsii in cutaneous lesions. Am J Clin Pathol 1978;69:619–623.

50. Fleisher G, Lennette ET, Honig P. Diagnosis of Rocky Mountain spotted fever by immunofluorescent identification of Rickettsia rickettsii in skin biopsy tissue. J Pediatr 1979;95:63–65.

51. Green WR, Walker DH, Cain BG. Fatal viscerotropic Rocky Mountain spotted fever: Report of a case diagnosed by immunofluorescence. Am J Med 1978;64:523–528.

52. Dumler JS, Gage WR, Pettis GL, et al. Rapid immunoperoxidase demonstration of Rickettsia rickettsii in fixed cutaneous specimens from patients with Rocky Mountain spotted fever. Am J Clin Pathol 1990;93:410–414.

53. Tzianabos T, Anderson BE, McDade JE. Detection of Rickettsia rickettsii DNA in clinical specimens by using polymerase chain reaction technology. J Clin Microbiol 1989;27:2866–2868.

54. Carl M, Tibbs CW, Dobson ME, et al. Diagnosis of acute typhus infection using the polymerase chain reaction. J Infect Dis 1990;161:791–793.

55. Horwitz MS, Grose C, Fisher M. Atypical measles rash mimicking Rocky Mountain spotted fever. N Engl J Med 1973;289:1203–1204.

56. Woodward TE. Rocky Mountain spotted fever: Epidemiological and early clinical signs are keys to treatment and reduced mortality. J Infect Dis 1984;150:465–468.

57. Raoult D, Drancourt M. Antimicrobial therapy of rickettsial diseases. Antimicrob Agents Chemother 1991;35:2457–2462.

58. Harrell GT. Treatment of Rocky Mountain spotted fever with antibiotics. Ann N Y Acad Sci 1952;55:1027–1029.

59. Raoult D, Walker DH. *Rickettsia rickettsii* and other spotted fever group rickettsiae (Rocky Mountain spotted fever and other spotted fevers). In: Mandell GL, Douglas RG, Bennett JE, eds. Principles and Practice of Infectious Diseases, 3rd edition. New York: Churchill Livingstone; 1990:1465–1471.

60. Walker DH. Rickettsioses of the spotted fever group around the world. J Dermatol 1989;16:169–177.

61. Font-Creus B, Bella-Cuets F, Espejo-Arenas E, et al. Mediterranean spotted fever: A cooperative study of 227 cases. Rev Infect Dis 1985;7:635–642.

62. Montenegro MR, Mansueto S, Hegary BC, et al. The histology of "taches noires" of boutonneuse fever and demonstration of *Rickettsia conorii* in them by immunofluorescence. Virchows Arch [Pathol Anat] 1983;400:309–317.

63. Kemper CA, Spivack AP, Deresinski SC. Atypical papulovesicular rash due to infection with *Rickettsia conorii*. Clin Infect Dis 1992;15:591–594.

64. Hudson BJ, McPetrie R, Kitchener-Smith J, et al. Vesicular rash associated with infection due to *Rickettsia australis* (letter). Clin Infect Dis 1994;18:118–119.

65. Brouqui P, Tissot Dupont H, Drancourt M, et al. Spotless boutonneuse fever. Clin Infect Dis 1992;14:114–116.

66. Raoult D, de Micco C, Gallais H et al. Laboratory diagnosis of Mediterranean spotted fever by immunofluorescent demonstration of *Rickettsia conorii* in cutaneous lesions. J Infect Dis 1984;150:145–148.

67. Raoult D, Weiller PJ, Chagnon A, et al. Mediterranean spotted fever: Clinical, laboratory and epidemiological features of 199 cases. Am J Trop Med Hyg 1986;35:845–850.

68. Walker DH, Gear JHS. Correlation of the distribution of *Rickettsia conorii*, microscopic lesions, and clinical features in South African tick bite fever. Am J Trop Med Hyg 1985;34:361–371.

69. Bella-Cueto F, Font-Creus B, Segura-Porta F, et al. Comparative, randomized trial of one-day doxycycline versus 10-day tetracycline therapy for Mediterranean spotted fever (letter). J Infect Dis 1987;155:1056–1058.

70. Raoult D, Gallais H, De Micco P, et al. Ciprofloxacin therapy for Mediterranean spotted fever. Antimicrob Agents Chemother 1986;30:606–607.

71. Ruiz Beltrán R, Herrero Herrero JI. Deleterious effect of trimethoprim-sulfamethoxazole in Mediterranean spotted fever (letter). Antimicrob Agents Chemother 1992;36:1342–1343.

72. Brettman LR, Lewin S, Holzman RS, et al. Rickettsialpox: Report of an outbreak and a contemporary review. Medicine 1981;60:363–372.

73. Wong B, Singer C, Armstrong D, et al. Rickettsialpox: Case report and epidemiologic review. JAMA 1979;242:1998–1999.

74. Rose HM. The clinical manifestations and laboratory diagnosis of rickettsialpox. Ann Intern Med 1949;31:871–883.

75. Burnett JW. Rickettsioses: A review for the dermatologist. J Am Acad Dermatol 1980;2:359–373.

76. Committee on Pathology, Division of Medical Sciences, National Research Council. Pathology of epidemic typhus: Report of fatal cases studied by United States of America Typhus Commission in Cairo, Egypt, during 1943–1945. Arch Pathol 1953;56:397–435.

77. Saah AJ. *Rickettsia prowazekii* (epidemic or louse-borne typhus). In: Mandell GL, Douglas RG, Bennett JE, eds. Principles and Practice of Infectious Diseases, 3rd edition. New York: Churchill Livingstone; 1990:1476–1478.

78. Perine PL, Chandler BP, Krause DK, et al. A clinico-epidemiological study of epidemic typhus in Africa. Clin Infect Dis 1992;14:1149–1158.

79. Bozeman FM, Masiello SA, Williams MS, et al. Epidemic typhus rickettsiae isolated from flying squirrels. Nature 1975;255:545–547.

80. Sonenshine DE, Bozeman FM, Williams MS, et al. Epizootiology of epidemic typhus *(Rickettsia prowazekii)* in flying squirrels. Am J Trop Med Hyg 1978;27:339–349.

81. McDade JE, Sehpard CC, Redus MA, et al. Evidence of *Rickettsia prowazekii* infections in the United States. Am J Trop Med Hyg 1980;29:277–284.

82. Ackley AM, Peter WJ. Indigenous acquisition of epidemic typhus in the eastern United States. South Med J 1981;74:245–247.

83. Russo PK, Mendelson DC, Etkind PH, et al. Epidemic typhus *(Rickettsia prowazekii)* in Massachusetts: Evidence of infection. N Engl J Med 1981;304:1166–1168.

84. Duma RJ, Sonenshine DE, Bozeman FM, et al. Epidemic typhus in the United States associated with flying squirrels. JAMA 1981;245:2318–2323.

85. Centers for Disease Control. Current trends: Epidemic typhus associated with flying squirrels—United States. MMWR 1982;31:555–561.

86. Bozeman FM, Sonenshine DE, Williams MS, et al. Experimental infection of ectoparasitic arthropods with *Rickettsia prowazekii* (GvF-16 strain) and transmission to flying squirrels. Am J Trop Med Hyg 1981;30:253–263.

87. Gelston AL, Jones TC. Typhus fever: Report of an epidemic in New York City in 1847. J Infect Dis 1977;136:813–821.

88. Riley HD. Rickettsial diseases and Rocky Mountain spotted fever—Part II. Curr Prob Pediatr 1981;11:3–38.

89. Boyd AS, Neldner KH. Typhus disease group. Int J Dermatol 1992;31:823–832.

90. Ormsbee R, Peacock M, Philip R, et al. Serologic diagnosis of epidemic typhus fever. Am J Epidemiol 1977;105:261–271.

91. Kaplan JE, McDade JE, Newhouse VF. Suspected Rocky Mountain spotted fever in the winter—epidemic typhus? (Letter.) N Engl J Med 1981;305:1648.

92. Perine Pl, Awoke S, Krause DW, et al. Single-dose doxycycline treatment of louse-borne relapsing fever and epidemic typhus. Lancet 1974;ii:742–744.

93. Huys J, Kayhigi J, Freyens P, et al. Single-dose treatment of epidemic typhus with doxycycline. Chemotherapy 1973;18:314–317.

94. Price WH. Studies on the interepidemic survival of louse borne epidemic typhus fever. J Bacteriol 1954;69:106–107.

95. Murray ES, Baehr G, Shwartzman G, et al. Brill's disease I: Clinical and laboratory diagnosis. JAMA 1950;142:1059–1066.

96. Green CR, Fishbein D, Gleiberman I. Brill-Zinsser: Still with us (letter). JAMA 1990;264:1811–1812.

97. Centers for Disease Control. Summary of notifiable diseases—United States, 1989. MMWR 1990;38:47–59.

98. Stuart BM, Pullen RL. Endemic (murine) typhus fever: Clinical observations of 180 cases. Ann Intern Med 1945;23:520–536.

99. Dumler JS, Taylor JP, Walker DH. Clinical and laboratory features of murine typhus in south Texas, 1980 through 1987. JAMA 1991;266:1365–1370.

100. Stasko T, De Villez RL. Murine typhus: A case report and review. J Am Acad Dermatol 1982;7:377–381.

101. Walker DH, Parks FM, Betz TG, et al. Histopathology and immunohistologic demonstration of the distribution of *Rickettsia typhi* in fatal murine typhus. Am J Clin Pathol 1989;91:720–724.

102. Strand O, Anders S. Ciprofloxacin treatment of murine typhus. Scand J Infect Dis 1990;22:503–504.

103. Binford CH, Ecker HD. Endemic (murine) typhus: Report of autopsy findings in three cases. Am J Clin Pathol 1947;17:797–806.

104. Berman SJ, Kundin WD. Scrub typhus in South Vietnam: A study of 87 cases. Ann Intern Med 1973;79:26–30.

105. Sheehy TW, Hazlett D, Turk RE. Scrub typhus: A comparison of chloramphenicol and tetracycline in its treatment. Arch Intern Med 1973;132:77–80.

106. Saah AJ. *Rickettsia tsutsugamushi* (scrub typhus). In: Mandell GL, Douglas RG, Bennett JE, eds. Principles and Practice of Infectious Diseases, 3rd edition. New York: Churchill Livingstone, 1990:1480–1481.

107. Chamberlain WP. Ocular findings in scrub typhus. Arch Ophthalmol 1953;48:313–321.

108. Kelly DJ, Wong PW, Gan E, et al. Comparative evaluation of the indirect immunoperoxidase test for the serodiagnosis of rickettsial disease. Am J Trop Med Hyg 1988;38:400–406.
109. McClain JB, Joshi B, Rice R. Chloramphenicol, gentamicin, and ciprofloxacin against murine scrub typhus. Antimicrob Agents Chemother 1988;32:285–286.
110. Sawyer LA, Fishbein DB, McDade JE. Q fever: Current concepts. Rev Infect Dis 1987;9:935–946.
111. Turck WPG, Howitt G, Turnberg LA, et al. Chronic Q fever. Q J Med 1976;45:193–217.
112. Kimbrough RC, Ormsbee RA, Peacock M, et al. Q fever endocarditis in the United States. Ann Intern Med 1979;91:400–402.
113. Varma MPS, Adgey AAJ, Connolly JH. Chronic Q fever endocarditis. Br Heart J 1980;43:695–699.
114. Fernández-Guerro ML, Muelas JM, Aguado JM, et al. Q fever endocarditis on porcine bioprosthetic valves. Ann Intern Med 1988;108:209–213.
115. Pellegrin M, Delsol G, Auvergnat JC, et al. Granulomatous hepatitis in Q fever. Hum Pathol 1980;11:51–57.
116. Spelman DW. Q fever: A study of 111 consecutive cases. Med J Aust 1982;1:547–553.
117. Srigley JR, Vellend H, Palmer N, et al. Q-fever: The liver and bone marrow pathology. Am J Surg Pathol 1985;9:752–758.
118. Ende N, Gelpi AP. Pathological changes noted in bone marrow in a case of Q fever. Arch Intern Med 1957;100:793–796.
119. Field PR, Hunt JG, Murphy AM. Detection and persistence of specific IgM antibody to *Coxiella burnetii* by enzyme-linked immunosorbent assay: A comparison with immunofluorescence and complement fixation tests. J Infect Dis 1983;148:477–487.
120. Maeda K, Markowitz N, Hawley RC, et al. Human infection with *Ehrlichia canis,* a leukocytic rickettsia. N Engl J Med 1987; 316:853–856.
121. Fishbein DB, Sawyer LA, Holland CJ, et al. Unexplained febrile illnesses after exposure to ticks: Infection with an *Ehrlichia?* JAMA 1987;257:3100–3104.
122. Dawson JE, Anderson BE, Fishbein DB, et al. Isolation and characterization of an *Ehrlichia* sp. from a patient diagnosed with human ehrlichiosis. J Clin Microbiol 1991;29:2741–2745.
123. Anderson BE, Dawson JE, Jones DC, et al. *Ehrlichia chaffeensis,* a new species associated with human ehrlichiosis. J Clin Microbiol 1991;2838–2842.
124. Anderson BE, Sumner JW, Dawson JE, et al. Detection of the etiologic agent of human ehrlichiosis by polymerase chain reaction. J Clin Microbiol 1992;30:775–780.
125. McDade JE. Ehrlichiosis—a disease of animals and humans. J Infect Dis 1990;161:609–617.
126. Eng TR, Harkess JR, Fishbein DB, et al. Epidemiologic, clinical and laboratory findings of human ehrlichiosis in the United States, 1988. JAMA 1990;264:2251–2258.
127. Mathisen GE, Weiss PJ, Kennedy CA. Pneumonia, aseptic meningitis and leukopenia in a 28-year-old man. Clin Infect Dis 1993;16:809–815.
128. Harkess JR, Ewing SA, Crutcher JM, et al. Human ehrlichiosis in Oklahoma. J Infect Dis 1989;576–679.
129. Dumler JS, Brouqui P, Aronson J, et al. Identification of ehrlichia in human tissue (letter). N Engl J Med 1991;325:1109–1110.
130. Harkess JR. Ehrlichiosis. Infect Dis Clin North Am 1991; 5:37–51.
131. Petersen LR, Sawyer LA, Fishbein DB, et al. An outbreak of ehrlichiosis in members of an army reserve unit. J Infect Dis 1989;159:562–568.

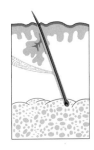

Bacillary Angiomatosis, Cat-Scratch Disease, and Bartonellosis

JORDAN W. TAPPERO and JANE E. KOEHLER

DEFINITION AND HISTORICAL ASPECTS

Our understanding of bacillary angiomatosis, cat-scratch disease, and bartonellosis has evolved rapidly over the past decade. The causative agents of all three zoonoses have been firmly established as closely related alpha-proteobacteria. In addition, the diseases resulting from infection with these organisms may share overlapping epidemiologic and clinical characteristics. These include transmission of infection to humans by an arthropod vector, resulting in a febrile illness accompanied by cutaneous lesions, or lymphadenopathy, or both (Table 115–1).

Bacillary Angiomatosis and Cat-Scratch Disease

In 1983, the illness that was later termed bacillary angiomatosis was first described by Stoler and colleagues, who reported on a patient with acquired immunodeficiency syndrome (AIDS) who developed subcutaneous vascular lesions containing bacilli visualized by Warthin-Starry silver staining and electron microscopy.[1] In the same year, bacilli were demonstrated within affected lymph nodes of patients with cat-scratch disease,[40] a disease first recognized by Debré in the 1940s.[2] The bacilli stained with the Warthin-Starry method, but not with conventional special stains, and despite numerous attempts, remained elusive to culture. In 1988, LeBoit and colleagues suggested a possible link between the causative agents of what was later to be called bacillary angiomatosis and cat-scratch disease.[3] These researchers based their suggestion on the histologic and electron microscopic

characteristics of these bacilli and on the immunoreactivity of bacilli in lesional tissue. Antisera raised against *Afipia felis*, the putative "cat-scratch disease bacillus," isolated from cat-scratch disease lymph nodes that same year were used in these studies.[3-5] In 1989, these investigators delineated histopathologic criteria separating the condition from other vascular proliferations, and proposed the name bacillary angiomatosis.[37] In 1990, Relman and associates used the polymerase chain reaction to amplify a bacterial 16S ribosomal gene fragment directly from bacillary angiomatosis tissue specimens.[6] DNA sequencing of this fragment established that the bacillary angiomatosis organism was closely related to *Rochalimaea quintana*, which caused trench fever, the scourge of World War I.[7,8]

In 1992, a new species, *R. henselae,* was isolated from blood of patients infected with human immunodeficiency virus (HIV) and from non–HIV-infected patients with fever and bacteremia.[9-11] The 16S ribosomal DNA sequence of this organism was found to be identical to that of the bacillary angiomatosis agent described by Relman. Interestingly, the newly named species, *R. henselae*, was shown to be quite distinct from *A. felis*, the purported cat-scratch disease bacillus.

In 1992, Koehler and colleagues isolated bacilli from cutaneous and osseous lesions of bacillary angiomatosis; surprisingly, either *R. henselae* or *R. quintana* was isolated from lesions obtained from different patients.[12] Subsequently, in 1993, *R. henselae* was isolated from the affected lymph nodes of two immunocompetent patients with cat-scratch disease.[13] In addition, the polymerase chain reaction was used to study multiple sources of cat-scratch disease skin test antigen prepared from purulent material aspirated from cat-scratch disease–affected

TABLE 115-1. Characteristic Features of Patients with Bacillary Angiomatosis, Cat-Scratch Disease, and Bartonellosis (Verruga Peruana)

Characteristic	Bacillary Angiomatosis	Cat-Scratch Disease	Bartonellosis (Verruga Peruana)
Age at onset	Children and adults	≥55% under 18 years	Children and adults
Sex	Male > female	Male = female	Male > female
Geographic setting	Worldwide	Worldwide	Latin America
Risk factors	Cat bite/cat scratch Immunodeficiency	Cat bite/cat scratch	Sandfly bite
Causative bacteria	*B. henselae* *B. quintana*	*B. henselae*	*B. bacilliformis*
Potential vector(s)	Cat flea, human body louse	Cat flea	Sand fly
Known reservoirs	Domestic cat	Domestic cat	Humans
Prominent clinical features	Vascular lesions (skin, liver/spleen, lymph nodes, and bone)	Lymphadenopathy, inoculation papule	Hemolytic anemia, vascular skin lesions
Treatment	Erythromycin or doxycycline	Usually self-limited	Chloramphenicol for Oroya fever

lymph nodes and used by some clinicians for establishing a diagnosis of cat-scratch disease. DNA sequences characteristic of *R. henselae* were amplified from each of the different skin test antigen preparations, but no *A. felis* DNA sequences could be detected.[14, 15] Accumulating evidence implies that the role played by *A. felis* in cat-scratch disease is probably minor, if any.

There are two other known species of *Rochalimaea: R. vinsonii,* which was isolated from voles and is not known to cause human disease; and *R. elizabethae,* which was isolated from a patient with endocarditis.[16]

Bartonellosis

Bartonellosis, or Carrión's disease, has been endemic in the Peruvian Andes since pre-Columbian times, as documented by numerous anthropoid ceramic artifacts (*huacas*) from the Inca dynasty depicting the cutaneous lesions of verruga peruana ("Peruvian wart").[17] The disease is characterized by two clinical phases: acute, with fever and hemolytic anemia (Oroya fever); and chronic, with cutaneous verruga, characterized by vascular papules and nodules that typically arise several weeks to months following the onset of febrile illness. In 1870, Oroya fever obtained its name following a severe outbreak of febrile anemia; the epidemic resulted in the death of over 7000 workers during the construction of a national railway from Lima to La Oroya, Peru. In 1909, *Bartonella bacilliformis* was identified as the cause of Oroya fever.[18] Barton demonstrated this organism within red blood cells obtained from febrile, anemic patients. In the same year, Daniel Carrión firmly established the link between the acute anemic phase and the chronic verruga phase when he inoculated himself with verruga material and developed a severe anemic fever to which he succumbed.[19, 20]

In 1993, Brenner proposed the unification of the genera *Bartonella* and *Rochalimaea* within the family Bartonellaceae, based on their genetic relatedness. He also proposed removing the family Bartonellaceae from the order Rickettsiales, because recent molecular evidence demonstrated that neither *Bartonella* nor *Rochalimaea* species was closely related to other organisms currently classified in the order Rickettsiales.[21] As this classification comes into general use, the causative agents of bacillary angiomatosis, cat-scratch disease, and Carrión's disease will become *Bartonella* (formerly *Rochalimaea*) *henselae, Bartonella* (formerly *Rochalimaea*) *quintana,* and *Bartonella bacilliformis,* respectively.

EPIDEMIOLOGY AND PATHOGENESIS

Bacillary Angiomatosis and Cat-Scratch Disease. Although five immunocompetent patients with bacillary angiomatosis have been reported,[22] the disease has been described predominantly in immunocompromised, HIV-infected men or in other immunosuppressed patients.[23, 24] In the United States, cat-scratch disease peaks seasonally during the fall and winter, with an annual incidence of 0.77 to 0.86 cases per 100,000 population. The disease affects an estimated 22,000 persons and accounts for roughly 2000 hospitalizations each year.[25] Cat-scratch disease occurs predominantly in children and young adults under 18 years of age (55% to 87% of reports) with an equal sex distribution.

Before the causative agents of bacillary angiomatosis and cat-scratch disease were isolated, Tappero and colleagues conducted a case control study of bacillary angiomatosis patients to identify a variety of exposures that might be risk factors for acquiring infection.[23] Traumatic contact with a cat (bite or scratch) was the only environmental exposure significantly associated with disease. Patients with bacillary angiomatosis were also more likely than controls to have a household kitten (a cat ≤1 year of age). A subsequent case control study of cat-scratch disease found that patients with cat-scratch disease were more likely than controls to have at least one kitten, to have recent traumatic contact with a kitten, and to have at least one kitten with fleas.[26]

Ensuing investigations by Koehler and coworkers established the pet cat, *Felis domesticus,* as a reservoir for *B. henselae* infection, and the cat flea, *Ctenocephalides felis*, as a possible vector for transmission of infection to humans.[27] Of the four patients with bacillary angiomatosis in this study, *B. henselae* was established as the cause of cutaneous bacillary angiomatosis in three individuals. *B. henselae* was subsequently isolated from the blood of all seven asymptomatic pet cats with which the bacillary angiomatosis patients had prolonged contact. This bacterium was also detected by both direct culture and polymerase chain reaction from several of the cat fleas combed from these bacteremic cats. In addition, the prevalence of infection among cats in the greater San Francisco Bay region was studied; 41% (25 of 61) of sampled pet or impounded cats had asymptomatic *B. henselae* bacteremia.[27] Although the reservoir(s) for the second causative agent of bacillary angiomatosis (*B. quintana*) remains unknown, the human body louse (*Pediculus humanus*) was established as a vector for *B. quintana* infections causing trench fever during the First World War.[8]

Bartonellosis. In Latin America, Carrión's disease has been reported predominantly in males. The incidence of disease is unknown. However, endemic and epidemic disease has been well documented throughout the Andean mountains of Peru, Ecuador, Colombia, Chile, and Bolivia, between the altitudes of 2500 and 8000 feet.[19, 28] The disease is transmitted to humans via the bite of a crepuscular *Phlebotomus* sand fly. In the Peruvian cordillera, sandflies are susceptible to arid conditions below 2500 feet and to cold temperatures above 8000 feet, thus explaining the unusual geographic distribution of bartonellosis.[29, 30] Except for humans, an animal reservoir for *B. bacilliformis* has not been identified.

CLINICAL FINDINGS

Bacillary Angiomatosis. Over the past decade, the clinical spectrum of bacillary angiomatosis has been expanded to include patients with single or multiple vascular lesions affecting virtually every organ system, including lymph node, bone, brain, and liver (peliosis hepatis) and spleen.[24, 31] However, skin lesions remain the most easily recognized and frequently reported clinical manifestation of bacillary angiomatosis. Of special significance among HIV-infected patients, cutaneous lesions of bacillary angiomatosis can be easily mistaken for Kaposi's sarcoma.[32]

Cutaneous lesions of bacillary angiomatosis begin as small, erythematous vascular papules, which may enlarge to form exophytic, friable nodules surrounded by a collarette of scale with or without erythema (Figs. 115–1 and 115–2; see color plate). Superficial subcutaneous lesions of bacillary angiomatosis have the appearance of flesh-colored cystic nodules or epidermal inclusion cysts (Fig. 115–3). They can also develop more deeply, presenting as soft tissue masses with or without overlying eruptive vascular lesions of cutaneous bacillary angiomatosis.[12] Among HIV-infected patients, bacillary angiomatosis usually develops in the late stages of infection, when CD4 counts are below 100 cells/mm[3].[24, 33]

Cat-Scratch Disease. Cat-scratch disease is typically a benign and self-limited illness lasting 6 to 12 weeks. Regional lymphadenopathy (axillary, head and neck, in-

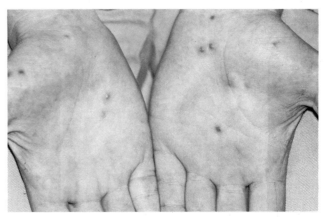

FIGURE 115–1. Small vascular papules of bacillary angiomatosis on the palms. (See color plate.)

guinal) is the predominant clinical feature of cat-scratch disease; affected nodes are often tender and occasionally suppurate.[26, 34, 35] Between 25% and 60% of patients report a primary cutaneous inoculation lesion (0.5- to 1-cm papule or pustule) at the site of a cat scratch or bite.[26, 35] The skin lesions typically develop 3 to 10 days after injury and precede the onset of lymphadenopathy by 1 to 2 weeks. Low-grade fever and malaise accompany lymphadenopathy in up to 50% of patients; headache, anorexia, weight loss, nausea and vomiting, sore throat, and splenomegaly may develop. In addition, short-lived, nonspecific maculopapular eruptions, erythema nodosum, figurate erythemas, and thrombocytopenic purpura have been observed.[2]

Unusual manifestations of cat-scratch disease, which occur in up to 14% of patients, include Parinaud's oculoglandular syndrome (6%), encephalopathy (2%), hepatic granulomas (0.3%), osteomyelitis (0.3%), and

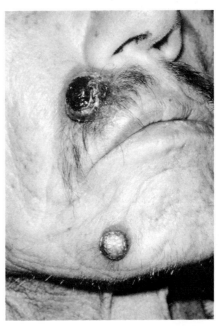

FIGURE 115–2. Characteristic exophytic angiomatous nodules of bacillary angiomatosis with and without surrounding cellulitic erythema. (See color plate.)

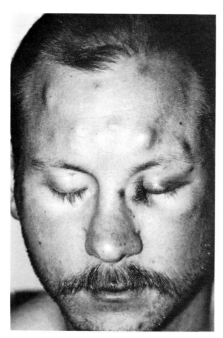

FIGURE 115-3. Multiple subcutaneous nodules of bacillary angiomatosis in a patient with concomitant Kaposi's sarcoma of the medial left eye canthus.

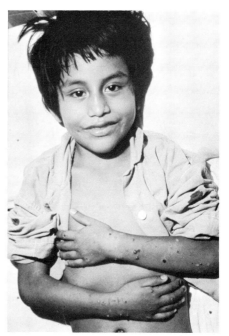

FIGURE 115-4. Verruga peruana of bartonellosis. There are erythematous papules that resemble those of bacillary angiomatosis. (Courtesy of F. Uriel Garcia, M.D., Department of Pathology, University of Kansas School of Medicine.)

pulmonary disease (0.2%).[2, 34, 35] In general, these complications resolve without sequelae. Parinaud's oculoglandular syndrome is manifested by conjunctival granuloma, periauricular lymphadenopathy, and nonsuppurative conjunctivitis. Encephalopathy, presenting as fever and coma with progression to convulsions, may last for days to weeks; cerebrospinal fluid is unremarkable.

Bartonellosis. Carrión's disease evolves in two phases: Oroya fever and verruga peruana. Following an incubation period of 3 to 4 weeks, a febrile illness accompanied by headache, chills, pallor, and severe hemolysis ensues, often complicated by concomitant *Salmonella* species bacteremia.[36] Historically, Oroya fever is associated with an exceedingly high mortality of 40% to 90%.[17] During the last documented Peruvian outbreak in 1987, the fatality rate among untreated patients was 88%.[28] Although Oroya fever and verruga peruana may develop concomitantly, the eruptive phase of bartonellosis typically develops several weeks to months following the onset of febrile illness, often signaling the resolution of hemolytic anemia. Verruga peruana is characterized by single to multiple cutaneous and subcutaneous vascular lesions that appear in successive crops (Fig. 115-4).

PATHOLOGY

Bacillary Angiomatosis. Routine hematoxylin and eosin staining of cutaneous bacillary angiomatosis tissue specimens reveals a characteristic lobular proliferation of small, capillary-sized blood vessels. These vessels have protuberant endothelial cells containing abundant cytoplasm with or without cytologic atypia.[4, 31, 37] The vessels are surrounded by a mixed inflammatory infiltrate with

neutrophils and leukocytoclasis (Fig. 115-5). Purple granular material, revealing clumps of tangled bacteria with Warthin-Starry silver staining, is scattered throughout the myxoid stroma between vessels. The organisms are often closely surrounded by neutrophilic debris. The bacilli are not demonstrable when stains for fungi, acid-fast stains for mycobacteria, or tissue Gram stains are used. With electron microscopy, these bacteria have a

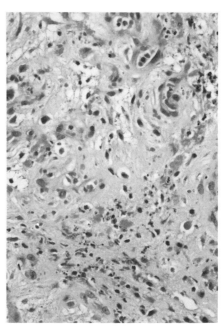

FIGURE 115-5. Bacillary angiomatosis is characterized by a densely cellular proliferation of endothelial cells and by infiltrates of neutrophils that surround clumps of bacilli.

trilaminar, gram-negative cell wall structure. Immunocytochemical staining that uses polyclonal rabbit antiserum to *B. henselae* may also demonstrate the presence of bacilli in tissue.[38]

With the exception of verruga peruana, the presence of bacilli clearly distinguishes bacillary angiomatosis from other cutaneous vascular lesions. The differential diagnosis, which includes lobular capillary hemangiomas (pyogenic granulomas), Kaposi's sarcoma, angiosarcoma, epithelioid (histiocytoid) hemangioma, and epithelioid hemangioendothelioma, can also be resolved using histopathologic criteria without resorting to special stains.[24,37]

Cat-Scratch Disease. With hematoxylin and eosin stains, the primary inoculation lesion of cat-scratch disease reveals small areas of necrosis and suppuration surrounded by concentric layers of histiocytes, giant cells, and lymphocytes.[39] Affected lymph nodes sometimes also show suppurative and granulomatous changes. Bacteria are frequently not demonstrable. When present, cat-scratch disease bacteria have identical staining and electron microscopic characteristics as the organisms seen within the lesions of bacillary angiomatosis.[2,3,40]

Bartonellosis. After hematoxylin and eosin staining, the lesions of verruga peruana closely resemble those of cutaneous bacillary angiomatosis.[3,41,42] However, the organisms seen in verruga peruana differ from those in bacillary angiomatosis in both their staining and electron microscopic characteristics; Rocha-Lima inclusions (endothelial phagocytic cells containing degenerating bacteria) are demonstrable only in the lesions of verruga peruana.[3,41,42]

DIAGNOSIS AND DIFFERENTIAL DIAGNOSIS (Table 115-2)

Bacillary Angiomatosis. Histopathologic features of bacillary angiomatosis establish the diagnosis in the vast majority of patients. However, a confirmatory diagnosis for patients whose lesions contain a paucity of organisms may require (1) the isolation of *Bartonella* species from blood or tissue, or (2) the amplification of *Bartonella* species DNA from tissue. The isolation of *Bartonella* species from infected tissue can be accomplished by direct plating of homogenized tissue onto chocolate or heart infusion agar containing 5% rabbit blood without antibiotics.[12, 24] Plates are incubated at 35° C with 5% CO_2 at high humidity for at least 4 weeks. Although patients with cutaneous bacillary angiomatosis are not always bacteremic, culturing of blood using either Isostat lysis centrifugation tubes (Wampole Laboratories, Cranbury, NJ)[9, 11, 12] or blood collection tubes containing ethylenediaminetetra-acetic acid (EDTA)[10] followed by direct plating may be an easier method for isolating *Bartonella* species from bacillary angiomatosis patients than culture from tissue. Amplification of *Bartonella* DNA from bacillary angiomatosis lesions with the use of polymerase chain reaction can be accomplished; however, the technique is labor intensive and its use has been restricted primarily to research studies for the detection of *Bartonella* DNA in archived paraffin-embedded tissue specimens and in human tissue specimens likely to be superinfected with other bacterial species.[6, 22-24]

Cat-Scratch Disease. Classically, the diagnosis of cat-

TABLE 115-2. Differential Diagnosis of Bacillary Angiomatosis, Cat-Scratch Disease, and Bartonellosis (Verruga Peruana)

Characteristic	Bacillary Angiomatosis*	Cat-Scratch Disease	Verruga Peruana*

Histologic differential diagnosis	Kaposi's sarcoma
	Angiosarcoma
	Pyogenic granuloma
	Verruga peruana
	Epithelioid (histiocytoid)
	  hemangioma
	Epithelioid
	  hemangioendothelioma
	Metastatic carcinoma
		Necrotizing granuloma
		Consistent with:
		  Tularemia
		  Brucellosis
		  Tuberculosis
		  Sarcoidosis
		Malignant disorders of histologic
		  origin
			Bacillary angiomatosis
			Kaposi's sarcoma
			Angiosarcoma
			Pyogenic granuloma
			Epithelioid (histiocytoid)
			  hemangioma
			Epithelioid
			  hemangioendothelioma
			Metastatic carcinoma

Clinical differential diagnosis	Kaposi's sarcoma
	Pyogenic granuloma
	Subcutaneous tumors
	Cellulitic plaques
	Verruga peruana
		Lymphadenopathy
		Consistent with:
		  Syphilis
		  Lymphogranuloma venereum
		  Tuberculosis
		  Sporotrichosis
		  Tularemia
		  Brucellosis
		  Histoplasmosis
		  Sarcoidosis
		  Toxoplasmosis
		  Infectious mononucleosis
		  Benign or malignant tumors
			Bacillary angiomatosis
			Kaposi's sarcoma
			Pyogenic granuloma

*Geographic setting may be helpful in defining the differential diagnosis of bacillary angiomatosis and verruga peruana.

scratch disease was made when three of the following four criteria were met in a patient with lymphadenopathy: (1) history of traumatic cat contact; (2) positive skin test response to cat-scratch disease skin test antigen; (3) characteristic lymph node pathology; and (4) negative laboratory investigation for unexplained lymphadenopathy.[2] However, because the cat-scratch disease skin test antigen is unlicensed and is prepared by the pasteurization of pus obtained from aspirated lymph nodes of patients with cat-scratch disease, there are concerns about its safety.

Alternatives for confirming the diagnosis of cat-scratch disease include the isolation of *B. henselae* from lymph nodes[13] and serologic testing. An indirect immunofluorescent antibody test is now available for the detection of antibodies to *B. henselae* and *B. quintana*.[43] This test is both sensitive (84%) and specific (96%) for diagnosing cat-scratch disease,[26] and it also appears promising for diagnosing bacillary angiomatosis in immunocompromised patients with bacillary angiomatosis.[44]

Bartonellosis. Isolation of *B. bacilliformis* from blood of a febrile patient confirms the diagnosis of Oroya fever.[18] A histologic diagnosis of verruga peruana may also be supported by a positive serologic test for *B. bacilliformis*.[45]

TREATMENT

Bacillary Angiomatosis. Although antibiotic therapy for patients with bacillary angiomatosis and bacillary peliosis has not been systematically evaluated, clinical experience for both *B. henselae* and *B. quintana* has established that erythromycin and doxycycline are the agents of first choice.[22, 24, 33] In general, patients with cutaneous bacillary angiomatosis in the absence of osseous and parenchymal disease or bacteremia have responded well to 8 to 12 weeks of oral antimicrobial therapy with one of these two agents (erythromycin, 500 mg four times per day, or doxycycline, 100 mg twice a day). The effectiveness of gentamicin, rifampin, trimethoprim-sulfamethoxazole, ceftriaxone, ceftizoxime, and ciprofloxacin has not been demonstrated; penicillin, penicillinase-resistant penicillins and aminopenicillins, and the first-generation cephalosporins have not been clinically efficacious.

Cat-Scratch Disease. For the vast majority of cat-scratch disease patients, no antimicrobial therapy is required because the adenopathy and associated symptoms will resolve without sequelae within 2 to 4 months.[2, 34, 35] Although not systematically evaluated, oral ciprofloxacin, trimethoprim-sulfamethoxazole, and rifampin have been found to be effective in some patients; parenteral gentamicin sulfate is recommended for severely ill patients.[34, 35] The apparent disparity between the currently recommended antimicrobial agents for bacillary angiomatosis and cat-scratch disease is of interest and requires further study.[46]

Bartonellosis. Anecdotal reports suggest that patients with Carrión's disease may respond favorably to antimicrobial therapy with chloramphenicol, tetracycline, penicillin, or streptomycin.[28, 42]

CONCLUSION

Although great strides have been made in increasing the knowledge of bacillary angiomatosis, cat-scratch disease, and bartonellosis in recent years, work remains to be done regarding the vectors, reservoirs, modes of transmission, prevention strategies, and clinical spectrum of disease for these rapidly emerging pathogens.

References

1. Stoler MH, Bonfiglio TA, Steigbigel RT, Pereira M. An atypical subcutaneous infection associated with acquired immune deficiency syndrome. Am J Clin Pathol 1983;80:714–718.
2. Warwick WJ. The cat-scratch syndrome, many diseases or one disease? Prog Med Virol 1967;9:256–301.
3. LeBoit PE, Berger TG, Egbert BM, et al. Epithelioid haemangioma-like vascular proliferation in AIDS: Manifestation of cat-scratch disease bacillus infection? Lancet 1988;1:960–963.
4. English CK, Wear DJ, Margileth AM, et al. Cat-scratch disease. Isolation and culture of the bacterial agent. JAMA 1988;259:1347–1352.
5. Brenner DJ, Hollis DG, Moss CW, et al. Proposal of *Afipia* gen. nov., with *Afipia felis* sp. nov. (Formerly the cat scratch disease bacillus), *Afipia clevelandensis* sp. nov. (Formerly the Cleveland Clinic Foundation strain), *Afipia broomeae* sp. nov., and three unnamed genospecies. J Clin Microbiol 1991;29:2450–2460.
6. Relman DA, Loutit JS, Schmidt TM, et al. The agent of bacillary angiomatosis: An approach to the identification of uncultured pathogens. N Engl J Med 1990;323:1573–1580.
7. Vinson JW, Varela G, Molina-Pasquel C. Trench fever. III. Induction of clinical disease in volunteers inoculated with *Rickettsia quintana* propagated on blood agar. Am J Trop Med Hyg 1969;18:713–722.
8. Strong RP (ed.). Trench fever: Report of Commission, Medical Research Committee, American Red Cross. Oxford: Oxford University Press, 1918:40–60.
9. Slater LN, Welch DF, Hensel D, Coody DW. A newly recognized fastidious gram-negative pathogen as a cause of fever and bacteremia. N Engl J Med 1990;323:1587–1593.
10. Regnery RL, Anderson BE, Clarridge JE III, et al. Characterization of a novel *Rochalimaea* species, *R. henselae*, sp. nov., isolated from blood of a febrile, human immunodeficiency virus–positive patient. J Clin Microbiol 1992;30:265–274.
11. Welch DF, Pickett DA, Slater LN, et al. *Rochalimaea henselae*, sp. nov., a cause of septicemia, bacillary angiomatosis, and parenchymal bacillary peliosis. J Clin Microbiol 1992;30:275–280.
12. Koehler JE, Quinn FD, Berger TG, et al. Isolation of *Rochalimaea* species from the cutaneous and osseous lesions of bacillary angiomatosis. N Engl J Med 1992;327:1625–1631.
13. Dolan MJ, Wong MT, Regnery RL, et al. Syndrome of *Rochalimaea henselae* adenitis suggesting cat scratch disease. Ann Intern Med 1993;118:331–336.
14. Perkins bacillary angiomatosis, Swaminathan B, Jackson LA, et al. Case 22-1992—pathogenesis of cat scratch disease (letter). N Engl J Med 1992;327:1599–1600.
15. Anderson B, Kelley C, Threlkel R, Edwards K. Detection of *Rochalimaea henselae* in cat-scratch disease skin test antigens. J Infect Dis 1993;168:1034–1036.
16. Daly JS, Worthington MG, Brenner DJ, et al. *Rochalimaea elizabethae* sp. nov. isolated from a patient with endocarditis. J Clin Microbiol 1993;31:872–881.
17. Schultz MG. A history of bartonellosis (Carrión's disease). Am J Trop Med Hyg 1968;17:503–515.
18. Noguchi H, Battistini TS. Etiology of Oroya fever. I. Cultivation of *Bartonella bacilliformis*. J Exp Med 1926;43:851–864.
19. Schultz MG. Daniel Carrión's experiment. N Engl J Med 1968;278:1323–1326.
20. Carrión D. Notes on verruga peruana. In: Buck C, Llopis A, Nájera E, Terris M, eds. The Challenge of Epidemiology: Issues and Selected Readings. Washington, DC: Pan American Health Organization, 1988:72–74.
21. Brenner DJ, O'Connor SP, Winkler HH, Steigerwalt AG. Propos-

als to unify the genera *Bartonella* and *Rochalimaea*, with descriptions of *Bartonella quintana* comb. nov., *Bartonella vinsonii* comb. nov., *Bartonella henselae* comb. nov., and *Bartonella elizabethae* comb. nov., and to remove the family *Bartonellaceae* from the order *Rickettsiales*. Int J Syst Bacteriol 1993;43:777–786.

22. Tappero JW, Koehler JE, Berger TG, et al. Bacillary angiomatosis and bacillary splenitis in immunocompetent adults. Ann Intern Med 1993;118:363–365.
23. Tappero JW, Mohle-Boetani J, Koehler JE, et al. The epidemiology of bacillary angiomatosis and bacillary peliosis. JAMA 1993;269:770–775.
24. Koehler JE, Tappero JW. AIDS commentary: Bacillary angiomatosis and bacillary peliosis in patients infected with human immunodeficiency virus. Clin Infect Dis 1993;17:612–624.
25. Jackson LA, Perkins BA, Wenger JD. Cat scratch disease in the United States: An analysis of three national databases. Am J Public Health 1993;83:1707–1711.
26. Zangwill KM, Hamilton DH, Perkins BA, et al. Epidemiology, risk factors, and evaluation of a new diagnostic test. N Engl J Med 1993;329:8–13.
27. Koehler JE, Glaser CA, Tappero JW. *Rochalimaea henselae* infection: A new zoonosis with the domestic cat as reservoir. JAMA 1994;271:531–535.
28. Gray GC, Johnson AA, Thornton SA, et al. An epidemic of Oroya fever in the Peruvian Andes. Am J Trop Med Hyg 1990;42:215–221.
29. Shannon RC. Entomological investigations in connection with Carrión's disease. Am J Hyg 1929;10:78–111.
30. Hertig M. Phlebotomus and Carrión's disease. Am J Trop Med 1942;22(Suppl.):1–80.
31. Perkocha LA, Geaghan SM, Yen TS, et al. Clinical and pathological features of bacillary peliosis hepatis in association with human immunodeficiency virus infection. N Engl J Med 1990;323:1581–1586.
32. Berger TG, Tappero JW, Kaymen A, LeBoit PE. Bacillary (epithelioid) angiomatosis and concurrent Kaposi's sarcoma in acquired immunodeficiency syndrome. Arch Dermatol 1989;125:1543–1547.
33. Mohle-Boetani J, Reingold A, LeBoit B, et al. Bacillary angiomatosis: Spectrum of disease and clinical characteristics in HIV+ Patients (abstract No. 372). In: Programs and Abstracts of the 32nd Interscience Conference on Antimicrobial Agents and Chemother-

apy. Washington, DC: American Society for Microbiology, 1992:173.
34. Carithers HA. Cat-scratch disease: An overview based on a study of 1,200 patients. Am J Dis Child 1985;139:1124–1133.
35. Margileth AM. Cat scratch disease. Adv Pediatr Infect Dis 1993;8:1–21.
36. Cuadra MC. Salmonellosis complications in human bartonellosis. Tex Rep Biol Med 1956;14:97–113.
37. LeBoit PE, Berger TG, Egbert BM, et al. Bacillary angiomatosis. The histopathology and differential diagnosis of a pseudoneoplastic infection in patients with human immunodeficiency virus disease. Am J Surg Pathol 1989;13:909–920.
38. Reed JA, Brigati DJ, Flynn SD, et al. Immunocytochemical identification of *Rochalimaea* in bacillary (epithelioid) angiomatous, parenchymal bacillary peliosis, and persistent fever with bacteremia. Am J Surg Pathol 1992;16:650–657.
39. Johnson WT, Helwig EB. Cat-scratch disease (histopathologic changes in the skin). Arch Dermatol 1969;100:148–154.
40. Wear DJ, Margileth AM, Hadfield TL, et al. Cat scratch disease: A bacterial infection. Science 1983;221:1403–1405.
41. Arias-Stella J, Lieberman PH, Erlandson RA, Arias-Stella J Jr. Histology, immunohistochemistry, and ultrastructure of the verruca in Carrión's disease. Am J Surg Pathol 1986;10:595–610.
42. Arias-Stella J, Lieberman PH, Garcia-Caceres U, et al. Verruga peruana mimicking malignant neoplasms. Am J Dermatol 1987;9:279–291.
43. Regnery RL, Olson JG, Perkins bacillary angiomatosis, Bibb W. Serological response to "Rochalimaea henselae" antigen in suspected cat-scratch disease. Lancet 1992;339:1443–1445.
44. Tappero J, Regnery R, Koehler J, Olson J. Detection of serologic response to *Rochalimaea henselae* in patients with bacillary angiomatosis (bacillary angiomatosis) by immunofluorescent antibody (IFA) testing (Abstract No. 674). In: Program and Abstracts of the 32nd Interscience Conference on Antimicrobial Agents and Chemotherapy. Washington, DC: American Society for Microbiology, 1992:223.
45. Knobloch J, Solano L, Alvarez O, Delgado E. Antibodies to *Bartonella bacilliformis* as determined by fluorescence antibody test, indirect hemagglutination and ELISA. Trop Med Parasitol 1985;36:183–185.
46. Tappero JW, Koehler JE. Cat scratch disease and bacillary angiomatosis (letter). JAMA 1991;266:1938–1939.

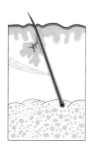

chapter 116

The Zoonoses

DALE R. WESTROM

Zoonotic infections encompass a large group of bacterial, viral, rickettsial, fungal, and parasitic diseases that are transmitted from animals to humans. Many of these diseases are described in other chapters, and some are so obscure or insignificant that they are not covered. A few zoonoses such as malaria and yellow fever have tremendous medical and historical importance but have no diagnostic cutaneous findings. There is, however, a small group of uncommon, but clinically relevant, zoonotic bacterial infections that have a wide variety of dermatologic manifestations. These diseases include anthrax, brucellosis, plague, and tularemia and are representative of the many ways humans can acquire zoonotic infections. Modes of transmission range from direct contact with infected animals, indirect contact with contaminated materials, inhalation and ingestion of organisms, and arthropod bite (vector borne).

Anthrax

DEFINITION

Anthrax is an uncommon bacterial disease of wild and domestic animals caused by *Bacillus anthracis* that is transmitted to humans by inoculation, inhalation, or ingestion.

CLINICAL DESCRIPTION

By far the most common route of infection is cutaneous, accounting for 95% of the cases seen in the United States.[1] Inhalation accounts for another 5%, and in other parts of the world gastrointestinal infection has been documented. The incidence of anthrax has declined rapidly in the United States, with only 231 cases reported between 1955 and 1986[2] and only four cases cited since 1979.[3] Nevertheless, worldwide it continues to be an important disease and at times can be epidemic, such as in Zimbabwe in the late 1970s when an estimated 6000 cases were reported.[4]

Animal reservoirs of anthrax include wild and domestic herbivores, including cattle, goats, sheep, and horses. Frequent sources of infection in humans are the hides, bristles, meat, and bones (bone meal fertilizer) of diseased animals. The majority of cases in the United States have been related to imported goat hairs. Vector-borne anthrax has also been reported.

After an incubation period of 2 to 5 days, the first symptom is pruritus at the site of a small erythematous papule, which soon vesiculates and becomes covered with an eschar. Occasionally, multiple vesicles coalesce into a larger bulla called a malignant pustule, which then forms a shallow crater and eventually heals with a scar. The lesions may be surrounded by nonpitting edema and, although not generally painful, may be accompanied by some discomfort and regional lymphadenopathy. There may be systemic manifestations, including fever, malaise, and, rarely, toxemia. Malignant edema has been used to describe an unusual type of cutaneous anthrax associated with significant local reaction, multiple bullae, induration, and septicemia.[1] The location of the lesions is generally on exposed skin, with the arms, face (Fig. 116–1), and trunk involved in that order.

Inhalation anthrax (woolsorters' disease) starts with a vague, nonspecific, systemic reaction 1 to 5 days after exposure. After a temporary improvement there is progression to severe respiratory distress characterized by dyspnea, diaphoresis, cyanosis, and stridor. Massive edema of the head and neck may also develop. Chest radiographs reveal mediastinal widening and pleural effusions with a nonspecific parenchymal infiltrate.[2] Gastrointestinal anthrax presents as abdominal pain, nausea, and vomiting and rapidly progresses to bloody diarrhea, prostration, toxemia, and shock. Oropharyngeal and

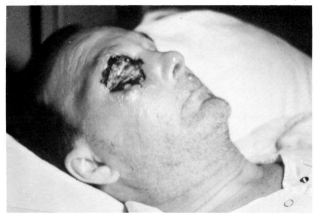

FIGURE 116–1. Cutaneous anthrax in the periorbital area.

pharyngeal anthrax have been associated with ingestion of contaminated meat.

PATHOLOGY

Anthrax causes hemorrhagic necrosis of the epidermis and superficial dermis, leading to ulceration. Inflammatory cells are scarce in some cases, but diffuse dermal infiltrates of neutrophils are present in others. Papillary dermal edema and spongiosis can occur adjacent to ulcerated lesions. Bacilli can be demonstrated by tissue Gram stain such as the Brown-Brenn method.

PATHOGENESIS AND ETIOLOGY

B. anthracis is a large, gram-positive, nonmotile, spore-forming, capsulated bacillus that occurs singly or in short chains in clinical specimens. Spores are resistant to heat and can remain viable for years in dry soil. Cattle have become infected by grazing in fields where animals died of anthrax decades before.

Infection follows introduction of the anthrax spores through the skin, respiratory tract, gastrointestinal tract, or oropharynx. Cutaneous anthrax results from introduction of spores through arthropod bite, abrasion of the skin, or scratching. The spores germinate, multiply, and produce a complex toxin. Hematogenous dissemination occurs in 5% to 20% of untreated cases.[2] Inhalation anthrax occurs when spores are inhaled, phagocytosed, and carried to regional lymph nodes where germination takes place. There the toxin produces hemorrhage and necrosis of mediastinal lymph nodes that can compromise the respiratory passages. Gastrointestinal anthrax results from germination of spores in the intestinal mucosa, leading to toxin production causing necrosis, ulcerative lesions, and hemorrhage, particularly in the terminal ileum and cecum.

DIAGNOSIS AND DIFFERENTIAL DIAGNOSIS

The clinical presentation of cutaneous anthrax is characteristic enough to raise a high index of suspicion, espe-

cially in patients with a history of industrial or agricultural exposure to the organism. The rapidly evolving ulcer and failure to respond to initial antibiotic therapy are highly suggestive. Inhalation anthrax may present as a nonspecific lower respiratory tract infection but soon evolves into respiratory distress and a clinical picture resembling congestive heart failure. Distinctive radiographic findings of mediastinal widening and parenchymal infiltrates are helpful in the diagnosis. Gastrointestinal anthrax is nonspecific clinically.

Laboratory diagnosis of anthrax is dependent on Gram stain and culture of blood, tissue, cerebrospinal fluid, or sputum. Serologic tests are retrospective and confirmatory of infection. The presence of large gram-positive rods on Gram stain is presumptive evidence of infection, and the definitive diagnosis is made by culture on nutrient agar. Identification of isolates can be made by specific bacteriophage lysis. A direct immunofluorescence antibody test is useful in making an early specific laboratory diagnosis. Many serologic tests are used for the diagnosis of anthrax, and they require a high degree of sensitivity since patients generally have a lower titer of antibody.[2] Complement fixation, agar gel, precipitation, and indirect microhemagglutination have been used in the past but either were too insensitive or lacked reproducibility. The enzyme-linked immunosorbent essay (ELISA) and the electrophoretic immunotransblot (EITB) are both sensitive and specific. The ELISA detects anticapsule antibodies, and the EITB detects lethal factor and protective antigen antibodies.

The differential diagnosis of cutaneous anthrax includes any disease process that causes a slowly developing ulcer that forms as a vesicle and heals with a scar (Table 116–1). The relative lack of pain, pitting edema, and systemic manifestations would be distinguishing features for anthrax.

TREATMENT

Untreated cutaneous anthrax can lead to serious complications and death in up to 20% of cases. Gastrointestinal and inhalation anthrax may be fatal even with antibiotic therapy. Mild cutaneous disease can be treated with potassium penicillin V, 30 mg/kg per day orally in four divided doses for 5 to 7 days (Table 116–2). Systemic disease requires procaine penicillin G, 20 to 30 mg/kg per day, intramuscularly in two equal doses for 5 to 7 days. Penicillin-allergic patients can be treated with tetracycline, 15 to 20 mg/kg per day, orally in four divided doses. Other forms of anthrax have been treated with massive doses of penicillin and streptomycin. Specific

TABLE 116–1. Differential Diagnosis of Anthrax
Cutaneous leishmaniasis
Ecthyma contagiosum (orf)
Staphylococcal abscess
Brown recluse spider bite
Tularemia

TABLE 116-2. Treatment of Anthrax

1. Penicillin
2. For penicillin-allergic patients: tetracycline
3. Alternative antibiotics:
   Erythromycin
   Chloramphenicol
   Cephalosporins
   Streptomycin
4. Specific antitoxin, when available

antitoxin, although available for animal infections in some countries, is not available in the United States. Incision and drainage or excision of cutaneous lesions is specifically contraindicated because of the risk of dissemination of the infection. Occasionally, the use of systemic corticosteroids may be useful for malignant edema, particularly of the thorax and neck when respiration may be compromised. It should be noted that the evolution of the anthrax pustule is not modified by appropriate antibiotic therapy because of the toxins elaborated in the early stages of infection. Although human transmission of anthrax has not been documented, careful handling and disposal with incineration of contaminated dressings are indicated.

PREVENTION

Although anthrax has become an increasingly rare disease in the United States, occasional outbreaks have occurred, especially in textile workers. Specific anthrax vaccines are available for immunization of those individuals at risk (i.e., textile workers, veterinarians, and military personnel). One case of human cutaneous anthrax in North Carolina in 1987[6] indicated that although only one person was infected at a textile mill, numerous samples of cashmere from western Asia were positive for *B. anthracis.*

Brucellosis

DEFINITION

Brucellosis is an uncommon systemic bacterial infection caused by *Brucella* species. In humans there is low incidence but a wide variety of cutaneous manifestations.

CLINICAL DESCRIPTION

Brucellosis is a zoonotic infection usually acquired from infected goats, cattle, pigs, or dogs. Dairy workers, shepherds, abattoir workers, meat packers, microbiologists, and veterinarians are especially at risk for infection. Milk and milk products have been increasingly impor-

tant sources of infection.[7] Open wounds are portals of entry for the organisms, but aerosols from infected material can invade through mucosal surfaces. Contamination of the environment may be a source of infection as well because *Brucella* can survive for up to 20 weeks in fetal organs left on the soil.[8] Blood transfusion, organ donation, placental transfer, and sexual transmission are all sources of infection. The organism has a worldwide distribution, and the disease affects about 500,000 persons. In the United States, the annual incidence of this disease decreased from 5000 to 200 since 1980.

The incubation period of brucellosis can be from a few days to a few weeks but most commonly is from 3 to 4 weeks.[9] In its acute form, the disease causes fever, sweats, chills, myalgia, lethargy, and headaches. The fever, which was once thought to be commonly undulating, usually does not have this characteristic feature. Lymphadenopathy and splenomegaly are also common, as are a wide variety of skeletal problems. Many neurologic, genitourinary, cardiovascular, gastrointestinal, pulmonary, and hematologic symptoms have been described. Cutaneous manifestations of brucellosis include primary, disseminated, and secondary (nonspecific) findings (Table 116-3). In a large review of patients with brucellosis 6% were found to have cutaneous lesions.[10] Twenty-one of the patients had positive blood cultures for *B. melitensis.* Widespread erythematous to violaceous papules and nodules, particularly on the lower extremities, are the most typical and frequent cutaneous manifestations of brucellosis. However, a wide variety of skin changes have been associated with this infection.[11, 12] Hypersensitivity reactions are believed to be the cause for the majority of these cutaneous reactions.

TABLE 116-3. Cutaneous Manifestations of Brucellosis

Primary (Direct Contact, Inoculation)
Abscesses
Brucella dermatitis

Disseminated
Subcutaneous papules
Multiple cutaneous abscesses
Multiple ulcers and eschars

Secondary/Nonspecific
Macular
Maculopapular
Urticarial/edematous
Vesicular
Eczematous
Psoriasiform
Pityriasis rosea-like
Erysipelas-like
Rubeoliform or scarlatiniform
Erythema nodosum
Petechial
Bronzing (photosensitive)

PATHOLOGY

Papules and nodules of brucellosis are due to infiltrates of lymphocytes and macrophages, which sometimes form small collections. A mixed septal and lobular panniculitis with plasma cells occurs in erythema nodosum–like lesions.[10, 12]

PATHOGENESIS AND ETIOLOGY

There are four species of *Brucella* that are capable of infecting humans: *B. melitensis, B. suis, B. abortus,* and the least common, *B. canis.* These organisms are gram-negative coccobacilli. They are small, aerobic, nonmotile, intracellular bacteria without spores or capsules. *B. melitensis* is the most virulent, followed by *B. suis, B. abortus,* and *B. canis.* These organisms grow slowly in culture, and they do best in liquid media such as trypticase soy broth in an atmosphere of 5% to 10% CO_2 at 37°C. *Brucella* organisms appear in peripheral blood within hours and are engulfed by polymorphonuclear leukocytes and monocytes, eventually being carried to lymph nodes, liver, spleen, and bone marrow. Infection caused by *B. abortus* produces noncaseating granulomas containing clusters of epithelioid histiocytes. In chronic brucellosis, abscesses may occur in multiple organs in subcutaneous tissue.

DIAGNOSIS AND DIFFERENTIAL DIAGNOSIS

History of exposure to contaminated animals, unpasteurized milk, dairy products, or travel to areas endemic for brucellosis can usually raise the suspicion of infection. Blood culture is most commonly used to isolate the organism. In patients with acute *B. melitensis* infections, culture of blood and bone marrow will be positive in 70% to 90% of cases.[13] Cultures must be retained up to 6 weeks to give the maximum chance of recovery of this slow-growing organism. The serum agglutination test is the most common serologic screening test, although complement fixation tests and radioimmune assay have also been used.[14] ELISA testing has also been used in the serodiagnosis of brucellosis. (Skin testing has also been used but is unreliable.) The differential diagnosis of brucellosis is presented in Table 116–4.

TABLE 116–4. Differential Diagnosis of Brucellosis
Typhoid fever
Tuberculosis
Q fever
Influenza
Tularemia
Mononucleosis
Malaria

TREATMENT

Tetracycline, either alone or in combination with streptomycin or rifampin, is used for periods of 3 to 6 weeks for acute and chronic infections, respectively. Rifampin is the drug of choice for treating brucellosis in pregnant women. Trimethoprim-sulfamethoxazole has been used to treat children with acute brucellosis.[8]

Plague

DEFINITION

Plague is a gram-negative bacterial infection caused by *Yersinia pestis* that is endemic in wild rodents and is transmitted to humans by fleas. Once established in humans, additional disease transmission can occur through the respiratory route.

CLINICAL DESCRIPTION

The three clinical forms of plague are bubonic, septicemic, and pneumonic. Bubonic plague is by far the most common form and results from direct contact with infected rodents or most frequently from the bite of fleas infesting infected animals. After an incubation period of 2 to 8 days there is fever, regional lymphadenopathy (bubo), and tenderness (Fig. 116–2). The lymphadenopathy is rapidly progressive and exquisitely tender, quickly followed by systemic symptoms and, if untreated, death. Although skin lesions are inconspicuous, one fourth of Vietnamese patients showed cutaneous changes including pustules, vesicles, eschars, or papules near the bubo or flea bite.[14a] Cellulitis with abscess formation and even ulceration have been reported.[15] Ecthyma gangrenosum has been described as a cutaneous manifestation of plague.[16] A striking cutaneous finding seen late in the course of infection is purpura and gangrene, which

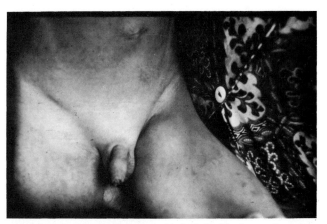

FIGURE 116–2. Matted lymph nodes (bubo) with surrounding edema in groin of patient with plague.

occurs as a result of endotoxin and probably accounts for the name "black death." The septicemic phase is characterized by fever, chills, prostration, shock, and coma. Blood cultures and, at times, even Gram stain of peripheral blood are positive for plague bacilli. Patients may be septicemic without lymphadenopathy. Pneumonic plague results from secondary hematogenous spread from infected buboes but can also occur directly by aerosol.

Plague has a worldwide distribution in temperate climates, particularly affecting North and South America, Africa, and Southeast Asia. In the United States it is especially established west of the 100th meridian (i.e., a line drawn south from North Dakota to Texas).[17] The reservoirs of *Y. pestis* are wild and commensal rodents usually with a relatively resistant host species in association with a highly susceptible group of animals such as ground squirrels that get infected and die in large numbers. Close contact with the epizootic leads to human infection, usually by flea bite but also by direct contact. Flea species vary in their ability to effectively transmit plague bacillus and may account for the geographic distribution of the disease.

PATHOGENESIS AND ETIOLOGY

Y. pestis is a gram-negative, aerobic, nonmotile, pleomorphic bacillus that may have a "safety pin" appearance on Giemsa- and Wright-stained smears but not usually on Gram stain. It grows well in most nutrient media, but growth is slow.[18] Various antigens, endotoxins, and exotoxins are responsible for the pathogenicity and virulence of the plague bacillus. Once the bacillus is ingested by the proper vector species of flea, the organisms multiply and eventually block the upper digestive tract of the flea (proventriculus), causing the insect to repeatedly bite its host. The blocking is caused by the product of a bacterial coagulant enzyme that is inactive above 28°C to 30°C, thus helping to account for the reduction in transmission of plague at high ambient temperatures. When the bacillus is introduced into humans by bite, contact, or inhalation, the organism is phagocytosed and destroyed by polymorphonuclear cells. However, macrophages may engulf bacilli, leading to resistant organisms that ultimately cause septicemia with or without lymphadenopathy.

DIAGNOSIS AND DIFFERENTIAL DIAGNOSIS

The presenting signs and symptoms of classic bubonic plague are sufficiently dramatic to strongly suggest a diagnosis, particularly in endemic areas. However, atypical syndromes and septicemic plague can often be missed. In New Mexico, 27 cases of plague were diagnosed between 1965 and 1989, and all 9 patients with classic plague were diagnosed and treated properly. Ten patients had fever, sore throat, or influenza-like symptoms, and 6 died, initially having been diagnosed with pharyngitis or influenza. The remaining patients had predominantly gastrointestinal symptoms or signs of menin-

TABLE 116-5. Treatment of Plague

Streptomycin, two divided intramuscular doses totaling
   30 mg/kg × 10 days
First alternative:
   Tetracycline, 2-4 g per day, four divided doses × 10 days
Other alternatives:
   Chloramphenicol
   Gentamicin
   Sulfamethoxazole-trimethoprim

Note: Penicillins and cephalosporins have not been proven effective.

gitis, and all survived because appropriate antibiotics were given even though the diagnosis was not entertained initially. It should be noted that only one patient gave a history of flea bite.[17]

TREATMENT

Because untreated plague is usually rapidly fatal, the use of an appropriate antibiotic is critical (Table 116-5).

Tularemia

DEFINITION

Tularemia is an uncommon zoonotic infection caused by *Francisella tularensis*. Humans become infected by a wide variety of routes.

CLINICAL DESCRIPTION

Tularemia has six clinical patterns: ulceroglandular, glandular, oculoglandular, oropharyngeal, typhoidal, and pneumonic. The clinical presentation depends on the route of exposure, with the ulceroglandular variety being most common, occurring in over 80% of the cases.[19] It is characterized by a small, pruritic, erythematous papule that proceeds to ulcerate, usually with an associated tender, regional lymphadenopathy. These lymph nodes may suppurate and drain. Fever, chills, and myalgias are commonly seen in infections of all types. Skin ulcers may be solitary or multiple and range from several millimeters to several centimeters in diameter.

The margins of the ulcer tend to be raised and chancre-like and ultimately form an eschar. Ulcers are most commonly found on the upper extremities when the patient has been exposed to infected animals or on the back, abdomen, and head when infected by arthropod bite.[20] Other cutaneous manifestations are unusual but include erythema nodosum, erythema multiforme, and rarely a diffuse, erythematous maculopapular rash.[21]

Glandular tularemia is identical to ulceroglandular tularemia but without any cutaneous lesions. This form of tularemia accounts for 10% to 15% of cases. Oculoglandular tularemia is even less common and results from the introduction of the infectious agent into the eye. Typically, conjunctivitis, pain, lacrimation, and edema are present. This can be followed by corneal ulceration and perforation. Oropharyngeal tularemia results from ingestion of contaminated meat and causes an ulcerative pharyngitis sometimes associated with a necrotic, gray membrane. Cervical lymph nodes are involved. Typhoidal tularemia occurs in approximately 15% of patients and usually presents as fever, chills, sore throat, and occasional abdominal pain and diarrhea. These patients are generally extremely ill, and the infection is probably acquired by inhalation of organisms during the ingestion of contaminated meat.[19] The clinical presentation of typhoidal tularemia may be difficult to differentiate from ulceroglandular tularemia until the latter stages of infection. Pulmonary tularemia is the most serious, but fortunately the least common, of the types of infection. Secondary pneumonia does result from hematogenous spread. Physical findings initially may be subtle, but eventually a nonproductive cough associated with rales and pleural effusions occurs. Radiographic findings include bronchopneumonia, hilar adenopathy, pleural effusions, and atypical infiltrates.

EPIDEMIOLOGY

Tularemia has been reported from North America, the Middle East, and Japan and infrequently from Africa and Central and South America. Most of the cases in the United States have been reported from Arkansas, Illinois, Missouri, Texas, Virginia, and Tennessee.[20] Less than 200 cases per year have been reported from the United States since 1967. Natural infections have been found in nearly 100 species of wild mammals, 9 species of domestic animals, 25 species of birds, and several species of fish and amphibians.[22] Wild rabbits are the major source of infections acquired from animals, although foxes, skunks, squirrels, and muskrats have also been implicated. Arthropods, particularly ticks, are the main vectors and reservoirs of tularemia. Two genera of ticks, *Amblyomma* and *Dermacentor*, are the chief vectors of tularemia. Transviral transmission occurs in *Amblyomma* ticks, increasing their significance as reservoirs of natural infection. Ticks are considered responsible for nearly 90% of human infections in North America.[23] The hematophagous deer fly, *Chrysops discalis*, has been associated with tularemia and accounts for the synonym deer fly fever.[24] In Finland and Sweden, the mosquito appears to be the main vector.[25]

PATHOLOGY

Tularemia results in a suppurative and granulomatous dermatitis. Secondary epidermal changes include spongiosis and psoriasiform epidermal hyperplasia. Bacilli can be demonstrated in tissue sections by immunofluorescence using specific antiserum but not by conventional special stains.

PATHOGENESIS AND ETIOLOGY

F. tularensis is a small pleomorphic gram-negative facultative aerobic coccobacillus that grows well in glucose-cystine blood agar but requires selective media for isolation from skin ulcers or respiratory secretions. Although all isolates of *F. tularensis* seem to be serologically identical, there appear to be two biotypes, a highly virulent form for humans (Jellison type A) and one that produces mild disease (Jellison type B). As few as 10 organisms injected subcutaneously or 10 to 50 organisms given by aerosol can cause infection in humans.[26] After the pathogen is introduced through arthropod bite or break in the skin, it is ingested by polymorphonuclear cells and macrophages. It then multiplies intracellularly and spreads to regional lymph nodes, distant lymph nodes, and ultimately liver, spleen, and lungs. Granulomatous inflammation and focal necrosis can occur in these organs[27] and may result in septic shock and death.

DIAGNOSIS

Gram stain of infected material is rarely useful in the diagnosis of tularemia and culture requires appropriate selective media and a great deal of caution because of the infectivity of the organisms. Diagnosis is generally made with serologic tests, especially serum agglutination (a titer greater than 1:160 or a fourfold increase). A skin test has been developed but is only available through the Centers for Disease Control and Prevention in Atlanta, Georgia.

The differential diagnosis for a cutaneous ulcer with associated lymphadenopathy is broad but would include the disorders listed in Table 116–6. Recent occupational or recreational exposure to wild game or arthropod bites are also suggestive of tularemia. Nevertheless, most of the time the diagnosis will be made retrospectively.

TREATMENT

Streptomycin, 7.5 mg/kg given intramuscularly every 12 hours for 10 days, remains the treatment of choice and is considered to be curative in the early stages of disease. Although tetracycline and chloramphenicol (2 g per day, orally) are as effective as streptomycin, relapses are likely if the drug is given for fewer than 14 days. Erythromycin has been used successfully for pleuropulmonary tularemia in children.[28]

TABLE 116-6. Differential Diagnosis of Tularemia
Anthrax
Pyogenic infections
Plague
Sporotrichosis
Cat-scratch fever
Lymphogranuloma venereum
Melioidosis

References

1. Brachman PS. Anthrax. In: Hoeprich PD, Jordan MC, eds. Infectious Diseases, 4th ed. Philadelphia: JB Lippincott, 1989: 1007–1013.
2. Longfield R. Anthrax. In: Strickland GT, ed. Hunter's Tropical Medicine, 7th ed. Philadelphia: WB Saunders Co., 1991:434–438.
3. Taylor J, Dimmitt D, Ezzell J, et al. Indigenous human cutaneous anthrax in Texas. South Med J 1993;86:1–4.
4. Knudson G. Treatment of anthrax in man: History and current concepts. Milit Med 1986;151:71–77.
5. Harrison L, Ezzell J, Abshire T, et al. Evaluation of serologic tests for diagnosis of anthrax after an outbreak of cutaneous anthrax in Paraguay. J Infect Dis 1989;1960:706–710.
6. Centers for Disease Control. Human cutaneous anthrax—North Carolina, 1987. MMWR 1988;37:413–414.
7. Thapar MK, Young EJ. Urban outbreak of goat cheese brucellosis. Pediatr Infect Dis 1986;5:640–643.
8. Mikolich DJ, Boyce JM. *Brucella* species. In: Mandell GL, Douglas RG Jr, Bennett JE, eds. Principles and Practice of Infectious Diseases, 3rd ed. New York: Churchill Livingstone, 1989: 1735–1742.
9. Spink WW. The Nature of Brucellosis. Minneapolis: Minnesota Press, 1956.
10. Ariza J, Servitje O, Pallares R. Characteristic cutaneous lesions in patients with brucellosis. Arch Dermatol 1989;125:380–383.
11. Gee-Lew BM, Nicholas EA, Hirose FM, et al. Unusual skin manifestations of brucellosis. Arch Dermatol 1983;119:56–58.
12. Berger TG, Guill MA, Goette DK. Cutaneous lesions in brucellosis. Arch Dermatol 1981;117:40–42.
13. Gutuzzo E, Carrillo C, Guerra J, et al. An evaluation of diagnostic methods for brucellosis: The value of bone marrow culture. Infect Dis 1986;153:122–125.
14. Buchanan TM, Selje CR, Frix MK, et al. Brucellosis in the United States, 1960–1972. An abattoir-associated disease: II. Diagnostic aspects. Medicine 1974;53:415–425.

14a. Butler T. A clinical study of bubonic plague: Observations of the 1970 Vietnam epidemic with emphasis on coagulation studies, skin histology, and electrocardiograms. Am J Med 1972; 53:268–276.
15. Butler T. Plague. In: Strickland GT, ed. Hunter's Tropical Medicine, 7th ed. Philadelphia: WB Saunders Co., 1991:408–416.
16. Wetty TK, Grabman J, Kompare E, et al. Nineteen cases of plague in Arizona. West J Med 1985;142:641–646.
17. Crook LD, Tempest B. Plague: A clinical review of 27 cases. Arch Intern Med 1992;152:1253–1256.
18. Poland JD. Plague. In: Hoeprick PD, Jordan MC, eds. Infectious Diseases, 4th ed. Philadelphia: JB Lippincott, 1989:1296–1306.
19. Hornick RB. Tularemia. In: Hoeprich PD, Jordan MC, eds. Infectious Diseases, 4th ed. Philadelphia: JB Lippincott, 1989: 1289–1295.
20. Evans MD, Gregory DW, Schaffner W, et al. Tularemia: A 30-year experience with 88 cases. Medicine 1985;64:251–269.
21. Warring WB, Ruffin JS. A tick-borne epidemic of tularemia. N Engl J Med 1946;234:137.
22. Hopla CE. The ecology of tularemia. Adv Vet Sci Comp Med 1974;18:25–53.
23. Lopez CE, Kornblatt AN, Sikes RK, et al. Tularemia: Review of eight cases of tick-borne infection and the epidemiology of the disease in Georgia. South Med J 1982;75:404–407.
24. Sanford JP. Tularemia. JAMA 1983;250:3225–3226.
25. Uhari M, Syrjala H, Salminen A. Tularemia in children caused by *Francisella tularensis* biovar *palaearctica*. Pediatr Infect Dis J 1990;9:80–83.
26. Brachman PS. *Francisella tularensis* in New England. N Engl J Med 1969;280:1296–1297.
27. Jacobs RF, Navair JP. Tularemia in children. Pediatr Infect Dis 1983;2:487–491.
28. Harrell RE, Simmons HF. Pleuropulmonary tularemia: Successful treatment with erythromycin. South Med J 1990;83: 1363–1364.

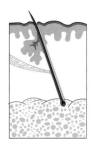

chapter 117

Common Superficial Mycoses

BONI E. ELEWSKI

Fungi that generally infect only the superficial layers of the hair or stratum corneum include (1) *Phaeoannellomyces werneckii* (*Exophiala werneckii*), which causes tinea nigra; (2) *Piedraia hortae*, which causes black piedra; (3) *Trichosporon beigelii* (*T. cutaneum*), which causes white piedra; and (4) *Malassezia furfur* (*Pityrosporum ovale*, *P. orbiculare*), which causes pityriasis versicolor.[1] Since some authors classify the folliculitis caused by *Malessezia furfur* as a variant of pityriasis (tinea) versicolor, a discussion of *"Pityrosporum"* folliculitis will also be included in this chapter.[2] All of these organisms typically produce a superficial cutaneous eruption; however, in immunodeficient hosts, opportunistic infection and systemic disease are possible. Little to no inflammatory response is generally elicited in the host.

Tinea Nigra

DEFINITION

Tinea nigra is a superficial, asymptomatic infection of the epidermis caused by *Phaeoannellomyces werneckii* (*Exophiala werneckii*). This condition is not caused by a dermatophyte and therefore should not be prefaced with the adjective "tinea," which refers to dermatophytosis; however, for traditional and historical reasons, *tinea nigra* is the accepted term.

CLINICAL DESCRIPTION

Patients usually present with asymptomatic, nummular, macular, brown to black patches with clearly delin-

eated margins on the palms, soles, or other areas of the integument. The typical presentation is a single lesion on the palm, without constitutional signs or lymphadenopathy. Infection is most common in tropical or subtropical climates and has been reported in North and South America, Africa, and Asia. The southeastern coastal areas of the United States have sporadic occurrences.[3] Most patients are in the teens, and females are more likely infected than males.[4, 5]

PATHOLOGY

The stratum corneum is hyperkeratotic and contains dematiaceous septate, short or elongated hyphae (Fig. 117–1). Occasionally, budding yeast cells are also noted. Large rounded or ovoid spaces are often evident in the cornified layer of specimens of tinea nigra.[6] The dermis is generally uninvolved. The dark color observed clinically is due to the dematiaceous fungus growing in the outer integument, rather than to changes in the melanocytes.

PATHOGENESIS AND ETIOLOGY

Phaeoannellomyces werneckii is a dematiaceous fungus found in nature as a soil saprophyte. Exposure to contaminated soil or vegetative matter may elicit infection. Human to human transmission is not known to occur. There are no known predisposing factors, and no information on immunity is available.[2]

DIAGNOSIS AND DIFFERENTIAL DIAGNOSIS

The diagnosis is based on the typical clinical presentation and can be confirmed by direct microscopy reveal-

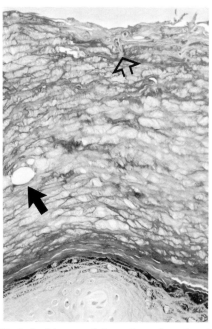

FIGURE 117-1. In this case of tinea nigra of a palm, there are pigmented hyphae (*open arrow*) within a compact cornified layer that also has ovoid spaces within it (*closed arrow*). These spaces are characteristic and can coalesce to become large and diamond shaped.

ing pigmented septate hyphae. Culture reveals a dematiaceous mold with characteristic one- or two-celled ellipsoidal conidia. Histopathologic study, although not necessary for diagnosis, also reveals the distinctive pigmented hyphae in the stratum corneum.

The differential diagnosis includes junctional nevus, lentigo, and melanoma (Table 117-1).

TREATMENT

Topical treatment with an antifungal agent in the imidazole class is generally curative.[7] Oral therapy with griseofulvin is ineffective.

TABLE 117-1. Differential Diagnosis of Common Superficial Mycoses	
Tinea Nigra	**Pityriasis Versicolor**
Junctional nevus	Pityriasis alba
Lentigo	Vitiligo
Melanoma	Seborrheic dermatitis
	Postinflammatory hyper/ hypopigmentation
	Cutaneous candidiasis
Piedra	**"Pityrosporum" Folliculitis**
Pediculosis	Bacterial or irritant folliculitis
Trichorrhexis nodosa	Acne vulgaris
Trichomycosis axillaris	Neurotic excoriations
Psoriatic or eczematous scales	Papular urticaria

Piedra

DEFINITION

Piedra, which is derived from the Spanish word for stone, refers to a superficial mycosis of the hair shaft. There are two varieties of piedra caused by two unrelated fungi. Black piedra is caused by *Piedraia hortae*, and white piedra is caused by *Trichosporon beigelii*.

CLINICAL DESCRIPTION

Black piedra is found on the scalp and occasionally facial hair and is prevalent in tropical climates of Central and South America, the South Pacific, and Asia. Asymptomatic, darkly colored nodules are firmly attached to the outer hair shaft without penetrating the cortex. Hair follicles and skin surface are unaffected. In white piedra, the concretions on the hair shaft are more amorphous, lighter in color, and softer than the nodules found in black piedra. Hairs in the genital area and facial area are commonly involved. White piedra of the scalp hair is rare. Although the carriage rate of *T. beigelii* in the anal area is higher in homosexual men,[8] white piedra does not appear to be transmitted by sexual contact.

PATHOLOGY

Direct microscopy or potassium hydroxide (KOH) preparation confirms the diagnosis of both black and white piedra. In black piedra, pigmented hyphae, arthroconidia, asci, and ascospores can be observed composing the nodule. The nodule of white piedra contains hyaline hyphae, blastoconidia, and arthroconidia.

PATHOGENESIS AND ETIOLOGY

Piedraia hortae is a dematiaceous fungus more prevalent in tropical climates. The natural habitat of this organism is not known,[2] although presumably infection is acquired by exposure to infected soil or vegetative matter. *T. beigelii* can occasionally be found in the normal flora of the skin, as well as in nature as a soil and plant saprophyte.

DIAGNOSIS AND DIFFERENTIAL DIAGNOSIS

The diagnosis of both black and white piedra is based on the typical clinical presentation and is confirmed by direct microscopy.

The differential diagnosis includes pediculosis, trichorrhexis nodosa, psoriatic or eczematous scales, and trichomycosis axillaris (see Table 117-1). Trichomycosis axillaris, caused by *Corynebacterium tenuis*, can easily be confused with white piedra. However, it can be differen-

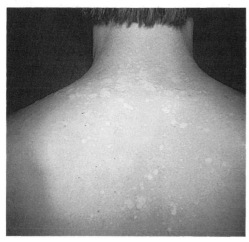

FIGURE 117-2. Pityriasis versicolor. Hyperpigmented and hypopigmented scaly patches on trunk and proximal extremities.

tiated by culture and by direct microscopy. The hair shaft concretion in trichomycosis axillaris is more amorphous than that of white piedra, and Gram stain reveals cocci and short bacilli.

TREATMENT

Cutting or shaving hairs is the definitive therapy for both black and white piedra. To prevent relapse, application of a topical imidazole preparation may be necessary. Recent data indicate that oral terbinafine is effective in black piedra.[8a]

Pityriasis Versicolor

DEFINITION

Pityriasis versicolor is a superficial fungal infection caused by the polymorphous endogenous yeast *Malasse-*

zia furfur. Infection typically occurs on the trunk and proximal upper extremities and is characterized by distinctive scaly, coalescent, hyperpigmented and/or hypopigmented to erythematous patches. Pityriasis versicolor was formerly referred to as tinea versicolor, but because the preface tinea is generally reserved for dermatophytosis the name was subsequently changed to reflect the correct etiology of this ubiquitous mycosis.

CLINICAL DESCRIPTION

Pityriasis versicolor generally presents as asymptomatic, slightly scaly, hypopigmented and/or hyperpigmented, erythematous, fawn or salmon-colored patches on the trunk and upper arms (Fig. 117-2). The most common areas of involvement are the upper back, shoulders, upper chest, and lateral upper arms (Fig. 117-3). Except in young children, the face is seldom involved. Lesions are initially discrete, scaly macules that coalesce into large patches. Most patients are asymptomatic and present because of cosmetic reasons. However, pruritus is occasionally encountered and is especially pronounced with sweating.

Pityriasis versicolor typically involves postpubertal, otherwise healthy persons and occurs worldwide. Both sexes are affected, and the male-to-female ratio is generally reported as equal or only slightly higher among males. There is no racial predilection. The highest incidence of infection occurs in tropical and subtropical climates. Most patients develop the disease during the summer months. If untreated, pityriasis versicolor tends to be chronic with periodic exacerbations or remissions often occurring with changes in climate.

PATHOLOGY

The diagnosis is generally based on cutaneous changes and can be confirmed by KOH preparation. Histopathologic studies are not needed if the condition is suspected clinically. The fungus is found in the stratum corneum where both short, stubby hyphae and yeast cells are often observed (Fig. 117-4). There are sometimes slight hy-

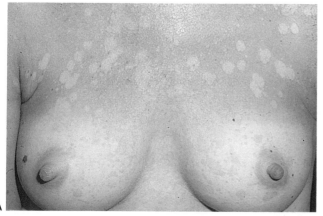

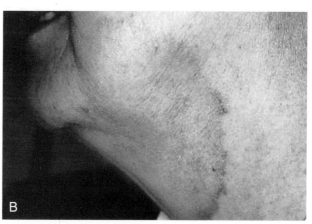

FIGURE 117-3. *A*, Anterior view of female chest with pityriasis versicolor. *B*, Pityriasis versicolor of the neck. (*A* and *B*, courtesy of June K. Robinson, M.D.)

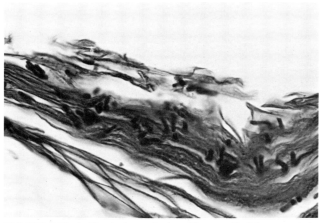

FIGURE 117-4. Pityriasis versicolor. The cornified layer contains large round spores and short, stubby hyphae.

perkeratoses and minimal epidermal hyperplasia with a sparse dermal lymphocytic infiltrate. One study from patients with hyperpigmented lesions showed an increase in melanosome size rather than numbers, which may explain the dark pigmentation change often observed.[9, 10] However, there have been patients with pityriasis versicolor who had vitiligo and therefore no melanosomes and who have hyperpigmented patches.[9, 10] The hypopigmentation may be explained by the presence of dicarbocyclic acids, which have a tyrosinase effect and are cytotoxic for melanocytes.[11, 12]

PATHOGENESIS AND ETIOLOGY

M. furfur is a polymorphous, lipophilic yeast and a member of the normal skin flora. It is a double-contoured yeast with spherical (globose) to oval or cylindrical cells that reproduce by unipolar budding.[2] Yeast cells can routinely be seen on scrapings from normal skin, but the filamentous form is uncommon on the normal skin surface. Under certain conditions, the fungus changes from the yeast form to the mycelial form and clinical disease ensues. Exogenous factors such as tropical ambient temperatures and increased humidity favor growth of this fungus and transformations to the mycelial state. Other factors that predispose to infection include hyperhidrosis, systemic corticosteroid therapy, Cushing's syndrome, immunodeficiency, malnutrition, and pregnancy.

M. furfur requires the addition of a lipid source to culture media for growth. Olive oil is often used for this purpose. The organism grows best at 32°C to 35°C.[2] *M. furfur* has not been isolated from lower animals or from nature as a saprophyte.

DIAGNOSIS AND DIFFERENTIAL DIAGNOSIS

The diagnosis of pityriasis versicolor is generally based on cutaneous changes and is confirmed by KOH preparation. Direct microscopy reveals short hyphae and yeast cells. Fungal cultures are seldom used for diagnosis. Histopathologic changes are characteristic and reveal the organism in the yeast and hyphal state.

The differential diagnosis includes pityriasis alba, vitiligo, seborrheic dermatitis, postinflammatory hyperpigmentation or hypopigmentation, and, occasionally, cutaneous candidiasis (see Table 117-1).

TREATMENT

Pityriasis versicolor is generally treated topically. In severe or extensive cases, and in patients who do not respond to topical medications, systemic therapy can be considered.

Topical medications effective against *M. furfur* are listed in Table 117-2. It is important to treat the entire trunk, upper extremities to the wrists, and lower extremities to the knees for the highest cure rate. Frequently, a prophylactic regimen is necessary to avoid recurrence of disease.

Oral medications effective against *M. furfur* include the azoles and triazoles. Interestingly, the allylamine terbinafine is effective when used topically and is ineffective if given orally. Studies are needed to confirm the dosage requirements with the newer triazoles fluconazole and itraconazole. An effective treatment schedule with itraconazole is 200 mg daily for 5 to 7 days.[13, 14] A single 400-mg dose of fluconazole has been shown to be effec-

TABLE 117-2. Treatment of Pityriasis Versicolor

Medication	Dosage and Duration
Topical Therapy	
2.5% selenium sulfide	Apply to skin for 10-15 minutes daily for 14 days.
50%-60% propylene glycol in water	Apply to skin for 10-15 minutes daily for 14 days.
Azoles:	
Clotrimazole Econazole Ketoconazole Miconazole Oxiconazole Sulconazole	Use twice daily for 2 weeks.
Allylamines:	
Naftifine Terbinafine	Use twice daily for 2 weeks.
Other Agents:	
Ciclopiroxolamine	Use twice daily for 2 weeks.
Zinc pyrithione	Available in over-the-counter shampoo for prophylactic use
Tolnaftate	Use twice daily until condition resolves
Systemic Therapy	
Imidazole:	
Ketoconazole	200 mg daily for 5-10 days (longer in severe infections); pulse dose of 400 mg initially, repeated in 7 days
Triazoles	
Fluconazole	Single 400-mg dose
Itraconazole	200 mg daily for 5-7 days

tive. Ketoconazole can also be dosed at 200 mg daily for 5 to 10 days.[14a]

Since *M. furfur* can change from saprophyte to pathogen depending on predisposing factors, a permanent cure is difficult to achieve. To avoid recurrence, prophylactic treatment regimens with oral or topical medications may be important.

"Pityrosporum" Folliculitis

DEFINITION

"Pityrosporum" folliculitis is folliculitis caused by the yeast *M. furfur*. Since the organism was formerly referred to as *Pityrosporum ovale (P. orbiculare)*, the designation *"Pityrosporum"* folliculitis rather than *"Malassezia"* folliculitis is based on tradition, rather than mycologic nomenclature.

CLINICAL DESCRIPTION

Although *Pityrosporum* folliculitis occurs in normal hosts, it may be more common in patients with seborrheic dermatitis. It also has been noted in pregnant patients, in patients receiving antibiotics, in immunocompromised patients such as recipients of bone marrow transplants, and in individuals with diabetes mellitus and Hodgkin's disease.[15, 16]

Pityrosporum folliculitis occurs in the same regions as does pityriasis versicolor. The upper back, chest, and lateral upper arms develop an acneiform eruption that may be associated with pruritus. Typically, the patient presents with a history of nonresponsiveness to systemic antibiotic therapy or with an incorrect diagnosis of acne vulgaris. *Pityrosporum* folliculitis can be differentiated from acne vulgaris by the lack of comedones.

PATHOLOGY

Since *M. furfur* is not routinely cultured in the laboratory, the diagnosis of *Pityrosporum* folliculitis is confirmed by histopathology. Yeast cells, rather than mycelial elements, are found in the hair follicle. Because *M. furfur* is part of the normal flora, the presence of a few yeast cells in a follicular infundibulum should be regarded as a normal finding. In *Pityrosporum* folliculitis there are large numbers of yeasts, and sometimes hyphae, in dilated follicular infundibula, often with attenuation of the follicular wall, which can be ruptured. Neutrophils, mononuclear cells, and foreign body giant cells surround extruded follicular contents, which sometimes include yeasts and hyphae of *Pityrosporum*. The organisms do not appear to invade the dermis except in immunosuppressed patients.

PATHOGENESIS AND ETIOLOGY

Predisposing factors for *M. furfur* infection have been addressed in the discussion of pityriasis versicolor. Although most authors favor the idea that the immune system modulates the number of yeasts in follicles, a study based on scanning electron microscopy suggested that occlusion of the pilar canal by keratin leads to overgrowth of yeasts and follicular rupture. The efficacy of ketoconazole in such cases could be due to its effect on follicular keratinization rather than to its antifungal activity.[17]

DIAGNOSIS AND DIFFERENTIAL DIAGNOSIS

The diagnosis is based on the clinical picture of a pruritic papular or pustular eruption on the trunk or proximal extremities and can be confirmed by histopathology. Since mycelial elements are not generally present, direct microscopy may be difficult to interpret. Culture is not routinely performed. The lack of comedones and the nonresponsiveness to systemic antibiotics should alert the clinician to the diagnosis of *Pityrosporum* folliculitis. The differential diagnosis includes bacterial or irritant folliculitis, acne vulgaris, neurotic excoriations, and papular urticaria (see Table 117–1).

TREATMENT

Treatment is similar to that used for pityriasis versicolor (see Table 117–2). Although many patients respond to topical therapy, those persons with extensive lesions and those who do not respond to topical agents may need a systemic antifungal agent. A 10-day course of 200 mg of ketoconazole is very effective, and generally improvement is dramatic.[18] Systemic fluconazole and itraconazole are also effective.

References

1. Elewski BE, Hazen PG. The superficial mycoses and the dermatophytes. J Am Acad Dermatol 1989;21:655–673.
2. Kwon-Chun KJ, Bennett JE. Medical Mycology. Philadelphia: Lea & Febiger, 1992.
3. Velsor HV, Singletary H. Tinea nigra palmaris. Arch Dermatol 1964;90:59–61.
4. Merwin CF. Tinea nigra palmaris: Review of the literature and case report. Pediatrics 1965;36:537–541.
5. Perret WJ, Henington VM, Kennedy B. Tinea nigra palmaris: Report of 14 cases. J La State Med Soc 1964;116:22–24.
6. Ackerman AB, Jacobson M, Vitale P. Clues to Diagnosis in Dermatopathology, vol I. Chicago: ASCP Press, 1991:1–4.
7. Pradinaud R. The treatment of two cases of tinea nigra by miconazole. Mycosen 1978;21:99–102.
8. Kalter DC. Genital white piedra: Epidemiology, microbiology, and therapy. J Am Acad Dermatol 1986;14:982–993.
8a. Gip L. Black piedra: The first case treated with terbinafine (Lamisil). Br J Dermatol 1994;130(Suppl. 43):26–28.
9. Dotz WI. Tinea versicolor: A light and electron microscopic study of hyperpigmented skin. J Am Acad Dermatol 1985;12:37–44.
10. Allen HB. Hyperpigmented tinea versicolor. Arch Dermatol 1974;112:1110–1112.
11. Nazzaro-Porro M, Passi S. Identification of tyrosinase inhibitors in cultures of *Pityrosporum*. J Invest Dermatol 1978;71:205–206.

12. Breathnach AS, Nazzaro-Porro M, Martin B. Ultrastructure of skin in pityriasis versicolor. Minerva Dermatol 1975;10:457–469.
13. Delescluse RCJ. Itraconazole in tinea versicolor: A review. J Am Acad Dermatol 1990;23:551–554.
14. Faergemann J. Treatment of pityriasis versicolor with itraconazole: A double-blind placebo-controlled study. Mycoses 1988;31: 377–379.
14a. Faergemann J. *Pityrosporum* infections. In: Elewski BE, ed. Cutaneous Fungal Infections. Tokyo: Igaku-Shoin, 1992:74.
15. Bufill JA, Lum LG, Caya JG. *Pityrosporum* folliculitis after bone marrow transplantation. Ann Intern Med 1988;108:560–563.

16. Helm KF, Lookingbill DP. *Pityrosporum* folliculitis and severe pruritus in two patients with Hodgkin's disease. Arch Dermatol 1993;129:380–381.
17. Hill MK, Goodfield MJD, Rodgers FG, et al. Skin surface electron microscopy in *Pityrosporum* folliculitis. Arch Dermatol 1990; 126:181–184.
18. Back O, Faergemann J, Hornquist R. *Pityrosporum* folliculitis: A common disease of the young and middle-aged. J Am Acad Dermatol 1985;12:56–61.

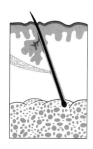

chapter 118

The Dermatophytoses

BONI E. ELEWSKI

DEFINITION

The dermatophytic fungi are a closely related group of molds that invade the stratum corneum of the epidermis and its keratinized appendages—the nail and hair.[1] Dermatophytes belong to three genera: *Epidermophyton*, *Microsporum*, and *Trichophyton*. Species in all genera are similar in physiology, morphology, and pathogenicity. Although there are over 40 known dermatophyte species, only about 10 are commonly encountered worldwide (Tables 118–1 and 118–2).[2]

Dermatophytoses are infections caused by dermatophytes. Infection can be transmitted from human to human (anthropophilic), animal to human (zoophilic), or soil to human (geophilic). The prevalence of organisms varies from country to country. However, the majority of infections worldwide are anthropophilic and caused by *T. rubrum* (see Tables 118–1 and 118–2).[2, 3]

CLINICAL DESCRIPTION

Dermatophytic infections are classified according to the anatomic site infected. The adjective tinea is generally added to the designated infected body site (in Latin). Although cutaneous changes resulting from fungal growth on the integument are protean and vary from exuberant inflammation to minimal inflammation, the prototypical lesion of dermatophytosis is an annular scaly patch.

Tinea Corporis

Tinea corporis is dermatophytosis of the trunk and extremities and can be caused by all species of dermatophytes. Infection can be spread human to human, animal to human, and soil to human.[1] The disease occurs worldwide and is generally more prevalent in tropical climates. *T. rubrum* is the most commonly encountered pathogen.

In general, tinea corporis caused by zoophilic dermatophytes such as *M. canis* is more inflammatory and more symptomatic than infections caused by anthropophilic dermatophytes. Additionally, animals with zoophilic dermatophytoses are a reservoir for human disease. Geophilic organisms rarely cause tinea corporis; the most common geophilic organism is *M. gypseum*.

The archetypical lesion of tinea corporis is an annular scaly patch, which may be single or multiple. The border of the lesion is generally most distinctive (Fig. 118–1). Follicular accentuation is common, and often follicular pustules occur. However, there is significant variation in presentation, which is often guided by the ecology of the infecting organism. For example, in infections in humans caused by zoophilic dermatophytes, pustules and even vesicles often occur. With anthropophilic fungi, slightly scaly, large patches with minimal erythema are typical. Geophilic human infections are generally more inflammatory than those caused by anthropophilic organisms (Fig. 118–2).

Risk factors for infection include exposure to infected animals, persons, and soil. Those at risk include athletes, veterinarians, animal handlers, and anyone who works outdoors. In addition, certain systemic diseases may predispose to infection, including Cushing's syndrome, diabetes mellitus, atopy, and most immunodeficiency conditions.

Tinea Capitis

Tinea capitis is dermatophytosis of the hair follicles of the scalp and is caused by dermatophytes in the genera *Microsporum* and *Trichophyton*. Most cases occur in children. The causative pathogens vary among countries. In the United States, *T. tonsurans*, an anthropophilic agent, predominates; however, in Europe the most common organism is *M. canis*. *T. violaceum* and *T. soudanense* are common in parts of Africa, whereas *M. ferrugineum* is prevalent in Southeast Asia (see Table

TABLE 118-1. Dermatophytes and Prevalence

Species	Prevalence and Region or Country
Microsporum Genus	
M. audouinii	Rare in North America
*M canis	Worldwide
*M. ferrugineum	Africa, Eastern Europe, Asia
*M. gypseum	Worldwide
*M. fulvum	Worldwide
M. nanum	Uncommon
M. gallinae	Uncommon
M. persicolor	Uncommon
M. cookei	Uncommon
M. vanbreuseghemii	Uncommon
M. racemosum	Worldwide, South America
M. praecoz	Uncommon
M. amazonicum	Uncommon
M. equinum	Uncommon
Trichophyton Genus	
*T. mentagrophytes var. mentagrophytes	Worldwide
*T. mentagrophytes var. interdigitale	Worldwide
*T. rubrum	Worldwide
*T. tonsurans	United States, Mexico, South America, Canada
*T. violaceum	South America, Central America, Asia, Africa
*T. verrucosum	Worldwide
T. schoenleinii	Eurasia, Africa, Eastern Europe
T. concentricum	Southern Asia, Pacific, Mexico
T. simii	Uncommon
T. equinum	Worldwide
T. megninii	Europe, Sardinia, Portugal
T. soudanense	Central, West Africa
T. gourvilii	West Africa
T. yaoundei	Equatorial Africa
T. ajelloi	Worldwide
T. terrestre	Uncommon
Epidermophyton Genus	
*E. floccosum	Worldwide, India, Southeast Asia

*Common dermatophytes.

TABLE 118-2. Ecology of Dermatophytes and Predominant Dermatophytic Infections

Organism	Predominant Infection
Anthropophilic Organisms	
Microsporum audouinii	Tinea capitis
M. ferrugineum	Tinea capitis
Epidermophyton floccosum	Tinea cruris, tinea pedis
Trichophyton concentricum	Tinea imbricata
T. mentagrophytes (var. interdigitale)	Tinea pedis
T. megninii	Tinea corporis
T. rubrum	Tinea pedis, tinea unguium, tinea cruris, tinea corporis
T. schoenleinii	Favus
T. soudanense	Tinea capitis
T. tonsurans	Tinea capitis
T. violaceum	Tinea capitis
T. yaoundei	Tinea capitis
Zoophilic Organisms	
M. canis	Tinea capitis
M. distortum	Tinea capitis
M. gallinae	Tinea corporis
T. verrucosum	Tinea corporis, tinea barbae
T. equinum	Tinea corporis
T. mentagrophytes (var. mentogrophytes)	Tinea barbae, tinea pedis
Geophilic Organisms	
M. cookei	Tinea corporis
M. gypseum	Tinea corporis
M. nanum	Tinea corporis
M. vanbreuseghemii	Tinea corporis
T. terrestre	Tinea corporis
T. ajelloi	Tinea corporis

118–2).[3] It is interesting that *T. rubrum* can be so prevalent worldwide and be the major causative agent in tinea corporis, tinea pedis, and tinea cruris but only sporadically causes tinea capitis.

There are three patterns of dermatophytic scalp infections: ectothrix, endothrix, and favus. Classification is

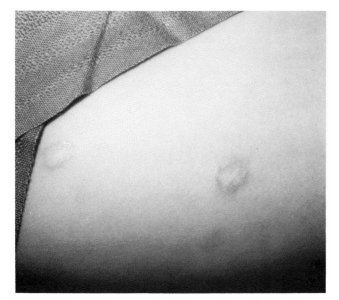

FIGURE 118-1. Tinea corporis. Anthropophilic infection. Annular patches are seen on upper extremity. *T. rubrum* was cultured.

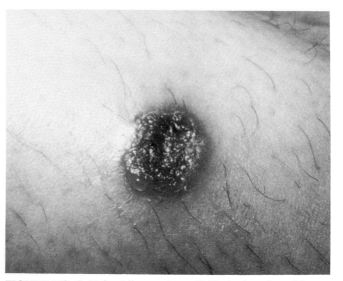

FIGURE 118-2. Majocchi's granuloma. Follicular invasion of dermatophytes may result in tinea folliculitis or Majocchi's granuloma. *T. rubrum* was cultured.

based on the pattern of arthroconidia (spore) location in relation to the hair shaft. In ectothrix invasion, arthroconidia form both inside and outside the hair shaft with the cuticle being destroyed. In endothrix invasion, arthroconidia formation occurs within the hair shaft and the cuticle remains intact. In favus, fragmented hyphae and air spaces occur within the hair shaft. The clinical presentation also varies among these patterns. In addition, the inflammatory reaction that occurs in some individuals with tinea capitis is determined by the immune response of the host (Fig. 118–3). In general, in endothrix invasion, hair breakage occurs at the scalp level, resulting in "black dots." Infection may be inflammatory or noninflammatory. Black children with endothrix *T. tonsurans* tinea capitis often present with prominent kerion, which is an exuberant inflammatory response to the dermatophyte and may resemble bacterial furunculosis (Fig. 118–4). In extensive infection, hair loss may be permanent. With ectothrix tinea capitis, hair generally breaks 1 to 2 mm above the scalp level and erythema and scale also occur. This is the presentation typically produced by the cat and dog dermatophyte *M. canis*. Kerion reaction may also occur.

Favus, caused by *T. schoenleinii*, occurs only sporadically, and there are occasional reports from Eastern Europe, North Africa, and the Middle East. Extensive crusts referred to as scutula, often intertwined with matted hair, are typical of infection. Scarring alopecia is a common sequela (Fig. 118–5), and both adults and children can be infected.

In addition to alopecia, crusting, scale, and kerion formation, cervical lymphadenopathy occurs in many patients with tinea capitis (see Fig. 118–4). Furthermore, a dermatophytid reaction may develop and often presents as lichenoid, pruritic papules progressing caudally from scalp to the trunk and extremities. Rarely, erythema nodosum may also occur and probably repre-

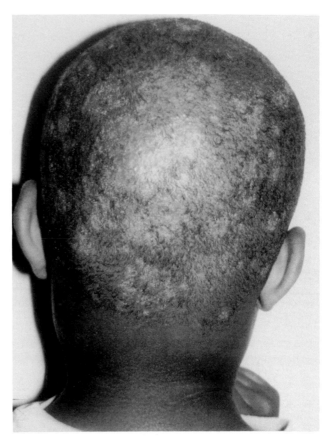

FIGURE 118–4. Tinea capitis. *T. tonsurans* infection. Note extensive patchy alopecia with scale. The patient also has prominent posterior cervical lymphadenopathy.

sents another dermatophytid reaction.[4] The immunologic basis for such reactions is unknown.

The diagnosis of tinea capitis can often be made by shining a filtered ultraviolet light (Wood's light) on the lesions. Certain species in the genus *Microsporum* fluoresce a yellow-green: *M. canis*, *M. distortum*, *M. audouinii*, *M. ferrugineum*, and, occasionally *M. gypseum*.[1, 3] This phenomenon is believed to be caused by a pteridine produced by the organism, occurs only in actively growing hair, and cannot be reproduced through artificial circumstances. Other than diagnostic implications, its significance is unknown. In the United States, the clinical usefulness of this procedure is less than in Europe, since *T. tonsurans*, the predominant pathogen in the United States, does not fluoresce. In addition, fluorescence needs to be cautiously interpreted, since crusts and scale occasionally yield false-positive results. Remember that fluorescent hair, rather than scale, is diagnostic.

Tinea Pedis and Tinea Manuum

Tinea pedis is a dermatophytic infection of the plantar surface and toe webs and is the most common dermatophyte infection. Tinea manuum is a similar process infecting the palm and interdigital spaces. Often, only one hand or foot is infected. Infection is rare before puberty.

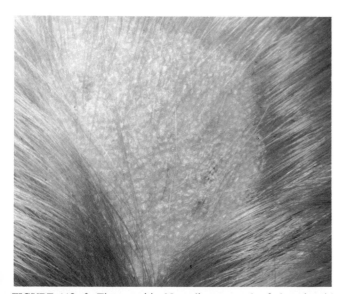

FIGURE 118–3. Tinea capitis. Note discrete patch of alopecia with scale, resembling alopecia areata. This pattern is often referred to as gray-patch tinea capitis. *T. tonsurans* was cultured, and no fluorescence can be seen.

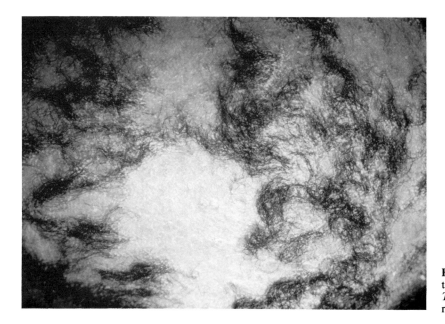

FIGURE 118–5. Tinea capitis. This patient has extensive alopecia and crusting resembling favus, but *T. tonsurans* was the pathogen. Scarring alopecia resulted.

Tinea pedis is generally caused by anthropophilic fungi. The most common organism is *T. rubrum*, followed by *T. mentagrophytes* and *E. floccosum*. Several nondermatophyte fungi may produce a syndrome clinically indistinguishable from tinea pedis that may lead to problems in therapy and diagnosis. These include *Scytalidium dimidiatum* (*Hendersonula toruloidea*), which has a pyknidial form known as *Nattrassia magnifera*, and *Scytalidium hyalinum*.[5]

There are three common presentations of tinea pedis: moccasin, interdigital, and inflammatory. In the interdigital variety, scale, crusting, and maceration develop in the interdigital spaces and predominantly in the fourth and fifth spaces (Fig. 118–6). Bacteria and the yeast *Candida* may be secondary invaders and produce moist, erosive, and often odiferous infections.[6, 7] The term *dermatophytosis complex* has been coined to describe this syndrome.[8] In moccasin tinea pedis, one or both plantar surfaces develop erythema, scale, and crusting. Chronic

infection is common. Inflammatory tinea pedis is generally caused by zoophilic strains of *T. mentagrophytes*. Vesicles and bullous lesions generally develop on the medial aspect of the plantar surface. Occasionally, a dermatophytid reaction resembling dyshidrotic eczema may be concurrent on one or both hands.

Nattrassia, a plant pathogen found in the western United States, Caribbean, and many other tropical and subtropical areas worldwide, causes infection that clinically mimics *T. rubrum* tinea pedis. When human infection occurs, this organism is generally referred to as *Scytalidium dimidiatum*. The albino variant, *S. hyalinum*, causes indistinguishable infections in humans but no plant diseases. A presentation resembling interdigital and moccasin tinea pedis, as well as tinea manuum, may occur. It is important to correctly diagnose infection since these nondermatophytes do not respond to currently available antifungal therapy.[5]

Tinea manuum generally occurs in association with

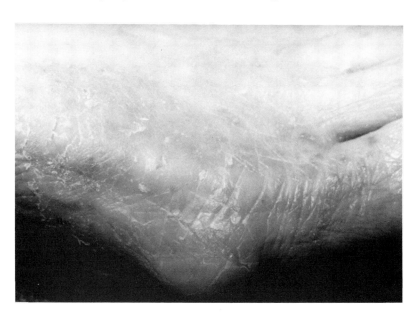

FIGURE 118–6. Tinea pedis. *T. rubrum* was cultured in this chronic infection that involved the entire plantar surface and extended on to the dorsum of the foot.

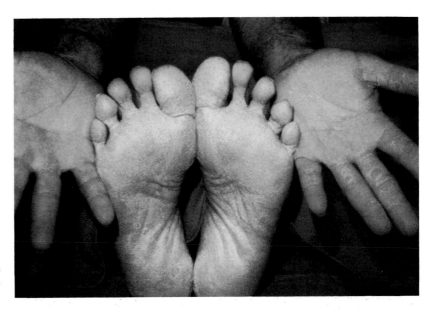

FIGURE 118-7. Both plantar and palmar involvement occur in this chronic and recalcitrant infection caused by *T. rubrum.*

tinea pedis (Fig. 118-7). Often one hand and both feet are involved. The presence of mycotic nail infection may help differentiate tinea manuum from keratoderma, eczema, and psoriasis.[9]

Tinea Unguium (Onychomycosis)

Tinea unguium (onychomycosis) is mycotic infection of the nail unit. When caused by dermatophytic fungi, tinea unguium is the correct name; the term *onychomycosis* is nonspecific and refers to nondermatophytes and dermatophytes causing infection of the nail unit. Tinea unguium is generally caused by members in the genera *Trichophyton* and *Epidermophyton* and is most common in adults. *T. rubrum* causes the majority of infection. Toenails are more commonly infected than fingernails. In a large study by Summerbell and associates, 2662 nail infecting fungi were identified among 10,000 fungal cultures. Of these, more than 90% were dermatophytes and 5.5% were *Candida albicans.* The nondermatophyte mold *Scopulariopsis brevicaulis* accounted for 1.6%, and a variety of other molds constituted the remaining, including *Scytalidium dimidiatum* and *S. hyalinum.*[10] With the exception of chronic mucocutaneous candidiasis, *C. albicans* invades the nail unit as a result of a paronychial infection and is generally more common on the fingernails of women. When the infection is cultured, other species of *Candida* must be interpreted cautiously since they are generally contaminants.

Onychomycosis causes about 50% of dystrophic nails, accounts for 30% of all mycotic skin infections, and occurs in about 3% of the population.[11] Predisposing factors include tinea pedis, communal bathing, hyperhidrosis, trauma, diabetes, advancing age, poor peripheral circulation, and immunodeficiency. Most disease occurs in men, and toenails are affected four times as often as fingernails.

Dermatophytes generally invade the nail plate from the nail bed. The distal and lateral margins of the nail bed develop hyperkeratosis, which eventuates in onycho-lysis, thickening, and discoloration of the nail plate. This pattern is referred to as distal subungual onychomycosis (Fig. 118-8). The nondermatophyte mold, *Scopulariopsis brevicaulis,* can produce a dystrophic nail resembling distal subungual onychomycosis. Features that point to this nondermatophyte include location on first toenail, a yellow to brown nail plate, a crumbly nail plate, and absence of tinea pedis. However, concurrent infection of a dermatophyte may occur. Fungal culture can determine the cause of the infection and guide therapy.

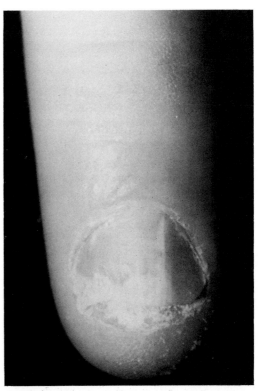

FIGURE 118-8. Distal subungual pattern of tinea unguium (onychomycosis).

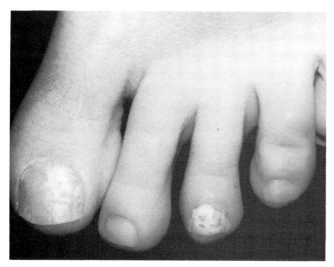

FIGURE 118–9. White superficial onychomycosis. The fungus directly invades into the nail plate, rather than through the nail bed. This pattern is generally caused by nondermatophytes and is usually limited to toenail involvement.

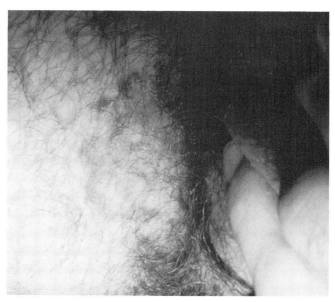

FIGURE 118–10. Tinea cruris. Annular scaly patch in proximal medial thigh. *E. floccosum* was cultured.

Proximal white subungual onychomycosis, while rare, is most common in persons infected with human immunodeficiency virus and is generally caused by *T. rubrum*.[12] Infection begins in the proximal nail fold, and the organism invades under the cuticle and first infects the proximal nail bed. A white color develops in the proximal nail plate, which may extend distally. A smooth, normal nail plate surface differentiates proximal white subungual onychomycosis from white superficial onychomycosis.

White superficial onychomycosis (leukonychia trichophytica) (Fig. 118–9) is caused by the dermatophyte *T. mentagrophytes*, as well as by several nondermatophytes, including *Aspergillus terreus*, *Fusarium oxysporum*, *Acremonium roseogriseum*, and, occasionally, *C. albicans*. These fungi have the ability to produce bore holes in the nail plate. As a result of infection, the nail plate becomes white, rough, and crumbly, resembling plaster. Toenails are more commonly infected than fingernails.[3]

Tinea Cruris

Tinea cruris refers to dermatophytosis of the groin, including the suprapubic area, perineum, proximal medial thighs, gluteal cleft, and buttocks. Infection is caused predominantly by *T. rubrum* and *E. floccosum* and typically occurs in men.[9] Male predominance may be explained by the propensity of moisture to accumulate in the crural folds. Erythema and scale develops in the proximal medial thighs and generally occurs bilaterally (Figs. 118–10 and 118–11). Pruritus is common. A

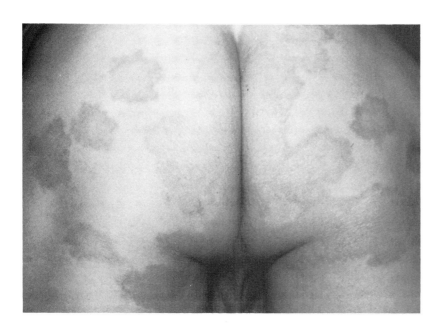

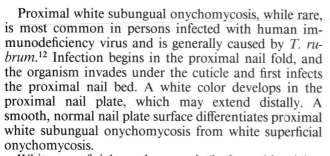

FIGURE 118–11. Tinea cruris. This patient has involvement of *T. rubrum* infection on proximal medial thighs, crural folds, perianal area, and buttocks. The scrotum was spared.

raised, often noninflammatory, erythematous advancing edge occurs and may be most prominent on the left thigh. Interestingly, the scrotal skin appears immune to infection. Women rarely develop tinea cruris. However, cutaneous candidiasis in women may resemble tinea cruris. In addition, *Candida* infection in the groin region of males often presents as scrotal dermatosis, which is a differentiating point from tinea cruris. There is no explanation for scrotal sparing in dermatophytic infections.

Tinea Barbae

Tinea barbae occurs in the beard area and neck and is caused predominantly by zoophilic fungi, including *T. verrucosum*, and *T. mentagrophytes*. Occasionally, *T. rubrum* can cause this infection. Men are generally infected, and infection may resemble bacterial folliculitis.

Tinea Facei

Tinea facei refers to dermatophytosis of the face other than the beard area. Annular lesions typical of tinea corporis may occur but may be difficult to appreciate. Children exposed to animals are at risk (Figs. 118–12 and 118–13). Additionally, *T. tonsurans* is a common culprit in infants.[13] Occasionally, tinea facei may flare with sunlight and thereby be confused with polymorphous light eruption or lupus erythematosus.

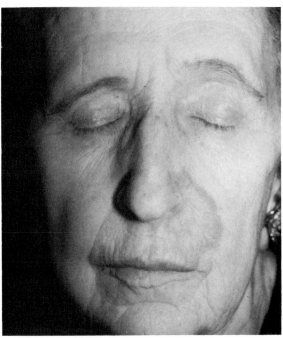

FIGURE 118–13. Tinea facei. Annular patch on face is seen in seborrheic area. *T. tonsurans* was cultured.

Tinea Imbricata

Tinea imbricata is caused by *T. concentricum* and occurs in certain geographic regions, including the South Pacific, Southeast Asia, and parts of South America. It is characterized by concentric annular rings, which are generally quite extensive. Susceptibility to infection may be inherited as an autosomal recessive trait.[3]

PATHOLOGY

Dermatophytosis is as variable in its histopathologic guises as in its clinical appearances. The most common findings on biopsy are those of a spongiotic dermatitis in which there are mounds of parakeratosis containing neutrophils ("neuts in the horn"). Hyphae are visible in hematoxylin and eosin–stained sections either as long, septated basophilic structures or as refractile spaces in the cornified layer. Although dermatophytosis commonly results in parakeratosis, the organisms eschew that material, perhaps because it is rapidly shed into the environment, favoring instead areas of compact orthokeratosis. Hyphae tend to be particularly numerous at the interface between different types of cornified material, a finding called the "sandwich sign" (Fig. 118–14).[14] The presence of dermatophytes can easily be confirmed by staining with periodic acid–Schiff (PAS) after diastase digestion.

Less common histopathologic findings in dermatophytosis of the skin surface include superficial and deep lymphocytic infiltrates accompanied by parakeratosis but without other epidermal changes, a psoriasiform dermatitis that can closely mimic psoriasis, spongiform or

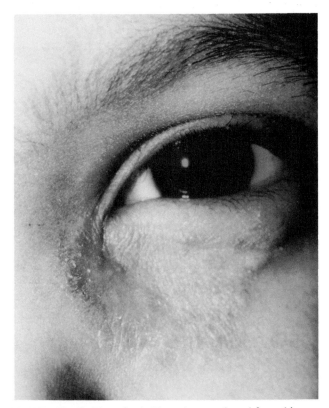

FIGURE 118–12. Tinea facei. *M. canis* was cultured from this young child.

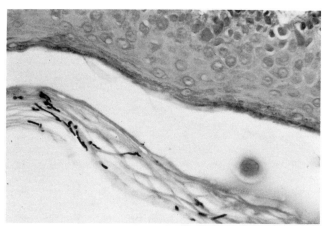

FIGURE 118-14. Dermatophytic hyphae are typically sandwiched between different types of cornified material, in this case compact and basketweave (PAS with diastase). (Courtesy of M. Tarif Zaim, M.D., Associate Professor of Dermatology and Pathology, Case Western Reserve University, Cleveland, Ohio.)

intraepidermal pustular dermatitis, bullous tinea resulting from marked papillary dermal edema, and intraepidermal vesiculation due to marked spongiosis.

Dermatophytic folliculitis results from fungi surrounding (ectothrix) or invading (endothrix) hair shafts or both (ectoendothrix). Although hyphae and spores are generally obvious, obtaining random sections during biopsy sampling for dermatophytic folliculitis can easily miss the infected hair follicle and level sections can be helpful. The infiltrates seen in dermatophytic folliculitis include neutrophils and lymphocytes; if follicular rupture occurs, granulomatous infiltrates can also be present. On occasion, eosinophils predominate, inviting misdiagnosis as eosinophilic pustular folliculitis.

Dermatophytosis of the nails is seldom diagnosed histopathologically. Since hyphae reside in the keratotic material beneath the nail plate, clippings of this debris can be submitted for rapid histopathologic confirmation of infection. This technique is sometimes diagnostic even when cultures are negative.[15] Dermatophytosis of the nail resembles psoriasis pathologically in that there are mounds of parakeratosis with neutrophils.[16] If these are present, a PAS stain with diastase should be obtained even if fungi are not discernible.

PATHOGENESIS AND ETIOLOGY

The dermatophytes are the largest group of fungi causing human cutaneous disease and have the unique ability among fungi to infect predominantly immunocompetent hosts. These organisms are skin pathogens of minimal virulence and generally invade the dead, cornified, keratinized layers of the integument. Although extracorporeal existence is the rule, dermatophytes produce considerable morbidity. Important in dermatophyte pathogenesis is their ability to become dormant and survive in the environment for years before transmission. The dormant form is referred to as arthroconidia (spores). Some dermatophytic fungi produce abundant infective arthro-

conidia and continually shower the environment with infected skin scales. Animal studies have shown that the arthroconidia are more virulent than other propagules. Fomites, including carpeting, furniture, shower stalls, and linen, can harbor infected squames.[2] This occurs with both *T. rubrum* and *T. tonsurans* infections.[17] Other dermatophytes, such as *E. floccosum*, may produce fewer arthroconidia, but these may remain viable in the environment for years. In certain chronic infections, such as moccasin tinea pedis, a host–parasite existence develops that promotes increased dissemination. Zoophilic strains harbor infective fungal elements in an animal host. This ability to produce infective, dormant arthroconidia is critical to their pathogenesis and ubiquity.

When infecting arthroconidia are exposed to skin, a variety of clinical presentations may ensue. Cutaneous changes resulting from growth of the fungal colony on the integument occur in three steps: (1) adherence to skin, (2) invasion into skin, and (3) disease produced by host factors.

Adherence of fungal elements to integumentary surface begins the cascade of events resulting in clinical cutaneous disease. Theoretically, the more capable the organism is of adhering to the stratum corneum, the more likely infection will ensue.[18] However, adherence of dermatophyte fungi to the stratum corneum has not been well studied. Host factors, such as atopy, probably mediate this process.

Invasion of fungal organism into the keratinized tissue is the next requirement for clinical dermatophytosis. Again, this area has not been well studied, although it may be mediated by enzymes such as dermatophyte keratinases. Unique among fungi, dermatophytes have the ability to produce keratinases and digest keratin in vitro, and this ability may be a virulence factor. Although the significance of keratinase production is unclear, the production of keratinases may allow the fungus to sustain itself in the keratinized tissue, provide an innate affinity for keratinized tissue, and promote invasion into keratin.[19, 20] Different keratinases are probably produced by different dermatophytes, which may directly affect the host inflammatory response. *Trichophyton mentagrophytes* has at least two keratinase isoenzymes.[21] In addition to digesting keratin, dermatophyte hyphae may be able to squeeze between epidermal keratinocytes, which differentiates them from other common cutaneous fungal pathogens, including *Candida* and *Malassezia*.

Host factors directly affect the clinical picture. These include protease inhibitors such as pepstatin, hormones such as progesterone, which inhibits fungal growth in vitro, skin surface factors such as pH, and carbon dioxide tension.[22] In addition, the presence or absence of immunodeficiency conditions may affect the extent of infection.

After the dermatophyte has made a home within a keratinized structure, a variety of host factors modulate the extreme variability in clinical disease. This may account for the protean manifestations that occur in different persons. Host factors responsible for divergent dermatophytic presentations include the location of infection (hair, nail, glabrous skin), the presence of sebum, concurrent cutaneous disease, systemic disease (immunodeficiency), and serum factors such as transferrin, which inhibits dermatophyte growth in vitro. In addition, if the epidermal surface is not intact, such as would occur if macerated from occlusion, dermatophyte invasion is more likely. This would account for the increased occurrence of tinea pedis in persons who wear shoes.

As discussed earlier, once invasion of dermatophyte hyphae into keratin is complete, a variety of host factors clearly mediate the spectrum of clinical disease. However, mannans elaborated by dermatophyte fungi may inhibit this step.[23] Mannans are a polymer of mannose sugar residues that when combined with protein result in a mannoprotein. Mannoproteins comprise about 20% of the fungal cell wall and structurally vary among dermatophyte species. In vitro, they are immunoinhibitory and may account for varying degrees of inflammation noted with different dermatophytes. Mannans may function to prevent elimination of dermatophytes from the host, thereby promoting chronicity. *T. mentogrophytes* also produces penicillin, which can influence the bacterial flora. This may give the fungus an advantage under some circumstances.

Dermatophytes are regarded as solely integumentary fungi. This unique extracorporeal existence cannot be well explained. Implicated in this regard is the temperature sensitivity that is shared by most dermatophytic fungi—normal body temperature inhibits their growth. It is not surprising that elevated body temperatures have been shown to kill dermatophytes in experimental situations.[24] Conversely, the dimorphic organisms have adapted to 37°C by changing in tissue from a hyphal to an alternate state (generally yeast).[2] Additionally, fresh serum may provide for dermatophytic growth inhibitory factors, such as unsaturated transferrin, which probably causes a toxic interaction with the dermatophyte or depletes essential true metal nutrients required for its growth and thereby restricts dermatophyte invasion beyond the keratinized tissue.

The integrity of the host immune system is pivotal in restricting dermatophyte growth to keratinized surfaces. With impaired cell-mediated immune function, atypical and locally aggressive presentations may occur,[25-27] and presentations include extensive cutaneous disease, subcutaneous abscesses, and even dissemination. *T. rubrum* has been implicated in most patients with defective cell-mediated immunity; however, *T. schoenleinii, E. floccosum,* and *T. violaceum* are also reported. Antigen-specific immunoreactivity may be demonstrated by delayed hypersensitivity reaction to *Trichophyton* skin test antigen. There is no evidence that specific humoral antibodies or lymphokines retard fungal growth. Although antibodies can damage dermatophytes in vitro, the clinical relevance is unclear. Additionally, locally aggressive dermatophytic infections may occur with neutropenia or in syndromes with impaired neutrophil function, suggesting that polymorphonuclear leukocytes also restrict dermatophyte growth to the stratum corneum.

In addition to immune dysfunction, a variety of systemic and cutaneous diseases may affect the extent of skin involvement. Patients with certain endocrinopathies, including Cushing's syndrome and diabetes mellitus, may have increased susceptibility to dermatophytic infection. Atopy appears to increase the prevalence of chronic dermatophytosis, particularly *T. rubrum* infection. Cutaneous disorders that involve increased epidermal cell turnover may also result in chronic dermatophytosis.

The etiologies of the various syndromes that comprise dermatophytosis are listed in Table 118-2.

DIAGNOSIS AND DIFFERENTIAL DIAGNOSIS

The diagnosis of dermatophytic infection can be confirmed by direct microscopic examination of skin scales and by fungal culture. Histopathology is required only in unusual cases. Direct microscopy is usually performed with a keratin clearing agent, such as potassium hydroxide. Septate, nondistinct hyphae that are 2 to 3 μm in diameter are visualized microscopically. Precise identification of a genus and species requires considerable expertise and can be accomplished by a fungal culture. Identification of the causative pathogen is important to determine the pattern of spread (anthropophilic, zoophilic, and geophilic).

The fungal colony morphology and its microscopic appearance will allow differentiation among dermatophytic species. The color of the colony obverse and reverse, presence or absence of diffusible pigments, texture, topography, and growth rate are important features to observe. Most dermatophytes grow quickly and can be identified within 2 weeks. An exception is *T. verrucosum,* which is slow growing and grows best at 37°C.[1]

Microscopic features of the colony generally begin with observation of conidia. Microconidia and macroconidia are asexual propagules that are formed by these fungi. The conidia may be unicellular or multicellular. These structures are observed only on microscopic examination of colony; they do not occur on tissue specimens. Features of conidia are relatively consistent within a particular genus. The genus *Epidermophyton* produces only large, club-shaped, septate conidia; *Microsporum* and *Trichophyton* feature both macroconidia and microconidia. Subtle features of these conidia may permit assignment of a genus and species.[1-3] In the genus *Trichophyton,* salient features of microconidia are diagnostic, including their arrangement and shape. In the genus *Microsporum,* distinctive echinulate macroconidia are noted and can be used for separation of species. Other microscopic features to observe for identification purposes include arthroconidia, chlamydoconidia, and specialized patterns of hyphae (pectinate, spiral, favic chandeliers).[1-3]

The nutrient requirements of the genus *Trichophyton* are important in their laboratory identification. *Trichophyton* test agars selectively isolate species of *Trichophyton* with particular vitamin requirements.[3] In vitro hair perforation is also useful in separating *T. mentagrophytes,* which perforates hair in vitro, from *T. rubrum.* Urea hydrolysis is another laboratory parameter that can differentiate these two common dermatophytes. *T. mentagrophytes* is urease positive, whereas *T. rubrum* is urease negative.

The clinician needs to be concerned about appropriate media selection and method of specimen collection. Dermatophytes are relatively unique in their ability to grow on media containing cycloheximide. This feature can differentiate dermatophytic fungi from many saprophytes. Media containing cycloheximide include Mycosel, Mycobiotic, and dermatophyte test medium (DTM). Appropriate media selection is especially critical in determining the etiology of nail infections, which can be caused by several nondermatophytes. In this circumstance, media with and without cycloheximide should be selected. Tinea pedis can also be caused by nondermatophytes and thereby requires the addition of media without cycloheximide. For determining the correct etiology of tinea capitis, tinea corporis, and tinea cruris, media with cycloheximide are generally sufficient. Caution must be exercised if *Candida* could be a potential pathogen, since not all species of this yeast reliably grow on cycloheximide-supplemented media.[3]

DTM is often used as a screen for dermatophytic infections. The phenol red indicator changes from yellow to red in the presence of the alkaline byproducts produced by dermatophyte fungi. Since false-positive reactions occur, the color change indicates only the possible presence of dermatophytes. Furthermore, the bright red color restricts visual colony identification. DTM contains cycloheximide and therefore has limited usefulness.[1]

To confirm the diagnosis, it is important to correctly select the appropriate site for specimen collection used for both direct microscopy and fungal culture. The materials obtained can be divided between direct microscopy and culture. In patients who present with a lesion with an advancing edge, as generally occurs in tinea corporis and cruris, this edge or border of the lesion is useful for sampling. In vesicular lesions, the roof of the vesicle generally has the highest fungal particles. Nail specimens can be especially challenging to correctly identify and isolate the causative pathogen. Since most mycotic nail infections occur in the nail bed, debris in the nail bed as proximal to the cuticle as possible generally has the highest number of viable fungi. The yield from culturing the nail plate is poor. Although fungi can often be observed in the nail plate, it is impossible to identify them or determine if they are viable without a fungal culture. Therefore, histopathology of the nail plate itself has limited usefulness. In scalp infection, several hairs from the infected sites should be epilated for culture. In certain *Microsporum* infections, the use of Wood's light might guide the selection of infected hairs.

Because dermatophyte fungi produce several clinical syndromes, the differential diagnosis of each entity is addressed in Table 118–3.

TREATMENT

From the historical perspective, antifungal agents can be divided into two groups, based on the method of derivation. One group includes those antifungal agents originally derived from microbes, and the second are those synthetically produced (Table 118–4). For almost

TABLE 118-3. Differential Diagnosis of Dermatophytoses

Disorder	Differential Diagnosis
Tinea corporis	Psoriasis, pityriasis rosacea, annular erythemas, granuloma annulare, eczema, and folliculitis; when disease is extensive, subacute cutaneous lupus erythematosus may be considered.
Tinea capitis	Noninflammatory disease: seborrheic dermatitis, psoriasis, alopecia areata, and trichotillomania. Inflammatory disease: bacterial furunculosis. A dermatophytid reaction may be a useful differentiating point.
Tinea pedis	Interdigital: erythrasma, bacterial infection, and candidiasis. Moccasin: other papulosquamous disorders, including psoriasis, pityriasis rubra pilaris, keratoderma, and eczematous dermatosis; onychomycosis may indicate a fungal infection. Inflammatory: dyshidrosis.
Tinea manuum	When bilateral, rule out keratodermas, psoriasis, and eczema.
Tinea unguium	Psoriasis, lichen planus, and nondermatophyte mycotic nails can be differentiated by fungal culture.
Tinea cruris	Candidiasis, neurodermatitis, erythrasma, eczema, and psoriasis; scrotal involvement generally indicates a nondermatophyte etiology.
Tinea barbae	Bacterial folliculitis, actinomycosis, eczema herpeticum, and inflammatory acne vulgaris; direct microscopy and fungal culture are diagnostic.
Tinea facei	Acne rosacea, folliculitis, lupus, and polymorphous light eruption
Tinea imbricata	Diagnosis is obvious in endemic countries; *T. concentricum* may be differentiated from other mycotic skin infections by fungal culture.

40 years, griseofulvin, available orally only, has been the mainstay of systemic dermatophytosis therapy. In addition, topical therapy has been monopolized by tolnaftate and the topical imidazoles.[28] More recently, new drugs have emerged that improve both cure and relapse rate.[29-33]

Mode of Action

Antifungal drugs target differences between mammalian and fungal cells.[34] The mode of action varies. The unique presence of the membrane sterol ergosterol, which is required for fungal cell membrane integrity, is a target site of many antimycotic agents (Table 118–5).

The allylamine terbinafine and the azole family, including ketoconazole and fluconazole, deplete the membrane sterol ergosterol. The azole family inhibits cytochrome P450–dependent lanosterol-N-demethylase, which converts lanosterol to 14-demethyl lanosterol. The allylamines inhibit ergosterol at an earlier stage with the

TABLE 118-4. Antifungal Agents for Cutaneous Mycoses

Agent	Availability	
	Oral	Topical
Antifungal Agents Derived from Microbes		
Griseofulvin (derived from *Penicillium griseofulvum*)	+	−
Polyenes (derived from *Streptomyces* sp.)		
Amphotericin B	−	+
Nystatin	+*	+
Natamycin	−	+
Antifungal Agents Synthetically Produced		
Imidazoles		
Ketoconazole	+	+
Clotrimazole	−	+
Oxiconazole	−	+
Sulconazole	−	+
Miconazole	−	+
Econazole	−	+
Triazoles		
Fluconazole	+	−
Itraconazole	+	−
Terconazole	−	+
Allylamines		
Terbinafine	+	+
Naftifine	−	+
Miscellaneous		
Ciclopirox olamine	−	+
Tolnaftate	−	+
Amorolfine	−	+
Selenium sulfide	−	+

*Denotes oral availability but not absorption.

enzyme squalene epoxidase, and this step does not involve cytochrome P450. The net result is depletion of ergosterol. Since mammalian cytochrome P450 enzymes are involved in the synthesis of important steroids, such as cortisol and testosterone, drugs with affinity with cytochrome P450 may be associated with toxicity. This toxicity is best illustrated by the reversible adverse effects observed in some patients on ketoconazole, including gynecomastia, impotence, and hypoadrenalism. The other members of the azole family are guilty by association and may cause similar reactions. However, no similar toxicity has yet been documented by the triazoles, which have less affinity for cytochrome P450 enzymes than does ketoconazole.[34]

Additionally, squalene accumulates with allylamine usage, and this is the presumed mechanism of the fungi-

TABLE 118-5. Mode and Site of Action of Antifungal Agents

Cell Membrane Level	Nuclear Level
Depletes ergosterol	Blocks microtubules
Azole family	Griseofulvin
Allylamines	Blocks DNA/RNA synthesis
Binds to cell membrane	Flucytosine
Polyenes	
Squalene accumulation	
Allylamines	

cidal action. The polyene antifungals are thought to bind and disrupt cell membrane integrity, leaving "holes" in the fungal membrane. Amphotericin B is thereby fungicidal.[34]

Antifungal Therapy for Cutaneous Mycoses: Special Considerations

Dermatophytes infect the stratum corneum and its keratinized appendages. In choosing an antifungal agent, the serum concentration is therefore of little relevance to treatment outcome and the primary determinant of therapeutic success is the level in the stratum corneum. Methods of antimycotic delivery to the stratum corneum include (1) passive diffusion; (2) eccrine sweat; (3) sebum; and (4) deposition in new cells of epidermis.[34] Drugs topically delivered can reach the stratum corneum in adequate concentration and, providing they persist for sufficient time to inhibit the target pathogen, are generally satisfactory (Table 118–6). Oral agents useful for

TABLE 118-6. Topical Treatment of Dermatophytes

Generic	Trade	Effectiveness
Imidazoles		
Bifonazole		+
Clotrimazole	Lotrimin, Mycelex	+
Econazole	Spectazole	+
Ketoconazole	Nizoral	+
Miconazole	Micatin, Monistat	+
Oxiconazole	Oxistat	+
Sulconazole	Exelderm	+
Tioconazole	Vagistat	+
Triazoles		
Terconazole	Terazol	+
Allylamines		
Naftifine	Naftin	+
Terbinafine	Lamisil	+
Miscellaneous		
Tolnaftate	Tinactin	+
	Footwork	+
	Aftate	
Compound undecylenic acid	Cruex, Desenex Pedi-Dri/Pedi-Pro	±
Benzoic acid, salicylic acid	Whitfield's ointment	±
Selenium sulfide	1% Selsun Blue 2.5% Selsun	
50%–60% propylene glycol		−
Zinc pyrithione	Head & Shoulders PHS Zincon	−
Sodium thiosulfate	Tinver	−
2% sulfur/2% salicylic	Antinea	−
Clinoquinol	Danex	−
	Vioform	±
Iodoquinol	Vytone	±
Polyene Antibiotics		
Amphotericin B	Fungizone	−
Nystatin	Mycolog, Mycostatin	−

+, Effective; ±, borderline effective; −, not effective.
Adapted from Elewski BE, Nagashima-Whalen L. Superficial fungal infections of the skin. In: Hoeprich PD, Jordan ME, Donald AR, eds. Infectious Disease, 5th edition. Philadelphia: JB Lippincott, 1994: 1029–1049.

TABLE 118-7. Systemic Treatment of Dermatophytes

Generic	Trade Name	Effectiveness
Griseofulvin	Grispeg Grifulvin V Fulvicin	+
Polyene Antibiotics		
Amphotericin B	Fungizone	–
Azoles		
Fluconazole	Diflucan	+
Itraconazole	Sporanox	+
Ketoconazole	Nizoral	+
Allylamines		
Terbinafine	Lamisil	+

+, Effective; –, ineffective; ±, borderline effective.
Adapted from Elewski BE, Nagashima-Whalen L. Superficial fungal infections of the skin In: Hoeprich PD, Jordan ME, Donald AR, eds. Infectious Disease, 5th edition. Philadelphia: JB Lippincott, 1994: 1029–1049.

dermatophytic infection include griseofulvin, the azole family (ketoconazole, itraconazole, and fluconazole), and the allylamine terbinafine (Table 118–7).

Management of Specific Dermatophytic Infection

Topical versus Systemic Therapy

Topical therapy is generally effective for uncomplicated tinea corporis, tinea cruris, and tinea pedis. It is ineffective as sole therapy in tinea capitis and tinea unguium. Additionally, in extensive dermatophytosis, in tinea folliculitis, and in immunocompromised patients, systemic therapy is indicated. The minimum duration of topical therapy has never been precisely established. Most patients with uncomplicated tinea corporis and tinea cruris experience clearance of their lesions within 2 weeks. However, therapy should be continued until the patient is clinically and mycologically clear of infection. An exception is topical terbinafine, which is effective after 1 week of usage probably because of its fungicidal action. Moccasin tinea pedis is generally recalcitrant to therapy and requires up to 8 weeks of topical agents to produce clearing, with a high relapse rate. In this circumstance, systemic therapy should be considered.

Oral Therapy

Griseofulvin. Available in the United States since 1958, griseofulvin has been extensively used to treat dermatophytosis of the skin, hair, and nails. The ultramicrosize and microsize forms are absorbed best, and a fatty meal may enhance absorption. A dosage of 10 to 15 mg/kg until the patient is clinically and mycologically cured is required. Griseofulvin is still one of the best oral agents for *M. canis* infection, an organism that is generally resistant to the azole family. It is therefore the most used therapy for tinea capitis worldwide. Treatment is disappointing for *T. rubrum* infection. Cure rate for tinea unguium is about 25% after 1 year of therapy for toenail

disease and slightly better for fingernail disease. Additionally, there are emerging resistant strains of *T. tonsurans*. The allylamine terbinafine and the triazole itraconazole are significantly more effective than griseofulvin in vitro against *T. rubrum* and *T. tonsurans* and may usurp the usage of griseofulvin in the near future.

Ketoconazole. Ketoconazole is the first oral broad-spectrum antifungal. It is effective for dermatophytic infections and, like griseofulvin, must be administered until the patient is clinically and mycologically normal. In patients allergic, intolerant, or nonresponsive to griseofulvin, ketoconazole may be an excellent alternative. Dosages of 200 mg daily are generally required. Use of this agent is limited by hepatotoxicity, which occurs in 1 in 10,000 patients.

Fluconazole. This triazole is indicated for candidiasis and cryptococcosis. Studies are underway to evaluate the effectiveness of this agent for dermatophytic nail disease. Dosages of 50 to 100 mg daily may be required, although pulse dosages of 150 mg per week to 450 mg per week (administered as a single dose) appear useful in tinea unguium of both fingernails and toenails. This drug has an excellent safety profile, is well tolerated, and may prove to be an excellent alternative to griseofulvin.

Itraconazole. This triazole is specifically indicated in therapy for blastomycosis and histoplasmosis. Preliminary data suggest this agent is an excellent alternative to griseofulvin in most dermatophytic infections. In patients with recalcitrant tinea pedis, a 1-week course of 200 mg twice daily is very effective. Additionally, a 30-day course of 100 mg daily in *T. tonsurans* tinea capitis is effective.[35] The usage in tinea capitis is restricted because it is available only in a 100-mg strength capsule and there is no liquid formula. For nail infections, two possible regimens are under investigation. The pulse dosage of 400 mg daily for 1 week, given 1 week per month for 3 to 4 months, has an 80% cure rate after 1 year of therapy. The alternative regimen has a similar cure rate and is given at a dosage of 200 mg daily for 12 weeks.[36] The pulse dosage is considered safer by its proponents, but there are no data to support this claim.

Terbinafine. The allylamine terbinafine is the only orally active fungicidal agent for dermatophytic infections. This agent is under investigation in the United States and is available in Canada, much of Europe, South America, and Asia. A dose of 250 mg daily is generally adequate. Six weeks of therapy is required for fingernail infections, and 12 weeks is needed for toenail infections.[32] Two weeks of therapy is adequate for extensive tinea corporis and cruris, and 2 to 4 weeks is needed for tinea capitis. The fungicidal mode of action may account for a very low relapse rate.

Other Therapies

Immunotherapy is used in veterinary medicine for prevention of dermatophytosis. There are no data on prevention of human disease, and this may be an area of research in the future.

References

1. Elewski BE, Hazen PG. The superficial mycoses and the dermatophytes. J Am Acad Dermatol 1989;21:655–673.
2. Rippon JW. Medical Mycology: The Pathogenic Fungi and the Pathogenic Actinomycetes, 3rd edition. Philadelphia: WB Saunders Co., 1988.
3. Elewski BE, ed. Cutaneous Fungal Infections. New York: Igaku-Shoin, 1992.
4. Martinez-Roig A, Llorens-Terol J, Torres JM. Erythema nodosum and kerion of the scalp. Am J Dis Child 1982;136:440–442.
5. Elewski BE, Greer DL. *Hendersonula toruloidea* and *Scytalidium hyalinum*: Review and update. Arch Dermatol 1991;127:1041–1044.
6. Kates SG, Nordstrom KM, McGinley KJ, et al. Microbiol ecology of interdigital infections of the web spaces. J Am Acad Dermatol 1990;22:578–582.
7. Leyden JJ, Kligman AM. Interdigital athlete's foot: The interaction of dermatophytes and resident bacteria. Arch Dermatol 1978;114:1466–1472.
8. Leyden JJ. Progression of interdigital infections from simplex to complex. J Am Acad Dermatol 1993;28:S7–S11.
9. Odom R. Pathophysiology of dermatophyte infections. J Am Acad Dermatol 1993;28:52–57.
10. Summerbell RC, Kane J, Krajden S. Onychomycosis, tinea pedis and tinea manuum caused by non-dermatophytic filamentous fungi. Mycoses 1989;32:609–619.
11. Jones HE, Reinhard JH, Rinaldi MG. A clinical, mycological and immunological survey for dermatophytosis. Arch Dermatol 1973;108:61–65.
12. Elewski BE. Proximal white subungual onychomycosis in acquired immunodeficiency syndrome. J Am Acad Dermatol 1993;29:631–632.
13. Raimer SS, Beightler EL, Hebert AA, et al. Tinea faciei in infants caused by *Trichophyton tonsurans*. Pediatr Dermatol 1986;3:452–454.
14. Gottlieb GJ, Ackerman AB. The "sandwich sign" of dermatophytosis. Am J Dermatopathol 1986;8:347–350.
15. Suarez SM, Silvers DN, Scher RK, et al. Histologic evaluation of nail clippings for diagnosing onychomycosis. Arch Dermatol 1991;127:1517–1519.
16. Scher RK, Ackerman AB. Histologic differential diagnosis of onychomycosis and psoriasis of the nail unit from cornified cells alone. Am J Dermatopathol 1980;2:255–257.
17. Babel DE, Baughman SA. Evaluation of the adult carrier state in juvenile tinea capitis caused by *Trichophyton tonsurans*. J Am Acad Dermatol 1989;21:1209–1212.
18. Zurita J, Hay RJ. Adherence of dermatophyte microconidia and arthroconidia to human keratinocytes in vitro. J Invest Dermatol 1987;89:529–534.
19. Jones HE. Immune response and host resistance of humans to dermatophyte infection. J Am Acad Dermatol 1993;28:S12–S18.
20. Dahl MV. Immunological resistance to dermatophyte infections. Adv Dermatol 1987;2:305–320.
21. Dahl MV. Suppression of immunity and inflammation by products produced by dermatophytes. J Am Acad Dermatol 1993;28:S19–S23.
22. Clemons KJ, Schar G, Stover EP, et al. Dermatophyte hormone relationships: Characterization of progesterone binding specificity in growth inhibition in the genera *Trichophyton* and *Microsporum*. J Clin Microbiol 1988;26:2110–2115.
23. Blake JS, Dahl MV, Herron MJ, et al. An immunoinhibitory cell wall glycoprotein (mannan) from *Trichophyton rubrum*. J Invest Dermatol 1991;96:651–661.
24. Lorincz AL, Sun SH. Dermatophyte viability at modestly raised temperatures. Arch Dermatol 1963;69:247–249.
25. Swart E, Smit FJA. *Trichophyton violaceum* abscesses. Br J Dermatol 1979;101:177–184.
26. Faergemann J, Gisslen H, Dahlberg E, et al. *Trichophyton rubrum* abscesses in immunocompromised patients. Acta Derm Venereol 1989;69:244–247.
27. Novick NL, Tapia L, Bottone EJ. Invasive *Trichophyton rubrum* infection in an immunocompromised host. Am J Med 1987;82:321–325.
28. Lesher JL Jr, Smith JG Jr. Antifungal agents in dermatology. J Am Acad Dermatol 1987;17:383–396.
29. Hay RJ, Clayton YM, Moore MK, et al. An evaluation of itraconazole in the management of onychomycosis. Br J Dermatol 1988;119:359–366.
30. Villars V, Jones TC. Clinical efficacy and tolerability of terbinafine (Lamisil): A new topical and systemic fungicidal drug for treatment of dermatomycoses. Clin Exp Dermatol 1989;14:124–127.
31. Zaias N, Serrano L. The successful treatment of fingernail *Trichophyton rubrum* onychomycosis with oral terbinafine. Clin Exp Dermatol 1989;14:120–124.
32. Goodfield MJD, Rowell NR, Forster RA, et al. Treatment of dermatophyte infection of the finger- and toe-nails with terbinafine (SF 86-327, Lamisil), an orally active fungicidal agent. Br J Dermatol 1989;12:1753–1757.
33. Walsoe I, Stangerup M, Svejgaard E. Itraconazole in onychomycosis. Acta Derm Venereol 1990;70:137–140.
34. Elewski BE. Mechanisms of action of systemic antifungal agents. J Am Acad Dermatol 1993;28:S28–S34.
35. Elewski BE. Tinea capitis: Itraconazole in *Trichophyton tonsurans* infection. J Am Acad Dermatol 1994;31:65–67.
36. Roseeuw D, DeDoncker P. New approaches to the treatment of onychomycosis. J Am Acad Dermatol 1993;29:S45–S50.

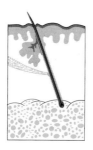

chapter 119

Cutaneous Candidiasis

GARY W. COLE

DEFINITION

Members of the genus *Candida* are unicellular, unencapsulated, budding fungi capable of forming germ tubes in serum at 37°C[1] and of producing skin and mucous membrane infections. In this genus the prototypical species, *C. albicans*, is by far the most common cause of human disease.

CLINICAL DESCRIPTION

The morphologic characteristics of candidiasis vary according to the affected anatomical area (Table 119–1).[2-4] On keratinized surfaces candidiasis appears as a pustular, red, scaling eruption that may be well marginated. On mucous membranes these infections produce a white, cheesy adherent mass surrounded by erythema (Fig. 119–1).

PATHOLOGY

Spongiform pustular dermatitis is the most frequent finding in specimens of superficial cutaneous candidiasis. In spongiform pustules neutrophils are interspersed between cells of the upper spinous and granular layers, sometimes accompanied by parakeratosis with neutrophils. In the adjacent stratum corneum are septate mycelia accompanied by an occasional ovoid yeast form (3 μm diameter).[5] In the subjacent dermis there is a sparse infiltrate of polymorphonuclear leukocytes and lymphocytes. In mucous membrane candidiasis a superficial mass of yeast and mycelial structures is accompanied by an infiltrate of lymphocytes and neutrophils beneath an epithelium that can show psoriasiform hyperplasia. The invasive mycelial forms appear to penetrate the epithelium vertically. In systemic candidiasis, yeast and mycelial forms are present in the dermis and within the lumina or walls of adjacent blood vessels, which can be

thrombosed. The epidermis is generally uninvolved. There is a minimal mononuclear inflammatory infiltrate,[6] and in some immunosuppressed patients, no inflammatory cells are present.

PATHOGENESIS AND ETIOLOGY

C. albicans is a normal commensal colonizing the mouth, gastrointestinal tract, and vaginal mucosa. About 25% of the normal adult population carry *Candida* orally, and about 20% of healthy women carry this yeast on their vaginal mucosa.[7] A variety of factors may perturb the local microenvironment to encourage the proliferation of *C. albicans* sufficient to produce a clinical infection. These include infancy, old age, pregnancy, local occlusion, epithelial destruction, diabetes mellitus, antibiotic or hormonal therapy, and immunosuppression.[7]

C. albicans exhibits attributes that enhance its virulence. The ability to adhere to an epithelial target cell is the first important step in the development of colonization and infection. The *C. albicans* cell surface possesses a complex molecule, a mannoprotein, composed of mannose, other hexoses, and a protein. This molecule, an adhesin, appears to mediate the yeast's adherence to epithelial tissues.[8] An extracellular proteolytic enzyme, *Candida* acid protease, can hydrolyze keratin, collagen, and a variety of other proteins of biologic significance. This protein could enhance the penetration of *C. albicans* into epithelial tissues.[9]

DIAGNOSIS AND DIFFERENTIAL DIAGNOSIS

If pustules are a component of any cutaneous eruption, the diagnosis of candidiasis should be suspected. The differential diagnosis of cutaneous candidiasis is listed in Table 119–2. Confusion with pyogenic bacterial infections or dermatophytosis would be expected. Lesions in flexural areas appear similar to dermatophytosis,

TABLE 119-1. Morphologic Characteristics of Candidiasis

Type	Description
Cutaneous disease	
Folliculitis	Pustules or inflammatory papules associated with hair follicles
Occlusive disease	Scaling, red eruption generally present on the back and most frequently noted in bedridden patients who have difficulty turning or moving spontaneously
Intertriginous disease	
Erosio interdigitalis blastomycetica	Scaling, red, eczematous inflammation of the finger webs generally involving the space between the middle and ring fingers
Diaper dermatitis	Involvement of the buttocks and crural areas of diapered infants with a pustular, papular, scaling dermatitis
Flexural disease	Involvement of the axilla, inframammary region, or groin with a pustular, papular dermatitis that occasionally may be sharply marginated
Nail disease	
Onychomycosis	White discoloration of the nail plate associated with distal onycholysis
Paronychia	Edema and redness of the proximal nail fold from which a purulent exudate may be expressed; often associated with nail dystrophy
Mucocutaneous disease	
Oral disease[2]	Acute pseudomembranous candidiasis is a whitish to yellowish, soft and creamy nonadherent plaque. When the oral commissures are involved the condition may be called angular cheilitis. Acute atrophic candidiasis presents as small or large erythematous painful areas on any mucous membranes. When the dorsal surface of the tongue is involved there is a loss of the lingual papillae, giving the appearance of atrophy, a condition called median rhomboid glossitis.
Balanitis	White, cheesy deposits on the glans penis that primarily affect uncircumsized, diabetic men
Vaginal disease	The appearance is identical to that of candidiasis of the oral mucous membranes.
Chronic mucocutaneous candidiasis[3]	Chronic and recurrent infections of the skin and/or mucous membranes. Prolonged infections may produce sheets of massive hyperkeratosis inappropriately named *Candida* granuloma. Chronic mucocutaneous candidiasis may be associated with multiple endocrine organ failure, thymoma, interstitial keratitis, chronic immunosuppression (acquired immunodeficiency syndrome) and KID (keratitis, ichthyosis, deafness) syndrome
Systemic candidiasis	Dissemination and invasion of major organ systems frequently associated with candidemia. This life-threatening condition occurs in the setting of immunosuppression or debilitation among patients who have hematologic malignancies or organ transplants. About 10% of patients with systemic candidiasis may exhibit cutaneous lesions characterized by painless, firm, pink, papules distributed discretely or diffusely on the trunk or extremities.[4]

pustular psoriasis, or even contact dermatitis and seborrheic dermatitis. Nail disease caused by *C. albicans* could be confused with dermatophytic onychomycosis or pyogenic bacterial infections. Mucous membrane candidiasis can resemble lichen planus, leukoplakia, or benign hyperkeratosis. Median rhomboid glossitis resembles geographic tongue. Chronic mucocutaneous candidiasis could be mistaken for a deep fungal infection.

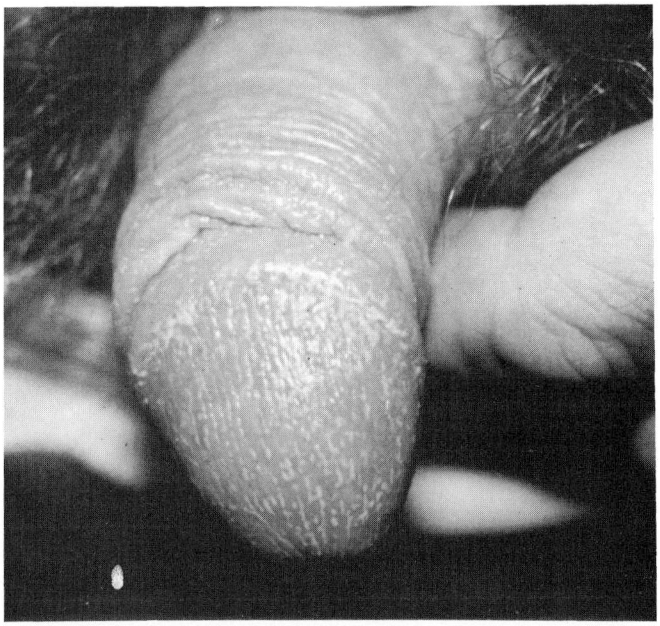

The diagnosis of cutaneous and mucous membrane candidiasis can be considered if scrapings reveal hyphae when examined by light microscopy after potassium hydroxide digestion. However, because yeast forms are difficult to visualize under these conditions, it is rarely possible to differentiate such findings from those seen in dermatophyte infections. In an exudate prepared using Gram stain, the presence of yeast forms producing germ tubes is confirmatory of the diagnosis of candidiasis (Fig. 119–2). The cultural isolation of *C. albicans* must be interpreted with some caution because this yeast can be part of the normal flora. Such a finding may be significant if this yeast is isolated in abundance from anatomic sites where it does not normally occur. *Candida* can also

FIGURE 119–1. Glans penis studded with pustules and a white, cheesy, adherent mass of yeast and mycelia.

TABLE 119-2. Differential Diagnosis of Cutaneous Candidiasis

Dermatophytosis
Bacterial skin infection
Herpes simplex
Seborrheic dermatitis
Contact dermatitis
Deep fungal infection

TABLE 119-3. Treatment of Cutaneous Candidiasis

Indication	Drug in Order of Preference*	Dosage and Duration	Dosage Form	Adjunctive Measures
Oral disease (acute)	Nystatin	5 mL in the mouth for 5 minutes tid for 10 days	Suspension	
	Clotrimazole	10 mg 10 times per day for 14 days	Troche	
Chronic mucocutaneous candidiasis	Itraconazole	100 mg per day for 2 to 4 weeks	Capsule	
	Ketoconazole	200–400 mg per day for 2 to 4 weeks	Tablets	Gastric acidity necessary for absorption
	Fluconazole	50–200 mg per day for 2 weeks, 50 mg per day for prophylaxis	Capsule	
Vaginal disease	Clotrimazole	Indefinite	Creams and inserts	
	Miconazole		Suppositories	
	Tioconazole		Cream	
Localized skin disease	Nystatin	Indefinite	Cream	Application of zinc oxide paste to the affected area
	Clotrimazole	Indefinite	Cream	
	Miconazole	Indefinite	Cream	
	Ketoconazole	Indefinite	Cream	
	Econazole	Indefinite	Cream	

*Based on cost and efficacy.
Data from Hay RJ, Kalter DC. Superficial *Candida* infections. In: Jacobs PH, Nall L, eds. Antifungal Drug Therapy. New York: Marcel Dekker, 1990:31–42; and Goldstein SM. Advances in the treatment of superficial *Candida* infections. Semin Dermatol 1993;12:315–330.

be visualized in routine histopathologic specimens. It is seen on hematoxylin and eosin–stained sections if the hematoxylin staining is sufficiently robust; staining with periodic acid–Schiff or Gomori methenamine silver more reliably demonstrates yeasts and pseudohyphae.

TREATMENT

Effective treatment of cutaneous candidiasis often requires simple changes in the local microenvironment. Replacement of poorly fitted dentures can result in the resolution of oral candidiasis. Control of the blood glucose level in diabetic patients can enhance their recovery from balanitis and vaginitis caused by *C. albicans*. Ending antibiotic or oral contraceptive therapy may be all that is needed to control candidiasis in certain patients. Diaper dermatitis caused by *Candida* can be prevented by the application of thick layers of zinc oxide paste to the perineal and perianal regions. Enhancing evaporation of water and sweat can aid the resolution of paronychia and truncal candidiasis.

Drugs useful in treating candidiasis belong to two chemical groups, the polyenes and the azoles. Nystatin and amphotericin B are polyenes. Ketoconazole and clotrimazole are members of the azole group. The indications for and dosages of specific anti-*Candida* drugs are found in Table 119–3.[10, 11]

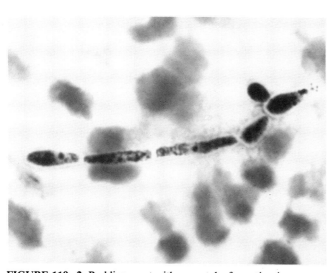

FIGURE 119–2. Budding yeast with germ tube formation in a purulent exudate from a patient with systemic candidiasis (Gram stain × 1000).

References

1. Cooper BH, Silva-Hunter M. Yeasts of medical importance. In: Lennette E, ed. Manual of Clinical Microbiology, 4th ed. Washington, DC: American Society for Microbiology, 1985:526–541.
2. Holmstrup P, Samaranayake LP. Acute and AIDS-related oral candidoses. In: Samaranayake LP, Macfarlane TW, eds. Oral Candidosis. London: Wright, 1990:133–155.
3. Kirkpatrick CH. Chronic mucocutaneous candidiasis. In: Bodey GP, ed. Candidiasis, 2nd ed. New York: Raven Press, 1993:167–184.
4. Bodey GP, Hematogenous and major organ candidiasis. In: Bodey GP, ed. Candidiasis, 2nd ed. New York: Raven Press, 1993:279–329.
5. Lever W, Lever G. Histopathology of the Skin, 7th ed. Philadelphia: JB Lippincott, 1990:368–370.
6. Luna MA, Tortoledo ME. Histologic identification and pathologic patterns of disease by *Candida*. In: Bodey GP, ed. Candidiasis, 2nd ed. New York: Raven Press, 1993:21–42.
7. Hay RJ. Fungi and fungal infections of the skin. In: Noble WC, ed. The Skin Microflora and Microbial Skin Disease. Cambridge, England: Cambridge University Press, 1992:249–252.
8. Edwards JE Jr, Mayer CL. Adherence of *Candida albicans* to mammalian cells. In: Ayoub EM, et al., eds. Microbial Determi-

nants of Virulence and Host Response. Washington DC: American Society for Microbiology, 1990:179–196.

9. Ray TL, Payne CD. *Candida albicans* acid proteinase: A role in virulence. In: Ayoub EM, et al., eds. Microbial Determinants of Virulence and Host Response. Washington DC: American Society for Microbiology, 1990:163–178.

10. Hay RJ, Kalter DC. Superficial *Candida* infections. In: Jacobs PH, Nall L, eds. Antifungal Drug Therapy. New York: Marcel Dekker, 1990:31–42.

11. Goldstein SM. Advances in the treatment of superficial *Candida* infections. Semin Dermatol 1993;12:315–330.

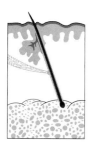

chapter 120

Deep Fungal and Opportunistic Mycoses

LIZA W. CHANG and KENNETH J. TOMECKI

Cryptococcosis

DEFINITION

Cryptococcosis is primarily an opportunistic systemic disease that affects the central nervous system (CNS). The causative agent is a yeast, *Cryptococcus neoformans.*

CLINICAL DESCRIPTION

C. neoformans has a worldwide distribution. Persons between the ages of 30 and 60 years are most often affected. Isolated from soil and abundant in pigeon droppings, the organism has an affinity for the immunocompromised host. Six to 10% of patients in the United States with the acquired immunodeficiency syndrome (AIDS) develop cryptococcosis.[1]

The organism, acquired by the respiratory route, can produce disseminated disease. The initial pulmonary infection is usually asymptomatic and self-limited. Disseminated disease typically involves the CNS, usually in the form of meningitis. Headache, malaise, and fever are the most common symptoms of meningeal infection,[2] although patients with AIDS may have few or no symptoms suggestive of meningitis. The prostate can be a site of silent persistent infection.[3] Skin involvement, the most common occurrence after CNS disease, occurs in 10% to 20% of patients with disseminated cryptococcosis.[4] Skin findings are varied and include papules, pustules, vegetative and infiltrated plaques, nodules, subcutaneous swellings and abscesses, cellulitis, acneiform eruptions, ulcers, granulomas, and palpable purpura.[4-6] The head and neck are most often affected. Disease is usually painless. In patients with AIDS, skin disease may resemble molluscum contagiosum,[7] herpes infection,[8] and Kaposi's sarcoma[9] (Fig. 120-1). Disseminated cryptococcosis is a sign of AIDS in the presence of laboratory evidence of human immunodeficiency virus (HIV) infection. Primary cutaneous infection occurring after injury to the skin is rare.[10] Even with seemingly isolated skin involvement, evaluation for systemic disease is necessary. Skin disease can precede CNS infection by 2 to 8 months.

PATHOLOGY

In general, two types of tissue reaction occur in the skin: gelatinous and granulomatous. More common is the gelatinous reaction, in which the inflammatory infiltrate is minimal and numerous organisms (4–12 μm in diameter) are encased by wide gelatinous capsules (Fig. 120-2). The granulomatous reaction has a polymorphous infiltrate of histiocytes, lymphocytes, and giant cells, with fewer organisms. The yeast (2–4 μm) is primarily located within giant cells and histiocytes; any capsule is negligible or absent. The organism stains with methenamine silver, as well as periodic acid–Schiff (PAS), and the staining is resistant to diastase (PAS-D); the capsule stains with mucicarmine, methylene blue, and alcian blue.

ETIOLOGY AND PATHOGENESIS

C. neoformans is the causative agent. In nature, it exists as a round unencapsulated yeast, is approximately 2 μm in diameter, and reproduces by narrow-based budding. Cryptococcosis is acquired through inhalation; subsequent hematogenous dissemination leads to systemic infection. Depressed cell-mediated immunity has occurred in affected patients. The polysaccharide capsule

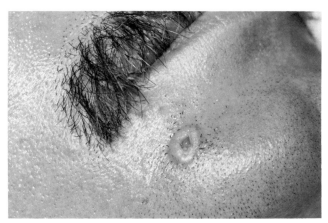

FIGURE 120-1. Cryptococcosis. Umbilicated plaque on the chin of patient with AIDS; the plaque resembles molluscum contagiosum, keratoacanthoma, and basal cell carcinoma.

may enhance the organism's virulence, possibly by inhibiting host phagocytosis.

DIAGNOSIS AND DIFFERENTIAL DIAGNOSIS

India ink examination of cerebrospinal fluid, pus, skin lesions, and other fluids may reveal the yeast. Culture is necessary for confirmation, and mouse inoculation can establish pathogenicity. *C. neoformans* grows on most fungal media without cycloheximide, which inhibits its growth. The cryptococcal latex agglutination test can detect capsular antigen in cerebrospinal fluid and/or blood; the test is positive in cerebrospinal fluid in more than

90% of patients with cryptococcal meningitis.[4] Anticryptococcal antibodies are not helpful diagnostically, and skin tests are primarily for epidemiologic use.

The differential diagnosis is extensive because skin findings are varied. The disease should be suspect in any immunocompromised patient with nondescript skin disease.

TREATMENT

Amphotericin B, with or without flucytosine, is the treatment of choice for cryptococcosis (Table 120-1).[1, 2, 11] Amphotericin B has been used in doses of 0.3 to 1.0 mg/kg per day intravenously for 6 weeks for a total dose of 1.5 to 3.0 g.[11, 12] Generally, a 1-mg test dose of amphotericin B is given first. If this test dose is tolerated, the dose is gradually increased. Administration is usually as a single daily dose or as a double dose on alternate days. Side effects of amphotericin B include fever, chills, and, most importantly, nephrotoxicity. Oral doses of flucytosine have ranged from 75 to 150 mg/kg per day.[11, 12] The use of flucytosine in patients with AIDS is still controversial; concerns regarding its benefit and toxicity (particularly bone marrow toxicity) in this setting exist.[1, 2, 11] Fluconazole and itraconazole, both triazole compounds, have been useful agents for systemic cryptococcosis.[11, 13] Fluconazole (100-400 mg per day, orally) is the agent of choice for chronic suppressive therapy in patients with AIDS. In selected patients, primary cutaneous cryptococcosis has responded to the use of fluconazole alone.[10, 14]

Sporotrichosis

DEFINITION

Sporotrichosis is a chronic subcutaneous infection arising from the traumatic inoculation of the dimorphic fungus *Sporothrix schenckii*.

CLINICAL DESCRIPTION

S. schenckii exists worldwide, especially in temperate and tropical regions. This yeast resides in soil, plants, and decaying vegetation; sources include rose thorns, sphagnum moss, and hay. Occupational and recreational exposure play a role, and humans and animals, particularly cats, can be infected.

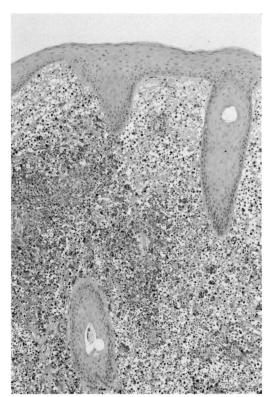

FIGURE 120-2. In the gelatinous form of cutaneous cryptococcosis, yeasts are surrounded by mucoid capsules (mucicarmine stain).

TABLE 120-1. Treatment of Cryptococcosis	
Condition	**Therapy**
Immunocompetent host	Amphotericin B ± flucytosine
AIDS	
Induction	Amphotericin B ± flucytosine
Maintenance	Fluconazole

Clinically, sporotrichosis has cutaneous and extracutaneous forms. The cutaneous form has three types: lymphocutaneous, fixed cutaneous, and disseminated cutaneous. Lymphocutaneous sporotrichosis is the classic presentation and accounts for up to 80% of cases,[15] with the dominant upper extremity most often affected. At the site of inoculation a painless, indurated nodule develops, which may ulcerate to form a sporotrichoid chancre; other asymptomatic nodules along the draining lymphatics and regional adenopathy may follow. This combination is known as sporotrichoid spread—a characteristic of sporotrichosis, though not unique (Fig. 120–3). The fixed cutaneous form occurs more often in endemic areas. Children commonly have this form, usually on the face,[16] with asymptomatic papules, ulcers, or verrucous plaques commonly localized to the site of inoculation. Disseminated cutaneous sporotrichosis is rare and may result from either hematogenous spread or autoinoculation. Extracutaneous sporotrichosis encompasses primary pulmonary sporotrichosis and systemic sporotrichosis; both are rare. Skin findings, usually absent in the former, include multiple papules, nodules, ulcers, or plaques. Disease can involve any organ in systemic sporotrichosis, with skin, bone and joints, and muscle most commonly affected; meningitis is uncommon. Disseminated disease has occurred in HIV-infected patients.[17, 18]

PATHOLOGY

Early lesions show a nonspecific mixed inflammation; later, granulomas, giant cells, and dermal and intraepidermal abscesses appear. The lymphatic nodules of lymphocutaneous sporotrichosis and the nodules of systemic sporotrichosis reveal a suppurative and granulomatous dermatitis. In the localized form, there is often pseudocarcinomatous hyperplasia overlying the infiltrates. In

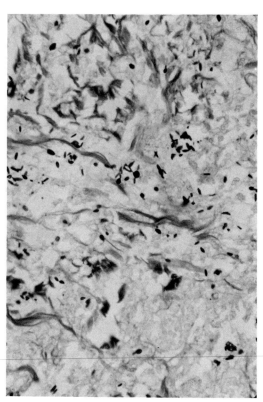

FIGURE 120–4. The cigar-shaped yeasts of sporotrichosis can be scarce in tissue sections (Gomori methenamine silver).

most biopsy specimens (except in systemic sporotrichosis) organisms are absent or sparse, even with the use of special stains, such as PAS-D or methenamine silver. In tissue, the yeast (4–6 μm in size) is cigar shaped with single, and occasionally multiple, buds (Fig. 120–4). Hyphae are rare. The asteroid body, a central oval basophilic spore surrounded by radiating eosinophilic material, may be present in the centers of suppurative foci; the entire body may be 25 μm in diameter.[19]

ETIOLOGY AND PATHOGENESIS

The causative organism of sporotrichosis is *S. schenckii*, a dimorphic fungus. Infection usually follows traumatic inoculation of the organism into the skin, classically through a rose thorn injury. The organism spreads through the draining subcutaneous lymphatics to produce a nodular lymphangitis. The fixed cutaneous form of disease, which lacks lymphatic spread, most likely represents increased host immunity to the organism. Inhalation of the fungus in a susceptible host may lead to extracutaneous sporotrichosis, a form with predilection for persons with decreased immunity (i.e., those with alcoholism, diabetes, and sarcoidosis). Patients with AIDS tend to have widely disseminated disease.

DIAGNOSIS AND DIFFERENTIAL DIAGNOSIS

Direct fluorescent antibody techniques help to identify the organism in histologic sections. Serial sections stained with PAS-D or methenamine silver can also be

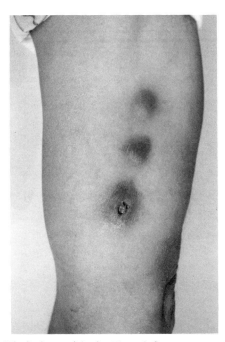

FIGURE 120–3. Sporotrichosis. Three inflammatory nodules in a linear distribution on the arm.

TABLE 120-2. Differential Diagnosis of Sporotrichosis	
Infections	

Atypical mycobacterioses (i.e., *Mycobacterium marinum*,
M. kansasii)
Tuberculosis
Furunculosis
Anthrax
Tularemia
Nocardia brasiliensis infection
Deep fungal infections
Majocchi's granuloma
Leishmaniasis
Cat-scratch disease
Syphilis

Other Disorders

Foreign body granuloma
Halogenoderma
Sarcoidosis
Pyoderma gangrenosum

used to detect organisms in cases in which the initial sections do not show them. Culture of the organism confirms the diagnosis. The fungus grows within 3 to 5 days on most fungal media and exhibits thermal dimorphism. At room temperature, early colonies are white; with time, they become wrinkled and brownish black. At 37° C, cream-colored colonies form. Microscopically, at room temperature, there are branching septate hyphae with a daisy-like arrangement of conidia. Serologic tests may be helpful, primarily in extracutaneous disease. Meningitis warrants a search for antibodies to *S. schenckii* within the cerebrospinal fluid.[18, 20] Skin testing has limited clinical value. The differential diagnosis is listed in Table 120-2.

TREATMENT

Despite a few reports of spontaneous resolution in cutaneous sporotrichosis, treatment is usually necessary (Table 120-3). For the cutaneous forms, saturated solution of potassium iodide is the agent of choice. It is given orally, usually beginning at a low dose (5 drops three times a day) and gradually increasing by 3 to 5 drops per day as tolerated to a maximum dose of 30 to 50 drops three times a day.[12, 15] The medication is given in water or juice, with treatment continued for 1 month beyond

TABLE 120-3. Treatment of Sporotrichosis	
Condition	**Therapy**
Cutaneous forms	Saturated solution of potassium iodide
Extracutaneous	
Primary pulmonary	Amphotericin B(± surgery)
Systemic	Amphotericin B

apparent clinical resolution. Locally applied heat may be helpful as adjunctive therapy. Ketoconazole, terbinafine, and itraconazole have been used with success in cutaneous sporotrichosis.

For extracutaneous disease, amphotericin B is usually necessary. In primary pulmonary sporotrichosis, complete surgical resection of localized diseased tissue, coupled with either perioperative saturated solution of potassium iodide or amphotericin B, may be necessary[21]; itraconazole has been effective therapy as well.[22] Amphotericin B, 0.4 to 1.0 mg/kg per day given intravenously for 2 to 3 months, is necessary for disseminated disease, either cutaneous or systemic. Treatment of sporotrichosis in patients with AIDS has involved multiple agents, including ketoconazole, amphotericin B, flucytosine, and fluconazole; all have only limited success.

Coccidioidomycosis

DEFINITION

Coccidioidomycosis is a systemic mycosis acquired by inhalation of the fungus *Coccidioides immitis*. It is usually a self-limited pulmonary infection but can occasionally disseminate hematogenously.

CLINICAL DESCRIPTION

C. immitis, a dimorphic fungus found in soil, is endemic to the desert regions of the southwestern United States, Mexico, and Central and South America. Disease in nonendemic areas may result from travel, past residence in endemic regions, or exposure to contaminated fomites (i.e., packing materials) from these places. Risk factors for dissemination include male sex, pregnancy, race (blacks, Filipinos, Hispanics), and immunosuppression (i.e., iatrogenic, AIDS). Reactivation of arrested disease may occur, particularly in immunosuppressed patients.

Coccidioidomycosis may appear as primary pulmonary disease (most common), disseminated disease, or, rarely, primary cutaneous disease. Primary pulmonary disease is asymptomatic in 60% of cases; in the remainder, symptoms are usually mild and flu-like. Skin findings of primary pulmonary infection include a generalized morbilliform eruption, seen in 10% to 15% of patients with symptomatic disease, erythema nodosum, and erythema multiforme. Valley fever is the combination of erythema nodosum or erythema multiforme, arthritis, and ocular symptoms (i.e., episcleritis) in the setting of primary pulmonary infection. Coccidioidomycosis is the main cause of erythema nodosum in endemic regions.[23] The initial pulmonary infection is usually self-limited but may progress to chronic pulmonary or disseminated disease. Dissemination is rare (less than 1% of all cases). Common sites for dissemination are the skin, bones and joints, and meninges. Skin findings consist of verrucous papules and nodules, pustules, subcutaneous abscesses, ulcers, and sinuses, with a predilection for the face, especially the nasolabial fold. HIV-associated infection is usually disseminated and associated with low CD4 counts.[24] In HIV-infected patients, skin findings may resemble molluscum contagiosum or acne.[23] Such patients may have a diffuse reticulonodular pattern on chest radiography.[25] In a patient with HIV infection, the presence of disseminated coccidioidomycosis establishes the diagnosis of AIDS.

PATHOLOGY

Histopathologic examination reveals a suppurative and granulomatous inflammatory infiltrate, within which are the tissue phase of the organism, termed *spherules*. Spherules can be recognized in hematoxylin and eosin–stained sections. They have a refractile capsule and often contain many endospores. They measure from 40 to 60 μm in diameter and can be found within giant cells and free in the dermis. Special stains, such as PAS, methenamine silver, and Gridley, may help to demonstrate the spherules.

ETIOLOGY AND PATHOGENESIS

The causative agent of coccidioidomycosis is the dimorphic fungus *C. immitis*. In nature, septate hyphae form and produce infective arthrospores, which, when inhaled, produce pulmonary infection, occasionally followed by hematogenous dissemination. T-cell immunity helps to limit the extent and progression of disease. Inoculum size may affect the severity and risk of dissemination. Human sex hormones have been found to promote the growth of *C. immitis;* this may be a factor in the increased risk of disseminated disease during pregnancy.

DIAGNOSIS AND DIFFERENTIAL DIAGNOSIS

Potassium hydroxide preparations of sputum, pus, and other body fluids may reveal the characteristic spherules. The organism grows readily at 30° C on most fungal media. Cultures are highly infective. Serologic testing is helpful for diagnosis. Precipitin antibodies (IgM) form early in the course of disease. Complement fixation antibodies of the IgG class appear slowly during infection. Complement fixation antibody quantitation has prognostic implications; a rising titer indicates a poor prognosis and probable dissemination. The presence of complement fixation antibodies in cerebrospinal fluid supports the diagnosis of coccidioidal meningitis. Skin test reactivity simply indicates exposure to the fungus, not necessarily active disease. Cutaneous anergy in the setting of known coccidioidomycosis is a poor prognostic sign. The differential diagnosis of skin disease is vast (Table 120–4).

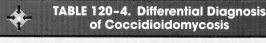

TABLE 120-4. Differential Diagnosis of Coccidioidomycosis
Infections
Other deep fungal
Bacterial (i.e., impetigo)
Mycobacterial (i.e., tuberculosis)
Tertiary syphilis
Viral (i.e., molluscum contagiosum)
Other Disorders
Warts
Prurigo nodularis
Keratoacanthoma
Halogenoderma
Rosacea

TREATMENT

Primary pulmonary infection is usually self-limited; bed rest, supportive therapy, and close follow-up are required (Table 120–5). Severe pulmonary disease or disease in pregnant women, in persons with an increased likelihood of dissemination, or in patients with diabetes, cancer, or other pulmonary disease deserves treatment, as does primary cutaneous coccidioidomycosis in children. Disseminated disease requires treatment. The mainstay of therapy is amphotericin B (0.5–1.0 mg/kg per day, given intravenously; total dose, 1.0–3.0 g).[12] Ketoconazole (400 mg per day, given orally) has shown mixed results. Fluconazole (200–400 mg per day, given orally) has been effective for both meningeal and nonmeningeal disease.[26] More recently, itraconazole (100–400 mg per day, given orally) has shown efficacy.[27-30] Relapse is common. Surgical therapy may be helpful in some cases of pulmonary and joint disease.

Histoplasmosis

DEFINITION

Histoplasmosis is a systemic fungal disease, primarily involving the reticuloendothelial system. The causative organism is *Histoplasma capsulatum*.

TABLE 120-5. Treatment of Coccidioidomycosis	
Condition	**Therapy**
Primary pulmonary infection	
Mild disease	Supportive therapy
Severe disease, or disease with increased risk of dissemination (including AIDS)	Amphotericin B
Disseminated disease	Amphotericin B

CLINICAL DESCRIPTION

Histoplasmosis has a worldwide distribution. Its main endemic area is the Ohio and Mississippi River valleys of the United States, where up to 80% of the residents may have positive histoplasmin skin tests. Immunosuppression predisposes to disseminated infection. The organism lives in the soil, particularly in association with bird droppings and bat guano.

The symptomatic forms of histoplasmosis include acute pulmonary histoplasmosis, disseminated histoplasmosis, chronic pulmonary histoplasmosis, and the rare primary cutaneous histoplasmosis. In most patients, primary pulmonary infection is asymptomatic and skin test conversion confirms exposure. Symptomatic acute pulmonary histoplasmosis exhibits flu-like symptoms and retrosternal or pleuritic chest pain; chest radiography may reveal hilar or mediastinal lymphadenopathy. Skin findings consist of erythema nodosum or erythema multiforme. Disseminated histoplasmosis is rare.[31] With dissemination, mucosal disease is more common than skin disease; common sites are the tongue, palate, buccal mucosa, and pharynx. Skin findings include erythematous macules, papules, nodules, pustules, petechiae, purpura, exfoliative erythroderma, granulomatous ulcerations, abscesses, cellulitis, and panniculitis.[32, 33] Adrenal gland involvement can result in Addison's disease. In patients with AIDS, histoplasmosis tends to be disseminated, with fever and weight loss the most common signs of disease.[34] A septic shock–like picture may occur in such patients, with multiorgan failure and a fulminant course. In one study, 11% of patients with HIV infection and disseminated histoplasmosis had skin involvement, which was much higher than the incidence in patients who are not infected with HIV.[35] Cutaneous findings in these patients also include eruptions resembling rosacea[36] and transepidermal elimination.[37] Disseminated histoplasmosis is an AIDS-defining infection. Chronic pulmonary histoplasmosis mimics tuberculosis and usually arises in the setting of emphysema.

PATHOLOGY

"Parasitized macrophages" arranged as nodular or diffuse dermal infiltrates are characteristic of histoplasmosis. Such macrophages have cytoplasm embedded with many round-to-oval 2- to 4-μm sized spores, with a surrounding clear space around the spores; in the past, this space was mistakenly thought to be a capsule. The organism is visible with hematoxylin and eosin stain but is more apparent with the methenamine silver or Giemsa stain.

ETIOLOGY AND PATHOGENESIS

Histoplasmosis is caused by the dimorphic fungus *H. capsulatum.* Acquired through inhalation of the infective spore, a large inoculum produces symptomatic disease. The organism has a predilection for the reticuloendothelial system, where it exists intracellularly. Cell-mediated immunity is important in limiting the extent of disease. In patients with HIV infection, it is unclear whether disseminated disease represents exogenous infection or endogenous reactivation of a latent focus.

DIAGNOSIS AND DIFFERENTIAL DIAGNOSIS

Examination of tissue, especially bone marrow or peripheral blood, with a silver stain may reveal the organism. Radiographs can detect calcified granulomas of resolved disease in affected organs. Culture of the fungus (i.e., from bone marrow) confirms the diagnosis, although growth may take 6 weeks. Incubation at room temperature yields a white colony, and microscopic examination reveals the diagnostic tuberculate macroconidia of *H. capsulatum.* The culture is highly infectious. Serologic testing is useful, specifically the use of complement fixation antibodies and immunodiffusion tests for H and M precipitins. A complement fixation antibody titer of 1:32 or higher suggests recent or current infection. Rapid diagnosis of histoplasmosis is possible with the detection of *H. capsulatum* polysaccharide antigen in urine, blood, and other body fluids.[34] Unlike cryptococcal antigen testing, this is not widely available yet.

Cutaneous disease is varied, and the differential diagnosis is extensive (Table 120–6).

TREATMENT

Generally, only bed rest and symptomatic treatment are needed for acute pulmonary histoplasmosis. For severe acute pulmonary disease and disseminated disease amphotericin B (0.5–0.6 mg/kg per day, given intravenously; total dose, 2.0–2.5 g), ketoconazole (400–800 mg per day, given orally), or itraconazole (200–400 mg per day, given orally) would be appropriate.[12, 38] Ketoconazole has been effective for some cases of chronic pulmonary histoplasmosis, although many cases are difficult to treat and fail to respond to ketoconazole. Some cases of chronic pulmonary histoplasmosis have responded to therapy with itraconazole. Determination of the role of fluconazole awaits further studies. In the immunosuppressed patient, amphotericin B is the drug of choice for induction therapy. Suppressive maintenance

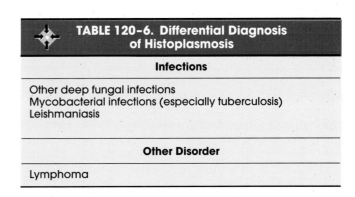

✦ TABLE 120–6. Differential Diagnosis of Histoplasmosis
Infections
Other deep fungal infections Mycobacterial infections (especially tuberculosis) Leishmaniasis
Other Disorder
Lymphoma

TABLE 120-7. Treatment of Histoplasmosis

Condition	Therapy
Primary pulmonary	
Mild	Symptomatic
Severe	Amphotericin B, ketoconazole, itraconazole
Chronic pulmonary	Ketoconazole
Disseminated	
Immunocompetent	Amphotericin B
AIDS	
Induction	Amphotericin B
Maintenance	Amphotericin B, ketoconazole, ? itraconazole

therapy requires amphotericin B, ketoconazole, or itraconazole (Table 120–7).[12, 31, 32, 34] In this setting, amphotericin B is given intravenously as weekly doses of 0.5 to 1.5 mg/kg per dose.

Blastomycosis

DEFINITION

Blastomycosis is a systemic mycosis caused by the dimorphic fungus *Blastomyces dermatitidis,* which primarily infects the lungs and occasionally the skin, bone, and genitourinary tract.

CLINICAL DESCRIPTION

The epidemiology of blastomycosis is ill-defined compared with other systemic mycoses, owing to lack of a reliable skin test antigen. Most cases have occurred in the areas bordering the Ohio and Mississippi Rivers and the Great Lakes. The southeastern states have also reported many cases. Soil is the organism's likely habitat, but recovery of the organism has been difficult. Exposure to soil and water probably predispose to infection. Both humans and animals (especially dogs) can acquire the disease, and sexual transmission has been reported. Unlike the case with other systemic mycoses, there is no increased incidence of disease in immunosuppressed patients, including patients with HIV infection.

Blastomycosis primarily infects the lungs, less so the skin, bone, and other organs. The initial pulmonary infection may be asymptomatic, but self-limited flu-like symptoms can occur. Pulmonary disease can become chronic, with signs and symptoms mimicking tuberculosis or malignancy. The skin is the most common extrapulmonary site of involvement. About 80% of patients have skin disease,[39] with exposed areas and mucous membranes as favored sites. Annular verrucous plaques studded with peripheral microabscesses are the hallmark of skin disease (Fig. 120–5). The plaques heal centrally

with atrophic scarring and may ulcerate; the active pustular border continues to advance. Asymptomatic bone and joint involvement occurs in approximately half of patients,[39] characterized by well-circumscribed osteolytic lesions on radiography. Genitourinary disease occurs in approximately 25% of men but rarely in women. CNS disease, usually meningitis and/or brain abscess, occurs in 5% to 10% of patients with disseminated disease.[40] In the few patients with AIDS and blastomycosis, both localized pulmonary disease and disseminated disease have occurred.[41] With disseminated disease, there is a much higher incidence of CNS involvement (40% in one study) compared with the immunocompetent population of patients.[41] The rare self-limited primary inoculation blastomycosis consists of a nodule at the site of inoculation and regional lymphadenopathy.

PATHOLOGY

Histology reveals marked pseudoepitheliomatous hyperplasia with scattered intraepidermal microabscesses and a mixed neutrophilic and granulomatous infiltrate in the dermis. Yeast organisms (8–15 μm in diameter) may lie either free in tissue or within giant cells; they have a double-contoured refractile wall and exhibit characteristic broad-based single budding. A silver or PAS-D stain facilitates visualization of the organism.

ETIOLOGY AND PATHOGENESIS

The causative agent of blastomycosis is the thermally dimorphic fungus *B. dermatitidis*. Disease begins after inhalation of spores that convert to yeast forms in the lungs. Extrapulmonary dissemination occurs hematogenously. Primary skin disease occurs mainly in laboratory workers through accidental inoculation. There is no increased incidence of blastomycosis among immunosuppressed persons. Endogenous reactivation, either pul-

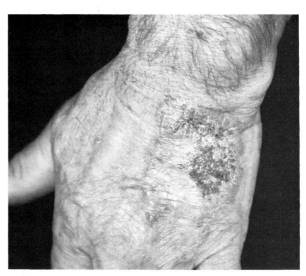

FIGURE 120-5. Blastomycosis. Large, verrucous, eroded plaque on dorsum of hand.

monary or extrapulmonary, may occur, even years after the initial infection has resolved.

DIAGNOSIS AND DIFFERENTIAL DIAGNOSIS

Potassium hydroxide examination of pus, sputum, and tissue may reveal the yeast. Culture of the organism at 30° C on routine fungal media yields a cottony white mold, and microscopic examination reveals round to pear-shaped conidia. Serologic tests are limited by low sensitivity and specificity. Skin testing has questionable value.

The differential diagnosis includes other infectious as well as noninfectious disorders (Table 120–8).

TREATMENT

Until recently, amphotericin B (0.3–0.6 mg/kg per day, given intravenously; total dose, 2.0 g) was the preferred treatment for blastomycosis (Table 120–9). Now, ketoconazole (400 mg per day, given orally) and itraconazole (200–400 mg per day, given orally) have proved to be effective agents for mild to moderate nonmeningeal blastomycosis in immunocompetent patients.[38, 42] Therapy should last for at least 6 months. For life-threatening or CNS disease and for disease in immunosuppressed patients, amphotericin B remains the preferred therapy.[40, 41, 43] Chronic administration of one of the oral azoles or amphotericin B is warranted in patients with AIDS. The efficacy of fluconazole remains to be determined. Other agents include 2-hydroxystilbamidine, terbinafine, and miconazole; in selected cases, surgery may be another option.[43]

The main characteristics of the systemic mycoses are summarized in Table 120–10.

TABLE 120-8. Differential Diagnosis of Blastomycosis

Infections
Warts
Tuberculosis
Leprosy
Nocardiosis
Actinomycosis
Mycetoma
Ecthyma
Tertiary syphilis
Granuloma inguinale
Leishmaniasis
Other deep fungal infections
Majocchi's granuloma

Other Disorders
Squamous cell carcinoma
Halogenoderma

TABLE 120-9. Treatment of Blastomycosis

Condition	Therapy
Nonmeningeal blastomycosis	
Immunocompetent and mild-to-moderate disease	Ketoconazole, itraconazole
Severe disease	Amphotericin B
AIDS	
Induction	Amphotericin B
Maintenance	Oral azole or amphotericin B
Meningeal blastomycosis	Amphotericin B

Chromoblastomycosis

DEFINITION

Chromoblastomycosis is a chronic dermal or subcutaneous infection characterized by the presence of pigmented sclerotic bodies in affected tissue. The causative agents are dematiaceous fungi.

CLINICAL DESCRIPTION

Chromoblastomycosis occurs worldwide, with the highest incidence in the tropics and subtropics. The causative organisms—the dematiaceous (pigmented) fungi—are saprophytes that are found in soil and decaying vegetation. Infection can occur in animals and humans (mainly men aged 30 to 40 years old involved in farm work). There is no evidence for human-to-human transmission.

Chromoblastomycosis primarily causes disease at the site of inoculation and differs from mycetoma, which is more invasive locally, often affecting underlying bone. Initially, a small scaly papule, usually on the exposed leg or foot develops, which, over time, enlarges as satellite papules appear. Through coalescence, multilobulated, verrucous, or smooth plaques develop, which can be pruritic and painful; plaques are often covered with "black dots" of purulent discharge. Secondary bacterial infection is common. Lymphatic obstruction can occur, sometimes followed by elephantiasis. Disease can remain indolent over many years. Dissemination and CNS disease are rare.

PATHOLOGY

Biopsy usually reveals pseudoepitheliomatous hyperplasia and suppurative and granulomatous dermal infiltrates. Organisms appear in tissue as characteristic sclerotic bodies (Medlar bodies, "copper pennies")—dark brown, round, thick-walled structures, 6 to 12 μm in diameter, usually found singly or in clusters, either free in tissue or within giant cells (Fig. 120–6). Morphologi-

TABLE 120-10. Characteristics of Systemic Mycoses

	Cryptococcosis	Coccidioidomycosis	Histoplasmosis	Blastomycosis
Organism	Cryptococcus neoformans	Coccidioides immitis	Histoplasma capsulatum	Blastomyces dermatitidis
Dimorphic	No	Yes	Yes	Yes
Distribution	Worldwide	California and southwestern US, Mexico, Central and South America	Eastern and central US	Ill defined; most cases in areas adjacent to Ohio and Mississippi Rivers, Great Lakes
Sites of Involvement	Central nervous system Lungs Skin	Lungs Skin Bone Meninges	Lungs Reticuloendothelial system Skin	Lungs Skin Bone Genitourinary tract
Skin Lesion Morphology	Varied	Varied	Varied; mucosal involvement common	Annular plaque with peripheral microabscesses
Histology	Gelatinous or granulomatous reaction	Granulomas	"Parasitized macrophages"	Pseudoepitheliomatous hyperplasia, microabscesses
Organism at 37° C	Gelatinous: 4–12 μm Granulomatous: 2–4 μm	Spherule (40–60 μm) containing endospores	Oval yeast (2–4 μm) with surrounding clear space	Thick-walled spore (8–15 μm), broad-based budding
Diagnostic Studies	Direct examination Culture Antigen detection	Direct examination Culture Serology Skin test	Direct examination Culture Serology Skin test Antigen detection	Direct examination Culture

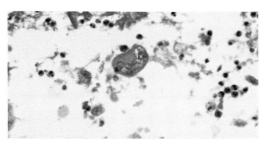

FIGURE 120-6. In chromoblastomycosis, diagnostic "sclerotic bodies" are evident as brown, septated yeast forms, seen here in a giant cell.

cally, the "black dots" are sites of transepidermal elimination of necrotic debris and sclerotic bodies.

ETIOLOGY AND PATHOGENESIS

Several dematiaceous fungi can produce chromoblastomycosis: *Fonsecaea compactum, F. pedrosoi, Phialophora verrucosa, Cladosporium carrionii,* and *Rhinocladiella aquaspersa.* Infection arises through accidental inoculation of the organism into the skin. Involvement of other organs, although rare, results from hematogenous spread.

DIAGNOSIS AND DIFFERENTIAL DIAGNOSIS

Both a potassium hydroxide examination of scrapings from "black dot" areas and a biopsy specimen will reveal characteristic sclerotic bodies. A culture of pus or tissue is essential for diagnosis. Good growth occurs at 25° C to 30° C on fungal media with chloramphenicol and cycloheximide after 6 weeks, yielding green-black colonies with a velvety surface. Precipitating and complement-fixing antibodies may be helpful in following the course of the disease. Skin testing is not helpful. The differential diagnosis includes blastomycosis, yaws, and leprosy (Table 120–11).

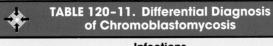

TABLE 120-11. Differential Diagnosis of Chromoblastomycosis

Infections
Blastomycosis
Lobomycosis
Mycetoma
Sporotrichosis
Tuberculosis verrucosa cutis
Mycobacterium marinum infection
Leprosy
Tertiary syphilis
Yaws
Leishmaniasis

Other Disorder
Halogenoderma

TABLE 120-12. Treatment of Chromoblastomycosis

Flucytosine
Amphotericin B
Ketoconazole
Itraconazole
Saperconazole
Thiabendazole
Physical modalities: cryosurgery, heat
Surgery

TREATMENT

Both surgical and nonsurgical modalities have been useful. For localized disease, wide surgical excision is warranted. Both cryosurgery and local heat therapy can be effective physical modalities.[44-46] Chemotherapy should begin with flucytosine (100–200 mg/kg per day, given orally) either alone or in combination with other agents.[12, 44] Other effective drugs include amphotericin B, ketoconazole (200–400 mg per day, given orally), thiabendazole, and, most recently, the newer triazoles itraconazole (200–400 mg per day, given orally)[47] and saperconazole[48] (Table 120–12). As a rule, prolonged administration of the medications is necessary.

Mycetoma

DEFINITION

Mycetoma is a chronic infection of subcutaneous tissue characterized by tumefaction, sinus tract formation, and the presence of grains.

CLINICAL DESCRIPTION

Mycetoma occurs worldwide, most commonly in tropical and subtropical regions, where etiologic agents reside in soil. Men between the ages of 20 and 40 years old are most frequently affected, and occupational exposure to soil predisposes to infection. Etiologically, mycetoma is either actinomycetoma, caused by the filamentous actinomycete bacteria, or eumycetoma, caused by true fungi. In the United States, mycetoma is uncommon; when it occurs, *Pseudoallescheria boydii* is the most frequently isolated organism. In Mexico and Central and South America, *Nocardia brasiliensis* accounts for almost 90% of cases. *Madurella mycetomi* and *Streptomyces somaliensis* predominate in Africa, and *M. mycetomi* and *N. madurae* are common in India.

The triad of tumefaction, sinus tracts, and grains is characteristic of mycetoma. After traumatic inoculation, a nodule slowly develops, enlarges, and may discharge serosanguineous or purulent material (Fig. 120–7). Other nodules appear in contiguous fashion. Sinus tracts

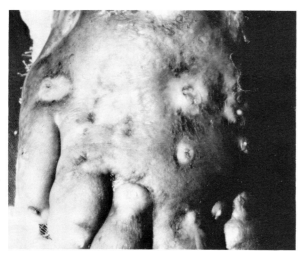

FIGURE 120–7. Mycetoma. Tumefaction and several draining nodules, many with visible grains, on the foot.

TABLE 120–13. Differential Diagnosis of Mycetoma

Infections

Botyromycosis
Actinomycosis
Cutaneous tuberculosis
Leprosy
Sporotrichosis
Chromoblastomycosis
Deep fungal infection
Syphilis
Yaws
Leishmaniasis

Other Disorders

Neoplasms
Foreign body granuloma
Kaposi's sarcoma

form and often interconnect. Grains, actually colonies of the causative organism, are hard concretions readily visible within drainage sites and affected tissue. Infection may spread to fascia, muscle, and bone. The repeated swelling, drainage, and subsequent fibrosis lead to enlargement and deformity of the affected site, usually an extremity. Mycetoma is generally painless; systemic symptoms usually occur only with secondary bacterial infection. The most common site of involvement is the dorsal foot. Mycetoma follows a chronic progressive course over years.

PATHOLOGY

Biopsy reveals suppurative granulomas and grains. The grains vary in size from 0.2 to 5 mm and are visible within abscesses. Eosinophilic "clubs," known as the Splendore-Hoeppli phenomenon, may surround the grains. The material in the clubs is derived in part from the granules of eosinophils. A Brown-Brenn, PAS-D, or silver stain provides better visualization of the organisms within the granules. True fungi appear as 3- to 5-μm wide septate hyphae. Actinomycetes appear as 1- to 2-μm wide branching filaments.

ETIOLOGY AND PATHOGENESIS

Both actinomycetes and true fungi can produce mycetoma. Causative agents of actinomycetoma include *N. brasiliensis*, *N. asteroides*, *N. madurae*, *S. somaliensis*, *S. pelletieri*, and *Actinomyces israelii*. Causative agents of eumycetoma include *M. mycetomi*, *M. grisea*, *P. boydii*, *Phialophora jeanselmi*, *Cephalosporium falciforme*, and *C. recifei*. Infection arises from repeated traumatic inoculation of the organism (i.e., via a thorn or splinter). The organism may ultimately invade underlying muscle and bone. Systemic infection is rare.

DIAGNOSIS AND DIFFERENTIAL DIAGNOSIS

The clinical triad establishes the diagnosis. Grain color, size, and shape help to identify an etiologic agent. Brown to black grains indicate true fungi only, such as *Madurella* species and *P. jeanselmi*. Red grains are characteristic of *S. pelletieri*. White to yellow granules are produced by the *Nocardia* species, *A. israelii*, *S. somaliensis*, *Pseudoallescheria boydii*, and *Cephalosporium* species. Radiography to evaluate bone involvement should be performed. Culture of pus, grains, or tissue helps to identify organisms. The true fungi grow on Sabouraud's medium with antibiotics; actinomycetes grow on Sabouraud's medium or brain-heart infusion agar without antibiotics. The differential diagnosis is listed in Table 120–13.

TREATMENT

The treatment of mycetoma is inexact and often problematic. In general, therapy is more successful for actinomycetoma than for eumycetoma. Surgery can be helpful, either through surgical excision of small nodules or through debridement of sinus tracts and diseased tissue in larger nodules and plaques.[49] Chemotherapy can be the main modality or adjunctive therapy with surgery. For actinomycetoma, streptomycin plus dapsone or trimethoprim-sulfamethoxazole (TMP-SMZ) has been effective therapy.[50] Doses used have included streptomycin, 1 g per day intramuscularly; dapsone, 200 mg per day orally; or TMP-SMZ (80 mg/400 mg), one to two tablets twice daily orally.[51] Other sulfonamides, tetracycline, erythromycin, rifampin, and amikacin have also been effective singly and in combination.[49, 51–53] Penicillin is the drug of choice for disease caused by *A. israelii*. For eumycetoma, griseofulvin, amphotericin B, flucytosine, miconazole, and oral azoles have yielded variable success (Table 120–14).

TABLE 120-14. Treatment of Mycetoma	
Actinomycetoma	**Eumycetoma**
Dapsone	Surgery
Trimethoprim-sulfamethoxazole	Amphotericin B
Other sulfonamides	Flucytosine
Streptomycin	Miconazole
Amikacin	Ketoconazole
Tetracyclines	Itraconazole
Isoniazid	Griseofulvin
Surgery	Thiabendazole
Penicillin (for *A. israelii*)	Penicillin

Table 120–15 summarizes the principal features of the subcutaneous mycoses.

Other Opportunistic Mycoses

Opportunistic fungal infections have become increasingly prevalent in patients debilitated and/or immunodeficient by either disease (e.g., AIDS, cancer, especially leukemia and lymphoma) or therapy. Despite prompt diagnosis and antifungal therapy, the mortality rate in affected patients is still high, ranging between 50% and 90%.[54] The most common opportunistic fungi are species of *Candida, Rhizopus, Aspergillus,* and *Cryptococcus,* although any fungus has the potential to produce invasive disease in a compromised host. Causative organisms, which can be molds (aspergillosis and zygomycosis), yeasts (cryptococcosis and candidiasis), or hyaline/dematiaceous fungi (hyalohyphomycosis and phaeohyphomycosis), thrive at 37° C, assume the same form in tissue and in vitro, and lack dimorphism. They are negligibly virulent and usually not contagious.

ASPERGILLOSIS

Aspergillosis is primarily a pulmonary infection of immunocompromised or chronically debilitated patients; with dissemination, skin disease can occur. Predisposing factors include neutropenia, hematologic malignancy, immunodeficiency (e.g., AIDS, organ transplantation), and corticosteroid or cytotoxic therapy.[55] *Aspergillus fumigatus* is the most common human pathogen, although *A. flavus, A. niger, A. terreus,* and *A. nidulans* can also cause disease.[55] Skin disease usually implies dissemination but may occur as a primary event in healthy or ill patients. *A. fumigatus* is the usual pathogen with dissemination, while *A. flavus* causes primary infection. Patients with disseminated disease may develop reddened macules, papules, pustules, nodules, or granulomas; cellulitis, purpura, and ulceration are less common. In primary aspergillosis, indurated purple plaques and nodules, hemorrhagic bullae, or cellulitis usually follows trauma; ulceration with a black eschar may develop.[55] Skin biopsy, with special staining (e.g., methenamine silver) to identify septated, branching hyphae, is necessary to establish diagnosis. Cultures, which are often negative, help to confirm the diagnosis.

TABLE 120-15. Subcutaneous Mycoses

	Sporotrichosis	Mycetoma	Chromoblastomycosis

Organism	*Sporothrix schenckii*	Actinomycetoma
		    Nocardia brasiliensis
		    N. asteroides
		    N. madurae
		    Streptomyces somaliensis
		    S. pelletieri
		    Actinomyces israelii
		Eumycetoma
		    Madurella mycetomi
		    M. grisea
		    Pseudoallescheria boydii
		    Phialophora jeanselmi
		    Cephalosporium falciforme
		    C. recifei
			Fonsecaea compactum
			F. pedrosoi
			Phialophora verrucosa
			Cladosporium carrionii
			Rhinocladiella aquaspersa

Distribution	Worldwide	Tropics, subtropics	Tropics, subtropics
Site of Involvement	Dominant Upper extremity	Foot/leg	Foot/leg

Clinical Findings	Nodule/chancre with
	    ascending nodular
	    lymphangitis
		Tumefaction
		Sinuses
		Grains
		Bone involvement
			Verrucous plaque with "black dots"

Histology	Acute and chronic
	    inflammation;
	    asteroid bodies
		Suppurative granulomas; grains:
		    0.2–5 mm
			Medlar bodies (6–12 µm);
			    mixed infiltrate

Diagnostic Studies	Culture Serology	Morphology of grains Culture Bone radiographs	Direct examination Culture Serology

ZYGOMYCOSIS

Zygomycosis represents a severe, often lethal, infection with a fungus from the genera *Absidia, Mucor, Rhizopus,* or *Cunninghamella*—"bread molds" of the class *Zygomycetes* that are ubiquitous. Infections, usually with a *Rhizopus* species, are most common in patients with diabetes, leukemia, and lymphoma[56]; disease rarely occurs in healthy persons. Rhinocerebral disease is the most common presentation and occurs most often in patients with diabetic ketoacidosis. Disease is invariably severe and fulminant. Patients have facial edema; often unilateral, bloody nasal discharge; ulcers of the septum and palate, usually with adherent, necrotic tissue; headache; and altered mental status. Infection can extend rapidly to produce ophthalmoplegia, orbital apex syndrome, thrombosis of the cavernous sinus and carotid artery, and brain abscess.[56] Skin disease can be a primary event, usually as a secondary infection of burns. With infection, healthy persons usually, after trauma or fracture, have superficial disease manifested by vesicles, pustules, or plaques. Compromised patients usually have gangrenous disease with purple-red plaques or indurated, dusky nodules that may be painful.[54] The pathologic hallmark of infection is hyphal invasion of blood vessels that yields thrombus formation, infarction of surrounding tissues, and necrotic black debris.

PHAEOHYPHOMYCOSIS AND HYALOHYPHOMYCOSIS

The phaeohyphomycoses are infections with fungi with septated hyphae that are dematiaceous (brown or pigmented) in tissue (e.g., species of *Alternaria, Bipolaris, Curvularia, Exserohilum,* and *Exophiala*). Organisms that cause chromoblastomycosis are also dematiaceous but have sclerotic bodies on biopsy. Classified as superficial, cutaneous and corneal, subcutaneous, or systemic,[57] skin disease, which is usually nonspecific and nondescript, can occur with dissemination or after primary inoculation. Invasive disease requires a compromised host or setting (e.g., burns).

The hyalohyphomycoses are infections with fungi with septated hyphae that are hyaline (nonpigmented) in tissue (e.g., species of *Acremonium, Chrysosporium, Fusarium, Paecilomyces, Penicillium, Pseudoallescheria, Scopulariopsis,* and *Sepedonium*). Opportunistic infections with these organisms are uncommon. Scopulariopsis can produce onychomycosis; *A. falciforme* is a frequent cause of mycetoma in the United States; and *Paecilomyces* and *Penicillium* rarely produce disease. *Fusarium* species, plant pathogens common in soil, have become serious and often fatal pathogens in patients with leukemia.[58] Skin disease is usually extensive, characterized by red, purple, or hemorrhagic papules or plaques that may ulcerate. *F. moniliforme* and *F. roseum* are the main cutaneous pathogens.

ALGAE

Algae, which are ubiquitous, unicellular, achloric organisms, rarely produce skin disease. *Prototheca* species,

specifically *P. wickerhami* and *P. zopfi,* can produce a nonspecific dermatitis or abscess in a compromised host.[59] Disease is chronic, and therapy is problematic, dependent on debridement and either amphotericin B or ketoconazole.

TREATMENT

Amphotericin B is the mainstay of treatment for these opportunistic mycoses, despite its limitations (i.e., toxicity) and limited success. The exact dose and duration are variable, with 1 g or more accepted as standard. Debridement is often necessary as adjunctive therapy in individual cases. Itraconazole, 200 to 400 mg per day, may soon be the accepted alternative to amphotericin, at least for aspergillosis,[60] and perhaps for the phaeohyphomycoses as well. Unfortunately, neither itraconazole nor fluconazole is effective against zygomycoses.

References

1. Powderly WG. Therapy for cryptococcal meningitis in patients with AIDS. Clin Infect Dis 1992;14(Suppl 1):S54–S59.
2. Chuck SL, Sande MA. Infections with *Cryptococcus neoformans* in the acquired immunodeficiency syndrome. N Engl J Med 1989;321:794–799.
3. Bozzette SA, Larsen RA, Chiu J, et al. A placebo-controlled trial of maintenance therapy with fluconazole after treatment of cryptococcal meningitis in the acquired immunodeficiency syndrome. N Engl J Med 1991;324:580–584.
4. Hernandez AD. Cutaneous cryptococcosis. Dermatol Clin 1989;7:269–274.
5. Barfield L, Iacobelli D, Hashimoto K. Secondary cutaneous cryptococcosis: Case report and review of 22 cases. Cutan Pathol 1988;15:385–392.
6. Anderson DJ, Schmidt C, Goodman J. Cryptococcal disease presenting as cellulitis. Clin Infect Dis 1992;14:666–672.
7. Rico MJ, Penneys NS. Cutaneous cryptococcosis resembling molluscum contagiosum in a patient with AIDS. Arch Dermatol 1985;121:901–902.
8. Manrique P, Mayo J, Alvarez JA, et al. Polymorphous cutaneous cryptococcosis: Nodular, herpes-like, and molluscum-like lesions in a patient with the acquired immunodeficiency syndrome. J Am Acad Dermatol 1992;26:122–124.
9. Blauvelt A, Kerdel FA. Cutaneous cryptococcosis mimicking Kaposi's sarcoma as the initial manifestation of disseminated disease. Int J Dermatol 1992;31:279–280.
10. Shuttleworth D, Philpot CM, Knight AG. Cutaneous cryptococcosis: Treatment with oral fluconazole. Br J Dermatol 1989; 120:683–687.
11. British Society for Antimicrobial Chemotherapy Working Party. Antifungal chemotherapy in patients with acquired immunodeficiency syndrome. Lancet 1992;340:648–651.
12. Drugs for treatment of fungal infections. Med Lett Drugs Ther 1992;34:14–16.
13. Denning DW, Tucker RM, Hanson LH, et al. Itraconazole in opportunistic mycoses: Cryptococcosis and aspergillosis. J Am Acad Dermatol 1990;23:602–607.
14. Feldman SR, Fleischer AB, Resnick SD. Fluconazole treatment of cutaneous cryptococcosis. Arch Dermatol 1992;128:1045–1046.
15. Belknap BS. Sporotrichosis. Dermatol Clin 1989;7:193–202.
16. Itoh M, Okamoto S, Kariya H. Survey of 200 cases of sporotrichosis. Dermatologica 1986;72:209–213.
17. Shaw JC, Levinson W, Montanaro A. Sporotrichosis in the acquired immunodeficiency syndrome. J Am Acad Dermatol 1989;21:1145–1147.
18. Penn CC, Goldstein E, Bartholomew WR. *Sporothrix schenckii* meningitis in a patient with AIDS. Clin Infect Dis 1992;15: 741–743.
19. Bullpitt P, Weedon D. Sporotrichosis: A review of 39 cases. Pathology 1978;10:249–256.

20. Scott EN, Kaufman L, Brown AC, et al. Serologic studies in the diagnosis and management of meningitis due to *Sporothrix schenckii*. N Engl J Med 1987;317:935–940.
21. Pluss JL, Opal SM. Pulmonary sporotrichosis: Review of treatment and outcome. Medicine 1986;65:143–153.
22. Breeling JL, Weinstein L. Pulmonary sporotrichosis treated with itraconazole. Chest 1993;103:313–316.
23. Hobbs ER. Coccidioidomycosis. Dermatol Clin 1989;7:227–239.
24. Fish DG, Ampel NM, Galgiani JN, et al. Coccidioidomycosis during human immunodeficiency virus infection: A review of 77 patients. Medicine 1990;69:384–391.
25. Galgiani JN, Ampel NM. Coccidioidomycosis in human immunodeficiency virus-infected patients. J Infect Dis 1990;162:1165–1169.
26. Robinson PA, Knirsch AK, Joseph JA. Fluconazole for life-threatening fungal infections in patients who cannot be treated with conventional antifungal agents. Rev Infect Dis 1990;12:S349–S363.
27. Tucker RM, Denning DW, Arathoon EG, et al. Itraconazole therapy for nonmeningeal coccidioidomycosis: Clinical and laboratory observations. J Am Acad Dermatol 1990;23:593–601.
28. Graybill JR, Stevens DA, Galgiani JN, et al. Itraconazole treatment of coccidioidomycosis. Am J Med 1990;89:282–290.
29. Diaz M, Puente R, de Hoyos LA, et al. Itraconazole in the treatment of coccidioidomycosis. Chest 1991;100:682–684.
30. Tucker RM, Denning DW, Dupont B, et al. Itraconazole therapy for chronic coccidioidal meningitis. Ann Intern Med 1990;112:108–112.
31. Wheat LJ. Histoplasmosis in Indianapolis. Clin Infect Dis 1992;14(Suppl 1):S91–S99.
32. Dijkstra JWE. Histoplasmosis. Dermatol Clin 1989;7:251–258.
33. Eidbo J, Sanchez RL, Tschen JA, et al. Cutaneous manifestations of histoplasmosis in the acquired immune deficiency syndrome. Am J Surg Pathol 1993;17:110–116.
34. Wheat LJ, Connolly-Stringfield PA, Baker RL, et al. Disseminated histoplasmosis in the acquired immune deficiency syndrome: Clinical findings, diagnosis, and treatment, and review of the literature. Medicine 1990;69:361–374.
35. Cohen PR, Bank DE, Silvers DN, et al. Cutaneous lesions of disseminated histoplasmosis in human immunodeficiency virus-infected patients. J Am Acad Dermatol 1990;23:422–428.
36. Wasserteil V, Jimenez-Acosta FJ, Kerdel FA. Disseminated histoplasmosis presenting as a rosacea-like eruption in a patient with the acquired immunodeficiency syndrome. Int J Dermatol 1990;29:649–651.
37. Mayoral F, Penneys NS. Disseminated histoplasmosis presenting as a transepidermal elimination disorder in an AIDS victim. J Am Acad Dermatol 1985;13:842–844.
38. Dismukes WE, Bradsher RW Jr, Cloud GC, et al. Itraconazole therapy for blastomycosis and histoplasmosis. Am J Med 1992;93:489–497.
39. Murphy PA. Blastomycosis. JAMA 1989;261:3159–3162.
40. Bradsher RW. Blastomycosis. Clin Infect Dis 1992;14(Suppl 1):S82–S90.
41. Pappas PG, Pottage JC, Powderly WG, et al. Blastomycosis in patients with the acquired immunodeficiency syndrome. Ann Intern Med 1992;116:847–853.
42. National Institute of Allergy and Infectious Diseases Mycoses Study Group. Treatment of blastomycosis and histoplasmosis with ketoconazole. Ann Intern Med 1985;103:861–872.
43. Steck WD. Blastomycosis. Dermatol Clin 1989;7:241–250.
44. Milam CP, Fenske NA. Chromoblastomycosis. Dermatol Clin 1989;7:219–225.
45. Tuffanelli L, Milburn PB. Treatment of chromoblastomycosis. J Am Acad Dermatol 1990;23:728–732.
46. Pimentel ERA, Castro LGM, Cuce LC, et al. Treatment of chromomycosis by cryosurgery with liquid nitrogen: A report on eleven cases. J Dermatol Surg Oncol 1989;15:72–77.
47. Queiroz-Telles F, Purim KS, Fillus JN, et al. Itraconazole in the treatment of chromoblastomycosis due to *Fonsecaea pedrosoi*. Int J Dermatol 1992;31:805–812.
48. Franco L, Gomez I, Restrepo A. Saperconazole in the treatment of systemic and subcutaneous mycoses. Int J Dermatol 1992;31:725–729.
49. Palestine RF, Rogers RS III. Diagnosis and treatment of mycetoma. J Am Acad Dermatol 1982;6:107–111.
50. Mahgoub ES. Medical management of mycetoma. Bull WHO 1976;54:303–310.
51. Magana M, Magana-Garcia M. Mycetoma. Dermatol Clin 1989;7:203–217.
52. McElroy JA, de Almeida Prestes C, Su WPD. Mycetoma: Infection with tumefaction, draining sinuses, and grains. Cutis 1992;49:107–110.
53. Welsh O. Mycetoma: Current concepts in treatment. Int J Dermatol 1991;30:387–398.
54. Radentz WH. Opportunistic fungal infections in immunocompromised hosts. J Am Acad Dermatol 1989;20:989–1003.
55. Rinaldi MG. Invasive aspergillosis. Rev Infect Dis 1983;5:1061–1077.
56. Parfrey NA. Improved diagnosis and prognosis of mucormycosis: A clinicopathologic study of 33 cases. Medicine 1986;65:13–23.
57. McGinnis MR. Chromoblastomycosis and phaeohyphomycosis: New concepts, diagnosis, and mycology. J Am Acad Dermatol 1983;8:1–16.
58. Anaissie E, Kantarjian H, Ro J, et al. The emerging role of *Fusarium* infections in patients with cancer. Medicine 1988;67:77–83.
59. Kuo T, Hsueh J, Wu J, Wang A. Cutaneous protothecosis. Arch Pathol Lab Med 1987;111:737–740.
60. Itraconazole. Med Lett Drugs Ther 1993;35:7–9.

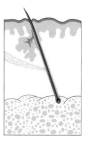

chapter 121

Herpesvirus Infections

ROY GULICK

Herpes Simplex Virus

DEFINITION

There are seven closely related human herpesviruses: herpes simplex virus (HSV) 1 and 2, varicella zoster virus (VZV), Epstein-Barr virus (EBV), cytomegalovirus (CMV), human herpesvirus 6 (HHV 6), and human herpesvirus 7 (HHV 7). HSV may be separated from the others by specific antigen analyses, and host cell infectivity and cytopathologic characteristics. HSV is subdivided into two closely related types: HSV 1 and HSV 2. HSV contains a double-stranded linear DNA genome with about 50% homology of nucleotide sequences occurring between HSV 1 and 2.[1] The viral genome is enclosed in a protein coat with an outer lipid envelope.

The HSV genome codes for a number of viral-specific proteins, including type-specific membrane glycoproteins, which mediate cell-cell fusion and which are recognized by specific neutralizing antibodies. The major glycoproteins of HSV 1 and 2 are closely related, with 80% homology.[2] Neutralizing antibodies induced to the glycoproteins are cross reactive between the two types.

Other specific proteins are involved in the replication of HSV DNA—viral thymidine kinase, viral DNA polymerase, and other specific enzymes. These HSV enzymes, which vary significantly from their host cell counterparts, serve as targets for the development of specific antiviral inhibitors. Completion of the viral replication process is associated with lysis of the infected cell.

CLINICAL DESCRIPTION

Epidemiology

HSV infection is one of the most common viral infections of man. Oral-labial HSV, most commonly caused by HSV 1, affects an estimated one third of the population of the United States. Worldwide, more than 85% of adult populations from both urban and rural areas show serologic evidence of prior HSV 1 exposure.[3] The disparity between viral exposure and frank clinical manifestations has been demonstrated in several studies: In one of these, 46% of graduating college students had a positive HSV 1 serology, whereas only 28% gave a history of cold sores.[4]

An estimated 25 million American adults have serologic evidence of exposure to HSV 2, the most common cause of genital herpes.[5] HSV infection accounts for an estimated 20% to 50% of genital lesions, and the incidence of genital herpes infections has increased markedly in recent years in the United States.[6] Holmberg and associates found that there is a higher prevalence of exposure to HSV 2 in those infected with human immunodeficiency virus (HIV) (68%) than in their seronegative counterparts (46%).[7] In fact, both a history of genital ulcer disease and the presence of antibody to HSV 2 have been associated with acquiring HIV infection in both heterosexual and homosexual groups in Africa,[8, 9] the United States,[10] and Europe.[11]

Primary herpes infection is defined as the first viral exposure in a seronegative individual. Most often this involves direct mucocutaneous contact between uninfected and infected individuals. There is no known transmission of HSV from respiratory contact or fomites. After primary infection, HSV establishes a latent infection in the nerve root ganglion,[12] and then may reactivate to cause disease recurrences.

Clinical Findings

Primary orofacial herpes infection manifests about 5 to 10 days after exposure to an infected individual. Primary infection is most common in children and young adults. Involvement varies from subclinical to severe, and there may be fever, pharyngitis, and painful vesicles

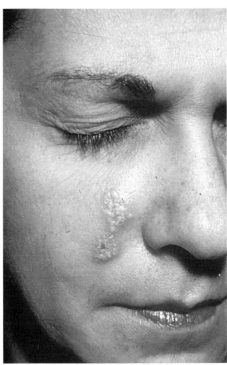

FIGURE 121–1. Orofacial herpes simplex virus (HSV). A cluster of tender vesicles on the face. (Courtesy of the Department of Dermatology, New York University.)

progressing to ulcers on the face, lips, tongue, and oral mucosa, accompanied by lymphadenopathy (Fig. 121–1). Primary HSV infection is a common cause of acute pharyngitis in college students.[13]

Primary genital herpes occurs 3 days to 2 weeks after exposure from an infected sexual partner, who often sheds the virus asymptomatically[14] (Fig. 121–2). Acute genital herpes manifests as a group of painful vesicles

that progress to ulcers over several days. Primary disease is typically severe, with large, multiple ulcerations, and tender inguinal lymphadenopathy. A minority of patients also have an aseptic meningitis.[15]

Up to 20% of patients with acute genital herpes have dysuria and some develop frank urinary retention, requiring intervention. Symptoms and the formation of the new lesions continue together with active viral shedding for 7 to 10 days, with compete resolution of lesions by about 3 weeks. HSV 2 is the etiologic agent in the majority of genital HSV cases. HSV 1 produces the same acute clinical syndrome, but is associated with fewer recurrences.

Neonatal HSV develops most frequently after exposure to infected maternal vaginal secretions during delivery, and, if left untreated, is associated with a significant mortality rate.[16] Most mothers of infants with neonatal herpes infection do not have a history of genital herpes, and are unaware of their prior exposure. Current data suggest that the risk to the newborn is highest when the mother acquires a primary genital herpes infection during pregnancy. Recommendations for the management of such women have been made recently.[17]

Herpes gladiatorum is the name given to cutaneous or ocular HSV 1 infections acquired in wrestlers and rugby players through sports contact.[18, 19] A recent outbreak at a wrestling camp demonstrated a high incidence of transmission in unusual locations including the head, trunk, and extremities.[20] This pattern was most consistent with transmission by direct skin-to-skin contact.

Recurrent herpes infections occur when latent virus is reactivated. Precipitating factors that promote viral protein synthesis and clinical recurrences are sunlight exposure, fatigue, menstruation, stress, trauma, and surgical manipulation. The mechanism of viral reactivation is not well understood. In general, recurrent infections with herpes are less severe than primary disease. Neutralizing

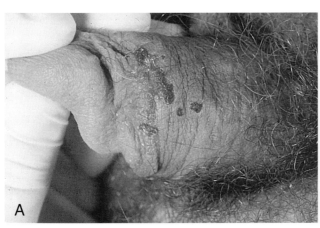
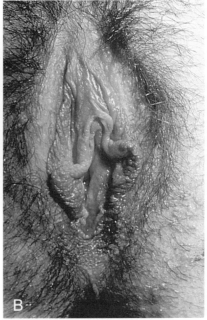

FIGURE 121–2. Genital HSV. *A,* Crusted vesicles on the shaft of the penis. *B,* Vesicles and erosions on the labia and perineum. (Courtesy of the Department of Dermatology, New York University.)

antibodies to HSV proteins do not protect against recurrent episodes.

Recurrent orofacial HSV manifests most commonly as oral or labial "cold sores" with an average of three to four episodes a year.[21] Local dysesthesias precede the appearance of a cluster of small papulovesicles that quickly ulcerate, often at the border of the lip. Crusting occurs in a few days, and viral shedding ceases. Complete healing of lesions occurs within about 10 days.

Recurrent genital herpes typically occurs within a year of primary infection. Individuals typically experience three to four recurrent outbreaks a year, although some will have eight or more. Recurrence is often heralded by prodromal symptoms of burning or tingling at the site of the outbreak. A cluster of painful vesicles appears with progression to ulceration and crusting. The lesions are typically fewer in number and smaller than in primary disease, and there are milder constitutional symptoms. Recurrent disease is more common with HSV 2 than HSV 1.

Many cases of erythema multiforme follow recurrent cutaneous herpes simplex. Herpetic DNA is detectable in the lesional keratinocytes of many cases of erythema multiforme associated with herpes simplex, as are viral antigens, and virions have actually been recovered from rare cases (see Chapter 22).

Herpetic whitlow refers to herpetic infection of the fingers or hands[22] (Fig. 121–3). Direct manual contact with oral or genital lesions[23] leads to infection with formation of painful vesicles, edema, and ulceration, which may be prolonged. Health care workers should wear latex gloves when contacting oral or genital lesions or saliva from patients to prevent such infections. HSV rarely causes noncutaneous systemic diseases including encephalitis, esophagitis, retinitis, pneumonitis, and disseminated cutaneous disease in immunosuppressed and less commonly, in immunocompetent hosts. Patients with severe preexisting cutaneous diseases, particularly atopic dermatitis and Darier's disease, are at risk to develop widespread HSV infection. This is most common in atopic patients, and is referred to as eczema leupeticum. It may resemble impetigo or be confused with a similar

clinical picture caused by infection with the vaccinia virus (eczema vaccination). Kaposi's varicelliform eruption refers to the localized or widespread cutaneous viral infection caused by either virus.

PATHOLOGY

Similar histopathologic findings are seen in cutaneous lesions of herpes simplex and herpes zoster. The earliest change in papular lesions seems to be in the nuclei of keratinocytes of the basal layer, which develop an homogeneous "steel gray" appearance, with peripheral margination of chromatin. In addition, herpetically infected keratinocytes can contain eosinophilic intranuclear inclusions, and some cells are multinucleated. To the side of these changes, and at the periphery of vesicular lesions, there is often an interface dermatitis that can resemble that of erythema multiforme, which is associated in many cases with herpes simplex viral DNA within the nuclei of lesional keratinocytes.

As papulovesicles develop, ballooning of keratinocytes occurs. Ballooning is intracytoplasmic edema, in contrast to spongiosis, or intracellular edema, and results in enlarged keratinocytes with pallid cytoplasm. As the cell membranes of keratinocytes rupture, reticular degeneration of the epidermis ensues, with strands of cytoplasmic membranes that are still interconnected. Intraepidermal vesiculation is usually present in vesicular lesions, although some herpetic vesicles are subepidermal as the result of "blow-out" of intraepidermal vesicles. Acantholytic keratinocytes often reside within vesicles, and can show the herpetic nuclear changes outlined above as well as multinucleation (Fig. 121–4). In late lesions of herpetic dermatitis, many neutrophils are present within blister cavities, along with nuclear dust, resulting in a "dirty" appearance. The nuclei of infected keratinocytes can dissolve, giving rise to nuclear ghosts, sometimes of multinucleated keratinocytes. Secondary vasculitis is sometimes present beneath late herpetic vesicles, with neutrophils and nuclear dust surrounding venules, some of which have endothelial cells with herpetic nuclear changes.

One variant of herpetic dermatitis occurs when follicular epithelium rather than surface epidermis is the major site of involvement. This results in a necrotizing folliculitis and ulceration, rather than intraepidermal vesicular dermatitis. Keratinocytes with viropathic changes and necrosis of keratinocytes occur in sebaceous as well as infundibular epithelium.

DIAGNOSIS AND DIFFERENTIAL DIAGNOSIS

Herpes infection is suspected when a patient presents with a cluster of small vesicles or erosions arising from erythematous, edematous skin on a mucocutaneous surface. To confirm the clinical impression, a Tzanck smear and/or viral culture of the lesion may be performed. A positive Tzanck smear (Fig. 121–5), indicated by the presence of multinucleated keratinocytic giant cells, signifies the presence of a herpesvirus family infection (ei-

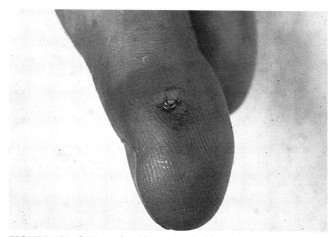

FIGURE 121–3. Herpetic whitlow. A painful vesicle and erythema on the fingertip. (Courtesy of the Department of Dermatology, New York University.)

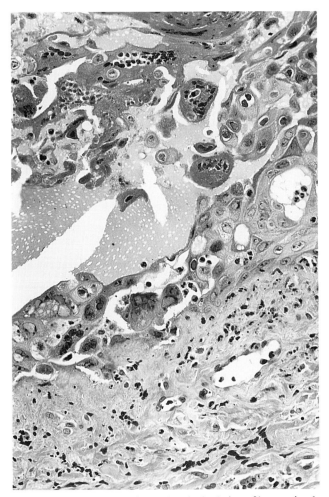

FIGURE 121–4. An intraepidermal vesicular lesion of herpes simplex featuring acantholytic keratinocytes, some of which are multinucleated.

✛ TABLE 121–1. Differential Diagnosis of Herpes Simplex Virus Infection	
Primary Herpetic Gingivostomatitis	

Bacterial pharyngitis
Enterovirus infection (e.g.,
  hand, foot, and mouth
  disease, herpangina)
Aphthous ulcers
Infectious mononucleosis
Primary human
  immunodeficiency virus
  infection
	Candidiasis
	Pemphigus
	Erythema multiforme
	Vincent's angina
	  (ulceromembranous
	  stomatitis)

Recurrent Orofacial Herpes Simplex	
Impetigo Aphthous stomatitis Erythema multiforme	
Primary and Recurrent Genital Herpes	
Syphilis Lymphogranuloma venereum Chancroid venereum Granuloma inguinale Trauma	Gonorrhea (vulvovaginitis) Candidiasis (vulvovaginitis)

ther HSV or VZV). To perform a Tzanck smear, one unroofs an active vesicular lesion, takes a sample of cells from the base or roof of the vesicle, and transfers it to a glass slide. The slide is stained with a Wright-Giemsa stain, and examined for the presence of characteristic

giant cells. Late lesions of herpes simplex often feature multinucleated "ghost cells," whose nuclei have largely dissolved, leaving behind empty spaces, and may have a background of neutrophilic debris. Their presence supports the diagnosis of herpesvirus infection.

The gold standard for diagnosis of HSV infections is viral culture of vesicular fluid or skin biopsy material. In clinical studies, viral culture from characteristic lesions is revealing in up to 90% of specimens. Serologic studies for the demonstration of antibodies to HSV 1 and HSV 2 are typically not warranted, since positivity simply implicates prior exposure. The differential diagnosis of HSV infections is noted in Table 121–1.

TREATMENT

Acyclovir is the treatment of choice for HSV infections.[24] As an analog of guanosine, it is specifically taken up by virally infected cells and subsequently phosphorylated to its monophosphate form by viral-specific thymidine kinase. Host cell enzymes produce acyclovir triphosphate, which both inhibits the viral DNA polymerase and functions as a viral DNA chain terminator. Due to its specific uptake, and viral enzyme inhibition,[25] acyclovir remains a remarkably safe and active drug with low toxicity.

The use of acyclovir in treating primary genital herpes infections is well established.[26, 27] Patients received oral acyclovir at a dose of 200 mg five times daily or placebo for a total of 10 days. Compared with placebo, acyclovir patients had decreased viral shedding, pain, and fewer new lesions and more rapid healing. The use of topical acyclovir in a controlled trial also reduced viral shedding

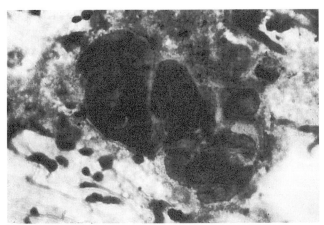

FIGURE 121–5. Tzanck smear. Material scraped from the base of a vesicle and stained with methylene blue reveals multinucleated giant cells, consistent with a herpesvirus infection. (Courtesy of the Department of Dermatology, New York University.)

and time to healing, but is less effective than the oral preparation.

The treatment of recurrent genital herpes with acyclovir was evaluated in a controlled clinical trial that compared patient-initiated acyclovir versus placebo.[28] Acyclovir therapy was most effective when initiated within 48 hours of prodromal symptoms, and resulted in decreased viral shedding, new lesion formation, and time to complete healing.

The treatment of orofacial herpes in immune competent hosts with topical acyclovir demonstrated decreased viral shedding but not a decrease in pain or an increased rate of healing.[29] In immunocompromised hosts with orofacial herpes, both topical and parenteral acyclovir therapy are beneficial.[30, 31]

Effectiveness in the prevention of recurrence of both orofacial and genital herpes infections with acyclovir has been shown in both immunocompetent and immunosuppressed hosts.[32-35] A dose of 400 mg of oral acyclovir twice daily markedly reduces recurrent epidsodes, without significant toxicity over literally years of treatment.

With the widespread use of repeated courses of acyclovir in immunocompromised hosts (with typically large viral loads), the development of acyclovir-resistant HSV disease, most commonly due to altered viral thymidine kinase activity, has occurred[36-38] (Fig. 121–6). Ehrlich and colleagues reported 12 patients with acquired immunodeficiency syndrome (AIDS) and severe mucocutaneous HSV infections (both oral and genital) that had previously responded to acyclovir, but subsequently developed evidence of clinical and laboratory resistance to acyclovir.[39] To date, immunocompetent hosts have not shown evidence of acyclovir-resistant HSV, despite widespread acyclovir usage.

The occurrence of acyclovir-resistant HSV disease prompted the search for other effective antiviral therapies. Foscarnet (phosphonoformic acid), an analogue of pyrophosphate that does not require viral thymidine kinase phosphorylation to its active form, directly inhibits viral DNA polymerase. At a dose of 40 mg/kg every 8 hours for 2 weeks, intravenous foscarnet demonstrated its effectiveness in treating acyclovir-resistant HSV infec-

tion in several clinical trials.[40, 41] Current clinical studies are assessing the need for maintenance antiviral therapy for resistant HSV infection.

Another potential treatment for acyclovir-resistant HSV is trifluorothymidine (trifluridine), which has been used as a topical solution for the treatment of HSV keratitis since the 1960s. Several reports suggest the effectiveness of the drug in resistant HSV lesions.[42, 43] Topical solution is applied directly to the lesion as a thin film, sealing with an occlusive dressing, twice daily. Prolonged treatment (up to 6 weeks or more) is required for complete healing.

Varicella-Zoster Virus (VZV)

DEFINITION

Varicella zoster virus (VZV) is a member of the human herpesvirus family and shares many properties with the other viruses. The virus consists of a double-stranded DNA genome enclosed by a protein core and a glycoprotein envelope.[44] The genome encodes more than 75 viral proteins.

Primary infection occurs in the nasopharynx via the respiratory route. Local viral replication in the upper respiratory tract leads to viremia,[45] with subsequent dissemination to the skin and viscera, causing primary VZV disease, varicella (chickenpox). VZV is intracellular and spreads by direct cell-to-cell contact. Only enveloped virus is infectious.

The sensory nerve ganglia are likely infected during the primary viremia, and become the site of latent VZV infection.[46, 47] The mechanism of latent VZV infection is poorly understood. At some point, the virus becomes reactivated, likely secondary to cellular immune system changes,[48] and manifests as secondary VZV disease, herpes zoster (shingles).

CLINICAL DESCRIPTION

Epidemiology

Exposure to VZV is nearly universal in developed countries.[49] In the United States, primary VZV infection, varicella, is primarily a disease of children, with up to 4 million annual cases. Ninety per cent of such cases occur in children ages 1 to 14. In tropical and subtropical climates, varicella occurs more frequently in older age groups.

Both sexes and all races are equally susceptible. Varicella infection is endemic in the population, with localized epidemics occurring in the winter and early spring in the United States. More than 90% of American adults show serologic evidence of previous VZV infection.

Varicella is highly infectious, with transmission likely to occur from an infected individual who has intimate contact with a susceptible host via the respiratory route.

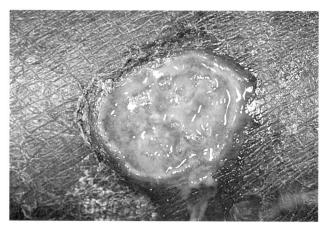

FIGURE 121–6. Resistant HSV. Persistent cutaneous erosion in an human immunodeficiency virus (HIV)-infected patient on chronic acyclovir therapy was culture positive for HSV. (Courtesy of the Department of Dermatology, New York University.)

The secondary attack rate in susceptible household contacts is over 70%.[50] This has implications for both day care and school-age children as well as susceptible health care workers. Prior to AIDS, about 100 annual deaths were attributed to varicella and its complications.[51]

Reactivated VZV infection, herpes zoster, occurs at all ages, though uncommonly under the age of 50. Zoster affects over 10% of the total population over their lifetimes.[52] Prior to the AIDS epidemic, an estimated 300,000 to 400,000 cases of zoster occurred annually in the United States. Reactivation of infection depends on the interaction of viral and host immune factors, though this is not well understood. There is little evidence to suggest that exposure to an active case of VZV infection causes VZV reactivation.

Patients with immune compromise from advanced age, malignancy, immunosuppressive medications, and HIV infection have significantly higher rates of herpes zoster infection.[48, 53-55] In a cohort of gay men, the age-adjusted relative risk of developing zoster was 17 times higher in HIV-infected men than in their seronegative counterparts.[56]

Although the incidence of zoster is increased in patients with malignancies, a population-based study demonstrated no increase in the incidence of cancer in individuals presenting with herpes zoster.[52] Several recent studies suggested that the occurrence of herpes zoster in populations at risk for HIV infection is highly predictive of HIV seropositivity.[57, 58] It is reasonable to suggest HIV testing in such patients.

Clinical Findings

Primary VZV infection manifests about 2 weeks after exposure to an infectious individual (range 10 to 20 days).[59] Clinical signs may be preceded by a prodrome of fever, chills, malaise, myalgias, and arthralgias for a day or two. The characteristic eruption begins as erythematous maculopapules that rapidly progress to vesicles. The classic description of "dew drop on a rose petal" describes a small fluid-filled vesicle on an erythematous base. Initially, lesions appear on the head or trunk, with subsequent crops of lesions extending centripetally over 2 to 4 days to involve the extremities, including the palms and soles, and less commonly, the oral and genital mucosa (Fig. 121-7). The fluid-filled vesicles progress from clear to cloudy fluid as inflammatory cells appear. The resultant pustules then begin to crust over, signaling the end of viral shedding and infectivity (Fig. 121-8). Characteristically, lesions at all stages of disease occur simultaneously during the illness.[60] The typical number of lesions may vary from 10 to 200. Constitutional symptoms of fever, malaise, pruritis, and anorexia are common. Crusted lesions ultimately resolve over 1 to 2 weeks.

In immunocompetent children, varicella most often is a benign, self-limited illness lasting under a week. The most common complication of varicella is secondary bacterial infection, most often with streptococcal or staphylococcal species, often prompted by excoriation. Immunocompromised hosts may have more severe dis-

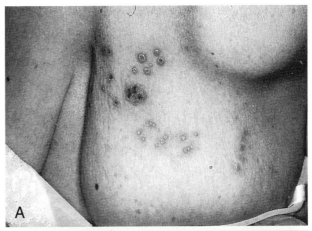

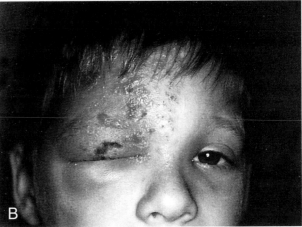

FIGURE 121-7. Herpes zoster. *A,* Thoracic zoster. *B,* Ophthalmic zoster: a recurrent infection with the varicella-zoster virus. The eruption is usually dermatomal but can become generalized. (From Callen JP, Greer KE, Hood AF, et al. Color Atlas of Dermatology. Philadelphia: WB Saunders Co., 1993:171.)

ease, characterized by greater numbers of lesions, prolonged healing time, visceral complications, and a resultant increased mortality.[61-63]

Visceral complications may affect multiple organs, with brain, lung, and liver manifestations occurring most commonly.[64] Neurologic complications of varicella occur with presentations of cerebellar ataxia, meningoencephalitis, transverse myelitis, and cerebral angitis. Pneumonitis presents with symptoms of dyspnea and cough, with interstitial or alveolar infiltrates on chest radiograph.[65] Varicella pneumonia has a high mortality rate, particularly in immunocompromised hosts.

Reye's syndrome has been linked with varicella infection and aspirin use.[66] The syndrome presents with the sudden onset of neurologic symptoms, signs of increased intracranial pressure with cerebral edema and signs of liver dysfunction, and is associated with significant mortality.[64] Because of this, salicylates are contraindicated in varicella infection.

Neonatal varicella results when maternal varicella occurs from 5 days before to 2 days after delivery, and is associated with visceral disease and significant mortality.[67] Maternal varicella occurring at 8 to 20 weeks of gestation causes the fetal varicella syndrome,[68] character-

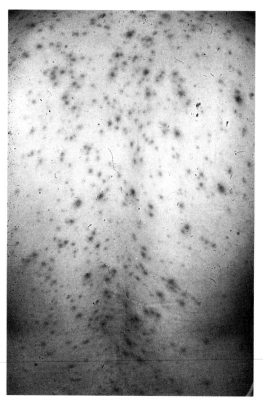

FIGURE 121-8. Varicella. Disseminated vesicles on erythematous bases with apparent early crusting. (Courtesy of the Department of Dermatology, New York University.)

ized by prematurity, low birth weight, hypoplasia, and ocular and neurologic abnormalities.

When latent VZV reactivates, it causes clinical herpes zoster. The typical presentation of zoster is the development of local radicular pain 2 to 3 days before the characteristic eruption occurs, involving one to three contiguous dermatomes. The thoracic dermatomes are most frequently involved, followed by the lumbar, trigeminal, cervical, and sacral dermatomes. The lesions begin as macules and papules, progressing to vesicles that may coalesce to bullae, and subsequently heal with crusting and reepithelialization. Up to one third of patients with herpes zoster have several vesicles found outside the affected dermatome, presumably from hematogenous dissemination. Widespread lesions (disseminated or generalized herpes zoster) are found most commonly in patients with malignancies (particularly lymphoma), other causes of immune suppression, or in the aged. Occasionally, the rash occurs without pain, and more rarely, dermatomal pain is recognized without skin lesions, "zoster sine herpete."

Herpes zoster ophthalmicus is the term used for zoster localized in the ophthalmic (V1) branch of the trigeminal nerve.[69] The presence of lesions on the tip of the nose reflects the V1 nerve distribution, and often indicates ocular involvement. Inflammation of the conjunctiva and cornea is common, and may lead to scarring and visual loss. Other structures of the eye are involved less commonly.

Herpes zoster oticus (Ramsay Hunt syndrome) occurs when zoster involves the geniculate ganglion. The syndrome is characterized by a polycranial neuropathy involving cranial nerves VI and VII. Lesions may appear on the face, neck, tongue, palate, ear, and in the auditory canal. Patients may develop ear pain, facial nerve palsy, or compromised hearing, balance, taste, or lacrimation. Sensory and motor deficits may persist following resolution of cutaneous lesions.

Postherpetic neuralgia is defined as debilitating pain at the site of previous zoster that persists more than 1 month. It may affect up to one half of patients over 50,[70] and is very common after trigeminal nerve zoster. Like varicella, herpes zoster may occasionally disseminate and/or involve extracutaneous sites such as the central nervous system, retina, lungs, and liver.

Immunocompromised hosts suffer more severe herpes zoster with prolonged lesion formation and reduced healing, and an increased risk of dissemination.[60, 71] More recently, a syndrome of atypical chronic herpes zoster has been described in HIV-infected patients receiving chronic acyclovir therapy.[72-74] The atypical lesions are verrucous, hyperkeratotic, ecthymatous, or pox-like papules or nodules or ulcerations with or without an eschar. These lesions are associated with acyclovir-resistant VZV.[73, 74]

PATHOLOGY

Biopsies of vesicles of varicella or herpes zoster show similar histopathologic changes to those of herpes simplex. The atypical verrucous lesions of herpes zoster seen in immunosuppressed patients are due to papillated epidermal hyperplasia and hyperkeratosis. Diagnostic herpetic nuclear changes are evident in circumscribed foci either in the epidermis or in adnexal epithelium. Irregular hyperplasia of adnexal epithelium can result in a profile simulating that of keratoacanthoma or squamous cell carcinoma.[74a]

DIAGNOSIS AND DIFFERENTIAL DIAGNOSIS

Both varicella and herpes zoster are most commonly diagnosed clinically on the basis of a compatible history and physical examination. The typical clinical presentation of fluid-filled cutaneous vesicles on an erythematous base in association with neuropathic pain occurring either diffusely in a child or dermatomally distributed in an adult is easily diagnosed as primary or reactivated VZV infection, respectively.

To confirm the clinical impression, a vesicle may be unroofed and the base scraped for cells to perform a Tzanck smear. A Wright or Giemsa stain of the vesicular cells will demonstrate characteristic multinucleated giant cells in a majority of patients.[75]

Serum sampling may define acute or previous exposure by showing new seroconversion or preexisting VZV antibody, respectively. Vesicular cells or tissue biopsy specimens may be directly stained for the presence of VZV antigen with specific VZV monoclonal antibody using newer immunohistochemical techniques. Finally, vesicular fluid and tissue biopsy specimens can be cul-

TABLE 121-2. Differential Diagnosis of Varicella Zoster Virus
Varicella
Disseminated herpes simplex Disseminated zoster Hand, foot, and mouth disease Other enteroviral infections Atypical measles Impetigo (Smallpox) (Vaccinia)
Zoster
Herpes simplex Cellulitis Erysipelas
Atypical Zoster
Ecthyma gangrenosum Disseminated fungal infection Disseminated mycobacterial infection Atypical herpes simplex

tured for VZV, although the virus is comparatively difficult to isolate. The differential diagnosis of VZV infection is noted in Table 121-2.

TREATMENT

Acyclovir is the antiviral of choice when the treatment of VZV infection is indicated.[76] The mechanism of action of the drug against VZV is identical to that for herpes simplex virus, as discussed earlier. The 50% inhibitory concentration of acyclovir in vitro is three to six times higher for VZV than for HSV,[77] and treatment doses must be increased accordingly.

Despite the availability of antiviral agents, uncomplicated varicella in children has historically been managed with supportive care: bathing, cutting fingernails short to prevent excoriation, and the use of antipruritics and antipyretics. Salicylates should not be given because of the risk of Reye's syndrome.[64, 66] More recent studies,[78, 79] have shown clinical benefits from the use of acyclovir in healthy children if started within 24 hours of the onset of rash. At a dose of 20 mg/kg, four times a day, acyclovir decreased the number and duration of formation of lesions, and the need for antipruritics. Similarly, the use of oral acyclovir at a dose of 800 mg five times daily for 7 days in immunocompetent adults with varicella within 24 hours of rash onset was associated with a reduction in the number and healing time of lesions, and the duration of fever and other symptoms.[80] Because of the severity of disease and the risk of complications, acyclovir is the treatment of choice for immunocompromised hosts with varicella,[81] at a dose of 500 mg/m^2 (or 10 mg/kg) intravenously every 8 hours for 10 days.

The current management of herpes zoster in immuno-

competent hosts often includes acyclovir. Several studies[82, 83] document increased healing and decreased acute pain using acyclovir at an oral dose of 800 mg five times daily or an intravenous dose of 10 mg/kg every 8 hours to 7 to 10 days. A recent study showed little benefit in terms of pain relief to prolonging the course of acyclovir to 3 weeks or adding steroids.[84] Recent reports of the use of a new antiviral, famciclovir (a precursor of penciclovir, a potent inhibitor of VZV) in acute zoster in normal hosts led to its recent FDA approval.[85] The dose of famciclovir is 500 mg three times daily. Acute neuritis and postherpetic neuralgia may be managed with traditional analgesics, or combinations of amitriptyline and perphenazine, topical capsaicin, or regional nerve blocks.

Acyclovir is the treatment of choice for herpes zoster in immunosuppressed hosts,[86, 87] including disseminated herpes zoster.[88] Acyclovir decreases viral shedding, new lesion formation, pain, and fever, and promotes cutaneous healing.

The use of chronic acyclovir therapy in immunocompromised hosts has been associated with atypical VZV lesions and laboratory and clinical resistance to acyclovir[72-74] (Fig. 121-9). Foscarnet (phosphonoformic acid) acts as an analogue of pyrophosphate to inhibit viral DNA polymerase and is not dependent on viral thymidine kinase. A recent small series in AIDS patients with resistant VZV infection demonstrated clinical benefits from a 10-day course of foscarnet at a dose of 40 mg/kg every 8 hours, with promotion of cutaneous healing.[89]

After a reported patient exposure to varicella, the benefits of administration of prophylactic varicella zoster immune globulin must be considered.[90] Varicella zoster immune globulin is administered via intramuscular injection at a recommended dose of 125 units (1 vial) per 10 kg, up to a maximum of 675 units (5 vials). Current recommendations for prevention consider the timing of the exposure, the likelihood of transmission, and the patient's history of VZV disease.[91] Up to 95% of adults with a negative or unknown history of VZV disease will be immune.

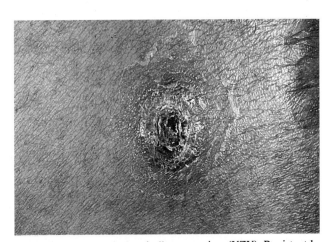

FIGURE 121-9. Atypical varicella zoster virus (VZV). Persistent hyperkeratotic papule in an HIV-infected patient on chronic acyclovir therapy was direct fluorescent antibody positive for VZV. (Courtesy of the Department of Dermatology, New York University.)

Epstein-Barr Virus

DEFINITION

The Epstein-Barr virus (EBV), the fourth human herpesvirus, was first identified in 1964 in cultured Burkitt's lymphoma cells by electron microscopy[92] and later identified and confirmed as the etiologic agent of infectious mononucleosis.[93-95] EBV is a member of the human herpesvirus family and is morphologically indistinguishable from the other herpesviruses. It is an enveloped virus containing double-stranded DNA that establishes a primary cellular infection followed by a latent infection.

EBV is distinguished from the other herpesviruses by its biologic properties. The virus is tropic for B lymphocytes and nasopharyngeal and salivary gland epithelial cells.[96, 97] More recently, cervical epithelium has also been identified as a site of EBV shedding.[98] The target cells are specifically recognized through the cell surface marker, the CR2 molecule[99] (also the receptor for complement component C3d[100]). EBV binds to this cellular receptor and gains entry into cells.

Whereas the other herpesviruses produce cytopathic changes in tissue culture cells, EBV has the unique property of establishing a latent state in infected B lymphocytes, and subsequently synthesizing viral proteins (Epstein-Barr nuclear antigens) that promote cellular proliferation and transform affected cells, conferring immortality.[101] This property likely gives EBV its oncogenic potential.

CLINICAL DESCRIPTION

Epidemiology

Infection with EBV, like other human herpesviruses, is ubiquitous in the population. Over 90% of adults will have a positive EBV serology.[102] EBV infection occurs worldwide, and once infection is established, it is lifelong. Primary infection with EBV occurs in two distinct age groups: young children and young adults.[102, 103] Lower socioeconomic status is associated with earlier acquisition of EBV infection. Reactivation infection occurs primarily in immunocompromised patients, with immunosuppression from exogenous agents of organ transplantation or infection with HIV.

The tropism for salivary and nasopharyngeal epithelial cells allows EBV excretion in saliva.[104, 105] Primary infection occurs most often with oral contact between a susceptible person and an asymptomatic person shedding EBV in the saliva. Asymptomatic shedding may occur up to 18 months after complete recovery from the acute syndrome.[106] Environmental exposures via fomites have not been implicated.

These factors explain the lack of EBV epidemics among populations, and inasmuch as intimate oral contact is necessary for transmission, isolation of the infected patient is not necessary.

Clinical Findings

Primary infection with EBV occurring in young children manifests most commonly as subclinical or mild nonspecific clinical findings of low-grade fever and pharyngitis.

Papular acrodermatitis of childhood or infantile papular acrodermatitis (Gianotti-Crosti syndrome) is a distinctive eruption occurring in children from 2 to 6 years old.[107] The syndrome presents acutely as symmetrical flat, 2-mm papules, localized to the face and extremities with sparing of the trunk. The lesions may be skin colored or erythematous and are nonpruritic. There is no associated fever although generalized lymphadenopathy is often present. The syndrome is self-limited and lasts about 3 weeks. Initially, Gianotti-Crosti syndrome was associated with hepatitis and hepatitis B surface antigenemia. Subsequent reports have documented cases without hepatitis B antigenemia but associated with primary viral infections including coxsackievirus, parainfluenza, and EBV,[108-110] documented by seroconversion indicated by viral antibody titers. In some cases of virally related Gianotti-Crosti syndrome, there was no evidence of an associated hepatitis or hepatomegaly.

Primary infection with EBV in young adults (age 15 to 25) manifests clinically in over one third of infected patients as infectious mononucleosis (glandular fever). Pharyngitis, fever, and cervical lymphadenopathy are the most common manifestations. Skin eruptions are rare with an estimated incidence of about 3%.[111] When present, eruptions consist of generalized macular erythema, urticaria (sometimes associated with the cold[112, 113]), or scarlatiniform eruptions. About 50% of all patients will have upper eyelid edema, and about 10% of patients will have a petechial palatal enanthem.[111] Symptoms of mononucleosis may last weeks to a few months and are most often self limited. Complications of mononucleosis are uncommon but may include hepatitis, splenic rupture, immune cytopenias, and neurologic syndromes.

There are a few well-documented cases of prolonged chronic active mononucleosis syndromes with persistent or progressive disease after an initial episode of EBV mononucleosis.[114, 115] Some investigators have related other skin lesions such as erythema multiforme to chronic fatigue syndrome attributed to Epstein-Barr virus.[116] A consensus case definition of chronic fatigue syndrome that focuses on symptoms and signs rather than EBV as the etiologic agent has been developed.[117] Epidemiologic and serologic studies have not confirmed the association of EBV and chronic fatigue.[118, 119]

Inadvertent treatment of acute EBV mononucleosis with antibiotics often results in a hypersensitivity eruption.[120, 121] Extensive pruritic maculopapular lesions occur with associated fever. The rash typically persists for a few days, occasionally progressing to desquamation. Ampicillin is the most frequently implicated antibiotic, with more than 90% of patients developing the hypersensitivity reaction. Penicillin, tetracycline, and other antibiotics have also been implicated.

Reactivation or secondary EBV infection occurs in patients with immune compromise from malignancy, immunosuppressive therapy for organ transplantation and autoimmune diseases, or HIV infection, causing EBV lymphoproliferative disorders.[122] Burkitt's (B-cell) lymphoma, nasopharyngeal (epithelial cell) carcinoma, and other B-cell lymphomas, including cutaneous B and T cell lymphomas occur in the setting of immune compromise.[123, 124]

HIV-infected patients also may develop EBV-related B-cell lymphomas. A more common EBV-related complication of HIV disease is oral hairy leukoplakia[125, 126] (Fig. 121–10). This lesion appears as raised, striated white areas on the sides of the tongue or, less commonly, on the buccal mucosa, which do not scrape off. EBV has been detected in affected tissues by electron microscopy and antigen and DNA detection techniques.

Oral hairy leukoplakia is a sign of compromised immune function in HIV disease and predicts progression to clinical AIDS.[127] In one study, about half of the patients developed AIDS an average of 16 months after the diagnosis of oral hairy leukoplakia, although this was prior to the widespread use of opportunistic infection prophylaxis and antiviral therapies.

Another manifestation of EBV infection reported in an immunocompromised patient is a widespread eruption of purpuric macules and papules in which viral genome was detected in lesional keratinocytes.[127a] Recurrent, necrotizing nodules on the face and oral mucosa have also been linked with elevated levels of EBV antibodies.[127b]

PATHOLOGY

The vesicles of the Gianotti-Crosti syndrome are intraepidermal, the result of spongiotic dermatitis. There are no discernible viropathic changes. Biopsies of the exanthem of mononucleosis are seldom performed, but reveal a sparse superficial perivascular dermatitis with minimal vacuolar change or spongiosis, or both. Histologic examination of the purpuric lesions reported in an immunocompromised patient revealed an interface dermatitis with parakeratosis. EBV was detected in the nuclei of basal keratinocytes.[127a] The ulcerating nodules reported in a patient with high levels of antibodies to EBV showed dense infiltrates of CD8+ lymphocytes around the area of necrosis.[127b]

DIAGNOSIS AND DIFFERENTIAL DIAGNOSIS

The diagnosis of one of the disease syndromes of primary or reactivation of EBV infection is often made clinically. Papular acrodermatitis has a characteristic appearance. The typical clinical syndrome of infectious mononucleosis occurring in the setting of a greater than 50% lymphocytosis with more than 10% atypical (large, activated) lymphocytes and a positive serum heterophile antibody test establishes the diagnosis.

The heterophile antibody test is positive in 70% of teenage and adult patients during the first week of illness and in 90% by 3 weeks. In children younger than 5 years old, less than 50% will develop a positive test. The positive serology will persist as long as 6 to 9 months after illness. False-positive tests occur with hepatitis and hematologic malignancies.

The diagnosis of lymphoproliferative syndromes due to EBV requires tissue diagnosis.

Oral hairy leukoplakia is currently most often diagnosed in an HIV-infected patient with a characteristic tongue lesion, particularly when fungal disease has been excluded. Biopsy is confirmatory and distinguishes the condition from other oral verrucous lesions.

EBV serologies are widely available although often not clinically useful to confirm diagnoses, except in unusual cases. The differential diagnosis of EBV infection is found in Table 121–3.

TREATMENT

EBV disease in the immunocompetent host is most often self limited and specific treatment is not required. Symptomatic therapy with analgesics, antipyretics, and bed rest is advisable initially. Limitation of exertion is warranted to avoid splenic rupture as a complication of acute mononucleosis.

The use of corticosteroids in acute infectious mononu-

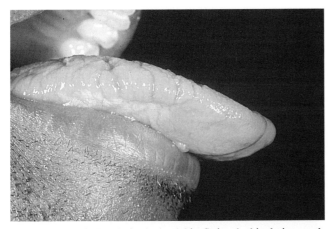

FIGURE 121–10. Oral hairy leukoplakia. Striated white lesion on the side of the tongue in a patient with HIV infection. (Courtesy of the Department of Dermatology, New York University.)

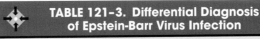

TABLE 121–3. Differential Diagnosis of Epstein-Barr Virus Infection
Infectious Mononucleosis
Cytomegalovirus (CMV) mononucleosis Viral hepatitis Toxoplasmosis Streptococcal pharyngitis Rubella
Oral Hairy Leukoplakia
Fungal infection (thrush) Lichen planus Geographic tongue

cleosis reduced the duration of both fever and pharyngitis in clinical trials.[128, 129] However, their routine use has not been widely accepted. Most clinicians reserve steroids for the treatment of certain complications of mononucleosis: severe pharyngitis with airway edema, or immune cytopenias.

Acyclovir treatment of infectious mononucleosis has been tested in a few clinical trials and shown to decrease viral replication transiently but with no effect on symptoms.[130, 131] Acyclovir has anecdotally reported benefit in EBV polyclonal lymphoproliferative disease[132] but, in general, chemotherapy or radiation therapy is required.[122, 133]

Acyclovir has been shown to cause regression of oral hairy leukopenia,[134] as have ganciclovir,[135] zidovudine (AZT),[136] and topical application of podophyllin. Others have advocated surgery,[137] although in the absence of pain or discomfort, specific treatment of leukoplakia is usually not necessary.

Cytomegalovirus

DEFINITION

Cytomegalovirus (CMV) is the most complex of the herpesviruses, with a genome 50% larger than that of herpes simplex. The original observations of unusual large cells with intranuclear and cytoplasmic inclusions in the tissues of autopsy specimens first led to the term *cytomegalic inclusion disease*. Weller and coworkers first identified the viral pathogen and named it cytomegalovirus.[138] Like the other herpesviruses, CMV is a double-stranded DNA virus that causes a primary infection, then establishes clinical latency, and subsequently may reactivate to cause secondary infection, particularly with immunosuppression. The site of clinical latency of CMV is unclear, though it is likely to be peripheral monocytes.[139, 140]

CLINICAL DESCRIPTION

Epidemiology

Serologic studies show that infection with CMV occurs worldwide, is widespread, and is most often clinically unrecognized.[141] Between 40% and 100% of adults are seropositive for CMV antibody, reflecting previous exposure. Ordinary transmission of CMV occurs in three distinct periods of life: perinatally from infected mother to child; in young childhood from other children in families or day care settings; and in the reproductive years from sexual contact. CMV transmission also occurs with blood transfusion[142] or tissue donation from a seropositive donor to a seronegative recipient. CMV has been isolated from many body fluids including urine, feces, saliva, semen, cervical secretions, breast milk, and lymphocytes.[143]

CLINICAL FINDINGS

Cytomegalovirus infection is most often clinically inapparent. CMV is responsible for distinct clinical entities: congenital CMV infection, CMV mononucleosis in the normal host, and reactivation of CMV causing disseminated or visceral disease in the immunocompromised host. Dermatologic manifestations of CMV are uncommon and nonspecific.

Congenital CMV infection may occur either as the result of primary CMV infection of the mother or reactivation of CMV infection in the mother. CMV is the most common congenital viral infection.[144] More than 90% of infants who acquire perinatal CMV infection have few or no clinical findings.

The similarity of congenital syndromes has led to the designation of the TORCH (Toxoplasma, Other [bacterial sepsis, syphilis, etc.], Rubella, Cytomegalovirus, Herpes simplex virus) syndrome. Clinical manifestations include hepatosplenomegaly with or without jaundice, neurologic abnormalities including microcephaly, encephalitis, and paralysis, ophthalmologic disease, including chronic chorioretinitis, and typical cutaneous lesions.

The classic dermatologic findings in congenital CMV disease are purple-red papules or nodules, "blueberry muffin" lesions. These are sites of extramedullary hematopoiesis in the dermis, and lesions may last from 4 to 6 weeks. Petechiae or purpura due to thrombocytopenia may be persistent. Jaundice may occur from direct hyperbilirubinemia.

CMV may present in the immunocompetent host as a syndrome resembling infectious mononucleosis due to Epstein-Barr virus with a uniformly negative monospot test.[145] CMV mononucleosis is a disease of young adults (average age 28 years) and most commonly presents with prolonged fever lasting up to 2 weeks, myalgias, malaise, pharyngitis, and headache.[146, 147] Splenomegaly, pharyngeal erythema, and lymphadenopathy, which typically accompany EBV mononucleosis, occur in about one third of patients. Frank exudative tonsillitis occurs in only about 6% of patients. Laboratory studies also are typical for mononucleosis: atypical lymphocytosis and elevations in liver enzymes.

A rash occurs in about one third of patients. Often, a generalized macular and papular eruption appears 7 to 9 days after nonspecific treatment with ampicillin, similar to that seen when a patient with EBV mononucleosis receives ampicillin.[148] These eruptions subside over 5 to 8 days. Similar rashes may appear in patients who receive other antibiotics, such as tetracycline. Other rashes that may be seen are described as rubelliform-like, scarlatiniform, maculopapular, follicular or urticarial, both generalized and localized to the lower extremities.

Systemic complications occur infrequently but may include pneumonitis, myocarditis, neurologic disorders (encephalitis, Guillain-Barré syndrome, cranial nerve palsies), jaundice, and granulomatous hepatitis, although the disease is usually self limited. Laboratory abnormalities may persist, particularly lymphocytosis and elevated transaminases.

Immunocompromised patients are at high risk for reactivation of latent CMV infection whether their immune compromise is caused by malignancy, burns, use of immunosuppressive agents, or HIV infection. In these populations, CMV may be reactivated to cause pneumonitis, hepatitis, colitis, retinitis, encephalitis, or adrenalitis.[149] Dermatologic manifestations of CMV disease, however, are uncommon.[143, 150] One early report detailed the case of an apparently healthy elderly woman who developed perianal ulcers with viral inclusion bodies on skin biopsy as part of fatal disseminated CMV infection.[151]

In the early 1980s, Pariser reviewed published cases of cutaneous CMV in immunocompromised individuals and noted two patterns: localized ulcerative lesions of the perianal or genital areas or extremities, and disseminated purpuric macules.[150] Lin attributed two cases of cutaneous CMV in immunocompromised hosts to antecedent penicillin or ampicillin therapy.[152]

In a review of unusual cutaneous lesions in AIDS, Penneys reported purpuric macules with characteristic CMV inclusion bodies and vasculitis on skin biopsy of a patient.[153] Subsequent reports of cutaneous CMV disease in HIV-infected patients[154, 155] have prompted debate of the viral etiology (CMV vs. VZV). A large natural history study of HIV-infected patients that monitored over 1000 patients with AIDS described a 21% incidence of CMV disease in patients with CD_4 cells less than 100/mm³ and no cases of dermatologic CMV disease.[156]

Several recent reports have documented cutaneous CMV disease in burn patients.[157, 158] Two patients had focal areas of poorly healing granulation tissue that on biopsy (performed in each case for suspected fungal infection) showed characteristic CMV inclusions. Neither patient in this report had evidence of disseminated CMV infection. Skin lesions in immunocompromised hosts may often signal disseminated infection, and a biopsy should be performed early to assist in identifying systemic diseases.

PATHOLOGY

The hallmark of cutaneous infection with CMV is enlargement of the nuclei of venular endothelial cells, which can contain either intranuclear or intracytoplasmic inclusions, or both (Fig. 121–11). Sparse infiltrates of neutrophils are sometimes present; rarely, a small vessel leukocytoclastic vasculitis occurs in lesional skin.

DIAGNOSIS AND DIFFERENTIAL DIAGNOSIS

The diagnosis of CMV infection is made by histopathologic demonstration of characteristic CMV viral inclusion bodies in tissue biopsy specimens (Fig. 121–12). Body fluid viral cultures (urine, blood, sputum) are often unreliable in distinguishing active disease from viral colonization and are not always predictive of visceral disease.[159] Serologic testing for CMV antibody demonstrates previous exposure to the virus without confirming active disease. The differential diagnosis of CMV disease is found in Table 121–4.

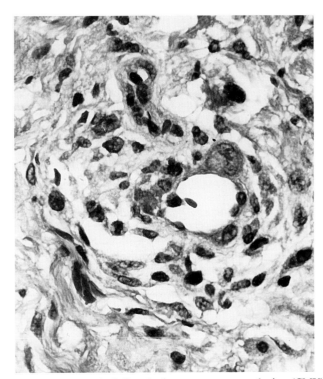

FIGURE 121–11. The hallmark of cutaneous cytomegalovirus (CMV) infection is enlarged endothelial cell nuclei, with intranuclear or cytoplasmic inclusions, or both.

TREATMENT

CMV disease in the normal host is most often a self-limited disease that does not require specific treatment. In the immunocompromised host, visceral or disseminated disease is treated with specific antiviral agents: ganciclovir or foscarnet. The role of therapy for isolated cutaneous CMV disease in the immunocompromised host is unclear.

Ganciclovir, a derivative of acyclovir, is an analogue of guanosine that is phosphorylated intracellularly to its active form and functions to inhibit viral DNA synthe-

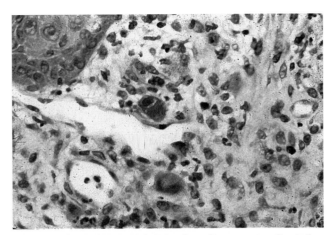

FIGURE 121–12. CMV. Typical "owl's eye" appearance of pathology of a cutaneous lesion of CMV. (Courtesy of the Department of Dermatology, New York University.)

TABLE 121–4. Differential Diagnosis of Cytomegalovirus Infection

Congenital Cytomegalovirus (CMV)
Toxoplasmosis
Syphilis
Bacterial sepsis
Listeria
Rubella
Herpes simplex

CMV Mononucleosis
EBV mononucleosis
Acute viral hepatitis
Drug reaction
Enteroviral exanthem

Cutaneous CMV in Immunocompromised Host
Disseminated fungal disease
Cryptococcus
Candida
Histoplasma
Disseminated mycobacterial disease
Tuberculosis
Atypical mycobacterial
Drug reaction
Herpes simplex virus
Varicella zoster virus

sis.[160] Early trials studied the use of ganciclovir at a dose of 5 mg/kg intravenously twice daily in CMV retinitis, pneumonitis, and enteritis in immunocompromised patients. With treatment, 70% to 80% of patients show decreases in CMV excretion and 50% to 70% show stabilization or improvement of disease. In contrast, 90% of untreated HIV-infected patients have progressive CMV disease.[161]

Because of high relapse rate, HIV-infected patients with CMV retinitis require maintenance, suppressive ganciclovir treatment (5 mg/kg daily).[162] This is less well established for other (gastrointestinal, pulmonary) CMV disease. CMV infection with both laboratory and clinical resistance to ganciclovir has led to the search for alternative active antiviral agents.[163] Foscarnet (phosphonoformate) is an analogue of pyrophosphate and acts to inhibit viral DNA synthesis. Clinical trials have demonstrated efficacy in CMV retinitis, including retinal disease unresponsive to ganciclovir.[164] In a trial of the initial treatment of CMV retinitis in HIV-infected patients, the viral efficacy of ganciclovir and foscarnet was no different, although a survival benefit was demonstrated for patients who received foscarnet.[165]

Prevention of primary and reactivation of CMV infections in immunocompromised hosts, notably transplant recipients and HIV-infected patients, has been difficult to achieve. Snydman and associates[166] showed that the use of cytomegalovirus hyperimmune globulin reduced the incidence of primary CMV disease in renal transplant recipients from 60% to about 20%. Balfour and colleagues[167] showed that high-dose prophylactic acyclovir prevented primary CMV disease in recipients of kidneys from CMV-seropositive donors.

Human Herpesvirus-6

DEFINITION

The sixth human herpesvirus was first isolated from the peripheral blood of patients immunocompromised due to HIV infection and/or hematologic malignancies in 1986 and was first called *human B-lymphotropic virus* (HBLV).[168] Further investigation found the virus to be tropic for T lymphocytes[169, 170] and to have morphologic and biologic similarities to the human herpesviruses,[171] leading to its designation as *human herpesvirus-6* (HHV-6).

HHV-6 is an enveloped virus with an icosahedral nucleocapsid enclosing a linear double-stranded DNA. HHV-6 shares genomic homology with other human herpesviruses coding for a set of conserved gene sequences.[172] Its closest homology is to human cytomegalovirus (CMV),[172] with 66% shared amino acid sequences. Despite genetic homology, they are serologically distinct.

HHV-6 has two closely related strains or genotypes, designated types A and B, distinguished by growth and immunologic properties, DNA analyses, and apparent pathogenic potential.[173]

CLINICAL DESCRIPTION

Epidemiology

Exposure to HHV-6 is ubiquitous and occurs worldwide, most frequently at an early age. Adults demonstrate HHV-6 antibody seroprevalence rates of 50% to 90%.[174–176] Infants less than 3 months of age have a similar seroprevalence to adults, with a subsequent decline in antibody most consistent with passive transfer of maternal antibody.[176, 177] Low seroprevalence in 4- to 6-month-old infants increases by 11 to 12 months of age. This rise in prevalence at the highest geometric mean titers of antibody, which occur in early childhood, suggests a rapid and early acquisition of HHV-6 infection in the first years of life.[175, 176, 178] Seroprevalence rates remain stable in children and young adults and then show a consistent age-related decline by the third and fourth decades of life. Over age 40, only about 60% of adults show antibody to HHV-6.[178]

The T-cell tropism of HHV-6 and laboratory evidence of its ability to activate HIV in vitro have prompted speculation as to its role as a possible cofactor of HIV infection.[179] Epidemiologic studies based on serology have not linked infection with HHV-6 and HIV.[180, 181]

Clinical Findings

Primary infection with HHV-6 in children causes exanthem subitum (roseola infantum, sixth disease), a common childhood illness, characterized by acute fever without localizing signs and the subsequent development of an erythematous macular rash as the fever subsides.

Yamanishi[182] first isolated HHV-6 from the peripheral blood lymphocytes of four infants with exanthum subitum. Serologic studies confirmed the findings with negative HHV-6 antibody titers in the acute illness, followed by an increased titer over 2 weeks, confirming acute seroconversion.

HHV-6 primary infection has also been described as the typical exanthem subitum rash without fever, and by others as fever without rash.[183] Pruksananonda and colleagues[184] studied children under 2 years of age who presented to a pediatric emergency room with an acute febrile illness. Thirty-four of 243 children had isolable HHV-6. The children presented after an average of about 3 days of symptoms with significant fever (65% over 40° C), irritability, and otitis media (in 21 of the 34). Only three HHV-6 positive children had the classic exanthem. The symptoms resolved after about 4 days. The authors concluded that HHV-6 is an important cause of acute febrile childhood illness and is not always associated with the typical exanthum subitum rash. Although in general, exanthem subitum is a benign, self-limited disease, reports of complications of primary infection include seizures (the most common complication), meningoencephalitis,[185] hepatitis,[186, 187] and intussusception.[188]

Primary infection with HHV-6 in immunocompetent adults produces a mononucleosis-like syndrome.[189, 190] In general, the characteristic clinical sign is enlarged, nontender, bilateral cervical lymphadenopathy that lasts 1 to 3 months without significant fever. Mild headache, fatigue, and malaise are also observed. Laboratory evaluation reveals a mild leukopenia with a prominent mononucleosis (about 40% to 60%) and atypical lymphocytes.

Akashi[190] reported a severe mononucleosis-like syndrome in a 43-year-old man who seroconverted for HHV-6 antibody and had evidence of HHV-6 by polymerase chain reaction of peripheral blood mononuclear cells and skin biopsy. His illness was characterized by high fever (40.6° C), cervical lymphadenopathy, mild splenomegaly, exudative pharyngitis, and erythematous maculopapular rash. Laboratory evaluation revealed a leukocytosis with 58% atypical lymphocytes and elevations of liver transaminases (300 to 400 IU/L) and creatinine (3.6 μg/dL). He experienced progression of the rash with lesion coalescence and total body erythema, prompting treatment with a brief course of corticosteroids. The skin eruption healed with prominent exfoliation and the patient eventually recovered.

After primary infection, HHV-6 presumably remains latent in the body. Several groups have isolated HHV-6 from the saliva[191, 192] and salivary gland tissue[193] of immunocompetent adults, suggesting transmission occurs commonly via this route. Other groups have demonstrated evidence of HHV-6 in lymph nodes[194] and monocytes and macrophages.[195] HHV-6 has also been identified in the cells of sinus histiocytosis with massive lymphadenopathy (see elsewhere in text) and Langerhans cell histiocytosis. Its pathogenic role in these conditions is unknown.

Reactivation of HHV-6 infection has been reported in organ transplant patients and linked to syndromes of fever and rash,[196] interstitial pneumonitis,[197, 198] bone marrow suppression,[199] and possibly correlated with transplant rejection.[200]

DIAGNOSIS AND DIFFERENTIAL DIAGNOSIS

The typical clinical syndrome of an infant or young child with acute fever followed by the development of an erythematous macular rash or an adult with a heterophile-negative mononucleosis-like illness not caused by cytomegalovirus (CMV) is most consistent with the diagnosis of (primary HHV-6) infection.

Serologic confirmation of seroconversion with appearance of HHV-6 IgG antibody by indirect immunofluorescence or enzyme immunoassay supports the clinical diagnosis. Demonstration of HHV-6 from tissues by viral culture or detection of viral proteins with specific monoclonal antibodies or of viral DNA by Southern blot or polymerase chain reaction[190, 198] implicates the virus in a causal role, although these techniques remain primarily research tools at present. The differential diagnosis of HHV-6 infection is found in Table 121–5.

PATHOLOGY

There are no specific histologic changes associated with HHV-6 infection. Biopsies are seldom performed on exanthem subitum, and it cannot be distinguished from other viral exanthemata. HHV-6 in other conditions has largely been detected by immunohistochemistry.

TABLE 121–5. Differential Diagnosis of Human Herpesvirus-6

Exanthem Subitum
Rubella
Measles
Erythema infectiosum
Scarlet fever
Drug eruption
Viral exanthem (adenovirus, echovirus, coxsackievirus, rotavirus)

Mononucleosis-like
EBV mononucleosis
CMV mononucleosis
Atypical drug reaction

TREATMENT

There is no specific treatment for primary HHV-6 infection in children or adults because this is in general a benign, self-limited viral illness. In vitro virologic susceptibility studies show HHV-6 to have a similar inhibitory pattern as CMV. HHV-6 replication is inhibited by ganciclovir and foscarnet, and high-dose acyclovir.[201-203] With additional case reports of more severe HHV-6 disease in immunocompetent patients, and particularly in diseases of immunocompromised patients, most notably transplant recipients, there may be a place for the clinical use of these antiviral agents for HHV-6 infections.

Carrigan et al[197] reported the use of foscarnet in a bone marrow transplant patient co-infected with HHV-6 and CMV with interstitial pneumonitis. Drobyski and colleagues[199] reported four cases of HHV-6–associated bone marrow suppression after bone marrow transplant where ganciclovir or foscarnet was used. Further clinical experience with these agents will be necessary to evaluate their efficacy in serious HHV-6 infections.

DNA sequences of a new human herpesvirus have recently been discovered in Kaposi's sarcoma (KS) lesions from patients with acquired immunodeficiency syndrome (AIDS). This finding lends support to epidemiologic evidence that KS may be sexually transmitted, and has implications for treatment options, perhaps with antiviral therapies.

References

1. Roizman B. The structure and isomerization of herpes simplex virus genomes. Cell 1979;16:481–494.
2. Pereira L, Dondero DV, Gallo D, et al. Serological analysis of herpes simplex virus types 1 and 2 with monoclonal antibodies. Infect Immun 1982;35:363–367.
3. Nahmias AJ. Sero-epidemiological and -sociological patterns of herpes simplex virus infection in the world. Scand J Infect Dis Supp 1990;69:19–36.
4. Gibson JJ, Hornung CA, Alexander GR, et al. A cross-sectional study of herpes simplex virus types 1 and 2 in college students: Occurence and determinants of infection. J Infect Dis 1990; 162:306–312.
5. Johnson RE, Nahmias AJ, Magder LS, et al. A seroepidemiologic survey of the prevalence of herpes simplex virus type 2 infection in the United States. N Engl J Med 1989;321:7–12.
6. Becker TM, Blount JH, Guinan ME. Genital herpes infections in private practice in the United States, 1966 to 1981. JAMA 1985;253:1601–1603.
7. Holmberg SD, Stewart JA, Gerber AR, et al. Prior herpes simplex virus type 2 infection as a risk factor for HIV infection. JAMA 1988;259:1048–1050.
8. Kreiss JK, Koech D, Plummer FA, et al. AIDS virus infection in Nairobi prostitutes. Spread of the epidemic to East Africa. N Engl J Med 1986;314:414–418.
9. Simonsen JN, Cameron DW, Gakinya MN, et al. Human immunodeficiency virus infection among men with sexually transmitted diseases. Experience from a center in Africa. N Engl J Med 1988;319:274–278.
10. Quinn TC, Glasser D, Cannon RO, et al. Human immunodeficiency virus infections among patients attending clinics for sexually transmitted diseases. N Engl J Med 1988;318:197–203.
11. Kuiken CL, van Griensven GJP, deVroome EMM, et al. Risk factors and changes in sexual behavior in male homosexuals who seroconverted from human immunodeficiency virus. Am J Epidemiol 1990;132:523–530.
12. Bastian FO, Rabson AS, Yee CL, et al. Herpesvirus hominis: Isolation from human trigeminal ganglion. Science 1972; 178:306–307.
13. Glezen WP, Fernald GW, Lohr JA, et al. Acute respiratory disease of university students with special reference to the etiologic role of herpesvirus hominis. Am J Epidemiol 1975; 101:111–121.
14. Mertz GJ, Benedetti J, Ashley R, et al. Risk factors for the sexual transmission of genital herpes. Ann Intern Med 1992; 116:197–202.
15. Corey L, Holmes KK. Genital herpes simplex virus infections: Clinical manifestations, course and complications. Ann Intern Med 1983;98:973–983.
16. Whitley RJ, Nahmias AJ, Visintine AM, et al. The natural history of herpes simplex virus infection of mother and newborn. Pediatrics 1980;66:489–494.
17. Prober CG, Corey L, Brown ZA, et al. The management of pregnancies complicated by genital infections with herpes simplex virus. Clin Infect Dis 1992;15:1031–1038.
18. Selling B. An outbreak of herpes simplex among wrestlers (herpes gladiatorum). N Engl J Med 1964;270:979.
19. White WB, Grant-Kels JM. Transmission of herpes simplex virus type 1 infection in rugby players. JAMA 1984; 252:533–535.
20. Belongia EA, Goodman JL, Holland EJ, et al. An outbreak of herpes gladiatorum at a high-school wrestling camp. N Engl J Med 1991;325:906–910.
21. Bader C, Crumpacker CS, Schnipper LE, et al. The natural history of recurrent facial-oral infection with herpes simplex virus. J Infect Dis 1978;138:897–905.
22. Feder HM Jr, Long SS. Herpetic whitlow: Epidemiology, clinical characteristics, diagnosis, and treatment. Am J Dis Child 1983;137:861–863.
23. Glogau R. Herpetic whitlow as part of genital viral infection. J Infect Dis 1977;136:689–692.
24. Dorsky DI, Crumpacker CS. Drugs five years later. Acyclovir. N Engl J Med 1987;107:859–874.
25. Elion GB, Furman PA, Fyfe JA, et al. Selectivity of action of an antiherpetic agent, 9-(2-hydroxyethoxymethyl) guanine. Proc Natl Acad Sci 1977;74:5716–5720.
26. Bryson YJ, Dillon M, Lovett M, et al. Treatment of first episodes of genital herpes simplex virus infection with oral acyclovir: A randomized double-blind controlled trial in normal subjects. N Engl J Med 1983;308:916–921.
27. Corey L, Nahmias AJ, Guinan ME, et al. A trial of topical acyclovir in genital herpes simplex virus infections. N Engl J Med 1982;306:1313–1319.
28. Reichman RC, Badger GJ, Mertz GJ, et al. Treatment of recurrent genital herpes simplex infections with oral acyclovir: A controlled trial. JAMA 1984;251:2103–2107.
29. Spruance SL, Crumpacker CS. Topical 5 percent acyclovir in polyethylene glycol for herpes simplex labialis: Antiviral effect without clinical benefit. Am J Med 1982;73:315–319.
30. Whitley RJ, Levin M, Barton N, et al. Infections caused by herpes simplex virus in the immunocompromised host: Natural history and topical acyclovir therapy. J Infect Dis 1984; 150:323–329.
31. Shepp DH, Newton BA, Dandliker PS, et al. Oral acyclovir therapy for mucocutaneous herpes simplex virus infections in immunocompromised marrow transplant recipients. Ann Intern Med 1985;102:783–785.
32. Douglas JM, Critchlow C, Benedetti J, et al. A double-blind study of oral acyclovir for suppression of recurrences of genital herpes simplex virus infection. N Engl J Med 1984;310:1551–1556.
33. Conant MA. Prophylactic and suppressive treatment with acyclovir and the management of herpes in acquired immunodeficiency syndrome. J Am Acad Derm 1988;18:186–188.
34. Kaplowitz LG, Baker D, Gelb L, et al. Prolonged continuous acyclovir treatment for normal adults with frequently recurring genital herpes simplex virus infection. JAMA 1991;265:747–751.
35. Rooney JF. Straus SE, Mannix ML, et al. Oral acyclovir to suppress frequently recurrent herpes labialis. Ann Intern Med 1993;118:268–272.
36. Crumpacker CS, Schnipper LE, Marlowe SI, et al. Resistance to antiviral drugs of herpes simplex virus isolated from a patient treated with acyclovir. N Engl J Med 1982;306:343–346.
37. Wade JC, McLaren C, Meyers JD. Frequency and significance

of acyclovir-resistant herpes virus isolated from marrow transplant patients receiving multiple courses of treatment with acyclovir. J Infect Dis 1982;148:1077–1082.

38. Ellis MN, Keller PM, Fyfe JA, et al. Clinical isolate of herpes simplex type 2 that induces a thymidine kinase with altered substrate specificity. Antimicrob Agents Chemother 1987; 31:1117–1125.

39. Ehrlich KS, Mills J, Chatis P, et al. Acyclovir-resistant herpes simplex virus infections in patients with the acquired immunodeficiency syndrome. N Engl J Med 1989;320:293–296.

40. Hardy D. Foscarnet treatment of acyclovir-resistant herpes simplex virus infection in patients with acquired immunodeficiency syndrome: Preliminary results of a controlled, randomized, regimen-comparative trial. Am J Med 1992;92:30S–35S.

41. Safrin S, Crumpacker C, Chatis P, et al. A controlled trial comparing foscarnet with vidarabine for acyclovir-resistant mucocutaneous herpes simplex in the acquired immunodeficiency syndrome. N Engl J Med 1991;325:551–555.

42. Murphy M, Morley A, Eglin RP, et al. Topical trifluridine for mucocutaneous acyclovir-resistant herpes simplex II in an AIDS patient. Lancet 1992;340:1040.

43. Kessler H, Weaver D, Benson C, et al. ACTG 172: Treatment of acyclovir-resistant mucocutaneous herpes simplex virus infection in patients with AIDS: Open label pilot study of topical trifluridine. Int Conf AIDS 1992;8:abstract WeB 1056.

44. Achong BG, Meurisse EV. Observations on the fine structure and replication of varicella virus in cultivated human amnion cells. J Gen Virol 1968;3:305–308.

45. Asano Y, Itakura N, Hiruishi Y, et al. Viremia is present in the incubation period in nonimmunocompromised children with varicella. J Pediatr 1985;106:69–71.

46. Hyman RW, Ecker JR, Tenser RB. Varicella-zoster virus RNA in human trigeminal ganglia. Lancet 1983;ii:814–816.

47. Mahalingam R, Wellish M, Wolf W, et al. Latent varicella-zoster viral DNA in human trigeminal and thoracic ganglia. N Engl J Med 1990;323:627–631.

48. Miller AE. Selective decline in cellular immune reponse to varicella-zoster in the elderly. Neurol 1980;30:582–587.

49. Straus SE, Ostrove JM, Inchauspe G, et al. Varicella-zoster virus infections. Ann Intern Med 1988;108:221–237.

50. Ross AH, Modification of chickenpox in family contacts by administration of gamma globulin. N Engl J Med 1962;267:369–376.

51. Preblud SR. Age-specific risks of varicella complications. Pediatrics 1981;68:14–17.

52. Ragozzino MW, Melton LJ, Kurland TL, et al. Population-based study of herpes zoster and its sequelae. Medicine 1982;51:310–316.

53. Burke B, Steele R, Beard O, et al. Immune responses to varicella-zoster in the aged. Arch Intern Med 1982;142:291–293.

54. Locksley RM, Flournoy N, Sullivan KM, et al. Infection with varicella zoster virus after marrow transplantation. J Infect Dis 1985;152:1172–1181.

55. Glesby NJ, Moore RD, Chaisson RE, et al. Herpes zoster in patients with advanced human immunodeficiency virus infection treated with zidovudine. J Infect Dis 1993;168:1264–1268.

56. Buchbinder SP, Katz MH, Hessol NA, et al. Herpes zoster and human immunodeficiency virus infection. J Infect Dis 1992;166:1153–1156.

57. Melbye M, Grossman RJ, Goedert JJ, et al. Risk of AIDS after herpes zoster. Lancet 1987;i:728–731.

58. Colebunders R, Mann JM, Francis H, et al. Herpes zoster in African patients: A clinical predictor of human immunodeficiency virus infection. J Infect Dis 1988;157:314–318.

59. Preblud SR. Orenstein WA, Bart KJ, et al. Varicella: Clinical manifestations, epidemiology and health impact in children. Pediatr Infect Dis J 1984;3:505–509.

60. Liesegang G. Varicella zoster virus: Systemic and ocular features. J Am Acad Dermatol 1984;11:165–191.

61. Feldman S, Hughes WT, Daniel CB. Varicella in children with cancer: Seventy seven cases. Pediatrics 1975;56:388–397.

62. Jura E, Chadwick EG, Josephs SH, et al. Varicella-zoster virus infections in children infected with human immunodeficiency virus. Pediatr Infect Dis J 1989;8:586–590.

63. Perronne C, Lazanas M, Leport C, et al. Varicella in patients infected with the human immunodeficiency virus. Arch Dermatol 1990;126:1033–1036.

64. Fleisher G, Henry W, McSorley M, et al. Life-threatening complications of varicella. Am J Dis Child 1981;135:896–899.

65. Schlossberg D, Littman M. Varicella pneumonia. Arch Intern Med 1988;148:1630–1632.

66. Linnemann CC Jr, Shea L, Partin JC, et al. Reye's syndrome: Epidemiologic and viral studies. Am J Epidemiol 1975; 101:517–526.

67. Preblud SR, Bregman DJ, Vernon LL, et al. Deaths from varicella in infants. Pediatr Infect Dis J 1985;4:503–507.

68. Alkalay AL, Pomerance JJ, Rimoin DL. Fetal varicella syndrome. J Pediatr 1987;111:320–323.

69. Karlin JD. Herpes zoster ophthalmicus: The virus strikes back. Ann Ophthal 1993;25:208–215.

70. Watson PN, Evans RJ. Postherpetic neuralgia: A review. Arch Neuro 1986;43:836–840.

71. Cohen PR, Beltrani VP, Grossman ME. Disseminated herpes zoster in patients with human immunodeficiency virus infection. Am J Med 1988;84:1076–1080.

72. Janier M, Hillion B, Baccard M, et al. Chronic varicella zoster infection in acquired immunodeficiency syndrome. J Am Acad Derm 1988;18:584–585.

73. Pahwa S, Biron K, Lim W, et al. Continuous varicella-zoster infection associated with acyclovir resistance in a child with AIDS. JAMA 1988;260:2879–2882.

74. Jacobson MA, Berger TG, Fikrig S, et al. Acyclovir-resistant varicella-zoster virus infection after chronic acyclovir therapy in patients with acquired immunodeficiency syndrome (AIDS). Ann Intern Med 1990;112:187–191.

74a. LeBoit PE, Limova M, Yen TSB, et al. Chronic verrucous varicella-zoster infection in patients with the acquired immunodeficiency syndrome. Histologic and molecular biologic findings. Am J Dermatopathol 1992;14:1–8, 1992.

75. Oranje AP, Folkers E. The Tzanck smear: Old, but still of inestimable value. Pediatr Derm 1988;5:127–129.

76. Whitley RJ. Therapeutic approaches to varicella-zoster virus infections. J Infect Dis 1992;166:S51–S57.

77. Biron KK, Elian GB. In vitro susceptibility of varicella-zoster virus to acyclovir. Antimicrob Agents Chemother 1980;18:443–447.

78. Balfour HH, Kelly JM, Suarez CS, et al. Acyclovir treatment of varicella in otherwise healthy children. J Pediatr 1990;116:633–639.

79. Dunkle LM, Arvin AM, Whitley RJ, et al. A controlled trial of acyclovir for chickenpox in normal children. N Engl J Med 1991;325:1539–1544.

80. Wallace MR, Bowler WA, Murray NB, et al. Treatment of adult varicella with oral acyclovir. Ann Int Med 1992;117:358–363.

81. Prober DG, Kirk LE, Keeney RE, et al. Acyclovir therapy of chickenpox in immunosuppressed children—a collaborative study. J Pediatr 1982;101:622–625.

82. Bean B, Braun C, Balfour HH. Acyclovir therapy for acute herpes zoster. Lancet 1982;ii:118–121.

83. McKendrick MW, McGill JI, White JI, et al. Oral acyclovir in acute herpes zoster. Br Med J 1986;293:1529–1532.

84. Wood MJ, Johnson RW, McKendrick MW, et al. A randomized trial of acyclovir for 7 days or 21 days with and without prednisolone for treatment of acute herpes zoster. N Engl J Med 1994;330:896–900.

85. Gnann JW, Jr. New antivirals with activity against varicella-zoster virus. Ann Neurol 1994;34:S69–S72.

86. Balfour HH, Bean B, Laskin OL, et al. Acyclovir halts progression of herpes zoster in immunocompromised patients. N Engl J Med 1983;308:1448–1453.

87. Shepp DH, Dandliker PS, Meyers JD. Treatment of varicella-zoster infection in severely immunocompromised patients. N Engl J Med 1986;314:208–212.

88. Whitley RJ, Gnann JW Jr, Hinthorn D, et al. Disseminated herpes zoster in the immunocompromised host: a comparative trial of acyclovir and vidarabine. J Infect Dis 1992;165:450–455.

89. Safrin S, Berger TG, Gilson I, et al. Foscarnet therapy in five patients with AIDS and acyclovir-resistant varicella-zoster virus infection. Ann Intern Med 1991;115:19–21.

90. Zaia JA, Levin MJ, Preblud SR, et al. Evaluation of varicella-

zoster immune globulin. Protection of immunosuppressed children after household exposure to varicella. J Infect Dis 1983;147:737–743.

91. Centers for Disease Control: Varicella-zoster immune globulin for the prevention of chickenpox. Recommendations of the Immunization Practices Advisory Committee. Ann Intern Med 1984;100:859–865.

92. Epstein MA, Achong BG, Barr YM. Virus particles in cultured lymphoblasts from Burkitt's malignant lymphoma. Lancet 1964;i:252–253.

93. Henle G, Henle W, Diehl V. Relation of Burkitt's tumor-associated herpes-type virus to infectious mononucleosis. Proc Natl Acad Sci 1968;59:94–101.

94. Evans AS, Niederman JC, McCollum RW. Seroepidemiologic studies of infectious mononucleosis with EB virus. N Engl J Med 1968;279:1121–1127.

95. Niederman JC, McCollum RW, Henle G, Henle W. Infectious mononucleosis: Clinical manifestations in relation to EB virus antibodies. JAMA 1968;203:205–209.

96. Sixbey JW, Nedrud JG, Raab-Traub M, et al. Epstein-Barr virus replication in oropharyngeal epithelial cells. N Engl J Med 1984;310:1225–1234.

97. Wolf H, Haus M, Wilmes E: Persistence of Epstein-Barr virus in the parotid gland. J Virol 1984;51:795–798.

98. Sixbey JW, Lemon SM, Pagano JS: A second site for Epstein-Barr virus shedding: The uterine cervix. Lancet 1986;ii:1122–1124.

99. Yang LS, Sixbey JW, Clark D, et al. Epstein-Barr virus receptor on human pharyngeal epithelia. Lancet 1986;i:240–242.

100. Fingeroth JD, Weiss JJ, Tedder TF, et al. Epstein-Barr virus receptor of human lymphocytes is the C3d receptor CR2. Proc Natl Acad Sci 1987;81:4510–4514.

101. Henderson E, Miller G, Robinson J, Heston L. Efficiency of transformation of lymphocytes by Epstein-Barr virus. Virology 1977;76:152–163.

102. Pereira MS, Blake JM, Macrae AD. EB virus antibody at different ages. Br Med J 1969;4:526–527.

103. Porter DD, Wimberly I, Benyesh-Melnick M: Prevalence of antibodies to EB virus and other herpesviruses. JAMA 1969;208:1675–1679.

104. Gerber P, Lucas S, Nonoyama M, et al. Oral excretion of Epstein-Barr virus by healthy subjects and patients with infectious mononucleosis. Lancet 1972;ii:988–989.

105. Niederman JC, Miller G, Pearson HA, et al. Infectious mononucleosis: Epstein-Barr virus shedding in saliva and the oropharynx. N Engl J Med 1976;294:1355–1359.

106. Miller G, Niederman JC, Andrews LL. Prolonged oropharyngeal excretion of Epstein-Barr virus following infectious mononucleosis. N Engl J Med 1973;288:229–232.

107. Crosti A, Gianotti F. Dermatosi infantile eruttiva acroesposta di probabile origine virosica. Minerva Dermatol 1956;31:483.

108. Labbe A, Goumy J, Peyrot P, et al. Syndrome acro papulovésiculeux de Gianotti-Crosti au cors d'une primo-infection à virus Epstein-Barr. Nouv Presse Med 1981;10:2992–2993.

109. Konno M, Kikuta H, Ishikawa N, et al. A possible association between hepatitis B antigen-negative infantile papular acrodermatitis and Epstein-Barr virus infection. J Pediatr 1982;101:222–224.

110. Spear K, Winkelmann RK. Gianotti-Crosti syndrome. A review of ten cases not associated with hepatitis B. Arch Dermatol 1984;120:891–896.

111. McCarthy JT, Hoagland RJ. Cutaneous manifestations of infectious mononucleosis. JAMA 1964;187:153–154.

112. Lemanske RF Jr, Bush RK. Cold urticaria in infectious mononucleosis. JAMA 1982;247:1604.

113. Mesko JW, Wu LYF: Infectious mononucleosis and cold urticaria. JAMA 1982;248:828.

114. Snydman DR, Rudders RA, Daoust P, et al. Infectious mononucleosis in an adult progressing to fatal immunoblastic lymphoma. Ann Intern Med 1982;96:737–742.

115. Jones JF, Shurin S, Abramowsky C, Tubbs RR, et al. T-cell lymphomas containing Epstein-Barr viral DNA in patients with chronic Epstein-Barr virus infections. N Engl J Med 1988;318:733–740.

116. Drago F, Romagnoli M, Loi A, Rebora A. Epstein-Barr virus-related persistent erythema multiforme in chronic fatigue syndrome. Arch Dermatol 1992;128:217–222.

117. Holmes GP, Kaplan JE, Gantz NM, et al. Chronic fatigue syndrome: A working case definition. Ann Intern Med 1988;108:387–389.

118. Horwitz CA, Henle W, Henle G, et al. Long term serological follow-up of patients for Epstein-Barr virus after recovery from infectious mononucleosis. J Infect Dis 1985;151:1150–1153.

119. Holmes GP, Kaplan JE, Stewart JA, et al. A cluster of patients with a chronic mononucleosis-like syndrome: Is Epstein-Barr virus the cause? JAMA 1987;257:2297–2302.

120. Pullen H, Wright N, Murdoch JM. Hypersensitivity reactions to anti-bacterial drugs in infectious mononucleosis. Lancet 1967;ii:1176–1178.

121. Patel BM. Skin rash with infectious mononucleosis and ampicillin. Pediatrics 1967;40:910–911.

122. Cohen JI. Epstein-Barr virus lymphoproliferative disease associated with acquired immunodeficiency. Medicine 1991;70:137–160.

123. Tsai TF, Su IJ, Lu Y-C, et al. Cutaneous angiocentric T-cell lymphoma associated with Epstein-Barr virus. J Am Acad Dermatol 1992;26:31–38.

124. McGregor JM, Yu CC, Lu QL, et al. Posttransplant cutaneous lymphoma. J Am Acad Dermatol 1993;29:549–554.

125. Greenspan D, Greenspan JS, Conant M, et al. Oral "hairy" leukoplakia in male homosexuals: Evidence of association with both papillomavirus and a herpes-group virus. Lancet 1984;ii:831–834.

126. Greenspan JS, Greenspan D, Lennette ET, et al. Replication of Epstein-Barr virus within the epithelial cells of oral "hairy" leukoplakia, an AIDS-associated lesion. N Engl J Med 1985;313:1564–1571.

127. Greenspan D, Greenspan JS, Hearst NG, et al. Relation of oral hairy leukoplakia to infection with the human immunodeficiency virus and the risk of developing AIDS. J Infect Dis 1987;155:475–481.

127a. Fermand J-P, Bendelac A, Delauche-Cavallier M-C, et al. Detection of Epstein-Barr virus in epidermal skin lesions of an immunocompromised patient. Ann Intern Med 1990;112:511–515.

127b. Okada N, Yamamura T, Sato K, et al. Recurrent mucocutaneous lymphocytic infiltration association with Epstein-Barr virus infection. Dermatologica 1991;183:139–142.

128. Bender CE. The value of corticosteroids in the treatment of infectious mononucleosis. JAMA 1967;199:529–531.

129. Bolden KJ. Corticosteroids in the treatment of infectious mononucleosis. J R Coll Gen Practice 1972;22:87–95.

130. Pagano JS, Sixbey JW, Lin J-C: Acyclovir and Epstein-Barr virus infection. J Antimicrob Chemother 1983;12(Suppl. B):113–121.

131. Andersson J, Britton S, Ernberg I, et al. Effect of acyclovir on infectious mononucleosis: A double-blind, placebo-controlled study. J Infect Dis 1986;153:283–290.

132. Sullivan JL, Byron KS, Brewster FE, et al. Treatment of life-threatening Epstein-Barr virus infections with acyclovir. Am J Med 1982;73:262–266.

133. Hanto DW, Najarian JS. Advances in the diagnosis and treatment of EBV-associated lymphoproliferative diseases in immunocompromised hosts. J Surg Oncol 1985;30:215–220.

134. Schöfer H, Ochsendorf FR, Helm EB, Millbrandt R. Treatment of oral "hairy" leukoplakia in AIDS patients with vitamin A acid (topically) or acyclovir (systemically) (letter). Dermatologica 1987;174:150–151.

135. Newman C, Polk BF. Resolution of oral hairy leukoplakia during therapy with 9-(1, 3-dihydroxy-2-propoxymethyl) guanine (DHPG). Ann Intern Med 1987;107:348–350.

136. Kessler HA, Benson CA, Urbanski P. Regression of oral hairy leukoplakia during zidovudine therapy. Arch Intern Med 1988;148:2496–2497.

137. Herbst JS, Morgan J, Raab-Traub N, et al. Comparison of the efficacy of surgery and acyclovir in the treatment of oral hairy leukoplakia. J Am Acad Dermatol 1989;21:753–756.

138. Weller TH, Hanshaw JB, Scott DE. Serologic differentiation of viruses responsible for cytomegalic inclusion disease. Virology 1960;12:130–132.

139. Rinaldo CR Jr, Black PH, Hirsch MS. Interactions of cytomegalovirus with leukocytes from patients with mononucleosis due to cytomegalovirus. J Infect Dis 1977;136:667–678.
140. Rice GPA, Schrier RD, Oldstone MBA. Cytomegalovirus infects human lymphocytes and monocytes: Virus expression is restricted to immediate early antigen products. Proc Natl Acad Sci 1984;81:6134–6138.
141. Kretch U. Complement-fixing antibodies against cytomegalovirus in different parts of the world. Bull WHO 1973;49:103–106.
142. Kaariainen L, Klemola E, Paloheimo J. Rise of cytomegalovirus antibodies in an infectious mononucleosis-like syndrome after transfusion. Br Med J 1966;2:1270–1272.
143. Lesher JL Jr. Cytomegalovirus infections and the skin. J Am Acad Dermatol 1988;18:1333–1338.
144. Fine JD, Arndt KA. The TORCH syndrome: A clinical review. J Am Acad Dermatol 1985;12:697–706.
145. Jordan MC, Rousseau WE, Stewart JA. Spontaneous cytomegalovirus mononucleosis. Ann Intern Med 1973;79:153–160.
146. Cohen JI, Corey GR. Cytomegalovirus infection in the normal host. Medicine 1985;64:100–114.
147. Horwitz CA, Henle W, Henle G, et al: Clinical and laboratory evaluation of cytomegalovirus-induced mononucleosis in previously healthy individuals. Medicine 1986;65:124–134.
148. Klemola E. Hypersensitivity reactions to ampicillin in cytomegalovirus mononucleosis. Scand J Infect Dis 1970;2:29–31.
149. Armstrong D, Gold JWM, Dryjanski J, et al. Treatment of infections in patients with acquired immunodeficiency syndrome. Ann Intern Med 1985;103:738–743.
150. Pariser RJ. Histologically specific skin lesions in disseminated cytomegalovirus infection. J Am Acad Dermatol 1983;9:937–946.
151. Nakoneczna I, Kay S. Fatal disseminated cytomegalic inclusion disease in an adult presenting with a lesion of the gastrointestinal tract. Am J Clin Pathol 1967;47:124–128.
152. Lin C-S, Penha PD, Krishnan MN, et al. Cytomegalic inclusion disease of the skin. Arch Dermatol 1981;117:282–284.
153. Penneys NS, Hicks B. Unusual cutaneous lesion associated with acquired immunodeficiency syndrome. J Am Acad Dermatol 1985;13:845–852.
154. Bournérias I, Boisnic S, Patey O, et al. Unusual cutaneous cytomegalovirus involvement in patients with acquired immunodeficiency syndrome. Arch Dermatol 1989;125:1243–1246.
155. Smith KJ, Skelton HG 3d, James WD, Angritt P. Concurrent epidermal involvement of cytomegalovirus and herpes simplex virus
in two HIV-infected patients. J Am Acad Dermatol 1991;25:500–506.
156. Gallant JE, Moore RD, Richman DD, et al. Incidence and natural history of cytomegalovirus disease in patients with advanced human immunodeficiency virus disease treated with zidovudine. J Infect Dis 1992;166:1223–1227.
157. Swanson S, Feldman PS. Cytomegalovirus infection initially diagnosed by skin biopsy. Am J Clin Pathol 1987;87:113–116.
158. Bale JF Jr, Kealey GP, Ebelhack CL, et al. Cytomegalovirus infection in a cyclosporine treated burn patient: Case report. J Trauma 1992;32:263–267.
159. Zurlo JJ, O'Neill D, Polis MA, et al. Lack of clinical utility of cytomegalovirus blood and urine cultures in patients with HIV infection. Ann Intern Med 1993;118:12–17.
160. Matthews T, Boehme R. Antiviral activity and mechanism of action of ganciclovir. Rev Infect Dis 1988;10(Suppl. 3):S490–S494.
161. Koretz SH, Buhles WC, Brewin A, et al. Treatment of serious cytomegalovirus infections with 9-(1,3-dihydroxy-2-propoxymethyl) guanine in patients with AIDS and other immunodeficiencies. N Engl J Med 1986;314:801–805.
162. Jacobson MA, O'Donnell JJ, Brodie HR, et al. Randomized prospective trial of ganciclovir maintenance therapy for cytomegalovirus retinitis. J Med Virol 1988;25:339–349.
163. Erice A, Chou S, Biron KK, et al. Progressive disease due to ganciclovir-resistant cytomegalovirus in immunocompromised patients. N Engl J Med 1989;320:289–293.
164. Jacobson MA, Drew WL, Feinberg J, et al. Foscarnet therapy for ganciclovir-resistant cytomegalovirus retinitis. J Infect Dis 1991;163:1348–1351.
165. Studies of Ocular Complications of AIDS Research Group. Mortality in patients with the acquired immunodeficiency syndrome treated with either foscarnet or ganciclovir for cytomegalovirus retinitis. N Engl J Med 1992;326:213–220.
166. Snydman DR, Werner BG, Heinze-Lacey B, et al. Use of cytomegalovirus immune globulin to prevent cytomegalovirus disease in renal transplant patients. N Engl J Med 1987;317:1049–1054.
167. Balfour HH, Chace BA, Stapleton JT, et al. A randomized, placebo-controlled trial of oral acyclovir for the prevention of cytomegalovirus disease in receipients of renal allografts. N Engl J Med 1989;320:1381–1387.
168. Salahuddin SZ, Ablashi DV, Markham PD, et al. Isolation of a new virus, HBLV, in patients with lymphoproliferative disorders. Science 1986;234:596–600.
169. Lusso P, Markham PD, Tschachler E, et al. In vitro cellular tropism of human B-lymphotropic virus (human herpesvirus-6). J Exp Med 1988;167:1659–1670.
170. Takahashi K, Sonoda S, Higashi K, et al. Predominant CD_4 T-lymphocyte tropism of human herpesvirus 6–related virus. J Virol 1989;63:3161–3163.
171. Tedder RS, Briggs M, Cameron CH, et al. A novel lymphotropic herpesvirus (letter). Lancet 1987;ii:390–392.
172. Lawrence GL, Chee M, Craxton M, et al. Human herpesvirus-6 is closely related to human cytomegalovirus. J Virol 1990;64:287–299.
173. Alblashi DV, Balachandran N, Josephs SF, et al. Genomic polymorphism, growth properties, and immunologic variations in human herpesvirus-6 isolates. Virology 1991;184:545–552.
174. Saxinger C, Polesky H, Eby N, et al. Antibody reactivity with HBLV (HHV-6) in U.S. populations. J Virol Methods 1988;21:199–208.
175. Briggs M, Fox J, Tedder RS. Age prevalence of antibody to human herpesvirus-6. Lancet 1988;i:1058–1059.
176. Knowles WA, Gardner SD. High prevalence of antibody to human herpesvirus-6 and seroconversion associated with rash in two infants. Lancet 1988;ii:912–913.
177. Takahashi K, Sonoda S, Kawakami K, et al. Human herpesvirus-6 and exanthem subitum. Lancet 1988;i:1463.
178. Brown NA, Sumaya CV, Liu C, et al. Fall in human herpesvirus-6 seropositivity with age. Lancet 1988;ii:396.
179. Ensoli B, Lusso P, Schachter F, et al. Human herpesvirus-6 increases HIV-1 expression in co-infected T cells via nuclear factors binding to the HIV-1 enhancer. EMBO J 1989;8:3019–3027.
180. Fox J, Briggs M, Tedder RS. Antibody to human herpesvirus-6 in HIV-1 positive and negative homosexual men (letter). Lancet 1988;ii:396–397.
181. Spira TJ, Bozeman LH, Sanderlin KC, et al. Lack of correlation between human herpesvirus-6 infection and the course of human immunodeficiency virus infection. J Infect Dis 1990;161:567–570.
182. Yamanishi K, Okuno T, Shiraki K, et al. Identification of human herpesvirus-6 as a causal agent for exanthem subitum. Lancet 1988;i:1065–1067.
183. Sura S, Yoshikawa T, Asano Y, et al. Human herpesvirus-6 infection (exanthem subitum) without rash. Pediatrics 1989;83:1003–1006.
184. Pruksananonda P, Hall CB, Insel RA, et al. Primary human herpesvirus-6 infection in young children. N Engl J Med 1992;326:1445–1450.
185. Yoshikawa T, Nakashima T, Suga S, et al. Human herpesvirus-6 DNA in cerebrospinal fluid of a child with exanthem subitum and meningoencephalitis. Pediatrics 1992;89:888–890.
186. Asano Y, Yoshikawa T, Suga S, et al. Fatal fulminant hepatitis in an infant with human herpesvirus-6 infection (letter). Lancet 1990;335:862–863.
187. Sobue R, Miyazaki H, Okamoto M, et al. Fulminant hepatitis in primary human herpesvirus-6 infection. N Engl J Med 1991;324:1290.
188. Asano Y, Yoshikawa T, Suga S, et al. Simultaneous occurrence of human herpesvirus-6 infection and intussusception of three infants. Pediatr Infect Dis J 1991;10:335–337.
189. Niederman JC, Liu C-R, Kaplan MH, et al. Clinical and serolo-

gical features of human herpesvirus-6 infection in three adults. Lancet 1988;ii:817–818.

190. Akashi K, Eizuru Y, Sumiyoshi Y, et al. Brief report: Severe infectious mononucleosis-like syndrome and primary human herpesvirus-6 infection in an adult. N Engl J Med 1993; 329:168–171.

191. Jarrett RF, Clark DA, Josephs SF, et al. Detection of human herpesvirus-6 DNA in peripheral blood and saliva. J Med Virol 1990;32:73–76.

192. Levy JA, Ferro F, Greenspan D, et al. Frequent isolations of HHV-6 from saliva and high seroprevalence of the virus in the population. Lancet 1990;335:1047–1050.

193. Fox JD, Briggs M, Ward PA, et al. Human herpesvirus-6 in salivary glands. Lancet 1990;336:590–593.

194. Maeda A, Sata T, Enzan H, et al. The evidence of human herpesvirus-6 infection in the lymph nodes of Hodgkin's disease. Virchows Archiv-A 1993;423:71–75.

195. Kondo K, Kondo T, Okuno T, et al. Latent human herpesvirus-6 infection of human monocytes/macrophages. J Gen Virol 1991;72:1401–1408.

196. Yoshikawa T, Suga S, Asano Y, et al. Human herpesvirus-6 infection in bone marrow transplantation. Blood 1991;78: 1381–1384.

197. Carrigan DR, Drobyski W, Russler SK, et al. Interstitial pneu-monitis associated with human herpesvirus-6 infection after marrow transplantation. Lancet 1991;338:147–149.

198. Cone RW, Hackman RC, Huang ML, et al. Human herpes-virus-6 in lung tissue from patients with pneumonitis after bone marrow transplantation. N Engl J Med 1993;329:156–161.

199. Drobyski WR, Dunne WM, Burd EM, et al. Human herpes-virus-6 (HHV-6) infection in allogeneic bone marrow transplant recipients: Evidence of a marrow-suppressive role for HHV-6 in vivo. J Infect Dis 1993;167:735–739.

200. Okuno T, Higashi K, Shiraki K, et al. Human herpesvirus-6 infection in renal transplantation. Transplantation 1990;49: 519–522.

201. Agut H, Collandre H, Aubin JT, et al. In vitro sensitivity of human herpesvirus-6 to antiviral drugs. Res Virol 1989;140: 219–228.

202. Burns WH, Sandford GR. Susceptibility of human herpesvirus-6 to antivirals in vitro. J Infect Dis 1990;162:634–637.

203. Agut H, Aubin JT, Huraux JM. Homogenous susceptibility of distinct human herpesvirus-6 strains to antivirals in vitro (letter). J Infect Dis 1991;163:1382–1383.

204. Chang Y, Cesarman E, Pessin MS, et al. Identification of her-pesvirus-like DNA sequences in AIDS-associated Kaposi's sarcoma. Science 1994;266:1865–1869.

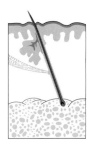

chapter 122

Poxviruses

RICHARD W. GROVES

Viruses of the family Poxviridae are large, ovoid or brick-shaped particles containing a double-stranded DNA genome. Members of the Poxviridae infect a variety of organisms from insects to mammals, but only those affecting humans are discussed here. These can be divided into two distinct genera: the orthopoxviruses (which cause smallpox, monkeypox, cowpox, and vaccinia) and the parapoxviruses (which cause orf and milker's nodule). The organism that causes molluscum contagiosum is also a poxvirus but is unclassified.

Orthopoxviruses are approximately 200×250 nm with randomly arranged surface tubules about 10 nm in diameter. Parapoxviruses are slightly narrower and have a single surface tubule that winds around the virus, giving rise to a criss-cross pattern on electron microscopy. The molluscum contagiosum virus is even larger than the orthopoxviruses, measuring 200×300 nm.

Smallpox

One of the greatest triumphs of modern medicine is the global eradication of smallpox, a disease that had plagued humanity for centuries. The last case occurred in Somalia in 1977, and global eradication was accepted by the World Health Organization in May 1980.[1] Thus this discussion focuses on a disease that no longer occurs, but because stocks of the virus are still held, and outbreaks related to these stocks have occurred,[2, 3] knowledge of the disease is still of benefit.

DEFINITION

Smallpox was caused by the orthopoxvirus variola. It was divided into two variants: variola major, which was associated with a high mortality, and variola minor (alastrim), which was rarely fatal.

CLINICAL DESCRIPTION

Epidemiology

Although smallpox was a worldwide disease, variola major and alastrim had distinct geographic characteristics, with the former found predominantly in Asia and the latter largely in southern Africa and South America. Furthermore, smallpox strains were identified in Africa that were distinct from variola major and minor,[1] and it is likely that a spectrum of virulence existed from high (variola major) to low (alastrim).

In the unvaccinated, smallpox was a disease of children, and transmission generally occurred through close physical contact, although spread from airborne particles and fomites was also suspected. Smallpox was considered to be a highly contagious disease, but it is likely that only about 30% of susceptible contacts became infected.[4]

Eradication of smallpox was possible because of a number of factors, including the existence of an effective vaccine, the absence of a carrier state, and the lack of any cultural or social barriers to case reporting. The eradication campaign, which was coordinated by the World Health Organization, was separated into three distinct phases. In the first, or "attack," phase, attention was given to mass vaccination together with improvement of reporting and case detection. In the second, or "consolidation," phase, the aim was elimination of smallpox in that area. Cases were recognized, patients were isolated, and their contacts were vaccinated. In this phase surveillance had to be sensitive enough to confirm the absence of cases. The final, or "maintenance," phase was intended to ensure that areas free of smallpox remained so, and every suspect case was extensively investigated. Eventually an area was declared "smallpox free" if no cases were detected over a 2-year period.

Smallpox virus exists in laboratories in Russia and in the United States, where its genome is being sequenced. It is debated as to whether, once sequencing is complete, the organism should be destroyed.[5, 6] Proponents of destruction of the virus argue that the disease is no longer a threat to humans and that there is therefore no rationale to maintain stocks of such a dangerous organism, which might in the future be misused. Those on the other side of the debate believe that the risk of maintaining virus stocks is far outweighed by the potential gains to humans from studying the ways in which smallpox became such a successful virus. Certainly there is evidence that other poxviruses have evolved highly sophisticated ways of defeating host immunity,[7, 8] and it is likely that the smallpox virus developed similar methods of enhancing its virulence.

Clinical Findings

Smallpox had an incubation period of 12 to 13 days during which massive viral replication occurred. This was followed by a severe prodromal illness characterized by malaise, high fever, and backache. Two to 4 days later the characteristic eruption appeared (Fig. 122–1), with successive macules, papules, vesicles, and pustules that crusted by about day 9 of the rash. At any time, all lesions were at the same stage of development, which is an important sign that helped to distinguish smallpox from infection with varicella-zoster. The patient was infectious from the start of the prodrome until the last crust had separated, although infection was most commonly transmitted 4 to 6 days after the onset of the prodrome.[9] The eruption was predominantly distal, affecting the face, forearms, and lower legs more than the trunk; and lesions often healed with considerable scarring.

A number of clinical variants of smallpox were described.[1] A hemorrhagic form was associated with very high mortality, and "modified" smallpox was milder than the classic form, occurring in those with immunity from previous vaccination. This form had a less severe prodrome, and the cutaneous lesions evolved more rapidly, frequently with crusting by the seventh day.

PATHOLOGY

Smallpox was an intraepidermal vesicular process in which ballooning of keratinocytes led to reticular alteration of the epidermis. Intracytoplasmic inclusions in keratinocytes called Guarnieri's bodies were a hallmark of the disease.[10]

DIAGNOSIS AND DIFFERENTIAL DIAGNOSIS

In endemic areas, the diagnosis of smallpox was generally a clinical one. Investigation of suspected cases now would involve intensive virologic study, because the identification of a case would have worldwide public health implications.

Routine laboratory investigations were of little diagnostic help in smallpox. The virus could be isolated from the blood during the prodrome and from vesicle fluid later in the disease. Electron microscopy and immunofluoresence were also of use in identifying the virus, although precise characterization depended on laboratory culture.

Prodromal smallpox had to be differentiated from other severe febrile illnesses, including dengue fever. The eruptive phase had to be distinguished from varicella-zoster infection (Table 122–1), and, if any hemorrhagic

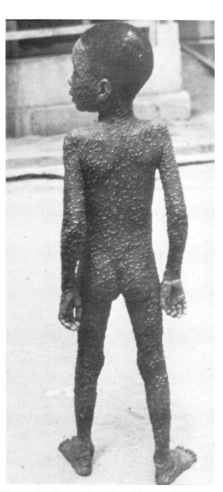

FIGURE 122–1. Smallpox. Note the widespread lesions, particularly over the limbs and face.

TABLE 122–1. Comparison of Varicella-Zoster (Chickenpox) and Smallpox

	Smallpox	Varicella-Zoster
Family	Poxvirus	Herpesvirus
Prodrome	Severe	Mild
Lesions	Peripheral, extensor	Central, flexor
Vesicle Formation	Reticular degeneration	Ballooning and reticular degeneration
Multinucleate Cells	No	Yes
Cytoplasmic Inclusions	Yes	No

component was present, from meningococcal septicemia, typhus, and other hemorrhagic fevers.

TREATMENT

No effective treatment for smallpox was available. General medical support, including attention to fluid and nutritional requirements, prevention of secondary infection, and expert nursing care, was essential. Vaccination has been generally discontinued, although military personnel and some others (e.g., those working with smallpox or related viruses) may still be vaccinated.

Vaccinia

DEFINITION

Vaccinia is an orthopoxvirus that was used for vaccination against smallpox. Jenner, who popularized vaccination in the late 18th century, is thought to have employed cowpox virus, but the current vaccinia virus is distinct from this and other poxviruses.[9] It is possible that vaccinia was derived from smallpox or cowpox by human or animal passage, by genetic hybridization between smallpox and cowpox, or from a now extinct animal poxvirus. The last possibility seems most likely because of the clear differences between vaccinia, cowpox, and smallpox.

Normal vaccination resulted in severe symptoms (fever, nausea, headache) in about 25% of persons and additional abnormal reactions occurred in up to 8% of vaccinees.[11] It is these responses that are discussed here.

CLINICAL DESCRIPTION

Abnormal reactions to smallpox vaccination could be either local or generalized (Table 122–2). Bacterial superinfection and accidental inoculation of virus to other body sites or individuals were the main local complications. Although these were generally trivial and avoidable, inoculation of vaccinia to certain sites (e.g., the eye)

TABLE 122-2. Classification of Abnormal Responses to Smallpox Vaccination

	Mild	Severe
Localized	Bacterial superinfection Autoinfection (some)	Autoinfection (some) Progressive vaccinia Eczema vaccinatum
Generalized	Erythema multiforme Generalized vaccinia	Congenital vaccinia Vaccinial encephalitis

or individuals (e.g., the immunosuppressed) could be dangerous. Eczema vaccinatum occurred in children with a history of atopic dermatitis and was acquired either through primary vaccination or by contact with a vaccinee. Lesions appeared at sites that were or had been involved by eczema. Patients were systemically unwell, and a case-fatality rate of 5% was reported.[12] For this reason, atopic dermatitis was regarded as a contraindication to vaccination. Progressive vaccinia occurred in immunodeficient patients and resulted in progressive enlargement of the inflammatory lesion at the vaccination site. Sometimes the entire upper arm and shoulder were involved, and distant secondary lesions developed. The disease was usually fatal.

Generalized reactions could be relatively benign or severe. Erythema multiforme could be associated with vaccination, and in generalized vaccinia a widespread eruption developed 6 to 9 days after vaccination. Both of these eruptions had a benign prognosis. Vaccinial encephalitis[13] and congenital vaccinia, in which virus was disseminated to the fetus from the mother, could be fatal.

PATHOLOGY

The histopathologic features of vaccinia were similar to those of variola.

PATHOGENESIS AND ETIOLOGY

During vaccination, live vaccinia virus was introduced into intact skin. Local multiplication of virus was followed by brief viremia, an antibody response, and resolution with immunity. Because live virus was used, individuals immunocompromised in either major (e.g., lymphoma, leukemia) or minor (e.g., atopy) ways were at risk of dissemination of the organism.

DIAGNOSIS

The diagnosis of vaccinia should be confirmed by virologic studies (culture, electron microscopy, and serology), and investigations to identify immunologic defects should be performed in persons with reactions other than simple secondary infection or autoinoculation. Human immunodeficiency virus has been associated with severe vaccination reactions.[14]

TREATMENT

Prevention of reactions by appropriate clinical screening for immunodeficiency and eczema was important, as was advice on appropriate care of the vaccination site. Those with severe reactions could be treated with hyperimmune globulin (VIG, vaccinia immune globulin) together with antiviral agents such as vidarabine or interferon.

Monkeypox

DEFINITION

The monkeypox agent is an orthopoxvirus that produces an eruption clinically indistinguishable from smallpox.[15, 16]

CLINICAL DESCRIPTION

Although the virus was first isolated from captive Asiatic monkeys, its natural animal reservoir remains uncertain. The disease is found exclusively in West and Central Africa. The mode of infection of index cases has been suggested to be close contact with or handling of infected animals. Person-to-person spread occurs but is uncommon, and smallpox vaccination appears to have a protective effect.[17]

Infection is most common among unvaccinated children. The rash is very similar to smallpox, but lymphadenopathy tends to be more severe and cropping of lesions is sometimes seen. The disease lasts 2 to 4 weeks, is occasionally complicated by gastrointestinal and respiratory problems, and has a mortality of approximately 10%.[16]

PATHOLOGY

The cutaneous pathology of monkeypox is the same as that of smallpox.

DIAGNOSIS AND DIFFERENTIAL DIAGNOSIS

Distinction of smallpox and monkeypox was important and clinically difficult. However, virologic studies such as the ability to form pocks at 39°C, and growth in RK13 cells pointed to a diagnosis of monkeypox rather than variola. Serologic tests are now available,[18] and the organism can be identified as an orthopoxvirus by electron microscopy.

TREATMENT

As with smallpox, treatment is essentially supportive. Persons working with monkeypox virus should be vaccinated.[19]

Cowpox

DEFINITION

Cowpox is an uncommon poxvirus zoonosis circulating in Europe that occasionally affects humans, generally causing a localized self-limiting inflammatory reaction.

CLINICAL DESCRIPTION

Although initially isolated from cows and farm workers, and hence named cowpox, this disease is rare in cattle.[9, 20] Its natural reservoir remains unknown but has been suggested to be a small mammal, and infection of domestic cats is not uncommon.[21, 22] Human infections occur at the site of minor trauma and are generally limited to the hands. The lesion starts as an inflammatory papule with associated erythema and hemorrhage and may ulcerate.[23, 24] Sporotrichoid spread has been reported.[25] Local lymph node enlargement and fever occur often, sometimes necessitating admission to a hospital. The lesion resolves in 4 to 6 weeks and may be complicated by secondary bacterial infection or, very rarely, encephalitis.[26]

PATHOLOGY

Like smallpox, early cowpox lesions show prominent reticular degeneration, and "A" type eosinophilic cytoplasmic inclusions are often present.[10, 24] There is marked epidermal hyperplasia and inflammatory cell infiltration.

DIAGNOSIS AND DIFFERENTIAL DIAGNOSIS

In the context of contact with an infected animal, clinical diagnosis is not difficult. However, in the absence of this history other diagnoses must be considered (Table 122–3) including orf, milker's nodule, and, if there are hemorrhagic lesions, anthrax. Investigations including electron microscopy and viral culture will establish the correct diagnosis.

TREATMENT

Because of the self-limiting and mild nature of the disease, no treatment is generally necessary. In severe

TABLE 122–3. Differential Diagnosis of Parapoxvirus Infections
Other Infections
Bacterial (e.g., anthrax, atypical mycobacteria, erysipeloid, primary syphilis, inoculation tuberculosis)
Fungal (e.g., sporotrichosis)
Viral (e.g, herpetic whitlow, cowpox, wart)
Epidermal Tumors
Keratoacanthoma
Squamous cell carcinoma
Melanoma
Miscellaneous Conditions
Pyoderma gangrenosum

cases, however, human cowpox should respond to vaccinia immune globulin.[26] Patients with infection should be warned about transferring it to other sites or persons.

Orf and Milker's Nodule

DEFINITION

Orf and milker's nodule are caused by closely related parapoxviruses[27] and are discussed here together because of their clinical, pathologic, and virologic similarities. The human diseases can generally only be distinguished by history, with orf resulting from contact with sheep and milker's nodule occurring in persons in contact with cattle. The collective term *farmyard pox* has been proposed.[28]

CLINICAL DESCRIPTION

These diseases are found in persons who have contact with sheep and cattle, on farms or in the meat trade. The virus is resistant to drying: infection may therefore be acquired indirectly from contaminated structures on farms.[29] The diseases are widely recognized by persons working with sheep or cattle, and it is likely that many cases go unreported. Infection occurs through small cuts and abrasions, and the site depends on local practice in handling animals. For example, in shepherds, the left hand, which is used for holding a sheep's mouth during dosing, is affected more commonly than the right. Lesions are generally solitary, although multiple lesions can occur and are found predominantly on the extremities. Lesions start as an erythematous papule that subsequently develops a white halo, becomes nodular, and may ulcerate (Fig. 122–2). Most cases resolve in about 6 weeks. Lesions average 1 to 2 cm in diameter, although giant orf has been reported in immunosuppressed indi-

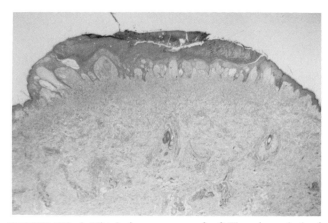

FIGURE 122–3. Histologic appearance of orf. There is marked epidermal hyperplasia, dermal vascular proliferation and dilatation, and a dense dermal inflammatory infiltrate.

viduals.[30] Systemic upset is uncommon, but erythema multiforme has been associated.[31]

PATHOLOGY

Orf and milker's nodule both begin with ballooning of keratinocytes, spongiosis, and epidermal hyperplasia. Small round eosinophilic viral inclusions are present in the cytoplasm of infected keratinocytes. Intraepidermal vesiculation, necrosis, and ulceration occur in later lesions, accompanied by dense dermal infiltrates of lymphocytes and plasma cells (Fig. 122–3). Marked vascular dilatation corresponds to the erythematous color of nodular lesions, and vascular proliferation simulating a neoplasm can occur. Electron microscopy demonstrates parapoxvirus (Fig. 122–4), and culture and DNA analysis can distinguish the ovine and bovine strains.

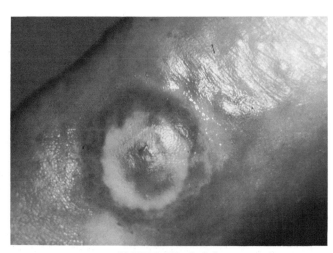

FIGURE 122–2. Orf.

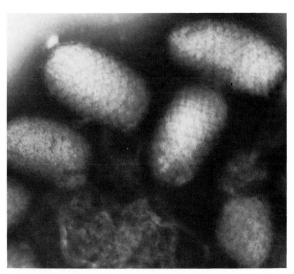

FIGURE 122–4. Electron micrograph of orf virus. Note the criss-cross pattern of surface tubules, characteristic of parapoxviruses.

DIAGNOSIS AND DIFFERENTIAL DIAGNOSIS

The diagnosis of orf and milker's nodule is generally a clinical one and is often suggested by the patient! However, in the absence of a history, diagnoses such as cowpox, herpetic whitlow, atypical mycobacterial infection, and pyogenic granuloma must be considered (see Table 122–3). The histologic features are generally sufficiently distinctive to differentiate these possibilities, and electron microscopy of scrapings from a lesion will provide conclusive evidence of parapox infection.

TREATMENT

Generally no treatment is required since both conditions are self-limiting. Correct diagnosis is important to avoid mutilating surgery on the assumption that the lesion represents a rapidly growing malignant tumor. Attention should be paid to the avoidance of secondary infection.

Molluscum Contagiosum

DEFINITION

Molluscum contagiosum is a common poxvirus infection of the skin and mucous membranes characterized by pearly umbilicated papules.

CLINICAL DESCRIPTION

The disease occurs throughout the world, and its prevalence in the United States has been estimated at 1%.[32] Although it may occur at any age, the majority of cases occur in childhood, with boys being more frequently affected than girls. Transmission is thought to be by person-to-person spread, and genital lesions in adults are probably transmitted sexually. The disease is more severe in the immunosuppressed, and giant lesions are a feature of human immunodeficiency virus infection.[33] Infection is more common in children with atopic eczema.[34] Lesions may occur at any site and start as grouped, flesh colored or pearly papules a few millimeters in diameter (Fig. 122–5). As they progress, they develop a distinct central depression (umbilication) and a white, curd-like core may easily be expressed. The lesions are generally asymptomatic, but occasionally there is surrounding eczematization and pruritus may then be a feature. Like virus warts, molluscum contagiosum exhibits the Koebner phenomenon. Individual lesions last about 2 months and resolve either spontaneously or after minor trauma, but the eruption as a whole frequently persists longer than this.

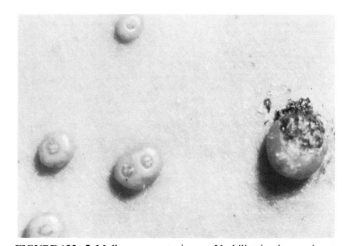

FIGURE 122–5. Molluscum contagiosum. Umbilication is prominent in these lesions.

PATHOLOGY

Molluscum contagiosum appears to infect follicular epithelium, because its viral inclusions are found within endophytic, bulbous lobules of keratinocytes attached to the epidermis, and not within the interfollicular epidermis itself. This propensity to infect follicular epithelium explains the rarity of cases of mucosal molluscum infection. The distinctive large, round molluscum bodies that are the hallmark of the condition form above the basal layer and are initially eosinophilic (Fig. 122–6). They consist of masses of brick-shaped viral particles. The nuclei of keratinocytes harboring these inclusions are compressed into crescentic remnants at their peripheries. As keratinocytes bearing inclusions ascend, the inclusions become basophilic and are discharged into a central channel, presumably the pilar canal of the infected follicle.

The pathologic diagnosis of molluscum contagiosum is usually easy. It can be difficult if the plane of sectioning includes only the edge of an infected follicle, in which case a lobule of keratinocytes with abundant pale cytoplasm and uniformly enlarged, vesicular nuclei can be a clue to the diagnosis even in the absence of inclusions. If

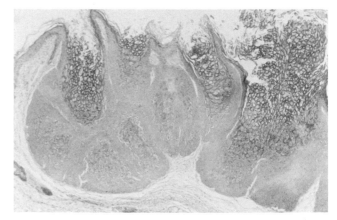

FIGURE 122–6. Histologic appearance of molluscum contagiosum.

rupture of a lesion occurs, dense, diffuse lymphocytic infiltrates with large lymphocytes can result in a picture simulating lymphoma.[35]

PATHOGENESIS AND ETIOLOGY

The molluscum contagiosum virus is one of the largest poxviruses (200 × 300 nm) and as mentioned earlier is generically distinct. Unlike other poxviruses it cannot be cultured in vitro. Although at least three strains have been distinguished on restriction enzyme analysis,[36] no clinical differences between these strains have been identified. Experimental transmission to humans has been achieved with an incubation period of 2 to 7 weeks.[37]

DIAGNOSIS AND DIFFERENTIAL DIAGNOSIS

The clinical appearance is generally characteristic, but in cases of doubt, histologic examination should be diagnostic. In human immunodeficiency virus infection, molluscum contagiosum must be distinguished from cutaneous cryptococcal infection.[33]

TREATMENT

Because the lesions are self-limiting, heal without scarring, and tend to occur in childhood, treatment is generally not required. However, if considered necessary, gentle manual expression of the central core or pricking with a sterile needle is effective. There is also some evidence that simple painting with iodine solutions is helpful. In adults, cryotherapy with liquid nitrogen using a cotton-wool bud or spray gun is the mainstay of treatment, although several sessions of therapy may be required to eradicate the numerous lesions.

References

1. Fenner F, Henderson DA, Arita I, et al. Smallpox and its Eradication. Geneva: World Health Organization, 1988.
2. Smallpox in Birmingham. Br Med J 1978;2:837.
3. Report of the investigation of the cause of the 1978 Birmingham Smallpox Occurrence. London: Her Majesty's Stationery Office, 1980.
4. Foege WH, Millar JD, Henderson DA. Smallpox eradication in West and Central Africa. Bull WHO 1975;52:209–222.
5. Mahey BWJ, Almond JW, Berns KI, et al. The remaining stocks of smallpox should be destroyed. Science 1993;262:1223–1224.
6. Joklik WK, Moss B, Fields BN, et al. Why the smallpox virus stocks should not be destroyed. Science 1993;262:1225–1226.
7. Ray CA, Black RA, Kronheim SR, et al. Viral inhibition of inflammation: Cowpox virus encodes an inhibitor of the interleukin-1 beta converting enzyme. Cell 1992;69:597–604.
8. Spriggs MK, Hruby DE, Maliszewski CR, et al. Vaccinia and cowpox viruses encode a novel secreted interleukin-1-binding protein. Cell 1992;71:145–152.
9. Baxby D. Poxviruses. In: Belshe RB, ed. Textbook of Human Virology, 2nd ed. St. Louis: Mosby–Year Book, 1991:930–946.
10. Strano AJ. Smallpox. In: Binford CH, Connor DH. Pathology of tropical and extraordinary diseases, vol. 1. Armed Forces Institute of Pathology, Washington DC, 1976: 65–67.
11. Baxby D. Indications for smallpox vaccination: Policies still differ. Vaccine 1993;11:395–396.
12. Waddington E, Bray PT, Evans AD, Richards IDG. Cutaneous complications of mass vaccination in South Wales. Trans St John's Hosp Dermatol Soc 1962;50:22–42.
13. Kaplan C. Vaccinia virus: A suitable vehicle for recombinant vaccines? Arch Virol 1989;106:127–139.
14. Redfield RR, Wright DC, James WD, et al. Disseminated vaccinia in a military recruit with human immunodeficiency virus (HIV) disease. N Engl J Med 1987;316:673–676.
15. Jezek Z, Fenner F. Human Monkeypox. Basel: Karger, 1988.
16. Jezek Z, Szczenikowski M, Paluku KM, Mutumbo M. Human monkeypox: Clinical features of 282 patients. J Infect Dis 1987;156:293–297.
17. Jezek Z, Marennikova SS, Mutumbo M, et al. Human monkeypox: A study of 2510 contacts of 214 patients. J Infect Dis 1986;154:551–555.
18. Hutchinson HD, Ziegler DW, Wells DE, Nakano JH. Differentiation of variola, monkeypox and vaccinia antisera by radioimmunoassay. Bull WHO 1977;55:613–623.
19. Baxby D. Human poxvirus infection after the eradication of smallpox. Epidemiol Infect 1988;100:321–334.
20. What's new pussycat? Cowpox. Lancet 1986;2:668.
21. Martland MF, Poulton GJ. Three cases of cowpox infection of domestic cats. Vet Rec 1985;117:231–233.
22. Gaskell RM, Gaskell CJ, Evans RJ, et al. Natural and experimental poxvirus infection in the domestic cat. Vet Rec 1983;112:164–172.
23. Baxby D. Is cowpox misnamed? A review of 10 human cases. Br Med J 1977;1:1379–1381.
24. Casemore DP, Emslie ES, Whyler DK, Baxby D, et al. Cowpox in a child, acquired from a cat. Clin Exp Dermatol 1987;12:286–287.
25. Vestey JP, Yirrell DL, Aldridge RD. Cowpox/catpox infection. Br J Dermatol 1991;124:74–78.
26. Baxby D. Poxviruses. In: Zuckerman AJ, Banatvala JE, Pattison JR, eds. Principles and Practice of Clinical Virology. Chichester, England: John Wiley & Sons, 1990:411–434.
27. Gassmann U, Wyler R, Wittek R. Analysis of parapoxvirus genomes. Arch Virol 1985;83:17–31.
28. Shelley WB, Shelley ED. Farmyard pox: Parapox virus infection in man. Br J Dermatol 1983;108:725–727.
29. Groves RW, Wilson-Jones E, MacDonald DM. Human orf and milkers' nodule: A clinicopathologic study. J Am Acad Dermatol 1991;25:706–711.
30. Savage J, Black MM, "Giant" orf of finger in a patient with a lymphoma. Proc R Soc Med 1972;65:766–768.
31. Agger WA, Webster SB. Human orf infection complicated by erythema multiforme. Cutis 1983;31:334–338.
32. Epstein WL. Molluscum contagiosum. Semin Dermatol 1992;11:184–189.
33. Schwartz JJ, Myskowski PL. Molluscum contagiosum in patients with human immunodeficiency virus infection: A review of twenty-seven patients. J Am Acad Dermatol 1992;27:583–588.
34. Pauly CR, Artis WM, Jones HE. Atopic dermatitis, impaired cellular immunity, and molluscum contagiosum. Arch Dermatol 1978;114:391–393.
35. Ackerman AB, Tanski EV. Pseudoleukemia cutis: Report of a case in association with molluscum contagiosum. Cancer 1977;40:813–817.
36. Porter CD, Archard LC. Characterisation by restriction mapping of three subtypes of molluscum contagiosum virus. J Med Virol 1992;38:1–6.
37. Postlethwaite R. Molluscum contagiosum. Arch Environ Health 1970;21:432–452.

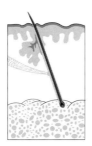

chapter 123

Human Papillomavirus Infection

ELLIOT J. ANDROPHY, KARL BEUTNER, and SUZANNE OLBRICHT

DEFINITION

The papillomaviruses cause a spectrum of epithelial diseases, ranging from cutaneous and genital warts to papillomas of the mucosal epithelium of the larynx and cervix. All papillomaviruses are composed of about 8000 deoxyribonucleotide bases on each of their two complementary strands of DNA. The differences in the specific order of their nucleotides, as determined by DNA sequencing, are used to distinguish human papillomavirus (HPV) types. HPV types are therefore referred to more accurately as genotypes. Nearly 70 different HPV genotypes have been isolated, although many are rare in the general population.[1] These differences in DNA sequence are responsible for their varying pathogenic outcomes. Infection with specific HPV types has been strongly associated with the development of epithelial cancers, most commonly those of the cervix. Most animal species are infected by papillomaviruses, all somewhat related; however, for unknown reasons, animal papillomaviruses are restricted to their species of origin, and infection of humans by other animal papillomaviruses has not been substantiated.

The HPV genotypes appear to have preferred sites of infection and lesion morphology, although the preferences are not strict and may reflect their route of spread rather than genetic predilection. Table 123-1 classifies the HPV types in three groups: cutaneous, mucosal, and those subtypes affecting the mucosal and cutaneous surfaces of patients with epidermodysplasia verruciformis (EV). HPV types 1, 2, 3, and 4 are the predominant isolates from cutaneous warts. A large number of rare genotypes have been found in EV, a heritable syndrome in which afflicted individuals have persistent flat warts, usually from an early age. EV was one of the earliest recognized examples of a viral infection leading to malignancy in humans. In EV, infection with specific HPV types (most commonly types 5 and 8) can result in progression from benign wart to squamous cell carcinomas. However, although an individual can have many warts infected with HPV 5 or 8, only a minority proceed to malignancy.

Of the HPVs that primarily infect mucosal epithelia such as the oropharynx and anogenital region, a subset has also shown a predilection to progress to squamous cell carcinoma. HPV 6 and 11 are commonly found in genital warts and cervical papillomas, whereas HPV 16 and 18 are less frequent. The incidence is reversed in cervical, penile, vulvar, and anal cancers. Because most cervical carcinomas contain types 16, 18, 31, and 35, these genotypes are referred to as "high risk," whereas HPV 6 and 11 are rare in cancers and termed "low risk."[2-4] A preponderance of biologic, experimental, and epidemiologic evidence confirms the causative role of HPVs in neoplastic progression in the cervix, as will be discussed later in this chapter. In addition, high-risk genital HPV types have been reported to infect nongenital epithelia, and the HPV genome has been isolated in a minority of the squamous cell carcinomas of the skin, oropharynx, and cornea, as well as other epithelia. Both the latent period (estimated to be 5 to 20 years) between infection and development of cancer and the fact that all infections do not induce malignancy, even with high-risk HPVs, indicate that infection with HPV is necessary but not sufficient for the manifestation of cancer. Under the influence of the viral genome, changes must be occurring within the cell during the progression from papilloma to neoplasia.

TABLE 123-1. Human Papillomavirus Genotypes and Their Most Common Clinical Manifestations

Clinical Lesions	HPV Genotypes
Cutaneous warts, including plantar, palmar, and flat	1–4, 10, 28, 29, 37, 41, 48, 60, 63, 65
Epidermodysplasia verruciformis; immunosuppression	5, 8, 9, 12, 14, 15, 17, 19–27, 36, 46, 47, 49, 50
Mucosal ("low risk"): Anogenital and cervical papillomas; oropharynx and respiratory tract papillomas	6, 11, 30, 34, 40, 42–44, 55, 57–59
Mucosal ("high risk"): Anogenital and cervical papillomas; bowenoid papulosis, cervical dysplasia; oropharynx, anogenital cancers including cervical	16, 18, 31, 33, 35, 39, 45, 51, 52, 56

HPV, human papillomavirus.

CLINICAL DESCRIPTION

Warts are the most common clinical manifestation of HPV infection, occurring on virtually any cutaneous or mucosal epithelial surface, most frequently on the hands, feet, face, legs, and external genital area. They are often classified based on anatomic distribution (face, hands, periungual, plantar, genital). Morphologically, cutaneous warts are of two major types, common warts (Fig. 123-1) and flat warts (Fig. 123-2). Common warts or verruca vulgaris are hard papules or plaques often with an irregular, spiked, scaly surface. Flat warts or verruca plana are small 2 to 4-mm slightly raised, slightly scaly papules.

The diagnosis of warts is based primarily on clinical morphology. Although classic verruca vulgaris is difficult to misdiagnose, other keratotic and papular lesions may mimic its appearance (Table 123-2). On the soles of the feet, there is particular difficulty distinguishing solitary

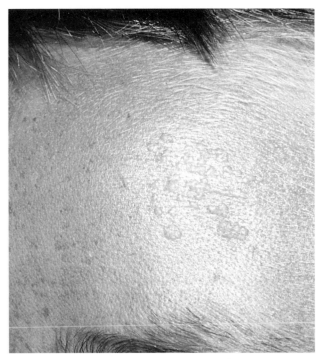

FIGURE 123-2. Flat warts on the forehead.

plantar warts from a clavus or corn. In general, viral warts lack dermatoglyphics and have small thrombosed capillaries that appear as punctate, blue/black stippling, whereas a clavus has dermatoglyphics but not the stippling.

Three types of skin are present in the genital area: keratinized hair-bearing skin, keratinized non–hair-bearing skin, and incompletely keratinized non–hair-bearing skin, corresponding in the male to the pubic area, shaft of the penis, and the perianal area or occluded prepuce, and in the female to the labia majora, lateral

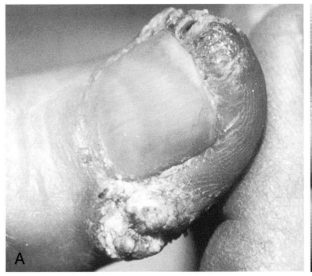
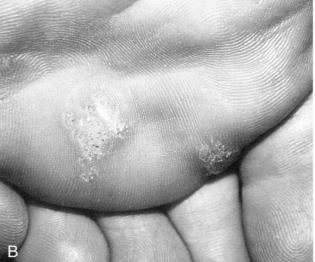

FIGURE 123-1. Common warts on the hands *(A)* and on the plantar aspect of the foot *(B).*

TABLE 123-2. Differential Diagnosis of Human Papillomavirus Infection

Common Warts

Molluscum contagiosum
Gottron's papules of dermatomyositis
Acrochordons
Perforating granuloma annulare
Acrokeratosis verruciformis
Lichen nitidus
Lichen planus
Seborrheic keratosis
Actinic keratosis
Squamous cell carcinoma

Flat Warts

Freckles
Lichen planus

Plantar Warts

Clavus
Acquired digital fibrokeratoma
Corn
Foreign body

Genital Warts

Condyloma latum
Lichen planus
Psoriasis
Bowenoid papulosis
Squamous cell carcinoma
Seborrheic keratosis
Pearly penile papules
Skin tags
Sebaceous (Tyson's) glands

labia minor, and introitus. These differences influence wart morphology. Condylomata acuminata are pedunculated cauliflower-like verrucous papules and nodules seen primarily on moist, non–hair-bearing, incompletely keratinized surfaces such as the vulvar labia, under the foreskin of the penis, and the perianal area (Fig. 123–3). Condyloma latum (Fig. 123–4) of secondary syphilis can be mistaken for condyloma acuminatum. Smooth papular (Fig. 123–5) and keratotic genital warts (Fig. 123–6) occur more commonly on keratinized genital skin. In the genital area, HPV DNA has also been found in keratotic verrucous plaques with a pasted-on appearance clinically consistent with seborrheic keratosis. Homosexual and heterosexual male and female patients may have perianal genital warts, but intra-anal warts occur most commonly in patients who have had receptive anal intercourse.

Flat or small papular genital warts observed after soaking with dilute acetic acid or vinegar, often with the aid of magnification, have been termed *acetowhite* or *subclinical warts*. Acetowhite warts represent a subtle manifestation of genital HPV infection. Unfortunately, not all genital warts will whiten with acetic acid, and, of perhaps greater significance, many acetowhite areas are not genital warts. Any condition involving disruption of the epithelial barrier can produce acetowhitening; these include lichen planus, atopic dermatitis, psoriasis, yeast and dermatophyte infection, as well as irritant dermatitis and intertrigo. There is no clear consensus on the indications for application of acetic acid in the detection of genital warts.

In addition to the genital tract, warts can occur on other mucous membranes, including nasal, conjunctival, oral, and laryngeal epithelial surfaces.[5] Respiratory papillomatosis is a serious disease that can lead to obstruction of the airway. Patients with genital warts and/or their

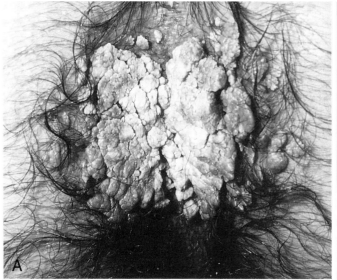
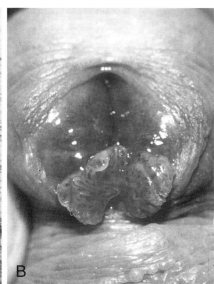

FIGURE 123–3. Condyloma acuminatum type of genital warts: *A*, perianal area; and *B*, urethral meatus.

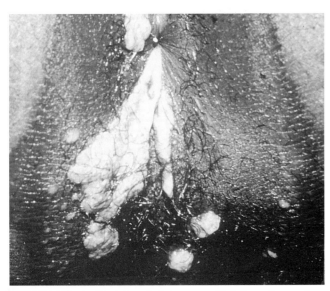

FIGURE 123-4. Condylomata lata, a manifestation of secondary syphilis.

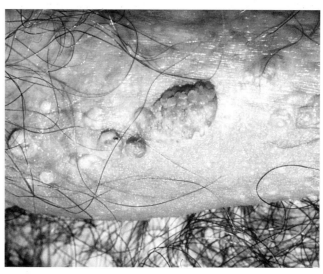

FIGURE 123-6. Keratotic genital warts on the shaft of the penis.

sexual partners have an increased frequency of oral condyloma acuminata.[6] In the oral cavity, HPV has also been associated with focal epithelial hyperplasia or Heck's disease. Focal epithelial hyperplasia is essentially a non-sexually transmitted oral infection with HPV. The characteristic morphology consists of multiple smooth, soft, whitish papules and small plaques on the oral mucosa (Fig. 123-7). Focal epithelial hyperplasia is most common in Native Americans, but has been reported in most races.[5, 7]

Common genital warts are usually the manifestation of infection with low-risk HPV types, most commonly types 6 and 11. On the external genital area, the high-risk HPV types have been associated with bowenoid papulosis or squamous cell carcinoma in situ.[8-11] Morphologically, this manifestation of HPV infection can present as small 1- to 4-mm dome-shaped papules (Fig. 123-8A)

or, at times, velvety, sometimes bluish patches or plaques (Fig. 123-8B). It is currently believed that squamous cell carcinoma in situ of the external genitalia rarely results in invasive squamous cell carcinoma of the external genitalia, which is relatively uncommon. Invasive squamous cell carcinoma of the penis, vulva and anus have been reported to contain HPV DNA. Whether these arise from bowenoid papulosis is unknown. However, women with vulvar bowenoid papulosis, or female partners of men with bowenoid papulosis, need to be monitored closely for cervical cancer because the risk of transition to cancer is much higher in the cervix then in the genital skin. Furthermore, in the genital area, clinical morphology may not always predict histopathology, particularly with the smooth papular genital warts that may, on biopsy, actually prove to be squamous cell carcinomas in situ or bowenoid papulosis. For this reason, one should perform biopsies on genital warts that are refractory to treatment because they may represent squamous cell carcinoma or Bowen's disease.

The most frequent site of HPV-related oncogenicity is the transformation zone of the uterine cervix. A majority

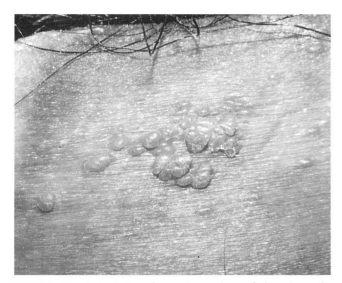

FIGURE 123-5. A cluster of smooth papular genital warts on the shaft of the penis.

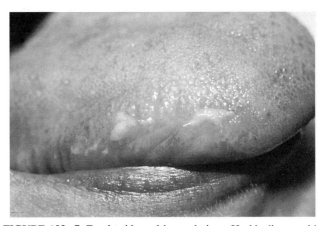

FIGURE 123-7. Focal epidermal hyperplasia or Heck's disease with white papules along the side of the tongue.

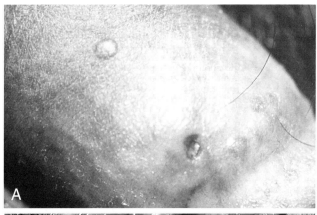

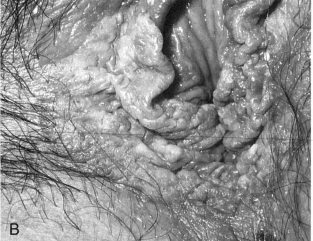

FIGURE 123–8. Bowenoid papulosis: *A*, as papules on the penis, ulceration is a biopsy site; *B*, as a vulvar patch.

Outside the genital area, HPV-induced squamous cell carcinoma may mimic the clinical appearance of a common wart.[13] Verrucous carcinoma is a locally invasive cytologically bland form of squamous cell carcinoma that does not metastasize unless transformation to high-grade carcinoma occurs. Early lesions may have the clinical morphology of a wart. There have been reports of verrucous carcinoma on fingers, toes, and genitalia, where it has been called "giant condyloma of Bushke and Lowenstein." Verrucous carcinomas may or may not contain HPV DNA. Genital verrucous carcinoma usually contains low-risk HPV, such as type 6 or 11.

Epidemiology of Nongenital Human Papillomavirus Infection

The incidence, frequency, and manifestations of nongenital HPV infection vary in different populations. Given their frequency, there is a striking lack of new epidemiologic information on the natural history of common warts. Most recent studies have focused on genital HPV infection. A major obstacle to the study of HPV epidemiology has been the lack of investigational tools. A serologic test to detect the presence of HPV-specific antibodies is not available. This, coupled with the inability to culture HPV, has greatly limited the nature of epidemiologic studies to little more than counting warts in different populations and to the detection of viral DNA. We will review the epidemiology of nongenital HPV infection in three populations: immunocompetent patients, immunosuppressed patients, and patients with EV.

Immunocompetent Patients

Approximately 8% of office visits to dermatologists are for warts, and only half of patients with warts are seen by dermatologists.[14] The remainder of these patients are cared for by general or family practitioners, internists, and pediatricians. In a general survey of skin diseases among 2180 adults, 3.5% were found to have warts. In a university pediatric dermatology clinic, verruca vulgaris was the fifth most common diagnosis and was noted in nearly 5% of patients.[15] In a study of school children, about 5% were found to have plantar warts.[16] In one study, 8% of patients referred to dermatologists for the treatment of warts had other dermatologic lesions that mimic warts, most commonly skin tags and corns.[17] Common and plantar warts were the most frequent warts, occurring in 40% and 38% of patients, respectively. Filiform (3%), periungual (2%), plaque (2%), and mosaic plantar (2%) warts were much less common. A combination of common warts and one or more of the other types was noted in 15% of patients. The age distribution was from 2 to 81 years, with children the most frequently affected. The median age at presentation was 11 years. Thirty per cent of patients were between 10 and 14 years, and 65% between 5 and 20 years. Only 16% of these patients were over 35 years of age.[17]

There are environmental factors associated with acquisition of warts. Frequent wet work involving the

of woman with external genital warts have vaginal or cervical HPV infection. Therefore, women with external genital warts and female sexual partners of men with genital warts should have a complete gynecologic examination. Because genital warts in adults are predominantly a sexually transmitted disease, they should be treated as such and sexual partners should be examined. This is complicated by the fact that incubation time from infection to clinical manifestation can range from months to years. After successful treatment of visible warts, it is not known whether a patient is rendered noninfectious or whether HPV DNA remains present. Additionally, it is becoming apparent that the anal mucosa is susceptible to the oncogenic potential of HPV.[12] Prior to the human immunodeficiency virus epidemic, anal cancer was predominantly a disease of women. Perianal and intra-anal condylomata are common sexually transmitted diseases in the homosexual population, and never-married men have experienced a 20-fold increase in anal cancer. Immunosuppressed patients should be carefully examined for the presence of perianal and intra-anal warts and need to be monitored for the development of anal carcinoma. Again, high-risk HPV types on a mucosal surface and with diminished host immune status are important risk factors for the manifestation of the oncogenic potential of HPV.

hands appears to be a risk factor for development of periungual warts.[17] Hyperhidrosis of the feet has been reported to increase the chance of development of plantar warts.[14] Butchers and slaughterhouse workers have an increased number of hand warts.[18-21]

Although the male-to-female ratio approached 1:1, women were more likely to have warts on their fingers and toes than were men, who more frequently had warts on their palms. Of interest, 78% of patients with periungual warts reported being nail biters, compared with 33% of patients with other nonplantar warts. Multiple (> 2) warts on the hands were associated with frequent immersion of hands into water. In this study, 19% of patients with plantar warts and 34% of patients with nonplantar warts reported a household contact with warts. The number of warts increased with duration of infection. Multiple warts were noted in 71% of patients having warts longer than 6 months, but in only 33% of patients having warts for less than 6 months.[17]

In a classic study, Massing and Epstein[22] studied the natural history of common warts. Over a 2-year period, 1000 institutionalized children were evaluated for warts on their hands and feet. At the time of initial evaluation, 18.3% of these children had warts, predominantly on the hands. Complete "spontaneous involution" was noted in 53% of 168 patients within 1 year and in 67% by 2 years. Involution was noted more frequently in male patients (56% [55 of 99]) than in female patients (32% [22 of 66]). Patients with warts at baseline were three times more likely to develop new warts than were subjects who were wart-free at the initial evaluation. Twelve per cent (80 of 690) of subjects who were wart-free at baseline developed warts during the first year. New warts were observed during the first year in 39% of subjects who had warts at the initiation of the study.

Immunocompromised Patients

Manifestations of nongenital HPV infection in the immunocompromised population have been well studied. It appears that HPV infection and HPV-associated carcinoma are common complications of chronic immunosuppression.[23-27] The best-studied immunocompromised population consists of renal allograft recipients. With each year of immunosuppression, there is an increase in the number of warts. The HPV types associated with these cutaneous lesions are of interest. These immunocompromised patients are infected by the same HPV types as seen in immunocompetent patients as well as by HPV types usually seen in patients with EV.[24, 28] It is not known whether immunocompromised patients develop verruca vulgaris because of an increased susceptibility to HPV infection or because of reactivation of subclinical HPV infection.

Warts are common in renal allograft recipients; reported incidences of warts range from 24% to 100%. The spectrum of HPV disease in allograft recipients ranges from verruca vulgaris to squamous cell carcinoma. In addition to immunosuppression, ultraviolet light may be a cofactor in the development of HPV-associated cutaneous malignancies.[29] Immunosuppressed patients also demonstrate an accelerated course from wart to carcinoma. Caution is necessary in the clinical evaluation of warts in these patients. Although in immunocompetent patients, the histology of common warts is quite predictable, this is not so in renal allograft recipients. Biopsy specimens from 59 lesions that clinically appeared to be common warts demonstrated 18 squamous cell carcinomas, 19 warts with dysplasia, and 16 simple warts.[13]

An increased incidence of warts has also been noted in patients with malignancy. In one study, 30% of patients with Hodgkin's disease, 20% of patients with lymphoma, and 18% of patients with chronic lymphatic leukemia had warts (compared with 2.3% of normal controls, 6.2% of patients with basal cell carcinoma, and 4.5% of patients with other systemic malignancies).[30] In addition to therapeutically challenging verrucae vulgares, patients with human immunodeficiency virus infection have been noted to have macular lesions similar to those noted in EV.[31]

Epidermodysplasia Verruciformis

Epidermodysplasia verruciformis is a rare disease, first described by Lewandowski and Lutz and characterized by chronic, extensive HPV-induced warts. In EV, the clinical morphology can be that of reddish, scaly papules that resemble other flat warts or scaly macules that have a striking resemblance to tinea versicolor (Fig. 123-9). There are no estimates of the incidence of this disease in the general population, although it is thought to be very low. Approximately 25% of reported cases are familial.[32, 33] Autosomal recessive inheritance appears to be the predominant mode,[34] although X-linked inheritance[35] has been reported. The male-to-female ratio approaches 1:1. The onset of warts most frequently occurs in early childhood, but adult onset has been reported. A serious complication of EV is the development of skin cancer, usually during the second decade of life or 2 to 20

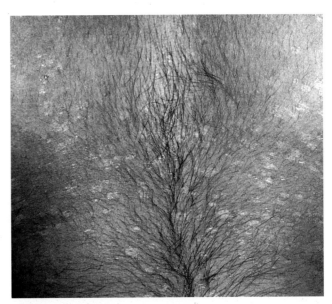

FIGURE 123-9. Multiple scaling plaques of epidermodysplasia verruciformis. Note the resemblance to lesions and distribution of pityriasis rosea.

years after the onset of warts. The reported incidence of skin cancer ranges from 30% to 100% and occurs most frequently on sun-exposed areas, suggesting that ultraviolet light acts as a cofactor.[10, 36] It is currently believed that EV is the result of HPV infection and a defect in cell-mediated immunity, specifically natural killer cell activity.[37]

Genital Human Papillomavirus Infections

Genital warts as a manifestation of HPV infection are very common in the sexually active population.[38-40] Asymptomatic infection appears to be far more common than symptomatic infection. It has been estimated that 1% of all sexually active adults in the United States have visible genital warts at any given time. Another 2% of the population have warts that can be detected after soaking with acetic acid, and 20% to 50% have infection of the genital tract based on detection of HPV DNA.

The natural history of genital HPV infection has not been defined. It is often quoted that, based on clinical trials, the short-term spontaneous resolution rate for genital warts is 20% to 25%.[39, 41] These trials have been predominantly studies where the placebo control is repetitive intralesional injections of saline. In clinical trials limited to topical agents, a much lower spontaneous resolution rate of less than 5% over several months was noted.[42]

Juvenile Laryngeal Papillomatosis

Juvenile laryngeal or respiratory papillomatosis is an HPV infection of the larynx, most commonly noted in young children.[43] It is thought to be transmitted via birth through an infected birth canal. Although potentially extensive and life-threatening, it is relatively rare compared with the number of children born through HPV-infected birth canals. These laryngeal papillomas are almost uniformly associated with low-risk mucosal HPV types such as 6 and 11.

Genital Human Papillomavirus Infection in Children

Although genital warts in adults appear to be a sexually transmitted disease, the exact route of transmission of genital papillomas in children is not certain. Whereas a proportion of children with genital warts have acquired these via sexual abuse, most probably have acquired the infection via other routes.[44-47] The papillomavirus is relatively resistant to physical and chemical destruction because it lacks a lipid envelope. In all likelihood, HPV can remain infectious for weeks or months at room temperature, and infection could be transmitted by fomites such as clothing, washcloths, towels, and the like. Although nonsexual modes of transmission of genital HPV infection to children exist, all children with genital warts need to be carefully evaluated for sexual abuse.

PATHOLOGY

A verruca vulgaris is elevated above the skin surface due to digitated epidermal hyperplasia (Fig. 123–10). Its papillations have convex surfaces, and often appear to radiate outward from a common point in the dermis, an appearance that is often accentuated by inwardly bowed rete ridges. Verrucae vulgares are commonly as tall as they are broad, and covered by compact orthokeratosis, features that contrast with seborrheic keratosis. Dilated, tortuous capillaries are present within dermal papillae inside the digitations. In many warts, tiers of parakeratotic cells with entrapped erythrocytes are present above the tips of digitations. As warts are pared down, coagulated blood in the cornified layer appears as minute black dots, and capillaries in dermal papillae within papillations result in small bleeding puncta as they are transected. HPV is demonstrable in young warts but not in older lesions. In warts that still harbor HPV, the granular layer in the dells between papillations contain cells with coarse keratohyaline granules, and vacuoles surround the wrinkled-appearing nuclei of these keratinocytes (Fig.

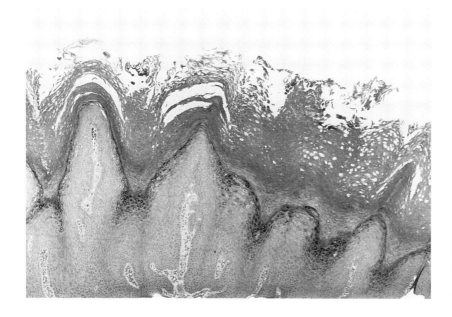

FIGURE 123–10. Verruca vulgaris is characterized by digitated epidermal hyperplasia with compact hyperkeratosis, and foci of parakeratosis and hemorrhage over the tips of papillations. Note hypergranulosis in the intervening dells.

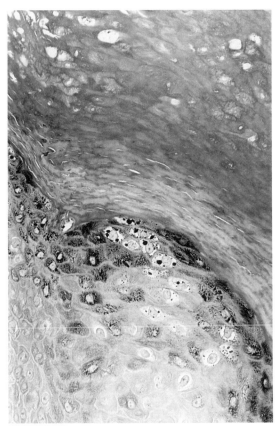

FIGURE 123-11. Keratinocytes in the granular layer of this verruca vulgaris show evidence of papillomavirus infection, namely perinuclear vacuoles and enlarged keratohyaline granules.

123-11). Viral particles can be detected within the nuclei of these cells by electron microscopy, immunoperoxidase staining, or in situ hybridization.

Old verrucae vulgares from which HPV has disappeared show a variety of appearances. Some have the architectural features of a younger wart, but are devoid of keratinocytes with viropathic changes. Irritated lesions feature squamous eddies, as do irritated seborrheic keratoses. Some old verrucae lose their distinctive silhouette, and become difficult to differentiate from seborrheic keratoses. Descriptive diagnoses such as verrucous keratosis, squamous papilloma, verrucous acanthoma, or basosquamous acanthoma are applied to such lesions. In some old warts, the papillary dermis becomes markedly fibrotic and contains dilated vessels, simulating an angiofibroma.

Palmar and plantar warts, or myrmecia, also feature papillated epidermal hyperplasia, inward bending of rete ridges, compact hyperkeratosis, and hypergranulosis. A distinctive feature of myrmeciae is the presence of polygonal, refractile-appearing eosinophilic cytoplasmic inclusions that are composed of keratin filaments (Fig. 123-12). Authentic viral inclusions can be present in myrmeciae, but are intranuclear and stain a light pink with hematoxylin and eosin.

Flat warts, or verrucae planae, have features that resemble those of verrucae vulgares but are muted in comparison. There is only slight papillated epidermal hyper-

plasia, and rete ridges are not centripetally inclined. Most flat warts have prominent perinuclear halos around nuclei of cells in the granular layer (so-called owl's eye cells).

Some sporadic flat warts, warts due to HPV 5 in familial EV, and multiple flat warts in some immunosuppressed patients feature another distinctive cytopathic change, with cells in the upper spinous and granular layer having pale basophilic granular cytoplasm and pleomorphic vesicular nuclei. Cells with this appearance have been referred to as "swollen keratinocytes" (Fig. 123-13).

Condyloma acuminatum demonstrates gently papillated epithelial hyperplasia, with thick, rounded rete ridges composed of spinous keratinocytes (Fig. 123-14). Perinuclear halos are present in granular and spinous keratinocytes in the dells between these knuckle-like papillations. Occasionally, horn pseudocysts are present in benign, gently papillated keratinocytic proliferations on genital or anal skin, resulting in confusion with seborrheic keratosis. One study used the polymerase chain reaction to prove that many such lesions harbor the HPV genome. The nature of these lesions is debated, but several findings, including the predominance of pale spinous rather than darker basaloid cells, imply that they are condylomata rather than seborrheic keratoses that harbor HPV. In condylomata that have been treated with

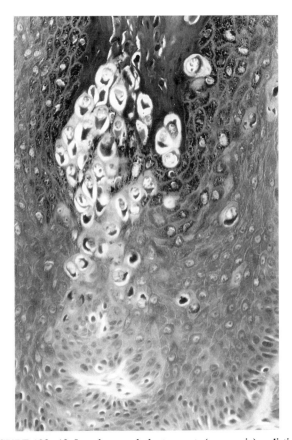

FIGURE 123-12. In palmar and plantar warts (myrmecia), a distinctive feature is the presence of large curved and angulated eosinophilic inclusions in the cytoplasms of keratinocytes in the granular layer. They often lie within perinuclear vacuoles.

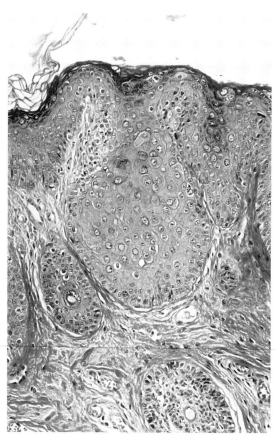

FIGURE 123-13. A flat wart from an immunosuppressed patient showing a bulbous rete ridge distended by keratinocytes with abundant pale basophilic cytoplasm and enlarged vesicular nuclei ("swollen keratinocytes"). This effect is usually the result of infection with HPV 5. Conventional flat warts feature perinuclear vacuoles.

podophyllin, the superficialmost layers of the epidermis are often necrotic, and there are many cells in mitosis figures arrested in metaphase. This appearance can be confused with those of squamous cell carcinoma in situ

or of bowenoid papulosis. Podophyllin-treated condylomata do not show the other features of these conditions.

Bowenoid papulosis often resembles condyloma acuminatum with respect to its microscopic profile, but differs in that there is crowding, enlargement, and hyperchromasia of keratinocyte nuclei. The degree of cytologic atypia is sometimes subtle, and maturation as evidenced by flattening of cells can be present in the superficial layers of the epidermis of such lesions. Viropathic changes are generally subtle.

Verrucous carcinoma typically is a vertically oriented, exoendophytic, slightly papillated proliferation of cytologically bland keratinocytes in which bulbous rete ridges can penetrate deeply within the dermis. Furrows containing necrotic debris are often present between papillations. Only in the basal layer of the thick, blunt-ended rete ridges of verrucous carcinoma are there crowding or atypia of keratinocyte nuclei, or mitotic figures. More anaplastic appearing squamous cell carcinoma can arise within verrucous carcinomas subjected to radiation therapy.

Dermatopathologists are sometimes called upon by clinicians to provide HPV typing on biopsy specimens. Several type-specific probes for in situ hybridization are available, including some of those for high-risk genital HPVs. At present, the clinical value of typing in specific cases is limited.

PATHOGENESIS, ETIOLOGY AND MOLECULAR BIOLOGY OF PAPILLOMAVIRUS INFECTION

Papillomaviruses gain access to the host by direct implantation through disruptions in the normal epithelial barrier. Infection is confined to the epithelium and does not lead to systemic dissemination of the virus. It is thought that viral infection begins in the basal cell layer. Viral DNA replicates extrachromosomally or episomally, as a covalently closed circle within the nucleus of

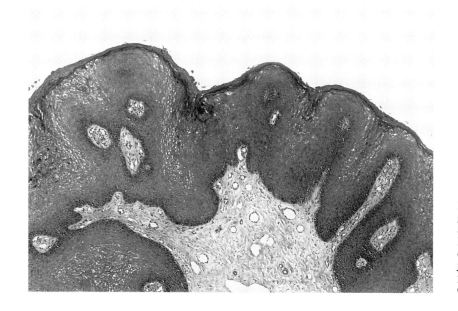

FIGURE 123-14. Condyloma acuminatum shows gently papillated epidermal hyperplasia resulting in a profile similar to that made by the condyles of the knuckles, hence its name. The granular layer in the dells between papillations is thickened, and the subjacent spinous layer contains many koilocytes (papillomavirus-infected cells with cave-like perinuclear vacuoles and wrinkled-appearing nuclei).

infected cells. Basal keratinocytes are assumed to be infected with one or two copies of the circular viral DNA per cell. The viral DNA is believed to replicate in concert with the host DNA, and the resulting copy of the viral genome is transported along with the daughter cells to upper levels of the epithelium. It is only in these highly differentiated keratinocytes that viral RNAs are expressed at substantial qualities.[48] Importantly, the viral DNA is replicated to high numbers only in these expendable, terminally differentiated cells that are destined to be sloughed off, and therefore there is no acute lytic infection. This relatively slow life cycle is reflected in the time from initial infection to clinically detectable papilloma, which can range from weeks to possibly years.

The viral genome encodes sufficient information to synthesize about 10 proteins. After entering the host cell, the virus must establish the proper order in which its own genes will be expressed. The precise determinants that regulate expression of the viral genome have yet to be resolved, but most likely involve complex interplay between differentiation-specific cellular factors and the viral E2 protein. This protein and the specific sequence of DNA it binds with high affinity[49] are found in all papillomaviruses (PVs). Binding of E2 to these specific sites can induce expression of nearby viral genes. Conversely, under certain circumstances E2 can act as a repressor. It is possible that differentiation-specific events induce E2 expression, which in turn establishes the proper order of viral gene expression and induces viral DNA replication.

The virus must later selectively replicate its own DNA in order to produce a large number of infectious progeny. The viral E1 protein also binds a specific sequence of the viral DNA, although with lower affinity than E2 recognizes its target sequences. E1 is required for replication of the viral DNA and initiates the process, probably involving unwinding of the duplex DNA, at the correct site in the viral genome.[50] Both E1 and E2 proteins are necessary for replication,[51] and a physical complex of these proteins has been identified.[52] However, E1 and E2 are not sufficient for DNA synthesis because PVs do not encode a DNA polymerase or the associated factors necessary to duplicate DNA. The paradox of PV replication is that it begins in a nonreplicating host epithelial layer in which the multitude of enzymes necessary for DNA synthesis are not present. It is likely that the viral oncogenes described below stimulate the cell to prepare for DNA synthesis, and the E2 and E1 proteins subsequently recruit these factors to the viral DNA.

The replicated DNA is packaged into a protein shell referred to as a capsid. The DNA-containing viral capsid is called a virion. Encapsidation occurs in the nuclei of the upper epithelial strata. The capsid, composed of the L1 and L2 proteins, serves several purposes. It protects the viral DNA for traversal through the epithelium and after being shed into the environment, and presumably recognizes a receptor on the host cell. In this manner the PV progeny are continuously released from a viable epithelium. Importantly, PV capsids do not bud from the cell's plasma membrane. It is this membrane-derived lipid envelope that encircles the virions of infectious agents such as herpesviruses and the human immunode-

ficiency virus and results in their susceptibility to environmental stresses such as heat, soaps, and desiccation. Because PVs have no envelope, they are very stable and can probably remain infectious for prolonged periods in the environment.

The L1 and L2 proteins have been expressed at high levels in several in vitro cell culture systems. L1 proteins self-assemble into virus-like particles, and the L2 protein can also enter this highly organized structure.[53-57] These virus-like particles resemble native PV capsids and have exposed specific epitopes found only in infectious viruses.[54] These in vitro assembled particles do not contain viral genes, and therefore are not transmissible.

Immune Response

Papillomavirus encoded proteins are present at exceedingly low levels in epithelium, and most viral encoded proteins, including the viral capsids, are localized to the nucleus. Although low-titer antibodies to HPV proteins have been reported, the significance of these results is uncertain. A serologic test to confirm exposure to HPV is not currently available. An enzyme-linked immunosorbent assay to detect HPV 16 virus-like particles appears to be promising,[58] and these particles may also be of utility for protective vaccination.

Models to Study Papillomavirus Biology

In vitro assays have been employed to understand the cellular events triggered by PV infection.[59] Using techniques of recombinant DNA technology, one can introduce any fragment of DNA into a cell and test the biologic consequences. Introduction of PV genes has been shown to alter cellular growth parameters in a variety of assays. One model incorporates the use of cells that stop growing when a monolayer is fully formed on a plastic dish. Introduction of an oncogene results in continuous proliferation of the cells, which also acquired the ability to form tumors in animals, whereas the original cell line without the oncogene did not. In another system normal cells from an animal are placed into culture. Human cells, such as keratinocytes, will proliferate in vitro for a limited number of generations, and their continuous growth in vitro is exceedingly rare. Introduction of specific PV genes causes cultured keratinocytes to become "immortal" although they appear morphologically unchanged and will not form tumors in susceptible animals.

The normal keratinocyte differentiation program can be more faithfully reproduced by cultivating the cells at the air-liquid interface. In this model, the epithelial cells are grown on a permeable collagen raft that may contain fibroblasts. Introduction by genetic techniques of either the whole viral genome or its oncogenes from the high-risk HPVs into these keratinocytes results in disruption of their normal maturation program, and the PV-containing epithelium histologically resembles in situ squamous cell carcinoma.[60-62] The low-risk HPVs do not induce this preneoplastic appearance.

Until recently it has not been possible to cultivate

HPV in vitro, even using the raft model. Recently, using the raft culture system, two groups have reported production of viral particles in vitro. In both, keratinocytes from an HPV-infected lesion were expanded in culture and placed onto the collagen matrix. One group, using cells from a cervical lesion that contained autonomously replicating HPV 31, found that treatment of the cells with phorbol ester induced expression of the viral capsid proteins, synthesis of viral DNA, and assembly of viral particles.[63] In the second system, infected cervical tissue was placed on a raft with embedded murine fibroblasts, and virus particles were detected.[64]

Animal-based models have yielded selected HPVs. Human cervix or skin cells were infected with HPV and placed under the renal capsule of an immunodeficient (nude) mouse for an extended period, usually several months.[65, 66] In this protected environment the epithelial cells differentiate and form a papilloma in which PV capsid proteins were detected. This has been successful for isolates of HPV 11 and HPV 1; however, production of high-risk genital HPV virions has not been reported. Another model utilized a cell line derived from an HPV 16 infected cervical lesion in which the viral DNA was maintained extra chromosomal. Incubation of these cells in a chamber on the back of a nude mouse has been reported to allow stratified differentiation and production of HPV 16 particles.[67]

Papillomavirus Oncogenes

The association of specific HPV types with the development of epithelial malignancies, such as in EV and cervical cancer, strongly support the causative role of HPV in cancer. A primary goal of the viral reproductive cycle cannot be oncogenesis, as inferred from the observation that virions are not detected in cervical dysplasias and other HPV-associated cancers.

Studies of the oncogenic potential of HPV began with the high-risk genital HPVs.[59] Introduction of both their E6 and E7 genes rendered human keratinocytes resistant to calcium- and serum-induced terminal differentiation.[68, 69] E6 and E7 cooperate in immortalization of rodent fibroblasts and human keratinocytes.[70-79] The high-risk genital E6 and E7 genes induce disorganized differentiation and abnormal mitoses in epithelial cells cultured in the raft model. Continued passage of HPV 18–containing immortal keratinocytes resulted in outgrowth of fully malignant cells.[80] This implies additional genetic changes occurred in the cells, events that may be accelerated by the PV oncogenes' mechanisms. Thus, at least for HPV 16 and 18, the E6 and E7 oncoproteins are able to oncogenically transform normal cells. Consistent with these observations, the E6 and E7 genes are always retained in HPV-associated cancers, whereas the remainder of the viral genes are either lost or mutated.

Important insights into the mechanism of action of the high-risk HPV E6 and E7 genes were gained from comparison with other DNA tumor viruses. The oncoproteins of adenovirus, simian virus (SV) 40, and polyomavirus were known to physically bind an overlapping set of cellular proteins. The identification of these common targets as tumor suppressor gene products led to the discovery, by analogy, that the PV-transforming proteins E6 and E7 complex in vitro with the p53 and retinoblastoma (Rb) proteins, respectively. The precise mechanisms by which p53 and Rb are involved in cell proliferation are not fully understood.[81] Mutations in p53 are the most common genetic abnormality identified in human cancers.[82] Expression of p53 is stimulated by DNA damage such as with ultraviolet or x-ray irradiation. Levels of p53 protein are elevated after ultraviolet irradiation of skin, and p53 mutations consistent with ultraviolet damage to DNA are found in cutaneous squamous cell carcinomas.[83, 84] Activation of p53 results in arrest of cell division, probably allowing time for repair of the DNA. Rb was first identified as a gene that was mutated in kindreds with hereditary risk of cancers, including retinoblastoma of the eye in early childhood. The Rb protein is a member of a family of proteins that appear to directly regulate entry into cell cycle division.

The high-risk genital HPV E6 gene products have been reported to complex with p53, as do SV40 large T and adenovirus E1a.[85] Formation of the E6-p53 complex induces the degradation of p53 in vitro[86] and in cultured cells.[79] Low-risk genital E6 proteins are not capable of inducing p53 degradation.[87] E6 proteins probably have other functions. Bovine papillomavirus (BPV) E6 does not bind p53, but transforms murine cells to a malignant phenotype.[88] HPV 5 and 8, which are found in cutaneous squamous cell carcinoma in immunosuppression and in EV, do not bind or degrade p53 in vitro.[89] BPV E6 and HPV 6 E6, which do not induce p53 degradation in vitro or in vivo, can immortalize human mammary epithelial cells, although they are much less efficient than HPV 16 E6.[90]

Recognition of the amino acid similarities between the HPV E7 proteins and other DNA tumor virus transforming proteins facilitated elucidation of the biochemical properties of E7. These similarity regions have been demonstrated to bind the tumor suppressor gene product Rb.[91-93] The amino terminal half of E7 also binds the Rb-related protein called p107.[94] Like Rb, p107 functions in regulation of cell growth, but acts at a different stage in the cell cycle. It is thought that when E7 binds Rb/p107, a transcription factor (called E2F) normally bound to Rb and p107 is released because E7 efficiently competes for the same binding pocket. As a consequence of its release, E2F activates expression of genes that are necessary for cell division.[95] Other regions of E7 bind additional growth related cellular factors. HPV 16 E7 has been identified in complexes with histone kinase,[96] p33cdk2 and cyclin A,[97] and casein kinase II,[98] which phosphorylates high-risk E7 more efficiently than low-risk E7. Rb preferentially binds to phosphorylated E7 protein, and this may in part relate to the oncogenic potential of high-risk E7.[99]

In murine cell line assays, both HPV 16 and 18 E7 induced morphologic transformation.[100, 101] Introduction of E7 alone into primary human keratinocytes resulted in these cells displaying an increased rate of proliferation for an extended period of time, although they eventually senesced.[102] Using high-efficiency retroviral mediated infection of primary human keratinocytes, low-risk HPV 6

E7 was found to cooperate with high-risk E6 in immortalization of primary human keratinocytes, and in the alternative mixing experiment, HPV 6 E6 cooperated with HPV 16 E7, although in both instances, the efficiency was less than with high-risk E6 and E7.[102] As with E6, there remain unidentified properties of E7 that are required for its transforming activities. For example, mutations in E7 that do not affect Rb/p107 association interfere with its ability to transform and immortalize cells.[103]

Some PVs have been found to encode a third oncogene. E5 is a very small PV protein, ranging from 44 amino acids in BPV type 1 to about 100 amino acids in some HPVs.[104-119] Most studies have been performed with BPV E5, introduction of which induces DNA synthesis and transformation of established mouse cell lines. The E5 proteins are believed to induce cell proliferation and transformation by stimulating the activation of endogenous growth factor receptors such as the platelet-derived and epidermal growth factor receptors. The molecular details of these interactions have been reported and reveal the ingenious interception of normal cellular pathways by a virus. For example, E5 stimulates the dimerization of monomeric receptors, a step necessary for their activation. In addition, E5 probably inhibits the normal down-regulation of other activated growth factor receptors.

The cottontail rabbit papillomavirus (CRPV) provides a unique tool to study the requirements for specific PV genes in vivo.[120] Remarkably, inoculation of CRPV DNA into the skin can reproduce the full viral life cycle with development of papillomas in which infectious virions are synthesized. Surprisingly, CRPV DNA with mutations in the E7 gene that inactivated its Rb-binding ability formed papillomas, indicating that the interaction with Rb was not absolutely necessary for development of a wart or for replication of the virus.[121, 122] The role of E5 in viral pathogenesis has also been examined using the CRPV inoculation model. Injection of DNA containing inactivating E5 mutations into the skin of domestic rabbits resulted in reduced efficiency of papilloma formation.[123]

Several lines of evidence support the role of HPV in causing cancer. As presented above, the E6 and E7 genes interact with multiple cellular proteins that control cell growth. E6 and E7 are potent oncogenes in transformation/immortalization assays in vitro. Insertion of HPV 16 E6 and E7 into the mouse genome (transgenic) leads to epithelial tumors in tissues that express the viral genes.[124, 125] HPV DNA is found in greater than 90% of cervical cancers, and metastases retain the HPV DNA, specifically the E6 and E7 genes. Treatment of cervical carcinoma cells with antisense oligonucleotides or genetic insertion of antisense DNA has been reported to inhibit E6 and E7 expression and resulted in decreased cell proliferation and loss of tumorigenicity.[126-128] Cell hybrids of normal fibroblasts crossed with HeLa cells (derived from a cervical cancer cell containing HPV 18) led to decreased expression of E6 and E7 and loss of HeLa tumorigenicity.[129] These observations imply that the continued expression of E6 and E7 in both fresh cervical cancers and cervical tumor cell lines is necessary

for the malignant state. Whereas ultraviolet light is a cofactor for development of cutaneous squamous cell carcinoma in EV, a cofactor in cervical cancer is not yet known, although cigarette smoking is suspected.

DIAGNOSIS AND DIFFERENTIAL DIAGNOSIS

The diagnosis of wart infection is usually not difficult and lesions most often appear as previously described. At times, however, many other conditions can resemble the cutaneous manifestations of HPV infection, and these disorders are detailed in Table 123–2.

TREATMENT

Overview

The ideal therapy would be effective, painless, safe, and inexpensive. The multiplicity of treatment methods used to treat warts (Table 123–3) supports the fact that reliable effective therapy does not currently exist. Therefore, it is important for both the clinicians and patients to have reasonable expectations of therapy: induction of a sustained, asymptomatic, wart-free remission. Warts should be treated for a variety of reasons. Warts may cause mechanical discomfort on sensitive areas such as hands, feet, and genitalia. Treatment should also reduce

TABLE 123–3. Treatment of Human Papillomavirus	
Nonsurgical Methods	**Surgical Methods**
Keratolytic	*Surgery*
Salicylic acid	Scissors excision
	Debulking large tumors
	Excision (not suggested)
	Curettage
	Blunt dissection
Cytotoxic Agents	
Podophyllin	
Podofilox	
DNA Inhibitors	
Bleomycin (intralesional)	
5-fluorouracil (intralesional)	
Vesicants	*Cryosurgery*
Cantharidin	
Caustic Agents	*Electrosurgery*
Trichloro- or bichloroacetic acid	
Immunotherapy	*Laser Surgery*
Dinitrochlorobenzene	
Diphenciprone	
Heat	*Infrared Coagulation*
Laser hyperthermia	
Immersion in 113°F water	
Interferons	
Intralesional	
Systemic	
Retinoids	
Topical	
Systemic	
Behavioral Techniques	
Hypnosis	

the risk of transmission. The presence of genital warts, which can be traumatized and bleed, may facilitate transmission of human immunodeficiency virus. Genital and cervical HPV infections have a finite risk of malignant progression. Detection of abnormal cervical cell pathology by Papanicolaou smear and early effective treatment have dramatically reduced the incidence and mortality of invasive cervical cancer.

Treatment of nongenital cutaneous warts has not been subjected to rigorous controlled clinical trials, so there is very little scientific basis for therapeutic recommendations. With genital and mucosal HPV infection, several therapies have been systematically studied, including podofilox and the interferon(s). The more commonly used modalities such as cryotherapy, podophyllin, and electrosurgery, laser surgery, and excisional surgery have not been prospectively and systematically evaluated.

The mainstay of treatments of nongenital warts are cryotherapy and topical keratolytics. Surgical modalities are employed less frequently.[130] Paring and use of salicylic acid plasters (sal-acid) or topical liquids containing salicylic acid and lactic acid (Duofilm, Duoplant) are popular, often effective, nontraumatic therapies that can be administered at home by the patient. Other treatments with low morbidity that may be particularly effective in children include hypnosis[130a] and oral cimetidine.[130b] Intralesional bleomycin has been shown to be effective for common warts.[131, 132] Topical agents such as podofilox, podophyllin resin, and trichloroacetic acid are of little value for nongenital, cutaneous warts. Immunotherapy by induction with dinitrochlorobenzene[133, 134] and diphenciprone[135, 136] has efficacy in the treatment of common warts for which other treatments have failed. A vesicant, cantharidin, has also been employed in the treatment of common warts, particularly of the hands and feet. Simple scissors excision, electrodesiccation and curettage, or laser surgery are all applicable to the treatment of genital and cutaneous warts. The surgical approach has advantage for large, bulky lesions. Patients with exceptionally large wart areas or those who have had frequent recurrences are a major clinical challenge. Patients with frequent recurrences need to be seen and treated promptly for their recurrences. Treatment of genital warts has been recently reviewed.[137-139] In alphabetical order, current therapies include caustic agents (trichloro or bichloro-acetic acid)[40-42] cryotherapy, 5-fluorouracil, interferons, podophyllin,[139, 140] podofilox,[42, 139] and retinoids, surgery (laser, cold steel, electrosurgery). Factors that influence selection of therapy include the clinician's experience, patient preferences,

the number of warts, anatomic location of warts, and morphologic type of wart. The same modalities employed for the treatment of genital warts are also used to treat bowenoid papulosis. These patients and their sexual partners require more intensive long-term follow-up than patients with routine genital warts.

All current treatments have about a 50% complete response rate and a 25% to 50% recurrence rate.[44] However, better results can be achieved if treatments are properly selected. All patients will not benefit equally from any given treatment (Table 123-4). Cryotherapy is applicable to all morphologic types of genital warts. Unless local anesthetic is used, this modality is difficult to use for patients with a large number of warts. Because of dose-dependent adverse reactions, the use of the interferons is restricted to patients with relatively small numbers of small warts. Properly performed surgical treatment has few limitations. Podophyllin resin and caustic agents such as trichloroacetic acid have the greatest utility for patients with a small number of warts on moist surfaces and are severely limited in efficacy for dry, smooth papular or keratotic warts. Podofilox offers the advantage of being a treatment patients can apply themselves. In addition to recurrence, a common problem is patients with a "partial response" to treatment. Patients with classic genital warts may also have other genital papules such as skin tags or keratoses that are incorrectly diagnosed as genital warts and may not respond to genital wart treatments.

Emotional Needs

When treating any patient with potentially sexually transmitted disease, in addition to addressing their medical and physical problems, one must be attuned to and acknowledge the existence of emotional issues. The emotional impact of HPV infection varies greatly from patient to patient, based not only on their perception of the problem but also often on the circumstances by which they believe they were infected. There are often feelings of uncleanliness, guilt, feelings of being wronged or tainted. Patients will often not vocalize these problems without prompting. Asking how they are doing emotionally with their wart infection will often be greeted by the patient with relief that the emotional component of their problem exists. At times, referral for professional counseling is helpful and other times support groups or physician counseling are adequate. In addition to having concerns about how and where they acquired the infection,

TABLE 123-4. Factors That Influence Selection of Treatment for Genital Warts

Modality	Wart Morphology	Wart Size	Total Wart Area/Count
Cryotherapy	All types	Small to average	Limiting
Interferon(s)	All types	All sizes	Limiting
Surgery (excision, electrodesiccation, curettage, laser)	All types	All sizes	Non-limiting
Trichloroacetic acid	Moist, nonkeratotic	Small	Limiting
Podophyllin	Moist, nonkeratotic	All sizes	All but very large
Podofilox	All types	All sizes	<10 cm^2

women and men are concerned about the impact of HPV on their ability to reproduce and to avoid the risk of cervical cancer. Other than the exceptional case of warts with extensive condylomata that impede vaginal delivery, HPV is not thought to have any direct adverse effect on reproductive capacity.

Physical Modalities for the Therapy of Warts

The primary physical modalities for the therapy of warts include cryosurgery, electrosurgery, blunt dissection surgical excision, and laser surgery. These modalities destroy or ablate visible warty tissue, but probably do not induce viral-free states. In an in vitro study detecting HPV DNA in genital warts by polymerase chain reaction, the DNA was found in 100% of untreated specimens, 92% of specimens treated with liquid nitrogen, and in 15% and 7% of specimens treated with podophyllin and trichloro-acetic acid respectively.[141] Detailed prospective randomized studies of these treatments are few and even fewer comparative trials have been done; nevertheless they are commonly used by both dermatologists and nonspecialists in the standard treatment of warts and are often quite effective.

Cryosurgery (see Robinson et al., *Atlas of Cutaneous Surgery,* Chapter 5) involves the application of liquid nitrogen (− 195° C) via cotton swabs or cryospray unit to the wart and a small 1- to 2-mm rim of surrounding normal tissue. The usual method involves applying the liquid nitrogen for 10 to 60 seconds until the wart and a 1- to 2-mm halo appear frozen and remain white for 10 to 30 seconds, depending on the size and thickness of the wart. After thawing, a second application is commonly applied. During freezing, the patient experiences a burning sensation that is usually tolerated without anesthesia. Throbbing occurs after thawing. Immediately after the treatment the site is red and swollen. Blistering may ensue within 24 hours but is not a necessary part of successful wart cryosurgery. Repeated rapid freezing and slow thawing disrupts living cells. Two to three weeks after treatment, the wart may be dry, crusted, dark, smaller, the same size, or eradicated completely. When the wart is completely eradicated, the skin at the site appears and feels completely normal. Overly vigorous treatment may leave persistent hypopigmentation, which is of greatest concern when treating darkly pigmented patients, or hypesthesia in sites of superficial nerves such as the sides of the fingers.

In a study[142] of 72 randomized patients with hand warts treated prospectively for 12 weeks at intervals of 2-week treatments, 3-week treatments, and 4-week treatments, 70% to 80% had eradication of their warts in three or more treatments if the interval between treatments was not more than 3 weeks. If the interval was 4 weeks, only 40% of hand warts resolved over the treatment period. When compared with a group of hand warts treated with a keratolytic paint containing salicylic acid and acetic acids, as well as a group receiving both treatments concurrently, there was no significant difference in the percentage cure. In another study[143] of 400 consecutive hand and foot warts, patients were treated for 3 months with cryotherapy and a keratolytic wart pain, curing 52% of patients. Paring improved the cure rate for plantar warts but not for hand warts. Cure was inversely related to both length of wart infection and to the diameter of the largest wart. Similar results have been reported for cryotherapy of genital warts; 88%[144] and 74%[145] were cured in 10 to 12 weeks with weekly treatments. Patients with a few small lesions were cleared in 4 to 6 weeks. Treatment regimens in which cryotherapy was used for genital warts in conjunction with local injection or systemic administration of interferon alfa[146] and inosine pranobex[143] have also been reported but without great success.

Electrosurgery (see *Atlas of Cutaneous Surgery,* Chapter 6) involves the use of an alternating electrical current to destroy warty tissue. Local anesthesia is required. The electrode tip is held either in contact to the wart surface or slightly away from the surface so that a spark extends across the gap. Energy is administered until the wart is desiccated and black. Treated tissue is removed by rough curettage and any remaining wart is again treated.[147] Treatment of 1 to 2 mm of normal skin surrounding the wart may decrease recurrences. Once the treatment is completed, a superficial ulcer is present. Re-epithelialization is promoted by keeping the wound covered and moist[148] either by topical antibiotic and bandaging or a semipermeable occlusive dressing. Time to heal depends upon the size and site of the wound. The final result is usually atrophic scarring. Hypertrophic scarring and nail dystrophy can also result.

Electrosurgery was used in the treatment of warts long before modern controlled trials. It is rarely used for plantar warts because slow healing and painful scarring often result. In other sites, if scarring is acceptable to the patient, electrosurgery may be highly effective in one treatment. For treatment of warts on genital skin, where healing is commonly uncomplicated, electrosurgery is often employed. In studies of fewer than 20 patients with genital warts, 84% were cured at 10 to 12 weeks with podophyllin[149] and 91%[150] with electrocautery. In a group of human immunodeficiency virus–seropositive patients,[151] electrocautery induced clearance in 90% to 100% of patients; addition of systemic interferon did not statistically improve the results.

Heat energy supplied by an infrared coagulator that delivers a narrow beam of incoherent infrared light may also be used to destroy wart tissue. A study of 31 warts treated with an infrared coagulator under local anesthesia produced a cure rate of 70%.[151a] Wounds and healing time are similar to those for electrocautery.

Surgical removal of warts has been performed ever since the advent of local anesthesia. Whereas filiform warts may be simply snipped and flat warts can sometimes be "flicked off" by a curette or blade, most procedures are done under local anesthesia. For blunt dissection, superficial callus and warty tissue is pared until a sharp demarcation between wart and normal skin is seen. With a blunt dissector or blunt-tipped scissors, the wart is dissected using firm pressure. A plane of cleavage becomes apparent and the base separates easily from its loose connection. Blunt dissection cured 85% of 60 plantar warts with minimal pain and scar formation.[152] Subungual and periungual warts can also be removed by a similar technique.[153] Standard full-thickness fusiform excision with repair can also be performed. In addition to the usual results and complications following excisional surgery including scarring, the risk of recurrence is not negligible.

Use of the Carbon Dioxide Laser for Treatment of Warts and Other Cutaneous Lesions

The carbon dioxide laser may also be used as a tool for the destruction of warts. This laser has been used clinically for almost 20 years. It produces an invisible beam of energy in the far infrared portion of the electromagnetic spectrum at 10,600 nanometers. This beam of energy may be emitted as a continuous wave, a shuttered continuous wave, or a pulsed wave (Superpulse, Ultrapulse). It is produced in a resonating cavity with carbon dioxide molecules excited by an electrical stimulus and then is delivered to the tissue via an articulated arm system with a terminal attachment that is a hand-held handpiece or a joystick-manipulated operating microscope. In some units producing low powers, the delivery system is a semiflexible thin tube called a wave guide. Also available is a desktop low-power model that incorporates the main resonating cavity within the handpiece itself. Carbon dioxide lasers have power outputs of 10 to 100 watts. The beam is focused through a lens in the handpiece and may have effective spot sizes at the tissue level of 0.2 mm to 0.5 mm. The beam can be used tightly focused at high-power densities for cutting or defocused at lower power densities for ablation through tissue vaporization and coagulation.

The tissue effect of the carbon dioxide laser energy[154] begins when the energy is absorbed by water in the tissues, producing heat. With a pulse energy greater than 5 J/cm^2, tissue water is heated instantaneously to greater than the boiling point. Rapid heating causes explosion of tissue structures by shock waves, cavitation, and rapid thermal expansion and thereby vaporizes tissue into a plume containing tissue components and water. The heat also diffuses through the adjacent tissues. Tissue immediately adjacent to the site of vaporization heats to between 50° C and 100° C. Depending upon the duration of exposure to heat at these temperatures, denaturation or irreversible coagulation of proteins may occur. Tissue heated to less than 50° C generally recovers completely. If the energy used is below the minimum necessary to induce vaporization, tissues will coagulate and desiccate. With prolonged exposure, heat will accumulate slowly and may result in temperatures of 300° C to 600° C, creating extensive peripheral thermal damage secondary to thermal diffusion. Char results from burning of tissue at greater than 300° C. Therefore, three zones of damage surrounding the site of vaporization are usually grossly and microscopically appreciable; carbonized eschar, coagulative necrosis, and a sheath of edema. Beyond the edema, there is a sharp transition to normal tissue. Thermal damage appears to be the most significant effect of the carbon dioxide laser energy. Tissue

affected by char and coagulative necrosis will slough or be reabsorbed and remodeled during the wound healing process. The repair processes are similar to that occurring after other thermal injuries. Clinically speaking, destruction of tissue occurs both through vaporization as well as coagulative necrosis and subsequent repair processes.

Carbon dioxide laser energy penetrates only about 20 microns into water. In tissue, however, penetration is affected by exposure spot size, duration of exposure, proportion of water within the tissue,[155] and scattering and is estimated to vary from 0.2 mm[156] to more than 1 mm.[155] The volume of tissue vaporized varies directly with power density at the tissue level. The width of the zone of thermal damaged adjacent tissue, however, varies directly in relationship to duration of exposure. If exposure times are shorter than the time it takes the heated tissue to cool, adjacent thermal damage is minimized because there is not excessive heat energy available for diffusion.[154] Therefore, short laser exposure with a high-power density vaporizes the same volume of tissue as a longer exposure at a lower power density but with much less adjacent thermal damage.[155] Tissue damage has been measured 50 microns to 2 mm beyond the site of vaporization.[157-159]

Tissue effects, both vaporization and adjacent tissue damage, are therefore related to absorption, heat diffusion, and the continuing process of vaporization and dehydration, allowing more absorption and diffusion. These factors are related to power density and duration of exposure. In practical terms, control of destruction, as well as control of the residual wound and partial control of the resulting scar, depend upon a variety of factors within the command of the surgeon. Power output is varied by knob or touch pad control on the main laser unit. The spot size may be altered by changing the handpiece and focusing lens or by modifying the distance the handpiece is held from the skin surface. The duration of exposure to the laser beam may be adjusted by shuttering and/or moving the handpiece more or less quickly across the skin surface. The pulse waveforms are further modifications of the duration of exposure such that for any given average power, laser energy with higher peak powers has been produced for a shorter period of time.

The most important advantage of the carbon dioxide laser for ablative therapy is its ability to produce limited destruction very rapidly. In addition, the continuous wave beam supplies relative hemostasis during the procedure. Blood vessels 0.5 mm in diameter and smaller are heated and sealed,[160] allowing procedures to be performed quickly with minimal blood loss.[161] Large vessels can be grasped with forceps and welded shut without difficulty. The pulse waveform minimizes adjacent thermal injury and also minimizes the hemostasis properties of the carbon dioxide laser so that wounds made with a pulsed carbon dioxide laser may bleed similarly to a scalpel cut wound. The laser also sterilizes as it vaporizes[162, 163] and does not interfere with pacemakers or monitoring devices. Nail and thick hyperkeratotic debris melt away and even bone can be ablated. The surgery is non-contact, thus theoretically limiting the transfer of infection or malignant cells from the surface of a surgical tool to the wound. The laser has been said to seal nerve endings,[164] but data documenting diminished pain in wounds are anecdotal. An early histologic study suggested that small lymphatics were sealed[165] and it had been assumed that the wound would, therefore, demonstrate less postoperative edema; however, two other ultrastructural studies[166, 167] reported patent lymphatic channels, and in a third study[168] technetium-labeled colloid placed in a laser-induced wound migrated into regional lymph nodes in a fashion similar to migration noted in scalpel wounds. Paired trials of the use of the scalpel and the carbon dioxide laser in blepharoplasties offers mixed reviews of whether postoperative edema and pain is diminished by the use of the laser.[169–171] In contrast to electrosurgical techniques for ablation, the carbon dioxide laser creates much less adjacent thermal tissue damage[159, 160] and shortens the length of the procedure.[172] Cryosurgery generally produces more edema and pain.[173, 174] In addition, blistering cannot develop after the use of the carbon dioxide laser because the epidermis will not be intact. Of note, when the carbon dioxide laser is used for ablation, there is no specimen to be sent to pathology. Any clinically nonpathognomic lesion requires biopsy prior to destruction.

Numerous applications have been described for the use of the carbon dioxide laser in cutaneous surgery as an ablating tool (Table 123–5). It is the instrument of choice for treating a variety of thin epidermal processes characterized by hyperplasia and/or atypia. Warts were one of the first disorders treated. The basic technique is detailed in Table 123–6. Vaporization of tissue is appreciated visibly when an opalescent bubbling of the skin surface is seen. If tissue fragments and their coagulum are wiped away, an intact pinkish-white base may be found in the epidermis if the lesion is thick or within the superficial dermis with normal dermatoglyphic markings visible if the lesion is thin. Subsequent passes over the same site may reveal visible contraction of tissue if the dermis is vaporized or heated or grape-like globules of yellowish fat from subcutaneous tissue.

The surgeon depends on visual feedback, either by gross inspection or through an operating microscope, to gauge depth of vaporization and the degree of surrounding tissue damage, and may continuously vary the power density by changing power output, spot size, duration of delivery, or speed of movement. He or she, therefore, has an instrument that is easily and rapidly adjusted to each specific site, lesion, or wound even as the wound changes throughout the procedure. In addition, without changing instruments, bulky or pedunculated warts may be removed by cutting with the laser using a tightly focused beam with high-power densities, then ablating flatter warts and coagulating the base with the beam defocused and lower power densities. Limitations of this technique include its dependence on the accuracy of the surgeon in judging the depth of the lesion, the skill with which he or she manipulates the handpiece, the lack of precise calculation of power densities and duration of exposure for each treatment, and the inability to reduplicate precisely the treatment at another time by the same surgeon, much less by readers of the surgeon's description of the procedure. Regardless, the endpoint of any ablative procedure is eradication of the lesion, and the optimal power

TABLE 123–5. Disorders for Which the Carbon Dioxide Laser Has Been Used As an Ablating Tool

I. Epidermal or mucosal disorders
  A. Actinic cheilitis*
  B. Erythroplasia of Queyrat*
  C. Oral florid papillomatosis*
  D. Sublingual keratosis*
  E. Bowenoid papulosis*
  F. Balanitis xerotica obliterans†
  G. Bowen's disease or squamous cell carcinoma in situ‡
  H. Superficial basal cell carcinomas‡
  I. Epidermal nevus†
  J. Nail ablation‡
  K. Lentigines§
  L. Lower labial macules§
  M. Lichen sclerosus et atrophicus§
  N. Zoon's balanitis§
  O. Hailey-Hailey disease§
  P. Darier's disease§
  Q. Porokeratosis§
II. Warts
  A. Verruca vulgaris‡
  B. Verruca plantaris‡
  C. Periungual warts‡
  D. Widespread condyloma acuminatum†
  E. Recalcitrant warts†
III. Dermal processes
  A. Syringomas†
  B. Granuloma faciale‡
  C. Trichoepitheliomas‡
  D. Neurofibromas‡
  E. Xanthelasma‡
  F. Adenoma sebaceum‡
  G. Myxoid cysts§
  H. Apocrine hydrocystoma§
  I. Angiolymphoid hyperplasia§
  J. Pearly penile papules§
  K. Cowden's disease§
  L. Chondrodermatitis nodularis helicis§
  M. Debridement of granulation tissue§
  N. Cutaneous infections (botryomycosis, leishmaniasis)§
IV. Vascular lesions
  A. Port-wine stains‖
  B. Telangiectasis‖
  C. Cherry angiomas‡
  D. Lymphangioma circumscriptum§
  E. Pyogenic granulomas§
  F. Angiokeratomas‡
  G. Angiosarcomas§
  H. Venous lakes‡
V. Miscellaneous
  A. Tattoos‖
  B. Red tattoo reactions†
  C. Cutaneous resurfacing§
  D. De-epithelialization before reconstructive surgical procedure§
  E. Aging hands§
  F. Sterilization of infected wounds§
  G. Debridement of burn wounds§

*Treatment of choice.
†Results often better than alternatives.
‡Results usually same as alternatives, use of the laser may facilitate procedure.
§Results may or may not be acceptable; current information cannot be easily evaluated.
‖Better results now obtained with newer laser systems.
Reprinted by permission of the publisher from Olbricht SO. Use of the carbon dioxide laser in dermatologic surgery, a clinically relevant update for 1993. J Dermatol Surg Oncol 1993;19:367. Copyright 1993 by Elsevier Science, Inc.

TABLE 123-6. Technique for Ablation

1. Surgical Plan: Determine desired endpoint.
2. Preparation of site: Lesion and necessary margins may be outlined with surgical marking pen and cleaned with normal saline.
3. Anesthesia: Local, regional, or general.
4. Draping: Wet sponges for prevention of inadvertent burns.
5. Power output setting: 4 to 30 watts depending on lesion and site.
6. Waveform: Continuous wave, shuttered beam, or super-pulsed beam.
7. Spot size at the tissue surface: 0.5- to 5-mm diameter defocused beam, depending on distance of handpiece from tissue surface.
8. Vaporization with beam defocused:
   a. Continuous wave beam or superpulsed beam used with air brush–like movements
   or
   b. Shuttered beam directed to single site
9. Debridement: Wipe with wet sponge (saline, sterile water, hydrogen peroxide) to clean off tissue fragments, char, or coagulum.
10. Repeat treatment: Vaporization and debridement repeated as necessary to achieve desired endpoint.
11. Surgical dressing: Appropriate for size and site of wound.
12. Postoperative instructions for wound care: Appropriate for size and site of wound.

density is that which is just high enough to achieve rapid vaporization of the complete lesion but low enough for the surgeon to control. Applying this principle, an experienced surgeon, using a laser model to which he or she is accustomed with manual control of the handpiece, is likely to achieve good, consistent results. This modified empirical technique has become a standard procedure because of its ease of use and flexibility.

Following ablation by the carbon dioxide laser, the wound heals by secondary intention. The zone of coagulation necrosis widens over the first few days[175] then begins to slough. Within 6 to 7 days, the wound has a bed of granulation tissue and re-epithelialization begins. The onset of epidermal migration is somewhat delayed but progresses normally once it begins.[176-179] Wound contraction may occur, similar to that of wounds created by other modalities.[180] Two studies on gynecologic tissues have demonstrated more rapid healing of pulsed carbon dioxide laser incisions compared with incisions created by continuous waveforms or electrosurgery.[181, 182] A comparison[183] of the epithelialization of mid-dermal wounds created by ablation with a pulsed carbon dioxide laser controlled by a mechanical scanning device with wounds produced by a dermatome documented a significant lengthening in re-epithelialization time for laser-created wounds as opposed to dermatome-cut wounds on day 3, but complete recovery by day 14. Of note, in the treatment regimen the surfaces of the laser-created wounds were dry and remained dry under a dressing, whereas the dermatome wounds were moist and probably remained moist under the dressing, despite the known effect of dryness on re-epithelialization. In addition, there was no comparison made with a similar wound created by controlled continuous wave energy. Although it seems apparent that the use of optimal treatment parameters would improve healing in wounds cre-

ated by ablation with the carbon dioxide laser, studies that document the presumption do not yet exist. Likewise, no improvement in tissue healing with a pulsed carbon dioxide laser as opposed to a continuous wave beam has been adequately demonstrated, even though a strong case can be made theoretically.

Attention to appropriate wound care will speed wound healing and minimize scarring. Appropriate wound care is especially important following wounds created by ablation by the carbon dioxide laser because secondary intention healing is intended and may require weeks if the defect is large or deep. Wound care should be simple for the patient to perform and repeat, and supply comfort and protection. Early wound care involves cleansing the wound twice a day with diluted hydrogen peroxide or mild soap and water followed by the application of an antibiotic such as bacitracin or Neosporin ointment in a thin layer. A moist wound heals faster than a dry wound[148] and bacitracin or Neosporin ointment is known to promote re-epithelialization, as opposed to petrolatum[184] or povidone-iodine.[185] The wound is then protected by a Telfa dressing and gauze. Alternatively, semipermeable occlusive dressings such as Vigilon, Duo-Derm, or OpSite can be used. A study[186] comparing some of these dressings to no treatment at all documents their effectiveness. Wound care is continued until complete re-epithelialization has occurred. Complete healing may require 2 to 8 weeks depending on the site of the wound and the extent of surgery. Wound care is continued after complete re-epithelialization to decrease or prevent hypertrophic scarring.[187] Moisturizing and massaging healed wounds for 2 to 6 months is standard advice. Constant pressure (tailor-made pressure garments, surgical compression earrings) and splints are effective deterrents to hypertrophic scarring. Intralesional corticosteroid injections (10 to 40 mg/cc triamcinolone diacetate or acetonide) at monthly intervals may be required if thick areas of scar develop.

A survey of laser surgeons concerning complications due to the use of the carbon dioxide laser[188] noted that complications are rare but included hypertrophic scarring, hemorrhage, unexpected pain, unexpected prolonged healing, and infection. Reactive benign growths following surgery such as mucocele, excessive granulation tissue, and pyogenic granuloma have been reported. Attention to safety issues is essential. Unintentional burns to the patients or personnel are not frequent. One physician and his assistant developed laryngitis attributed to aspiration of laser plume when their smoke evacuation system failed. Certainly, viable infectious agents[189-191] and lung-damaging dust[192] may be present in the plume, and adequate plume evacuation systems must be used intraoperatively. Infectious PV has been documented in the plume of warts treated with electrocoagulation as well as with the carbon dioxide laser.[193]

The early studies of the treatment of warts with the carbon dioxide laser were encouraging.[194-196] However, more recent data suggest that this procedure is not without its difficulties. In a study[197] of 18 patients with persistent warts on the hands and feet, 56% were cured at follow-up (minimum 6 months), 17% patients achieved partial clearance, and 27% relapsed. Considerable morbidity including postoperative pain, temporary loss of function, and scarring was associated with the procedure. In another study,[197] of 25 patients with warts resistant to other therapies, 32% were cured, 20% improved, and 48% relapsed completely. In 17 patients[198] with 24 periungual warts resistant to other therapy, vaporization of the entire wart with the partial or complete avulsion of the nail led to a 71% cure rate with one or two treatments and 94% cure rates with an adjacent use of other therapeutic modalities. Time for complete re-epithelialization was approximately 2 months. Complications reported include significant pain (12%), postoperative numbness (18%), and nail dystrophy (29%). In 46 patients with 300 warts, use of continuous wave carbon dioxide and Superpulse carbon dioxide energy produced clearing in 68% of treatments, whereas the Ultrapulse carbon dioxide laser produced clearing in 90%.[199] Scarring differed by wave form used and was 54%, 33%, and 7%, respectively. All procedures were designed to ablate all appreciable warty tissue.

The reason for the relatively moderate cure rate after vigorous therapy with its attendant morbidity is not known. However, it probably relates to viral persistence in adjacent, yet clinically uninvolved areas. Persistent subclinical infection has been documented in HPV-related diseases of the female genital tract, in which 50% of patients had viral genome found by Southern blot hybridization in normal appearing skin 5 to 10 mm away from visible lesions.[200] Detection of persistent viral genome was associated with a 67% incidence of recurrence following laser surgery. In a study[201] of 25 women with recalcitrant and widespread genital disease, the carbon dioxide laser was used to destroy the entire epithelial/mucosal surface from the cervix to the anal canal and the entire perineum whether or not it appeared involved with condylomatous changes. Thirteen of 19 male consorts were also treated vigorously, including the entire penile shaft. As expected, the morbidity was high. At 3 months, there was also histologic evidence of persistent wart virus in 88% of patients, and 23 of the 25 women had clinically apparent HPV lesions. In other studies, the success rates in treating genital warts in women have ranged from 65% to 100%,[202-204] and more than one procedure was required in some patients. Cure rates may be enhanced by treating the male partner simultaneously.[204] Because women generally have warts in more than one perineal location, colposcopy to detect the presence of vaginal or cervical warts should be carried out prior to treatment of external genital or perianal warts.

Results of treating male patients with HPV-induced condyloma are similar. One study[205] of 119 patients achieved an 82.3% cure rate of lesions treated in one session, but new areas of involvement appeared in 5 patients. Two thirds of the patients healed within 3 to 4 weeks, whereas the remainder required up to 6 weeks. Thirteen per cent of patients developed complications such as local infection and cellulitis. In another study of 43 male patients,[206] acetowhite lesions thought to be characteristic of HPV were treated by the carbon dioxide laser with or without intraurethral 5-fluorouracil with a 50% cure rate. Other adjuvant therapies such as interferon-alfa-2b local injections[207] or systemic administration[208] may reduce the risk of recurrence.

The wide difference reported in response rates may be related to differences in warts chosen for reporting (recalcitrant or previously untreated, localized or diffuse, small or large, of long duration or short), different HPV subtypes, different anatomic sites, and different host immune status, but differences in technique are also apparent. Some authors used low-power densities,[197] others used much higher powers,[205] and some debrided hyperkeratotic material first.[199] The margin of normal skin treated is often not mentioned, but when reported varies from 2 to 10 mm. The use of different waveforms in a comparative trial[199] illustrates the influence of treatment parameters used. Morbidity also varies, probably for the same reasons. The procedure generally produces a wound that requires a healing time of 1 to 2 months, induces some pain, and sometimes results in scarring. These anticipated results of surgery are complicated by the (nearly universal) expectation of patients and referring physicians that laser surgery is easy and painless (without anesthesia), involves no postoperative care, leaves no scar, and guarantees a cure. Recurrence is further complicated by the oncogenic potential of some HPV types (16, 18, 31–35, 39, 42, 48, 51),[209] which may be associated with squamous cell carcinoma of the skin,[210, 211] as well as bowenoid papulosis, cervical dysplasia, cervical cancer, and anogenital carcinoma.[209] Successful laser ablation of cervical intraepithelial neoplasia associated with HPV infection may not preclude development of invasive cancer of the cervix.[212]

Inasmuch as warts are frequently associated with dilated blood vessels in the papillary dermis, a trial[213] using a laser with selective absorption by hemoglobin, the pulsed-dye laser (see Chapter 146) was performed. Of 39 patients with recalcitrant warts, treatment with the pulsed-dye laser at 585 mm, 450 m/sec pulse duration, and spot size of 5 mm (fluences 6.25–7.5 J/cm^2) cleared 28 (72%) in an average of 1.68 treatments. Only 1 of the 28 patients had a recurrence after 3 months. These excellent preliminary results have not been confirmed in other centers to date.

It is clear that any of several modalities may induce complete clearing of clinical lesions. Laser therapy is best reserved for those warts that are recalcitrant to less morbid treatments and those that are bulky, painful, or histologically atypical. In addition, the treatment of warts in sites difficult to treat by other modalities may be facilitated by use of the carbon dioxide laser. Thick plantar warts can be treated faster than by electrosurgical devices. Periungual warts and overlying nail can be ablated easily without avulsion of the nail plate. Laser treatment does not preclude the use of other adjuvant therapies or the use of less morbid treatments for small recurrences, and certainly must be associated with rigorous and long-term follow-up for any lesion with a potential for malignant degeneration. Follow-up for female partners of male patients with genital lesions associated with HPV infection must include yearly surveillance for cervical disease regardless of whether the therapy clears visible lesions in either partner.

References

1. De Villiers E. Heterogeneity of the human papillomavirus group. J Virol 1989;63:4898–4903.
2. Durst M, Gissmann L, Ikenberg H, zur Hausen H. A papillomavirus DNA from a cervical carcinoma and its prevalence in cancer biopsy samples from different geographic regions. Proc Natl Acad Sci 1983;80:3812–3815.
3. zurHausen H. Human papillomaviruses in the pathogenesis of anogenital cancer. Virology 1991;184:9–13.
4. Lorincz AT, Reid R, Jenson AB, et al. Human papillomavirus infection of the cervix: Relative risk associations of 15 common anogenital types. Obstet Gynecol 1992;79:328–337.
5. Syrjanen S, Kellokoski J. Oral manifestations of HPV infection. In: Gross G, et al., eds. Genital Papillomavirus Infection: Modern Diagnosis and Treatment. Berlin, Heidelberg: Springer-Verlag, 1990:209–223.
6. Panici P, Scambia G, Perrone L, et al. Oral condyloma in patients with extensive genital human papillomavirus infection. Am J Obstet Gynecol 1992;167:451–458.
7. Cohen P, Hebert A, Adler-Storthz K. Focal epithelial hyperplasia: Heck's disease. Pediatr Dermatol 1993;10:245–251.
8. Gross G, Jablonska S, Pfister H, et al., eds. Genital Papillomavirus Infection: Modern Diagnosis and Treatment. Berlin, Heidelberg: Springer-Verlag, 1990:209–223.
9. Wade TR, Ackerman AB. Bowenoid papulosis of the genitalia. Arch Dermatol 1979;115:306.
10. Obalek S, Jablonska S, Beaudenon S, et al. Bowenoid papulosis of the male and female genitalia: Risk of cervical neoplasia. J Am Acad Dermatol 1986;14:433–443.
11. Patterson J, Kao G, Graham J, et al. Bowenoid papulosis: A clinicopathologic study with ultrastructural observations. Cancer 1986;57:823–836.
12. Palefsky J. Natural history of anal cytologic abnormalities and papillomavirus infection among homosexual men with Group IV HIV disease. J Acquir Immune Defic Synd 1992;5:1258–1266.
13. Blessing K, McLaren K, Benton E, et al. Histopathology of skin lesions in renal allograft recipients: An assessment of viral features and dysplasia. Histopathology 1989;14:129–139.
14. Stern R, Johnson M, DeLozier J. Utilization of physician services for dermatologic complaints. Arch Dermatol 1987;113:1062–1066.
15. Schachner L, Ling N, Press S. A statistical analysis of a pediatric dermatology clinic. Pediatr Dermatol 1983;1:157–164.
16. Grigg W, Wilhelm G. Epidemiological study of plantar warts among school children. Public Health Rep 1953;68:985–988.
17. Steele K, Irwin W, Merrett J. Warts in general practice. Ir Med J 1989;82:122–124.
18. Finkel M, Finkel D. Warts among meat handlers. Arch Dermatol 1984;120:1314–1317.
19. Jablonska S, Obalek S, Golebiowska A, et al. Epidemiology of butchers' warts. Arch Dermatol Res 1988;280(Suppl):S24–S28.
20. Keefe M, Al-Ghamdi A, Coggon D, et al. Cutaneous warts in butchers. Br J Dermatol 1994;130:9–14.
21. Keefe M, Al-Ghamdi A, Coggon D, et al. Butchers' warts: No evidence for person to person transmission of HPV7. Br J Dermatol 1994;130:15–17.
22. Massing AM, Epstein WL. Natural history of warts: A two year study. Arch Dermatol 1963;87:306.
23. Bergfeld E, Roenigk H. Cutaneous complications of immunosuppressive therapy: A review of 215 renal transplant patients. Cutis 1978;22:169–172.
24. Gassenmaier A, Fuchs P, Schell H, et al. Papillomavirus DNA in warts of immunosuppressed renal allograft recipients. Arch Dermatol Res 1986;278:219–223.
25. Ingelfinger J, Grupe W, Topor M, et al. Warts in a pediatric renal transplant population. Dermatologica 1977;155:7–12.
26. Spencer E, Andersen A. Clinically evident, non-terminal infections with herpesviruses and the wart virus in immunosuppressed renal allograft recipients. Br Med J 1970;1:251–254.
27. Rudlinger R, Smith I, Bunney M, et al. Human papillomavirus infections in a group of renal transplant recipients. Br J Dermatol 1986;115:681–692.
28. Van der Leest R, Zachow K, Ostrow R, et al. Human papillomavirus heterogeneity in 36 renal transplant recipients. Arch Dermatol 1987;123:354–357.
29. Boyle J, Briggs J, MacKie R, et al. Cancer, warts, and sunshine in renal transplant patients: A case control study. Lancet 1984;1:702–705.
30. Morison W. Viral warts, herpes simplex and herpes zoster in patients with secondary immune deficiencies and neoplasms. Br J Dermatol 1975;92:625.
31. Berger T. Epidermodysplasia verruciformis: Associated papillomavirus infection complicating human immunodeficiency virus disease. Br J Dermatol 1991;124:79–83.
32. Jablonska S, Orth G, Jarzabek-Chorzelska M, et al. Twenty-one years of follow-up of studies of familial epidermodysplasia verruciformis. Dermatologica 1979;158:309–327.
33. Lutzner M, Blanchet-Bardon C. Epidermodysplasia verruciformis. Curr Probl Dermatol 1985;13:164–185.
34. Lutzner M. Epidermodysplasia verruciformis: An autosomal recessive disease characterized by viral warts and skin cancer, a model for viral oncogenesis. Bull Cancer (Paris) 1978;65:269–282.
35. Androphy EJ, Dvoretzky I, Lowy DR. X-linked inheritance of epidermodysplasia verruciformis. Genetic and virologic studies of a kindred. Arch Dermatol 1985;121:864–868.
36. Ostrow R, Bender M, Niimura M, et al. Human papillomavirus DNA in cutaneous primary and metastasized squamous cell carcinomas from patients with epidermodysplasia verruciformis. Proc Natl Acad Sci USA 1982;79:1634–1638.
37. Jablonska S, Orth G, Jarzabek-Chorzelska, et al. Immunological studies in epidermodysplasia verruciformis. Bull Cancer (Paris) 1978;65:183–190.
38. Koutsky LA, Galloway DA, Holmes KK. Epidemiology of genital human papillomavirus infection. Epidemiol Rev 1988;10:122–63.
39. Beutner K, Becker T, STone K. Epidemiology of human papillomavirus infections. Dermatol Clin 1991;9:211–218.
40. Chuang T, Perry H, Kurlanc L, et al. Condyloma acuminatum in Rochester, Minnesota, 1950–1978. Arch Dermatol 1984;120:469–475.
41. Friedman-Kien A, Eron L, Conant M, et al. Natural interferon alfa for treatment of condylomata acuminata. JAMA 1988;259:533–538.
42. Beutner KR, Friedman-Kien AE, Artman NN, et al. Patient-applied podofilox for treatment of genital warts. Lancet 1989;1:831–834.
43. Mounts P, Shah K, Kashima H. Viral etiology of juvenile and adult onset squamous papilloma of the larynx. Proc Natl Acad Sci USA 1982;79:5425–5429.
44. Boyd A. Condylomata acuminata in the pediatric population. Am J Dis Child 1990;144:817–824.
45. Padel A, Venning V, Evans M, et al. Human papillomaviruses in anogenital warts in children: Typing by in-situ hybridization. Br Med J 1990;300:1491–1494.
46. Cohen BA, Honig P, Androphy E. Anogenital warts in children. Clinical and virologic evaluation for sexual abuse. Arch Dermatol 1990;126:1575–1580.
47. Obalek S, Jablonska S, Favre M, et al. Condylomata acuminata in children: Frequent association with human papillomaviruses responsible for cutaneous warts. J Am Acad Dermatol 1990;23:205–213.
48. Stoler MH, Wolinsky SM, Whitbeck A, et al. Differentiation-linked human papillomavirus types 6 and 11 transcription in genital condylomata revealed by in situ hybridization with message-specific RNA probes. Virology 1989;172:331–340.
49. Androphy EJ, Lowy DR, Schiller JT. Bovine papillomavirus E2 trans-activating gene product binds to specific sites in papillomavirus DNA. Nature 1987;325:70–73.
50. Lambert PF. Papillomavirus DNA replication. J Virol 1991;65:3417–3420.
51. Ustav M, Stenlund A. Transient replication of BPV-1 requires two viral polypeptides encoded by the E1 and E2 open reading frames. EMBO J 1991;10:449–457.
52. Mohr IJ, Clark R, Sun S, et al. Targeting the E1 replication protein to the papillomavirus origin of replication by complex

formation with the E2 transactivator. Science 1990;250: 1694–1699.

53. Hagensee ME, Yaegashi N, Galloway DA. Self-assembly of human papillomavirus type 1 capsids by expression of L1 protein alone or by co-expression of the L1 and L2 capsid proteins. J Virol 1993;67:315–322.

54. Kirnbauer R, Booy F, Cheng N, et al. Papillomavirus L1 major capsid protein self-assembles into virus-like particles that are highly immunogenic. Proc Natl Acad Sci USA 1992;89: 12180–12184.

55. Kirnbauer R, Taub J, Greenstone H, et al. Efficient self-assembly of human papillomavirus type 16 L1 and L1-L2 into virus-like particles. J Virol 1993;67:6929–6936.

56. Rose RC, Bonnez W, Reichman RC, Garcea RL. Expression of human papillomavirus type 11 L1 protein in insect cells: In vivo and in vitro assembly of virus like particles. J Virol 1993;67:1936–1944.

57. Zhou J, Sun XY, Stenzel J, Frazer IH. Expression of vaccinia recombinant HPV 16 L1 and L2 ORF proteins in epithelial cells insufficient for assembly of HPV virion-like particles. Virology 1991;185:251–257.

58. Kirnbauer R, Hubbert N, Wheeler C, et al. A virus-like particle enzyme-linked immunosorbent assay detects serum antibodies in a majority of women infected with human papillomavirus type 16. J Natl Cancer Inst 1994;86:494–499.

59. Mansur C, Androphy E. Cellular transformation by papillomavirus oncoproteins. Biochim Biophys Acta Reviews in Cancer 1993;1155:323–345.

60. McCance DJ, Kopan R, Fuchs E, Laimins LA. Human papillomavirus type 16 alters human epithelial cell differentiation in vitro. Proc Natl Acad Sci 1988;85:7169–7173.

61. Hudson JB, Bedell MA, McCance DJ, Laimins LA. Immortalization and altered differentiation of human keratinocytes in vitro by the E6 and E7 open reading frames of human papillomavirus type 18. J Virol 1990;64:519–526.

62. Blanton RA, Perez RN, Merrick DT, McDougall JK. Epithelial cells immortalized by human papillomaviruses have premalignant characteristics in organotypic culture. Am J Pathol 1991;138:673–685.

63. Meyers C, Frattini MG, Hudson JB, Laimins L. Biosynthesis of human papillomavirus from a continuous cell line upon epithelial differentiation. Science 1992;257:971–973.

64. Dollard SC, Wilson JL, Demeter LM, et al. Production of human papillomavirus and modulation of the infectious program in epithelial raft cultures. Genes Dev 1992;6:1131–1142.

65. Kreider JW, Howett MK, Leure-Dupree AE, et al. Zaino RJ, Weber JA. Laboratory production in vivo of infectious human papillomavirus type 11. J Virol 1987;61:590–593.

66. Stoler MH, Whitbeck A, Wolinksy SM, et al. Infectious cycle of human papillomavirus type 16 in human foreskin xenografts in nude mice. J Virol 1990;64:3310–3318.

67. Sterling J, Stanley M, Gatward G, Minson T. Production of human papillomavirus type 16 virions in a keratinocyte cell line. J Virol 1990;64:6305–6307.

68. Schlegel R, Phelps WC, Zhang YL, Barbosa M. Quantitative keratinocyte assay detects two biological activities of human papillomavirus DNA and identifies viral types associated with cervical carcinoma. EMBO J 1988;7:3181–3187.

69. Barbosa MS, Schlegel R. The E6 and E7 genes of HPV-18 are sufficient for inducing two-stage in vitro transformation of human keratinocytes. Oncogene 1989;4:1529–1532.

70. Pirisi L, Yasumoto S, Feller M, et al. Transformation of human fibroblasts and keratinocytes with human papillomavirus type 16 DNA. J Virol 1987;61:1061–1066.

71. Pecoraro G, Morgan D, Defendi V. Differential effects of human papillomavirus type 6, 16, and 18 DNAs on immortalization and transformation of human cervical epithelial cells. Proc Natl Acad Sci 1989;86:563–567.

72. Kaur P, McDougall JK. HPV-18 immortalization of human keratinocytes. Virology 1989;173:302–310.

73. Munger K, Phelps WC, Bubb V, et al. The E6 and E7 genes of the human papillomavirus type 16 together are necessary and sufficient for transformation of primary human keratinocytes. J Virol 1989;63:4417–4421.

74. Kaur P, McDougall JK, Cone R. Immortalization of primary human epithelial cells by cloned cervical carcinoma DNA containing human papillomavirus type 16 E6/E7 open reading frames. J Gen Virol 1989;70:1261–1266.

75. Woodworth CD, Waggoner S, Barnes W, et al. Human cervical and foreskin epithelial cells immortalized by human papillomavirus DNAs exhibit dysplastic differentiation in vivo. Cancer Res 1990;50:3709–3715.

76. Sedman SA, Barbosa MS, Vass WC, et al. The full-length E6 protein of human papillomavirus type 16 has transforming and trans-activating activities and cooperates with E7 to immortalize keratinocytes in culture. J Virol 1991;65:4860–4866.

77. Pecoraro G, Lee M, Morgan D, Defendi V. Evolution of in vitro transformation and tumorigenesis of HPV16 and HPV18 immortalized primary cervical epithelial cells. Am J Pathol 1991; 138:1–8.

78. Barbosa MS, Vass WC, Lowy DR, Schiller JT. In vitro biological activities of the E6 and E7 genes vary among human papillomaviruses of different oncogenic potential. J Virol 1991; 65:292–298.

79. Hubbert NL, Sedman SA, Schiller JT. Human papillomavirus type 16 increases the degradation rate of p53 in human keratinocytes. J Virol 1992;66:6237–6241.

80. Hurlin PJ, Kaur P, Smith PP, Perez RN, Blanton RA, McDougall JK. Progression of human papillomavirus type 18-immortalized human keratinocytes to a malignant phenotype. Proc Natl Acad Sci USA 1991;88:570–574.

81. Levine AJ, Momand J. Tumor suppressor genes: The p53 and retinoblastoma sensitivity genes and gene products. Biochim Biophys Acta 1990;1032:119–136.

82. Vogelstein B, Kinzler KW. p53 function and dysfunction. Cell 1992;70:523–526.

83. Brash DE, Rudolph JA, Simon JA, et al. A role for sunlight in skin cancer. UV-induced p53 mutations in squamous cell carcinoma. Proc Natl Acad Sci 1991;88:10124–10128.

84. Hall PA, Mckee PH, Menage H, et al. High levels of p53 protein in UV-irradiated normal human skin. Oncogene 1993;8: 203–207.

85. Werness BA, Levine AJ, Howley PM. Association of human papillomavirus types 16 and 18 E6 proteins with p53. Science 1990;248:76–79.

86. Scheffner M, Werness BA, Huibregtse JM, et al. The E6 oncoprotein encoded by human papillomavirus types 16 and 18 promotes the degradation of p53. Cell 1990;63:1129–1136.

87. Crook T, Tidy J, Vousden K. Degradation of p53 can be targeted by HPV E6 sequences distinct from those required for p53 binding and trans-activation. Cell 1991;67:547–556.

88. Schiller JT, Vass WC, Lowy D. Identification of a second transforming region in bovine papillomavirus DNA. Proc Natl Acad Sci USA 1984;81:7880–7884.

89. Steger G, Pfister H. In vitro expressed HPV 8 E6 protein does not bind p53. Arch Virol 1992;125:355–360.

90. Band V, Dalal S, Delmolino L, Androphy EJ. Enhanced degradation of p53 protein in HPV-6 and BPV-1 E6-immortalized human mammary epithelial cells. EMBO J 1993;12: 1847–1852.

91. DeCaprio JA, Ludlow JW, Figge J, et al. SV40 large tumor antigen forms a specific complex with the product of the retinoblastoma susceptibility gene. Cell 1988;54:275–283.

92. Dyson N, Howley PM, Munger K, Harlow E. The human papilloma virus-16 E7 oncoprotein is able to bind to the retinoblastoma gene product. Science 1989;243:934–937.

93. Munger K, Werness BA, Dyson N, et al. Complex formation of human papillomavirus E7 proteins with the retinoblastoma tumor suppressor gene product. EMBO J 1989;8:4099–4105.

94. Dyson N, Guida P, Munger K, Harlow E. Homologous sequences in adenovirus E1a and human papillomavirus E7 proteins mediate interaction with the same set of cellular proteins. J Virol 1992;66:6893–6902.

95. Nevins JR. E2F: A link between the Rb tumor supressor protein and viral oncoproteins. Science 1992;258:424–429.

96. Davies R, Hicks R, Crook T, et al. Human papillomavirus type 16 E7 associates with a histone H1 kinase and with p107

through sequences necessary for transformation. J Virol 1993; 67:2521–2528.

97. Tommasino M, Adamczewski JP, Carlotti F, et al. HPV 16 E7 protein associates with the protein kinase p33-cdk2 and cyclin A. Oncogene 1993;8:195–202.

98. Barbosa MS, Edmonds C, Fisher C, et al. The region of the HPV E7 oncoprotein homologous to adenovirus E1a and Sv40 large T antigen contains separate domains for Rb binding and casein kinase II phosphorylation. EMBO J 1990;9:153–160.

99. Imai Y, Matsushima Y, Takashi S, Terada M. Purification and characterization of human papillomavirus type 16E7 protein with preferential binding capacity to the underphosphorylated form of retinoblastoma gene product. J Virol 1991;65: 4966–4972.

100. Vousden KH, Doniger J, DiPaolo JA, Lowy DR. The E7 open reading frame of human papillomavirus type 16 encodes a transforming gene. Oncogene Res 1988;3:167–175.

101. Tanaka A, Noda T, Yajima H, et al. Identification of a transforming gene of human papillomavirus type 16. J Virol 1989;63:1465–1469.

102. Halbert CL, Demers GW, Galloway DA. The E7 gene of human papillomavirus type 16 is sufficient for immortalization of human epithelial cells. J Virol 1991;65:473–478.

103. Jewers RJ, Hildebrandt P, Ludlow JW, et al. Regions of human papillomavirus type 16 E7 oncoprotein required for immortalization of human keratinocytes. J Virol 1992;66:1329–1335.

104. Schiller JT, Vass WC, Vousden KH, Lowy DR. E5 open reading frame of bovine papillomavirus type 1 encodes a transforming gene. J Virol 1986;57:1–6.

105. Burkhardt A, DiMaio D, Schlegel R. Genetic and biochemical definition of the bovine papillomavirus E5 transforming protein. EMBO J 1987;6:2381–2385.

106. Burkhardt A, Willingham M, Gay C, et al. The E5 oncoprotein of bovine papillomavirus is oriented asymmetrically in Golgi and plasma membranes. Virology 1989;170:334–339.

107. Goldstein DJ, Schlegel R. The E5 oncoprotein of bovine papillomavirus binds to a 16 kd cellular protein. EMBO J 1990;9:137–145.

108. Halbert CL, Galloway DA. Identification of the E5 open reading frame of human papillomavirus type 16. J Virol 1988;62:1071–1075.

109. Horwitz BH, Burkhardt AL, Schlegel R, DiMaio D. 44-amino-acid E5 transforming protein of bovine papillomavirus requires a hydrophobic core and specific carboxyl-terminal amino acids. Mol Cell Biol 1988;8:4071–4078.

110. Horwitz BH, Settleman J, Prakash SS, DiMaio D. Structure, activity, and regulation of the bovine papillomavirus E5 gene and its transforming protein product. Curr Top Microbiol Immunol 1989;144:143–151.

111. Jareborg N, Alderborn A, Burnett S. Identification and genetic definition of a bovine papillomavirus type 1 E7 protein and absence of a low-copy-number phenotype exhibited by E5, E6, or E7 viral mutants. J Virol 1992;66:4957–4965.

112. Leechanachai P, Banks L, Moreau F, Matlashewski G. The E5 gene from human papillomavirus type 16 is an oncogene which enhances growth factor-mediated signal transduction to the nucleus. Oncogene 1992;7:19–25.

113. Leptak C, Ramon y Cajal S, Kulke R, et al. Tumorgenic transformation of murine keratinocytes by the E5 genes of bovine papillomavirus type 1 and human papillomavirus type 16. J Virol 1991;65:7078–7083.

114. Martin P, Vass WC, Schiller JT, et al. The bovine papillomavirus E5 transforming protein can stimulate the transforming activity of EGF and CSF-1 receptors. Cell 1989;59:21–32.

115. Petti L, Nilson LA, DiMaio D. Activation of the platelet-derived growth factor receptor by the bovine papillomavirus E5 transforming protein. EMBO J 1991;10:845–855.

116. Petti L, DiMaio D. Stable association between the bovine papillomavirus E5 transforming protein and activated platelet-derived growth factor receptor in transformed mouse cells. Proc Natl Acad Sci USA 1992;89:6736–6740.

117. Pim D, Collins M, Banks L. Human papillomavirus type 16 E5 gene stimulates the transforming activity of the epidermal growth factor receptor. Oncogene 1992;7:27–32.

118. Schlegel R, Wade Glass M, Rabson MS, Yang YC. The E5

119. Settleman J, Fazeli A, Malicki J, et al. Genetic evidence that acute morphologic transformation, induction of cellular DNA synthesis, and focus formation are mediated by a single activity of the bovine papillomavirus E5 protein. Mol Cell Biol 1989;9:5563–5572.

120. Brandsma JL, Yang ZH, Barthold SW, Johnson EA. Use of a rapid, efficient inoculation method to induce papillomas by cottontail rabbit papillomavirus DNA shows that the E7 gene is required. Proc Natl Acad Sci USA 1991;88:4816–4820.

121. Meyers C, Harry J, Lin Y-L, Wettstein FO. Identification of three transforming proteins encoded by cottontail rabbit papillomavirus. J Virol 1992;66:1655–1664.

122. Defeo-Jones D, Voucolo GA, Haskell KM. Papillomavirus E7 protein binding to the retinoblastoma protein is not required for viral induction of warts. J Virol 1993;67:716–725.

123. Brandsma JL, Yang Z-H, DiMaio D, et al. The putative E5 open reading frame of cottontail rabbit papillomavirus is dispensable for papilloma formation in domestic rabbits. J Virol 1992;66:6204–6207.

124. Lambert PF, Pan H, Pitot H, et al. Epidermal cancer associated with expression of papillomavirus type 16 E6 and E7 oncogenes in the skin of transgenic mice. Proc Natl Acad Sci USA 1993;90:5583–5587.

125. Griep AE, Herber R, Jeon S, et al. Tumorigenicity by human papillomavirus type 16 E6 and E7 in transgenic mice correlates with alterations in epithelial cell growth and differentiation. J Virol 1993;67:1373–1384.

126. Storey A, Oates D, Banks L, et al. Anti-sense phosphorothioate oligonucleotides have both specific and non-specific effects on cells containing human papillomavirus type 16. Nucleic Acids Research 1991;19:4109–4114.

127. Steele C, Cowsert LM, Shillitoe EJ. Effects of human papillomavirus type 18-specific antisense oligonucleotides on the transformed phenotype of human carcinoma cell lines. Cancer Res 1993;53:2330–2337.

128. von Knebel Doeberitz M, Oltersdorf T, Schwarz E, Gissmann L. Correlation of modified human papilloma virus early gene expression with altered growth properties in C4-1 cervical carcinoma cells. Cancer Res 1988;48:3780–3786.

129. Bosch F, Schwarz E, Boukamp P, et al. Suppression in vivo of human papillomavirus type 18 E6-E7 gene expression in nontumorigenic HeLa x fibroblast hybrid cells. J Virol 1990;64: 4743–4754.

130. Bunney M, Benton C, Cubie H. Viral Warts: Biology and Treatment, 2nd edition. Oxford University Press, 1992.

130a. Spanos NP, Williams V, Gwynn MI. Effects of hypnotic, placebo, and salicylic acid treatments on wart regression. Psychosom Med 1990;52:109–114.

130b. Choi YS, Hann SK, Park YK. The effect of cimetidine on verruca plana juvenilis: Clinical trials in six patients. J Dermatol 1993;20:497–500.

131. Hayes M, O'Keefe E. Reduced dose of bleomycin in the treatment of recalcitrant warts. J Am Acad Dermatol 1986;15: 1002–1006.

132. Shelley W, Shelley E. Intralesional bleomycin sulphate therapy for warts. Arch Dermatol 1991;127:234–236.

133. Buckner D, Price N. Immunotherapy of verrucae vulgaris with dinitrochlorobenzene. Br J Dermatol 1977;98:451–455.

134. Dunagin W, Millikan L. Dinitrochlorobenzene immunotherapy for verrucae resistant to standard treatment modalities. J Am Acad Dermatol 1982;6:40–45.

135. Naylor M, Neldner K, Yarborough G, et al. Contact immunotherapy of resistant warts. J Am Acad Dermatol 1988;19: 679–683.

136. Orecchia G, Douville H, Santagostino L. Treatment of multiple relapsing warts with diphenciprone. Dermatologica 1988;177: 225–231.

137. Kraus S, Stone K. Management of genital infection caused by human papillomavirus. Rev Infect Dis 1990;12(Suppl 6): S620–S632.

138. Kling A. Genital warts-therapy. Semin Dermatol 1992;11: 247–255.

139. Centers for Disease Control and Prevention. Sexually transmit-

transforming gene of bovine papillomavirus encodes a small, hydrophobic polypeptide. Science 1986;233:464–467.

ted diseases: Treatment guidelines. MMWR 1993;42 (#RR-14):83–91.

140. Marcus J, Camisa C. Podophyllin therapy for condyloma acuminatum. Int J Dermatol 1990;29:693–698.

141. Zhu W, Blauvelt A, Goldstein B. Detection with the polymerase chain reaction of human papillomavirus DNA in condyloma acuminata treated in vitro with liquid nitrogen, trichloroacetic acid, and podophyllin. J Am Acad Dermatol 1992;26:710–714.

142. Bunney M, Nolan M, Williams D. An assessment of methods treating viral warts by comparative treatment trials based on a standard design. Br J Dermatol 1976;94:667–679.

143. Berth-Jones J, Hutchinson P. Modern treatment of warts: Cure rates at 3 and 6 months. Br J Dermatol 1992;127:262–265.

144. Goodley M. A comparison of cryotherapy with trichloroacetic acid in the treatment of genital warts. Genitourin Med 1987;63:390–392.

145. Damstra R, WA. Cryotherapy in the treatment of condyloma acuminata: A controlled study of 64 patients. J Dermatol Surg Oncol 1991;17:273–276.

146. Handley J, Maw R, Horner T, et al. Non-specific immunity in patients with primary anogenital warts treated with interferon alpha plus cryotherapy or cryotherapy alone. Acta Derm Venereol 1992;72:39–40.

147. Arndt K. Manual of Dermatologic Therapeutics. Boston: Little, Brown, 1989;177–179.

148. Winter G. Formation of the scab and the rate of epithelialization of superficial wounds in the skin of the young domestic pig. Nature 1962;4812:292–294.

149. Simmons P, et al. Podophyllin 10% and 25% in the treatment of anogenital warts. Br J Vener Dis 1981;57:208–209.

150. Simmons P, et al. Cryotherapy versus electrocautery in the treatment of genital warts. Br J Vener Dis 1981;57:273–274.

151. Orani A, Fossati M, Bolis D, et al. Efficacy and safety evaluation on combination therapy with systemic interferon beta and electrocautery in the anogenital warts treatment of HIV-seropositive patients. Int Conf AIDs 1993;9:356.

151a. Halasz CL. Treatment of common warts using the infrared coagulator. J Dermatol Surg Oncol 1994;20:252–256.

152. Pringle W, Helms D. Treatment of plantar warts by blunt dissection. Arch Dermatol 1973;108:79–82.

153. Habif T, Graf F. Extirpation of subungual and periungual warts by blunt dissection. J Dermatol Surg Oncol 1981;7:553–555.

154. Anderson R, Parrish J. Selective photothermolysis: Precise microsurgery by selective absorption of pulsed radiation. Science 1983;220:524–527.

155. Schomacker K, Walsh J, Flotte T, et al. Thermal damage produced by high-irradiance continuous wave CO_2 laser cutting of tissue. Lasers Surg Med 1990;10:74–84.

156. Kamat B, Tang S, Arndt K, et al. Low fluence CO_2 laser irradiation: Selective epidermal damage to human skin. J Invest Dermatol 1985;85:274–278.

157. Mihaslin S, Jako G, Incze J, et al. Laser surgery in otolaryngology: Interaction of CO_2 laser and soft tissue. Ann NY Acad Sci 1976;267:264–294.

158. Walsh J, Flotte T, Anderson R, Deutsch T. Pulsed CO_2 laser tissue ablation: Effect of tissue type and pulse duration on thermal damage. Lasers Surg Med 1988;8:108–118.

159. Montgomery T, Sharp J, Bellina J, et al. Comparative gross and histologic study of the effects of scalped, electric knife, and carbon dioxide laser on skin and uterine incisions in dogs. Laser Surg Med 1983;3:9–15.

160. Hall R. Haemostatic incisions of the liver. CO_2 laser compared with surgical diathermy. Br J Surg 1971;58:538–541.

161. Slutzki S, Shafir R, Bornstein L. Use of the carbon dioxide laser for large excisions with minimal blood loss. Plast Reconstr Surg 1977;60:250–257.

162. Reid A, Stranc M. Healing of infected wounds following iodine scrub or CO_2 laser treatment. Lasers Surg Med 1991;11:475–480.

163. Mullarky M, Norris C, Goldberg I. The efficacy of the CO_2 laser in the sterilization of skin seeded with bacteria: Survival at the skin surface and in the plume emissions. Laryngoscope 1985;95:186–187.

164. Aschler P, Ingolitsch E, Walter G, et al. Ultrastructural findings in CNS tissue with CO_2 laser. In: Kaplan I, ed. Laser Surgery. Jerusalem: Academic Press, 1976.

165. Ben-Bassat M, Ben Bassat J, Kaplan I. An ultrastructural study of the cut edges of skin and mucous membrane specimens excised by carbon dioxide laser. In: Kaplan I, ed. Laser Surgery. Jerusalem: Academic Press, 1976.

166. Ehrenberger KJI. The effect of carbon dioxide laser on skin lymphatics. Wien Klin Wochenschr 1978;90:307–309.

167. Schenk P. Ultrastructure of skin and mucous membranes after incision with a CO_2 laser. Laryngol Rhinol Otol (Stuttg) 1979;58:770–777.

168. Fruhling J, Lejoune E, Van Hoof G, Gerard A. Lymphatic migration after laser surgery. Lancet 1977;2:973–974.

169. Morris D, Morrow L. CO_2 laser blepharoplasty. A comparison with cold-steel surgery. J Dermatol Surg Oncol 1992;18:307–313.

170. David L, Sanders G. CO_2 laser blepharoplasty: A comparison to cold steel and electrocautery. J Dermatol Surg Oncol 1987;13:110–114.

171. Mittelman H, Apfelberg D. Carbon dioxide laser blepharoplasty—advantages and disadvantages. Ann Plast Surg 1990;24:1–6.

172. Becker D. Use of the carbon dioxide laser in treating multiple cutaneous neurofibromas. Ann Plast Surg 1991;26:582–586.

173. Stanley T, Roenigk R. The carbon dioxide laser treatment of actinic cheilitis. Mayo Clin Proc 1988;63:230–235.

174. Kardos T, Ferguson M. Comparison of cryosurgery and the carbon dioxide laser in mucosal healing. Int J Oral Maxillofac Surg 1991;20:108–111.

175. Weigel J, Dolmaniecki J, Orlowski I, et al. Healing of liver wounds inflicted with CO_2 lasers. Acta Med Pol 1981;22:105–118.

176. Carney J, Kamat B, Stern R, et al. Cutaneous tissue repair after focused CO_2 laser irradiation. Lasers Surg Med 1985;5:180–181.

177. Hall R. The healing of tissues incised by a carbon dioxide laser. Br J Surg 1971;58:222–227.

178. Hishimoto K, Rockwell J, Epstein R, et al. Laser wound healing compared with other surgical modalities. Burns 1973;1:13–21.

179. Moreno R, Hebda P, Zitelli J, et al. Epidermal cell outgrowth from CO_2 laser- and scalpel-cut explants: Implications for wound healing. J Dermatol Surg Oncol 1984;10:863–869.

180. Fry T, Gerba R, Bostros S, et al. Effects of laser, scalpel and electrosurgical excision on wound contracture and graft "take." Plast Reconstr Surg 1980;65:729–731.

181. Badawy S, Mohammed E, Baggish M. Comparative study of continuous and pulsed CO_2 laser on tissue healing and fertility outcome in tubal anastomosis. Fert Steril 1987;47:843–847.

182. Baggish M, Mohamed M. Comparison of electronically superpulsed and continuous wave CO_2 laser on the rate of uterine horn. Fertil Steril 1986;45:120–125.

183. Green H, Burd E, Nishioka N, et al. Middermal wound healing: A comparison between dermatomal excision and pulsed carbon dioxide laser ablation. Arch Dermatol 1992;639–642.

184. Eaglstein W, Mertz P. "Inert" vehicles do affect wound healing. J Investig Dermatol 1980;74:90–91.

185. Geronemus R, Mertz P, Eaglstein W. Wound healing. The effects of topical antimicrobial agents. Arch Dermatol 1979;115:1311–1314.

186. Chan P, Vincent J, Wangemann R. Accelerated healing of carbon dioxide laser burns in rats treated with composite polyurethane dressing. Arch Dermatol 1987;123:1042–1045.

187. Larson D, Abston S, Evans E, et al. Techniques for decreasing scar formation and contractions in the burned patient. J Trauma 1971;11:807–823.

188. Olbricht S, Stern R, Tang S, et al. Complications of cutaneous laser surgery. A Survey. Arch Dermatol 1987;123:345–349.

189. Kashima H, Kessis T, Mounts P, et al. Polymerase chain reaction identification of human papillomavirus DNA in CO_2 laser plume from recurrent respiratory papillomatosis. Otolaryngol Head Neck Surg 1991;104:191–195.

190. Ferenczy A, Bergeron C, Richart R. Carbon dioxide laser energy disperses human papillomavirus deoxyribonucleic acid onto treatment fields. Am J Obstet Gynecol 1990;163:1271–1274.

191. Matchette L, Faaland R, Royston D, et al. In vitro production of viable bacteriophage in carbon dioxide laser. Am J Obstet Gynecol 1984;148:9–12.

192. Nezhat C, Winer W, Nezhat F, et al. Smoke from laser surgery: Is there a health hazard? Lasers Surg Med 1987;7:376–382.

193. Sawchuk W, Weber P, Lowy D, et al. Infectious papillomavirus in the vapor of warts treated with carbon dioxide laser or electrocoagulation: Detection and protection. J Am Acad Dermatol 1989;21:41–49.

194. Bailin P. CO_2 laser therapy for non-PWS lesions. In: Arndt KA, Noe JM, Rosen S, eds. Cutaneous Laser Therapy: Principles and Methods. New York: John Wiley & Sons, 1983;195–196.

195. Mueller T, Carlson B, Lundy M. The use of the carbon dioxide surgical laser for treatment of verrucae. J Am Pediatr Assoc 1980;70:136–141.

196. McBurney E, Rosen D. Carbon dioxide laser treatment of verrucae vulgares. J Dermatol Surg Oncol 1984;10:45–48.

197. Logan R, Zachary C. Outcome of carbon dioxide laser therapy for persistent cutaneous viral warts. Br J Dermatol 1989; 121:99–105.

198. Street M, Roenigk R. Recalcitrant periungual verrucae: The role of carbon dioxide laser vaporization. J Am Acad Dermatol 1990;23:115–120.

199. Fitzpatrick R, Goldman M. CO_2 laser surgery. In: Goldman MP, Fitzpatrick RE, eds. Cutaneous Laser Surgery: The Art and Science of Selective Photothermolysis. St. Louis: Mosby, 1994;198–258.

200. Ferenczy A, Mitao M, Nagai N, et al. Latent papilloma virus and recurring genital warts. N Engl J Med 1985;313:784–788.

201. Riva J, Sedlacek T, Cunhane M, et al. Extended carbon dioxide laser vaporization in the treatment of subclinical papilloma virus infection of the lower genital tract. Obstet Gynecol 1989;73:25–30.

202. Calkins J, Masterson B, Magrina J, et al. Management of condyloma acuminata with the carbon dioxide laser. Obstet Gynecol 1982;59:105–108.

203. Baggish M. CO_2 laser surgery for condyloma acuminata venereal infection. Obstet Gynecol 1980;55:711–715.

204. Bellina J. The use of the CO_2 laser in management of condyloma acuminata with eight year follow-up. Am J Obstet Gynecol 1983;147:375–378.

205. Bar-Am A, Shilon M, Peyser M, et al. Treatment of male genital condylomatous lesions by carbon dioxide laser after failure of previous nonlaser methods. J Am Acad Dermatol 1991;24: 87–89.

206. Carpiniello V, Schoenberg M, Malloy T. Longterm follow-up of subclinical human papillomavirus infection treated with the carbon dioxide laser and intraurethral 5-fluorouracil: A treatment protocol. J Urol 1990;143:726–728.

207. Vance J, Davis D. Interferon alpha-2b infections used as an adjuvant therapy to carbon dioxide laser vaporization of recalcitrant ano-genital condylomata acuminata. J Invest Dermatol 1990;95:146S–148S.

208. Reid R, Greenberg M, Pizzuit D, et al. Superficial laser vulvectomy. V. Surgical debulking is enhanced by adjuvant systemic interferon. Am J Obstet Gynecol 1992;166:815–820.

209. Cobb M. Human papillomavirus infection. J Am Acad Dermatol 1990;22:547–566.

210. Moy R, Eliezri Y, Nuovo G, et al. Human papillomavirus type 16 DNA in periungual squamous cell carcinomas. JAMA 1989;261:2669–2673.

211. Kawashima M, Jablonska S, Favre M, et al. Characterization of a new type of human papillomavirus found in a lesion of Bowen's disease of the skin. J Virol 1986;57:688–692.

212. Pearson S, Whittaker J, Ireland D, et al. Invasive cancer of the cervix after laser treatment. Br J Obstet Gynecol 1989;96: 486–488.

213. Tan O, Hurwitz R, Stafford T. Pulsed dye laser treatment of recalcitrant verrucae; a preliminary report. Lasers Surg Med 1993;13:127–137.

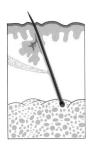

chapter 124

Viral Exanthems

RENÉE HOWARD and ILONA J. FRIEDEN

Viral exanthems are acute, generalized cutaneous eruptions due to viral infection. They may result from either direct viral invasion of the skin or host immune response to viral assault. Because patterns of cutaneous response to viral and other systemic infections are limited, totally unrelated infectious agents may cause similar exanthems. Conversely, identical agents may cause eruptions with different appearances, depending on the patient's age or duration of infection. Exanthems from bacterial and rickettsial infections, as well as drug eruptions, may mimic viral rashes. This makes the evaluation of the patient with a possible viral exanthem a formidable task (Table 124–1).[1]

Because many viral exanthems are not instantly recognizable, the approach to diagnosis involves consideration of other physical and laboratory findings, as well as the epidemiologic and historic features of the case (Table 124–2). Potentially life-threatening or treatable illnesses such as bacterial or rickettsial infections should be considered first. Diagnoses with important public health implications, such as rubella or measles, should not be overlooked.

Clinical Approach

EPIDEMIOLOGY

Epidemiologic data may provide important clues to the diagnosis of a viral exanthem. The patient's age may determine whether he or she is at risk for a particular viral infection and how that infection presents in the skin. For example, 95% of roseola occurs between ages 6 months and 3 years, and most cases occur in the last half of the first year.[2] Infectious mononucleosis in preschoolers is commonly associated with a mild papular eruption, whereas exanthems are rare later in life unless ampicillin is administered.[3, 4] The season of the year may also be helpful in making a diagnosis. Enteroviruses are the most common cause of viral exanthems in the summer and autumn in temperate climates, while those due to respiratory viruses are more common in winter.[5] Geography may be significant: where the patient lives or has traveled may alter the spectrum of viral agents that one considers in the differential diagnosis. Travel to India, for example, may result in exposure to measles or other viral agents better controlled in the United States because of immunization.

HISTORY

A careful history can help narrow the differential diagnosis. The evolution of the rash can point to its cause. Varicella begins as a papular eruption that becomes vesicular and then crusted. The rash of measles begins at the hairline and then spreads centrifugally.

The presence and evolution of any associated symptoms is important. Some exanthems have characteristic prodromes: the exanthem of measles is preceded by 3 to 4 days of fever, cough, coryza, and conjunctivitis. A known outbreak of a viral illness (e.g., varicella) in the patient's school or workplace may provide an important clue. The patient's medical history may reveal underlying illnesses, such as human immunodeficiency virus (HIV) infection, which predisposes the patient to more severe manifestations of usual viral infections and to unusual infections, prompting a more aggressive diagnostic and therapeutic approach. A history of any previous allergies or adverse reactions to drugs should be elicited, including history of exposure to prescription or over-the-counter medications. Distinguishing the patient with a drug eruption from one with a viral exanthem who was treated with antibiotics is a common dilemma. Written immunization records can be useful, but histories of "baby shots" from patients or their parents are often unreliable. Even a documented record of an immu-

TABLE 124–1. Exanthems

Disease (Etiology)	Usual Age	Season	Prodrome	Morphology
Viral Causes				
Measles (rubeola virus)	Infants to young adults	Winter/spring	High fever, signs and symptoms of upper respiratory tract infection, conjunctivitis	Erythematous macules and papules become confluent
Rubella (rubella virus)	Adolescents/ young adults	Spring	Absent or low-grade fever, malaise	Rose pink papules that are not confluent
Erythema infectiosum (parvovirus B19)	5–15 y	Winter/spring	Usually none	Slapped cheeks: reticulate erythema or maculopapular
Roseola (herpesvirus 6)	6 mo–3 y	Spring/fall	High fever for 3–5 days	Maculopapular rash appears after fever declines
Human Immunodeficiency virus	Adults	Any season	Fever, malaise, sore throat, diarrhea	Roseola-like hemorrhagic macules
Chickenpox (varicella-zoster virus)	1–14 y	Late Fall/winter/ spring	Usually none	Macules, papules rapidly become vesicles on erythematous base, then crusts
Enteroviral exanthems (coxsackie viruses, echo viruses, other enteroviruses)	Young children	Summer/fall	Fever (occasional)	Extremely variable; maculopapular, petechial, purpura, vesicular
Epstein-Barr exanthems (Epstein-Barr virus)	Young children/ adolescents	Any season	Fever, adenopathy, sore throat	Maculopapular or morbilliform
Gianotti-Crosti syndrome (Hepatitis B, coxsackie virus infection, Epstein-Barr virus, etc.)	1–6 y	Any season	Usually absent	Papules/paulovesicles; may become confluent
Bacterial and Rickettsial Causes				
Staphylococcal scalded skin syndrome (*S. aureus*/epider molytic toxin)	Neonates and infants	Any season	None	Abrupt onset, tender erythroderma
Toxic shock syndrome (staphylococcal toxin)	Adolescents/ young adults	Any season	None	Macular erythroderma
Scarlet fever (β-*Streptococcus*)	School-age children	Fall to spring	Acute onset with fever, sore throat	Diffuse erythema with sandpaper texture
Meningococcemia (meningococcus)	<2 y	Winter/spring	Malaise, fever, upper respiratory tract infection symptoms	Papules, petechiae, purpura
Rocky mountain spotted fever (*Rickettsia rickettsii* carried by ticks)	Any age	Summer	Fever, malaise	Maculopapular/ petechial rash
Unknown Cause				
Kawasaki disease (etiology unknown)	6 mo–6 y	Winter/spring	Irritability	Polymorphous-papular, morbilliform, erythema with desquamation

Adapted from Williams ML, Frieden IJ. Dermatologic disorders. In: Grossman M, Dieckman RA, eds. Pediatric Emergency Medicine: A Clinician's Reference. Philadelphia: JB Lippincott, 1991.

TABLE 124–1. Exanthems (*Continued*)

Distribution	Associated Findings	Diagnosis	Special Management
Begins on face and moves downward over whole body	Koplik's spots, toxic appearance, photophobia, cough, adenopathy, fever	Clinical; acute/convalescent hemagglutinin serology	Report to public health. Oral vitamin A therapy
Begins on face and moves downward	Postauricular and occipital adenopathy; headache, malaise	Rubella IgM or acute/convalescent hemagglutinin serology	Report to public health; check for exposure to pregnant women
Usually arms/legs; may be generalized	Rash waxes/wanes several weeks; occasional arthritis, headache, malaise	Usually clinical; acute/convalescent serology	
Trunk, neck; may be generalized; lasts hours to days	Cervical and postauricular adenopathy	Usually clinical	
Upper body predominates, palm, soles	Adenopathy	Acute and convalescent HIV-1 serologies	Counseling, referral for consideration of antiviral therapy and follow-up
Often begins on scalp/face; more profuse on trunk than extremities	Pruritic, fever, oral	Usually clinical; Tzanck prep, direct immunofluorescence or viral culture	Antihistamines for itching; aspirin contraindicated (Reye's syndrome); acyclovir
Usually generalized, may be acral	Low-grade fever; occasional myocarditis, aseptic meningitis, pleurodynia, malaise	Usually clinical; viral culture from throat, rectal swabs in selected cases	If petechiae or purpura, must consider meningococcemia
Trunk, extremities	Cervical adenopathy Liver/spleen enlarged	Mono spot; Epstein-Barr nuclear antigen acute/convalescent; IgG-Viral Capsid antigen	
Face, arms, legs, buttocks, spares torso	Occasional lymphadenopathy, hepatomegaly, splenomegaly	Clinical; hepatitis B and Epstein-Barr serologies	
Diffuse with perioral, perinasal scaling	Fever, conjunctivitis rhinitis	Clinical; culture of *S. aureus* from systemic site (not skin)	Neonate: if blistering present, hospitalize for intravenous nafcillin and fluid/electrolyte therapy
Generalized	Hypotension; fever, myalgias, diarrhea/vomiting	Clinical case definition criteria isolation *S. aureus* cervix, etc.	Treatment of hypotension, admit to hospital; antibiotics to eradicate *S. aureus*
Facial flushing with circumoral pallor, linear erythema in skin folds	Exudative pharyngitis, palatal petechiae, abdominal pain	Throat culture	Penicillin, intramuscularly or orally Penicillin or erythromycin
Trunk, extremities, palms, soles	Temp > 40˚C Meningismus, circulatory collapse	Clinical blood culture, spinal tap	Immediate intravenous penicillin in emergency department, treatment for shock, if present
Wrists, ankles, palms, soles; trunk later	Central nervous system, pulmonary, cardiac lesions	Serology	Treat on presumptive clinical grounds
Generalized, often with perineal accentuation	Conjunctivitis, cheilitis, glossitis, peripheral edema, adenopathy	Clinical	Admit to hospital for intravenous gamma globulin, salicylates

TABLE 124-2. Clinical Evaluation of the Patient with a Viral Exanthem

Epidemiology

Age of the patient
Season of the year
Travel history
Geography

History

Nature and evolution of the rash
Associated symptoms or prodrome
Contacts
Underlying illnesses
Medications (prescription or over-the-counter)
Allergies or adverse reactions to drugs
Immunizations
Previous exanthems

Physical Examination

Exanthem: morphology, distribution
Enanthem: location, type, pharyngitis
Other physical findings: general appearance, vital signs, organomegaly, adenopathy, joints, meningismus

nization to a given illness (e.g., measles) does not completely exclude that illness, because primary vaccine failure and waning immunity may occur. Similarly, a history of previous exanthems, such as varicella, may not help, since recurrent episodes have been reported.

PHYSICAL EXAMINATION

A thorough physical examination is required for any patient with a viral exanthem. The goal is to look for signs of specific viral infections and to exclude treatable or life-threatening illnesses (see Table 124–2).

A general impression of how ill the patient appears can dictate how aggressively one pursues the cause of the illness. Vital signs such as temperature and blood pressure should be noted. Fever makes an infectious disease or drug reaction more likely. One may be more concerned about bacterial sepsis or toxic shock syndrome in a hypotensive patient. The presence of lymphadenopathy or hepatosplenomegaly would lead one to consider not only infectious causes such as Epstein-Barr infection but also causes such as Epstein-Barr infection and immunologic (Still's disease) or neoplastic (leukemia) conditions. The presence of an enanthem or pharyngitis may narrow the differential diagnosis.

The morphology of the rash can be nonspecific. Macular, papular, vesicular, and even petechial eruptions occur in viral infection. A lateralized eczematous or scarlatiniform eruption of the thorax and of flexural areas has been described.[6, 7] The eruption became generalized in some patients and resolved within 3 to 6 weeks without response to antibiotics. A zoster-like unilateral vesiculobullous eruption due to echovirus-6 has also been reported.[8]

PATHOPHYSIOLOGY

Viruses produce exanthems in a variety of ways.[9] They can disseminate from blood to skin, inducing rash as a result of direct invasion of and damage to dermal blood vessels or the epidermis. For example, endothelial damage may result in perivascular edema or infiltrate, resulting in a papule, or leakage of red blood cells, leading to petechiae. Alternatively, the host cellular or humoral immune response to the virus may indirectly result in skin changes, such as urticarial eruptions.

Measles (Rubeola)

Until the introduction of measles vaccines in the mid 1960s, measles was a common childhood exanthem. Epidemics in the 1980s and 1990s have re-emphasized its importance in the differential diagnosis of childhood exanthems. It is caused by a paramyxovirus that is closely related to the canine distemper virus.[10] There is only one antigenic type, and humans are the natural hosts and only reservoir of the infection.

EPIDEMIOLOGY

Most cases in the United States occur in infants younger than 15 months of age, with a second peak in incidence in adolescence. Measles has continued to be a major health problem in many developing countries. The disease is most prevalent in winter and spring. It is spread by droplets from respiratory secretions. The incubation period is from 9 to 12 days from the time of exposure to the onset of symptoms.[11, 12]

CLINICAL DESCRIPTION

The prodrome of measles lasts from 2 to 4 days. Fever as high as 38.5°C to 40°C, nasal congestion, sneezing, rhinitis, conjunctivitis, and cough are nearly always present.[10, 12] A transitory macular or urticarial rash has been described early in the prodrome. Koplik spots, which are pathognomonic of measles, develop during the prodrome, consisting of tiny white or bluish-gray specks approximately 1 mm in size, superimposed on an erythematous, granular base, beginning on the buccal mucosa, opposite the lower molars, and then spreading to involve other parts of the buccal mucosa and the palate. The pharynx is frequently infected.[10, 12]

The exanthem begins behind the ears and at the hairline (Fig. 124–1; see color plate) and spreads centrifugally from head to foot, so that by the third day of the rash the whole body is involved. Lesions begin as discrete, erythematous papules, which gradually coalesce. They are occasionally purpuric, but pruritus is uncommon.[12, 13] The rash fades after 3 to 4 days but may persist for 6 to 7 days.

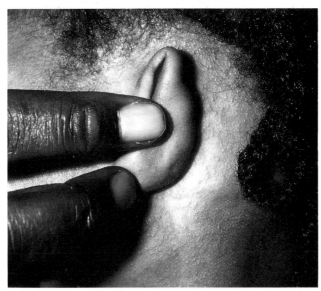

FIGURE 124–1. The rash of measles begins behind the ears. (See color plate.) (From Frieden IJ, Penneys N. In: Schachner L, Hansen R, eds. Pediatric Dermatology. New York: Churchill Livingstone, 1988.)

Most children with typical measles appear ill. Complications are more common in children in developing countries and in immunocompromised hosts and include pneumonia, otitis media, laryngotracheobronchitis, encephalitis, myocarditis, and pericarditis.[12] In "black measles," a rare form, the abrupt onset of fever and delirium are followed by respiratory distress and an extensive confluent hemorrhagic eruption resembling disseminated intravascular coagulation.[13] Infection during pregnancy is associated with a high incidence of fetal wastage and in some cases congenital malformations.[12]

A milder form of measles, "modified measles," usually occurs in partially immune hosts, such as infants younger than 9 months of age and in cases in which partial vaccine failure has occurred. The prodrome may be shortened, and cough, congestion, and fever may be less severe. The presence of Koplik spots is variable. The skin eruption is usually less confluent.[12, 14] "Atypical measles," due to infection with wild-type virus after vaccination with killed virus vaccine is extremely rare. Its main characteristics are fever, onset of an acrally located hemorrhagic rash, and pneumonia.

PATHOLOGY

The pathologic findings in measles are characterized by the presence of multinucleated giant cells of two types: the Warthin-Finkeldey cell, found in lymphoid tissue, and epithelial giant cells, present in the skin, mucosa, and respiratory epithelium. Biopsy specimens of lesional skin show a slight spongiotic, psoriasiform dermatitis with occasional dyskeratotic cells and parakeratosis. The epidermis also contains syncytial keratinocytic giant cells that have from 3 to 26 nuclei. Nuclear and cytoplasmic inclusions are often present. Koplik spots show similar findings, but more giant cells are present.[15]

DIAGNOSIS AND DIFFERENTIAL DIAGNOSIS

Virus may be isolated from the blood, respiratory tract, skin, and other organs, but acute and convalescent serologic samples for hemagglutination inhibition or measles IgM are reliable and usually more practical. Typical measles usually is not difficult to distinguish from other childhood exanthems, especially early in the course of infection when Koplik spots are present, but it may be confused with drug eruptions and other exanthems, particularly Kawasaki disease.[16]

TREATMENT

High oral doses of vitamin A significantly decrease morbidity and mortality in hospitalized children with measles.[17, 18] Vitamin A can be given as retinyl palmitate in two doses of 200,000 IU each separated by 24 hours.[19] No specific antiviral therapy is available.

Rubella

Rubella, an RNA virus and member of the Togaviridae, generally produces a mild exanthematous illness except when it is transmitted in utero when it may result in severe congenital infection.

EPIDEMIOLOGY

Rubella was once a common exanthematous disease of childhood, but after the use of vaccine the number of cases has dropped precipitously. Epidemics of rubella occasionally occur in developed countries, and rubella infection continues to be common in countries where vaccinations are not widely available.

Most cases occur in the spring. The incubation period ranges from 12 to 23 days but is between 15 and 21 days in most cases. The period of communicability is from 5 to 7 days before the appearance of the rash until 3 to 5 days after its appearance. Spread is probably through the respiratory route.[20]

CLINICAL DESCRIPTION

Inapparent infection is common and may represent 50% to 80% of actual infections.[21] A prodrome of malaise, cough, sore throat, eye pain, headache, swollen glands, red eyes, runny nose, fever, aches, chills, anorexia, and nausea may be present for 1 to 5 days before onset of rash. Pain on lateral and upward eye movement is a common and at times distressing symptom.

The progression, extent, and duration of the exanthem are variable. The rash, consisting of discrete pink macules and papules, begins on the face and progresses downward to the trunk, then to the extremities. In typical cases, the rash covers the entire body in the first 24 hours, then fades on the face on the second day, and disappears entirely by the end of the third day, but it may last less than 24 hours.[20] An enanthem consisting of pinhead-sized, rose-red macules or petechiae on the soft palate and uvula (Forscheimer spots) is seen occasionally.[20]

Suboccipital and posterior auricular adenopathy occurs in 50% to 100% of patients with rash. Generalized adenopathy may also occur. The presence of low-grade fever is variable. Arthritis and arthralgia are well-described complications of rubella, and their incidence increases with age.

DIAGNOSIS AND DIFFERENTIAL DIAGNOSIS

Virus may be isolated from the throat, urine, and other body fluids, but the availability of specific serologic tests usually makes this unnecessary. Hemagglutination inhibition is sensitive and can determine whether an individual has had prior exposure to rubella.[22] Rubella-specific IgM or acute and convalescent hemagglutination inhibition titers are helpful if the suspicion for infection is high (particularly in pregnant women).

The exanthem of rubella is not specific and may resemble viral exanthems produced by many other viruses (including enteroviruses, reoviruses, adenoviruses, rubeola) as well as streptococcal scarlet fever. The nearly universal presence of rash of the face may be helpful, though this may have disappeared by the time of examination.[20, 21] The presence of suboccipital adenopathy is helpful, but this may be present with enteroviral, adenoviral, Epstein-Barr virus (EBV), and other infections.

TREATMENT

There is no specific treatment, but live viral vaccine is now widely administered to prevent disease. The disease should be reported to the local public health department. Hospitalized patients should be placed in respiratory isolation. All hospital personnel who may come in contact with pregnant patients with rubella should be screened for immunity to rubella. Specific measures for care of exposed pregnant women are outlined in several references.[11, 20]

Erythema Infectiosum

Erythema infectiosum (fifth disease) is a well-described childhood exanthem, caused by parvovirus B19, a single-stranded encapsulated DNA virus. In addition to rashes, the virus causes several other forms of clinical illness, including acute arthritis in adults, aplastic crises in patients with hereditary hemolytic anemias, chronic anemia in immunodeficient hosts, and hydrops fetalis or fetal death in some women infected during pregnancy.

EPIDEMIOLOGY

Infection is year-round and may be sporadic or occur in large outbreaks. The exanthem is most common in school-aged children. The virus is spread through respiratory secretions, usually through close contact (e.g., within households, school, or health care settings). The incubation period is usually between 4 and 14 days.

CLINICAL DESCRIPTION

The primary manifestation of erythema infectiosum is its distinctive exanthem. Prodromal symptoms such as low-grade fever, malaise, and headache may be present for 1 or 2 days before the exanthem. Typically, the exanthem has three stages. First, a fiery red, macular erythema appears on the cheeks. Within days, discrete erythematous macules and papules appear on the proximal extremities, sometimes involving the trunk as well. The eruption may evolve into a characteristic lacy or reticulate pattern (Fig. 124–2; see color plate). The third stage of the exanthem, a waxing and waning of the eruption varies in duration from one to several weeks, brought about by changes in environmental temperature, exposure to sunlight, exercise, crying, and emotional factors.[23, 24] Pruritus is occasionally present. The slapped cheeks may be present without the reticulate eruption and vice versa.

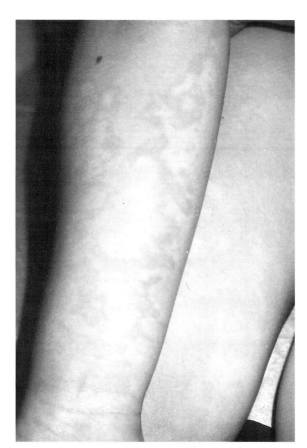

FIGURE 124–2. Erythema infectiosum: Characteristic reticulate pattern on the arm. (See color plate.) (From Frieden IJ. Viral exanthems. In: Sams W, Lynch P, eds. Principles and Practice of Dermatology. New York: Churchill Livingstone, 1990.)

Recent studies show that the classic rash of erythema infectiosum is seen in a minority of individuals with acute parvovirus B19 infections; most have either no rash or a generalized maculopapular rash. Morbilliform, urticarial, hemorrhagic, and vesicular eruptions have all been reported in the context of epidemics of erythema infectiosum.[25] The presence of petechiae or purpura in a glove and sock distribution has been emphasized.[26-29] Enanthem is rarely seen.[25]

Most children with erythema infectiosum appear well. Headache, fever, sore throat, coryza, sore eyes, abdominal pain, anorexia, and joint pain occur in from 5% to 15% of children. These symptoms are more common in adults. Arthritis, the most common complication in adults, is present in only 5% of children. Encephalitis is extremely rare.[30]

Multiple cases of intrauterine infection with acute maternal parvovirus B19 infection, resulting in hydrops fetalis and fetal death, have been described.[31-33] The risk of developing hydrops is greatest if infection occurs in the first trimester, with fetal wastage as high as 19%. The risk in the second half of pregnancy is considerably lower.

DIAGNOSIS AND DIFFERENTIAL DIAGNOSIS

Laboratory tests are rarely necessary in typical cases of erythema infectiosum, but diagnosis of acute parvovirus B19 infection can be confirmed by the presence of specific IgM antibodies or seroconversion with specific IgG antibodies. The reticulocyte count may be low even in patients without anemia due to the effect of the virus on erythroid precursors. The leukocyte count is usually normal. Mild eosinophilia may be present.[24]

When the typical exanthem is present, the findings are usually distinct enough to establish a diagnosis. Other diagnostic considerations include juvenile rheumatoid arthritis.

TREATMENT

No specific treatment is available. Patients with the rash can return to school, since viral shedding is generally over at the time of appearance of rash.[11] Patients with aplastic crises or chronic B19 infection should have respiratory isolation and not be cared for by pregnant women. Exposed pregnant women may have serologic testing and if found to be infected can be evaluated with ultrasound, α-fetoprotein levels (which may be elevated in infection), and other diagnostic tests.[31, 34, 35]

Roseola

Roseola (exanthem subitum) is a common, self-limited illness of infancy characterized by 3 to 5 days of high fever followed by an exanthem. First characterized as a distinct exanthem by Zahorsky in 1911,[36] the search for a viral cause continued for decades. In 1988, Yama-nishi and coworkers[37] implicated human herpesvirus 6 (HHV-6), as the etiologic agent, a finding subsequently corroborated by others.[38] HHV-6 is a member of the Herpesviridae, and like other herpesviruses it is an enveloped, double-stranded DNA virus. It is similar to cytomegalovirus in its morphology and DNA sequences.[39]

EPIDEMIOLOGY

Roseola is primarily an illness of infancy, but cases in the first months of life are rare.[2, 40, 41] Most newborns have transplacental maternal antibody that wanes by 5 to 6 months of age.[42] By 1 year of age, 86% of infants have reacquired antibodies presumably due to primary infection with HHV-6.[43] The exact mode of spread is not yet known, but acquisition from asymptomatic adults with salivary shedding is suspected.[44, 45] Although most cases are sporadic, an outbreak in an orphanage in Japan suggests that the virus can be transmitted horizontally.[46]

After initial infection, the virus may persist in a latent state in salivary glands,[45] or in blood monocytes or tissue macrophages.[47] Thus HHV-6 may be reactivated later and be shed or produce disease, especially in the setting of immune deficiency. Viremia has been detected in 20% to 40% of transplant recipients 10 to 24 days after surgery.[48]

CLINICAL DESCRIPTION

Roseola typically begins with the sudden onset of high fever (up to 40°C) in an infant 6 months to 3 years of age.[2] The fever persists for 3 to 5 days, usually with no other symptoms, although occipital adenopathy and/or mild pharyngitis may be present.[40, 49] Many infants with roseola appear happy and well. The rash, characterized by discrete, irregular, 2- to 5-mm, rose-pink macules and papules appearing on the trunk and neck,[2, 41] typically develops after defervescence, either on the same day or 1 to 2 days later (Fig. 124–3). It fades completely within hours or days without desquamation.[36]

Since the discovery that HHV-6 causes roseola, serologic testing for that agent has shown that there are several variations of this typical clinical picture. The rash may develop without fever,[49, 50] fever may occur without the rash,[51, 52] and asymptomatic infection can occur. HHV-6 has also been implicated in a wide range of diseases other than roseola, including a mononucleosis-like illness,[53, 54] pneumonitis,[55] and a fatal disseminated infection.[56] Although most cases have a benign course, neurologic complications include febrile seizures, a relatively common problem, and encephalitis, a rare one.[57, 61] Other rare complications include hemophagocytic syndrome[62] and immune thrombocytopenic purpura.[63]

DIAGNOSIS AND DIFFERENTIAL DIAGNOSIS

In most cases of self-limited roseola, a clinical diagnosis based on a typical clinical picture is sufficient. Complete blood cell count will show a relative neutro-

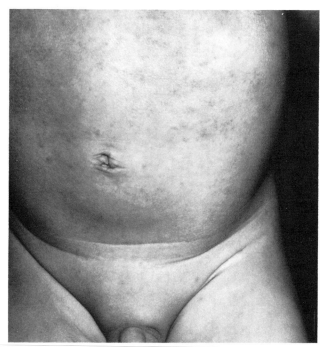

FIGURE 124–3. Roseola: Fine maculopapular rash usually develops after defervescence. (From Frieden IJ. Update on childhood exanthems. In: Dahl MV, Lynch P, eds. Current Opinion in Dermatology. Philadelphia: Current Science, 1993.)

these potentially toxic drugs, which will certainly be reserved for severe cases with complications.

Human Immunodeficiency Virus

Primary infection with human immunodeficiency virus (HIV) is sometimes associated with an acute illness consisting of fever, exanthem, malaise, sore throat, and diarrhea.[68–70] The exanthem may be roseola-like,[70] erythematous papules, or macules with hemorrhagic centers (Fig. 124–4; see color plate).[69] It is located predominantly on the upper body but may involve palms and soles, and there may be lymphadenopathy, mimicking secondary syphilis.[69] Because this acute illness is associated with seroconversion, HIV antibody tests will not be positive until weeks later. Clinical diagnosis of this exanthem may lead to early detection of HIV infection. Dermatopathology of the exanthem shows superficial perivascular lymphocytic infiltrates; occasionally, vacuolar change at the dermoepidermal junction or slight spongiosis is noted.[69, 71]

penia and lymphocytosis.[49] Since the diagnosis of roseola is usually made clinically, skin biopsy is rarely performed.

If complications are present, specific diagnostic tests for HHV-6 can be done, although these may not be available in all laboratories. Acute and convalescent antibody titers can be measured by immunofluorescent antibody test, enzyme-linked immunosorbent assay, and neutralizing antibody test; the latter two are more sensitive.[39, 42] IgM antibodies to HHV-6 may take 3 to 5 days to develop and reach a maximum at 2 to 3 weeks.[64, 65] Polymerase chain reaction has been used to detect HHV-6 in peripheral blood mononuclear cells from patients with exanthem subitum.[64] Viral culture from peripheral blood mononuclear cells is most sensitive during the febrile part of the illness.[65] Because of the potential for viral latency and re-activation, identification of virus by culture or polymerase chain reaction does not necessarily confirm the presence of acute infection.

The differential diagnosis of roseola includes other viral exanthems, especially enteroviruses, rubella, and measles. In young infants presenting with high fever and no obvious source, pursuit of a possible bacterial infection is warranted.

TREATMENT

Treatment is usually limited to supportive measures, such as control of fever with acetaminophen. In vitro data suggest that HHV-6 is sensitive to ganciclovir and foscarnet,[39] but there are as yet no published trials using

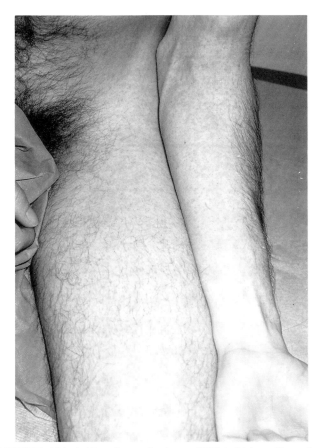

FIGURE 124–4. Exanthem of primary HIV infection. (See color plate.)

Varicella

Varicella (chickenpox) is one of the most common childhood exanthems. It is caused by the varicella-zoster virus, a double-stranded DNA virus that is a member of the Herpesviridae.

EPIDEMIOLOGY

Varicella is a highly contagious disease: 96% of susceptible children will develop the disease within 1 month of exposure. Both airborne and direct person-to-person contact can result in infection. The average incubation period is 14 to 16 days, with a range from 11 to 20 days. Although later winter and early spring peaks of infection are common, the disease can occur at any time of the year.[11, 66, 67]

CLINICAL DESCRIPTION

A mild prodrome of fever and malaise may occur 1 to 2 days before onset of the rash. A transient maculopapular or urticarial phase before vesicular eruption has also been reported. Typically, the exanthem begins on the scalp or trunk. Lesions occur in crops as erythematous macules and papules that rapidly evolve into vesicles, said to resemble "a dew-drop on a rose petal." They spread to involve nearly any part of the body, usually with centrifugal spread, and may be accentuated in areas of friction or previous skin injury such as a sunburn. The average number of skin lesions is approximately 500. Younger children generally have milder disease than adolescents and adults.[72] As the lesions evolve they form crusts and then generally begin to heal. Pruritus is variable but can be severe. The rash usually resolves over 4 to 6 days. Patients are considered infectious until all lesions have crusted over.

In some patients, particularly immunocompromised hosts, skin lesions may be bullous and/or hemorrhagic, with less rapid crusting, resulting in a more monomorphous appearance of the rash.[73-75] Mucous membrane lesions are common, typically involving the palate and uvula, but may also occur on the conjunctiva, vulva, and other sites.

Complications of varicella occur in a small percentage of cases, the most common being secondary bacterial skin infections and scarring. Others include otitis media, pneumonia, hepatitis, purpura fulminans, carditis, encephalitis, and Reye's syndrome. Severe, life-threatening varicella has been well documented in immunocompromised hosts but can occur in others, particularly those receiving systemic corticosteroids, even only briefly.[76]

PATHOLOGY

Skin biopsy of primary varicella is rarely performed; but if it is done, the specimen shows features indistinguishable from those of vesicular lesions of herpes zoster or those caused by herpes simplex (see Chapter 121).

DIAGNOSIS AND DIFFERENTIAL DIAGNOSIS

The diagnosis of varicella is usually made clinically. Further documentation can be obtained by viral culture (though less sensitive than cultures of herpes simplex), by Tzanck preparation, by demonstrating multinucleated giant cells, or by fluorescent or immunoperoxidase antibody slide tests, which are both sensitive and specific in early lesions.

The differential diagnosis includes other vesicular viral exanthems, particularly those caused by enteroviruses, herpes simplex infection, insect bite reactions, pityriasis lichenoides et varioliformis acuta, and autoimmune blistering diseases, such as chronic bullous dermatosis of childhood. Recurrent varicella-zoster virus infection in apparently immunocompetent children has been reported, so previous history of varicella does not exclude the diagnosis.[77]

TREATMENT

Oral acyclovir, 20 mg/kg given four times per day (up to 800 mg qid) has been demonstrated to be moderately effective in decreasing time to new lesion formation and total number of skin lesions if given within 24 hours of the onset of rash, but its routine use is controversial. It should probably be used in adolescents and adults, in whom varicella is known to be more severe, but its routine use in otherwise healthy children is controversial.[72, 78] A preliminary report suggests that the prophylactic use of acyclovir begun 7 to 9 days after a known exposure to chickenpox is also effective in preventing significant clinical disease.[79] Intravenous acyclovir is the treatment of choice for immunocompromised hosts, although in some cases with relatively mild immune deficit, oral therapy may be employed.[80]

Oral antihistamines may be helpful in patients with severe pruritus. Bland shake lotions such as calamine may also help, but those with topical diphenhydramine should be avoided.

Enteroviral Infection

Enteroviruses are the most common cause of viral exanthems in the summer and fall in temperate climates.[81] Members of the Picornaviridae, they are single-stranded, unenveloped RNA viruses. Based on specific antigenic and other characteristics, enteroviruses were once classified as coxsackievirus, echovirus, or poliovirus. These viruses were subsequently grouped together, and although previously identified viruses retained names such as "echo" or "coxsackie," those subsequently identified are labeled numerically.[72-74]

EPIDEMIOLOGY

Infection is spread by the fecal-oral and, more rarely, the respiratory route. The incubation period is 4 to 7 days, and the majority of infections are asymptomatic. When symptoms are present, they are highly variable, depending on the host and the serotype of enterovirus.[81]

CLINICAL DESCRIPTION

Enteroviruses can cause virtually any type of exanthem, but the hand-foot-and-mouth syndrome is the most distinctive of these. After 1 or 2 days of fever, small vesicles develop on the gingivae and lingual and buccal mucous membranes. The cutaneous lesions then appear as multiple, 3- to 7-mm usually oval vesicles. They develop on the dorsa and, less commonly, on volar hands and feet (Fig. 124–5). Buttock lesions also occur in younger children. The exanthem resolves spontaneously within days. Coxsackievirus A16 is the most common cause of hand-foot-and-mouth disease, but many other enteroviruses have been implicated.[82]

Enteroviruses can also cause macular, papular,[83] morbilliform, vesicular,[82–85, 88] urticarial,[85, 86] petechial,[87] rubelliform,[82] and roseola-like eruptions.[44, 89] Echoviruses 25 and 32 have caused hemangioma-like lesions, which are small papules with a dilated vessel in the center that blanch with pressure and have surrounding white halos.[90]

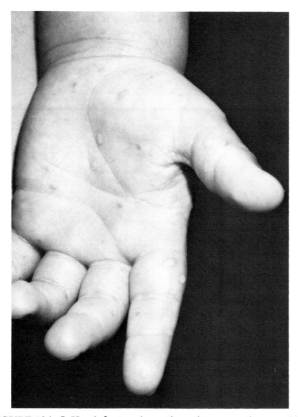

FIGURE 124–5. Hand, foot, and mouth syndrome may be caused by several different enteroviruses.

These papules resolve spontaneously within days. Echovirus 16 causes outbreaks of an acute febrile illness with a roseola-like exanthem known as Boston exanthem.[44] Other eruptions caused by enteroviruses include Kaposi's varicelliform eruption in patients with preexisting skin disease (e.g., atopic dermatitis or Darier's disease) and a zosteriform eruption.[8] A fatal dermatomyositis-like syndrome caused by echovirus 24 has been described in a patient with hypogammaglobulinema.[91] Herpangina, an enanthem characterized by small papulovesicles on the soft palate, uvula, and tonsils, is caused by several different enteroviruses.[81, 85]

Systemic involvement in enteroviral infection may include mild fever, vomiting and diarrhea, and respiratory symptoms. Myocarditis and aseptic meningitis are less common complications.[92–94]

DIAGNOSIS AND DIFFERENTIAL DIAGNOSIS

Enteroviral exanthems are usually diagnosed clinically, based on morphology and the time of year; but when a specific diagnosis is required, viral cultures from rectum, eye, nose, and oropharynx may be obtained. The results of serologic tests are usually not helpful, owing to the large number of enteroviral serotypes. Because enteroviral infections are frequently diagnosed clinically, skin biopsy is only performed if other conditions are suspected. The blisters show intraepidermal vesiculation secondary to ballooning and reticular degeneration of the epidermis, along with superficial perivascular lymphocytic infiltrates and papillary dermal edema. Inclusions and giant cells are absent.

The differential diagnosis is broad and, depending on the presentation, includes herpes stomatitis, varicella-zoster infection, aphthous stomatitis, roseola, group A streptococcal infection, and meningococcemia.

TREATMENT

There is no specific antiviral therapy for enteroviral infections. Supportive measures, such as administration of acetaminophen for fever and fluids to prevent dehydration, are indicated. Local measures, such as rinsing the mouth with antacids, may alleviate discomfort associated with oral lesions.

Epstein-Barr Virus

Epstein-Barr virus (EBV) is a double-stranded DNA virus and a member of the Herpesviridae. Its clinical manifestions are protean and depend on the age of the patient at the time of infection. EBV causes infectious mononucleosis in adolescents, but it causes rash and upper respiratory tract symptoms with only mild adenopathy in young children.[3]

EPIDEMIOLOGY

No seasonal pattern is seen.[3] Infection is spread by close interpersonal contact.

CLINICAL DESCRIPTION

Young adults with primary EBV infection present with an acute illness consisting of fever, sore throat, and fatigue known as infectious mononucleosis. A striking, frequently exudative, tonsillopharyngitis is seen, often with a characteristic petechial enanthem at the junction of the hard and soft palate. Adenopathy (particularly posterior cervical), hepatosplenomegaly, and jaundice are not uncommon.[95] Periorbital edema has been reported[96] and may be the presenting symptom.[97] Rash occurs in a minority of patients in this age group. However, if amoxicillin is given, a morbilliform exanthem may develop.[4] This resolves within 5 days and does not represent a true drug allergy.

Children younger than 5 years old may present with an acute illness similar to infectious mononucleosis, with fever, malaise, pharyngitis, and cervical adenopathy.[13] In addition, many of these younger patients have prominent upper respiratory tract symptoms, such as runny nose, cough, and otitis media. Younger children are more likely to have rash, which may be maculopapular, petechial, papulovesicular, or erythema multiforme-like.[3] EBV may also cause Gianotti-Crosti syndrome (see later).

Complications of acute EBV infection include upper airway obstruction due to markedly swollen lymphoid tissue, co-infection with group A *Streptococcus,* and pneumonia. Neurologic disturbances (seizures, encephalitis) and hematologic abnormalities (thrombocytopenia with bleeding) occur occasionally. Most patients recover without treatment within a month, although it may be several months before they feel normal.[95]

PATHOLOGY

Although the common exanthem of mononucleosis shows only sparse lymphocytic infiltrates, minimal vacuolar change, and papillary dermal edema, a severe eruption due to EBV has been described in immunosuppressed patients, in whom an interface reaction with many necrotic keratinocytes and parakeratosis can occur. EBV can be demonstrated in the nuclei of lesional keratinocytes in this eruption.[98] Another unusual finding in adults is a granuloma annulare–like eruption in which there is granulomatous dermatitis that does not show palisading and mucin deposition, as does authentic granuloma annulare.[99]

DIAGNOSIS AND DIFFERENTIAL DIAGNOSIS

Routine laboratory assessment of patients with infectious mononucleosis will show absolute lymphocytosis, prominent atypical lymphocytes, mild thrombocytopenia, and mildly to moderately elevated results of liver function tests.[13] In adolescents and young adults, heterophil antibody tests are usually positive, but they are often negative in younger children. Specific serologic tests, such as IgM and IgG to the viral capsid antigen, may be done but should be reserved for diagnostic enigmas, particularly in patients with severe or prolonged illness. Measurement of acute and convalescent titers to the Epstein-Barr nuclear antigen (EBNA) may also be helpful. The differential diagnosis of adolescents with infectious mononucleosis includes adenoviral infection, rubella, cytomegalovirus infection, acute toxoplasmosis, streptococcal pharyngitis, and scarlet fever. An infectious mononucleosis–like illness due to HHV-6 has been described.[53, 54] EBV infection in young children is difficult to diagnose since nonspecific cold symptoms and exanthems can be caused by a variety of viruses that affect the respiratory tract.

TREATMENT

Treatment of acute EBV infection is supportive. Patients with upper airway obstruction may be helped by administration of prednisone.[95] Antibiotics should be reserved for those patients with proven bacterial superinfection, such as streptococcal pharyngitis. There are no specific antiviral drugs clinically proven effective in EBV infection, although high doses of acyclovir have been used in immunosuppressed patients with some effect. More effective antiviral agents may soon be available.[95]

Gianotti-Crosti Syndrome

Several viral infections are associated with erythematous papular rashes affecting primarily the face and extremities, with relative sparing of the chest, abdomen, and back. In 1955, Gianotti and Crosti described a distinctive eruption characterized by the presence of multiple, discrete, nonpruritic, erythematous papules located exclusively on the face, neck, and extremities. The rash, called "papular acrodermatitis of childhood," was later found to be caused by hepatitis B.[100] Subsequently, many other infectious agents have been found to cause similar rashes.[101, 102] The forms caused by other agents have sometimes been called "papulovesicular acro-located syndrome" to distinguish them from the hepatitis B–associated exanthem.[103]

EPIDEMIOLOGY

The age of affected children varies from 3 months to 15 years, with a peak incidence at 2 to 5 years of age. Both sexes are affected equally. Most cases associated with hepatitis B infection are due to the ayw subtype. Most children in the United States do not have hepatitis

B infection. Epstein-Barr virus and enteroviruses are the most common causes, but cases have been reported due to poliovaccine virus, cytomegalovirus, hepatitis A, and parainfluenza virus.[101]

CLINICAL DESCRIPTION

The distribution of Gianotti-Crosti syndrome is distinctive and usually the first clue to diagnosis. Whereas most exanthems have significant involvement of the torso, this syndrome spares the torso, with most lesions being noted on the face and extremities with occasional involvement of the buttocks. Lesions may vary from flat-topped papules to "juicy," papulovesicular lesions resembling insect bites (Fig. 124–6; see color plate). Pruritus is variable. Hepatomegaly and lymphadenopathy may be present, depending on the etiology. The rash persists longer than most exanthems, often lasting from 2 to 4 weeks.[103]

DIAGNOSIS AND DIFFERENTIAL DIAGNOSIS

Evaluation of children with papular acral eruptions should include a history of exposure to hepatitis and other infectious illnesses. Evaluation should include a careful examination for lymphadenopathy, hepatomegaly, and splenomegaly.

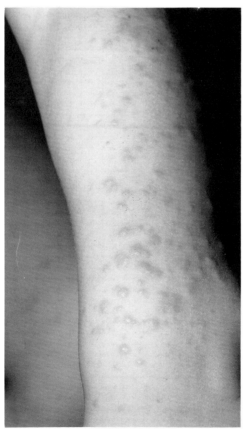

FIGURE 124–6. Gianotti-Crosti syndrome due to Epstein-Barr virus infection. (See color plate.)

If an exposure history suggests the possibility of hepatitis B infection, laboratory evaluation including a complete blood cell count, liver function tests, and hepatitis B surface antigen should be obtained. Because ayw hepatitis B is quite rare in the United States, such serologic testing is probably not necessary in all cases.

The differential diagnosis includes papular urticaria, erythema multiforme, and frictional lichenoid dermatitis.

PATHOLOGY

The cutaneous lesions of Gianotti-Crosti syndrome are produced by spongiotic dermatitis, sometimes accompanied by superficial and deep lymphocytic infiltrates. Fully developed lesions can show marked edema of the papillary dermis and psoriasiform epidermal hyperplasia.

TREATMENT

There is no specific treatment. Oral antihistamines are occasionally necessary. The prognosis is generally good, although some children with hepatitis B–associated disease go on to develop chronic hepatitis.[100]

References

1. Goodyear HM, Laidler PW, Price EH, et al. Acute infectious erythemas in children: A clinico-microbiological study. Br J Dermatol 1991;124:433–438.
2. Berenberg W, Wright S, Janeway CA. Roseola infantum (exanthem subitum). N Engl J Med 1949;241:253–259.
3. Sumaya CV, Ench Y. Epstein-Barr virus infectious mononucleosis in children: I. Clinical and general laboratory findings. Pediatrics 1985;75:1003–1010.
4. Patel BM. Skin rash with infectious mononucleosis and ampicillin. Pediatrics 1967;40:910.
5. Cherry JD. Cutaneous manifestations of systemic infections. In: Feigen RD, Cherry D, eds. Textbook of Pediatric Infectious Disease, 3rd ed. Philadelphia: WB Saunders Co., 1992:775–781.
6. Bodemer C, de Prost Y. Unilateral laterothoracic exanthem in children: A new disease? J Am Acad Dermatol 1992;27:693–696.
7. Taieb A, Megraud F, Legrain V, et al. Asymmetric periflexural exanthem of childhood. J Am Acad Dermatol 1993;29:391–393.
8. Meade RH, Chang T. Zoster-like eruption due to echovirus 6. Am J Dis Child 1979;133:283–284.
9. Cherry JD. Viral exanthems. Curr Probl Pediatr 1983;13:1–55.
10. Gershon AA: Measles virus (rubeola). In: Mandell GL, Douglas RG, Bennett JE, eds. Principles and Practice of Infectious Diseases, 3rd ed. New York: John Wiley & Sons, 1990:1279–1285.
11. Committee on Infectious Diseases: Report of the Committee on Infectious Diseases, 21st ed. Elk Grove, IL: Am Academy of Pediatrics, 1988:277–289.
12. Cherry JD: Measles. In: Feigin RD, Cherry JD, eds. Textbook of Pediatric Infectious Diseases, 3rd ed. Philadelphia: WB Saunders Co., 1992:1591–1609.
13. Krugman S, Katz SL: Infectious Diseases of Children, 7th ed. St. Louis: CV Mosby, 1981.
14. Cherry JD, Feigin RD, Shackelford PG, et al. A clinical and serologic study of 103 children with measles vaccine failure. J Pediatr 1973;82:802–808.
15. Suringa DWR, Bank LJ, Ackerman AB: Role of measles virus in skin lesions and Koplik's spots. N Engl J Med 1970;283:1139–1142.
16. Burns JC, Mason WH, Glode MP, et al. Clinical and epidemiologic characteristics of patients referred for possible Kawasaki disease. J Pediatr 1991;118:680–686.

17. Barclay AJ, Foster A, Sommer A. Vitamin A supplements and mortality related to measles: A randomized clinical trial. Br Med J 1987;294:294–296.
18. Hussey GD, Klein M. Measles-induced vitamin A deficiency. Ann NY Acad Sci 1992;669:188–194.
19. Committee on Infectious Diseases, American Academy of Pediatrics. Vitamin A treatment of measles. Pediatrics 1993;91:1014–1015.
20. Cherry JD. Rubella. In: Feigin RD, Cherry JD, eds. Textbook of Pediatric Infectious Diseases, 3rd ed. Philadelphia: WB Saunders Co., 1992;1792–1817.
21. Horstmann DM. Rubella. In: Evans AS, ed. Viral Infections of Humans. Epidemiology and Control. New York: Plenum, 1976:409.
22. Gershon AA. Rubella virus (German measles). In: Mandell GL, Douglas RG, Bennett JE, eds. Principles and Practice of Infectious Diseases, 3rd ed. New York, John Wiley & Sons, 1990:1242–1247.
23. Dolin R. Parvoviruses (erythema infectiosum, aplastic crisis). In: Mandell GL, Douglas RG, Bennett JE, eds. Principles and Practice of Infectious Diseases, 3rd ed. New York: John Wiley & Sons, 1990:1231–1232.
24. Wadlington WB. Erythema infectiosum. JAMA 1965;192:58–60.
25. Grimmer H, Joseph A. An epidemic of infectious erythema in Germany. Arch Dermatol 1959;80:283–285.
26. Zerbini M, Musiani M, Gallinella G, et al. Different syndromes associated with B19 parvovirus viraemia in paediatric patients: Report of four cases. Eur J Pediatr 1992;151:815–817.
27. Pillay D, Patou G, Hurt S, et al. Parvovirus B19 outbreak in a children's ward. Lancet 1992;339:107–109.
28. Evans LM, Grossman ME, Gregory N. Koplik spots and a purpuric eruption associated with parvovirus B19 infection. J Am Acad Dermatol 1992;27:466–467.
29. Charles L, Halasz G, Cormier D, et al. Petechial glove and sock syndrome caused by parvovirus B19. J Am Acad Dermatol 1992;27:835–838.
30. Cherry JD. Parvoviruses. In: Feigin RD, Cherry JD, eds. Textbook of Pediatric Infectious Diseases, 3rd ed. Philadelphia: WB Saunders Co., 1981:1626.
31. Centers for Disease Control. Risks associated with human parvovirus B19 infection. MMWR 1989;38:81–88, 93–97.
32. Anand A, Gray ES, Brown T, et al. Human parvovirus infection in pregnancy and hydrops fetalis. N Engl J Med 1987;316:183–186.
33. Anderson LJ, Hurwitz ES. Human parvovirus B19 and pregnancy. Clin Perinatology 1988;15:273–286.
34. Anderson MJ, Jones SE, Fischer-Hoch SP, et al. Human parvovirus, the cause of erythema infectiosum (fifth disease)? Lancet 1983;1:1378.
35. Torok TJ, Wang Q, Gary GW, et al. Prenatal diagnosis of intrauterine infection with parvovirus B19 by the polymerase chain reaction technique. Clin Infect Dis 1992;14:149–155.
36. Zahorsky J. Roseola infantalis. Pediatrics 1910;22:60–64.
37. Yamanishi K, Kondo T, Kondo K, et al. Exanthem subitum and human herpesvirus 6 (HHV-6) infection. Adv Exp Med Biol 1990;278:29–37.
38. Ueda K, Kusuhara K, Hirose M, et al. Exanthem subitum and antibody to human herpesvirus-6. J Infect Dis 1989;159:750–752.
39. Leach CT, Sumaya C, Brown NA. Human herpesvirus-6: Clinical implications of a recently discovered, ubiquitous agent. J Pediatr 1992;121:173–181.
40. Kempe CH, Shaw EB, Jackson JR, et al. Studies on the etiology of exanthema subitum (roseola infantum). J Pediatr 1950;37:561–568.
41. Juretic M. Exanthema subitum: A review of 243 cases. Helv Pediatr Acta 1963;1:80–95.
42. Yamanishi K. Human herpesvirus 6. Microbiol Immunol 1992;36:551–561.
43. Yoshikawa T, Suga S, Asano Y, et al. Distribution of antibodies to a causative agent of exanthem subitum (human herpesvirus-6) in healthy individuals. Pediatrics 1989;84:675–677.
44. Hall CB, Cherry JD, Hatch MH, et al. The return of Boston exanthem. Am J Dis Child 1977;131:323–326.
45. Fox JD, Briggs M, Ward PA, et al. Human herpesvirus 6 in salivary glands. Lancet 1990;336:590–593.
46. Okuno T, Mukai T, Baba K, et al. Outbreak of exanthem subitum in an orphanage. J Pediatr 1991;119:759–761.
47. Kondo K, Kondo T, Okuno T, et al. Latent human herpesvirus 6 infection of human monocytes/macrophages. J Gen Virol 1991;72:1401–1408.
48. Chou S. Human herpesvirus 6 infection and associated disease. J Lab Clin Med 1993;121:388–393.
49. Okada K, Ueda K, et al. Exanthema subitum and human herpesvirus 6: Clinical Observations in fifty-seven cases. Pediatr Infect Dis J 1993;12:204–208.
50. Asano Y, Suga S, Yoshikawa T. Human herpesvirus 6 infection (exanthem subitum) without fever. J Pediatr 1989;115:264–265.
51. Suga S, Yoshikawa T, Asano Y, et al. Human herpesvirus-6 infection (exanthem subitum) without rash. Pediatrics 1989;83:1003–1006.
52. Pruksananonda P, Hall CB, Insel RA, et al. Primary human herpesvirus 6 infection in young children. N Engl J Med 1992;326:1445–1450.
53. Steeper TA, Horwitz CA, Ablashi DV, et al. The spectrum of clinical and laboratory findings resulting from human herpesvirus-6 (HHV-6) in patients with mononucleosis-like illnesses not resulting from Epstein-Barr virus or cytomegalovirus. Am J Clin Pathol 1990;93:776–783.
54. Akashi K, Eizuru Y, Sumiyoshi Y, et al. Severe infectious mononucleosis-like syndrome and primary human herpesvirus 6 infection in an adult. N Engl J Med 1993;329:168–171.
55. Cone RW, Hackman RC, Huang ML, et al. Human herpesvirus 6 in lung tissue from patients with pneumonitis after bone marrow transplantation (comments). N Engl J Med 1993;329:156–161.
56. Prezioso P, Caniarella J, Lee M, et al. Fatal disseminated infection with human herpesvirus-6. J Pediatr 1992;120:921–923.
57. Yoshikawa T, Nakashima T, Suga S, et al. Human herpesvirus-6 DNA in cerebrospinal fluid of a child with exanthem subitum and meningoencephalitis. Pediatrics 1992;89:888–890.
58. Suga S, Yoshikawa T, Asano Y, et al. Clinical and virological analyses of 21 infants with exanthem subitum (roseola infantum) and central nervous system complications. Ann Neurol 1993;33:597–603.
59. Yamanishi K, Kondo K, Mukai T. Human herpesvirus-6 in the central nervous system. Acta Paediatr Jpn 1992;34:337–343.
60. Kondo K, Nagafuji H, Hata A, et al. Association of human herpesvirus 6 infection of the central nervous system with recurrence of febrile convulsions. J Infect Dis 1993;167:1197–1200.
61. Asano Y, Yoshikawa T, Kajita Y, et al. Fatal encephalitis/encephalopathy in primary human herpesvirus-6 infection. Arch Dis Child 1992;67:1484–1485.
62. Huang LM, Lee CY, et al. Human herpesvirus-6 associated with fatal hemophagocytic syndrome (letter). Lancet 1990;336:60–61.
63. Nishimura K, Igarashi M. Thrombocytopenic purpura associated with exanthem subitum. Pediatrics 1977;60:260.
64. Kondo K, Hayakawa Y, Mori H, et al. Detection by polymerase chain reaction amplification of human herpesvirus 6 DNA in peripheral blood of patients with exanthem subitum. J Clin Microbiol 1990;28:970–974.
65. Asano Y, Yoshikawa T, Suga S, et al. Viremia and neutralizing antibody response in infants with exanthem subitum. J Pediatr 1989;114:535–539.
66. Brawley RL, Wenzel RP. An algorithm for chickenpox exposure. Pediatr Infect Dis 1984;3:502–504.
67. Preblud SR, Oreinstein WA, Bart KJ. Varicella: Clinical manifestations, epidemiology and health impact in children. Pediatr Infect Dis 1984;3:505–509.
68. Cooper DA, Maclean P, Finlayson R, et al. Acute AIDS retrovirus infection: Definition of a clinical illness associated with seroconversion. Lancet 1985;1:537–540.
69. Hulsebosch HJ, Claessen FA, van Ginkel, CJ, et al. Human immunodeficiency virus exanthem. J Am Acad Dermatolol 1990;23:483–486.
70. Wantzin L, Lindhardt O, Weismann K, et al. Acute HTLV III infection associated with exanthema, diagnosed by seroconversion. Br J Dermatol 1986;115:601–606.
71. LeBoit PE. Dermatopathologic findings in patients infected with HIV. Dermatol Clin 1992;10:59–71.
72. Balfour HH, Kelly JM, Suarez CS, et al. Acyclovir treatment of varicella in otherwise health children. J Pediatr 1990;116:633–639.

73. Srugo I, Israele V, Wittek AE, et al. Clinical manifestations of varicella-zoster virus infections in human immunodeficiency virus-infected children. Am J Dis Child 1993;147:742–745.

74. Fleisher G, Henry W, McSorley M, et al. Life-threatening complication of varicella. Am J Dis Child 1981;135:896–899.

75. Lynfield R, Herrin JT, Rubin RH. Varicella in pediatric renal transplant recipients. Pediatrics 1992;90:216–220.

76. Kasper WJ, Howe PM. Fatal varicella after a single course of corticosteroids. Pediatr Infect Dis J 1990;9:729–732.

77. Junker AK, Angus E, Thomas EE. Recurrent varicella-zoster virus infections in apparently immunocompetent children. Pediatr Infect Dis J 1991;10:559–575.

78. Committee on Infectious Diseases. The use of oral acyclovir in otherwise healthy children with varicella. Pediatrics 1993;91: 674–676.

79. Asano Y, Yoshikawa T, Suga Sadao, et al. Postexposure prophylaxis of varicella in family contact by oral acyclovir. Pediatrics 1993;92:219–222.

80. Balfour HH. Intravenous acyclovir therapy for varicella in immunocompromised children. J Pediatr 1984;104:134–136.

81. Cherry JD. Enteroviruses: Polioviruses (poliomyelitis), coxsackieviruses, echoviruses, and enteroviruses. In: Feigen RD, Cherry JD, eds. Textbook of Pediatric Infectious Diseases, 3rd ed. Philadelphia: WB Saunders Co., 1992:1705–1753.

82. Cherry JD, Lerner AM, Klein JO, et al. ECHO 11 virus infections associated with exanthems. Pediatrics 1963;32:509–516.

83. Lepow ML, Carver DH, Robbins FC. Clinical and epidemiologic observations on enterovirus infection in a circumscribed community during an epidemic of echovirus 9 infection. Pediatrics 1960;26:12–26.

84. Deseda-Torres J, Byatt PH, Cherry JD. Vesicular lesions in adults due to echovirus 11 infections. Arch Dermatol 1977;113: 1705–1706.

85. Forman JL, Cherry JD. Enanthems associated with uncommon viral syndromes. Pediatrics 1968;41:873–882.

86. Cherry JD, Lerner AM, Klein JO, et al. Coxsackie A9 infections with exanthems with particular reference to urticaria. Pediatrics 1963;31:819–823.

87. Frothingham TE. ECHO virus type 9 associated with three cases of stimulating meningococcemia. N Engl J Med 1958;259: 484–485.

88. Gohd RS, Faigel HC. Hand-foot-and-mouth-disease resembling measles: A life-threatening disease: Case report. Pediatrics 1966; 37:644–648.

89. Cherry JD, Lerner AM, Klein JO, et al. Coxsackie B5 infections with exanthems. Pediatrics 1963;31:455–462.

90. Cherry JD, Bobinski JE, Horvath FL, et al. Acute hemangioma-like lesions associated with ECHO viral infections. Pediatrics 1969;44:498–502.

91. Bardelas JA, Winkelstein JA, Seto DSY, et al. Fatal ECHO 24 infection in a patient with hypogammaglobulinemia: Relationship to dermatomyositis-like syndrome. J Pediatr 1977;90: 396–399.

92. Ishimaru Y, Nakano S, Yamaoka K, et al. Outbreaks of hand, foot, and mouth disease by enterovirus 71. Arch Dis Child 1980; 55:583–588.

93. Gilbert G, Dickson KE, Waters M, et al. Outbreak of enterovirus 71 infection in Victoria, Australia, with a high incidence of neurologic involvement. Pediatr Infect Dis J 1988;7:484–488.

94. Karzan DT, Hayner NS, Winkelstein W, et al. An epidemic of aseptic meningitis syndrome due to echovirus type 6: II. A clinical study of ECHO 6 infection. Pediatrics 1962;29:418–431.

95. Sumaya CV. Epstein Barr virus. In: Feigen RD, Cherry JD, eds. Textbook of Pediatric Infectious Disease, 3rd ed, vol II. Philadelphia: WB Saunders Co., 1992;1547–1557.

96. McCarthy JT, Hoagland RJ. Cutaneous manifestations of infectious mononucleosis. JAMA 1964;187:153–154.

97. Decker GR, Berberian BJ, Sulica VI. Periorbital and eyelid edema: The initial manifestation of acute infectious mononucleosis. Cutis 1991;47:323–324.

98. Fermand J-P, Gozlan J, Bendelac A, et al. Detection of Epstein-Barr virus in epidermal skin lesions of an immunocompromised patient. Ann Intern Med 1990;112:511–515.

99. Spencer SA, Fenske NA, Espinoza CG, et al. Granuloma annulare-like eruption due to chronic Epstein-Barr virus infection. Arch Dermatol 1988;124:250–255.

100. Gianotti F. Papular acrodermatitis of childhood: An Australia antigen disease. Arch Dis Child 1973;48:794–799.

101. Draelos ZK, Hansen RC, James WD. Gianotti-Crosti syndrome associated with infections other than hepatitis B. JAMA 1986; 256:2386–2388.

102. Caputo R, Gelmetti C, Ermacora E, et al. Gianotti-Crosti syndrome: A retrospective analysis of 308 cases. J Am Acad Dermatol 1992;26:207–210.

103. Gianotti F: Papular acrodermatitis of childhood and other papulovesicular acro-located syndromes. Br J Dermatol 1979;110: 49–59.

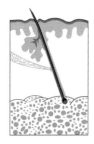

chapter 125

Human Immunodeficiency Virus Infection and the Cutaneous Complications of Immunosuppression

TIMOTHY G. BERGER and JORDAN W. TAPPERO

In this chapter we discuss those conditions associated with immunosuppression from human immunodeficiency virus (HIV) infection, malignancies, and congenital immunodeficiency states. Most of this discussion is on HIV infection and its cutaneous manifestations. Conditions seen in both HIV infection and other forms of immunosuppression are reviewed, and conditions seen with immunosuppression (but not so common in HIV infection) are also outlined. Because the manifestations of certain conditions (e.g., herpesvirus infections) are different in HIV disease from the same condition in other forms of immunosuppression, these conditions are discussed in two sections of this chapter.

Human Immunodeficiency Virus Infection and Its Cutaneous Complications

Clinical Description

HIV is spread by exchange of body fluids. The most common modes of transmission are sexual contact (both homosexual and heterosexual), intravenous drug use, blood or blood product transfusion, and spread from mother to child during birth (perinatal transmission). Since HIV-infected persons are frequently asymptomatic but infectious for many years before they develop clinical disease, large numbers of persons may become infected before the presence of an epidemic is recognized. In general, in an established epidemic, persons with acquired immunodeficiency syndrome (AIDS) represent 10% or less of the HIV-infected population.

Human immunodeficiency virus type 1 (HIV-1) infects cells that bear surface CD4 receptors: helper T cells and members of the monocyte/macrophage system. HIV binds to CD4 receptors through its surface glycoprotein, gp 120. The enumeration of helper T cells has become the most frequently used and reliable marker of progression of HIV disease.

During initial infection, there is transient viremia, but HIV is rapidly cleared from the circulation by the immune response. During the initial viremia, CD4 cells fall abruptly. This phase is called primary HIV disease. After the primary stage, the immune system appears to largely contain the virus within the reticuloendothelial system, primarily in lymph nodes. Viremia is no longer detectable, and the helper T cells initially return to normal levels. This second phase is called the asymptomatic stage because the infected person usually has no symptoms (except perhaps generalized lymphadenopathy). There is a gradual depletion of helper T cells in most persons, while HIV proliferates within lymph nodes. Symptomatic HIV disease (the third phase of infection) begins on the average about 10 years after infection and is often manifested by fever, night sweats, diarrhea, or weight loss. Helper T-cell counts are variable, but usually less than 400 cells/mm³. Everyone who develops symptomatic HIV disease progresses to AIDS, the fourth stage of infection. AIDS is diagnosed by the presence of certain neoplastic, infectious, or laboratory (a helper T-cell count < 200 cells/mm³) complications of infection. Once the infected person develops AIDS there is a gradual deterioration of his or her health as a result of recurrent infectious and/or neurologic complications. The final stage of HIV infection occurs at a helper T-cell count less than 50 cells/mm³ (advanced AIDS). At this stage, certain chronic infections reactivate, therapy for infections becomes more difficult, and death supervenes.

Over 90% of persons who seroconvert for HIV suffer an acute mononucleosis-like illness.[1-5] The incubation period ranges from 11 to 28 days, with a median of 14 days.[2] The most characteristic symptoms are fever, sore throat, malaise, myalgias, and headache. Enlarged lymph nodes are found in 50% to 90% of patients, as well as an inflamed throat. A cutaneous eruption occurs in 25% to 75% of patients and consists of either a diffuse morbilliform or papular exanthem or 5- to 10-mm oval, papulosquamous, maculopapular lesions sometimes with central petechiae predominantly over the upper trunk. The palms and soles may be involved. Skin biopsy specimens show a sparse mononuclear cell upper dermal infiltrate with slight exocytosis and occasionally hemorrhage.[5]

An enanthem is seen in about one third of patients with primary HIV disease. Oral candidiasis may be present.[4] Oral, genital, anal, and esophageal ulcerations are frequent, and odynophagia and/or retrosternal pain may occur. HIV has been identified in these ulcerations.[3] The acute illness lasts 1 to 2 weeks. Most patients recover within 4 weeks, but lymphadenopathy and lethargy may persist. Acute hepatitis may occur.[4] Neurologic disease in the form of encephalitis, neuritis, or myelitis may develop 2 to 3 weeks after the acute illness[2] and in persons at risk is highly suggestive of acute HIV infection.

The diagnosis of group I, or primary, HIV disease is confirmed by detecting HIV seroconversion, an IgM antibody response in the second to tenth week, and isolation in the blood of HIV virus or antigens during the acute episode. IgG antibodies detected by Western blot analysis may be present at the onset of the illness although enzyme-linked immunosorbent assays are negative.[4] There is a reversal of the helper/suppressor T-cell ratio, which is normally 2:1.

Bacterial Infections

The nasal carriage rate of *Staphylococcus aureus* is approximately 50% in HIV-infected persons of all stages

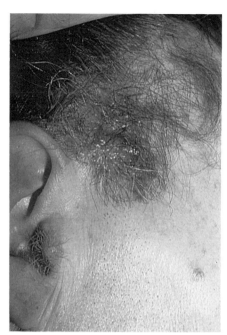

FIGURE 125-1. Crusted plaques due to *Staphylococcus aureus.*

of disease, and staphylococcal pyodermas are very common. Staphylococcal infections manifest as folliculitis, ecthyma, abscess, or tender boggy plaques (Fig. 125-1). Pruritus may complicate staphylococcal folliculitis.[6] Secondary infection of pruritic inflammatory skin disorders with *S. aureus* is frequent. Treatment of staphylococcal pyoderma is with oral antibiotics, and prolonged courses may be required. Ablation of nasal carriage with topical mupirocin or oral rifampin may benefit patients with recurrent episodes.

S. aureus folliculitis may be extremely pruritic in the setting of HIV infection.[6] As in atopic dermatitis, staphylococcal infection frequently complicates and exacerbates eczematous eruptions in HIV infection.

Viral Infections

MOLLUSCUM CONTAGIOSUM

Clinical Description

Molluscum contagiosum affects between 10% and 20% of patients with AIDS. Eighty percent of patients with molluscum contagiosum have a helper T-cell count (CD4) below 200 cells/mm³. Patients with extensive molluscum usually have fewer than 50 helper T cells/mm³.[7] Subclinical infection is probably common in patients with advanced HIV disease, as evidenced by the finding of microscopic changes of molluscum contagiosum on routine biopsy samples in the absence of visible lesions and the finding by electron microscopy of molluscum contagiosum virus in apparently normal skin.

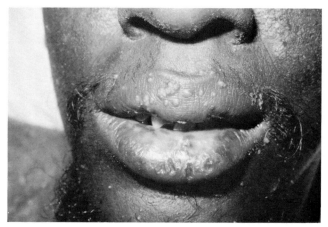

FIGURE 125–2. Extensive cutaneous and mucosal molluscum contagiosum in a patient with advanced AIDS.

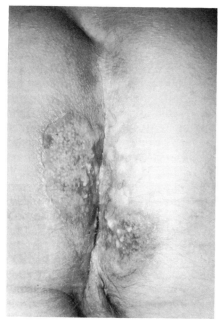

FIGURE 125–3. Extensive perianal erosions due to herpes simplex virus type 2 in a patient with AIDS.

Molluscum contagiosum preferentially affects the genital area and face, especially around the eyes.[8] In the beard area, lesions begin at the follicular opening as barely visible skin-colored papules. Lesions may number in excess of 100, and individual lesions may become greater than 1 cm in diameter (Fig. 125–2). A large solitary lesion may simulate a basal cell carcinoma.[9] Disseminated fungal infections, especially cryptococcosis, may mimic molluscum contagiosum, but in these cases the onset is usually more rapid, and the lesions tend to be of a uniform size.[10]

Treatment

Cryotherapy is the usual method of treatment. Alternative methods of therapy include gentle electrosurgery, cantharidin, and removal by curette. Recurrence is almost universal. Shaving with razor blades should be stopped if lesions are in the beard area. The nightly application of topical retinoic acid at the highest strength tolerated appears to reduce the rate of appearance and size of new lesions.

HERPES SIMPLEX VIRUS INFECTION

Clinical Description

Early in the course of HIV disease herpes simplex virus (HSV) infection is often a self-limited disorder.[11] Once significant immunosuppression occurs, however, lesions persist. The presence of mucocutaneous HSV infection for more than 1 month is an indicator disease for AIDS.[12] Tender, often painful, ulcerative lesions of the penis, perianal area, and lip are the hallmark.[13] Less commonly, periungual lesions (herpetic whitlow)[14] or follicular facial lesions (herpetic folliculitis) occur. Without treatment, lesions may continue to enlarge peripherally, sometimes reaching over 100 cm² (Fig. 125–3). Multiple scattered lesions in one area are not uncommon, but widespread dissemination of HSV even in AIDS is unusual. Related to CD4 count, only 13% of ulcerative lesions in HIV-infected patients with CD4

counts greater than 400 cells/mm³ are HSV related, whereas in persons with CD4 counts less than 50 cells/mm³, 58% of all ulcerations and 67% of perianal ulcerations contain HSV.[15] *Any ulcerative or erosive lesion in a patient with HIV disease should be considered HSV until proven otherwise.*

The diagnosis of HSV infection is by Tzanck smear, viral culture, and/or direct fluorescent antibody staining of scrapings from lesions. If these tests are negative, a skin biopsy specimen from the edge of the ulcer will usually demonstrate typical herpetic effect in epithelial cells of the skin, mucosa, or adnexal structures or yield HSV on tissue culture.[16] Staining of the histologic specimen with antibodies to HSV or searching for HSV DNA by polymerase chain reaction may help in those unusual culture-negative cases in which typical cytopathic changes are not found.[17] A viral isolate is required when acyclovir therapy fails and acyclovir resistance is suspected. Serologic tests are of no value in the diagnosis of cutaneous HSV infection. It is not uncommon to find evidence of cytomegalovirus (CMV) expression in chronic perianal ulcerative (and occasionally oral) lesions in patients with advanced HIV disease.[17–19] Herpes simplex is often coexistent. CMV cytopathic changes may also rarely be seen in normal skin, and CMV is known to be expressed preferentially in areas of active inflammation.[18, 19] For this reason it is unclear whether CMV causes cutaneous ulceration or is simply expressed in lesions induced by herpes simplex.

Treatment

For active mucocutaneous lesions therapy consists of 200 to 400 mg of acyclovir five times daily until the lesions have healed. If ineffective, increased oral doses (up to 800 mg five times daily) or intravenous acyclovir (5 mg/kg three times daily) may be used. Since the likelihood of recurrence is high, chronic suppressive acyclovir (400 mg twice daily) is given indefinitely, once lesions have healed.

Any documented herpetic lesion that fails to heal appropriately should be cultured and sampled and the isolate tested for resistance to acyclovir. Evaluation for additional infectious processes that might explain the failure of the lesion to heal is recommended. Although virtually all acyclovir-resistant mutants lack thymidine kinase, alterations of the viral DNA polymerase can also lead to drug resistance.[20, 21]

The therapy for acyclovir-resistant HSV infection is with trisodium phosphonoformate (foscarnet).[22-25] Once lesions heal, acyclovir suppression may be reinstituted, although suppressive foscarnet may be required.[26, 27] In solitary, smaller lesions topical treatment with (S)-1-(3-hydroxy-2-phosphonylmethoxypropyl) cystosine (HPMPC) or trifluorothymidine with or without topical interferon alfa may be successful.[28, 29] Ablation with electrocautery or excision may eradicate smaller lesions.

VARICELLA-ZOSTER VIRUS

Clinical Description

In HIV-infected hemophiliacs, the cumulative 10-year risk of varicella-zoster virus (VZV) infection is 12% in adults and 14% in children; in HIV-infected homosexual men the cumulative 12-year risk is 30%.[30, 31] The mean CD4 count for HIV-infected hemophiliacs (children and adults) with zoster was 315 cells/mm^3,[31] that is, many HIV-infected persons develop zoster before they have other symptoms of HIV disease. Zoster has also been reported to follow rapidly primary varicella in HIV-infected children.[32]

HIV-infected persons when exposed to VZV for the first time may develop varicella.[33, 34] Although varicella may follow a benign course, resolving without therapy, pulmonary involvement and fatal disease may occur, even in patients with asymptomatic HIV infection. Complications appear to be more common in HIV-positive children than in adults.[33, 34] Serum antibodies to VZV do not appear to prevent varicella in HIV-infected persons, and recurrent varicella can occur.

In the HIV-infected patient with few or no HIV-related symptoms, herpes zoster usually follows a course similar to that seen in healthy persons.[11] Lesions resolve over 2 to 3 weeks, often without specific therapy.[35] Severe ulceration with pain and post-herpetic neuralgia are not uncommon, however.[36, 37] Recurrences are seen in between 10% and 20% of HIV-infected persons with herpes zoster. Disseminated zoster is uncommon and usually seen in HIV-infected persons with advanced disease.[38-41] Because in HIV disease disseminated VZV is much more common than disseminated HSV, patients with disseminated herpetic lesions must be assumed to have VZV and treated appropriately.

In addition to the typical vesiculobullous lesions com-

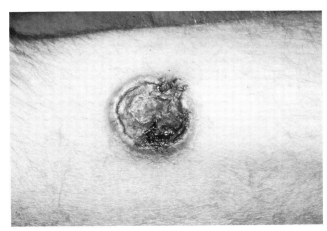

FIGURE 125–4. Ecthymatous varicella-zoster virus infection that was acyclovir resistant.

monly seen with disseminated VZV, patients with AIDS develop two unusual clinical patterns: ecthymatous, crusted, punched-out ulcerations (Fig. 125–4)[41-43] or true verrucous lesions that may be seen alone or in association with vesicular or ecthymatous lesions (Fig. 125–5).[44, 45] These patterns may be associated with acyclovir resistance.[45] In one study polymerase chain reaction demonstrated VZV in all verrucous herpetic lesions tested.[46]

Diagnosis

In typical varicella or herpes zoster, a confirming Tzanck smear is usually all that is required. In unusual patterns of infection such as ecthymatous, verrucous, or disseminated lesions, definitive tests such as viral culture or fluorescent antibody testing should be performed to establish the diagnosis. Fluorescent antibody testing is preferred in the setting of VZV since the result is much more rapid than viral culture, and results confirm immediately not only the presence of a herpesvirus infection but also the species (HSV vs. VZV). Skin biopsy may be required in unusual patterns of VZV infection. When acyclovir resistance is suspected a viral isolate is required.

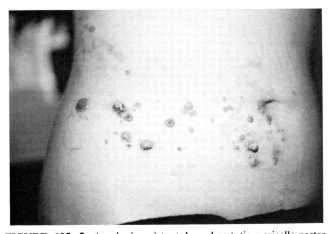

FIGURE 125–5. Acyclovir-resistant hyperkeratotic varicella-zoster virus infection.

Treatment

HIV-infected persons with varicella, either as a primary infection, a second episode, or a reactivation, should be evaluated carefully for evidence of systemic involvement. If evidence of pulmonary, hepatic, or other systemic disease is found, intravenous acyclovir at a dosage of 10 mg/kg every 8 hours, adjusted for renal function, should be given. Oral acyclovir at a dosage of 800 mg every 4 hours may be used in persons without evidence of visceral disease, but these patients should be followed carefully, and if evidence of visceral disease occurs, intravenous acyclovir therapy should be instituted.

The management of herpes zoster is determined by two factors: (1) the overall immune status of the patient and (2) the location of the VZV infection. First and foremost, since herpes zoster is a common presenting sign in HIV disease, all persons with herpes zoster should be questioned about HIV risk factors and examined for other manifestations of HIV disease. HIV serologic testing should be considered. Most patients with herpes zoster as a manifestation of early HIV disease do well without therapy.[36, 37] Nonetheless, oral acyclovir in the dose of 800 mg five times daily for 7 to 10 days is recommended. Since complications due to herpes zoster ophthalmicus are common even early in HIV infection, all HIV-infected persons with herpes zoster ophthalmicus should be given intravenous acyclovir, in a dose of 10 mg/kg three times daily, adjusted for renal function. Other indications for intravenous acyclovir are uncontrollable pain, Ramsay Hunt syndrome, dissemination, visceral disease, and failure of oral treatment.

The chronic forms of cutaneous VZV infection may require prolonged therapy. Ecthymatous lesions may respond to oral or intravenous acyclovir therapy,[41] but they may relapse or recur.[42] In the case of verrucous lesions, therapy with intravenous acyclovir may fail,[44, 45] indicating the presence of acyclovir resistance. As with HSV, acyclovir-resistant isolates of VZV are deficient in thymidine kinase.[45] Foscarnet is recommended in a dose of 40 mg/kg every 8 hours.[47] Healing is much slower than in acyclovir-resistant HSV, sometimes exceeding 3 weeks.

Systemic Fungal Infections

A number of systemic fungal infections have been reported in patients with symptomatic HIV disease and AIDS, most notably cryptococcosis, histoplasmosis, sporotrichosis, coccidioidomycosis, candidiasis, aspergillosis, and actinomycosis.[48-80]

CRYPTOCOCCOSIS

Clinical Description

Cryptococcus neoformans infections occur in nearly 10% of patients with AIDS. Virtually all infections in-

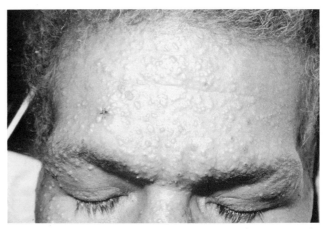

FIGURE 125–6. Extensive facial pearly papules of cryptococcosis.

volve the central nervous system, with meningitis the most frequent manifestation.[48] The disease is subacute, and often mild headache, fever, and malaise are the predominant features. Lesions outside the central nervous system occur in about half of patients with AIDS with cryptococcosis. In non–HIV-infected immunosuppressed persons with cryptococcosis 10% to 15% have specific cutaneous lesions. In patients with AIDS the frequency of cutaneous cryptococcosis is much less.[48]

Cutaneous cryptococcosis in HIV infection usually presents as 0.2- to 1-cm papules with a central umbilication or crust and have been described as resembling molluscum contagiosum or herpes simplex (Fig. 125–6).[49-53, 55] The face is most often involved. Tumors and ulcerative lesions of the skin or mucous membranes are also seen (Fig. 125–7).[56] In the setting of renal transplantation and other forms of immunosuppression, cutaneous cryptococcosis may present as a cellulitis.[71] Biopsy

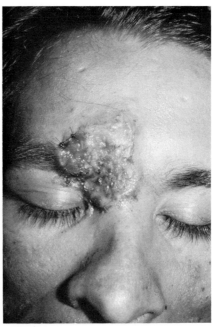

FIGURE 125–7. Chronic ulcerative cryptococcosis.

specimens usually show the gelatinous rather than the granulomatous pattern of infection.

Diagnosis

The possibility of cutaneous cryptococcosis must be considered when evaluating any HIV-infected person with lesions resembling molluscum contagiosum. The diagnosis can be made by a potassium hydroxide examination or a skin biopsy. A serum cryptococcal antigen will confirm the diagnosis of cryptococcosis. The finding of cutaneous cryptococcosis in a patient with AIDS has always been associated with systemic infection, usually of the central nervous system but less commonly of the lungs.[48-54] A lumbar puncture and chest roentgenogram are required.

Treatment

Amphotericin B or fluconazole is the initial therapy. Lifelong maintenance therapy, usually with fluconazole, is required. In the setting of cryptococcal cellulitis the diagnosis is confirmed by skin biopsy. Visceral disease may not be present in HIV-seronegative immunosuppressed patients. Amphotericin or fluconazole is recommended, and patients frequently do not require maintenance therapy.[71]

HISTOPLASMOSIS

Clinical Description

In the central United States disseminated histoplasmosis is a common opportunistic infection of patients with AIDS.[57, 58] In Houston, at the edge of the endemic area for histoplasmosis, 5% of all patients with AIDS develop disseminated histoplasmosis, and in three fourths it was the initial manifestation of AIDS. In Indianapolis, up to two thirds of patients with AIDS develop disseminated histoplasmosis.

Ten per cent of patients with AIDS with disseminated histoplasmosis have skin lesions.[57-65] Cutaneous histoplasmosis may present as many different types of lesions. Papular and papulonecrotic skin lesions appear to be most common.[59-62] Other morphologies include exanthematous, scaling maculopapular lesions resembling a dermatitis,[63] cup-shaped papules, vegetative plaques, and diffuse purpura. Diffuse purpura may be associated with disseminated intravascular coagulopathy and is usually fatal.[57] Oral ulcerations may also be seen.[59, 60] Biopsy of skin lesions confirms the diagnosis in over 80% of cases.[57] Amphotericin B is the treatment of choice, and maintenance therapy, usually with fluconazole or itraconazole, is required.

SPOROTRICHOSIS

In patients with AIDS, characteristic skin lesions of sporotrichosis are chronic ulcerations with crusting.[66-69]

Multiple visceral organ involvement may occur, characteristically including septic arthritis.[66, 67] Amphotericin B or itraconazole, not saturated solution of potassium iodide, should be used for treatment in immunosuppressed patients with sporotrichosis.

ASPERGILLOSIS

Rare cases of cutaneous aspergillosis have been reported in patients with AIDS.[53] They have presented as umbilicated crusted papules at sites of central venous catheters. In one patient, cultures of the tape used to dress the site yielded *Aspergillus fumigatus.* Histologically, hyphae were seen in dilated follicular lumina associated with pseudoepitheliomatous hyperplasia of the surrounding epidermis. In one patient an associated pulmonary focus was found at autopsy.

Cutaneous Mycobacterial Infection

Infections with *Mycobacterium avium – intracellulare* and *M. tuberculosis* are frequent in patients with HIV disease. These infections may be disseminated, unusual, and severe.[72] Cutaneous lesions are unusual and present as chronic sinuses over involved lymph nodes (scrofula), chronic ulcerations, or hemorrhagic macules.[73] All specimens showing either suppurative or granulomatous inflammation from HIV-infected patients should be examined with appropriate stains for mycobacteria. When present, organisms are usually abundant.[74]

In most cases the presence of acid-fast bacilli in skin lesions indicates disseminated mycobacterial disease, usually from *M. avium – intracellulare.* Rarely, however, abscesses or sporotrichoid lesions due to mycobacteria may represent localized disease.[75] *M. avium – intracellulare* causes most cases of isolated lymph node or sporotrichoid disease. Treatment with effective antimycobacterial agents may result in cure in HIV-infected patients with localized disease.

M. haemophilum is a rare cause of mycobacterial infection in immunosuppressed persons. It commonly presents as cutaneous abscesses or ulcerations and tenosynovitis or arthritis. In HIV-infected patients, lesions have been widespread and blood cultures and/or pulmonary studies have demonstrated evidence of disseminated disease. This organism should be suspected if skin or joint lesions yield acid-fast bacilli on smears, yet standard acid-fast bacilli cultures are negative. Hemin supplementation may result in positive cultures.[76, 77]

Rarely *M. kansasii* can cause skin-colored papules and plaques with a spindle cell proliferation resembling Kaposi's sarcoma in HIV-infected persons.[78] Localized *M. marinum* that responded to therapy has also been reported.[79] Bacille Calmette-Guérin (BCG) immunization is probably contraindicated in HIV-infected persons since disseminated *M. bovis* may result.[80]

Scabies

Clinical Description

Most cases of scabies are associated with close personal contact, including sexual exposure. In the setting of advanced HIV infection, however, a source of infection is frequently not found. Virtually all patients with a helper T-cell count over 200 cells/mm³ have typical scabies and a normal response to therapy; unusual manifestations and treatment failures are seen in patients with fewer than 200 CD4-positive cells/mm³.[81]

Most patients with HIV infection, independent of CD4 count, have a clinical presentation similar to HIV-seronegative persons. Staphylococcal pyoderma complicates at least 50% of all scabies cases. Atypical variants of scabies include bullous scabies, exaggerated scabies,[82] papular scabies, and crusted scabies.[81] Exaggerated scabies is a widespread eruption that may spare the typical scabies areas and involve the head and neck. Individual lesions are small papules, and scrapings are positive from many of the lesions. Exaggerated scabies is frequently misdiagnosed as an inflammatory dermatosis or drug eruption and treated with corticosteroids. Papular scabies is an eruption consisting solely of papules on the trunk. Each papule is the site of a burrow, and there is no associated hypersensitivity reaction. Pruritus may be minimal. Crusted (Norwegian, or hyperkeratotic) scabies is usually nonpruritic and is characterized by sand-like, thick, tan crusts that flake off, revealing underlying normal skin.[81, 83, 84] Lesions are usually generalized. Fissures may be the source of fatal septic events.[84] Localized lesions of the feet are rarely seen (Fig. 125–8).[85] Crusted scabies appears to be associated with HIV-neuropathy or dementia.[81] Patients with crusted scabies may be the source of epidemics of scabies in hospices and nursing homes.[83]

Treatment

Virtually all patients with a CD4-positive count over 200 cells/mm³ will respond to standard therapy with lindane. Failure to respond to lindane is seen in patients with lower CD4-positive counts with and without atypical features. There is no evidence that the mites are resistant to treatment since nonimmunosuppressed persons infected by these patients respond normally to standard treatment. Treatment failure appears to be related to immunosuppression, high mite burden, and, perhaps, associated central nervous system disease. For AIDS patient with scabies permethrin 5% lotion is initial therapy. The head and neck are also treated. Patients may require multiple treatments. Crusted scabies is extremely difficult to eradicate and may require repeated applications of scabicides for weeks to months. In addition, since patients with crusted scabies shed mite-infested scale into their environments, extensive housekeeping measures are required, including treatment of bedding, carpets, drapes, clothing, and furniture. A patient with crusted scabies should never be transferred to a hospice or long-term care facility until cure is complete, since the risk of a scabies epidemic is high.

Other Parasitic Infections

In endemic areas both visceral and disseminated cutaneous leishmaniasis may complicate HIV disease.[86-90] Visceral disease may be asymptomatic, present with hepatosplenomegaly or hematologic abnormalities, and be fatal. Skin lesions may be present. The diagnosis may be difficult because patients may have negative *Leishmania* serology and negative bone marrow examinations, but cultures of the bone marrow are positive. Disseminated cutaneous leishmaniasis presents as widespread plaques or nodules. Skin biopsy specimens demonstrate organisms. Treatment of both forms of leishmaniasis is difficult. Antimonial therapy may fail.

Disseminated strongyloidiasis (hyperinfection) rarely occurs in the setting of AIDS and other immunosuppressed states, even in endemic areas.[91-94] Patients usually have far advanced disease and another cause of immunosuppression, usually sepsis. Pneumonia is the most frequent complication, and sputum examination is often positive for larvae. Cutaneous lesions may be either generalized urticarial migratory lesions (larva currens) or periumbilical purpura.

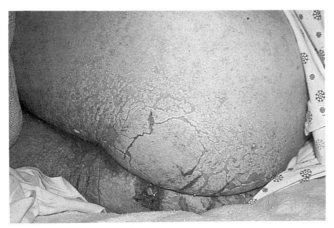

FIGURE 125–8. Norwegian scabies in AIDS.

Superficial Fungal Infections (Tinea and Candidiasis)

Clinical Description

Trichophyton rubrum causes almost all dermatophytoses in HIV-infected persons. Tinea pedis is the most common pattern in patients with asymptomatic HIV disease, usually manifested by the typical interdigital maceration and scale and by hyperkeratosis diffusely of the sole. Bullous lesions, two foot–one hand involvement, or onychomycosis is sometimes also seen. The rate of dermatophytosis is not increased in this group over control groups of athletes.[95]

Once patients develop AIDS the pattern of dermatophytosis appears to change. Dystrophy of a few or many toenails frequently occurs. Proximal subungual onychomycosis represents 90% of onychomycosis in patients with AIDS.[96] Patients with toenail onychomycosis may not have evidence of tinea elsewhere on the feet. Fingernail onychomycosis is one tenth as frequent as toenail involvement and is virtually always limited to, begins, or is worse on one hand. *Candida albicans* alone may be the cause of onychomycosis of the fingernails and should be suspected if "two feet – one hand" dermatophytosis is not seen.

Tinea cruris follows tinea pedis and onychomycosis in frequency presenting as an expanding scaling plaque of the upper thighs, with central clearing and a red, elevated border. Scrapings are mandatory in groin rashes since seborrheic dermatitis of the groin is common and may simulate tinea. Tinea corporis in the setting of HIV disease virtually always represents tinea cruris that has extended beyond the groin onto the trunk. This extensive form of tinea occurs in hot, humid climates.[97] It may be seen at all levels of immunosuppression. In severely immunosuppressed patients with AIDS lesions may have little inflammation and often lack the elevated border and central clearing typical of tinea. They are recognized as sharply marginated areas of hyperkeratosis resembling dry skin. Tinea capitis (*T. tonsurans*) in the adult and tinea facei (*T. rubrum*) can occur.

In pediatric HIV infection, candidal diaper dermatitis is frequent. *T. rubrum* may also cause eruptions in the diaper area. Tinea capitis due to *T. tonsurans* is seen in HIV-infected children.

Over 70% of women with AIDS suffer recurrent vaginal candidiasis, and it is the presenting sign in 24% of women.[98] Intermittent or prophylactic therapy is usually required.

Treatment

For uncomplicated tinea pedis, a topical imidazole or allylamine is effective. Tinea corporis, if extensive, often requires systemic therapy with oral griseofulvin, an imidazole, or an allylamine. As in non – HIV-infected persons, fingernail infection can usually be cured with 3 to 6 months of an oral agent. Toenail infection requires longer treatment. Low gastric acidity in patients with AIDS may reduce absorption of ketoconazole, decreasing efficacy.[99] For candidiasis of the intertriginous areas, drying the skin is most important. Topical nystatin or imidazoles are effective. In women, vaginal candidiasis is usually the source of groin candidiasis.

Inflammatory Cutaneous Complications of HIV Infection

During all stages of HIV infection inflammatory conditions of the skin occur. HIV infection is characterized by anergy against infection and hyperinflammation simultaneously. This is analogous to atopic patients who are at increased risk for herpes and warts in their inflamed, sensitive skin. The frequency of pruritus and inflammatory dermatoses increases as the helper T-cell count falls; most patients with severe pruritic eruptions have fewer than 200 helper T cells per cubic millimeter. HIV infection appears to facilitate the expression of conditions to which the person is predisposed. Atopic manifestations (dermatitis, sinusitis) increase as HIV disease advances.

EOSINOPHILIC FOLLICULITIS

Most patients with AIDS with a chronic, pruritic, follicular eruption of the central trunk or face have eosinophilic folliculitis. The primary lesion is an edematous, almost urticarial, follicular papule often *without* a central pustule.[100] The most common areas of involvement are the forehead, cheeks, central back, and chest (Fig. 125 – 9). The eruption classically waxes and wanes independent of treatment. It does not respond to antistaphylococcal antibiotics, but because of scratching, patients may have coexistent staphylococcal infection. The pathogenesis of eosinophilic folliculitis is unknown. Routine bacterial cultures are negative. *Demodex* is found in some lesions, and may be pathogenically related. The diagnosis is established by skin biopsy, which shows in early lesions perifollicular inflammation with eosinophils at the level of the sebaceous glands extending into the surrounding dermis and in late lesions an intrafollicular abscess with many eosinophils. Treatment options include class I topical corticosteroids, antihistamines, ultraviolet B (UVB) light or psoralens and ultraviolet A light (PUVA) phototherapy,[101] and itraconazole.[102] Many patients require maintenance therapy.

INSECT BITE REACTIONS

Hypersensitivity to insect bites is extremely common in HIV disease.[103, 104] Patients note exaggerated and per-

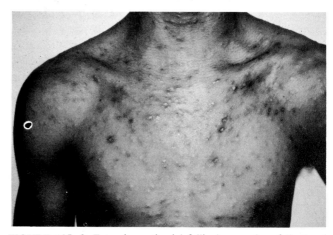

FIGURE 125–9. Extensive urticarial follicular papules of the trunk characteristic of eosinophilic folliculitis.

sistent lesions after bites of potentially sensitizing insects. Mosquitoes probably represent a common cause of pruritic papular eruptions found on exposed sites, especially the arms, legs, and face. Other causes of pruritic papules can be ruled out by a skin biopsy. Treatment consists of the extermination of biting insects from the patient's environment, insect repellents and clothing to deter the insects, topical corticosteroids to the individual lesions, and chronic potent antihistamines to reduce the hypersensitivity. Intralesional triamcinolone may be used in persistent lesions.

GRANULOMA ANNULARE

Granuloma annulare can occur at all stages of HIV disease. Three patterns of granuloma annulare are seen in HIV disease: typical localized lesions, in sun-exposed areas only (actinic granuloma), and, frequently, generalized granuloma annulare.[105] Generalized granuloma annulare is relatively more common in HIV disease and is not associated with diabetes mellitus.

ANETODERMA

Anetoderma is not an uncommon finding in HIV-infected persons and is usually seen in early HIV disease.[106] A preceding inflammatory condition may or may not exist. It may be an autoimmune phenomenon of early HIV disease.

PAPULAR MUCINOSIS

In advanced HIV disease, patients may present with small noninflammatory papules of the trunk or extremities.[107] On biopsy, scant inflammation and increased amounts of hyaluronic acid in the mid-dermis are seen. A paraprotein spike is not usually found. Scleromyxedema and visceral involvement is rare.

Drug Reactions

Clinical Description

The frequency of drug reactions is increased in HIV-infected patients, especially to certain medications: trimethoprim-sulfamethoxazole (37%–45%), antituberculosis regimens (10%), and amoxicillin-clavulanate.[108] Patients with AIDS receiving trimethoprim-sulfamethoxazole as treatment or prophylaxis for *Pneumocystis* pneumonia have a higher rate of reaction than similarly treated HIV-negative immunosuppressed patients. Patients with AIDS have more frequent reactions if their CD4 count is less than 200 cells/mm³. The rate of reaction is dose dependent and increased in certain groups (e.g., white patients with AIDS have more frequent reac-

tions to trimethoprim-sulfamethoxazole than African, Haitian, and African-American patients with AIDS). This suggests that not only immune status but also other genetically determined factors such as drug metabolism are pathogenically related to drug reactions in the setting of HIV.

Most adverse reactions in HIV disease occur to antibiotics, especially sulfonamides. The patterns of cutaneous reactions to medications that are increased in HIV-infected persons are morbilliform reactions, fixed drug reactions, erythema multiforme major (Stevens-Johnson syndrome), and toxic epidermal necrolysis. Morbilliform drug reactions usually begin during the second week of treatment. Pruritus is usually moderate to severe, necessitating discontinuation of the offending medication in about 20% of patients. In those in whom the eruption is mild and controllable with topical and systemic therapy, the medication may be continued to the end of the course. No maculopapular drug reaction has converted to a more severe form *during the same course of treatment*. Rechallenge with the drug at a later date may, however, result in a more severe reaction (e.g., Stevens-Johnson syndrome). Desensitization can be considered if the medication is required.[109] A small subset of patients with AIDS have multiple, sequential, morbilliform reactions to unrelated medications.[110] Some of these patients will have ascendingly severe reactions with each exposure, which may culminate in Stevens-Johnson syndrome or toxic epidermal necrolysis.

Fixed drug reactions are most frequently seen with trimethoprim-sulfamethoxazole and can be to either component. Most HIV-infected patients with Stevens-Johnson syndrome or toxic epidermal necrolysis have AIDS. Long-acting sulfonamides are the most common cause. Most patients with Stevens-Johnson syndrome survive, but the mortality in toxic epidermal necrolysis in patients with HIV infection is about 50%.

Foscarnet causes penile ulcerations, most commonly in uncircumcised patients. It appears to be a direct toxic effect of the medication.[111] Zidovudine causes pigmentation of the nails and oral mucosa, especially in pigmented races.[112] The nail pigmentation appears as blue lunulae, as longitudinal pigmented bands, or as diffuse blue or black pigmentation. It is dose dependent and resolves with discontinuation of the medication. The oral mucosa is pigmented on the lateral tongue most commonly, but the buccal mucosa is also pigmented. Similar oral hyperpigmentation may be seen in the setting of HIV infection without zidovudine administration. In all cases the pigment is due to increased melanin deposition.

Eczematous Eruptions

When viewed as a group, HIV-infected patients, especially those with CD4 counts less than 200 cells/mm³ have elevated levels of IgE.[113] This may be related to a change in the cytokine environment of advanced disease with a decrease in the capacity to produce interleukin-2

(TH1 pattern) and an increase in interleukin-4 and interleukin-10 (TH2 pattern). TH2-derived cytokines stimulate IgE production by B cells and down-regulate TH1-type responses.[114] It is unknown if the elevated IgE and sometimes eosinophilia seen in advanced HIV disease is related to atopy, the presence of skin disease, or as a reaction to infectious agents or medications.

Dry skin (xerosis, asteatosis) is extremely common in HIV disease, especially AIDS. The cause is unknown. Dry skin frequently accompanies or is the basis for eczematous eruptions. In addition, in AIDS patients, any pruritic eruption may induce scratching and secondary eczematous eruptions of the skin, so eczematous plaques may accompany scabies, staphylococcal folliculitis, or eosinophilic folliculitis.

ATOPIC DERMATITIS

Atopic eczema is common in children with HIV disease. In addition, in HIV-infected adults atopic dermatitis may appear in those with a prior history of atopy (allergic rhinitis, asthma).[115]

ASTEATOTIC ECZEMA (DRY SKIN ECZEMA, WINTER ITCH)

The underlying xerosis of HIV disease is a major cause of pruritus as it is in the geriatric population. Many HIV-infected patients bathe excessively, either to prevent folliculitis or to soothe their itching skin. There may be little erythema. The skin is slightly scaly and shiny. Small fissures filled with fine crusts may be seen on the most severely affected areas. These fissures characteristically form small (0.5–1.0 cm) circles. Untreated xerotic eczema may progress to nummular dermatitis.

NUMMULAR DERMATITIS

In HIV disease, nummular dermatitis is usually a consequence of atopic dermatitis, xerotic eczema, or seborrheic dermatitis and appears similar in HIV infection as in the normal population. Secondary infection with *S. aureus* is often present.

ATYPICAL SEBORRHEIC DERMATITIS

An unusual form of seborrheic dermatitis seen in HIV infection is a pattern resembling nummular eczema. The seborrhea spills down the central back and chest, forming confluent plaques and down the forearms as scattered annular lesions. Itching is more severe than with typical seborrhea. The diagnosis is made by the distribution and confirmed histologically if necessary.

Photosensitivity

Photosensitivity in various forms is extremely common in HIV-infected persons, despite the scant reports in the literature.[116]

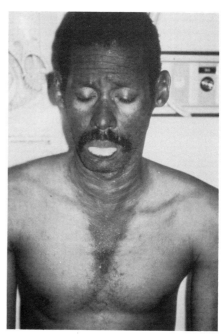

FIGURE 125–10. Photosensitivity (chronic actinic dermatitis) in AIDS.

PHOTODERMATITIS

HIV-infected patients may develop dermatitis from ultraviolet light exposure due to medications (drug-induced photosensitivity) or as polymorphous light eruption or actinic prurigo (with prurigo nodularis). Chronic actinic dermatitis may develop. Histologically, most patients with photosensitivity have features of chronic spongiotic dermatitis or polymorphous light eruption. Occasionally lichen planus– or lichen nitidus–like patterns are seen. Except for the lichen nitidus–like pattern, which is not related to medication, the other forms of photodermatitis can be drug induced. The most frequent offending medications are sulfonamides and nonsteroidal anti-inflammatory agents. Many patients are sensitive only to UVB, but some also have UVA sensitivity and require more broad sun protection. Black men with CD4 counts of less than 50 cells/mm³ are at particular risk for chronic actinic dermatitis (Fig. 125–10).

PORPHYRIA CUTANEA TARDA

Porphyria cutanea tarda is the most common form of porphyria. It is expressed in persons with hepatocellular injury from alcohol and infectious hepatitis. HIV-infected persons with the genetic tendency and these risk factors also develop porphyria cutanea tarda. Porphyria cutanea tarda in HIV disease is typical and responds identically to therapy.

ACNE ROSACEA

Rosacea occurs in both children and adults with HIV.[117] In some patients it may be severe and difficult to manage. Oral metronidazole may be beneficial in refractory cases that fail topical measures and tetracyclines.

Papulosquamous Eruptions

Papulosquamous eruptions are very common in HIV-infected persons. Seborrheic dermatitis, the most common, is seen in up to 80% of patients with AIDS. It does not appear to be related to overgrowth of *Pityrosporum ovale.*[118] Whether the other papulosquamous diseases are increased in HIV disease is unknown, but 1% to 2% of HIV-infected persons have psoriasis and 0.5% to 1.7% have Reiter's syndrome, usually in an incomplete form.[119, 120] The three papulosquamous disorders form a spectrum of disease, and patients may be found at any point along the disease continuum.[121]

SEBORRHEIC DERMATITIS

Seborrhea usually affects hair-bearing areas, especially the scalp, eyebrows, moustache, and beard, as well as the nasolabial fold and behind and in the ears. Involvement of the axillae and groin are not uncommon (Fig. 125–11). Red, nonscaling patches with no central clearing and involvement of the scrotum and penis are characteristic. Lesions may extend from the scalp onto the central back and mid chest. Pruritus is variable; it is usually absent or mild, but it occasionally is severe on the scalp. Standard therapy is usually effective.

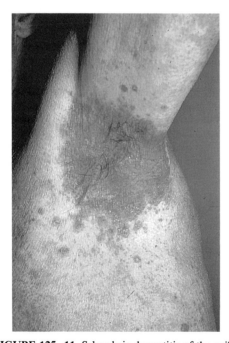

FIGURE 125–11. Seborrheic dermatitis of the axilla.

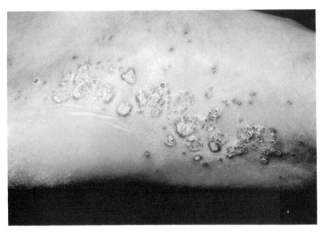

FIGURE 125–12. Keratotic pustular lesions of the side of the sole in HIV-associated psoriasis.

PSORIASIS

Psoriasis is seen in HIV-infected persons with at least as great a frequency as the general population (1%–2%). About one third of persons with psoriasis and HIV have clinical evidence of psoriasis before HIV infection, and two thirds note skin lesions only after they are HIV infected.[120] This suggests that HIV permits or enhances expression of psoriasis in an at-risk person. HIV-infected persons with psoriasis often have either HLA-B27 or a B27 cross-reactive CREG antigen.[121] All clinical patterns of psoriasis may be seen in HIV-infected persons, but axillary and groin involvement (inverse pattern) and palm and sole involvement (similar to Reiter's syndrome) seem to be especially common (Fig. 125–12).[120]

HIV-associated psoriasis is clinically similar to psoriasis seen in uninfected persons. Factors that exacerbate common psoriasis may flare HIV-associated psoriasis as well (i.e., streptococcal colonization or infection of the throat and certain medications, such as lithium and beta-blockers). HIV-associated psoriasis may flare severely in association with staphylococcal sepsis, and in any HIV-infected person with sudden worsening of psoriasis this must be considered, even if the patient does not appear severely ill.[122]

Psoriasis may appear at any stage of HIV disease and may worsen as HIV disease progresses. Most patients with HIV disease and severe psoriasis seem to have more advanced HIV disease. About 10% of HIV-infected patients with psoriasis have some joint involvement. This is higher than in non–HIV-infected persons with psoriasis. The arthritis seen in HIV-infected patients with psoriasis is similar to the joint disease seen in psoriasis unassociated with HIV disease.

Treatment of psoriasis in patients with HIV disease uses standard modalities. Zidovudine, but not didanosine or zalcitabine (DDI or DDC), improves psoriasis and may be added or increased as a part of psoriasis treatment.[123] Etretinate is safe and effective. When topical measures fail, UVB alone or in combination with tar (Goeckermann regimen) or PUVA is useful. The risk of ultraviolet light exposure in HIV-infected persons is unknown, but only in vitro activation of HIV by ultraviolet light has been documented. Light therapy has not seemed to enhance HIV expression in HIV-infected persons.[124] Immunosuppressive agents such as methotrexate and cyclosporine must be considered experimental in the setting of HIV disease and are of potentially high risk.

REITER'S SYNDROME

The characteristic skin lesions of Reiter's syndrome, keratoderma blenorrhagica and circinate balanitis, may be seen in HIV-infected persons in association with arthritis, urethritis, and conjunctivitis. Most patients have only some of these features at one time (incomplete Reiter's syndrome). Persons with Reiter's syndrome and HIV disease are HLA-B27 positive between 30% and 70% of the time. The arthritis of HIV-associated psoriasis and Reiter's syndrome may be quite difficult to manage. Etretinate and sulfasalazine have anecdotally been reported as useful.

PITYRIASIS RUBRA PILARIS

Rare cases of pityriasis rubra pilaris have been reported in HIV disease.[125-127] Typical cases with widespread red scaling plaques may be seen. Many cases, however, have marked follicular plugging, giving the patient a lichen spinulosus–like appearance.[128, 129] Unique to HIV-associated pityriasis rubra pilaris, and perhaps caused by the marked follicular plugging, is the simultaneous onset of severe cystic acne with pityriasis rubra pilaris.[126-129]

Oral Manifestations of HIV Disease

HIV-associated oral findings are common and may be early markers of HIV infection. Both oral candidiasis and oral hairy leukoplakia are predictors of more rapid progression to AIDS.[130]

ORAL CANDIDIASIS

Thrush affects most HIV-infected persons at some time during the course of their disease. The most common pattern is the pseudomembranous type. The erythematous or atrophic type appearing as denuded red areas may be seen alone or in combination with the more common pattern. Angular cheilitis (perlèche) often accompanies oral thrush. Candidiasis may extend into the posterior pharynx and down the esophagus. Candidal esophagitis is the most common cause of dysphagia in HIV disease and is an AIDS-defining illness.

Treatment options for oropharyngeal candidiasis include clotrimazole troches or vaginal suppositories; nystatin suspension, lozenges, or vaginal pastilles; and systemic imidazoles. Higher-dose products are better for active disease. For candidiasis the efficacy of oral imidazoles appears to be fluconazole→ketoconazole→itraconazole. Recurrence within 3 months is universal in all patients with CD4 counts less than 200 cells/mm³. Prophylaxis with topical or systemic agents may be required. Increasing numbers of imidazole-resistant cases are being reported, due most frequently to *C. glabrata,* and *C. kruseii,*[131] but also to *C. albicans.* The treatment is amphotericin B.

ORAL HAIRY LEUKOPLAKIA

Oral hairy leukoplakia is caused by Epstein-Barr virus infection of the oral epithelium.[132] It presents as adherent corrugated white plaques on the lateral aspects of the tongue. Lesions may extend onto the dorsum or ventral surface of the tongue and less commonly on other mucosal surfaces. The typical corrugated pattern is not seen at other sites, and a biopsy may be required to establish the diagnosis. Lesions are usually asymptomatic and do not require therapy. A single application of 25% podophyllin for 30 seconds to 1 minute, topical retinoic acid twice daily, and high doses of oral acyclovir are effective treatments.[133] Recurrence is expected. Oral hairy leukoplakia is occasionally seen in other immunosuppressed persons.[134] Lesions identical to oral hairy leukoplakia (pseudo-oral hairy leukoplakia) have been reported in nonimmunosuppressed persons.[135] These do not contain Epstein-Barr virus, however.

RECURRENT APHTHOUS ULCERATION

HIV-infected persons may develop recurrent aphthous ulceration at any stage of HIV disease. Lesions may be of the minor, major, or herpetiform types.[136, 137] Involvement of the posterior pharynx and esophagus may cause dysphagia. In most cases the clinical morphology is typical and lesions are smaller than infectious ulcerations. Larger lesions should be cultured for herpes simplex; and if lesions persist or are atypical, they should be sampled. Potent topical corticosteroid ointments, intralesional corticosteroids, steroid oral suspension (dexamethasone [Decadron]), and systemic steroids are effective. These therapies should be accompanied by good oral hygiene and anticandidal prophylaxis.

HIV Salivary Gland Disease (Sicca Syndrome)

A small subset of adult and pediatric HIV-infected patients early in disease develop swelling of the salivary glands, especially the parotid glands.[138, 139] This may be accompanied by symptoms of dry mouth (xerostomia) and lymphocytic interstitial pneumonitis. These patients have increased CD8 counts. Biopsy of the salivary glands shows lymphocytic infiltrates identical to those of Sjögren's syndrome. Unlike sporadic Sjögren's syndrome, HIV-infected patients with this condition have HLA-DR5 or DR6 whereas those with sporadic Sjögren's syndrome have HLA-B8, or DR2, DR3, DR4, or DRw52.[138] Patients with HIV salivary gland disease are at lower risk for progression to AIDS but have a high risk of lymphoma.

Other oral findings in HIV include mucosal warts, molluscum contagiosum, periodontal disease, histoplasmosis, cryptococcosis, herpes simplex, herpes zoster, Kaposi's sarcoma, lymphoma, and squamous cell carcinoma.[140]

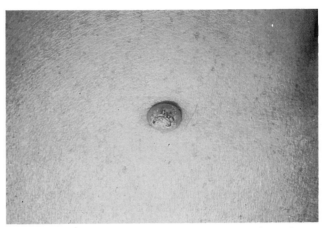

FIGURE 125-13. Squamous cell carcinoma resembling a keratoacanthoma in an HIV-infected man.

Inflammatory Vascular Complications of HIV Disease

Although uncommon, vasculitis may complicate HIV infection, even during the asymptomatic phase. Small vessel vasculitis presenting as palpable purpura or Henoch-Schönlein purpura may occur in adults or children.[141, 142] Systemic vasculitis involving arteries resembling polyarteritis nodosa or lymphomatoid granulomatosis can also be seen. Erythema elevatum diutinum, presenting as vascular or fibrotic nodules with characteristic histology, has been reported.[142, 143] The vascular nodules closely resemble Kaposi's sarcoma or bacillary angiomatosis. The vascular nodules, but not the fibrotic ones, respond to dapsone therapy.

Neoplastic Complications of HIV Disease

NONMELANOMA SKIN CANCER

Basal cell carcinomas are extremely common in HIV-infected white men, occurring in nearly 5% of whites in one cohort in a 3-year period.[144] They are most frequently located on the trunk and are commonly of the superficial type. Treatment is by standard modalities with similar cure rates.[145] Squamous cell carcinomas in sun-exposed sites are seen in the setting of HIV disease (Fig. 125-13). Patients with squamous cell carcinomas in general have had greater sun exposure than those with basal cell carcinomas. Unlike renal transplant patients, the ratio of squamous cell carcinoma to basal cell carcinoma is not reversed in most HIV-infected persons.[145] Genital squamous cell carcinomas of the rectum in homosexual men and of the cervix in women who are HIV infected are increased.[146-148] These are related to human papillomavirus infection, analogous to cervical cancer in the immunocompetent population. In the setting of HIV infection, however, the progression from human papillomavirus infection to dysplasia and then to carcinoma appears accelerated.[147, 148]

MELANOMA

There are scattered reports of malignant melanoma in the setting of HIV disease.[149] It has been suggested that there is a diminished host response in comparison to melanomas in immunocompetent persons. Melanoma may have a worse prognosis in the setting of HIV disease. The sudden onset of atypical nevi has been reported in HIV infection, but it has not been associated with the development of melanoma.[150]

KAPOSI'S SARCOMA

In 1872, Moritz Kaposi described five elderly patients with idiopathic multiple pigmented sarcoma, later designated Kaposi's sarcoma.[151] During the following century, this unusual tumor was also described in isolated, endemic African populations and among immunosuppressed organ transplant recipients.[152] In 1981, Kaposi's sarcoma emerged from relative obscurity as a predominant feature of the AIDS epidemic.[153, 154] The study of Kaposi's sarcoma in patients with AIDS has had a profound impact on our understanding of this fascinating tumor.[155, 156]

Epidemiology

The descriptive epidemiology of Kaposi's sarcoma has been outlined in four relatively distinct populations (Table 125-1). Classic Kaposi's sarcoma is primarily a skin disease of the lower extremities affecting predominantly elderly men of Mediterranean, East European, or

TABLE 125-1. Epidemiology of Kaposi's Sarcoma Variants

Type	Population at Risk	Age at Onset (years)	Male:Female Ratio
Classic	Persons of Eastern European Jewish and Mediterranean backgrounds	50–80	10–15:1
Endemic Africa			
1. Benign nodular	Black African adults	25–40	17:1
2. Aggressive	Black African adults	25–40	17:1
3. Florid	Black African adults	25–40	17:1
4. Lymphadenopathic	Black African children	2–15 (mean: 3)	3:1
Iatrogenic immunosuppression	Patients on azathioprine, cyclosporine, and corticosteroids; renal transplant recipients; those with systemic lupus erythematosus; those with temporal arteritis	20–60 (mean: 42)	2.3:1
Epidemic AIDS-related	Homosexual men (95%); other risk groups (5%)	18–65 (mean: 37)	106:1

From Friedman-Kien AE. Color Atlas of AIDS. Philadelphia: WB Saunders Co., 1989:44.

Jewish heritage.[156, 157] The disease course is typically indolent, with patients surviving an average of 10 to 15 years before dying of unrelated causes; secondary malignancies (primarily lymphomas) develop in more than one third of cases.[158, 159] African-endemic Kaposi's sarcoma has been described in two age groups: (1) young adults with generally benign cutaneous nodular disease but sometimes aggressive or florid disease fatal within 5 to 8 years and (2) young children with fulminant lymphadenopathic disease, typically fatal within 2 to 3 years.[160] Iatrogenic, immunosuppressive drug-associated Kaposi's sarcoma is frequently seen among organ transplant recipients, accounting for 3.4% of all neoplasms (with an average of 16.5 months after transplantation[161]). Spontaneous remission after discontinuation of immunosuppressive therapy may occur.[162] Kaposi's sarcoma associated with AIDS occurs predominantly among homosexual men (Table 125–2).

Additional epidemiologic features suggest that Kaposi's sarcoma in AIDS is caused by a sexually transmissible infectious agent more likely to induce vascular lesions with advancing immunosuppression (Table 125–3).[163, 164] Early in the AIDS epidemic, as many as 60% of homosexual men with AIDS developed Kaposi's sarcoma, and this population is still the most likely to develop AIDS-associated Kaposi's sarcoma.[163] In addition to finding an increased risk of developing AIDS-

associated Kaposi's sarcoma with an increasing number of sex partners, some investigators have found the risk of developing AIDS-associated Kaposi's sarcoma to increase with a prior history of oropharyngeal gonorrhea and with increasing contact with a sex partner's feces through oral-anal contact ("rimming").[156, 164–166]

Since the onset of the AIDS epidemic, there has been a gradual decline in the proportion of HIV-infected homosexual men presenting with AIDS-associated Kaposi's sarcoma, suggesting that changes in sexual behavior and sexual practices may have reduced the risk of Kaposi's sarcoma for men not already infected with both HIV and the proposed Kaposi's sarcoma agent.[156, 164] Nevertheless, Kaposi's sarcoma remains a major clinical manifestation of AIDS in the United States, accounting for more than 15% of all AIDS diagnoses reported to the Centers for Disease Control and Prevention.[163, 164] A sexually transmissible Kaposi's sarcoma agent may also account for increasing reports of Kaposi's sarcoma among young, HIV-negative homosexual men at increased risk for acquiring HIV infection.[156, 167]

Despite these epidemiologic clues, a causative agent of Kaposi's sarcoma has not been identified. During the past 2 decades, several studies have implicated CMV and other herpesviruses as possible co-factors for the development of Kaposi's sarcoma, but no consistent association has been established.[156] Recent studies suggest that

TABLE 125-2. Percentage of Adult Patients with AIDS with Kaposi's Sarcoma by HIV Transmission Group and Sex—United States

HIV Transmission Group	Sex	No. of Patients with Kaposi's Sarcoma/Total	%
Homosexual/bisexual	M	24,160/122,170	19.8
Homosexual/bisexual and intravenous drug user	M	2,244/13,094	17.1
Born in Caribbean/Africa	M	110/1,849	6.0
	F	27/741	3.6
Heterosexual partner of person born in Caribbean/Africa	M	6/97	6.2
	F	4/78	5.1
Injecting drug user	M	909/33,276	2.7
	F	192/10,608	1.8
Blood transfusion	M	98/2,689	3.6
	F	35/1,647	2.1
Hemophilia	M	19/1,717	1.1

From Peterman TA, Jaffe HW, Beral V. Epidemiologic clues to the etiology of Kaposi's sarcoma. AIDS 1993;7:605–611.

TABLE 125-3. Summary of Epidemiologic Characteristics of the Kaposi's Sarcoma Agent

Factor	Comment
Incubation period	Usually remains silent until immunosuppression develops; then lesions develop within a few months to a few years.
Percentage of infected persons who develop disease	Sixty to 80% among homosexual men with AIDS; unknown with other types of immunosuppression. Most infection is likely to be asymptomatic.
Period of communicability	Unknown
Portal of entry	Unknown, probably genital or rectal mucosa; possibly fecal-oral.
Transmissibility	
Sexual	Most common mode of transmission, but probably less than HIV because prevalence is declining in the presence of increasing HIV prevalence.
Blood	Much less than HIV: 15%–20% of blood recipients with AIDS received blood from donors who developed Kaposi's sarcoma, but only 2% of recipients developed Kaposi's sarcoma.
Factor concentrate	Very rare, if at all; much less than HIV. Among the HIV transmission groups, hemophiliacs have the highest risk of HIV infection.
Perinatal	Some transmission has occurred. Rates are unknown.

From Peterman TA, Jaffe HW, Beral V. Epidemiologic clues to the etiology of Kaposi's sarcoma. AIDS 1993;7:605–611.

human papillomavirus may play a role, but the virus is only present in a minority of cases.[168, 169]

Clinical Description

Classic Kaposi's sarcoma is predominantly a cutaneous disease of the lower extremities, although lymph node and visceral disease may occur. Iatrogenic Kaposi's sarcoma is primarily a cutaneous complication of immunosuppressive drug therapy. African-endemic Kaposi's sarcoma presents in one of four clinically distinct patterns: (1) benign nodular cutaneous disease mimicking the classic form of the disease; (2) aggressive localized cutaneous disease invading soft tissue and bone; (3) florid mucocutaneous and visceral disease; and (4) lymphadenopathic disease, rapidly disseminating to lymph nodes and visceral organs, usually in the absence of skin disease. AIDS-associated Kaposi's sarcoma is characterized by a broad clinical disease spectrum with overlapping features of all patterns of the non–AIDS-associated disease; therefore, the following discussion will focus on the clinical presentation of the AIDS-associated form.

Presentation. Although Kaposi's sarcoma may first appear at any stage of HIV disease,[170] fewer than one sixth of patients with AIDS and Kaposi's sarcoma present with CD4 counts exceeding 500 cells/mm³.[156] Common cutaneous sites include the oral cavity, face, trunk, penis, and the lower extremities. Approximately 50% of patients with cutaneous lesions will develop lymph node disease.[171, 172]

Cutaneous lesions may arise singly or multiply at any site. New lesions may develop rapidly over a few days, frequently in a symmetrical distribution. The progression of each individual lesion is unpredictable, and lesions in one area may involve while similar lesions at more distant sites may enlarge. The progression of the disorder roughly correlates with the overall activity of the patient's HIV disease; patients with aggressive AIDS-associated Kaposi's sarcoma generally have symptomatic HIV infection with CD4 counts below 200 cells/mm³.[173, 174]

Macular, Papular, and Nodular Lesions. Macular lesions are faint, are red to purple, and vary from several millimeters to several centimeters. These lesions are usually asymptomatic and are frequently seen on the soles of the feet, the hard palate, and the tip of the nose. Macular lesions are rarely accompanied by edema. Papular lesions of the face are usually oval and less than 1 cm in size; papular lesions on the nose may expand, forming large plaques covering the entire nasal bridge. Lesions on the neck, trunk, and lower extremities are typically papular and oblong, following skin tension lines (Fig. 125–14).

Lesions of the gums, hard palate, and distal extremities may progress from macules and papules to form exophytic friable nodules (Figs. 125–15 and 125–16). Confluence of leg lesions frequently results in painful, edematous, ulcerative disease. Pseudomonas and anaerobic bacteria may colonize chronically ulcerated lesions. Penile lesions are characterized by papules and nodules

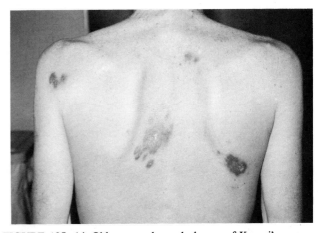

FIGURE 125–14. Oblong papules and plaques of Kaposi's sarcoma following skin tension lines.

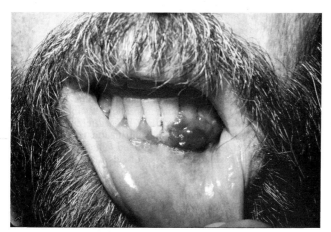

FIGURE 125–15. Gingival infiltration by Kaposi's sarcoma.

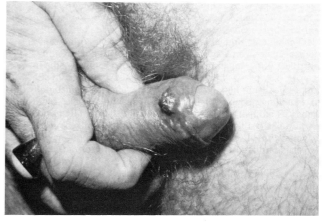

FIGURE 125–17. Papulonodular lesion of Kaposi's sarcoma on the penis.

often accompanied by edema (Fig. 125–17). Trauma or prior cutaneous disease may give rise to Kaposi's sarcoma (Koebner's phenomenon).[156, 175] Subcutaneous nodules in the absence of overlying dermal disease are uncommon.

Plaques and Lymphatic Disease. AIDS-associated Kaposi's sarcoma of the distal extremities may present as grouped papules expanding peripherally and forming large plaques (Fig. 125–18). Lymphatic involvement may occur at any site but is most commonly seen in the inguinal region, giving the skin a doughy or woody texture, with or without overlying cutaneous lesions. Extensive lymphatic infiltration may lead to severe cutaneous and subcutaneous complications, including severe pain, maceration, and ulceration. Even without extensive lymphatic infiltration, lymph node involvement may cause edema of the genitalia and intermittent or chronic edema of the lower extremities.

Mucocutaneous and Ocular Lesions. Among patients with AIDS-associated Kaposi's sarcoma, oral lesions are the clinical manifestation among 22% of patients and oral lesions arise concomitantly with skin lesions among 45% of patients.[176, 177] The palate is the most common site for oral disease, which occurs in about 50% of patients. Oral AIDS-associated Kaposi's sarcoma may be a

marker for more advanced HIV infection, because patients with this condition usually present with CD4 counts below 200 cells/mm³.[178] Kaposi's sarcoma involving ocular adnexal structures is reported to occur in up to 20% of patients; benign lesions of the conjuctiva are the most common site of ocular involvement.[179] Periorbital edema may be present in conjunction with periocular lesions.

Visceral Lesions. Visceral lesions are extremely common among patients with AIDS-associated Kaposi's sarcoma. Postmortem studies suggest that less than 25% of these patients have lesions limited to skin or mucosae.[172, 180] Although usually asymptomatic, common sites of visceral involvement include the lungs, bowel, liver, and spleen. Visceral lesions may also be found in the pharynx, heart, bone marrow, genitourinary tract, brain, kidney, and adrenal glands.[156] Death can be attrib-

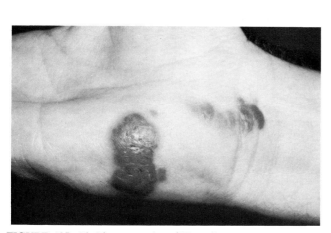

FIGURE 125–16. Linear papules of Kaposi's sarcoma on the wrist and palm.

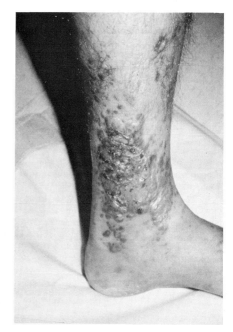

FIGURE 125–18. Characteristic coalescent papules forming a plaque of Kaposi's sarcoma on the leg.

uted to visceral disease in 10% to 20% of patients with AIDS-associated Kaposi's sarcoma.[180]

Pathology

The three histologic stages of Kaposi's sarcoma are patch, plaque, and nodular disease. These patterns often correlate with the clinical appearance of lesions.[156, 181] Patch-stage disease occurs in the reticular dermis of macules. There is proliferation of small, irregular and jagged endothelial-lined spaces lined by cytologically bland spindled cells surrounding normal dermal vessels and adnexal structures. A normal vessel or adnexal structure protruding into an ectatic vascular space (promontory sign) is a hallmark for patch-stage disease. Plaque-stage disease, the histologic correlate for some papules and plaques, is a spindle-celled vascular process that permeates dermal collagen bundles, forming irregular, cleft-like, angulated vascular channels containing erythrocytes. Periodic acid–Schiff-positive, diastase-resistant, eosinophilic hyaline globules representing degenerating erythrocytes are found within cells of the plaque and nodular stages. Nodular-stage lesions correspond to nodules and some papules. These lesions are composed of sheets and fascicles of spindled cells with mild to moderate cytologic atypia, single cell necrosis, and trapped erythrocytes within an extensive network of slit-like vascular spaces. All three patterns are usually accompanied by an inflammatory lymphocytic infiltrate with or without plasma cells.

The histologic differential diagnosis for cutaneous Kaposi's sarcoma includes targetoid hemosiderotic hemangioma, benign lymphangioendothelioma, acro-angiodermatitis, cutaneous angiosarcoma, spindle cell hemangioendothelioma, angiolipoma, aneurysmal fibrous histiocytoma, bacillary angiomatosis, and scar.

Pathogenesis

The cell of origin of Kaposi's sarcoma remains elusive. Studies suggest that the disease may arise from mesenchymal cells of vascular or lymphatic endothelium, factor XIIIa–expressing dermal dendrocytes, or vascular smooth muscle cells expressing α-actin.[156, 171, 182] Immunophenotypic studies show that the spindle cells that actually line vascular spaces in Kaposi's sarcoma are endothelial. Cell culture lines derived from tissues of patients with the classic form and the AIDS-associated form have identical cytochemical and molecular properties,[183] suggesting a common etiology for Kaposi's sarcoma regardless of the population at risk for disease.

Laboratory studies suggest that long-term growth of Kaposi's sarcoma–derived cell cultures obtained from patients with AIDS-associated lesions is facilitated by the HIV *tat* gene product (Tat) and by cytokines demonstrating both autocrine and paracrine function produced by retrovirally infected cells, such as fibroblast growth factors, tumor necrosis factor–α, interleukin-1, interleukin-6, and oncostatin M.[184, 185] Oncostatin M, a cytokine produced by activated T lymphocytes, appears to be the major cytokine responsible for maintaining the long-term growth of AIDS-associated Kaposi's sarcoma cells in culture.[185-187] Transgenic mice containing both the HIV transactivating gene (*tat*) and the long terminal repeat sequence, which controls the viral regulatory region of the HIV genome, provide evidence for a direct role for HIV in the development of AIDS-associated Kaposi's sarcoma.[188] These mice produce both male and female offspring expressing *tat* messenger RNA (mRNA), and 15% of male offspring develop vascular spindle cell tumors suggestive of patch-type Kaposi's sarcoma and lacking *tat* mRNA expression. Finally, DNA hybridization studies demonstrate the presence of HIV RNA transcripts in tissues of patients with AIDS-associated disease.[189]

Differential Diagnosis

Clinical lesions that can mimic AIDS-associated Kaposi's sarcoma include dermatofibroma, hemangioma, scar, bacillary angiomatosis, acroangiodermatis, pyogenic granuloma, ruptured epidermoid cysts, postinflammatory hyperpigmentation, prurigo nodularis, blue nevi, malignant melanoma, and cutaneous lymphoma.[156] These lesions are easily distinguished histopathologically.

Treatment

No cure for AIDS-associated Kaposi's sarcoma exists, and palliative therapy, either alone or in combination with zidovudine antiviral therapy, has not been shown to prolong survival.[156] In addition, because the majority of patients with AIDS-associated Kaposi's sarcoma die of opportunistic infection rather than from Kaposi's sarcoma, the primary goal of treatment is to provide safe and effective palliation. Specific indications for treatment include cosmetic control of disfiguring Kaposi's sarcoma lesions, shrinkage of problematic oral lesions, abatement of pain and edema associated with lymphadenopathy or extensive cutaneous disease, and alleviation of symptomatic visceral disease.

The dermatologist is capable of treating many patients, because most patients present with cutaneous lesions amenable to common dermatologic therapies, including cryotherapy, intralesional therapy, and simple excision (Table 125–4). Standardized staging criteria for Kaposi's sarcoma[190] can help the clinician to determine the subset of patients requiring more aggressive local therapy, such as with radiation, or systemic therapies, such as interferon alfa or antineoplastic chemotherapy.[156, 191] In general, local therapies are effective for patients with a "good risk" staging classification.

Local Treatment. Several local modalities have been evaluated for the control of AIDS-associated Kaposi's sarcoma. Clinicians administering cryotherapy, intralesional injections, radiation therapy, and laser treatments to these patients should take precautions to prevent unnecessary exposure to HIV, as well as potential side effects associated with these modalities.[156, 192-194]

TABLE 125-4. Treatment of AIDS-associated Kaposi's Sarcoma

Limited Intervention	Aggressive Intervention
Local therapy	Single-agent chemotherapy
Radiation therapy	Doxorubicin
Liquid nitrogen	Vinblastine
Intralesional therapy	Etoposide
Surgery	Multiagent chemotherapy
Interferon alfa	Vincristine/vinblastine
Interferon alfa + zidovudine	Doxorubicin + vincristine + bleomycin

Adapted from Kahn JO. AIDS-associated Kaposi's sarcoma. In: Volberding PA, Jacobson MA, eds. AIDS Clinical Review 1990. New York: Marcel Dekker, 1990:121. Reprinted by courtesy of Marcel Dekker, Inc.

Cryotherapy. Among patients with limited numbers of macular and papular lesions, liquid nitrogen cryotherapy has demonstrated an 85% complete or partial clinical response rate following an average of three treatments.[156, 192] Cosmetic improvement is a direct consequence of acceptable superficial scarring that camouflages persistent Kaposi's sarcoma in the reticular dermis.

Intralesional Therapy. Intralesional antineoplastic chemotherapy of cutaneous Kaposi's sarcoma with vinblastine or vincristine has demonstrated complete or partial clinical response rates of up to 88%.[156, 195] Visibly recurrent disease is seen in approximately 40% of lesions within 6 months after therapy. Although experience is limited, iontophoresis with 1% vinblastine has shown similar results to that of intralesional therapy in five patients with AIDS-associated disease.[196] Advantages of intralesional chemotherapy over cryotherapy include higher response rates for papulonodular lesions greater than 1 cm in diameter and the ability to treat symptomatic oral lesions to reduce pain and to prevent ulceration and bleeding.

A variety of other agents have also shown promise when administered by the intralesional route. Approximately 85% of nodular intraoral lesions will also respond to intralesional sclerotherapy with 3% sodium tetradecyl sulfate.[197] Intralesional interferon alfa has demonstrated similar results.[155, 198] Intralesional therapy with tumor necrosis factor$-\alpha$ and recombinant granulocyte-macrophage colony–stimulating factor are also effective[199, 200]; however, the former is associated with significant local and systemic side effects and the latter has not been systematically evaluated.

Radiation Therapy. Before the AIDS epidemic, radiation therapy was considered the treatment of choice for symptomatic Kaposi's sarcoma. Based on experience gained during the past 10 years, recommendations for dosage and guidelines for the selection of patients for radiation therapy are now available.[156, 201, 202] In the largest retrospective series on radiation therapy for AIDS-associated Kaposi's sarcoma (187 patients treated with 375 fields), there was no difference in clinical response or duration of response regardless of the fractionation regimen used (8 Gy in a single fraction, up to 15 to 40 Gy in 5 to 10 fractions).[203] Patients receiving single fractions of 8 Gy to cutaneous fields are less likely to experience severe toxic reactions (cellulitis, blistering, desquamation) than patients receiving multiple fractions, but single-fraction therapy may have a shorter duration of response.[203] Radiation therapy appears best suited for symptoms due to mass effects, including large intraoral lesions and localized disease resulting in pain, extensive lymphadenopathy, or lymphedema of the extremities and penis.[156]

Laser and Surgical Treatment. Carbon dioxide and argon lasers and photodynamic therapy have been used successfully to treat large oral lesions.[204] Pulsed-dye laser therapy is effective for cutaneous macular lesions, but lesions typically recur within 12 weeks.[194] Local excision can be beneficial for troublesome lesions at selected sites.

Systemic Treatment. Patients with disease that is not easily managed with local treatment frequently respond to systemic therapy, despite the increased risk of significant side effects. Systemic treatment can be divided into limited intervention (interferon ± zidovudine) and aggressive intervention (chemotherapy ± zidovudine).

Systemic Interferon. Early studies evaluating systemic interferon alfa for the treatment of AIDS-associated Kaposi's sarcoma defined minimum dose requirements of greater than 20 million units/m^2 (5 to 7 days per week) for objective response rates of 20% to 50%.[156, 191] Gradual escalation of the dosage was shown to reduce the acute, flu-like toxicity associated with the relatively high-doses of interferon alfa required for acceptable clinical response rates. In general, pretreatment CD4 counts appear to be the best independent predictor of response.[156, 191] Patients with CD4 counts of greater than 400 cells/mm^3, 200 to 400 cells/mm^3, and less than 200 cells/mm^3 have objective response rates of 40% to 50%, 30%, and 10%, respectively.

Systemic Chemotherapy. Before the AIDS epidemic, excellent results were obtained using cytotoxic chemotherapy for patients with widespread Kaposi's sarcoma.[156, 191] For AIDS-associated disease, single-agent regimens for patients with minimal disease and extensive disease have demonstrated response rates of about 40% and 80%, respectively. Because these patients frequently develop cytotoxic drug toxicity at dosages required for clinical response when administered as single agents, multiagent cytotoxic regimens that reduce the cumulative toxicities of drugs administered as single agents are generally preferred. Frequently used multidrug regimens include combinations of *Vinca* alkaloids (vincristine and vinblastine) or a *Vinca* alkaloid combined with one or more of the following: bleomycin, an anthracycline, or etoposide. These regimens have shown promising results in patients with extensive cutaneous and visceral disease, and even in patients with severely compromised immune function.[156, 191] Finally, experience with liposomally encapsulated anthracyclines suggests that targeted drug delivery systems may be a less toxic and more effective method for cytotoxic drug administration.[155, 205]

Systemic Treatment in Combination with Zidovudine. Several clinical studies have evaluated the synergistic antiviral effect of combination zidovudine with interferon alfa demonstrated in vitro.[156, 191] In general, clinical response rates range from 30% to 60%, and antiviral effects can be demonstrated by peripheral blood HIV cultures and tests for HIV p24 antigen. In addition, response rates of up to 30% have been demonstrated in patients with CD4 counts less than 200 cells/mm^3. The recommended maximum dose for either agent (zidovudine, 600 mg; interferon alfa, 9 – 18 million units) is roughly half the maximum tolerated dose for either agent used alone. Systemic cytotoxic chemotherapy in combination with reduced doses of zidovudine is safe when closely monitored.[206] Finally, future studies employing granulocyte-macrophage colony stimulating factor in combination with cytotoxic chemotherapy and interferon alfa may prevent the severe additive myelotoxicities currently reported with the combination of the later two agents.[156]

Promising therapies for the future include new antiangiogenic drugs, for example, recombinant human platelet factor-4, synthetic analogues of fumagillin, synthetic heparin substitutes, vitamin D$_3$ analogues, bacterial cell wall compounds, and the development of inhibitors to both cytokine growth factors and Kaposi's sarcoma cell-specific cytokine receptors.[155, 156]

Cutaneous Complications of Immunosuppression

NEOPLASTIC COMPLICATIONS

Neoplasia is an important complication of the immunosuppression of congenital immunodeficiency states (primary immunodeficiency), of immunosuppressive agents for organ transplantation or other diseases, or in the setting of HIV infection. These complications are greatest in those situations where the cellular immune system is impaired. Three classes of tumors are especially increased in the setting of immunosuppression: lymphoreticular malignancies, Kaposi's sarcoma (not in primary immunodeficiency states), and squamous cell carcinomas of the skin and genital tract.

Non-Hodgkin's lymphoma is the lymphoreticular malignancy most frequently reported in the setting of immune suppression, although Hodgkin's disease is also seen. It is characterized by extranodal location (especially central nervous system), by high grade, and by presentation at an advanced stage. These tumors are primarily of the B-cell type, but T-cell lymphomas also occur (including cutaneous T-cell lymphoma).[207] B-cell lymphomas may be monoclonal or polyclonal, and the Epstein-Barr virus genome may be found in the lymphomas. In the setting of HIV it appears that prognosis is predicted by the health of the patient at presentation.

In organ transplant recipients, nonmelanoma skin cancers represent between 38% and 77% of the cancers that develop in these patients. These tumors occur primarily on sun-exposed skin, although genital squamous cell carcinomas are also increased. In Australia 10 years after transplantation, 29% of patients have developed skin cancer.[208] Squamous cell carcinomas are the most frequent tumor, occurring 3 to 15 times more frequently

than basal cell carcinomas.[209, 210] These actinic lesions can be aggressive; they metastasize in 5% to 12% of patients and cause death in as many as 5%. Cutaneous squamous cell carcinoma represents 82% of skin cancer metastases and 64% of skin cancer deaths in organ transplant patients.[210, 211] The incidence of malignant melanoma is also increased.

HUMAN PAPILLOMAVIRUS INFECTION

Epidemiology

Immunosuppressed patients have greater numbers of warts than the general population,[212] and many demonstrate multiple DNA types.[213] Numerous studies have linked certain human papillomavirus (HPV) types (types 16, 18, and 33 through 35) with cervical, anal, penile, and subungual squamous cell carcinoma.[214–216] Anal squamous cell carcinoma is more common in homosexual men.[217–219]

Anogenital warts occur in 20% of HIV-infected homosexual men and 27% of homosexual men with AIDS.[220] When anal swabs are examined by the dot blot technique, 48% of HIV-negative homosexual men and 54% of homosexual men with AIDS show evidence of HPV infection.[221–223] Combined infections were common.[221] Of greatest importance was the finding of anal intraepithelial neoplasia in 38% of anal swabs (Papanicolaou smear equivalent) and in 15% of biopsy specimens from patients with AIDS. Cervical dysplasia/neoplasia related to HPV infection is more common in women who are immunosuppressed as a result of organ transplantation, lymphoreticular malignancy (especially Hodgkin's disease), and HIV disease.[222] Cervical carcinoma is an index AIDS diagnosis. Genital warts and cervical dysplasia/neoplasia increase in frequency and severity with advancing immunosuppression.[224, 225] Noncervical cancers of the anogenital area are also increased in immunosuppressed transplant patients.[226]

Patients receiving immunosuppressive therapy to prevent organ transplant rejection are at high risk of developing nongenital warts. Both the prevalence of wart infection and the number of warts increases with length of immunosuppression, so that by 5 years after transplantation, 90% patients have warts.[227] HIV infection also predisposes patients to cutaneous warts. Most nongenital warts in the setting of immunosuppression are of the common "benign" types.[213] Some patients are infected with epidermodysplasia verruciformis "specific" HPV types. As in classic epidermodysplasia verruciformis, immunosuppressed patients with warts are at increased risk of developing cutaneous squamous cell carcinomas, especially on sun-exposed skin.[210] These carcinomas have been shown to contain the DNA of epidermodysplasia verruciformis "specific" HPV types.[209]

Clinical Description

Common warts of the hands and plantar warts are frequent in immunosuppressed persons. Multiple, large, and treatment-resistant warts are the hallmark of symptomatic HIV infection, especially in patients with AIDS. Flat warts of the beard area may also be seen. In the anogenital area, typical condylomata to large vegetating masses occur, especially if there is a history of receptive anal intercourse. Lesions may extend into the anal canal, requiring anoscopy to evaluate the full extent of the infection. Typical condylomatous papules are most common on the penile shaft and vulvar skin and may be few or quite numerous.

Flat lesions of HPV infection (often hyperpigmented) may histologically demonstrate features similar or identical to squamous cell carcinoma in situ (bowenoid papulosis).[228-230] In HIV infection these hyperpigmented plaques may involve substantial portions of the genital area. Although the natural history of such lesions is unknown, it is hypothesized that the associated immunosuppression may lead to more frequent development of genital squamous cell carcinoma. The transition zones of the cervix and anus are at highest risk for malignancy. One case of squamous cell carcinoma of the anus has developed in an HIV-infected man with bowenoid papulosis.[230] HPV 16 is the most common HPV type associated with bowenoid papulosis.[230]

Treatment

As in other infectious conditions in the immunosuppressed host, treatment of warts is difficult and recurrence is to be anticipated. Although not yet documented, experience suggests that failure of therapy is highest in persons with the most advanced immunosuppression. The management of common and plantar warts is by the usual methods. Flat warts of the beard area may respond to topical 13-*cis*-retinoic acid or 5-fluorouracil. Shaving using razor blades should be discontinued until the beard area is free of lesions.

The most effective treatment of condylomata appears to be frequent (weekly) destructive therapy with liquid nitrogen, trichloroacetic acid, podophyllin, or electrocautery. 5-Fluorouracil can be used topically to treat bowenoid dysplasia of the genitalia and to reduce recurrence of treated lesions.[231-233] Interferon appears to have less efficacy in the setting of immunosuppression.[234] In immunosuppressed patients, treatment of genital warts by any method is often followed by recurrence. Refractory lesions should be sampled. Histology is the best predictor of biologic behavior, and lesions with atypical histology should be considered for more aggressive management. At a minimum, patients with atypical biopsy specimens require regular evaluation. Due to the high risk of cervical dysplasia in immunosuppressed women, annual Papanicolaou smears are recommended. Once cervical dysplasia is detected or the patient develops AIDS the frequency of Papanicolaou smears should increase to every 3 or 6 months, respectively.

HERPES SIMPLEX INFECTION

Suppression of cell-mediated immunity with organ transplantation, bone marrow transplantation, hematologic malignancy, or the immunosuppressive agents used to treat these conditions frequently leads to reactivation of herpes simplex. The degree of immunosuppression correlates with the likelihood of reactivation, with positive oral cultures in 80% of bone marrow transplant patients, 70% of acute leukemia patients receiving chemotherapy, 50% of lymphoma patients on chemotherapy, and 50% of renal transplant patients.[235, 236] The greater the degree of immunosuppression, the more likely a positive oral culture will be associated with painful clinical disease (i.e., 100% in bone marrow transplantation and leukemia patients and 32% in transplant patients). Since the seroprevalence for HSV type 1 is higher than HSV type 2, most reactivations are in the orolabial area. They represent 80% of severe, painful orolabial lesions in this population. Clinically, they present as erosions or ulcerations that may be extensive, destructive, and persistent. Acyclovir is effective both in prevention and treatment.[236]

VARICELLA-ZOSTER VIRUS

Varicella is substantially more severe in immunosuppressed persons, especially those in whom the cell-mediated immune system is impaired by malignancy or chemotherapy, including corticosteroids alone. Children with no prior history of varicella are at particularly high risk. The rash is more extensive and lasts longer, and visceral disease and death are much more common. In untreated children with cancer, about one third will develop varicella pneumonitis and up to 25% of those affected will die if untreated.[237] Lymphopenia (<500 lymphocytes) is the major risk factor for dissemination and death. Varicella pneumonia is the most common complication, but encephalitis, hepatitis, and purpura fulminans can also occur. The most effective management strategy is to prevent or attenuate disease with the appropriate use of varicella-zoster immune globulin and varicella vaccination in at-risk persons.[238] Acyclovir given intravenously at a dose of 500 mg/m^2 every 8 hours is effective treatment, especially if instituted in the first 72 hours.[239]

Recurrence of VZV in the form of herpes zoster is a common complication of immunosuppression, especially hematologic malignancies and particularly Hodgkin's disease. The cumulative risk over 5 years for the development of zoster is 14% for Hodgkin's disease, 10% for leukemia, 5% for non-Hodgkin's lymphoma, and about 2% for solid tumors.[240] Thoracic dermatomal involvement is most common overall, but patients with hematologic malignancy have relatively more frequent trigeminal involvement (16% vs. 9%). In solid tumors there is a correlation between the dermatome involved and the site of the malignancy, with breast and lung cancer having thoracic involvement most commonly, whereas sacral and lumbar involvement is relatively more common in genituourinary and gynecologic malignancies. Approximately 70% of patients with cervical, thoracic, lumbar, and sacral zoster had previously received radiation therapy to that region. Approximately one third of bone marrow transplant patients develop zoster in the first year after transplantation.

In the immunosuppressed person herpes zoster tends to last longer and be more painful, is frequently hemorrhagic, and often scars. Dissemination occurs in between 12% and 45% of patients, depending on the degree of immunosuppression. Between 10% and 20% of immunosuppressed patients with disseminated zoster die if their disease is not treated.[240] Fatal complications include pneumonitis, encephalitis, and hepatitis.

Uncomplicated herpes zoster in the immunocompromised host should be treated with acyclovir. Only intravenous acyclovir (10 mg/kg every 8 hours) can reach adequate blood levels to inhibit all VZV strains, so it is the treatment of choice for patients with severe immunosuppression. Mildly immunosuppressed patients may be managed with oral acyclovir (800 mg orally five times daily) if there is no evidence of dissemination and if they are observed closely. Dissemination, ophthalmic involvement, Ramsay Hunt syndrome, and failure of oral acyclovir are all indications for intravenous use of acyclovir. Zoster–immune globulin prevents dissemination.[241] After bone marrow transplantation prophylactic acyclovir may be used to prevent herpes zoster.[242]

PSEUDOMONAS INFECTION

Pseudomonas aeruginosa rarely causes systemic infection in the immunocompetent host. Immunosuppression, especially neutropenia, is associated with the development of life-threatening infection with this organism. Ecthyma gangrenosum is the most common cutaneous manifestation of *Pseudomonas* infection. It may be associated with *Pseudomonas* sepsis or may be seen in neutropenic patients without sepsis.[243] Lesions usually occur in the groin as red plaques that develop a pseudobullous violaceous center and eventually ulcerate. A rarer cutaneous manifestation of *Pseudomonas* sepsis is red subcutaneous nodules.

FUNGAL INFECTIONS

Candidiasis is the most common fungal infection complicating immunosuppression. It usually presents as oral, vaginal, or intertriginous lesions. The combination of impaired mucosal barriers in the mouth and gastrointestinal tract plus neutropenia may be associated with candidal septicemia. *Candida albicans* is the most common cause, but *C. krusei, C. tropicalis,* and others are also pathogenic in this setting. Skin lesions are present in at least 13% of patients with candidal sepsis, most frequently appearing as 0.5- to 1.0-cm erythematous, sometimes purpuric papules with central pallor or pustulation.[244] Less commonly, necrotic skin lesions are seen.[245, 246] Histologically, the dermal infiltrate may be scarce, but yeast forms and pseudohyphae are abundant. Increasing imidazole resistance by non–*C. albicans* species is being noted in immunosuppressed persons.

Aspergillus species are the most common cause of noncandidal fungal infections in the immunosuppressed patient.[247] *Aspergillus* is most frequently a pulmonary pathogen that disseminates hematogenously in 20% to 50% of immunosuppressed patients. Metastatic skin lesions are seen in less than 5% of patients with disseminated aspergillosis.[248] Primary cutaneous aspergillosis is also seen. Lesions occur at the sites of intravenous catheters[249-251] or more commonly at sites of minor trauma around catheters, such as tape or armboard erosions. *Aspergillus niger, A. flavus,* and *A. fumigatus* have all been implicated. These organisms have occasionally been cultured from tape and armboard material. Most patients are leukopenic and on broad-spectrum antibiotic therapy. Erythema, induration and pustulation, or hemorrhagic bullae progressing rapidly to necrosis are characteristic. The diagnosis may be established by identifying hyphae on potassium hydroxide preparations or by skin biopsy. Disease may remain limited to the skin or may disseminate. Treatment optimally involves the reversal of leukopenia, amphotericin B (or possibly itraconazole), and local care.

Immunosuppressed persons are at risk from infection with other normally nonpathogenic fungi, including *Trichosporon, Fusarium,* zygomycetes, *Drechslera,* and others. Risk factors for these infections include profound neutropenia (<100 cells/mm³), antibacterial antibiotics, and central venous catheters. Infections are most frequently disseminated, with the lungs the most common site of involvement. Skin lesions are present in about 15% of patients and are more frequent with some pathogens, especially *Fusarium.* About two thirds of patients die, half from the fungal infection. Disseminated infection and profound neutropenia without recovery are associated with a poor prognosis.

References

1. Tindall B, Barker S, Donova B, et al. Characterization of the acute clinical illness associated with human immunodeficiency virus infection. Arch Intern Med 1988;148:945–949.
2. Gaines H. Primary HIV infection: Clinical and diagnostic aspects. Scand J Infect Dis 1989;S61:1–46.
3. Rabeneck L, Mikulas P, Gartner S, et al. Acute HIV infection presenting with painful swallowing and esophageal ulcers. JAMA 1990;263:2318–2322.
4. Sinicco A, Palestro G, Caramello P, et al. Acute HIV-1 infection: Clinical and biological study of 12 patients. J Acquir Immune Defic Syndr 1990;3:260–265.
5. Hulsebosch HJ, Claessen FAP, van Ginkel CJW, et al. Human immunodeficiency virus exanthem. J Am Acad Dermatol 1990;23:483–486.
6. Duvic M. Staphylococcal infections and the pruritus of AIDS-related complex. Arch Dermatol 1987;123:1599.
7. Schwartz JJ, Myskowski PL. Molluscum contagiosum in patients with human immunodeficiency virus infection. J Am Acad Dermatol 1992;27:583–588.
8. Kohn SR. Molluscum contagiosum in patients with acquired immunodeficiency syndrome. Arch Ophthalmol 1987;105:458.
9. Fivenson DP, Weltman RE, Gibson SH. Giant molluscum contagiosum presenting as basal cell carcinoma in an acquired immunodeficiency syndrome patient. J Am Acad Dermatol 1988; 19:912–914.
10. Picon L, Vaillant L, Duong T, et al. Cutaneous cryptococcosis resembling molluscum contagiosum: A first manifestation of AIDS. Acta Derm Venereol 1989;69:365–367.
11. Crowe SM. Unusual features of herpes simplex or zoster infection that suggest HIV infection. Med J Aust 1993;158:186–187.
12. Centers for Disease Control: Revision of the CDC surveillance case definition for acquired immunodeficiency syndrome. MMWR 1987;36(1S):3S–15S.
13. Siegal FP, Lopez C, Hammer GS, et al. Severe acquired immunodeficiency in male homosexuals, manifested by chronic perianal ulcerative herpes simplex lesions. N Engl J Med 1981;305:1439–1444.

14. Glickel SZ. Hand infections in patients with acquired immunodeficiency syndrome. J Hand Surg 1988;13A:770–775.

15. Bagdades EK, Pillay D, Squire SB, et al. Relationship between herpes simplex virus ulceration and CD4 + cell counts in patients with HIV infection. AIDS 1992;6:1317–1320.

16. Kory WP, Rico MJ, Gould E, Penneys NS. Dermatopathologic findings in patients with acquired immunodeficiency syndrome. South Med J 1987;80:1529–1532.

17. Horn TD, Hood AF. Cytomegalovirus is predictably present in perineal ulcers from immunosuppressed patients. Arch Dermatol 1990;126:642–644.

18. Heinic GS, Northfelt DW, Greenspan JS, et al. Concurrent oral cytomegalovirus and herpes simplex virus infection in association with HIV infection: A case report. Oral Surg Oral Med Oral Pathol 1993;75:488–494.

19. Garcia-Patos V, Pujol RM, Curell R, et al. Cytomegalovirus-induced cytopathic changes in skin biopsy specimens: Clinicopathologic study in patients with the acquired immunodeficiency syndrome and an active extracutaneous cytomegalovirus infection. Arch Dermatol 1992;128:1552–1553.

20. Hirsch MS, Schooley RT. Resistance to antiviral drugs: The end of innocence. N Engl J Med 1989;320:313–314.

21. Erlich KS, Mills J, Chatis P, et al. Acyclovir-resistant herpes simplex virus infections in patients with the acquired immunodeficiency syndrome. N Engl J Med 1989;320:293–296.

22. Youle MM, Hawkins DA, Collins P, et al. Acyclovir-resistant herpes in AIDS treated with foscarnet. Lancet 1988;2:341–342.

23. Chatis PA, Miller CH, Schrager LE, Crumpacker CS. Successful treatment with foscarnet of an acyclovir-resistant mucocutaneous infection with herpes simplex virus in a patient with acquired immunodeficiency syndrome. N Engl J Med 1989;320:297–300.

24. MacPhail LA, Greenspan D, Schiodt M, et al. Acyclovir-resistant, foscarnet-sensitive oral herpes simplex type 2 lesion in a patient with AIDS. Oral Surg Oral Med Oral Pathol 1989;67:427–432.

25. Erlich KS, Jacobson MA, Koehler JE, et al. Foscarnet therapy for severe acyclovir-resistant herpes simplex virus type-2 infections in patients with the acquired immunodeficiency syndrome (AIDS): An uncontrolled trial. Ann Intern Med 1989;110:710–713.

26. Safrin S, Crumpacker C, Chatis P, et al. A controlled trial comparing foscarnet and vidarabine for acyclovir-resistant mucocutaneous herpes simplex in the acquired immunodeficiency syndrome. N Engl J Med 1991;325:551–555.

27. Hardy WD. Foscarnet treatment of acyclovir-resistant herpes simplex virus infection in patients with acquired immunodeficiency syndrome: Preliminary results of a controlled, randomized, regimen-comparative trial. Am J Med 1992;92:30S–35S.

28. Birch CJ, Tyssen DP, Tachedjian G, et al. Clinical effects and in vitro studies of trifluorothymidine combined with interferon-a for treatment of drug-resistant and -sensitive herpes simplex virus infections. J Infect Dis 1992;16:108–112.

29. Snoeck R, Andrei G, De Clercq E, et al. A new topical treatment for resistant herpes simplex infections. N Engl J Med 1993;329:968–969.

30. Buchbinder SP, Katz MH, Hessol NA, et al. Herpes zoster and human immunodeficiency virus infection. J Infect Dis 1992;166:1153–1156.

31. Eyster ME, Rabkin CS, Hilgartner MW, et al. Human immunodeficiency virus–related conditions in children and adults with hemophilia: Rates, relationship to CD4 counts, and predictive value. Blood 1993;81:828–834.

32. Patterson LE, Butler KM, Edwards MS. Clinical herpes zoster shortly following primary varicella in two HIV-infected children. Clin Pediatr 1989;28:354.

33. Perronne C, Lazanas M, Leport C, et al: Varicella in patients infected with the human immunodeficiency virus. Arch Dermatol 1990;126:1033–1036.

34. Jura E, Chadwick EG, Josephs SH, et al. Varicella-zoster virus infections in children infected with human immunodeficiency virus. Pediatr Infect Dis J 1989;8:586–590.

35. Colebunders R, Mann JM, Francis H, et al. Herpes zoster in African patients: A clinical predictor of human immunodeficiency virus infection. J Infect Dis 1988;157:314–318.

36. Melbye M, Grossman RJ, Goedert JJ, et al. Risk of AIDS after herpes zoster. Lancet 1987;1:728–730.

37. De Perre PV, Bakkers E, Batungwanayo J, et al. Herpes zoster in

African patients: An early manifestation of HIV infection. Scand J Infect Dis 1988;20:277–282.

38. Safrin S, Berger TG, Gilson I, et al. Foscarnet therapy in five patients with AIDS and acyclovir-resistant varicella-zoster virus infection. Ann Intern Med 1991;115:19–21.

39. Williamson BC. Disseminated herpes zoster in a human immunodeficiency virus–positive homosexual man without complications. Cutis 1987;40:485–486.

40. Cohen PR, Beltrani VP, Grossman ME. Disseminated herpes zoster in patients with human immunodeficiency virus infection. Am J Med 1988;84:1076–1080.

41. Cohen PR, Grossman ME. Clinical features of human immunodeficiency virus–associated disseminated herpes zoster virus infection: A review of the literature. Clin Exp Dermatol 1989;14:273–276.

42. Gilson IH, Barnett JH, Conant MA, et al. Disseminated ecthymatous herpes varicella-zoster virus infection in patients with acquired immunodeficiency syndrome. J Am Acad Dermatol 1989;20:637–642.

43. Alessi E, Cusini M, Zerboni R, et al. Unusual varicella-zoster virus infection in patients with the acquired immunodeficiency syndrome. Arch Dermatol 1988;124:1011–1012.

44. Pahwa S, Biron K, Lim W, et al. Continuous varicella-zoster infection associated with acyclovir resistance in a child with AIDS. JAMA 1988;260:2879–2882.

45. Jacobson MA, Berger TG, Fikrig S, et al. Acyclovir-resistant varicella zoster virus infection after chronic oral acyclovir therapy in patients with the acquired immunodeficiency syndrome (AIDS). Ann Intern Med 1990;112;187–191.

46. LeBoit PE, Limova M, Yen TSB, et al. Chronic verrucous varicella-zoster infection in patients with the acquired immunodeficiency syndrome: Histologic and molecular biologic findings. Am J Dermatopathol 1992;14:1–8.

47. Safrin S, Berger TG, Gilson I, et al. Foscarnet therapy in five patients with AIDS and acyclovir-resistant varicella-zoster virus infection. Ann Intern Med 1991;115:19–21.

48. Panther LA, Sande MA. Cryptococcal meningitis in AIDS. In: Sande MA, Volberding PA, eds. The Medical Management of AIDS, 2nd ed. Philadelphia: WB Saunders Co., 1990:265–279.

49. Picon L, Vaillant L, Duong T, et al. Cutaneous cryptococcosis resembling molluscum contagiosum: A first manifestation of AIDS. Acta Derm Venereol 1989;69:365–367.

50. Borton LK, Wintroub BU. Disseminated cryptococcosis presenting as herpetiform lesions in a homosexual man with acquired immunodeficiency syndrome. J Am Acad Dermatol 1984;10:387–390.

51. Rico MJ, Penneys NS. Cutaneous cryptococcosis resembling molluscum contagiosum in a patient with AIDS. Arch Dermatol 1985;121:901–902.

52. Concus AP, Helfand RF, Imber MJ, et al. Cutaneous cryptococcosis mimicking molluscum contagiosum in a patient with AIDS. J Infect Dis 1988;158:897–898.

53. Hunt SJ, Nagi C, Gross KG, et al. Primary cutaneous aspergillosis near central venous catheters in patients with the acquired immunodeficiency syndrome. Arch Dermatol 1992;128:1229–1232.

54. Libow LF, Dobert D, Sibulkin D. Co-existent cutaneous cryptococcosis and Kaposi's sarcoma in a patient with the acquired immodeficiency syndrome. Cutis 1988;41:159–162.

55. Jimenez-Acosta F, Casado M, Borbujo J, et al. Cutaneous cryptococcosis mimicking molluscum contagiosum in a haemophiliac with AIDS. Clin Exp Dermatol 1987;12:446–450.

56. Glick M, Cohen SG, Cheney RT, et al. Oral manifestations of disseminated *Cryptococcus neoformans* in a patient with acquired immunodeficiency syndrome. Oral Surg Oral Med Oral Pathol 1987;64:454–459.

57. Johnson PC, Khardori N, Najjar AF, et al. Progressive disseminated histoplasmosis in patients with acquired immunodeficiency syndrome. Am J Med 1988;85:152–158.

58. Wheat LJ, Slama TG, Zeckel ML. Histoplasmosis in the acquired immune deficiency syndrome. Am J Med 1985;78:203–210.

59. Cohen PR, Bank DE, Silvers DN, et al. Cutaneous lesions of disseminated histoplasmosis in human immunodeficiency virus–infected patients. J Am Acad Dermatol 1990;23:422–428.

60. Penneys NS. Disseminated fungal and protozoal infections. In:

Mark R, ed. Skin Manifestations of AIDS. Philadelphia: JB Lippincott, 1990:23–24.

61. Hazelhurst JA, Vismer HF. Histoplasmosis presenting with unusual skin lesions in acquired immunodeficiency syndrome (AIDS). Br J Dermatol 1985;113:345–348.

62. Bonner JR, Alexander WJ, Dismukes WE, et al. Disseminated histoplasmosis in patients with the acquired immune deficiency syndrome. Arch Intern Med 1984;144:2178–2181.

63. Greenberg RG, Berger TG. Progressive disseminated histoplasmosis in acquired immune deficiency syndrome: Presentation as a steroid-responsive dermatosis. Cutis 1989;43:535–538.

64. Kalter DC, Tschen JA, Klima M. Maculopapular rash in a patient with acquired immunodeficiency syndrome. Arch Dermatol 1985;121:1454.

65. Mayoral F, Penneys NS. Disseminated histoplasmosis presenting as a transepidermal elimination disorder in an AIDS victim. J Am Acad Dermatol 1985;13:842–844.

66. Lipstein-Kresch E, Isenberg HD, Singer C, et al. Disseminated *Sporothrix schenckii* infection with arthritis in a patient with acquired immunodeficiency syndrome. J Rheumatol 1985;12:805–808.

67. Bibler MR, Luber HJ, Glueck HI, et al. Disseminated sporotrichosis in a patient with HIV infection after treatment for acquired factor VIII inhibitor. JAMA 1986;256:3125–3126.

68. Kurosawa A, Pollock SC, Collins MP, et al. *Sporothrix schenckii* endophthalmitis in a patient with human immunodeficiency virus infection. Arch Ophthalmol 1988;106:376–380.

69. Bronnimann DA, Adam RD, Galgiani JN, et al. Coccidioidomycosis in the acquired immunodeficiency syndrome. Ann Intern Med 1987;106:372–379.

70. Prichard JG, Sorotzkin RA, James RE III. Cutaneous manifestations of disseminated coccidioidomycosis in the acquired immunodeficiency syndrome. Cutis 1987;39:203–205.

71. Carlson KC, Mehlmauer M, Evans S, et al. Cryptococcal cellulitis in renal transplant recipients. J Am Acad Dermatol 1987;17:469–472.

72. Sunderam G, McDonald RJ, Maniatis T, et al. Tuberculosis presenting as a manifestation of the acquired immunodeficiency syndrome (AIDS). JAMA 1986;256:362–366.

73. Penneys NS, Hicks B. Unusual cutaneous lesions associated with acquired immunodeficiency syndrome. J Am Acad Dermatol 1985;13:845–852.

74. Kaplan MH, Sadick N, McNutt NS, et al. Dermatologic findings and manifestations of acquired immunodeficiency syndrome (AIDS). J Am Acad Dermatol 1987;16:485–506.

75. Barbaro DJ, Orcutt VL, Coldiron BM. *Mycobacterium avium–Mycobacterium intracellulare* infection limited to the skin and lymph nodes in patients with AIDS. Rev Infect Dis 1989;11:625–628.

76. Rogers PL, Walker RE, Lane HC, et al. Disseminated *Mycobacterium haemophilum* infection in two patients with the acquired immunodeficiency syndrome. Am J Med 1988;84:640–642.

77. Males BM, West TE, Bartholomew WR. *Mycobacterium haemophilum* infection in a patient with acquired immunodeficiency syndrome. J Clin Microbiol 1987;25:186–190.

78. Brandwein M, Choi H-SH, Strauchen J, et al. Spindle cell reaction to nontuberculous mycobacteriosis in AIDS mimicking a spindle cell neoplasm. Virchows Arch Pathol Anat 1990;416:281–286.

79. Lambertus MW, Mathisen GE. *Mycobacterium marinum* infection in a patient with cryptosporidiosis and the acquired immunodeficiency syndrome. Cutis 1988;41:38–40.

80. Boudes P, Sobel A, Deforges L, Leblic E. Disseminated *Mycobacterium bovis* infection from BCG vaccination and HIV infection. JAMA 1989;262:2386.

81. Funkhouser M, Omohundro C, Ross A, et al. Management of scabies in patients with HIV disease. Arch Dermatol 1993;129:911–913.

82. Sadick N, Kaplan MH, Pahwa SG, et al. Unusual features of scabies complicating human T-lymphotropic virus type III infection. J Am Acad Dermatol 1986;15:482–486.

83. Moss VA. Scabies in an AIDS hospice unit. Br J Clin Pathol 1991;45:35–36.

84. Hulbert TV, Larsen RA. Hyperkeratotic (Norwegian) scabies

with gram-negative bacteremia as the initial presentation of AIDS. Clin Infect Dis 1992;14:1164–1165.

85. Arico M, Noto G, La Rocca E, et al. Localized crusted scabies in the acquired immunodeficiency syndrome. Clin Exp Dermatol 1992;17:39–41.

86. Berenguer J, Moreno S, Cercenado, et al. Visceral leishmaniasis in patients infected with human immunodeficiency virus (HIV). Ann Intern Med 1989;111:129–132.

87. Condom MJ, Clotet B, Sirera G, et al. Asymptomatic leishmaniasis in the acquired immunodeficiency syndrome (AIDS). Ann Intern Med 1989;111:767–768.

88. Jeannel D, Tuppin P, Brucker G, et al. Leishmaniasis in France. Lancet 1989;2:804.

89. Yebra M, Segovia J, Manzano, et al. Disseminated-to-skin kala-azar and the acquired immunodeficiency syndrome. Ann Intern Med 1988;108:490–491.

90. Rosenthal PJ, Chaisson RE, Hadley WK, et al. Rectal leishmaniasis in a patient with acquired immunodeficiency syndrome. Am J Med 1988;84:307–309.

91. Neto VA, Pasternak J, Mopreira AA, et al. *Strongyloides stercoralis* hyperinfection in the acquired immunodeficiency syndrome. Am J Med 1989;87:602–603.

92. Gompels MM, Todd J, Peters B, et al. Disseminated strongyloidiasis in AIDS: Uncommon but important. AIDS 1991;5:329–332.

93. Kramer MR, Gregg PA, Goldstein M, et al. Disseminated strongyloidiasis in AIDS and non-AIDS immunocompromised hosts: Diagnosis by sputum and bronchoalveolar lavage. South Med J 1990;83:1226–1229.

94. Maayan S, Wormser GP, Widerhorn J, et al. *Strongyloides stercoralis* hyperinfection in a patient with the acquired immune deficiency syndrome. Am J Med 1987;83:945–948.

95. Di Silverio A, Brazzelli V, Brandozzi G, et al. Prevalence of dermatophytes and yeasts—(*Candida* spp., *Malassezia furfur*) in HIV patients: A study of former drug addicts. Mycopathologia 1991;114:103–107.

96. Dompmartin D, Dompmartin A, Deluol AM, et al. Onychomycosis and AIDS: Clinical and laboratory findings in 62 patients. Int J Dermatol 1990;29:337–339.

97. Wright DC, Lennox JL, James WD, et al. Generalized chronic dermatophytosis in patients with human immunodeficiency virus type 1 infection and CD4 depletion. Arch Dermatol 1991;127:265–266.

98. Laurence J. Women and AIDS: An overview and specific disease manifestations. AIDS Reader 1991:153–159.

99. Lake-Bakaar G, Tom W, Lake-Bakaar D, et al. Gastropathy and ketoconazole malabsorption in the acquired immunodeficiency syndrome (AIDS). Ann Intern Med 1988;109:471–473.

100. Rosenthal D, LeBoit PE, Klumpp L, et al. Human immunodeficiency virus–associated eosinophilic folliculitis: A unique dermatosis associated with advanced human immunodeficiency virus infection. Arch Dermatol 1991;127:206–209.

101. Buchness MR, Lim HW, Hatcher VA, et al. Eosinophilic pustular folliculitis in the acquired immunodeficiency syndrome. N Engl J Med 1988;318:1183–1186.

102. Berger TG, Heon V, King C, et al. Itraconazole therapy for HIV-associated eosinophilic folliculitis. Arch Dermatol, submitted for publication.

103. Diven DG, Newton RC, Ramsey KM. Heightened cutaneous reactions to mosquito bites in patients with acquired immunodeficiency syndrome receiving zidovudine. Arch Intern Med 1988;148:2296.

104. Penneys NS, Nayar JK, Bernstein H, et al. Chronic pruritic eruption in patients with acquired immunodeficiency syndrome associated with increased antibody titers to mosquito salivary gland antigens. J Am Acad Dermatol 1989;21:421–425.

105. Ghadially R, Sibbald RG, Walter JB, et al. Granuloma annulare in patients with human immunodeficiency virus infections. J Am Acad Dermatol 1989;20:232–235.

106. Ruiz-Rodriguez R, Longaker M, Berger TG. Anetoderma and HIV infection. Arch Dermatol 1992;128:661–662.

107. Ruiz-Rodriguez R, Maurer TA, Berger TG. Papular mucinosis and human immunodeficiency virus infection. Arch Dermatol 1992;128:995–996.

108. Bayard P, Berger TG, Jacobson MA. Drug hypersensitivity reac-

tions and human immunodeficiency virus disease. J AIDS 1992;5:1237–1257.

109. Finegold I. Oral desensitization to trimethoprim-sulfamethoxazole in a patient with acquired immunodeficiency syndrome. J Allergy Clin Immunol 1986;78:905–908.

110. Ong ELC, Mandal BK. Multiple drug reactions in a patient with AIDS. Lancet 1989;2:976–977.

111. Moyle G, Barton S, Gazzard BG. Penile ulceration with foscarnet therapy. AIDS 1993;1:140–141.

112. Greenberg RG, Berger TG. Nail and mucocutaneous hyperpigmentation of azidothymidine therapy. J Am Acad Dermatol 1990;22:327–330.

113. Wright DN, Nelson RP, Ledford DK, et al. Serum IgE and human immunodeficiency virus (HIV) infection. J Allergy Clin Immunol 1990;85:445–452.

114. Clerici M, Shearer GM. A $T_H1 \rightarrow T_H2$ switch is a critical step in the etiology of HIV infection. Immunol Today 1993;14:107–111.

115. Parkin JM, Eales L-J, Galazka AR, et al. Atopic manifestations in the acquired immune deficiency syndrome: Response to recombinant interferon gamma. Br Med J 1987;294:1185–1186.

116. Toback AC, Longley J, Cardullo AC, et al. Severe chronic photosensitivity in association with acquired immunodeficiency syndrome. J Am Acad Dermatol 1986;15:1056–1057.

117. Vin-Christian K, Maurer TA, Berger TG. Acne rosacea as a cutaneous manifestation of human immunodeficiency virus (HIV) infection. J Am Acad Dermatol 1994;30:139–140.

118. Wikler JR, Nieboer C, Willemze R. Quantitative skin cultures of *Pityrosporum* yeasts in patients seropositive for the human immunodeficiency virus with and without seborrheic dermatitis. J Am Acad Dermatol 1992;27:37–39.

119. Calabrese LH, Kelley DM, Myers A, et al. Rheumatic symptoms and human immunodeficiency virus infection. Arthritis Rheum 1991;34:257–263.

120. Obuch ML, Maurer TA, Becker B, et al. Psoriasis and human immunodeficiency virus infection. J Am Acad Dermatol 1992;27:667–673.

121. Reveille JD, Conant MA, Duvic M. Human immunodeficiency virus–associated psoriasis, psoriatic arthritis, and Reiter's syndrome: A disease continuum? Arthritis Rheum 1990;33:1574–1578.

122. Jaffe D, May LP, Sanchez M, et al. Staphylococcal sepsis in HIV antibody seropositive psoriasis patients. J Am Acad Dermatol 1991;24:970–972.

123. Kaplan MH, Sadick NS, Wieder J, et al. Antipsoriatic effects of zidovudine in human immunodeficiency virus–associated psoriasis. J Am Acad Dermatol 1989;20:76–82.

124. Meola T, Soter NA, Ostreicher, et al. The safety of UVB phototherapy in patients with HIV infection. J Am Acad Dermatol 1993;29:216–220.

125. Menni S, Brancaleone W, Grimalt R. Pityriasis rubra pilaris in a child seropositive for the human immunodeficiency virus. J Am Acad Dermatol 1992;27:1009.

126. Martin AG, Weaver CC, Cockerell CJ, et al. Pityriasis rubra pilaris in the setting of HIV infection: Clinical behaviour and association with explosive cystic acne. Br J Dermatol 1992;126:617–620.

127. Auffret N, Quint L, Domart P, et al. Pityriasis rubra pilaris in a patient with human immunodeficiency virus infection. J Am Acad Dermatol 1992;27:260–261.

128. Resnick SD, Murrell DF, Woosley J. Acne conglobata and a generalized lichen spinulosus–like eruption in a man seropositive for human immunodeficiency virus. J Am Acad Dermatol 1992;26:1013–1014.

129. Cohen SJ, Dicken CH. Generalized lichen spinulosus in an HIV-positive man. J Am Acad Dermatol 1991;25:116–118.

130. Katz MH, Greenspan D, Westenhouse J, et al. Progression to AIDS in HIV-infected homosexual and bisexual men with hairy leukoplakia and oral candidiasis. AIDS 1992;6:95–100.

131. Wingard JR, Merz WG, Rinaldi MG, et al. Increase in *Candida krusei* infection among patients with bone marrow transplantation and neutropenia treated prophylactically with fluconazole. N Engl J Med 1991;325:1274–1277.

132. Greenspan JS, Greenspan D, Lennette ET, et al. Replication of Epstein-Barr virus within the epithelial cells of oral "hairy" leukoplakia, an AIDS-associated lesion. N Engl J Med 1985;313:1564–1571.

133. Lozada-Nur F, Costa C. Retrospective findings of the clinical benefits of podophyllum resin 25% sol on hairy leukoplakia. Oral Surg Oral Med Oral Pathol 1992;73:555–558.

134. Greenspan D, Greenspan JS, De Souza YG, et al. Oral hairy leukoplakia in an HIV-negative renal transplant recipient. J Oral Pathol Med 1989;18:32–34.

135. Fisher DA, Daniels TE, Greenspan JS. Oral hairy leukoplakia unassociated with human immunodeficiency virus: Pseudo oral hairy leukoplakia. J Am Acad Dermatol 1992;27:257–258.

136. MacPhail LA, Greenspan D, Feigal DW, et al. Recurrent aphthous ulcers in association with HIV infection: Description of ulcer types and analysis of T-lymphocyte subsets. Oral Surg Oral Med Oral Pathol 1991;71:678–683.

137. Bach MC, Valenti AJ, Howell DA, et al. Odynophagia from aphthous ulcers of the pharynx and esophagus in the acquired immunodeficiency syndrome (AIDS). Ann Intern Med 1988;109:338–339.

138. Itescu S, Brancato LJ, Buxbaum J, et al. A diffuse infiltrative CD8 lymphocytosis syndrome in human immunodeficiency virus (HIV) infection: A host immune response associated with HLA-DR5. Ann Intern Med 1990;112:3–10.

139. Itescu S, Winchester R. Diffuse infiltrative lymphocytosis syndrome: A disorder occurring in human immunodeficiency virus-1 infection that may present as a sicca syndrome. Rheum Dis Clin North Am 1992;18:683–697.

140. Silverman S Jr, Migliorati CA, Lozada-Nur F, et al. Oral findings in people with or at high risk for AIDS: A study of 375 homosexual males. J Am Dent Assoc 1986;112:187–192.

141. Chren M-M, Silverman RA, Sorensen RU, et al. Leukocytoclastic vasculitis in a patient infected with human immunodeficiency virus. J Am Acad Dermatol 1989;21:1161–1164.

142. Requena L, Yus ES, Martin L, et al. Erythema elevatum diutinum in a patient with acquired immunodeficiency syndrome. Arch Dermatol 1991;127:1819–1822.

143. LeBoit PE, Cockerell CJ. Nodular lesions of erythema elevatum diutinum in patients infected with the human immunodeficiency virus. J Am Acad Dermatol 1993;28:191–922.

144. Smith KJ, Skelton HG, Yeager J, et al. Cutaneous neoplasms in a military population of HIV-1–positive patients. J Am Acad Dermatol 1993;29:400–406.

145. Lobo DV, Chu P, Grekin RC, et al. Non-melanoma skin cancer and infection with the human immunodeficiency virus. Arch Dermatol 1992;128:623–627.

146. Schafer A, Friedmann W, Mielke M, et al. The increased frequency of cervical dysplasia-neoplasia in women infected with the human immunodeficiency virus is related to the degree of immunosuppression. Am J Obstet Gynecol 1991;164:593–599.

147. Vermund SH, Kelley KF, Klein RS, et al. High risk of human papillomavirus infection and cervical squamous intraepithelial lesions among women with symptomatic human immunodeficiency virus infection. Am J Obstet Gynecol 1991;165:392–400.

148. Palefsky JM, Gonzales J, Greenblatt RM, et al. Anal intraepithelial neoplasia and anal papillomavirus infection among homosexual males with group IV HIV disease. JAMA 1990;263:2911–2916.

149. McGregor JM, Newell M, Ross J, et al. Cutaneous malignant melanoma and human immune virus: A report of 3 cases. Br J Dermatol 1992;126:516–519.

150. Duvic M, Lowe L, Rapini RP, et al. Eruptive dysplastic nevi associated with human immunodeficiency virus infection. Arch Dermatol 1989;125:397–401.

151. Kaposi M. Idiopathic multiple pigmented sarcoma of the skin. Arch Dermatol Syph 1872;4:265–273; translated in CA 1982;32:342–347.

152. Wahman A, Melnick SL, Rhame FS, et al. The epidemiology of classic, African, and immunocompromised Kaposi's sarcoma. Epidemiol Rev 1991;13:178–199.

153. Centers for Disease Control. Kaposi's sarcoma and *Pneumocystis* pneumonia among homosexual men: New York City and California. MMWR 1981;30:305–308.

154. Centers for Disease Control. Follow-up on Kaposi's sarcoma and *Pneumocystis* pneumonia. MMWR 1981;30:409–410.

155. Myskowski PL. Kaposi's sarcoma: Where do we go from here? Arch Dermatol 1993;129:1320–1323.

156. Tappero JW, Conant MA, Wolfe SF, Berger TG. Kaposi's sarcoma: Epidemiology, pathogenesis, histology, clinical presenta-

tion, staging criteria and therapy. J Am Acad Dermatol 1993;28:371–395.

157. Friedman-Kien AE, Saltzman BR. Clinical manifestations of classical, endemic African, and epidemic AIDS-associated Kaposi's sarcoma. J Am Acad Dermatol 1990;22:1237–1250.

158. Safai B, Mike V, Giraldo G, et al. Association of Kaposi's sarcoma with second primary malignancies: Possible etiopathogenic implications. Cancer 1980;45:1472–1479.

159. Piette WW. The incidence of second primary malignancies in subsets of Kaposi's sarcoma. J Am Acad Dermatol 1987;16:855–861.

160. Olweny CLM. Epidemiology and clinical features of Kaposi's sarcoma in tropical Africa. In: Friedman-Kien AE, Laubenstein LJ, eds. AIDS: The Epidemic of Kaposi's Sarcoma and Opportunistic Infections. New York: Masson Publishing, 1984:35–40.

161. Penn I. Kaposi's sarcoma in organ transplant recipients. Transplantation 1979;27:8–11.

162. Harwood AR, Osoba D, Hofstader SL, et al. Kaposi's sarcoma in recipients of renal transplants. Am J Med 1979;67:759–765.

163. Beral V, Peterman TA, Berkelman RL, et al. Kaposi's sarcoma among persons with AIDS: A sexually transmitted infection? Lancet 1990;335:123–128.

164. Peterman TA, Jaffe HW, Beral V. Epidemiologic clues to the etiology of Kaposi's sarcoma. AIDS 1993;7:605–611.

165. Beral V, Bull D, Darby S, et al. Risk of Kaposi's sarcoma and sexual practices associated with faecal contact in homosexual or bisexual men with AIDS. Lancet 1992;339:632–635.

166. Jacobson LP, Munoz A, Fox R, et al. Incidence of Kaposi's sarcoma in a cohort of homosexual men infected with the human immunodeficiency virus type I. J AIDS 1990;3(Suppl 1):S24–S31.

167. Friedman-Kien AE, Saltzman BR, Cao Y, et al. Kaposi's sarcoma in HIV-negative homosexual men. Lancet 1990;335:168–169.

168. Huang YQ, Li JJ, Rush MG, et al. HPV-16–related DNA sequences in Kaposi's sarcoma. Lancet 1992;339:515–518.

169. Nickoloff BJ, Huang YQ, Li JJ, et al. Immunohistochemical detection of papillomavirus antigens in Kaposi sarcoma. Lancet 1992;339:548–549.

170. Lane HC, Masur H, Gelmann EP, et al. Correlation between immunologic function and clinical subpopulations of patients with the acquired immune deficiency syndrome. Am J Med 1985;78:417–422.

171. Welch K, Finkbeiner W, Alpers CE, et al. Autopsy findings in the acquired immune deficiency syndrome. JAMA 1984;252:1152–1159.

172. Lemlich G, Schwan L, Lebwohl M, et al. Kaposi's sarcoma and acquired immunodeficiency syndrome: Postmortem findings in twenty-four cases. J Am Acad Dermatol 1987;16:319–325.

173. Taylor J, Afrasiabi R, Fahey JL, et al. A prognostically significant classification of immune changes in AIDS with Kaposi's sarcoma. Blood 1986;67:666–671.

174. Vadhan-Raj S, Wong G, Gnecco C, et al. Immunological variables as predictors of prognosis in patients with Kaposi's sarcoma and the acquired immunodeficiency syndrome. Cancer Res 1986;46:417–425.

175. Janier M, Morel P, Civatte J. The Koebner phenomenon in AIDS-related Kaposi's sarcoma. J Am Acad Dermatol 1990;22:125–126.

176. Silverman S, Migliorati CA, Lozada-Nur F, et al. Oral findings in people with or at risk for AIDS: A study of 375 homosexual males. J Am Dent Assoc 1986;112:187–192.

177. Ficarra G, Berson AM, Silverman S, et al. Kaposi's sarcoma of the oral cavity: A study of 134 patients with a review of the pathogenesis, epidemiology, clinical aspects, and treatment. Oral Surg Oral Med Oral Pathol 1988;66:543–550.

178. Feigal DW, Katz MH, Greenspan D, et al. The prevalence of oral lesions in HIV-infected homosexual and bisexual men: Three San Francisco epidemiological cohorts. AIDS 1991;5:519–525.

179. Shuler JD, Holland GN, Miles SA, et al. Kaposi sarcoma of the conjuctiva and eyelids associated with the acquired immunodeficiency syndrome. Arch Ophthalmol 1989;107:858–862.

180. McKenzie R, Travis WD, Dolan SA, et al. The causes of death in patients with human immunodeficiency virus infection: A clinical and pathologic study with emphasis on the role of pulmonary diseases. Medicine 1991;70:326–343.

181. Chor PJ, Santa Cruz DJ. Kaposi's sarcoma: A clinicopathologic review and differential diagnosis. J Cutan Pathol 1992;19:6–20.

182. Nickoloff BJ, Griffiths CEM. Factor XIIIa expressing dermal dendrocytes are increased in AIDS-associated cutaneous Kaposi's sarcoma. Science 1989;243:1736–1737.

183. Werner S, Hofschneider PH, Roth WK. Cells derived from sporadic and AIDS-related Kaposi's sarcoma reveal identical cytochemical and molecular properties in vitro. Int J Cancer 1989;43:1137–1144.

184. Ensoli B, Barillari G, Buonaguro L, Gallo RC. Molecular mechanisms in the pathogenesis of AIDS-associated Kaposi's sarcoma. Adv Exp Med Biol 1991;303:27–38.

185. Miles SA, Martinez-Maza O, Rezai A, et al. Oncostatin M as a potent mitogen for AIDS–Kaposi's sarcoma–derived cells. Science 1992;255(SOSO):1432–1434.

186. Gearing DP, Comeau MR, Friend DJ, et al. The signal transducer, gp130: An Oncostatin M receptor and affinity converter for the LIF receptor. Science 1992;255:1434–1437.

187. Nai BC, DeVico AL, Nakamura S, et al. Identification of a major growth factor for AIDS–Kaposi's sarcoma cells as Oncostatin M. Science 1992;255:1430–1432.

188. Vogel J, Hinrichs SH, Reynolds RK, et al. The HIV *tat* gene induces dermal lesions resembling Kaposi's sarcoma in transgenic mice. Nature 1988;335:606–611.

189. Mahoney SE, Duvic M, Nickoloff BJ, et al. Human immunodeficiency virus (HIV) transcripts in HIV-related psoriasis and Kaposi's sarcoma. J Clin Invest 1991;88:174–185.

190. Krown SE, Metroka C, Wernz JC. Kaposi's sarcoma in the acquired immunodeficiency syndrome: A proposal for uniform evaluation, response, and staging criteria. J Clin Oncol 1989;7:1201–1207.

191. Krown SE, Myskowski PL, Paredes J. Kaposi's sarcoma: Medical management of AIDS patients. Med Clin North Am 1992;76:235–257.

192. Tappero JW, Berger TG, Kaplan LD, et al. Cryotherapy for cutaneous Kaposi's sarcoma (KS) associated with acquired immune deficiency syndrome (AIDS): A phase II trial. J AIDS 1991;4:839–846.

193. Tappero JW, Berger TG. Caution in the use of local therapies for Kaposi's sarcoma. Arch Dermatol 1993;129:42.

194. Tappero JT, Grekin RC, Zanelli GA, Berger TG. Pulsed-dye laser therapy for cutaneous Kaposi's sarcoma associated with acquired immunodeficiency syndrome. J Am Acad Dermatol 1992;27:526–530.

195. Boudreaux AA, Smith LL, Cosby CD, et al. Intralesional vinblastine for cutaneous Kaposi's sarcoma associated with acquired immunodeficiency syndrome: A clinical trial to evaluate efficacy and discomfort associated with injection. J Am Acad Dermatol 1993;28:61–65.

196. Smith KJ, Konzelman JL, Lombardo FA, et al. Iontophoresis of vinblastine into normal skin and for treatment of Kaposi's sarcoma in human immunodeficiency virus–positive patients. Arch Dermatol 1992;128:1365–1370.

197. Muzyka BC, Glick M. Sclerotherapy for the treatment of nodular intraoral Kaposi's sarcoma in patients with AIDS. N Engl J Med 1993;328:210–211.

198. Sulis E, Floris C, Sulis ML, et al. Interferon administered intralesionally in skin and oral cavity in heterosexual drug-addicted patients with AIDS-related Kaposi's sarcoma. Eur J Cancer Clin Oncol 1989;25:759–761.

199. Kahn J, Kaplan L, Volberding P, et al. Intralesional tumor necrosis factor–α for AIDS-associated Kaposi's sarcoma. J AIDS 1989;2:217–223.

200. Boente P, Sampiaio C, Brandao MA, et al. Local perilesional therapy with rhGMCSF for Kaposi's sarcoma. Lancet 1993;341:1154.

201. Chak LY, Gill PS, Levine AM, et al. Radiation therapy for acquired immunodeficiency syndrome–related Kaposi's sarcoma. J Clin Oncol 1988;5:863–867.

202. Cooper JS. Optimal treatment of epidemic Kaposi's sarcoma. Int J Radiat Oncol Biol Phys 1990;19:807–808.

203. Berson AM, Quivey JM, Harris JW, et al. Radiation therapy for AIDS-related Kaposi's sarcoma. Int J Radiat Oncol Biol Phys 1990;19:569–575.

204. Schweitzer VG, Visscher D. Photodynamic therapy for treatment

of AIDS-related Kaposi's sarcoma. Otolaryngol Head Neck Surg 1990;102:639–649.

205. Present CA, Scolaro M, Kennedy P, et al. Liposomal daunorubicin treatment in HIV-associated Kaposi's sarcoma. Lancet 1993;341:1242–1243.

206. Brunt AM, Goodman AG, Phillips RH, et al. Short communication: The safety of intravenous chemotherapy and zidovudine when treating epidemic Kaposi's sarcoma. AIDS 1989;3:457–460.

207. Burns MK, Cooper KD. Cutaneous T-cell lymphoma associated with HIV infection. J Am Acad Dermatol 1993;29:394–399.

208. Sheil AGR, Flavel S, Disney APS, et al. Cancer development in patients progressing to dialysis and renal transplantation. Transplant Proc 1985;17:1685–1688.

209. Barr BBB, McLaren K, Smith IW, et al. Human papillomavirus infection and skin cancer in renal allograft recipients. Lancet 1989;1:124–129.

210. Sheil AGR, Mahoney JF, Horvath JS, et al. Cancer following renal transplantation. Aust NZ J Surg 1979;49:617–620.

211. Penn I. Why do immunosuppressed patients develop cancer? In Pimental E, ed. CRC Critical Reviews in Oncogenesis. Boca Raton, FL: CRC Press, 1989:27–52.

212. Briggaman RA, Wheeler CE. Immunology of human warts. J Am Acad Dermatol 1979;1:297–304.

213. Van der Leest RJ, Zachow KR, Ostrow RS, et al. Human papillomavirus heterogeneity in 36 renal transplant recipients. Arch Dermatol 1987;123:354–357.

214. Gissman L, Schwarz E. Persistence and expression of human papillomavirus DNA in genital cancer. In: Evered D, Clark S, eds. Papillomaviruses, Ciba Foundation symposium 120. Chichester, England, John Wiley & Sons, 1986: 190–197.

215. Macnab JCM, Walkinshaw SA, Cordiner JW, et al. Human papillomavirus in clinically and histologically normal tissue of patients with genital cancer. N Engl J Med 1986;315:1052–1058.

216. Gal AA, Meyer PR, Taylor CR. Papillomavirus antigens in anorectal condyloma and carcinoma in homosexual men. JAMA 1987;257:337–340.

217. Austin DF. Etiological clues from descriptive epidemiology: Squamous carcinoma of the rectum or anus. NCI Monogr 1982;62:89–90.

218. Daling JR, Weiss NS, Klopfenstein LL, et al. Correlates of homosexual behaviour and the incidence of anal cancer. JAMA 1982;247:1988–1990.

219. Peters RK, Mack TM. Patterns of anal carcinoma by gender and marital status in Los Angeles County. Br J Cancer 1983;48:629–636.

220. Matis WL, Triana A, Shapiro R, et al. Dermatologic findings associated with human immunodeficiency virus infection. J Am Acad Dermatol 1987;17:746–751.

221. Palefsky JM, Gonzales J, Greenblatt RM, et al. Anal intraepithelial neoplasia and anal papillomavirus infection among homosexual males with group IV HIV disease. JAMA 1990;263:2911–2916.

222. Rudlinger R, Grob R, Buchmann P, et al. Anogenital warts of the condyloma acuminatum type in HIV-positive patients. Dermatologica 1988;176:277–381.

223. Syrjanen SM, von Krogh G, Syrjanen KJ. Anal condylomas in men: I. Histopathological and virological assessment. Genitourin Med 1989;65:216–224.

224. Schafer A, Friedmann W, Mielke M, et al. The increased frequency of cervical dysplasia-neoplasia in women infected with the human immunodeficiency virus is related to the degree of immunosuppression. Am J Obstet Gynecol 1991;164:593–599.

225. Vermund SH, Kelley KF, Klein RS, et al. High risk of human papillomavirus infection and cervical squamous intraepithelial lesions among women with symptomatic human immunodeficiency virus infection. Am J Obstet Gynecol 1991;165:392–400.

226. Blohme I, Brynger H. Malignant disease in renal transplant patients. Transplant 1985;39:23–35.

227. Rudlinger R, Smith IW, Bunney MH, et al. Human papillomavirus infections in a group of renal transplant recipients. J Dermatol 1986;115:681–692.

228. Ikenberg H, Gissman L, Gross GT, et al. Human papillomavirus type 6–related DNA in genital Bowen's disease and bowenoid papulosis. Int J Cancer 1983;32:563–565.

229. Patterson JW, Kao GFR, Graham JH, et al. Bowenoid papulosis: A clinicopathologic study with ultrastructural observations. Cancer 1986;57:823–836.

230. Rudlinger R, Buchmann P. HPV 16–positive bowenoid papulosis and squamous cell carcinoma of the anus in an HIV-positive man. Dis Colon Rectum 1989;32:1042–1045.

231. Goette DK. Topical chemotherapy with 5-fluorouracil. J Am Acad Dermatol 1981;4:633–649.

232. Ferenczy A. Comparison of 5-fluorouracil and CO_2 laser for treatment of vaginal condylomata. Obstet Gynecol 1984;64:773–778.

233. Silman FH, Sedlis A, Boyce JG. A review of lower genital intraepithelial neoplasia and the use of topical 5-fluorouracil. Obstet Gynecol Survey 1985;40:190–220.

234. Douglas JM, Rogers M, Judson FN. The effect of asymptomatic infection with HTLV-III on the response of anogenital warts to intralesional treatment with recombinant alfa$_2$ interferon. J Infect Dis 1986;154:331–334.

235. Greenberg MS, Friedman H, Cohen SG, et al. A comparative study of herpes simplex infections in renal transplant and leukemic patients. J Infect Dis 1987;156:280–287.

236. Wade JC, Newton B, Fluornoy N, et al. Oral acyclovir for prevention of herpes simplex virus reactivation after marrow transplantation. Ann Intern Med 1984;100:823–828.

237. Feldman S, Lott L. Varicella in children with cancer: Impact of antiviral therapy and prophylaxis. Pediatrics 1987;80:465–472.

238. Centers for Disease Control. Varicella-zoster immune globulin for the prevention of chickenpox. Ann Intern Med 1984;100:859.

239. Whiteley RJ. Therapeutic approaches to varicella-zoster virus infections. J Infect Dis 1992;166(Suppl 1):851.

240. Rusthoven JJ, Ahlgren P, Alhakim T, et al. Varicella-zoster infection in adult cancer patients. Arch Intern Med 1988;148:1561–1566.

241. Stevens DA, Merigan TC. Zoster immune globulin prophylaxis of disseminated zoster in compromised hosts. Arch Intern Med 1980;140:52–54.

242. Perren TJ, Powles RL, Easton, D, et al. Prevention of herpes zoster in patients by long-term oral acyclovir after allogeneic bone marrow transplantation. Am J Med 1988;85(Suppl 2A):99–101.

243. Huminer D, Siegman-Igra Y, Morduchowicz G, et al. Ecthyma gangrenosum without bacteremia: Report of six cases and review of the literature. Arch Intern Med 1987;147:299–301.

244. Bodey GP, Luna M. Skin lesions associated with disseminated candidiasis. JAMA 1974;229:1466–1468.

245. File TM, Marina OA, Flowers FP. Necrotic skin lesions associated with disseminated candidiasis. Arch Dermatol 1979;115:214–215.

246. Fine JD, Miller JA, Harrist TJ, et al. Cutaneous lesions in disseminated candidiasis mimicking ecthyma gangrenosum. Am J Med 1981;70:1133.

247. Morrison VA, Haake RJ, Weisdorf DJ. The spectrum of non-*Candida* fungal infections following bone marrow transplantation. Medicine 1993;72:78–89.

248. Findlay G, Roux H, Simson I. Skin manifestations in disseminated aspergillosis. Br J Dermatol 1971;85(Suppl 7):94–97.

249. Allo MD, Miller J, Townsend T, et al. Primary cutaneous aspergillosis associated with Hickman intravenous catheters. N Engl J Med 1987;317:1105–1108.

250. Grossman ME, Fithian EC, Behrens C, et al. Primary cutaneous aspergillosis in six leukemic children. J Am Acad Dermatol 1985;12:313–318.

251. Estes SA, Hendricks AA, Merz WG, et al. Primary cutaneous aspergillosis. J Am Acad Dermatol 1980;3:397–400.

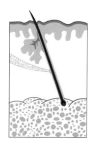

chapter 126

Leishmaniasis

ETHAN A. LERNER and SUZANNE A. GREVELINK

DEFINITION

Leishmaniasis is a protozoal disease whose diverse clinical manifestations are dependent both on the infecting species of *Leishmania* and the immune response of the host. Transmission of the disease occurs by the bite of a sandfly infected with *Leishmania* parasites. Infection may be restricted to the skin in cutaneous leishmaniasis (CL), limited to the mucous membranes in mucosal leishmaniasis (ML), or spread throughout the reticuloendothelial system in visceral leishmaniasis (VL) or kala-azar. Three rare clinical variants of cutaneous leishmaniasis include diffuse cutaneous leishmaniasis (DCL), leishmaniasis recidivans, and post–kala-azar dermal leishmaniasis (PKADL). The disease in its various forms affects at least 12 million persons worldwide, with 400,000 new cases per year.[1]

The cutaneous afflictions of leishmaniasis have been known since antiquity. Descriptions of the cutaneous disease in the Old World are found from the first century A.D. New World pottery from Peru and Ecuador dating from A.D. 400 to 900 is illustrated with faces afflicted with a process consistent with leishmaniasis. The first description in English of a lesion resembling leishmaniasis was made in 1756 by Russell, who described the "Aleppo evil" from Turkey. In 1885, Cunningham observed organisms in macrophages from lesions of "Delhi boil" in India. A Russian army physician named Borovsky noted the protozoal nature of the organism in 1898 in biopsy specimens from skin lesions. In 1903, Leishman identified the parasite in the spleen of an English private who had died of Dum-Dum fever in Dum-Dum, India. A few months later Donovan described identical organisms in a splenic puncture specimen from a living child. The distinctive histologic feature of this 2- to 5-μm parasite was the presence of both a nucleus and a smaller rod-shaped structure called the kinetoplast, which has since proven to consist of mitochondrial DNA. Ross named the parasite *Leishmania donovanii* later the same year.[2] Synonyms for the disease include

oriental sore, Baghdad sore, chiclero's ulcer, uta, espundia (mucosal form), and forest yaws.

CLINICAL DESCRIPTION

Leishmaniasis in its various forms is present on all continents except Australia and Antarctica (Table 126–1).[3, 4] Localized cutaneous leishmaniasis (LCL) is widespread throughout the Old World and is primarily caused by the organism *L. major.* New World LCL is endemic in Central and South America. Two independent species or "complexes" of parasites are responsible for New World LCL, including *L. braziliensis* and *L. mexicana.*

LCL usually affects unclothed parts of the body easily bitten by the sand fly vector, including the face, neck, and arms. New World leishmaniasis commonly presents as a solitary primary lesion, while multiple primary lesions are often found in Old World disease. After an incubation period of 1 week to 3 months, a red papule appears that enlarges to a plaque or nodule. The lesion often develops into an ulcer, which is well circumscribed with a violaceous border. The ulcer base is granular appearing and crusted, and the margins are raised but without extensive undermining (Fig. 126–1). Painless rubbery subcutaneous nodules or cords may develop around the ulcer owing to local lymphangitic spread of the organism. Draining lymph nodes may be enlarged and reveal parasites on biopsy. Inflammatory satellite papules and subcutaneous induration may develop around the primary lesion representing a reaction to local dissemination of the parasite or its antigenic products. A generalized papular eruption may also develop, representing a hypersensitivity reaction. Areas of trauma may "koebnerize." Itching and pain are mild, if present. The wound may become superinfected, leading to misdiagnosis. After 6 to 12 months the ulcer spontaneously regresses leaving a scar with hypopigmentation or hyperpigmentation. Immunity is not always complete, and

TABLE 126-1. Clinical Forms of Leishmaniasis, Associated Parasites, and Geographic Location

Form of Disease	New World Parasite	Old World Parasite	Geography
Cutaneous			
Localized	L. braziliensis braziliensis	L. major	Northern Africa, India
	L. braziliensis guyanensis	L. tropica	Middle East, China
	L. braziliensis panamensis	L. aethiopica	Southern Russia, Pakistan
	L. mexicana mexicana	L. infantum	Mediterranean countries
			Central and South America
			Texas, Caribbean islands
Diffuse	L. amazonensis	L. aethiopica	Venezuela, Bolivia, Mexico
	L. mexicana		Dominican Republic, Brazil
	L. pifanoi		Ethiopia
Recidivans	L. braziliensis	L. tropica	Central and South America
			Middle East
Post kala-azar		L. donovani	India, Bangladesh
		L. tropica	Eastern Africa, Sudan
Mucocutaneous	L. braziliensis braziliensis		Brazil, Venezuela
	L. braziliensis panamensis		Peru, Ecuador
			Colombia
Visceral	L. donovani chagasi	L. donovani	China, India, Bangladesh
		L. infantum	Asia, Sudan, Africa
		L. tropica	Eastern Russia, Mediterranean countries
			South America

secondary infection may occur in up to 10% of individuals.

Diffuse cutaneous leishmaniasis (DCL) is an anergic variant of LCL in which lesions are disseminated, resembling lepromatous lepropsy. Infection is primarily caused by *L. aethiopica* in the Old World and *L. amazonensis* in Central and South America. The disease usually begins with an initial primary lesion and then disseminates to involve other areas of the skin. The lesions are nonulcerative nodules that are often scattered over the limbs, buttocks, and face. Unlike lepromatous leprosy, there is no nerve involvement. The disease responds partially to treatment and often relapses, becoming chronic.

Leishmaniasis recidivans or "recurrent leishmanisias" refers to the development of new lesions in the center or periphery of a scar of a healed acute lesion of leishmaniasis. Clinically, leishmaniasis recidivans commonly presents as scaly, erythematous papules within scars of healed lesions, although ulcers, psoriasiform lesions, and verrucous forms have also been described. The active disease is confined to the scar and immediate contiguous area. The causative organism is usually *L. tropica* in the Middle East and less commonly *L. braziliensis* in South America. Lesions tend to resist treatment and become chronic. The mechanism postulated for recurrent disease is reactivation of "dormant" organisms, with the period of dormancy ranging from 1 to 15 years. Characterization of the species in initial and recurrent lesions, however, has revealed that 50% of the recurrent strains differed from the initial strain, suggesting exogenous reinfection as a mechanism in many of the cases rather than reactivation.[5]

Post–kala-azar dermal leishmaniasis (PKADL) generally occurs 1 to 3 years after recovery from visceral leishmaniasis. This disease is primarily caused by *L. donovani* and is endemic in India and Bangladesh. Dermatologic manifestations of PKADL consist of hypopigmented macules, erythematous macules, and nodules. Hypopigmented macules are usually the first manifestation of PKADL, beginning as very small macules that enlarge to form large irregular patches. Lesions are often bilateral and symmetrical, appearing primarily on the chest and back, anterior thighs, arms, and neck. The pigmentary loss is never complete, and there is no pigment change in the hair overlying the lesions. Erythematous macules develop next, often on the face in a malar distribution, but they may also develop in other areas, especially in the hypopigmented patches. Finally, soft, painless, nonulcerative, yellowish-pink nodules replace the hypopigmented and erythematous macules and sometimes develop de novo. Nodules most commonly affect the face, earlobes, trunk, and genitalia and less frequently occur on the hands and feet. Cases of PKADL are more resistant to

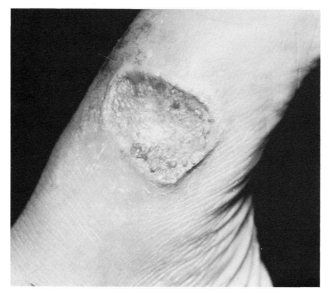

FIGURE 126-1. Ulcer of the lower extremity caused by *L. braziliensis braziliensis.*

treatment, requiring higher doses of systemic medication. Hypopigmented areas almost never completely repigment.

Mucocutaneous leishmaniasis (MCL) is most commonly reported in the New World. *L. braziliensis braziliensis* is the most common etiologic agent, although cases due to other *Leishmania* subspecies have been reported. In particular, there has been a recent increase in mucocutaneous disease due to *L. braziliensis panamensis,* increasing the risk that travelers to Central America could potentially develop MCL. The disease usually presents 2 years to decades after the initial cutaneous lesions but may occur within the first year (Fig. 126-2). This form of leishmaniasis typically affects a small percentage (approximately 3%) of individuals previously infected with *L. braziliensis* subspecies, although a prevalence as high as 34% in endemic areas has been reported. Mucous membrane involvement probably develops due to hematogenous or lymphatic dissemination or occasionally from direct extension of nearby skin lesions. Factors associated with the development of MCL include male gender, large or multiple primary lesions, persistent lesions lasting longer than 1 year, and inadequate treatment for the primary skin lesions. The disease often begins in the nasal septum, which becomes inflamed and infiltrated and subsequently perforates. MCL has a predilection for the distal cartilaginous part of the nose, and the resulting deformation has been named "tapir's nose," "parrot's beak," and "camel's nose." Mutilation of the nasal septum, palate, pharynx, tonsils, gums, and/or lip may ensue, whereas bony structures remain intact. Rarely, dissemination to the mucous membranes of the eye and genitalia is seen. Invasion of the respiratory tract, including the larynx, trachea, and bronchi, may lead to compromised respiration and swallowing (Fig. 126-3). Malnutrition and acute respiratory pneumonia are the leading causes of death in patients with MCL.

Kala-azar or visceral leishmaniasis (VL) is a systemic disease caused by the dissemination of *L. donovani*

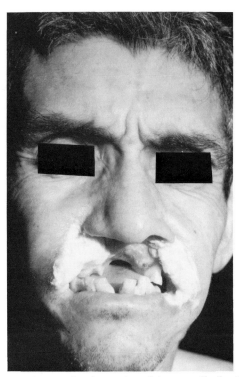

FIGURE 126-3. Extensive destruction of the upper lip due to mucocutaneous infection with *L. braziliensis braziliensis.*

throughout the reticuloendothelial system. Recently, *L. tropica,* which almost exclusively causes cutaneous disease, was found to be the causative organism in several cases of VL reported in soldiers of Operation Desert Storm returning from Saudi Arabia.[6] Characteristic signs and symptoms include fever, splenomegaly, emaciation, pancytopenia, and hyperglobulinemia. The primary lesion of VL is a small erythematous papule usually seen on the legs, sometimes referred to as a "leishmanioma." During the active period of VL, a patchy blackening of the skin appears that is the origin of the name *kala-azar,* meaning "black fever." This hyperpigmentation is secondary to increased melanocytic activity as well as an enhancement of the natural skin color due to xerosis. The skin in general becomes very dry and rough, and the hair becomes so brittle that a complete alopecia may ensue. An impairment in wound healing is often seen. After an incubation period of 2 to 4 months, VL runs an insidious chronic course until treated. Treatment is successful in 95% to 98% of cases, and relapses are uncommon.

PATHOLOGY

The histopathologic findings in leishmaniasis reflect the immunity of the host, the stage of the infection, and, to a lesser extent, the infecting species.[7]

In LCL there are nodular and diffuse infiltrates of lymphocytes, plasma cells, and macrophages parasitized with the amastigotes, termed *Leishman-Donovan bodies.* These are 2 to 4 μm, are round to oval, and have a large peripheral nucleus and a smaller rod-shaped kinetoplast

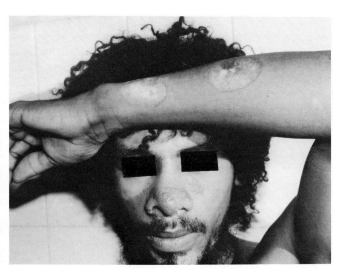

FIGURE 126-2. Young man with healed prior lesions of cutaneous leishmaniasis on the arms caused by *L. braziliensis braziliensis,* now presenting with new lesions of the nasal mucosa.

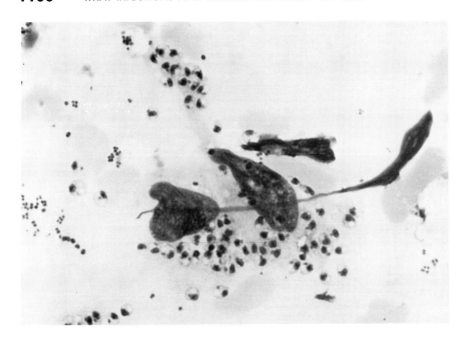

FIGURE 126–4. Smear from ulcerated lesion revealing diagnostic Leishman-Donovan bodies of *L. major* within macrophages.

of mitochondrial DNA (Fig. 126–4). The kinetoplast is generated from the base of the flagellum, which is lost during conversion from the promastigote to the amastigote. Leishman-Donovan bodies are faintly visible in hematoxylin and eosin–stained sections, but their appearance is enhanced by the Giemsa stain.

Variable features of early LCL include epidermal atrophy or hyperplasia and neutrophils in either the dermal infiltrate or within the epidermis, especially in those patients who develop sporotrichoid lesions.

As lesions of LCL age, signs of chronicity appear, such as tuberculoid granulomas with Langhans' giant cells.[8] The number of organisms decreases.

In lesions from anergic patients who develop DCL, there are dense, diffuse infiltrates of heavily parasitized, foamy macrophages throughout the dermis, with thinning of the epidermis.

In the cicatricial stage of LCL, the dermis is replaced by scar and organisms are not identifiable. If relapse occurs adjacent to the scar (leishmaniasis recidivans or recurrent leishmaniasis), the epidermis is often hyperplastic and the dermis contains tuberculoid granulomas, with or without necrosis. The number of organisms is highly variable in recurrent leishmaniasis.

In MCL, lesions initially are edematous, with superficial and deep infiltrates of lymphocytes, plasma cells, and macrophages. Organisms are few. In older lesions of MCL there is often pseudocarcinomatous hyperplasia of the epidermis, with many more organisms despite the presence of tuberculoid granulomas. In destructive lesions of MCL, there are areas of necrosis in the dermal infiltrates, with neutrophils and many organisms. Although patients with destructive lesions often have concomitant tuberculosis, acid-fast bacilli are not evident in the necrotic foci.[8]

In PKADL there are dermal infiltrates of lymphocytes, plasma cells, and macrophages that vary in density, from scant in macular lesions to dense in nodular ones. The number of organisms is also variable. The basal layer of

the epidemis often has diminished melanin, reflecting the hypopigmented clinical appearance of clinical lesions.[9]

Immunophenotypic analysis of cell subsets in LCL lesions reveals an abundance of T cells with an activated phenotype, expressing interleukin (IL)-2 (CD25-positive), transferrin receptors (CD71-positive), or major histocompatibility complex class II molecules on their surface.[10] Approximately equal numbers of helper/inducer (CD4-positive) and suppressor/cytotoxic (CD8-positive) lymphocytes are present in LCL lesions. In addition, while the majority of T cells in control skin biopsy specimens bear the TCR $\alpha\beta$ complex, 20% to 30% of the T cells in early LCL lesions bear the TCR $\gamma\delta$ complex. $\gamma\delta$ T cells also accumulate in skin lesions of leprosy and in active granulomas and are thought to participate in the early stages of immune defense.[11]

Analysis of the cytokine profiles in three different clinical forms of cutaneous leishmaniasis suggests that the host's immune system plays an immunoregulatory role in disease expression. In LCL the primary cytokines are IL-2 and interferon gamma, whereas in MCL and DCL IL-4 and IL-10 predominate.[12] These data correlate well with studies of leishmaniasis in murine models where the production of IL-2 and interferon gamma mediates healing of disease while IL-4 and IL-10 are associated with disease progression and dissemination.[13] Two distinct subsets of T-helper cells in the murine immune system are critical in inducing resistance or susceptibility to infection. One subset of cells called T-helper cells type 1 (Th1) produce IL-2 and interferon gamma, and augment cell-mediated immune responses by activating macrophages. Th1 cells thus mediate a clinically mild or spontaneously resolving disease. In contrast, Th2 cells, which secrete IL-4, IL-5, and IL-10, augment humoral responses and inhibit some cell-mediated immune responses, resulting in disseminated infection. The use of interferon gamma with antimony in the treatment of VL and DCL is based on data showing that exogenous interferon gamma enhances resistance to leishmania in vivo.[14] Studies demonstrate that distinct lymphokine patterns have also been associated with the response to infection in humans.[15] In conclusion, although disease expression largely depends on the species of infecting parasite, the course of infection is also based on the specific host immune response.

PATHOGENESIS AND ETIOLOGY

The arthropod vector of all forms of leishmaniasis is the female sand fly. In the Old World the disease is transmitted by flies of the genus *Phlebotomus,* and in the New World it is transmitted primarily by *Lutzomyia* and rarely by *Psychodopygus.* Specific vectors include *P. papatasi* for *L. major, Lutzomyia olmeca* for *L. mexicana, Lutzomyia wellcomei* for *L. braziliensis,* and *Lutzomyia trapidoi* for *L. panamensis.*

Adult female sand flies require a blood meal as a stimulus for oviposition. During blood feeding, infected sand flies regurgitate saliva containing *Leishmania* organisms through the proboscis into the wound. There are at least two reasons why the sand fly and not another arthropod is the vector for the disease. The first is that the environment in the gut of the fly is necessary for a portion of the life cycle of the parasite. The second is that there is evidence that certain components of sand fly saliva enhance the development of leishmanial lesions. Investigations into salivary gland extracts of *Lutzomyia longipalpis* have identified a vasodilatory peptide called maxadilan that aids in blood feeding.[16] Maxadilan or another substance in sand fly saliva contains infection-enhancing properties. In nature, sand flies inject 10 to 100 parasites to induce a lesion, while in laboratory models, injection of 10^6 parasites is necessary to generate a lesion. The co-injection of salivary gland extracts along with as few as 10 organisms allows the establishment of lesions, reflecting the natural situation.[17] This observation suggests the possibility of vaccinating against the arthropod vector to prevent transmission of the disease.

The transmission cycle of *Leishmania* organisms requires an arthropod vector and a mammalian reservoir (Fig. 126–5). The parasite assumes two distinct forms during the life cycle: (1) an extracellular, flagellated promastigote form and (2) a nonflagellated obligate intracellular form called the amastigote. During the course of probing the skin, the sand fly injects saliva containing the promastigote form of *Leishmania.* The promastigote is taken up by macrophages and transformed into the round, nonflagellated amastigote form. The parasite then resides in the phagolysosome of the macrophage and proliferates despite the presence of lysosomal enzymes. When a sand fly bites an infected host, amastigotes taken up during the blood meal transform back to the promastigote form in the gut of the fly, completing the life cycle. In hyperendemic regions such as Israel, Jordan, and Saudi Arabia, *L. major* promastigotes are recoverable from 20% to 50% of female sand flies, but in other areas less than 1% of sandflies are infected.[18] Humans are accidental hosts of leishmaniasis because they live in endemic zones and are thereby exposed to infected sand

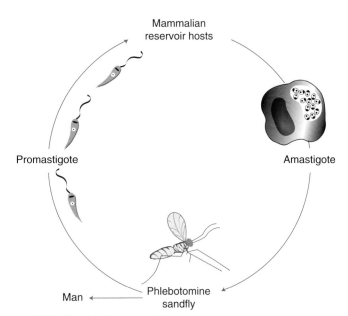

FIGURE 126–5. Transmission cycle of *Leishmania* parasites.

flies. The zoonotic reservoir includes sloths, anteaters, rodents, foxes, and dogs.

Transmission of leishmaniasis occurs almost exclusively through the bite of an infected sand fly; however, other possible modes of transmission have been reported. Direct transmission of CL through skin contact was suggested by the discovery of *Leishmania* parasites in a lesion on the upper lip of a 3-month old infant who was nursing from a mother with a lesion on the nipple.[19] With regard to VL, several cases of congenital transmission have been reported in which infants were born to women with VL during the pregnancy. *Leishmania* parasites have also been found in the placenta of a woman who spontaneously aborted after the diagnosis of VL.[20] Venereal transmission of VL has also been reported.

Leishmaniasis is characterized by a spectrum of disease phenotypes that correspond to the strength of the host's cell-mediated immune response. Both susceptible and resistant phenotypes exist within human populations. For example, many persons in endemic regions develop positive skin tests without ever manifesting signs of clinical disease. Clinical cutaneous disease ranges from a few spontaneously healing lesions to diffuse external or internal disease to severe mucous membrane involvement. Spontaneously healing lesions are associated with positive antigen-specific T-cell responsiveness, diffuse cutaneous and visceral disease with T-cell nonresponsiveness, and mucocutaneous disease with T-cell hyper-responsiveness.[21] Current research is focused on determining the extent to which this spectrum of host response to leishmanisis is genetically determined.

DIAGNOSIS AND DIFFERENTIAL DIAGNOSIS

The differential diagnosis for leishmaniasis is extensive (Table 126–2). The diagnosis is often made on clinical grounds alone, especially in endemic areas. However,

TABLE 126-2. Differential Diagnosis of Leishmaniasis

Infections

Fungal
  Paracoccidioidomycosis
  Chromoblastomycosis
  Sporotrichosis
Bacterial
  Mycobacterioses
    Leprosy
    Lupus vulgaris
    Tuberculosis verrucosa cutis
    Other mycobacterioses
  Treponematoses
    Pinta
    Yaws
    Syphilis
  Staphylococcal/streptococcal pyodermas
    Impetigo, ecthyma, furunculosis
    Insect bite (superinfected)
Parasitic
  Amebiasis
  Malaria
Viral
  Orf

Inflammatory

Psoriasis
Lichen planus
Sarcoidosis
Foreign body granuloma

Neoplastic

Cutaneous T-cell lymphoma
Basal cell carcinoma
Squamous cell carcinoma
Keratoacanthoma

multiple diagnostic techniques are available. A punch or wedge biopsy may be performed, preferably from the indurated border of a lesion and not from a necrotic center. A touch prep or tissue impression slide may be done on excised tissue, scapel scrapings, slit skin smears, or dental scrapings. Fine-needle aspiration of a lesion may be done after injection of sterile saline. Specimens from a biopsy or aspirate may be cultured on NNN blood agar (Nicolle's modification of Novy and McNeal's medium) or rabbit blood agar, with the growth of promastigotes apparent between 2 days and 2 weeks (Fig. 126–6). Alternatively, biopsy or aspirate specimens may be inoculated into hamster footpads for in vivo culture. In addition, blood samples may be examined for anti-leishmania antibodies by direct agglutination test (DAT), enzyme-linked immunosorbent agglutination (ELISA), or indirect fluorescent antibody test (IFA).

The intradermal leishmanin (Montenegro) test is useful in nonendemic areas as a diagnostic tool and in endemic areas as a test for survey work. This test consists of the intradermal injection of 0.10 to 0.20 mL of a suspension of antigen prepared from dead promastigotes (2 to 3 million promastigotes in 1 mL of phenolized saline solution). The reaction is read at 48 to 72 hours, and a positive reading consists of bright erythema with an inflammatory halo over 10 mm in diameter. A positive test indicates that a patient has, or has had, leishmaniasis but cannot distinguish between active and quiescent disease. The test is positive in 90% to 98% of patients with LCL and MCL and is negative in patients with disseminated disease. A survey in an endemic area revealed that two thirds of persons had a positive skin test, and the risk of developing a positive skin test is directly related to amount and duration of exposure to heavily forested areas. In addition, 50% of persons without any signs of past or present disease had positive skin tests, suggesting

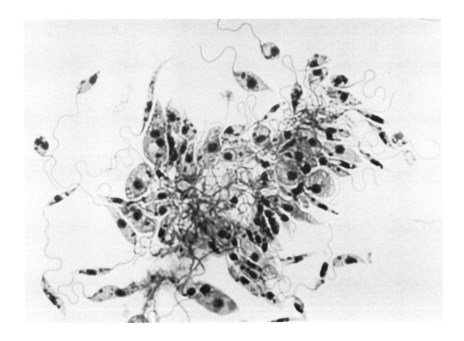

FIGURE 126-6. Culture of *L. major* in rabbit blood agar revealing multiple promastigotes.

past or active subclinical infection.[22] The test is not available in the United States.

The identification of the specific species of parasite responsible for infection is important for the diagnosis of disease, evaluation of therapy, and prognosis. Consequently, a number of laboratory techniques have been developed designed for species-specific identification of parasites within the genus Leishmania. Monoclonal antibodies to parasite surface antigens and isoenzyme analysis have been used to identify Leishmania species. Other methods of characterization involve molecular analysis of kinetoplast DNA (kDNA), a complex network of concatenated maxicircle and minicircle double-stranded DNA. Determination of the buoyant density of kDNA has been used successfully, as well as DNA hybridization using species-specific oligonucleotide probes for kDNA sequences. Oligonucleotide primers based on kDNA sequences have been used in the polymerase chain reaction to aid in determination of species. Finally, restriction endonuclease digestion of kDNA has been shown to be one of the most sensitive procedures for species and strain identification.[23] The molecular techniques can sometimes be performed on miniscule amounts of material, such as tissue sections or touch preparations, rather than on the cultured organisms needed for the other analyses.

TREATMENT

The natural history of leishmaniasis must be considered when evaluating therapeutic agents. Lesions of cutaneous leishmaniasis heal spontaneously over 1 month to 3 years, while lesions of mucocutaneous and visceral disease rarely, if ever, heal without treatment. Consequently, all cases of MCL and VL require treatment, but therapy is not always essential in LCL. Patients with LCL should, however, be treated in two occasions. Patients with lesions on the face or other cosmetically important area should be treated to reduce the size of the resultant scar. In addition, the species of parasite should be identified so that infection with *L. braziliensis braziliensis* and *L. braziliensis panamensis* can be treated to reduce the risk of development of mucocutaneous disease.

The pentavalent ammonial compound sodium stibogluconate (Pentostam), introduced in 1935, is still the conventional therapeutic agent.[24] Ironically, the exact structure of this drug remains unknown. The drug appears to inhibit amastigote glycolytic activity and fatty acid oxidation. It is available from the Centers for Disease Control and Prevention (404) 639-3670 to treat cases diagnosed in the United States. The accepted dose for the treatment of leishmaniasis is 20 mg/kg given intravenously or intramuscularly daily, without an upper limit on the daily dose. Cutaneous disease is treated for 20 days, and visceral and mucosal disease is treated for 28 days. Side effects associated with parenteral antimonial administration include arthralgias, myalgias, abdominal discomfort, reversible elevations of hepatocellular enzymes, and occasional anemia, leukopenia, or thrombocytopenia. Changes in the electrocardiogram also may develop and occur more frequently the higher the daily

dose and the longer the duration of therapy. The electrocardiographic abnormalities include T wave inversion, ST segment elevation or depression, and prolongation of the QT interval.

A review of the use of Pentostam for the treatment of leishmaniasis has generated several recommendations with regard to these side effects.[25] All patients receiving 20 mg/kg per day of Pentostam should ideally have an electrocardiogram, serum chemistries, and complete blood cell counts before treatment and weekly during treatment. However, healthy children receiving only 20 days of therapy may not require electrocardiographic monitoring. If more than 20 days of therapy are required, an electrocardiogram should be performed biweekly. Elderly patients or patients with underlying cardiac, hepatic, or renal disease should be monitored more frequently. Therapy should be discontinued if one of the serum aminotransferase values reaches five times the upper limit of normal, or if patients develop concave ST segments, prolongation of the QT interval to more than 0.5 second, or significant arrhythmias. Deaths due to antimony-induced cardiotoxicity have been reported in a few patients receiving very high daily doses of drug (30–60 mg/kg per day). However, other patients have received high and even toxic doses of antimony without untoward effects.[26]

In the United States, most patients are admitted for cardiac monitoring during treatment with Pentostam. In South America, where a slightly different pentavalent ammonial, meglumine antimoniate (Glucantine), is available, the drug is often administered at home. Glucantine is administered at 85% of the dose of Pentostam, and both drugs have similar efficacy. From 1985 through April 1990, Pentostam was released by the Centers for Disease Control and Prevention for the treatment of 129 patients.[27] The antimonials have a reported efficacy of more than 90% in most studies, although cure rates ranging from 34% to 100% have been reported, depending on the parasite species and the dose and duration of treatment.

A wide variety of alternative systemic and topical treatments have been used to treat leishmaniasis (Table 126–3). Most of these treatments have not been analyzed with randomized, placebo-controlled trials, making it difficult to accurately evaluate their effectiveness. A few conclusions, however, may be drawn: both pentamidine[28] and amphotericin B have been used successfully as second-line agents for VL and New World CL, and amphotericin B has some effectiveness in mucosal disease. Allopurinol[29] and ketoconazole[30] may have some effectiveness against VL and New and Old World CL, and in one study ketoconazole was more effective than antimony in the treatment of *L. mexicana* infection. The combination of antimony and interferon gamma has been used effectively in the treatment of refractory VL in Brazil.[31] Finally, immunotherapy consisting of three vaccinations of live bacille Calmette Guérin (BCG) with killed *Leishmania* promastigotes was comparable in efficacy to three standard courses of antimony in Venezuelan LCL.[32] With regard to topical therapy, a controlled trial revealed that paromomycin ointment is effective in the treatment of Old World LCL.[33]

TABLE 126-3. Treatment of Leishmaniasis

Systemic

*Antimonials
  Sodium stibogluconate (Pentostam)
  Meglumine antimoniate (Glucantime)
*Pentamidine
*Amphotericin B
*Interferon gamma and antimonials
  Allopurinol and allopurinol riboside
*Ketoconazole
  Itraconazole
  Rifampin
  Dapsone
  Monomycine and methyluracil
*Immunotherapy with heat-killed promastigotes of
  L. mexicana and live bacille Calmette Guérin (BCG)
†Liposome-encapsulated antimony or amphotericin B
†WR 6026

Topical

*Paromomycin sulfate 15% and methylbenzethonium
  chloride 5%–12%
 Antimony potassium tartrate 5% cream
 Clotrimazole
 Chlorpromazine ointment
 Heat
 Cautery/excision
 Intralesional antimony injection

*Believable effectiveness.
†Investigational.

Two new potential agents for the treatment of leishmaniasis in the future include WR 6026, and drug-encapsulated liposomes. WR 6026 is a primaquine analogue that has shown effectiveness in animal models of VL and is undergoing phase I (safety and tolerance) clinical trials. Liposomes are artificial lipid particles that are primarily phagocytized by macrophages. The administration of drug-containing liposomes in theory delivers the therapeutic agent of choice directly to macrophages in which amastigotes reside. Although antimonials and amphotericin B encapsulated in liposomes have proven more effective than free drug in in vitro systems, liposomes have not yet been tried in clinical trials.[34]

Methods of prevention or control of leishmaniasis have included eradication of the vector or its habitat, destruction of animal reservoirs, treatment of human reservoirs, and vaccination. Technical difficulties such as drug resistance, drug toxicity, insecticide resistance, financial constraints, and operational difficulties have impaired progress toward effective control of leishmaniasis. Vaccination trials in animal models and/or humans have been performed using virulent promastigotes; promastigotes attenuated or killed with either γ-irradiation, heat, or a mutagen; and specific antigens purified from promastigotes. Vaccination with virulent promastigotes, a practice called "leishmanization" was performed on at least 10,000 individuals in the Soviet Union and on about 5,000 individuals in Israel.[35] Reduced rates of subsequent infection were noted, but owing to side effects including secondary infection and even immunosuppression, this practice has been discontinued. Moreover, the spread of human immunodeficiency virus infection and the common use of immunosuppressive drugs makes the development of a live vaccine less attractive. Trials in Brazil and Venezuela using killed promastigotes,[36] and a trial in Brazil[37] using a partially purified promastigote fraction have been some promise, but longer follow-up is necessary to determine the degree and duration of protection. The development of an effective, noninfectious vaccine is problematic. A study revealed that live parasites could be recovered from the site of immunization as well as from draining lymph nodes of animals inoculated with promastigotes rendered "nonpathogenic" through high doses of γ-radiation.[38] In addition, it may be more feasible to develop several species-specific vaccines, rather than one broadly protective vaccine. Cross-species protection in humans with different species of *Leishmania* is rare and has been documented only between *L. tropica* and *L. major*. The difficulty associated with the development of a vaccine directed against the parasite suggests that evaluation of a vaccine based on the vector should be attempted. Control and prevention of leishmaniasis in the future depends on the development of more efficacious vaccines and convenient, nontoxic therapeutic agents.

References

1. Control of the leishmaniases. WHO Tech Rep Ser 1990; 793:50–52.
2. Peters WJ, Killick-Kendrick R. The Leishmaniases in Biology and Medicine. San Diego: Academic Press, 1987:1–120.
3. Lerner EA, Von Lichtenburg FC. Case records of the Massachusetts General Hospital: A 21-year-old woman with a persistent rash on the elbow after a sojourn in Central America (leishmaniasis). N Engl J Med 1991;324:476–485.
4. Kalter DC. Cutaneous and mucocutaneous leishmaniasis. Prog Dermatol 1989;23:1–11.
5. Saravia NG, Weigle K, Segura I, et al. Recurrent lesions in human *Leishmania braziliensis* infection: Reactivation or reinfection? Lancet 1990;336:398–402.
6. Magill AJ, Grögl M, Gasser RA Jr, et al. Visceral infection caused by *Leishmania tropica* in veterans of Operation Desert Storm. N Engl J Med 1993;328:1383–1387.
7. Ridley DS, Ridley MJ. The evolution of the lesion in cutaneous leishmaniasis. J Pathol 1983;141:83–96.
8. Sangueza OP, Sangueza JM, Stiller MJ, Sangueza P. Mucocutaneous leishmaniasis: A clinicopathological classification. J Am Acad Dermatol 1993;28:927–932.
9. Girgla HS, Marsden RA, Singh GM, et al. Post–kala-azar dermal leishmaniasis. Br J Dermatol 1977;97:307–311.
10. Esterre P, Dedet JP, Fremay C, et al. Cell populations in the lesion of human cutaneous leishmaniasis: A light microscopical, immunohistochemical and ultrastructural study. Virchows Arch [Pathol Anat] 1992;421:239–247.
11. Modlin RL, Pirmez C, Hofman FM, et al. Lymphocytes bearing antigen-specific γδ T-cell receptors accumulate in human infectious disease lesions. Nature 1989;339:544–548.
12. Pirmez C, Yamamua M, Uyemura K, et al. Cytokine patterns in the pathogenesis of human leishmaniasis. J Clin Invest 1993; 91:1390–1395.
13. Scott P. The role of TH1 and TH2 cells in experimental cutaneous leishmaniasis. Exp Parasitol 1989;68:369–372.
14. Bardaró R, Johnson WD Jr. The role of interferon-γ in the treatment of visceral and diffuse cutaneous leishmaniasis. J Infect Dis 1993;167(Suppl 1):S13–S17.
15. Kemp M, Kurtzhals JAL, Bendtzen K, et al. *Leishmania donovani*–reactive Th1- and TH2-like T-cell clones from individuals who have recovered from visceral leishmaniasis. Infect Immun 1993;61:1069–1073.

16. Lerner EA, Ribeiro JMC, Nelson JR, et al. Isolation of maxadilan, a potent vasodilatory peptide from the salivary glands of the sand fly *Lutzomyia longipalpis*. J Biol Chem 1991;266:11234–11236.
17. Titus RG, Ribeiro JM. Salivary gland lysates from the sand fly enhance *Leishmania* infectivity. Science 1988;239:1306–1308.
18. Norton SA, Frankenburg S, Klaus SN. Cutaneous leishmaniasis acquired during military service in the Middle East. Arch Dermatol 1992;128:83–87.
19. Nanji AA, Greenway DC. *Leishmania braziliensis* infection of the nipple. Br Med J 1985;290:433–434.
20. Eltoum IA, Zijlstra EE, Ali MS, et al. Congenital kala-azar and leishmaniasis in the placenta. Am J Trop Med Hyg 1992;46:57–62.
21. Blackwell JM. Leishmaniasis epidemiology: All down to the DNA. Parasitology 1992;104:S19–S34.
22. Marrano NM, Mata LJ, Durack DT. Cutaneous leishmaniasis in rural Costa Rica. Trans R Soc Trop Med Hyg 1989;83:340.
23. Barker DC, Butcher J. Molecular approaches to DNA diagnosis. Parasitology 1989;99(Suppl):S125–S146.
24. Drugs for parasitic infections. Med Lett 1992;34:21.
25. Herwaldt BL, Berman JD. Recommendations for treating leishmaniasis with sodium stibogluconate (Pentostam) and review of pertinent clinical studies. Am J Top Med Hyg 1992;46:296–306.
26. Herwaldt BL, Kaye ET, Lepore TJ et al. Sodium stibogluconate (Pentostam) overdose during treatment of American cutaneous leishmaniasis. J Infect Dis 1992;165:968–971.
27. Herwaldt BL, Stokes SL, Juranek DD. American cutaneous leishmaniasis in U.S. travelers. Ann Intern Med 1993;118 (10):779–784.
28. Soto-Mancipe J, Grogl M, Berman JD. Evaluation of pentamidine for the treatment of cutaneous leishmaniasis in Colombia. Clin Infect Dis 1993;16:417–425.
29. Martinez S, Marr JJ. Allopurinol in the treatment of American cutaneous leishmaniasis. N Engl J Med 1992;326:741–744.
30. Navin TR, Arana BA, Arana FE, et al. Placebo-controlled clinical trial of sodium stibogluconate (Pentostam) versus ketoconazole for treating cutaneous leishmaniasis in Guatemala. J Infect Dis 1992;165:528–534.
31. Badaro R, Falcoff E, Badaro FS, et al. Treatment of visceral leishmaniasis with pentavalent antimony and interferon gamma. N Engl J Med 1990;322:16–21.
32. Convit J, Rondon A, Ulrich M, et al. Immunotherapy versus chemotherapy in localised cutaneous leishmaniasis. Lancet 1987:401–405.
33. El-On J, Halevy S, Grunwald MH, et al. Topical treatment of Old World cutaneous leishmaniasis caused by *Leishmania major*. A double-blind control study. J Am Acad Dermatol 1992;27:227–231.
34. Berman JD. Chemotherapy for leishmaniasis: Biochemical mechanisms, clinical efficacy, and future strategies. Rev Infect Dis 1988;10:560–586.
35. Higashi GI. Vaccines for parasitic diseases. Ann Rev Public Health 1988;9:483–501.
36. Playfair JHL, Blackwell JM, Miller HRP. Modern vaccines: Parasitic diseases. Lancet 1990;335:1263–1266.
37. Monjour L, Silva OA, Vouldoukis I, et al. Immunoprophylaxis in cutaneous leishmaniasis. Lancet 1992;340:1098–1099.
38. Rivier D, Shah R, Bovay P, et al. Vaccine development against cutaneous leishmaniasis: Subcutaneous administration of radioattenuated parasites protects CBA mice against virulent *Leishmania major* challenge. Parasite Immunol 1993;15:75–84.

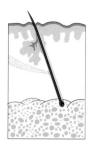

chapter 127

Parasitic Diseases

DEBRA CHESTER KALTER,* TERRI LYNN MEINKING,
EDITH GARCIA, and MOHAMED AMER

PROTOZOAN INFECTIONS

Amebiasis

Amebiasis is a cosmopolitan gastrointestinal infection caused by *Entamoeba histolytica*, which affects over 500 million people worldwide.[1] These parasitic protozoans of the class Sarcodina have pseudopods that provide motility and enable them to capture food. *E. histolytica* has the unique capability of erythrophagocytosis; ingested red blood cells in the trophozoites often aid in diagnosis. Although approximately 90% of those infected are asymptomatic, invasive intestinal and extraintestinal disease may occur. Prevalence of infection in the United States is approximately 4%, but may be over 50% in less developed, tropical countries. Humans are the reservoir, with asymptomatic carriers sporadically excreting up to 45 million cysts in a day.[2] Cyst-contaminated hands, water, drinks, or food, and oral-anal sex, may be sources of transmission. The hardy ingested (10–20 μm) cysts survive gastric digestion, multiplying and dwelling in the cecum and colon as trophozoites. These may be seen in watery stools; however, it is usually only the cyst form, which the trophozoites produce by binary fission, that is excreted.[2] High-risk groups include the institutionalized, mentally retarded, promiscuous male homosexuals ("gay bowel syndrome"), acquired immune deficiency syndrome and other immunocompromised individuals, and immigrants from endemic areas, such as Mexico, South America, Africa, and South Asia.[3] Symptomatic infection typically presents as colitis, abdominal pain, bloody diarrhea, and mucosal ulcerations. Extraintestinal complications of hepatic abscess, empyema, pericardial effusion, ameboma, and cutaneous disease (0.3% of cases) are rare. The skin of the anus, buttocks, and perineum is

involved by direct extension from the rectum. Draining abscesses, fistulae, and abdominal surgery may result in skin disease elsewhere. Ill-defined erythematous, raised, or overhanging borders surround painful ulcers, which are covered in exudate (Fig. 127–1). Tissue destruction may advance rapidly postoperatively, simulating synergistic gangrene of Meleney and provoking extensive surgical debridement in place of appropriate therapy.[4]

Diagnosis may be made upon identifying cysts or trophozoites in freshly passed stools. Trichrome stain of stool smears and concentration techniques may help. False negatives are common, and nonpathogenic amebae must be distinguished from *E. histolytica*. Histologic examination of biopsy specimens from the rectum or perianal skin is of more value. Ulcers caused by *E. histolytica* are often flanked by pseudocarcinomatous epidermal hyperplasia, and have bases of granulation tissue above which is a neutrophilic infiltrate containing trophozoites. The organisms range from 12 to 20 μm in diameter, and have large central karyosomes that exceed the size of and stain more brightly than the nuclei of macrophages, which can also be present in the beds of ulcers. The abundant cytoplasm of trophozoites sometimes contains phagocytized erythrocytes, highlighted in periodic acid–Schiff–stained sections. In rare cases, pseudocarcinomatous hyperplasia can dominate the picture, and ulceration can be quite focal, resulting in a picture resembling that of squamous cell carcinoma.[5] Inasmuch as amebae adhere to cotton swabs, a stick or curette is preferable in obtaining material, which should then be suspended in saline and examined under high power. A drop of iodine on the slide often facilitates detection. The ENZYMEBA test, an enzyme immunoassay, has been shown to be a simple, effective method of determining *E. histolytica* infections and may be easily used in the field.[1] Polymerase chain reaction (PCR) discriminates *E. histolytica* from nonpathogenic amebae. The cutaneous differential diagnosis includes: herpes simplex, tuberculosis, atypical

---

*Deceased.

1172

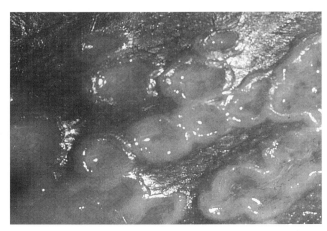

FIGURE 127-1. Ulcers of cutaneous amebiasis.

mycobacteria, syphilis, chancroid, ecthyma, squamous cell carcinoma, and metastases.

Therapy for invasive disease is metronidazole, 750 mg, or diloxanide, 500 mg three times per day for 10 days, tinidazole, 2 g once a day for 2 days for adults and 50 to 60 mg/kg per day in a single dose for children, or alternatively emetine hydrochloride, 1 to 1.5 mg/kg per day (maximum 90 mg per day), subcutaneously or intramuscularly for 5 to 10 days. To eradicate cyst carriage, any of the above regimens should be followed by iodoquinol, 650 mg three times per day for 20 days, or paromomycin, 25 to 30 mg/kg per day in 3 doses for 7 days.[6] Some controversy exists regarding the necessity of treating asymptomatic "cyst passers." This condition may spontaneously resolve and rarely progresses, although treatment would control spread or prevent infections in contacts.

American Trypanosomiasis

American trypanosomiasis, commonly termed Chagas' disease, occurs only in the Western hemisphere and is caused by the protozoan *Trypanosoma cruzi (Schizotrypanum cruzi)*. It is estimated that between 10 and 20 million individuals are infected worldwide.[2] Chagas' disease occurs in Central America, Mexico, and South America. The greatest prevalence is found in Brazil, where it was first described in 1909 by Chagas, who found that the thatched roof houses were infested with flagellate-infected, large, bloodsucking insects of the family Reduviidae.[7] Almost 5% of Central American migrants living in the Washington, DC, area are infected with *T. cruzi*.[8] A few vector-borne cases have been acquired in the United States as well as a few from blood transfusions. Humans as well as over 150 species of wild and domestic animals are reservoirs for *T. cruzi*. Transmission may occur by intrauterine infections, transfusions, or triatomine insect species.

The disease usually occurs in three phases. The *acute* or *primary stage* is characterized by the "chagoma of inoculation," a board-like induration with edema, erythema, and tenderness at the bite site. This often occurs at an early age when the reduviid bugs, attracted to CO_2,

bite sleeping children on the face, hence the term *kissing bugs*. The infected bug feces are scratched or rubbed into the bite or skin wound, conjunctiva, lips, or mucous membranes. The resulting chagoma appears within 5 to 14 days and is usually accompanied by regional adenopathy. Chagas' disease may begin without a primary chagoma, but this is rare. Romana's sign (oculoglandular syndrome) is a unilateral bipalpebral edema, seen in about 80% of infected individuals (Fig. 127-2), and often accompanied by preauricular adenopathy (Parinaud's syndrome). Malaise, variable fever, and lymphadenopathy are common in the primary stage; however, a macular rash, hepatosplenomegaly, thrombocytosis, leukocytosis, and eosinophilia may also be present. Many infected individuals are asymptomatic. The acute symptoms and chagoma usually last 2 months, and may result in a hyperpigmented and depressed area at the bite site. In most cases the patient recovers, but myocarditis and meningoencephalitis are life-threatening complications that may require pacemaker insertion, and result in a 10% fatality rate in the acute stage.[9] In the *intermediate phase*, the patient is clinically symptom-free, but serologically positive. *T. cruzi*, measuring 20 μm long, is found in the blood in early stages of the disease but does not divide there. Instead the trypanosomes penetrate into the cells of heart and other voluntary muscles where they lose their flagellae and become *amastigotes*. These multiply by binary fission while destroying organ tissue, with each producing a flagellum and transforming into *epimastigotes*. These give rise to *trypomastigotes*, which enter the blood, and the cycle continues over and over. Years to decades may pass before the *third-stage* clinical symptoms appear. The most common sequela of chronic Chagas' disease is cardiac damage. Cardiac failure, sudden cardiac death, heart block, arrhythmias, embolic phenomena, and intestinal tract involvement with megaesophagus and megacolon may occur.

Diagnosis in the acute stage is made by detection of

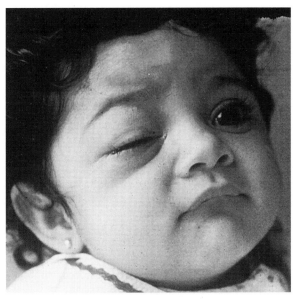

FIGURE 127-2. Romana's sign of Chagas' disease. (Courtesy of the Armed Forces Institute of Pathology.)

trypanosomes in blood either from a fresh smear or after hemoconcentration, culture, intracerebral inoculation of suckling mice, or by xenodiagnosis (the feeding of uninfected triatomid bugs on the patient and demonstrating the organism in insect feces a month later). Serologic tests, which include complement fixation, indirect fluorescent antibody, and indirect hemagglutination, are of considerable value during the subacute and chronic stages. Diagnosis using PCR has been shown to be 100% effective and far superior to serologic tests and xenodiagnosis.[10]

Treatment is useful only in the acute stage and consists of oral therapy using nifurtimox, 8 to 10 mg/kg per day in four doses for 60 to 120 days, or benznidazole, 5 to 7 mg/kg per day for 30 to 120 days. Both drugs have serious side effects and are of little or no value in the chronic stage. Transfusion acute disease can be prevented by better screening techniques such as PCR or by treating blood with gentian violet (1:4000) for 24 hours.

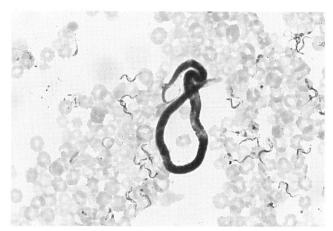

FIGURE 127–3. Wright-Giemsa blood smear of African sleeping sickness (*T. brucei* species) parasitemia. The large filarial worm *Wuchereria bancrofti* is also seen in this field (× 1000).

African Trypanosomiasis

African trypanosomiasis, commonly called African sleeping sickness, is a systemic protozoan disease transmitted by an infected tsetse fly (*Glossina* sp.). This disease is endemic in a belt running through tropical Africa between 15° north and 15° south latitude, which corresponds to the distribution of the vector, the tsetse fly. Two subspecies of the genus *Trypanosoma* are responsible for disease in humans: *Trypanosoma brucei gambiense* and *T. b. rhodesiense*. Six species of *Glossina* are known to be principal vectors of African trypanosomiasis. Gambian sleeping sickness is found in Central and West Africa, occurring mainly in Uganda and southern Sudan, and is associated with rivers and lakes. The principal vector is the riverine tsetse (*Glossina palpalis*). Humans are the main reservoir of Gambian trypanosomiasis, which is often chronic, running a protracted course for several years. Rhodesiense sleeping sickness is associated with savanna and woodland regions of East Africa. Domestic cattle and wild animals, especially antelopes and bushbuck, are the chief reservoir of *T. b. rhodesiense*. Because this trypanosome is less well adapted to humans, it causes a more aggressive disease, often resulting in death within 6 months.[9]

T. brucei are elongated, wriggling, somewhat eel-like parasites 10 to 30 μm in length and 1.5 to 3.5 μm in width, each containing a nucleus and kinetoplast (Fig. 127–3). Their body is like a curved, flattened blade with a single flagellum projecting from the posterior end of the body and running along the undulating membrane to the anterior end, often extending beyond this point as a "free flagellum." They always swim in the direction of the anterior end, while being propelled by the ripples produced by their undulating membrane. It is impossible to differentiate the two subspecies morphologically; however, they differ in their epidemiologic and clinical features. When a tsetse fly bites a patient with parasitemia, trypanosomes are sucked into the gut of the fly with the bloodmeal, reaching the salivary glands, where they develop into "metacyclic" infective forms within 2 to 5 weeks. The *first stage* occurs when the fly's saliva, containing infected trypanosomes, is injected into the subcutaneous tissues of the host, usually resulting in local inflammation, with a "chancre" appearing at the bite site within 4 to 10 days. The chancre spontaneously resolves in about 2 weeks, and the *second stage* soon follows, with the trypanosomes invading the peripheral blood, resulting in irregular fevers and symmetrical adenopathy. Possible cutaneous symptoms include edema of the hands, feet, or eyelids, erythema nodosum, and annular or serpiginous erythemas that often resemble erythema multiforme. The trypanosomal rash is present in about 50% of patients and appears about 10 days after infection. It may take up to a month before there are sufficient numbers of organisms in the blood for direct examination, by which time the lymph nodes are involved. Nonspecific neurologic manifestations, such as headache, insomnia, and a delayed deep hyperesthesia (*Kerandel's* sign), may occur at this stage.[2] The *third stage* of African sleeping sickness consists of progressive deterioration due to central nervous system (CNS) involvement. Symptoms associated with CNS invasion by the protozoans are paresis, seizures, ataxia, and personality changes. Blindness, myocarditis and heart failure may occur. Rarely are cutaneous signs present, but xerosis and pruritus may be present. In the rhodesiense disease, the parasites invade the CNS in 3 to 6 weeks. The disease is lethal within a few weeks to 9 months. The Gambian form may exist as a chronic condition for years before the parasites enter the CNS. Other modes of transmission include direct inoculation with infected material, blood transfusions, and intrauterine infection. Both forms of African trypanosomiasis are fatal without treatment.

Diagnosis is made by finding trypanosomes in blood, lymph or cerebral spinal fluid, or in Giemsa-stained smears made from the exudates of chancres. They are difficult to detect in tissue sections. Concentration techniques and lymph node aspirates are especially helpful in the diagnosis of Gambian sleeping sickness. Inoculation of blood or tissue fluids into laboratory rats or mice may be useful in the diagnosis of the Rhodesian form. Specific antibodies may be demonstrated by the card agglutination test (CATT), indirect fluorescent antibody test, and enzyme-linked immunosorbent assay (ELISA). Immunoglobulins, especially IgM, are commonly elevated. An important diagnostic tool, PCR has been successfully used to detect *Trypanosoma brucei* subspecies.[11]

Because treatment depends on the stage of the disease, the cerebral spinal fluid should be examined prior to treatment. If there is any abnormality, the patient is treated as having advanced disease.

Suramin is the drug of choice for the early stages of either form of African trypanosomiasis, providing the CNS shows no changes in either protein or cellular content.[8] A test dose of 100 to 200 mg (or 5 mg/kg) should be given intravenously to determine if the patient has an idiosyncratic reaction to suramin. The treatment regimen consists of 20 mg/kg intravenously to a 1-g maximum single dose on days 1, 3, 7, 14, and 21. Close supervision is necessary when using this toxic drug, whose most significant side effect is kidney damage. Pentamidine isethionate, 3 to 4 mg/kg intramuscularly for 10 days or every other day for a 10-dose total, is the alternative therapy. Melarsoprol (Mel B, Arsobal), given intravenously at 3.6 mg/kg per day for four injections over 1 week, is highly effective for either type and all stages of African sleeping sickness, even in cases of treatment failure with suramin or pentamidine. The World Health Organization's Technical Report Series, No. 739, 1986, offers various other treatment schedules. Melarsoprol, which contains 18.8% arsenic, has significant side effects, which occur in 5% to 10% of patients, and should not be used in early stages of disease.

Eflornithine (DFMO; Ornidyl), an ornithine decarboxylase inhibitor, is effective and possibly the preferable drug of choice for Gambian disease with CNS involvement. Initial administration of the drug should be given either intravenously or intramuscularly in four divided doses of 400 mg/kg per day for 2 weeks, followed by 2 to 4 weeks of oral therapy. Eflornithine has few side effects; however, further studies are required to determine the efficacy of this drug for early-stage disease, *rhodesiense* infections, and possible synergism with other anti-trypanosome compounds. In November of 1990, the U.S. Food and Drug Administration approved eflornithine as the first therapy in 40 years for sleeping sickness. In 1991, it was approved by the World Health Organization and the European Community regulatory authority.

All patients, regardless of the type of therapy or disease form, should be seen at 3, 6, 12, and 24 months after treatment to check the possibility of relapsed infections.

Toxoplasmosis

Humans acquire infection with the obligate intracellular protozoan *Toxoplasma gondii*, congenitally or at any age, by ingesting oocysts shed in cat feces or tissue cysts in undercooked meat. Iatrogenic infection may result from transfusion, transplantation, or laboratory inoculation. This zoonosis is worldwide; adult seroprevalence ranges from 3% to 90%. Acute infection in the immunocompetent human is underdiagnosed because it is of short duration and may be asymptomatic or nonspecific

in presentation. Infection persists, latently, as cysts in tissue, kept in check by both humoral and cellular immunity, but can reactivate if the host becomes immunocompromised.

Congenital infection occurs only if the mother becomes infected during pregnancy and has not been previously exposed. Antibodies developed from a previous *T. gondii* encounter provide protection. Although the risk of fetal transmission increases during the pregnancy, the severity of infection decreases after the first trimester. Acute maternal infection has been estimated to occur in 1 to 6 in 1000 pregnancies, with a fetal transmission rate of 25% to 65%, depending upon trimester of infection.[12] Manifestations may not be present in the neonatal period, but eventually, chorioretinitis or neurologic sequelae develop in the majority of congenitally infected individuals. Affected neonates may suffer from chorioretinitis, microphthalmia, blindness, seizures, microcephaly, hydrocephalus, intracerebral calcifications, encephalitis, mental retardation, lymphadenopathy, hepatosplenomegaly, myocarditis, and interstitial pneumonitis.[13] The skin findings are nonspecific, and include jaundice, petechiae, ecchymoses, and the bluish macules or plaques of dermoerythropoiesis (Fig. 127–4). "Blueberry muffin" lesions are also seen in congenital cytomegalovirus and rubella infections, and in leukemia. Diagnosis depends upon clinical presentation and the presence of specific IgM antibodies directed against *Toxoplasma*. Serial titers at 3 weeks are helpful.

Skin lesions are very uncommon in acquired toxoplasmosis, and are pleomorphic. They have been described as resembling erythema multiforme or roseola, or as telangiectatic or hemorrhagic macules, lichenoid or erythematous papules, pustules, vesicles, or purpuric nodules.[14] Clinical symptoms are variable and nonspecific. Lymphadenopathy, especially of the head and neck, fever, headache, malaise, arthralgia, and bone pain may be present. A number of cases of polymyositis-dermatomyositis have been diagnosed as toxoplasmosis, or have responded to therapy directed against this parasite.[15] Patients immunocompromised by steroids, cytotoxic agents, or acquired immunodeficiency syndrome are highly susceptible to toxoplasmosis, probably by reactivation more often than acute infection. Encephalitis and chorioretinitis are the most common manifestations, but

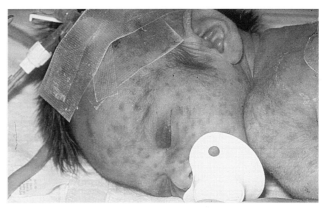

FIGURE 127–4. "Blueberry muffin" lesions of congenital *Toxoplasma gondii* in an infant.

the skin may be rarely involved in disseminated disease.[16] The histology of the lesion depends upon the clinical nature, and organisms are rarely found. When present, organisms are seen as pseudocysts within the cytoplasms of macrophages that comprise sparsely cellular dermal infiltrates. They can also lie freely within the dermis as 3- to 4-mm oval to cigar-shaped trophozoites. Rarely, trophozoites can be present within the cytoplasms of keratinocytes in the epidermis in immunosuppressed patients.[17] Organisms stain with periodic acid–Schiff and Giemsa, and pseudocysts must be differentiated from other intracellular parasites. Their identification may be facilitated by electron microscopy (Fig. 127–5).[17] The histopathology of the dermatomyositis-like eruption is that of a sparsely cellular vacuolar interface dermatitis.

Combined therapy with sulfadiazine, 1 to 2 g per day, and pyrimethamine, 25 to 100 mg per day, with folinic acid for 3 to 4 weeks is standard.[5] Spiramycin, 3 to 4 g per day is less active, but also less toxic than the above, and has been used effectively in pregnant women and infants.

Early therapy may prevent late sequelae.[12] Steroids are indicated for inflammatory eye disease. Instruct pregnant women to eat well-cooked meats, and to avoid kittens and any contact with cat feces, such as changing litter boxes; frequent handwashing helps to prevent infections.

Trichomoniasis

Trichomonas vaginalis produces a genitourinary infection of both sexes, which may or may not be symptomatic. Trichomoniasis is one of the most common sexually transmitted diseases, estimated to have a prevalence of 180 million cases per year worldwide.[18] Infection is found in association with an infected sexual partner, other sexually transmitted diseases, multiple sexual partners, and the use of contraception other than hormonal or barrier-type. Infection may rarely be transmitted perinatally.

The most common clinical complaint by women is of vaginal discharge, which is typically malodorous, frothy, and yellow-green. Pruritus and irritation are also common, followed by dysuria and dyspareunia; infection may be asymptomatic. Other findings include vulvar or vaginal erythema. Visualization reveals a "strawberry" cervix, but its detection may require colposcopic examination. Infection in males is symptomatic in approximately 50%, with complaints of a small to moderate, usually clear, urethral discharge. Persistent infection has been associated with infertility, preterm labor, premature rupture of membranes, low birth weight, increased postsurgical infection of the reproductive tract, urethritis, epididymitis, and prostatitis. Infection in men may spontaneously clear by 2 weeks after exposure.[18]

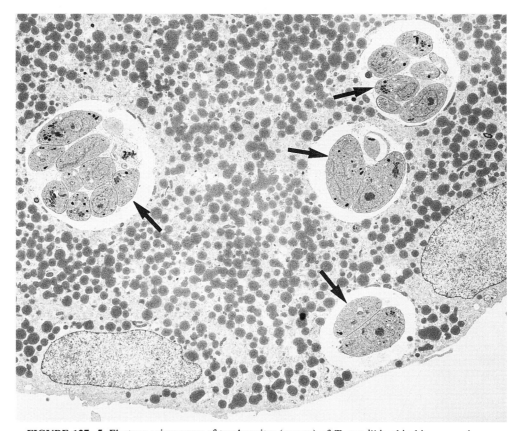

FIGURE 127–5. Electron microscopy of trophozoites (*arrows*) of *T. gondii* in skin biopsy specimen. (From Leyva WH, Santa Cruz DJ. Cutaneous toxoplasmosis. J Am Acad Dermatol 1986;14:600–605.)

The causative agent is a motile, 10 to 20 μm, oval protozoan. It bears four anterior flagella, and a flagellum attached to an undulating membrane. Its movement is readily detected in saline wet mounts of vaginal or urethral discharge. Although this method provides an immediate and unquestionable diagnosis, sensitivity is only 60% to 80%. Potassium hydroxide (10%) examination is often performed concurrently in the evaluation of vaginal discharge, and a characteristic odor may be associated with trichomonas-positive samples. Culture of vaginal or urethral discharge is the most accurate method of diagnosis, when available. Examination and culture of the first-voided urine sediment may enhance sensitivity. Smears can be stained with Giemsa, Papanicolaou's stain, acridine orange, or fluorescent monoclonal antibody. Differential diagnosis includes bacterial and candidal vaginoses.

Treatment with metronidazole, 2 g orally once, or in a split dose the same day, is effective in the majority of cases. Dosing with 250 mg three times daily for 7 days is an alternative. Sexual partners need to be treated concurrently, as recurrent infection is common. Relative metronidazole resistance occurs, and responds to prolonged high-dose treatment. Other nitroimidazoles are also effective: tinidazole 2 g orally once, or nimorazole, 2 g per day orally for 2 days. Local agents are used in pregnancy, such as tinidazole vaginal suppositories, which are available in some countries, metronidazole gel, or nonoxynol-9; however, they are less effective. Condom use is preventative.

TISSUE NEMATODE INFECTIONS

Onchocerciasis

Onchocerciasis, due to infection by *Onchocerca volvulus*, may be the most important parasitic infection primarily involving the skin, inasmuch as dermatitis is the most common manifestation of this high morbidity disease affecting at least 18 million people. It is the second leading cause of infectious blindness globally, and second only to polio as a cause of long-term disability.[19] The bulk of disease is found in equatorial Africa, with smaller foci in Yemen, Saudi Arabia, Guatemala, Mexico, Ecuador, Venezuela, Brazil, and Colombia. Transmission occurs from the bite of the female black fly of *Simulium* species within a few kilometers of river banks, where breeding occurs. Prolonged exposure with repeated bites of infected flies is required to produce clinical disease, unlike leishmaniasis. Fertile river valleys in Africa have been deserted in favor of less productive lands because of the severity of onchocerciasis. Eye disease is more prevalent in savanna compared with forest areas, due to parasite strain differences. In hyperendemic villages, 15% to 40% of adults in their most productive years may be blind.[20]

The hematophagous black fly vector ingests microfilariae present in the upper dermis of infected humans, the reservoir. Maturation into infective larvae occurs within the fly over 6 to 8 days. When the fly next feeds, these are passed to another person, who may or may not already be infected. The larvae molt twice to become adults during a 9- to 18-month period. Adult females may reach 70 mm in length, whereas males may grow to 30 mm; the life span is up to 15 years. Adults are usually localized in small groupings within a fibrotic capsule (onchocercoma), releasing large numbers of microfilariae into the surrounding skin. It is the microfilariae, not the adults, that lead to clinical disease. The immune response of the individual determines the extent of the disease. Those with mild disease tend to be hyporesponsive to parasite antigens. Hyperreactive individuals may have severe dermatitis and pruritus, as in sowda (described below).

The skin manifestations range from no obvious disease to generalized atrophy. Pruritus is the most common complaint, and may be so severe as to disturb sleep and, anecdotally, lead to suicide. Initial skin findings are nonspecific and relate to scratching and a transient maculopapular rash. An acute papular to nearly vesicular eruption may be scattered on the upper body or in patches. This type of reaction can follow use of diethylcarbamazine (DEC) as a treatment or as a provocative diagnostic test (Mazzotti reaction). Other early changes are urticarial, eczematous, or lichenified; hyperpigmentation is common. Localized limb swelling with tender adenopathy may rarely occur. More specific but subtle fullness may be seen on the upper chest and back, appearing shiny, "plump and juicy," or even sclerodermatous.[21] The nonpitting interfollicular turgidity produces a peau d'orange texture, which over time regresses to leave patulous follicles and interfollicular sag (Fig. 127–6). In the New World, *erisipela de la costa* refers to edematous erythema of the face with fever, photophobia, and headache. Thickening of the ears and facial skin results in leonine facies. *Mal de morado* describes lichen planus–like plaques.

Chronic onchodermatitis develops after years of disease, and may be manifest as lizard skin, crushed tissue paper skin, atrophy, pachydermia, leopard skin, pigmentary changes, and doughy abdomen. An individual may have a combination of various acute and chronic signs. Lizard skin is lustrous and darkened, with a smooth surface and fine epidermal markings. It is most obvious

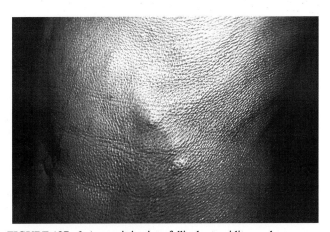

FIGURE 127–6. A nonpitting interfollicular turgidity produces a peau d'orange texture in onchocerciasis.

in a diamond-shaped area over the lumbar spine. Crushed tissue paper skin is atrophic, dry, and lusterless with exaggerated skin lines, easily crinkling with gentle traction. On the lower legs the atrophic skin is plate-like, making a "crazy pavement" or craquelle pattern. Redundant pachydermatous skin folds are common over the knees, where oval atrophic scars suggest those seen in Ehlers-Danlos syndrome. The abdominal wall may appear doughy in some older individuals. Severe generalized atrophy, or presbydermia, may involve most of the body, which appears at a distance to be coated with a fine gray dust. Depigmentation is seen in chronic disease, especially involving the shins, where sparing of the follicular pigment has led to the descriptive term *leopard skin* (Fig. 127–7). Milder hypopigmentation and hyperpigmentation are common as well. *Sowda* (Arabic for black) is a form of onchocerciasis with intense pruritus, lichenification, and hyperpigmentation. The affected limb may be swollen, with reactive adenopathy. Although most common in Yemen, sowda is seen globally.

Onchocercomas are asymptomatic, rubbery subcutaneous nodules, usually felt over bony prominences. In Africa, they localize to the sacrum, coccyx, iliac crest, and greater trochanter. In the New World, the head and shoulder girdle as well as the pelvic girdle are common sites. The biting habits of local vectors appear to influence the site. Nontender, fibrotic adenopathy is typical, especially in the inguinal and femoral nodes of affected Africans, and in the head and cervical nodes in Central America. Adenocele formation follows; folds of skin may droop in the groin and genital area as an end stage called *hanging groin*. Hernias are common. Back, joint, and muscle pains are frequent systemic complaints.

Both anterior and posterior segments of the eye can eventually be affected by onchocerciasis. Corneal opacities are initially punctate, termed *fluffy* or *snowflake*. These can resolve without scarring. Anterior uveitis and iridocyclitis occur early, and may become chronic, resulting in secondary glaucoma and pupillary distortion. Sclerosing keratitis results in blindness over a period of many years and is more common in savanna regions. Optic atrophy and chorioretinitis contribute to eye disease.

The skin histopathology varies with the diverse clinical manifestations. Of note is the presence of microfilariae in the upper dermis between collagen fibers with no surrounding inflammation. A sparse infiltrate of lymphocytes and eosinophils may be seen perivascularly. Less commonly, granuloma formation occurs. In severe end-stage atrophy, there is a marked loss of elastic fibers. Onchocercomas reveal multiple cross sections of the tightly coiled worms within a sclerotic capsule.

Diagnosis is not typically made by punch biopsy, but by skin snips. These can be obtained by tenting the skin with a needle and slicing off a 2-mm section through the dermal papillae. A corneoscleral punch is superior for obtaining a uniform, painless sample. The best sites are over the scapulae, the posterior iliac crests, the calves, and over any nodules. Each skin snip is placed on a glass slide or in a microtiter well with 0.1 ml saline. Microfilariae will leave the skin within a few hours, but samples should be allowed to sit at room temperature for 24 hours before discarding as negative. *Mansonella streptocerca*, which also produces a pruritic eruption due to migration of microfilariae through the skin, must be distinguished morphologically. Serology may be helpful in nonendemic exposure, but does not distinguish the filarids. An eye examination is essential in evaluating the possibility of onchocerciasis. The best way to find onchocerciasis is by asking the patient, although some are clearly visible. Ultrasound has been helpful at localizing deeper nodules. Use of the Mazzotti test for diagnosis is controversial because severe eye disease may flare with the test dose of DEC, 50 mg. In general, it is reserved for individuals thought to have onchocerciasis, but with repeatedly negative skin snips and eye examination. Within 15 minutes to 24 hours, the infected patient will develop severe pruritus and erythema or a papular eruption over involved skin, as a reaction to dying microfilariae.

Oral ivermectin, 150 to 200 µg/kg is the treatment of choice, given every 6 months. It is microfilaricidal only, so therapy may need to be given as long as the adult worms survive. Side effects are less severe than with DEC, but hypotension, although rare, may occur. DEC, 6 mg/kg, for 11 days following an initial dose of 3 mg/kg per day, is reserved for situations in which ivermectin cannot be given, such as meningitis, pregnancy, the first month of breast feeding, drug allergy, or age younger than 5 years, because toddlers cannot successfully swallow the pills. Suramin, the only available macrofilaricide, is quite toxic and requires prolonged parenteral administration. It is rarely indicated, but may be helpful in the expatriate who remains debilitated after multiple courses of ivermectin. Nodulectomy is reasonable for accessible onchocercomas, especially in the head region. Disease prevention for the traveler includes protective clothing,

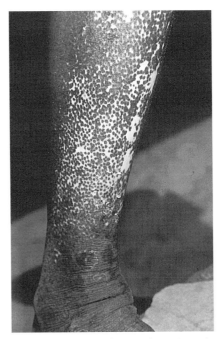

FIGURE 127–7. Depigmentation in chronic onchocerciasis results in "leopard skin."

insect repellent, and avoidance of the vector habitat, if possible.

Streptocerciasis

Mansonella streptocerca microfilariae migrate through the dermis, producing a pruritic dermatitis that must be differentiated from onchocerciasis and leprosy. The main importance of the disease lies in this distinction, inasmuch as a skin snip yielding microfilariae may well lead the clinician to erroneously diagnose onchocerciasis. Streptocerciasis is endemic to western and central Africa, where it is transmitted by the bite of the midge *Culicoides grahami*.[22] The worms are found in the skin of the upper trunk and shoulder girdle, where hypopigmentation is the main manifestation, but papules and lichenification may occur. Fibrotic axillary and inguinal adenopathy is common. Skin snip reveals sluggish microfilariae, with characteristic "shepherd's crook" tails, which are distinguishable from *O. volvulus*. A Mazzotti reaction occurs following treatment with DEC, which is macrofilaricidal and microfilaricidal, and is given in the same dosage as for onchocerciasis.

Filariasis

Filariasis affects over 90 million people worldwide, with the preponderance of infections in China, India, and Indonesia. *Wuchereria bancrofti* is found in Africa, Asia, Oceania, Latin America, and the Caribbean, and accounts for over 90% of the cases (see Fig. 127–3). *Brugia malayi* is found in Southeast Asia, India, and Indonesia, and is the only form that also has a zoonotic component, with a reservoir in monkeys, macaques, and felines. *Brugia timori* is found in foci of Indonesia. Mosquitoes are the vectors, ingesting the L_1 microfilariae in the blood meal from an infected human host. The larvae develop through the L_2 stage into infective larvae, L_3, during 1 to 3 weeks. The L_3 are passed with subsequent feedings into a new human host, where they develop into L_4 and adult forms over a period of 4 to 6 months. The adults dwell within the lymphatics adjacent to lymph nodes and genitalia, shedding microfilariae into the peripheral blood. Although the presence of the adults results in lymphatic dilation and thickening of the walls, obstruction occurs primarily due to the host's immune reaction to dead worms, with inflammation, granuloma formation, and fibrosis.

Exposure to infective larvae must be intense and prolonged for infection to occur.[23] Response to infection varies between endemic and nonendemic individuals, and varies according to specific immune responsiveness to the parasites. Most individuals in filarial-endemic regions are asymptomatic and microfilaremic, and are considered to be immunologically tolerant or hyporesponsive.[24] Responders have eventual disease manifestations such as elephantiasis and hydrocele, despite often being amicrofilaremic. Acute attacks of retrograde lymphangitis, fever, and malaise lasting 3 to 15 days are irregularly recurrent. Lymphadenitis affects the groin or axilla, and may suppurate. Recurrent orchitis, funiculitis, and epididymitis may lead to hydrocele. Eosinophilia and high levels of IgE are found. Reversible pitting edema of the legs, scrotum, or arms results from acute attacks, but may linger in resolution, becoming eventually nonpitting and persistent. The breast, penis, and labia are involved less frequently.[25] Progression of disease appears to be more rapid in nonendemic individuals. Cutaneous changes of elephantiasis are secondary to the chronic lymphedema, with thickening of the skin that can be smooth or verrucous and nodular over many years. Transverse skin folds are typical between the foot and ankle. Infections, fissures, and ulcers may develop in the fibrotic skin. Elephantiasis due to *Brugia* is softer, producing a "water bag" deformity of the lower legs. Rarely, individuals develop a hyper-responsive state manifest as tropical pulmonary eosinophilia, which is more common in young men, with asthma-like wheezing, adenopathy, and marked eosinophilia.

Diagnosis depends upon epidemiology, the clinical picture, and, if possible, the demonstration of the microfilaria in the peripheral blood. Thick blood smears are insensitive except in infections with more than 100 mf/ml. Serial blood samples for concentration (1 to 10 ml anticoagulated blood) should be obtained around midnight to identify the nocturnally periodic *W. bancrofti*. Afternoon sampling is additionally indicated in individuals exposed in the South Pacific or Southeast Asia, where periodicity has presumably adapted to coincide with peak feeding times of the local vector. Parasites are susceptible to jet lag as are humans, and may delay during travel in establishing their characteristic periodicity.[23] Microfilariae found in the blood should be stained with Giemsa or hematoxylin to identify the morphologic features that allow differentiation of the various blood-dwelling filariae. Serology may be required to identify infection in amicrofilaremic individuals; unfortunately, endemic exposure, current infection, and past infections are indistinguishable. Cross-reaction between all filariae is typical. More specific antigen-detection assays are being developed; however, sensitivity is not yet enhanced. Lymphoscintigraphy has demonstrated the presence of lymphatic abnormalities in early disease, and can be performed and repeated safely.

Standard therapy for filariasis is with oral microfilaricidal DEC, 6 mg/kg for 12 days, preceded by a single dose of 3 mg/kg. The Mazzotti reaction does not occur in filariasis as in onchocerciasis, and the drug is well tolerated. Mass treatment with a single yearly dose appears to be efficacious in reducing transmission. In China, low-dose DEC is administered in medicated salt for mass therapy. Aggressive repeated therapy with DEC is macrofilaricidal to *W. bancrofti*.[23] Ivermectin, 200 to 400 μg/kg in a single oral dose, is microfilaricidal and has similar efficacy to DEC with fewer side effects. Although ivermectin is promising for the treatment of lymphatic filariasis, it seems to be microfilaricidal only, but clinical investigations are in progress.[25] Dosing schedules for both drugs are being reevaluated. Surgery is indicated in moderate to advanced cases of elephantiasis, by lymph nodovenous shunt or an excisional operation.[26]

Trichinosis

Humans become accidentally infected with *Trichinella spiralis* by ingesting raw or insufficiently cooked meat, usually from wild carnivores or swine. Trichinosis is found worldwide, except for Australia and some Pacific islands.[27] Formerly, pigs had been the main source of infection; however, this has changed in the United States with improved meat inspections and the regulation to boil any garbage or food scraps fed to pigs. Now infections are most likely to come from eating undercooked or microwaved bear, wild boar, bush pig, wart hog, polar bear, walrus, or homemade sausage of wild animal meat or noncommercial pork.[28] Raw horse meat has been a source in France, presumably through contamination of the feed. Carnivores eat the muscles of infected animals, and the larvae excyst in the stomach and mature into adults in the small intestine epithelium. Mating of adult worms results in discharge of live larvae within a week. The larvae migrate into the circulation and invade striated skeletal muscle. Within the muscle cell, the larvae coil and a cyst forms around them by 3 weeks after infection. The encysted larvae may survive for years in this state, although calcification can eventually occur.

Gastrointestinal complaints are predominant during the first week, followed by the classic features associated with encystment of the larvae: fever, myalgia, periorbital edema, and eosinophilia. A macular or petechial rash may also occur, simulating a viral exanthem. Subungual or retinal splinter hemorrhages and subconjunctival hemorrhage and chemosis can sometimes be seen. Severity of disease relates to larval burden and parasite strain.

Diagnosis is made from the clinical picture with a history of questionable meat ingestion, especially if others who consumed the same meat are similarly affected. Pronounced eosinophilia is typical beginning the tenth day, and muscle enzymes may be elevated. Antibodies develop by 4 weeks, and acute and convalescent titers may help distinguish new from old infection. Analysis of a muscle biopsy specimen from a tender swollen muscle may reveal coiled larvae within the fiber, surrounded by eosinophils and lymphocytes. The differential diagnosis includes viral infections, dermatomyositis, and typhoid.

Treatment is suboptimal. Thiabendazole, 25 mg/kg/day for 1 week, is larvacidal if started within 24 hours of ingesting contaminated meat. Thereafter, mebendazole, 200 to 400 mg three times daily for 3 days, followed by 400 to 500 mg three times daily for 10 days, may be used in conjunction with prednisone, 40 to 60 mg/day, especially if symptoms are severe.[6] Disease is self-limited. Prevention is easy by heating meat to 77° C or freezing for 3 weeks.

Loiasis

Loa loa is a filarial nematode infecting humans in equatorial rain forests of West and Central Africa. Transmission from infected human to human is mediated by female tabanid fly vectors of the genus *Chrysops*, which bite during the day, ingesting the diurnal microfilariae from the bloodstream. Infective filariform larvae develop in 10 to 12 days and are released from the proboscis in subsequent feedings. Maturation results in adult worms, surviving up to 17 years and producing sheathed microfilariae that circulate in the peripheral blood by 1 year after infection. The microfilariae are not considered to be pathogenic, except following treatment with DEC, when large numbers may die and block cerebral vessels. Clinical manifestations relate to movement of the adults through the subcutaneous tissues and subconjunctivae. Recurrent subcutaneous swellings 10 to 20 cm in diameter, termed *Calabar swellings*, are most common on the forearms, wrists, ankle, and face. The Calabar swellings are the result of allergenic response to the worm's by-products released into the dermis, and may last for hours or days, recurring at irregular intervals of weeks or months for up to 15 years.[9] Although *L. loa* usually does not cause serious harm, the lumps can be painful, erythematous, and pruritic. If located near a joint or eye, they can be incapacitating.[9]

DEC is effective against developing larvae, microfilariae, and adult worms and should be administered at the same doses recommended for filariasis. Repeated courses may be necessary. In severe cases, 1 mg/kg of prednisone for the first week to 10 days with DEC has been advised.[9] A single dose of oral ivermectin, 300 to 400 μg/kg, has been shown to be effective for 3 months in the treatment of loiasis and has fewer and less severe side effects than DEC.[29] Because ivermectin kills only the microfilariae and not the adult worm, further dosing regimens need to be investigated.

Dracunculosis

Human infection with *Dracunculus medinensis*, the guinea worm, results from ingestion of drinking water containing infected *Cyclops* copepods. Disease is encountered in parts of India, Pakistan, Asia, Africa, and the Middle East. Larvae are released in the human intestinal tract, and migrate into the abdominal or thoracic cavity, where they mature and mate. The 60- to 120-cm long, thin, gravid female migrates into the lower extremities usually, after a 10- to 14-month silent incubation. Prior to emergence, the undulating course of the worm's body may be appreciated within the skin. At the time of cutaneous rupture, a marked allergic prodrome develops with local erythema, generalized urticaria, itching, dyspnea, gastrointestinal upset, and mild fever. Within hours, a papule forms over the female worm, which enlarges to vesicle or bulla on an inflammatory base. Often triggered by contact with water, rupture through the skin in this area allows the release of millions of larvae from the worm's uterus. An ulceration remains at this site, where traditionally the body of the female worm may be slowly extracted from the tissues by slow, gentle traction made by winding onto a stick over a several-week period. Infection is associated with significant morbidity as a result of cutaneous ulceration, necrosis, abscess formation, secondary bacterial infections, tetanus, and subsequent contractures or ankylosis of the lower extremities. Inability to work for 1 to 2 months is typical.[30] Multiple infections are common, and immunity to reinfection does not develop.

Oral medication has been found to be helpful with metronidazole, 250 mg three times daily for 10 to 20 days, thiabendazole, 50 to 75 mg/kg per day in 2 doses for 3 days, or niridazole, 25 mg/kg per day for 10 days. Surgical extraction of the worm is still advocated prior to spontaneous rupture through the skin. Extraction must be done with great care so as not to disrupt the body of the female, because the release of the larvae is thought to elicit the marked inflammatory reaction and sequelae.[30] Prevention of disease is obtainable with the provision of clean drinking water.

Dirofilariasis

Zoonotic infection of man with *Dirofilaria* species is usually manifest by pulmonary or subcutaneous lesions. Cases are described worldwide, wherever people live in proximity to the definitive hosts: dogs, coyotes, wolves, cats, foxes, raccoons, opossums, bears, and otters.[31] Mosquitoes are the vector and intermediate host. Blood containing microfilaria (mf) is ingested from an infected animal. Infective third-stage larvae develop in the mosquito over a 2-week period, and are deposited with subsequent feedings on the animal or human host. In animals, the mf mature over several months, migrating through venous channels to lodge and reproduce in the right ventricle. The gravid female produces several thousand mf per day, and eventually the animal succumbs to right-sided heart failure.

In humans, maturation and propagation do not occur, and the mf die. Prior to death, the mf may migrate through subcutaneous tissues, provoking a local reaction anywhere in the body, or into the venous system, where embolization to the lungs may be detected as a "coin" lesion on chest roentgenogram. This event may be asymptomatic or accompanied by cough, hemoptysis, pleuritic pain, and is usually due to infection with *D.*

immitis, the dog heartworm. Other species may produce subcutaneous masses, which may be asymptomatic, firm, and cystic, or migratory, erythematous, and pruritic. The breast, head, neck, and eye are common sites of involvement.[34] *D. tenuis* (*D. conjunctivae*) (raccoon) and *D. ursi* (bear) are the agents most often encountered in the United States, whereas *D. repens* (dog or cat) is found in Europe. Eosinophilia, if present, is mild. Diagnosis is usually made upon identifying the nematode in the dermis or subcutaneous tissues, often surrounded by a granulomatous reaction. The differential diagnosis is primary or metastatic cancer, cutaneous cysts, and other skin tumors. The diagnosis is rarely entertained prior to biopsy. Specific therapy in humans is seldom necessary; DEC and ivermectin have been used anecdotally.

INTESTINAL NEMATODE INFECTIONS

Cutaneous Larva Migrans

Cutaneous larva migrans (CLM), also known as creeping eruption or sandworm disease, is a self-limited cutaneous eruption caused by larvae of roundworms that do not normally parasitize humans (Table 127–1).[33–35] *Ancylostoma braziliense*, the dog and cat hookworm, is the most common agent. Larvae of several other nematode species, including *A. tubaeforme, A. caninum, A. ceylonicum, Uncinaria stenocephala, Bunostomum phlebotomum, Gnathostoma spinigerum, Dirofilaria conjunctivae (D. tenuis), Capillaria* species, *Strongyloides myopotami, S. papillosus,* and *S. westeri* may also cause creeping eruption, but are less common.[2, 36] *Strongyloides stercoralis* can produce CLM, although it is usually associated with larva currens, a more rapidly migratory condition. Larvae of *Necator americanus* and *A. duodenale,* human hookworm, can cause abortive forms of creeping eruption. CLM has a worldwide distribution, including the Caribbean, the southeastern United States, Central and South America, Africa, and Southeast Asia.[33] CLM is

TABLE 127-1. Causes of Cutaneous Larva Migrans

Species	Primary Host	Clinical Features
Ancylostoma braziliense, A. tubaeforme	Dog and cat hookworm	Thread-like, slightly raised, pruritic, migratory burrow, may persist for 3 months or more; moves 1–2 cm/day
Ancylostoma caninum, A. ceylonicum	Dog hookworm	Papular, rarely linear lesions; atypical CLM; disappears in 2 weeks
Uncinaria stenocephala	European dog hookworm	Similar clinical appearance to *Ancylostoma braziliense*
Bunostomum phlebotomum	Cattle hookworm	Papules with a few millimeters' migration; disappears in 2 weeks
Strongyloides stercoralis (cause of larva currens)	Human (strongylid)	Urticarial band in perianal or buttocks area; rapid migration up to 10 cm/hr; chronic and intermittent for years
Strongyloides animal species	Sheep, goat, cattle, horse, raccoon, and nutria parasite (strongylid)	Macule papular serpiginous lesions
Capillaria species	Rodents, cats, dogs, foxes, poultry (whipworm)	Linear track; extremely severe pruritus
Gnathostoma species	Cat, dog, pig, and wild feline nematodes	Intermittent episodes of red, edematous, subcutaneous nodules; limited migration of individual lesions; may be recurrent for years

CLM, cutaneous larva migrans.

found in the coastal areas of the United States from New Jersey to Texas, with a high incidence in Florida.[33] Beaches tend to be the most common reservoir of CLM, although it may result from contact with sand in children's sandboxes or in construction sites. To limit transmission, dogs are prohibited from roaming on many beaches in Florida. Physicians from nonendemic regions should question patients about travel because the rash may not appear until the vacationer returns home.

Nematode eggs are passed in the feces of infected animals, which hatch into filariform larvae in soil or sand. Humans become accidentally infected upon exposure to the larvae, capable of quickly penetrating skin. Patients recall a tingling or stinging sensation upon initial penetration of the larvae, and an erythematous papule or nonspecific dermatitis may develop within hours.[36] Migration of larvae usually occurs within a week, although it can be delayed for several weeks or months.[35] As the larvae migrate in human skin, they produce an intensely pruritic, 2- to 4-mm wide, erythematous, slightly elevated, vesicular, serpiginous track (Fig. 127–8). The larvae are restricted to the epidermis, where they wander aimlessly, unable to penetrate the basement membrane or complete their life cycle. The larva is found in normal skin 1 to 2 cm beyond the track, which marks the host's allergic reaction to the larva or its products. The larvae travel at a rate of several millimeters to 2 cm per day.[2] Untreated, lesions spontaneously resolve within weeks to months, following the eventual death of the larvae. The feet are the most common site for CLM, followed by the hands, arms, and buttocks. Diagnosis is based upon clinical findings with an appropriate history. Secondary bacterial infection, usually yielding *Streptococcus pyogenes*, may result in cellulitis and edema, making the tracks difficult to see, and may lead to the misdiagnosis of acute or secondarily infected tinea pedis.

Treatment with ethyl chloride spray, carbon dioxide slush, and liquid nitrogen have all been used in the past, but may be ineffective and scarring. Oral thiabendazole at 25 mg/kg twice a day for 2 days is usually effective, but has a high incidence of side effects including nausea, vomiting, and diarrhea. Topical thiabendazole liquid at 10% to 15% applied topically two to four times daily for a week is a safe and highly effective therapy for CLM. Oral albendazole, 400 mg a day for 3 days, is effective and side effects are rare. Ivermectin in a single dose of 200 μg/kg appears to be well tolerated and effective.[37]

Strongyloidiasis

Larva currens, or "running larva," is the cutaneous manifestation of intestinal infection and autoinfection with the human nematode *Strongyloides stercoralis*, and rarely, *S. fulleborni*.[38] It is found in feces-contaminated, moist, tropical and subtropical soil, where it may be free-living. Infection follows skin penetration by filariform larvae measuring 500 × 16 μm. These larvae enter the bloodstream and exit via the lungs, to ascend to the glottis and be swallowed. Maturation and reproduction occur in the upper small bowel. This organism is unusual in that rhabditiform (noninfective) larvae hatch from ova within the gastrointestinal tract. These larvae may transform into infectious filariform larvae, which reinfect the host by penetrating the intestinal mucosa (internal autoinfection) or the skin of the perianal and perineal areas, and occasionally the buttocks, abdomen, and thighs (external autoinfection). Infection can be persistent, with recurrences reported over a 40-year period in men who were prisoners of war in Southeast Asia.[2] Chronic steroid use, immunodepressed states, achlorhydria, nephrosis, burns, leprosy, and institutionalization predispose to chronic infection and to hyperinfection, where the larvae are widely disseminated (Fig. 127–9; see color plate).[39]

Reminiscent of CLM, pruritic, erythematous, serpiginous tracks migrate through the skin, but at the alarming rate of up to 10 cm per hour. Nonspecific rash, urticaria, papules, and vesicles can also be seen; individual lesions persist only about 48 hours. Cutaneous lesions are more widespread in hyperinfection, and may be petechial or purpuric in a reticulated pattern, especially in the periumbilical area.[40] Gram-negative bacteremia is common. Mortality is high in these patients (86%). Löffler's syndrome, shortness of breath with wheezing,

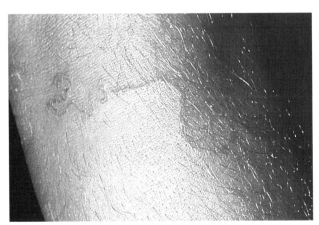

FIGURE 127–8. Cutaneous larva migrans, "creeping eruption." (Courtesy of the Harvey Blank, M.D. collection.)

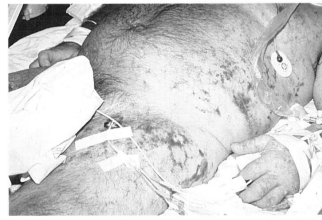

FIGURE 127–9. Premorbid strongyloidiasis in a case of superinfection. (See color plate.) (Courtesy of the Armed Forces Institute of Pathology.)

transient pulmonary infiltrates, fever, and eosinophilia, may accompany the migration of larvae through the lungs.

Except in the extreme immunocompromised patient, eosinophilia is common, in association with gastrointestinal complaints. Diagnosis is made upon identification of *S. stercoralis* ova or larvae in the stool. Since excretion of larvae is sporadic, multiple samples should be obtained and examined after Baermann-type concentration. Worms may also be recovered by oral passage and recovery of a string attached to a gelatin capsule (Enterotest, Hedeco, Palo Alto, CA). Immunofluorescent antibody assay and ELISA may be useful in nonendemic settings. A biopsy is likely to be diagnostic only in hyperinfection, where larvae are numerous.

Oral thiabendazole, 25 mg/kg twice daily for 2 to 5 days, is the drug of choice; a 2-day course may be repeated 1 week later. Mebendazole, 100 mg twice daily for 4 days, is an alternative, but may be poorly absorbed. Albendazole, 400 mg daily for 3 days, and ivermectin, 200 μg/kg daily for 1 to 2 days, have also been used.[6] Surprisingly, cyclosporine is active against *Strongyloides*.[39] Eradication of infection may be extremely difficult in immunocompromised individuals, in whom prolonged therapy is recommended.

Uncinarial Dermatitis

Human hookworm disease is caused by infection of the small intestine with *Ancylostoma duodenale*, the Old World hookworm, or *Necator americanus*, the New World hookworm.[36] *A. duodenale* is found in southern Europe, North Africa, and Asia with foci in the Caribbean and South and Central America. *N. americanus* is predominant in the New World, including the southeastern United States. *A. ceylonicum* may cause infection in the Philippines and India.[38] Adult female worms may lay 10,000 to 25,000 eggs per day, which are excreted in the feces and, under proper sand or soil conditions, hatch in approximately 1 day. Rhabditiform larvae emerge, and undergo two molts to become the infective filariform larvae. These larvae are thermotropic, causing them to seek a higher temperature than soil.[2] The warmer temperature of the skin is attractive to these filariform larvae, because they cannot survive for long without finding a mammalian host. Penetration of human skin may occur within 10 minutes of exposure to contaminated soil, and produces an immediate stinging sensation, especially by *N. americanus.*

A local pruritic dermatitis known as "ground itch" or "dew itch," with erythematous papules on the feet or ankles, follows penetration and persists up to 2 weeks. Urticaria, punctate hemorrhage, vesicles, or bullae can sometimes be seen, as can edema and regional adenopathy. Secondary bacterial infection is not uncommon, and may obscure the diagnosis. Symptoms are more severe and persistent in repeated infections. Spontaneous resolution occurs following the migration of larvae through the bloodstream to the lungs, then the gastrointestinal tract. Wheezing, cough, and eosinophilia often accompany this progression. Iron deficiency anemia follows

chronic infection. Diagnosis depends upon demonstration of ova in the stool.

The cutaneous lesions are treated symptomatically and for any concurrent bacterial infection. Mebendazole, 100 mg twice a day for 3 days, is the treatment of choice. Alternatives include albendazole, 400 mg as a single oral dose, pyrantel pamoate, 11 mg/kg (maximum 1 g) for 3 days, and thiabendazole, 25 mg/kg twice daily (maximum 3 g) for 2 days.

Toxocariasis

Visceral larva migrans is caused by the migration of zoonotic helminth larvae, most commonly the dog and cat ascarids, *Toxocara canis* and *T. cati*, in human eyes or tissues other than the skin. Infection occurs following ingestion of embryonated eggs from contaminated soil or hands. Cutaneous manifestations include generalized pruritus, urticaria, or urticarial papules of the trunk and extremities. A panniculitis consisting of firm, tender, subcutaneous nodules lasting 1 to 2 weeks and resembling erythema nodosum has been reported.[2] Eosinophilia is typical; ELISA can be diagnostic. Infection is self-limited, usually running a chronic benign course for up to 18 months. The treatments of choice are DEC, 2 mg/kg three times a day for 7 to 10 days, thiabendazole, 25 mg/kg twice daily for 5 days, or mebendazole, 100 to 200 mg twice daily for 5 days.[6] Visceral larva migrans will spontaneously remit without therapy; however, the duration of the disease may last up to 18 months.

Enterobiasis

Enterobiasis is the most common helminth infection in the United States and Western Europe, especially among school-age children. It occurs worldwide, and humans are the only host. Adult pinworms attach to the mucosa of the cecum, appendix, and nearby bowel, living up to 13 weeks.[41] The females, 8 to 13 mm in length, migrate nightly to the anus and perineum for oviposition. The eggs are ovoid, 55 $\times$ 25 μm, flattened on one side, and embryonate in 6 hours. Transmission is usually from the hands of infected individuals, but may be from fomites. After ova are ingested, the larvae hatch in the duodenum, and develop through two molts into adults by 1 to 2 months.

Pruritus ani, especially at night, is the most common clinical presentation. Although frequently asymptomatic, anorexia, abdominal pain, irritability, restlessness, insomnia, dysuria, and enuresis have been attributed to infection. Rarely, ectopic infection results in vaginitis, endometritis, salpingitis, epididymitis, urethritis, or pyelitis.[42]

Diagnosis is made by applying adhesive tape to the anal area in the early morning, and affixing this to a microscope slide to identify the ova; sensitivity increases up to five examinations.[28] Ova or larvae may rarely be detected in urine. Eosinophilia occurs only in invasive disease. The differential diagnosis includes idiopathic pruritus ani and localized disease as suggested by physical examination.

Therapy is effective with mebendazole, 100 mg, pyrantel pamoate, 11 mg/kg (maximum 1 g), and albendazole, 400 mg. Second-line drugs are piperazine, 65 mg/kg (maximum 2.5 g) for 7 days, and pyrvinium pamoate, 5 mg/kg (maximum 350 mg). All but piperazine are given as a single oral dose, best repeated in 2 weeks. Reinfection is frequent; treatment of the entire household is often indicated.

Gnathostomiasis

Gnathostomiasis is a zoonosis due to infection with *Gnathostoma spinigerum*, or less often *G. hispidum, G. doloresi,* or *G. nipponicum.* Infection is endemic in Southeast Asia, especially Thailand and Japan, where it is common to eat raw freshwater fish, a second intermediate host. Numerous cases have been reported from Ecuador, where raw freshwater fish are used in the preparation of ceviche, and the disease is called nodular migratory eosinophilic panniculitis.[43] Gnathostomiasis has also been diagnosed in Mexico, Australia, the Philippines, and Ceylon. Cases described in Europe and the United States did not originate there.

The definitive hosts are wild and domestic carnivores: cats, dogs, pigs, tigers, leopards, lions, minks, weasels, opossums, raccoons, and otters. Adult nematodes live within a tumor they induce in the host's gastric wall, from which ova are discharged and passed in the feces. In fresh water, the first-stage larvae hatch and are consumed by *Cyclops*, the first intermediate host, within whom the second-stage and early third-stage larvae develop.

These copepods are ingested by the second intermediate hosts: fish, frogs, snakes, chickens, rabbits, rodents, and pigs. The larvae penetrate the gastric wall, migrate to the musculature, and encyst there as advanced third-stage larvae. When the infected tissues are eaten by the definitive host, the larvae excyst in the stomach, penetrate the gastric wall, migrate through the liver and to the muscles of the host. After a 4-week period, the larvae return to the gastric mucosa to form the surrounding tumor, and reproduce after 6 to 8 months' maturation into the adult forms.

Humans become infected by ingesting a raw or undercooked second intermediate host, most often freshwater fish, poultry, or pork. The third-stage larvae excyst in the stomach, penetrate the gastric wall, and begin the migration through the accidental host, which may continue up to 12 years.[44] Fish and meat handlers are potentially at risk for percutaneous penetration of the larvae from infected second intermediate hosts. Initial symptoms relate to gastric penetration and migration through the liver, including abdominal pain, fever, nausea, vomiting, diarrhea, malaise, pruritus, and urticaria. Eosinophilia is pronounced at this stage, and may exceed 50% of the white blood cell count. Involvement of the lungs, gastrointestinal tract, genitourinary tract, eyes, ears, or central nervous system is called visceral gnathostomiasis. Migration through subcutaneous tissues has two clinical presentations: the deeper form is manifest by intermittent migratory urticarial plaques; the less common form presents as creeping eruption.[45] Rarely, it may present as an abscess or nodule. The edematous swellings are nonpitting, most often of the trunk or face, and may be associated with pain, pruritus, and erythema. They persist for 1 to 2 weeks, and with time, episodes become shorter, less frequent, less intense, and eventually disappear. Facial involvement is more often associated with the far more serious disease of the ocular, auditory, or central nervous system. Subconjunctival edema and hemorrhage with swelling of the eyelids may be seen in ocular gnathostomiasis.

Diagnosis requires suspicion of gnathostomiasis, or chance inclusion of the organism in the biopsy specimen. Highest yield has been at the swelling edge of linear erythema or discrete papules.[45] Sections of the parasite may be seen in the dermis or subcutaneous fat, surrounded by eosinophilic panniculitis. Blind biopsies or surgical explorations are rarely rewarding. Occasionally, extrusion of the nematode will occur through the skin or biopsy site. The worm may be a third-stage larva or a reddish adult, 1 to 3 cm long; the cephalic bulb has four to eight rows of transverse hooklets, followed by rows of cuticular spines to the middle of the body. Eosinophilia and leukocytosis are common. ELISA, indirect immunofluorescence, and skin test are helpful, but may not distinguish between other parasitic infections. The differential diagnosis includes panniculitis, urticaria, cellulitis, loiasis, and other ectopic larval helminthic infections: paragonimiasis, sparganosis, and fascioliasis.

Surgical removal of the worm is the only specific and effective therapy, but it may not be feasible. Numerous antihelminthic drugs have been used with limited success including albendazole, 400 mg per day for 2 weeks, mebendazole, 200 mg every 3 hours for 6 days, praziquantel, 25 mg/kg three times a day for 1 day, and thiabendazole, 25 mg/kg twice daily for 5 days. Anti-inflammatory agents, such as steroids and phenylbutazone, 200 mg twice daily for 5 days, have been used. Boiling fish for 5 minutes, freezing for 5 days, or marinating in vinegar (but not lime juice) for 6 hours, or soy sauce for 12 hours will kill larvae.[44]

TREMATODE INFECTION

Schistosomiasis

Human schistosomiasis is caused by blood flukes of the superfamily Schistosomatoidea. They differ from the other trematodes that infect man, because the sexes are separate and the adults inhabit the blood, being parasitic in the portal system.[9] The three schistosomes that cause disease in humans are *Schistosoma haematobium* (prevalent from Africa to Iran), *S. mansoni* (found in Africa and South America), and *S. japonicum* (which occurs in the Far East). Humans and animals are the definitive hosts of schistosomes, with a variety of snail genera as intermediate hosts. Approximately 200 million people in 71 countries are infected with human blood flukes.[2] Other related trematodes that may cause skin lesions, however, cannot mature in humans and, therefore, do not produce disease (see "Cercarial Dermatitis").

Schistosomiasis has been endemic in Egypt for thousands of years. Ancient Egyptian medical papyri describe the disease, noting that hematuria was common, and calcified ova of *S. haematobium* have been found in the kidneys of Egyptian mummies. In 1851, Bilharz described the adult worm found in the portal vein of an Egyptian man, hence the common term *Bilharzia*.

The fork-tailed cercaria (immature form), which are found in fresh water contaminated with snails, penetrate exposed skin or mucous membranes (Fig. 127–10). They enter the lymphatics and the bloodstream, reaching the liver, which is the site of maturation and sexual differentiation. The adult male is shorter and wider with a "gynaecophoric canal" that holds the female. They exist in monogamous harmony for life, which may be up to 30 years. The adult parasites move to various sites. *S. haematobium* migrates down the portal vein and mesenteric branches to the rectal plexus, which communicates freely with the vesical plexus and the prostatic or interovaginal plexi. *S. mansoni* and *S. japonicum* migrate via the portal vein down to the ileocolic and colic branches of the superior and inferior mesenteric veins. Less than one fifth of the production capacity of the females manage to leave the body; the rest are either retained in place or carried by the bloodstream to different organs.[46] The eggs of *S. haematobium* are spindle-shaped, large (140 × 50 µm), with a short terminal spine, and contain highly organized miracidium. The eggs of *S. haematobium* do not hatch in the urine, nor do *S. mansoni* or *S. japonicum* hatch in human feces, instead the eggs rupture when exposed to fresh water, releasing ciliated miracidium (Fig. 127–11). These can survive for 30 hours while in search of a suitable snail intermediate host, usually *Bulinus* species. The miracidium penetrates the soft tissue of the snail and migrates to the snail's digestive system where it looses its cilia and becomes a sporocyst. After several weeks, the sporocyst multiplication ceases, giving rise to cercaria, which are released from the sporocyst, escaping from the snail host (family Planorbidae) into the water. Humans become infected from drinking, swimming, bathing, or wading in cercaria-infested water.

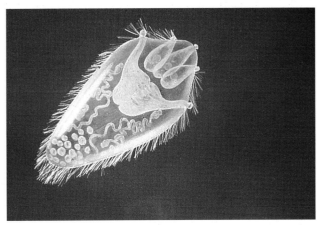

FIGURE 127–11. Ciliated miracidia of *S. japonicum* are released into fresh water and penetrate the snail intermediate host. (Courtesy of the Armed Forces Institute of Pathology.)

If the cercaria are unable to find a human host in 2 to 3 days, they die. When the cercaria penetrate human skin, which occurs in less than 30 minutes, the cercarial tails fall off and they become "schistosomulae." These penetrate human tissue by a combination of active movement and secretions.[9] If the cercariae are ingested from contaminated water, they attach and bore into the mucous membranes of the mouth and throat.[7] In *S. mansoni*, the eggs are 150 × 60 µm, have a lateral spine, with the adult male measuring 1 cm and female 1.4 cm. The eggs of *S. japonicum* are considerably smaller than the other two species (90 × 50 µm) with a small knob on the side and near the pole; however, it is not as predominant as the other species and often difficult to see. After the embryo has matured, an enzyme is secreted from the egg, resulting in necrosis of blood vessels and tissue. If the ovum does not find its way outside the body, the embryo inside becomes calcified and the tissues react to it as a foreign body.[46]

Symptomatology is related to the location and number of eggs in the host. *S. haematobium* produce urinary tract manifestations, such as dysuria, hematuria, and urinary frequency. *S. mansoni* and *S. japonicum* produce intestinal and hepatic symptoms, which include abdominal pain, hepatosplenomegaly, and diarrhea.[8]

Cutaneous manifestations of schistosomiasis can be divided into four types depending upon the stage of development of the parasite and the chronicity of the systemic disease: (1) *Dermatitis schistosomica* is caused by skin penetration by cercaria; (2) *bilharzides* represent the allergic anaphylactoid reactions that occur when large quantities of eggs (new antigenic material) are released and antibodies cross-react; (3) *bilharziasis cutanea tarde* is the specific schistosomal skin lesion caused by the deposit of eggs in the dermis; (4) lesions are related to complications of schistosomiasis.[47] *Schistosomal dermatitis* refers to exposure to human blood flukes cercariae. The first exposure may go unnoticed; however, the host becomes more sensitized with repeated encounters, resulting in pruritic papules to hive-like swellings. *S. haematobium* reactions are less severe than those of *S. mansoni* or *S. japonicum*. *Bilharzides* may develop early in

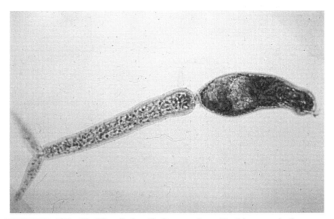

FIGURE 127–10. The fork-tailed cercariae of schistosomiasis penetrate human skin. (Courtesy of the Armed Forces Institute of Pathology.)

the invasive and development stage, or late in oviposition, when tissue reaction to eggs occurs. In this acute stage, lasting 2 to 10 weeks after cercaria penetration, cutaneous manifestations occur and may consist of urticaria, edema, purpura, and wheals. This syndrome is termed *Yangtze River fever* in China and *Katayama fever* in Japan. Clinical findings consist of fever, transient edema (face, trunk, limbs, or genitals), chills, joint pain, malaise, diarrhea, abdominal cramps, bronchitis, and pneumonitis. Hepatomegaly, splenomegaly, and lymphadenitis may occur, and there is leukocytosis, eosinophilia, and an elevated sedimentation rate. *Bilharziasis cutanea tarda* is usually manifested by granulomatous anogenital lesions. Extragenital or papular ectopic lesions are less common and are found on the trunk and umbilical area, often in a zosteriform distribution. Primary lesions are 2- to 3-mm flesh-colored, asymptomatic, firm papules that develop into irregular plaques, that may darken, become scaly, and occasionally ulcerate.[2] The eggs, not the adult worms, cause the pathologic changes associated with schistosomiasis.

With respect to systemic manifestations, visceral *S. haematobium* infection is characterized by terminal hematuria, bladder papilloma, and ulceration. Intestinal schistosomiasis, caused by *S. mansoni* or *S. japonicum*, produces dysenteric symptoms and leads to cirrhosis of the liver, ascites, and splenomegaly.

Diagnosis of *S. haematobium* infection is made by identifying eggs in centrifuged urine. Egg output is increased with physical exercise and fluid intake just prior to the urinalysis, which should be obtained about noon, the peak excretion time for *S. haematobium*. In suspected cases with negative urine samples, rectal biopsies are highly diagnostic. For diagnosis of *S. mansoni* and *S. japonicum*, fecal samples should be examined for eggs using either a direct smear procedure or the Kato thick smear technique. Among serologic tests, the complement fixation fluorescence test is the most sensitive and has the advantage of early detection and the disadvantage of being impractical for field use. PCR has also been used in *S. mansoni* infections.[48]

The treatment of choice for schistosomiasis is praziquantel administered in the following dose regimens: for *S. haematobium* and *S. mansoni*, 40 mg/kg per day in 2 doses × 1 day; for *S. japonicum*, 60 mg/kg per day in 3 doses × 1 day.

Cercarial Dermatitis

Cercarial dermatitis, commonly known as swimmer's itch, is a distinctive papular eruption caused by penetration of the skin by cercariae of nonhuman schistosomes. This cutaneous schistosomiasis is usually limited to the exposed areas of the body. It is associated with freshwater lakes, although "clam digger's itch" has been reported from the saltwater tributaries of Long Island Sound, New York.[2] There are approximately 20 species of these flukes worldwide that have been implicated in human disease. The cercariae responsible infect birds, rodents, or ungulates, and belong to the species *Schistosoma, Ornithobilharzia, Gigantobilharzia, Austrobilharzia, Trichobilhar-*

zia, and *Orientobilharzia*.[49] Cercarial dermatitis is a potential hazard worldwide, wherever people share an aquatic environment with vertebrates and mollusks harboring schistosomes.

These blood flukes require an intermediate snail host and a definitive vertebrate host to complete the life cycle. Inasmuch as man is an accidental host, development cannot proceed, and clinical manifestations of cercarial penetration resolve spontaneously within a week. A prickling sensation lasting minutes to an hour results from exposure to cercariae-infested water. Pruritic erythematous macules, papules, and occasionally, papulovesicles and wheals can be seen soon thereafter. Postinflammatory hyperpigmentation is a common sequela. Edema, lymphangitis, and regional adenopathy develop in some individuals, as may eosinophilia and systemic symptoms of generalized urticaria, nausea, and vomiting.[2] The nonhuman schistosomes incite a greater inflammatory reaction from penetration, although this varies among individuals. Repeated exposures produce more severe insect bite reaction, with perivascular lymphocytes, histiocytes, and eosinophils.[49]

Treatment is oriented toward the relief of symptoms. Oral antihistamines, topical steroids, and topical antipruritic agents may be helpful. The rash may be prevented by toweling off vigorously and showering promptly after freshwater bathing. Copper salts have been used effectively for decades to eliminate snail populations; however, this practice is now environmentally questionable. Niclosamide is effective, but rarely necessary.

Seabather's Eruption

Because seabather's eruption is often confused with swimmer's itch, we mention it here, despite its more appropriate categorization among stinging invertebrates rather than parasitic infections.

Seabather's eruption is a highly pruritic cutaneous eruption that occurs primarily under swimwear after bathing in the ocean. It is caused by the stinging nematocysts of the larvae of the phylum Cnidaria (formerly Coelenterata), which includes jellyfish, Portuguese man-of-war, sea anemones, hydroids, and fire coral. These pinhead-sized larvae become trapped between the skin and bathing apparel. Pressure or exposure to freshwater elicits the release of the coiled nematocysts, which fire irritating toxins into the skin. The larva of *Edwardsiella lineata*, a sea anemone, is the probable cause of seabather's eruption in the North Atlantic coastal states and occurs from August through October.[50] The larva of *Linuche unguiculata*, the thimble jellyfish, is the cause on the southern Atlantic coast, especially Florida and the Caribbean, and has been reported from March to August, usually peaking in late May.[51, 52] Seabather's eruption is often inappropriately termed *sea lice*. "Sea lice" refer to metazoan parasites of fish and do not affect humans (Table 127–2).

Exposure to cnidarian larvae is associated with stinging or prickling under swimwear upon exiting the ocean. Lesions appear within a few hours of exposure and con-

TABLE 127-2. Characteristics of Cercarial Dermatitis,
Seabather's Eruption, and "Sea Lice"

	Cercarial Dermatitis ("Swimmer's Itch")	Seabather's Eruption (Northern)	Seabather's Eruption (Southern)	"Sea Lice"
Location	Worldwide distribution, highly endemic in Canada & Great Lakes, and U.S. northern mid-west lakes	North Atlantic coast from Massachusetts to South Carolina	Southern Atlantic coast, especially S. Florida and the Caribbean	Worldwide distribution
Type of water	Fresh water (predominantly), occasionally saltwater tributaries	Salt (ocean)	Salt (ocean)	Salt (ocean)
Affects	Humans	Humans	Humans	Fish
Skin involved	Exposed	Covered	Covered	N/A
Etiology	Schistosome cercariae, usually of birds, rodents, or ungulates	Cnidarian larvae of the sea anemone, *Edwardsiella lineata*	Cnidarian larvae of the thimble jellyfish, *Linuche unguiculata*	Parasitic crustaceans

N/A, not applicable.

sist of pruritic erythematous papules and wheals, often developing into pustules or vesicles (Fig. 127-12). Although lesions usually resolve in a few days, some patients have a delayed hypersensitivity that occurs about 10 days after the initial exposure and is often more severe, extending to exposed areas of the body, which were not previously affected. Fever (101° F to 104° F), nausea, vomiting, and diarrhea may occur, with frequency and severity more common in children. Recent history of ocean exposure is the most important diagnostic aid. Oral antihistamines, systemic and medium to high-strength topical corticosteroids, and antipruritic agents are effective in most cases. Bathing suits should be washed in fresh water and detergent and dried prior to reuse; otherwise unreleased nematocysts will fire, producing the eruption without additional exposure to ocean water.

Paragonimiasis

Paragonimiasis is caused by infection with lung flukes of the genus *Paragonimus*. Migratory subcutaneous nodules are common in 20% to 60% of patients infected with *P. skrjabini* in China, and in 10% of those with *P. westermani* infection.[53] The nodules are firm, slightly mobile, and may be tender or irritating, growing up to 10 cm in diameter. They are found usually over the lower abdomen, inguinal area, thigh, or postauricularly. Clinical presentation usually relates to pulmonary disease, but diagnosis can be made following surgical excision of a nodule. Treatment is with praziquantel, 75 mg/kg per day in 3 doses for 2 days.

LARVAL CESTODE INFECTION

Cysticercosis

Humans are the definitive host for gastrointestinal infection with the adult pork tapeworm, *Taenia solium*. Cysticercosis, however, is caused by infection with the larval stage, cysticercus cellulosae, in which humans are an incidental intermediate host, usually transmitted by oral-fecal contamination or by eating inadequately cooked "measly pork." Ingested eggs hatch in the stomach, penetrating the intestinal wall and developing into oncospheres, then infective larval cysts. Cysts are viable up to 5 years, and elicit little reaction until death and subsequent calcification. Cysticercosis is encountered most often in Mexico, South America, and parts of Europe, Asia, and Africa.

Cysticercus cysts may develop anywhere in the body, but show predilection for the brain, meninges, eyes, muscle, heart, liver, lungs, oral cavity, and skin.[54] Clinical disease usually relates to the central nervous system involvement. Subcutaneous nodules are round, rubbery, and asymptomatic, reaching 1- to 2-cm size, and eventually calcifying. Diagnosis is made after excision or roentgenogram, with confirmatory serology. Treatment has been surgical, but can be accomplished with praziquantel, 50 mg/kg per day in 3 divided doses for 2 weeks, or alternatively albendazole, 15 mg/kg per day in 3 divided

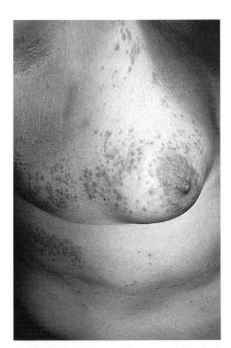

FIGURE 127-12. Seabather's eruption caused by the larvae of the thimble jellyfish, *Linuche unguiculata*.

doses for 8 days. Seizure control and steroids may be required concurrently.

Sparganosis

Humans become infected with the zoonotic, plerocercoid larva of *Spirometra* species by (1) drinking water containing infected *Cyclops*, the first intermediate host; (2) eating raw or poorly cooked flesh of the second intermediate host (fish, snake, frog, rodent, raccoon, opossum); or (3) percutaneous penetration upon applying infected flesh as a poultice to wounds or the eyes, a practice more common to the Orient. Cases are most often reported from Southeast Asia, but also have been found in the southeastern United States, the Caribbean, South America, Africa, and Australia.

The adult tapeworm infects the gastrointestinal tract of small carnivores, and eggs are passed in the feces. The first larval form, coracidia, are released in fresh water and are consumed by *Cyclops*. They, in turn, are consumed by the second intermediate host. The larvae penetrate the bowel wall, then migrate through the gut wall to anywhere in the body. The most common clinical presentation is that of a subcutaneous nodule; however, the mass can be tender, pruritic, and occasionally migratory. The differential diagnosis includes lipoma, abscess, fat necrosis, and neoplasm. Other sites of involvement include the eye, brain, lung, epididymis, urethra, bowel, skeletal muscle.[55] An unusual form of infection is human proliferative sparganosis, in which large numbers of vermiform or vesicular larva are encountered, having reproduced asexually by budding or branching.[56] The prognosis is poor.

Diagnosis is usually made following surgical resection of the mass, upon encountering sections of the parasite. A marked granulomatous inflammation with eosinophils may surround the larva. Eosinophilia may be present. ELISA may be helpful in endemic areas, if the diagnosis is suspected. Rarely, the live sparganum, a glistening white, thread-like worm up to 50 cm long, resembling a guinea worm, is discharged. Surgical excision is the treatment of choice. Praziquantel, mebendazole, and neoarsphenamine use has been reported.[56]

References

1. Luaces AL, Osorio LM, Barrett AJ. A new test for infection by *Entamoeba histolytica*. Parasitology Today 1993;9(2):69–71.
2. Pardo RJ, Kerdel FA. Parasites, arthropods, and hazardous animals of dermatologic significance. In: Moshella SL, Hurley HJ, eds. Dermatology, 3rd edition. Philadelphia: WB Saunders Co., 1992:1923–2003.
3. Ravdin JI. *Entamoeba histolytica*: From adherence to enteropathy. J Infect Dis 1989;159:420–429.
4. Davson J, Jones DM, Turner L. Diagnosis of Meleney's synergistic gangrene. Br J Surg 1988;75:267–271.
5. Fujita WH, Barr RJ, Gotschalk MR. Cutaneous amebiasis. Arch Dermatol 1981;117:309–310.
6. Drugs for parasitic infections. Med Lett Drugs Ther 1992;34:17–26.
7. Chandler AC, Read CP. Introduction to Parasitology, 10th edition. New York: John Wiley & Sons, 1961.
8. Benenson AS. Control of Communicable Diseases in Man, 15th edition. Washington, DC: American Public Health Association, 1990.
9. Crewe W, Haddock DRW. Parasites and Human Diseases. New York: John Wiley & Sons, 1985.
10. Avila HA, Pereira JB, Thiemann O, et al. Detection of *Trypanosoma cruzi* in blood specimens of chronic chagasic patients by polymerase chain reaction amplification of kinetoplast minicircle DNA: Comparison with serology and xenodiagnosis. J Clin Microbiol 1993;31(9):2421–2426.
11. Moser DR, Cook GA, Baileys CP, et al. Detection of *Trypanosoma congolense* and *Trypanosoma brucei* subspecies by DNA amplification using the polymerase chain reaction. Parasitology 1989;99:57.
12. McCabe RE, Remington JS. *Toxoplasma gondii*. In: Mandell GL, Douglas RG, Bennett JE, eds. Principles and Practice of Infectious Diseases, 3rd edition, vol. 2. New York: Churchill Livingstone, 1990:2090–2103.
13. Fine JD, Arndt KA. The TORCH syndrome: A clinical review. J Am Acad Dermatol 1985;12:697–706.
14. Leyva WH, Santa Cruz DJ. Cutaneous toxoplasmosis. J Am Acad Dermatol 1986;14:600–605.
15. Harland CC, Marsden JR, Vernon SA, et al. Dermatomyositis responding to treatment of associated toxoplasmosis. Br J Dermatol 1991;125:76–78.
16. Hirschman JV, Chu AC. Skin lesions with disseminated toxoplasmosis in a patient with acquired immunodeficiency syndrome. Arch Dermatol 1988;124:1446–1447.
17. Leyva WH, Santa Cruz DJ. Cutaneous toxoplasmosis. J Am Acad Dermatol 1986;14:600–605.
18. Heine P, McGregor JA. *Trichomonas vaginalis*: A reemerging pathogen. Clin Obstet Gynecol 1993;36:137–144.
19. Greene BM. Modern medicine versus an ancient scourge: Progress toward control of onchocerciasis. J Infect Dis 1992;166:15–21.
20. Kalter DC, Freedman DO. Onchocerciasis. Semin Dermatol 1994: in press.
21. Reber EW, Hoeppli R. The relationship between macroscopic skin alterations, histological changes and microfilariae in one hundred Liberians with onchocercal dermatitis. Z Tropenmed Parasitol 1964;15:153–163.
22. Meyers WM, Neafie RC. Streptocerciasis. In: Strickland GT, ed. Hunter's Tropical Medicine, 7th edition. Philadelphia: WB Saunders Co., 1991:746–749.
23. Freedman DO, Nutman TB. Filariasis. In: Balows A, Hawker WJ, Ohashi M, et al., eds. Laboratory Diagnosis of Infectious Diseases. New York: Springer-Verlag, 1988:863–871.
24. King CL, Nutman TB. Regulation of the immune response in lymphatic filariasis and onchocerciasis. Immunol Today 1991; 12:A54–58.
25. Buck AA. Filariasis. In: Strickland GT, ed. Hunter's Tropical Medicine, 7th edition. Philadelphia: WB Saunders Co., 1991:713–727.
26. Dandapat MC, Mohapatro SK, Mohanty SS. Filarial lymphoedema and elephantiasis of lower limb: A review of 44 cases. Br J Surg 1986;73:451–453.
27. Mahmoud AAF. Intestinal nematodes (roundworms). In: Mandell GL, Douglas RG, Bennett JE, eds. Principles and Practice of Infectious Diseases, 3rd edition. New York: Churchill Livingstone, 1990:2135–2140.
28. Walrus without tears (editorial). Lancet 1990;i:202.
29. Martin-Prevel Y, Cosnefroy JY, Tshipamba P, et al. Tolerance and efficacy of a single high-dose ivermectin for the treatment of loiasis. Am J Trop Med Hyg 1993;48:186–192.
30. Rohde JE, Sharma BL, Patton H, et al. Surgical extraction of Guinea worm: Disability reduction and contribution to disease control. Am J Trop Med Hyg 1993;48:71–76.
31. MacDougall LT, Magoon CC, Fritsche TR. *Dirofilaria repens* manifestating as a breast nodule. Am J Clin Pathol 1992;97:625–630.
32. Finkel LJ, Headington JT. Subcutaneous dirofiliasis in a raccoon keeper. Clin Cases Dermatol 1990;2:2–4.
33. Davies HD, Sakuls P, Keystone JS. Creeping eruption. Arch Dermatol 1993;129:588–591.
34. Stein D. Fungal, protozoa, and helminth infections. In: Schachner LA, Hansen RC, eds. Pediatric Dermatology, 1st edition, vol. 2. New York: Churchill Livingstone, 1988:588–591.
35. Scheiner RB, Griffin TD, Lattanand A, et al. Lesions on the feet of a scuba diver. Arch Dermatol 1990;126(8):1095–1096.

36. Chaudhny AZ, Longworth DL. Cutaneous manifestations of intestinal helminth infections. Dermatol Clin 1989;7(2):275–290.
37. Caumes E, Datry A, Paris L, et al. Efficacy of ivermectin in the therapy of cutaneous larva migrans (Letter to the Editor). Arch Dermatol 1992;128:994–995.
38. Pearson RD, Guerrant RL. Intestinal nematodes that migrate through skin and lung. In: Strickland GT, ed. Hunter's Tropical Medicine, 7th edition. Philadelphia: WB Saunders Co., 1991: 700–711.
39. Purvis RS, Beightler EL, Sanchez RL, et al. *Strongyloides stercorales* hyperinfection. Int J Dermatol 1992;31:160–164.
40. Purvis RS, Beighler EL, Diven DG, et al. Strongyloides hyperinfection presenting with petechiae and purpura. Int J Dermatol 1992;31:169–171.
41. Pearson RD, Schwartzman JD. Nematodes limited to the intestinal track. In: Strickland GT, ed. Hunter's Tropical Medicine, 7th edition. Philadelphia: WB Saunders Co., 1991:689–700.
42. Kollias G, Kyriakopoulos M, Tiniakos G. *Enterobius vermicularis*: A case report. J Urol 1992;147:1114–1116.
43. Ollaque W, Ollaque J, Guevara de Veliz A, et al. Human gnathostomiasis in Ecuador (nodular migratory eosinophilic panniculitis). Int J Dermatol 1984;23:647–651.
44. Rusnak JM, Lucey DR. Clinical gnathostomiasis. Clin Inf Dis 1993;16:33–50.
45. Taniguchi Y, Ando K, Isoda K, et al. Human gnathostomiasis. Int J Dermatol 1992;31:175–177.
46. Amer M. Cutaneous schistosomiasis. Int J Dermatol 1982;21:44.
47. Amer M. Cutaneous schistosomiasis. In: Canizares D, Harman R, eds. Clinical Tropical Dermatology. Boston, London: Blackwell Scientific Publications, 1992:363.
48. Gasser RB, Morahan C, Mitchell GF. Sexing single larval stages of schistosoma mansori by polymerase chain reaction. Mol Biochem Parasitol 1991;255.
49. Kullavanijaya P, Wongwaisayawan H. Outbreak of cercarial dermatitis in Thailand. Int J Dermatol 1993;32:113–115.
50. Freudenthal AR, Joseph PR. Seabather's eruption. N Engl J Med 1993;329:542–544.
51. Tomchik RS, Russell MT, Szmant AM, et al. Clinical perspectives on seabather's eruption, also known as "Sea Lice." JAMA 1993;269:1669–1672.
52. Wong DE, Meinking TL, Rosen LB, et al. Seabather's eruption: Clinical, histological and immunological features. J Am Acad Derm 1994: in press.
53. Goldsmith R, Bunnag D, Bunnag T. Lung fluke infections: Paragonimiasis. In: Strickland GT, ed. Hunter's Tropical Medicine, 7th edition. Philadelphia: WB Saunders Co., 1991:827–831.
54. Sarti E, Schantz PM, Plancarte A, et al. Prevalence and risk factor for Taenia solium taeniasis and cysticercosis in humans and pigs in a village in Morelos, Mexico. Am J Trop Med Hyg 1992;46: 677–685.
55. Sarma DP, Wibaecher TG. Human sparganosis. J Am Acad Dermatol 1986;15:1145–1148.
56. Nakamura T, Hara M, Matsuoka M, et al. Human proliferative sparganosis. Am J Clin Pathol 1990;94:224–228.

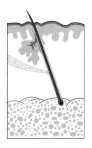

chapter 128

Body Lice, Head Lice, Pubic Lice, and Scabies

JAMES E. RASMUSSEN

Pediculosis Corporis (Body Lice)

DEFINITION

Pediculus humanus corporis is similar in many aspects to the human head louse *Pediculus humanus capitis*, and some authors believe the body louse evolved from the head louse when humans began wearing clothing.

CLINICAL DESCRIPTION

Although there are no exact population statistics, some investigators believe that body lice infestations are less common than head and pubic lice infestations. During times of social unrest, poverty, and war, large epidemics of body lice have been reported in humans in over-crowded living conditions. The organism feeds on the body but lives on clothes and lays its eggs near the seams. This location has given rise to some of their nick-names, such as seam squirrels, cooties, and gray backs.[1] The body louse is anatomically indistinguishable from the head louse, but it has important physiologic distinctions.

In most instances fewer than 10 adult organisms are present, but this number may range up to 200 or more. The lice move freely about on the body and are blood-sucking insects. This gives rise to the clinical features of pruritus and excoriations. Because infestation with body lice tends to be a chronic problem, the long-term scratching can contribute to formation of the multiple scarring lesions on the upper back that is sometimes referred to as vagabond's disease.[2]

PATHOLOGY

It is generally presumed that the initial bite of the louse produces only a small red punctum and that once sensitization has occurred the cellular response becomes more pronounced, with perivascular infiltration of lympho-cytes, eosinophils, and plasma cells.

PATHOGENESIS AND ETIOLOGY

The human body louse is indistinguishable anatomi-cally from the human head louse. Infestations are passed from person to person through direct physical contact or through fomites such as blankets, pillows, and sleeping bags. Huge epidemics have been reported in times of famine and war. In this situation, body lice may transmit the rickettsial diseases epidemic typhus and trench fever.[3] These diseases are uncommonly reported today in the United States.

DIAGNOSIS AND DIFFERENTIAL DIAGNOSIS

The diagnosis of pediculosis corporis should be sus-pected in anyone who has a chronic pruritic disease, particularly affecting the upper back and chest. This is an uncommon area for an adult to have impetigo, and re-peated episodes of impetigo in this area should encourage the physician to search through the clothing. The cloth-ing should be examined with particular attention paid to the seams of those garments worn closest to the patient's body, such as underwear and shirts. Unfortunately for the diagnostician, patients who are likely to be infested with lice will often shed their frequently worn clothing

TABLE 128-1. Differential Diagnosis of Pediculosis Corporis

Impetigo
Simple excoriations
Delusions of parasitosis
Acne, folliculitis
Grover's disease
Dermatitis herpetiformis

when visiting their physician in favor of their "Sunday best," which will not be infected.

The differential diagnosis (Table 128–1) consists of entities that make the back itch, such as Grover's disease, acne, xerosis, dermatitis herpetiformis, and delusions of parasitosis.

TREATMENT

The most important point of the treatment of patients with body lice is to sanitize the clothing, bedding, and immediate environment by thorough washing with hot water. This is often difficult to do since many of these patients are homeless or live in areas with very rudimentary sanitary facilities. Many of the over-the-counter or prescription agents mentioned in the section on head lice can be used successfully but probably require several treatments separated over a period of 7 to 10 days.

Pediculosis Capitis (Head Lice)

DEFINITION

Pediculosis capitis represents infestation of scalp hair with the human head louse *Pediculus humanus capitis.*

CLINICAL DESCRIPTION

Infestation with head lice is quite common in the United States.[4, 5] Schoolaged children are affected more often than adults, with most publications suggesting that girls are slightly more susceptible than boys. The head louse has no respect for an individual's economic position and probably is seen commonly in all levels of society.

At least in the United States head lice infection is very uncommon in blacks. The exact reasons for this are not known, although the speculation has ranged from hair grooming products (oils) to hair styles and hair shape. There are, however, many reports of head lice in blacks occurring in countries other than the United States.

Since the disease is usually not reportable, exact population statistics are difficult to assess and a clinician's impression of the prevalence of the disease varies widely

from practice to practice. Most cases of pediculosis are detected by the patient, parent, or teacher and usually treated with over-the-counter remedies. Consequently, those cases that are actually detected in the physician's office represent only a very small percentage of the total number of cases.

The disease is spread from person to person through direct physical contact or through the use of fomites such as combs or other toilet articles, hats, scarves, and towels. Overcrowding in the home leads to rapid transmission to all members of the family. Previous infection probably does not convey any degree of resistance, although this has not been well studied.

Adult lice live for 1 to 2 months, and the female deposits four to six eggs per day on the most proximal part of the hair shaft, cementing them at an oblique angle with chitin. These eggs sacks are referred to as nits. An unhatched nit has a characteristic white to tan color, while a hatched nit is seen as gray.

The first sign of clinical involvement occurs when the lice move about on the scalp or take a blood meal, often from around the margins of the scalp and above the ears. This produces a sensation of pruritus. Therefore, any child with an itchy scalp that does not have an obvious cause such as psoriasis should receive a vigorous search for nits. The adult lice move freely about on the scalp and are usually not seen unless present in great numbers. After a period of a few days to several weeks the pruritus increases and is often accompanied by excoriations and secondary infection. Consequently, cervical and occipital adenopathy is quite common. More advanced cases feature lesions over the neck, ears, and upper back. Chronic scratching as well as serous exudate often produces matted clumps of hair that are difficult to untangle and occasionally must be removed with scissors.

The extent of the problem has never been ascertained on a national basis. However, several large epidemics have been reported and one paper described the results of therapy in more than 30,000 patients collected from a multicenter trial.[6] In some Third World countries 50% to 100% of the population of all ages may be infected.

PATHOLOGY

The histopathology is not characteristic and depends on the degree of excoriation and secondary impetiginization. Ackerman[7] reports a superficial and deep perivascular mixed cell infiltrate with occasional eosinophils. Since the organism and its eggs live on but not in the skin, the biopsy specimen usually shows only secondary characteristics; thus biopsy is not usually indicated.

PATHOGENESIS AND ETIOLOGY

The etiologic agent of head lice is *Pediculus humanus capitis.* It is a species-specific human parasite that is not known to have any other host. On rare occasions, closely related animal species have been transmitted from monkeys to humans, but in general this is not a problem.

The pruritus and many of the primary lesions are caused by the blood-sucking activities of the insect. Some researchers believe that the saliva produces a hypersensitivity reaction that is most marked by urticarial papules and wheals.

DIAGNOSIS AND DIFFERENTIAL DIAGNOSIS

The diagnosis should be considered in any patient who complains of itching near the scalp, ears, neck, and upper back. The presence of impetigo or exudative eczematous lesions should suggest this diagnosis, particularly in a child. The diagnosis is confirmed by finding the adult mite or the nits. Adult head lice can move surprisingly rapidly over the scalp. Consequently, it is much easier to detect nits, which are gray to white ellipsoidal objects that are cemented to the side of the hair shaft. The distance from the surface of the scalp indicates the duration of the infection and how recently the eggs were laid. As a general rule, eggs more than 4 cm from the scalp have probably hatched and the absence of eggs any closer to the scalp indicates that the infestation has been terminated.

If the diagnosis is in doubt, plucked hair can be evaluated microscopically for the presence of nits. Confusing artifacts consist of hair spray, hair scale, trichorrhexis nodosa, and piedra. Nits are cemented to the shaft and will not slide with gentle traction.

Other important considerations in the differential diagnosis (Table 128–2) are conditions that produce an itchy scalp or impetiginization of the ears, neck, and shoulders. Seborrheic dermatitis is characterized by a typical scale and distribution. True seborrheic dermatitis is uncommon in the prepubertal age group, which is the population commonly infected with head lice.

Impetigo in the scalp of a child should always make one consider the possibility of an inflammatory fungal infection. This is much more common in blacks, in whom hair loss is usually quite noticeable. A potassium hydroxide mount and fungal culture will help separate the difficult cases.

TREATMENT

The standard of care involves eradication of all live lice, destroying the incubating larvae, nit removal, and treatment of secondary infection (Table 128–3). Pyrethrins and synthetically related compounds are one of the mainstays in the treatment of head lice. Pyrethrins are an extract of a specific type of chrysanthemum often

TABLE 128-3. Treatment of Pediculosis Capitis

Lindane (Kwell)*
Permethrin (Nix)[†]
Pyrethrins/piperonyl butoxide (RID, A-200, others)[†]
Crotamiton 10% (Eurax)*
Malathion 0.5% (Ovide)*
Sulfur creme, 6%–12%*

*Available only by prescription.
[†]Available without prescription.

coupled with piperonyl butoxide to potentiate their effect and provide stability.[8, 9]

These compounds are all sold without prescription and come in a variety of creams, lotions, shampoos, and rinses (RID, A-200 and many others). All require a second application approximately a week after the first, since they are not ovicidal.

Pyrethroids are synthetic derivatives of pyrethrins. Permethrin (Nix) is a member of this class of drugs that has a residual activity of 7 to 10 days and is also ovicidal.[10, 11] It is used as a 1% cream rinse and is available without prescription. Because of its ovicidal effectiveness, permethrin can be used as a single 10-minute treatment application, although I recommend applying it a second time after 1 week just to make certain.

Lindane (Kwell) is available as a 1% solution in the form of a shampoo. It is effective against adults but not against the nits. Consequently, a second application is necessary after a week's interval. Although lindane is safe when applied topically, with abuse (frequent repeat applications) or with ingestion it can produce considerable neurotoxicity. This usually takes the form of seizures. With proper use all the popular remedies are safe, as was demonstrated in a multicentered study[6] in which there were no significant differences in medically important events in over 30,000 patients treated with either permethrin, lindane, or pyrethrins.

Malathion has been irregularly marketed in the United States but is commonly used throughout the rest of the world.[12] At the present time I am not aware of its commercial availability in the United States. Precipitated sulfur 2% to 6%, benzyl benzoate, disulfiram, thiabendazole, and crotamiton have been used in other countries but are not marketed in the United States for this indication.[13]

Each product except malathion and sulfur needs an 8- to 10-minute contact time. Malathion and sulfur require overnight (8-hour) application.

The question of resistance to any of these pediculicides is both a theoretical and a real problem in certain parts of the world.[14, 15] It is difficult to find documented instances of resistance that have occurred in the United States. More often "resistance" represents failure to treat all affected family members.

General Guidelines

It is appropriate that all family members be treated even if they do not exhibit signs or symptoms of the

TABLE 128-2. Differential Diagnosis of Pediculosis Capitis and Scalp Itching

Nits	Scalp Itching
Hair spray	Tinea capitis
Scale	Seborrheic dermatitis
Trichorrhexis nodosa	Atopic dermatitis
Piedra	Delusions of parasitosis

disease. Patients who are clinically infected should be treated a second time after an interval of a week. Although this is probably not necessary with use of permethrin, I still make it a rule to do so. It is also important that all of the patient's household personal use items and bedding be deloused. Combs, brushes, caps, scarves, and sheets, pillow cases, and other bedding should be thoroughly washed in hot water. Articles of personal hygiene can be soaked in rubbing alcohol or may be washed in a kitchen dishwasher.

It is not necessary to disinfect the entire house, and the use of sprays on carpets, drapes, and furniture is not recommended.

Nit Removal

Most modern pediculicides come with a scientifically designed nit comb that is somewhat effective for removing eggs from the hair. Fifty to 85% of nits can be removed with a conventional nit comb, but parents should not be made to feel guilty if this goal is not achieved. As previously mentioned, nits further than 4 cm from the scalp will probably not be viable and the absence of nits on the more proximal hair shaft indicates the infection has been eradicated.

A commercial preparation containing formic acid combined with an extra-fine nit comb has been marketed intermittently in the United States.[16] It is clearly more effective than the nit comb and a regular pediculicide used by itself, but it is not widely available.

Systemic agents have also been used in the treatment of head lice. It is difficult to envision a situation in which one or more of the topically applied pesticides is not effective, but if this should arise then cotrimoxazole (80 mg trimethoprim and 400 mg sulfamethoxazole [Bactrim or Septra]) has been used effectively. Patients should be treated twice a day for 3 days, and according to one study the lice will soon leave the head and later die. Neither trimethoprim nor sulfamethoxazole shows any effect on the lice when used separately. A second course given at a week's interval is probably necessary since this agent does not have effect on the viability of nits. Although its mechanism of action is speculative, it probably decreases the bacterial flora that are necessary for the louse's digestion of its human blood meal.

Shaving the head is mentioned only to condemn it. Except in the severe and neglected case in which hair matting makes hair combing impossible, this therapy should never be considered.

Pediculosis Pubis (Pubic Lice)

DEFINITION

Pediculosis pubis is a condition of infestation of the pubic hair with *Phthirus pubis*. It is unique among the diseases described in this chapter because it is spread primarily through sexual contact.

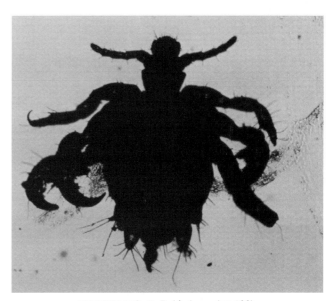

FIGURE 128–1. Pubic louse (× 100).

CLINICAL DESCRIPTION

Phthirus pubis, commonly called the pubic or crab louse, is morphologically distinct from the somewhat cylindrically shaped head and body lice (Fig. 128–1).[17] *P. pubis* is shorter and more rounded and has the compact shape of a crab, from which it takes its name. The second and third pairs of legs are developed into heavy pincers, which it uses to move about in the region of sparsely populated pubic hair. The disease is seen almost exclusively in men and women who are sexually active. Two to 5% of patients at sexually transmitted disease clinics have been reported to be infected with this organism.[18, 19] General population statistics are not known since this is not a reportable entity. Of considerable importance is the fact that other venereal diseases commonly accompany pediculosis pubis. One survey reported that one third of patients with pediculosis pubis had a second venereal disease.[20]

The disease is usually self-diagnosed because of the pruritus in the genital area and a sensation of insects' crawling over the skin. There are usually many organisms and nits present, and because of the sparsity of the pubic hair they are often easy to see (Fig. 128–2). In men with heavier body hair the infestation may extend in a broad area outside the pubic region, including the axillae and fringes of the scalp hair. Because of the ease of self-diagnosis, pediculosis pubis is not commonly seen in a dermatologist's office. Although symptoms of chronic scratching and multiple bites can produce pyoderma with underlying lymphadenopathy, this situation is usually not as common as is seen in head lice.

In children who have been exposed to adults with pubic lice, the organisms will frequently take up residence in the eyelashes if the patient lacks appropriate pubic hair (Fig. 128–3). In this situation the child will complain of itching and discharge from the eyes and without a close examination may be diagnosed as having blepharitis.

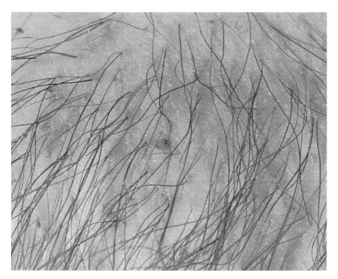

FIGURE 128–2. Pubic lice and nits.

Another clue to the diagnosis, although it is uncommonly seen, is the presence of blue macules (maculae ceruleae) on the lower abdomen, thighs, and lateral aspects of the trunk. These represent minute hemorrhages caused by the bite of the crab louse when it is foraging far from the pubic hair.

Pubic lice are not known to transmit any serious diseases, although impetigo normally accompanies their infestation.

PATHOLOGY

Although I am not aware of any published reports of the pathology of infestation with *P. pubis*, I presume it is similar to that of the head louse. The maculae ceruleae represent very scant hemorrhage in the upper dermis.

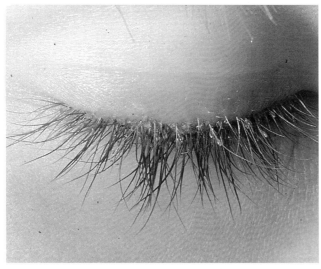

FIGURE 128–3. Lice on eyelashes.

PATHOGENESIS AND ETIOLOGY

This infestation is usually transmitted through sexual activities and is frequently accompanied by other diseases, such as gonorrhea, scabies, herpes, and trichomoniasis, and in certain populations by infection with the human immunodeficiency virus.[20, 21] In addition to direct physical contact the louse can also be transmitted by fomites such as bedding, sleeping bags, and articles of clothing. Other than impetigo no diseases are known to be transmitted by the louse itself.

DIAGNOSIS AND DIFFERENTIAL DIAGNOSIS

The diagnosis is usually made by the patient. Itching in the groin and a sensation of something crawling in the pubic area usually alerts all but the most naive patients to their predicament. With an index of suspicion the diagnosis can easily be confirmed by seeing the pubic lice, which often remain motionless during an examination. Nits always outnumber adults, and consequently a hair from a patient suspected of having this problem can be plucked and examined under a microscope.

The differential diagnosis (Table 128–4) is similar to that for head lice. Lint, scale, and pus may collect around hairs, giving the casual appearance of a nit. Trichorrhexis nodosa can be induced by scratching. White piedra is rare in North America, is not symptomatic, and does not usually occur in the groin.

Other pruritic conditions of the groin include tinea cruris, candidiasis, and simple intertrigo. These can all be distinguished on the basis of their morphology and lack of involvement of the hair-bearing areas in the pubic region.

TREATMENT

The choice of agents is similar to that listed in the section for head lice (Table 128–5): over-the-counter pyrethrins, synthetic pyrethroids (1% permethrin [Nix]), and lindane (Kwell) shampoo or lotion. Less commonly used are crotamiton 10% (Eurax), benzyl benzoate (only approved for veterinary use), and malathion (not currently marketed in the United States).

Published trials indicate that none of these agents works reliably with a single application.[22, 23] Although studies in the early 1980s indicated a single application of lindane or pyrethrin product was 100% effective,[23] more recent reports comparing lindane with permethrin

TABLE 128–4. Differential Diagnosis of Pediculosis Pubis	
Nits	**Itching**
Lint	Lichen simplex chronicus
Scale	Allergic eczematous dermatitis
Trichorrhexis nodosa	Candidiasis
White piedra	Scabies

TABLE 128-5. Treatment of Pediculosis Pubis
Pyrethrins (RID, A-200, others)*
Permethrin (Nix)
Lindane (Kwell)†
2%–6% Sulfur
Crotamiton
Malathion

*Available without prescription.
†Available only by prescription.

showed 60% to 65% cure rate for each agent.[22] Consequently, I believe it prudent to treat all body surface areas from the neck to the toes with a single application, followed by a second after a period of 7 to 10 days. Removal of nits with nit combs is also advisable.

In some young persons infestation of the scalp has been documented, and I have seen a case in the beard. The treatment of choice for eyelash lice (usually pubic, but may be head lice) is to treat the eyelashes with petrolatum three times a day for 3 days. Other treatments include fluorescein,[24] yellow oxide of mercury, and physostigmine.[25] Of course the source of these eyelash lice should be identified and eliminated.

Scabies

DEFINITION

Scabies is infestation with the human itch mite *Sarcoptes scabiei*. The correct biological name is *Sarcoptes scabiei* var. *hominis*. When this mite was discovered in the 17th century, it became the first infectious disease of humans with a known cause.[26] "Scabies" may have originally referred to the scabs from scratching and infection.

CLINICAL DESCRIPTION

Infestation with the human itch mite is fairly common in the United States. Although public health statistics are not kept, it is not uncommon for a dermatologist to see several cases a month. When an initial case is found, many family members with close physical contact may also be infected. Physicians may also have the unfortunate opportunity to encounter scabies first hand when a patient is admitted with an incorrect diagnosis of psoriasis, eczema, or some other itchy disease, with subsequent infection of many members of the health care team.

The adult female mite measures 0.4×0.3 mm, and the adult male is approximately half this size.[27] Fertilization takes place on the surface of the skin, and the male subsequently dies. The fertilized female burrows into the stratum corneum at the rate of 2 to 4 mm per day, laying 2 to 3 eggs per day for a total 10 to 25 eggs. The six-legged larvae emerge after 3 to 4 days, going through several moltings and maturing in approximately 2 weeks.

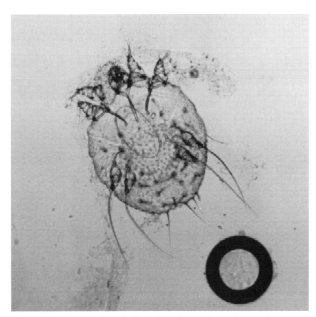

FIGURE 128-4. Female mite with egg ($\times 100$).

The adult female is an oval, whitish arthropod with four pairs of legs. These legs are quite stubby in comparison with the body size, and the posterior pairs have long spines protruding from them (Fig. 128–4).

The clinical manifestations begin some weeks after infestation, in part because it takes the host this long to become sensitized to the mite's excreta and saliva.[28] It also takes the mites a significant period of time to reach a noticeable population. The chief clinical symptom is notorious pruritus, which can occur on any part of the body but most occurs commonly on the hands, waist, and genital area. It is reported that this itching is worse at night, but this is not much help in the diagnosis. Almost all diseases itch more at night when there is less distraction.

Repeated scratching produces widespread weeping eczematous patches that are frequently secondarily infected with *Staphylococcus*. In addition, because of persistent mite parts and host immunologic responses, red-brown hyperkeratotic scaling nodules commonly develop near the axilla, on the genitalia, and on the trunk (Fig. 128–5).

The distribution of these lesions depends on the age and immunologic status of the patient. In infants, lesions may be distributed on all body parts, but in patients older than age 3 or 4 years lesions are usually confined from the neck to the toes. Patients with immunologic suppression such as in the acquired immunodeficiency syndrome may have lesions over the entire body.

Many variations of this pattern have been noted[29]: scabies in the clean, crusted (Norwegian) scabies,[30] scabies incognito (findings obscured by corticosteroid use), and scabies in adopted foreign children. Patients who have very good hygiene usually have only a few lesions, particularly around the hands and genitalia. Patients who are immunologically suppressed or who have a variety of neurologic disorders such as Down syndrome or severe depression often develop tremendous numbers of mites

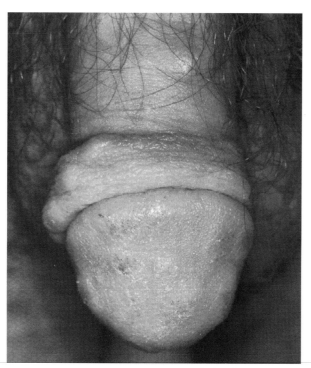

FIGURE 128-5. Nodules on the genitalia of an adult.

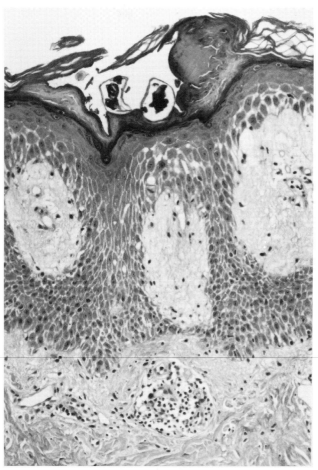

FIGURE 128-7. Scabies. Biopsy specimen reveals mites within a burrow in the cornified layer. Lesions show variable degrees of epidermal hyperplasia, hyperkeratosis, and inflammation depending in part on the immune status of the patient.

that live in a honeycomb of crust, serum, and debris. These crusted lesions may simulate psoriasis, lichenified eczema, and hyperkeratosis palmaris et plantaris.

In another variant the lesions may become bullous and have actually been mistaken for pemphigoid and dermatitis herpetiformis (Fig. 128-6).[31] It is not certain whether these bullae are a result of the scabies or of secondary bacterial infection with *S. aureus*.

PATHOLOGY

The pathology of scabies is usually diagnostic (Fig. 128-7).[32] In a classic case, mites will be found from the stratum corneum throughout the upper layers of the

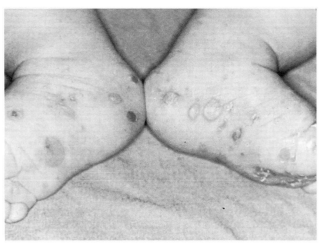

FIGURE 128-6. Bullous scabies in an infant.

epidermis in their burrows usually sliced in some tangential or oblique section. The burrows are often diamond shaped, and fortuitous sections may include the feces (scybala) of the mite or its body. The accompanying inflammatory response usually features superficial and deep perivascular and interstitial collections of lymphocytes, histiocytes, eosinophils, and plasma cells. In some immunosuppressed patients, inflammatory cells are few. In some crusted or nodular lesions mites may not be seen, and in this situation pathologic findings resemble those of a chronic insect bite, with a predominance of plasma cells and eosinophils. Serial sections sometimes reveal parts of mites, implying that scabietic nodules are due to persistent scabietic antigens.[33] It is normally not necessary to biopsy a lesion to establish the diagnosis, however.

PATHOGENESIS AND ETIOLOGY

The disease is caused only by the human itch mite *Sarcoptes scabiei* var. *hominis*. It is spread primarily by person-to-person contact, with fomites playing a lesser role. The mite is relatively immobile at room temperature and cannot survive for long off the host. Mellanby[28] inoculated mites into volunteers and noted that while the organisms lived and reproduced, symptoms did not become apparent for approximately a month. Reinfestation, however, in a patient previously cured of scabies produced symptoms within 1 to 2 days. This suggests an immunologic factor such as cell-mediated immunity. Other authors have noted the presence of IgM, IgA, and C3 in the cornified layer of the epidermis, at the dermoepidermal junction, and in the papillary vessels.[34-37] An alternative explanation for the presence of immunoreactants in scabies is that damage to the epidermis from scratching exposes antigens, which then elicit antibodies.[31]

There are numerous case reports and epidemics of canine scabies occurring in humans.[38, 39] *Sarcoptes scabiei* var. *canis* has produced epidemics in children and adults in contact with heavily infested dogs and other pets. In this situation, mites do not reproduce on human skin and lesions are found mostly at points of contact, such as the abdomen, arms, and anterior thighs.

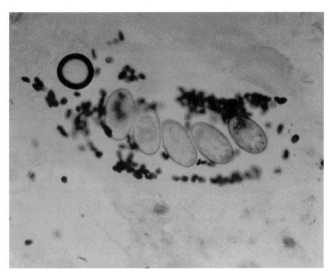

FIGURE 128–8. Eggs and scybala (× 100).

DIAGNOSIS AND DIFFERENTIAL DIAGNOSIS

The only way to make a diagnosis of scabies is to suspect it in every patient who presents to the physician's office with a complaint of itching. If no obvious cause for the itching is found, then a diligent search should be made for the signs of scabies. The most diagnostic lesions are the burrows (see Fig. 128–7). It is often stated that burrows are not seen in a majority of patients with scabies. While this is true, it reflects the inadequacy of the observer because burrows are actually present in nearly all patients with scabies. Burrows are small, crooked lines 4 to 6 mm in length that are most common in the web spaces of the fingers, sides of the hands, flexor surfaces of the wrist, and (especially in the children) the lateral and medial surfaces of the foot nearest the heel. Mellanby[28] has shown that the number of mites an individual harbors is far fewer than the number of clinical lesions the patient has. Therefore, randomly scraping excoriated papules over the trunk, back, and genitalia usually produces negative results.

The best technique used to demonstrate the mite is to first identify a burrow with good light and magnification. The mite is at the limit of human vision so good magnification is essential. It is also important to remember that older patients cooperate much better with the scraping than younger patients do; that is, if parents and children have the disease, scrape the skin of the parent first. After a burrow is identified the lesion should be moistened with alcohol, water, or mineral oil. (I prefer not to use mineral oil.) The burrow is then scraped vigorously until it is deroofed. This may produce bleeding, but it is not necessary to make a patient bleed to make a positive diagnosis on potassium hydroxide examination. Material from as many burrows as can be found should be scraped. If burrows are not found, scaling papules on the hands can be scraped. After each scraping the material is transferred to a slide, which is then covered with potassium hydroxide (or mineral oil if it was used). Scanning

should be done under low power since with higher magnification the mite will fill up half or more of the field. Diagnostic findings are of the mite itself (see Fig. 128–4), one of the graceful spined legs, eggs, egg cases, or the golden-brown fecal pellets (scybala) (Fig. 128–8).[40, 41] In some situations the scraping may be negative, and in this case treatment should be instituted without proof of the existence of the mite. The ink burrow test may help identify infected patients.[42]

The differential diagnosis (Table 128–6) consists of other pruritic diseases such as atopic dermatitis, insect bites, nummular eczema, psoriasis, prurigo nodularis, and delusions of parasitosis. None of these diseases features manifestations in common sites such as the genitalia, webbed spaces, and axillary folds. Also, the history of the disease spreading from family member to family member is very suggestive of scabies and not any of the other choices.

TREATMENT

Treatment is divided into four areas: (1) eradication of the mites on the patient; (2) treatment of associated problems such as pruritus, scabietic nodules, and impe-

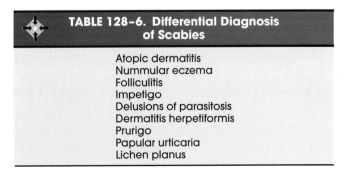

✛ TABLE 128–6. Differential Diagnosis of Scabies
Atopic dermatitis
Nummular eczema
Folliculitis
Impetigo
Delusions of parasitosis
Dermatitis herpetiformis
Prurigo
Papular urticaria
Lichen planus

tigo; (3) treatment of personal contacts; and (4) destruction of the mite in the patient's surroundings.

Permethrin 5% (Elimite) and lindane (Kwell) are the mainstays of therapy.[43, 44] I do not believe that either of these agents is 100% effective with a single application. Consequently, I encourage all patients to treat themselves from their neck to their toes, with particular attention to the crusted areas and around the fingernails. Applications should remain on 8 to 12 hours and then rinsed off. Applications for less than 2 hours are not as effective.[44] This treatment should be repeated in a week in all patients who have itching and visible lesions. Exposed but asymptomatic patients should be treated only once. Intermediate-potency topical steroids help decrease pruritus and should be used in most cases after the first application of a scabicide.

Patients should be told that while this will produce a gradual decrease in itching, the itching may continue for a period of weeks and occasionally months but that this rarely indicates the presence of active scabies. Post-scabietic nodules should be treated with intermediate- to high-potency topical steroids and may require intralesional corticosteroid injections.

Used properly, both permethrin and lindane are safe, but lindane has the greatest potential for adverse reaction if it is misused (e.g., used on a daily basis, used two or three times a day).[45, 46] Toxicity from lindane poisoning usually takes the form of seizures. Consequently, patients who are prone to seizures should not be treated with this agent. Neither of these agents is proven safe in the treatment of pregnant women, but there have been no reported adverse fetal effects in widespread laboratory investigation and in clinical use.

Alternate scabicides are crotamiton 10%[47] and 6% to 10% sulfur ointments.[48] These have considerably less efficacy than the previously mentioned agents and must be applied on a daily basis for 5 to 10 days. There are no data suggesting that these agents are any safer.

It is not uncommon for children to continue to develop small vesicles and pustules on the sides of the hands and feet without burrows that are repeatedly negative on scraping and do not respond to further applications of lindane or permethrin.[49] This has been termed the *post-scabietic syndrome* and it appears similar if not identical to infantile acropustulosis. Scabies in the United States is rarely reported in black patients, whereas infantile acropustulosis is more commonly reported in blacks.

Since the scabies mite is not very mobile, it is not necessary to fumigate the entire house. Routine cleaning of the bedding, clothes, and personal articles using hot water washing cycles is probably all that is required.

The treatment of animal scabies should be left to an experienced veterinarian since the agents commonly used in humans will be licked off by pets, producing toxicity.

Crusted scabies that does not respond to repeated applications of topical medications may occasionally be treated with oral methotrexate or thiabendazole. Hyperkeratotic lesions may be treated with keratolytics, and it may be important to use a brisk scrub brush for the fingernail area.

References

1. Pediculosis pubis poster, circa World War I. Courtesy Gerard Tilles, M.D., Hopital Saint Louis, Paris, France. Int J Dermatol 1992;32:300.
2. Maunder J. Parasites and man: Human lice—biology and control. R Soc Health J 1977;97:29–32.
3. Burnett J. Rickettsioses: A review for the dermatologist. J Am Acad Dermatol 1980, 2:359–373.
4. Rasmussen J. Pediculosis and the pediatrician. Pediatr Dermatol 1984;2:74–79.
5. Janniger C, Kuflik A. Pediculosis capitis. Pediatr Dermatol 1993;51:407–408.
6. Gronzick J, Voorhees J, Coleman, et al. A multicenter comparison of head lice treatments. Am J Public Health 1992;82:857–861.
7. Ackerman A. Histologic Diagnosis of Inflammatory Skin Diseases: A Method by Pattern Analysis. Philadelphia: Lea & Febiger, 1978: 294–302.
8. Brandenburg R, Deinard A, DiNapoli J, et al. 1% Permethrin cream rinse vs 1% lindane shampoo in treating pediculosis capitis. Am J Dis Child 1986;140:894–896.
9. Carson D, Tribble P, Weart C. Pyrethrins combined with piperonyl butoxide (RID) vs 1% permethrin (Nix) in the treatment of head lice. Am J Dis Child 1988;142:768–769.
10. Bowerman J, Gomez M, Austin R, et al. Comparative study of permethrin 1% creme rinse and lindane shampoo for the treatment of head lice. Pediatr Infect Dis J 1987;6:252–255.
11. Taplin D, Meinking T, Castillero P, et al. Permethrin 1% creme rinse for the treatment of *Pediculus humanus* var *capitis* infestation. Pediatr Dermatol 1986;3:344–348.
12. Taplin D, Castillero P, Spiegel J, et al. Malathion for treatment of *Pediculus humanus* var *capitis* infestation. JAMA 1982;247: 3103–3105.
13. Brinck-Lindroth G, Lundqvist L, Nilsson A. Control of the human head louse with disulfiram and benzyl benzoate emusions. Acta Derm Venereol 1984;64:325–330.
14. Kucirka S, Parish L, Witkowski J. The story of lindane resistance and head lice. Int J Dermatol 1983;22:551–555.
15. Parish L, Witkowski J, Kucirka A. Lindane resistance and pediculosis capitis. Int J Dermatol 1983;22:572–574.
16. DeFelice J, Rumsfield J, Bernstein J, et al. Clinical evaluation of an after-pediculicide nit removal system. Int J Dermatol 1989; 28:468–470.
17. Burns D, Sims T. A closer look at *Phthirus pubis*. Br J Dermatol 1988;118:497–503.
18. Centers for Disease Control. Non-reported sexually transmitted diseases: United States. MMWR 1979;28:61–63.
19. Judson F, Penley K, Robinson M, et al. Comparative prevalence rates of sexually transmitted disease in heterosexual and homosexual men. Am J Epidermiol 1980;112:836–843.
20. Chapel T, Katta T, Kuszmar T, et al. Pediculosis pubis in a clinic for treatment for sexually transmitted disease. Sex Transm Dis 1979;257–260.
21. Orkin M, Maibach H. Current views of scabies and pediculosis pubis. Cutis 1984;33:85–96.
22. Kalter, D, Sperber J, Rosen T, et al. Treatment of pediculosis pubis. Arch Dermatol 1987;123:1315–1319.
23. Smith D, Walsh J. Treatment of pubic lice infestation: A comparison of two agents. Cutis 1980;26:618–619.
24. Mathew M, D'Souza P, Mehta D. A new treatment of pthiriasis palpebrarum. Ann Ophthalmol 1982;68:439–441.
25. Couch J, Green W, Hirst L, et al. Diagnosing and treating *Phthirus pubis* palpebrarum. Surv Ophthalmol 1982;26:219–225.
26. Parish LC. History of scabies. In: Orkin M, Maibach H, Parish LC, Schwartzman RM, eds. Scabies and Pediculosis. Philadelphia: JB Lippincott, 1977:1–7.
27. Mellanby K. Biology of the parasite. In: Orkin M, Maibach H, Parish LC, Schwartzman RM, eds. Scaabies and Pediculosis. Philadelphia: JB Lippincott, 1977:8–16.
28. Mellanby K. The development of symptoms, parasitic infection and immunity in human scabies. Parasitology 1944;35:197–206.
29. Orkin M. Special forms of scabies. In: Orkin M, Maibach H, Parish LC, Schwartzman RM, eds. Scabies and Pediculosis. Philadelphia: JB Lippincott, 1977:23–28.
30. Epsy PD, Jolly HW Jr. Norwegian scabies. Arch Dermatol 1976;112:193–196.

31. Bhawan J, Milstone E, Malhotra R, et al. Scabies presenting as bullous pemphigoid–like eruption. J Am Acad Dermatol 1991; 24:179–181.
32. Ackerman AB. Histopathology of human scabies. In: Orkin M, Maibach H, Parish LC, Schwartzman RM, eds. Scabies and Pediculosis. Philadelphia: JB Lippincott, 1977:88–95.
33. Liu H-N, Sheu W-J, Chu T-L. Scabietic nodules: A dermatopathologic and immunofluorescent study. J Cutan Pathol 1992; 19:124–127.
34. Van Neste D. Immunologic studies in scabies. Int J Dermatol 1981;20:264–269.
35. Ratanen T, Bjorksten F, Reunala T, et al. Serum IgE antibodies to scabies mite. Acta Derm Venereol 61:358–360.
36. Hoefling KK, Schroeter AL. Dermatoimmunopathology of scabies. J Am Acad Dermatol 1980;3:237–240.
37. Dahl MV. The immunology of scabies. Ann Allergy 1983; 51:560–566.
38. Charlesworth EN, Johnson JL. An epidemic of canine scabies in man. Arch Dermatol 1974;110:572–574.
39. Arlian LG, Runyan RA, Estes SA. Cross-infestivity of *Sarcoptes scabies*. J Am Acad Dermatol 1984;10:979–986.
40. Muller GH. Laboratory diagnosis of scabies. In: Orkin M, Maibach H, Parish LC, Schwartzman RM, eds. Scabies and Pediculosis. Philadelphia: JB Lippincott, 1977:99–104.
41. Eaglstein WH, Pariser DM. Ectoparasite demonstration. In: Office Techniques for Diagnosing Skin Disease. Chicago: Year Book Medical Publishers, 1978:45–48.
42. Woodley D, Saurat JH. The burrow ink test and the scabies mite. J Am Acad Dermatol 1981;4:715–722.
43. Taplin D, Meinking TL, Chen JA, et al. Comparison of crotamiton 10% cream (Eurax) and permethrin 5% cream (Elimite) for the treatment of scabies in children. Pediatr Dermatol 1990;7:67–73.
44. Taplin D, Rivera A, Walker JG. A comparative trial of three treatment schedules for the eradication of scabies. J Am Acad Dermatol 1983;9:550–554.
45. Ginsburg CM, Lowry W, Reisch JS. Absorption of lindane (gamma benzene hexachloride) in infants and children. J Pediatr 1977;91:998–1000.
46. Rasmussen JE. The problem of lindane. J Am Acad Dermatol 1981;5:507–516.
47. Konstantinov D, Stanoeva L. Crotamiton cream and lotion in the treatment of infants and young children with scabies. J Int Med Res 1979;7:4438.
48. Hurwitz S. Scabies in infants and children. In: Orkin M, Maibach H, Parish LC, Schwartzman RM, eds. Scabies and Pediculosis. Philadelphia: JB Lippincott, 1977:31–38.
49. Bjornbert A. Recidiverande pustulo hos adoptivbarn fran syd-och Ostabsien. Lakartidningen 1975;72:5142.

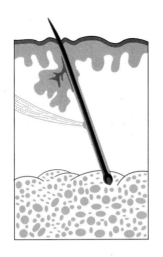

What Diseases Alter Skin Color?

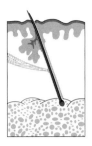

chapter 129

Biology of Melanocytes

RAYMOND E. BOISSY and JAMES J. NORDLUND

The melanocyte comprises approximately 5% of the cellular component of the interfollicular epidermis and an equal component of the hair bulb. In spite of a limited number of melanocytes, the major synthetic product of this cell, pigment, is the primary determinant of the coloration for the skin and hair. The type and amount of pigment produced by the melanocyte varies considerably in humans, accounting for racial and ethnic skin differences and all hair color differences. In addition, the capacity of the melanocyte to up-regulate or down-regulate the production of pigment in response to physiologic, environmental, or pathologic stimuli varies considerably. The major role of melanin, primarily deposited in the keratinocytes of the interfollicular epidermis, is to absorb incident ultraviolet light and protect the genome of the dividing basal keratinocytes and melanocytes. In addition, melanin has been shown to be an effective free oxygen radical scavenger, and thus one could speculate that its transfer to the keratinocytes of the skin protects these metabolically active cells from the damaging effects of an abundant amount of oxygen radicals that are generated.

In addition to its role of providing pigment for the skin and hair, the role of the melanocyte in contributing to epidermal homeostasis especially during an inflammatory process has also been suggested. Data demonstrating the production of many cytokines and lymphokines by these cells have been investigated.[1, 2] The embryologic development, histologic aspects, the current status on the cell biology of the melanocyte, and the biochemistry of melanin synthesis are discussed in this chapter.

EMBRYOLOGIC ORIGIN

In the 1930s and 1940s, elegant embryonic neural tube transplantation studies in amphibians, birds, and mammals demonstrated that the cutaneous melanocyte population originates from the neural tube.[3-5] A group of cells within the forming neural tube emigrate dorsally from the lateral ridges of the neural plate as the ridges join during the closure of the neural tube (Fig. 129-1). This group of cells forms a defined population called the neural crest cells.[6] These cells are the precursors of a multitude of cell and tissue types, which include most of the neurons of the peripheral nervous system, glial and Schwann cells, skeletal and connective tissue elements of the head and face, cells of the aorticopulmonary septum of the heart, chromaffin cells of the adrenal medulla, as well as virtually all the melanocytes of the skin, uveal tract, ear, and leptomeninges.[7-11] In contrast, the ocular layer of melanocytes of the retinal pigment epithelium arises from an outgrowth of the primitive forebrain (i.e., neural endoderm) as it invaginates to form the outer wall of the eye cup.[12]

Melanoblasts travel from the neural crest to their target site in the skin by a route that is not clearly defined, owing to the lack of specific markers for this early stage of melanocyte differentiation.[13] However, when neural crest cell migration is analyzed using an antibody against an early differentiation marker expressed by all neural crest cells (i.e., *HNK-1*),[14, 15] a small population of HNK-1 positive cells migrate dorsolaterally through the mesenchyme beneath the developing ectoderm.[16] These are thought to be melanoblasts, as opposed to the majority of the HNK-1–positive neural crest cells that migrate ventrolaterally along the dermatome or ventrally along the side of the neural tube and somites.[17] The dorsally migrating group of HNK-1–positive cells (presumptive melanoblasts) migrate through the mesenchyme to the dermis.

It was originally speculated that melanocytes migrate from the dermis into the developing epidermis at about 11 weeks of gestation.[18] Once they enter the epidermis the melanoblasts are initially localized suprabasally, and only after a few weeks do they settle on the basal lamina beneath the basal epithelial layer of the epidermis.[19, 20] Late-stage melanoblasts had originally been identified either by their preferential staining for reduced silver (i.e., for melanin), histochemical reaction after DOPA

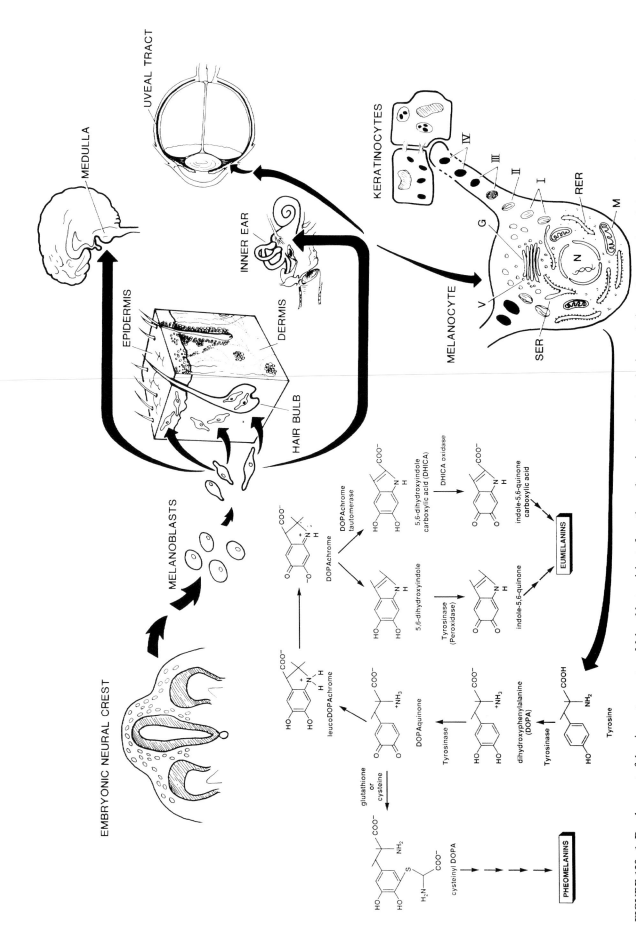

FIGURE 129-1. Development of the pigmentary system. Melanoblasts originate from the embryonic neural crest and migrate during embryogenesis to their target sites in the skin, eye, ear, and brain. The melanocytes in the skin synthesize melanosomes, which are transferred to keratinocytes of the interfollicular epidermis and the hair. The biochemical synthesis of melanins begins with the amino acid substrate tyrosine and progresses through many regulated and spontaneous steps. N, nucleus; RER, rough endoplasmic reticulum; SER, smooth endoplasmic reticulum; G, Golgi apparatus; V, vesicles; M, mitochondria; I–IV, numerical stages of melanosomes.

incubation (i.e., for tyrosinase), or ultrastructural appearance of melanosomes (i.e., a specific organelle). These techniques revealed melanoblasts immediately after they had been committed to synthesizing melanin precursors, the tyrosinase enzyme, or melanosomes and immediately before the synthesis of visible melanin. A monoclonal antibody, HMB-45, has been developed that recognizes melanoblasts at an earlier stage. This antibody was originally made against an extract of melanoma and was shown to recognize a cytoplasmic product of melanoma cells, junctional nevi, and fetal and neonatal melanocytes but not adult melanocytes.[21] The use of this antibody in immunolocalization studies on developing fetal skin has demonstrated that melanoblasts appear in the epidermis as early as approximately 7 weeks of gestation.[22] The initial population density is 50% of the density at birth, and the cells are distributed in a nonrandom pattern.[22] Melanin synthesis becomes microscopically apparent by 15 to 16 weeks of gestation, and melanosomal transfer appears to begin at around 20 weeks.[23] The melanocytes of the hair follicle appear to originate from the epidermal melanoblast population by traveling along with the epithelial cells that grow down into the dermis to form the hair germ.[19, 24]

Regulation of embryonic cell migration and differentiation for any cell system including melanocytes is an extremely complex and poorly described process. However, analysis of mutations affecting the ability of melanoblasts to successfully reach their target site and complete their differentiation has provided some molecular clues to this process. The c-kit proto-oncogene, which encodes a tyrosine kinase cell surface receptor,[25, 26] and its corresponding ligand, steel factor (also known as hematopoietic growth factor or murine stem cell factor,[27-30] form an important molecular signal system that appears essential for the development of the melanocyte as well as possibly other cell types. Mutations affecting the function of the c-kit receptor or its ligand result in altered melanoblast migration or development and the subsequent appearance of white hair and skin as exemplified by the dominant spotting (W) white and the steel (Sl) mouse models, respectively.[31] Mice expressing genomic mutations in either the dominant spotting/c-kit locus or the steel locus also develop defects in erythropoiesis and gametogenesis.[31] In some humans, the congenital depigmentation known as piebaldism represents the human homologue to mutations in the kit gene.[32-35] The functional role of this specific receptor/ligand system in the embryonic migration and/or development of melanoblasts and melanocytes remains to be defined.

Two other genes in which mutations appear to affect embryonic melanocyte development have been cloned. The mouse gene, microphthalmia (mi), consists of over one dozen alleles, which variably affect the successful migration of melanoblasts to their target sites of the skin, hair, and/or eye.[31, 36] In addition, defects within mast cells,[37] osteoclasts,[38, 39] and retinal cells[40-43] are associated with some of the microphthalmia alleles. Deduction of the putative gene product suggests that it is a novel basic helixloop–helix-zipper protein and a member of a family of transcription factors.[44, 45] The human homology of the mouse microphthalmia gene, MITF, has recently been cloned and assigned to chromosome 3.

The mutations in the pax gene, associated with the Splotch (Sp) locus in mice[46, 47] and in the pax3 human homologue associated with Waardenburg's syndrome,[48] result in congenital depigmentation and abnormalities in neural development. As in microphthalmia, mutations at this gene prevent the successful migration and differentiation of melanoblasts during embryogenesis. The gene product of pax belongs to a paired domain family of DNA binding proteins.[49, 50] How the mi and pax gene products function in the embryonic development of the melanocyte system, as well as possibly other systems, remains to be determined.

MELANOCYTE HISTOLOGY

Once the melanocytes set up residency in the basal epithelial layer of the interfollicular epidermis, they appear to remain there for the life of the individual at a density range of 1000 to 1500/mm².[51] It is thought that melanocytes rarely proliferate or die under normal conditions. However, melanocytes can be induced to proliferate by stimuli such as ultraviolet light or during an inflammatory process. Also, melanocytes decrease in number with age and there is a decrease in number of melanocytes per surface area with age over approximately 50.[52] Melanocytes in the hair bulb dramatically differ in that they are not static in their behavior.[51] When the hair follicle begins to enter catagen, the melanocyte halts melanin synthesis and disappears until early anagen, at which point melanin synthesis is reinitiated. It is uncertain whether during this period the melanocyte dedifferentiates and undergoes subsequent reactivation or dies and is replaced by cells from a stem reservoir of melanoblasts.

The interfollicular melanocytes reside on the basement membrane at the dermoepidermal junction. However, unlike the basal keratinocytes or Merkel cells, the melanocyte is not riveted to the basement by hemidesmosomal complexes. It is uncertain how the melanocyte remains adherent to the basal lamina as the keratinocyte population streams dorsally. Whether adhesive-like molecules facilitate the maintenance of the melanocyte on the basement membranes is being addressed. It has been demonstrated that the extracellular matrix components, laminin and fibronectin, are expressed on the cell surface of cultured human melanocytes. In addition, these molecules appear to affect the adhesion and motility of cultured melanocytes.[53]

There is approximately one melanocyte per 36 keratinocytes[54] in all races and ethnic groups[55] in what is termed the *epidermal melanin unit*. Numerous dendrites of the melanocyte interweave among the keratinocytes. Melanosomes (i.e., pigment granules) are transferred to the keratinocytes, presumably through these dendrites, by phagocytosis of dendritic tips by the keratinocytes (see Fig. 129–1).[56-58] The outcome of pigment transfer from the melanocyte to the keratinocytes differs dramatically between races. Melanosomes within the cytoplasm of the keratinocytes of black skin exist individually, whereas in white skin these melanosomes are clustered into groups of four to eight and are membrane bound.[59] It is this keratinocyte distribution difference and its effect on light absorption and reflection that account for most of the dramatic skin coloration difference between black and white skin.[60] However, differences in size of the melanosome and in the amount and type of melanin produced by melanocytes of various races also appear to play a role in complexion differences.[61] The amount of melanin and of tyrosinase activity correlates clearly with skin color.[62] However, protein and mRNA transcript levels for tyrosinase appear to be equally abundant in melanocytes cultured from black and white races.[63] These data suggest that post-translational regulation of preexisting enzyme controls the extent of tyrosinase activity and melanin synthesis.

MELANOCYTE BIOLOGY

The process of melanosome/melanin synthesis has been called a bipartite system. The structural framework onto which melanin is eventually deposited (i.e., the melanosome) is synthesized independently from the enzymes responsible for melanin synthesis (i.e., predominantly tyrosinase) (Fig. 129–2; see also Fig. 129–1). The premelanosome, which contains a uniquely organized matrix of melanofilaments, is believed to originate from the smooth endoplasmic reticulum.[64] A melanosomal matrix glycoprotein has been identified.[65] The biosynthetic processing of this glycoprotein is not affected by enzymes housed in the Golgi apparatus, which is consistent with the hypothesis that the premelanosome is generated from the smooth endoplasmic reticulum. In contrast, tyrosinase, and probably other enzymes involved in

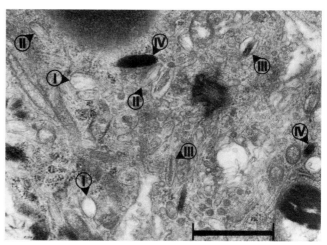

FIGURE 129–3. Electron micrograph of melanosomes. Melanosomes are categorized into four transitional stages: stage I, premelanosome; stage II, unpigmented melanosome; stage III, minimally pigmented melanosome; and stage IV, completely melanized melanosome; bar = 1.0 μm.

melanin synthesis, are translated at the rough endoplasmic reticulum and shuttled to the Golgi apparatus for final maturation.[66, 67] Eventually the mature, functional form of tyrosinase leaves the trans-Golgi network through coated vesicles and is translocated to the neighboring premelanosomes.[68] At this stage, melanin synthesis and melanosome maturation can proceed to completion (Fig. 129–3).[69] New data suggest that initiation of melanin synthesis (i.e., the hydroxylation of tyrosine and dihydroxylation of DOPA) occurs within the coated vesicles before their convergence with the premelanosome.[70]

For many years, the biochemistry of melanin synthesis was considered to be relatively simple. The initial catalytic enzyme in this process is tyrosinase, which is an approximately 75-kd molecule[71] coded for by its gene on human chromosome 11 (q14→q21).[72] Tyrosinase hydroxylates the amino acid substrate tyrosine to DOPA, then converts DOPA to DOPAquinone (see Fig. 129–1). Formerly, the remaining molecular alterations in the elaborate and somewhat undefined pathway to melanin were thought to be spontaneous.[73] However, data from numerous investigators for the past decade or more have demonstrated that the post-DOPAquinone steps are enzymatically regulated by tyrosinase in addition to other enzymes and cofactors such as metal cations, which are involved in modulation (see Fig. 129–1). DOPAquinone appears to spontaneously progress to leucaDOPAchrome and then DOPAchrome. At this stage a diversion can occur. In the presence of a newly identified melanocyte-specific enzyme, DOPAchrome tautomerase (also called tyrosinase-related protein 2 [TRP-2])[74–76] and/or divalent metal cations,[77] DOPAchrome is converted to dihydroxyindole carboxylic acid (DHICA), which in turn is enzymatically oxidized by a DHICA oxidase to indole-5,6-quinone-carboxylic acid before progressing to form eumelanins.[78] DOPAchrome tautomerase is a 75 to 80-kd molecule.[79, 80] In contrast, without the catalytic contribution of DOPAchrome tautomerase, DOPAchrome can spontaneously oxidize to 5,6-dihydroxyindole, which in turn is converted to indole-5,6-quinone,

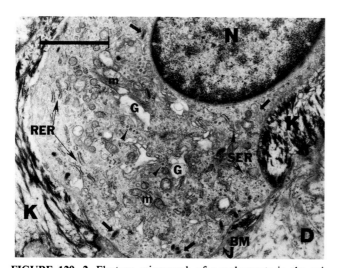

FIGURE 129–2. Electron micrograph of a melanocyte in the epidermis. The melanocyte resides among keratinocytes (K) in the basal layer of the epidermis. It rests on the basement membrane (BM) of the dermoepidermal junction (D). The cytoplasm contains organelles involved in the synthesis of pigment granules/melanosomes (*arrows*), RER, rough endoplasmic reticulum; SER, smooth endoplasmic reticulum; G, Golgi apparatus; arrowheads indicate coated vesicles emigrating from the trans-Golgi network; N, nucleus of the melanocyte; m, mitochondria; bar = 2.0 μm.

putatively by the catalytic activity of tyrosinase[81] or peroxidase.[82] The molecule progresses to form eumelanins in the absence of a stablin/inhibitor.[83] Hence, there are now more regulatory steps and respective genes and gene products known to be involved in the synthesis of melanin.

The previous discussion on the biochemical synthesis of melanins pertains particularly to the synthesis of what is classified as eumelanins. Eumelanins are the black and brown polymers. There is a second group of pigments called pheomelanins that are the yellow and red polymers predominantly apparent in hair. The synthesis of pheomelanins is initiated by the same mechanism as eumelanins up to the production of DOPAquinone (see Fig. 129–1). At this point, a high intracellular or intramelanosomal concentration of glutathione or cysteine, provided by glutamyl transpeptidase/glutathione reductase, will divert DOPAquinone to cysteinyl DOPA.[84–86] This alternate pathway proceeds by largely unknown mechanisms to the pheomelanins contributing to the red and yellow coloration of hair. Whether a single melanocyte is programmed to synthesize either eumelanin or pheomelanin in contrast to its ability to synthesize both types of melanin or mixed melanins[87] is not known.[88] Of interest is the agouti pattern of hair pigmentation, found on many mammalian species, which exhibits a terminal or sub-terminal band of yellow pheomelanin on an otherwise black or brown eumelanin hair shaft.[88a] The product of the murine agouti locus,[89] which acts as an agonist of the melanocyte stimulating hormone receptor,[90] permits the switch in coloration of each individual hair from pheomelanin to eumelanin. It has been proposed that an individual melanocyte in the agouti hair bulb can switch the type of melanin it can manufacture.[91, 92]

Additional melanocyte-specific genes and/or gene products have been identified that significantly contribute to the process of melanization; however, their mechanism of action is not yet conclusively elucidated. The murine pink-eye dilution gene product is a protein synthesized by the pink-eye dilution locus (p) at which there exists at least 16 alleles.[93] Defects in this protein prevent normal melanin synthesis to occur within the melanosome, although a functional tyrosinase enzyme has been histochemically demonstrated.[31] The human homologue for this gene has been identified, and it resides on chromosome 15 (15q11.2-13), an area affected in patients with Angelman's syndrome and Prader-Willi syndrome.[94] It is proposed that the hypomelanosis of these syndromes results from defects in the pink-eye component of this chromosomal area. In addition, a form of tyrosinase-positive oculocutaneous albinism appears related to defects in this gene.[95, 96] The p locus protein is a relatively large molecule (approximately 110 kd) with 12 putative membrane spanning regions.[94] This gene codes for a putative tyrosine transporter localized to the limiting membrane of the premelanosome.[96]

Tyrosinase-related protein-1 is also a novel melanocyte-specific protein.[97, 98] It was serendipitously identified by investigators attempting to clone the tyrosinase gene.[99] This 75-kd glycoprotein has a strong molecular similarity to the tyrosinase. Specifically it has 40% to 52%

amino acid homology to tyrosinase.[97] Significantly, these similarities are highly conserved and/or common in the copper-binding domains, the cysteine and tryptophan residues, the transmembrane domains, the signal sequence, and the glycosylation sites.[100] However, this molecule has very little if any tyrosine hydroxylase activity[101, 102] and is coded independently from tyrosinase on human chromosome 9 (9p23).[103–105] Therefore, the primary function of this protein, which appears to be the most abundant melanocyte-specific protein synthesized by the melanocyte, remains unknown. Defects in TRP-1 are responsible for the production of brown as opposed to black pelage in the mouse.[98, 106] It has been demonstrated that melanocytes cultured from a patient with the Brown form of tyrosinase-positive oculocutaneous albinism lack transcript and protein for TRP-1 and exhibit brown soluble melanin and an altered tyrosinase function.[107, 108]

Pmel-17 is also a new melanocyte-specific gene product that has been cloned and mapped to the silver (si) locus of the mouse and to human chromosome 12 (12pter-q21).[109] Defects in this molecule also inhibit the complete synthesis of melanin. It has been speculated that this protein may be "stablin" (indole blocking factor), which regulates the conversion of 5,6-dehydroxyindole/indole-5,6-quinone toward melanins.[83]

The cell biology of melanization is going through a renaissance in respect to the current understanding of this elaborately regulated process. The complete list of melanocyte-specific proteins that participate in melanin synthesis and melanosome formation, as well as their interaction and regulation by cytokines and environmental cues, is far from complete, and undiscovered gene products and functions await documentation.

References

1. Zachariae COC, Thestrup-Pedersen K, Matsushima K. Expression and secretion of leukocyte chemotactic cytokines by normal human melanocytes and melanoma cells. J Invest Dermatol 1991;97:593–599.
2. Swope VB, Sauder DN, McKenzie RC, et al. Differential synthesis of IL-1α and IL-1β by neonatal and adult human melanocytes. J Invest Dermatol 1994;102:749–753.
3. DuShane GP. An experimental study of the origin of pigment cells in Amphibia. J Exp Zool 1935;72:1–31.
4. Dorris F. The production of pigment by chick neural crest in grafts to the 3-day limb bud. J Exp Zool 1939;80:315–345.
5. Rawles ME. Origin of pigment cells from the neural crest in the mouse embryo. Physiol Zool 1947;20:248–266.
6. His W, ed. Unterschungen uber die erst Anlage des Wirbeltierleibes: Die erste Entwicklung des Huhnchens im Ei. Leipzig: Vogel, 1868.
7. Weston JA. The migration and differentiation of neural crest cells. Adv Morphogen. 1970;8:41–114.
8. Weston JA. Motile and social behavior of neural crest cells. In: Bellairs R, Curtis A, Dunn G, eds. Cell Behavior. Cambridge, England: Cambridge University Press, 1982:429–470.
9. Noden DM. Interactions directing the migration and cytodifferentiation of avian neural crest cells. In: Garrod D, ed. Specificity of Embryological Interactions. London: Chapman & Hall, 1978:5–49.
10. Le Douarin NM, ed. The Neural Crest. Cambridge, England: Cambridge University Press, 1982.
11. Kirby ML, Gale TF, Stewart DE. Neural crest cells contribute to normal aorticopulmonary septation. Science 1983;220:1051–1061.

12. Feeney-Burns L. The pigments of the retinal pigment epithelium. Curr Top Eye Res 1980;2:119–178.

13. Erickson CA. From the crest to the periphery: Control of pigment cell migration and lineage segregation. Pigment Cell Res 1993;6:336–347.

14. Vincent M, Duband J-L, Thiery J-P. A cell surface determinant expressed early on migrating neural crest cells. Dev Brain Res 1983;9:235–238.

15. Tucker GC, Aoyuma H, Lipinski M, et al. Identical reactivity of monoclonal antibodies HNK-1 and NC-1: Conservation in vertebrates on cells derived from the neural primordium and on some leukocytes. Cell Differentiation 1984;14:223–230.

16. Bhattacharyya A, Frank E, Ratner N, et al. Po is an early marker of the Schwann cell lineage in chickens. Neuron 1991;7:831–844.

17. Loring JF, Erickson CA. Neural crest cell migratory pathways in the trunk of the chick embryo. Dev Biol 1987;121:220–236.

18. Zimmerman AA, Becker SW Jr. Melanoblasts and melanocytes in fetal Negro skin. In: Illinois Monographs in Medical Sciences, 3rd ed, vol VI. Urbana, IL: University of Illinois Press, 1959:1–59.

19. Mishima Y, Widlan S. Embryonic development of melanocytes in human hair and epidermis. J Invest Dermatol 1966;46:263–277.

20. Breathnach AS, Wyllie LM. Electron microscopy of melanocytes and Langerhans cells in human fetal epidermis at fourteen weeks. J Invest Dermatol 1965;44:51–60.

21. Gown AM, Vogel AM, Hoak D, et al. Monoclonal antibodies specific for melanocytic tumors distinguish subpopulations of melanocytes. Am J Pathol 1986;123:195–203.

22. Holbrook KA, Underwood RA, Vogel AM, et al. The appearance, density and distribution of melanocytes in human embryonic and fetal skin revealed by the antimelanoma monoclonal antibody. Anat Embryol Berl 1989;180:443–455.

23. Zimmerman AA, Cornbleet T. The development of epidermal pigmentation in the Negro fetus. J Invest Dermatol 1948;11:383–395.

24. Hashimoto K. The ultrastructure of the skin of human embryos: VIII. Melanoblast and intrafollicular melanocyte. J Anat 1971;108:99–108.

25. Geissler EN, Ryan MA, Housman DE. The dominant-white spotting (W) locus of the mouse encodes the c-*kit* proto-oncogene. Cell 1988;55:185–192.

26. Chabot B, Stephenson DA, Chapman VM, et al. The proto-oncogene c-*kit* encoding a transmembrane tyrosine kinase receptor maps to the mouse W locus. Nature 1988;335:88–89.

27. Williams DE, Eisenman J, Baird A, et al. Identification of a ligand for the c-*kit* proto-oncogene. Cell 1990;63:167–174.

28. Flanagan JG, Leder P. The *kit* ligand: A cell surface molecule altered in steel mutant fibroblasts. Cell 1990;63:185–194.

29. Zsebo KM, Williams DA, Geissler EN, et al. Stem cell factor is encoded at the Sl locus of the mouse and is the ligand for the c-*kit* receptor. Cell 1990;63:213–214.

30. Huang E, Nocka K, Beler DR, et al. The hematopoietic growth factor KL is encoded by the Sl locus and is the ligand of the c-*kit* receptor, the gene product of the W locus. Cell 1990;63:225–233.

31. Silvers WK, ed. The Coat Colors of Mice: A Model for Mammalian Gene Action and Interaction. New York: Springer-Verlag, 1979.

32. Hoo JJ, Haslam RH, van Orman C. Tentative assignment of piebald trait gene to chromosome band 4q12. Hum Genet 1986;73:230–231.

33. Yarden Y, Kuang W-J, Yang-Feng T, et al. Human proto-oncogene c-*kit*: A new cell surface receptor tyrosine kinase for an unidentified ligand. EMBO J 1987;6:3341–3351.

34. Giebel LB, Spritz RA. Mutation of the *kit* (mast/stem cell growth factor receptor) proto-oncogene in human piebaldism. Proc Natl Acad Sci USA 1991;88:8696–8699.

35. Fleischman RA, Saltman DL, Stastny V, et al. Deletion of the c-*kit* proto-oncogene in the human developmental defect piebald trait. Proc Natl Acad Sci USA 1991;88:10885–10889.

36. Green MC. Catalog of mutant genes and polymorphic loci. In: Lyon MF, Searle AG, eds. Genetic Variants and Strains of the Laboratory Mouse. New York: Oxford University Press, 1989:8–278.

37. Stechschulte DJ, Sharma R, Dileepan KN, et al. Effect of the *mi* allele on mast cells, basophils, natural killer cells, and osteoclasts in C57BL/6J mice. J Cell Physiol 1987;132:565–570.

38. Walker DG. Bone resorption restored in osteoporotic mice by transplants of normal bone marrow and spleen cells. Science 1975;190:784–785.

39. Marks SC Jr, Walker DG. The hematogenous origin of osteoclasts: Experimental evidence from osteopetrotic (microphthalmic) mice treated with spleen cells from beige mouse donors. Am J Anat 1981;161:1–10.

40. Konyukhov BV, Osipov VV. Interallelic complementation of microphthalmia and white genes in mice. Sov Genet 1968;4:1457–1465.

41. West JD, Fisher G, Loutit JF, et al. A new allele of microphthalmia induced in the mouse: Microphthalmia-defective iris (*mi^di^*). Genet Res Camb 1985;46:309–324.

42. Scholtz CL, Chan KK. Complicated colobomatous microphthalmia in the microphthalmic (*mi/mi*) mouse. Development 1987;99:501–508.

43. Sidman RL, Neuman P. Vitiligo: A new retinal degeneration mutation. Mouse Newsl 1988;81:60.

44. Hodgkinson CA, Moore KJ, Nakayama A, et al. Mutations at the mouse microphthalmia locus are associated with defects in a gene encoding a novel basic helix-loop–helix-zipper protein. Cell 1993;74:395–404.

45. Hughes MJ, Lingrel JB, Krakowsky JM, et al. A helix-loop-helix transcription factor–like gene is located at the *mi* locus. J Biol Chem 1993;268:20687–20690.

45a. Tachibana M, Perez-Jurado LA, Nakayama A, et al. Cloning of MITF, the human homolog of the mouse microphthalmia gene, and assignment to human chromosome 3 region. Hum Mol Genet 1994;3:553–557.

46. Asher JH, Friedman TB. Mouse and hamster mutants as models for Waardenburg syndrome in humans. J Med Genet 1990;27:618–626.

47. Moase CE, Trasler DG. Splotch locus mouse mutants: Models for neural tube defects and Waardenburg syndrome type 1 in humans. J Med Genet 1992;29:145–151.

48. Tassabehji M, Read AP, Newton VE, et al. Waardenburg's syndrome patients have mutations in the human homologue of the *Pax*-3 paired box gene. Nature 1992;355:635–636.

49. Epstein DJ, Vekemans M, Gros P. Splotch (Sp2H), a mutation affecting development of the mouse neural tube, shows a deletion within the paired homeodomain of *Pax-3*. Cell 1991;67:767–774.

50. Baldwin CT, Hoth CF, Amos JA, et al. An exonic mutation in the *HuP2* paired domain gene causes Waardenburg's syndrome. Nature 1992;355:637–638.

51. Quevedo WC Jr, Fitzpatrick TB, Szabo G, et al. Biology of melanocytes. In: Fitzpatrick TB, Eisen AZ, Wolff K, et al., eds. Dermatology in General Medicine, 3rd ed, vol 1. New York: McGraw-Hill, 1987:224–251.

52. Gilchrest BA, Blog FB, Szabo G. Effects of aging and chronic sun exposure on melanocytes in human skin. J Invest Dermatol 1979;73:141–143.

53. McClenic BK, Mitra RS, Riser BL, et al. Production and utilization of extracellular matrix components by human melanocytes. Exp Cell Res 1989;180:314–325.

54. Frenk E, Schellhorn JP. Zur morphologie der epidermalen Melanineinheit. Dermatologica 1969;139:271–277.

55. Fitzpatrick TB, Breathnach AS. Das epidermale melamim-einheit system. Derm Wochenschr 1963;147:481–489.

56. Mottaz JM, Zelickson AS. Melanin transfer: A possible phagocytic process. J Invest Dermatol 1967;49:605–610.

57. Wolff K, Jimbow K, Fitzpatrick TB. Experimental pigment donation in vivo. J Ultrastruct Res 1974;47:400–419.

58. Okazaki K, Uzuka M, Morikawa F, et al. Transfer mechanism of melanosomes in epidermal cell culture. J Invest Dermatol 1976;57:541–547.

59. Szabó G, Gerald AB, Pathak MA, et al. Racial differences in the fate of melanosomes in human epidermis. Nature 1969;222:1081–1082.

60. Szabo G, Hirobe T, Flynn EA, et al. The biology of the melanocyte. In: Bagnara JT, ed. Advances in Pigment Cell Research. Progress in Clinical and Biological Research, vol 256. New York: Alan R. Liss, 1988:463–474.

61. Quevedo WC Jr, Fitzpatrick TB, Pathak MA, et al. Light and skin color. In: Fitzpatrick TB, Pathak MA, Harber LC, et al., eds. Sunlight and Man. Tokyo: University of Tokyo Press, 1974:165–194.

62. Iwata M, Corn T, Iwata S, et al. The relationship between tyrosin-

ase activity and skin color in human foreskins. J Invest Dermatol 1990;95:9–15.

63. Iozumi K, Hoganson GE, Pennella R, et al. Role of tyrosinase as the determinant of pigmentation in cultured human melanocytes. J Invest Dermatol 1993;100:806–811.

64. Seiji M, Fitzpatrick TB, Birbeck MSC. The melanosome: A distinctive subcellular particle of mammalian melanocytes and the site of melanogenesis. J Invest Dermatol. 1961;36:243–252.

65. Orlow SJ, Zhou B-K, Boissy RE, et al. Identification of a mammalian melanosomal matrix glycoprotein. J Invest Dermatol. 1993;101:141–144.

66. Maul GG. Golgi–melanosome relationship in human melanoma in vitro. J Ultrastruct Res 1969;26:163–176.

67. Maul GG, Brumbaugh JA. On the possible function of coated vesicles in melanogenesis of the regenerating fowl feather. J Cell Biol 1971;48:41–48.

68. Tomita Y, Hariu A, Kato C, et al. Transfer of tyrosinase to melanosomes in Harding-Passey mouse melanoma. Arch Biochem Biophys 1983;225:75–85.

69. Jimbow K, Takeuchi T. Ultrastructural comparison of pheo- and eu-melanogenesis in animals. In: Klaus SN, ed. Pigment Cell 1979: Biologic Basis of Pigmentation, vol. 4. Basel: Karger, 1979:308–317.

70. Hatta S, Mishima Y, Ichihashi M, et al. Melanin monomers within coated vesicles and premelanosomes in melanin synthesizing cells. J Invest Dermatol 1988;91:181–184.

71. Jiménez M, Kameyama K, Maloy WL, et al. Mammalian tyrosinase: Biosynthesis, processing and modulation by melanocyte stimulating hormone. Proc Natl Acad Sci USA 1988;85:3830–3834.

72. Barton DE, Kwon BS, Francke U. Human tyrosinase gene, mapped to chromosome 11 (q14→q21), defines second region of homology with mouse chromosome 7. Genomics 1988;3:17–24.

73. Lerner AB, Fitzpatrick TB. Biochemistry of melanin formation. Physiol Rev 1950;30:91–126.

74. Korner AM, Pawelek J. Dopachrome conversion: A possible control point in melanin biosynthesis. J Invest Dermatol 1980;75:192–195.

75. Barber JI, Townsend D, Olds DP, et al. Dopachrome oxidoreductase: A new enzyme in the pigment pathway. J Invest Dermatol 1984;83:145–149.

76. Aroca P, Garcia-Borron JC, Solano F, et al. Regulation of distal mammalian melanogenesis: I. Partial purification and characterization of a dopachrome converting factor: Dopachrome tautomerase. Biochem Biophys Acta 1990;1035:266–275.

77. Palumbo A, d'Ischia M, Misuraca G, et al. Effect of metal ions on the rearrangement of dopachrome. Biochem Biophys Acta 1987;925:203–209.

78. Pawelek JM. After dopachrome? Pigment Cell Res 1991;4:53–62.

79. Tsukamoto K, Jackson IJ, Urabe K, et al. A second tyrosinase-related protein, TRP-2, is a melanogenic enzyme termed dopachrome tautomerase. EMBO J 1992;11:519–526.

80. Jackson IJ, Chambers DM, Tsukamoto K, et al. A second tyrosinase-related protein, TRP-2, maps to and is mutated at the mouse slaty locus. EMBO J 1992;11:527–535.

81. Korner AM, Pawelek JM. Mammalian tyrosinase catalyzes three reactions in the biosynthesis of melanin. Science 1982;217:1163–1165.

82. d'Ischia M, Napolitano A, Prota G. Peroxidase as an alternative to tyrosinase in the oxidative polymerization of 5,6-dihydroxyindoles to melanin(s). Biochim Biophys Acta 1991;1073:423–430.

83. Chakraborty AK, Park KC, Kwon BS, et al. Stablin activity is associated with Pmel-17 gene expression. Pigment Cell Res 1992;5:84.

84. Mojamdar M, Ichihashi M, Mishima Y. Tyrosinase and τ-glutamyl transpeptidase in 5-S-cysteinyldopa genesis within melanotic and amelanotic melanomas. J Dermatol 1982;9:73–77.

85. Jiménez M, García-Cánovas F, García-Carmona F, et al. Kinetics and stoichiometry of cysteinylDOPA formation in the first steps of melanogenesis. Int J Biochem 1986;18:161–166.

86. Jara JR, Aroca P, Solano F, et al. The role of sulfhydryl compounds in mammalian melanogenesis: The effect of cysteine and glutathione upon tyrosinase and the intermediates of the pathway. Biochem Biophys Acta 1988;967:296–303.

87. Wick MM, Hearing VJ, Rorsman H. Biochemistry of melanization. In: Fitzpatrick TB, Eisen AZ, Wolff K, et al., eds. Dermatology in General Medicine, 3rd ed, vol 1. New York: McGraw-Hill, 1987:251–258.

88. Thody AJ, Higgins EH, Wakamatzu K, et al. Pheomelanin as well as eumelanin is present in human epidermis. J Invest Dermatol 1991;97:340–344.

88a. Searle AG, ed. Comparative Genetics of Coat Colour in Mammals. London: Logos Academic Press, 1968.

89. Bultman SJ, Michaud EJ, Woychik RP. Molecular characterization of the mouse agouti locus. Cell 1992;71:1195–1204.

90. Jackson IJ. Molecular genetics: Colour-coded switches. Nature 1993;362:587–588.

91. Granholm NH, Japs RA, Kappenman KE. Differentiation of hairbulb pigment cell melanosomes in compound agouti and albino locus mouse mutants (A^y, a, c^{2J}; C57BL/6J). Pigment Cell Res 1990;3:16–27.

92. Sakurai T, Ochiai H, Takeuchi T. Ultrastructural change of melanosomes associated with agouti pattern formation in mouse hair. Dev Biol 1975;47:466–471.

93. Lyon MF, King TR, Gondo Y, et al. Genetic and molecular analysis of recessive alleles at the pink-eyed dilution(p) locus of the mouse. Proc Natl Acad Sci USA. 1992;89:6968–6972.

94. Gardner JM, Nakatsu Y, Gondo Y, et al. The mouse pink-eyed dilution gene: Association with human Prader-Willi and Angelman syndromes. Science 1992;257:1121–1124.

95. Ramsay M, Colman MA, Stevens G, et al. The tyrosinase-positive oculocutaneous albinism locus maps to chromosome 15q11.2-q12. Am J Hum Genet 1992;51:879–884.

96. Rinchik EM, Bultman SJ, Horsthemke B, et al. A gene for the mouse pink-eyed dilution locus and for human type II oculocutaneous albinism. Nature 1993;361:72–76.

97. Jackson IJ. A cDNA encoding tyrosinase-related protein maps to the brown locus in mice. Proc Natl Acad Sci USA 1988;85:4392–4396.

98. Jackson IJ, Chambers DM, Rinchik EM, et al. Characterization of TRP-1 mRNA levels in dominant and recessive mutations at the mouse brown (b) locus. Genetics 1990;126:451–459.

99. Shibahara S, Tomita Y, Sakakura T, et al. Cloning and expression of cDNA encoding mouse tyrosinase. Nucl Acids Res 1986;14:2413–2427.

100. Hearing VJ, Jiménez M. Analysis of mammalian pigmentation at the molecular level. Pigment Cell Res 1989;2:75–85.

101. Jiménez M, Tsukamoto K, Hearing VJ. Tyrosinases from two different loci are expressed by normal and by transformed melanocytes. J Biol Chem 1991;266:1147–1156.

102. Vijayasaradhi S, Houghton AN. Purification of an autoantigenic 75-kDa human melanosomal glycoprotein. Int J Cancer 1991;47:298–303.

103. Abbott C, Jackson IJ, Carritt B, et al. The human homolog of the mouse Brown gene maps to the short arm of chromosome 9 and extends the known region of homology with mouse chromosome 4. Genomics 1991;11:471–473.

104. Chintamaneni CD, Ramsay M, Colman M-A, et al. Mapping the human CAS2 gene, the homologue of the mouse brown (b) locus, to human chromosome 9p22-pter. Biochem Biophys Res Commun 1991;178:227–235.

105. Murty VV, Bouchard B, Mathew S, et al. Assignment of the human TYRP (brown) locus to chromosome region 9p23 by nonradioactive in situ hybridization. Genomics 1992;13:227–229.

106. Zdarsky E, Favor J, Jackson IJ. The molecular basis of *brown*, an old mouse mutation, and of an induced revertant to wild type. Genetics 1990;126:443–449.

107. Zhao H, Boissy Y, Nordlund JJ, et al. Melanocytes cultured from a patient with tyrosinase-positive albinism lack TRP-1 (abstract). Mol Biol Cell 1992;3:85.

108. Boissy RE, Zhao H, Boissy YL, et al. Melanocytes from a Brown oculocutaneous albino lack expression of TRP-1 and exhibit reduced insoluble melanin and aberrant tyrosine hydroxylase activity (abstract). Pigment Cell Res 1993;6:275–276.

109. Kwon BS, Chintamaneni CD, Kozak CA, et al. A melanocyte-specific gene, Pmel-17, maps near the silver coat color locus on mouse chromosome 10 and is a syntenic region on human chromosome 12. Proc Natl Acad Sci USA 1991;88:9228–9232.

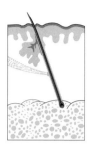

chapter 130

Vitiligo

RAYMOND E. BOISSY and JAMES J. NORDLUND

DEFINITION

Vitiligo is an acquired depigmentary disorder characterized by loss of melanocytes from the epidermis, the mucous membranes, and other tissues. Vitiligo affects primarily melanocytes in the interfollicular epidermis, and to a lesser degree the melanocytes in the hair bulb.

CLINICAL FEATURES

Vitiligo generally begins between the ages of 2 and 40 years, but it has been reported to begin as late as 85 years of age.[1, 2] The initial presentation of a lesion or lesions and the subsequent progression of the disease are extremely variable. A lesion of vitiligo is initially noticed as either a hypopigmented or snow white macule or patch, usually 1 to 3 cm in diameter (Fig. 130–1). The margins of the lesion are distinct. The lesions are most easily noticed in dark skin and/or tanned individuals. In fairskinned individuals, the sharp border of the lesions becomes apparent with Wood's light examination. Variations in the color of the lesion and its margin can occur. There can be a trichrome appearance in which almost the entire lesion or a narrow peripheral area within its margin may be light brown or tan, presumably as a result of partial progressive elimination of interfollicular epidermal melanocytes. The margin of the lesion is hyperpigmented in approximately 5.5% of cases[3] or, less frequently, exhibits erythema, suggesting an inflammatory process (Fig. 130–2).

In three fourths of cases a single lesion is initially noticed, while in the remaining cases multiple initial lesions that are bilateral and often remarkably symmetrical are observed.[4] The face, joints, hands, and legs are the most initially common affected sites, although no area on the body, including the mucous membranes, is exempt from developing vitiligo. New lesions can develop immediately after the initial macule, or there may be an extended period of time—up to years—before additional lesions develop. Lesions progress in size and number, sometimes at a slow rate and in some patients very rapidly. Adjacent lesions will frequently coalesce. In the course of the disease, periods of slow or rapid enlargement of the lesion, arrest in depigmentation, and spontaneous or partial repigmentation can occur. Eventually the number and size of vitiligo lesions on a patient become extremely heterogeneous (Fig. 130–3). In addition, the extent and patterns of vitiligo between patients are extremely variable.

Vitiligo can be classified by its extent and distribution of cutaneous depigmentation (Table 130–1). *Focal vitiligo* is defined as a single or a few depigmented macules that are located in a discrete area. *Segmental vitiligo* is the unilateral localization of one or more macules to one area of the body. Segmental vitiligo has been classified as Type B by Koga,[5] in contrast to Type A, which includes all other forms of vitiligo. *Generalized vitiligo*, the most common variant, is defined as widespread distribution of numerous macules over the integument in a random pattern.[1] *Universal vitiligo* is complete depigmentation of the epidermis and is fairly rare. This latter form need not include depigmentation of the hair. A classification that recognizes the most common patterns for the expression of vitiligo has been succinctly presented with illustrations by Ortonne[1] (see Table 130–1).

Although the cutaneous depigmentation is almost always the primary and initial symptom in vitiligo, other symptoms and medical problems may be associated with this disease. The ocular and auditory changes observed in patients with vitiligo suggest that extracutaneous melanocytes may also be affected. In the eye, there are neural crest–derived melanocytes within the uveal tract (i.e., choroid, ciliary bodies, and iris) and retinal pigment epithelium. Uveitis, chorioretinal depigmentation, iris and conjunctival depigmentation, and retinitis pigmentosa frequently occur in patients with vitiligo.[6–8] In addition, some animal models of vitiligo have demonstrated cellular abnormalities and destruction of ocular melanocytes associated with the cutaneous depigmentation.[9–11]

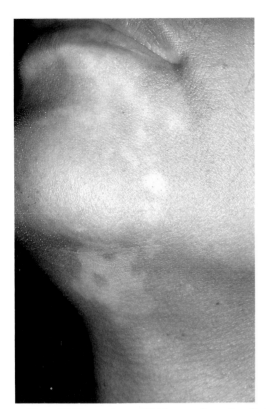

FIGURE 130–1. Vitiligo patient exhibiting small amelanotic lesions at onset.

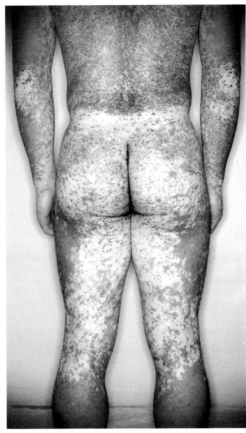

FIGURE 130–3. Patient exhibiting typical generalized vitiligo.

Melanocytes exist within the stria vascularis of the cochlea in the inner ear.[12] Although the function of otic melanocytes is not known, it has been proposed that they contribute to the developmental or functional role of hearing.[13-15] There have been a few reports of partial loss in sensorineural hearing[16] and bilateral and unilateral hypoacusis in patients with vitiligo.[17]

Melanocytes also reside in the leptomeninges of the brain stem.[18] Whether anecdotal reports of migraine headaches in vitiligo patients are associated with the destruction of this population of melanocytes or are a coincidence remains undetermined.

Many diseases are associated with vitiligo. Significantly, most of these have a putative immune mecha-

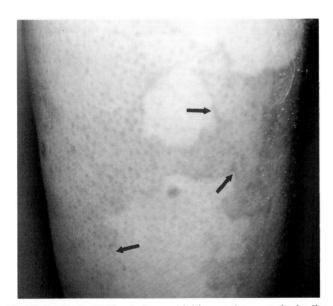

FIGURE 130–2. Vitiligo lesions exhibiting erythema at the leading edge *(arrows)* suggestive of an inflammatory process.

TABLE 130-1. Classification of Patterns of Vitiligo Expression

Localized
Focal: One or more macules in one area, but not clearly in a segmental or zosteriform distribution Segmental: One or more macules in a dermatomal pattern Mucosal: Mucous membrane involvement alone

Generalized
Acrofacial: Distal extremities and face (possibly early vitiligo vulgaris) Vulgaris: Scattered macules Mixed: Acrofacial and vulgaris, or segmental and acrofacial and/or vulgaris

Universal
Complete or nearly complete depigmentation

nism. The hypothesis that vitiligo is an autoimmune disease is based in part on this association. Thyroid diseases (both hypothyroidism and hyperthyroidism as well as Graves' disease), diabetes mellitus, pernicious anemia, Addison's disease, multiglandular insufficiency syndrome, and alopecia areata all occur in patients with vitiligo.[1] The evidence verifying that an autoimmune mechanism does indeed play an important role in the pathogenesis of vitiligo is discussed below. In addition, vitiligo has also been reported in patients with Hodgkin's disease,[19] multiple myeloma,[20] dysgammaglobuline-mia,[21] cutaneous T-cell lymphoma,[22] thymoma,[23,24] and immune deficiency diseases such as AIDS.[25]

PATHOLOGY

Vitiligo is caused by a loss of melanin from the epidermis, coupled with a decrease in the numbers of melanocytes in affected areas. In biopsy specimens that span the erythematous edge of a lesion, or in very early lesions, there may be a few lymphocytes near the basal layer of the epidermis, with some in seeming contact with melanocytes. Ultrastructural examination supports the contention that lymphocytes exert cytotoxic effects on melanocytes; indeed, a few keratinocytes may also suffer damage. As melanocytes diminish in number, their place in the basal layer appears to be taken by Langerhans cells, which are normally found only in the midspinous zone. This electron microscopic finding can be of use in the differential diagnosis of leukoderma.[26]

PATHOGENESIS AND ETIOLOGY

No definitive precipitating factor responsible for initiating vitiligo has been established. Anecdotal correlations of the onset of depigmentation with psychologic stress, physical trauma, pregnancy and oral contraceptives, and sunlight and artificial ultraviolet radiation have been described.[1] However, these associations are frequently observed in a high percentage of normal individuals and have not been epidemiologically shown to occur more frequently in patients with vitiligo.

There appears to be a genetic component that predisposes one to vitiligo. Although it is clear that vitiligo is not inherited by a simple mendelian mechanism, studies on familial inheritance patterns in India suggest a complex inheritance pattern.[27, 28] More extensive analysis of families in a larger population suggested that a minimum of three unlinked diallelic genes might be involved[29] and is consistent with a polygenic disorder.[30] Most vitiligo patients do not relate a family history of hypopigmentation.

The basic pathogenesis of vitiligo in general, or for any of the putative subsets of vitiligo, still remains unknown. Although much information on the cellular pathophysiology of vitiligo is unknown, the molecular aspects of the disease are virtually unexplored.

Current hypotheses for the pathogenesis of vitiligo have been classified into two broad, and probably overlapping, categories—that is, an intrinsic melanocyte

dysfunction and/or death and an autoimmune-mediated destruction. It is generally agreed that by whatever the mechanism, melanocytes are completely eliminated from the amelanotic lesions. Immunocytochemical analysis using a battery of antibodies to melanocyte-specific proteins has demonstrated that none of these antigens are detectable in vitiligo lesions.[31] In addition, skin biopsied from a macule of vitiligo does not yield melanocytes in culture as does skin biopsied from the pigmented areas of vitiligo patients (personal observations). One study has demonstrated that repigmentation induced by psoralens and ultraviolet A light (PUVA) therapy begins with melanocytes migrating from terminal hair follicles in a radial pattern.[32] These latter data suggest two important points: (1) the depigmented interfollicular epidermis in the vitiligo lesions does not contain a stem population of melanoblasts, and (2) the stem reservoir of melanocytes for repigmentation originates from follicular melanocytes.

It has been controversial whether melanocytes in vitiligo intrinsically malfunction or are susceptible to autodestruction and subsequently eliminated or both. Histologic examination of early lesions and ultrastructural analysis of melanocytes at the border of vitiliginous macules have not revealed conclusive evidence. On occasion, researchers have documented enlarged melanocytes with numerous irregular dendrites at these sites.[33] The major ultrastructural abnormality reported consists of extracellular granular material present between keratinocytes and occasionally melanocytes in nearby pigmented foci.[34] Defects of keratinocytes in vitiligo patients may also exist. It has been reported that the epidermis of vitiligo lesions has reduced thioredoxin reductase activity,[35] defective calcium uptake,[36] low catalase activity,[37] and high expression of beta-adrenoreceptors.[38] However, these findings need confirmation.

Melanocytes from the pigmented regions of vitiligo patients have been established in culture and subsequently analyzed. Vitiligo melanocytes behave differently than melanocytes from control donors in various ways, suggesting that the vitiligo melanocyte may harbor an intrinsic problem. Vitiligo melanocytes demonstrate a lag in proliferation at the onset of primary cultures and are less able to survive subculturing.[39] These abnormal characteristics of cultured vitiligo melanocytes are reversible in patients successfully repigmenting (either spontaneously or after therapy) or when fetal lung fibroblast-derived growth factor is added to the melanocyte cultures.[40] In a separate study, melanocytes cultured from numerous vitiligo patients did not demonstrate any gross abnormalities—that is, their morphology and proliferation in culture appeared to be normal.[41] However, when viewed with the electron microscope, cultured melanocytes from 78.6% of the patients demonstrated dilated or circular profiles of rough endoplasmic reticulum and/or autophagosomes, indicating an intrinsic abnormality of some form.[42]

It has been proposed that melanocyte death in vitiligo may be the consequence of the cells' susceptibility to environmentally induced or self-generated chemical toxicity. Many people exposed to derivatives of hydroquinones such as monobenzyl ether of hydroquinone, para-tert-butyl phenol,[43] 4-isopropyl catechol,[44] and similar compounds[45, 46] have been noted to develop depigmentation, primarily at sites of contact with the chemical. In addition, intermediates in the biosynthesis of melanin, particularly the indole quinones, are thought to be cytotoxic to melanocytes if present in elevated amounts.[47] The hypothesis that melanocyte death results from sensitivity to toxic substances that build up in the cells has been proposed for the feather amelanosis in the White Leghorn and the Barred Plymouth Rock chicken models of depigmentation.[48]

Many studies suggest that an autoimmune response is a significant component of the pathogenesis of vitiligo. This idea was proposed because many vitiligo patients also exhibit other autoimmune types of disorders—that is, multiple glandular insufficiencies, thyroid diseases, pernicious anemia, type I diabetes mellitus, Addison's disease, alopecia areata, and autoimmune hypoparathyroidism.[49] Circulating antimelanocyte antibodies were first identified in vitiligo patients in the mid-1970s.[50] More recently, serum antibodies to antigens on melanocytes or melanoma cells have been repeatedly identified in vitiligo patients[51-55] and animal models of vitiligo.[56-58] The presence of serum melanocyte-specific autoantibodies appears to correlate with the extent of the disease.[55, 59, 60] Five vitiligo antigens of approximately 35, 40 to 45, 75, 90, and 150 kd molecular weight, respectively, frequently react against vitiligo serum.[61] The functional ability of serum from some vitiligo patients to destroy cultured melanocytes by complement-mediated damage and antibody-dependent cellular cytotoxicity has also been demonstrated.[62, 63] Whether intrinsic abnormalities of the vitiligo melanocyte stimulate melanocyte-specific antibody production and cell destruction or whether melanocyte defects and autoimmune reactions are separate entities in different patients needs to be determined. Aberrancies in T-cell subset populations and functions have also been demonstrated to exist in vitiligo patients.[64-68] However, many of these studies are contradictory and highly variable.

In addition to the question of how the immune system is involved in the pathophysiology of vitiligo, it has been shown that the immune function of the depigmented vitiligo skin is ultimately compromised. Specifically, contact sensitivity reactions to sensitizing agents (dinitrochlorobenzene, poison ivy, etc.) are diminished or nonexistent in the lesions of vitiligo patients.[69-71]

DIFFERENTIAL DIAGNOSIS

Skin diseases that produce depigmentation and/or hypopigmentation (Table 130–2) should be considered when evaluating for vitiligo.

Piebaldism is a genetic disorder in which there is a complete absence of melanocytes in the skin and hair. Areas of absent pigmentation are usually apparent at or soon after birth, especially in dark-skinned neonates. It might not be obvious for several weeks or months in fair-skinned infants. Leukoderma at birth or shortly after is the most important distinguishing feature of piebaldism. Congenital vitiligo is extremely rare, and a review of the few reported cases raises the possibility that the in-

TABLE 130–2. Differential Diagnosis of Vitiligo

Cutaneous Disorders with Depigmentation or Hypopigmentation
Piebaldism
Lupus erythematosus
Tinea versicolor
Pityriasis alba
Lichen sclerosus et atrophicus
Cutaneous T-cell lymphoma
Sarcoidosis
Scleroderma
Nevus anemicus
Postinflammatory hypopigmentation
Idiopathic guttate hypomelanosis
Pityriasis lichenoides chronica
Chédiak-Higashi syndrome
Tuberous sclerosis
Hypomelanosis of Ito
Nevus depigmentosus
White fibrous papulosis of the neck

fants might have had piebaldism. Several other features help in differentiating the two disorders. There usually is a strong family history of piebaldism, since it is transmitted as an autosomal trait. A parent and several other sibs are usually affected. Vitiligo is probably polygenic, and the family history is negative or inconclusive.[30] The findings of piebaldism are usually located on the ventral surface of the body and classically include a depigmented patch on the forehead and a white forelock. The latter can be very subtle or at times absent. In contrast, vitiligo usually affects both the dorsal and ventral surfaces and a depigmented forelock is almost never seen. The pigmented skin in piebaldism usually exhibits hyper- and hypopigmented patterns. The depigmented patches of piebald skin can show, at the edges, minimal pigment spread or regression. However, the depigmentation usually is stable throughout life. Vitiligo typically spreads widely or occasionally spontaneously repigments. Piebaldism in some animals and about a third of affected humans is caused by a defect in the gene for the c-kit proto-oncogene, which has been cloned and sequenced.[72] Genetic analysis rarely is needed to differentiate the two disorders. The family history, the presence of depigmentation at birth, and the distribution of depigmentation and hyperpigmentation are usually sufficient to distinguish piebaldism from vitiligo.

Lupus erythematosus, systemic or cutaneous, can present as depigmented patches. Erythema is especially prominent in white skin. The edges of the depigmentation often are hyperpigmented, although this can be observed in vitiligo as well. Meticulous examination usually reveals a few typical red plaques, scaly patches, periungual erythema, or other signs of lupus. At times, the two are not readily distinguishable on clinical findings. Biopsies for routine history or immunofluorescence or both and serologic tests for lupus are on occasion necessary to resolve this differential diagnosis. This is particularly important because the major treatment for vitiligo is phototherapy.

Tinea versicolor is sometimes confused with vitiligo. The distribution of lesions on the trunk, the slight scale, and positive KOH preparation readily distinguish the two disorders.

Pityriasis alba is a patchy form of hypopigmentation located commonly on the arms and legs. The patches have poorly defined borders and are scaly. The two disorders are usually not difficult to differentiate.

Lichen sclerosus et atrophicus, especially when it begins around the vulva or perirectal area, might be indistinguishable from vitiligo. Atrophy may not be apparent clinically, and a biopsy may be required. Lichen sclerosus on other parts of the body is easy to diagnose.

Both cutaneous T-cell lymphoma and sarcoid can present as hypopigmented macules or patches that can be difficult to distinguish from early onset, localized vitiligo. Biopsy reveals typical changes of sarcoidosis or of mycosis fungoides.[73]

Scleroderma, nevus anemicus, postinflammatory depigmentation, and similar disorders should be considered when evaluating a patient with vitiligo.

TREATMENT

Treatment for vitiligo is important.[74] The epidermis is devoid of one of its three main cell types and functions abnormally. The goal of treatment differs for the patient and physician. The patient wishes to eradicate the severe disfigurement and the resulting embarrassment. The physician wishes to restore the normal morphology and function of the epidermis.

Therapy can be divided into two general types: medical and surgical (Table 130–3).[75] Medical therapies include topical steroids and phototherapy. Surgical treatments include various forms of melanocyte grafts and tattooing. Each therapy has specific indications.

Medical Therapies

Repigmentation requires proliferation and migration of melanocytes from a reservoir into the depigmented skin. The melanocytes will migrate only a few milli-

TABLE 130–3. Treatment of Vitiligo
Medical Therapies
Topical steroids
Phototherapy
Topical PUVA
Systemic PUVA
Depigmentation
Surgical Therapies
Punch grafts
Minigrafts
Blister grafts
Autologous cultured composite skin substitutes
Autologous cultured melanocyte grafts
Micropigmentation (tattooing)

meters from the pigmented edge. The main reservoir is the hair follicle. Glabrous skin cannot respond to medical therapy. Similarly, hair-bearing skin in which terminal hairs are clearly depigmented does not respond because the reservoir in the follicle has been destroyed.

Topical Steroids. Steroids have been used for years to treat vitiligo. Because treatment must be continued for many months, systemic steroids are not considered appropriate because of the numerous side effects. Topically applied steroids avoid systemic toxicity.

Topical steroids can be useful in children under the age of 10 years or for those with limited depigmentation. A low-potency (class 4 or 5) preparation applied only once daily for several months or longer is the optimal therapy. More potent steroids produce significant side effects when applied for several months and are unnecessary. Frequent applications of the agents do not seem to improve results. About 50% of individuals will note significant return of pigment in treatable areas. If repigmentation is not observed within 3 months, the applications should be discontinued and tried again 6 months later or another treatment tried.

Phototherapy. Psoralens and exposure to ultraviolet light in the 320 to 400 nm spectrum (PUVA) is the most common treatment for vitiligo. It can be employed on individuals aged 10 years or older. Generally the psoralens are taken by mouth, although topical psoralens are also used by some practitioners.

TOPICAL PUVA. For topical use, 8-methoxypsoralen (8-MOP) or trimethylpsoralen (TMP) is dissolved in petrolatum or ethanol. The commercially available 1% solution of 8-MOP is too potent. It should be dissolved at least 1:10 or preferably 1:100 prior to application by the physician or trained nurse. Thirty minutes later, the treated skin is exposed to UVA beginning at 0.12 joule (J). Treatments are repeated twice weekly but never on consecutive days. The dose of UVA is increased 0.12 J per session until a slight erythema is produced. Treatment is continued for 3 months after the erythema dose is reached. If no evidence of repigmentation is observed by this time, treatment should be discontinued and tried again 6 months later.

The window of safety for topical psoralens is very small. Almost all individuals will develop painful blisters during this therapy. Topical psoralens should never be used with direct sunlight. The patient should not be given the medication or allowed to apply it because small errors produce severe second-degree burns. The patient must apply a UVA sunscreen immediately after treatment is complete. The individual must avoid all sun exposure for the remainder of the day, including that obtained through the windows of an office or car. Topical PUVA is the most difficult of available treatments and should be utilized only by those who are well trained in its use, indications, contraindications, and toxicities.

SYSTEMIC PUVA. Psoralens taken by mouth have a wider margin of safety, although they can produce severe burns or even death if not used with caution. In general, the source of UVA is a medical phototherapy unit, although there are alternative sources of UVA. Physicians using alternative sources of UVA should have specific training in their use.

The standard recommendation is for the patient to take 0.25 to 0.4 mg/kg of 8-MOP 1 hour before exposure to UVA. With larger doses of psoralens, the dose of UVA is low, usually 1 to 2 J for the first exposure. The dose is increased by 1 J at each treatment until erythema is noted.

More recently, some vitiligo experts have used smaller doses of 8-MOP and larger doses of UVA (called low-dose psoralen therapy). Individuals take only 10 mg of 8-MOP 1 hour before exposure to 4 J of UVA. At each treatment, the dose is increased by 2 to 3 J. If erythema is not reached by 20 J, the patient takes 20 mg of 8-MOP and starts at 2 J, which increases until erythema is noted, often around 6 to 8 J. The use of smaller doses of psoralens and large doses of UVA significantly widens the safety margin. Patients rarely burn, and those with erythema note only mild discomfort. Nausea from the medication is rare.

Systemic therapy is continued for 3 to 4 months. If no response is noted, treatment should be stopped and tried again in 6 months. It is continued as long as repigmentation is observed. Generally, 100 treatments given two to three times per week (never on consecutive days) are required. The dose of psoralens and UVA must be individualized for each patient to achieve mild erythema. Patients will exhibit a wide range of sensitivity to the treatments. PUVA will not repigment glabrous skin or skin with white terminal hair. Appropriate laboratory data include a serum antinuclear antibody assay prior to therapy. Those using larger doses of psoralens should monitor liver functions.

Patients taking oral psoralens should wear UVA-absorbent eyeglasses at least until that evening, and some investigators recommend that patients wear the glasses for 24 hours. An eye examination by an ophthalmologist should be performed annually.

Depigmentation. Some patients have vitiligo that is too extensive to repigment by medical or surgical therapies. Depigmentation that involves more than half of the integument is an indication that attempts to regain the color will not be successful, at least within a period of 1 to 2 years. For such individuals, depigmentation therapy should be considered. The optimal goal is to repigment the patient. The worst option is to ignore the depigmentation, leaving the patient significantly disfigured. The second best option is for the skin to be one color—that is, completely depigmented. For patients who desire this option and have thought it through carefully, depigmentation is an excellent treatment. Monobenzone is applied to the skin twice daily. The residual pigment disappears gradually, leaving the individual with an excellent outcome. Such individuals have the appearance of a person with a type 1 skin (i.e., the most lightly pigmented of the skin tones).

Depigmentation does require the full informed consent of the patient. It is permanent, and the patient will be photosensitive for life. It is good practice to have the individual consider the option with the family members because the individual will undergo a significant alteration in his or her bodily image. Once he or she has emotionally accepted the concept of a permanently altered appearance, the patient will be ready to undertake the treatment. Some patients will not accept this option, and their feelings should be respected.

Depigmentation requires application of monobenzone to the affected areas twice daily. Patients with treated skin must be careful not to touch other individuals for 1 to 2 hours, lest they inadvertently apply the drug to a spouse or child and cause depigmentation. The cream should be applied sparingly and rubbed into the skin to avoid spreading it to others. The only other toxicity is a mild dermatitis, which is readily treated with topical steroids. An occasional patient is allergic to monobenzone.

Surgical Therapies

The best and most rapid therapies today are medical. However, there is a small population of patients who are candidates for surgical transplants. In general, this population has small areas of vitiligo, the disease is stable, and the individuals are willing to undergo the numerous procedures needed to complete repigmentation.

The techniques differ, but the concept underlying the different procedures is the same—that is, transplant of autologous melanocytes into an area that has no pigment cells and cannot be repigmented by medical therapies. The different approaches will be described briefly.

Punch Grafts. This technique is essentially the same as hair transplants. Punch biopsy specimens from a pigmented donor site are transplanted into depigmented sites.[76] The donor punch generally is slightly larger than the recipient site. Preparation of the site with sterilizing scrubs and local anesthesia are the same as those for hair transplants. The grafts are held in place by pressure dressings. Repigmentation and spread of color begin about 4 to 6 weeks post-graft. The color match is good. The major problem is a residual pebbled or shagreen-like surface because the grafts do not necessarily remain perfectly positioned. Ambient lighting will highlight the uneven surface. Pebbled skin is cosmetically unacceptable on the face for some individuals. It is recommended to try three or four test spots on skin near the hair line before proceeding with larger areas. This allows the patient to determine whether the repigmentation is desirable even if some pebbling is present. In two patients, this author (James J. Nordlund) thought that the use of grafts was less successful in repigmenting piebald skin than skin depigmented by vitiligo.

Minigrafts. This is a variant of the preceding technique and minimizes the problem of an uneven surface texture. Donor grafts, usually 4 mm in diameter, are bisected into four quadrants.[77, 78] The recipient site is prepared and anesthetized. A No. 11 blade is used to make 2- to 3-mm stab incisions about 3 to 4 mm apart. The small grafts are inserted into the incisions and held in place by a pressure dressing. The grafts heal readily and begin to repigment within 4 to 6 weeks. Some pebbling persists but is minimal and the cosmetic result excellent. The procedure is tedious and very time consuming. Because the area that repigments is small, a few millimeters in diameter, the number of grafts is large. As many as 50 to 100 grafts can be placed at one visit, but the process takes several hours. Several or many visits usually are needed to repigment even moderately sized areas of pigment loss.

Suction Blisters. Epidermal grafts can be obtained by vacuum suction,[79, 80] usually about 150 mm Hg. It takes several hours to raise the blister from the donor site. The blister roof can be removed in toto and used as a graft. The recipient site can be prepared by suction, freezing, or dermabrasion[81] of the site 24 hours prior to grafting. The depigmented blister roof is discarded and the epidermal donor graft placed on the vitiliginous area. Freezing should not be used for the donor site, as depigmentation of donor skin can result. Larger areas can be repigmented by suction blister grafts. Freezing is a good method to produce blisters on recipient sites such as the dorsum of the hands and fingers. The preparation of sites and anesthetic methods are similar to those for other procedures. The repigmentation from suction blisters tends to be mottled compared with that from punch or minigrafts. Blisters from freezing can be painful. (For further information see the Atlas of Cutaneous Surgery, Chapter 17.)

Autologous Cultures. A variation on the blister technique requires the culture of mixed populations of keratinocytes and melanocytes.[82, 83] Small shave biopsy specimens from pigmented skin serve as a source for the cells. The cells are trypsinized to make a single cell suspension and placed in culture where a mixture of keratinocytes and melanocytes forms a composite skin substitute. Cultures expand the quantity of donor skin by a large factor. Recipient sites are prepared by removal of the epidermis with suction, freezing, or dermabrasion. The keratinocyte/melanocyte composite skin culture is placed onto the denuded depigmented skin and covered with a dressing to hold the graft in place. The melanocytes will engraft, and repigmentation occurs. Like blister grafts, the color tends to be mottled. This technique has the advantage that only small amounts of donor skin are needed. Its major disadvantage is that the operator needs access to a pathogen-free culture facility that can grow the composite grafts in sufficient quantities to repigment the various sites. Such cultures are expensive to prepare and maintain and require trained personnel.

Autologous Melanocyte Grafts. A variation on composite skin grafts is the culture of melanocytes alone for injection into the skin,[84, 85] or alternatively on superficially dermabraded skin.[86, 87] In the former technique, small blisters raised by freezing of depigmented sites serve as a recipient site. In the latter technique, dermabrasion of the recipient site is used. The donor site can be a small shave biopsy from which melanocytes can be grown and expanded in number by a very large factor. The culture of melanocytes is not difficult but does require a trained technician and considerable expense for ingredients; also, it is very slow, requiring months. The original techniques for culture required the addition of tumor promoters like phorbol esters for the cells to grow. Cells from cultures prepared under these conditions might not be suitable for human use. However, newer techniques are now under study to replace artificial mitogens with basic fibroblast growth factor, endothelin, and/or hepatocyte growth factor, which might be more acceptable.[88-90] The success of autologous melanocyte

grafts is not perfect. However, over half of the recipient sites show regrowth of melanocytes, but spread of pigment is minimal. The other sites seem to be failures. The technology for this procedure should improve rapidly in the near future.

Problems. All of these techniques have advantages and disadvantages. Failure of the graft to "take" and produce pigment is common to all of the techniques. Vitiligo is a disease that exhibits the isomorphic response. Donor sites can become depigmented. Infection is always a risk. Scarring at the donor or recipient site can occur if the techniques for removal of the epidermis are not sufficiently gentle. The techniques take experience to achieve the optimal result. For all of them, the cost can be prohibitive. Cultures are very expensive and require special facilities and technical help. Suction systems require several hours for blister formation. Not all blisters are large, tense bullae. Some are small and irregular and are not useful for transplant even after the long preparation. The operator and patient must be very dedicated to undergo these techniques if the areas of treatment are large or numerous. If small, success is more easily achieved.

Micropigmentation (Tattooing). Tattooing can be used to repigment depigmented skin in dark-skinned individuals.[91] A special large, nine-prong needle is used in order to decrease the number of sticks necessary. The colored pigments can be purchased commercially but must be mixed to match the patients' natural color. Matching is difficult, and the color tends to fade. It often has a bluish discoloration. Lips are best treated by this technique, especially in African-Americans, although the color is not entirely normal. It is better than the pink color that is often characteristic of individuals with dark skin who have vitiligo of the lips. Herpes simplex labialis is a common sequela and is easily treated with acyclovir. If vitiligo spreads after the tattooing, the patient must be retreated.

References

1. Ortonne JP, Mosher DB, Fitzpatrick TB, eds. Vitiligo and Other Hypomelanosis of Hair and Skin. New York: Plenum Press, 1983.
2. Nordlund JJ, Ortonne JP. Vitiligo and depigmentation. In: Weston WL, MacKie RM, Provost TT, eds. Current Problems in Dermatology, vol. 4. St. Louis: Mosby–Year Book, 1992:3–30.
3. Seghal VN. A clinical evaluation of 202 cases of vitiligo. Cutis 1974;14:439–445.
4. Levai M. A study of certain contributory factors in the development of vitiligo in South Indian patients. Arch Dermatol 1958;78:364–370.
5. Koga M. Vitiligo: A new classification and therapy. Br J Dermatol 1977;97:255–261.
6. Albert DM, Wagoner MD, Pruett RC, et al. Vitiligo and disorders of the retinal pigment epithelium. Br J Ophthalmol 1983;67:153–156.
7. Wagoner MD, Albert DM, Lerner AB, et al. New observations on vitiligo and ocular disease. Am J Ophthalmol 1983;96:16–26.
8. Cowan CL Jr, Halder RM, Grimes PE, et al. Ocular disturbances in vitiligo. J Am Acad Dermatol 1986;15:17–24.
9. Boissy RE, Smyth JR Jr, Fite KV. Progressive cytologic changes during the development of delayed feather melanosis and associated choroidal defects in the DAM chicken line. A vitiligo model. Am J Pathol 1983;111:197–212.
10. Boissy RE, Moellmann GE, Lerner AB. Morphology of melanocytes in hair bulbs and eyes of vitiligo mice. Am J Pathol 1987;127:380–388.

11. Smith SB. C57BL/6J-vit/vit mouse model of retinal degeneration: Light microscopic analysis and evaluation of rhodopsin levels. Exp Eye Res 1992;55:903–910.
12. Hilding D, Ginzberg R. Pigmentation of the stria vascularis. Acta Otolaryngol 1977;84:24–37.
13. Yanz JL, Herr LR, Townsend D, et al. The questionable relation between cochlear pigmentation and noise-induced hearing loss. Audiology 1985;24:260–268.
14. Steel KP, Barkway C. Another role for melanocytes: Their importance for normal stria vascularis development in the mammalian inner ear. Development 1989;107:453–463.
15. Garber SR, Turner CW, Creel D, et al. Auditory system abnormalities in human albinos. Ear Hear 1982;3:207–210.
16. Thurmon TF, Jackson J, Fowler CG. Deafness and vitiligo. Birth Defects 1976;12:315–320.
17. Tosti A, Bardazzi F, Tosti G, et al. Audiologic abnormalities in cases of vitiligo. J Am Acad Dermatol 1987;17:230–233.
18. Goldgeier M, Klein LE, Klein-Angerer S, et al. The distribution of melanocytes in the leptomeninges of the human brain. J Invest Dermatol 1984;82:235–239.
19. Nordlund JJ, Lerner AB. Vitiligo: Its relationship to systematic disease. In: Moschella SL, ed. Dermatology Update. Amsterdam: Elsevier–North Holland, 1979:411–432.
20. Gomez Ar, Harley JB. Multiple myeloma and pernicious anemia. W VA Med J 1970;66:38–41.
21. Bader PI, Biegel A, Epinette WW, et al. Vitiligo and dysgammaglobulinemia. A case report and family study. Clin Genet 1975;7:62–76.
22. Marsh JH, Colbourn DS, Donovan V, et al. Systemic Castelman's disease in association with Evans' syndrome and vitiligo. Med Pediatr Oncol 1990;18:169–172.
23. Durance RA. Myasthenia gravis, rheumatoid arthritis, vitiligo and autoimmune heamolytic anaemia. Proc R Soc Med 1971; 64:7–8.
24. Thivolet J, Ortonne JP, Monier JC, et al. Vitiligo, Thymusdefekt und autoimmunitateine hypothetische pathogenese. Der Hautarzt 1975;26:50–51.
25. Duvic M, Rapimi R, Hoots WK, et al. Human immunodeficiency virus–associated vitiligo: Expression of autoimmunity with immunodeficiency? J Am Acad Dermatol 1987;17:656–662.
26. Zelickson AS. The clinical use of electron microscopy in dermatology. Minneapolis: Bolger Publications, 1985:41.
27. Shah VC, Mojamdar MV, Sharma KS. Some genetic, biochemical and physiological aspects of leucoderma vitiligo. J Cytol Genet Congr 1975(Suppl):173–178.
28. Shah VC, Haribhakti PB, Mojamdar MV, et al. Statistical study of 600 vitiligo cases in the city of Ahmedabad. Gujarat Med J 1977;42:51–59.
29. Majumder PP, Das DK, Li CC. A genetical model for vitiligo. Am J Hum Genet 1988;43:119–125.
30. Majumder P, Nordlund JJ, Nath SK. Pattern of familial aggregation of vitiligo. Arch Dermatol 1993;129:994–998.
31. Le Poole IC, van den Wijingaard RMJGJ, Westerhof W, et al. Presence or absence of melanocytes in vitiligo lesions: An immunohistochemical investigation. J Invest Dermatol 1993; 100:816–822.
32. Cui J, Shan L, Wang G. Role of hair follicles in the repigmentation of vitiligo. J Invest Dermatol 1991;97:410–416.
33. Bleehen SS. Histology of vitiligo. In: Klaus SN, ed. Pigment Cell 5: Part II of Proceedings of the Xth International Pigment Cell Conference, Cambridge, Massachusetts, 1977. Basel/New York: S. Karger, 1979:54–61.
34. Moellmann G, Klein-Angerer S, Scollay D, et al. Extacellular granular material and degeneration of keratinocytes in the normally pigmented epidermis of patients with vitiligo. J Invest Dermatol 1982;79:321–330.
35. Schallreuter KU, Pittelkow MR, Wood JM. Free radical reduction by thioredoxin reductase at the surface of normal and vitiliginous human keratinocytes. J Invest Dermatol 1986;87:728–732.
36. Schallreuter KU, Pittelkow MR. Defective calcium uptake system in vitiligo. Arch Dermatol Res 1988;280:137–139.
37. Schallreuter KU, Levenig C, Berger J. Vitiligo and cutaneous melanoma: A case study. Dermatologica 1991;183:239–245.
38. Schallreuter KU, Pittelkow MR, Swanson N, et al. High expression of beta 2-adrenoreceptors in vitiligo (abstract). J Invest Dermatol 1992;98:542.
39. Puri N, Mojamdar M, Ramaiah A. In vitro growth characteristics of melanocytes obtained from adult normal and vitiligo subjects. J Invest Dermatol 1987;88:434–438.
40. Puri N, Mojamdar M, Ramaiah A. Growth defects of melanocytes in culture from vitiligo subjects are spontaneously corrected in vivo in repigmenting subjects and can be partially corrected by the addition of fibroblast-derived growth factors in vitro. Arch Dermatol Res 1989;281:178–184.
41. Medrano EE, Nordlund JJ. Successful culture of adult human melanocytes from normal and vitiligo donors. J Invest Dermatol 1990;95:441–445.
42. Boissy RE, Liu Y-Y, Medrano EE, et al. Structural aberration of the rough endoplasmic reticulum and melanosome compartmentalization in long-term cultures of melanocytes from vitiligo patients. J Invest Dermatol 1991;97:395–404.
43. Bajaj AK, Gupta SC, Chatterjee AK. Contact depigmentation from free para-tertiary-butylphenol in bindi adhesive. Contact Dermatitis 1990;22:99–102.
44. Bleehen SS. The treatment of hypermelanosis with 4-isopropylcatechol. Br J Dermatol 1976;94:687–694.
45. Gellin GA, Possick PA, Perone VB. Depigmentation from 4-tertiary butyl catechol: An experimental study. J Invest Dermatol 1970;55:190–197.
46. Malten KE, Seutter E, Hara I, et al. Occupational vitiligo due to paratertiary butylphenol and homologues. Trans St. John's Hosp Dermatol Soc 1971;57:115–134.
47. Hochstein P, Cohen G. The cytotoxicity of melanin precursors. Ann N Y Acad Sci 1963;100:876–881.
48. Bowers RR, Harmon J, Prescott S, et al. Fowl model for vitiligo: Genetic regulation on the fate of the melanocytes. Pigment Cell Res 1992(Suppl. 2):242–248.
49. Cunliffe WJ, Hall R, Newell DJ, et al. Vitiligo, thyroid diseases and autoimmunity. Br J Dermatol 1968;80:135–139.
50. Hertz K, Gazze L, Kirkpatrick C, et al. Autoimmune vitiligo. Detection of antibodies to melanin-producing cells. N Engl J Med 1977;297:634–637.
51. Naughton GK, Eisinger M, Bystryn J-C. Antibodies to normal human melanocytes in vitiligo. J Exp Med 1983;158:246–251.
52. Xia P, Geoghegan WD, Duvic M, et al. Western blot analysis of vitiligo and alopecia areata autoantibody reactivity with cultured normal human melanocytes (abstract). J Invest Dermatol 1992;98:630.
53. Bystryn JC, Naughton GK. The significance of vitiligo antibodies. J Dermatol 1985;12:1–19.
54. Bystryn JC, Pfeffer S. Vitiligo and antibodies to melanocytes. In: Bagnara JT, ed. Advances in Pigment Cell Research. New York: Alan R. Liss, 1988:195–206.
55. Harning R, Cui J, Bystryn JC. Relationship between the incidence and level of pigment cell antibodies and disease activity in vitiligo. J Invest Dermatol 1991;97:1078–1080.
56. Naughton GK, Mahaffey M, Bystryn J-C. Antibodies to surface antigens of pigmented cells in animals with vitiligo. Proc Soc Exp Biol Med 1986;181:423–426.
57. Austin LM, Boissy RE, Jacobson BS, et al. The detection of melanocyte autoantibodies in the Smyth chicken model for vitiligo. Clin Immunol Immunopathol 1992;64:112–120.
58. Searle EA, Austin LM, Boissy YL, et al. Smyth chicken melanocyte autoantibodies: Cross-species recognition, in vivo binding, and plasma membrane reactivity of the antiserum. Pigment Cell Res 1993;6:145–157.
59. Aronson PJ, Hashimoto K. Association of IgA anti-melanoma antibodies in the sera of vitiligo patients with active disease (abstract). J Invest Dermatol 1987;88:475.
60. Naughton GK, Reggiardo MD, Bystryn JC. Correlation between vitiligo antibodies and extent of depigmentation in vitiligo. J Am Acad Dermatol 1986;15:978–981.
61. Cui J, Harning R, Henn M, et al. Identification of pigment cell antigen defined by vitiligo antibodies. J Invest Dermatol 1992;98:162–165.
62. Norris DA, Kissinger GM, Naughton GM, et al. Evidence for immunologic mechanisms in human vitiligo: Patients' sera induce damage to human melanocytes in vitro by complement-mediated damage and antibody-dependent cellular cytotoxicity. J Invest Dermatol 1988;90:783–789.
63. Cui J, Arita Y, Bystryn J-C. Cytolytic antibodies to melanocytes in vitiligo. J Invest Dermatol 1993;100:812–815.

64. Ghoneum M, Grimes PE, Gill G, et al. Natural cell-mediated cytotoxicity in vitiligo. J Am Acad Dermatol 1987;17:600–605.
65. Halder RM, Walters CS, Johnson BA, et al. T-lymphocytes and interleukin 2 activity are decreased in vitiligo. Presented at the XIIIth International Pigment Cell Conference, Tucson, 1986.
66. Grimes PE, Ghoneum M, Stockton T, et al. T-cell profiles in vitiligo. J Am Acad Dermatol 1986;14:196–201.
67. D'Amelio R, Frati C, Fattorossi A, et al. Peripheral T-cell subset imbalance in patients with vitiligo and in their apparently healthy first-degree relatives. Ann Allergy 1990;2:143–145.
68. Abdel Nasser MB, Ludwig WD, Gollnick H, et al. Non-segmental vitiligo: Decrease of the CD45RA$^+$ T-cells subset and evidence for peripheral T-cell activation. Int J Dermatol 1992;31:321–326.
69. Hatchome N, Aiba S, Kato T, et al. Possible functional impairment of Langerhans cells in vitiliginous skin: Reduced ability to elicit dinitrochlorobenzene contact sensitivity reaction and decreased stimulatory effect in the allogeneic mixed skin cell lymphocyte culture reaction. Arch Dermatol 1987;123:51–54.
70. Uehara M, Miyauchi H, Tanaka S. Diminished contact sensitivity response in vitiliginous skin. Arch Dermatol 1984;120:195–198.
71. Nordlund JJ, Forget B, Kirkwood J, et al. Dermatitis produced by applications of monobenzone in patients with active vitiligo. Arch Dermatol 1985;121:1141–1145.
72. Spritz RA. The molecular basis of human piebaldism. Pigment Cell Res 1992;5:340–343.
73. Zackheim HS, Epstein EH Jr, Grekin DA, McNutt NS. Mycosis fungoides presenting as areas of hypopigmentation. J Am Acad Dermatol 1982;6:340–345.
74. Nordlund JJ, Halder RM, Grimes P. Management of vitiligo. Dermatol Clin 1993;11:27–33.
75. Plott RT, Wagner RF. Modern treatment approaches to vitiligo. Cutis 1990;45:311–316.
76. Suvanprakorn P, Dee-Ananlap S, Pongsomboon C, et al. Melanocyte autologous grafting for the treatment of leukoderma. J Am Acad Dermatol 1985;13:968–974.
77. Falabella R. Repigmentation of segmental vitiligo by autologous minigrafting. Arch Dermatol 1988;9:514–521.
78. Falabella R. Treatment of localized vitiligo by autologous minigrafting. Arch Dermatol 1988;124:1649–1655.
79. Koga M. Epidermal grafting using the tops of suction blisters in the treatment of vitiligo. Arch Dermatol 1988;124:1656–1658.
80. Zachariae H, Zachariae C, Deleuran B, et al. Autotransplantation in vitiligo: Treatment with epidermal grafts and cultured melanocytes. Acta Derm Venereol (Stockh) 1993;73:46–48.
81. Kahn AM, Cohen MJ, Kaplan L, et al. Vitiligo: Treatment by dermabrasion and epithelial sheet grafting—a preliminary report. J Am Acad Dermatol 1993;28:773–774.
82. Brysk MM, Newton RC, Rajaraman S, et al. Repigmentation of vitiliginous skin by cultured cells. Pigment Cell Res 1989;2:202–207.
83. Plott RT, Brysk MM, Newton R, et al. A surgical treatment for vitiligo: Transplantation of autologous cultured epithelial grafts. J Dermatol Surg Oncol 1989;15:1161–1166.
84. Lerner AB, Halaban R, Klaus SN, et al. Transplantation of human melanocytes. J Invest Dermatol 1987;89:219–224.
85. Lerner AB. Repopulation of pigment cells in patients with vitiligo. Arch Dermatol 1988;124:1701–1702.
86. Olsson MJ, Juhlin L. Repigmentation of vitiligo by transplantation of cultured autologous melanocytes. Acta Derm Venereol (Stockh) 1993;73:49–51.
87. Olsson MJ, Juhlin L, Lerner AB. Repigmentation in vitiligo by pigment cell transplantation (abstract). Pigment Cell Res 1993;6:286.
88. Halaban R, Langdon R, Birchall N, et al. Basic fibroblast growth factor from human keratinocytes is a natural mitogen for melanocytes. J Cell Biol 1988;107:1611–1619.
89. Halaban R, Rubin JS, Funasaka Y, et al. Met and hepatocyte growth factor/scatter factor signal transduction in normal melanocytes and melanoma cells. Oncogene 1992;7:2195–2206.
90. Imokawa G, Yada Y, Miyagishi M. Endothelins secreted from human keratinocytes are intrinsic mitogens for human melanocytes. J Biol Chem 1992;267:24675–24680.
91. Halder RM, Pham HN, Breadon JY, et al. Micropigmentation for the treatment of vitiligo. J Dermatol Surg Oncol 1989;15:1092–1098.

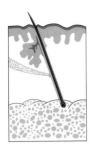

chapter 131

Albinism and Other Disorders of Hypopigmentation

JEAN L. BOLOGNIA and PHILIP E. SHAPIRO

The clinical findings in disorders of hypopigmentation other than vitiligo are the focus of this chapter. These diseases can be divided into several categories, including diffuse versus circumscribed, inherited versus acquired, and amelanotic (complete lack of melanin) versus hypomelanotic (partial decrease in melanin). An absence of melanocytes, a decrease in the number of melanocytes, and a decrease in the function of melanocytes are three major explanations for the observed decrease or absence of pigmentation.

Application of the tools of molecular biology has led to significant advances in understanding the types of genetic mutations that can give rise to diseases such as oculocutaneous albinism and piebaldism. A specific genetic abnormality has been identified in patients with type I Waardenburg's syndrome, and there has been exciting progress in the areas of clinical criteria and pathogenesis for two other diseases, tuberous sclerosis and hypomelanosis of Ito. Although perhaps less profound, new information is available as well on more common disorders such as idiopathic guttate hypomelanosis and hypopigmentation secondary to inflammation or infections. The major goal of this chapter is to simplify the approach to a patient with a disorder of hypopigmentation while at the same time providing insight into pathophysiology.

Oculocutaneous and Ocular Albinism

In oculocutaneous albinism (OCA), reduced or absent melanin production leads to pigmentary dilution of the eyes, hair, and skin. The degree of diffuse hypopigmentation that is observed is dependent on the specific type of OCA as well as the racial background of the patient. In the past, OCA was divided into two major clinical categories: tyrosinase-negative and tyrosinase-positive. This distinction was based on the presence or absence of melanin pigment and tyrosinase activity in the hair or skin of these patients.[1] Tyrosinase is the major enzyme in the melanin biosynthetic pathway and therefore plays a key role in determining the degree of pigmentation.

At birth, individuals with albinism often have a similar appearance: the hair is white, the eyes are gray to blue, and the skin is pink to white. If the parents and siblings are skin type I or even II,[2] the pigmentary dilution may go unnoticed. Individuals with tyrosinase-positive OCA may have lightly pigmented hair at birth, but as they age there is darkening of hair, eye, and skin color, the degree of which is dependent on racial background and the particular subtype of OCA (Table 131–1).[1] For example, a person with OCA and skin types IV or V can develop lentigines (Fig. 131–1) and red to light brown hair and, if seen in the absence of their relatives, can be mistaken for an unaffected person with skin type I or II. However, a major clue to the diagnosis of OCA is the presence of ophthalmic abnormalities including nystagmus, decreased visual acuity, monocular vision, and photophobia. The decreased visual acuity is thought to be related to hypoplasia of the fovea (a relatively hyperpigmented portion of the retina), and the monocular vision is a reflection of a decrease in the ipsilateral fibers that run from the temporal retina to the visual cortex through the lateral geniculate body.[3]

With the advent of molecular biology, there have been further refinements in the categorization of patients with OCA. One major group is now referred to as type I

TABLE 131-1. Clinical Characteristics of the Different Forms of Oculocutaneous Albinism

Characteristic	Type IA, ty-neg	Type IB, Ym	Type I, Ts	Type I, Minimal Pigment
Hair	White throughout life	White at birth; yellow-red by 6 months	White at birth; develops slight yellow tint (scalp); lower leg hair dark brown*	White at birth to white or very slight yellow in adults
Skin color	Pink to red	White at birth; cream, slight tan on exposed skin	Creamy white; slight tan	Pink-white, no tan
Pigmented nevi and freckles	Absent (nevi are nonpigmented)	Present	Present	Absent
Susceptibility to skin neoplasia	++++	++	Unknown, probably ++++	Unknown, probably ++++
Eye color	Gray to blue	Blue in infancy; darkens with age	Blue	Gray to blue
Transillumination of iris	No pigment	Cartwheel in adults	No pigment	Pigment in pupil, clumps at limbus
Red reflex	Present	Present	Present	Present
Fundal pigment	0	Present	0	0 to ? in adults
Nystagmus	++++	+ to +++	++++	++++
Photophobia	++++	+ to ++	++++	++++
Visual acuity	Most legally blind; constant or worse with age; 20/200 to 20/400+	20/90 to 20/400	20/200	20/160 to 20/200
Melanosomes in hair bulbs	Stages I and II only	To stage III pheomelanosomes	Stages I, II (scalp hair); stages II, III, IV (leg hair)	Late stage II, some with melanin
Incubation of hair bulbs in tyrosine	No pigmentation	None to questionable	None (scalp hair)	Unknown
Gene mutations	Tyrosinase gene (>35 different mutations lead to absence of enzymatic activity)[13] (t-/t-)	Tyrosinase gene (1 allele as in IA and 1 allele decreased enzyme activity vs two alleles decreased enzyme activity) (t-/y vs y/y)	Tyrosinase gene (1 allele as in IA and 1 allele enzyme less active at higher temperatures)[‡]	Tyrosinase gene (1 allele as in IA and 1 allele decreased enzyme activity)
Other	Heterozygotes have near zero tyrosinase activity; prenatal diagnosis possible by biopsy of scalp[17,18]	Hair bulb test shows increased red or yellow with tyrosine-cysteine incubation	Hair bulb tyrosinase assay; loss of activity above 35°C–37°C; temperature-sensitive mutation	Heterozygotes have zero to normal tyrosinase activity

Ym, yellow mutant; Ts, temperature sensitive; ty-pos, tyrosinase positive; HPS, Hermansky-Pudlak syndrome; CHS, Chédiak-Higashi syndrome.
  * Axillary hair remains white; pubic hair dark yellow to light brown color; forearm hair reddish blond; relatively warm body parts (eyes, skin, hair of the scalp and axilla) remained unpigmented, but less warm parts (facial and pubic hair) developed slight pigmentation and relatively cool parts (arm and leg hair) became well pigmented.
  †Differential diagnosis of silver hair includes Griscelli/PAID, Elejalde's and pseudothalidomide syndromes.
  ‡Human homologue of the Siamese cat and Himalayan mouse.
  §Human homologue of the pink-eyed dilution (p) locus in the mouse.
  Adapted from Witkop CJ, Quevedo WC, Fitzpatrick TB, et al. Albinism. In: The Metabolic Basis of Inherited Disease, 6th ed. New York: McGraw-Hill, 1989:2905–2947. Reproduced with permission of McGraw-Hill.

Type II, ty-pos	Type IV, Brown OCA	Type V, Rufous OCA	Type VIA, HPS	Type VIB, CHS	Type VII, Autosomal Dominant OCA
White, yellow tan; darkens with age	Beige to light brown in Africans	Mahogany red to deep red	White, red, brown	Blond to dark brown; steel-gray tint†	White to cream with reddish tint
Pink-white to cream, lentigines but no tan	Cream to light tan on exposed skin; tans lightly	Reddish brown	Cream-gray to light normal	Pink to pink-white	White to cream
May be present and numerous	Uncommon	May be present	Present	Present	May be present
++++	Similar to whites in Africa+	Low	+++	++	Unknown
Blue, yellow-brown; age and race dependent	Hazel to light tan	Reddish brown to brown	Blue-gray to brown; age and race dependent	Blue to dark brown	Gray to blue
Pigment at pupil and limbus or cartwheel	Cartwheel effect	Slight	None to cartwheel effect	Cartwheel effect to normal	Translucent to cartwheel effect
May be absent in darker-race adults	Present in children; may be absent in adults	Unknown	Present in fair-skinned individuals; not in dark races	Present, less after 5 years	Present in children
0 to + in adults	+ to +++ in adults	+ to +++	0 to + in adults	+ to +++	0 to +
++ to +++	+ to ++	0 to ++	+ to +++	+ to ++	++ to +++
++ to +++	+ to ++	0 to ++	+ to ++++	+ to ++	++ to +++
Children, severe defect; adults, same or better; 20/200 to 20/400+	20/30 to 20/150	Normal to 20/100, most 20/30	20/70 to 20/400	Normal to moderate decrease	20/70 to 20/200
To stage III, eumelanosomes	Stage I to Stage II, some lightly pigmented stage IV	Unknown	To stage III, pheomelanosomes and eumelanosomes	Macromelanosomes and normal to stage IV	Stage I to early stage III; no structural abnormality
Pigmentation marked	Slight to no pigment increase	Pigmentation	Pigmentation slight increase	Pigmentation	Pigmentation; increased tyrosinase activity in Golgi bodies
P gene (chromosome 15q)§	Unknown	Unknown	? pallid gene	Unknown	Unknown
³Tyrosinase assay suggests heterogeneity	Tyrosinase activity normal; seen in New Guineans, Africans, and black Americans	Seen in New Guineans and Africans	Lysosomal disease, platelet-dense granules absent; ceroid storage (symptomatic in lungs and gastrointestinal tract); heterozygotes detected by low thioredoxin reductase; more common in Puerto Ricans and Dutch	Lysosomal disease; susceptibility to infection; giant lysosomal granules; platelet-dense granules can be absent; lymphoreticular malignancy	

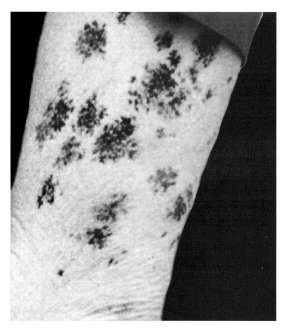

FIGURE 131-1. Lentigines in a patient with type II (tyrosinase-positive) OCA. (Courtesy of Odette Fournier-Blake, M.D.)

OCA or tyrosinase-related OCA; the latter name reflects the identification of abnormalities in the tyrosinase gene in these patients. Under the new classification, type I OCA encompasses tyrosinase-negative (type IA), yellow mutant (Ym; type IB), temperature-sensitive (Ts), and minimal pigment OCA (see Table 131-1).[4-9] Persons previously referred to as tyrosinase positive are now categorized primarily as type II OCA,[10, 11] but a number of whites have been reclassified as type IB (Ym). One clinical clue that points to the diagnosis of type IB (Ym) OCA rather than type II OCA is the history of white hair at birth (type II patients have pigmented hair at birth [King R, personal communication]). Because it is important to identify those individuals with Hermansky-Pudlak syndrome or Chédiak-Higashi disease (see Table 131-1), the evaluation of a patient with OCA should include ancestry as well as the possible history of a bleeding diathesis, recurrent infections, or shortness of breath.[12]

Because OCA is inherited as an autosomal recessive trait, both parents are presumed to be carriers of an abnormal gene. In patients with type I OCA (see Table 131-1), molecular studies have shown mutations in both copies of the tyrosinase gene (located on chromosome 11q); these mutations are the same (homozygous) in some patients, while in the majority they are different (compound heterozygotes).[13] For example, in a compound heterozygote, one copy of the tyrosinase gene may have a single nucleotide substitution that leads to an amino acid substitution (missense mutation) while the second copy may have a base deletion that leads to premature termination (frameshift mutation; Fig. 131-2).[14, 15] When the sites of the mutations are mapped, there is clustering at the putative copper-binding sites and in exon 1 and 4[16]; the tyrosinase gene has 5 exons (regions of the DNA that are transcribed into mRNA as opposed to regions that are spliced out called introns).

Diagnosis of OCA at an early age is important so that recommendations can be made regarding daily sunscreen use and limited sun exposure. Referral to an ophthalmologist for longitudinal care is also indicated. For an improved cosmetic appearance, the patient can try creams that contain dihydroxyacetone. As patients enter their 20s, they need to have total-body skin examinations on a regular basis to detect cutaneous malignancies, especially squamous cell carcinoma. In regions near the equator, squamous cell carcinoma is a leading cause of morbidity and mortality in individuals with OCA.[19]

Pigmentary dilution of the hair, eyes, and skin can also be seen in patients with phenylketonuria. Because of a deficiency in phenylalanine hydroxylase, the enzyme that converts phenylalanine to tyrosine, there is an accumulation of the former metabolite. Possible explanations for the associated pigmentary dilution include a decrease in the amount of tyrosine available for melanin production, an inhibition of tyrosinase by phenylalanine, and the possibility that phenylalanine hydroxylase is involved in melanin biosynthesis.[20, 21] In the United States, however, it is unusual to see such patients because of mandatory screening for phenylketonuria in infants.

Generalized pigmentary dilution (eye, skin, hair) can also be seen in patients with the Prader-Willi syndrome, Angelman's syndrome, histidinemia, homocystinuria, and Apert's syndrome.[20-24] Deletions in the *P* gene (human homologue for the pink-eyed dilution gene [*p*] in the mouse) on chromosome 15q have been identified in the first two entities and therefore explain their overlap with type II OCA.[10, 25] Hypopigmentation of the hair and skin can be seen in individuals with copper deficiency, Menkes' kinky hair syndrome, malabsorption secondary to chronic pancreatic disease, selenium deficiency,

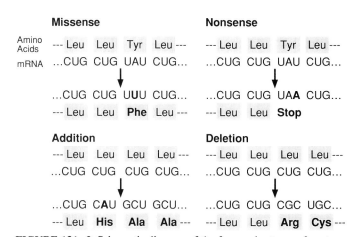

FIGURE 131-2. Schematic diagram of the four major types of mutations seen in the tyrosinase gene in patients with type I OCA. Because nonsense mutations cause premature chain termination, the remaining polypeptide fragment is almost always nonfunctional. An addition or deletion of any number of nucleotides that is not a multiple of three will produce a frameshift, hence the term *frameshift mutation*. Unless this occurs near the carboxyl terminus of a protein, a nonfunctional protein results. (Adapted from Hartl DL. Basic Genetics, 2nd ed. © 1991, Boston: Jones & Bartlett Publishers. Reprinted with permission.)

kwashiorkor, and the EEC (ectrodactyly, ectodermal dysplasia, and clefting) syndrome.[20, 26-28] Generalized vitiligo is distinguished by its progressive nature, lack of eye findings characteristic of OCA, and, if present, prematurely gray (not lightly colored) hair. In addition, biopsy specimens of skin from patients with OCA contain a normal number of melanocytes.

Individuals with ocular albinism (OA) have the same eye findings as in OCA, but pigmentary dilution of the hair and skin is either absent or more subtle. There are cutaneous clues that aid in the diagnosis of the correct subtype (e.g., hypopigmented macules in individuals with X-linked Nettleship OA and multiple lentigines in the autosomal dominant form of OA [Table 131–2]).[29, 30] Two forms of OA are inherited in an X-linked recessive pattern, and the female carriers are mosaics for the mutation as a result of the Lyon phenomenon.[31] This is reflected in a striated pigmentary pattern in the peripheral retina[32] as well as an alternating spokewheel-like pattern in the iris (alternating normal and hypopigmentation).[33] In the two X-linked variants, both affected males and female carriers have macromelanosomes in the melanocytes, keratinocytes, and dermal macrophages of normal skin.[29, 34]

Piebaldism

In this autosomal dominant disorder, the areas of leukoderma are congenital and, in the majority of cases, stable in relative size and configuration. There are a few case reports of spontaneous expansion and contraction of the leukoderma.[35, 36] The cutaneous lesions favor the midforehead, the ventral trunk, and the midportions of the extremities but routinely spare the midline of the back.[37, 38] Within the patches of leukoderma, macules of normal and hyperpigmented skin 1 to 5 cm in diameter are often seen; the latter are frequently aligned at the border of involved and uninvolved skin (Fig. 131–3). Poliosis (circumscribed area of white hair) is seen most commonly in the midline of the frontal scalp as a white forelock (80%–90% patients; Table 131–3), but white hairs can also be found in the eyelashes, eyebrows, and areas of hypopigmentation. Multiple café-au-lait spots are often seen in uninvolved skin, and their presence does not require the diagnosis of a second genodermatosis.

TABLE 131–2. Comparison of the Characteristics of the Various Forms of Ocular Albinism

Characteristic	X-Linked (Nettleship)	X-Linked with Deafness	Autosomal Recessive Ocular Albinism	Ocular Albinism– Lentigines–Deafness
Hair color	Normal to slight lightening	Normal to slight lightening	Normal to slight lightening	Normal
Skin color	Normal to mild lightening	Normal to mild lightening	Normal to mild lightening	Normal
Pigmented nevi and freckles	Present	Present	Present	Lentigines
Susceptibility to skin neoplasia	No	No	No	Unknown
Eye color	Normal range	Normal range	Normal range	Normal range
Transillumination of iris	Cartwheel, females; diaphanous, males	Cartwheel, females; diaphanous, males	Cartwheel to diaphanous	Cartwheel to diaphanous
Red reflex	Present, males	Present, males	Present, males and female	Present
Fundal pigment	Males, 0; females, mosaic fundus	Males, 0; females, mosaic fundus	Males and females, 0 to +	0
Nystagmus	++ to ++++	++ to ++++	++ to ++++	+++
Photophobia	++ to +++	++ to +++	++ to +++	+++
Visual acuity	Moderate to severe decrease; 20/50 to 20/400	Moderate to severe decrease; 20/50 to 20/400	Moderate to severe decrease; 20/100 to 20/400	20/200
Melanosomes	Macromelanosomes in normal skin of hemizygotes and heterozygotes	Macromelanosomes in normal skin of hemizygotes and heterozygotes	Normal	Macromelanosomes in lentigines
Incubation of hair in tyrosine	Pigmentation	Pigmentation	Pigmentation	Unknown
Other	Hypomelanotic macules and patches in some individuals	High-frequency hearing loss; onset puberty to age 40 years	Males and females equally affected	Congenital sensorineural deafness; autosomal dominant

Adapted from Witkop CJ, Quevedo WC, Fitzpatrick TB, et al. Albinism. In: Scriver CR, Beaudet AL, Sly WS, et al., eds. The Metabolic Basis of Inherited Disease, 6th ed. New York: McGraw-Hill, 1989:2905–2947. Reproduced with permission of McGraw-Hill.

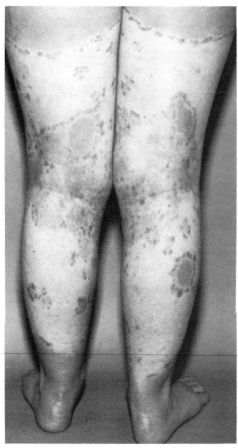

FIGURE 131–3. Leukoderma of the midportion of the lower extremities that had been present since birth in a patient with piebaldism. Note the sparing of the feet and the macules of hyperpigmentation at the border between involved and uninvolved skin. (From Pinto FJ, Bolognia JL. Disorders of hypopigmentation in children. Pediatr Clin 1991;38:991–1017.)

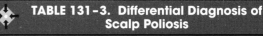

TABLE 131–3. Differential Diagnosis of Scalp Poliosis
Inflammatory or Autoimmune[20]
Alopecia areata (primarily initial cycle of regrowth) Post inflammation (e.g., discoid lupus, trauma) Halo nevus Vitiligo Vogt-Koyanagi-Harada syndrome Alezzandrini's syndrome
Inherited
Tuberous sclerosis Piebaldism (primarily midline frontal) Waardenburg's syndrome (primarily midline frontal) Isolated white forelock[38]* Isolated occipital white lock—X-linked recessive[38] White forelock with osteopathia striata—autosomal or X-linked dominant[39] White forelock with multiple malformations—autosomal or X-linked recessive†[40]
Nevoid
Associated with nevus comedonicus[41]
Idiopathic

*Possible forme fruste of piebaldism.

The majority of investigators have noted an absence of melanocytes or a markedly reduced number of melanocytes in the amelanotic areas.[36, 37, 42] However, in one study, melanocytes were observed in the areas of leukoderma,[43] but the argument was raised that biopsies were performed in the border zones between uninvolved and involved skin.[44] The consensus that there is a lack of melanocytes in the areas of leukoderma has led to the debate as to whether the cause of piebaldism is an abnormal melanocyte with aberrant migration or a normal melanocyte that cannot survive in an abnormal environment. Evidence existed for both theories from transplant experiments in mouse homologues (i.e., an abnormal melanocyte in the dominant white spotting [*W*] mouse and a hostile environment in the steel [*Sl*] mouse).[45]

Subsequent molecular characterization of the defect in the *W* mouse demonstrated point mutations or deletions in the *KIT* proto-oncogene.[46, 47] The *KIT* gene was first described as an oncogene in the feline sarcoma virus; it encodes for a cell-surface transmembrane receptor that when activated attaches phosphate groups to itself as well as to other proteins (sites of attachment are the amino acids serine and tyrosine). For this reason, the receptor is referred to as a tyrosine kinase receptor (Fig. 131–4). It

was later shown that the ligand for this receptor is the steel factor (i.e., a protein encoded by the *steel* locus and therefore abnormal in the *Sl* mutant mouse).[48] The steel factor has several names that reflect its biologic properties; these include mast cell growth factor, stem cell growth factor, and melanocyte growth factor.

In subsequent studies performed in human piebaldism, deletions in the *KIT* gene (chromosome segment 4q12) were observed as were at least nine different pathologic point mutations.[47, 49] As in the *W* mouse, the missense mutations favor the kinase domain of the receptor, which is responsible for the placement of phosphate groups onto amino acids. To date, no mutations in

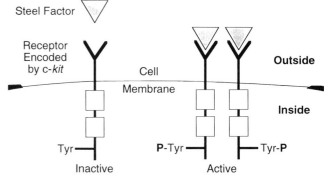

FIGURE 131–4. Schematic diagram of the c-*kit* receptor. When the ligand (steel factor) binds to the receptor, it is activated and phosphate groups are attached to tyrosine residues on the receptor and other proteins.

the *steel* locus have been described in patients with piebaldism.[47] However, there are individuals with this disease in whom no abnormalities in the *KIT* gene have been observed. In these cases, there may be involvement of the promoter region for the gene, its introns, or perhaps other "spotting genes."[47]

Treatment options in piebaldism are limited; psoralens and ultraviolet A light (PUVA) therapy[36, 43, 50] and grafts of cultured melanocytes[51] have been tried, but neither has produced cosmetically significant results.[52] In addition, tissue culture of melanocytes requires specialized facilities and is fairly expensive. Greater success has been reported with minigrafts of normally pigmented, autologous skin.[52, 53] It is important to screen patients with piebaldism for possible deafness and to be aware, especially in infants, of the association with Hirschsprung's disease (congenital megacolon; Table 131–4).[37, 54–62] The latter association is also seen in at least three strains of mice with white spotting[63] and reflects an abnormality in the embryonic migration of two neural crest–derived elements: melanocytes and myenteric ganglion cells. In Woolf's syndrome (which is limited to one family of Native Americans), the changes of piebaldism were seen in addition to deafness.[55]

Waardenburg's Syndrome

The classic sextad of Waardenburg's syndrome consists of dystopia canthorum, a broad nasal root, confluent eyebrows, iris heterochromia (total or partial), congenital sensorineural hearing loss (unilateral or bilateral), and a white forelock or piebaldism.[64] In addition to the latter cutaneous findings (seen in 15% to 60% of patients depending on the series), premature graying of the hair has also been reported.[38] Dystopia canthorum is defined as lateral displacement of the inner canthi in the presence of a normal interpupillary distance; clinically, this translates into a decrease in the extent of the medial portion of the sclerae that is visible. Although Waardenburg[64] reported an incidence of 99% for dystopia canthorum in his original series, the incidence in subsequent

TABLE 131–5. Three Types of Waardenburg's Syndrome*

Type	Features
Waardenburg's syndrome I	Piebaldism, heterochromic irides, dystopia canthorum, deafness
Waardenburg's syndrome II	Piebaldism, heterochromic irides, no dystopia canthorum, deafness (more common than in type I)
Klein-Waardenburg syndrome (WS III)	Piebaldism, heterochromic irides, dystopia canthorum, deafness, plus congenital anomalies of the upper limbs (hypoplasia of muscles, flexion contractures, axillary webs, fusion of carpal bones, syndactyly)

*Patients may have all or some of the physical findings listed.
Adapted from Gomez MR. Other autosomal dominant disorders. In: Neurocutaneous Disease: A Practical Approach. Stoneham, MA: Butterworth, 1987:91.

studies was significantly less.[65] These discrepancies have been resolved by dividing Waardenburg's syndrome into several forms (Table 131–5).[66] In addition, one family has been described in which members had ocular albinism plus a white forelock, congenital sensorineural hearing loss, and premature graying of the hair.[67]

In 1992, three groups of investigators reported mutations in the *Pax-3/HuP2* gene (chromosome 2q37) in families with type I Waardenburg's syndrome.[68–70] Other members of the *Pax* gene family were already known to be involved in embryogenesis and regulation of gene expression, and defects in *Pax* genes had been shown to cause developmental anomalies such as aniridia.[71, 72] As a group, *Pax* genes share a conserved sequence (the paired-box domain) that encodes a DNA-binding motif.[71] More recently, a mutation in the paired domain of the *Pax-3* gene was also found in a family with Klein-Waardenburg syndrome (see Table 131–5).[73] Waardenburg's syndrome, like piebaldism, can be associated with congenital megacolon (Hirschsprung's disease).[63, 74]

TABLE 131–4. Associated Findings in Patients with Piebaldism

Heterochromic irides[37,54*†]
Deafness[55–57*‡]
Mental retardation[56,58–61§]
Cerebellar ataxia[56]
Hirschsprung's disease[57‖]
Chondrodysplasia[62]
Pulmonic stenosis[57]

*Some cases may represent forme fruste of Waardenburg's syndrome.
†Includes isohypochromia (bilateral pale blue eyes).
‡Includes patients with Woolf's syndrome.
§Of five patients reported, four had deletions on chromosome 4.
‖Congenital megacolon secondary to underdevelopment of Auerbach's plexus (hypoganglionosis).

Nevus Depigmentosus

Nevus depigmentosus is a common birthmark, occurring in approximately 1 in 125 neonates.[75] There is usually a single, well-demarcated hypomelanotic macule or patch ranging in size from 0.5 to 10 cm. Less often, the distribution will be segmental or systematized (multiple streaks along the lines of Blaschko), raising the possibility of a somatic mutation early in embryogenesis.[20, 76] It is fairly simple to distinguish nevus depigmentosus from nevus anemicus because the boundary of the former does not disappear with diascopy. However, the ash-leaf spot of tuberous sclerosis can have the same clinical and histologic appearance as nevus depigmentosus with partial loss of pigment and a decreased to normal number of melanocytes.[42, 77]

In studies utilizing electron microscopy, a defect in the transfer of normal melanosomes from melanocytes to keratinocytes was reported in biopsy specimens of nevus depigmentosus whereas ash-leaf spots of tuberous sclerosis contained a decreased number of melanosomes that were poorly melanized.[42] Unfortunately, these ultrastructural differences may sometimes be subtle, and with the cost and limited availability of electron microscopy, the diagnosis is usually made clinically. If there is a single lesion and the child is asymptomatic, longitudinal observation is indicated; if there are multiple lesions or additional signs or symptoms suggestive of tuberous sclerosis (Table 131–6), then diagnostic imaging can be performed.

In African-Americans, group E pigmentary demarcation lines (hypopigmented bands or "lanceolate" areas on the upper chest) may be confused with nevus depigmentosus or ash-leaf spots. However, the demarcation lines tend to be bilaterally symmetrical and obliquely oriented.[78] Persons with multiple streaks of hypopigmentation must be evaluated for associated systemic abnormalities to exclude hypomelanosis of Ito (Table 131–7).

Hypomelanosis of Ito

Patients with hypomelanosis of Ito have multiple streaks of hypopigmentation in addition to systemic abnormalities, especially neurologic, musculoskeletal, and ocular. Associated findings include mental retardation, seizures, craniofacial dysmorphism, triphalangeal thumbs, and hypertelorism.[20, 79–82] The streaks of hypopigmentation can be unilateral (Fig. 131–5) or bilateral; and although the majority follow Blaschko's lines, lesions can also be patchy.[83] The lesions are usually present at birth but may appear in early childhood[79]; an increase in the extent of lesions during infancy can be followed by spontaneous repigmentation at a later age. Histologically, there is a reduction in the melanin content of the basal layer of the epidermis in association with either a normal or a decreased number of melanocytes; and in one report, the melanocytes were reduced in size with small dendrites.[79, 84, 85] In contrast to incontinentia pigmenti, no dermal melanophages are seen, and this is one of the reasons that the name hypomelanosis of Ito is favored over that of incontinentia pigmenti achromians.

Because the diagnosis of hypomelanosis of Ito must be made clinically, there has been an attempt to establish clinical criteria (see Table 131–7),[83] as was done in neurofibromatosis and tuberous sclerosis. One of the minor criteria listed in Table 131–7 is chromosomal mosaicism, which is detected by examination of peripheral lymphocytes and dermal fibroblasts. This association has been reported in more than 20 cases of hypomelanosis of

TABLE 131-6. Diagnostic Criteria for Tuberous Sclerosis Complex

Primary Features

Facial angiofibromas*
Multiple ungual fibromas*

Cortical tuber (histologically confirmed)
Subependymal nodule or giant cell astrocytoma (histologically confirmed)
Multiple calcified subependymal nodules protruding into the ventricle (radiographic evidence)
Multiple retinal astrocytomas*

Secondary Features

Shagreen patch*
Forehead plaque*

Affected first-degree relative
Cardiac rhabdomyoma (histologic or radiographic confirmation)
Cerebral tubers (radiographic confirmation)
Noncalcified subependymal nodules (radiographic confirmation)
Other retinal hamartoma or achromic patch*
Pulmonary lymphangiomyomatosis (histologic confirmation)
Renal angiomyolipoma (radiographic or histologic confirmation)
Renal cysts (histologic confirmation)

Tertiary Features

Hypomelanotic macules*
"Confetti" skin lesions*
Gingival fibromas*

Renal cysts (radiographic evidence)
Randomly distributed enamel pits in deciduous and/or permanent teeth
Hamartomatous rectal polyps (histologic confirmation)
Bone cysts (radiographic evidence)
Pulmonary lymphangiomyomatosis (radiographic evidence)
Cerebral white matter "migration tracts" or heterotopias (radiographic evidence)
Hamartoma of other organs (histologic confirmation)
Infantile spasms

Definite:

Either one primary feature, two secondary features, or one secondary plus two tertiary features

Probable:

Either one secondary plus one tertiary feature or three tertiary features

Suspect:

Either one secondary feature or two tertiary features

*Histologic confirmation is not required if the lesion is clinically obvious.

Adapted from Roach ES, Smith M, Huttenlocher P, et al. Report of the Diagnostic Criteria Committee of the National Tuberous Sclerosis Association. J Child Neurol 1992;7:221-224.

TABLE 131-7. Diagnostic Criteria for Hypomelanosis of Ito

Criterion	Features
1. Sine qua non	Congenital or early acquired nonhereditary cutaneous hypopigmentation in linear streaks or patches involving more than two body segments
2. Major	One or more nervous system anomalies; one or more musculoskeletal anomalies
3. Minor	Two or more congenital malformations other than nervous or musculoskeletal system; chromosomal anomalies
Definitive diagnosis	Criterion 1 plus one or more criterion 2 or two or more criterion 3
Presumptive diagnosis	Criterion 1 alone or in association with one minor criterion

Adapted from Ruiz-Maldonado R, Toussaint S, Tamayo L, et al. Hypomelanosis of Ito: Diagnostic criteria and report of 41 cases. Pediatr Dermatol 1992;9:1-10. Reprinted by permission of Blackwell Scientific Publications, Inc.

Ito, and the most common anomalies were diploid/triploid, trisomy 18, and tetrasomy 12p (Pallister).[83, 86-93] Chromosomal mosaicism provides an explanation for the hypothesis that hypomelanosis of Ito reflects the migration during embryogenesis of two clones of cells with different pigmentary potential.

Although chromosomal translocations have also been detected,[94, 95] a number of patients with hypomelanosis

of Ito do have normal karyotypes.[83, 96] Two explanations exist: (1) only lymphocytes, and not dermal fibroblasts, were examined (in one series, 61% [22/36] of the cases of mosaicism were abnormal only in the skin fibroblasts[86]), and (2) the patients with normal karotypes are mosaics, but for point mutations or deletions of a few base-pairs that were not detected by currently available techniques. Interestingly, Turleau and colleagues[97] reported one patient with hypomelanosis of Ito who had mosaicism for a microdeletion of 15q1, which is the location of the *P* gene that is involved in type II OCA.[10, 11, 98]

In the differential diagnosis, the major consideration is systematized nevus depigmentosus, and the distinction is made by the lack of associated systemic abnormalities. Of note, however, some clinicians prefer to categorize patients as manifesting hypomelanosis of Ito either with or without systemic abnormalities. Table 131-8 is a list of additional disorders in which linear lesions of hypopigmentation can be found; pigmentary demarcation lines, group C and group E, are included in that list because the former represent longitudinal hypopigmented bands on the chest that result from two side-by-side pigmentary demarcation lines and the latter can resemble nevus depigmentosus.[78] Although the majority of the cases of hypomelanosis of Ito are sporadic,[92] confusion has arisen as a result of several families who were misdiagnosed as having hypomelanosis of Ito because the authors were unaware of the fourth, hypopigmented phase of incontinentia pigmenti.[99]

Tuberous Sclerosis

As reported in 1968, one of the earliest clinical signs of tuberous sclerosis is multiple hypopigmented macules (approximately 10% of patients have only one hypopigmented macule).[20, 100] The most common locations for these lesions are the trunk and lower extremities, and the most common shapes are polygonal, oval, and lance-ovate (round at one end and pointed at the other); it is this last shape that led to the name "ash-leaf spot" because of the resemblance to the leaflet of the Eastern mountain ash tree.[100] In addition, patients with tuberous

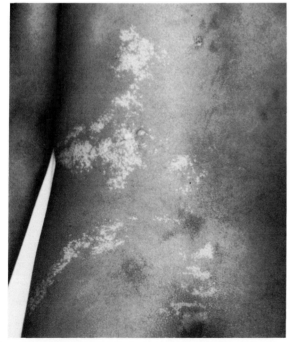

FIGURE 131-5. Streaks and splashes of hypopigmentation on the left side of the trunk in a patient with hypomelanosis of Ito. (Courtesy of Yale Dermatology Residents' Slide Collection.)

TABLE 131-8. Disorders with Linear Lesions of Hypopigmentation

Lesions follow Blaschko's lines
Hypomelanosis of Ito
Nevus depigmentosus
Mosaicism
Focal dermal hypoplasia (Goltz syndrome)
Menkes' kinky hair disease (female carriers)
Lichen striatus
Lesions may follow Blaschko's lines
Segmental vitiligo
Segmental ash-leaf spot
Fourth stage of incontinentia pigmenti
Lesions do not follow Blaschko's lines
Pigmentary demarcation lines, group C and E

sclerosis can have multiple 1- to 3-mm hypopigmented macules that are referred to as "confetti-like," poliosis of scalp hair, eyebrows, and eyelashes,[75, 101, 102] and hypopigmented spots of the iris and fundus.[102]

Histologically, in comparison to uninvolved skin, there is a decrease in the pigment content of the epidermis; however, a complete loss of pigment is not observed and melanocytes are present. By electron microscopy, the melanosomes in the melanocytes are decreased in number and poorly melanized[42, 103]; although distinctions have been made between these electron microscopic findings and those of nevus depigmentosus (the major entity in the differential diagnosis), the differences are not always clear cut. For this reason plus the cost and limited availability of electron microscopy, the diagnosis of ash-leaf spot of tuberous sclerosis versus nevus depigmentosus is usually made clinically based on longitudinal observation and the clinical criteria for tuberous sclerosis (see Table 131–6).[104] The incidence of tuberous sclerosis is less than 1 in 30,000 as compared with 1 in 120 for nevus depigmentosus.

Both the hypopigmented macules and the confetti-like lesions are considered tertiary features of tuberous sclerosis (see Table 131–6) and therefore raise the possibility of this genodermatosis, but do not by themselves fulfill the clinical criteria. In light-skinned persons, detection of these lesions can be enhanced by illumination with Wood's lamp. Multiple facial angiofibromas and multiple ungual fibromas represent the primary cutaneous features of tuberous sclerosis, and the presence of either of these in a patient is sufficient to make a definite diagnosis of tuberous sclerosis. Shagreen patch and forehead plaque[105] are secondary features of tuberous sclerosis and, histologically, altered collagen can be seen in both. Although nevus depigmentosus is the major consideration in the differential diagnosis of oval or polygonal ash-leaf spots, there are several disorders in which guttate hypomelanotic macules are seen (Table 131–9).[106-111]

As a result of advances in the field of diagnostic imaging, cardiac rhabdomyomas as a manifestation of tuberous sclerosis have been detected by echography prenatally as early as 22 weeks of gestation.[112] Approximately 50% of asymptomatic cardiac rhabdomyomas are associated with tuberous sclerosis[113]; therefore, if such lesions are detected on routine prenatal screening, complete skin examination of family members is indicated.[114] Up to 58% (25/43) of children (defined as younger than 18 years of age) with tuberous sclerosis have evidence of cardiac rhabdomyomas by echography,[115] and this represents a noninvasive procedure for children with multiple hypopigmented macules or the diagnosis of probable or suspect tuberous sclerosis by clinical criteria (see Table 131–6). If further evaluation is indicated, computed tomography and magnetic resonance imaging are sensitive in the detection of associated calcifications or cerebral tubers, 96% and 94%, respectively.[116, 117] In addition, magnetic resonance imaging of a fetus can be performed and the diagnosis of tuberous sclerosis by this method has been made in utero.[118]

Idiopathic Guttate Hypomelanosis

Idiopathic guttate hypomelanosis is a very common disorder, affecting approximately 50% of individuals in their 40s and more than 70% of those in their 60s.[119] The lesions are well demarcated, range in size from 2 to 6 mm, and favor the extensor surfaces of the upper and lower extremities. Because of this distribution, sun exposure is assumed to play a role in this disorder. However, the lack of involvement of the face has led to alternative explanations, such as somatic mutations.[120] The characteristic sharply angulated outlines are a reflection of the borders respecting skin lines. In biopsy specimens, there is also a sharp demarcation in the melanin content of the basal layer between uninvolved and involved skin and there is epidermal atrophy. Melanocytes may be reduced in number but are not completely gone, which contrasts with the absence of melanocytes seen in fully developed lesions of vitiligo.[121]

Treatment options are limited, but successful results were reported in 79 of 87 lesions of idiopathic guttate hypomelanosis in 10 patients after a light freeze with liquid nitrogen.[122] This may seem somewhat ironic, given the observation that melanocytes are more sensitive to freezing than are other cell types of the skin. Although patients and nondermatologists sometimes confuse idiopathic guttate hypomelanosis with vitiligo, the major differential diagnosis is the confetti-like lesions of tuberous sclerosis. Occasionally, guttate hypomelanotic lesions can be seen in patients with Darier's disease,[106] with biphasic amyloidosis,[107] and after PUVA therapy (see Table 131–9).[110]

TABLE 131–9. Differential Diagnosis of Multiple Guttate Hypomelanotic Macules

Idiopathic guttate hypomelanosis*
Confetti-like lesions of tuberous sclerosis
Pityriasis lichenoides chronica
Pityriasis alba
Darier's disease (admixed with keratotic lesions)[106]
Biphasic amyloidosis[107]
In association with keratosis punctata[108]
In association with chromosomal abnormalities[109]
Leukoderma punctata (after PUVA therapy)[110]
Disseminated hypopigmented keratoses[111†]
Lichen sclerosus et atrophicus‡

*Also referred to as angulated hypopigmented macules.
†Flat-topped papules.
‡Epidermal atrophy and follicular plugging.

Hypopigmentation Secondary to Inflammation or Neoplasms

Several common inflammatory disorders such as psoriasis and atopic dermatitis can resolve leaving areas of postinflammation hypopigmentation. The diagnosis is usually not difficult because of the presence of primary lesions. It is important to realize, however, that there are several disorders that can present as just hypopigmentation in the absence of classic primary lesions; these include atopic dermatitis (pityriasis alba), sarcoidosis (Fig. 13–6), mycosis fungoides (Fig. 131–7), pityriasis lichenoides chronica, lichen sclerosus et atrophicus, and alopecia mucinosa.[12, 123–126] In general, performing a biopsy in this group of diseases will provide more diagnostic information than in the primary disorders of hypopigmentation.

Pityriasis alba is a common disorder in children that favors the face[127]; histologically there is slight spongiosis and parakeratosis, and clinically fine scale is often seen. One theory for the associated hypopigmentation in pityriasis alba is a block in the transfer of melanosomes from melanocytes to keratinocytes as a result of inflammation and edema.[128] Treatment options include mild topical corticosteroids and emollients, but the response to therapy can be variable. In patients with extensive pityriasis alba, PUVA therapy has been used successfully.[129]

Hypopigmented lesions of sarcoidosis may be macular or papular, and biopsy specimens usually demonstrate dermal granulomas.[123] One patient with sarcoidosis did experience repigmentation of facial lesions following an 8-month course of PUVA.[130] Hypopigmented mycosis fungoides clinically consists of patches or slightly scaly plaques and histologically resembles early mycosis fungoides that is not hypopigmented;[124] by electron micros-

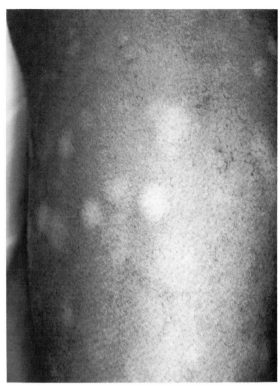

FIGURE 131–7. Hypopigmented macules and patches in a patient with mycosis fungoides, at the time of presentation. (Courtesy of Irwin M. Braverman, M.D.)

copy, degenerative changes in the melanocytes have been observed, as has disordered melanogenesis with spherical melanosomes.[124] Treatment with PUVA and topical alkylating agents has led to a reversal of the hypomelanosis.[131] In children with multiple, widespread hypopigmented macules, it is essential to search for the red-brown, slightly scaly papules that are characteristic of pityriasis lichenoides chronica.[125] Treatment options include topical corticosteroids, oral erythromycin, and ultraviolet B light.

Hypopigmentation Secondary to Infectious Diseases

Hypopigmentation of the skin is associated with several infectious agents, including the bacteria *Treponema pertenue*, *Treponema carateum*, and *Mycobacterium leprae*; the yeast *Pityrosporum orbiculare*; the protozoan *Leishmania donovani*; and the helminth *Onchocerca volvulus*. Hypomelanotic lesions are seen primarily in the tuberculoid and indeterminate forms of leprosy and perhaps a factor or factors released from histiocytes affects pigment production in this disease as well as sarcoidosis.[130] One possible explanation for the hypopigmented variant of pityriasis versicolor is the production of azelaic acid (an inhibitor of tyrosinase) from the breakdown of

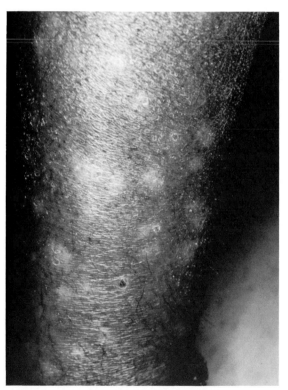

FIGURE 131–6. Hypopigmented macules and papules on the lower extremity of an individual with sarcoidosis. (From Bolognia JL. Disorders of hypopigmentation. Curr Concepts Skin Dis 1993;13:7–11; 16–17.)

fatty acids by the lipophilic yeast *Pityrosporum*.[132] Although the presence of hypopigmentation has no effect on the diagnostic pathologic findings or culture results in any of these infectious diseases, the hypomelanosis may persist despite an adequate response to appropriate therapy.

Acknowledgments

We wish to thank Seth Orlow, M.D., for helpful discussion, Donna Carroll for her excellent secretarial skills, and Steven R. Kohn, M.D., for his editorial suggestions.

References

1. Witkop CJ Jr, Quevedo WC Jr, Fitzpatrick TB, et al. Albinism. In: Scriver CR, Beaudet AL, Sly WS, et al., eds. The Metabolic Basis of Inherited Disease, 6th ed. New York: McGraw-Hill, 1989:2905–2947.
2. Melski JW, Tanenbaum L, Parrish JA, et al. Oral methoxsalen photochemotherapy for the treatment of psoriasis: A cooperative clinical trial. J Invest Dermatol 1977;68:328–335.
3. Witkop CJ, King RA, Creel DJ. The abnormal albino animal. Pigment Cell 1976;3:201–210.
4. Giebel LB, Strunk KM, King RA, et al. A frequent gene mutation in classic, tyrosinase-negative (type IA) oculocutaneous albinism. Proc Natl Acad Sci USA 1990;87:3255–3258.
5. Nance WE, Jackson CE, Witkop CJ Jr. Amish albinism: A distinctive autosomal recessive phenotype. Am J Hum Genet 1970;22:579–586.
6. Giebel LB, Tripathi RK, Strunk KM, et al. Tyrosinase gene mutations associated with type IB ("yellow") oculocutaneous albinism. Am J Hum Genet 1991;48:1159–1167.
7. King RA, Townsend D, Oetting W, et al. Temperature-sensitive tyrosinase associated with peripheral pigmentation in oculocutaneous albinism. J Clin Invest 1991;87:1046–1053.
8. Giebel LB, Tripathi RK, King RA, et al. A tyrosinase gene missense mutation in temperature-sensitive type I oculocutaneous albinism: A human homologue to the Siamese cat and the Himalayan mouse. J Clin Invest 1991;87:1119–1122.
9. King RA, Wirtschafeter JD, Olds DP, et al. Minimal pigment: A new type of oculocutaneous albinism. Clin Genet 1986;29:42–50.
10. Rinchik EM, Bultman SJ, Horsthemke B, et al. A gene for the mouse pink-eyed dilution locus and for human type II oculocutaneous albinism. Nature 1993;361:72–76.
11. Ramsay M, Colman MA, Stevens G, et al. The tyrosinase-positive oculocutaneous albinism locus maps to chromosome 15q11.2-q12. Am J Hum Genet 1992;51:879–884.
12. Bolognia JL, Pawelek JM. Biology of hypopigmentation. J Am Acad Dermatol 1988;19:217–255.
13. Oetting WS, King RA. Molecular basis of type I (tyrosinase-related) oculocutaneous albinism: Mutations and polymorphisms of the human tyrosinase gene. Hum Mutat 1993;2:1–6.
14. Harl DL. The molecular basis of mutation. In: Basic Genetics, 2nd ed. Boston: Jones & Barlett, 1991:365–367.
15. Oetting WS, Mentink MM, Summers CG, et al. Three different frameshift mutations of the tyrosinase gene in type IA oculocutaneous albinism. Am J Hum Genet 1991;49:199–206.
16. King RA, Mentink M, Oetting WS. Non-random distribution of missense mutations within the human tyrosinase gene in type I (tyrosinase-related) oculocutaneous albinism. Mol Biol Med 1991;8:19–29.
17. Eady RAJ, Gunner DB, Garner A, et al. Prenatal diagnosis of oculocutaneous albinism by electron microscopy of fetal skin. J Invest Dermatol 1983;80:210–212.
18. Shimizu H, Ishiko A, Kikuchi A, et al. Prenatal diagnosis of tyrosinase-negative oculocutaneous albinism. Lancet 1992;340:739–740.
19. Luande J, Henschke CI, Mohammed N. The Tanzanian human albino skin: Natural history. Cancer 1985;55:1823–1828.
20. Ortonne J-P, Mosher DB, Fitzpatrick TB. Genetic and congenital disorders. In: Ortonne J-P, Mosher DB, Fitzpatrick TB, eds. Viti-

ligo and Other Hypomelanoses of Hair and Skin. New York: Plenum Medical Book Co., 1983:59–466.
21. Breakefield XO, Castiglione CM, Halaban R, et al. Phenylalanine hydroxylase in melanoma cells. J Cell Physiol 1978;94:307–314.
22. Creel DJ, Bendel CM, Wiesner GL, et al. Abnormalities of the central visual pathways in Prader-Willi syndrome associated with hypopigmentation. N Engl J Med 1986;314:1606–1609.
23. Shapiro Fryburg J, Breg WR, Lindgren V. Diagnosis of Angelman syndrome in infants. Am J Med Genet 1991;38:58–64.
24. Margolis S, Siegel IM, Choy A, et al. Depigmentation of hair, skin, and eyes associated with the Apert syndrome. Birth Defects 1978;14:341–360.
25. Gardner JM, Nakatsu Y, Gondo Y, et al. The mouse pink-eyed dilution gene: Association with human Prader-Willi and Angelman syndromes. Science 1992;257:1121–1124.
26. Klaus SN. Acquired pigment dilution of the skin and hair: A sign of pancreatic disease of the tropics. Int J Dermatol 1980;19:508–509.
27. Vinton NE, Dahlstrom KA, Strobel CT, et al. Macrocytosis and pseudoalbinism: Manifestations of selenium deficiency. J Pediatr 1987;111:711–717.
28. Pries C, Mittelman D, Miller M, et al. The EEC syndrome. Am J Dis Child 1974;127:840–844.
29. O'Donnell FE, Hambrick GW, Green WR, et al. X-linked ocular albinism: An oculocutaneous macromelanosomal disorder. Arch Ophthalmol 1976;94:1883–1892.
30. Lewis RA. Ocular albinism and deafness. Am J Hum Genet 1978;30:57A.
31. Lyon MF. Gene action in the X-chromosome of the mouse. (*Mus musculus* L.). Nature 1961;190:372–373.
32. Lang GE, Rott H-D, Pfeiffer RA. X-linked ocular albinism: Characteristic pattern of affection in female carriers. Ophthalmol Paediatr Genet 1990;11:265–271.
33. Maguire AM, Maumenee IH. Iris pigment mosaicism in carriers of X-linked ocular albinism cum pigmento. Am J Ophthalmol 1989;107:298–299.
34. Yoshiike T, Manabe M, Hayakawa M, et al. Macromelanosomes in X-linked ocular albinism (XLOA). Acta Derm Venereol 1985;65:66–69.
35. Davis BK, Verdol LD. Expansion and contraction of hypomelanotic areas in human piebaldism. Hum Genet 1976;34:163–170.
36. Campbell B, Swift S. Partial albinism: Nine cases in six generations. JAMA 1962;181:1103–1106.
37. Comings DE, Odland GF. Partial albinism. JAMA 1966;195:519–523.
38. Ortonne J-P. Piebaldism, Waardenburg's syndrome, and related disorders. "Neural crest depigmentation syndromes?" Dermatol Clin 1988;6:205–216.
39. Whyte MP, Murphy WA. Osteopathia striata associated with familial dermopathy and white forelock: Evidence for postnatal development of osteopathia striata. Am J Med Genet 1980;5:227–234.
40. Goodman RM, Yahav J, Frand M, et al. A new white forelock (poliosis) syndrome with multiple congenital malformations in two sibs. Clin Genet 1980;17:437–442.
41. Paige TN, Mendelson CG. Bilateral nevus comedonicus. Arch Dermatol 1967;96:172–175.
42. Jimbow K, Fitzpatrick TB, Szabo G, et al. Congenital circumscribed hypomelanosis: A characterization based on electron microscopic study of tuberous sclerosis, nevus depigmentosus, and piebaldism. J Invest Dermatol 1975;64:51–62.
43. Hayashibe K, Mishima Y. Tyrosinase-positive melanocyte distribution and induction of pigmentation in human piebald skin. Arch Dermatol 1988;124:381–386.
44. Mosher DB, Fitzpatrick TB. Piebaldism (editorial). Arch Dermatol 1988;124:364–365.
45. Mayer TC, Green MC. An experimental analysis of the pigment defect caused by mutations at the *W* and *Sl* in mice. Dev Biol 1968;18:62–75.
46. Tan JC, Nocka K, Ray P, et al. The dominant *W*42 *spotting* phenotype results form a missense mutation in the *c-kit* receptor kinase. Science 1990;247:209–212.
47. Spritz RA. The molecular basis of human piebaldism. Pigment Cell Res 1992;5:340–343.
48. Zsebo KM, Williams DA, Geissler EN, et al. Stem cell factor is

encoded at the *Sl* locus of the mouse and is the ligand for the *c-kit* tyrosine kinase receptor. Cell 1990;63:213–224.

49. Giebel LB, Spritz RA. Mutation of the *KIT* (mast/stem cell growth factor receptor) protooncogene in human piebaldism. Proc Natl Acad Sci USA 1991;88:8696–8699.

50. Fukai K, Hamada T, Ishii M, et al. Acquired pigmented macules in human piebald lesions: Ultrastructure of melanocytes in hypomelanotic skin. Acta Derm Venereol 1989;69:524–527.

51. Lerner AB, Halaban R, Klaus SN, et al. Transplantation of human melanocytes. J Invest Dermatol 1987;89:219–224.

52. Bolognia JL. Therapeutics in pigmentary disorders: Medical, surgical, and physical approaches. In: Levine N, Maibach H, eds. Pigmentation and Pigmentary Disorders. Boca Raton, FL: CRC Press, 1993;491–524.

53. Falabella R. Repigmentation of leukoderma by minigrafts of normally pigmented, autologous skin. J Dermatol Surg Oncol 1978;4:916–919.

54. Cockayne EA. A piebald family. Biometrika 1914;10:197–200.

55. Woolf CM, Dolowitz DA, Aldous HE. Congenital deafness associated with piebaldness. Arch Otolaryngol 1965;82:244–250.

56. Telfer MA, Sugar M, Jaegar EA, et al. Dominant piebald trait (white forelock and leukoderma) with neurological impairment. Am J Hum Genet 1971;23:383–389.

57. Kaplan P, de Chaderévian J-P. Piebaldism-Waardenburg syndrome: Histopathologic evidence for a neural crest syndrome. Am J Med Genet 1988;31:679–688.

58. Funderburk SJ, Crandall BF. Dominant piebald trait in a retarded child with a reciprocal translocation and small intercalary deletion. Am J Hum Genet 1974;26:723–726.

59. Lacassie Y, Thurmon TF, Tracy MC, et al. Piebald trait in a retarded child with interstitial deletion of chromosome 4. Am J Hum Genet 1977;29:641–642.

60. Hoo JJ, Haslam RHA, van Orman C. Tentative assignment of piebald trait gene to chromosome band 4q12. Hum Genet 1986;73:230–231.

61. Yamamoto Y, Nishimoto H, Ikemoto S. Interstitial deletion of the proximal long arm of chromosome 4 associated with father–child incompatibility within the Gc-system: Probable reduced gene dosage effect and partial piebald trait. Am J Med Genet 1989;32:520–523.

62. Beylot C, Bioulac P, Verger P, et al. Une famille de piebaldisme: Association dans un cas à une dystrophie osseuse: Étude ultrastructurale. Ann Pediatr 1975;22:341–348.

63. Badner JA, Chakravarti A. Waardenburg syndrome and Hirschsprung disease: Evidence for pleiotropic effects of a single dominant gene. Am J Med Genet 1990;35:100–104.

64. Waardenburg PJ. A new syndrome combining developmental anomalies of the eyelids, eyebrows, and nose root with pigmentary defects of the iris and head hair and with congenital deafness. Am J Hum Genet 1951;3:195–253.

65. Reed WB, Stone VM, Boder E, et al. Pigmentary disorders in association with congenital deafness. Arch Dermatol 1967; 96:176–186.

66. Gomez MR. Other autosomal dominant disorders. In: Gomez MR, ed. Neurocutaneous Diseases: A Practical Approach. Boston: Butterworth 1987:91.

67. Bard LA, Heterogeneity in Waardenburg's syndrome: Report of a family with ocular albinism. Arch Ophthalmol 1978;96: 1193–1198.

68. Tassabehji M, Read AP, Newton VE, et al. Waardenburg's syndrome patients have mutations in the human homologue of the *Pax-3* paired box gene. Nature 1992;355:635–636.

69. Baldwin CT, Hoth CF, Amos JA, et al. An exonic mutation in the *HuP2* paired domain gene causes Waardenburg's syndrome. Nature 1992;355:637–638.

70. Morell R, Friedman TB, Moelijopawiro S, et al. A frameshift mutation in the HUP2 paired domain of the probable human homolog of murine *Pax-3* is responsible for Waardenburg syndrome type I in an Indonesian family. Hum Mol Genet 1992;1:243–247.

71. Walter MA, Goodfellow PN. Disease and development. Nature 1992;355:590–591.

72. Pierpont JW, Erickson RP. Invited editorial: Facts on *PAX*. Am J Hum Genet 1993;52:451–454.

73. Hoth CF, Milunsky A, Lipsky N, et al. Mutations in the paired domain of the human PAX3 gene cause Klein-Waardenburg syndrome (WS-III) as well as Waardenburg's syndrome type I (WS-I). Am J Hum Genet 1993;52:455–462.

74. Mallory SB, Wiener E, Nordlund JJ. Waardenburg's syndrome with Hirschsprung's disease: A neural crest defect. Pediatr Dermatol 1986;3:119–124.

75. Alper JC, Holmes LB. The incidence and significance of birthmarks in a cohort of 4,641 newborns. Pediatr Dermatol 1983;1: 58–68.

76. Coupe RL. Unilateral systematized achromic naevus. Dermatologica 1967;134:19–35.

77. Takaiwa T, Mishima Y. Population density of intraepidermal dendritic cells in nevus depigmentosus. Jpn J Clin Electron Microsc 1970;3:367–377.

78. Selmanowitz VJ, Krivo JM. Pigmentary demarcation lines: Comparison of Negroes with Japanese. Br J Dermatol 1975; 93:371–377.

79. Takematsu H, Sato S, Igarashi M, et al. Incontinentia pigmenti achromians (Ito). Arch Dermatol 1983;119:391–395.

80. Pascual-Castroveijo I. Hypomelanosis of Ito. In: Gomez MR, ed. Neurocutaneous Diseases: A Practical Approach. Boston: Butterworth, 1987;85–90.

81. Stricker M, Meley M, Chassane JF, et al. Congenital cranio-facial dysmorphosis associated with Ito's syndrome (incontinentia pigmenti achromians): A case report. Br J Plast Surg 1984;37: 472–476.

82. Stewart RE, Funderburk S, Setoguchi Y. A malformation complex of ectrodactyly, clefting and hypomelanosis of Ito (incontinentia pigmenti achromians). Cleft Palate J 1979;16:358–362.

83. Ruiz-Maldonado R, Toussaint S, Tamayo L, et al. Hypomelanosis of Ito: Diagnostic criteria and report of 41 cases. Pediatr Dermatol 1992;9:1–10.

84. Grosshans EM, Stoebner P, Bergoend H, et al. Incontinentia pigmenti achromians (Ito): Étude clinique et histo-pathologique. Dermatologica 1971;142:65–78.

85. Morohashi M, Hashimoto K, Goodman TF, et al. Ultrastructural studies of vitiligo, Vogt-Koyanagi syndrome, and incontinentia pigmenti achromians. Arch Dermatol 1977;113:755–766.

86. Thomas IT, Frias JL, Cantu ES, et al. Association of pigmentary anomalies with chromosomal and genetic mosaicism and chimerism. Am J Hum Genet 1989;45:193–205.

87. Chitayat D, Friedman JM, Johnston MM. Hypomelanosis of Ito: A nonspecific marker of somatic mosaicism: Report of case with trisomy 18 mosaicism. Am J Med Genet 1990;35:422–424.

88. Ishikawa T, Kanayama M, Sugiyama K, et al. Hypomelanosis of Ito associated with benign tumors and chromosomal abnormalities: A neurocutaneous syndrome. Brain Dev 1985;7:45–49.

89. Golden SE, Kaplan AM. Hypomelanosis of Ito: Neurologic complications. Pediatr Neurol 1986;2:170–174.

90. Sybert VP, Pagon RA, Donlan M, et al. Pigmentary abnormalities and mosaicism for chromosomal aberration: Association with clinical features similar to hypomelanosis of Ito. J Pediatr 1990; 116:581–586.

91. Ritter CL, Steele MW, Wenger SL, et al. Chromosome mosaicism in hypomelanosis of Ito. Am J Med Genet 1990;35:14–17.

92. Vormittag W, Ensinger C, Raff M. Cytogenetic and dermatoglyphic findings in a familiar case of hypomelanosis of Ito (incontinentia pigmenti achromians). Clin Genet 1992;41:309–314.

93. Ohashi H, Tsukahara M, Murano I, et al. Pigmentary dysplasias and chromosomal mosaicism: Report of 9 cases. Am J Med Genet 1992;43:716–721.

94. Miller CA, Parker WD Jr. Hypomelanosis of Ito: Association with a chromosomal abnormality. Neurology 1985;5:607–610.

95. Bernstein R, Dawson B, Kohl R, et al. X;15 translocation in a retarded girl: X inactivation pattern and attempt to localise the hexosaminidase A and other loci. J Med Genet 1979;16: 254–262.

96. Hall BD. Invited editorial: Of mice, persons, and pigment. Am J Hum Genet 1989;45:191–192.

97. Turleau C, Taillard F, Doussau de Bazignan M, et al. Hypomelanosis of Ito (incontinentia pigmenti achromians) and mosaicism for a microdeletion of 15q1. Hum Genet 1986;74: 185–187.

98. Brilliant MH. The mouse pink-eyed dilution locus: A model for aspects of Prader-Willi syndrome, Angelman syndrome, and

a form of hypomelanosis of Ito. Mammal Genome 1992;3: 187–191.

99. Sybert VP. Hypomelanosis of Ito. Pediatr Dermatol 1990; 7:74–76.

100. Fitzpatrick TB, Szabó G, Hori Y, et al. White leaf-shaped macules: Earliest visible sign of tuberous sclerosis. Arch Dermatol 1968;98:1–6.

101. McWilliam RC, Stephenson JBP. Depigmented hair: The earliest sign of tuberous sclerosis. Arch Dis Child 1978;53:961–963.

102. Park S, Albert DM, Bolognia JL. Ocular manifestations of pigmentary disorders. Dermatol Clin 1992;10:609–622.

103. Ruiter DJ, van Duinen SG, Peters ACB, et al. Hypomelanotic macules in tuberous sclerosis: An ultrastructural and enzymehistochemical study. Arch Dermatol Res 1981;271:171–182.

104. Roach ES, Smith M, Huttenlocher P, et al. Report of the diagnostic criteria committee of the National Tuberous Sclerosis Association. J Child Neurol 1992;7:221–224.

105. Fryer AE, Osborne JP, Schutt W. Forehead plaque: A presenting skin sign in tuberous sclerosis. Arch Dis Child 1987;62:292–293.

106. Cornelison RL, Smith EB, Knox JM. Guttate leukoderma in Darier's disease. Arch Dermatol 1970;102:447–450.

107. Piamphongsant T, Kullavanijaya P. Diffuse biphasic amyloidosis. Dermatologica 1976;152:243–248.

108. Cole LA. Hypopigmentation with punctate keratosis of the palms and soles. Arch Dermatol 1976;112:998–1000.

109. Atnip RL, Summitt RL. Tetraploidy and 18-trisomy in a six-year-old triple mosaic boy. Cytogenetics 1971;10:305–317.

110. Falabella R, Escobar CE, Carrascal E. Leukoderma punctata. J Am Acad Dermatol 1988;18:485–494.

111. Morison WL, Kerker BJ, Tunnessen WW, et al. Disseminated hypopigmented keratoses. Arch Dermatol 1991;127:848–850.

112. Crawford DC, Garrett C, Tynan M, et al. Cardiac rhabdomyomata as a marker for the antenatal detection of tuberous sclerosis. J Med Genet 1983;20:303–304.

113. Hausdorf G, Schroeder S, Sieg K, et al. Diagnose des kardialen rhabdomyoms im neugeborenenalter. Z Kardiol 1983;72:57–60.

114. Journel H, Roussey M, Plais MH, et al. Prenatal diagnosis of familial tuberous sclerosis following detection of cardiac rhabdomyoma by ultrasound. Prenat Diagn 1986;6:283–289.

115. Smith HC, Watson GH, Patel RG, et al. Cardiac rhabdomyomata in tuberous sclerosis: Their course and diagnostic value. Arch Dis Child 1989;64:196–200.

116. Altman NR, Purser RK, Donovan Post MJ. Tuberous sclerosis: Characteristics at CT and MR imaging. Radiology 1988;167: 527–532.

117. Kingsley DPE, Kendall BE, Fitz CR. Tuberous sclerosis: A clinicoradiological evaluation of 110 cases with particular reference to atypical presentation. Neuroradiology 1986;28:38–46.

118. Mirlesse V, Wener H, Jacquemard F, et al. Magnetic resonance imaging in antenatal diagnosis of tuberous sclerosis. Lancet 1992;340:1163.

119. Cummings KI, Cottel WI. Idiopathic guttate hypomelanosis. Arch Dermatol 1966;93:184–186.

120. Wilson PD, Lavker RM, Kligman AM. On the nature of idiopathic guttate hypomelanosis. Acta Derm Venereol 1982; 62:301–306.

121. Savall R, Ferrandiz C, Ferrer I, et al. Idiopathic guttate hypomelanosis. Br J Dermatol 1980;103:635–642.

122. Ploysangam T, Dee-Ananlap S, Suvanprakorn P. Treatment of idiopathic guttate hypomelanosis with liquid nitrogen: Light and electron microscopic studies. J Am Acad Dermatol 1990; 23:681–684.

123. Clayton R, Breathnach A, Martin B, et al. Hypopigmented sarcoidosis in the Negro: Report of eight cases with ultrastructural observations. Br J Dermatol 1977;96:119–125.

124. Breathnach SM, McKee PH, Smith NP. Hypopigmented mycosis fungoides: Report of five cases with ultrastructural observations. Br J Dermatol 1982;106:643–649.

125. Clayton R, Warin A. Pityriasis lichenoides chronica presenting as hypopigmentation. Br J Dermatol 1979;100:297–302.

126. Locker E, Duncan WC. Hypopigmentation in alopecia mucinosa. Arch Dermatol 1979;115:731–733.

127. Bassaly M, Milae A, Prasad AS. Studies on pityriasis alba. Arch Dermatol 1963;88:272–275.

128. Klaus SN. The biologic basis of eight unusual hypopigmentary disorders. Ala J Med Sci 1979;16:290–305.

129. Zaynoun S, Jaber LAA, Kurban AK. Oral methoxsalen photochemotherapy of extensive pityriasis alba. J Am Acad Dermatol 1986;15:61–65.

130. Patterson JW, Fitzwater JE. Treatment of hypopigmented sarcoidosis with 8-methoxypsoralen and long wave ultraviolet light. Int J Dermatol 1982;21:476–480.

131. Zackheim HS, Epstein EH, Grekin DA, et al. Mycosis fungoides presenting as areas of hypopigmentation. J Am Acad Dermatol 1982;6:340–345.

132. Nazzaro-Porre M, Passi S. Identification of tyrosinase inhibitors in cultures of *Pityrosporum*. J Invest Dermatol 1978;81:205–208.

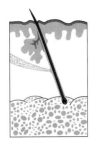

chapter 132

Melasma and Other Disorders of Hyperpigmentation

JORGE E. TORRES and JORGE L. SÁNCHEZ

Pigmentary changes, causing emotional and social problems in those affected, can be classified into two main groups: (1) hypomelanosis or leukoderma and (2) disorders of hyperpigmentation. Disorders of hyperpigmentation have common clinical, histopathologic, and etiologic factors (Table 132–1). Clinically, either brown hyperpigmentation or slate-gray hyperpigmentation is present. Brown hyperpigmentation or hypermelanosis results from increased melanin in the basal layer melanocytes and keratinocytes. Some hypermelanosis may be associated with dermal macrophages containing melanin. Slate-gray to blue pigmentation of the skin results from the Tyndall effect on pigment deposits in the dermis.

Since melasma constitutes a common and important dermatologic problem, emphasis will be placed on this disorder of hyperpigmentation. Selected examples of other diseases that cause hyperpigmentation are also discussed.

Melasma

DEFINITION

Melasma is an acquired, brown hypermelanosis of the face that develops slowly and symmetrically.[1] Although it has been associated with multiple etiologic factors (pregnancy, genetic, racial, and endocrine), sunlight appears to be one of the primary causes of its exacerbation.[2]

CLINICAL DESCRIPTION

Melasma is more common in women and persons of Latino origin living in tropical areas. It has been reported in 50% to 70% of pregnant women and in 8% to 29% of nonpregnant women taking birth control pills.[2, 3] Pregnancy- and contraceptive-related melasma are more common during the summer and in southern latitudes, probably secondary to sunlight exposure. Melasma in men shares the same clinicopathologic characteristics as in women, but hormonal factors do not seem to play a significant role.[4]

Melasma presents as a symmetrical, irregular light to dark brown hyperpigmentation of the face with three different clinical patterns: centrofacial, malar, and mandibular.[2] In the centrofacial location (Fig. 132–1), which is the most common (63%), melasma involves the cheeks, forehead, upper lip, nose, and chin. The malar pattern (Fig. 132–2) occurs in 21% of the patients and refers to melasma localized to the cheeks and nose. The mandibular pattern (16%) involves the ramus of the mandible. Melasma can be also classified on the basis of Wood's light (320–400 nm) examination. Four types are recognized: (1) an epidermal type, which shows enhancement of the pigmentation; (2) a dermal type, with no enhancement of color; (3) a mixed type that shows no or slight enhancement; and (4) a type seen in type V to VI skin in which the lesions are not discernible under a Wood's light. The epidermal type is the most common, occurring in 70% of patients.

PATHOLOGY

An epidermal and a dermal type of melasma can be observed histopathologically.

TABLE 132-1. Disorders of Hyperpigmentation

Hereditary or Developmental Disorders

Incontinentia pigmenti
Dyskeratosis congenita
Poikiloderma congenitale (Rothmund-Thompson syndrome)
Reticulate acropigmentation of Kitamura
Familial progressive hyperpigmentation
Acromelanosis progressiva
Dowling-Degos disease
Dermal melanocytosis
   Nevus of Ota
   Nevus of Ito
   Mongolian spot

Metabolic Disorders

Hemochromatosis
Niemann-Pick disease
Gaucher's disease
Macular and lichenoid amyloidosis
Ochronosis (endogenous)
Porphyria cutanea tarda
Wilson's disease

Endocrine Disorders

Melasma (and other facial melanoses)
Addison's disease
MSH-producing neoplasm
Exogenous ACTH therapy

Inflammatory Disorders

Erythema dyschromicum perstans
Lichen planus and variants
Lupus erythematosus
Pigmented contact dermatitis
Fixed drug eruption
Postinflammatory hyperpigmentation

Chemically Induced Disorders

Antimalarial agents
Tetracyclines
Heavy metals
Chemotherapeutic agents
Corticosteroids
Phenothiazides
Tar melanosis
Arsenic intoxication
Exogenous ochronosis
Berloque dermatitis
Amiodarone

Nutritional Disorders

Pellagra
Vitamin B_{12} deficiency
Kwashiorkor

Neoplastic Disorders

Metastatic melanoma
Mastocytosis

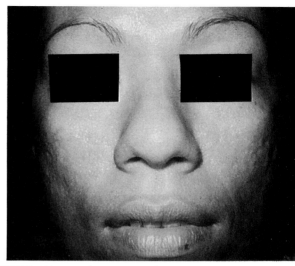

FIGURE 132-1. Melasma (centrofacial). Brown hyperpigmentation on the cheeks, upper lip, and nose.

In the epidermal type, melanin is deposited mainly in the basal and suprabasal layers but can also be seen throughout the other layers of the epidermis. The melanocytes, demonstrated best with the Fontana-Masson stain, are highly dendritic and filled with pigment (Fig. 132-3).

The dermal type is characterized by melanophages in the superficial and deep dermis in addition to the epidermal hyperpigmentation. Parenthetically, many cases of the so-called dermal melasma may represent examples of poikiloderma of Civatte or pigmented contact dermatitis.

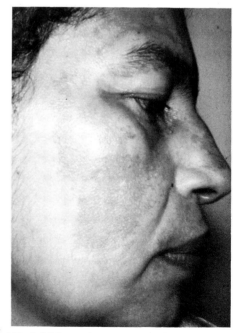

FIGURE 132-2. Melasma (malar pattern). Brown hyperpigmentation localized to the cheeks and nose.

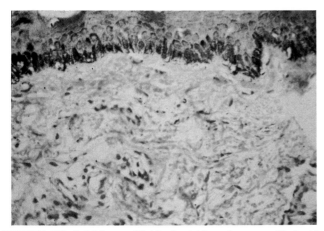

FIGURE 132–3. Melasma. Highly dendritic melanocytes filled with melanin in the basal layer (Fontana-Masson stain, ×100).

✦ **TABLE 132–2. Differential Diagnosis of Melasma**
Drug-induced hyperpigmentation
Riehl's melanosis
Poikiloderma of Civatte
Lichen planus pigmentosus
Exogenous ochronosis
Pigmented contact dermatitis
Postinflammatory hyperpigmentation
Nevus of Ota

PATHOGENESIS AND ETIOLOGY

Electron microscopic studies have revealed that the pigmentation in melasma is secondary to an increase in the number and activity of melanocytes, which appear highly dendritic with highly melanized melanosomes.[2] Multiple etiologic factors are probably responsible for these alterations in melanocytes, including oral contraceptives,[3] pregnancy, cosmetics (by a phototoxic mechanism), and genetic, endocrine, racial, nutritional, and metabolic factors. Sunlight is one of the most important factors in the pathogenesis of melasma,[5] as suggested by its increased incidence in southern latitudes and during the summer. Ultraviolet light (290–400 nm) is known to increase melanocytic activity, with resulting hyperpigmentation.[5] Further evidence of the role of ultraviolet light in the pathogenesis of melasma is the improvement obtained by using a broad-spectrum sunscreen (UVA and UVB)[6] and the recurrence of the hyperpigmentation on re-exposure to sunlight.

Although their mode of action is not known, progesterone and estrogen stimulate melanogenesis and have been implicated in the pigmentation seen in pregnancy and oral contraceptive use.[7, 8] Plasma levels of immunoreactive β-melanocyte-stimulating hormone (MSH),[9, 10] plasma α-MSH, urine 17-hydroxysteroids and 17-ketosteroids, serum cortisol, follicle-stimulating hormone, and adrenocorticotropin are normal in patients with melasma.[10] Pérez and Sánchez found statistically significant increased levels of luteinizing hormone and lower levels of serum estradiol in patients with melasma, which may represent evidence of a mild ovarian dysfunction.

A genetic predisposition has been suggested by its occurrence in twin sisters[11] and its positive family history in some cases.[2]

DIAGNOSIS AND DIFFERENTIAL DIAGNOSIS

In most of the cases, a diagnosis of melasma can be made clinically. Melasma has to be differentiated from other facial melanoses, including Riehl's melanosis, poikiloderma of Civatte, berloque dermatitis, postinflammatory hyperpigmentation, drug-induced hyperpigmentation, actinic lichen planus, exogenous ochronosis, and pigmented contact dermatitis (Table 132–2).

Riehl's melanosis refers to an acquired spotty brown, gray, or bluish pigmentation mostly on the face, especially prominent on the forehead and malar regions, behind the ears, and on the sides of the neck.[12, 13] A phototoxic contact dermatitis to fragrances seems to be the most likely cause of this condition. In fact, it has been called pigmented cosmetic dermatitis by the Japanese[14] because they obtained positive patch tests to cosmetics or their ingredients. Also, Sudan I dye, found in the cosmetic coloring agent Brilliant Lake Red R, has been found to be the cause in some cases.[15] Riehl's melanosis is differentiated clinically from melasma by its different distribution, often grayish or bluish color, and the history of the use of cosmetics. The histopathology is that of a vacuolar interface dermatitis with melanophages, in contrast to melasma, which is noninflammatory.

Poikiloderma of Civatte refers to a reticulated, brownish pigmentation with telangiectases limited to sunexposed areas such as the face, sides of neck, and the "V" of the chest. The most likely cause is chronic sun exposure as well as endocrine dysfunction.[16] Biopsy specimens show solar elastosis, epidermal atrophy, telangiectases, and melanophages.

Berloque dermatitis, probably related to Riehl's melanosis, is an irregular ("hanging drop") hyperpigmentation of the sides of the neck and in the retroauricular areas of women. It may also occur in men in the bearded area after using after-shave lotion containing bergamot oil. The most likely cause of berloque dermatitis is a contact photodermatitis caused by furocoumarin-containing compounds (such as perfumes and bergamot oil).[17]

Exogenous ochronosis refers to the pigmentary changes that occur after prolonged topical application of hydroquinones, phenol, or resorcinol. A blue-black pigmentation develops on the face, sides and back of the neck, upper aspects of the chest, and the extensor aspect of the extremities. The histopathologic changes are characteristic and consist of yellow-brown, bizarre-shaped collagen bundles with jagged, sharp edges that result from pigment deposits within the bundles.

Postinflammatory hyperpigmentation, chemically induced hyperpigmentation, and lichen planus pigmentosus are discussed later in this chapter.

TREATMENT

Therapy for melasma should begin with the identification and elimination of causative factors such as oral contraceptives and other hormone-containing drugs, photosensitizing drugs and cosmetics, and sunlight.[16]

Broad-spectrum sunscreens with ultraviolet A (UVA) and ultraviolet B (UVB) light protection should be used daily. The compound PARSOL 1789, which is present in several sunscreens, absorbs throughout the UVA spectrum. Opaque formulations containing titanium dioxide and zinc oxide are effective in blocking both UVA and UVB light.

Hydroquinone, alone or in combination with topical steroids and retinoic acid, is the most commonly used agent in the treatment of melasma. Hydroquinone inhibits melanogenesis in vivo and in vitro through inhibition of tyrosinase and by exhibiting cytotoxicity toward melanocytes (Table 132–3).[18]

In 1975, Kligman and Willis[19] introduced a formula that combined 5% hydroquinone, 0.1% tretinoin, 0.1% dexamethasone, and ascorbic acid. Tretinoin, which causes mild irritation, enhances the epidermal penetration of hydroquinone. In addition, retinoic acid has been shown to reduce the activity of the melanocytes. This formula can be modified by changing the retinoic acid concentration, the steroid potency, and the hydroquinone concentration. When therapy is started with this formula, lower hydroquinone concentrations should be used, which can be increased subsequently if necessary. The medication should be used twice daily—once in the morning and before bedtime. A broad-spectrum sunscreen (UVA, UVB) should be applied in the morning, since its combination with hydroquinone has been demonstrated to be more effective than hydroquinone alone.[6]

Patients with few lesions should be started on preparations with low concentrations of hydroquinone (3%). Higher concentrations should be reserved for patients with extensive lesions. Buthionine sulfoximine seems to enhance the depigmenting effect of hydroquinone, but results remain preliminary.[18]

Side effects of hydroquinone therapy include irritant contact dermatitis, exogenous ochronosis, and brown discoloration of the nails due to the deposition of hydroquinone oxidation products. The frequency of irritant reactions depends on the hydroquinone concentration and its combination with retinoic acid.

Topical steroids alone may cause hypopigmentation.[20] This hypopigmenting ability depends on the chemical structure of the steroid. The pigmentary change occurs rapidly, is never total, and regresses after discontinuation.[16]

4-Isopropylcatechol was used in 54 patients with melasma, 66% of whom experienced significant improvement.[21] However, the use of this drug was associated with a high incidence of irritant and allergic contact dermatitis.[21]

Patients with actinically damaged skin and melasma showed a marked improvement in their melasma if they were first given a 2-week course of 5-fluorouracil,[22] with subsequent use of a bleaching cream. There have been no controlled clinical trials evaluating the combination of 5-fluorouracil and hydroquinone.

Azelaic acid is a naturally occurring dicarboxylic acid that causes a reversible inhibition of tyrosinase.[16, 23, 24] It has been used to treat melasma, acne, and other disorders of hyperpigmentation such as postinflammatory melanoderma and hypermelanosis caused by physical agents.[23] When combined with a 2% hydroquinone cream, azelaic acid was found to yield "good results" in 73% of patients with melasma.[24] The definite efficacy of this compound alone in melasma is still in doubt.

N-Acetyl-4,5-cysteaminylphenol, a phenolic thioether amine, is melanocytotoxic and affects only active melanocytes.[21] This compound seems to be more stable and less irritating than hydroquinone.[25] Jimbow used this compound in 12 patients with melasma, and 9 patients had complete loss of pigment.

Limited chemical peeling with 25% trichloroacetic acid or 95% phenol solution may induce temporary improvement of selected patches. Bleaching is usually seen after a week.

Several lasers, including Q-switched ruby, Q-switched neodymium:yttrium-aluminum-garnet, and 510-nm pulsed dye lasers, have been used in the treatment of melasma with variable results.[26-28] The most effective appears to be the Q-switched ruby laser used in patients with epidermal melasma.

Before starting any of the previously mentioned therapies it is important to perform a Wood's light examination to determine the type of melasma. The epidermal form, which is the more common, is more responsive to therapy than the dermal type. The mixed type is also less responsive to treatment.

Chemically Induced Hyperpigmentation

DEFINITION

Hyperpigmentation of the skin has long been associated with exposure to a variety of chemicals (see Table 132–1). The pigmentation may be induced by direct deposition of the chemical, stimulation of melanin formation, binding to melanin, and production of metabolites or nonmelanin pigments. Exposure to ultraviolet light seems to enhance hyperpigmentation in some of the cases. Offending agents include antimalarial agents, anti-

---

◄ TABLE 132–3. Treatment of Melasma

Eliminate inciting agents: drugs, cosmetics
Hydroquinone alone >3%
Hydroquinone with retinoic acid
Broad-spectrum sunscreen
Topical steroids
5-Fluorouracil
4-Isopropylcatechol
Chemical peeling
Laser surgery

biotics, heavy metals, cancer chemotherapeutic agents, and topical preparations such as tar-containing compounds.

CLINICAL DESCRIPTION

The clinical presentation of chemically induced hyperpigmentation is highly variable. The pigmentation may be localized or diffuse; may involve hair, nails, and mucosa; and may vary from red, bright yellow to brown, blue-gray, to black.[29]

The antimalarial agents, including chloroquine, hydroxychloroquine, and quinacrine, are a group of 4-aminoquinolones and acridines that have been reported as the cause of bluish black to slate-gray pigmentation of the face, extremities, oral mucosa, and nails.[29] Those changes may be limited to the cartilaginous structures (pseudo-ochronosis). Mepacrine is known for its ability to produce a yellowish discoloration of the skin.[30]

Pigmentary change is a rare but well-documented side effect of prolonged high-dose administration of minocycline, particularly in the treatment of severe acne and chronic bronchitis (Fig. 132–4). The pigmentation may involve the skin, nails, bones, teeth, aorta, endocardium, and sclerae.[30-32] These pigmentary changes may occur in three different forms: (1) blue-black pigmentation in the areas of previous inflammatory lesions, such as acne lesions; (2) involvement of the sun-exposed areas; and (3) diffuse "muddy brown" pigmentation that can affect the entire skin. Rarely, there is generalized hyperpigmentation with involvement of the sclerae and nail beds.[31]

Heavy metals, such as gold, silver, and mercury, may cause skin pigmentation. Gold produces a characteristic slate-gray pigmentation in sun-exposed skin, while silver-induced pigmentation affects both sun-exposed and nonexposed areas, including sclerae, nails, and mucous membranes. Mercury-induced pigmentation usually involves the skin folds.[30]

Cancer chemotherapeutic agents, particularly the alkylating agents and the antibiotics, are well recognized as a cause of hyperpigmentation.[29] Alkylating agents include, among others, cyclosphosphamide and busulfan.

Cyclophosphamide produces transverse or longitudinal brown to black pigmentation of the nails and teeth.[31] Busulfan may cause a dusky pigmentation of the face, forearms, chest, and abdomen, without a predilection for sun-exposed areas.[30]

Chemotherapeutic antibiotics that may cause hyperpigmentation include bleomycin, daunorubicin, and doxorubicin. Bleomycin causes the characteristic linear or "flagellate" hyperpigmentation in areas of trauma. Daunorubicin has been reported to produce a brown-black transverse hyperpigmentation of the fingernails and toenails.[29] Doxorubicin may cause mucosal hyperpigmentation.

Phenothiazines, particularly chlorpromazine, may cause skin hyperpigmentation after prolonged use. It most commonly involves the sun-exposed areas. Amiodarone, a cardiac antiarrhythmic agent, may cause, in addition to photosensitivity, a striking slate-gray pigmentation in sun-exposed areas.[29, 30]

Clofazimine, a commonly used antileprosy agent, usually causes a generalized redness that is followed by a dark-brown pigmentation.[32]

PATHOLOGY AND PATHOGENESIS

The pathology and pathogenesis of chemically induced hyperpigmentation depend on the etiologic agent.

Hyperpigmentation caused by antimalarial agents appears in the dermis as a dense amorphous material, probably composed of melanin and hemosiderin.[30] In minocycline pigmentation, the nature of the pigment differs depending on the clinical presentation. In hyperpigmented acne scars, hemosiderin and ferritin are present in macrophages. The blue-gray patches that occur on extremities have pigmented macrophages that stain for both melanin and iron. The "muddy brown" pigmentation that can affect the entire skin is chiefly due to basilar epidermal melanin. The iron-containing granules in minocycline-induced hyperpigmentation seem to be due to drug metabolite complexes.

The pigment in heavy metal pigmentation is the chemical itself. Black granules may be seen in macrophages in gold pigmentation and extracellularly in silver-induced pigmentation.

The pigmentation seen with chlorpromazine use appears to be due to melanin or a complex of melanin with chlorpromazine.[30] Many pigment-containing macrophages are seen throughout the dermis.

DIAGNOSIS

The diagnosis of chemically induced hyperpigmentation is often difficult to make. A thorough history and physical examination, and possibly a skin biopsy, may aid in making a correct diagnosis.

TREATMENT

Chemical-induced hyperpigmentation is often persistent. The most effective treatment is stopping the offend-

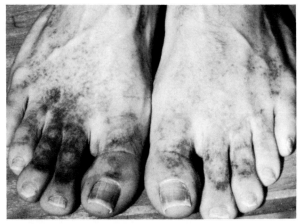

FIGURE 132–4. Minocycline-induced pigmentation. Note irregular hyperpigmented patches on the dorsa of the feet.

ing drug. Prevention appears to be an effective way of managing these patients. This can be achieved by having knowledge of the chemicals that may cause hyperpigmentation and then taking preventive measure, such as the use of sunscreens.

Erythema Dyschromicum Perstans (Ashy Dermatosis)

DEFINITION

Erythema dyschromicum perstans, first described by Ramirez[33] in 1957, is a cutaneous disorder of unknown etiology characterized by widespread gray-brown pigmented macules and patches that have an erythematous, raised border in the early stages.

CLINICAL DESCRIPTION

Erythema dyschromicum perstans has been reported most commonly in people of Spanish or Indian descent.[34, 35] In its early stages, the lesions are characterized by blue-gray macules and patches with a raised, erythematous border. The most common locations are the face, neck, trunk, and upper limbs. In the late stage, the patches are gray-blue with an ill-defined border. The lesions are usually asymptomatic, and the disease has a chronic, insidious course.

PATHOLOGY

Histopathologic examination of the active red border reveals vacuolar alteration of the basal layer, necrotic keratinocytes in the basal layer, and a sparse superficial perivascular lymphocytic infiltrate with many melanophages.[36, 37] In subsequent stages, melanophages remain in the papillary dermis but the other components may be minimal or absent. At this stage it cannot be differentiated from any other disease causing postinflammatory hyperpigmentation.

PATHOGENESIS AND ETIOLOGY

The etiology of erythema dyschromicum perstans is unknown. There is controversy as to whether it is a variant of lichen planus, particularly lichen planus pigmentosus.[35-38]

Erythema dyschromicum perstans has been considered a variant of lichen planus because of their similar histopathology.[38] Also, immunofluorescence studies on a patient with what was believed to be ashy dermatosis revealed a pattern commonly seen in lichen planus.[35]

Nevertheless, the histopathologic findings in erythema

dyschromicum perstans and lichen planus pigmentosus are also seen in other inflammatory conditions.

On the basis of its unique clinical characteristics in the early stages, the distribution, and the chronic, asymptomatic course, it appears that erythema dyschromicum perstans is not a variant of lichen planus.

DIAGNOSIS AND DIFFERENTIAL DIAGNOSIS

In its early stages, erythema dyschromicum perstans can be accurately diagnosed clinically. In subsequent stages it must be differentiated from lichen planus pigmentosus, postinflammatory hyperpigmentation, and macular amyloidosis.

Erythema dyschromicum perstans has been differentiated from lichen planus pigmentosus mostly on clinical grounds. Lichen planus pigmentosus is a variant of lichen planus that largely affects dark-skinned patients and that, like erythema dyschromicum perstans, results in hyperpigmented lesions. In erythema dyschromicum perstans there is an active border in some cases, blue-gray macules and patches, a symmetrical distribution, and a chronic, insidious course. On the other hand, lichen planus pigmentosus is characterized by dark brown macules with occasional papules, no active border, a sun-exposed distribution, and a chronic course with relapses and remissions.[36]

TREATMENT

There is no effective treatment for erythema dyschromicum perstans. Even the use of potent depigmenting creams has been unsuccessful.

Postinflammatory Hyperpigmentation

DEFINITION

Postinflammatory hyperpigmentation refers to the brown macules and patches that may be seen after any inflammatory condition of the skin, either endogenous or exogenous.[39] Exogenous causes include physical and chemical agents that are used topically or systemically. Endogenous causes include lichen planus, discoid lupus erythematosus, macular amyloidosis, and other primary inflammatory conditions of the skin.

CLINICAL DESCRIPTION

Postinflammatory hyperpigmentation is characterized by macules and patches of different shades of brown in sites of previous inflammation. In some cases, as in lichen planus, the pigmentation is so distinctive that a retrospective diagnosis can be made. In most cases, however, the cause of the hyperpigmentation is not known.

The pigmented macules or patches of fixed drug eruption are recognized by their bluish hue and the occurrence of erythema and vesiculation on each exposure to the offending agent.

PATHOLOGY

In late stages, postinflammatory hyperpigmentation is characterized histologically by a sparse, superficial perivascular infiltrate with melanophages. In earlier stages, one may find changes suggestive of the etiology. For example, if there is vacuolar alteration of the basal layer, then lichen planus, fixed drug eruption, and erythema dyschromicum perstans are suggested.

The different shades of brown seen clinically correlate with the amount and distribution of melanin pigment seen in macrophages and within the basal layer of the epidermis.

PATHOGENESIS AND ETIOLOGY

Epidermal melanocytes may increase in size, number, and activity after being stimulated by chemical irritation, ultraviolet light irradiation, and many diverse inflammatory conditions. The melanin produced by these melanocytes, which is subsequently found in the dermis, is the cause of the hyperpigmentation seen clinically.

The term *postinflammatory hyperpigmentation* describes the end stage of a prior inflammatory process but most of the time provides no clues to the nature of the original dermatitis.

DIAGNOSIS

The diagnosis of postinflammatory hyperpigmentation is made clinically. In some cases, a biopsy may help in identifying the primary process.

TREATMENT

Treatment of postinflammatory hyperpigmentation is often inadequate. Bleaching creams, as described in the melasma section, may be tried in those cases in which the pigment is more superficially located. Topical tretinoin (0.1% retinoic acid cream) has been shown to significantly lighten postinflammatory hyperpigmentation in black persons.[40]

The Q-switched ruby and 510-nm dye lasers have been used to treat postinflammatory hyperpigmentation. In a study by Fitzpatrick and colleagues,[41] lesions in 8 of 10 patients cleared by 75% or more with the 510-nm pulsed dye laser.

Nevus of Ota and of Ito

DEFINITION

Nevus of Ota and nevus of Ito are hamartomas of dermal melanocytes. These lesions may be present at birth or appear during the first year of life or adolescence.[42] They rarely occur in childhood. Some investigators consider them to be congenital forms of blue nevus.

CLINICAL DESCRIPTION

Nevus of Ota (nevus fuscoceruleus ophthalmomaxillaris) presents itself as a unilateral blue-brown speckled patch usually involving the malar region, periorbital area, temple, and forehead. Other areas that may be affected include the sclera, conjunctiva, retina, cornea, ocular muscles, periosteum, oral and buccal mucosa, and the retrobulbar fat. These lesions enlarge slowly, become deeper in color, and persist throughout life. They are more common in females (80%), and 5% to 10% are bilateral rather than unilateral. Nevus of Ota is benign, but in rare cases melanoma can arise within it.[43, 44]

Nevus of Ito (nevus fuscoceruleus acromiodeltoides) differs from nevus of Ota only by the location in the supraclavicular, side of the neck, shoulder, and scapular areas. Although rare, melanoma has also been reported in nevus of Ito.[45]

PATHOLOGY

Nevus of Ota and nevus of Ito show similar histopathologic changes, namely, an increased number of elongated, dendritic melanocytes scattered throughout the dermis. Unlike with most common blue nevi, the dermal collagen pattern is unaffected. A fibrous sheath can be found surrounding dermal melanocytes on ultrastructural examination.[46, 47]

PATHOGENESIS AND ETIOLOGY

Nevus of Ota and nevus of Ito are hamartomas of dermal melanocytes, probably due to faulty migration of melanoblasts from the neural crest to the skin.

DIAGNOSIS AND DIFFERENTIAL DIAGNOSIS

Nevus of Ota and nevus of Ito can usually be accurately diagnosed clinically. They differ from the mongolian spot by their characteristic location.

Histopathologically, nevus of Ota and nevus of Ito have a greater number of dendritic melanocytes than do mongolian spots. On the other hand, blue nevi are characterized by a much greater number of melanocytes than are nevus of Ota and nevus of Ito.

TREATMENT

For many years, treatment of nevus of Ota and nevus of Ito was unsatisfactory. Recently, the Q-switched ruby and Q-switched neodymium:yttrium-aluminum-garnet (1064 nm) lasers, through selective photothermolysis of melanosomes, have been shown to be effective in lightening or removing the lesions.[48, 49] (For further information see Atlas of Cutaneous Surgery, Chapter 23.)

Mongolian Spot

DEFINITION

The mongolian spot is a congenital blue-gray patch usually localized in the sacral region. It is common in Asian and black infants.

CLINICAL DESCRIPTION

Mongolian spots characteristically occur in the lumbosacral region as blue-gray patches of variable size (2 to 8 cm). They rarely occur at other sites such as the middle or upper back or as multiple lesions.[50] Mongolian spots usually disappear spontaneously during childhood, although they rarely persist into adulthood.[51]

PATHOLOGY

Histopathologic examination of mongolian spots shows elongated dendritic melanocytes widely scattered between collagen bundles in the reticular dermis.

PATHOGENESIS AND ETIOLOGY

Mongolian spots result from the delayed disappearance of dermal melanocytes. The blue color results from the Tyndall effect.

DIAGNOSIS AND DIFFERENTIAL DIAGNOSIS

The diagnosis of mongolian spot is usually evident clinically. Histopathologically, nevus of Ota and nevus of Ito and blue nevi show a greater number of dendritic melanocytes.

TREATMENT

There is no effective treatment of persistent mongolian spots.

References

1. Newcomer VD, Lindbert MC, Stenbert TH. A melanosis of the face ("chloasma"). Arch Dermatol 1961;83:284–297.
2. Sánchez NP, Pathak MA, Sato S, et al. Melasma: Clinical, light microscopic, ultrastructural, and immunofluorescence study. J Am Acad Dermatol 1981;4:698–710.
3. Resnick S. Melasma induced by oral contraceptive drugs. JAMA 1967;199:95–99.
4. Vázquez M, Maldonado H, Benmamán C, et al. Melasma in men: A clinical and histologic study. Int J Dermatol 1988;27:25–27.
5. Pathak MA, Riley FC, Fitzpatrick TB. Melanogenesis in skin following exposure to long-wave ultraviolet and visible light. J Invest Dermatol 1962;39:435–443.
6. Vázquez M, Sánchez JL. The efficacy of a broad spectrum sunscreen in the treatment of melasma. Cutis 1983;32:92–96.
7. Snelle RS, Bischitz PG. The effect of large doses of estrogen and progesterone on melanin pigmentation. J Invest Dermatol 1960;35:73–81.
8. Snell RS. The pigmentary changes occurring in the breast skin during pregnancy and following estrogen treatment. J Invest Dermatol 1964;43:181–186.
9. Smith AG, Shuster S, Thody AJ. Chloasma, oral contraceptives and plasma immunoreactive beta-melanocyte stimulating hormone. J Invest Dermatol 1977;68:169–170.
10. Pérez M, Sánchez JL, Aguiló F. Endocrinologic profiles of patients with idiopathic melasma. J Invest Dermatol 1983;81:543–545.
11. Hughes BR. Melasma occurring in twin sisters. J Am Acad Dermatol 1987;17:841.
12. Rorsman H. Riehl's melanosis. Int J Dermatol 1982;21:75–78.
13. Serrano G, Pujol L, Cuadra J, et al. Riehl's melanosis: Pigmented contact dermatitis caused by fragrances. J Am Acad Dermatol 1989;21:1057–1060.
14. Nakayama H, Harada R, Toda M. Pigmented cosmetic dermatitis. Int J Dermatol 1976;15:673.
15. Kozuka T, Tashiro M, Sano S, et al. Brilliant Lake Red R as a cause of pigmented contact dermatitis. Contact Dermatitis 1979;5:297.
16. Benmamán O, Sánchez JL. Treatment and camouflaging of pigmentary disorders. Clin Dermatol 1988;6:50–61.
17. Harber LC, Harris H, Leider M, et al. Berloque dermatitis. Arch Dermatol 1964;90:572–576.
18. Lubell A. Controversies of pigmentation disorders discussed. Cosmet Dermatol 1993;6:32–34.
19. Kligman AM, Willis I. A new formula for depigmenting human skin. Arch Dermatol 1975;111:40–48.
20. Neering H. Treatment of melasma (chloasma) by local application of the steroid cream. Dermatologica 1975;151:349–353.
21. Bleehen SS. The treatment of hypermelanosis with 4-isopropylcatechol. Br J Dermatol 1976;94:687–694.
22. Milstein HG. 5-Fluouracil as an aid in management of acne and melasma. J Am Acad Dermatol 1981;4:97–98.
23. Nazzaro-Porro M. Azelaic acid. J Am Acad Dermatol 1987;17:1033–1041.
24. Breathnach AC, Nazzaro-Porro M, Passi S, et al. Azelaic acid therapy in disorders of hyperpigmentation. Clin Dermatol 1989;7:106–119.
25. Jimbow K. N-acetyl-4-5-cysteaminylphenol as a new type of depigmenting agent for the melanoderma of patients with melasma. Arch Dermatol 1991;127:1528–1534.
26. Hruza GJ, Geronemus RG, Dover JS, Arndt KA. Lasers in dermatology. Arch Dermatol 1993;129:1026–1035.
27. Dover JS, Linsmeier Kilmer S, Anderson RR. What's new in cutaneous laser surgery. J Dermatol Surg Oncol 1993;19:295–298.
28. Goldberg DJ. Benign pigmented lesions of the skin: Treatment with the Q-switched ruby laser. J Dermatol Surg Oncol 1993;19:376–379.
29. Hendrix JD, Greer KE. Cutaneous hyperpigmentation caused by systemic drugs. Int J Dermatol 1992;31:458.
30. Ferguson J, Fraia-Bell W. Pigmentary disorders and systemic drug therapy. Clin Dermatol 1989;7:44–54.
31. Pepine M, Flowers FP, Ramos-Caro FA. Extensive cutaneous hyperpigmentation caused by minocycline. J Am Acad Dermatol 1993;28:292–295.
32. Olumide YM, Odunowo BD, Odiase AO. Regional dermatoses

in the African. I. Facial hypermelanosis. Int J Dermatol 1991; 30:186–189.

33. Ramirez CO. Los cenicientos, problema clinico. Memoria del Primer Congreso Centroamericano de Dermatología, San Salvador, El Salvador, December 5, 1957.

34. Kark EC, Litt JZ. Ashy dermatosis: A variant of lichen planus? Cutis 1980;25:631–633.

35. Arenas R, Hojyo T, Dominguez-Soto L. Ashy dermatosis and lichen planus pigmentosus: A clinicopathologic study of 31 cases. Int J Dermatol 1992;31:90–94.

36. Arenas R, Hojyo T, Dominguez-Soto L. Ashy dermatosis versus lichen planus pigmentosus: A controversial matter. Int J Dermatol 1992;31:87–88.

37. Sánchez NP, Pathak MA, Sato S, et al. Circumscribed dermal melaninoses, classification, light and ultrastructural studies of the erythema dyschromicum perstans type. Int J Dermatol 1982;21:25.

38. Bhutani LK. Ashy dermatosis or lichen planus pigmentosus: What is in a name? Arch Dermatol 1986;122:133.

39. Epstein JH. Post-inflammatory hyperpigmentation. Clin Dermatol 1989;7:55–65.

40. Bulengo-Ransby SM, Griffiths C, Kimbrough-Green C, et al. Topical tretinoin (retinoic acid) therapy for hyperpigmented lesions caused by inflammation of the skin in black patients. N Engl J Med 1993;328:1438–1443.

41. Fitzpatrick RE, Goldman MP, Ruiz-Esparza J. Laser treatment of benign pigmented epidermal lesions using a 300-ns pulse and 510-nm wavelength. J Dermatol Surg Oncol 1993;19:341–347.

42. Hidano A, Kajima H, Ikedea S, et al. A natural history of nevus of Ota. Arch Dermatol 1967;95:187–195.

43. Halasa A. Malignant melanoma in a case of bilateral nevus of Ota. Arch Ophthalmol 1970;84:176–178.

44. Jay B. Malignant melanoma of the orbit in a case of oculodermal melanocytosis. Br J Dermatol 1965;49:389.

45. Van Krieken J, Boom B, Scheffer E. Malignant transformation in a naevus of Ito: A case report. Histopathology 1988;12:100–112.

46. Okawa Y, Yokata R, Yamanchi A. On the extracellular sheath of dermal melanocytes in nevus fuscocaeruleus acromio deltoideus and mongolian spot: An ultrastructural study. J Invest Dermatol 1979;73:224–230.

47. Hori Y, Ouhara K, Miimura M, et al. Electron microscopy: Ultrastructural observations of the extracellular sheath of dermal melanocytes in nevus of Ota. Am J Dermatopathol 1982;4:245–251.

48. Lowe NJ, Wieder JM, Sawcer D, et al. Nevus of Ota: Treatment with high energy fluences of the Q-switched ruby laser. J Am Acad Dermatol 1993;29:997–1001.

49. Geronemus RG. Q-switched ruby laser therapy of nevus of Ota. Arch Dermatol 1992;128:1618–1622.

50. Bashiti HM, Blair JD, Triska RA, et al. Generalized dermal melanocytosis. Arch Dermatol 1981;117:791–793.

51. Hidano A. Persistent mongolian spot in the adult. Arch Dermatol 1971;103:680–681.

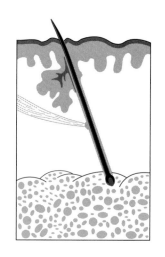

What Diseases Alter Hair, Nails, and Sweat Glands?

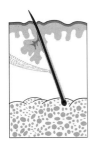

chapter 133

Biochemistry and Control of Hair Growth

Anatomy

Marty E. Sawaya

IMPORTANCE OF HAIR

In mammals, hair is for thermal regulation, involving a "moulting process" for the organism to adapt to changing environments. In some species it is also correlated with their sexual cycle, and survival by camouflage.[1]

In humans, hair is a means of social and sexual communication and has become important to the cosmetic and pharmaceutical industries.[2] Our "self-image" and appearance depend a lot on our hair—styles, color, length, fullness, texture, and so forth.

Medically, hair can be an indicator of physiologic changes within an individual. For example, an increase in hair shedding can be attributed to nutritional changes, hormone fluctuations (e.g., postpartum pregnancy), or side effects noted with taking certain drugs and medications. Women complaining of frontal hair loss and/or hirsutism may have an underlying endocrine problem.[3]

Hair growth in certain areas of the body that may be unwanted by some people, such as on the legs, face, abdomen, and axilla, can only partially be explained from an evolutionary standpoint. Hair in those locations was important for protection, sexual signaling, and thermal regulation, as it still remains for other mammals. It is important to emphasize that cellular mechanisms mediating hair growth may be similar or identical in all follicles, but that the "molecular genetic message" each hair follicle carries may be different depending on location on the body. In any case, the role of androgens is important for understanding follicular growth and cycling. Androgens have a "dual" effect of stimulating hair growth on the body while eventually mediating hair loss on the scalp.[3-6] The hair follicle is studied for its many physiologic processes, including control of cell growth, mesenchymal-epithelial interactions, epithelial differentiation, and hormone-endocrine influences.

Physiologically, the hair follicle cycle varies from species to species,[4] and within species by various regions of the body (e.g., the cycle varies between scalp and body hair).[4, 5] Hair dynamics (see Table 133–1), the hair cycle, and what structurally takes place in each phase of the cycle in humans contribute to the wide variety in hair growth.

ANATOMY AND PHYSIOLOGY OF THE HAIR FOLLICLE

The hair follicle is composed of epidermal and dermal tissue (Fig. 133–1). The dermal components—namely the dermal papilla and dermal sheath—are derived from an aggregate of mesenchymal cells that forms directly beneath the epithelial hair germ at the onset of follicular development. The epidermal hair germ grows in a downward progression to form the hair peg, which becomes a bulbous hair peg where all elements of the hair follicle are present. Experiments involving tissue recombination using embryonic skin have shown that follicular development depends on a series of messages between dermis and epidermis.

Each of the various compartments or cell layers is important in understanding hair follicle growth[1, 7] (Fig. 133–1). Specific messages relayed between dermis and epidermis are transmitted to all parts of the follicle for continuous cycling and growth to occur.

TABLE 133-1. Hair Dynamics

Scalp hairs range from 100,000 to 150,000 in number in red-heads, brunettes, and blondes; 90% in anagen/10% telogen in spring, 80% in anagen/20% telogen in late summer-fall

Anagen hair follicles grow 2-8 years
Telogen hair follicles rest 1-4 months

Body hair (trunk, eyelashes, extremities)
    Anagen hair follicles grow 1-6 months
    Telogen hair follicles rest 1-4 months

Outer Root Sheath

The hair follicle produces keratinized hair, which is seen emerging from the skin. Underneath the skin surface, the follicle has many cell layers that enclose the hair shaft, called outer root sheath cells. The outer root sheath layer surrounds the hair, making up several layers of cells continuous with the epidermis. It is divided into two parts—the short lower part surrounding the outer part of the bulb, and the upper part from the neck of the bulb to the level of sebaceous duct. The area surrounding the hair bulb is one to two cells thick, the outer layer being elongated and the inner layer markedly flattened. In the suprabulbar area, it is three cell layers thick and becomes multilayered half way up along the follicle. The outer cell layer is the germinative layer continuous with the epidermal basal cells.

The outer root sheath differs from the follicular canal in containing prominent Golgi vesicles associated with well-developed rough endoplasmic reticulum producing

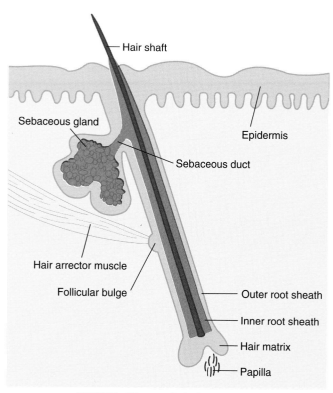

amorphous cytoplasmic granules during differentiation. The overall function of the outer root sheath is not known; however, during the early anagen phases of the hair cycle, the outer root sheath elongates rapidly because of a high rate of mitotic activity, which ceases when the follicle reaches its full length. It is also during this phase that steroid enzymes such as aromatase is detected, which may play a role in follicular differentiation and growth.[8, 9] The outer root sheath is not a static structure as it was once thought to be, but a dynamic structure participating in follicular growth.

Inner Root Sheath

The inner root sheath consists of three layers, from within outward, the cuticle, Huxley's, and Henle's layers; the cuticle being one cell layer thick, while Huxley's layer is several cells deep. All three layers are formed from the peripheral mass of matrix cells in the hair bulb. The primary function of the inner root sheath is to mold the hair by hardening in advance of the hair so that full keratinization takes the shape of the root sheath.[1, 7]

Hair Matrix: Cuticle/Cortex/Medulla

The keratogenous zone of the hair follicle is formed from the hair matrix. This area is made up of rapidly dividing cells in the lower and upper bulb surrounding the dermal papilla. Between the epithelial cells melanocytes can be seen, and they are scattered throughout the lower part of the bulb and extend into the outer root sheath. It is the matrix cells that give rise to the cuticular, cortical, and medullary layers of hair.

Cuticle

The human hair is surrounded by 6 to 10 layers of cuticle cells, each being approximately 0.2 to 0.5 μm thick, varying in number of layers from coarse to fine hairs. The cuticle may account for up to 10% of the fiber by weight. The cuticular cells overlap similar to tiles on a roof, imbricated, with the free margins pointing to the tip of the follicle. Each cuticular cell is composed of lamellar components with major layers consisting of a cystine-rich layer, the exocuticle, and the endocuticle. It is the exocuticle that consists of the "strong" high-sulfur protein that migrates to the outer part of each cuticular cell.[10] The mechanism controlling the production and migration of these proteins is under genetic control and may be lost in hair diseases such as trichothiodystrophy.

Cortex/Hair Keratins

The cortex is the main bulk of hair and contributes to the mechanical properties of the fibers. The hair fiber that emerges from the follicular shaft is composed primarily of cortical cells filled with 10-nm keratin filaments.

Biochemical studies have shown that hair is made of three major classes of keratin proteins:[11] (1) the low-sul-

FIGURE 133-1. Hair follicle anatomy.

fur keratins designated 40 to 60 kd; (2) the high-sulfur protein keratins, 10 to 25 kd; and (3) the high-glycine/tyrosine proteins, which are 6 to 9 kd. It is believed that the low-sulfur keratins form the 10-nm filaments and that the latter two groups of proteins form interfilamentous matrix. The low-sulfur proteins are further subdivided to type I, acidic proteins, and type II, basic proteins. The hair keratins are among the most acidic.

Keratins are also described as being "hard" and "soft," in a classic sense, to describe the alpha-keratins of the hardened, cornified tissues that comprise hair and nail, versus those of the "soft," mucosal-type epithelia.[11]

Cortical cells consist of closely packed macrofibrils within, and overall they are closely packed to one another and are oriented to the axis of the hair, being approximately 3 to 6 μm in diameter and up to 100 μm long.[10]

The macrofibrils are composed of rod-like microfibrils of approximately 7 nm in diameter arranged in whorls embedded in a intermicrofibrillar matrix. Between the macrofibrils is a variable amount of intermacrofibrillar matrix and melanin pigment granules, similar to the cuticular endocuticle.

Medulla

The medulla constitutes a continuous central part of fiber usually found only in terminal hair and has been described as being continuous, discontinuous, or even absent in hair. The medulla in all keratin fibers consists of a cortex-like framework of spongy keratin supporting thin shells of an amorphous material bounding air spaces of variable size. The medullary protein is known as being insoluble and difficult to isolate; therefore, analytical studies have not been possible. The medulla has a very low cystine and sulfur content and contains large quantities of acidic and basic amino acids and hydroxy amino acids.

Follicular Stem Cells

Another follicular structure has been shown to be important in growth. It had been assumed that the germinative center of the follicle was in the bulb, and that the only follicular stem cells were located in the matrix. Some investigators now believe that there are follicular stem cells located in the "bulge" area, where the arrector pili muscle inserts just below the sebaceous gland.[12] This site is located near the bottom of the permanent portion of the follicle in the outer root sheath. The "bulge" area is not always apparent on cross-section and varies in prominence depending on the site of the follicle.

Basal cells in the bulge region express keratin 19, which has been associated with regions containing stem cells and increased proliferative activity.[13] Also, morphologic irregularities are seen with expression of keratin 19 during epidermal regeneration.

Follicular stem cells from the bulge reportedly replenish matrical keratinocytes in early anagen. They may also be involved in skin carcinogenesis.[12] Further work to better understand the importance of these cells is needed.

The concept that stem cells reside in the bulge explains certain aspects of hair pathology. In alopecia areata, a nonscarring alopecia, the inflammatory infiltrate is concentrated in and around the hair bulb. In scarring alopecias, the inflammatory infiltrate affects the upper follicle including the stem cell region.

The "bulge hypothesis" implies that cell movement in the outer root sheath is downward rather than in an upward direction from the matrix, a concept difficult to confirm by direct examination.[7]

Dermal Papilla Cells

The papilla plays a major role in inducing follicular differentiation into anagen.[1, 10] Interactions between the papilla and neighboring matrix cells are involved in regulating the hair growth cycle. Once established during embryogenesis, the cellular population of the papilla is thought to be constant during successive hair growth cycles. The changes that do take place in the dermal papilla during the hair growth cycle are cell morphologic changes, vascularization, and the composition and volume of the extracellular matrix.

The size of the dermal papilla and surrounding bulb are thought to be directly related to the size of the hair produced.[10] In anagen follicles, the papilla is attached to a basal plate of connective tissue by a narrow stalk. In smaller hair follicles, there may be no visible vasculature, but terminal hair follicles show variable numbers of papillary blood vessels. There is a close relationship between the mitotic activity of papillary cells and the matrix cells. In human hair follicles, the ratio of papillary cells to matrix cells is approximately 1:9.

HAIR DYNAMICS

The anagen phase of the hair cycle varies in follicles. The normal duration of anagen in human scalp hairs is genetically determined and ranges from 2 to 8 years, versus 1 to 6 months for body hair, (eyelashes, trunk, extremities)[5] (Table 133–1). The resting, telogen phase lasts approximately 100 days or 1 to 4 months in follicles regardless of their location.[1, 5]

The ratio of anagen to telogen hairs is therefore approximately 90:10, since the percentage of hairs in catagen at any given moment is small. The average number of hairs shed per day is 100. The human scalp has approximately 100,000 follicles, with blondes having more and redheads fewer.[1] Seasonal variation in human scalp hair follicles growth indicates that over 90% of hair follicles are in anagen in the spring, decreasing to about 80% at the end of summer.[6] These are approximate figures representing the dynamics of follicular activity.

HAIR GROWTH CYCLE

The growth cycle of the human hair follicle is subdivided into various complex stages.[1] The biochemical signals that control the follicular cycle are not well understood. From the time the follicle is first formed, it undergoes repeated cycles of active growth and rest, called anagen and telogen, respectively.

Anagen

Anagen, or the active growth phase of the hair cycle, can be subdivided into six stages.[1] In stage I, cells of the dermal papilla increase in size and show increased RNA synthesis; at the same time, the germinal cells at the base of the follicle show increased mitotic activity (see Fig. 133-1). In stage II, the follicular bulb grows downward, enclosing the dermal papilla. In stage III, the follicle reaches its maximum length and the matrix cells give rise to the base of the internal root sheath. In stage IV, bulbar melanocytes develop dendrites and start to form melanin. The hair shaft is forming but still within the base of the internal root sheath. In stage V, the hair shaft starts to emerge from the internal root sheath. Stage VI is when the hair emerges from the skin surface and continues to grow until the onset of catagen. This stage has also been called *metanagen*. The stages I to V are known as *proanagen*.

Catagen

In the catagen phases of the hair cycle, mitosis in the matrix decreases and then stops completely, usually within a few days.[1] The melanocytes in the bulb resorb their dendrites, and keratinization of hair and inner root sheath continues. The terminal portion of the hair, which becomes club shaped, loses pigment, and more keratinized fibers extend between epithelial cells. Mitosis finally ceases in the inferior portion of the follicle, and the inner root sheath disintegrates and disappears. The dermal papilla moves upward as the follicle shortens. The club is surrounded by a partially keratinized capsule and enters telogen.

Telogen

Telogen is the resting phase of the cycle, in which the club hair is unpigmented and held in a sac by the intercellular junctions and kept in the follicle until the next cycle of anagen takes place spontaneously, or sometimes induced if the resting club hair is plucked.

It is important to combine individual stages of the hair cycle with our understanding of the anatomy to gain some understanding of the biochemistry and control of the cycle. In the past, it was thought that the dermal papilla produced the potent proliferative and morphogenic stimuli to signal hair growth. Today, it is believed that many structural areas of the follicle participate together in these complex signals, and that one area cannot function without the others.

BIOCHEMISTRY AND CONTROL OF HAIR FOLLICLE GROWTH

Hair Types

In humans, hair follicles are classified into three types: nonsexual hair, ambosexual hair, and male sexual hair.[2] Nonsexual hair is hair that grows independent of the presence of steroid hormones. These follicles are located on eyebrows, eyelashes, occipital scalp, forearms, and lower legs. Ambosexual hair is dependent on female levels of steroid hormones, localized in lower pubic triangle, axilla, and other parts of the body. Male sexual hair is dependent on androgens and is localized to the beard, ears, nasal tip, pubis, and frontal to vertex scalp.

Hormonal Effects

The effects of hormones on the hair cycles have been studied in both humans and animals. Cortisol has been found to inhibit the initiation of anagen in the resting follicle, and gonadectomy and adrenalectomy accelerate it.[1] Estrogens have been found to delay the initiation of follicular activity, retard the rate of growth during anagen, and prolong the duration of anagen.[1, 10] Thyroid hormones stimulate follicular activity, advancing the onset of anagen in resting follicles and increasing hair length. Thyroidectomy slightly reduces the rate of hair growth and the shaft diameter[1, 10] (Table 133-2).

Androgens have the most profound effect on follicles. Male hormones such as testosterone and dihydrotestosterone have "dual" effects of stimulating and inhibiting hair growth. Follicles on axillary, pubic, and beard hair grow in response to androgens, yet those on the scalp regress and recede in genetically susceptible men and women.[2-7]

Androgen Biochemistry

The way that androgens exert their effect on hair growth is still not totally clear (Fig. 133-2). The target

TABLE 133-2. Hormonal Effects on Hair Growth*

	Hair Growth Effects	
Hormone	*Scalp*	*Body*
Androgens	−	+
Cortisol	+/−	−
Estrogens	+/−	−
Progestins	+/−	+
Thyroid	+	+
Adrenalectomy	+	−
Gonadectomy	+	−
Thyroidectomy	−	−

*Systemic or topical treatment of hormones and their effects on human hair growth, (+) indicating a positive hair growing effect, and (−) no growth indicated, while (+/−) indicates either effect depending on the specfic hormone derivative given.

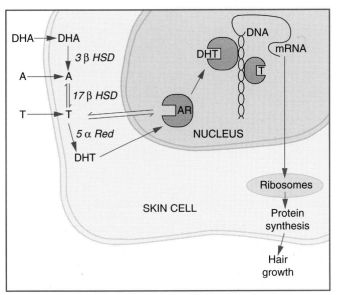

FIGURE 133-2. Mechanism of action of androgens. DHA, dehydro-epiandrosterone; A, androstenedione; T, testosterone; 5αRed, 5α-reductase; DHT, dihydrotestosterone; HSD, hydroxysteroid dehydrogenase; AR, aromatase. (Adapted from Simpson NB, Barth JH. Hair patterns in hirsuties and baldness. In: Rook A, Dawber R (eds.). Diseases of Hair and Scalp, 2nd edition. Oxford: Blackwell Scientific Publications, 1991:71–135.)

tissue androgens testosterone and dihydrotestosterone have an effect on shortening the length of anagen; ironically, in other areas of the body, they stimulate hair growth. Androgens stimulate the production of growth factors and proteases, and have an effect on the vascularization, basement membrane proteins, and other metabolic cycles that alter the levels of vital cofactors, thus affecting hair growth.

Enzymes

Each hair follicle is genetically regulated depending on location—for example, frontal versus occipital scalp. Previous investigators have shown that follicles as well as sebaceous glands can metabolize weak androgens (Fig. 133–2), such as dehydroepiandrosterone and 4-androstenedione, to testosterone and dihydrotestosterone via important enzymes in the steroid cascade.[2-6] These enzymes, δ-5-3β-hydroxysteroid dehydrogenase (3β-HSD), 17β-HSD, and 5α-reductase, have been localized and quantitated in isolated hair follicles and sebaceous glands and have been found to vary in quantity depending on location of the pilosebaceous structure.[2, 8, 9]

There are two forms of the 5α-reductase enzyme: type I in skin and type II in prostate.[2-6] Many antiandrogen compounds may not work as well in treating androgen-related skin conditions, such as hair loss or acne, because they are more specific for the type II enzyme found in prostate and are not as effective for the type I skin enzyme.

Another enzyme in the pathway is called "aromatase," a cytochrome P-450 enzyme that has been specifically located in the outer root sheath[8] and found at higher levels in hair follicles from the scalps of women than men.[9] This enzyme is responsible for converting 4-androstenedine and testosterene to estrogens, such as estrone and estradiol, respectively. It has been hypothesized that aromatase may be important in mediating a balance of androgens in the hair follicle, thus regulating the hair cycle.[8, 9]

Immunohistochemical studies reveal that aromatase is located in the lower portion of the outer root sheath, suggesting that circulating hormones are metabolized or processed prior to entry into the hair bulb or dermal papilla cells,[8, 9] where receptors are most concentrated and are likely to be the target area stimulating gene expression.

Finding aromatase as well as the other steroid enzymes suggests that the outer root sheath may play an important role in hormone metabolism to maintain a "balance" of hormones entering the bulbar dermal papilla cells, therefore regulating hair cycles. Therefore, each component of the follicle plays a vital role in maintaining follicular homeostasis.

Androgen Receptor

Once dihydrotestosterone or testosterone is formed, it binds to a specific intranuclear receptor protein, namely the androgen receptor, which then forms an "activated" hormone-receptor complex. This "activation" is dependent on other cellular factors, such as a specific phosphokinase that phosphorylates the androgen receptor (since the androgen receptor is a phosphoprotein) and a sulfhydryl-reducing enzyme (since the androgen receptor must also be sulfhydryly reduced for optimum hormone binding to occur).[14-16]

Receptor/Nuclear Factors

The sulfhydryl-reducing factor is believed to be a thioredoxin enzyme system that influences intramolecular disulfide bonding of the androgen receptor, which affects hormone binding to its binding site.[14-16] The thioredoxin enzyme is found in high levels in anagen follicles, but is diminished in balding areas.[14-16] It is uncertain if thioredoxin in low amounts is a reflection of the balding process, or if it represents hair follicles that are in a metabolically resting telogen state.

A 12-kd nuclear matrix acceptor protein (NAP) has been found to be important for mediating high-affinity binding of the hormone-receptor complex to DNA. The NAP was found in scalp follicles of both men and women.[2, 17] Characterizing the DNA fragments associated with the NAP will be important for finding the specific DNA sequences involved with hormone-receptor complex binding to androgen-regulated genes signaling synthesis or inhibition of cellular proteins affecting hair growth in beard or scalp hair, respectively.[17]

CONCLUSIONS

Each compartment of the hair follicle is important in regulating events during the hair growth cycle. We are beginning to understand the molecular basis of hair growth control with the use of embryonic skin culture, in vitro recombinant cultures, organ cultures, and transgenic constructs. Recent findings on androgen-regulated biochemical processes altering hair growth have furthered our understanding of hair disorders. Other fundamental questions still remain unanswered with regard to "the" gene sequence controlling or signaling the growth cycle, and why this control or signal is different for hair follicles in different body sites. By answering these questions, perhaps better treatments may be found to treat the millions of men and women who suffer from hair disorders or diseases.

Androgenetic Disorders

Maria K. Hordinsky

DEFINITION

Androgenetic alopecia is an inherited, androgen-dependent form of hair loss. Orentreich first used this term in 1960 to take into account that both genes and hormones play a role in this hair disorder.[18] However, many investigators use other synonyms, such as common baldness, male-pattern baldness, female-pattern baldness, and diffuse alopecia of women, to describe androgenetic alopecia.[19]

CLINICAL DESCRIPTION

The prevalence of androgenetic alopecia has not been accurately recorded in any population. However, in contrast to other races, the development of androgenetic alopecia may approximate 100% in Caucasians.[20]

In 1951, Hamilton proposed a classification system for male androgenetic alopecia. This system evolved from a study of 312 white males and 214 white females between the ages of 20 and 89 years.[21] The types of male androgenetic alopecia in the Hamilton classification system are presented in Figure 133–3. Hamilton described Type I as normal scalp before puberty, after which it is replaced by Type II in 96% of men. Over one half of men in his study who were 50 years of age and older had Type V to Type VIII, and the extent of baldness was noted to increase with aging. The Hamilton Baldness Scale was modified by Norwood to a more comprehensive 12-point scale and is also presented in Figure 133–3.[22]

Though the pattern of male androgenetic alopecia has been well documented, only recently have the changes in the affected areas been followed quantitatively. Rushton and colleagues followed a cohort of men and age- and sex-matched controls between the ages of 20 and 30 years for 24 months. They compared several parameters and over a 24-month period found a continuing decrease in the percentage of hairs in the anagen phase, total hair density, and meaningful hair density. A greater than 15% decrease in hair density had to take place before patients became aware of a change in hair density. A large proportion of hairs less than or equal to 40 mm in length with diameters similar to those of longer hair fibers were also found. When the vellus hair frequency was subtracted, the percentage of these nonvellus hairs less than or equal to 40 mm in length was 12.2% (range, 5.7% to 21.5%), whereas in the men with androgenetic alopecia, the mean frequency of this type of hair was 48% (range, 8.0% to 84.2%). The authors postulated that if these hairs could be induced to grow longer, the aesthetic profile could be changed significantly.[23]

The "male" pattern of alopecia does occur in women, but a more common presentation is widening of the part width associated with a diffuse pattern of scalp hair loss on the crown.[24, 25] Ludwig described three grades of balding patterns in women (Fig. 133–4). Women with Grade I show perceptible thinning of hair on their crown with no loss of the frontal hairline and a relatively normal part width. In contrast, women with Grade II have pronounced thinning of the hair on the crown and an increase in their part width diameter. Those with Grade III show extreme baldness on the crown and further widening of their part width.

In Hamilton's study, 79% of women developed Type II androgenetic alopecia after puberty and about 25% of women had Type IV androgenetic alopecia by the age of 50.[26] A correlation between decreased circulating estrogen levels and an increased presentation of patterned androgenetic alopecia was first described by Binazzi.[26] Venning and Dawber found that all of the women that they studied experienced a change in their scalp hair

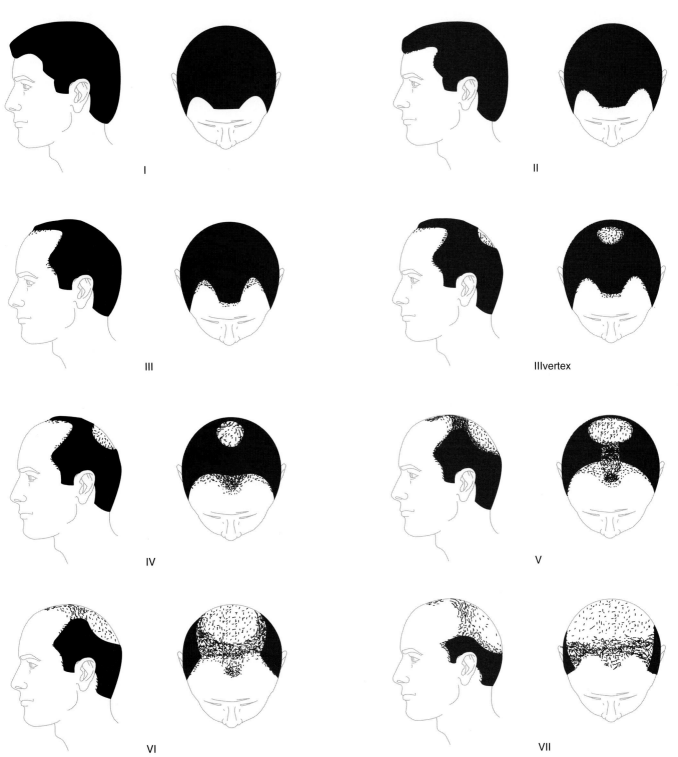

FIGURE 133-3. Hamilton's classification of androgenetic alopecia. The modifications made by Nor-wood are presented in bold font. Type I, Full hair. Type II, Bitemporal recession. **Type IIa.** Type III, Borderline. **Type IIIa.** Type IV, Deep frontotemporal recession; usually also some midfrontal recession. **Type IVa.** Type V, Increased frontotemporal recession and marked denudation of vertex. **Type Va.** Type VI, Increased loss from the vertex and frontotemporal region with the areas becoming confluent. Type VII, Frontotemporal and vertical balding with only a band of sparse hair. Type VIII, Complete loss of hair between the frontotemporal and vertical regions (not shown). (Reprinted by permission from the SOUTHERN MEDICAL JOURNAL, 1975; 68:1359–1365.)

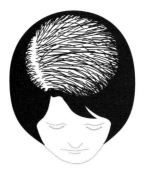 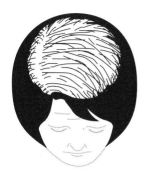 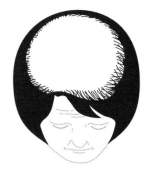

FIGURE 133-4. Ludwig's classification of female androgenetic alopecia. *A*, Grade I female androgenetic alopecia. *B*, Grade II female androgenetic alopecia. *C*, Grade III female androgenetic alopecia. (From Ludwig E. Classification of the types of androgenetic alopecia arising in the female sex. Br J Dermatol 1977;97:249-257.)

pattern after puberty, and classic male-type Hamilton patterns were frequently noted in women after they experienced menopause.[27]

Recent investigations have focused on the psychologic effects of androgenetic alopecia on men and women. Cash first investigated the psychologic effects of androgenetic alopecia in men. He studied 145 men: 63 with modest balding, 40 with more extensive balding, and 42 nonbalding controls. Study subjects completed a battery of standardized psychologic measures. Cash found that men with more extensive balding, younger men, single men, and those with an earlier hair-loss onset had less body image satisfaction, were considerably preoccupied with their hair problem, and had moderate stress or distress, and that these individuals developed several adjustive strategies to cope with, compensate for, or conceal their hair loss.[28]

In a subsequent study, Cash and colleagues studied 96 women and 60 men with androgenetic alopecia and 56 female control patients. Subjects completed standardized questionnaires in which psychologic reactions to their hair loss and measurements of body image, personality, and adjustment were examined.[29] The presence of androgenetic alopecia was found to be a stressful experience for both sexes, but especially so for women. Affected women were found to have a more negative body image and a pattern of less adaptive functioning. In still another study, Van der Donk and colleagues found that women with androgenetic alopecia had more psychosocial problems than women with other dermatologic complaints.[30]

The presence of androgenetic alopecia in males has been hypothesized to be a predictor of cardiovascular disease including myocardial infarction.[31] The presence of gray hair in both black and white males has also been hypothesized to be a possible risk factor in coronary artery disease.[32] In a major study examining the relationship between male androgenetic alopecia and the risk of myocardial infarction in men under the age of 55 years, Lesko and colleagues conducted a hospital-based case-control study in eastern Massachusetts and Rhode Island.[31] Six hundred and sixty-five men admitted to the hospital for a first nonfatal myocardial infarction and 772 men admitted to the same hospitals with noncardiac diagnoses were studied. The risk of myocardial infarction was found to significantly increase as the degree of vertex baldness increased. For severe vertex baldness, the relative risk was 3.4 (95% confidence interval, 1.7 to 7.0) in men under the age of 55 years. This association was present regardless of the presence of other risk factors for

coronary artery disease such as smoking, hypertension, hypercholesterolemia, or family history of myocardial infarction. The mechanism responsible for this association is not clear but is postulated to be related to the presence of dihydrotestosterone, the active metabolite of testosterone produced in tissue by the enzyme 5α-reductase. A similar study examining females with androgenetic alopecia and the relationship to cardiovascular disease remains to be undertaken.

PATHOLOGY

The main histopathologic findings in male androgenetic alopecia derive from shortening of the anagen stage of the hair cycle. With each successive cycle, anagen resumes in follicles whose bulbs are smaller and more superficially situated, producing progressively more narrow hair shafts.[33] Thus in biopsy specimens of evolving androgenetic alopecia, there are anagen follicles (recognizable by the formation of both inner and outer root sheaths, the former marked by trichohyalin granules) of sizes intermediate between terminal hairs whose bulbs reside in the subcutis and vellus hairs whose much smaller bulbs are found in the superficial dermis. Increased numbers of catagen and telogen follicles may also be seen. Vellus hairs occur in normal scalp, so that their mere identification does not signify androgenetic alopecia. All of these findings are best appreciated in transverse sections, which demonstrate many more follicles than do routine vertical sections (Fig. 133-5). Female androgenetic alopecia has not been studied as comprehensively, but similarities to male androgenetic alopecia have been suggested.[34]

Eventually, the delicate and highly vascularized collagen bundles of the fibrous tracts are replaced by sclerosis, limiting the potential for regrowth. Staining for elastic tissue by the orcein method demonstrates Arao-Perkins bodies, which derive from condensed elastic fibers at the sites of previously present hair papillae.[33] These elastic fibers can later be found aligned vertically within the previously present tracts.

There are a number of other microscopic findings in androgenetic alopecia.[34-36] Thinning of the epidermis, degeneration of the lower connective tissue sheath, perivascular basophilic changes, a decrease in the upper dermal capillary network, and increased dermal glycosaminoglycans and mucopolysaccharides have all been noted in male androgenetic alopecia. While some studies have

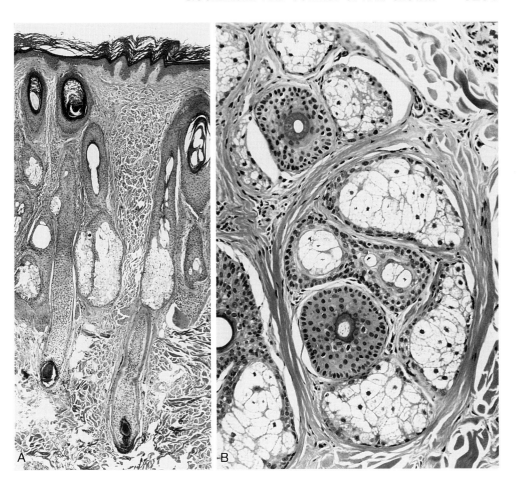

FIGURE 133–5. A vertical section of a 4-mm punch biopsy of a male with evolving androgenetic alopecia shows anagen follicles with bulbs in the dermis rather than in the subcutis (*A*). Transverse section (*B*) shows normally sized sebaceous glands next to anagen and vellus hairs in a follicular unit.

claimed that sebaceous glands are enlarged, morphometry has proven that their enlarged appearance is due only to their comparatively large size in relation to the diminished hair bulbs that they are associated with. Changes in cutaneous innervation have also been described.[37]

Dystrophic hair follicles also occur in the scalp with advancing age. However, follicular degenerative changes or abnormalities in the surrounding tissue are not routinely seen.[38]

Inflammation has been described as being significant, minor, or absent in male androgenetic alopecia.[35, 36, 39–42] Lattanand and Johnson examined 347 tissue specimens from 23 patients and 10 control samples taken from the posterior scalp of donors undergoing hair transplants. They found inflammation in almost one half of the specimens.[36] Abell found an inflammatory reaction in 75% of the specimens studied.[39] Whiting described inflammation or fibrosis in 70% of cases, in contrast to the 40.9% found in his normal control population.[40] Jaworsky reported the inflammatory reaction to be restricted to the region around the sebaceous glands and infundibulum.[41] Whiting also noted that the inflammatory process was more common around the upper than the lower follicle.[40]

Immunopathologic studies of androgenetic alopecia suggest an immunopathologic process. Bystryn examined skin samples from 19 patients with androgenetic alopecia. Ten patients donated biopsy specimens from both normal and involved scalp. Samples from involved scalp only were obtained from 6 patients; from 3 patients, samples were obtained only from uninvolved skin. In 3 patients, the third component of complement, C3, was found in a discontinuous pattern along the basement membrane zone of the hair follicle and, in one case, in the epidermis. Two of the patients showed the same findings in involved and uninvolved skin, one only in involved skin. One patient showed immunoglobulin (Ig) G in both involved and uninvolved skin and IgM deposition only in the balding area.[43]

Young and colleagues examined specimens from 26 patients and 8 controls. Nineteen patients had male androgenetic alopecia, and seven had female androgenetic alopecia. Tissue sections were stained with goat antihuman antibodies to IgM, IgG, IgA, C3, and fibrinogen. IgM or C3 (or both) was detected at the basement membrane in 96% or 25 of 26 patients and in 12% or one of eight control specimens. No immunoreactants were found in any of the other control specimens. Interestingly, *Propionibacterium acnes* was found in the pilosebaceous canal in 58% of patients and in 12% of the control subjects. Young and colleagues postulated that since *Propionibacterium acnes* produces porphyrins, ultraviolet light directed at scalp skin could possibly activate microbial porphyrins as it does human porphyrins, thereby activating C3 and the complement cascade.[42]

PATHOGENESIS AND ETIOLOGY

In 1942, Hamilton linked a genetic predisposition and androgens with the development of androgenetic alopecia.[44] The genetic inheritance in both men and women is believed to be autosomal dominant with variable penetrance, but a multifactorial inheritance has not been excluded.[45-46]

Hamilton's description of the association of androgens with androgenetic alopecia has since been supported by several studies. In the original studies, Hamilton described the absence of baldness in 10 eunuchoids — 10 men castrated before puberty — and in 34 men who had undergone orchiectomy during adolescence. When testosterone was administered, androgenetic alopecia developed only in those presumed to be genetically predisposed. When administration of the hormone testosterone was discontinued, the balding process did not progress but it was also not reversed.[44]

In the absence of ovarian or adrenal gland disease, levels of circulating free or total androgens are usually normal in individuals predisposed to developing androgenetic alopecia. Individuals with complete androgen insensitivity syndrome also have relatively normal testosterone levels but lack functional androgen receptors.[47] Such 46 chromosome, XY individuals exhibit a female phenotype but at adolescence do not develop any terminal body hair or pubic or axillary hair. They also do not develop balding.

Localization studies of androgen receptors in the skin have shown that the number of receptors varies with anatomic site.[47, 48] Follicular receptivity and reactivity to androgens in androgenetic alopecia are believed to be localized to the papilla/matrix unit.[49] Studies with ^{3}(H)-testosterone have localized the radioactivity only to the dermal papilla and not in follicular epithelial cells.[50]

In target tissues, testosterone is reduced by the enzyme 5α-reductase to 5α-dihydrotestosterone. Earlier studies showed that 5α-reductase enzyme activity is increased in hair follicles of balding scalp but not in nonbalding scalp. This observation, along with the observation that 5α-reductase–deficient individuals have less temporal hair regression, suggested early on that the synthesis of dihydrotestosterone is associated with the development of androgenetic alopecia.[51]

Two steroid 5α-reductase enzymes, called types 1 and 2, are recognized.[52] The 5α-reductase type 1 gene (SRD5A1) encodes an isozyme with an alkaline pH optimum, and the 5α-reductase type 2 gene (SRD5A2) encodes an isozyme with an acidic pH optimum. The activity of the 5α-reductase type 2 enzyme can be blocked by finasteride (Proscar), a drug currently marketed in the United States for the therapy of benign prostatic hypertrophy and which is in clinical trials for the treatment of androgenetic alopecia.

No genetic mutations of the type 1 enzyme in humans have been reported. Mutations in the type 2 gene are associated with decreased synthesis of dihydrotestosterone.[53] Affected 46, XY males are born with normal internal reproductive structures (epididymes, seminal vesicles, and vasa deferentia) but have a hypoplastic prostate and female-appearing external genitalia. During puberty, varying degrees of virilization occur but secondary sexual hair remains sparse and less acne or androgenetic alopecia develops.

The expression of 5α-reductase type 1 activity in the scalp of balding and nonbalding men has been examined.[52] All but one of five individuals were comprehensively studied and found to have no significant differences in 5α-reductase activity between balding and non-balding scalp. The one exception was an obese male (>400 pounds) with Hamilton Type II balding. This male had a marked decrease in the expression of type 1 5α-reductase activity not only in his scalp skin but also in his liver.[52] The significance of this latter finding is unclear.

Examination for 5α-reductase type 2 activity in samples taken from the crown to the hairline to the peripheral region of the scalp from a Caucasian male with Hamilton Type VIII baldness revealed no activity in any of the samples. In still other experiments, Thigpen and coworkers described the expression of type 1 5α-reductase activity in female scalp skin to be qualitatively equivalent to that of male scalp.[52]

It is postulated that androgens are regulators of hair growth and either directly or indirectly alter the activity of many components of the hair follicle, including melanocytes, epithelial cells, and dermal papilla cells. One hypothesis is that androgens act on the cells of the dermal papilla, which in turn secrete paracrine factors that influence other follicular components. This hypothesis is based on the concept that the dermal papilla plays an essential role in inducing and maintaining epithelial differentiation.[49]

Biochemical advances in androgenetic alopecia suggest that when testosterone or dihydrotestosterone diffuses into and binds to hair follicle cells, an "activated" complex is formed. This complex is translocated into the nucleus, where it binds to specific nuclear chromatin acceptor sites that affect the rate of transcription by altering levels of RNA polymerase II and subsequently protein synthesis.[54] The number, type, and affinity of androgen receptor proteins are postulated to differ depending on endogenous regulatory peptides found in the hair follicle cell. Sawaya has described two such endogenous factors, which she has called "inhibitor protein" and "converting factor." Both of these endogenous factors have been found in microdissected anagen scalp hair follicles. When the androgen receptor is in its monomeric form in contrast to a larger, tetrameric form, dihydrotestosterone is able to bind and form an "activated" hormone-receptor complex that can translocate to the nucleus. Once in the nucleus, this hormone-receptor complex is postulated to bind to specific sites on the DNA called *hormone response elements*. These are presumed to be upstream from neighboring structural genes that can influence hair growth.[54-56]

Very few biochemical studies on female androgenetic alopecia have been performed. Type 1 5α-reductase activity in female androgenetic alopecia is reportedly equivalent to that of male scalp.[52] Sawaya reported regional differences in enzyme levels of aromatase, 3β-dehydrogenase, 17β-dehydrogenase, and 5α-reductase between involved balding and uninvolved male and female and scalp skin. Involved scalp skin showed decreased enzyme levels as compared with unaffected scalp in both sexes. Since aromatase is needed to convert androstenedione and testosterone to estrone and estradiol, respectively, she postulated that the maintenance of the frontal hairline in women may be related to a higher concentration of these estrogens in this region.[57]

Hormones and genes have both been accepted as playing a role in adrogenetic alopecia. However, the presence of an inflammatory infiltrate and its role in the pathogenesis of androgenetic alopecia still remain to be explained. A hypothetical sequence of events for the role of inflammation in progressive male androgenetic alopecia has been proposed by Jaworsky and colleagues.[41] They postulate that normal anagen follicles become infiltrated with activated T cells that preferentially distribute within the epithelium and the adventitial sheath at the level of the lower infundibulum near the putative stem cell population of the hair bulge. Mast cell degranulation occurs, and collagen synthesis is induced by sheath fibroblasts. The end-stage follicle becomes characterized by a fibrous tract whose delicate structure is replaced by sclerosis and an infundibular region incapable of hair growth.[40]

DIAGNOSIS AND DIFFERENTIAL DIAGNOSIS

Hyperandrogenism implies an elevated androgen concentration or an exaggerated clinical response to androgen action. Clinical features may include any of the following: hirsutism, acne, primary or secondary amenorrhea, increased libido and muscle mass, loss of breast tissue, deepening of the voice, infertility, and clitoral enlargement (overall size > 35 mm^2), as well as androgenetic alopecia[58] (Fig. 133–6). Androgenetic alopecia not associated with an underlying endocrinologic disturbance is considered "idiopathic" and is the main presentation of androgen excess in the majority of women.[59] However, between 30% and 40% of women with andro-

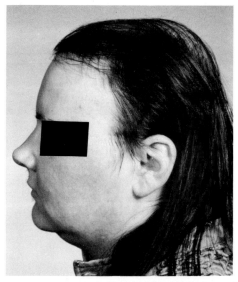

FIGURE 133–6. Female patient presenting with signs of androgen excess including acne, hirsutism, and androgenetic alopecia.

genetic alopecia will have an underlying adrenal or ovarian disorder to explain their androgenetic alopecia.[60] In women, the major sources of androgens are the ovaries and adrenal glands, with many of the same compounds produced by the ovaries also produced by the adrenal glands.[61] In men, the major source of androgens is the adrenal gland. The same enzymatic pathways are used by the ovaries and the adrenal glands for the production of androgens. However, the ovaries do not produce cortisol or aldosterone and the adrenal gland does not produce estrogen or progesterone. Seventy per cent of dehydroepiandrosterone (DHEA) and over 95% of the sulfated form (DHEA-S) are derived from the adrenal gland. Testosterone and androstenedione are derived in approximately equal amounts from the ovary and the adrenal gland.[58] Extraglandular production of circulating androgens occurs and includes the conversion of androgens to estrogens and the conversion of relatively weak androgens into more potent forms such as testosterone and dihydrotestosterone at the level of target organs as in the skin.[58] When androgens are released into the bloodstream, only a small fraction exists as free steroid. About 80% of circulating testosterone is bound to sex hormone–binding globulin (SHBG), 19% to albumin, and only about 1% remains unbound.[62] Estrogen binds to SHBG and various factors can influence SHBG levels. Estrogen and excessive thyroid hormone are associated with increases in SHBG, whereas obesity, hyperinsulinemia, and elevated androgen levels decrease SHBG.

The main causes of androgen dysfunction in females include abnormalities in the pituitary/adrenal and pituitary/ovarian axes or abnormal target cell hormone metabolism and utilization.[58] However, it has also been noted that subtle defects can exist in the adrenal steroidogenic pathway and that these can contribute to androgen-mediated diseases. Abnormalities in the enzyme pathway can be diagnosed only by adrenocorticotropic hormone (ACTH) stimulation tests because basal blood hormone levels do not usually reveal these subtle abnormalities.[63]

The hormonal status of postmenopausal women with androgenetic alopecia has been examined. Conflicting results are reported. Gourgiotou and colleagues measured circulating concentrations of testosterone, SHBG, and estradiol in 10 postmenopausal women with androgenetic alopecia and 10 normal controls. They found no significant differences, in contrast to other reported studies in which circulating androgen excess was reported.[64]

The evaluation of the male or female patient who presents with hair loss should include taking a good medical history and a careful assessment of drug use. The appearance of thin, sparse hair on the crown of the head of women has been associated not only with androgen excess but also thyroid disease, particularly hypothyroidism, and abnormal iron metabolism.[65, 66] Serum ferritin levels have been found to be low in some women with hair loss. Therefore, if indicated, the laboratory evaluation should consist of assessing thyroid function, serum ferritin, and other parameters of iron metabolism, and an assessment of androgen metabolism.

What constitutes a necessary and sufficient evaluation of hyperandrogenism? Sperling divided affected women and their laboratory evaluation into four major categories based on their clinical presentations.[62] Category IA, called "simple," includes women with treatment-resistant acne or hirsutism or alopecia. Category IB, called "sudden," includes women with severe treatment-resistant acne, hirsutism, and/or alopecia. Women in Category II are patients with menstrual dysfunction and signs of hyperandrogenism as acne, hirsutism, and alopecia. Women in Category III have frank virilization.

The laboratory assessment of women in Category 1A could range from assessing DHEA-S and free testosterone levels to including SHBG and total testosterone levels. As patients in Category 1B have more severe clinical symptoms, these patients can be evaluated as those in Category 1A, but if Cushing's syndrome is suspected, an ACTH stimulation test is recommended. 17-Hydroxyprogesterone has been used as a screening test for late-onset congenital adrenal hyperplasia. However, it is now recommended this test be checked (if used at all) in conjunction with an ACTH stimulation test.[67, 68]

Patients in Category II who have menstrual dysfunction and acne, hirsutism, or alopecia need to be evaluated in greater depth. The presence of irregular or infrequent periods, amenorrhea, and infertility are examples of menstrual dysfunction. These can be associated with both adrenal and ovarian abnormalities. In addition to assessing a DHEA-S level and free and total testosterone levels, a prolactin level should be checked, as a serum prolactin–secreting tumor can cause both hyperandrogenism and menstrual dysfunction.[67] A prolactin level determination should always be ordered if there is a history of galactorrhea. Luteinizing hormone and follicle-stimulating hormone levels should also be obtained and when amenorrhea is present, a serum estradiol level should be checked.[67, 68] Patients in Category III who show frank virilization in addition to acne and androgenetic alopecia most likely have a significant abnormality in androgen metabolism. The presence of an underlying tumor must be ruled out in such patients. Patients in Categories II and III should probably also be followed in conjunction with an endocrinologist or gynecologist.

TREATMENT

Treatments for androgenetic alopecia range from nonhormonal therapy with topical minoxidil to the experimental use of antiandrogens and various combinations of medical and surgical treatment (Table 133–3). (Surgical treatment is discussed in a separate section.) Topical 2% minoxidil (Rogaine) is a piperidinopyrimidine derivative, nonhormonal therapy that is effective in the treatment of androgenetic alopecia. Minoxidil has been widely tested in multicenter trials and in the United States is approved by the Food and Drug Administration for the therapy of androgenetic alopecia in both men and women. Hair growth appears to peak at 1 year, but maintenance of nonvellus hair beyond that seen at baseline can still be found in patients on long-term therapy—up to 5 years.[69–71] Discontinuing therapy is associated with loss of the hair gained within 4 to 6 months of stopping the drug.[72] The best responders are those in whom the

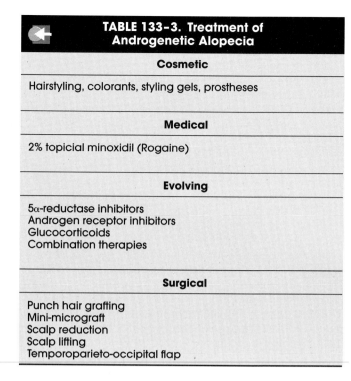

TABLE 133–3. Treatment of Androgenetic Alopecia
Cosmetic
Hairstyling, colorants, styling gels, prostheses
Medical
2% topical minoxidil (Rogaine)
Evolving
5α-reductase inhibitors Androgen receptor inhibitors Glucocorticoids Combination therapies
Surgical
Punch hair grafting Mini-micrograft Scalp reduction Scalp lifting Temporoparieto-occipital flap

balding process is relatively early, the pretreatment hair density is greater than 20 hairs/cm^2, and the maximum diameter of the bald area is less than 10 cm.[73] The mechanism by which minoxidil induces hair regrowth remains to be elucidated but may be related to the drug having a direct effect on the proliferation of follicular cells. Side effects are minimal and include local irritation and facial hypertrichosis.

Examination of horizontal sections of scalp biopsy specimens in male androgenetic alopecia provides not only diagnostic information but also predictive information about the potential to respond to topical minoxidil therapy.[40] An average 4-mm horizontal section contains a 2:1 ratio of terminal to vellus hairs, in contrast to 7 terminal:1 vellus hair ratio in normal control subjects. Forty-four patients treated with 2% topical minoxidil were observed for 1 year or slightly longer. Five patients with fewer than two follicular structures/mm^2 showed no hair regrowth, 32 with two to four follicular structures/mm^2 showed regrowth, and 7 with more than four follicular structures/mm^2 showed regrowth in 86% of cases.[40] Such information may be useful to both the patient and physician who are considering embarking on a course of topical minoxidil therapy for the treatment of androgenetic alopecia.

Antiandrogens have been used topically and administered orally or intralesionally to retard the extension of androgenetic alopecia. Investigators have focused on finding an antiandrogen that will give significant hair regrowth.[60] Antiandrogens used to manage androgenetic alopecia either inhibit the conversion of testosterone to dihydrotestosterone by 5α-reductase or inhibit dihydrotestosterone binding to the steroid receptors. Still other agents affect the binding of testosterone or dihydrotestosterone by binding to different areas on the enzyme or receptor and thereby affecting either the reaction rate of the enzyme or binding of hormone to the receptor protein.[60]

Nonsteroidal drugs such as flutamide and cimetidine have been used to treat androgenetic alopecia.[74, 75] Flutamide was marketed in 1989 in the United States for patients with metastatic prostate cancer and for patients who responded to or were beginning treatment with an analogue of luteinizing hormone–releasing hormone (LHRH). Its use; however, for the treatment of hyperandrogenism has not been approved by Food and Drug Administration. Furthermore, some patients taking this drug may develop serious hepatotoxicity.[76]

Cimetidine, a gastric H_2-receptor antagonist, has been found to act as a weak antiandrogen by competitively inhibiting dihydrotestosterone. Its use as an antiandrogen has been examined in the management of hirsutism, but its effectiveness in the management of androgenetic alopecia has not been established.[77]

The competitive inhibitors—those compounds structurally similar to testosterone or dihydrotestosterone such as progesterone and 17α-hydroxyprogesterone—have been used to treat androgenetic alopecia. However, these antiandrogens also have the potential to provoke the process because of their androgenic potential.[60] Progesterone has been used orally and in 1% and 5% topical and intralesional solutions. Oral contraceptives have also been used to suppress systemic androgen production by the progestin in the particular oral contraceptive. The results of using progestins to treat androgenetic alopecia have reportedly been somewhat successful, but no controlled, large-scale studies have been performed to confirm the efficacy of this approach.[18, 60, 78]

When choosing an oral contraceptive, not only the progestational agent needs to be considered but also the estrogen component. The estrogen component decreases ovarian and adrenal androgen production and stimulates SHBG from the liver. SHBG binds to free circulating androgens and decreases the amount of active free androgen.[60] Although there is evidence that higher dose estrogen pills and mid-potency oral contraceptives containing 35 to 50 μg of ethinyl estradiol and 0.5 to 1.0 mg of norethindrone are effective in treating hirsutism, there are no well-controlled studies to support one product over another in treating androgenetic alopecia.[67, 79, 80]

In postmenopausal women, estrogen supplementation (without progestin) has been suggested as a useful therapy for androgenetic alopecia as well as acne and hirsutism.[81] Topical estrogen-containing hair preparations have also been used to treat androgenetic alopecia. However, no topical estrogen-containing hair preparations are approved for the treatment of androgenetic alopecia in

the United States. In addition, no controlled studies are available on the usefulness of this modality, and therapy can be complicated by the development of gynecomastia in males and abnormal uterine bleeding in both pre- and postmenopausal women.[82–84]

Another group of drugs that have been used to suppress adrenal and ovarian androgen production are the glucocorticoids. Typically, dexamethasone is prescribed.

Spironolactone (Aldactone) is another steroid that is best known for its use in the management of primary aldosteronism and conditions such as congestive heart failure and hypertension. This drug also decreases testosterone production by the adrenal gland. It affects the cytochrome P-450 enzyme system, a system necessary for the 17-hydroxylase and desmolase enzymes to synthesize androgens. Spironolactone is also a mild competitive inhibitor of dihydrotestosterone binding to the androgen receptor and interferes with the translocation of the receptor complex to the nucleus.[60]

A compound that inhibits 5α-reductase activity has been examined for its effect on the development of baldness in the stumptail macaque (*Macaca speciosa*), an animal model for male androgenetic alopecia. As compared with the control group, treated monkeys did not show a change in the percentage of actively growing hair follicles in the frontal scalp, whereas a significant decrease occurred in the control group.[85] The oral administration of finasteride, a 5α-reductase inhibitor, alone or in combination with topical 2% minoxidil to the balding stumptail macaque resulted in an increase in hair weight. The combination of finasteride and minoxidil generated an additive effect, suggesting that the inhibition of the conversion of testosterone to dihydrotestosterone by finasteride reverses the balding process and enhances hair regrowth by topical minoxidil in the male balding stumptail macaque.[86] Clinical trials assessing the safety and efficacy of oral finasteride for the therapy of male androgenetic alopecia are currently in progress.

Another combination treatment that has been used to treat male androgenetic alopecia is the combination of 0.5% topical minoxidil with .025% tretinoin. Results of preliminary studies show that moderate to good hair regrowth can occur with this combination in over 50% of treated patients.[87, 88] However, additional studies are needed to confirm the efficacy of this approach.

Still other approaches to the management of androgenetic alopecia include wearing creative hairstyles and using correct shampoos and conditioners, mousses, colorants, and styling gels. Surgical removal of the affected area and replacement with hair-bearing skin offers still another approach to the treatment of androgenetic alopecia in both men and women.[56]

Hair Replacement Surgery

Dominic A. Brandy and Kathryn L. Brandy

While medical management of hair loss may slow the inevitable progression of androgenetic alopecia, enhance hair regrowth, or camouflage the loss, there are still individuals who have experienced such significant loss that they are not substantially benefited by medical management. For these individuals, a variety of hair replacement surgical techniques may offer a permanent solution. The underlying principle of hair replacement surgery is the concept of donor dominance. Donor dominance refers to skin flaps or characteristics regardless of the properties of the recipient site on to which they are placed. In early work with androgenetic alopecia, small hair-bearing grafts from the occiput retained the characteristic hair growth of the occiput after transplantation to the bald scalp. Although this basic tenet has remained unchanged, various refinements and modifications continue to evolve and improve the final result of hair replacement surgery. Punch hair grafting is the base upon which mini-micrografts, scalp reduction, scalp lifting, and temporoparieto-occipital flaps build.

PUNCH HAIR GRAFTING

Description

Punch hair transplantation is a technique, based on the theory of donor dominance, that was introduced by Orentreich in 1959.[89] The initial phase of this method involves the harvesting of donor-dominant scalp at the proper angle with a motor-driven, cylindrical, carbon-steel trephine (4.0 to 5.0 mm in diameter, which yields 15 to 25 hairs per graft). In the developmental years, these punch grafts were removed randomly and allowed to heal by secondary intention; but the procedure has evolved to the point at which the donor-dominant grafts are now harvested in a cluster fashion (Fig. 133–7A) with the remaining defect being repaired with a interdigitated closure. After excising these donor punch grafts, including hair bulbs, the fat of the graft is trimmed and stray hairs are removed under magnification. Trimming fat from donor grafts prevents later cobblestoning at the recipient site. The grafts are then placed into slightly smaller holes (0.5 to 0.75 mm differential) that are created with trephines directed at a 45-degree anterior angle. A circumferential bandage is recommended for compression and the absorption of blood.

The most common sequencing utilized for the recipient area is a systematic four-step approach that ensures that each alopecic area will be covered with hair upon completion of the hair transplantation sessions (Fig. 133–8). Once the graft congeals with the recipient area and revascularizes, the hair in that graft begins growing approximately 3 months from the point of implantation. In regard to timing between transplantation sessions, 4 months is probably ideal because it allows the scalp to regain full laxity and gives the surgeon the ability to analyze the growth of the previous session.

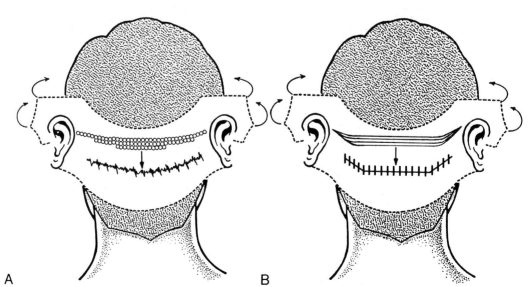

A   B

FIGURE 133–7. *A,* Schematic demonstrating the cluster harvesting technique followed by an interdigitated closure. *B,* Schematic demonstrating the strip harvesting technique followed by a straight line closure.

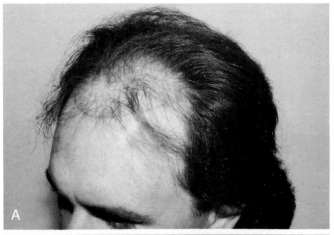

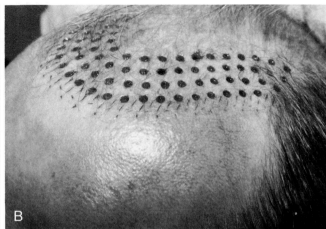

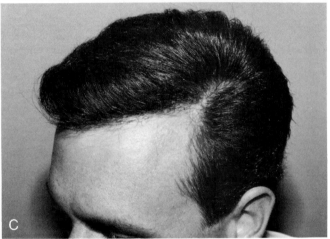

FIGURE 133-8. The first session of punch hair grafting intraoperatively. The holes are arranged circumferentially, with each hole being separated from the adjacent hole by one hole size (3.0 to 3.5 mm). The spaces between rows 1, 3, 5, and 7 are also separated by one hole size. The second session is performed in rows 2, 4, 6, and 8 in the same fashion. The third session is performed in between the first session of growing grafts, and the fourth session between the second session. *A*, Before surgery. *B*, During surgery. *C*, Long-term follow-up with hair growth.

Indications

The most popular usage of punch hair transplantation is for the correction of male pattern baldness. Although this method is still used today, it is beginning to fall out of favor because of the more natural results that can be achieved with smaller grafts (i.e. mini and micrografts). The procedure's best results are accomplished on patients with gray, blonde, or red hair. Its worst results are on patients with dark brown or black hair on light skin.

The procedure has also been described to be beneficial for various types of cicatricial alopecia[90] (i.e., burns, inactive lupus). The surgeon must, however, be certain that the area being transplanted is not recipient dominant; and should refer to Orentreich's original paper on this topic to help make that determination.[89]

Contraindications

It is the authors' opinion that dark-haired individuals (with white skin) and women with female-pattern baldness should be treated with slit mini-micrografting instead of punch grafting. Other contraindications to punch grafting are recipient-dominant diseases such as active discoid lupus, alopecia areata, active skin infections, lichen planus, and so forth.[89]

Risks

The risks for punch hair transplantation include infection, postoperative bleeding, temporary hypoesthesia, arteriovenous fistula, arterial aneurysm, temporary and permanent hair loss, abnormal hair texture, hyperpigmentation of the hair, and scarring. Because of the excellent circulation of the scalp, infection is extremely rare. Hematoma may develop at the donor site, but this is usually self-limiting. Hypoethesia will usually occur postoperatively in the areas adjacent to the operative sites; however, this usually resolves within a 3- to 6-month period. Arteriovenous fistula and arterial aneurysm are both extremely rare complications. Each has occurred only once in the authors' series of over 6000 cases. An arteriovenous fistula can result when a severed end of an artery abnormally heals into the severed end of a vein. It will usually present as a pulsating bluish area and can be treated by placing a figure-of-eight suture around the area. Rarely, it may need to be excised. An aneurysm, on the other hand, has no discoloration but also presents as a pulsating mass. It is most likely caused by intraoperative arterial injury and can be treated rather easily with a figure-of-eight suture.

Another common sequela of hair transplantation is telogen effluvium in the areas adjacent to the operation, which is most likely caused by trauma and slight impairment of the vasculature. If the blood supply is further embarrassed, permanent hair loss and even necrosis can result. This occurrence, however, is rare and usually involves the donor site, when too much tension is applied to the closure. Additionally, a "kinkiness" can sometimes occur to the newly grafted hair. This has been shown by electron microscopy to be caused by an abnormal cuticle on the transplanted hair shaft.[91] This coarseness will usually improve with time, but the hair may take years to regain its former texture. Hyperpigmentation of the hair shaft has also been described as a sequela to hair transplantation.[92] This, too, will usually revert to normal, but may take several years to do so. Finally, abnormal scarring may occur as a result of (1) a tendency to form keloids, (2) Ehlers-Danlos syndrome, or (3) poor technique. If an innate scarring abnormality is suspected, a test graft can be performed in an inconspicuous area.

Benefits

The benefits can be extraordinary if the patient is chosen properly. The donor-dominant hair that is transplanted is permanent and can evoke a much greater sense of confidence and self-esteem in the properly chosen patient.

MINI-MICROGRAFTS

Description

Minigrafts are smaller than punch grafts (3 to 8 hairs per graft) and can be created in several different ways. The approach that Bradshaw[93] described was that of quartering 4.5-mm punch grafts (Fig. 133–9A). This required the surgeon to harvest several 4.5-mm punch grafts with a motor-driven trephine and then quadrasect these under magnification with a blade. Other described methods have included bisecting 4.0-mm grafts, trisecting 3.0-mm grafts, and similar dissecting approaches. With all of these techniques, 1- to 2-hair micrografts are also usually excised from edge of the conventional grafts and used later to refine the hairline.

More recently, the authors[94] have recommended utilizing a triple- or quadruple-bladed knife to excise two or three 3.0-mm strips (ear to ear) from the donor area (see Fig. 133–7B) and subsequently transecting these into 3.0-mm × 1.5-mm rectangular minigrafts and 1- to 2-hair micrografts (Fig. 133–9B). Each strip will normally yield 80 minigrafts (6 to 8 hairs per graft), which fit very nicely into No. 15 Bard-Parker incisions. Although the authors utilize slits as recipient sites, some surgeons feel that holes (1.0 to 2.0 mm in diameter) make better recipient sites because bald skin is removed with this approach. That opinion, however, has been heavily debated, primarily because the slit method is easier to perform, requires less cost and maintenance of instrumentation, compresses bald skin, causes less trauma, causes less scarring, and does not permanently destroy previously placed, growing hair grafts.

In regard to the organization of the recipient sites for

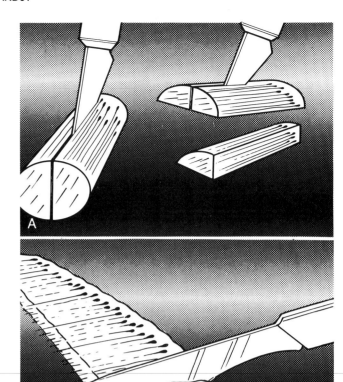

FIGURE 133–9. *A,* Bradshaw's original technique involved quadrasecting 4.5-mm grafts to create minigrafts containing 6 to 8 hairs per graft. *B,* With the strip technique, each 3.0-mm strip is transected into 3.0 mm × 1.5 mm rectangular minigrafts with each minigraft containing 6 to 8 hairs.

mini-micrografting, the most common approach is to make random incision or holes, then continue to randomly fill in the spaces during subsequent sessions. The authors agree that randomness is essential at the hairline, but believe strongly that order should be the goal posterior to the hairline. To achieve this order, the authors draw three or four horizontal reference lines on the patient preoperatively. These lines will guide a systematic three-step approach that will allow the surgeon to cover all alopecic areas with hair.[95] The initial set of incisions are placed 6.0 mm apart and are organized in a fully staggered pattern (Fig. 133–10A). Four months after the first session, the second session is performed 2.0 mm to the right of the first session of growing minigrafts (Fig. 133–10B). Four months after the second session, the third session is performed 2.0 mm to the right (and slightly posterior) to the second session of growing minigrafts (Fig. 133–10C). If a fourth session is desired by the patient, 3- to 4-hair minigrafts placed into random 16-gauge NoKor needle incisions are used. During all of these sessions, fifty to one hundred 1- to 2-hair micrografts are inserted into random 18-gauge NoKor needle incisions at the hairline. A stencil[96] (Robbins Instruments, Chatham, NJ) is utilized before the first session and has been found to keep the first session extremely

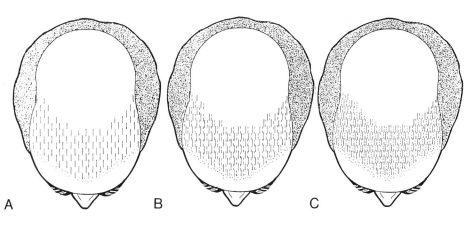

FIGURE 133–10. *A*, The first step of a systematic three-step slit-minigrafting approach involves No. 15 blade slits separated by 6.0 mm and arranged in a full staggered pattern. Micrografts are placed anteriorly in a random fashion with all sessions. *B*, The second step involves placing incisions 2.0 mm to the right of the first growing session. *C*, The third step is performed 2.0 mm to the right (and slightly posterior) of the second session of growing minigrafts. Each session is separated by 4 months.

well organized (Fig. 133–11). This is extremely important because all secondary procedures will be based on this initial session. During the second session, the surgeon simply makes a small dot over each growing graft from the first session, then makes his or her No. 15 blade incisions 2.0 mm to the right of these marks. During the third session, the surgeon likewise makes larger dots encompassing the first and second sessions of growing grafts, then makes the intraoperative incisions in between (and slightly posterior) to these dots.

Indications

This method of hair transplantation is the method of choice for the vast majority of patients wanting to improve the problem of cicatricial alopecia and pattern baldness. This approach does not usually give the density of conventional punch hair grafting, but it yields results that are consistently more natural appearing. Minimicrografting is also the method of choice for those with dark hair on light skin and for female pattern baldness.

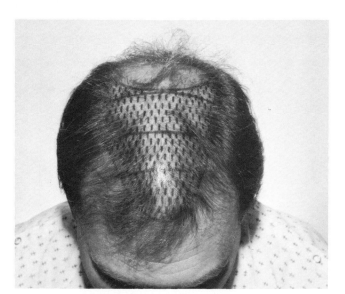

FIGURE 133–11. A stencil is used during the first session to meticulously organize the foundation for the three-step approach. Notice the important circular configuration posteriorly.

Contraindications

The contraindications are the same as conventional punch hair grafting in regard to transplanting into recipient-dominant conditions. As far as esthetics are concerned, there are minimal to no contraindications. Dark-haired individuals can achieve extremely natural results; however, it is a good idea to use extremely small 3- to 4-hair minigrafts in these individuals. Some investigators also believe that holes should be utilized on these patients to avoid compression of the grafts. The authors use 3- to 4-hair minigrafts into 16-gauge NoKor incisions on these individuals and have found no problem with compression. One precaution about using these small 3- to 4-hair minigrafts is that, because it is not unusual to insert 40 of these grafts per square inch, sessions of over 600 grafts are not uncommon.

Risks

The risks are identical to those of the conventional punch hair grafting technique. There is usually less scarring at the recipient area if slits are utilized. On the converse, cyst formation, ingrown hair, and a "pitted" appearance of an occasional graft can occur with this technique. All three of these problems usually result when the mini-micrograft (with its intact epidermis) falls below the skin surface. If "pitting" occurs, the normal treatment is to have the patient apply hot compresses; if a cyst persists, one must surgically remove it. If the skin heals in an inverted fashion, an esthetically displeasing "pitted" appearance results. These grafts should be bored out with a small hand-held trephine and replaced with another graft.

Benefits

The primary benefit of mini-micrografting is that the patient looks extremely natural even during the early stages of transplantation. This observation is especially true when 3- to 4-hair minigrafts are utilized. As with conventional grafting, the improved self-esteem that this procedure can generate is truly amazing.

SCALP REDUCTION

Description

Scalp reduction involves the treatment of alopecia by excision, rather than by hair grafting. After undermining the entire scalp above the nuchal ridge, the surgeon overlaps the undermined scalp to estimate a safe margin for excision. The overlapping bald skin is then excised with a scalpel and is sutured with a two-layered closure. A secure closure at the galea aponeurotica is essential to ensure fine healing at the skin surface. The types of scalp reductions are classified into four basic patterns: (1) the midline sagittal ellipse (Fig. 133–12*A*), (2) the Y pattern (Fig. 133–12*B*), (3) the paramedian pattern (Fig. 133–12*C*), and (4) the circumferential pattern (Fig. 133–12*D*). All of these procedures, except for the circumferential pattern, involve the undermining of bald skin and placing that bald skin under tension.

Indications

Midline, Y-pattern, and paramedian scalp reduction procedures are usually recommended for patients desiring elimination of cicatricial alopecia, mild posterior-pattern alopecia, or the partial reduction of extensive baldness. All scalp reductions advance hair with its normal uniformity and hair texture—they therefore should usually be performed posteriorly whenever the circumstances are amenable to the technique.

Circumferential scalp reduction, unlike midline, Y-pattern, and paramedian scalp reductions, can be utilized for the complete elimination of both mild and extensive forms of male-pattern baldness. The primary reasons for this fact are (1) stretch-back (the stretching back of the alopecic skin) is virtually eliminated because the central bald skin is not undermined, and (2) the posterior donor fringe is elevated approximately 1.5 cm with each procedure (significantly reducing the chances of inferior slot formation).

Contraindications

In the authors' view, midline or paramedian scalp reductions should not be utilized for the attainment of closure on extensively bald individuals. This is due to the reality that the bald area increases by approximately 10% of its total length with each scalp reduction.[92] Therefore, with each successive surgery the bald area progresses inferiorly, leaving the patient with what is commonly referred to as *slot formation*. This deformity has a very sharp divergence of hair inferiorly and can present as a significant cosmetic defect for the patient. Although a Frechet Z-plasty procedure[98] can help correct this deformity, it is not a panacea because approximately three times as much scar tissue is created by this operation. Conversely, Y-pattern scalp reduction does not form a deep central slot, but it does form two smaller slots inferolaterally. Therefore, if midline, paramedian, or Y-pattern scalp reductions are the only tools in the surgeon's armamentarium, and the patient is extensively bald, it is the authors' opinion that one should partially resect the posterior baldness with scalp reductions and hair graft the remaining area of baldness. This will prevent slot formations from becoming excessive.

Risks

The risks include infection, hematoma, temporary hypoesthesia, stretch-back, slot formation, and diverging hair direction. Infection is highly unusual, owing to the excellent blood supply of the scalp. Hematoma can occur, but it is usually self-limiting as a result of the limited undermining to the nuchal ridge. If this does occur, the surgeon can aspirate blood with a 14-gauge needle and subsequently apply pressure. Temporary hypoesthesia can occur with all scalp reductions but tends to be more severe with paramedian and circumferential reductions, primarily because the vertex is cut off from the posterolateral nerve supply. This hypoesthesia will usually abate after 3 to 6 months. Stretch-back occurs when alopecic skin is undermined and is then placed on tension adjacent to the incision line. It has been demonstrated by Nordstrom that the majority of the stretch-back occurs within 1.0 cm of the incision line and that,

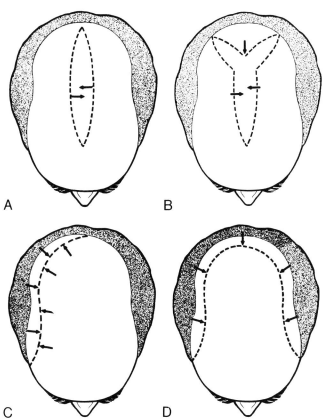

FIGURE 133–12. *A*, The midsagittal reduction undermines bald skin and has two primary vectors. *B*, The Y-pattern reduction also undermines alopecic skin, but has three primary vectors. *C*, The paramedian reduction involves the undermining of bald skin on just one side and has two primary vectors, except for the posterior aspect. *D*, The circumferential reduction undermines no bald skin and has multidirectional vectors throughout its entire length.

on average, 50% of what is gained with scalp reduction is lost over the ensuing 3 months.[99] This problem (associated with midline, paramedian, and Y-pattern scalp reductions) can now be partially ameliorated with either intraoperative retention sutures placed into the galea underlying the donor fringes[100] or with scalp extension techniques.[100-101]

Benefits

The midline, Y-pattern, and paramedian scalp reductions can be beneficial for moderate forms of posterior baldness. Using these procedures advances uniform hair that has normal texture. This eliminates the need to totally graft the posterior scalp. This fact allows the surgeon to focus on grafting to a smaller area anteriorly, thereby achieving a better cosmetic result at the hairline. The other advantage is that the procedure raises the lateral parietal hairline on extensively bald patients, which allows the temporal angle to be in a vertical line with the lateral canthus.

Circumferential scalp reduction[102] has all the same benefits of midline, Y-pattern, and paramedian scalp reductions with the added benefit of being able to "close" extensively bald patients with three to five procedures (Fig. 133–13). This reality is primarily due to the lack of stretch-back with this procedure (bald skin is not undermined), an upward posterior movement, many different vectors, and the visibility to sever the occipitalis and postauricular muscles. Additionally, this improved visualization allows for more aggressive undermining lateral to the occipital neurovascular bundles into the postauricular skin. This extra undermining, of course, leads to improved superior and medial movement of the scalp.

The other benefit of circumferential scalp reduction is that it gives the surgeon the technical ability to use sutured scalp extension techniques[100] to increase scalp laxity rather than being forced to use premade hook devices[10] (as is necessary with midline, paramedian, and Y-pattern scalp reductions). The main contrast between these two approaches is that it is much less expensive to use a suturing technique.

SCALP LIFTING

Description

Scalp lifting[103] consists of five basic techniques: (1) the Marzola lateral scalp lift (Fig. 133–14A), (2) the bilateral occipitoparietal scalp lift (Fig. 133–14B), (3) the bitemporal scalp lift (Fig. 133–14C), (4) the modified bitemporal scalp lift, and (5) the frontoparietal advancement scalp lift (Fig. 133–14D).

The primary difference between these procedures and scalp reduction is that the undermining proceeds down to the hairline of the nape. This extra undermining is important because it gives approximately 60% more stretch (Fig. 133–15), primarily owing to the fact that the area below the nuchal ridge is devoid of restrictive galea.

The incision and configuration of this procedure are exactly the same as those of the circumferential scalp reduction. It begins at the mid-sideburn anterior to the

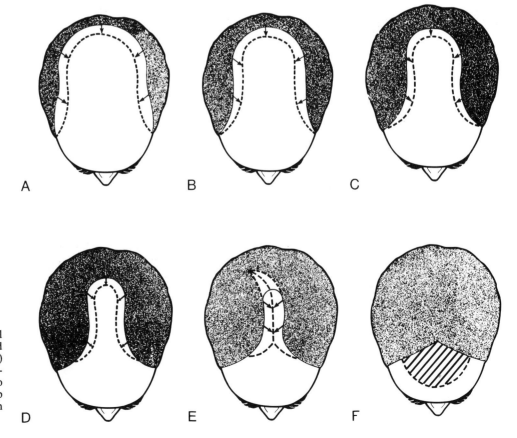

FIGURE 133–13. Circumferential scalp reductions (A to D) followed by a bitemporal scalp reduction (E) will accomplish closure on most extensively bald patients with three to five procedures, depending on scalp laxity. Mini-micrografting can then be performed frontally (F).

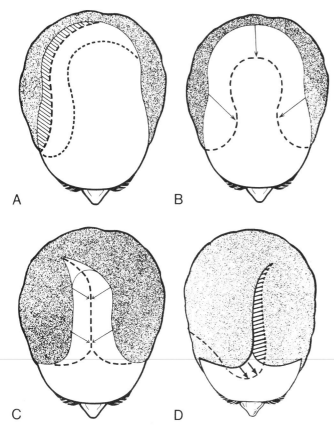

FIGURE 133-14. *A*, The Marzola lateral scalp, the lift compared with a paramedian scalp reduction. The significant extra movement of the Marzola lift is accomplished without undermining bald skin. *B*, The bilateral occipitoparietal scalp lift. *C*, The bitemporal scalp lift. The vectors can be shifted anteriorly for the treatment of bitemporal recessions (modified bitemporal lift). *D*, The frontoparietal advancement scalp lift. This procedure is delayed 2 weeks before the actual lift and must usually be performed two times for hairline development.

superficial temporal artery, proceeds around the entire donor dominant fringe, and ends at the mid-sideburn on the opposite side. This incision give the surgeon tremendous visualization and the ability to easily undermine down to the hairline of the nape.

Indications

This procedure is primarily indicated for those patients with extensive baldness. Because of the much greater advancements accomplished with these procedures, most Norwood Type VI extensively bald patients can be closed posteriorly with just two procedures (i.e., a bilateral occipitoparietal scalp lift and a bitemporal scalp lift).

For those with lesser forms of baldness, a modified bitemporal scalp lift works exceptionally well as a one-step treatment for bitemporal recessions and stable posterior hair. The excision of this procedure is shaped somewhat like a conventional bitemporal lift, but the vectors are shifted anteriorly so that more is advanced anteriorly and less medially. A conventional bitemporal scalp lift can be used as an excellent treatment for those with Type IV baldness that will not progress in the fu-

ture. In most cases, however, it is used as a closure procedure 3 months after the bilateral occipitoparietal scalp lift. The frontoparietal advancement lift is used for hairline development for those who wish to forego hair transplantation frontally. A delay is performed 2 weeks before the actual lift, and two are usually necessary for the hairline to be fully developed.

Contraindications

The procedure should not be used on patients with thin, sparse hair below the nuchal ridge. Since 60% of the stretch comes from this area, significant thinning can occur in this region if the patient is not carefully chosen. In these situations, successive circumferential scalp reductions would be the protocol of choice. The procedure should also not be performed on patients with an extremely narrow donor fringe. These patients would benefit more from the creation of a hairline with mini-micrografting, forgoing the posterior crown. Additionally, patients with a high periauricular hairline preoperatively should be "lifted" cautiously, because the hairline will usually elevate approximately 0.5 mm with each procedure. If the patient is exceptionally motivated, grafting in this area with 3- to 4-hair micrografts can accomplish an excellent correction.

Risks

The primary feared risk of scalp lifting is necrosis at the nuchal ridge. When occipital artery ligations are not performed 2 to 6 weeks prior to the actual lifting surgery, the necrosis rate on virgin scalps was found to be 6.5%.[104] Since ligations have been performed through vertical incisions 2 to 6 weeks before the surgery, the rate has been 0.42% on 235 consecutive virgin scalps at the time of this writing. Other precautions concerning necrosis are as

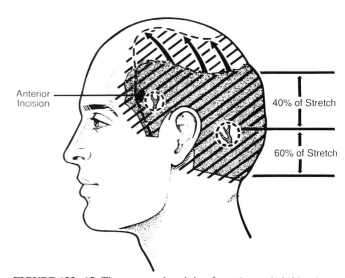

FIGURE 133-15. The extra undermining from the nuchal ridge down to the hairline of the nape contributes approximately 60% of the stretch with scalp lifting.

follows: (1) use lateral procedure on patients with prior hair grafting, (2) split the fascia of the trapezius muscle deep to the nuchal ridge (proper plane), (3) use Doppler imaging to identify the superficial temporal arteries preoperatively, and (4) advance with minimal tension. Besides the normal risks of infection, scarring, and hematoma (as with scalp reduction), all patients will develop hypoesthesia at the vertex. This sequela must be explained explicitly on the consent form. Usually, a significant degree of sensation will return over a 1- to 2-year period, but in most cases there will still remain a lessened sensitivity to touch at the vertex. This has not presented as a problem for the authors as long as it was thoroughly explained preoperatively to the patient.

Benefits

The most important benefit aesthetically is the 4.0- to 5.0-cm elevation in the crown. This feature helps to significantly reduce slot formation, as the final scar will end up on the top of the head instead of down the back of the head. The other benefits of this procedure are (1) the elimination of the temporal recessions, (2) minimal to no stretch-back owing to the lack of undermining of bald skin, (3) a prodigious elimination of bald skin, and (4) a significant reduction in the area needing grafting.

TEMPOROPARIETO-OCCIPITAL FLAPS

Description

The temporoparieto-occipital flap (TPO, or Juri flap) is a pedicled transposition flap based on the superficial temporal artery.[104] Before one plans this 4.0-cm-wide flap, the superficial temporal artery must be identified by Doppler imaging, making certain that the artery traverses the center of the flap. The base of the flap should begin approximately 3.0 cm above the root of the helix and should incline about 40 degrees in a posterior-superior direction. The flap is designed to mildly arch superiorly into the parietal scalp and then curve posteriorly and inferiorly toward the hairline of the nape, making certain not cross the midline. The flap length is determined by measuring the base of the flap to the distal end of the hairline and adding approximately 4.0 cm to adjust for dog-ear formation.

There are four stages to performing this procedure. The first stage involves the incising of the proximal three fourths of the flap (without elevation). One week later, the distal 5.0 cm of the flap is incised, elevated, and sutured back down into place. The occipital neurovascular bundle that lies under this distal end is cauterized or ligated at this time. One week after the second delay, the flap is elevated in a subgaleal plane and is transposed to lie across the frontal area. Undermining adjacent to the donor site is performed superiorly as far as needed, laterally to the postauricular sulcus and inferiorly past the hairline of the nape toward the clavicle. After it is determined that a loose closure is achievable, the wound is closed in a double layer and the flap is transposed anteriorly (Fig. 133–16). It is important to bevel the forehead skin edge and de-epithelialize the anterior 1.0 mm of the flap edge so that hair grows through the anterior scar. Any overlapping alopecia posterior to the flap is then excised, making certain to avoid tension on the flap. The dog-ear that develops at the transposition site is revised 6 weeks after rotating the flap. If a second flap is desired, it is placed 4.0 cm behind the first flap in 3 months. The bald space between the two flaps can then be reduced with scalp reductions.

Indications

This flap is usually indicated when a patient has absolutely no desire for hair grafting, wants an instant hairline, wants to avoid the change in hair texture that can occur with hair grafting, or wants more density at the hairline. It should be utilized only in limited cases, when the surgeon is certain that only the frontal area is going to recede.

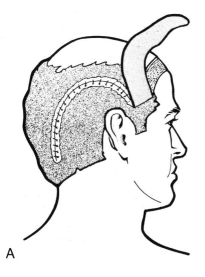
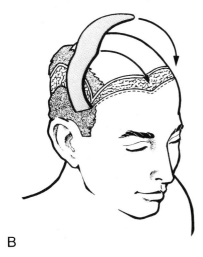

FIGURE 133–16. *A*, The donor site of the temporoparieto-occipital flap is closed after extensive undermining to the postauricular sulcus and past the hairline of the nape. Tissue expanders can be used preoperatively to lessen the degree of undermining. *B*, The flap is then transposed anteriorly. The anterior 1.0 mm of the flap is de-epithelialized and the posterior alopecia excised. The dog-ear is revised 6 weeks after the actual transposition.   A   B

Contraindications

This procedure should not be utilized on patients who are predicted to lose significant hair at the posterior crown. This progression can usually be predicted by wetting the hair with alcohol. Hair that is androgen sensitive will usually have a finer consistency and be less pigmented than androgen-insensitive hair. This characteristic is intensified when the hair is wet. If a flap is performed on a patient who develops posterior thinning in the future, what the patient is left with is "disproportionate density" (tremendous density at the hairline, no hair at the crown, and then density at the donor site). TPO flaps should also be approached with caution on those patients who have had previous punch hair grafting. These patients will incur a higher necrosis rate as a result of the scarring in the donor and flap areas. Also, patients who fear a scar at the hairline should be operated on with caution. These patients should also be told that hair styling may be a problem because the hair is flowing in the wrong (posterior) direction.

Risks

The primary tasks of TPO flaps are donor site and distal flap necrosis, elevated periauricular and nape hairline, scarring, abnormal hair direction, hypoesthesia, and spinal accessory nerve damage. All flaps incur the risk of necrosis. However, if there is the proper delay and minimal tension is placed, on both the donor and recipient sites, this occurrence should be rare. An elevated periauricular hairline ipsilateral to the donor site will always occur; therefore, the patient should be forewarned about this normal sequela. When undermining must proceed beyond the hairline of the nape, an elevated nape hairline will normally result and damage to the spinal accessory nerve becomes a possibility. This latter occurrence is extremely rare and would, of course, lead to weakness of the trapezius muscle ipsilaterally.

Benefits

The primary benefits of any flap procedure are instant, uniform, and thick hair and retention of the normal texture of the hair. These benefits must, of course, be weighed against the aforementioned risks and contraindications.

References

1. Dawber RA. The comparative physiology, embryology and physiology of human hair. In: Rook A, Dawber R, eds. Diseases of Hair and Scalp, 2nd edition. Oxford: Blackwell Scientific Publications, 1991:1–27.
2. Sawaya ME, Hordinsky MK. Advances in alopecia areata and androgenetic alopecia. In: Callen JP, Dahl MV, Golitz LE, et al., eds. Advances in Dermatology, vol. 7. St. Louis: Mosby–Year Book, 1992:211–227.
3. Sawaya ME, Hordinsky MK. The antiandrogens. In: Madden S, McLean DI, eds. Dermatologic Therapy, vol. 11, no. 1. Philadelphia: WB Saunders Co., 1993:65–72.
4. Uno H. The histopathology of hair loss. In: Current Concepts: A Scope Publication. Kalamazoo, MI: Upjohn, 1988:25–33.
5. DeVillez RL. The growth and loss of hair. In: Current Concepts: A Scope Publication. Kalamazoo, MI: Upjohn, 1986:1–27.
6. Randall VA, Thornton MJ, Hamada K, et al. Androgens and the hair follicle. Am N Y Acad Sci 1992;642:355–375.
7. Messenger AG. The control of hair growth: An overview. J Invest Dermatol 1993;101:4s–9s.
8. Sawaya ME, Penneys NS. Immunohistochemical distribution of aromatase and 3b-hydroxysteroid dehydrogenase in human hair follicle and sebaceous gland. J Cutan Pathol 1991;19:309–314.
9. Sawaya ME, Price VH, Harris KA, et al. Human hair follicle aromatase activity in females with androgenetic alopecia. J Invest Dermatol 1990;94:575.
10. Dawber RA. Hair follicle structure, keratinization and the physical properties of hair. In: Rook A, Dawber R, eds. Diseases of Hair and Scalp, 2nd edition. Oxford: Blackwell Scientific Publications, 1991:18–50.
11. Lynch MH, O'Guinn WM, Hardy C, et al. Acidic and basic hair/nail ("hard") keratins: Their colocalization in upper cortical and cuticle cells of the human hair follicle and their relationship to "soft" keratins. J Cell Biol 1986;103:2593–2606.
12. Cotsarelis G, Sun TT, Lavker RM. Label retaining cells reside in the bulge area of pilosebaceous unit: Implications for follicular stem cells, hair cycle, and skin carcinogenesis. Cell 1990;61:1329–1337.
13. Lane EB, Wilson CA, Hughes BR, Leigh IM. Stem cells in hair follicles. Cytoskeletal studies. Ann N Y Acad Sci 1991;642:197–213.
14. Sawaya ME. Androgen receptor regulation in human hair follicles and sebaceous glands. In: Matias J, ed. Androgens and Antiandrogens. Proc Terra Symposia, 1993;1:111–118.
15. Sawaya ME. Purification of androgen receptors in human sebocytes and hair. J Invest Dermatol 1992;98:92–96.
16. Sawaya ME, Lewis LA, Hsia SL. Presence of a converting factor for androgen receptor proteins in isolated human hair follicles and sebaceous glands. FASEB J 1989;2:4765.
17. Sawaya ME, Kraffert CA, Hsia SL. A nuclear matrix associated acceptor protein involved in the chromatin binding of the androgen receptor regulating human hair follicle growth in androgenetic alopecia. J Invest Dermatol 1991;96:595.
18. Orentreich N. Pathogenesis of alopecia. J Soc Cosmet Chem 1960;11:479–486.
19. Dawber RP. Aetiology and pathophysiology of hair loss. Dermatologica 1987;175(Suppl. 2):23–28.
20. Dawber RPR, Ebling FJG, Wojnarowska FT. Disorders of hair. In: Champion RH, Burton JL, Ebling FJG, eds. Textbook of Dermatology, 5th edition, vol. IV. Oxford: Blackwell Scientific Publications, 1992:2533–2638.
21. Hamilton JB. Patterned long hair in man: Types and incidence. Ann N Y Acad Sci 1951;53:708–714.
22. Norwood OT. Male pattern baldness: Classification and incidence. South Med J 1975;68:1359–1365.
23. Rushton D, Ramsay I, Norris M, et al. Natural progression of male pattern baldness in young men. Clin Exp Dermatol 1991;16:188–192.
24. Ludwig E. Classification of the types of androgenetic alopecia arising in the female sex. Br J Dermatol 1977;97:249–257.
25. Spindler J, Data J. Female androgenetic alopecia: A review. Dermatol Nurs 1992;4:93–99.
26. Binazzi M, Wierolis T. Les alopecies feminines hypooetrogeniques. Ann Dermatol Syphil 1962;89:382–385.
27. Venning VA, Dawber R. Patterned androgenic alopecia. J Am Acad Dermatol 1988;18:1073–1078.
28. Cash T. The psychological effects of androgenetic alopecia in man. J Am Acad Dermatol 1992;26:926–931.
29. Cash TF, Price VH, Savin RC. Psychological effects of androgenetic alopecia on women: Comparisons with balding men and with female control subjects. J Am Acad Dermatol 1993;29:568–575.
30. Van der Donk J, Passchier J, Knegt-Junk C, et al. Psychological characteristics of women with androgenetic alopecia: A controlled study. Br J Dermatol 1991;125:248–252.
31. Lesko S, Rosenberg L, Shapiro S. A case-control study of baldness

in relation to myocardial infarction in men. JAMA 1193; 269:998–1003.

32. Eisenstein I, Edelstein J, Gray hair in black males: A possible risk factor in coronary artery disease. Angiology 1982;33:652–654.

33. Montagna W. Morphology of the aging skin: The cutaneous appendages. In: Montagna W, ed. Advances in Biology of Skin, vol. 6. New York: Pergamon Press, 1965:1–6.

34. Scott GS, Stenn KS, Savin R. Diffuse female pattern alopecia—a histological study of 40 cases (abstract). J Cutan Pathol 15:348.

35. Bergfeld WF. Alopecia: Histologic changes. In: Callen JP, Dahl MV, Golitz LE, et al, eds. Advances in Dermatology, vol. IV. Chicago: Year Book Medical Publishers, 1989:301–322.

36. Lattanand A, Johnson WC. Male pattern alopecia. A histopathologic and histochemical study. J Cutan Pathol 1975;2:58–70.

37. Giacometti L, Montagna W. The nerve fibers in male pattern alopecia. In: Baccaredda-Boy A, Mooretti G, Frey JR, eds. Biopathology of Pattern Alopecia. Basel: S Karger, 1968:208–219.

38. Kligman AM. The comparative histopathology of male-pattern baldness and senescent baldness. Clin Dermatol 1988;6:108–118.

39. Abell E. Histologic response to topically applied minoxidil in male-pattern alopecia. Clin Dermatol 1988;6:191–194.

40. Whiting D. Diagnostic and predictive value of horizontal sections of scalp biopsy specimens in male pattern androgenetic alopecia. J Am Acad Dermatol 1993;28:755–763.

41. Jaworsky C, Kligman AM, Murphy GF. Characterization of inflammatory infiltrates in male pattern alopecia: Implications for pathogenesis. Br J Dermatol 1992;127:239–246.

42. Young J, Conte E, Leavitt M, et al. Cutaneous immunopathology of androgenetic alopecia. J Am Osteopath Assoc 1991;81: 765–771.

43. Bystryn J-C,Orentreich N, Stengel F, Direct immunofluoresence studies in alopecia areata and male pattern alopecia. J Invest Dermatol 1979;73:317–320.

44. Hamilton JB. Male hormone stimulation is a prerequisite and an incitant in common baldness. Am J Anat 1942:71:451–479.

45. Kuster W, Happle R. The inheritance of common baldness: Two B or not two B. J Am Acad Dermatol 1984;11:921–926.

46. Smith M, Wells R. Male-type alopecia, alopecia areata, and normal hair in women. Arch Dermatol 1964;89:155–158.

47. Griffin JE, Wilson JD. The syndrome of androgen resistance. N Engl J Med 1980;302:198–209.

48. Krieg M, Voigl KD. *In vitro* binding and metabolism of androgens in various organs: A comparative study. J Steroid Biochem 1976;7:1005–1012.

49. Randall VA, Thornton MJ, Hamada K, et al. Androgens and the hair follicle: Cultured human dermal papilla cells as a model system. Ann N Y Acad Sci 1991;642:355–375.

50. Stumpf WE, Sar M. Autoradiographic localization of estrogen, androgen, progestin, and glucocorticosteroid in "target tissues" and "non-target tissues." In: Pasqualini J, ed. Modern Pharmacology-Toxicology, vol 8. Mechanism of Action of Steroid Hormones. New York: Marcel Dekker, 1976:41–84.

51. Schmidt JA, Schweikert HU. Testosterone and epitestosterone metabolism of single hairs in 5 patients with 5α-reductase deficiency. Acta Endocrinol 1986;113:588–592.

52. Thigpen A, Silver R, Guileyardo J, et al. Tissue distribution and ontogeny of steroid 5 α-reductase isozyme expression. J Clin Invest 1993;92:903–910.

53. Anderson S, Berman DM, Jenkins EP, Russell DW. Deletion of steroid 5α-reductase 2 gene in male pseudohermaphroditism. Nature 1991;354:159–161.

54. Sawaya ME, Lewis LA, Hsia SL. Presence of a converting factor for androgen receptor proteins in isolated human hair follicles and sebaceous glands. FASEB J 1989;2:4765.

55. Sawaya ME, Mendez AJ, Hsia SL. Presence of an inhibitor to androgen binding to receptor protein in human sebaceous gland and hair follicle. J Invest Dermatol 1988;90:605.

56. Sawaya M, Hordinsky M. Advances in alopecia areata and androgenetic alopecia. Adv Dermatol 1992;7:211–227.

57. Sawaya ME, Price VH, Harris KA, et al. Human hair follicle aromatase activity in females with androgenetic alopecia. J Invest Dermatol 1990;94:575.

58. Sperling L, Heimer W. Androgen biology as a basis for the diag-

nosis and treatment of androgenic disorders in women. I. J Am Acad Dermatol 1993;28:669–683.

59. Kasick JM, Bergfeld WF, Steck WD, et al. Adrenal androgenic female-pattern alopecia, sex hormones and the balding women. Cleve Clin Q 1983;50:111–122.

60. Sawaya M, Hordinsky M. The antiandrogens. Dermatol Clin 1993;11:65–72.

61. Cumming DC. Androgenesis and androdynamics in normal women. Cleve Clin J Med 1990;57:161–166.

62. Selby C. Sex hormone binding globulin: Origin, function, and clinical significance. Ann Clin Biochem 1990;27:532–541.

63. Siegel SF, Finegold DN, Lanes R, et al. ACTH stimulation tests and plasma dehydroepiandrosterone sulfate levels in women with hirsutism. N Engl J Med 1990;323:849–854.

64. Gourgiotou K, Kassoulli S, Stratigos J. Hormonal status in postmenopausal androgenetic alopecia. Int J Dermatol 1992;31: 858–859.

65. Rushton DH, Ramsay ID, James KC, et al. Biochemical and trichological characterization of diffuse alopecia in women. Br J Dermatol 1990;123:187–197.

66. Freinkel RK, Freinkel N. Hair growth and alopecia in hypothyroidism. Arch Dermatol 1972;106:349–352.

67. Sperling L, Heimer W. Androgen biology as a basis for the diagnosis and treatment of androgenic disorders in women. II. J Am Acad Dermatol 1993;28:901–916.

68. Nestler JE. Evaluation and treatment of the hirsute woman. Va Med Q 1989;116:310–315.

69. Katz HI, Kien NT, Prawer SE, et al. Long-term efficacy of topical minoxidil in the treatment of male pattern baldness. J Am Acad Dermatol 1987;16:696–704.

70. Olsen EA, Weiner MS, Amara I. Five-year follow-up of men with androgenetic alopecia treated with topical minoxidil. J Am Acad Dermatol 1990;22:643–646.

71. Savin RC. Use of topical minoxidil in the treatment of male pattern baldness. Am Acad Dermatol 1987;16:696–704.

72. Olsen EA, Weiner MS. Topical minoxidil in male pattern baldness: Effects of discontinuation of treatment. J Am Acad Dermatol 1987;17:97–101.

73. DeVillez RI. Topical minoxidil therapy in hereditary androgenetic alopecia. Arch Dermatol 1985;121:197–202.

74. Aram H. Treatment of female androgenetic alopecia with cimetidine. Int J Dermatol 1987;26:128–133.

75. Cusan L. Dupont A, Belanger A, et al. Treatment of hirsutism with the pure antiandrogen flutamide. J Am Acad Dermatol 1990;23:462–469.

76. Wysowski D, Freiman J, Tourtelot, J, Horton M. Fatal and nonfatal hepatotoxicity associated with flutamide. Ann Intern Med 1993;118:860–864.

77. Vigersky RA, Mehlman I, Glass AR, et al. Treatment of hirsute women with cimetidine. N Engl J Med 1980;303:1042.

78. Orentreich N. Medical treatment of baldness. Ann Plast Surg 1978;116–118.

79. Maroulis GB. Evaluation of hirsutism and hyperandrogenemia. Fertil Steril 1981;36:273–305.

80. Griffing GT, Melby JC. Hirsutism: Causes and treatments. Hosp Pract 1991;30:43–58.

81. Redmond GP, Bergfeld WF. Treatment of androgenic disorders in women: Acne, hirsutism, and alopecia. Cleve Clin J Med 1990;57:428–432.

82. Orfanos DE, Wustner H. Penetration und Nebenwirkungen lokala Ostrogen—Applikation bei Alopecia androgenetica. Hautarzt 1975;26:367–369.

83. Emons G, Diedrich K, Krebs D, Knuppen R. Postmenopausenblutung nach Anwendung eines ostrogenhaltigen Haarwassers-begleitende endokrine Veranderungen. Geburtshilfe Frauenheilkd 1984;44:460–462.

84. Gottswinter JM, Korth-Schutz S, Ziegler R. Gynecomastia caused by estrogen containing hair lotion. J Endocrin Invest 1984;7:383–386.

85. Rittmaster R, Uno H, Povar M, et al. The effects of N, N-diethyl-4-methyl-3-oxo-4-aza-5α-androstane-17β-carboxamide, a 5-α-reductase inhibitor and antiandrogen, on the development of baldness in the stumptail macaque. J Clin Endocrinol Metab 1987;65:188–193.

86. Diani A, Mulholland MJ, Shull K, et al. Hair growth effects of oral administration of finasteride, a steroid 5α-reductase inhibitor, alone and in combination with topical minoxidil in the balding stumptail macaque. J Clin Endocrin Metab 1992; 74:345–350.

87. Bazzano GS, Terezakis N, Galen W. Topical tretinoin for hair growth promotion. J Am Acad Dermatol 1986;15:880–883.

88. Terezakis N, Bazzano G. Retinoids: Compounds important to hair growth. Clin Dermatol 1988;4:129–131.

89. Orentreich N. Autographs in alopecias and other selected dermatological conditions. Ann N Y Acad Sci 1959;83:463.

90. Stough DB III, Berger RA, Orentreich N. Surgical improvement of cicatricial alopecia of diverse etiology. Arch Dermatol 1968;97:331.

91. Stough DB IV. Why does transplanted hair have a different quality? The electron microscope gives the answer. The First World Congress of the International Society of Hair and Scalp Surgery, Dallas, April 30–May 2, 1993.

92. Nordstrom REA. Hyperpigmentation of transplanted terminal hairs after punch hair grafting. J Dermatol Surg Oncol 1982;8:787–789.

93. Bradshaw W. Quarter grafts. International Congress on Hair Replacement Surgery, American Academy of Cosmetic Surgery, New York, 1984.

94. Brandy DA. A new instrument for the expedient production of minigrafts. J Dermatol Surg Oncol 1992;18:487–492.

95. Brandy DA. A three-step systematic incisional-slit minigrafting approach. J Dermatol Surg Oncol 1993;19:421–426.

96. Brandy DA. A stencil for the improved accuracy, speed and aesthetics in slit-minigrafting. J Dermatol Surg Oncol, in press.

97. Nordstrom REA. Scalp kinetics in multiple excisions for correction of male pattern baldness. J Dermatol Surg Oncol 1984;10:991–995.

98. Frechet P. A new method for correction of the vertical scar observed following scalp reduction for extensive alopecia. J Dermatol Surg Oncol 1990;16:640–644.

99. Nordstrom REA. Stretch-back in scalp reductions for male pattern baldness. Plast Reconstr Surg 1984;73:422–426.

100. Brandy DA. The use of retention sutures and tensed Silastic-Dacron strips for the prevention of stretch-back after alopecia reducing procedures. J Dermatol Surg Oncol, in press.

101. Frechet P. Scalp extension. J Dermatol Surg Oncol 1993;19: 616–622.

102. Brandy DA. Circumferential scalp reduction: The application of the principles of extensive scalp-lifting for the improvement of scalp reduction surgery. J Dermatol Surg Oncol 1994;20: 217–284.

103. Brandy DA. Scalp-lifting: An 8 year experience with 1,231 cases. J Dermatol Surg Oncol 1993;19:1009–1014.

104. Juri J. Use of parieto-occipital flaps in the surgical treatment of baldness. Plast Reconstr Surg 1975;55:456.

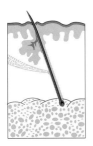

chapter 134

Alopecia Areata and Other Nonscarring Alopecias

VIRGINIA C. FIEDLER

Nonscarring alopecia is potentially reversible if the inciting factors can be eliminated and/or if appropriate therapy can be found. The most common causes of reversible alopecia are alopecia areata and diffuse alopecia, which usually results from telogen hair shedding or, less commonly, from some forms of anagen hair shedding.

ALOPECIA AREATA

DEFINITION

Alopecia areata is clinically recognized as patchy hair loss that may occur in any hair-bearing area on the body surface. The process is mediated by lymphocytic infiltrates in and around hair bulbs. Extensive involvement may result in total scalp hair loss (alopecia totalis), total body hair loss (alopecia universalis), diffuse scalp hair loss (diffuse alopecia areata), or localized hair loss along the scalp margin (ophiasis).

CLINICAL DESCRIPTION

In alopecia areata, extensive body hair loss may be present, sometimes for many years, before the onset of patchy loss of scalp hair. Nail abnormalities, predominantly nail pitting, may precede or occur in conjunction with active alopecia areata.

Itching, tingling, burning, or painful sensations frequently occur at the sites of hair loss. These sensations may begin 1 to 2 weeks before or during the time of active hair shedding; thus, patients can often predict where their next areas of hair loss will occur. In rare instances the sensation of pain is severe. Occasionally, patients with alopecia universalis have associated diffuse pruritus with no other etiology.

Exclamation point hairs, when present, are diagnostic of alopecia areata (Fig. 134–1). These characteristic hairs fracture at their distal end as they taper and lose pigment proximally toward the scalp, giving them the appearance of an exclamation point. During periods of active disease, telogen hairs are readily pulled from the periphery of patches. In diffuse alopecia areata or disease rapidly progressing to alopecia totalis or universalis, telogen and rarely anagen hairs may be easily pulled anywhere on the scalp surface. The skin surface in involved areas may appear normal, slightly erythematous and/or scaly, slightly hyperpigmented, and rarely depigmented.

Autoimmune diseases, especially thyroid disease and vitiligo, appear to be more common in patients with alopecia areata.[1] The incidence of alopecia areata has been found to be increased in patients with lupus erythematosus,[2] lichen planus,[3] and Down syndrome.[4] Nuchal nevus flammeus has been reported to be frequently associated with severe alopecia areata.[5]

Alopecia areata affects males and females equally. Approximately 1% of the population will have had a patch of alopecia areata by the age of 50 years. Although it may occur at any age, approximately 60% of affected persons will develop the disease before the age of 20.[6]

A positive family history of alopecia areata occurs in about 20% of patients.[6] Studies of HLA association have not been consistent.[7–9]

The course of alopecia areata is difficult to predict.

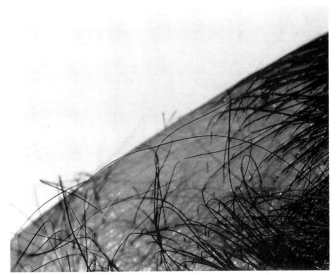

FIGURE 134–1. Exclamation point hairs of alopecia areata.

Some patients have minimal transient hair loss followed by spontaneous regrowth and no further hair loss. Other patients have a few chronic stable patches of hair loss that may last many years. Patients with extensive disease usually have a chronic or chronically recurrent problem with hair loss. The alopecia may be extensive from its onset or may evolve to a more extensive form with repeated flares of hair loss. Pigmented hairs may be shed while white hairs are spared. Regrowing hairs may initially be white and later darken to a normal shade. Regrowing hair is usually but not always of normal texture.

Poor prognosis of alopecia areata is associated with childhood onset of disease, atopy, ophiasis, and/or onychodystrophy.[10] In my own experience, most patients with severe chronically treatment-resistant disease are atopic.[11] Many of these atopic patients experience predictable cyclic, seasonal episodes of hair loss that correlate with flares in atopic symptoms[11, 12] and/or positive responses to immediate hypersensitivity skin tests of related seasonal allergens.[11]

Although stress is commonly stated to be a trigger factor for flares of the disease, there is no good evidence to support that notion.[13] The disease itself, especially in its severe forms, is significantly stressful. Patients report a range of feelings such as loss of control, helplessness, cosmetic concerns, vulnerability (nakedness), loss of self-esteem, altered self-image, and/or self-identity, grief, and guilt.[14]

PATHOLOGY

Patches of active alopecia areata show increased numbers of catagen and telogen hairs, with infiltrates of mononuclear cells in and around hair bulbs (Fig. 134–2). Helper T cells predominate at sites of active loss.[15, 17] Degeneration of lower follicular keratinocytes and matrix cells as well as melanocytes, Langerhans' cells, and dermal papilla cells are reported.[18, 19]

Areas of spontaneous regrowth[17] as well as areas of "normal" scalp[19, 20] of patients with alopecia areata may also show dense peribulbar accumulations of infiltrating mononuclear cells although the CD4/CD8 ratio may differ from that in active disease.[17] The clinically "normal" scalp of affected patients can also show changes in the dermal papilla and at the dermoepithelial junction of the hair bulb similar to those in areas of active disease.[19] These findings support the notion of a subclinical phase of alopecia areata.

Persistent areas of baldness may show follicles in late-stage telogen arrest, and rarely there may be evidence of follicular attrition.[20] Because peribulbar lymphocytic infiltrates are necessary for a definitive diagnosis of alopecia areata and do not occur or persist around every follicle, transverse sections that demonstrate all of the hair bulbs in a given specimen are often useful (see Fig. 134–2). Transverse sections can be used to estimate disease activity.

PATHOGENESIS AND ETIOLOGY

Alopecia areata is thought to be an autoimmune disorder. Atopy, autoimmune thyroid disease, vitiligo, and other autoimmune disorders may be associated with alopecia areata. Antibodies to thyroid, gastric parietal cells,

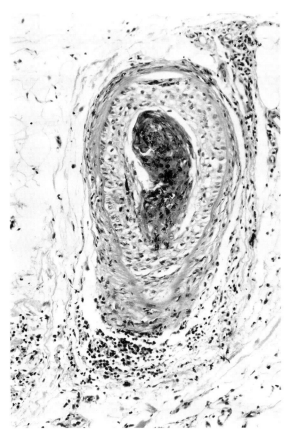

FIGURE 134–2. A transverse section from alopecia areata showing a peribulbar lymphocytic infiltrate. Some of the bulbar keratinocytes are necrotic, a finding seen in the "nanogen" follicles of this disorder.

smooth muscle, and adrenal are more commonly present in affected patients than in normal controls.[1] Antinuclear and other antibodies may also be present. The majority of patients who develop these antibodies do not subsequently develop any associated autoimmune disease.

Changes in number and function of circulating T cells have been variably reported in patients with alopecia areata. Decreased suppressor T-cell numbers and/or function in patients with active disease have been reported.[11, 21, 22] Some studies have found evidence of activated T cells in the peripheral blood of patients with active disease.[23, 24]

Lesional biopsy specimens show a predominance of CD4-positive cells that are greatest in sites of active hair loss.[15, 17] CD8-positive cells, Langerhans' cells, and monocytes are also present.[16, 17] Autoreactive T cells that proliferate in response to autologous irradiated peripheral blood mononuclear cells are variably enriched in scalp biopsy specimens relative to peripheral blood.[25] Aberrant intercellular adhesion molecule-1 (ICAM-1) expression by hair follicle epithelial cells and endothelial leukocyte adhesion molecule-1 (ELAM-1) expression by vascular cells are seen in lesional biopsy specimens.[26]

Biopsy specimens from involved skin of patients with alopecia areata and alopecia universalis show regrowth of hair after being grafted onto nude mice. Passive transfer of serum from the patients to the nude mice does not inhibit hair growth in these transplants.[27] These data support the notion that cellular, not humoral, immune mechanisms are involved in the pathogenesis of alopecia areata.

Data suggest there is inhibition of keratinocyte proliferation in the bulb of lesional anagen follicles.[28] Ultrastructure of exclamation point hairs shows evidence of cortex disintegration just below the frayed brush-like top,[29] and the medulla may show low-density features as well.[30]

Human hair follicle mesenchyme contains a distinctive extracellular matrix that varies in volume and composition in concert with the hair growth cycle. Some large anagen follicles in lesional biopsy specimens show evidence of disturbed mesenchymal function with loss of the normal staining pattern for chondroitin-6-sulfate in the dermal papilla. Increased peribulbar urokinase-dependent fibrinolytic activity has been demonstrated in lesional skin as well.[31]

Although numerous data are now available, the pathogenesis of alopecia areata remains to be elucidated.

DIAGNOSIS AND DIFFERENTIAL DIAGNOSIS

The patchy as well as total and universal forms of alopecia areata are usually distinctive and easily recognizable. At times the clinical picture may be confusing and a scalp biopsy may be necessary to distinguish alopecia areata from trichotillomania, tinea capitis, syphilis, telogen effluvium, androgenetic alopecia, and loose anagen syndrome. Distinctive features of each form of alopecia are outlined in Table 134–1.

TREATMENT

Because of the enormous psychosocial significance of alopecia areata, *key elements to treat it effectively* include (1) helping the patient understand the disease, (2) encouraging the patient to share his or her feelings about the disease, and (3) helping the patient to maintain a sense of hope for future scientific knowledge and treatment of the disease.[14, 32]

Mild patchy alopecia areata may demonstrate spontaneous regrowth. Persistent patchy disease usually responds readily to a variety of treatments (Table 134–2).[14]

Severe forms of alopecia areata are extensive and/or rapidly progressive and are likely to be chronic or at least chronically recurrent and often resistant to treatment. There is no good evidence to suggest that treatment induces remission or affects the ultimate course of the disease. Since treatment is only suppressive of the underlying process, and since individuals with severe disease often require long-term treatment to maintain cosmetically adequate hair growth, treatment must be not only effective but also safe for long-term use.[14] Of the large number of treatments tried for severe alopecia areata, none is uniformly effective and some are not safe for long-term use (Tables 134–3 and 134–4).[14]

All topical treatments for alopecia areata must be tried for a minimum of 3 months since early hair regrowth may not occur before that time.[14]

Mild disease, defined as stable patches involving less than 25% of the scalp, can be treated successfully with intralesional or topical steroids. Topical steroids offer an advantage in that treatment is painless and the patient can begin to treat patches as they arise. Topical betamethasone dipropionate cream 0.05% in the nonoptimized vehicle (Diprosone) may be applied to the patch and 1 cm of adjacent scalp skin twice daily. Daily shampoos are recommended to minimize the potential for folliculitis. The patient may be re-evaluated at 3-month intervals. If the response is progressively better, then the same treatment may be continued until adequate regrowth has been obtained, which can take many months. If no response is obtained or if the response plateaus, topical anthralin cream 1.0% (Drithocreme) can often be effectively substituted. It is applied for 10 to 20 minutes daily to the patch and 1 cm of adjacent scalp skin and then shampooed off the scalp.[14] Combining steroids and anthralin seems to decrease the efficacy of each of them. Some patients will also respond to topical minoxidil (Rogaine).[14]

Extensive disease, defined as greater than 25% scalp hair loss, can respond to topical steroids or anthralin. Because these patients often develop new patches during treatment, medication should be applied to the entire scalp to maximize the likelihood of cosmetically adequate regrowth. Treatment of only patches often results in "chasing" the disease and is less likely to elicit a cosmetic effect.[14] When using cream over the entire scalp, the patient should part the hair approximately every $\frac{1}{2}$ inch and rub a very small amount of cream into the part.

Rapidly progressive disease, defined by the light hair

TABLE 134–1. Differential Diagnosis of Alopecia Areata

Disease	Clinical Features	Histologic Features	Serologic Findings	Other Findings
Alopecia areata	Patches or diffuse Exclamation point hairs Hair pull test often positive, usually telogen hairs	Miniaturized follicles Peribulbar and intrabulbar inflammation	Autoantibodies may be present	Atopy common in early onset and severe disease
Trichotillomania	Patches Broken hairs of different lengths Hair pull test negative Folliculitis	Increased catagen follicles Increased telogen follicles Folliculitis Melanin pigment casts and granules Trichomalacia		History may or may not be helpful
Tinea capitis	Patches	Suppurative and granulomatous folliculitis; hyphae in and around hair shafts		Potassium hydroxide and culture positive
Syphilis	Patches or diffuse	Dense band-like infiltrates of plasma cells and histiocytes in adventitial dermis	Fluorescent treponemal antigen positive Rapid plasmid reagin positive	Possible relevant history
Telogen effluvium	Diffuse Hair pull test usually positive, telogen hairs May show diffuse early regrowth	Variable		History of associated factors
Androgenetic alopecia	Male pattern or female pattern or diffuse Hair pull test often positive, telogen hairs	Increased telogen follicles Decreased anagen follicles Decreased terminal follicles Increased vellus follicles Increased telogen germinal units Decreased follicular density—late stage		Positive family history
Loose anagen syndrome	Patches or diffuse Hair pull test positive, anagen hairs, painless Hair does not grow long	Small follicles Premature keratinization of Huxley's and Henle's layers		Improves over time

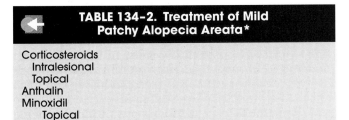

TABLE 134-2. Treatment of Mild Patchy Alopecia Areata*

Corticosteroids
 Intralesional
 Topical
Anthalin
Minoxidil
 Topical

*Not all studies were controlled, but the data suggest efficacy.
 Data from Fiedler VC. Alopecia areata: A review of therapy, efficacy, safety and mechanism. Arch Dermatol 1992;128:1519–1520. Copyright 1992, American Medical Association.

TABLE 134-4. Combination Treatment of Severe Alopecia Areata

Treatment	Cosmetic Efficacy (% of Total with Severe Disease)	No. of Patients with Severe Disease
Systemic + local steroids	25–87	19
Systemic steroid + systemic sulfones	36	11
Systemic steroid + systemic cyclosporine	100	2
Topical minoxidil + topical steroid*	31	78
Topical minoxidil + systemic steroid*	?, poor	75
Topical minoxidil + topical anthralin	11	45
Topical minoxidil + topical sensitizer*	?, no synergistic effect	15
PUVA + topical sensitizer*	?, no synergistic effect	3
Topical estrogen + UVB	67	3

*Controlled studies.
 Data from Fiedler VC. Alopecia areata: A review of therapy, efficacy, safety and mechanism. Arch Dermatol 1992;128:1519–1520. Copyright 1992, American Medical Association.

pull test eliciting four or more hairs, may initially be treated as for extensive disease. It is important to re-evaluate these patients after 4 weeks. If the light hair pull test has decreased to three or fewer hairs, the same treatment may be maintained. If the pull test is unchanged or greater, a higher potency steroid cream may be tried for a time. Local tolerance for the higher-potency topical steroid creams is highly variable (weeks to months). If the pull test is diminished, the patient may gradually be switched back to the well-tolerated betamethasone di-

TABLE 134-3. Single-Agent Treatment of Severe Alopecia Areata*

Treatment	Cosmetic Efficacy (% of Total with Severe Disease)	Side Effects
Corticosteroids		
Intralesional	Poor	Pain, local atrophy, decreased cortisol levels
Topical	33–100	Local folliculitis, acne
		Telangiectasia and local atrophy with super high-potency steroids
Systemic	11–100	Diabetes, striae, acne, hypertrichosis, purpura, pseudoacanthosis nigricans, dysmenorrhea, weight gain, abdominal pain, hypertension, psychosis and other psychological difficulties, lenticular opacities, knee pain, cataracts, osteoporosis, decreased cortisol levels, aseptic necrosis of the hip, gastrointestinal bleeding
Anthralin	25–66	Pruritus, erythema, scaling, folliculitis, local pyoderma, regional lymphadenopathy
Minoxidil		
Topical	0–53	Mild local irritation, rare allergic contact dermatitis, very rare photoallergic contact dermatitis, hypertrichosis
Oral	18	Edema, headaches, depression, lethargy, palpitations, tachycardia, hypertrichosis, T-wave changes
Phototherapy		
UVB	18	Erythema
Psoralens and UVA	19–65	Nausea, pigmentary changes, risk of skin cancers and cataracts
Sensitizers	4–50	Mild to severe local and disseminated dermatitis, itching, sleep disturbances, regional lymphadenopathy, shivering, fever, arthralgia, fainting, contact urticaria, erythema multiforme, vitiligo
Cyclosporine		
Topical	Poor	Folliculitis from the vehicle, increased white blood cells, increased lymphocytes
Oral	~50	Fatigue, myalgias, flushing, paresthesias, headache, dysesthesia, diarrhea, gingival hyperplasia, cutaneous lymphocytic infiltrates, increased blood urea nitrogen and creatinine levels
Dapsone	54	Hemolysis, leukopenia[†]
Nitrogen mustard	64	Local hyperpigmentation, contact sensitization
Zinc	15–75	Nausea, vomiting, diarrhea, gastrointestinal ulceration, anemia

*The majority of these studies were not controlled.
†Author's unpublished data.
 Data from Fiedler VC. Alopecia areata: A review of therapy, efficacy, safety and mechanism. Arch Dermatol 1992;128:1519–1520. Copyright 1992, American Medical Association.

propionate. If the hair pull test is not diminished, the patient may be treated as if his or her disease is resistant to treatment.

Treatment of resistant disease is very difficult. Some combination therapies such as topical minoxidil plus topical steroid[2, 14] or topical minoxidil plus topical anthralin[14, 33] appear to offer a therapeutic advantage. Other combinations such as topical minoxidil plus topical sensitizer,[14, 34] psoralens and ultraviolet light (PUVA) plus topical sensitizer,[35] and topical steroid plus topical anthralin show no synergistic effect. It is often a temptation to use systemic steroids to treat these patients. Experience suggests, however, that if appropriate combinations of topical treatments cannot control a flare of the disease or enhance regrowth, then the patient will often require either lengthy or frequent courses of systemic steroids exposing the patient to the attendant risks of such treatment.[14] Other treatments that have been tried for these patients are listed in Tables 134–3 and 134–4.

DIFFUSE ALOPECIA

DEFINITION

Excessive telogen (club) hair shedding usually produces a diffuse alopecia that may or may not be clinically obvious. A variety of hormonal and nutritional factors, ingestion of various drugs, exposure to certain chemicals, systemic and local cutaneous disease, as well as psychological stress have all been associated with telogen hair shedding. Prognosis for hair regrowth is usually good if the cause can be found and eliminated and if the patient does not have associated androgenetic alopecia.

CLINICAL DESCRIPTION

Telogen hair shedding may be intermittent or constant. Apparent hair thickness depends on hair density, hair shaft width, and hair length, all of which vary considerably among individuals. A decrease of at least 25% of scalp hairs may be necessary for an objective observer to consistently diagnose diffuse alopecia.[36] The physician may be uncertain, therefore, if hair loss has occurred or is occurring. The patient's perceptions regarding hair loss are probably more valid than the physician's.

Assessment includes a thorough history of the evolution of the hair loss, review of systems, review of exposure to drugs and chemicals, dietary history, history of recent illnesses, family history of hair loss (e.g., androgenetic alopecia), and hair grooming procedures. Evaluation of a possible etiologic role for psychological stress is complicated by the fact that hair loss usually provokes at least a moderate stress reaction.

Examination of scalp and body hair for density and distribution as well as comparative assessment of part width at several sites on the scalp should be done. The parts should be observed from a tangential vantage point for evidence of short hairs of normal texture (e.g., regrowing hairs) versus short hairs of visibly diminished shaft diameter (e.g., indeterminate hairs of androgenetic alopecia). Evidence of underlying scalp and/or other cutaneous or systemic disease or nail changes should be sought.

The light hair pull test should be performed at several sites on the scalp by pinching approximately 20 hairs between the thumb and index finger and gently pulling. If any anagen hairs are extracted, then further evaluation is definitely warranted. In a normal situation fewer than two telogen (club) hairs are extracted per light pull. If more hairs are pulled, abnormal telogen shedding is likely (Fig. 134–3). The light pull test may be falsely negative if the patient's hair has recently been combed, brushed, or shampooed.

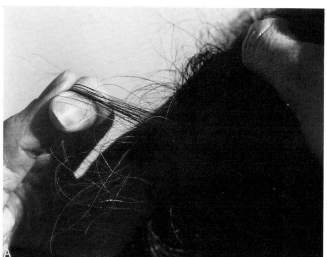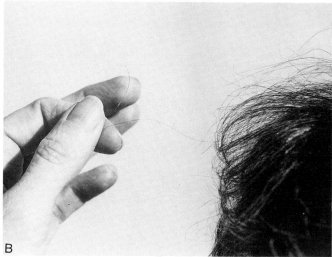

FIGURE 134–3. *A,* Hair pull test. *B,* Abnormal hair pull test with more than two hairs per pull.

Daily hair collections from the comb, brush, pillow case, sink, shower, and collar can be placed in separate envelopes and marked with the date, number of hairs collected, and whether the patient shampooed his or her hair on that day. Normally 50 to 100 telogen hairs are shed per day. Hair shafts collected should be examined to determine if they are telogen, anagen, or broken; if they are structurally normal; and if they are of similar or variable diameter.

Hair plucking[37] provides the most accurate measure of anagen–telogen ratios, although it often significantly distorts anagen hair morphology.[38] This test causes discomfort and is usually not necessary. Telogen counts obtained by hair plucking vary widely, ranging from 4% to 37% and averaging 13% to 15% in healthy adults.[36, 37] The data are conflicting regarding similarities versus differences in men versus women and changes with advancing age.[37, 39] Kligman[36] has defined telogen counts higher than 25% as being diagnostic of telogen effluvium and counts above 20% as presumptively abnormal.

PATHOLOGY

In classic telogen effluvium, shed telogen hairs are reported to derive exclusively from follicles that are generating new anagen hairs.[36] Biopsy specimens taken during the stage of hair shedding show a decreased percentage of telogen follicles. The latency between the inciting event, which precipitates anagen follicles to enter catagen, and the onset of hair loss reflects the duration of catagen and telogen (2 to 4 months). Other mechanisms of telogen hair shedding may be associated with an increased percentage of telogen follicles or the presence of inflammation or both. The timing of the biopsy critically determines the histologic picture.[40] Transverse sections are preferable to routine vertical sections for enumerating catagen and telogen follicles.

PATHOGENESIS AND ETIOLOGY

Hormones and Alopecia

Hypothyroidism. Diffuse hair loss may be the only symptom of hypothyroidism,[41] and it has been reported to be present in 18% to 50% of patients with myxedema.[42, 43] No correlations between the degree or extent of hair loss and duration or severity of myxedema[43] or the thyroid hormone levels have been made.[44] Deficiency of thyroid hormone, whether disease-associated or drug-induced, is apparently responsible for a decrease in the anagen–telogen ratio.[44, 45] Why some individuals develop alopecia and some do not is unknown.

Hyperthyroidism. Short, scanty, or thin scalp hair has been reported in about half of 40 cases of diffuse toxic and toxic multinodular goiter.[46]

Pregnancy. Postpartum alopecia is probably the most commonly recognized form of telogen hair shedding. During the second and third trimesters of pregnancy there is a marked increase in the percentage of anagen hairs.[47, 48] After delivery there is a rapid decrease in the percentage of anagen hairs with an associated increase in the percentage of telogen hairs, ranging as high as 65%.[49] Hair shedding begins from less than a month to 4 months postpartum[36, 50] and typically lasts less than 6 months,[36, 51] although it can last as long as 1 year.[36, 50] Basal metabolic rate and 17-ketosteroid excretion have been found to be normal.[51] It is widely thought that the high estrogen levels of pregnancy prolong the anagen phase and that after delivery decreases in circulating estrogens are responsible for the increases in telogen follicles. An alternative explanation is that a more rapid shedding of telogen hairs during the first trimester of pregnancy accounts for the higher percentages of anagen hairs observed in subsequent trimesters.[47] Additional factors that may be relevant to postpartum hair loss may include stress, blood loss, and other hormonal factors such as prolactin secretion with nursing.

Androgenetic Alopecia. Distinct patterns of hair thinning in men (male pattern baldness) and women (female pattern hair thinning) (Fig. 134–4) are characteristic of androgenetic alopecia. Diffuse alopecia over the entire scalp with increased telogen shedding may also be a manifestation of androgenetic alopecia in women and rarely also in men. It may be confused clinically with other causes of telogen hair shedding. The diagnosis is usually made by exclusion of other causes, a positive family history of androgenetic alopecia, and microscopic hair assessment that reveals marked variability in hair shaft diameters. A biopsy is necessary in men and may be necessary in women to clarify the diagnosis in cases of diffuse alopecia.[40, 52, 53]

Involutional Alopecia. Diffuse hair thinning after age 50 with a negative family history of male pattern baldness is termed *involutional (senescent, senile) alopecia.*[54] Histology shows an increase in telogen follicles, decreased follicular size,[54] and variably diminished follicular density.[54, 55] Much remains to be learned to further refine the concept of involutional alopecia and whether it may actually be a more subtle expression of androgenetic alopecia or be entirely unrelated.

Oral Contraceptives. Diffuse alopecia may occur in some women after they stop taking oral contraceptives. Telogen counts have been variable, as has a history of postpartum hair loss.[49, 56] Studies of the effects of oral contraceptives on the hair cycle have not shown consistent effects.[57–59]

Hair loss during oral contraceptive use has been documented.[56, 60] One report of six such patients is suggestive of the possibility that contraceptives of moderate androgenic potency may exacerbate an underlying androgenetic alopecia although no characteristic histologic changes were seen on biopsy specimens from these patients.[60] Increased telogen percentages have been documented in some women during early months of contraceptive use.[57, 58]

Nutrition and Alopecia

Weight Loss. Stringent dieting may result in diffuse hair shedding within 1 to 6 months. Hair loss has been reported with calorie deprivation of 0 to 1000 K cal/d.[61–64] It has been suggested that hair loss is seen

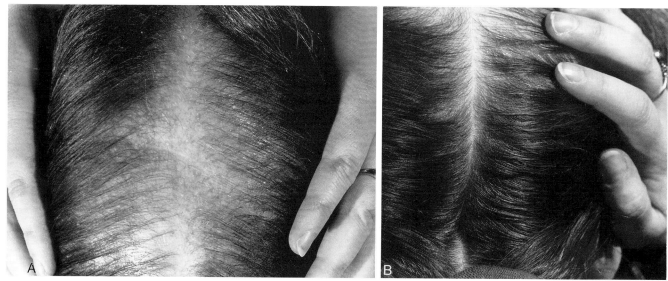

FIGURE 134–4. *A*, Abnormally wide center part over crown in Ludwig pattern female androgenetic alopecia. *B*, Occipital part in same patient.

only in those persons with negative nitrogen balance (i.e., loss of lean body mass). Increased protein intake or re-feeding results in reduction or cessation of hair loss.[65, 66] Stringent dieting has been shown to decrease basal metabolic rate below levels that would be predicted by loss of lean body mass. These patients were found to have significant reductions in triiodothyronine levels, which were thought to be diet related.[67] Such triiodothyronine reductions may also contribute to diet-related hair loss. Fasting has also been shown to increase the biologic half-life of dehydroepiandrosterone sulfate, which could exacerbate an underlying androgenetic alopecia.[68]

Protein–Calorie Malnutrition. Marasmus is a chronic deficiency of protein and calories beginning in the first year of life. Marasmus can result from poor nutrition, or it can occur after gastroenteritis, parasitic infections, or glomerulonephritis.[69] Hair is thin, sparse, straight, light, and easily plucked. Kwashiorkor is due to acute or chronic protein deficiency in an otherwise calorically adequate diet. Acute deficiency results in dark hair with bands of red or white, termed the *flag sign.* Advanced protein deficiency results in fine, sparse, brittle hair. The rate of proliferation of hair root cells is one of the most rapid in the body. Deficient protein intake correlates positively with protein content of anagen roots.[70] During relative depletion of protein stores, impairment of hair root protein synthesis apparently occurs before a decrease in synthesis of serum albumin that serves a more vital function.[70, 71] Protein deprivation results in hair bulb atrophy[71] and an increase in telogen hairs.[70, 72]

Essential Fatty Acid Deficiency. After 2 to 4 months of inadequate intake of essential fatty acids, the scalp and eyebrows become red and scaly and significant telogen hair shedding begins. The remaining hair is dry, unruly, and light. Serum levels of eicosatrienoic acid (20:3, N-9) are high, and levels of arachidonic acid are low.[73–75]

Iron Deficiency. As many as 72% of women with diffuse telogen hair shedding have been found to have iron deficiency with or without associated anemia.[76] Oral iron therapy has been shown to result in cessation of hair loss followed by regrowth as iron levels returned to normal.[77] Current data suggest that ferritin levels of 40 μg/L or greater may be necessary for optimal hair growth.[78] It is thought that iron deficiency results in decreased depot iron and tissue iron much earlier than anemia is manifest. It is likely that iron availability limits DNA synthesis in proliferating cells.[79]

Zinc Deficiency. Symptoms of hereditary or acquired zinc deficiency include hair loss, acral and periorificial dermatitis, diarrhea, susceptibility to infection and altered cellular immunity, mood changes, anorexia, neurologic disturbances, and growth retardation. Acquired zinc deficiency has been described in association with inadequately supplemented parenteral nutrition,[80, 81] pancreatitis, and intestinal bypass surgery.[82] Hairs are white, sparse, short, and brittle and appear defective when polarized.[83] A variety of hair shaft abnormalities have been described.

Biotin Deficiency. Symptoms of congenital or acquired biotin deficiency include dermatitis, alopecia, seizures, hypotonia, ataxis, sensorineural hearing loss, visual pathway defects, mental retardation, and recurrent infections. Acquired biotin deficiency has been reported in association with parenteral alimentation[84] or excessive ingestion of raw egg white.[85] Scalp hair is diffusely sparse and finely textured. No hair shaft abnormalities have been noted.[86] Anagen–telogen ratios have not been measured, and no scalp biopsies have been performed.

Physiologic Stress and Alopecia

Fever. Telogen hair shedding has been described 2 to 5 months after febrile illnesses. In many instances other factors such as weight loss and malnutrition may contribute to the alopecia.[36, 87] Fever, which augments metabolic demands, might impair the ability of rapidly multiplying follicular matrix cells to proliferate normally in a nutritionally compromised host. It is also possible that fever from one of the endogenous pyrogens[88] may directly down-regulate follicular matrix cell proliferation. Both interferon alfa and gamma have been shown to decrease epithelial proliferation in tissue culture,[89, 90] and both have caused hair loss after intravenous infusion into humans.[91, 92] Biopsies of postfebrile alopecia showed an increased number of normal telogen follicles with no other significant changes noted.[36]

Systemic Illness. Chronic illness such as systemic lupus erythematosus, terminal carcinoma, ulcerative colitis, leukemia, tuberculosis, and malnutrition have all been associated with diffuse alopecia. Kligman[36] found that telogen counts in patients with debilitating disease correlated with morbidity; that is, the less "sick" patients had normal telogen counts. Other reports suggest that telogen hair shedding may herald the onset of some systemic diseases and that indeed the patients may not be "sick" at the onset of the hair loss. Diseases associated with telogen hair shedding include syphilis, lymphoproliferative disorders, inflammatory bowel disease, hepatic disease, systemic amyloidosis, and eosinophilia-myalgia syndrome.[93]

Surgery. Postoperative hair loss consistent with telogen effluvium has been described. The cause of this hair loss may well be multifactorial and has not been well studied. Postoperative localized pressure alopecia probably caused by pressure-induced ischemia may occur as well.[93]

Psychological Stress and Alopecia

Although the literature supports the notion of psychogenic telogen effluvium,[36] the paucity of reports and my experience suggest that it is uncommon. Eckert[94] studied 32 women complaining of diffuse hair loss. Seven of the 32 women did have evidence of psychiatric disturbance, but they did not have evidence of greater daily hair loss or telogen counts than did women with alopecia and no psychiatric disturbance.

Drugs and Alopecia

A large number of drugs have been reported to cause telogen hair shedding and diffuse alopecia (Table 134–5).[93, 95] Mechanisms for drug-induced hair loss are generally only speculative. Antimetabolites are known to produce necrosis of follicular keratinocytes resulting in anagen effluvium.

Local Cutaneous Disease

Acute, chronic, or chronically recurrent alopecia may occur in association with the scalp inflammation of psoriasis, seborrheic dermatitis, allergic contact dermatitis, and pemphigus vulgaris or foliaceus. Most commonly telogen hairs are shed, but very active inflammation may be associated with anagen hair shedding.[93]

TABLE 134–5. Diffuse Alopecia

Hormonal Causes	Drugs
Hypothyroidism	Allopurinol
Hyperthyroidism	Androgens (Danazol)
Postpartum alopecia	ACE inhibitors
Androgenetic alopecia	Captopril
Normal androgen levels	Enalapril
Abnormal androgen levels	Anticholesterolemics
Involutional alopecia	Anticoagulants
	Antimitotics
	Colchicine
Nutritional Causes	Methotrexate
	Antithyroid medications
Stringent weight loss diet	Benzimidazoles
Protein–calorie malnutrition	β-Blockers
Essential fatty acid deficiency*	Systemic
Iron deficiency	Topical ophthalmic
Zinc deficiency*	Borates
Biotin deficiency*	Bromocriptine
	Cimetidine
	Gold
Physiologic Stressors	Intravenous immunoglobulin
	Interferon alpha and gamma
Fever	Levodopa
Systemic illness	Minoxidil†
Eosinophilia-myalgia	Oral contraceptives
syndrome	During use
Hepatic disease	After discontinuation
Inflammatory bowel disease	Proguanil
Leukemia/	Psychotropics
lymphoproliferative	Amphetamines
disorders	Antidepressants
Systemic lupus	Dixyrazine
erythematosus	Lithium
Syphilis	Tranylcyprimine
Systemic amyloidosis	Valproic acid
Terminal carcinoma	Pyridostigmine bromide
Tuberculosis	Retinoids
Surgery	Sulfasalazine
	Terfenadine
	Vitamin A

Local Cutaneous Diseases
Psoriasis
Seborrheic dermatitis
Allergic contact dermatitis
Pemphigus vulgaris
Pemphigus foliaceus

*These are rare causes of alopecia; see text for details.
†Patients with androgenetic alopecia may have telogen hair shedding for a few weeks after initiation of minoxidil and at cyclic intervals during treatment. Regrowth of hair follows the shedding.

DIFFERENTIAL DIAGNOSIS

The differential diagnosis of diffuse alopecia includes hormonal causes, nutritional causes, physiologic stress, drugs, local cutaneous disease, and, rarely, psychological stress (see Table 134–5).

TREATMENT

Identification and elimination of the etiologic factors responsible for hair loss is the best treatment if possible.

Prognosis for hair regrowth is generally good if the cause of the alopecia can be found and eliminated or adequately treated and if the patient does not have associated androgenetic alopecia.

References

1. Bystryn JC, Tamesis J. Immunologic aspects of hair loss. J Invest Dermatol 1991;21:88S.
2. Werth VP, White WL, Sanchez MR, et al. Incidence of alopecia areata in lupus erythematosus. Arch Dermatol 1992;128:368–371.
3. Italian Group of Epidemiological Studies in Dermatology. Study of lichen planus conducted by the IGESDA: Results, implications for clinical practice, prospects. G Ital Dermatol Venereol 1990; 125:563–567.
4. Scherbenske JM, Benson PM, Rotchford JP, et al. Cutaneous and ocular manifestations of Down syndrome. J Am Acad Dermatol 1990;22:933–938.
5. Camacho F, Nevas J. Nuchal nevus flammeus in alopecia areata. Dermatology 1992;184:158.
6. Price VH. Alopecia areata: Clinical aspects. J Invest Dermatol 1991;96:68S.
7. Zlotogorski A, Weinrauch L, Brautbar C. Familial alopecia areata: No linkage with HLA. Tissue Antigens 1990;36:40–41.
8. Odum N, Morling N, Gorgsen J, et al. HLA-DP antigens in patients with alopecia areata. Tissue Antigens 1990;35:114–117.
9. Duvic M, Hordinsky MK, Fiedler VC, et al. HLA-D locus associations in alopecia areata: DRw52a may confer disease resistance. Arch Dermatol 1991;127:64–68.
10. DeWaard-van der Spek FB, Oranje AP, De Raeymaecker DM, et al. Juvenile versus maturity-onset alopecia areata: A comparative retrospective clinical study. Clin Exp Dermatol 1989;14:429–433.
11. Fiedler VC. Alopecia areata: Current therapy. J Invest Dermatol 1991;96:69S–70S.
12. Crosby DL, Gammon WR. Seasonal alopecia areata with atopy. J Am Acad Dermatol 1989;21:806–807.
13. van der Steen P, Boezeman J, Duller P, et al. Can alopecia areata be triggered by emotional stress? An uncontrolled evaluation of 178 patients with extensive hair loss. Acta Derm Venereol 1992;72:279–280.
14. Fiedler VC. Alopecia areata: A review of therapy, efficacy, safety and mechanism. Arch Dermatol 1992;128:1519–1520.
15. Perret C, Wiesner-Menzel L, Happle R. Immunohistochemical analysis of T-cell subsets in the peribulbar and intrabulbar infiltrates of alopecia areata. Acta Derm Venereol 1984;64:26–30.
16. Wiesner-Menzel L, Happle R. Intrabulbar and peribulbar accumulation of dendritic OKT6-positive cells in alopecia areata. Arch Dermatol Res 1984;276:333–334.
17. Fiedler VC, Buys CM. Immunohistochemical characterization of the cellular infiltrate in severe alopecia areata before and after minoxidil treatment. Dermatologica 1987;175(S2):29–35.
18. Tobin DJ, Fenton DA, Kendall MD. Cell degeneration in alopecia areata: An ultrastructural study. Am J Dermatopathol 1991; 13:248–256.
19. Hull SM, Nutbrown M, Pepall L, et al. Immunohistologic and ultrastructural comparison of the dermal papilla and hair follicle bulb from "active" and "normal" areas of alopecia areata. J Invest Dermatol 1991;96:673–681.
20. Headington JT. The histopathology of alopecia areata. J Invest Dermatol 1991;96:69S.
21. Hordinsky MK, Hallgren H, Nelson D, et al. Suppressor cell number and function in alopecia areata. Arch Dermatol 1984; 120:188–194.
22. Valsecchi R, Bontempelli M, Vicari O, et al. Peripheral T-cell subsets in patients with alopecia areata in different clinical phase. Dermatologica 1985;171:170–174.
23. Imai R, Miura J, Takamori K, et al. Increased HLA-DR+ T-lymphocyte population in peripheral blood of alopecia areata. Clin Exp Dermatol 1991;16:176–180.
24. Valsecchi R, Imberti G, Martino D, et al. Alopecia areata and interleukin-2 receptor. Dermatology 1992;184:126–128.
25. Kalish RS, Johnson KL, Hordinsky MK. Alopecia areata: Autoreactive T cells are variably enriched in scalp lesions relative to peripheral blood. Arch Dermatol 1992;128:1072–1077.
26. Nickoloff BJ, Griffiths CE. Aberrant intercellular adhesion molecule-1 (ICAM-1) expression by hair-follicle epithelial cells and endothelial leukocyte adhesion molecule-1 (ELAM-1) by vascular cells are important adhesion-molecule alterations in alopecia areata. J Invest Dermatol 1991;96:91S–92S.
27. Gilhar A, Pillar T, Assay B, et al. Failure of passive transfer of serum from patients with alopecia areata and alopecia universalis to inhibit hair growth in transplants of human scalp skin grafted onto nude mice. Br J Dermatol 1992;126:166–171.
28. van Baar HM, Perret CM, van Vlijmen IM, et al. Abnormal expression of Ki-67 antigen in hair follicle of alopecia areata. Acta Derm Venereol 1992;72:161–164.
29. Tobin DJ, Fenton DA, Kendall MD. Ultrastructural study of exclamation-mark hair shafts in alopecia areata. J Cutan Pathol 1990;17:348–354.
30. Peereboom-Wynia JD, Koerten HK, van Joost T, et al. Scanning electron microscopy comparing exclamation mark hairs in alopecia areata with normal hair fibres, mechanically broken by traction. Clin Exp Dermatol 1989;14:47–50.
31. Lotti T, Teofoli P, Senesi C, et al. The role of plasminogen activators in alopecia areata. Int J Dermatol 1991;30:19–21.
32. Beard HO. Social and psychological implications of alopecia areata. J Am Acad Dermatol 1986;14:697–700.
33. Fiedler VC, Wendrow A, Szpunar GJ, et al. Treatment-resistant alopecia areata: Response to combination therapy with minoxidil plus anthralin. Arch Dermatol 1990;126:756–759.
34. Shapiro J, Tan J, Tron V. Diphencyprone and minoxidil in alopecia areata: A clinical and immunopathologic evaluation. J Invest Dermatol 1992;98:562.
35. Orecchia G, Perfetti L, Borroni G, et al. Photochemotherapy plus squaric acid dibutylester in alopecia areata treatment. Dermatologica 1990;181:167–169.
36. Kligman AM. Pathologic dynamics of human hair loss. Arch Dermatol 1961;83:175–198.
37. Van Scott EJ, Reinertson RP, Steinmuller R. The growing hair roots of the human scalp and morphologic changes therein following amethopterin therapy. J Invest Dermatol 1957;29:197–204.
38. Maguire HC, Kligman AM. Hair plucking as a diagnostic tool. J Invest Dermatol 1964;43:77–79.
39. Barman JM, Astore I, Pecoraro V. The normal trichogram of the adult. J Invest Dermatol 1965;44:233–236.
40. Headington JT. Telogen effluvium: New concepts and review. Arch Dermatol 1993;129:356–363.
41. Church RE. Hypothyroid hair loss. Br J Dermatol 1965; 77:661–662.
42. Watanakunakorn C, Hodges RE, Evans TC. Myxedema. Arch Intern Med 1965;116:183–190.
43. Saito R, Hori Y, Kuribayashi T. Alopecia in hypothyroidism. In: Kobori T, Montagna W, eds. Biology of Diseases of the Hair. Tokyo: University of Tokyo Press, 1976:279–285.
44. Freinkel RK, Freinkel N. Hair growth and alopecia in hypothyroidism. Arch Dermatol 1972;106:349–352.
45. Smith JG, Weinstein GD, Burr JM. Hair roots of the human scalp in thyroid disease. J Invest Dermatol 1959;32:35–38.
46. Famuyiwa OO, Bella AF. Thyrotoxicosis in Nigeria. Trop Geogr Med 1990;42:248–254.
47. Pecoraro V, Barman JM, Astore I. The normal trichogram of pregnant women. Adv Biol Skin 1967;9:203–210.
48. Lynfield YL. Effect of pregnancy on the human hair cycle. J Invest Dermatol 1960;35:323–327.
49. Dawber RPR, Connor BL. Pregnancy, hair loss and the pill. Br Med J 1971;4:234.
50. Skelton JB. Postpartum alopecia. Am J Obstet Gynecol 1966; 94:125–129.
51. Schiff BL, Pawtucket RI, Kern AB. Study of postpartum alopecia. Arch Dermatol 1963;87:609–611.
52. Headington JT. Transverse microscopic anatomy of the human scalp. Arch Dermatol 1984;120:449–456.
53. Fiedler VC, Storrs PA, Abell E. Histologic evaluation of the evolution and response to treatment of female pattern androgenetic alopecia. J Invest Dermatol 1994;102:566.
54. Kligman AM. The comparative histopathology of male-pattern baldness and senescent baldness. Clin Dermatol 1988;6:108–118.
55. Pinkus H. Alopecia: Clinopathologic correlations. Int J Dermatol 1980;19:245–253.

56. Cormia FE. Alopecia from oral contraceptives. JAMA 1967; 201:635-637.

57. Zaun H, Gerber T. Die Wirkung Monophasischer Ovulationshemmer auf das Wachstum der Kopfhaare. Arch Klin Exp Dermatol 1969;234:353-361.

58. Zaun H, Ruffing H. Untersuchungen über den Einfluß Antikonzeptiver Zweiphasen-Hormonpräparate auf das Wachstum der Kopfhaare. Arch Klin Exp Dermatol 1970;238:197-206.

59. Tronnier H. Dermatologische Nebenwirkungen von Ovulationshemmern. Arch Klin Exp Dermatol 1970;237:197-200.

60. Griffiths WAD. Diffuse hair loss and oral contraceptives. Br J Dermatol 1973;88:31-36.

61. Goette DK, Odom RB. Profuse hair loss. Arch Dermatol 1975;111:930.

62. Krusinski PA. Telogen effluvium secondary to weight loss and therapy with chorionic gonadotropin. Arch Dermatol 1976; 112:556.

63. Kaufman JP. Telogen effluvium secondary to starvation diet. Arch Dermatol 1976;112:731.

64. Goette DK, Odom RB. Alopecia in crash dieters. JAMA 1976;235:2622-2623.

65. Blackburn GL, Bistrain BR, Hoag C. Hair loss with rapid weight loss. JAMA 1976;236:252.

66. Rooth G, Carlström S. Therapeutic fasting. Acta Med Scand 1970;187:455-463.

67. Cavallo E, Armellini F, Zamboni M, et al. Resting metabolic rate, body composition and thyroid hormones. Horm Metab Res 1990;22:632-635.

68. Hendrikx A, Heyns W, Moor PD. Influence of a low-calorie diet and fasting on the metabolism of dehydroepiandrosterone sulfate. J Clin Endocrinol 1968;28:1525-1533.

69. Johnson AA, Latham MC, Roe DA. An evaluation of the use of changes in hair root morphology in the assessment of protein-calorie malnutrition. Am J Clin Nutr 1976;29:502-511.

70. Jordan VE. Protein status of the elderly as measured by dietary intake, hair tissue and serum albumin. Am J Clin Nutr 1976;29:522-528.

71. Bradfield RB. Protein deprivation: Comparative response of hair roots, serum protein, and urinary nitrogen. Am J Clin Nutr 1971;24:405-410.

72. Bradfield RB, Cordano A, Graham GG. Hair root adaptation to marasmus in Andean Indian children. Lancet 1969;2:1395-1397.

73. Caldwell MD, Jonsson HT, Othersen HB. Essential fatty acid deficiency in an infant receiving prolonged parenteral alimentation. J Pediatr 1972;81:894-898.

74. Riella MC, Broviac JW, Wells M, et al. Essential fatty acid deficiency in human adults during total parenteral nutrition. Ann Intern Med 1975;83:786-789.

75. Skolnik P, Eaglstein WH, Ziboh VA. Human essential fatty acid deficiency. Arch Dermatol 1977;113:939-941.

76. Rushton DH, Ramsay ID, James KC, et al. Biochemical and trichological characterization of diffuse alopecia in women. Br J Dermatol 1990;123:187-197.

77. Hård S. Non-anemic iron deficiency as an etiologic factor in diffuse loss of hair of the scalp in women. Acta Derm Venereol 1963;43:562-569.

78. Rushton DH, Ramsay ID. The importance of adequate serum ferritin levels during oral cyproterone acetate and ethinyl oestradiol treatment of diffuse androgen-dependent alopecia in women. Clin Endocrinol 1992;36:421-427.

79. Laskey J, Webb I, Schulman HM, et al. Evidence that transferrin supports cell proliferation by supplying iron for DNA synthesis. Exp Cell Res 1988;176:87-95.

80. Kay RG, Tasman-Jones C. Acute zinc deficiency in man during intravenous alimentation. Aust NZ J Surg 1975;45:325-330.

81. Tucker SB, Schroeter AL, Brown PW, et al. Acquired zinc deficiency. JAMA 1976;235:2399-2402.

82. Weisman K, Wadskov S, Mikkelsen HI, et al. Acquired zinc deficiency dermatosis in man. Arch Dermatol 1978;114:1509-1511.

83. Dupré A, Bonafé JL, Carriere JP. The hair in acrodermatitis enteropathica: A disease indicator? Acta Derm Venereol 1979;59: 177-178.

84. Mock DM, Baswell DL, Baker H, et al. Biotin deficiency complicating parenteral alimentation: Diagnosis, metabolic repercussions, and treatment. J Pediatr 1985;106:762-769.

85. Sydenstricker VP, Singal SA, Briggs AP, et al. Observations on the "egg white injury" in man. JAMA 1942;118:1199-1200.

86. Williams ML, Packman S, Cowan MJ. Alopecia and periorificial dermatitis in biotin-responsive multiple carboxylase deficiency. J Am Acad Dermatol 1983;9:97-103.

87. Bernstein GM, Crollick JS, Hassett JM. Postfebrile telogen effluvium in critically ill patients. Crit Care Med 1988;16:98-99.

88. Dinarello CA, Cannon JG, Wolff SM. New concepts on the pathogenesis of fever. Rev Infect Res 1988;10:168-189.

89. Yaar M, Karassik RL, Schnipper LE, et al. Effects of alpha and beta interferons on cultured human keratinocytes. J Invest Dermatol 1985;85:70-74.

90. Tabibzadeh SS, Satyaswaroop PG, Rao PN. Antiproliferative effect of interferon-γ in human endometrial epithelial cells in vitro: Potential local growth modulatory role in endometrium. J Clin Endocrinol Metab 1988;67:131-138.

91. Brown TD, Koeller J, Beougher K, et al. A phase I clinical trial of recombinant DNA gama interferon. J Clin Oncol 1987; 5:790-798.

92. Olsen EA, Rosen ST, Vollmer RT, et al. Interferon alpha-2a in the treatment of cutaneous T cell lymphoma. J Am Acad Dermatol 1989;20:395-407.

93. Fiedler VC, Hafeez A. Diffuse alopecia: Telogen hair loss. In: Olsen EA, ed. Disorders of Hair Growth: Diagnosis and Treatment. New York: McGraw-Hill, 1994:241-255.

94. Eckert J. Diffuse hair loss and psychiatric disturbance. Acta Derm Venereol 1975;55:147-149.

95. Brodin MB. Drug-related alopecia. Dermatol Clin 1987; 5:571-579.

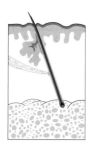

chapter 135

Scarring Alopecia

STEPHEN F. TEMPLETON and ALVIN R. SOLOMON

The scarring alopecias are a diverse group of diseases that are characterized by the common endpoint of obliteration of the hair follicle. The terms *scarring* and *cicatricial* have been historically used to describe this group of permanent alopecias, but these terms may be misleading in that true dermal scarring is not always present.

Clinically, scarring alopecias are characterized by permanent hair loss with partial or complete loss of follicular orifices. It may be difficult to determine if alopecia is scarring on clinical grounds alone because some alopecias that have not been traditionally classified as scarring may also cause some degree of permanent hair loss with loss of follicular orifices. The early stages of scarring alopecias have distinguishing clinical characteristics that aid in diagnosis. In addition, some scarring alopecias are accompanied by cutaneous findings that aid in diagnosis (e.g., lesions of lichen planus on the wrist of a patient with lichen planopilaris).

DEFINITION

The defining characteristic of all scarring alopecias is follicular destruction. Scarring alopecias may be either primary or secondary, depending on the pattern of follicular destruction. Primary scarring alopecia is defined as preferential destruction of hair follicles and/or associated adventitial dermis.[1] In primary scarring alopecias, the hair follicle is the primary target of destruction and alteration as the result of inflammation, interface alteration, infection, and/or vesicle formation. The interfollicular epidermis may be affected in some primary scarring alopecias (e.g., discoid lupus erythematosus and lichen planopilaris), but the epidermal changes in and of themselves do not result in follicular destruction.

The destruction of hair follicles in secondary scarring alopecia results from nonfollicular events that impinge on the follicular unit (e.g., alteration of the reticular dermis, epidermis, or subcutis that eventually eradicates the follicle).[1] Examples of pathomechanisms resulting in secondary scarring alopecia include reticular dermal sclerosis, neoplasia, and nonfolliculocentric inflammation (i.e., sarcoidosis).

Permanent "scarring" alopecia may also occur in diseases that have not been traditionally considered cicatricial. This group of alopecias generally results from persistence of abnormalities of follicular dynamics, eventually causing "dropout" of affected follicles. Examples of this type of permanent alopecia include chronic, ongoing traction alopecia and trichotillomania, as well as persistent, nonremitting alopecia areata, androgenetic alopecia, and telogen effluvium. In addition, certain hair shaft abnormalities may result in permanent partial alopecia. These latter groups of potentially permanent "scarring" alopecias are fully discussed elsewhere in this text. Finally, permanent scarring alopecia may be a feature of several inherited genodermatoses. This group of alopecias are poorly characterized pathogenetically and are therefore difficult to classify as either primary or secondary scarring alopecias.

Primary Scarring Alopecias

Primary scarring alopecias have been grouped and classified according to clinical, microscopic, and proposed pathogenic criteria. No one classification schema is ideal. Classification according to the predominate inflammatory cell has been proposed, and this classification system correlates well with the clinical feature of presence or absence of a pustulofollicular component (Table 135–1).[1–3]

TABLE 135-1. Primary Scarring Alopecia

Pustulofollicular primary scarring alopecias
Lymphocyte associated primary scarring alopecias
Vesiculobullous primary scarring alopecias
Uncategorized primary scarring alopecias

PUSTULOFOLLICULAR PRIMARY SCARRING ALOPECIAS

The term *pustulofollicular primary scarring alopecia* is used to classify a group of alopecias that have some clinical and microscopic similarities on the basis of clinical and microscopic pustules and purulent follicular infiltrates (Table 135-2). Both infectious and noninfectious processes comprise the pustulofollicular scarring alopecias. There may be some clinical and microscopic overlap between some of the early noninfectious pustulofollicular alopecias; however, the fully developed pustulofollicular alopecias are usually quite distinctive.

Dissecting Cellulitis of the Scalp (Perifolliculitis Capitis Abscedens et Suffodiens)

Clinical Description. This pustulofollicular scarring alopecia was named perifolliculitis capitis abscedens et suffodiens by Hoffman in 1908 and later renamed dissecting cellulitis of the scalp.[4, 5] Other synonyms are dissecting folliculitis of the scalp or dissecting perifolliculitis of the scalp. The lesions most commonly begin on the vertex or occiput as relatively painless, deep-seated, firm to fluctuant nodules and abscesses. The nodules and deep abscesses commonly extend to form a complex serpiginous or reticulate pattern of interconnecting sinuses and abscesses filled with purulent, seropurulent, or hemopurulent material (Fig. 135-1). Pressure applied to one nodule or abscess can cause purulent exudate to emerge several centimeters away. The epidermal surface overlying the sinuses and nodules may or may not be erythematous and scaly. Scattered superficial follicular pustules are frequently present on the surface of the nodules. Hypertrophic and keloidal scarring may occur in affected areas.

Dissecting cellulitis of the scalp is more common in young to middle-aged black men. It may occur simultaneously with acne conglobata and hidradenitis suppurativa. This complex is known as the follicular occlusion triad.

Pathology. Acneiform dilatation of the follicular in-

TABLE 135-2. Pustulofollicular Primary Scarring Alopecias

Dissecting cellulitis of the scalp
Acne keloidalis nuchae
Folliculitis decalvans
Erosive pustular dermatosis of the scalp
Tinea capitis

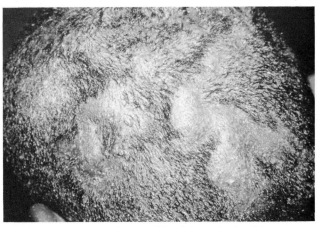

FIGURE 135-1. Dissecting cellulitis of the scalp showing numerous interconnected fluctuant abscesses and sinus tracts with overlying crusts and pustules.

fundibulum with intrafollicular and perifollicular accumulation of neutrophils and subsequent follicular perforation are the earliest microscopic findings. Biopsy specimens from well-developed fluctuant nodules and sinuses reveal large, perifollicular, mid to deep reticular dermal abscesses often rich in plasma cells. Abscesses are located immediately adjacent to follicles, between follicles in the mid and deep reticular dermis, and subjacent to follicles within the superficial subcutis. In well-developed lesions of dissecting cellulitis, the abscesses are partially lined with squamous epithelium derived from the overlying epidermis or adjacent follicular epithelium. Dense dermal fibrosis eventually surrounds the sinus tracts and the affected follicles are destroyed by the fibroinflammatory process. Bacteria may be present within dilated follicular infundibula but are not routinely observed within the dermal abscesses.[2]

Pathogenesis and Etiology. The pathophysiology of dissecting cellulitis of the scalp is poorly understood but may involve a combination of factors, including recurrent bacterial infections and abnormal follicular keratinization.[6]

Diagnosis and Differential Diagnosis. Patients with well-developed nodules, abscesses, and sinuses are easily diagnosed clinically. The presence of deep fluctuant sinuses differentiates this disease from the more superficial pustulofollicular alopecias: folliculitis decalvans, acne keloidalis nuchae, and erosive pustular dermatosis of the scalp. Keloidal scarring may occur in dissecting cellulitis of the scalp, but the scarring is more broad, deep seated, and less exophytic than in acne keloidalis. The scarring in dissecting cellulitis of the scalp also has a lattice-like clinical appearance occurring in the areas of the abscess and sinus formation.

Bacterial culture of abscess fluid and overlying pustules is frequently sterile but may yield *Staphylococcus epidermidis* or *S. aureus*. The pathogenic role of these organisms is uncertain because chronic antibiotic therapy is frequently not curative. Fungal culture is indicated to exclude dermatophyte infection.[7] Rarely, squamous cell carcinoma may arise in long-standing dissecting cellulitis of the scalp.[8]

Treatment. A permanent cure is rarely achieved in patients with dissecting cellulitis of the scalp. Initial therapy frequently involves oral antibiotics such as tetracycline (1–2 g per day), doxycycline (200 mg per day), and minocycline (50–200 mg per day) (Table 135–3). Combination antibiotic therapy of cephalexin (1 g per day) and rifampin (600 mg per day) has been helpful in our experience. Intralesional corticosteroid injections (triamcinolone acetonide, 40 mg/mL) can be helpful in noninfectious nodules and sinuses. Oral corticosteroids tapered to low-dose alternate-day usage may also be helpful.[9] Isotretinoin (1 mg/kg per day) has been effective in some reported cases.[10, 11] Dapsone may be helpful in some patients.[12] Assessment of glucose-6-phosphate dehydrogenase level and follow-up evaluation for hemolytic anemia and methemoglobinemia are essential in dapsone-treated patients. Oral zinc has also been reported to be effective.[13]

Surgical therapy may be considered in advanced cases but is usually quite deforming. Complete scalp excision,[14] carbon dioxide laser excision,[15] or more conservative local incision and drainage of individual lesions may be considered.

Acne Keloidalis Nuchae

Clinical Description. Acne keloidalis nuchae was described separately by Kaposi in 1869 (dermatitis papillaris capillitis)[16] and by Bazin in 1872 (acne cheloidique).[17] It is a destructive pustulofollicular process that invariably occurs on the occipital scalp and posterior neck and primarily affects young black men. The lesions begin as discrete follicular pustules and papules (Fig. 135–2) but progress to form less discrete, large, exophytic keloidal nodules and plaques largely devoid of hair. The severity of involvement is variable and ranges from

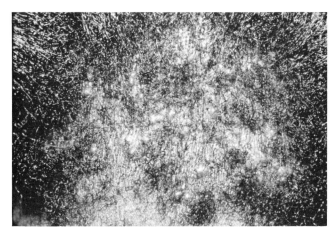

FIGURE 135–2. Acne keloidalis nuchae with many follicular and perifollicular keloidal papules located on the occipital scalp.

few small follicular pustules and papules with minimal alopecia to extensive keloidal plaque formation with prominent patterned alopecia.[18] Similar lesions may occur in the beard area of patients with pseudofolliculitis barbae.

Pathology. Early lesions are characterized by comedonal dilatation of the follicular infundibulum similar to that seen in folliculitis decalvans and dissecting cellulitis of the scalp. Intrafollicular neutrophils fill the infundibulum and isthmus in pustular and inflammatory papular lesions and spill out into the adjacent dermis when follicles rupture. The inflammation in older lesions consists of perifollicular and perivascular predominantly lymphoplasmacytic infiltrates more prominent in the upper and mid reticular dermis with fewer neutrophils. Perifollicular granulomatous inflammation may also be present. Perifollicular fibrosis involving the adventitial and reticular dermis is characteristic of acne keloidalis nuchae. "Naked" hair shafts, devoid of surrounding follicular epithelium but surrounded by histiocytes and giant cells, are embedded within dermal fibrosis. The extent of true keloid formation may vary.[19]

Pathogenesis and Etiology. The etiology of this common condition is unknown. Some have suggested that acne keloidalis nuchae is a variant of acne vulgaris. Early lesions are characterized by follicular and perifollicular inflammation with acneiform dilatation of the follicular infundibulum similar to that seen in acne vulgaris. Bacteria may be cultured from lesions of acne keloidalis nuchae, but it is unclear whether these organisms are pathogenic or represent superinfection.[18] Repetitive low-grade trauma and friction by football helmets, other headware, and collars have been reported in association with acne keloidalis nuchae and may help explain the restricted distribution to the posterior scalp.[20] Close shaving of posterior scalp and neck hair may initiate or exacerbate acne keloidalis nuchae as in pseudofolliculitis barbae and may be due to curved ingrown hairs.

Diagnosis and Differential Diagnosis. The typical distribution and morphology of acne keloidalis nuchae readily suggest the correct diagnosis. Bacterial folliculitis of the scalp does not typically result in scarring papules and is not restricted to the occipital scalp. Cylindroma,

---

> **TABLE 135–3. Treatment of Dissecting Cellulitis of the Scalp**

1. Oral antibiotics
   a. Tetracycline, 1–2 g per day
   b. Doxycycline, 200 mg per day
   c. Minocycline, 50–200 mg per day
   d. Cephalexin, 1 g per day
   e. Rifampin, 600 mg per day
   f. Combination oral antibiotic therapy with cephalexin and rifampin
2. Intralesional corticosteroids (triamcinolone acetonide 40 mg/mL)
3. Oral corticosteroids (tapering dosage of prednisone, 40–60 mg per day)
4. Isotretinoin, 1 mg/kg per day
5. Dapsone, 50–100 mg per day (must check glucose-6-phosphate dehydrogenase level)
6. Oral zinc supplements
7. Surgical therapies
   a. Local incision and drainage of individual lesions
   b. Complete scalp excision, carbon dioxide laser excision (only in extremely severe cases may this be considered)

TABLE 135-4. Treatment of Acne Keloidalis Nuchae

1. Oral antibiotics
  a. Tetracycline, 1 g per day
  b. Doxycycline, 200 mg per day
  c. Minocycline, 50-100 g per day
  d. Erythromycin, 1 g per day
2. Topical antibiotics
  a. Erythromycin solution 2%
  b. Clindamycin solution 1%
3. Tretinoin cream or gel 0.025%-0.1%
4. Benzoyl peroxide gel or lotion 5%-10%
5. Intralesional corticosteroid injections (triamcinolone acetonide, 3-40 mg/mL)
6. Surgical excision for large exophytic keloidal nodules and plaques

trichilemmal cyst, proliferating pilar tumor, cutaneous metastasis, and other tumors may be considered in more exophytic keloidal nodules. However, a background of follicular pustules and papules in acne keloidalis nuchae aids in diagnosis.

Treatment. Long-term oral antibiotics such as tetracycline (1 g per day), doxycycline (200 mg per day), minocycline (50–100 mg per day), or erythromycin (1 g per day) are useful in inflammatory pustular lesions (Table 135–4). Topical antibiotics in a drying vehicle (2% erythromycin and 1% clindamycin) are also helpful. The combination of oral or topical antibiotics with tretinoin cream or gel is helpful for preventing formation of new lesions and fairly effective for resolution of minimally scarred lesions. Topical benzoyl peroxide and sulfurated solutions may also be used.

Intralesional corticosteroid injections into large and small papules and plaques are helpful in reducing inflammation and size of the lesions. Superpotent corticosteroids may also reduce inflammation but may exacerbate the acneiform component of this disorder.

Large, keloidal nodules and plaques are generally unresponsive to medical therapy and require surgical excision for removal. However, keloid recurrence at the site of excision may recur, and therefore close clinical follow-up and prophylactic intralesional corticosteroid injections into the surgical excision site are recommended.

Folliculitis Decalvans

Clinical Description. In 1888, Quinquaud first described the classic findings of this pustulofollicular alopecia, which later became known as folliculitis decalvans.[21] Folliculitis decalvans occurs in both sexes. Onset of disease in men ranges from puberty to advanced age, while in women the age at onset ranges from young to older adults.[22] Folliculitis decalvans primarily affects the scalp and results in patches of patterned alopecia, but involvement of beard, axillary, pubic, and inner thigh hair has also been reported.[23, 24] In classic folliculitis decalvans, well-developed clinical lesions consist of irregular- to oval-shaped atrophic patches of alopecia with small follicular pustules present at the advancing edge of the patch of alopecia (Fig. 135–3). In progressive folliculitis decalvans, the area of scalp affected by the scarring alopecia gradually enlarges and multiple sites of involvement are present. Extensive scarring alopecia may result. Older, inactive patches of folliculitis decalvans in which pustules are not present closely resemble pseudopelade of Brocq.

A variant of folliculitis decalvans, termed *epilating folliculitis of glabrous skin,* may involve large areas of nonscalp, glabrous skin and result in permanent hair loss with perifollicular atrophy.[23]

Pathology. The earliest finding in folliculitis decalvans is comedonal follicular infundibular dilatation similar to that seen in acne keloidalis nuchae and dissecting cellulitis of the scalp. Variably dense infiltrates composed primarily of neutrophils are present in perifollicular and intrafollicular areas. In more advanced lesions, follicular destruction is evident and large numbers of admixed lymphocytes and plasma cells are present around the affected follicles. The adventitial dermis associated with residual follicles is fibrosed. In addition, "naked" hair shafts surrounded by granulomatous infiltrates are often present and, as in all other types of scarring alopecia, residual fibrous tracts (stele) mark the sites of destroyed follicles.[2]

The perifollicular fibrosis is much more limited in extent than in acne keloidalis nuchae. No hypertrophic or keloidal fibrosis is noted. The infiltrate in folliculitis decalvans does not significantly extend away from the follicle to form dermal and subcutaneous abscesses as in dissecting cellulitis of the scalp. Periodic acid–Schiff and tissue Gram stains are helpful to rule out dermatophyte and staphylococcal infections.

Pathogenesis and Etiology. The pathogenesis of folliculitis decalvans is unknown. Although bacteria may be cultured from some pustules, other pustules have been reported to be sterile, and only limited improvement with oral and topical antibiotics is seen.

Diagnosis and Differential Diagnosis. Although folliculitis decalvans is rare, the classic presentation of a

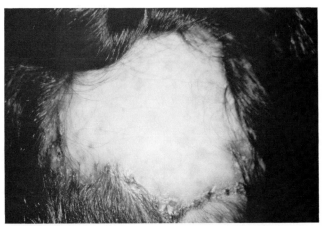

FIGURE 135–3. Folliculitis decalvans showing a large patch of atrophic scarring alopecia with numerous superficial, peripherally located perifollicular crusts and pustules. (Courtesy of Robert A. Swerlick, M.D.)

TABLE 135-5. Treatment of Folliculitis Decalvans

1. Oral antibiotics
   a. Tetracycline, 1-2 g per day
   b. Doxycycline, 200 mg per day
   c. Minocycline, 100 mg per day
   d. Erythromycin, 1 g per day
   e. Dicloxacillin, 1 g per day
   f. Cephalexin, 1 g per day
2. Topical antibiotics
   a. Erythromycin solution 2%
   b. Clindamycin solution 1%

scarring patch of alopecia with a peripheral rim of follicular pustules is diagnostic clinically. Scalp folliculitis with few scattered follicular pustules and minimal if any alopecia is common. This limited scalp folliculitis is not true folliculitis decalvans but is usually a bacterial folliculitis responsive to topical or oral antibiotics. Occasionally, scalp folliculitis may also occur as the result of occlusion by hair care products that contain heavy oils or ointments. Fungal culture is indicated to rule out dermatophyte infection. Inactive, end-stage folliculitis decalvans in which pustules are no longer present may closely resemble pseudopelade.

Treatment. Oral and topical antibiotics are the mainstay of therapy as in dissecting cellulitis of the scalp (Table 135-5).

Erosive Pustular Dermatosis of the Scalp

Clinical Description. Erosive pustular dermatosis of the scalp was first described by Pye and associates in 1979.[25] It is an uncommon erosive and pustular process affecting the scalp that is most commonly found in elderly white females.[26] The age at onset is usually in the sixth to ninth decades. Most reports in the literature are from England.

The process typically begins on the crown, vertex, or lateral scalp as pustules and erosions with gradual increase in size over a period of months to years. Thick purulent crusts frequently overlie erosions (Fig. 135-4).

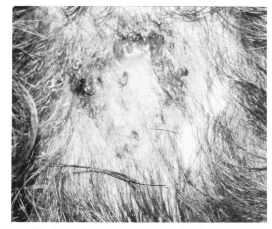

FIGURE 135-4. Erosive pustular dermatosis of the scalp showing a localized patch of alopecia with pustular erosions and crusts occurring throughout the area of alopecia.

The process is limited to the scalp. The lesions frequently occur in areas of recent or remote trauma to the scalp.

Pathology. The microscopic features of erosive pustular dermatosis of the scalp are not specific. Epidermal and superficial dermal ulceration with subjacent mixed inflammatory infiltrates and abscesses have been reported. Direct immunofluorescence microscopy of lesional and perilesional skin is negative. No circulating autoantibodies are seen by indirect immunofluorescence microscopy.

Pathogenesis and Etiology. The pathogenesis of erosive pustular dermatosis of the scalp is unknown. Numerous types of bacteria and fungi have been cultured from lesions of this disorder including *Staphylococcus* species, *Pseudomonas aeruginosa*, *Proteus mirabilis*, *Candida* species, and *Aspergillus ochraceus*. However, the lack of clinical response to systemic and topical antibiotics and antifungal agents suggests that these organisms are not pathogenic but represent secondary colonization.[26] In addition, many cases of erosive pustular dermatosis of the scalp have been reported to have sterile pustules and exudates.

Diagnosis and Differential Diagnosis. The diagnosis is established by exclusion of other pustulofollicular processes on the basis of clinical, microscopic, and microbiologic criteria. Other primary pustulofollicular scarring alopecias such as dissecting cellulitis of the scalp, folliculitis decalvans, and tinea capitis must be considered. Erosive pustular dermatosis of the scalp lacks the deepseated fluctuant nodules and sinuses typically seen in dissecting cellulitis of the scalp. Folliculitis decalvans and erosive pustular dermatosis of the scalp have some clinical similarities. However, folliculitis decalvans is more characterized by an atrophic sclerotic plaque of scarring alopecia with advancing, peripherally located pustules, whereas erosive pustular dermatosis of the scalp is more characterized by inflammatory erosions, crusts, and pustules distributed throughout the affected area.

Infectious pustulofollicular processes such as tinea capitis, bacterial pyoderma, and herpes simplex virus infection must be excluded by culture and/or microscopic evaluation. Finally, neutrophilic dermatoses such as Sweet's syndrome and pyoderma gangrenosum may be considered in the clinical differential diagnosis.

Treatment. Treatment of erosive pustular dermatosis of the scalp is difficult (Table 135-6). If bacterial cultures are positive, appropriate oral antibiotics are suggested. However, even prolonged oral antibiotic therapy is usually only minimally beneficial. Oral, intralesional, and potent topical corticosteroids seem to be the most efficacious therapy, but full control or resolution of the pustular inflammatory process does not typically occur.

TABLE 135-6. Treatment of Erosive Pustular Dermatosis of the Scalp

1. Class I topical corticosteroid cream or ointment
2. Oral prednisone, 40 mg per day, tapered over 6-8 weeks
3. Intralesional triamcinolone acetonide, 10-40 mg/mL
4. Appropriate oral antibiotics if bacterial culture is positive
5. Dermatophyte infection ruled out with appropriate culture

Oral zinc sulfate and isotretinoin have been reported to be effective in a small number of patients.[27, 28] Dapsone was ineffective in one of Pye's original patients.

Tinea Capitis, Kerion, Favus

Follicular dermatophyte infections lead to a permanent scarring alopecia. Other scalp infections that may lead to a scarring alopecia such as herpes zoster are not folliculocentric and therefore are considered secondary scarring alopecias.

Uncomplicated tinea capitis is a common childhood infection and does not cause a scarring alopecia. However, two subtypes of tinea capitis—kerion and favus—may result in permanent hair loss (Fig. 135–5). Kerion is a very inflammatory form of tinea capitis that is most commonly caused by a zoophilic or geophilic dermatophyte infection. Kerions are characterized by well-circumscribed, crusted, boggy plaques with decreased follicular density and numerous broken hair shafts. Cervical adenopathy and an accompanying eczematous "id" eruption are common.[29]

Favus is an uncommon chronic dermatophyte infection of the scalp seen in rural areas and associated with poor hygiene and poor nutrition. Clinical lesions are characterized by cup-shaped yellow crusts (scutula) that may progress to patches of scarring alopecia. The etiologic agent is usually *Trichophyton schoenleinii*.[30]

Pathology. The follicular infundibula are dilated and filled with keratin and neutrophils. The infundibular epithelium is frequently ruptured and surrounded by dense perifollicular mixed inflammation consisting of neutrophils, lymphocytes, plasma cells, and histiocytes. Endothrix (hyphae within hair shafts) and ectothrix (hyphae around hair shafts) dermatophyte infections are usually detectable on routine hematoxylin and eosin–stained sections but are best seen in periodic acid–Schiff-stained or silver-impregnated sections. In older, advanced lesions complete follicular destruction with "naked" hair shafts and dermal fibrosis is present.[2]

Scutula of favus are characterized by thick parakeratotic and orthokeratotic hyperkeratosis overlying a thinned epidermis. Similar follicular changes as in kerion are seen. Biopsy specimens of kerions show marked dermal edema and dense mixed infiltrates that include neutrophils. Hyphae are often rare. In well-developed lesions the inflammation may have a more prominent lymphoplasmacytic and granulomatous component. Dermal fibrosis in areas of destroyed follicles is present.

LYMPHOCYTE-ASSOCIATED PRIMARY SCARRING ALOPECIAS

Pseudopelade of Brocq, discoid lupus erythematosus, lichen planopilaris, and alopecia mucinosa are the most common lymphocyte-associated primary scarring alopecias. In contrast to the pustulofollicular primary scarring alopecias, no clinical pustules or prominent neutrophilic infiltrates are seen in this group of alopecias, but perifollicular lymphocytic infiltrates are present. Each lymphocyte-associated primary scarring alopecia has particular clinical and microscopic features that facilitate diagnosis. The etiologies of these diseases are not fully understood, and whether the perifollicular lymphohistiocytic inflammation is a primary or a secondary phenomenon remains to be established (Table 135–7).

Pseudopelade of Brocq

Clinical Description. Brocq introduced the term *pseudopelade* in 1885 to describe a clinically noninflammatory, progressive, idiopathic scarring alopecia. The alopecia is usually patterned and consists of round to irregularly shaped patches of complete or near-complete alopecia most commonly on the vertex or crown. In classic cases of pseudopelade of Brocq, the skin in the patches of alopecia is smooth, shiny, and atrophic. Scattered isolated hairs may be present in the patches of alopecia. In addition, minimal perifollicular erythema and scale may be present at the periphery of some of the alopecic patches (Fig. 135–6). However, lichenoid papules or follicular spinous lesions are absent. Onset is usually between 25 and 45 years of age, and there is a female predominance.[31]

A common presentation of pseudopelade of Brocq occurs in adult black women, begins on the crown, and expands centrifugally in a relatively symmetrical fashion (Fig. 135–7). In early cases, the alopecia is not as patterned but is characterized by more diffuse follicular dropout on the vertex and crown. In more advanced cases, patches of near-complete alopecia with few remaining follicles are present on the crown. LoPresti and colleagues initially described this condition as *hot comb*

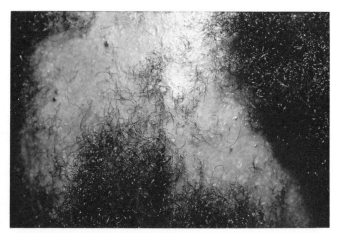

FIGURE 135–5. Tinea capitis with fairly extensive hair loss and few scattered perifollicular pustules and crusts.

TABLE 135–7. Lymphocyte-Associated Primary Scarring Alopecias

Pseudopelade of Brocq
Lichen planopilaris
Discoid lupus erythematosus
Alopecia mucinosa

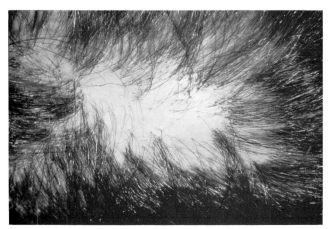

FIGURE 135-6. Pseudopelade of Brocq with irregular patches of scarring alopecia and only minimal perifollicular erythema and scale. Some follicular orifices are dilated and contain multiple hair shafts. There are a few, isolated follicles remaining within the patches of scarring alopecia.

alopecia.[32] However, hot comb usage has never been confirmed as the cause of this condition. Sperling and associates[33] reported a series of black patients with this form of scarring alopecia and termed it *the follicular degeneration syndrome.* Others consider this form of scarring alopecia commonly seen in black patients to be a variant of pseudopelade of Brocq.[2, 34, 35]

Some authors believe that pseudopelade of Brocq is not a distinct clinicopathologic entity but only represents a form of end-stage alopecia caused by other scarring alopecias such as discoid lupus erythematosus, lichen planopilaris, and folliculitis decalvans.[36-38] However, as described earlier, there are patients who exhibit this par-

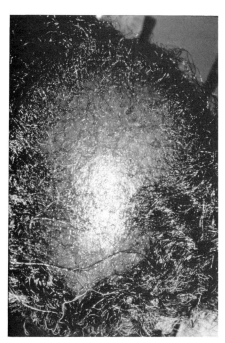

FIGURE 135-7. Pseudopelade of Brocq/follicular degeneration syndrome commonly seen in black females with prominent follicular dropout over the crown and vertex.

ticular pattern of alopecia without a history of preceding characteristics of those disorders. In addition, lesions of pseudopelade of Brocq may have relatively distinct histologic features.

Pathology. Early lesions are characterized by perifollicular and perivascular lymphocytic infiltrates of variable density *without* associated interface alteration. The lymphocytic inflammation is found primarily at the level of the follicular infundibulum but may occur at all levels of the follicle. Disruption of the usual follicular unit anatomy with a prominent decrease in follicular density is observed best in transverse sections obtained from well-developed lesions.[1] As the alopecia develops, the infundibular epithelium becomes atrophic and consists of only one- to two-cell layers. Often this epithelial atrophy results in an eccentric location of the follicular canal and fusion of multiple infundibula to form a common canal. In advanced lesions the follicular epithelium is entirely destroyed and only naked hair shafts surrounded by histiocytic and foreign body giant cell inflammation remain. Residual fibrous tracts of hair follicles (stele) located in the reticular dermis and within the superficial subcutis also mark the sites of the destroyed follicles.[39] Characteristic concentric lamellar fibroplasia is present in early lesions but is more prominent in well-established patches of alopecia. Often some degree of miniaturization of hair follicles is present and may represent the result of chronic follicular damage.

Immunohistologic findings have revealed only occasional, minimal IgM deposits at the level of the follicular infundibular basement membrane zone. No immunoreactants consistent with discoid lupus erythematosus or lichen planopilaris at the level of the follicular infundibulum or epidermis are seen.[31, 40]

Pathogenesis and Etiology. The etiology of pseudopelade of Brocq is unknown. Sperling and associates[33] have suggested that the pathogenesis may be related to premature inner root sheath desquamation leading to subsequent follicular infundibular epithelial atrophy, perifollicular fibroplasia, and eventual follicular dropout.

Diagnosis and Differential Diagnosis. As described earlier, some researchers prefer not to regard pseudopelade as an autonomous disease and instead recognize a "pseudopeladic state" resulting from discoid lupus erythematosus, lichen planopilaris, or folliculitis decalvans.[36, 37] End-stage, inactive lesions of these disorders may clinically resemble pseudopelade of Brocq. However, the combination of clinical and microscopic features of this form of scarring alopecia without preceding cutaneous lupus erythematosus, lichen planus, or folliculitis warrants the designation of a separate scarring alopecia termed *pseudopelade of Brocq.*

Treatment. Topical corticosteroid cream or solution may be used as a palliative treatment (Table 135–8). No effective therapy exists for pseudopelade of Brocq, and

TABLE 135-8. Treatment of Pseudopelade of Brocq
Palliative therapy only with midpotency topical corticosteroid cream or solution

irreversible scarring alopecia results. The progression of pseudopelade of Brocq is slow, and its course may be protracted. In one study, disease activity was noted to subside between 2 and 18 years after onset.[31]

Lichen Planopilaris (Follicular Lichen Planus)

Clinical Description. In 1895, Pringle first described the association of lichen planus and spinous follicular lesions as "lichen planopilaris."[41] In 1915, Graham-Little described a patient with a similar pattern of cicatricial alopecia and spinous follicular lesions at other body sites.[42] These two variants of lichen planopilaris may also be referred to as follicular lichen planus.

Lichen planopilaris is more common in women between 30 and 70 years of age. Early lesions consist of acuminate, spinous, and hyperkeratotic follicular papules with perifollicular erythema (Fig. 135–8). The hair follicles are subsequently destroyed, yielding atrophic, irregular, especially angular or polygonal shaped patches of alopecia with similar follicular papules at the periphery of the patch of alopecia. In addition, similar spinous follicular papules as well as more typical lichen planus lesions are frequently present elsewhere on the body, including mucous membranes and nails.

The clinical triad of classic plaque-type lichen planus, spinous or acuminate lesions, and alopecia of the scalp or other hairy areas has been described as the Graham-Little syndrome. Fifty to 70% of patients with lichen planopilaris have been reported to have lichen planus elsewhere on the body.[43, 44] The main symptom is pruritus. Acuminate lesions, the most consistent clinical feature, are dilated hair follicles filled with keratin plugs and perifollicular erythema occurring at any hair-bearing site, including the scalp, chest, back, axillae, and groin. The other manifestations may or may not be present. When scalp involvement occurs, initial perifollicular erythema is often followed by the follicular acuminate papules. The lesions progress to smooth patches of hair loss, and in the scalp, scarring alopecia is a common sequela. End-

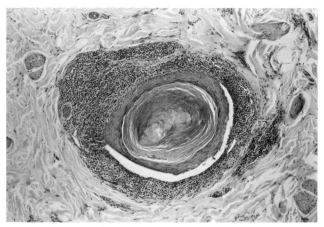

FIGURE 135–9. Lichen planopilaris with prominent lichenoid interface alteration surrounding a dilated follicular infundibulum (hematoxylin-eosin, original magnification ×200).

stage lesions frequently exhibit a permanent loss of pilosebaceous units and may clinically resemble pseudopelade of Brocq.

Pathology. Lichenoid interface alteration of the epidermis and follicular epithelium is characteristic of lichen planopilaris (Fig. 135–9). Lichenoid interface change can be defined as disruption of the epithelial-adventitial dermal junction with prominent dyskeratosis with individually necrotic, brightly eosinophilic, polygonal basal keratinocytes. A linear, variably dense lymphocytic infiltrate abuts the follicular infundibular epithelium. Dyskeratotic keratinocytes may be present within the follicular epithelium, epidermis, and perifollicular adventitial dermis as well. Focal areas of vacuolar interface alteration may be present in lichen planopilaris, but lichenoid dermatitis predominates. In many cases of lichen planopilaris, the interfollicular epidermis is uninvolved.[43] Perivascular and perieccrine lymphocytic infiltrates of the mid and deep reticular dermis that are typically seen in discoid lupus erythematosus are not present in lichen planopilaris.

Later lesions are characterized by perifollicular fibrosis, near-complete or complete absence of follicles with scattered "naked" hair shafts surrounded by foreign body histiocyte and giant cell inflammation. End-stage changes are identical to end-stage pseudopelade of Brocq and end-stage discoid lupus erythematosus.

In lichen planopilaris, globular IgM deposits are present on cytoid bodies at the dermoepidermal junction, papillary dermis, follicular infundibulum, and associated adventitial dermis. In addition, heavy deposits of fibrin are commonly seen within the papillary and adventitial dermis.[40, 45] A linear deposition of immunoglobulin restricted to the basement membrane of the hair follicle and sparing the overlying epidermis was observed in one study.[46]

Pathogenesis and Etiology. The pathogenesis of lichen planopilaris is unknown. Since lichen planopilaris is regarded as a follicular variant of lichen planus by most authors, the pathogenesis of lichen planopilaris is likely the same as that of lichen planus and is discussed in detail in Chapter 20.

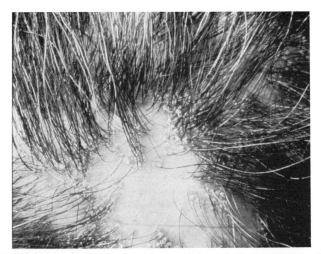

FIGURE 135–8. Lichen planopilaris with irregularly shaped areas of scarring alopecia, perifollicular erythema, scale, and some hyperkeratotic follicular acuminate papules.

Diagnosis and Differential Diagnosis. The combination of acuminate follicular papules in an area of alopecia and signs of lichen planus elsewhere on the body is virtually diagnostic of lichen planopilaris. Inactive, noninflammatory areas of alopecia without evidence of lichen planus elsewhere may mimic pseudopelade of Brocq. Chronic cutaneous lupus erythematosus is generally not confused with lichen planopilaris. Lesions of discoid lupus erythematosus frequently exhibit follicular plugging and follicular accentuation, but the interfollicular skin is more inflamed and sclerotic than in lichen planopilaris.

Treatment. The course of lichen planopilaris usually resembles that of typical lichen planus and can last several months to several years. If the perifollicular inflammatory reaction can be controlled early in the course of the disease, preservation of follicular units and regrowth may be possible. However, most patients suffer from cosmetically significant permanent alopecia.

Therapy (Table 135–9) is directed at controlling perifollicular inflammation and pruritus. High-potency topical corticosteroids and oral corticosteroids are the most effective therapies in lichen planopilaris. Oral corticosteroids (30 to 40 mg per day) with subsequent taper have been reported to be the most efficacious therapy for controlling pruritus and hair loss. However, relapse is common. Other oral medications that have been used for typical lichen planus may be tried (i.e., griseofulvin and hydroxychloroquine) but have not been very effective.[43]

Discoid Lupus Erythematosus

Clinical Description. Discoid lupus erythematosus is a common form of chronic cutaneous lupus erythematosus and is typically found in young to middle-aged adults with a 2:1 female to male predominance. Age at onset is usually between 20 and 60 years of age. Lesions are most commonly located on the face, scalp, and inner ear. Approximately 50% of patients have scalp lesions, and in 10% of patients, scalp involvement may be the sole manifestation of discoid lupus.[47] Patients with discoid lupus uncommonly progress to involvement with systemic lupus erythematosus.[48] Approximately 15% of patients with systemic lupus may exhibit discoid lesions at some point in their illness.[49]

Early lesions consist of small erythematous papules or irregular small, scaly plaques that expand to form round to irregular shaped atrophic, sclerotic plaques. Thick, adherent scale frequently develops that when removed reveals keratinous plugs on its undersurface. These follicular plugs are the mirror image of dilated follicular orifices. When active, the peripheral borders are erythema-

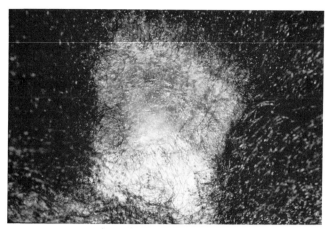

FIGURE 135–10. Discoid lupus erythematosus showing an inflammatory, sclerotic plaque of scarring alopecia with postinflammatory pigmentary alteration.

tous or violaceous and continue to enlarge to involve other areas of the scalp (Figs. 135–10 and 135–11). Active lesions are symptomatic and patients complain of lesional pruritus, burning, and pain. Multifocal involvement is also common. Postinflammatory pigmentary alteration, both hypopigmentation and hyperpigmentation, is frequently seen. Central atrophy and telangiectasia eventually becomes prominent. Advanced plaques are scarring both clinically and histologically.

Hypertrophic discoid lupus, a less common but very destructive variant of discoid lupus erythematosus, may occur on the scalp. The greatly elevated, verrucous, red-violet plaques with thick adherent scales result in tender inflammatory lesions, severe tissue destruction, and scarring alopecia. Hypertrophic discoid lupus lesions typically occur in patients with a long history of more typical

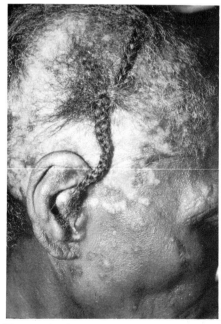

FIGURE 135–11. Discoid lupus erythematosus with more extensive scalp and facial involvement.

TABLE 135–9. Treatment of Lichen Planopilaris

1. Class I or II topical corticosteroid cream
2. Oral prednisone, 30–40 mg per day tapered over 6 to 12 weeks
3. See therapy options in Chapter 20.

discoid lupus but may present in the scalp as a sole cutaneous manifestation of systemic lupus erythematosus.[3]

Pathology. Vacuolar interface alteration of the epidermis and follicular epithelium is characteristic of discoid lupus. Dyskeratotic keratinocytes are often seen at the dermoepidermal junction and within the outer follicular epithelium, but the dyskeratosis is usually not as conspicuous as in lichen planopilaris. The epidermis ranges from atrophic to acanthotic (hypertrophic discoid lupus). Overlying orthokeratotic hyperkeratotic stratum corneum with focal parakeratosis is usually present. Laminated keratin fills and expands follicular ostia corresponding to the clinical follicular plugs.

Relatively dense lymphocytic infiltrates with occasional admixed plasma cells are present in both perivascular and periadnexal locations. The perifollicular infiltrates are most prominent at the level of the follicular infundibulum. Increased dermal mucin is commonly seen both superficially and deep and is best detected in colloidal iron– or alcian blue–stained sections. Reticular dermal sclerosis is present in advanced lesions.

Dense granular deposition of immunoglobulin (most commonly IgG, but IgM and IgA may also be seen) and complement at the dermoepidermal junction is seen in 75% to 90% of cases. Occasional IgM deposits on cytoid bodies within the epidermis and papillary dermis may also be seen.[40, 45, 50]

Pathogenesis and Etiology. Lupus erythematosus is considered to be an autoimmune disease, and the pathophysiology is discussed in detail in Chapter 24.

Diagnosis and Differential Diagnosis. The clinical diagnosis of discoid lupus involving the scalp is usually not difficult. The previously described clinical features and distribution of lupus lesions are usually quite characteristic. The presence of classic lesions at other sites (ears, face, neck, chest, and arms) can aid in the diagnosis. A routine skin biopsy for hematoxylin and eosin staining should be performed to confirm the clinical diagnosis. A lesional skin biopsy for immunofluorescence microscopy can be done but in most cases is usually not necessary. A clinical history and physical and laboratory examinations are indicated to rule out systemic involvement.

Psoriatic plaques of the scalp may be considered in the differential diagnosis, but lesions of psoriasis lack follicular plugging and have characteristic silvery micaceous scale. In addition, psoriatic involvement of other sites is usually present. Lichen planopilaris may present a diagnostic challenge both clinically and histologically. Distinguishing characteristics have been described earlier. End-stage "burned out" lesions of discoid lupus erythematosus, lichen planopilaris, and folliculitis decalvans may be clinically and histologically indistinguishable from pseudopelade of Brocq.

Treatment. Treatment of cutaneous lupus erythematosus including discoid lupus is discussed in detail in Chapter 24 (Table 135–10). Topical and intralesional corticosteroids are the mainstays of conservative local therapy in patients with relatively limited involvement. Intralesional injections of triamcinolone acetonide, 3 to 10 mg/mL, into active erythematous and violaceous lesions

TABLE 135–10. Treatment of Discoid Lupus Erythematosus

1. See Chapter 24 for full therapeutic options
2. Intralesional triamcinolone acetonide, 10–40 mg/mL
3. Class I or II topical corticosteroid cream or ointment
4. Antimalarial agents
5. Oral corticosteroids

are frequently quite effective for local control of discoid lupus lesions.

If extensive scalp or cutaneous involvement is present and is not responding to local therapy, consideration may be given to systemic therapy. Effective systemic medications include oral prednisone and the antimalarial drugs: chloroquine diphosphate (Aralen), hydroxychloroquine sulfate (Plaquenil), and quinacrine hydrochloride (Atabrine).[3] Patients on antimalarial therapy must be monitored for possible side effects. Ocular toxicity is the greatest concern, and regular ophthalmologic examinations are essential. Hematologic side effects are rare with antimalarial drugs but include leukopenia, thrombocytopenia, and agranulocytosis. Hemolysis in glucose-6-phosphatase dehydrogenase–deficient patients is a potentially serious problem. Therefore, measurement of glucose-6-phosphate dehydrogenase levels before initiation of antimalarial therapy is indicated.

Alopecia Mucinosa (Follicular Mucinosis)

Clinical Description. Pinkus[51] initially described alopecia mucinosa in 1957. This clinical syndrome of patches and plaques of alopecia occurs as a result of mucin deposition and subsequent degeneration of hair follicles. Alopecia mucinosa most commonly involves the face, scalp, and neck, but involvement of extremities may also occur. Clinically detectable alopecia is most often present in those lesions involving the scalp and face. Scalp lesions have variable morphology ranging from scaling erythematous infiltrated plaques and nodules to noninflammatory circular patches resembling alopecia areata (Fig. 135–12).[52] Age at onset ranges from 2 to 80 years. Alopecia mucinosa usually does not result in permanent alopecia unless mucin deposition completely destroys the follicular epithelium. Follicular mucinosis is considered to be a synonym by some authors but more correctly describes the microscopic finding of follicular mucin deposition with or without clinical alopecia.[53]

Two clinically distinct groups of alopecia mucinosa (follicular mucinosis) exist: lymphoma associated and non–lymphoma associated. Mycosis fungoides is the most common lymphoproliferative disorder associated with alopecia mucinosa and follicular mucinosis and usually occurs in patients 30 years of age and older. The reported incidence of lymphoma in alopecia mucinosa (follicular mucinosis) ranges from 9.4% to 60%, with a recent study citing an incidence of approximately 30%.[52, 54] The lymphoma is diagnosed before or at the time of diagnosis of alopecia mucinosa (follicular mucin-

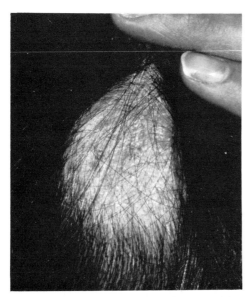

FIGURE 135–12. Alopecia mucinosa showing a circumscribed, scaling, slightly infiltrated plaque of alopecia. (Courtesy of S. Wright Caughman, M.D.)

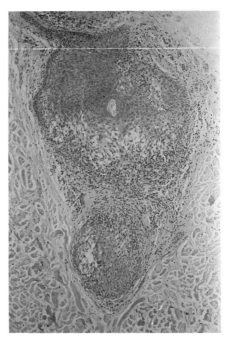

FIGURE 135–13. Alopecia mucinosa showing mucin within follicular epithelium and perifollicular lymphocytic infiltrates (hematoxylin-eosin, original magnification ×100). (From Templeton SF, Solomon AR. Scarring alopecia: A classification based on microscopic criteria. J Cutan Pathol 1994;21:97–109. © 1994, Munksgaard International Publishers Ltd., Copenhagan, Denmark.)

osis) in only a minority of cases. Since no reproducible histologic criteria can predict the development of future lymphoma, close follow-up of patients with repeat biopsy studies when clinically indicated is essential.

The non–lymphoma-associated alopecia mucinosa (follicular mucinosis) frequently occurs in children and young adults and is usually self-limiting without resultant permanent alopecia. However, occasionally permanent patches of alopecia may result from mucinous degeneration of follicles. In addition, Hodgkin's lymphoma may rarely occur in association with childhood alopecia mucinosa (follicular mucinosis).[52, 55–57]

Pathology. The earliest findings are mucin deposition within the outer root sheath (Fig. 135–13). The keratinocytes of the outer root sheath are splayed apart by the mucin and may appear stellate. Mucin is usually detected in routine hematoxylin and eosin–stained sections but is best appreciated with stains such as colloidal iron and consists primarily of hyaluronic acid.[58] In more advanced lesions the entire follicular epithelium may be altered with large mucin-filled intrafollicular cystic spaces. Variably dense perivascular and perifollicular lymphocytic infiltrates with occasional admixed eosinophils are present in most cases. Some degree of folliculotropism of lymphocytes may be seen in follicular mucinosis both with and without associated lymphoma. Although no single histologic criterion has been shown to predict the future development of lymphoma with statistical significance, the presence of a band-like, atypical lymphocytic infiltrate near the dermoepidermal junction with significant epidermotropism is more commonly seen in lymphoma-associated follicular mucinosis.[52, 55]

Pathogenesis and Etiology. The pathogenesis of follicular mucin deposition is unknown. See Chapter 158 for full discussion of mycosis fungoides.

Diagnosis and Differential Diagnosis. Infiltrative erythematous plaques with associated alopecia are clinically suggestive of alopecia mucinosis (follicular mucinosis). Microscopic examination and close clinical follow-up are essential given the potential association with cutaneous lymphoma.

Treatment. Non–lymphoma-associated alopecia mucinosis (follicular mucinosis) usually resolves spontaneously. In children and young adults, permanent scarring alopecia is uncommon. Topical and intralesional corticosteroids may be of some therapeutic benefit (Table 135–11). The treatment of lymphoma-associated alopecia mucinosis (follicular mucinosis) is that of the underlying cutaneous T-cell lymphoma in general and is discussed in Chapter 158.

VESICULOBULLOUS DISEASE CAUSING ALOPECIA

Cicatricial pemphigoid and certain forms of epidermolysis bullosa may cause a primary permanent scarring alopecia. Other bullous diseases, unless complicated by extensive secondary impetiginization, do not typically result in a scarring alopecia.

TABLE 135–11. Treatment of Alopecia Mucinosa

1. Non–lymphoma-associated alopecia mucinosa is usually self-limiting.
2. Topical and intralesional corticosteroids may be of some benefit.
3. See Chapter 158 for therapeutic options of lymphoma-associated alopecia mucinosa.

Cicatricial Pemphigoid

Clinical Description. Cicatricial pemphigoid is a rare chronic scarring immunobullous disease characterized by recurrent blisters primarily involving mucosal surfaces. The conjunctiva and oral mucosa are most commonly involved.[59] Blisters occur on the skin in 10% to 30% of cases and are most commonly located on the scalp and face.[60] Brunsting and Perry[61] described a form of cicatricial pemphigoid that spared mucous membranes and involved only skin. In both mucosal and nonmucosal variants of cicatricial pemphigoid, recurrent blisters of the scalp may eventuate in scarring alopecia.

Pathology. The histologic hallmark of pemphigoid, both bullous pemphigoid and cicatricial pemphigoid, is an inflammatory subepidermal vesicle with numerous eosinophils within the vesicle cavity and superficial dermal infiltrate. The subepidermal vesicle may extend down follicular infundibula. Involvement of the follicular infundibulum by this inflammatory vesicular process may result in follicular destruction and perifollicular fibrosis.

Linear immunoglobulin deposits, most commonly IgG, and complement are usually present at the dermoepidermal junction in perilesional skin.[62]

Pathogenesis. Cicatricial pemphigoid is considered an autoimmune primary immunobullous disease. See Chapter 76 for discussion of pathogenesis.

Diagnosis and Differential Diagnosis. Routine and immunofluorescence microscopy coupled with indirect immunofluorescence microscopy of serum on normal salt-split skin aids in laboratory diagnosis of cicatricial pemphigoid and exclusion of other primary immunobullous diseases. Other blistering diseases that may be considered are pemphigus vulgaris that often involves the scalp but does not typically result in permanent scarring alopecia, bullous pemphigoid, and epidermolysis bullosa acquisita, which are more easily distinguished clinically.

Treatment. Immunosuppressive therapy primarily with systemic corticosteroids is the treatment of choice. Other steroid-sparing immunosuppressive agents may be used. See Chapter 76 for a full discussion of therapy for this disorder.

Epidermolysis Bullosa

Clinical Description. Epidermolysis bullosa is a mechanicobullous disease. Numerous subtypes exist that are based on clinical, pathologic, ultrastructural, and immunopathologic criteria. Patients with the more severe subtypes such as junctional epidermolysis bullosa, dominant dystrophic epidermolysis bullosa, or recessive dystrophic epidermolysis bullosa may develop a scarring alopecia.

Pathology. Early lesions of epidermolysis bullosa consist of noninflammatory or pauci-inflammatory subepidermal vesicles. As in cicatricial pemphigoid, the subepidermal clefting may extend down follicular epithelium, resulting in separation of the epithelium from the adventitial dermis. The amount of clefting and the depth of extension down the follicle may be extensive in epidermolysis bullosa. The chronic vesicular process leads to follicular dropout and superficial and perifollicular fibrosis.[2]

Pathogenesis, Diagnosis and Differential Diagnosis, and Treatment. See Chapter 78.

Secondary Scarring Alopecias

The hair loss of secondary scarring alopecias occurs as a result of nonfolliculocentric skin disease, genetic defect, or external injury (Table 135–12). Follicular destruction is only incidental in secondary scarring alopecias.[1] The clinical and histologic features of secondary scarring alopecias are typical for the specific disease involved. Nonfolliculocentric sclerosing diseases (e.g., linear morphea) and infections (e.g., herpes zoster) may cause secondary scarring alopecia. Sarcoidosis, with extensive non–follicular-associated granulomas, may cause secondary scarring alopecia. Benign and malignant neoplasms, both primary and metastatic, may involve the scalp and cause clinical alopecia. External injury in the form of mechanical trauma, thermal injury, radiation (Fig. 135–14), and chemical damage may cause secondary scarring alopecia.

TABLE 135–12. Secondary Scarring Alopecia

I. Sclerosing Disorders
   A. Morphea
   B. Sclerodermoid porphyria cutanea tarda
   C. Lichen sclerosus et atrophicus
   D. Parry-Romberg syndrome
II. Physical and Chemical Agents
   A. Mechanical trauma, laceration
   B. Thermal burns
   C. Chemical burns
   D. Radiation dermatitis
III. Dermal Infiltrative Processes
   A. Tumors
      1. Basal cell carcinoma
      2. Squamous cell carcinoma
      3. Metastatic carcinoma
      4. Lymphoma
      5. Adnexal tumors
      6. Dermatofibrosarcoma protuberans
      7. Others
   B. Granulomatous
      1. Sarcoidosis
      2. Necrobiosis lipoidica
      3. Actinic granuloma
      4. Infections
         a. Syphilis (tertiary)
         b. Tuberculosis
         c. Viral
         d. Protozoal
         e. Other
   C. Amyloidosis

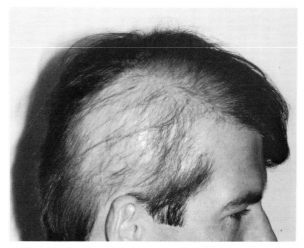

FIGURE 135–14. Secondary scarring alopecia due to orthovoltage radiation. (Courtesy of S. Wright Caughman, M.D.)

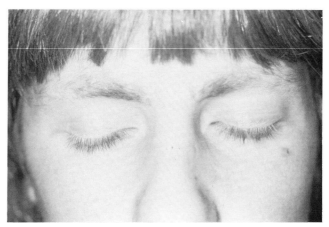

FIGURE 135–15. Keratosis pilaris atrophicans with hair loss in the lateral portion of both eyebrows. (Courtesy of S. Wright Caughman, M.D.)

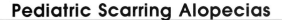

Pediatric Scarring Alopecias

Many of the previously described alopecias, both primary and secondary, begin in childhood. In addition, there are several scarring alopecias that almost always present in childhood. Many of these latter pediatric scarring alopecias are thought to be due to genetic defects. Some of the pediatric scarring alopecias affect only the integumentary system while others have multiorgan system involvement, but variable degrees of permanent scarring alopecia may be seen in association with certain hereditary disorders and developmental defects. The etiology of most pediatric scarring alopecias is unknown, but both primary and secondary types of scarring alopecia exist.

SCARRING FOLLICULAR KERATOSIS

Clinical Description. Several hereditary syndromes involving follicular dilatation, hyperkeratosis, and ultimate follicular destruction associated with keratosis pilaris have been described. The three major variants of the scarring follicular keratosis are keratosis pilaris decalvans (keratosis pilaris spinulosa decalvans), keratosis pilaris atrophicans (ulerythema ophryogenes), and atrophoderma vermiculata (acne vermiculata, folliculitis ulerythematosa reticulata).

Scarring alopecia of the scalp is generally seen only in keratosis pilaris decalvans. In this entity, lesions of keratosis pilaris begin in childhood. Similar dilated hair follicles with hyperkeratosis and focal surrounding erythema occur throughout the scalp and lead to scarring alopecia. Facial involvement with keratosis pilaris–like lesions also frequently occurs. Palmar and plantar hyperkeratosis, photophobia, keratoconjunctivitis, cataracts, and other corneal abnormalities may also be associated with keratosis pilaris decalvans.[22, 63, 64]

Keratosis pilaris atrophicans begins in childhood with keratosis pilaris–like lesions of the lateral portion of the eyebrow (Fig. 135–15). Follicular destruction with permanent loss of the lateral eyebrows occurs. Similar lesions may also be present to a variable degree on the cheeks. Scarring alopecia of the scalp does not usually occur.

Atrophoderma vermiculata consists of follicular plugging of the cheeks and preauricular area with subsequent follicular destruction and resultant reticulate atrophy. The scalp is generally not involved.

Pathology. The microscopic findings are not specific. Common features to all of the follicular scarring keratoses include follicular infundibular dilatation and follicular plugging with hyperkeratosis. Inflammatory infiltrates are perifollicular and perivascular and usually consist primarily of lymphocytes. Admixed neutrophils may be present. Over time, there is fibrosis of the perifollicular adventitial dermis and sclerosis of underlying fibrous tracts.

Pathogenesis and Etiology. The cause of the follicular scarring keratosis is unknown.

Diagnosis and Differential Diagnosis. The clinical features are usually diagnostic. The alopecia in keratosis pilaris decalvans may resemble pseudopelade; however, the presence of lesions of keratosis pilaris on the scalp and elsewhere as described earlier aids in the diagnosis. Spinous follicular papules of keratosis pilaris decalvans may be reminiscent of those seen in lichen planopilaris. However, in keratosis pilaris decalvans, no typical lesions of lichen planus are present, and the histology of the spinous follicular lesions is not characterized by lichenoid interface dermatitis as seen in lichen planopilaris.

TABLE 135–13. Treatment of Scarring Follicular Keratosis

1. No effective therapy
2. Palliative therapy
   a. Midpotency topical steroid cream or solution
   b. Tretinoin cream
   c. Systemic retinoids

TABLE 135-14. Pediatric Scarring Alopecias

Presumed Primary Scarring Alopecias

Scarring follicular keratosis
Generalized follicular hamartoma
Marie-Unna hypotrichosis
Hallerman-Streiff syndrome
Ectodermal dysplasia

Presumed Secondary Scarring Alopecias

Aplasia cutis congenita
Incontinentia pigmenti
Polyostotic fibrous dysplasia
Conradi's syndrome
Icthyosis
Epidermal nevus
Nevus sebaceous

Treatment. There is no effective therapy (Table 135-13).

OTHER PEDIATRIC SCARRING ALOPECIAS

Most other pediatric scarring alopecias are rare to uncommon. They are listed in Table 135-14.

References

1. Solomon AR. The transversely sectioned scalp biopsy specimen: The technique and an algorithm for its use in the diagnosis of alopecia. Adv Dermatol 1994;9:127-158.
2. Templeton SF, Solomon AR. Scarring alopecia: A classification based on microscopic criteria. J Cutan Pathol 1994;21:97.
3. Newton RC, Hebert AA, Freese TW, et al. Scarring alopecia. Dermatol Clin 1987;5:603-618.
4. Hoffman E. Perifolliculitis capitis abscedens et suffodiens: Case presentation. Derm Ztschr 1908;15:122.
5. Wise F, Parkhurst HJ. A rare form of suppurating and cicatrizing disease of the scalp. Arch Dermatol Syph 1921;4:750.
6. C.-W.Yu C, Cook MG. Hidradenitis suppurativa: A disease of follicular epithelium, rather than apocrine glands. Br J Dermatol 1990;122:763.
7. Padilha-Goncalves A. Inflammatory tinea capitis (kerion) mimicking dissecting cellulitis (letter). Int J Dermatol 1992;31:66.
8. Curry SS, Gaither DH, King LE. Squamous cell carcinoma arising in dissecting perifolliculitis of the scalp. J Am Acad Dermatol 1981;4:673-678.
9. Adrian RM, Arndt KA. Perifolliculitis capitis: Successful control with alternate-day corticosteroids. Ann Plast Surg 1980;4:166-169.
10. Bjellerup M, Wallengren J. Familial perifolliculitis capitis abscedens et suffodiens in two brothers successfully treated with isotretinoin. J Am Acad Dermatol 1990;23:752-753.
11. Schewach-Millet M, Ziv R, Shapira D. Perifolliculitis capitis abscedens et suffodiens treated with isotretinoin (13-*cis*-retinoic acid). J Am Acad Dermatol 1986;6:1291-1292.
12. Shelley WB, Shelley ED. Perifolliculitis capitis. In: Advanced Dermatologic Therapy. Philadelphia: WB Saunders Co., 1987:368-369.
13. Bern B, Venge P, Ohman S. Perifolliculitis capitis abscedens et suffodiens (Hoffman): Complete healing associated with oral zinc therapy. Arch Dermatol 1985;121:1028-1030.
14. Moschella SL, Klein MH, Miller RJ. Perifolliculitis capitis abscedens et suffodiens: Report of a successful therapeutic scalping. Arch Dermatol 1967;96:195-197.
15. Glass LF, German B, Laub D. Treatment of perifolliculitis capitis abscedens et suffodiens with the carbon dioxide laser. J Dermatol Surg Oncol 1989;15:673-676.
16. Kaposi M. Ueber die sogennante framboesia und mehrere andere Arten von papillaren Neubildungen der Haut. Arch Dermatol Syph 1869;1:382.
17. Cosman B, Wolff M. Acne keloidalis. Plast Reconstr Surg 1972;50:25.
18. Dinehart SM, Herzberg AJ, Pollack SV, et al. Acne keloidalis: A review. J Dermatol Surg Oncol 1989;15:642.
19. Herzberg AJ, Dinehart SM, Pollack SV, et al. Acne keloidalis: Transverse microscopy, immunohistochemistry, and electron microscopy. Am J Dermatopathol 1990;12:109.
20. Harris H. Acne keloidalis aggravated by football helmets. Cutis 1992;50:154.
21. Quinquaud E. Folliculite épilante et destructive des régions velues. Bull Mem Soc Hop Paris 1888;5:395.
22. Rook A, Dawber R. Cicatricial alopecia. In: Rook A, Dawber R, eds. Diseases of the Hair and Scalp. Oxford: Blackwell Scientific Publications, 1982:307-341.
23. Miller RF. Epilating folliculitis of the glabrous skin. Arch Dermatol 1961;83:777.
24. Bogg A. Folliculitis decalvans. Acta Derm Venereol 1963;43:14.
25. Pye RJ, Peachey RDG, Burton JL. Erosive pustular dermatosis of the scalp. Br J Dermatol 1979;100:559-566.
26. Caputo R, Veraldi S. Erosive pustular dermatosis of the scalp. J Am Acad Dermatol 1993;28:96-98.
27. Ikeda M, Arata J, Isaka H. Erosive pustular dermatosis of the scalp successfully treated with oral zinc sulphate. Br J Dermatol 1982;106:742-743.
28. Moisson YF, Janier M, Le Bozec P, et al. Pustulose érosive du cuir chevelu. Ann Dermatol Venereol 1991;118:899-901.
29. Daaman T, Torssander J. Dermatophytid—a mistaken diagnosed entity? Acta Derm Venereol 1983;63:404.
30. Dvoretzky I, Fisher BK, Movshovitz M, et al. Favus. Int J Dermatol 1980;19:89.
31. Braun-Falco O, Imai S, Schmoeckel C, et al. Pseudopelade of Brocq. Dermatologica 1986;172:18-23.
32. LoPresti P, Papa CM, Kligman AM. Hot comb alopecia. Arch Dermatol 1968;98:234-238.
33. Sperling LC, Sau P. The follicular degeneration syndrome in black patients: "Hot comb alopecia" revisited and revised. Arch Dermatol 1992;128:68-74.
34. Price VH. Hair loss in cutaneous disease. In: Baden HP, ed. Symposium on Alopecia. New York: HP Publishing, 1987;6:3-11.
35. Whiting DA. Current Concepts: The Diagnosis of Alopecia. Kalamazoo, MI: Upjohn, 1990:24.
36. Degos R, Rabut R, Duperrat B, et al. L'état pseudopéladique. Ann Dermatol Syph 1954;81:5.
37. Prieto JG. Pseudopelade of Brocq: Its relationship to some forms of cicatricial alopecias and to lichen planus. J Invest Dermatol 1955;24:323.
38. Anderton RL, Cullen SI. Pseudopelade of Brocq secondary to lichen planus. Cutis 1976;17:916.
39. Headington JT. Transverse microscopic anatomy of the human scalp: A basis for a morphometric approach to disorders of the hair follicle. Arch Dermatol 1984;120:449.
40. Abell E. Immunofluorescent staining technics in the diagnosis of alopecia. South Med J 1977;70:1407.
41. Pringle JJ: Cited in Adamson HG. Lichen pilaris seu spinulosus. Br J Dermatol 1905;17:77.
42. Little EG. Folliculitis decalvans et atrophicans: Report of a case. Br J Dermatol 1915;27:183-185.
43. Mehregan DA, Van Hale HM, Muller SA. Lichen planopilaris: Clinical and pathologic study of forty-five patients. J Am Acad Dermatol 1992;27:935-942.
44. Braun-Falco O, Bergner T, Heilgemeir GP. Pseudopelade Brocq-Krankheitsbild oder Krankheitsentitat. Hautarzt 1989;40:77-83.
45. Jordon RE. Subtle clues to diagnosis by immunopathology: Scarring alopecia. Am J Dermatopathol 1980;2:157.
46. Ioannides D, Bystryn JC. Immunofluorescence abnormalities in lichen planopilaris. Arch Dermatol 1992;128:214-216.
47. Callen JP. Chronic cutaneous lupus erythematosus. Arch Dermatol 1982;118:412.

48. Callen JP. Chronic cutaneous lupus erythematosus. Arch Dermatol 1982;118:412.
49. Estes D, Christian CL. The natural history of systemic lupus erythematosus by prospective analysis. Medicine 1971;50:85–95.
50. Tuffanelli DL. Lupus erythematosus. J Am Acad Dermatol 1981;4:137–142.
51. Pinkus H. Alopecia mucinosa: Inflammatory plaques with alopecia characterized by root-sheath mucinosis. Arch Dermatol 1957;76:419.
52. Gibson LE, Muller SA, Leiferman KM, et al. Follicular mucinosis: Clinical and histopathologic study. J Am Acad Dermatol 1989;20:441.
53. Hempstead RW, Ackerman AB. Follicular mucinosis: A reaction pattern in follicular epithelium. Am J Dermatopathol 1985;7:245.
54. Mehregan DA, Gibson LE, Muller SA. Follicular mucinosis: Histopathologic review of 33 cases. Mayo Clin Proc 1991;66:387.
55. Logan RA, Headington JT. Follicular mucinosis: A histologic review of 80 cases (abstract). J Cutan Pathol 1988;15:324.
56. Gibson LE, Muller SA, Peters MS. Follicular mucinosis of childhood and adolescence. Pediatr Dermatol 1988;5:231.
57. Raab B, Soltani K, Medenica M. Follicular mucinosis in childhood. Cutis 1982;2:201.
58. Ishibashi A. Histogenesis of mucin in follicular mucinosis: An electron microscopic study. Acta Derm Venereol 1976;56:163–171.
59. Hardy KM et al. Benign mucous membrane pemphigoid. Arch Dermatol 1971;104:467.
60. Lever WF. Pemphigus and Bullous Pemphigoid. Springfield, IL: Charles C Thomas, 1965:103.
61. Brunsting LA, Perry HO. Benign pemphigoid? A report of seven cases with chronic, scarring, herpetiform plaques about the head and neck. Arch Dermatol 1957;75:489.
62. Rogers RS III, et al. Immunopathology of cicatricial pemphigoid: Studies of complement deposition. J Invest Dermatol 1977;68:39.
63. Rand R, Baden HP. Keratosis follicularis spinulosa decalvans: Report of two cases and literature review. Arch Dermatol 1983;119:22–26.
64. Eramo LR, Esterly NB, Zieserl EJ, et al. Icthyosis follicularis with alopecia and photophobia. Arch Dermatol 1985;121:1167–1174.

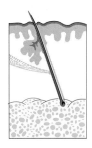

chapter 136

Biology and Disorders of Nails

PAUL KECHIJIAN and STUART SALASCHE

THE NAIL UNIT

Abnormalities of the nail unit are common and can be due to a large number of local and systemic disorders.[1-7] Phylogenetically related to claws in lower animals, human nails are ornamental yet can act as offensive and defensive weapons, enhance fingertip sensitivity, protect the fingertip from injury, and, most importantly, provide counterpressure, a function that facilitates fine tactile movements such as buttoning and picking up tiny objects. This last function is impossible without the nail.

Formation and Growth

The nail plate is largely formed by the germinative nail matrix. Matrix cells lose their nuclei, cornify, flatten, and migrate distally to generate the nail plate. The proximal nail matrix forms the dorsal nail plate; the distal matrix forms the ventral portion. A lesser contribution is made by the nail bed epithelium (Fig. 136–1).

Fingernails continuously grow on average 0.1 mm per day (3 mm per month). Knowledge of growth rate is often helpful in establishing disease onset and in predicting resolution time (see Beau's lines later). Nails grow faster during the day, in the summer, on the dominant hand, and on longer fingers. Although pregnancy and hyperthyroidism increase growth rate, serious systemic illness and hypothyroidism slow growth rate. Minor trauma such as nail biting stimulates nail growth; immobilization, malnutrition, and fever inhibit growth. The nails of men and younger individuals grow faster than those of women and older individuals. Fingernails grow twice to three times as quickly as toenails. In one study, biotin in a dose of 2.5 mg per day was reported to speed nail plate formation.[8] Supporting data are limited.

The hard keratin of the nail lies perpendicular to the nail's growth axis and parallel to the surface of the nail plate. The nail combines a high tensile strength with a low lipid content; the latter makes it more permeable than the stratum corneum to water. When hydrated, nail plates are softer, less brittle, and easier to clip and file.

Nail Unit Anatomy (Fig. 136–2)

The *nail plate* is a translucent rectangular structure that extends past the free edge of the digit. It adheres tightly to the nail bed and proximal nail fold. The richly vascularized *nail bed* lies under the nail plate. It is bordered proximally by the lunula, laterally by the *lateral nail folds*, and distally by the hyponychium. Elongated longitudinal epidermal ridges in the nail bed interdigitate with the ventral surface of the overlying nail plate and hold the nail plate firmly in place. The arrangement of these longitudinal ridges accounts for the linearity of splinter hemorrhages by providing grooves in which small amounts of extravasated blood collect. The opaque, white *lunula* comprises the most distal and visible portion of the boomerang-shaped germinative *matrix*. Melanocytes are most abundant in the distal matrix and absent from the nail bed. The *proximal nail fold* overlies the matrix (except for the lunula) and is continuous with the lateral fold. The *cuticle* originates at the distal margin of the proximal nail fold and extends to the lateral nail folds that border both sides of the nail plate. The cuticle adheres to the surface of the nail plate and prevents foreign material from entering the cleft between the nail plate and proximal nail fold. Removing or altering the cuticle is a common cause of paronychias. Normally seen only in nail biters, the *hyponychium* constitutes the most distal portion of the nail unit. Unlike the nail bed, the hyponychium is covered by epidermis. It

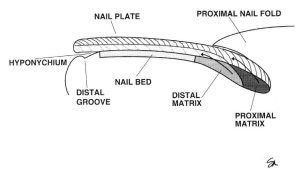

FIGURE 136–1. Representation of nail unit. The ventral nail plate is formed by the distal matrix. The dorsal nail plate is formed by the proximal matrix.

begins at the nail bed and ends at the *distal groove*, the most distal component of the nail unit.

Blood Supply

Dorsal and ventral digital arteries run parallel to the ulnar and radial sides of the phalanges and supply blood to the finger and nail unit. The dorsal arteries terminate near the distal interphalangeal joint; the ventral arteries extend beyond this joint distally and dorsally to supply blood to the fingertip and nail unit. Numerous anastomoses ensure an adequate blood supply. With sufficient magnification (e.g., by using an ophthalmoscope), the clinician can visualize capillary loops in the proximal nail fold; alterations in these loops are useful in the diagnosis of systemic disorders. The nail bed is richly supplied with arteriovenous anastomoses regulated by glomus bodies. These tiny organs help preserve an adequate blood supply when the digits are exposed to cold; glomus bodies occasionally produce benign tumors.

Innervation

The nail unit and finger have a rich nerve supply that is crucial to the finger's tactile sensitivity. The ulnar, radial, and median nerves innervate the hand; the fourth

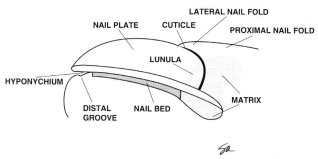

FIGURE 136–2. Median sagittal section through the nail unit. Important components of the nail unit are represented. Note in particular the boomerang-shaped matrix that generates the nail plate. Its most anterior portion may be visible as the lunula.

and fifth lumbar, and first sacral nerves innervate the foot. The nail unit is supplied by dorsal and ventral nerves that accompany the dorsal and ventral digital arteries. Analogous to blood vessels, tiny branches from the ventral nerves innervate the dorsal and ventral regions of the second, third, and fourth fingers. In contrast to finger vasculature, the dorsal nerves in the first and fifth digits extend distally and innervate the dorsal distal finger and nail unit, rather than stopping at the distal interphalangeal joint (R. Baran, personal communication, January 1993).

CLINICAL DESCRIPTION

Clinical changes in the nail unit result from alterations in blood supply and connective tissue, hemorrhage, inflammation, infection, epidermal proliferation, scarring, and tumor formation. Systemic diseases as well as localized dermatologic disorders produce changes that may arise in more than one area of the nail unit simultaneously. Recognizing the etiology of these clinical changes facilitates diagnosis and treatment.

When a patient presents with a nail disorder, the relevant history includes (1) onset, duration, and pattern of nail involvement; (2) previous nail, skin, and/or hair problems; (3) response to past treatments; (4) family history of skin, hair, or nail disorders; (5) the patient's drug history; (6) history of past and present medical conditions; (7) careful system review; and (8) the patient's occupation, hobbies, grooming habits, topical exposures, and habit tics.

Examination is performed with nonglaring light using a suitable magnifying lens. The nail may be viewed from above, from the side (to pick up subtle alterations in the surface of the nail plate), and/or from below by shining a penlight dorsally through the distal finger. All fingernails and toenails should be examined. The skin, scalp, hair, and oral cavity are also included in a complete examination.

Because onychomycosis is common, a potassium hydroxide (KOH) preparation is often the most useful test that is performed in patients with nail disorders. Pathogenic fungi are best detected in the most proximal portion of the affected nail bed—not at the distal end of the nail plate or bed. Accordingly, optimal test results are obtained by removing the entire affected nail plate; double-action nail clippers (Figs. 136–3 and 136–4) facilitate relatively painless and complete nail plate removal. Once exposed, the most proximal portion of involved nail bed is scraped with a No. 15 scalpel blade or curette. "Fresh" material obtained for microscopic examination is prepared with 1 or 2 drops of KOH mixed with dimethylsulfoxide (60 mL of 20% KOH mixed with 40 mL technical-grade dimethylsulfoxide)[1] to "clear" epidermal cells and make hyphae more visible. Scrapings may be cultured on (1) Sabouraud's medium containing no antimicrobial agents; (2) Mycosel, a selective medium that contains chloramphenicol and cyclohexamide; and/or (3) dermatophyte test medium (DTM), a selective medium that contains a color indicator to facilitate identification of pathogenic dermatophytes.

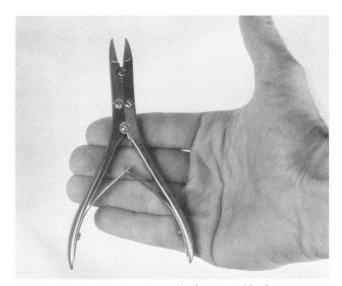

FIGURE 136–3. Double-action nail clippers enable the operator to apply considerable force to clip thick nails.

When a dystrophy is severe and bony involvement is likely or a fracture or osteomyelitis is suspected, radiographs should be obtained.

DIAGNOSIS AND TREATMENT (Tables 136–1 and 136–2)

Nail Bed and Hyponychial Disorders

Often, nail bed and hyponychial disorders appear as changes in nail color. The "shape" of the dyschromia is helpful in determining whether the color change is systemic or external. If the color change is convex distally (parallel to the lunula), the dyschromia originates in the nail unit. If the color change is convex proximally (parallel to the cuticle and proximal nail fold), the dyschromia originates externally.

Anemic pallor is visible as a paleness of the normally pink nail bed; it may be accompanied by onycholysis or koilonychia in cases of iron deficiency anemia. *Cyanosis*

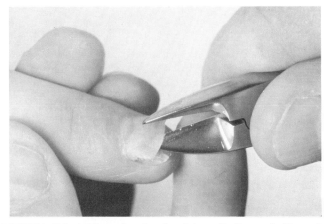

FIGURE 136–4. The pointed ends of the nail clippers facilitate the ability to work painlessly in difficult to reach areas.

is visible as a bluish color of the nail bed and reflects disorders of the cardiopulmonary system.

"Salmon patch" macule, seen in psoriasis, appears as erythema of the nail bed or as punctuate erythematous dots in the lunula. Erythematous dots within the lunula also occur in alopecia areata and are seen more frequently in this disorder. The erythema results from vasodilation of capillaries in the nail bed and lunula. In psoriasis, this sign is often accompanied by the *"oil drop" sign*, visible through the nail plate as a yellow "oil drop" on the nail bed surface. Focal parakeratosis, neutrophil migration, and serous exudate produce these changes, which are analogous to those that arise in psoriatic skin. *Microabscess formation*, which represents a yet more advanced exudative process, appears as a greenish-white dot under the nail plate and is characterized by a preponderance of neutrophils; it is seen in psoriasis and Reiter's syndrome. Since these alterations occur in the nail bed and lie under the nail plate, they do not respond favorably to local therapy.

Onycholysis (Fig. 136–5) is a common disorder characterized by the formation of a distal or lateral cleft between the nail plate and bed.[9] The affected plate usually appears white but may appear yellow, brown, or green, depending on the degree of subungual hyperkeratosis, inflammation, and secondary bacterial or yeast proliferation. Onycholysis may be congenital or "idiopathic." Usually, the etiology can be established.

Onycholysis is often caused by overhydration (e.g., in bartenders, cooks, and homemakers whose hands are immersed in water throughout the day). Nail enamel use, particularly in women with long or acrylic nails, is another frequent cause of onycholysis. Nail enamel and acrylics are occlusive and prevent evaporation of water through the nail plate. Moisture that remains trapped under the nail encourages overgrowth of yeast and bacteria that in many persons eventuates in chronic infection. Long nails further enhance the likelihood of onycholysis; longer nails are more subject to trauma and separation from the underlying bed. Acrylics applied to the nail plate as wraps or as artificial nails may cause allergic contact dermatitis–induced onycholysis; acrylics have also been reported to cause long lasting pain and even permanent absence of nails long after their use is discontinued.[10, 11]

In addition, onycholysis occurs in dermatophyte infections, as a result of drug ingestion (both phototoxic and nonphototoxic), and in a number of dermatologic disorders including eczema, hyperhidrosis, lichen planus, and pachyonychia congenita. Psoriasis is the most common "dermatologic" cause of onycholysis and often occurs in the absence of other signs of psoriasis (Fig. 136–6). Nail biopsy may be helpful in distinguishing onychomycotic from psoriatic onycholysis. Since the histology of the two disorders is nearly identical, the absence of hyphae is more compatible with the diagnosis of psoriasis. The presence of hyphae, however, does not necessarily rule out psoriasis since fungi can superinfect psoriatic nails. Onycholysis is unlikely to occur as an isolated finding in skin disorders other than psoriasis. Systemic diseases or conditions that cause onycholysis include diabetes mellitus, porphyria, pellagra, pregnancy, thyroid

TABLE 136-1. Differential Diagnosis of Nail Disorders

Nail Bed and Hyponychium

Onycholysis
  Overhydration
  Nail enamel, acrylics, long fingernails
  Onychomycosis
  Drug reactions
  Psoriasis, eczema, lichen planus
  Allergic contact dermatitis
  Systemic disorders and states: diabetes mellitus, porphyria, pellagra, pregnancy, thyroid disease
  Single digit, squamous cell carcinoma in situ
Splinter hemorrhage and subungual hematoma
  Single digit
    Trauma
    Several digits
    Systemic disorders: subacute bacterial endocarditis, collagen vascular disease, scurvy, blood dyscrasias
    Dermatologic disorders: eczema, psoriasis, exfoliative dermatitis, cutaneous T-cell lymphoma, Darier-White disease
Subungual hyperkeratosis
  Psoriasis
  Onychomycosis
  Darier-White disease
  Lichen planus
  Norwegian scabies
  Pityriasis rubra pilaris
  Reiter's syndrome
Ventral pterygium
  Raynaud's disease
  Progressive systemic sclerosis
  Trauma
  Familial and idiopathic
Nail dyschromias
  White or red longitudinal streaks: Darier-White disease, squamous cell carcinoma in situ
  Proximal nail bed white, absent lunula: Terry's nail—cirrhosis, chronic congestive heart failure, diabetes mellitus, normal in elderly
  Double white translucent bands: Muehrcke's lines—hypoalbuminemia
  Distal brown: Lindsay's nail—chronic renal failure
Periungual and subungual fibromas
Glomus tumors
Subungual exostoses

Lunula

Absent: endocrine, collagen vascular, reticuloendothelial, normal variant
Dyschromia
 Azure: hepatolenticular degeneration (Wilson's disease)
  Blue: argyria
  Red: heart failure, collagen vascular disease
  White: ischemia
  Yellow: tetracycline
Punctate erythematous macules: alopecia areata, psoriasis
Triangular: nail-patella syndrome
Ulceration: graft-versus-host disease

Nail Plate

Clubbing: pachydermoperiostosis; pulmonary, cardiovascular, gastrointestinal, and endocrinologic disorders; intrathoracic neoplasms
Koilonychia: Plummer-Vinson syndrome, normal neonates, onychomycosis, occupational nail softening, iron-deficiency anemia
Nail plate thickening (differentiate from subungual hyperkeratosis): chronic trauma, onychomycosis, psoriasis, Darier-White disease, lichen planus, pityriasis rubra pilaris, Norwegian scabies, pachyonychia congenita
Onychogryphosis: trauma from footwear, poor hygiene, impaired circulation, ichthyoses, psoriasis, onychomycosis
Pincer (trumpet) nail: subungual exostoses, footwear pressure, osteoarthritis
Ridging: lichen planus, mild ridging normal in elderly
Dorsal pterygium: lichen planus, vascular insufficiency, trauma
Median nail dystrophy: habit tic, mucous cyst
Beau's lines: systemic illness as measles, myocardial infarction; cytotoxic drugs
Brittle nails: elderly, onychomycosis, psoriasis, lichen planus
Pitting: psoriasis, alopecia areata, eczema, normal variant
Leukonychia: see text

TABLE 136-1. Differential Diagnosis of Nail Disorders (*Continued*)

Nail Plate

Longitudinal melanonychia: hyperplasia of normal or abnormal melanocytes; multiple bands suggest benign cause; single band suggests melanoma
Melanoma

Proximal and Lateral Nail Folds

Dilated capillary loops: progressive systemic sclerosis, lupus erythematosus, dermatomyositis
Paronychia
 Acute: trauma, bacterial infection
 Chronic: absent cuticle, chronic bacterial or yeast infection, food allergy
Ingrown nail: improper nail trimming, tight-fitting shoes, hyperhidrosis, abnormally wide or curved nail plate
Periungual warts
Mucous (myxoid) cysts
Acquired digital fibrokeratomas
Squamous cell carcinoma in situ (Bowen's disease)
Squamous cell carcinoma

TABLE 136-2. Treatment of Nail Disorders

Onycholysis

Overhydration
 Remove nail plate.
 Curtail water immersion.
 Stop use of nail enamel.
 Apply clear tincture of iodide 1:1 with 70% isopropyl alcohol.
Psoriatic: topical or intralesional corticosteroids

Hyperkeratosis, White Longitudinal Streaks

Darier-White disease, retinoids

Onychogryphosis

Nail plate trimming, footwear alteration, nail avulsion, matricectomy

Ridging

Intralesional corticosteroids

Median Nail Dystrophy

Avoid trauma.

Brittle Nails

Minimize water immersion.
Use emollient lotions after washing.
Clip while nail is hydrated
?Biotin
Limit acrylic and nail enamel application and removal.

Paronychia

Acute
 Incise and drain.
 Send for culture.
 Prescribe systemic antibiotics.
Chronic
 Rule out food allergy.
 Rule out osteomyelitis.
 Apply emollient lotions to cuticles.
 Minimize cuticle trauma.
 Apply clear tincture of iodide with 70% isopropyl alcohol.
 Apply Lotrisone.
 Inject corticosteroid into proximal nail fold.
 Surgically resect proximal nail fold.

Ingrown Nail

Nail trimming, antibiotics for infection, lateral matricectomy

Periungual Warts

Prevent wart proliferation with 5-fluorouracil application of involved area(s), nail avulsion, topical salicylic acid and paring, cryotherapy, intralesional bleomycin or interferon, electrodesiccation, and curettage

Mucous (Myxoid) Cysts

Incision and drainage, intralesional corticosteroids, cryotherapy, surgical excision

Acquired Digital Fibrokeratomas

Surgical excision

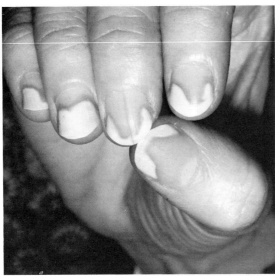

FIGURE 136-5. Onycholysis. All five nail plates are separated from the nail bed. Slight erythema at the proximal margin of the onycholysis is evident. Subungual hyperkeratosis, debris, and discoloration, however, are absent from all onycholytic clefts.

disease, and impaired circulation. Finally, squamous cell carcinoma in situ may cause onycholysis and should always be included in the differential diagnosis of onycholysis involving a single digit. The pathogenesis of onycholysis is as varied as the local and systemic disorders that cause it.

To treat onycholysis, one must identify its cause. Overhydration is best managed by removing the overlying onycholytic nail plate to facilitate nail bed debridement and expose the nail bed to air. Whenever possible, the patient's exposure to water is curtailed. Nail enamel use must be stopped. In yeast and bacterial infections, the most common cause, the overlying plate, must be removed. Clear tincture of iodide mixed 1:1 with 70% isopropyl alcohol is applied to the nail bed repeatedly throughout the day and at bedtime. Therapy for psoriatic onycholysis is usually unrewarding. One may treat the nail bed with subungual applications of topical corticosteroids; in stoic patients intralesional triamcinolone

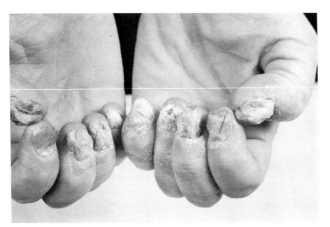

FIGURE 136-6. Psoriasis. All of the fingernails demonstrate similar clinical features. The nail plates are thickened, yellow-brown, and friable. The proximal and lateral nail folds are erythematous and scaly.

acetonide, 1.5 mg/mL, may be injected into the nail bed after frosting the skin with FluoroEthyl. Systemic antipsoriatic agents often clear psoriatic nails; nevertheless, they are not indicated for psoriasis confined to the nail unit. Other causes of onycholysis are treated according to the underlying diagnosis.

Splinter hemorrhage and *subungual hematoma* differ in the extent of nail bed hemorrhage. In splinter hemorrhage, blood that is confined to thin grooves between the nail bed's longitudinal epidermal ridges adheres to the nail plate and grows out with time. Splinter hemorrhages appear as thin black lines, 1 to 2 mm long, located in the distal third of the nail bed.

Once considered a sign pathognomonic of subacute bacterial endocarditis, splinter hemorrhage in several fingers is associated with a large number of systemic disorders. Trauma, the most frequent cause, probably accounts directly or indirectly for most cases of splinter hemorrhage. Whether from a variety of systemic disorders that increase capillary fragility or from primary nail bed involvement in dermatologic disorders (e.g., cutaneous T-cell lymphoma, Darier-White disease, eczema, exfoliative dermatitis, onychomycosis, or psoriasis), the cause of splinter hemorrhage can usually be established by careful history and physical examination.

Subungual hematoma may be caused by blood dyscrasias, collagen vascular disorders, emboli, and scurvy. The most common cause is also trauma. Subungual hematoma may mimic longitudinal melanonychia and often presents an important diagnostic dilemma. History, location, and clinical appearance will usually help distinguish between the two. Biopsy is occasionally necessary; however, surgery may be required to drain blood from the nail unit. When trauma is severe, radiographs should be considered to rule out fracture of the distal phalanx.

Subungual hyperkeratosis results from epidermal hyperplasia of the nail bed or hyponychium. Psoriasis, subungual onychomycosis, Darier-White disease, lichen planus, Norwegian scabies, pityriasis rubra pilaris, and Reiter's syndrome are noteworthy causes of subungual hyperkeratosis. KOH and mycologic cultures should always be performed when hyperkeratosis is encountered; biopsy may be required to establish the diagnosis.

Red longitudinal streaks, white longitudinal streaks, and *wedge-shaped distal subungual hyperkeratotic papules* occur in Darier-White disease. Additional findings in Darier-White disease include splinter hemorrhages, flat keratotic papules in the proximal nail fold, and nail plate fragility. Mild epithelial hyperplasia and vasodilation of the nail bed account for the red streaks of Darier-White disease. Red streaks may also occur as an isolated finding in Bowen's disease. More florid hyperplasia with multinucleated epithelial cells accounts for the white streaks (longitudinal leukonychia) in Darier-White disease. Subungual hyperkeratotic papules in Darier-White disease are due to hyperplasia of the hyponychial epithelium. Oral retinoids improve the skin and nails of patients with Darier-White disease.

Three distinctive signs of systemic disease are reflected in the nail unit. In *Terry's nail,* the proximal nail bed is white, the lunula is obscured, and the distal pink nail bed is preserved. Although commonly associated with cirrhosis, Terry's nail may also be seen in chronic congestive heart failure, in diabetes mellitus, and as a normal finding in the elderly. Overgrowth of connective tissue in the proximal nail bed in conjunction with diminished vascularity is the postulated cause of this nail sign. *Muehrcke's lines* are characterized by double, white, translucent bands separated from one another and from the lunula by the normal pink nail bed. Muehrcke's lines, which are associated with hypoalbuminemia, resolve when the serum albumin level returns to normal. Edema of the nail bed is the probable cause of this sign, which disappears when pressure is exerted on the nail bed. In *Lindsay's half and half nail*, the proximal nail bed is often dull white and obscures the lunula; the nail bed may, however, be normal. Probably the result of increased melanin deposition, the distal fourth (or more) of the nail bed is usually brown and represents the important criterion of this sign. Lindsay's nail is a sign of chronic renal failure. These three signs represent examples of pseudoleukonychia.

In *ventral pterygium*, the hyponychial groove is obliterated by scarring; the nail bed and hyponychium fuse with the overlying nail plate. Hypoxia causes necrosis and the scarring of ventral pterygium that is encountered in Raynaud's disease and progressive systemic sclerosis. Trauma, from nail biting for example, may also cause ventral pterygium. Idiopathic and familial varieties also occur. The hyponychial groove may also be obliterated by hyperkeratosis as a normal variant that may be confused with ventral pterygium. The absence of scar tissue distinguishes prominent hyponychium from ventral pterygium.

Glomus tumors are uncommon painful tumors that may appear as a blue-red macule of the nail bed, may extend through the nail plate as a papule or nodule, or may erode the underlying distal bony phalanx. These benign neoplasms of the glomus body may be diagnosed with magnetic resonance imaging.[12] Complete extirpation is mandatory for cure.

Periungual and subungual fibromas are important because they develop in 50% of patients with tuberous sclerosis. They usually appear between the ages of 12 and 14. Trauma appears to play a role in their induction. They appear as pink linear lesions with a hyperkeratotic tip that protrudes from the undersurface of the nail fold or plate. Fibromas often originate deep under the proximal nail fold. Displacing the nail plate, they cause a groove in the nail plate.

Subungual exostoses are benign painful osteocartilaginous overgrowths of the terminal phalanx that usually occur on the great toe. Trauma and/or infection are postulated to play a role in their pathogenesis. Beginning as small elevations, they enlarge and eventually emerge from under the nail plate. The surface overlying the exostosis takes many clinical forms and is not diagnostic. The diagnosis must be suspected and radiographs obtained to confirm the diagnosis.

Disorders of the Lunula

Changes of the lunula[2, 3, 13, 14] are summarized in Table 136–1.

Nail Plate Disorders

Loss of the normal inverted 160-degree angle (Lovibond's angle) between the nail plate and the proximal nail fold defines *clubbing* where the angle is everted and exceeds 180 degrees. Increase in connective tissue under the matrix elevates and "frees" the nail plate, leading to abnormal nail mobility and a fusiform enlargement of the distal digit. The pathogenesis of the connective tissue alteration is not understood. Clubbing occurs in pachydermoperiostosis and as an autosomal dominant trait. More common is acquired secondary clubbing, which has been observed in a number of pulmonary, cardiovascular, gastrointestinal, and endocrinologic disorders as well as with intrathoracic neoplasms. Clubbing may revert to normal with successful treatment of the underlying disease.

In *koilonychia* the nails are spoon shaped and concave; the edges evert upward. Koilonychia occurs in normal neonates, is associated with nail thinning in the elderly, occurs in the Plummer-Vinson syndrome (sideropenic dysphagia), and is found in onychomycosis. The two conditions most frequently associated with koilonychia are occupational nail plate softening and iron deficiency anemia, particularly in children. The pathogenesis has not been established.

Anonychia, partial or complete loss of the nail plate, may be congenital or may result from permanent damage to the nail matrix from trauma and from destructive disorders such as lichen planus.

Nail plate thickening derives from epithelial hyperplasia within the matrix. Often, however, the nail plate appears thickened when, in fact, it is normal in thickness (0.5 mm in the fingernails). Accordingly, nail plate thickening must be differentiated from subungual hyperkeratosis, which simulates thickening. Subungual hyperkeratosis is characterized by a thin rim of "normal" nail overlying a hyperkeratotic nail bed. In true thickening, the nail plate is homogeneously thickened; the thin nail "rim" is absent. True nail thickening is produced by chronic trauma and occurs in onychomycosis, psoriasis, Darier-White disease, lichen planus, pityriasis rubra pilaris, and Norwegian scabies. Pachyonychia congenita is associated with both true thickening and subungual hyperkeratosis.

Thick nails are caused by inflammation and/or trauma that stimulates hyperplasia of the matrical epithelium.

Onychogryphosis, an extreme form of nail thickening, usually occurs in the great toenails of the elderly and infirm. The hypertrophic nail plate is shaped like a ram's horn. In part due to pressure from footwear, the nail curves ventrally. Poor hygiene, disease-induced matrical hyperplasia, and impaired circulation also appear to play a pathogenic role. Onychogryphosis is also seen in ichthyoses, psoriasis, and onychomycosis.

Therapy consists of nail plate trimming, avulsion, total matricectomy for permanent removal, and/or appropriate footwear alterations. Onychomycosis may be treated with systemic antifungal agents.

In *pincer (trumpet) nail*, the nail is overly curved transversely, a curve that is accentuated distally. The shape is similar to a transected ice cream cone, the apex of the cone corresponding to the distal nail. The pincer nail tip, which rarely closes completely, may constrict tissues of the distal nail unit, causing intense pain. In some persons, subungual exostoses and pressure from tight shoes cause pincer nails. Osteoarthritis usually accompanies pincer nails of the fingers; fibrous deposits that extend from the joint appear to compress the lateral matrix, causing the pincer effect in these persons. A developmental anomaly of the matrix is another postulated cause of pincer nail. Therapy, which is often unsatisfactory, is directed at the underlying cause when discernable.

In *ridging (onychorrhexis)*, thin longitudinal elevations/ridges alternate with depressions or grooves along the nail plate surface. In *beading*, linear "rain drops" form partial ridges along the nail surface. Ridges may develop from bead coalescence. Mild ridging occurs as a normal finding in the elderly.

Severe ridging is prototypic of lichen planus. Other nail changes occur in lichen planus.[15] Matrix destruction may lead to complete absence of the nail. Partial matrix obliteration leads to shortening and/or thinning of the nail. Splitting may occur when longitudinal segments of the matrix are destroyed. Lichen planus may also involve isolated foci within the matrix, producing small papules under the nail fold.

In addition to nail loss, matrix destruction in lichen planus may lead to scarring and atrophy; adherence of the nail fold to the underlying nail bed produces *dorsal pterygium*. Depending on the width of the pterygium, nail plate remnants of varying size, "angel wings," may be present on either side of the pterygium. Other conditions that lead to matrix destruction, including peripheral vascular insufficiency, Raynaud's disease, inflammatory dermatoses, burns, and trauma, cause dorsal pterygia as well.

In "reversible" matrix disorders, early treatment with corticosteroids often clears matrix inflammation, preventing destruction and scar formation. Triamcinolone acetonide, 1.5 mg/mL, may be administered by injection into the skin of the proximal nail fold after light anesthesia with FluoroEthyl; injecting less than 0.1 mL will cause a peau d'orange effect, blanching the skin and flooding the underlying matrix with corticosteroids. Higher corticosteroid concentrations are accompanied by greater risk of atrophy; doses in excess of 10 mg/mL should not be administered. Systemic prednisone in doses of 1 mg/kg may also be used; because of side effects and the likelihood of recurrence once treatment is discontinued, systemic corticosteroids are not indicated for routine therapy.

Median nail dystrophy is characterized by an irregular longitudinal depression in the midportion of the nail plate. Often symmetrical, the dystrophy usually occurs on the thumbs. Clinical features are variable: the band may be wide or thin and the plate split or intact. Typically, the dystrophy is caused by pressure from the index finger nail; the patient has a habit or tic of pressing the sharp end of the index nail into the nail of the thumb at the proximal nail fold margin. Pressure on the underlying, newly formed, relatively soft nail leads to transverse indentations or depressions in the surface of the thumb nail. The differential diagnosis includes space-occupying lesions of the matrix such as a mucous cyst. If the patient can be persuaded to avoid trauma, the affected nail will return to normal.

Beau's lines are transverse grooves or ridges in the nail plate that, unlike median nail dystrophy, traverse the entire width of the nail plate. A transient, diminished production of nail by the matrix causes this dystrophy; the width of the depression corresponds precisely to the duration of diminished matrix activity. The distance of the line from the proximal nail fold corresponds to the time when nail production was impaired. Produced by illness that diminishes matrix function, the line appears from under the cuticle after onset of the illness. A groove clinically similar to Beau's line may be produced by localized nail fold trauma. In contradistinction to Beau's line, this pseudo-Beau's line neither extends across the full width of the nail nor involves all nails. Common causes of Beau's lines include acute febrile illnesses, measles, myocardial infarction, menstrual cycle changes in otherwise normal women, pulmonary embolism, and cytotoxic drugs. Beau's lines are "story tellers."

The term *brittle fingernails* means different things to different persons. Generally, brittleness is characterized by nail thinning, some degree of ridging, and *onychoschizia* (distal splitting and lamellar [layered] separation of thin sheets of nail plate). Brittle nails are encountered most commonly in the elderly, in individuals who repeatedly immerse their hands in water throughout the day, and in women who continually wear nail enamel or use acrylics. Less commonly, brittleness results from fungal infections and from systemic disorders, including anemia, vascular insufficiency, and endocrine and metabolic disorders; it may be encountered in psoriasis, lichen planus, and retinoid therapy. Brittleness may also be "idiopathic," presenting as an acquired or congenital disorder that presents at birth or develops spontaneously in middle age.

The pathogenesis is variable. In the elderly, brittleness probably results from "normal" changes in the matrix; nail formation becomes slower and production defective. In the elderly when nails take longer to grow, they are subject for more prolonged periods of time to trauma. More rapidly growing nails in younger persons encounter less trauma because nail replacement time is more brief. Nails in the elderly are thinner and have less cohesive onychocytes.

Repeated water immersion exacerbates brittleness. When nails absorb water, nail volume expands; evaporation leads to volume contraction. Over the course of time, repeated expansions and contractions weaken the nail by inducing latent "fracture planes," which eventually become permanent.

Nail enamel generally protects the nails, "shielding" them with protective coats of polish. Enamel removal, however, enhances brittleness. Applications of enamel removers (acetone and ethyl acetate) not only remove enamel but also dehydrate the nail and (probably) dissolve cellular and intercellular elements of the nail as well. In time, the nail succumbs to repeated solvent-induced injury. Why brittleness does not develop in everyone who uses enamels and removers remains an open question.

Little can be done to clear brittleness in all situations. Several measures are beneficial, however. Liberal application of emollient lotions after hand washing helps keep the nail hydrated. Clipping immediately after bathing when the plate is hydrated and soft is less traumatic to the nail than clipping when it is dry and brittle. Filing rough edges reduces the likelihood of the edge being caught and tearing the nail further. Filing in one direction rather than back and forth is less traumatic. One report suggests that biotin, a vitamin, in doses of 2.5 mg per day helps brittleness and makes nails grow faster.[8] A retrospective study without controls or quantitative brittleness criteria purports to lend credence to biotin therapy.[16] Controlled trials will probably not show significant benefit from this therapy. Gelatin and calcium supplements have no effect on brittleness.

In those instances when the source of the problem can be identified, an improvement in brittleness is likely to occur.

Pitting derives from the proximal matrix; loosely adherent, immature onychocytes are displaced from the dorsal nail plate, leaving pits in the surface of the nail. The surface of the nail plate is occupied by cup-shaped depressions that vary in size, number, depth, and pattern—all dependent on the degree of proximal matrix alteration. Severe pitting can so roughen the surface of the nail plate that it takes on the appearance of sandpaper, developing features of *trachyonychia* (rough nail). Psoriasis and alopecia areata, common causes of pitting, may develop the extensive surface alteration of rough, brittle, ridged nails. Deep pits are diagnostic of psoriasis.

In addition to psoriasis and alopecia areata, pitting may appear as a normal variant. Other causes include Reiter's syndrome, eczema, occupational trauma, and lichen planus.

Treatment is rewarding in the sense that pitting usually clears with injections of triamcinolone acetonide. Although clearing may be temporary, the benefits of properly performed treatment far outweigh the risk of atrophy.

Pigmentary Disorders

The nail appears white in *leukonychia* (Fig. 136–7). Leukonychia may be divided into two types. True leukonychia originates in the nail matrix. Onychocytes from the midportion of the matrix remain cornified and give the nail a white color. The white appearance is due to the diffraction of light by "immature," nucleated onychocytes located in the mid (vs. dorsal or ventral) portion of the nail plate. In pseudoleukonychia, the nail appears white. The color alteration derives not from matrix alteration but from changes in nail bed connective tissue and vasculature that simulate nail plate whitening.

Leukonychias can be transient or permanent, acquired or congenital, and total, subtotal, or partial. Partial leukonychias can be striated, punctate, or variegated. Baran and Dawber[3] offer an excellent discussion of leukonychias and their causes.

Longitudinal melanonychia[17] is characterized by a longitudinal band of brown melanin pigment that ex-

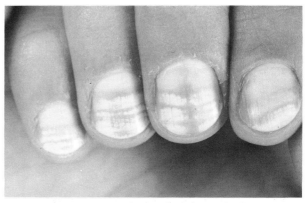

FIGURE 136–7. Leukonychia. Varying widths of striate leukonychia alternate with bands of normal nail plate. All conform to the shape of the lunula. Intermittent production of parakeratotic corneocytes produces the wave-like effect.

tends from the cuticle to the distal edge of the nail plate. Longitudinal melanonychia is important because it may indicate *melanoma*. It usually originates in the distal matrix where melanocytes are most abundant. Increased pigment in longitudinal melanonychia may be due to increased melanin production by normal melanocytes as well as by hyperplasias or proliferations of normal or abnormal melanocytes.

Differentiating longitudinal melanonychia from subungual hematomas may be difficult: subungual hematomas usually migrate distally with time; longitudinal melanonychia does not. Differentiating among the various benign and malignant causes of longitudinal melanonychia on clinical grounds alone can be difficult; biopsy is often necessary. Clinical clues that suggest a benign etiology are multiple bands of longitudinal melanonychia as opposed to a single band. Very pale tan bands are unlikely to be caused by melanoma. Longitudinal melanonychia arising in children is distinctly unlikely to represent melanoma. *Melanoma*, on the other hand, (1) may be associated with periungual pigmentation; (2) usually begins in older persons; (3) is usually subject to clinical change as opposed to being morphologically static; (4) often becomes wider or darker with time; (5) may occur in the presence of a history of trauma; (6) is often characterized by ill-defined, blurred lateral margins; (7) should be suspected if the band is black or variegated in color; (8) may be accompanied by nail dystrophy; and (9) often occurs in the thumb, great toe, or index finger.

A large variety of causes of longitudinal melanonychia other than melanoma have been reported.[17] Multiple bands may be caused by a number of systemic and dermatologic conditions. Infections and racial variations also account for longitudinal melanonychia; dark-skinned individuals are more likely than fair persons to develop longitudinal melanonychia. Longitudinal melanonychia occurs in essentially all blacks by age 70. Single bands are usually caused by a localized growth of normal or abnormal melanocytes. Melanocytic and non-melanocytic neoplasms, postinflammatory changes, and trauma cause single bands of longitudinal melanonychia. Although a single band is not necessarily due to melanoma, this possibility must *always* be included in the differential diagnosis of longitudinal melanonychia.

Once it has been determined that melanoma is strongly considered in the differential diagnosis of a pigmented streak, an adequate biopsy is required. Since pigment is transferred to the nail plate only from nail matrix cells, it is this tissue that must be sampled. The streak itself acts as the road map leading back to the pathologic process just proximal to where the pigmented portion of the plate begins. A biopsy sample may be obtained with a sharp 3- to 4-mm punch that extends through the nail plate and matrix down the periosteum of the underlying phalanx. A split or deformed nail may result from this biopsy. A more controlled biopsy is performed by first gently avulsing the nail plate and then exposing the entire matrix area by reflecting the proximal nail fold. The latter is achieved by making bilateral relaxing incisions at the lateral portions of the proximal nail folds. Scalpel biopsy of the affected area is then possible under direct vision. If possible, the biopsy sample should be about 3 mm in width, oriented transversely with respect to the matrix, and taken from tissue as far down as the periosteum; the wound is then closed primarily with absorbable sutures. Closure prevents a split or deformed nail. Avulsion of the nail may produce an area of denudation, roughly outlining the nail plate, in which the epidermis of the nail bed and hyponychium is lost. If preservation of the epidermis is important to pathologic diagnosis, as it is in a pigmented streak, then the punch biopsy method through the nail plate and matrix is a better way of ensuring preservation of the epidermis. (For further information, see Robinson et al., *Atlas of Cutaneous Surgery*, Chapter 18.)

Proximal and Lateral Nail Fold Disorders

Within the proximal nail fold, increased numbers of dilated and tortuous *capillary loops*, often located adjacent to scarred, avascular areas, may be found in patients with a variety of connective tissue disorders, including progressive systemic sclerosis, lupus erythematosus, and dermatomyositis. Similar alterations have been reported in patients with diabetes mellitus, cystic fibrosis, congenital heart disease, and Down syndrome. Unlike the fine linear capillaries found in normal persons, the capillaries in patients with these disorders are altered by fibrosis and vasoconstriction. Although these alterations typically occur late in the natural course of these disorders, their early recognition may be an important diagnostic clue in patients who present with undiagnosed systemic complaints.

Paronychia is characterized by erythema, edema, and tenderness of the proximal and lateral nail folds. Paronychia may be divided into two types: acute and chronic. Acute paronychia is usually caused by bacteria. Injury to the cuticle or nail folds enables bacteria to enter the nail unit, proliferate, and produce infection. If the infection is not deep seated, the abscess should be incised and drained and the pus submitted for culture.

Chronic paronychia is characterized by erythema and edema as well as by retraction of the proximal nail fold.

The onset is much more insidious, and pain tends to appear later in the course of the disease. Absence of the cuticle in chronic paronychia tends to perpetuate the inflammation because foods,[18] chemicals, and microbes continue to enter the cleft between the nail plate and nail fold.

Effective management of chronic paronychia can be achieved when the cause is identified. The possibility of osteomyelitis should be considered and appropriate radiographs obtained when deep-seated infection is suspected. Chronic hydration and dehydration of the cuticle and nail fold as occurs in bartenders, homemakers, and others who work in a waterborne environment is best addressed by limiting as much as possible the cycle of hydration and dehydration. A careful history with respect to contact with foods and patch testing (when indicated) to rule out food contact dermatitis may also be necessary.[18] Frequent application of emollient lotions will help to hydrate the cuticle, enabling it to re-form and protect the nail unit. Wearing cotton gloves inside rubber gloves also offers important protection for the hand and cuticle.

Clear tincture of iodide mixed with equal parts of 70% isopropyl alcohol and applied under the cleft between the nail fold and plate will destroy yeast and bacteria that often perpetuate chronic paronychia. Application of the combination of clotimazole and betamethasone (Lotrisone) in conjunction with emollient lotions will diminish irritation caused by iodine or alcohol and simultaneously inhibit the growth of yeast. Subsequent application of emollient lotions will lubricate the nascent cuticle as well as the hands. Bacterial infection of the paronychia is treated with antibiotics.

When the paronychia is more acutely inflamed and/or slow to respond to conservative measures, intralesional corticosteroid administration is indicated. Triamcinolone acetonide, 1.5 mg/mL, is injected into the proximal nail fold after light anesthesia with FluoroEthyl; less than 0.1 mL will blanch the area and provide enough stimulus to help resolve the inflammation. Application of potent topical corticosteroids is likely to cause atrophy of the nail fold without having a significant impact on the more deep-seated paronychia. Occasionally, a crescent of nail fold will be excised if more conservative measures fail.

Trauma is the initiating event in essentially all cases of *ingrown nail*. The nail plate either encroaches on or actually pierces the lateral nail fold, causing injury either by constriction or laceration. Edema, erythema, and infection commonly ensue. Excess granulation tissue (pyogenic granuloma) may also be produced at the site of injury. The great toe nails are usually affected, and toenails are involved more commonly than fingernails.

Causes of ingrown nails include (1) pressure from tight-fitting shoes, (2) leaving spicules of nail that injure the nail fold after improper nail trimming or tearing the nail, (3) overly curved or acquired wider-than-normal nails, (4) onychomycosis, and (5) hyperhidrosis. Early stages of ingrown nails are best treated by removing the ingrown portion of nail with double-action nail clippers. Trimming should bevel the nail at an angle (much like a snow sled), which will enable the nail to grow without repiercing the lateral nail fold. Infection is treated with antibiotics after assessing the degree of infection and obtaining cultures. Repeatedly inserting a hydrogen peroxide–saturated cotton-tipped applicator between the nail plate and nail fold during the period of nail regrowth helps prevent recurrence and keeps the area free of debris. Properly fitting shoes must also be worn and onychomycosis treated by regular trimming or systemic antifungal therapy.

In some instances, the above measures will fail because the nail is overly curved or too wide. In this situation, lateral matricectomy must be performed to remove the offending nail. The purpose of lateral matricectomy is to permanently destroy that portion of the nail matrix and diminish the width of the nail plate. Although surgical techniques have been described, chemical matricectomy using 88% liquefied phenol is easier to learn and perform. After securing adequate digital nerve block anesthesia with 2% lidocaine without epinephrine, the embedded portion of the lateral nail plate is avulsed with the aid of an English anvil nail splitter. This must be complete and carried back under the proximal nail fold to the most proximal portion of the nail plate. A channel is formed, allowing direct application of a phenol-soaked cotton-tipped toothpick to the matrix surface. Matrix cells are denatured and destroyed by firm application of the phenol for 30 seconds. The area is flushed with alcohol and dried with a cotton-tipped applicator, and the entire procedure is repeated once more. The phenol-treated area frosts a white color. Postoperative care includes antibiotic ointment, a nonadherent pad, and a bulky expansile dressing, which is changed daily. (For further information, see Robinson et al., *Atlas of Cutaneous Surgery*, Chapter 18.)

Warts of the nail unit are difficult to manage. In addition to arising in the proximal and/or lateral nail folds, warts develop under the nail plate, which necessitates removal of the nail plate to ensure adequate exposure. Warts tend to penetrate deep into thickened epidermis, enabling the virus to extend beyond the wart into surrounding noninvolved skin. The germinative matrix must always be guarded to prevent permanent nail dystrophy. Since periungual and subungual warts are often multiple, treatment is more difficult because one must attempt to prevent further wart proliferation while simultaneously treating clinically visible warts. The presence of multiple warts implies inadequate patient immunity to the wart virus, which makes clearing more difficult.

The application of 1% or 5% 5-fluorouracil cream to areas surrounding the warts assists in preventing wart proliferation. The application of salicylic acid preparations in conjunction with podofilox (Condylox) and home paring with a scalpel will help diminish wart volume and make warts more responsive to liquid nitrogen cryotherapy, interferon, and bleomycin.[19] Before removing warts surgically, medical therapy should be exhausted.

Since squamous cell carcinoma may masquerade as a wart, biopsy should be performed on "resistant" warts.

Mucous (myxoid, synovial) cysts develop as small pink semi-translucent nodules gradually enlarging in the skin overlying the distal interphalangeal joint or proximal nail fold. These relatively common lesions may first be de-

tected by the presence of a longitudinal groove in the nail plate produced by the cyst's pressure on the underlying matrix. Mucoid cysts usually arise in association with osteoarthritis. Some authorities believe mucoid cysts develop from localized mucinous degeneration within the proximal nail fold, while others believe that all cysts connect with the synovial joint by a thin pedicle of tissue. Therapeutic modalities include incision and drainage followed by intralesional corticosteroid injections, cryotherapy, and surgical excision of arthritic osteophytes.

Acquired digital fibrokeratomas are asymptomatic tumors that present as pink, slow-growing, hyperkeratotic projections. Unlike fibromas, they do not protrude from under the nail plate or fold. They may be related to angiofibromas, and the history of trauma may be coincidental. They usually develop on the sides of fingers and become caught on clothing. Although they share some features with warts, fibrokeratomas differ clinically in that they are more protuberant, surrounded at their base by a collarette of smooth epidermis, and arise from either the nail bed or the proximal nail fold.

Squamous cell carcinoma in situ (Bowen's disease) may involve the nail bed or periungual tissues. The clinical presentation is variable, depending on location and degree of hyperkeratosis. The tumor may appear as a recalcitrant periungual erythematous scaly plaque, a verrucoid neoplasm, subungual hyperkeratosis, or onycholysis. The nail plate may be present or absent. The tumor generally arises in the elderly and is more common on the fingers than toes. Polydactylous involvement is not uncommon.[20]

Suggested factors contributing to the formation of this neoplasm include trauma, chronic infection, radiation, and human papillomavirus infection. "Genital" human papillomavirus types 16, 18, and 32 are commonly found in the neoplastic keratinocytes of subungual Bowen's disease.

Squamous cell carcinoma of the nail unit is usually a low-grade malignancy that is slow-growing, is nonaggressive, rarely metastasizes, and occurs predominantly in males. Contributing factors are similar to squamous cell carcinoma in situ. Most often the patient is believed to have a chronic infection, eczema, wart, or paronychia. Squamous cell carcinoma arises most frequently on the thumb and index finger and presents as swelling, bleeding, ulceration, pain, drainage, and nail deformity. The tumor is often friable and simulates a pyogenic granuloma. Whenever a single digit presents as a nonhealing persistent lesion, squamous cell carcinoma should be suspected and biopsy performed.

References

1. Baden HP. Diseases of the Hair and Nails. Chicago: Year Book Medical Publishers, 1987.
2. Baran R, Barth J, Dawber R. Nail Disorders: Common Presenting Signs, Differential Diagnosis and Treatment. New York: Churchill Livingstone, 1991.
3. Baran R, Dawber RPR, eds. Diseases of the Nails, 2nd ed. Oxford: Blackwell Scientific Publications, 1993.
4. Daniel CR, ed. Symposium on the nail. Dermatol Clin 1985; 3:371–559.

5. Samman PD, Fenton DA. The Nails in Disease, 4th ed. London: William Heinemann Medical Books, 1986.
6. Scher RK, Daniel CR, eds. Nails: Therapy, Diagnosis, Surgery. Philadelphia: WB Saunders Co., 1990.
7. Zaias N. The Nail in Health and Disease, 2nd ed. Norwalk, CT: Appleton & Lange, 1990.
8. Colombo VE, Gerber F, Bronhofer M, Floersheim GL. Treatment of brittle fingernails and onychoschizia with biotin: Scanning electron microscopy. J Am Acad Dermatol 1990;23:1127–1131.
9. Kechijian P. Onycholysis. J Am Acad Dermatol 1985;12:552–560.
10. Baran R, Schibli H. Permanent paresthesia to sculptured nails: A distressing problem. Dermatol Clin 1990;8:139–141.
11. Fisher AA. Allergic reactions to cyanoacrylate "Krazy Glue" nail preparations. Cutis 1987;40:475–476.
12. Holzberg M. Glomus tumor of the nail. A "red herring" clarified by magnetic resonance imaging. Arch Dermatol 1992;128:160–162.
13. Cohen PR. Red lunulae: Case report and literature review. J Am Acad Dermatol 1992;26:292–294.
14. Hendricks AA. Yellow lunulae with fluorescence after tetracycline therapy. Arch Dermatol 1980;116:438–440.
15. Tosti A, Peluso AM, Fanti PA, Piraccini BM. Nail lichen planus: Clinical and pathologic study of twenty-four patients. J Am Acad Dermatol 1993;28:724–730.
16. Hochman LG, Scher RK, Meyerson MS. Brittle nails: Response to daily biotin supplementation. Cutis 1993;51:303–305.
17. Baran R, Kechijian P. Longitudinal melanonychia (melanonychia striata): Diagnosis and management. J Am Acad Dermatol 1989;21:1165–1175.
18. Tosti A, Guerra L, Morelli R, et al. Role of foods in the pathogenesis of chronic paronychia. J Am Acad Dermatol 1992;27:706–710.
19. Shelley WB, Shelley ED. Intralesional bleomycin sulfate therapy for warts: A novel bifurcated needle puncture technique. Arch Dermatol 1991;127:234–236.
20. Baran R, Gormley DE. Polydactylous Bowen's disease of the nail. J Am Acad Dermatol 1987;17:201–204.

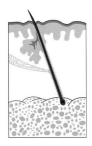

chapter 137

Biology and Disorders of Sweat Glands

Sweat Gland Science

Kenzo Sato, Neal Kane, Gyula Soos,
Takashi Toyomoto, and Fusako Sato

Eccrine sweating is unique to humans and apes and enables them to regulate rising body temperature due to heat or physical activity through the evaporative heat loss of eccrine sweating. Inability to regulate body temperature leads to hyperthermia and death. Patients with anhidrotic ectodermal dysplasia are unable to perspire, and their plight exemplifies the importance of an efficient method for evaporative heat loss. Likewise, poorly acclimatized individuals, such as infants or elderly persons who are sedentary, were the most vulnerable to the heat waves that attacked the midwestern United States in the 1980s. The eccrine sweat gland is a secretory as well as an excretory organ. Sweat is a dilute electrolyte solution containing mainly sodium, chloride, potassium, proteins, peptides, and inorganic compounds such as lactate, urea, and ammonia. Since profuse sweating causes an obligatory loss of water and electrolytes, the conservation of electrolytes by ductal reabsorption with the resultant secretion of hypotonic sweat is a vital function of the eccrine sweat gland. Patients with cystic fibrosis, whose eccrine sweat ducts are defective in reabsorbing sodium chloride, are also intolerant of heat because of their excessive loss of sodium chloride in sweat. In addition to electrolytes and small organic molecules, sweat also contains a number of biologically active agents such as interleukins[1] and proteolytic enzymes.[2]

Clinical problems of eccrine sweating include hyperhidrosis, hypohidrosis, and sweat retention syndromes. Sweat retention syndromes consist of miliaria rubra, miliaria crystallina, miliaria pustulosa, and tropical anhidrotic asthenia. There is good evidence from serial sections that dyhidrotic dermatitis is unrelated to eccrine

ducts. It is puzzling that heat stroke is always associated with anhidrosis in the face of hyperthermia.[3] Interestingly, serum interleukin concentrations are markedly increased during heat stroke.[4] Although the pathogenesis of anhidrosis during heat stroke is unknown, it is tempting to speculate that sweat retention, not sweat gland exhaustion resulting in unresponsiveness, is the cause of anhidrosis in heat stroke and that the migration of sweat-derived cytokines could contribute to elevated serum levels of cytokines and recalcitrant hyperthermia.

Hypohidrosis is common, but patients rarely seek medical attention unless it is severe enough to cause heat intolerance. It is evident from experience that the hyperhidrosis is often localized and secondary to generalized anhidrosis. It is the localized hyperhidrosis that brings the patient to the physician's office.

Eccrine sweating is controlled by sympathetic nervous system activity. The sympathetic nervous system involves the central autonomic network,[5] preganglionic efferent sympathetic pathways, sympathetic ganglions, postganglionic sympathetic fibers, neurotransmitters released from the terminals of periglandular sympathetic C fibers, and pharmacologic receptors.[2] Thus, it is tempting to assume that hyperhidrosis is due to increased sympathetic activity and that examination of the sympathetic nervous system alone will help clarify the pathogenesis of hyperhidrosis and hypohidrosis. Whereas this may be true in certain types of hyperhidrosis, we have come to realize that glandular factors, such as glandular hypertrophy, also influence the degree of sweating in physiologic and pathologic conditions.[6, 7] Although glandular hypertrophy may be important in some types of hyperhidrosis, we know very little about what causes the hypertrophy and what regulates the reactivity of the sweat gland to agonists. Furthermore, it is also unknown to what extent periglandular vascular activity is involved in regulation of sweating and how the sweat gland interacts with periglandular blood vessels.[8]

AUTONOMIC NERVOUS SYSTEM

The eccrine sweat gland is innervated by the sympathetic nervous system. Its principal terminal neurotransmitter is acetylcholine. In contrast to the classic dogma that the hypothalamus is the sole control center of the autonomic nervous system and so controls the sweat gland, more recent studies show that both the sympathetic nervous system and the parasympathetic nervous system are closely integrated and regulated by the central autonomic neuronal network.[5] The single most important structure of the central autonomic neuronal network is the nucleus tractus solitaris located in the dorsomedial region of the medulla oblongata. The nucleus tractus solitaris is reciprocally controlled or influenced by neocortical regions, nuclei of the forebrain, the higher brain stem, the diencephalon, and the cerebellum. The central autonomic neuronal network has both direct and indirect reciprocal connections with parasympathetic and sympathetic cranial and spinal cord outflow, as well as with more rostral neuronal aggregates located in the hypothalamus, the amygdala, and the forebrain.[5] The exact location and function of the so-called sweat center, presumed to be present in the anterior hypothalamus, has not yet been defined. Axons originating from the nucleus tractus solitaris form the reticular formations in the ventral medullary region, from which nerve fibers arise that innervate intermediolateral neurons in the lateral horn of the spinal cord. Although the presence of a descending spinal sympathetic tract has been postulated for decades,[9] no studies have identified it.[10]

New neurons arising from the lateral horns of the spinal cord constitute sympathetic preganglionic fibers, which change synapses in the sympathetic ganglions. The postganglionic sympathetic C fibers arising from the sympathetic ganglions mix with other sensory and motor nerves to form peripheral nerves and supply the eccrine sweat gland. The sympathetic nerves to the skin of the upper limbs are supplied by T-2 to T-9 and the face and the eyelids by T-1 to T-4. Resection of T-2 for the treatment of palmar hyperhidrosis is likely to cause Horner's syndrome. The trunk is supplied by T-4 to T-12, and the lower limbs by T-10 to L-2. Unlike the sensory dermatomes, a significant overlap of innervation occurs in the sympathetic dermatome. This is because a single preganglionic fiber can synapse with several postganglionic fibers. In other words, sharply demarcated localized hyperhidrosis, as in idiopathic unilateral circumscribed hyperhidrosis, cannot be due to lesions in the sweat center or in preganglionic sympathetic fibers.

Although epinephrine is the universal neurotransmitter released from postganglionic sympathetic fibers, those fibers supplying the sweat gland largely release acetylcholine and, to a lesser extent, epinephrine.[11] In addition

to acetylcholine and epinephrine, many neuropeptides have been localized to the spinal and peripheral autonomic nervous system, including vasoactive intestinal peptide (VIP), substance P, adenosine triphosphate (ATP), neuropeptide Y, enkepharine, and calcitonin gene-related substance.[2] The significance of the presence of multiple neurotransmitters in the periglandular nerves relative to the regulation of glandular function remains to be studied.

ANATOMY OF THE SWEAT GLAND

There are three histologically and functionally distinguishable types of sweat glands: the eccrine, apocrine, and apoeccrine (Fig. 137–1).[12, 13] Of these three types, it is the eccrine sweat gland that is primarily involved in thermoregulation. In humans, 2 to 3 million eccrine sweat glands are distributed over nearly all parts of the body. The eccrine sweat gland consists of two components: (1) the secretory coil, which secretes a nearly isotonic primary fluid, and (2) the duct, which reabsorbs sodium chloride in excess of water, releasing hypotonic sweat onto the skin surface. The size of the sweat gland varies as much as fivefold among different individuals, with gland size largely correlated with individual differences in the rate of sweating. When the maximal rate of sweating is measured, it ranges from 2 to 20 nL/min per gland.[6] Sweat gland size and rate of sweating may vary among regions of the body.

The secretory coil is composed of three distinct cell types: clear, dark (mucoid), and myoepithelial cells.[14] The fine morphology of the clear cell is characterized by the presence of intricate basal infoldings and intercellular canaliculi. The basal infoldings stain densely with ouabain-sensitive sodium-potassium–dependent p-nitrophenyl phosphatase (which reflects the catalytic activity of sodium-potassium ATPase).[15] In contrast, the intercellular canaliculus, which is actually a pouch opening into the lumen and thus corresponds to the luminal membrane, is free of p-nitrophenyl phosphatase activity.[15] Mitochondria are more numerous near the basal side of the clear cells, especially in the basal labyrinth. However, they are absent or very scarce near the intercellular canaliculi, suggesting that energy-requiring membrane transport is more active in the basal side of the cell. These morphologic characteristics support the notion that the basolateral membrane, but not the luminal membrane or the membrane forming the intercellular canaliculi, has sodium pumps. The dark cells are easily discernible because of the presence of many electron-dense "dark cell granules" in the cytoplasm. Although the function of the dark cells is unknown, periodic acid–Schiff-positive sweat glycoproteins have been traced to dark cell granules.[16]

Myoepithelial cells are located at the periphery of the secretory tubule. They are spindle shaped and contract in response to cholinergic, but not adrenergic, stimulation.[17] The cytoplasm is filled with dense myofilaments that react to antiactin antibodies. The function of the myoepithelium may be to provide mechanical support for the secretory coil wall against increasing luminal hy-

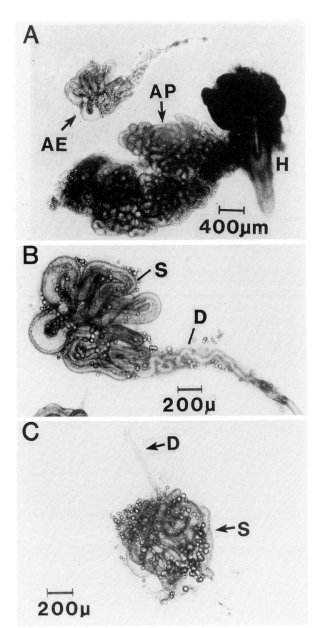

FIGURE 137-1. Human axillary apocrine (AP in *A*), apoeccrine (AE in *A* and in *B*), and eccrine (*C*) sweat glands isolated from a 22-year-old man. Note the magnification for *B* and *C* is twice that of *A*. The apoeccrine gland in *A* is the same gland shown in *B*. D, duct; S, secretory coil; H, hair follicle. The bar is 400 µm for *A* and 200 µm for *B* and *C*.

drostatic pressure.[17] The duct is composed of two morphologically and functionally distinct layers of cells, the basal (or peripheral) and the luminal ductal cells. A basal ductal cell is replete with mitochondria, and the entire cell membrane is rich in ouabain-sensitive sodium-potassium–dependent *p*-nitrophenyl phosphatase activity, the catalytic subunit of sodium-potassium ATPase,[15] suggesting that the entire basal cell membrane is involved in sodium pumping for ductal sodium absorption. In contrast, the luminal ductal cells have fewer mitochondria, much less ouabain-sensitive *p*-nitrophenyl phosphatase activity, and a dense layer of tonofilaments near

the luminal membrane. This membrane is often referred to as the cuticular border because, at the light microscopic level, it resembles a cuticle. Due to the abundance of tonofilaments, the cuticular border provides a structural resilience to the otherwise very friable tubular wall. The entire structural organization of the duct is well designed for efficient sodium reabsorptive function since the luminal membrane serves as an absorptive surface by housing both sodium and chloride channels and the basal membrane provides maximally expanded sodium pumping sites that are supplied with efficient energy metabolism.

MECHANISM OF SWEAT SECRETION

Stimulation of sympathetic neuronal outflows results in the release of periglandular neurotransmitters, especially acetylcholine, and perhaps also epinephrine and ATP. These mediators interact with their special receptors in the secretory cell membrane, triggering a sequence of events leading to sweat secretion. The immediate consequence of cholinergic receptor stimulation may be an increase in cytosolic calcium concentration (Fig. 137-2).[18] ATP significantly elevates cytosolic calcium (see Fig. 137-2) in a dose-dependent fashion.[19] VIP, which increases tissue cyclic adenosine monophosphate (AMP) levels in the sweat gland,[20] elevates calcium very slightly. This effect of VIP may not be mediated by cyclic AMP because forskolin, which also elevates tissue cyclic AMP levels to a similar extent, has no effect on cytosolic calcium concentration. Thus, the main cytosolic second messengers are calcium, which is regulated by acetylcholine or ATP stimulation, and cyclic AMP, which is affected by stimulation with β-adrenergic agonists or VIP. Studies from our laboratory have disclosed that methacholine, an analogue of acetylcholine, stimulates both calcium-dependent potassium and chloride channels presumably due to an increase in cytosolic calcium concentration,[21] inducing transient potassium chloride loss from the cell[22] and causing cell shrinkage by as much as 40% (Fig. 137-3).[23] The decreased cytosolic potassium and chloride concentrations favor the movement of ions into the cell through sodium-potassium-chloride co-transporters (see Fig. 137-3*C*). More recently, we have observed that increased cyclic AMP levels achieved by periglandular epinephrine and VIP stimulation also activate these co-transporters. The activated co-transporters (which are inhibited by loop diuretics bumetanide and furosemide) carry sodium, potassium, and chloride from outside into the cell interior in an electrically neutral fashion without the expenditure of energy. This partially replenishes the lost cytosolic potassium and chloride and increases cytosolic sodium. The latter activates sodium–potassium exchange pumps that dislocate the ions against their electrochemical gradients at the expenditure of energy (i.e., cytosolic metabolically generated ATP). During the steady state of cholinergic sweating, ionic movement takes place as shown in cell III in Figure 137-3. This model is analogous to that proposed for a variety of secretory epithelia, including the salivary acinar cell.[24] Thus, for each molecule of cytosolic ATP

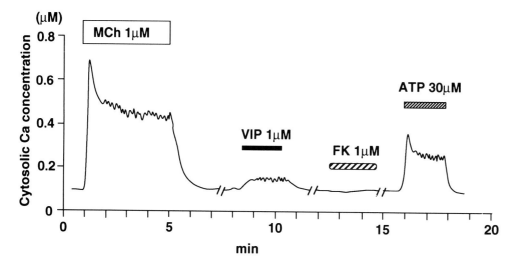

FIGURE 137-2. Illustrative examples of changes in cytosolic calcium concentration during stimulation with various agonists. MCh, methacholine; VIP, vasoactive intestinal peptide; FK, forskolin (which elevates cyclic AMP by directly stimulating the catalytic subunit of adenylate cyclase); ATP, adenosine triphosphate. Cytosolic calcium concentration was determined in dissociated rhesus palm eccrine secretory coil cells using the fura-2 method.[19] Note that resting cytosolic calcium concentration was approximately 0.1 μM.

hydrolyzed by sodium–potassium ATPase, the sodium pump translocates two potassium ions into the cytoplasm and pumps three sodium ions out of the cell. Five potassium ions diffuse out of the cell through potassium channels, generating a membrane potential and allowing potassium to completely recycle across the basolateral membrane (BL) (Fig. 137–3). Likewise, sodium also recycles across the basolateral membrane. However, for each ATP molecule hydrolyzed, all six of the chloride ions that had moved into the cell through the co-transporter pass into the lumen across the luminal membrane through calcium-dependent chloride channels.[21] This movement of chloride ions generates a lumen-negative electrical potential of −6 to −10 mV,[25, 26] which attracts sodium ions and water across the intercellular junctions to form primary sweat. In contrast, cyclic AMP–elevating agents fail to induce cell shrinkage because, although cyclic AMP stimulates cyclic AMP-dependent chloride channels in the luminal membrane, it has either no effect or an inhibitory effect on basolateral potassium channels.[21, 23]

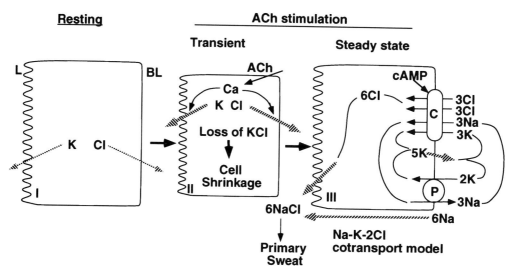

FIGURE 137-3. Ionic movement in an eccrine clear cell during cholinergic stimulation. Cell I: resting cell with minimal potassium and chloride channel activity. Cell II: immediately after stimulation with acetylcholine (ACh), cytosolic calcium concentration rises (see Fig. 137–2), which activates both calcium-stimulated potassium and chloride channels, causing massive loss of cellular potassium chloride and dramatic cell shrinkage. This cell shrinkage is partially balanced by an influx of sodium, potassium, and chloride through a co-transporter (C in cell III). Data suggest that cyclic AMP stimulates the co-transporter. Note that both sodium and potassium completely recycle across the basolateral membrane (BL). In contrast, only chloride moves across the luminal membrane (L). For each adenosine triphosphate molecule hydrolyzed, six chloride ions move into the lumen across the cell, which depolarizes the luminal membrane, attracting six sodium ions across the cell junction. Cell II is consistent with the traditional co-transport model widely employed for a variety of secretory cells.

Pathology and Surgery

William P. Coleman, III, Kenzo Sato, Neal Kane,
Gyula Soos, Takashi Toyomoto, and Fusako Sato

Hyperhidrosis

DEFINITION

In hyperhidrosis the eccrine glands produce excessive sweat in one or more anatomic locations.[27] The axillae, palms, soles, and groin are commonly affected.

CLINICAL DESCRIPTION

Hyperhidrosis, or excessive sweating, is a source of great embarrassment to individuals afflicted with this condition. Millions of dollars are spent annually on antiperspirants and deodorants to control both the amount of axillary sweat and the accompanying odor.

Hyperhidrotic patients are at particular risk for heat prostration when they are exposed to excessively high temperatures.[27] This often occurs in athletic situations such as football training camps when proper attention to fluid and electrolyte replacement is not provided.

A number of systemic or local disorders can produce or accompany hyperhidrosis. Neurologic injury or disease affecting the autonomic system can overstimulate the eccrine sweat gland. Vascular disorders or injury can have the same effect. Metabolic disorders including diabetes mellitus, gout, hyperthyroidism, and porphyria, as well as hormonal disorders, fever, and shock, can also cause hyperhidrosis.

PATHOGENESIS

Although heat is usually responsible for an increase in sweating of the hairy surfaces, emotional stimuli control sweating of the palms and soles, and in some patients the axillae. It has been postulated that the hypothalamic sweat centers for the palms, soles, and axillae are under control of the cortex and independent of temperature stimulation.[2] There is evidence that patients with palmar and plantar hyperhidrosis have overstimulation of the sympathetic nerves. During sleep, hyperhidrotic individuals sweat normally.[28] Patients with axillary hyperhidrosis usually do not have bromhidrosis (abnormal sweat odor).

Patients with palmoplantar hyperhidrosis are reported to have less reflex bradycardia than control groups in response to the Valsalva maneuver or facial immersion, but they have a higher degree of cutaneous vasoconstriction in response to finger immersion in cold,[29] indicating that there is an increased sympathetic outflow passing through the T-2 to T-3 ganglia. Excessive palmoplantar sweating lowers the skin temperature of the hands and fingers by evaporative cooling, which may then increase reflexive sympathetic outflow and further aggravate the hyperhidrosis. Interestingly, successful treatment of palmoplantar hyperhidrosis elevates palmar skin temperature by 2.5°C,[30] which may also help alleviate the vicious cycle of sympathetic reflex.

Damage to the spinal cord results in sudden loss of physiologic (thermally induced) sweating below the level of the lesion. In contrast, local sweating due to intradermal injection of cholinergic agents gradually declines within a few weeks to several months after damage to postganglionic fibers. When the damage occurs at the preganglionic level, the loss of the sweating response to a local injection of acetylcholine lasts several months to 2 years.[31] However, some patients with a past history of spinal cord injury experience episodes of profuse sweating over periods of months or years after injury with the area of hyperhidrosis not related to any sensory or sympathetic dermatomes. Hyperhidrosis due to spinal cord injury can be associated with autonomic dysreflexia,[32-34] triggered by orthostatic hypotension,[35] or due to posttraumatic syringomyelia.[36, 37]

Paraplegic patients with a spinal cord lesion at or above T-6 may have hyperhidrosis that is ascribed to exaggerated autonomic responses to innocuous stimuli such as distention of the bowel or urinary bladder, visceral inflammation, or skin irritation.[32-34] The clinical triads include episodic profuse sweating on the face, neck, and upper trunk; vasodilatation resulting in flushing of the face and congestion of the nasal passages; and throbbing headaches. In addition, other signs of sympathetic hyperactivity, such as piloerection and hypertension, may coexist with signs of increased parasympathetic activity such as bradycardia and vasodilatation. Its pathogenesis is best explained by the increased axon reflex at the level of the spinal cord (i.e., afferent stimuli arising from the bladder or bowel travel to the spinal cord in the caudal stump causing reflex anterior spasm of the skin and splanchnic vessels through the efferent sympathetic motor fibers). As a result, severe paroxysmal hypertension ensues, followed by compensatory vasodilation (and bradycardia in some patients) most likely mediated by the action of the carotid and aortic body. Despite the concomitant compensatory activation of parasympathetic nerves, the hypertension persists. The mechanism of hyperhidrosis in autonomic dysreflexia (usually above the spinal cord lesions) is not well understood. The beneficial effect of oral propoxyphene (Darvon) on hyperhidrosis in autonomic dysreflexia has been reported in a few patients.[34] It is not clear why hyperhidrosis in autonomic dysreflexia occurs several weeks after spinal injury in some patients but as late as 13 years after injury in others or why it occurs in certain patients but not others. The differential diagnoses include pheochromocytoma, toxemia of pregnancy, intracranial posterior fossa neoplasms, migraine, cluster headaches, and primary hypertension.

DIFFERENTIAL DIAGNOSIS

Systemic and local causes of hyperhidrosis should be considered (Table 137–1).[38-50] In addition, there are variants of hyperhidrosis that are episodic or localized to specific regions, such as night sweats.

Night sweats are occasionally associated with tuberculosis, endocarditis, lymphoma, hyperthyroidism, diabetes mellitus, hypoglycemia due to insulin overdose or insulinoma, systemic vasculitis, pheochromocytoma, carcinoid syndrome, drug withdrawal, dysautonomic states, other chronic infectious diseases, dumping syndrome, acromegaly, and Prinzmetal's angina.[51] A beneficial effect of indomethacin in apparently idiopathic night sweats was reported in a patient in 1982,[52] but similar reports have not appeared since then. Treatment of the underlying disorders, if known, is of primary importance.

Hodgkin's disease is characterized by the triad of fever, night sweating, and weight loss.[53] The increased sweating in this disease may be due to a fluctuating fever and an instability of the thermoregulatory hypothalamic center. Gobbi and associates[54] reported that many patients with Hodgkin's disease initially present with night sweats as the only symptom. When their body temperature was monitored during sleep, a sudden drop of body temperature was found to coincide with the onset of profuse night sweats. The ultimate cause of fever in Hodgkin's disease is still unknown, but the production of interleukin-1 by activated macrophages has been implicated as the cause of body temperature instability.[54] Interleukin-1 is known to induce an abrupt increase in the synthesis of prostaglandin E_2 in the preoptic anterior hypothalamic region, resulting in an elevation of the temperature "set point" and the generation of fever.[54, 55]

The concept of compensatory hyperhidrosis is relatively new and is not clearly defined. We often use the term *compensatory hyperhidrosis* when we describe the occurrence of hyperhidrosis on the trunk and legs after a thoracic sympathectomy for the treatment of palmar hyperhidrosis, of facial hyperhidrosis in patients with generalized sweat retention syndrome, or of hyperhidrosis of the face and the upper trunk in patients with widespread diabetic neuropathy. Sweating is usually triggered by thermal stimuli or by physical exercise. It is presumably due to an increased thermoregulatory need resulting from anhidrosis. The sweat glands in a specific area of the body hypertrophy and become more pharmacologically sensitive. Interestingly, it is the hyperhidrosis that causes a patient to seek medical advice. Thus, it is important to detect coexisting anhidrosis in such patients. The most frequent causes of anhidrosis in such patients include diabetic neuropathy,[56] lesions in the spinal cord or sympathetic trunk, and widespread portal occlusion in atopic dermatitis or in extensive miliaria.[57]

Unilateral circumscribed hyperhidrosis is not an uncommon condition, and in fact a number of cases have been reported in the dermatologic literature over the past 40 years.[58-62] The hyperhidrotic area is usually sharply demarcated, measures no larger than 10 × 10 cm², and is present mainly on the face and upper extremities of otherwise healthy persons (Fig. 137–4A). The age at onset varies between 7 and 67 years. Patients typically notice a sudden onset of profuse sweating that lasts 15 to 120 minutes. Sweating is precipitated by heat or physical exercise. The attacks occur more frequently in summer than in winter. Characteristically, there is no accompanying sensory or motor neuropathy. Sweating is not accompanied by flushing of the face, headaches, excessive salivation, lacrimation, vasodilation, or piloerection. The pathogenesis of circumscribed hyperhidrosis is unknown. Increased sweat rates in response to intradermal cholinergic agents have been reported.[58, 61] Hypertrophy of the sweat gland has also been suggested on routine histologic

---

TABLE 137–1. Differential Diagnosis of Hyperhidrosis

Neurologic injury or disease
  Spinal cord injury
    At or above T-6—automatic dysreflexia
    Cervical—orthostatic hypotension in quadriplegics with
      secondary hyperhidrosis
    Post-traumatic syringomyelia[38]
  Peripheral neuropathies
    Familial dysautonomia (Riley-Day syndrome or
      hereditary sensory neuropathy type III)[39]
  Brain lesions
    Episodic hypothermia with hyperhidrosis (Hines and
      Bannick syndrome)[40,41]
    Parkinson's disease[42]
Vascular
  Raynaud's disease
  Erythromelalgia
  Arteriovenous fistula
  Cold injury
Intrathoracic neoplasms of lesions[43,44]
Systemic diseases
  Rheumatoid arthritis
  Diabetes mellitus
  Congestive heart failure
  Thyrotoxicosis[45]
  Hyperpituitarism
  Pheochromocytoma[46]
Drugs or poisoning
  Antidepressants
    Cyclobenzaprine (Flexeril)[47]
    Fluoxetine[48]
  Acrodynia (mercury)[49]
Dermatologic conditions sometimes associated with
    palmoplantar hyperhidrosis
  Nail-patella syndrome[50]
  Keratosis palmaris et plantaris with clinodactyly
  Unna-Thost keratoderma

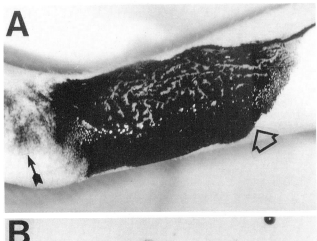

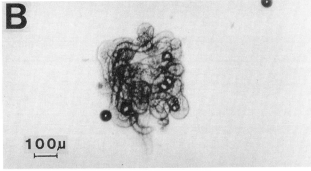

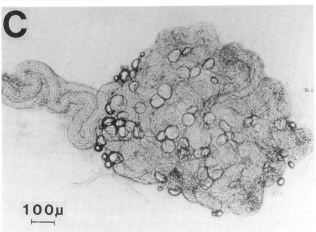

FIGURE 137–4. Idiopathic unilateral circumscribed hyperhidrosis in a 16-year-old boy. The involved area on the left forearm is visualized with iodinated starch (large arrow in *A*). His parents report that the area of involvement has gradually enlarged over the past 11 years and now partially involves the dorsum of the hand (small arrow in *A*). *B*, A normal sweat gland isolated from the contralateral side in the right forearm. *C*, A representative hypertrophic sweat gland isolated from the hyperhidrotic skin in the left forearm.

sections, but direct quantitation of glandular size has not been reported. In the patient shown in Figure 137–4*A*, a dramatic glandular hypertrophy was noted (see Fig. 137–4*C*). The pore density was not increased in the lesion as compared with the control site, indicating that it is not a hamartoma. It is not clear whether glandular hypertrophy simply represents glandular growth due to repeated episodes of sweating or is secondary to unidentified local tropic factors and/or abnormal nerve activity. Long-term follow-up of these patients has not been documented. Sweating may be partially controlled by local

application of 25% aluminum salts, topical anticholinergic agents, or systemic clonidine, inhibiting central sympathetic outflow.[60] Local tap water iontophoresis may also be tried. As a last resort, total excision of the affected area could be considered.

Localized hyperhidrosis has been reported in association with a variety of skin diseases, but the association of hyperhidrosis may be only coincidental. Localized hyperhidrosis has been observed in association with blue rubber-bleb nevus,[63] glomus tumors,[64] POEMS syndrome,[65] Goplan's disease (burning feet syndrome),[66] causalgia,[66] and pachydermoperiostosis.[67] Association of local sweating with these and other cutaneous lesions may be either a rare coincidental phenomenon or due to axon-reflex sweating. Two cases of spontaneous hyperhidrosis limited to painful pretibial myxedema lesions were reported by Gitter and Sato.[7] The sweat rate induced by local injection of methacholine was two to four times greater in the hyperhidrotic area. Interestingly, sweat glands isolated from the hyperhidrotic myxedematous sites were significantly larger than those in the perilesional normal sites.

Physiologic gustatory sweating occurs in normal persons while eating certain hot, spicy foods. Although pathologic gustatory sweating is also precipitated by gustatory stimulation, it is usually unilateral, involving the preauricular or infra-auricular areas of the face. It can be mild or embarrassingly profuse. Pathologic gustatory sweating can be classified into several types according to its etiology.

Gustatory sweating due to hyperactivity of sympathetic function is also reported to occur in association with encephalitis, syringomyelia, or Pancoast's syndrome (invasion of the cervical sympathetic trunk by a tumor).[68, 69] This condition must be differentiated from Frey's syndrome because episodes of hyperhidrosis are not always triggered by gustatory stimuli. Gustatory sweating is also reported to occur in 73% of patients who have had an upper dorsal sympathectomy. Its pathogenesis is explained on the basis of preganglionic sympathetic regeneration or collateral sprouting resulting in aberrant synapses with postganglionic fibers in the superior cervical ganglion.[70, 71] This is of interest because ipsilateral gustatory sweating occurs in the presence of other signs of Horner's syndrome (full Horner's syndrome includes ipsilateral anhidrosis, ptosis, miosis, and enophthalmos) but sweating is more intense in their absence.[71]

Gustatory sweating associated with peripheral autonomic and sensory neuropathy due to diabetic neuropathy is rare.[72] Sweating is bilateral and widespread on the face, resembling exaggerated physiologic gustatory sweating. However, diabetic gustatory sweating is often painful due to the abnormal sprouting of unmyelinated fibers. It has been suggested that axonal degeneration of the parasympathetic fibers with abnormal sprouting into the sympathetic fibers may be involved as its pathogenesis.[73] Clonidine has been reported to control the sweating in a patient with diabetic gustatory sweating.[74] Gustatory sweating has also been observed in association with post–herpes zoster neuralgia.[75]

Auriculotemporal (or Frey's) syndrome occurs in 37% to 100% of patients within 1 month to 5 years after having surgery of the parotid gland or preauricular area or after sustaining an injury to the preauricular region.[76-79] The syndrome results from injury to the auriculotemporal nerve, which carries sensory fibers from the skin, parasympathetic fibers to the salivary glands, and sympathetic fibers to the sweat glands in the preauricular region. The misdirection hypothesis holds that the severed parasympathetic fibers in the auriculotemporal nerve regenerate and migrate into the postganglionic sympathetic fibers to reach the sweat glands as well as the blood vessels in the preauricular area. When the greater auricular nerve is damaged together with the parotid gland, the parasympathetic fibers regenerating from the damaged parotid gland migrate into the distal segment of the greater auricular nerve to innervate the sweat glands in the infra-auricular area. In fact, surgical destruction of the tympanic plexus abolishes gustatory sweating in patients with Frey's syndrome, supporting the misdirection hypothesis. Gustatory sweating in Frey's syndrome is usually mild; that is, only 10% of the patients may require treatment. Topical scopolamine cream (3% to 5%) and 20% aluminum chloride in ethanol have been used with variable success.[79-81] Injecting alcohol around the auriculotemporal nerve has been reported to eliminate symptoms for several months.[79] Tympanic neurectomy[80] and interpositional fascia graft[82, 83] may offer permanent relief.

Patients with Raeder's syndrome (Horner's syndrome plus temporal and frontal headaches)[84] may note continuous profuse sweating in the right supraorbital region. The term *lacrimal sweating* was so coined because sweating is often suggestive of lacrimation. The etiology of this rare condition is unknown, but the presence of Horner's syndrome suggests that it is due to the localized neuropathy of sympathetic fibers supplying the orbital area.

Lance and colleagues[85] reported five patients, aged 27 to 64 years, who developed a sudden onset of unilateral facial flushing and sweating. Brain stem infarct was suspected as the cause in one patient. In the other four patients, occlusion of the anterior radicular artery due to strenuous exertion with consequent damage to the third thoracic segment was suspected as the cause. The flushing side showed increased sympathetic activity that was abolished by ipsilateral stellate ganglionectomy, whereas contralateral sympathetic activity was found to be deficient. Sweating was aggravated by heat or exercise in all the patients, but in four of the five patients gustatory stimuli also triggered sweating. The authors speculated that ipsilateral hyperhidrosis represented a compensatory mechanism since the contralateral side was completely anhidrotic and sympathetic activity was deficient.

TREATMENT

Once systemic or local causes of hyperhidrosis are ruled out, choosing among treatment options depends on the severity, location of the problem, and the impact on activities of daily living.

On the soles excessive sweating is annoying. Simply changing socks more frequently and using absorptive powder may be sufficient. Likewise, continually drying the palms throughout the day is a simple approach favored by many patients. Those with more difficult sweating problems can be treated with 0.1% formalin soaks several times a week, but there is a risk of producing contact dermatitis. Alternatively, 2% to 10% glutaraldehyde or 10% tannic acid in 70% alcohol can be painted on the involved areas daily. These topical approaches can also cause an irritant contact dermatitis. Perhaps the most practical approach is to employ powders containing tannic acid, salicylic acid, and talc frequently during the day to minimize the embarrassment of the "wet handshake."

Tap or deionized water iontophoresis can be used successfully in some patients for localized hyperhidrosis of the palms and soles.[86-88] A number of different units are being marketed. The more powerful models decrease the time needed for treatment. Cessation of sweating usually requires treatment of each palm or sole with 20 mA of current for 30 minutes daily. This approach may work by inducing plugging of the sweat gland pore. In an attempt

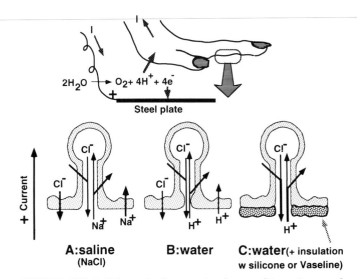

FIGURE 137–5. Schematic diagram showing possible pathways of ionic movement during iontophoresis. The equation for hydrolysis of water resulting in the generation of hydrogen ions is shown in the upper panel. The electrode plate should be made of an inert metal such as stainless steel and connected to the positive output of the galvanic unit. The hydrogen ion carries the positive current across the skin toward its interior. The lower panel shows the ionic movement across the sweat duct and the skin in three different conditions. *A,* Saline is used as the anodal solution. In this setting, galvanic current does not effectively induce anhidrosis. *B,* Water is used as the anodal solution but without silicone coating of the skin as in the conventional protocol for tap water iontophoresis. Although this setting is generally efficacious, some patients fail to respond adequately. *C,* Water is used as the anodal solution with the skin coated with silicone (or any insulating material such as petrolatum), the most effective setting. When saline is in the bath, as in *A,* the positive current is carried by the forward movement of sodium across the epidermis as well as through the sweat pores and the backward movement of chloride. *B,* Immersion of the skin in water causes swelling of the stratum corneum, narrowing of the sweat pores, and an increase in shunting current across the epidermis. *C,* Additional insulation of the stratum corneum with silicone grease or petrolatum minimizes swelling of the stratum corneum, occlusion of the pores, and the swelling-associated increase in shunt conductance across the epidermis. Thus, the positive current that is carried by hydrogen and is most critical in induction of anhidrosis is maximized.

to more thoroughly understand the mechanism of action of tap water iontophoresis and improve its therapeutic efficacy, investigators in the author's (KS) laboratory studied the detailed mechanism of action of tap water iontophoresis using well-defined experimental conditions and quantitative measures.[89] The summary of the study is as follows (Fig. 137–5). We confirmed that anodal current is superior to cathodal current, that water is superior to saline, and that the efficacy of tap water iontophoresis is a function of the amperage used. A layer of silicone grease placed on the skin prevented swelling of the stratus corneum without occluding the sweat pores (Fig. 137–6). The silicone grease reduced the total skin conductance by 60% and improved the efficacy of the tap water iontophoresis, probably due to an increase in the current flowing through the pores. The pH of the anodal water, but not saline, dropped to 3, whereas that of cathodal water increased to 10 during iontophoresis. Acidi-

fied anodal water was more efficacious than alkaline water. Sweat glands isolated from the treated anhidrotic palmar skin responded to methacholine in vitro with slightly lowered sweat rates and pharmacologic sensitivity. Thus we concluded that the strong acidity generated by the hydrolysis of water in the anodal bath is of critical importance. Hydrogen ions may further accumulate in the sweat duct by anodal current and produce unknown lesions in ducts or sweat pores resulting in ductal blockade. Secretory coil function may also be partially altered owing to exposure to intense acidity during tap water iontophoresis, but it does not appear to be the main mechanism for tap water iontophoresis–induced inhibition of sweating (Table 137–2).[89]

Axillary hyperhidrosis sometimes responds to potent topical antiperspirants. Antiperspirants contain acidic salts of aluminum or zinc that function by temporarily occluding the sweat ducts. Deodorants contain various

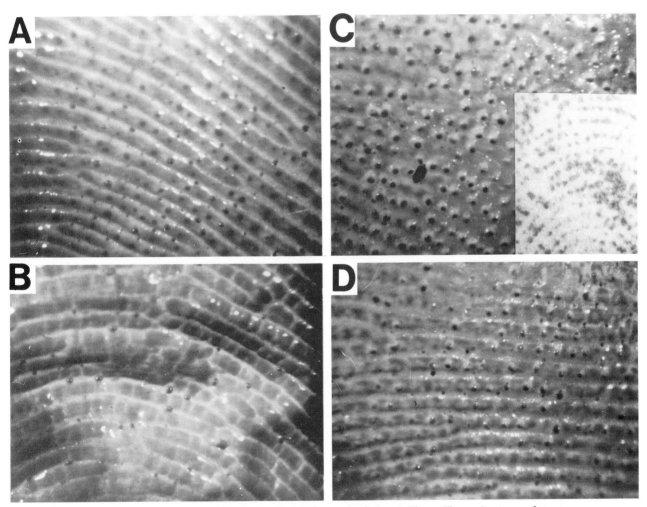

FIGURE 137–6. Effect of silicone coating on immersion-induced skin swelling and patency of sweat pores in the finger tips. Silastic imprints taken before (*A*) and after 30-minute immersion in distilled water (*B*) in a control (non–silicone-coated) finger. Note the marked swelling of the ridges (dermatoglyphs) and the disappearance of active sweat pores in *B*. *C* shows the imprint from a finger coated with silicone grease before water immersion and *D*, after 30 minutes of immersion. Imprints in *A* and *C* were taken simultaneously, as were those in *B* and *D*. The Silastic imprints were photographed under magnification. The inset in *C* is a sweat imprint of a silicone-coated fingertip done on iodinated paper. Note the presence of active pores in *D*, but not in *B*, where the sweat pores have been occluded by maceration of the skin. Inhibition of sweating due to maceration of skin is usually transient, and sweating recurs after completely drying the skin.

TABLE 137-2. Treatment of Hyperhidrosis

Medical Management

1. Frequent replacement of saturated clothing
   20% aluminum chloride hexahydrate in absolute alcohol topical application
   0.1% formalin soaks
   2%–10% glutaraldehyde or 10% tannic acid in 70% alcohol topical application
2. Systemic anticholinergic drugs
3. Tap water iontophoresis

Surgical Management

1. Ablation of lumbar and supraclavicular sympathetic ganglia
2. Excision of sweat glands
3. Liposuction

perfumes and antibacterial agents that are designed to mask the offending odors. Regular use of deodorant soaps helps to reduce the bacterial count and reduces the odor. For most people these simple hygienic approaches are sufficient. Aluminum chloride hexahydrate 20% in absolute alcohol is more effective than the commercial deodorants but may be irritating to axillary skin.[90, 91] This can be minimized by drying the axillae with a hair dryer before and immediately after application. Other antiperspirants must be avoided initially until the patient is accustomed to using the aluminum chloride. Baking soda can be substituted for other antiperspirants for its soothing and deodorant effects. After a few weeks of use at bedtime, this agent can be used in conjunction with commercial preparations. To minimize irritation the solution is applied once or twice a week, as infrequently as possible, to avoid dryness or irritation while still maintaining the anhidrotic effect. If simple application of aluminum chloride hexahydrate 20% is insufficient, then occlusion with plastic wrap nightly for two to three nights a week is performed.

In some cases, however, sweating is so copious that these measures do not work. Systemic measures may be used initially in combination with or without topical agents. This involves the use of anticholinergic drugs. Complications include decreased salivation, loss of urinary bladder sphincter control, and reduction of gastrointestinal peristalsis. Propantheline bromide and glycopyrrolate have been used successfully in many patients. To minimize side effects, anticholinergics can be used periodically, before stressful situations.

For resistant localized axillary hyperhidrosis, direct excision of the sweat glands under visualization has been performed for years. Simple surgical excision of the axillary vault can be employed to eliminate most sweating.[92, 93] It is not uncommon for eccrine sweat glands outside the original hyperhidrotic area to overcompensate gradually after surgery with increased sweating. This can become as severe as the original problem. The permanent axillary scar and hair loss may be disturbing to some persons.

Before performing surgical excision for hyperhidrosis, it is important to delineate the location of excess eccrine glands. The starch iodine technique can be used to identify the areas of most severe sweating. The starch is painted on a carefully dried axilla. When sweating resumes, a blue color appears on the areas of the greatest eccrine activity. This section of axillary skin can then be marked with a surgical pen and excised. Usually an area 7 to 10 cm long and 2 cm or more wide must be removed. These wounds are under tension, so extensive undermining must be performed. To minimize the scar, a layered closure with subcutaneous absorbable sutures is preferred. A running subcuticular suture works well to close the skin. Axillary surgical wounds are subject to maceration and are quite prone to infection and delayed healing. Meticulous postoperative care with topical antibiotics and proper wound management is important.

The newest surgical technique for treatment of hyperhidrosis of the axilla was developed from a modification of liposuction.[94–96] A blunt cannula is used to suction out sweat glands residing in the subcutaneous tissue. Additionally, superficial liposuction just under the dermis causes lower dermal inflammation and subsequent fibrosis. This technique has the advantage of reducing the number of eccrine glands without the significance of scarring axillary resections. Only two 4-mm incisions are required and axillary hair is preserved.

Liposuction, like any other surgical procedure of the axilla, must be performed carefully to avoid injury to the underlying nervous and vascular structures. The brachial plexus resides in the vault of the axilla; consequently, tunneling must be superficial. In contradistinction to the usual principles of liposuction, tunneling is performed in the most superficial portion of the subcutaneous layer. The aperture of the cannula is also directed up toward the dermis to remove as much fat, and sweat glands, as possible. Scraping the overlying dermis with the open end of the cannula promotes additional dermal fibrosis and sweat gland injury.

The tumescent anesthetic technique is particularly appropriate for liposuction of the axilla. By using very dilute solutions of lidocaine and epinephrine, excellent vasoconstriction as well as local anesthesia can be obtained. Furthermore, the swollen subcutaneous tissue resulting from injection of large volumes of this fluid provides an additional buffer to protect underlying nerves and vessels. Usually about 100 mL of a solution of 0.05% lidocaine and 1 : 1,000,000 epinephrine with 10 mEq of sodium bicarbonate is injected into a single axilla. Enough fluid must be injected to make the overlying skin quite firm. As with other procedures using tumescent anesthesia, it is very easy to maintain an appropriate plane when tunneling through the engorged fat.

After liposuction, the axilla is dressed with loose gauze fluffs overlying topical antibiotic ointment and nonstick pads. The axillary skin must be observed closely postoperatively for the possibility of localized necrosis since the liposuction dissection is carried up to the dermal subcutaneous junction. It is wise to perform this elective axillary surgical procedure one axilla at a time, allowing the patient a few weeks to recover completely from one surgery before proceeding to the opposite side. This avoids the inconvenience of being completely immobilized without the use of either arm postoperatively. (For further information, see Robinson et al., *Atlas of Cutaneous Surgery*, Chapter 28.)

As a last resort, patients with severe hyperhidrosis can also be treated by surgical ablation of the lumbar and supraclavicular sympathetic ganglia (usually second to fourth thoracic ganglia) that control the specific sweating sites.[97] Attendant side effects include postsympathetic neuralgia, phrenic nerve paralysis, Horner's syndrome, and compensatory hyperhidrosis in other areas.

Bromhidrosis

DEFINITION

Bromhidrosis, also referred to as bromidosis or osmidrosis, is a condition of excess, abnormal, or offensive body odor whether either apocrine or eccrine secretion is implicated.

Apocrine bromhidrosis (exaggerated and offensive odor) is confined to the axilla and results from excessive apocrine sweat. Eccrine bromhidrosis usually affects the feet due to maceration from excessive sweating. Apocrine bromhidrosis appears after puberty with the enlargement of apocrine glands, while eccrine bromhidrosis may appear early in childhood.[98]

PATHOGENESIS

Although freshly secreted eccrine and apocrine sweat is odorless, it provides a ready environment for the growth of bacteria, especially aerobic diphtheroids and micrococci.[99] Odor results from bacterial degradation of short-chain fatty acids. The odor of plantar skin bromhidrosis results from decomposition of keratin by bacteria. It appears that the major odor-causing substance in axillary sweat is 5α-androstenone, which has been known as the "boar taint" ketone or boar pheromone.[100, 101] Valeric acid (C5) and enanthic acid (C7) have also been observed by some to produce an odor resembling axillary odor.[102] The controlling role of diphtheroids in producing axillary odor has been established by Labows and co-workers.[101] Other common cutaneous flora such as *Staphylococcus epidermidis* and *Propionibacterium* species do not appear to play a major role in producing axillary odor. A study by Kanda and colleagues[102] suggests that isovaleric acid (iso C5), a short-chain fatty acid, is a principal foot-odor–causing chemical. *Trans*-3-methyl-2-hexenoic acid has been reported to be present in the sweat of schizophrenic patients and implicated in their characteristic body odor.[103] However, a subsequent study failed to confirm that trans-3-methyl-2-hexenoic acid is increased in patients with schizophrenia.[104]

DIFFERENTIAL DIAGNOSIS

The two significant disorders that the clinician should consider are psychiatric disorders and olfactory lobe brain tumors. Some patients with psychiatric disorders believe that they have offensive body odor in the absence of bromhidrosis. They may resort to excessive bathing and deodorant use. Psychiatric help may be required to solve their emotional problems.

TREATMENT

The treatment approach for bromhidrosis is the same as for hyperhidrosis.

References

1. Sato K, Sato F. Interleukin-1a in human sweat is functionally active and derived from the eccrine sweat gland. Am J Physiol 1994;266(Reg Integ Comp Physiol 35):R950–R959.
2. Sato K, Kang HW, Saga K, et al. Biology of the eccrine sweat gland: I. Mechanism of sweat secretion. J Am Acad Dermatol 1989;20:537–565.
3. Tucker LE, Stanford J, Graves B, et al. Classical heat stroke: Clinical and laboratory assessment. South Med J 1985;78:20–25.
4. Bouchama A, Al-Sedairy S, Siddiqui S, et al. Elevated pyrogenic cytokines in heat stroke. Chest 1993;104:1498–1502.
5. Barron KD, Chokroverty S. Anatomy of the autonomic nervous system: Brain and brainstem. In: Low PA, ed. Clinical Autonomic Disorders. Boston: Little, Brown & Co, 1993:3–15.
6. Sato K, Sato F. Individual variations in structure and function of human eccrine sweat gland. Am J Physiol 1983;245:R203–R208.
7. Gitter D, Sato K. Localized hyperhidrosis over pretibial myxedema associated with glandular hypertrophy. J Am Acad Dermatol 1990;23:252–254.
8. Hibino T, Takemura T, Sato K. Human eccrine sweat contains tissue kallikrein and kininase II. J Invest Dermatol 1994; 102:214–220.
9. List CF, Peet MM. Sweat secretion in man: II. Anatomic distribution of disturbances in sweating associated with lesions of the sympathetic nervous system. Arch Neurol Psychiatry 1938; 40:27–43.
10. Harati Y. Anatomy of the spinal and peripheral autonomic nervous system. In: Low PA, ed. Clinical Autonomic Disorders. Boston: Little, Brown & Co, 1993:17–37.
11. Uno H. Sympathetic innervation of the sweat glands and piloerector muscle of macaques and human beings. J Invest Dermatol 1977;69:112–130.
12. Sato K, Ledial R, Sato F. Morphology and development of an apoeccrine sweat gland in human axillae. Am J Physiol 1987;251(Reg Integ Comp Physiol 21):R160–180.
13. Sato K, Sato F. Sweat secretion by human axillary apoeccrine sweat gland in vitro. Am J Physiol 1987;251(Reg Integ Comp Physiol 21):R181–R187.
14. Ellis RA. Eccrine sweat glands. In: Jadassohn J, ed. Handbuch der Haut und Geschlechtskrankheiten, 1 Band, Nomale und Pathologische Antaomie der Haut. Berlin: Springer-Verlag, 1967: 224–266.
15. Saga K, Sato K. Ultrastructural localization of ouabain-sensitive, K-dependent *p*-nitrophenyl phosphatase activity in monkey eccrine sweat gland. J Histochem Cytochem 1988;36:1023–1030.
16. Yanagawa S, Yokozeki H, Sato K. Origin of periodic acid-Schiff-reactive glycoprotein in human eccrine sweat. J Appl Physiol 1986;60:1615–1622.
17. Sato K, Nishiyama A, Kobayashi M. Mechanical properties and function of the eccrine myoepithelium. Am J Physiol 1979; 237:C179–C184.
18. Sato K, Sato F. Relationship between quin2-determined cytosolic (Ca^{2+}) and sweat secretion. Am J Physiol 1988;254(Cell Physiol 23):C310–C317.

19. Grynkiewicz G, Poemie M, Tsien RY. A new generation of Ca^{2+} indicators with greatly improved fluorescence properties. J Biol Chem 1985;260:3440–3450.
20. Sato K, Sato F. Effect of VIP on sweat secretion and cAMP accumulation in simian eccrine glands. Am J Physiol 1987; 353(Reg Integ Comp Physiol 22):R935–R941.
21. Sato K, Ohtsuyama M, Sato F. Whole cell K and Cl currents in dissociated eccrine secretory coil cells during stimulation. J Membr Biol 1993;134:93–106.
22. Saga K, Sato K, Sato F. K^+ efflux from monkey eccrine secretory coil during the transient stimulation with agonists. J Physiol 1988;405:205–217.
23. Suzuki Y, Ohtsuyama M, Samman G, et al. Ionic basis of methacholine-induced shrinkage of dissociated eccrine clear cells. J Membr Biol 1991;123:33–41.
24. Cook DI, Young JA. Fluid and electrolyte secretion by salivary glands. In: Schultz SG, Forte JG, eds. Handbook of Physiology: The Gastrointestinal System III. Bethesda, MD: American Physiological Society, 1989:1–23.
25. Sato K, Sato F. Transepithelial p.d. during Sr^{2+}-induced spontaneous sweat secretion. Am J Physiol 1982;242:C360–C365.
26. Sato K. Differing luminal potential difference of cystic fibrosis and control sweat secretory coils in vitro. Am J Physiol 1984;247:R646–R649.
27. Sturm HM. Hyperhidrosis. In Demis DJ, ed. Clinical Dermatology, 17th revision, unit 9-3. Philadelphia: JB Lippincott, 1990:1–5.
28. Hurley HJ. The eccrine sweat glands. In: Moschella SL, Pillsbury DM, Hurley HJ, eds. Dermatology. Philadelphia: WB Saunders Co., 1975:1167–1175.
29. Shih CJ, Wu JJ, Lin MT. Autonomic dysfunction in palmar hyperhidrosis. J Auton Nerv Syst 1983;8:33–43.
30. Holzle E, Alberti N. Long-term efficacy and side effects of tap water iontophoresis of palmoplantar hyperhidrosis: The usefulness of home therapy. Dermatologica 1987;175:126–135.
31. Faden AI, Chan P, Mendoza E. Progressive isolated segmental anhidrosis. Arch Neurol 1982;39:172–175.
32. Jane MJ, Freehafer AA, Hazel C, et al. Autonomic dysreflexia: A cause of morbidity and mortality in orthopedic patients with spinal cord injury. Clin Orthop Rel Res 1982;169:151–154.
33. Kewalramani LS. Autonomic dysreflexia in traumatic myelopathy. Am J Phys Med 1980;59:1–21.
34. Tashjian EA, Richter KJ. The value of propoxyphene hydrochloride (Darvon) for the treatment of hyperhidrosis in the spinal cord injured patient: An anecdotal experience and case reports. Paraplegia 1985;23:349–353.
35. Khurana RK. Orthostatic hypotension–induced autonomic dysreflexia. Neurology 1987;37:1221–1224.
36. Streeten DHP, Kerr LP, Kerr CB, Prior JC. Hyperbradykininism: A new orthostatic syndrome. Lancet 1972;2:1048–1053.
37. Ottomo M, Heimburger RF. Alternating Horner's syndrome and hyperhidrosis due to dural adhesions following cervical spinal cord injury. J Neurosurg 1980;53:97–100.
38. Stanworth PA. The significance of hyperhidrosis in patients with post-traumatic syringomyelia. Paraplegia 1982;20:282–287.
39. Axelrod FB, Pearson J. Congenital sensory neuropathies: Diagnostic distinction from familial dysautonomia. Am J Dis Child 1984;138:947–954.
40. Sandel ME, Abram PL, Horn LJ. Hypertension after brain injury: Case report. Arch Phys Med Rehabil 1986;67:469–472.
41. Cunliffe WJ, Johnson CE, Burton JL. Generalized hyperhidrosis following epilepsy. Br J Dermatol 1971;85:186–188.
42. Turkka JT, Myllylä VV. Sweating dysfunction in Parkinson's study. Eur Neurol 1987;26:1–7.
43. McCoy BP. Apical pulmonary adenocarcinoma with contralateral hyperhidrosis. Arch Dermatol 1981;117:659–661.
44. McEvoy M, Ryan E, Neal G, Prichard J. Unilateral hyperhidrosis: An unusual presentation of bronchial carcinoma. Ir J Med Sci 1982;151:51–52.
45. Allen JA, Lowe DC, Roddie IC, Wallace WFM. Studies on sweating in clinical and experimental thyrotoxicosis. Clin Sci Mol Med 1973;45:765–773.
46. Bravo EL, Gifford RW. Pheochromocytoma: Diagnosis, localization, and management. N Engl J Med 1984;311:1298–1303.
47. Heckerling PS, Bartow TJ. Paradoxical diaphoresis in cyclobenzapine poisoning (letter). Ann Intern Med 1987;101:881.
48. Cohen JB, Wilcox C. A comparison of fluoxepine, imipramine, and placebo in patients with major depressive disorder. J Clin Psychiatry 1985;46:26–31.
49. Agos MM, Etzel RA, Parrish RG, et al. Mercury exposure from interior latex paint. N Engl J Med 1990;323:1096–1101.
50. Pechman KJ, Bergfeld WF. Palmar-plantar hyperhidrosis occurring in a kindred with nail-patella syndrome. J Am Acad Dermatol 1980;3:627–632.
51. Becker RC, Alpert JS. Nocturnal diaphoresis in Prinzmetal angina (letter). Ann Intern Med 1987;107(1):121.
52. Tkach JR. Indomethacin treatment of generalized hyperhidrosis (letter). J Am Acad Dermatol 1982;6:545.
53. Carbone PP, Kaplan HS, Musshoff K, et al. Report of the committee on Hodgkin's disease staging classification. Cancer Res 1971;31:1860–1861.
54. Gobbi PG, Pieresca C, Ricciarde L, et al. Night sweats in Hodgkin's disease. Cancer 1990;65:2074–2077.
55. Dinarello CA. Interleukin-1 and the pathogenesis of the acute phase response. N Engl J Med 1984;311:1413–1418.
56. Realey RD, Low PA, Thomas JE. Thermoregulatory sweating abnormality in diabetes mellitus. Mayo Clin Proc 1989;64: 617–628.
57. Sulzberger MB, Zimmerman HM, Emerson K Jr. Tropical anhidrotic asthenia (thermogenic anhidrosis) and its relationship to prickly heat. J Invest Dermatol 1946;7:153–164.
58. Cunliffe WC, Johnson CE, Williamson DW. Localized unilateral hyperhidrosis: A clinical and laboratory study. Br J Dermatol 1972;86:374–378.
59. Fernandez G, Armijo M. Unilateral facial circumscribed hyperhidrosis. Acta Derm Venereol 1985;65:445–447.
60. Chan P, Kao GF, Pierson DL, Rodman OG. Episodic hyperhidrosis on the dorsum of hands. J Am Acad Dermatol 1985; 12:937–942.
61. Van De Kerkhof PCM, Den Arend JAJC, Bousema MT, Stolz E. Localized unilateral hyperhidrosis. Br J Dermatol 1987; 117:779–782.
62. Kuritzky A, Hering R, Goldhammer G, Becher M. Clonidine treatment in paroxysmal localized hyperhidrosis. Arch Neurol 1984;41:1210–1211.
63. Tschernjawski J. Komplizierte Schweissdrüsennaevi mit Hyperfunktion derselben. Arch Dermatol Syph 1931;162:762–770.
64. Cooke SAR. Misleading features in the clinical diagnosis of the peripheral glomus tumour. Br J Surg 1971;58:602–606.
65. Kanitakis J, Roger H, Soubrier M, et al. Cutaneous angiomas in POEMS syndrome. Arch Dermatol 1988;124:695–698.
66. Allen JA, Armstrong JE, Roddie IC. Sweat responses of a hyperhidrotic subject. Br J Dermatol 1974;90:277–281.
67. Sirinavin C, Buist NRM, Mokkhaves P. Digital clubbing, hyperhidrosis, acro-osteolysis and osteoporosis: A case resembling pachydermoperiostosis. Clin Genet 1982;22:83–89.
68. McGibbon BM, Patetta FX. Further concepts in gustatory sweating. Plast Reconstr Surg 1972;49:639–642.
69. Friedman JH. Hemifacial gustatory sweating due to Pancoast's tumor. Am J Med 1987;82:1269–1271.
70. Kux M. Thoracic endoscopic sympathectomy in palmar and axillary hyperhidrosis. Arch Surg 1978;113:264–266.
71. Kurchin A, Adar R, Zweig A, Mozes M. Gustatory phenomena after upper dorsal sympathectomy. Arch Neurol 1977; 34:619–623.
72. Stuart DD. Diabetic gustatory sweating. Ann Intern Med 1978; 89:223–224.
73. Bronshvag MM. Spectrum of gustatory sweating, with especial reference to its presence in diabetics with autonomic neuropathy. Am J Clin Nutr 1978;31:307–309.
74. Janka HU, Standl E, Mehnert H. Clonidine effect on diabetic gustatory sweating (letter). Ann Intern Med 1979;91:130.
75. Drummond PD, Boyce GM, Lance JW. Postherpetic gustatory flushing and sweating. Ann Neurol 1987;21:559–563.
76. Kornblut AD, Westphal P, Miehike A. A reevaluation of the Frey's syndrome following parotid surgery. Arch Otolaryngol 1977;103:258–261.
77. Myers EN, Conley J. Gustatory sweating after radical neck dissection. Arch Otolaryngol 1970;91:534–542.
78. Gordon AB, Fiddian RV. Frey's syndrome after parotid surgery. Am J Surg 1976;132:54–58.

79. Harper KH, Spielvogel RL. Delayed onset of Frey's syndrome following trauma. J Assoc Milit Dermatol 1983;9:32–34.
80. Thomas RL. Tympanic neurectomy and chorda tympani section. Aust NZ J Surg 1980;50:352–355.
81. Bednarek J, Reid W, Matsumoto T. Frey's syndrome. Am J Surg 1976;1331:592–594.
82. Sessions RB, Roark DT, Alford BR. Frey's syndrome: A technical remedy. Ann Otol 1976;85:734–739.
83. Baddour HM, Ripley JF, Cortez EA, et al. Treatment of Frey's syndrome by an interpositional fascial graft: Report of case. J Oral Surg 31980;8:778–781.
84. Van Weerden TW, Houtman WA, Schweitzer NMJ, Minderhout JM. Lacrimal sweating in a patient with Raeder's syndrome. Clin Neurol Neurosurg 1979;81:119–121.
85. Lance JW, Drummond PD, Gandevia SC, Morris JGL. Harlequin syndrome: The sudden onset of unilateral facial flushing and sweating. J Neurol Neurosurg Psychiatry 1988;51:635–642.
86. Levit F. A simple device for the treatment of hyperhidrosis by iontophoresis. Arch Dermatol 1967;98:505–507.
87. Bouman HD, Grunewald-Lentzer EM. The treatment of hyperhidrosis of the hands and feet with constant current. Am J Phys Med 1952;31:158–169.
88. Shelley W, Horvath P, Weidman F, Pillsbury DM. Experimental miliaria in man: I. Production of sweat retention anhidrosis and vesicles by means of iontophoresis. J Invest Dermatol 1948; 11:275–291.
89. Sato K, Timm DE, Sato F, et al. Generation and transit pathway of H^+ is critical for inhibition of palmar sweating by iontophoresis in water. J Appl Physiol 1993;75:2258–2264.
90. Shelley WB, Hurley HJ. Studies of topical antiperspirant control of axillary hyperhidrosis. Acta Derm Venereol 1975;55:241–260.
91. Brandrup F, Larsen PO. Axillary hyperhidrosis: Local treatment with aluminum chloride hexahydrate 25% in absolute ethanol. Acta Derm Venereol 1978;58:461–465.
92. Bretteville-Jensen G, Mossing N, Albrechtsen R. Surgical treatment of axillary hyperhidrosis in 123 patients. Acta Derm Venereol 1975;55:73–77.
93. Hurley HJ. Local surgical management of axillary hyperhidrosis. In Epstein E, ed. Skin Surgery, 3rd ed. Springfield, IL: Charles C Thomas, 1970:587–597.
94. Shenaq SM, Spira M. Treatment of bilateral axillary hyperhidrosis by suction assisted lipolysis technique. Ann Plast Surg 1987;19:548–551.
95. Coleman WP III. Noncosmetic applications of liposuction. J Dermatol Surg Oncol 1988;14:1085–1090.
96. Lillis PJ, Coleman WP III. Liposuction for treatment of axillary hyperhidrosis. Dermatol Clin 1990;8:479–482.
97. Bogokowsky H, Slutzki S, Bacalu L, et al. Surgical treatment of primary hyperhidrosis: Bilateral, superclavicular, extrapleural sympathectomy. Arch Surg 1983;118:1065–1067.
98. Hurley HJ, Rosen MW. Apocrine bromhidrosis. In: Demis DJ, ed. Clinical Dermatology, 17th revision, unit 9-11. Philadelphia: JB Lippincott, 1990:1–3.
99. Shelley WB, Hurley HJ, Nichols AC. Axillary odor: The role of apocrine sweat, bacteria and deodorants. Arch Dermatol 1953; 68:430–446.
100. Gower DB. 16-Unsaturated C19 steroids: A review of their chemistry, biochemistry, and possible physiological role. J Steroid Biochem 1972;3:45–103.
101. Labows JN, McGinley KJ, Kligman AM. Perspectives on axillary odor. J Soc Cosmet Chem 1982;34:193–202.
102. Kanda F, Yagi E, Fukuda M, et al. Elucidation of chemical compounds responsible for foot malodour. Br J Dermatol 1990;122:772–776.
103. Smith K, Thompson GF, Koster HD. Sweat in schizophrenia patients: Identification of odorous substance. Science 1969; 166:398–399.
104. Gordon SG, Smith K, Rabinowitz JL, Vagelos PR. Studies of trans-3-methyl-2-hexenoic acid in normal and schizophrenic humans. J Lipid Res 1973;14:495–503.

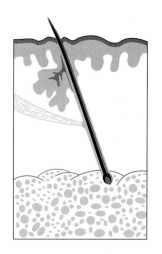

What Diseases Alter Mucous Membranes?

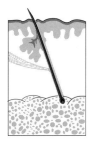

chapter 138

Disorders of Oral Mucous Membranes

DRORE EISEN and JOHN SEXTON

Oral medicine has evolved into a complex field that encompasses a variety of local and systemic neoplasms and diseases. Research has focused not only on the clinical manifestations of these conditions but, more importantly, also on the pathogenesis. Accurate diagnosis and effective therapy for stomologic diseases are more widespread than a decade ago.

The oral cavity displays evidence of cutaneous and systemic disorders that are often unappreciated. An oral cavity evaluation not uncommonly uncovers benign and malignant neoplasms or the first manifestation of a systemic disease. Mucosal abnormalities can only be identified if the normal state of oral health is recognized. Incorporation of an oral cavity examination into the routine practice of dermatology would accomplish this task. Additionally, tooth abnormalities requiring dental evaluation are frequently observed in a large number of dermatologic disorders (Table 138–1 and Fig. 138–1).

This chapter provides brief descriptions of various oral diseases of interest to dermatologists. For completeness, oral pathology and oral medicine textbooks as well as the references at the end of this chapter should be consulted.

BENIGN NEOPLASMS, REACTIVE PROCESSES, AND SYSTEMIC DISORDERS AFFECTING THE ORAL CAVITY

Blue and Black Lesions

Pigmentation of the oral cavity may be due to a variety of causes.[1] Antimalarials, minocycline, adrenocorticotropic hormone, oral contraceptives, phenolphthalein, and zidovudine are a few of the common medications that cause localized or diffuse hyperpigmentation of the oral mucosa. Heavy metals, although no longer used therapeutically, may account for gingival and diffuse oral pigmentation through accidental exposure. Systemic illnesses, including Addison's disease, neurofibromatosis, hemochromatosis, and Peutz-Jeghers disease, may be accompanied by various degrees of oral pigmentation. Diffuse patches of pigmentation on the buccal mucosa and gingiva are commonly present in dark-skinned persons.

Amalgam Tattoo. The most common cause of exogenous oral pigmentation is due to particles of amalgam fillings accidentally introduced into oral soft tissues. Clinically, macular lesions in shades of blue, gray, or black of varying sizes and configurations appear most commonly on the gingiva and alveolar mucosa. In most instances, amalgam tattoos can be recognized clinically and the diagnosis supported by dental history. Radiographs demonstrate radiopacities in fewer than 25% of cases. If there is uncertainty regarding the diagnosis, biopsy is needed. Histologically, amalgam appears as discrete, yellow to brown granules that coat connective tissue fibers.

Oral and Labial Melanotic Macules. In 1976, Weathers and coworkers[2] originally described the "labial melanotic macule," and Page and associates[3] subsequently described the "oral melanotic macule." Clinically, pigmented macules on the lips and in the oral cavity occur predominantly in women in the 20- to 30-year age group. In 80%, the lesions are usually solitary, well circumscribed, and either brown or black.[4] Histologically, keratinocytes of the basal cell layer are hyperpigmented and there is pigmentary incontinence. In contrast to simple lentigines, melanotic macules do not exhibit elongation of the rete ridges, nor are melanocytes markedly increased in number. Immunohistochemical studies of intralesional melanocytes are HMB-45 negative, in contrast to junctional melanocytes of nevi of melanomas.[4] These lesions are completely innocuous and have no malignant potential, although some lesions cannot be clinically differentiated from incipient mela-

TABLE 138-1. Abnormalities of Teeth in Dermatologic Diseases

Disease	Tooth Abnormalities	Other Oral Features
Ectodermal dysplasia	Hypodontia; conical or peg-shaped teeth of both dentitions	
Papillon-LeFevre syndrome	Premature loss of deciduous and permanent teeth	Childhood periodontal disease
Rothmund-Thomson syndrome	Dysplastic teeth	
Erythropoietic porphyria	Reddish-brown teeth that fluoresce under Wood's light	
Pachyonychia congenita	Natal teeth (erupted teeth at birth)	
Incontinentia pigmenti	Hypodontia; conical teeth of both dentitions	
Focal dermal hypoplasia	Hypodontia; enamel dysplasia; malocclusion	Oral papillomas of mucosa and lips
Tricho-dento-osseous syndrome	Small, pitted teeth with enamel defects	
Premolar aplasia, hyperhidrosis, and canities prematura	Hypodontia of bicuspid teeth and sometimes third molars	
Tuberous sclerosis	Enamel pitting most commonly affecting the bicuspids	Pigmented papillomas of the oral cavity
Acrodynia	Premature tooth loss	Stomatitis and gingivitis
Congenital syphilis	Hutchison's incisors (crescentic notch of incisal edge) in 50% of permanent maxillary incisors; mulberry molars (multiple conical and poorly developed cusps) in 20% to 50% of permanent mandibular molars	
Epidermolysis bullosa	Enamel and cementum defects in some types	Oral blisters that ulcerate and scar; common in dystrophic and lethal forms
KID syndrome	Dental dysplasia	Chronic oral ulcerations and oral candidiasis
Histiocytosis X	"Floating teeth" (loosening of teeth within lytic bone lesions)	Oral ulcers, stomatitis, and gingivitis
Gardner's syndrome	Supernumerary teeth (extra teeth embedded in the mandible and maxilla)	Osteomas of mandible
Lipoid proteinosis	Aplasia or hypoplasia of upper incisors and cuspids	Pink and flesh-colored papules and nodules on lips; tongue often thickened and bound down to floor of mouth

nomas and other causes of pigmentation. Atypical or progressive lesions should be excised.

Oral Melanoacanthoma. This rare cause of oral pigmentation occurs almost exclusively in young black females and is believed to be a reactive phenomenon to trauma.[5] Clinically, oral melanoacanthomas appear

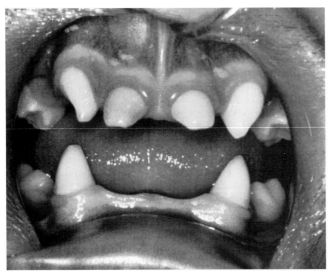

FIGURE 138-1. Ectodermal dysplasia: conical shaped and missing teeth are commonly observed.

as darkly pigmented, unilateral, sharply demarcated patches or plaques with a rough, irregular surface. Histologically, large, dendritic melanocytes are uniformly distributed through all layers of the epithelium and underlie a hyperplastic and spongiotic epithelium.[6] These benign lesions require a biopsy to differentiate them from other causes of oral pigmentation. Many but not all have regressed after performance of biopsy or removal of irritants.

Oral Nevi. Fewer than 300 oral melanocytic nevi have been documented in the literature. They are diagnosed most frequently during the third and fourth decades of life, and most are less than 1 cm in size.[7] The significance of oral nevi lies in their predilection for the palate, a characteristic shared by oral melanomas. The majority of oral nevi are raised, which helps differentiate them from macular pigmentation caused by melanotic macules, amalgam tattoos, and physiologic pigmentation. Histologically, half are of the intramucosal type and up to one third are common blue nevi.[7] Junctional, combined, congenital, and nonpigmented nevi occur less commonly. All oral nevi should be excised since their malignant potential is unknown and they cannot be clinically differentiated from oral melanomas.

Laugier-Hunziker Syndrome. This rare cause of oral pigmentation affects white exclusively. Multiple pigmented macules that may become confluent and appear in various shades of gray, brown, and black arise most commonly on the lips, buccal mucosa, and palate.[8] Patients often demonstrate pigmented, longitudinal streaks of the fingernails and less frequently streaks of the toenails. Pigmentation of the genitalia and neck occurs infrequently. Histologically, there is an accumulation of melanin in the basal keratinocytes and an increase in the number of melanophages in the papillary dermis. Mature melanosomes in the cytoplasm of the keratinocytes can be demonstrated by electron microscopic studies.[8] No therapy is required, since the lesions are asymptomatic. However, other causes of diffuse oral pigmentation, including Addison's disease and Peutz-Jeghers syndrome, should be excluded.

Acanthosis Nigricans. The oral manifestations of acanthosis nigricans have been reported in all forms of the disease but occur with the greatest frequency in the malignant form.[9] The tongue, lip, and buccal mucosa are most commonly involved, although lesions may appear on any mucosal surface. Velvety, papillomatous growths producing a verrucous, shaggy appearance of the mucous membranes are most characteristic of oral acanthosis nigricans. Varying degrees of hyperpigmentation may also be present. Histologically, marked acanthosis and parakeratosis are noted. The recognition of these oral lesions should prompt an investigation of an underlying internal malignancy.

White and Yellow Lesions

Fordyce's Spots. Fordyce's spots are small, white or yellow papules usually appearing in clusters at various sites in the oral cavity. A normal finding in approximately 80% of patients, these spots represent heterotopic sebaceous glands. They affect the sexes equally and are rarely seen before puberty. On occasion they may form large plaques. They are most frequently seen on the buccal mucosa and in the retromolar area.[10] Histologically, normal sebaceous glands are seen but they are devoid of a hair follicle. No treatment is indicated.

White Sponge Nevus. This autosomal dominant disorder is characterized by the development of oral white plaques that may vary in their severity. Mucous membrane involvement may be present at birth or develop during adolescence. The mucosa appears thickened and folded with a spongy texture, although the lesions are generally asymptomatic. Some patients exhibit involvement of isolated mucosal surfaces, most commonly the buccal mucosa, whereas others have widespread lesions affecting all of the oral mucous membranes. Extraoral lesions may involve the vagina, labia, anorectal mucosa, and nasal cavity. Histologically, the epithelium shows hyperkeratosis and acanthosis with parakeratotic cells extending into the spinous layer, where there are clusters of cells with abundant pale cytoplasm and pyknotic nuclei. The lesions are benign and do not undergo malignant transformation. Various treatment modalities have been used, with varying success, including penicillin and retinoids. Several case reports have documented the benefits of a tetracycline rinse.[11]

Pachyonychia Congenita (see Chapter 164). The oral manifestations in this rare disorder are almost always present and appear at birth.[12] Oral leukokeratosis characterized by white, opaque thickenings occurs most often on the tongue and buccal mucosa. The plaques may be discrete or confluent, covering the entire oral mucosa. These lesions are asymptomatic, and no therapy is required since they do not have any potential to undergo malignant transformation. Additional oral features of pachyonychia congenita include congenital and neonatal teeth, malformed and carious teeth, and angular cheilosis.[13]

Hereditary Benign Intraepithelial Dyskeratosis. This autosomal dominant disorder affecting the mouth and eyes is rare and found predominantly in families from a heterogeneous ethnic background residing in North Carolina.[14] Oral lesions appear in childhood and are characterized by asymptomatic, white, thickened plaques on the buccal mucosa, lips, and tongue. Histologically, "tobacco cells," described as eosinophilic cells within vacuolated prickle cells, are pronounced along with epithelial hyperplasia and acanthosis. Ocular lesions that arise in infancy are characterized by gelatinous plaques on a reddened conjunctiva. A biopsy may be required to differentiate this condition from other causes of leukoplakia.

Keratosis Follicularis (Darier-White Disease) (see Chapter 162). Oral lesions are present in 15% to 50% of patients from reported series with this autosomal dominant condition.[15] Clinically, white papules measuring 1 to 3 mm appear most commonly on the palate, followed by gingiva, buccal mucosa, and tongue. These lesions are often covered by pink mucosa and may appear similar to those of nicotine stomatitis. Coalescing lesions often result in a "cobblestoning" appearance, giving the palate a sandpaper surface. Parotid swelling is infrequently observed. The histology of oral Darier-White disease is identical to that of cutaneous lesions.

Psoriasis (see Chapter 27). Oral lesions occur infrequently or, as some argue, are nonexistent in patients with psoriasis. Those oral cases that have been described are poorly documented, and the lesions are characterized by red plaques covered with white scales. Many investigators have confirmed a high frequency of geographic tongue in patients with psoriasis, especially in those with a pustular flare.[16] Ectopic geographic tongue, which appears on mucosal surfaces other than the dorsal tongue, also has a high prevalence in psoriatic patients when compared with the general population.[17] Histologically, both of these conditions are identical to the cutaneous lesions of psoriasis, supporting studies that document a close association of these entities.

Red and Pink Lesions

Pyogenic Granuloma. Pyogenic granuloma or lobular capillary hemangioma may represent a response to chronic irritation such as sepsis, trauma, or a poorly fitting prosthesis. It presents as an intensely red, sometimes ulcerated, pedunculated mass that bleeds easily on provocation. Although the lesion may occur at any oral site, there is a predisposition for the maxillary anterior gingiva. A variant of the pyogenic granuloma known as the pregnancy tumor or epulis gravidarum may be seen in gravid patients.[18] Histologically, early lesions of pyogenic granuloma as well as the pregnancy tumor display granulation tissue in a polypoid configuration. Mature lesions feature lobular clusters of capillaries separated by intersecting bands of fibrosis. Treatment involves removal of the irritating stimulus and excision of the granuloma. Pregnancy tumors tend to regress after delivery.

Papillary Hyperplasia. Papillary hyperplasia is a benign condition of the palate seen frequently in denture wearers. It represents a reactive response to irritation due to poorly fitting dentures or dentures that are infrequently removed. Clinically, papillary hyperplasia shows diffuse red, papillary projections that bleed easily on provocation. They are confined to the hard palate, especially near the midline. Chronic lesions may appear pink and fibrotic.[19] The histology of papillary hyperplasia is consistent with an inflammatory process and features short, blunt papillations, hyperkeratosis and parakeratosis, and infiltrates of mononuclear cells that ascend to the suprabasilar layer of the hyperplastic epithelium. Treatment consists of prosthetic adjustment, removal of the denture at night, or surgical excision of fibrotic lesions.

Mucocele. The mucocele is one of the most common entities encountered in the oral cavity. Some traumatically induced lesions are the results of damage to the small duct of an accessory salivary gland, the so-called mucous extravasation phenomenon, which results in a pink, yellow, or slightly bluish, dome-shaped, fluctuant mass. The vast majority of this form of mucocele occur on the lower lip. Another type of mucocele is the mucous retention cyst, or ranula, which occurs in the buccal mucosa and on the floor of the mouth.[20] Histologically, mucoceles show a collection of mucus surrounded by fibrosis, foamy macrophages, and neutrophils. Ductular epithelium lines mucous retention cysts. The treatment of both types of mucocele is surgical excision. Care must be taken to include adjacent minor salivary gland tissue in addition to the damaged gland.

Fibroma. The fibroma is the most common oral mucosal lesion and represents a hyperplastic response to trauma (Fig. 138–2). Clinically, fibromas are firm, exophytic, nodular or pedunculated lesions covered by normal pink mucosa, most commonly seen in areas subjected to trauma (e.g., lips and tongue).[21] Histologically, the fibroma shows a dense, fibrous connective tissue core covered by normal or hyperkeratotic epithelium. Occasionally there may be calcifications, especially in gingival lesions, and sparse giant cells.[22] Treatment of fibromas consists of simple excision. Recurrence is rare unless the traumatic cause of the lesion is not eliminated.

Vascular Lesions. Hemangiomas and vascular malformations are frequently encountered in the oral cavity. Hemangiomas can be classified into capillary (red appearing) or cavernous (purple appearing) types. Vascular malformations, including the lymphangioma, include the capillary, venous, lymphatic, and arterial types. They occur most often in the tongue, lips, and cheek, where they may affect function. If superficial, they will be raised, red-blue nodules, while deep lesions have nondistinctive features until aspirated. A bruit or thrill is not evident.

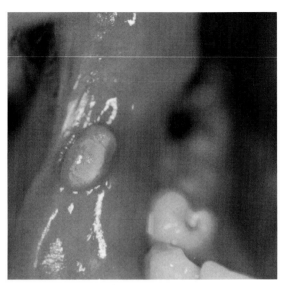

FIGURE 138–2. The oral fibroma is a reactive phenomenon found commonly on mucosa subjected to trauma.

Vascular malformations will range from life-threatening, large arterial abnormalities to innocuous, small venous ectasias. Like the hemangioma, lesions may be present at birth or arise thereafter. Clinically, vascular malformations will vary from pink to purple. The soft tissue lesions will be compressible, and many will exhibit a thrill. The Valsalva maneuver may cause the lesion to increase in size.[23]

Intraoral vessel ectasia and hemangiomas may be seen in a number of conditions, including Osler-Rendu-Weber syndrome, Sturge-Weber syndrome, Klippel-Trenaunay-Weber syndrome, blue rubber bleb nevus syndrome, and Maffucci's syndrome.

Hereditary Mucoepithelial Dysplasia. The oral lesions of this autosomal dominant disease arise in infancy and persist indefinitely.[24] The hard palate and gingiva display red macules or micropapules that are asymptomatic. Dyshesion and dyskeratosis seen histologically may be the result of a defect in the gap junction and desmosomal formation.[24] Associated findings include alopecia, follicular keratosis, and various cardiac and pulmonary disorders.

Mixed and Miscellaneous

Cowden's Disease. Oral lesions are present in virtually all cases, and Cowden's disease may occur with oral lesions unaccompanied by cutaneous tricholemmomas.[25] Papillomatosis, clinically characterized by a cobblestoning appearance of white and pink coalescing papules, occurs on the lips, tongue, palate, gingiva, and buccal mucosa. Histologically, these are benign fibromas that have a distinctive pattern. Other oral manifestations of Cowden's disease include a high-arched palate, fissured tongue, hypoplasia of the soft palate and uvula, and an increased incidence of caries and periodontal disease.[26]

Multiple Endocrine Neoplasia (Type 3) (see Chapter 175). The recognition of the oral features of this autosomal dominant condition should prompt an investigation for the presence of pheochromocytomas and medullary thyroid carcinomas. Oral mucosal neuromas are usually present at birth or develop shortly thereafter.[27] The lips are most commonly affected and are covered with flesh-colored papules resulting in their enlargement. The tongue and buccal mucosa are also frequently involved.

Histologically, these tumors are neural hamartomas consisting of myelinated and unmyelinated neuro-fibers.[27]

A high-arched palate is commonly observed in patients with multiple endocrine neoplasia.

Miescher-Melkersson-Rosenthal   Syndrome   and Cheilitis Granulomatosa. The Miescher-Melkersson-Rosenthal syndrome consists of a triad of recurrent orofacial swelling, relapsing facial paralysis, and fissured tongue. The complete triad, however, is found in only 10% to 20% of patients.[28] Cheilitis granulomatosa, described by Miescher in 1945, is an entity consisting of swelling of one or both lips and is considered an oligosymptomatic form of the syndrome.[29]

Labial swelling is often the initial sign and the most consistent feature of these conditions. The swelling develops suddenly and is often unilateral and asymmetrical. Recurrent, painless episodes are usual and increase in duration as the disease progresses. Intraoral involvement and swelling of the buccal mucosa, gingiva, and tongue are frequently observed and occasionally associated with erythema, erosions, and pain.

The facial paralysis may be the initial symptom in 30% to 50% of patients, although it may follow or occur concomitantly with labial swelling.[28] Facial swelling, paresthesias, and paralysis are usually unilateral and episodic, although they may be persistent.

Fissured tongue is found in approximately 50% of patients and may be associated with burning and swelling.[28] The onset of this condition occurs most commonly in the second and third decades of life and is more frequent among females.

Histologically, the classic features consist of small, noncaseating granulomas accompanied by edema, lymphangiectasia, and a perivascular lymphocytic infiltrate. However, in 40% to 50% of patients with clinical features of Miescher-Melkersson-Rosenthal syndrome, only nonspecific inflammation is noted, which has caused confusion regarding the etiology and epidemiology of this syndrome.[28]

Patients with orofacial swelling and histologic features demonstrating granulomatous inflammation should be evaluated for Crohn's disease and sarcoid. Although the oral manifestations of these diseases usually coincide with systemic symptoms, they may precede them. Rare identifiable causes of orofacial granulomatosis have included hypersensitivity reactions to cobalt[30] and monosodium glutamate.[31]

Because the etiology of Miescher-Melkersson-Rosenthal syndrome is obscure, various treatment regimens have been employed with multiple outcomes. Occasionally, dental foci of infection may be identified and, when corrected, result in marked improvement. Systemic and

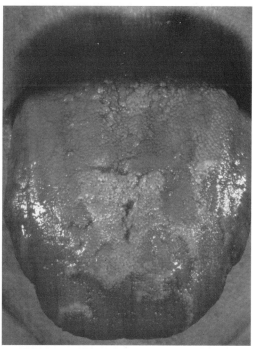

FIGURE 138–3. Geographic tongue: red areas devoid of papillae with white hyperkeratotic margins are characteristic of this condition in which the patterns may change daily.

intralesional corticosteroids are most commonly employed and produce adequate results in the majority. Systemic therapies with clofazimine, minocycline, and hydroxychloroquine sulfate have been reported to be beneficial.[28]

Geographic Tongue (Benign Migratory Glossitis). Geographic tongue (Fig. 138–3) has been estimated to occur in about 2% of the general population and is often associated with a fissured tongue and sometimes psoriasis.[32]

It presents as irregular areas of denuded, atrophic mucosa on the dorsum and lateral borders of the tongue. These areas are outlined by white or yellow elevated margins. In a cycle of healing and recurrence, the lesions migrate over the surface of the tongue, assuming constantly new configurations, thus leading to the term *migratory glossitis*. Histologically, the glossitis demonstrates a loss of the filiform papillae with marginal hyperkeratosis. There may be an intense inflammatory cell infiltrate. Also noted is microabscess formation near the epithelial surface, a feature noted in psoriasis.[43] Some patients undergo spontaneous regression. Symptomatic patients may respond to topical steroids, such as dexamethasone (Decadron).

Hairy Tongue. Clinically, a matted layer appears on the dorsal surface of the tongue due to hypertrophy of the filiform papillae and a lack of normal desquamation. The papillae appearing as elongated hairs may be yellow, white, brown, and often black, depending on their staining by foods, tobacco, medication, and organisms.

Hairy tongue is frequently seen in patients who have undergone radiation therapy for head and neck malignancies. It also occasionally follows the use of broad-spectrum antibiotics when they are employed for an unrelated infection. In both circumstances, overgrowth of *Candida albicans* and chromogenic bacteria may occur and may be causative factors.

The disorder is rarely symptomatic. The lesions will generally disappear when the tongue is brushed with a toothbrush causing desquamation of the papillae. Topical antifungal therapy and topical retinoids may hasten resolution.

Tori. Tori are simple, bony protuberances occurring on either the upper or lower jaw (Fig. 138–4). They are frequently seen in the midline of the hard palate and on the medial aspect of the lower jaw under the tongue. They occur in both sexes and are usually discovered in early adulthood. They may also be called exostoses and are bony hard and covered by normal, albeit thinned mucosa. No treatment is indicated unless the entity interferes with function. Tori are formed by normal cortical bone.

Burning Mouth Syndrome. Burning mouth syndrome may be associated with a large number of disorders, including infection, vitamin deficiency, and neurologic and metabolic disorders. Most cases, however, are found in postmenopausal women. The cause is unclear, and two studies conducted by Gorsky and colleagues have indicated that burning mouth syndrome may be a functional disorder.[33] Although the entire mouth may be involved, patients complain predominantly of tongue burning. There is associated xerostomia in up to a third of the cases. Clinically, the tissues appear normal. The only effective treatment for burning mouth syndrome is the use of mood-altering medications. Some cases resolve spontaneously.

Amyloid. Oral cavity involvement occurs in 20% to 40% of patients with systemic amyloidosis.[34] Both primary and secondary amyloidosis exhibit oral changes, and rarely the disease may be localized to the oral cavity. The most characteristic oral feature of systemic amyloidosis is macroglossia resulting from amyloid deposits in the tongue. Indentations along the lateral border of the tongue are frequently noted, as are nodules and ulcer-

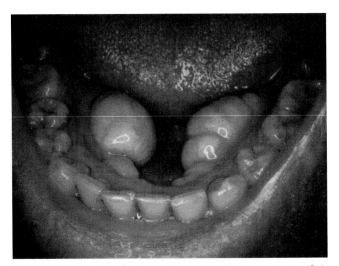

FIGURE 138–4. Mandibular tori present as bony exostoses of the lingual mandibular ridge and require no treatment.

ations on the dorsal surface. The gingiva is also commonly affected, and petechiae and purpura similar to periorbital cutaneous lesions are encountered.

Xerostomia. The causes of dry mouth are as diverse as the clinical signs and symptoms that result from this condition. Xerostomia is prevalent in the elderly. This may in part be due to reduced saliva production by the submandibular and minor salivary glands, although the saliva flow rate is not diminished by the aging process.[35] Systemic disorders and their therapies are more likely to produce dry mouth. These include diabetes and the use of diuretics or drugs with anticholinergic actions. Chemotherapy for malignancies, radiation therapy for head and neck cancers, and immunosuppressive agents, as well as sarcoid and Sjögren's syndrome all may produce salivary gland dysfunction. Salivary gland disease may also result from direct human immunodeficiency virus (HIV) infection characterized by persistent glandular enlargement and secretory hypofunction.[36]

Aside from a dry or burning sensation of the oral mucosa, patients with xerostomia may complain of difficulty eating, diminution of taste acuity, and discomfort when speaking. Additionally, there is an increased rate of mucosal infections, dental caries, periodontal disease, and intolerance of dentures. Sugar-free, flavored chewing gum can stimulate salivation and reduce caries by neutralizing acid production in dental plaque. Saliva substitutes are beneficial, as are sialagogues. Pilocarpine, which has been studied extensively as a therapy for xerostomia, promotes salivation as long as there is sufficient exocrine tissue capable of being stimulated.[37]

Gingival Hyperplasia. Gingival hyperplasia may result from the chronic administration of drugs such a phenytoin, cyclosporine, nifedipine, and diltiazem. Poor oral hygiene causes a greater degree of gingival enlargement. Hereditary disorders (fibromatosis gingivae) may uncommonly cause gingival enlargement in childhood and may interfere with tooth eruption. Acute periodontal disease results in erythematous, hemorrhagic enlargement, while chronic disease is manifest by hyperplastic pink gingiva. Mouth breathers frequently display enlarged maxillary gingiva. Inflammatory gingival hyperplasia may be noted during pregnancy or may be a manifestation of a systemic illness such as leukemia.[38] An allergic contact stomatitis to gum, dentrifices, and other agents may result in plasma cell gingivostomatitis characterized by bright red, swollen, and edematous gingiva.

PREMALIGNANT AND MALIGNANT ORAL DISORDERS

Leukoplakia and Erythroplakia. *Leukoplakia* and *erythroplakia* are descriptive terms for white and red plaques, respectively, that cannot be scraped off.[39] Common causes of leukoplakia include chronic irritation from smoking or chewing tobacco, sharp dental restorations, and cheek biting. Fewer than 10% of biopsy specimens of leukoplakia will reveal dysplasia or carcinoma. Leukoplakia that is verrucous and nodular, speckled with erythroplakia, or recurring in locations prone to the development of oral carcinoma (floor of mouth) is more likely to undergo malignant transformation.[40] Most erythroplakic lesions, when examined histologically, reveal carcinoma in situ or frank carcinoma. Thus, all red plaques should be viewed with suspicion and subjected to biopsy.

Dyskeratosis Congenita (see Chapter 175). The oral findings in this genodermatosis are characterized by oral leukoplakia. The onset of vesicles and ulcerations appears between the age of 5 and 15 and is followed by diffuse white patches and plaques. Involvement of the tongue and buccal mucosa is especially common and is almost always present by age 20. The hyperkeratotic lesions have a high propensity to undergo malignant change, frequently with fatal results.[41] Histologic examination of oral lesions reveals slight thickening of the epithelium with atypia of keratinocytic nuclei, and hyperkeratosis and parakeratosis. Cytokeratin profiles of tissue biopsy specimens from oral lesions reveal an unusually immature and disturbed state of tissue differentiation, which may indicate early malignant transformation.[42] Caries and severe gingival and periodontal destruction with tooth abnormalities have also been reported in patients with dyskeratosis congenita.[43]

Nicotine Stomatitis. Patients who smoke pipes or cigars may occasionally develop this characteristic alteration of the oral mucosa. Multiple white papules with tiny, red, depressed craters coalesce on the palate, producing fissuring and a wrinkled, irregular surface. The red dots represent dilated and sometimes occluded orifices of accessory palatal salivary glands surrounded by a keratotic surface epithelium.[44] In reverse smokers, who hold the burning end of a cigarette inside the mouth, dysplasia and foci of squamous cell carcinoma are not uncommonly found. Most lesions will regress with cessation of smoking, but careful follow-up is needed.

Cheilitis Glandularis. This uncommon disorder is characterized by enlargement of the lower lip, which eventually results in eversion. Excessive mucus secretion of the salivary glands occurs from orifices, which appear red and swollen. With advanced disease, the lip becomes painful and permanently enlarged. Ulcerations, which heal with scarring and secondary bacterial infections, eventually result in ectropion of the lip. The etiology of this condition is unknown and perhaps multifactorial. Actinic damage, bacterial infections, use of tobacco products, and oral habits have all been implicated as causes. Some authors consider this condition premalignant since a number of squamous cell carcinomas have arisen in cheilitis glandularis.[45] Intralesional corticosteroids may be helpful, but if the etiology is believed to be secondary to actinic damage, then a vermilionectomy is warranted.

Squamous Cell and Verrucous Carcinoma. Data from the National Institutes of Health indicate that approximately 30,000 people in the United States are diagnosed with oral cancer each year, an incidence of 7.7 cases per 100,000. The tongue appeared to lead the sites of involvement with 30% of reported cases, followed by lip (17.4%) and floor of the mouth (16.4%). Tobacco and alcohol, especially in combination, are major causes of oral carcinoma. Excessive exposure to ultraviolet light is now also known to be a factor.[46]

The classic appearance of a painless, nonhealing ulcer with elevated, rolled margins and induration is not always seen, especially in the early stages of the disease. Small areas of erythema, erosion, hyperkeratosis, or leukoplakia, if persistent, should be biopsied. Toluidine blue staining and exfoliative cytology aids in the identification of dysplastic areas.

Treatment of oral squamous cell carcinoma is complex and controversial. Mainstays of treatment (radiation therapy, chemotherapy, surgery, or combinations thereof) have failed to significantly improve outcome over the past 10 years. Progress has, however, been made in reconstruction for patients having ablative surgery.

Oral verrucous carcinoma is a slow-growing malignancy characterized by a white, warty, friable lesion with little tendency to metastasize. It is frequently observed in patients who chew tobacco and is seen most commonly on the alveolar ridge and buccal mucosa.

Kaposi's Sarcoma. In contrast to the classic and African forms of Kaposi's sarcoma, intraoral involvement is frequent in patients with acquired immunodeficiency syndrome (AIDS). As many as 50% of patients with AIDS may have oral involvement, and in 25% of cases the oral lesions represent the initial sign of HIV infection.[47] Oral Kaposi's sarcoma may be associated with an advanced stage of AIDS, since the patients have a CD4-positive cell count below 200/mm^3.[48]

Clinically, purple, blue, and red macules appear in the early stages, and darkly pigmented nodules and plaques occur in the advanced stages. As the tumors enlarge, they can cause interference in speech and mastication and result in episodes of hemorrhage and obstruction. Most lesions occur on the palate and gingiva. Multiple lesions are common, and nonpigmented tumors of oral Kaposi's sarcoma have been reported, requiring a high index of suspicion. Histologically, early macular lesions are composed of endothelial-lined vessels with jagged shapes, and late nodular lesions are dominated by spindle cells with interspersed, blood-filled clefts.

The therapeutic modalities used to manage oral Kaposi's sarcoma have varying degrees of success. Radiation therapy, laser surgery, systemic chemotherapy, immunotherapy, and intralesional vinblastine are the most commonly employed.[49] The use of 3% sodium tetradecyl sulfate, a sclerosing agent, was shown to be most effective in lesions less than 2.5 cm in size with no adverse consequences.[50]

Cutaneous T-Cell Lymphoma (see Chapter 158). Oral lesions are rare in cutaneous T-cell lymphomas, with only 30 cases reported worldwide. Involvement occurs late in the course of the disease, and most patients die within 3 years of the diagnosis of oral lesions.[51] Ulcerated, solitary plaques or tumors occur most commonly on the gingiva, palate, and tongue. Histologically, a dense, mixed cellular infiltrate with atypical lymphocytes and Pautrier microabscesses is noted. Local irradiation of oral lesions is usually effective, but recurrences can occur.

Oral Malignant Melanoma (see Chapter 151). Oral melanomas are rare and have been reported to constitute a range as broad as 0.1% to 8% of all melanomas.[1] A high incidence occurs in Japanese, Ugandans, southwestern

Native Americans, and Latinos. Oral melanomas occur most frequently in the fourth to seventh decades of life, and most studies support equal sexual predilection.

The lesions arise in the palate and maxillary gingiva in more than two thirds of cases. Asymptomatic oral pigmentation at the site of oral melanomas is noted before diagnosis by approximately one third of all patients. These pigmented macules and plaques represent the radial growth phase of the tumor and often go unrecognized for months or years before tumor invasion.[52]

Clinically, oral melanomas appear as asymptomatic pigmented macules, patches, plaques, and nodules. As they enlarge, they may cause ulceration, bleeding, pain, and loosening of teeth. Amelanotic lesions account for 5% to 15% of all oral melanomas.

Histologically, melanoma of the oral cavity is similar to its cutaneous counterpart, and especially resembles melanomas on acral skin in its growth pattern. Intraepithelial melanoma tends to have cells with angulated, hyperchromatic nuclei in the basal layer of the epithelium, and invasive melanoma of the oral cavity is often composed of spindled melanocytes.

The dismal prognosis of patients with a median survival of 1 to 2 years after diagnosis is partly due to patients' delayed recognition of signs of early disease and delayed diagnosis by physicians. The detection of oral melanomas with advanced Breslow depth of invasion and the difficulty of achieving wide radical excisions because of the anatomically imposed limitations of the oral cavity also account for the high mortality.

All oral pigmented lesions should be viewed with suspicion, and biopsies are indicated when the clinical diagnosis is uncertain.

Leukemia. Oral lesions occur commonly in all forms of leukemia. During the acute stage, oral lesions may be found in up to 90% of patients and are manifested as petechiae and ulceration of the mucosa. The most constant oral feature, however, is gingival hyperplasia, characterized by swollen, edematous, and deeply red gums that bleed easily. Oral necrosis and extensive periodontal disease with premature loss of teeth are not unusual. Patients with monocytic leukemia exhibit the highest frequency of oral disease, and thus children, whose leukemia is most commonly of the acute lymphocytic type, are less frequently affected.[53]

ULCERATIVE DISORDERS OF THE ORAL CAVITY

Oral ulcers result from a wide variety of causes. Traumatic ulcers are commonly observed and may be easily diagnosed by the history preceding their onset. For example, sharp dental restorations, cheek biting, hot foods, aspirin and other chemical burns, denture irritation, and iatrogenic injury resulting from a dental procedure may produce oral ulcerations that heal rapidly. Allergic contact stomatitis is commonly due to toothpaste, chewing gum, oral hygiene rinses, cinnamates. Stomatitis medicamentosa resulting from systemic medications, most commonly antibiotics, chemotherapy, and cardiac drugs, presents as erythema, blisters, and erosions. Those ulcer-

ations that persist require a biopsy to exclude other causes, such as malignancies.

Recurrent Aphthous Stomatitis. Recurrent aphthous stomatitis, also known as canker sores, is the most common cause of oral ulcerations, affecting approximately 25% of the general population. Although the disorder is observed during childhood and increases into adulthood, the severity of recurrent aphthous stomatitis decreases with aging. Clinically, recurrent aphthous stomatitis has been divided into three types.[54] Minor aphthous ulcerations are the most common form, accounting for 80% of cases. Episodes of single or multiple ulcerations, generally less than 1.0 cm, develop recurrently, with healing of lesions occurring in 7 to 14 days. Pain is minimal to moderate, and scarring does not usually occur. Major aphthous ulcerations (Sutton's disease), which comprise 10% of all cases, are characterized by larger and deeper ulcerations greater than 2.0 cm. The pain that results is usually severe, and healing, which takes 2 to 4 weeks, often leads to scarring. Herpetiform aphthae, accounting for the remaining 10% of cases, are similar to minor aphthae, with the exception of exhibiting large numbers (10–100) of 1- to 2-mm ulcerations.

Recurrent aphthous stomatitis occurs on the nonkeratinized mucosal surfaces. Whereas minor aphthae are observed most commonly on the labial and buccal mucosa, tongue, and floor of the mouth, major aphthae frequently involve the soft palate and oropharynx. There are considerable overlapping clinical features of these types of recurrent aphthous stomatitis.

The severity of aphthous ulcerations varies greatly among affected patients. Some may experience only a few recurrent episodes, while others may develop continuous and debilitating ulcerations. Many factors may induce recurrences, including trauma and possibly stress, illnesses, and menses. Nicotine in cigarettes and smokeless tobacco may reduce the prevalence of recurrences.[55]

The etiology of recurrent aphthous stomatitis remains obscure. The prevalence of aphthae is increased by a positive family history, and some investigators have demonstrated an association with HLA-B12 and HLA-B51.[56] An infectious etiology with various bacterial and viral agents has been suggested, but there have been no studies that have conclusively demonstrated this as the cause. An immune-mediated mechanism is strongly supported by numerous investigations[57, 58] and the response of recurrent aphthous stomatitis to immunosuppressive agents.

Histologically, the ulcerative stage consists of a nonspecific inflammatory infiltrate and mononuclear cells and polymorphonuclear leukocytes. Focal necrosis of the epithelium, an increased number of plasma cells, eosinophils, and mast cells may be seen.

Recurrent ulcerations may be a manifestation of a systemic illness. Various nutritional deficiencies of iron, folate, and vitamin B_{12} may be found, and correction results in clinical improvement.[59] Patients with inflammatory bowel disease, AIDS, systemic lupus erythematosus, and viral infections may all exhibit ulcerations that are clinically indistinguishable from recurrent aphthous stomatitis. Patients with Behçet's disease or complex aphthosis (oral and genital ulcerations) demonstrate ulcers identical to recurrent aphthous stomatitis, and the three disease processes may actually represent a spectrum of one disease.

The diagnosis of recurrent aphthous stomatitis is made clinically and supported by a history of spontaneously healing ulcerations. When other causes are suspected, in atypical cases, or when clinical differentiation from vesicular or erosive disease cannot be made, a biopsy should be performed.

No treatment of recurrent aphthous stomatitis is uniformly effective or results in permanent remission. Over-the-counter preparations containing benzocaine (Oragel) or tannic acids (Zilactin) may be all that is needed for many patients. Topical medications, including viscous lidocaine and tetracycline, may alleviate the discomfort, as do potent topical corticosteroids if therapy is initiated at the onset of lesion formation. In severe cases, systemic therapy with antibiotics, colchicine, and dapsone may be beneficial. Patients with AIDS and major aphthae respond well to thalidomide.[60] Prednisone should be reserved for acute exacerbations, since relapses occur when it is discontinued.

Oral Lichen Planus (see Chapter 20). Oral lichen planus is as common as cutaneous psoriasis, affecting approximately 1% of the general population. Only 10% to 20% of patients with oral lesions will exhibit cutaneous evidence of lichen planus, whereas more than two thirds of patients examined for cutaneous lichen planus will demonstrate oral lesions (Fig. 138–5). Oral lichen planus affects women twice as frequently as men and occurs most commonly during the fifth to sixth decades of life. It is a chronic disorder, and spontaneous, long-term remissions are almost nonexistent.

Clinically, the oral lesions can be divided into three groups[61]: reticular (white lesions appearing linear, papular, or as plaques), atrophic (erythematous lesions), and erosive (ulcerative and bullous lesions). Reticular lesions are easily recognized and require no therapy since they are generally asymptomatic. Atrophic and erosive oral

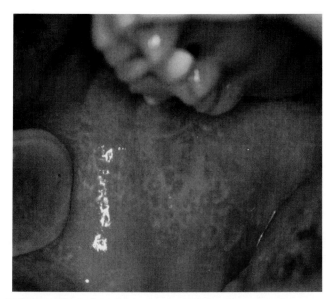

FIGURE 138–5. Oral lichen planus: white, reticulated lesions on the buccal mucosa are the most consistent finding.

lichen planus can be a source of significant pain and morbidity and should be differentiated from other oral vesiculoerosive diseases. Several morphologic types of oral lesions frequently coexist in different locations of the oral cavity.

Any mucosal surface may be involved, including the larynx and esophagus, but lesions have a predilection for the buccal mucosa and tongue. Gingival lesions present in women should prompt a search for lichen planus lesions on the vulva and vagina. Patients may rarely present with a desquamative gingivitis as the sole manifestation of the disease.

Lichenoid stomatitis represents a heterogeneous group of disorders. In some patients, the oral lesions are a result of a drug reaction, most commonly to nonsteroidal antiinflammatory or antihypertensive agents. In others, resolution of oral lesions may occur after replacement of amalgam restorations in patients allergic to mercury compounds.[62] In the majority, classified as oral lichen planus, the etiology is obscure, although there is strong evidence that an immunologically mediated process is pathogenic. The association of diabetes with oral lichen planus is supported by the results of several studies but disputed by most authors.

Histologically, liquefication degeneration of the basal cell layer is accompanied by a band-like lymphocytic infiltrate in the upper submucosa. Parakeratosis is common, as are cytoid bodies within the lamina propria. These histologic features can best be demonstrated from a white, reticular lesion. Immunofluorescent findings, which are nonspecific but help exclude other diagnoses, include fibrin deposition at the mucosal-submucosal junction and the nonspecific absorption of immunoreactants by cytoid bodies.

Malignant transformation of oral lichen planus has been reported to occur with frequencies ranging from 0.4% to 5.6%.[63] Considerable controversy exists regarding these figures and the premalignant nature of oral lichen planus. Failure to recognize lichenoid dysplasia (i.e., band-like lymphocytic infiltrates beneath an epithelium that shows disorderly maturation and keratinocytes with atypical nuclei) as a distinct histologic entity and precursor or oral carcinoma may account for some of the confusion.[64]

All therapy for oral lichen planus is palliative. Potent topical corticosteroids applied to the oral mucosa supplemented with intralesional corticosteroids, especially for erosive lesions, are the most frequently employed agents. In those patients whose disorder is refractory to this regimen, topical and systemic retinoids and cyclosporine may induce clinical remission. Hydroxychloroquine sulfate[65] or combinations of retinoids and corticosteroids[60] have been reported to be beneficial in open trials.

Pemphigus (see Chapter 74). The recognition of oral lesions in patients with pemphigus vulgaris and pemphigus vegetans is of paramount importance, since they are the initial manifestation of these diseases in over 75% of cases. Oral lesions develop insidiously, often contributing to a delay of 6 to 12 months in the correct diagnosis. Although intact blisters may occur, they are rarely observed, since they rupture rapidly and form large erosions with ragged borders. Pain, bleeding, swelling, and difficulty in mastication develop as the disease progresses. Any mucosal surface may be involved, but the soft palate is affected in over 80% of cases, followed in frequency by the buccal mucosa and tongue.[66] The oral lesions of pemphigus vegetans are similar to those of pemphigus vulgaris, although in the former a serpiginous pattern of pustules occurring on the palate and gingiva and a cerebriform tongue have been described.[67] Oral lesions are rare in pemphigus foliaceus and pemphigus erythematosus.

The clinical diagnosis of pemphigus should always be confirmed by direct and indirect immunofluorescence. A wedge biopsy from a single oral perilesional site provides tissue for both routine light microscopy and direct immunofluorescence.[68] Immunoglobulins predominantly of the IgG type are bound to the intercellular spaces of the oral mucosa.

Most patients with oral lesions can have their disease controlled with corticosteroids at doses of 40 to 120 mg per day, depending on the severity of the lesions. Some patients may require additional immunosuppressive therapy with azathioprine, cyclophosphamide, oral and parenteral gold, plasmapheresis, or cyclosporine. Potent topical corticosteroids are of great benefit. However, with the chronic use of these agents, treatment of secondary candidiasis becomes necessary. Serial indirect immunofluorescent titers are valuable in monitoring the response to therapy for oral lesions.[65]

Paraneoplastic Pemphigus (see Chapter 74). Paraneoplastic pemphigus is an autoimmune mucocutaneous disorder associated with an underlying neoplasm.[69] Oral involvement is often severe and characterized by widespread erosions and hemorrhagic crusting of the lips. Although systemic corticosteroids and other immunosuppressive agents have been employed for the mucocutaneous lesions, patients are usually refractory to therapy.

Pemphigoid (see Chapters 75 and 76). Oral lesions in bullous pemphigoid occur in 10% to 30% of reported series. Usually, small bullae and ulcerations are observed and, unlike pemphigus, are rarely the initial presenting features.

Oral manifestations of cicatricial pemphigoid (benign mucous membrane pemphigoid) are almost always encountered, and the disease may be confined entirely to the oral mucosa.[70] Desquamative gingivitis characterized by erythema, bleeding, swelling, and ulceration of the gums is the most common and characteristic presentation.[71] Nongingival involvement is frequent and appears as bullae and ulcerations.

Physicians and dentists often fail to recognize the oral manifestations and mistakenly attribute the gingival findings to poor oral hygiene. A definitive diagnosis of cicatricial pemphigoid requires a positive direct immunofluorescence test, since routine histology often yields nondiagnostic results. The technique that utilizes detached gingival epithelium obtained by rubbing an erythematous, nonulcerated surface procures mucosal tissue for direct immunofluorescence.[72] A positive test will reveal deposits of immunoglobulins and complement components on the basilar pole of the basal epithelial cells, most commonly C3 and IgG.

Localized oral disease may be treated with potent topical and intralesional corticosteroids. When these agents fail to control the diseases, systemic corticosteroids may need to be administered. Dapsone, azathioprine, and cyclophosphamide are often employed in more severe cases and act as steroid-sparing agents.

Epidermolysis Bullosa (see Chapter 78). Oral involvement is common in all forms of inherited epidermolysis bullosa, as reported in detail by Wright and colleagues.[73] Patients with recessive dystrophic epidermolysis bullosa have the highest frequency of oral disease (90%–100%) and the most severe involvement. In addition to widespread oral ulcerations, intraoral scarring often results in complete vestibular obliteration, ankyloglossia, and microstomia. Although 90% of patients with dominant dystrophic epidermolysis bullosa exhibit oral lesions, scarring does not occur. Patients with junctional epidermolysis bullosa and epidermolysis bullosa simplex demonstrate ulcerations frequently (90% and 50%, respectively). Intraoral milia are present in all major epidermolysis bullosa categories, most prevalently in the dystrophic form.

All therapies for epidermolysis bullosa are palliative. Minimizing chemical and physical oral trauma may reduce the frequency of oral blisters. Patients with recessive dystrophic epidermolysis bullosa are at an increased risk for the development of tongue carcinomas and should undergo routine oral examinations.

Lupus Erythematosus (see Chapter 24). Oral ulceration is one of the criteria for the diagnosis of systemic lupus erythematosus. Ulcers occur in 20% to 25% of patients with systemic lupus erythematosus, most commonly on the hard palate, and are associated with active systemic disease.[74] The lesions are usually asymptomatic. The histology of mucosal ulcerations is an interface reaction similar to that seen in cutaneous lesions of systemic lupus erythematosus. Patients with systemic lupus also manifest oral discoid lupus lesions more so than oral ulcerations.[75] These are clinically characterized by patches of erythema with white striae at the periphery and show identical histologic features as discoid lesions of the skin. Nonspecific erythema accompanied by edema and petechial reddening of the hard palate is the most frequent oral finding in patients with systemic lupus erythematosus.

Patients with discoid lupus erythematosus exhibit oral discoid lesions in approximately 25% of cases.[76] These are observed mainly on the buccal mucosa and vermilion border, although any mucosal surface may be involved. The lesions are chronic, and they are often asymptomatic.

Direct immunofluorescence studies from oral lesions correspond to lesional skin biopsy specimens from patients with systemic lupus erythematosus, and nonlesional oral mucosal changes are similar to those obtained from non–sun-exposed skin.

Topical corticosteroids are useful in alleviating the discomfort when oral ulcerations and discoid lesions are painful. Systemic therapy with antimalarial agents and other immunosuppressive agents is of greater value when needed.

Erythema Multiforme (see Chapter 22). The oral lesions in this mucocutaneous disorder usually occur simultaneously with skin lesions.[77] In general, the more severe the cutaneous disease, the higher the likelihood that oral mucous membranes are affected.

Oral lesions are characterized by diffuse areas of erythema and bullae, which rapidly appear and rupture, forming ulcerations. A distinctive, whitish gray pseudomembrane of necrotic epithelium covers the ulcerations. Hemorrhagic crusting of the lips and severe oral pain causing inability to eat or swallow are features of erythema multiforme major. The oral cavity almost always displays widespread erosions in toxic epidermal necrolysis.

Histologically, oral lesions and cutaneous lesions of erythema multiforme are identical.

Topical corticosteroids may hasten the resolution of oral lesions. Levamisole has been used to reduce the severity and frequency of oral lesions in patients with chronic or recurring erythema multiforme.[78] Additionally, extensive oral disease necessitates optimal oral hygiene to prevent secondary infections.

Dermatitis Herpetiformis and Linear IgA Disease (see Chapters 79 and 80). Vesicles and bullae, which rupture and result in superficial ulcerations, are the oral manifestations of dermatitis herpetiformis. Since the lesions are generally asymptomatic, a careful inspection of the oral cavity is required to detect these changes. Sites of oral trauma, including the buccal mucosa and tongue, are especially prone to develop oral ulcerations. In one study, 16 of 30 patients with dermatitis herpetiformis were found to exhibit enamel defects of the teeth similar to those observed in patients with celiac disease.[79]

The oral cavity is much more commonly affected in linear IgA disease than in dermatitis herpetiformis. Rarely is the oral cavity the initial site of presentation, although skin and mouth lesions usually occur simultaneously. Painful vesicles and erosions are frequently observed on any mucosal surface. Up to 15% of patients have gingival involvement, with clinical characteristics indistinguishable from cicatricial pemphigoid necessitating direct immunofluorescence studies.[80, 81] The oral lesions of dermatitis herpetiformis and linear IgA disease respond to treatment of skin lesions with sulfones.

Chronic Ulcerative Stomatitis with Stratified Epithelium-Specific Antinuclear Antibody. This entity is clinically and histologically similar to erosive lichen planus.[82] Both diseases demonstrate erosions, chronic stomatitis, or desquamative gingivitis. A distinctive immunofluorescence pattern from perilesional mucosa consisting of a particulate antinuclear antibody has been reported in all cases and is a necessary finding to establish this diagnosis.[83] The antinuclear antibody reacts predominantly with the lower third of the substrate epithelium and only on stratified epithelial substrates, such as esophagus of a monkey or guinea pig. Circulating antinuclear antibodies detected by indirect immunofluorescence are present in

high titers. Topical corticosteroids are of value, and in unresponsive cases hydroxychloroquine sulfate can be employed.

Angina Bullosa Hemorrhagica. This benign condition of the oral cavity occurs most commonly in the elderly. Blood-filled blisters appear rapidly and are seen predominantly at the junction of the hard and soft palate.[84] After several minutes or hours, the blisters spontaneously rupture to form ulcerations that heal without scarring. Patients with oral blood blisters have no underlying hematologic abnormalities. Although the exact etiology is unknown, many cases have been precipitated by trauma and some by the use of steroid inhalers.[85] No treatment is necessary, and recurrences are not uncommon.

Necrotizing Sialometaplasia. Necrotizing sialometaplasia is an uncommon, benign, inflammatory process of the salivary glands. Clinically, unilateral, painful, deep-seated ulcerations are observed in the majority of patients.[86] Approximately 70% of all cases occur on the hard and soft palate, although any mucosal site may be involved including the nasal cavity, maxillary sinus, and larynx.

Although a spectrum of histologic findings has been reported, frequent observations include acinar necrosis, squamous metaplasia of the ducts, pseudoepitheliomatous hyperplasia of the surface epithelium, and mucous pooling with granulation tissue.[86]

The exact etiology of necrotizing sialometaplasia is unknown, but it is believed that a traumatic episode causes compromised blood supply to salivary gland lobules, which results in ischemic necrosis or infarction.[87]

Necrotizing sialometaplasia is a benign, self-limited condition that heals spontaneously within 5 to 6 weeks. Unfortunately, misinterpreted biopsy specimens and unfamiliarity with the benign nature of this lesion often result in unnecessary surgical procedures.

Eosinophilic Ulcer of the Oral Mucosa. Eosinophilic ulcer of the oral mucosa, also known as traumatic granuloma and Rege Fede disease, is a benign reactive lesion. Clinically, the majority of lesions present as asymptomatic ulcerations with indurated borders, although nonulcerated submucosal masses have been reported.[88] Eosinophilic ulcers occur mostly on the tongue, followed by the buccal mucosa, and have a peak onset in the fifth to sixth decades of life.

Microscopically, a mixed, dense, cellular infiltrate composed of predominantly T lymphocytes and eosinophils extends from the ulcer base into skeletal muscle. This is accompanied by muscle degeneration, necrosis, and regenerative myocytes. Mitotically active, large mononuclear cells are characteristically observed in the infiltrate and have been defined as a mixture of CD68-positive macrophages, factor XIIIa-positive "dendrocytes," and S-100–positive connective tissue cells.[89] The pathogenesis of eosinophilic ulcer remains unknown, although trauma is believed to be an important etiologic factor.[88]

Spontaneous healing may take weeks to months and is hastened by the administration of either topical or systemic corticosteroids. Since eosinophilic ulcer of the oral mucosa may clinically and histologically mimic malignant neoplasms, recognition will prevent unnecessary surgical treatments.

Crohn's Disease. Oral involvement of patients with Crohn's disease occurs in approximately 15% of patients, with a greater prevalence in young, adolescent males.[90] Clinically, diffuse swelling of one or both lips identical to granulomatous cheilitis is the most constant oral feature. Mucosal cobblestoning of the buccal mucosa and lips, linear or extensive ulcerations indistinguishable from recurrent aphthous stomatitis, and mucosal tags are additional oral manifestations of Crohn's disease.[91] Oral lesions may occur simultaneously with, follow, or predate the appearance of intestinal lesions, with the latter occurring in 9 of 29 patients studied with oral Crohn's disease.[91] Histologically, oral Crohn's disease is characterized by a chronic, inflammatory cell infiltrate and noncaseating granulomas. Differentiation from other granulomatous lesions, including sarcoid and tuberculosis, can be achieved by histochemical stains and clinical and laboratory evaluation.

Oral Crohn's disease may require no therapy and undergo spontaneous remission. More commonly, pain produces significant morbidity and generally responds to systemic and topical corticosteroids. A significantly greater number of dental infections are observed in patients whose disease is active when compared with those whose disease is inactive.[92]

Pyostomatitis Vegetans. Pyostomatitis vegetans is considered to be a marker highly specific for inflammatory bowel disease.[93] In the majority of patients, bowel disease precedes the oral lesions and the severity of the oral disease parallels the activity of the gastrointestinal symptoms. In addition, 25% of patients with pyostomatitis vegetans have various liver diseases and several cases have been associated with Crohn's disease.[94]

Multiple, yellow pustules on an erythematous base coalesce to form the pathognomonic "snail track" appearance. Lesions show a predilection for the gingiva, buccal mucosa, and palate.[95] Oral vegetative nodules and hypertrophic gingiva may occur. Histologic features include intraepithelial and subepithelial abscesses containing eosinophils and neutrophils. A peripheral eosinophilia is found in more than half of the patients. Systemic and topical corticosteroids are most commonly employed, with generally poor results. Treatment of the underlying gastrointestinal disease will usually cause oral erosions to resolve.

Cyclic Neutropenia. In this uncommon disorder, oral aphthous-like ulcerations appear at regular intervals of 2 to 4 weeks accompanied by neutropenia in the peripheral blood and bone marrow.[96] Fever, malaise, gingivitis, and lymphadenopathy are often present and suggest the correct diagnosis. Although the cause is unknown, an immunologic defect has been postulated. Ulcerations respond to systemic corticosteroids, and an optimal oral hygiene program should be maintained to prevent secondary infection. A high index of suspicion is needed to establish this diagnosis in patients who have aphthous ulcerations with regular frequency.

Wegener's Granulomatosis (see Chapter 59). Oral lesions may be seen in as many as 60% of patients and may occasionally be the presenting sign of Wegener's granulomatosis.[97] The majority of patients will exhibit oral ulcerations on the buccal mucosa. A pathognomonic feature of oral Wegener's granulomatosis is the gingivitis that is commonly observed in the early stages of the disease. Painful and bleeding gingivitis starting in the interdental papillae progresses and results in exophytic, friable, and granular gingival tissue.[98] Biopsy specimens show a nonspecific inflammatory infiltrate, which may be accompanied with microabscesses and necrosis. The oral disease usually correlates with the systemic disease activity and resolves with treatment.

Graft-versus-Host Disease (see Chapter 19). Ulcerations are frequently noted and are accompanied by significant discomfort. *Candida*, herpes simplex virus, and oral microflora containing α-streptococci are sources of infection in bone marrow transplant recipients. Painful cytotoxic lesions that develop as a result of chemotherapy used as prophylaxis before transplantation are seen in approximately 40% of patients.[99] The elimination of T cells before the infusion of bone marrow has been shown to decrease the severity of oral mucosal lesions, diminish oral discomfort, and reduce nutritional deficiencies.[91]

Chronic graft-versus-host disease displays oral findings indistinguishable from oral lichen planus. However, biopsy specimens of oral mucosa from patients with chronic graft-versus-host disease exhibit a low number of infiltrating T lymphocytes when compared with those from patients with oral lichen planus.[100] Xerostomia is frequently noted early in the disease and may be a result of irradiation. Abnormalities in the salivary glands can be demonstrated by lip biopsy specimens, which also aid in establishing a diagnosis of chronic graft-versus-host disease.[101] Allogenic bone marrow transplant patients may show significant hypogeusia for salt and sour taste before clinical manifestations of oral graft-versus-host disease.[102]

Therapy with psoralens and ultraviolet A light, which has been shown to be effective for skin lesions of graft-versus-host disease, is also beneficial for oral lesions.[103]

INFECTIONS OF THE ORAL CAVITY

Viral Infections

A number of viral infections exhibit oral manifestations in which the oral cavity is often the initial site of involvement (Table 138–2).

Human Papillomavirus Infections. Human papillomavirus (HPV) has been associated with a number of oral lesions, including common warts, condylomata, focal epithelial hyperplasia, and precancerous and cancerous oral lesions.

WARTS. Oral verruca vulgaris are common lesions, especially in patients who exhibit extensive perioral warts. Single or multiple exophytic growths occur most often on the palate and lips. Oral warts may be extensive in immunocompromised patients and are a common oral manifestation of HIV infection. HPV-7, a genotype usually detected in butchers, has been identified in a large number of oral warts from patients with HIV infec-

TABLE 138-2. Viral Infections of the Oral Cavity

Infection	Virus	Oral Lesions	Location
Acute herpetic gingivostomatitis	Herpes simplex virus	Painful ulcerations, edema, and stomatitis	Interdental papilla first, then diffuse involvement
Herpangina	Coxsackievirus A	Multiple 1 to 2-mm shallow ulcers	Soft palate, uvula, tonsils, pharynx
Acute lymphonodular pharyngitis	Coxsackievirus A10	White, nonvesicular papules with surrounding erythema	Uvula, pharynx
Hand, foot, and mouth disease	Coxsackievirus A16; type B	1 to 3-mm vesicles that ulcerate	Any, but tongue and hard palate most common
Infectious mononucleosis	Epstein-Barr virus	Palatal petechiae, ulcerations, exudative pharyngitis, gingivitis	Soft palate, pharynx, tonsils
Chickenpox	Varicella	Painless vesicles that ulcerate	Palate, tongue, gingiva, buccal mucosa
Herpes zoster	Varicella	Painful unilateral ulcerations	Ulcers distributed along mandibular or maxillary division of trigeminal nerve
German measles	Rubella	Pinhead, red macules	Soft palate
Measles	Rubeola	Koplik spots (bright red macules with blue-white center)	Buccal mucosa opposite second molars, also on palate
Cytomegalovirus infection	Cytomegalovirus	Nonspecific oral ulcerations, gingival hyperplasia	Any gastrointestinal site, oral and esophageal common

tion.[104] Treatment is by excision, cryosurgery, or laser therapy.

Oral condylomata acuminata are believed to be much less common than verruca vulgaris. However, when patients with genital condylomata were examined for the presence of oral warts, a surprisingly large number (48%) were detected, predominantly by colposcopy.[105] Oral condylomata are transmitted by sexual contact or autoinoculation and occur most commonly on the lips and tongue. Recurrences are common, despite therapy with cryosurgery or excision.

CARCINOMA. The association of specific HPV genotypes with carcinoma of the anogenital region has been established. Although HPV has been recovered in precancerous and cancerous oral lesions,[106] its oncogenic potential is under investigation and remains unknown. The carcinogenicity of HPV may be greater in the oral cavity than elsewhere owing to the synergistic effects of other known oral carcinogens, including tobacco and alcohol.

FOCAL EPITHELIAL HYPERPLASIA (HECK'S DISEASE). Focal epithelial hyperplasia is an uncommon oral disorder that most commonly affects Native American children and adult Eskimos. Asymptomatic, multiple, soft papules and nodules occur on the lips, buccal mucosa, and tongue. A viral etiology for Heck's disease has been substantiated by the high percentage of cases demonstrating HPV-13 and HPV-32 in oral lesions.[107] In most cases, no therapy is required since the oral lesions regress spontaneously.

Herpes Simplex Virus Infections (see Chapter 121). Recurrent intraoral herpes simplex virus infection is an uncommon entity. Localized and grouped vesicles that ulcerate appear most often on the mucosa bound to bone, such as the hard palate and attached gingiva. In immunocompetent patients the lesions are mildly symptomatic and heal within 7 to 10 days, whereas in im-

munosuppressed patients the ulcers may be chronic. The combined effect of acyclovir and chlorhexidine mouthrinse (Peridex) may be beneficial in controlling intraoral herpetic infections.[108]

Bacterial

A number of bacterial infections demonstrate oral lesions (Table 138-3).

Mycotic (see Chapter 120)

Several of the systemic mycoses exhibit a high frequency of oral lesions that may assist in establishing their diagnoses. For example, in 50% of patients with disseminated histoplasmosis, painful oral nodules and ulcers are detected.[109] Thirty-six patients with oral lesions as the first sign of paracoccidioidomycosis have been described.[110] All had chronic, proliferative, mulberry-like, ulcerated lesions, most commonly on the gingiva and alveolar process. The vast majority of patients with oral mucormycosis have painful palatal ulcerations and demonstrate extension into adjacent vital structure.[111] In patients with AIDS, cryptococcosis is a major opportunistic infection and oral ulcerations and nodules occur.

Candidiasis and Related Disorders (see Chapter 119). *Candida* is demonstrated in the oral cavity of more than 50% of healthy persons. Therefore, it is imperative to differentiate between commensalism and mucosal disease. This can best be achieved by positive cytologic and culture results from patients demonstrating clinical features of candidiasis.

Some of the more common factors that predispose to the development of oral candidiasis include immunosuppression (AIDS, transplants, immunotherapy), malnutri-

TABLE 138–3. Oral Manifestations of Bacterial Infections

Infection	Organism	Oral Findings
Acute necrotizing ulcerative gingivitis	*Fusobacterium nucleatum; Borrelia vincentii*	Gingiva has characteristic punched-out and blunted interdental papillae that ulcerate, bleed, and are painful.
Noma	*Fusobacterium nucleatum; Borrelia vincentii*	In debilitated patients, gangrenous necrosis of the oral cavity may be fatal.
Leprosy	*Mycobacterium leprae*	Yellow-pink nodules that ulcerate or macroglossia occurs most commonly in the lepromatous form.
Tuberculosis	*Mycobacterium tuberculosis* and *M. bovis*	Oral lesions are rare and occur as chronic and nonspecific ulcers or nodules, most commonly on the tongue, pharynx, and gingiva.
Actinomycosis	*Actinomyces israelii*	Red nodules eventually form abscesses and sinus tracts over the cervical and submandibular regions.
Tularemia	*Francisella tularensis*	Painful, necrotic ulcers, and stomatitis
Gonorrhea	*Neisseria gonorrhoeae*	Ulcerations similar to oral erythema multiforme or herpetic stomatitis
Granuloma inguinale	*Calymmatobacterium granulomatis*	Ulcerations with or without genital lesions can occur; extensive scarring may limit mouth mobility.
Syphilis	*Treponema pallidum*	Primary: oral chancres are indurated ulcerations Secondary: mucous patches Tertiary: chronic interstitial glossitis and gummas

tion and debilitation, malignancy, dental prosthetic devices, antibiotic therapy, infancy, elderly and pregnancy, chronic oral diseases, xerostomia, and genetic and metabolic diseases. Oral candidiasis is an early and common manifestation of patients infected with HIV.

Clinically, candidiasis may appear in one of several forms, and the wide diversity can often make diagnosis difficult.[112] Thrush and pseudomembranous candidiasis are diagnosed by white, curd-like plaques, which can be partially removed. Atrophic candidiasis appears as mucosal erythema most frequently on the tongue and palate. Diffuse reddening of the hard palate in individuals who wear dentures continuously represents a form of atrophic candidiasis and has been termed *denture sore mouth*. Hyperplastic candidiasis may clinically present as leukoplakia and resemble squamous cell carcinoma, necessitating a biopsy.

Chronic mucocutaneous candidiasis is a rare entity with involvement of the mucous membranes, skin, and nails (see Chapter 119). Enamel defects are commonly observed.

Median rhomboid glossitis is characterized clinically by a smooth erythematous plaque on the posterior mid-dorsal surface of the tongue. Once considered to be a developmental defect, it is now recognized as a form of localized, chronic candidiasis.[113]

Angular stomatitis characterized by red, fissured crusts with or without ulceration at the labial commissures is a disorder with multiple causes. Infections with candidiasis and staphylococci have been demonstrated, especially in edentulous patients. Noninfectious causes include nutritional deficiencies, excessive salivation, and loss of vertical dimension in denture wearers, resulting in an overclosure of their bite.

The diagnosis of oral candidiasis is often made clinically and should be confirmed by cytology and culture.

Atrophic, ulcerative, and hyperplastic forms may be confused with other causes of stomatitis and neoplasia and may require biopsy.

Antifungal treatment for oral candidiasis consists of nystatin suspension (400,000–600,000 units four times a day swish and swallow) or clotrimazole troches (10 mg dissolved in the mouth five times daily). Chlorhexidine 0.12% (3 teaspoonfuls as a rinse and expectorate) is useful as maintenance therapy rather than as a first-line antimycotic agent. Systemic therapy with ketoconazole, fluconazole, or itraconazole is also commonly employed, especially in immunocompromised patients. Treatment with oral antifungal agents should extend beyond clinical resolution to minimize recurrences. It is essential to identify and correct predisposing causes leading to candidiasis.

Acquired Immunodeficiency Syndrome. Oral lesions are common at all stages of HIV infection (Table 138–4). Their recognition may lead to a positive diagnosis of AIDS, allowing early institution of therapy with antiretroviral agents.

Oral Hairy Leukoplakia. Oral hairy leukoplakia, described as an oral marker of HIV in 1984, represents one of the most common oral lesions in patients with AIDS. It is the first clinical sign of HIV infection in 6% of cases, and its prevalence in asymptomatic HIV-infected patients may be as high as 20%.[114] The presence of oral hairy leukoplakia in HIV-infected patients usually indicates severe immunodeficiency (helper T-cell reduction) and progression to AIDS.[115] The lesions may occur in immunocompromised patients who are HIV seronegative and rarely in healthy persons. Oral hairy leukoplakia is most likely caused by repeated direct infection of superficial epithelial cells by Epstein-Barr virus from saliva.[116]

Clinically, white patches and plaques that cannot be

**TABLE 138-4. Oral Manifestations of
Patients with AIDS**

Disorder	Examples
Candidiasis	Four variants: pseudomembranous, erythematous, hyperplastic, angular cheilitis; early manifestation present in 90% of patients with AIDS
Severe periodontal disease	Severe gingival erythema, extensive soft tissue necrosis, and destruction of alveolar bone predisposing to necrotic lesions that devastate adjacent oral mucosa
Aphthous ulcerations	Herpetiform and major aphthous ulcers greater than 0.5 cm most commonly on the soft palate and oropharynx
Malignancies	Oral Kaposi's sarcoma; aggressive, high-grade, non-Hodgkin's lymphomas; squamous cell carcinomas
Viral infections	Primary herpetic gingivostomatitis and intraoral herpes, varicella zoster, cytomegaloviral oral ulcers, human papillomavirus, and molluscum contagiosum
Fungal infections	Oral cryptococcosis, oral histoplasmosis, and oral geotrichosis
Miscellaneous	Parotid swelling and xerostomia, oral hyperpigmentation, and oral petechiae

Data from Scully C, Laskaris G, Pindborg J, et al. Oral manifestations of HIV infection and their management: I. More common lesions. II. Less common lesions. Oral Surg Oral Med Oral Pathol 1991;71:158-166; 167-171.

scraped off occur on the lateral margin of the tongue, frequently bilaterally. Involvement of the dorsal and ventral surfaces of the tongue and of other mucosal sites has been reported.

Histologically, oral hairy leukoplakia is characterized by acanthosis, hyperparakeratosis, and a band of ballooning cells resembling koilocytes in the upper third of the prickle cell layers. Nuclear inclusions that contain Epstein-Barr virus can be found in routinely processed material.

Oral hairy leukoplakia should be differentiated from leukoplakia, candidiasis, lichen planus, geographic tongue, white sponge nevus, and other conditions appearing as leukokeratosis. A presumptive diagnosis in HIV-infected patients may be corroborated by the clinical findings and histologic features showing intranuclear viral inclusions. In HIV-negative patients or when uncertainty exists, a definitive diagnosis requires identification of Epstein-Barr virus by electron microscopic, molecular, or immunocytochemical techniques.

Most patients require no therapy, since the lesions spontaneously remit. In those patients who are symptomatic, treatment with acyclovir or desciclovir, topical vitamin A analogues, and 25% podophyllum induces temporary remissions.[117]

Odontogenic-Cutaneous Fistula. Although the majority of tooth abscesses drain intraorally, on occasion chronic dental infections may result in a cutaneous fistula. These lesions, which occur most commonly on the chin and cheek, are asymptomatic, although patients often have a history of tooth pain or facial swelling before the onset of the fistula. The involved tooth is identified by probing the fistula under radiographic technique. Extraction of the infected tooth will result in resolution of the fistula.

References

1. Eisen D, Voorhees JJ. Oral melanoma and other pigmented lesions of the oral cavity. J Am Acad Dermatol 1991;24:527-537.
2. Weathers DR, Corio RL, Crawford BE, et al. The labial melanotic macule. Oral Surg 1976;42:196-205.
3. Page IR, Corio RL, Crawford BE, et al. The oral melanotic macule. Oral Surg 1977;44:219-226.
4. Ho KKL, Dervan P, O'Loughlin S, et al. Labial melanotic macule: A clinical, histopathologic, and ultrastructural study. J Am Acad Dermatol 1993;28:33-39.
5. Tomich CE, Zunt SI. Melanoacanthosis (melanoacanthoma of the oral mucosa). J Dermatol Surg Oncol 1990;16:231-236.
6. Sexton FM, Maize JC. Melanotic macules and melanoacanthomas of the lip: A comparative study with census of the basal melanocyte population. Am J Dermatopathol 1987;5:438-444.
7. Buchner A, Hansen LS. Pigmented nevi of the oral mucosa: A clinicopathologic study of 36 new cases and review of 155 cases from the literature: II. Analysis of 191 cases. Oral Surg 1987;63:676-682.
8. Veraldi S, Cavicchini S, Benelli C, et al. Laugier-Hunziker syndrome: A clinical, histopathologic, and ultrastructural study of four cases and review of the literature. J Am Acad Dermatol 1991;25:632-636.
9. Sedano HO, Gorlin RJ. Acanthosis nigricans. Oral Surg Oral Med Oral Pathol 1987;68:74-79.
10. Shafer W, Hine MK, Levy A. Developmental disturbances of oral and paraoral structures. In: A Textbook of Oral Pathology. Philadelphia: WB Saunders Co., 1983:22.
11. Lim J, Ng SK. Oral tetracycline rinse improves symptoms of white sponge nevus. J Am Acad Dermatol 1992;26:1003-1015.
12. Su WPD, Chun SI, Hammond DE, et al. Pachyonychia congenita: A clinical study of 12 cases and review of the literature. Pediatri Dermatol 1990;7:33-38.
13. Feinstein A, Friedman J, Schewach-Millet M. Pachyonychia congenita. J Am Acad Dermatol 1988;19:705-711.
14. Witkop CJ, Shankle CM, Graham JB. Hereditary benign intraepithelial dyskeratosis: Oral manifestations and hereditary transmission. Arch Pathol 1960;70:696-711.
15. Burge SM, Wilkinson JD. Darier-White disease: A review of the clinical features in 163 patients. J Am Acad Dermatol 1992;27:40-50.
16. Hubler WR. Lingual lesions of generalized pustular psoriasis: Report of five cases and a review of the literature. J Am Acad Dermatol 1984;11:1069-1076.
17. Morris LF, Phillips, CM, Binnie WH, et al. Oral lesions in patients with psoriasis: A controlled study. Cutis 1992;19:339-344.
18. Daley TD, Nartey NO, Wysocki GP. Pregnancy tumor: An analysis. Oral Surg Oral Med Oral Pathol 1991;72:196-199.
19. Shafer W, Hine MK, Levy A. Physical and chemical injuries of the oral cavity. In: A Textbook of Oral Pathology. Philadelphia: WB Saunders Co., 1983:552-556.
20. Peterson LJ, Indresano AT, Marciani RD, et al. Prinicples of Oral and Maxillofacial Surgery. Philadelphia: JB Lippincott 1992:862-865.
21. Pindborg JJ. Atlas of Diseases of the Oral Mucosa. Philadelphia: WB Saunders Co., 1993:124.
22. Bhaskar SN. Synopsis of Oral Pathology. St. Louis. CV Mosby, 1981:485-489.
23. Kaban LB, Mulliken JB. Vascular anomalies of the maxillofacial region. J Oral Maxillofac Surg 1986;44:203-213.
24. Scheman AJ, Roy DJ, Witkop CJ, et al. Hereditary mucoepithelial dysplasia. J Am Acad Dermatol 1989;21:351-357.
25. Starink TM. Cowden's disease: Analysis of fourteen new cases. J Am Acad Dermatol 1984;11:1127-1140.
26. Swart JGN, Lekkas C, Allard RHB. Oral manifestations in Cow-

den's syndrome: Report of four cases. Oral Surg Oral Med Oral Pathol 1985;59:264–268.

27. Carney JA, Sizemore GW, Lovestedt SA. Mucosal ganglioneuromatosis, medullary thyroid carcinoma and pheochromocytoma: Multiple endocrine neoplasia type 2b. Oral Surg Oral Med Oral Pathol 1976;41:739–743.

28. Zimmer WM, Rogers RS, Reeve CM, et al. Orofacial manifestations of Melkersson-Rosenthal syndrome. Oral Surg Oral Med Oral Pathol 1992;74:610–619.

29. Allen CM, Camisa C, Hamzeh S, et al. Cheilitis granulomatosa: Report of six cases and review of the literature. J Am Acad Dermatol 1990;23:444–450.

30. Pryce DW, King CM. Orofacial granulomatosis associated with delayed hypersensitivity to cobalt. Clin Exp Dermatol 1990; 15:384–386.

31. Oliver AJ, Rich AM, Reade PC, et al. Monosodium glutamate–related orofacial granulomatosis. Oral Surg Oral Med Oral Pathol 1991;71:560–564.

32. Pogrel MA, Cram D. Intraoral findings in patients with psoriasis with a special reference to ectopic geographic tongue (erythema circinata). Oral Surg Oral Med Oral Pathol 1988;44:184–189.

33. Gorsky M, Silverman S, Chinn H. Clinical characteristics and management outcome in the burning mouth syndrome. Oral Surg Oral Med Oral Pathol 1991;44:192–195.

34. Al-Hashimi I, Drinnan AJ, Uthman AA, et al. Oral amyloidosis: Two unusual case presentations. Oral Surg Oral Med Oral Pathol 1987;63:586–591.

35. Persson RE, Izutsu KT, Truelove EL, et al. Differences in salivary flow rates in elderly subjects using xerostomatic medications. Oral Surg Oral Med Oral Pathol 1991;72:42–46.

36. Gillespie GM, Marino R. Oral manifestations of HIV infection: A Panamerican perspective. J Oral Pathol Med 1993;22:2–7.

37. Ferguson MM. Pilocarpine and other cholinergic drugs in the management of salivary gland dysfunction. Oral Surg Oral Med Oral Pathol 1993;75:186–191.

38. Shafer W, Hine MK, Levy A. Diseases of the periodontium. In: A Textbook of Oral Pathology. Philadelphia: WB Saunders Co., 1983:781–787.

39. Silverman S, Gorsky M, Lozado S. Oral leukoplakia and malignant transformation. Cancer 1984;53:563–568.

40. Browne RM, Potts AJC. Dysplasia in salivary gland ducts in sublingual leukoplakia and erythroplakia. Oral Surg Oral Med Oral Pathol 1986;62:44–49.

41. Cannell H. Dyskeratosis congenita. Br J Oral Surg 1971;9:8–20.

42. Ogden GR, Chishold DM, Leigh IM, et al. Cytokeratin profiles in dyskeratosis congenita: An immunocytochemical investigation of lingual hyperkeratosis. J Oral Pathol Med 1992;21:353–357.

43. Yavuzyilmaz E, Yamalik N, Yetgin S, et al. Oral-dental findings in dyskeratosis congenita. J Oral Pathol Med 1992;21:280–284.

44. Reddy CR, Kameswari VR, Ramulu PG. Histopathological study of stomatitis nicotina. Br J Cancer 1971;25:403–407.

45. Swerlick RA, Cooper PH. Cleilitis glandularis: A re-evaluation. J Am Acad Dermatol 1984;10:466–472.

46. Walton L, Masouredis C. The epidemiology of maxillofacial malignancy. Oral Maxillofac Surg Clin North Am 1993;5:189–198.

47. Ficarra G, Berson AM, Silverman S, et al. Kaposi's sarcoma of the oral cavity: A study of 134 patients with a review of the pathogenesis, epidemiology, clinical aspects, and treatment. Oral Surg Oral Med Oral Pathol 1988;66:543–550.

48. Feigal DW, Katz MH, Greenspan D, et al. The prevalence of oral lesions in HIV-infected homosexual and bisexual men: Three San Francisco epidemiological cohorts. AIDS 1991;5:519–525.

49. Epstein JB, Scully C. HIV infection: Clinical features and treatment of 33 homosexual men with Kaposi's sarcoma. Oral Surg Oral Med Oral Pathol 1991;71:38–41.

50. Lucatorto FM, Sapp JP. Treatment of oral Kaposi's sarcoma with a sclerosing agent in AIDS patients. Oral Surg Oral Med Oral Pathol 1993;75:192–198.

51. Sirois DA, Miller AS, Harwick RD, et al. Oral manifestations of cutaneous T-cell lymphoma. Oral Surg Oral Med Oral Pathol 1993;75:700–705.

52. Rapini RP, Golitz LE, Greer RO, et al. Primary malignant melanoma of the oral cavity: A review of 177 cases. Cancer 1985;55:1543–1551.

53. Driezen S, McCredie KB, Keating MJ, et al. Malignant gingiva and skin infiltrates in adult leukemia. Oral Surg Oral Med Oral Pathol 1983;55:572–578.

54. Brice SL, Jester JD, Huff JC. Recurrent aphthous stomatitis. Curr Probl Dermatol 1991;3:113–127.

55. Grady D, Ernster VL, Stillman L, et al. Smokeless tobacco use prevents aphthous stomatitis. Oral Surg Oral Med Oral Pathol 1992;74:463–465.

56. Shohat-Zabarski R, Kalderon S, Klein T, et al. Close association of HLA-B51 in persons with recurrent aphthous stomatitis. Oral Surg Oral Med Oral Pathol 1992;74:455–458.

57. Hayrinen-Immonen R. Immune-activation in recurrent oral ulcers (ROU). Scand J Dent Res 1992;100:222–227.

58. Pedersen A, Houghen HP, Kenrad B. T-lymphocyte subsets in oral mucosa in patients with recurrent aphthous ulceration. J Oral Pathol Med 1992;21:176–180.

59. Porter S, Flint S, Scully C, et al. Recurrent aphthous stomatitis: The efficacy of replacement therapy in patients with underlying hematinic deficiencies. Ann Dent 1992;51:14–16.

60. Gunzler V. Thalidomide in human immunodeficiency virus (HIV) patients: A review of safety considerations. Drug Saf 1992;7:116–134.

61. Eisen D. The therapy of oral lichen planus. Crit Rev Oral Biol Med 1993;4;141–158.

62. Laine J, Kalimo K, Forssell, et al. Resolution of oral lichenoid lesions after replacement of amalgam restorations in patients allergic to mercury compounds. Br J Dermatol 1992;126:10–15.

63. Holmstrup P. The controversy of a premalignant potential of oral lichen planus is over. Oral Surg Oral Med Oral Pathol 1992; 73:704–706.

64. Eisenberg E, Krutchkoff DJ. Lichenoid lesions of oral mucosa: Diagnostic criteria and their importance in the alleged relationship to oral cancer. Oral Surg Oral Med Oral Pathol 1992; 73:699–704.

65. Eisen D. Hydroxychloroquine sulfate (Plaquenil) improves oral lichen planus: An open trial. J Am Acad Dermatol 1993; 28:609–612.

66. Lamey PJ, Rees TD, Wright JM, et al. Oral presentation of pemphigus vulgaris and its response to systemic steroid therapy. Oral Surg Oral Med Oral Pathol 1992;74:54–57.

67. Premalatha S, Jayakumar S, Yesudion D, et al. Cerebriform tongue: A clinical sign in pemphigus vegetans. Br J Dermatol 1981;104:587–591.

68. Siegel MA. Intraoral biopsy technique for direct immunofluorescence studies. Oral Surg Oral Med Oral Pathol 1991;72:681–684.

69. Anhalt LJ, Kim SC, Stanley JR, et al. Paraneoplastic pemphigus. N Engl J Med 1990;323:1729–1735.

70. Lamey PJ, Binnie WH, Rankin KV. Mucous membrane pemphigoid. Oral Surg Oral Med Oral Pathol 1992;74:50–53.

71. Ahmed AR, Kurgis BS, Rogers RS. Cicatricial pemphigoid. J Am Acad Dermatol 1991;24:987–1001.

72. Siegel MA, Anhalt GJ. Direct immunofluorescence of detached gingival epithelium for diagnosis of cicatricial pemphigoid. Oral Surg Oral Med Oral Pathol 1993;75:296–302.

73. Wright JT, Fine JD, Johnson LB. Oral soft tissues in hereditary epidermolysis bullosa. Oral Surg Oral Med Oral Pathol 1991; 71:440–446.

74. Urman JD, Lowenstein MB, Abeles M, et al. Oral mucosal ulceration in systemic lupus erythematosus. Arthritis Rheum 1978; 21:58–61.

75. Jonsson R, Heyden G, Westberg NG, et al. Oral mucosal lesions in systemic lupus erythematosus: A clinical, histopathological and immunopathological study. J Rheumatol 1984;11:38–42.

76. Schiødt M, Halberg P, Hentzner B. A clinical study of 32 patients with oral discoid lupus erythematosus. Int J Oral Surg 1978; 7:85–94.

77. Lozada-Nur F, Gorsky M, Silverman S. Oral erythema multiforme: Clinical observations in 95 patients. Oral Surg Oral Med Oral Pathol 1989;67:36–40.

78. Lozada-Nur F, Cram D, Gorsky M. Clinical response to levamisole in thirty-nine patients with erythema multiforme: An open prospective study. Oral Surg Oral Med Oral Pathol 1992; 74:294–298.

79. Aine L, Maki M, Reunala T. Coeliac-type dental enamel defects in patients with dermatitis herpetiformis. Acta Derm Venereol 1992;72:25–27.

80. Leonard JN, Wright P, Williams, DM, et al. The relationship between linear IgA disease and benign mucous membrane pemphigoid. Br J Dermatol 1984;110:307–314.

81. Porter SR, Scully CM. Linear IgA disease manifesting as recalcitrant desquamative gingivitis. Oral Surg Oral Med Oral Pathol 1992;74:179–182.

82. Beutner EH, Chorzelski TP, Parodi A, et al. Ten cases of chronic ulcerative stomatitis with stratified epithelium–specific antinuclear antibody. J Am Acad Dermatol 1991;24:781–782.

83. Church LF, Schosser RH. Chronic ulcerative stomatitis associated with stratified epithelial specific antinuclear antibodies. Oral Surg Oral Med Oral Pathol 1992;73:579–582.

84. Stephenson P, Lamey PJ, Scully C, et al. Angina bullosa haemorrhagica: Clinical and laboratory features in 30 patients. Oral Surg Oral Med Oral Pathol 1987;63:560–565.

85. Higgins EM, DuVivier AW. Angina bullosa haemorrhagica: A possible relation to steroid inhalers. Clin Exp Dermatol 1991; 16:244–246.

86. Brannon RB, Fowler CB, Hartman KS. Necrotizing sialometaplasia. Oral Surg Oral Med Oral Pathol 1991;72:317–325.

87. Arguelles MT, Viloria JB, Talens MC, et al. Necrotizing sialometaplasia. Oral Surg Oral Med Oral Pathol 1976;42:89–90.

88. El-Mofty SK, Swanson PE, Wick MR, et al. Eosinophilic ulcer of the oral mucosa. Oral Surg Oral Med Oral Pathol 1993; 75:716–722.

89. Regezi JA, Zarbo RJ, Daniels TE, et al. Oral traumatic granuloma. Oral Surg Oral Med Oral Pathol 1993;75:723–727.

90. Basu MK, Asquit P. Oral manifestations of inflammatory bowel disease. Clin Gastroenterol 1980;9:307–321.

91. Williams AJK, Wray D, Ferguson A. The clinical entity of orofacial Crohn's disease. Q J Med 1991;79:451–458.

92. Halme L, Meurman JH, Laine P, et al. Oral findings in patients with active or inactive Crohns' disease. Oral Surg Oral Med Oral Pathol 1993;76:175–181.

93. Van Hale HM, Rogers RS, Zone JJ, et al. Pyostomatitis vegetans: A reactive mucosal marker for inflammatory disease of the gut. Arch Dermatol 1985;121:94–98.

94. Philpot HC, Elewski BE, Banwell JG, et al. Pyostomatitis vegetans and primary sclerosing cholangitis: Markers of inflammatory bowel disease. Gastroenterology 1992;103:668–674.

95. Chan SWY, Scully C, Prime SS, et al. Pyostomatitis vegetans: Oral manifestation of ulcerative colitis. Oral Surg Oral Med Oral Pathol 1991;72:689–692.

96. Rodenas JM, Ortego N, Herranz MT, et al. Cyclic neutropenia: A cause of recurrent aphthous stomatitis not to be missed. Dermatology 1992;184:205–207.

97. Walton EW. Giant-cell granuloma of the respiratory tract (Wegener's granulomatosis). Br Med J 1958;2:265–270.

98. Scott J, Finch L. Wegener's granulomatosis presenting as gingivitis: Review of the clinical and pathologic features and report of a case. Oral Surg 1972;34:920–33.

99. Mattsson T, Heimdahl A, Dahllöf G, et al. Oral and nutritional status in allogenic marrow recipients treated with T-cell depletion or cyclosporine combined with methotrexate to prevent graft-versus-host disease. Oral Surg Oral Med Oral Pathol 1992; 74:34–40.

100. Mattsson T, Sundqvist KG, Heimdahl A, et al. A comparative immunological analysis of the oral mucosa in chronic graft-versus-host disease and oral lichen planus. Arch Oral Biol 1992; 37:539–547.

101. Sale GE, Shulman HM, Schubert MM. Oral and ophthalmic pathology of graft-versus-host disease in man: Predictive value of the lip biopsy. Hum Pathol 1981;12:1022–1030.

102. Marinone MG, Rizzonoi D, Ferremi P, et al. Late taste disorders in bone marrow transplantation: Clinical evaluation with taste solutions in autologous and allogeneic bone marrow recipients. Haematological 1991;76:519–522.

103. Atkinson K, Weller P, Ryman W, et al. PUVA therapy for drug resistant graft-versus-host disease. Bone Marrow Transplant 1986;1:227–236.

104. Greenspan D, de Villiers EM, Greenspan JS, et al. Unusual HPV types in oral warts in association with HIV infection. J Oral Pathol 1988;17:482–488.

105. Panici PB, Scambia G, Perrone L, et al. Oral condyloma lesions in patients with extensive genital human papillomavirus infection. Am J Obstet Gynecol 1992;167:451–458.

106. Watts SL, Brewer EE, Fry TL. Human papillomavirus DNA types in squamous cell carcinomas of the head and neck. Oral Surg Oral Med Oral Pathol 1991;71:701–707.

107. Henke RP, Guerin-Reverchon I, Milde-Langosch K, et al. In situ detection of human papillomavirus types 13 and 32 in focal epithelial hyperplasia of the oral mucosa. J Oral Pathol Med 1989;18:419–421.

108. Park NH, Park JB, Min BM, et al. Combined synergistic antiherpetic effect of acyclovir and chlorhexidine in vitro. Oral Surg Oral Med Oral Pathol 1991;71:193–196.

109. Young LL, Dolan CT, Sheridan PJ, et al. Oral manifestations of histoplasmosis. Oral Surg Oral Med Oral Pathol 1972;33: 191–196.

110. Sposto MR, Scully C, Paes de Almeida O, et al. Oral paracoccidioidomycosis. Oral Surg Oral Med Oral Pathol 1993;75: 461–465.

111. Jones AC, Bentsen TY, Freedman PD. Mucormycosis of the oral cavity. Oral Surg Oral Med Oral Pathol 1993;75:455–460.

112. Fotos PG, Vincent SD, Hellstein JW. Oral candidosis. Oral Surg Oral Med Oral Pathol 1992;74:41–49.

113. van der Waal N. *Candida albicans* in median rhomboid glossitis: A post-mortem study. Int J Maxillofac Surg 1986;15:322–325.

114. van der Waal I, Schulten EA, Pindborg JJ. Oral manifestations of AIDS: An overview. Int Den J 1991;41:3–8.

115. Greenspan D, Greenspan GS. Significance of oral hairy leukoplakia. Oral Surg Oral Med Oral Pathol 1992;73:151–154.

116. Rabanus JP, Greenspan D, Petersen V, et al. Subcellular distribution and life cycle of Epstein-Barr virus in keratinocytes of oral hairy leukoplakia. Am J Pathol 1991;130:185–197.

117. Lozada-Nur F, Costa C. Retrospective findings of the clinical benefits of podophyllum resin 25% solution on hairy leukoplakia. Oral Surg Oral Med Oral Pathol 1992;73:555–558.

118. Scully C, Laskaris G, Pindborg J, et al. Oral manifestations of HIV infection and their management: I. More common lesions. Oral Surg Oral Med Oral Pathol 1991;71:158–166.

119. Scully C, Laskaris G, Pindborg J, et al. Oral manifestations of HIV infection and their management: II. Less common lesions. Oral Surg Oral Med Oral Pathol 1991;71:167–171.

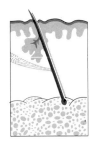

chapter 139

Genital Disorders

MARIA L. CHANCO TURNER

In this chapter guidelines are presented for the diagnosis and treatment of genital disorders. Advances made by other specialities such as the system of nomenclature for the more common genital disorders (Table 139–1)[1] and vulvar intraepithelial neoplasia (Table 139–2)[2] are integrated with dermatologic concepts. Finally, the common complaint of chronic vulvar burning pain or vulvodynia is discussed in depth.[3]

GENITAL EMBRYOLOGY AND ANATOMY

The urorectal septum divides the cloaca into the posterior anorectal canal and anterior urogenital sinus.[4] The cephalic portion of the urogenital sinus is known as the vesicourethral canal, from which arise the bladder, the entire female urethra, and the intramural and prostatic segments of the male urethra. The caudal end of the urogenital sinus is further subdivided into a deeper pelvic part, which in females eventually becomes the vulvar vestibule into which the urethra and vagina open. The superficial end of the urogenital sinus is known as the phallic part. This consists of an anterior genital tubercle that continues posteriorly toward the perineal body as paired genital folds that are separated from each other by the urogenital slit. Lateral to the genital folds are genital swellings. The genital tubercle gives rise to the clitoris (analogous to the glans penis), the genital folds to the labia minora (analogous to part of the penile shaft), and the genital swellings to the labia majora (analogous to the scrotum). Dihydrotestosterone (DHT) is responsible for differentiation of the urogenital sinus into male external genitalia. This causes fusion of the genital folds to form the penile shaft and fusion of the genital swellings to form the scrotum. DHT is derived from the conversion of testosterone (secreted by fetal testes) through the ac-

tion of 5α-reductase, an enzyme found in the cells derived from the urogenital sinus in both male and female fetuses.[5] Despite the fact that the external genitalia of female fetuses contain 5α-reductase, there is no testosterone in the milieu that could be converted to DHT, allowing the structures of the urogenital sinus to differentiate into the female phenotype.

The complexity of the embryologic development of the genitalia and the multiplicity of points at which sexual differentiation can be influenced accounts for a variety of congenital anomalies, ranging from relatively simple developmental cysts to indeterminate external genitalia. When the sex of the neonate cannot be clearly defined, karyotyping and a detailed examination of the entire genital tract are required. A detailed history may pinpoint exogenous hormones or maternal tumors that may have influenced the direction of sexual differentiation.

The pubic symphysis and coccyx form the anterior and posterior boundaries of the perineum with the ischial tuberosities and the sacrospinous ligaments forming the lateral boundaries. The pelvic diaphragm, which forms the roof of the perineum, is made up of the levator ani and the coccygeus muscles. It supports the pelvic contents against the inferior thrust caused by increases in intra-abdominal pressure. A contiguity of structures and shared vascular and nerve supplies helps explain why diseases, dysfunctions, and painful conditions of the structures of the urogenital triangle may involve the structures within the anal triangle.

Lymphatic drainage from one labium majorum will drain into the regional nodes on the same and opposite sides, which is important in planning the treatment of invasive cancers. The regional nodes in the femoral triangle below the inguinal fold drain into the para-aortic lymph nodes.

The cutaneous innervation of the perineum is supplied by the ilioinguinal nerve (L-1), the genitofemoral nerve (L-1, L-2), the perineal branch (S-1) of the posterior cutaneous nerve of the thigh, the perineal branch of S-4,

---

All material in this chapter is in the public domain, with the exception of any borrowed figures or tables.

TABLE 139-1. Nonneoplastic Epithelial Disorders of Genital Skin and Mucosa*

Lichen sclerosus (formerly lichen sclerosus et atrophicus)

Squamous cell hyperplasia (formerly hyperplastic lichen sclerosus et atrophicus)
Refers to hyperkeratosis *without cellular atypia* and may be seen independently or in association with lichen sclerosus or other dermatoses. Equivalent to lichen simplex chronicus.

Other dermatoses
Lichen planus, psoriasis, condylomata, acuminata, etc.
May be accompanied by squamous cell hyperplasia.

*Terminology adopted by International Society for the Study of Vulvar Diseases, 1987.

and the pudendal nerve (S-2, S-3, S-4). The muscles of the perineum are innervated by the pudendal nerve, which may be damaged in traumatic vaginal delivery, causing problems with incontinence.[6] Parasympathetic fibers (derived from S-2, S-3, and S-4) together with the hypogastric sympathetic nerves form the autonomic pelvic plexus that supplies vasodilator fibers to erectile tissue of the clitoris and penis.

The external genitalia are mainly covered by keratinizing stratified squamous epithelium (epidermis), with the exception of the vulvar vestibule. Genital epidermis contains hair, arrector pili, and sebaceous, sweat, and apocrine glands except over the medial aspects of the labia majora, the labia minora, the distal half of the penis, and the glans where there is no hair (Fig. 139-1). In general,

TABLE 139-2. Classification of Vulvar Intraepithelial Neoplasia (VIN)*

Squamous

VIN I   Mild dysplasia (formerly mild atypia)

Nuclear hyperchromasia present; cellular disarray in lower third of the epithelium; mitoses—often seen and usually abnormal in lower third of the epithelium.

VIN II   Moderate dysplasia (formerly moderate atypia)

Nuclear hyperchromasia present; cellular disarray—up to lower two thirds of the epithelium; mitoses—often seen and usually abnormal in lower two thirds of epithelium.

VIN III   Severe dysplasia (formerly severe atypia)

Nuclear hyperchromasia present; cellular disarray affects more than two thirds of the epithelium; mitoses usually abnormal throughout epithelium.

VIN III   Carcinoma in situ (formerly carcinoma in situ)

Term is reserved for cases that have nearly-full or full-thickness epithelial changes. The term bowenoid papulosis is not acceptable as a pathologic term; diagnosis of condyloma acuminatum should not influence diagnosis or grading of VIN.

Nonsquamous

Paget's disease
Melanoma in situ

*Terminology adopted by International Society for the Study of Vulvar Diseases, 1986.

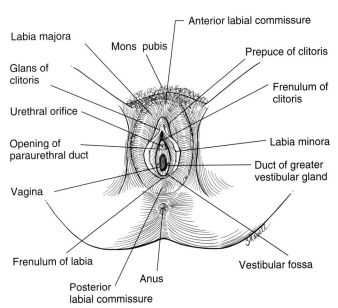

FIGURE 139-1. Topography of the female genitalia. (From Greenway HT, Breisch EA. Superficial cutaneous anatomy. In: Robinson JK, Arndt KA, LeBoit PE, Wintroub BU, eds. Atlas of Cutaneous Surgery. Philadelphia: WB Saunders Co., 1996:18.)

the labia minora are devoid of glandular structures, although occasionally small sebaceous glands that open directly to the surface may be seen as tiny yellowish white flat papules called Fordyce spots. The genital epidermis tends to have more melanocytes, which are hormone responsive such that the genital skin darkens early in pregnancy and in Addison's disease. Genital epithelium also contains Langerhans' and Merkel's cells and is richly supplied with nerve endings.

The vulvar vestibule and the structures within it are lined by modified squamous epithelium (mucosa) that lacks a stratum corneum and a granular layer. This mucosa is similar to the lining of the mouth, the conjunctiva, and the upper respiratory tract, which may explain the frequent simultaneous involvement of these structures in oro-oculogenital syndromes such as cicatricial pemphigoid. Like the vaginal and cervical mucosa, the vulvar mucosa becomes glycogenated and thickened in response to estrogen, as occurs during the early neonatal period (caused by maternal estrogen), during the reproductive years, and during estrogen replacement therapy. Conversely, a lack of estrogen causes this mucosa to atrophy, as can be seen during the prepubertal and postmenopausal years. Because the urethral orifice (see Fig. 139-1) in females is located within the vulva, its mucosal lining is similarly sensitive to estrogen levels. Besides the vaginal and urethral openings, the vulvar vestibule contains the openings of two pairs of major mucus-secreting glands, Bartholin's and Skene's glands, as well as the openings of numerous minor vestibular glands that are essentially simple tubular glands that open directly into the vestibule. Thus, the vulvar vestibule is affected by exudates coming from one or all of these openings.

DIAGNOSIS

History and Physical Examination

Pertinent information should include a gynecologic and obstetric history, a sexual history including types of sexual practices, a history of sexually transmitted diseases in the patient and his or her partner(s) and their therapy, the presence and character of abnormal discharges, and any symptoms referable to other structures in the perineum, such as abnormalities associated with urination and defecation. The two most common complaints are genital pruritus and pain. The description of these complaints is often imprecise, and pruritus must be differentiated from paresthetic symptoms such as formication (a sensation of insects crawling under the skin), stinging, and pricking. True pruritus is accompanied by objective evidence: punctate and linear excoriations, lichenification, hyperpigmentation, and broken-off hairs. The absence of these findings raises suspicion of a paresthetic condition. Pruritus must also be distinguished from pain, which, in this area is almost always described as stinging or burning. An overview of the likely causes of pruritus is presented in Table 139–3 and the causes of vulvodynia are given in Table 139–4. With minor variations, the differential diagnosis of vulvodynia applies to chronic genital pain in males.

When a patient presents to a dermatologist with a problem relating to genital skin, a total skin examination should be performed. A conscious effort needs to be made to examine the vulvar vestibule because it is hidden from view unless the lips of the labia minora are parted (see Fig. 139–1). The vulvar vestibule is also obscured by the vaginal speculum. When possible, the status of the cervix and vagina should be ascertained by a speculum examination because the vulva is contiguous with these structures and can be irritated by secretions coming from above.

Visual examination of the external genitalia allows for the morphologic classification of lesions. The differential diagnosis of macular lesions is given in Table 139–5,

---

TABLE 139–4. Differential Diagnosis of Vulvodynia

A. With visible lesions on mucocutaneous surfaces
   1. Vesiculopustules—recurrent herpes simplex, recurrent candidiasis, pustular psoriasis, Reiter's, chronic aphthosis, Behçet's disease, poststeroid vulvitis
   2. Ulcers—recurrent herpes simplex, chronic aphthosis, Behçet's disease, deep fungal infections, tuberculosis, pyoderma gangrenosum, Crohn's, malignant neoplasms
   3. Bullae—Hailey-Hailey disease, pemphigus vulgaris cicatricial pemphigoid, benign bullous dermatosis of childhood, recurrent bullous drug eruptions
   4. Erosions—all of No. 3 above; lichen sclerosus, lupus erythematosus, desquamative lichen planus, desquamative vulvitis, atrophic vulvovaginitis
B. With tender, red spots in vestibule only
   1. Vulvar vestibulitis*
   2. Zoon's vulvitis
C. Without visible lesions
   1. Pudendal neuralgia—with demonstrable sensory alterations such as allodynia and hyperalgesia
        Microneuromas, neurofibromas
        Post-nerve trauma, straddle injuries
        Post-zoster neuralgia; herpes simplex virus neuralgia
        Idiopathic
   2. Other perineal pain syndromes—?sensory findings
        Levator syndrome
        Perineal descent syndrome
        Proctalgia fugax
        Dysesthetic vulvodynia

*Except for vulvar vestibulitis syndrome, all of the above conditions may be seen in the male genitalia also.

TABLE 139–3. Differential Diagnosis of Pruritus in the Genital Area

A. With minimal visible changes
   1. Associated with generalized pruritus from:
        Systemic disease—diabetes, chronic renal and hepatic diseases, Sjögren's, malignancy
        Paresthesias
        Psychogenic—delusions of parasitosis
   2. Localized to genital area
        Infestation—pediculosis pubis, early scabies
        Dermatitis—early irritant/allergic contact
B. With scaling/maceration/crusting or thickening of cutaneous/mucosal surfaces
   1. Infections—erythrasma, superficial dermatophyte, candidiasis, tinea versicolor, human papillomavirus
   2. Dermatitis—intertrigo, seborrheic dermatitis, allergic/irritant contact, lichen simplex chronicus
   3. Papulosquamous dermatoses—psoriasis, Reiter's, lichen planus, Darier's, lichen sclerosus/balanitis xerotica obliterans
   4. Neoplasias—VIN I to III; PIN I to III; squamous cell carcinoma, extramammary Paget's disease
C. With vaginal/urethral discharge
   1. Vulvovaginitis—from estrogen deprivation; candidiasis; from cervicitis caused by herpes simplex, gonorrhea, *Trichomonas*, and bacterial vaginosis
   2. Balanoposthitis—in uncircumcised males from accumulation of smegma; candidiasis, from urethral discharge caused by gonorrhea, *Trichomonas*, and nonspecific urethritis

---

TABLE 139–5. Differential Diagnosis of Nonpalpable Genital Color Changes

A. Loss of pigment
   1. Vitiligo
   2. Early lichen sclerosus (balanitis xerotica obliterans)
   3. Postinflammatory scars
B. Increased pigmentation
   1. Diffuse
        Endocrine—Cushing's disease, Addison's disease, pregnancy
        Acanthosis nigricans
        Postinflammatory
   2. Patchy
        Postinflammatory
        Lentigines
        Melanosis
        Benign junction nevi
        Early seborrheic keratoses
        Human papillomavirus
        Intraepithelial neoplasia—Bowen's disease
        Melanoma in situ
C. Red discoloration
   1. Port-wine stain
   2. Telangiectasia
   3. Poststeroid rebound erythema
D. Yellow discoloration
   1. Fordyce spots—ectopic sebaceous glands

TABLE 139-6. Differential Diagnosis of Genital Papules and Nodules

A. Infections
1. Viral—human papillomavirus, molluscum contagiosum
2. Bacterial—syphilis, tuberculosis
3. Deep fungal
4. Miscellaneous—lymphogranuloma venereum
B. Noninfectious granulomas—sarcoid, paraffinomas
C. Benign cyst, hyperplasia, and tumors
1. From keratinocyte—seborrheic keratoses, milia, epidermoid and pilar cysts
2. From connective tissue—acrochordons, fibromas, dermatofibromas, lipomas
3. From nerves—neurofibromas, granular cell tumor
4. From blood vessels—varicosities, angiokeratomas, pyogenic granuloma, cherry angiomas, hemangiomas, lymphangioma circumscriptum, *sclerosing lymphangitis*
5. From muscle—leiomyomas
6. From adnexae—Bartholin's cyst, syringomas, hidradenoma papilliferum
7. Miscellaneous—developmental cysts, endometrial cysts, *pearly penile papules, hydrocele, hernia*
D. Malignant neoplasms
1. Basal cell carcinoma
2. Squamous cell carcinoma
3. Melanoma
4. Miscellaneous—Kaposi's sarcoma, adnexal carcinomas, metastatic lesions, *testicular carcinoma*

Note: Terms in italics are specific to male genitalia.

while that for papules and nodules is presented in Table 139–6.

Laboratory Examinations

Examinations that are done in the dermatologist's office include pH determinations, cultures, wet mounts, Gram stains, and Tzanck smears. Microscopic examination of vaginal secretions dissolved in 10% potassium hydroxide solution may be necessary to make a diagnosis of vulvovaginitis secondary to *Candida*. A vaginal culture that is positive for *Candida* in an asymptomatic woman will have to be evaluated in light of the finding that about 20% of normal, asymptomatic women may harbor *Candida* species in their vaginas.[7] Microscopic examination of vaginal secretion dissolved in normal saline (wet smear) is used to determine the presence and relative numbers of white blood cells, trichomonads, and "clue cells" of bacterial vaginosis and to ascertain the predominant vaginal flora. The differential diagnosis of vulvovaginitis based on examination of vaginal secretions is presented in Table 139–7.

TABLE 139-7. Differential Diagnosis of Vaginitis by Wet Smear

	Candida	Trichomonas	Bacterial Vaginosis
pH	4–5	5–7	>4.5
Pseudohyphae	+	−	−
Trichomonads	−	+	−
Clue cells	−	−	+

Biopsy

Although physicians may be hesitant to obtain tissue from the genitalia, histopathologic evaluation is sometimes necessary to establish the correct diagnosis. Biopsy of mucosal surfaces and the shaft of the penis is best accomplished by gently lifting the tissue with fine forceps and snipping the base with iris scissors. This results in an elliptical defect that is easily closed with 5-0 absorbable catgut. Although mucosal biopsy wounds heal well by second intention, suturing the defect decreases the healing time by several days, thus diminishing patient discomfort. Local anesthesia is achieved by injecting 1% lidocaine, with or without epinephrine, using a 30-gauge needle. Lidocaine without epinephrine is used in older men and in those suspected of having a compromised peripheral vascular circulation (i.e., from diabetes mellitus, arteriosclerosis). To minimize burning, the lidocaine solution may be buffered with sodium bicarbonate (1 mEq/L) using 10 parts anesthetic to 1 part bicarbonate.[8] Mucosal specimens should be laid out flat with the dermal side against a piece of filter paper and carefully slid into formalin. This preserves tissue orientation and prevents specimens from curling.

INFECTIONS IN THE GENITAL AREA

Bacterial Infections

Pyodermas

Staphylococcus aureus and group A hemolytic *Streptococcus* can cause the usual range of cutaneous pyodermas (i.e., impetigo, folliculitis, cellulitis, and abscesses) and may, in fact, do so more often because of the warmth and moisture in the area. *S. aureus* frequently infects Bartholin's glands. An abscess of Bartholin's gland may require marsupialization in addition to systemic antibiotics. Staphylococcal vulvovaginitis in menstruating women has been associated with toxic shock syndrome.

The genital area in young children is frequently involved in staphylococcal scalded skin syndrome, which is caused by an exotoxin (exfoliatin) of penicillin-resistant *S. aureus* phage group II.[9] Systemic antibiotics for penicillin-resistant *S. aureus* help this syndrome to resolve in 5 to 10 days.

An increasing incidence of vulvovaginitis caused by group A hemolytic *Streptococcus* has been reported in girls younger than 15 years of age.[10] A vaginal discharge with erythema and labial swelling are presenting signs. Diagnosis is made by culturing vaginal swabs.

Erythrasma

Corynebacterium minutissimum, a gram-positive rod, causes erythrasma, which appears as a well-demarcated patch that may be seen in the inguinal and intergluteal folds. It is diagnosed by the demonstration of a coral-red fluorescence on examination under a Wood's light. This fluorescence is due to coproporphyrin III, which is water soluble. It is easiest to demonstrate this if the patient is told not to shower for 24 hours before examination. A gram a day of erythromycin or tetracycline for 7 to 10 days is the usual therapy. Topical azoles and clindamycin in addition to measures aimed at keeping the involved areas clean and dry help to prevent recurrences.

Trichomycosis

Two or three other species of corynebacteria have been implicated as the etiologic agent for trichomycosis,[11] a condition characterized by the presence of yellow or red nodules along the hair shafts that may stain clothing. Nits of pediculosis can easily be differentiated from trichomycosis by the fluorescence of trichomycosis under Wood's light examination. Therapy consists of shaving the hair from the involved area. Washing with an antiseptic and keeping the involved area dry help prevent recurrences.

Syphilis

The chancre, the primary lesion of syphilis, starts as a painless papule that enlarges and becomes an indurated ulcer. The bases of these ulcers teem with the etiologic spirochete, *Treponema pallidum,* which cannot be cultured but is easily seen on darkfield examination. Although typically single and painless, multiple chancres may occur and secondary pyogenic infection may render these chancres painful. These ulcers may be located anywhere on the genitalia and are frequently missed when they occur on the cervix or vagina. Nontender, unilateral or bilateral inguinal adenopathy accompanies the chancre.

The secondary stage of syphilis is characterized by the appearance of a generalized, asymptomatic eruption consisting of erythematous macules, papules, or papulosquamous lesions with accompanying adenopathy. These lesions may be seen on the drier surfaces of the genitalia, while grayish white, round, thin papules known as mucous patches are seen on the moist surfaces. Thicker, discrete to confluent, flat-surfaced, white papules known as condylomata lata are also encountered in the moist genital and perianal areas in the second stage of syphilis. Like the chancre, these lesions teem with spirochetes and are very infectious (see Chapter 105).

Nongonococcal Urethritis and Mucopurulent Cervicitis

In 50% of cases, nongonococcal urethritis and mucopurulent cervicitis are caused by *Chlamydia trachomatis* types D to K.[12] These chlamydial infections are now considered to be the most common sexually transmitted diseases. Although chlamydial infection of the lower genital tract in women may cause an irritating vaginal discharge, it is more often asymptomatic. Besides the cervix and urethra, the ducts of Bartholin's glands in women and the epididymis in men may also become infected. In the female, ascending infection of the genital tract accounts for almost half the cases of pelvic inflammatory disease and 25% of subsequent cases of infertility.[13]

A rapid direct immunofluorescent test utilizing a monoclonal antibody that recognizes the major outer-membrane protein of 15 immunotypes of *C. trachomatis* was shown to be nearly as sensitive and specific as cultures.[14]

Bacterial Vaginosis (Nonspecific Vaginitis)

Bacterial vaginosis is not a true infection but is a disturbance of the normal vaginal flora.[15] About half of affected women are asymptomatic. The other half have a foul-smelling discharge that can cause vulvar irritation. For various reasons, such as chronic cervicitis or estrogen deficiency, the normal peroxide-producing *Lactobacillus*-dominated vaginal flora is replaced by anaerobic gram-positive streptococci and other anaerobes belonging to the *Gardnerella, Bacteroides, Mycoplasma,* and *Mobiluncus* species. Although initially considered a sexually transmitted disease, currently this is not considered to be true.

Three of the following four criteria are necessary for diagnosis[16]: (1) a gray-white homogeneous discharge at the introitus; (2) a pH of greater than 4.5; (3) a "fishy," amine odor intensified by adding 10% potassium hydroxide; and (4) presence of "clue cells" on microscopic examination. "Clue cells" are desquamated vaginal epithelial cells whose surfaces are covered with bacteria so as to obscure their margins.

Bacterial vaginosis may remit spontaneously. The standard therapy is a week's course of metronidazole, 800 to 1200 mg in divided doses.[17] Single-dose therapy with 2-g metronidazole results in a comparable response rate, although the recurrence rate may be higher.[18] An alternative to metronidazole is a week's course of clindamycin in a 2% cream or suppository.[19] Both of these treatments are aimed at eradicating the anaerobic bacteria that have taken over the vaginal flora.

Necrotizing Fasciitis

This rare but rapidly spreading, frequently fatal, deep subcutaneous infection is most often seen in diabetics after trauma to the genitalia such as an episiotomy.[20] Its origins may be polymicrobial (combination of aerobic and anaerobic organisms) or streptococcal (usually group A β-hemolytic). Fournier's gangrene is necrotizing fasciitis of the scrotum.[21] Clinically, the findings are consistent with a combination of cellulitis and infarction, with the cutaneous changes frequently lagging behind the subcutaneous necrosis so that, eventually, the overlying skin may even become anesthetic. Histologically, noninflammatory intravascular thrombosis is present at all levels of the skin. Bacteria can usually be demonstrated by special stains.[22] Early diagnosis is of the essence for the early institution of appropriate antibiotics and wide surgical debridement of necrotic tissue.

Mycotic Infections

Dermatophyte Infection

Dermatophyte infection of the labia minora, penis, or scrotum almost never occurs. When it involves the intergluteal and inguinal areas, the differential diagnosis includes flexural psoriasis, seborrheic dermatitis, erythrasma, and candidiasis. Fungal folliculitis may occur, especially where topical steroids have erroneously been used.

Genital White Piedra

White piedra may involve the genital area alone or may involve other warm and moist areas of the body. It is thought to be caused by *Trichosporon beigelii,* although different groups of coryneform bacteria have been cultured from hairs that grew *Trichosporon.* Although frequently asymptomatic, this mycosis may be the cause of recalcitrant intertrigo. Diagnosis is best established by performing a potassium hydroxide preparation of genital hairs. Topical therapy with econazole or systemic therapy with ketoconazole is temporarily effective, but resistance follows quickly.[23] Spontaneous remissions occur.

Candidiasis

Because of the warm and damp environment of this region, *Candida* infection in the genital area frequently manifests as an erythematous, macerated intertrigo with classic "satellite" pustules along the periphery. Most of these infections are caused by *C. albicans* strains, while the rest are due to other species, such as *Torulopsis glabrata.*

Acute *Candida* infections tend to be more severe in the uncircumcised male and in women with undiagnosed, clinical diabetes. Other predisposing conditions are systemic antibiotic therapy, vulvar candidiasis in a sexual partner, or topical steroid therapy to the area. The genitalia become erythematous and swollen, with erosions and pustules. In the chronic form of penile candidiasis, the glans appears glazed and may progress to sclerosis and fissuring. Erythema and pruritus of the penis have been reported in some males, minutes or hours after unprotected intercourse with women who carry *Candida* in their vaginas. These men do not harbor *Candida,* and this phenomenon is thought to be a type of hypersensitivity reaction.[24]

Approximately three fourths of adult women have vulvovaginal candidiasis at least once in their life. A few women with vulvovaginal candidiasis will have chronic, recurrent, symptomatic, vulvovaginal candidiasis. Approximately 20% of healthy asymptomatic women in the childbearing age have *Candida* in their genital tract.[7] This vaginal carriage rate and the incidence of symptomatic vulvovaginal candidiasis are higher in pregnant women, in diabetics, in users of antibiotics and high estrogen oral contraceptives, and in women frequenting clinics for treatment of sexually transmitted diseases.[25]

Several studies have failed to implicate subclinical diabetes, an intestinal reservoir, partner transmission, iron deficiency, and clothing and personal habits as predisposing factors in chronic or recurrent vulvovaginal candidiasis.[26] The role, if any, that candidal virulence factors, local and systemic immunity, and normal vaginal flora play remains to be determined.[25]

The clinical hallmark of infection of the female genitalia with *Candida* is the presence of pruritus and vulvitis, which may be erosive (Fig. 139–2). Symptoms vary from pruritus to burning and dyspareunia. Candidiasis can present acutely as edema, erythema, white mucosal plaques, and a "cheesy" discharge at the vulva with "satellite" pustules on surrounding skin. As the condition becomes chronic, the surrounding skin becomes lichenified. Many patients with the recurrent, incapacitating form show only marked erythema, some edema, and minimal discharge.

Diagnosis can be made in the office by microscopic examination of potassium hydroxide–treated vaginal discharge or skin scrapings. The presence of budding yeast and mycelia confirms the diagnosis. When candidiasis is suspected but the microscopic examination is negative, a culture is necessary.

Topical therapy is generally sufficient for *Candida* balanitis and vulvitis. In the presence of candidal vulvitis, the vagina also needs to be treated because the condition is a vulvovaginitis. There are several effective topical preparations (tablets, suppositories, creams and lotions) so that patient preference may guide the choice. Nystatin, a polyene antibiotic, and the numerous azole derivatives are beneficial. For the uncomplicated, episodic cases, azole derivatives in short courses or even single-dose regimens have been proven effective.[27] Daily consumption of *Lactobacillus acidophilus*–containing yogurt was found to decrease candidal colonization and infection in 33 patients with chronic vulvovaginal candidiasis, seeming to confirm existing folklore,[28] but corroboration of this research is necessary.

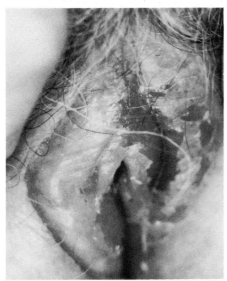

FIGURE 139–2. Acute, *Candida* vulvitis in a recently diagnosed diabetic. Note labial edema, erosions, and discharge at introitus.

Systemic anticandidal therapy tends to be reserved for patients who have chronic recurrent vulvovaginal candidiasis or who are immunosuppressed. In a prospective, placebo-controlled study, Sobel[29] demonstrated that maintenance prophylactic treatment with oral ketoconazole (100 mg daily for 6 months) was effective in preventing recurrent episodes of vulvovaginal candidiasis but that relapse occurred after withdrawal of the drug. Because of idiosyncratic hepatitis associated with systemic ketoconazole, its use should be limited to symptomatic culture-positive patients, who should be monitored frequently. Monthly doses of 125 mg of fluconazole are not as effective as daily doses of ketoconazole.[30] Treatment of the partner or the daily oral use of nystatin is not recommended.[25]

Viral Infections

Molluscum Contagiosum

This infection is caused by a poxvirus, and classic lesions are dome-shaped, shiny or white papules with central umbilication. An 11-fold increase in adult cases was noted in the years between 1966 and 1983.[31] This infection has joined the ranks of sexually transmitted diseases and can be quite extensive in persons with human immunodeficiency virus infection. Irritated lesions may be mistaken for furunculosis and early ones, particularly on the shaft of the penis, might be mistaken for flat warts.

Herpes Simplex

Genital herpes simplex virus (HSV) infection may be caused by HSV-1 or HSV-2. This infection is one of the most common and important sexually transmitted diseases, as demonstrated by the results of a seroepidemiologic survey encompassing the years 1976 to 1980 in which 16.4% of the U.S. population from 17 to 74 years of age was found to be infected with HSV-2. The prevalence of type-specific antibody increases from 1% in individuals younger than 15 years of age to 20.2% in women between ages 30 and 34.[32] At the same time, between 1961 and 1981, the incidence of neonatal HSV infection increased from 2 to 12 cases per 100,000 live births.[33] More important, as many as 50% of women whose sera were positive for HSV-2 antibodies were not aware of having genital lesions.[34] Asymptomatic viral shedding occurs in persons with known genital HSV infection.[35] Although HSV-1 infections occur in the genital area, most genital outbreaks are caused by HSV-2.[36] It is thought that HSV-1 genital infection is caused by orogenital sex.

Genital herpes infection may be primary or recurrent. Primary infection occurs in individuals with no history of previous outbreaks and absence of antibodies to HSV in their sera. After the primary infection, the virus remains latent in the sensory sacral ganglia and recurrences result from reactivation of these latent viruses by yet unclear mechanisms.

Primary infections have an incubation period of 3 to 7 days. Paresthesias may precede the eruption by 2 to 3 days. The eruption consists of erythematous papules on a diffusely edematous and tender base. The papules develop into vesicles and pustules, coalescing and breaking down into ulcers that take as long as 2 to 4 weeks to heal. On average, virus may be cultured from these lesions for around 12 days. In severely immunocompromised patients, extensive, persistent, phagedenic, perianal herpetic ulcers are not uncommon. Primary genital HSV infections (Fig. 139–3) are more likely to be accompanied by systemic symptoms, cover a wider area (cervix, vagina, urethra, bladder, anus), and take longer to heal than a recurrence. The eruption may assume a zosteriform or segmental distribution, making it difficult to differentiate from herpes zoster on clinical grounds alone. Systemic symptoms include low-grade fever, malaise, urinary retention, and regional lymphadenopathy. Urinary retention is secondary to lesions in the urethra and bladder. Dysuria may be secondary to urethral and bladder involvement or may result from urine touching ulcerated vulvar mucosa. The cervix is frequently involved in primary infections, as evidenced by viral recovery from 80% of the cervices of patients who did not have visible lesions on the cervix.[37] Primary HSV infections are also likely to be accompanied by other sexually transmitted diseases, which should be checked for. Within a year of recovering from primary genital HSV infection, 50% to 80% of patients develop a recurrence.[38] Recurrences are more frequent during the 2 years after a primary infection and generally tend to taper off with time. Recurrent genital HSV infection is much milder than the primary infection. The lesions are fewer, smaller, and less painful and heal in 7 to 10 days.[39] Viral shedding is reduced to 4 days, with a peak at 48 hours. Lesions consist of localized groups of vesicles, pustules, and shallow ulcers anywhere on the genital area. Occasionally, recurrences may occur only on the buttocks. Systemic symptoms are less likely to occur. One study has shown

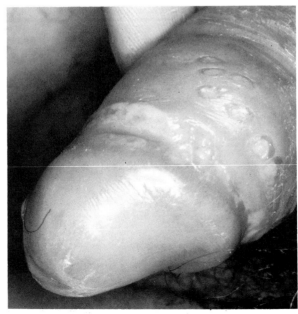

FIGURE 139–3. Primary herpes simplex infection involving the penis with multiple ulcers and marked edema of the distal shaft and glans.

that symptoms such as perigenital aching, itching, burning, or paresthesias are frequently missed as indicators of recurrent genital HSV infection.[34]

The differential diagnosis of genital HSV includes all the other sexually transmitted diseases that give rise to ulcers—syphilis (primary and secondary), chancroid, lymphogranuloma venereum, and granuloma inguinale. Zosteriform primary HSV infection needs to be differentiated from herpes zoster. Herpes zoster that recurs in the same sacral dermatomes is occurring with more frequency in immunocompromised patients. Recurrent genital ulcers may be a manifestation of recurrent genital aphthosis, inflammatory bowel disease, or Behçet's disease. In the latter two conditions, the ulcers tend to be larger, deeper, and more persistent.

The gold standard for diagnosis is a positive culture that may yield results in 24 to 48 hours, depending on the size of the inoculum. Direct immunofluorescence, indirect immunoperoxidase, and viral isolation techniques yielded 71%, 76%, and 90% positive results when specimens and smears were collected at the vesicular stage of the disease.[40] Currently available commercial serologic tests are not reliably able to distinguish between HSV-1 and HSV-2 infection. A Western blot technique for differentiating HSV-1 and HSV-2 infections is expensive and time consuming and is useful only for research purposes. For most clinical situations, a rapid, inexpensive, and fairly accurate test is a well-done Tzanck smear demonstrating multinucleated giant cells, intranuclear inclusions, or both. A comparison of Tzanck smears and viral cultures taken from vesicular lesions showed that Tzanck smears had a 90% predictive value when compared with positive cultures.[41]

The treatment of choice for primary genital HSV is systemic acyclovir, an analogue of deoxyguanidine that interferes with viral thymidine kinase. Widespread clinical use has confirmed its generally safe profile, with toxicities seemingly limited to reversible renal dysfunction in patients with preexisting renal disease and leukopenia in those with compromised bone marrow. Except for severely immunocompromised persons or those who have systemic involvement, acyclovir is given orally, 200 mg five times a day for 10 days.[42] When indicated, acyclovir may be given intravenously at a dose of 5 mg/kg every 8 hours for 7 days.[43] Treatment of primary genital HSV infection does not prevent recurrences. Ancillary therapy during the acute stage of a primary infection includes bed rest as needed, baths or open-wet dressings, and pain management.

The indications for treatment of recurrent genital HSV infection with acyclovir are not so clear cut since there is only a slight decrease in the duration of symptoms and lesions when therapy is initiated during the prodromal phase.[44] The Acyclovir Study Group[45] has been following the effects of long-term, oral acyclovir, 400 mg twice a day, on patients with an average of 12 recurrences a year. At the end of 3 years, 60% of those who completed the study did not have recurrences during the third year of the trial. Continuous therapy reduced signs and symptoms of recurrent disease but did not totally eliminate viral shedding and, hence, possible transmission.[46] Acyclovir-resistant strains are beginning to be seen in the

immunocompromised group of patients.[47] In an uncontrolled trial, foscarnet has shown therapeutic benefit.[48]

The most important aspect of genital HSV infection is the prevention of neonatal herpes infection. Untreated neonatal HSV infection most often results in death or severe central nervous system disease.[49] One study has shown that the presence of maternal antibodies specific to HSV-2 appears to reduce the neonatal transmission of this virus.[50] Because of these findings, new algorithms with regard to management of this problem are being evaluated.

Although there is seroepidemiologic evidence showing that antibodies to HSV-2 are more prevalent in patients with cervical cancer compared with normal controls, the role of HSV-2 in the pathogenesis of cervical cancer is not known.[51]

Patients with genital HSV infection frequently need counseling and reassurance regarding their disease. They especially need to be given up-to-date and correct information about transmission, about protection afforded by the use of barrier contraceptives, and about the importance of alerting their obstetricians if one or both of the partners have had genital HSV infection.

Varicella Zoster Virus

Although zoster is more common on the trunk, the lumbosacral nerves may sometimes be involved. Motor disturbances resulting in urinary retention and bowel dysfunction may accompany the cutaneous lesions.[52] As in other parts of the body, post-herpetic neuralgia may occur.

Human Papillomavirus

Genital human papillomavirus (HPV) infection is most often a sexually transmitted disease with an incubation period of 2 to 3 months.[53] The incidence of clinically evident HPV infection of the genital tract has increased remarkably in the past 2 decades, coincident with the increasing incidence of sexually transmitted diseases.[54, 55] The prevalence of subclinical HPV carriage has been demonstrated to be as high as 43% when the very sensitive, polymerase chain reaction (PCR) technique was used on samples from vulvar scrapings acquired from college students coming for routine gynecologic examinations.[56] Similarly, HPV DNA was detected by PCR in 41% of the semen samples obtained from men attending an infertility clinic who had no clinical evidence of genital warts.[57] There is strong epidemiologic[58, 59] and molecular biologic evidence[60] of an association between genital HPV and carcinoma.

HPV infection of the genitalia may be viewed as *clinical, subclinical,* or *latent.*[61] *Condylomata acuminata,* also known as genital warts, are the classic manifestation of HPV infection anywhere in the genital area and the urethral meatus. They are visible clinically and are so typical and recognizable that patients seek therapy for them. Single or multiple, discrete or coalescent, soft, cauliflower-like growths are most commonly seen on the moist, mucosal surfaces of the anogenital areas of both males and females (Fig. 139–4). On nonmucosal areas,

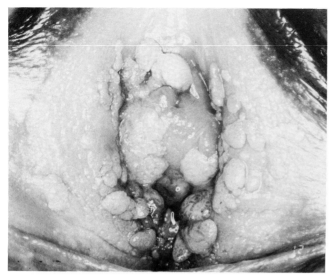

FIGURE 139-4. Multiple condylomata acuminata on the mucosal surface of the vulva involving the urethral orifice and hymen. Note scattered, discrete "satellite" papules along the edges of the main mass.

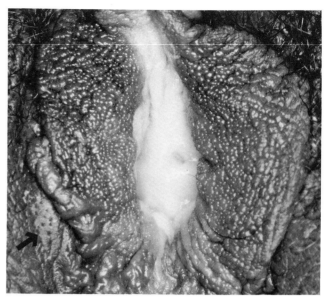

FIGURE 139-5. Confluent, cobblestoned appearance of mucosal surface of labia minora and vulvar vestibule, samples of which were positive for HPV-DNA, type 6, on dot blot hybridization. Arrow points to small white plaque that was positive for vulvar intraepithelial neoplasia type III (bowenoid papulosis).

they become less papilliferous and more keratotic. Condylomata are most often associated with HPV types 6 and 11[62] and are more likely to undergo spontaneous regression and run a benign course. Condylomata become more numerous and more resistant to therapy in immunosuppressed states such as pregnancy and acquired immunodeficiency syndrome, and during chemotherapy. The most important differential diagnosis of condylomata acuminata is the condylomata lata of secondary syphilis. Larger and more florid warts may need to be differentiated from verrucous carcinoma, particularly, if they are recalcitrant to therapy.

Flat papules and plaques may be solitary or multiple, discrete or confluent, skin colored, erythematous, or hyperpigmented. Their surfaces may be smooth, cobblestoned (Fig. 139-5), velvety, or verrucous. These lesions are analogous to flat warts on glabrous skin. The differential diagnosis includes vulvar intraepithelial neoplasia III (carcinoma in situ) (see Table 139-2), lichen simplex chronicus, Paget's disease, psoriasis, and lichen planus.

Micropapillary forms are small, soft, smooth, pink papillations of the vulvar vestibule, and their relationship to HPV is controversial. Keeping in mind that 43% of vulvar scrapings from college students were positive for HPV DNA, it is probably best to adopt a position of watchful waiting when these lesions are encountered in asymptomatic women, unless examination of the rest of the genital tract reveals clinical evidence of HPV. Similar-looking lesions that encircle the corona of the penis (pearly penile papules) are universally accepted as not related to HPV (Fig. 139-6).

Subclinical or latent infection is said to be present when the skin or mucosa appears normal by colposcopy, cytology, and histology. However, HPV DNA can be demonstrated by using molecular biologic techniques, particularly the extremely sensitive PCR. Latent infection is thought to be responsible for recurrences at and around treatment sites as demonstrated by the presence of HPV DNA in normal-appearing skin beyond the mar-

gins of laser treatment for anogenital condylomata and intraepithelial neoplasia.[63] Another study demonstrated that 36% of women who were positive for HPV DNA on routine screening did not have clinically evident warts.[64] The mechanisms by which a latent HPV infection becomes clinically manifest are not completely known, but impaired host immune response likely plays a role. Another unanswered question is whether latent infection is transmissible, and the theoretical evidence is that it is not.

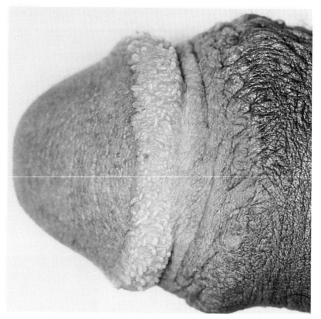

FIGURE 139-6. Pearly penile papules: confluent micropapillations encircling the coronal sulcus of the penis. This is considered to be a type of angiofibroma and is not HPV related.

Diagnosis of less typical, flat lesions may be aided by the application of 3% to 5% acetic acid before examination with a magnifying glass or colposcope. Acetic acid turns these papules white (acetowhitening), making them easier to see. Not all acetowhite areas denote HPV-infected sites. Colposcopy after application of acetic acid is most useful in the detection of subclinical infection in the cervix and vagina where it is helpful for directed biopsies.

The Papanicolaou smear is a very useful tool for screening the cervix and vagina for HPV infection. A positive result depends on the presence of "koilocytes," which are pathognomonic for HPV infection. On a Papanicolaou smear, koilocytes are easily recognized as abnormally enlarged epithelial cells with abundant basophilic cytoplasm and hyperchromatic single or multiple nuclei that contain granular or densely staining chromatin. These cells have a perinuclear halo that occupies a fourth to two thirds of the total cytoplasmic surface.[65]

The histopathology of papillomavirus infection is reviewed in Chapter 123. Histology is not very reliable in the diagnosis of subclinical HPV infection of the vulva because of marked interobserver and intraobserver variability.

Molecular biologic techniques, such as Southern blotting and its variations as well as the supersensitive PCR, may be applied to biopsy samples, scrapes, and washings. Depending on the sensitivity of the test, they will detect subclinical and latent infections. At present, they are mainly used as research tools.

Treatment. Treatment of clinically evident genital HPV infection is destructive, nonspecific, and not reliably effective. These treatments in themselves can cause a lot of morbidity, and the virus is unlikely to be totally eradicated. In a study of 400 consecutive patients treated with 16.5% salicylic acid and cryotherapy, the cure rate at 3 months was 52%. This fell to 41% after another 3 months of follow-up.[66] Before embarking on treatment, it is important to remember that spontaneous regression occurs about 30% of the time, that genital HPV infection is most often multifocal, involving contiguous structures, and that both local and systemic immunity play important roles. The indications for treatment are to (1) prevent spread (typical condylomata acuminata are vegetative lesions that shed infectious, intact virions); (2) alleviate symptoms such as itching and burning; (3) preserve normal function (e.g., urination, defecation, and coitus without bleeding); (4) treat concomitant, dysplastic changes; and (5) alleviate disfigurement caused by the presence of clinical lesions.

Podophyllin is used as 20% to 25% solutions in tincture of benzoin. The active ingredient is podophyllotoxin, which arrests mitosis in metaphase. It is painted on, allowed to dry, and washed off in 4 to 6 hours. Tissue necrosis occurs, followed by a slough in 4 to 5 days. Purified podophyllotoxin, 0.5% in ethanol has become available. This may be self-applied on the penis, twice daily for 3 days with the possibility of extending another 2 days if necessary. Podophyllotoxin is teratogenic and toxic to fetuses, kidney, brain, and myocardium when absorbed in sufficient quantities.

Depending on the site to be treated, a 30% to 85% solution of trichloroacetic acid may be used. On careful application, the mucosa turns white. Depending on response, treatment may be repeated weekly.

5-Fluorouracil is a fluorinated pyrimidine analogue that blocks DNA synthesis and cell division. It is effective for vaginal and vulvar warts especially when applied more than once at weekly intervals.[67] This chemical causes severe mucosal irritation and is not to be used during pregnancy. Genital intraepithelial neoplasia are also responsive.[68]

If the condylomata are large and extensive, a loop electrode may be used. A local anesthetic is needed, and healing occurs in 10 to 14 days.

Liquid nitrogen is commonly used and may be administered with a spray, a cotton-tipped swab, or a probe, as in the cervix. Treatment may be repeated every 3 weeks, as needed. Its main disadvantages are pain and frequent recurrences. It may be used in combination with 5-fluorouracil. As a single agent, it is safe to use during pregnancy.

LASER. The CO_2 laser is used for extensive lesions. Its major disadvantage is its cost. When it is used on the vulva, the postoperative course is marked by severe discomfort, lasting for about 3 weeks after the procedure.

INTERFERONS. Interferons are a group of biologically active glycoproteins with antiviral, antiproliferative, and immunomodulating properties. Recombinant interferon alfa is somewhat successful in the treatment of recalcitrant genital warts when injected intralesionally[69, 70] or when given systemically.[71] Similar treatment successes have been reported after the use of systemic interferon gamma.[72] The major reported side effects were flu-like symptoms experienced within the first 24 hours after administration.

OTHER THERAPIES. There have been anecdotal reports of temporary benefits from oral retinoid therapy of common warts[73] and nongenital warts in epidermodysplasia verruciformis.[74] However, isotretinoin by itself did not cause clearing of treatment-resistant condylomata acuminata.[75]

Combination of several modalities of therapy such as laser-interferon or laser–5-fluorouracil is thought to decrease the recurrence rate after cessation of therapy.

There is active research going on to develop a vaccine against papillomavirus and, indeed, there have been some reports of success in vaccinating rabbits and cattle.[76, 77] Even more tantalizing is Food and Drug Administration approval to begin human clinical trials using antisense compounds designed to inhibit the growth of warts.[78]

There is general agreement that currently available therapies, no matter how aggressive, do not result in eradication of latent HPV infection.[79] The use of proper barrier contraceptives is an important preventive measure. Once the presence of HPV infection is documented, regular surveillance such as by yearly or twice-yearly Papanicolaou smears and colposcopy is recommended.

DERMATOSES

These disorders are more fully described in specific chapters, and only those aspects with particular relevance to their occurrence on the genital area are addressed here.

Intertrigo

Intertrigo usually appears as an erythematous, moist, macerated, and frequently malodorous dermatitis affecting flexural areas in the obese person during hot, humid weather. There is frequently superinfection with *Candida*. The differential diagnosis includes psoriasis, seborrheic dermatitis, erythrasma, and, in infants, histiocytosis X. It is responsive to a combination of open wet dressings or tub baths followed by a combination of 1% hydrocortisone mixed with either 2% precipitated sulfur, miconazole, or iodoquinol in a light, greaseless base.

Psoriasis

Psoriasis may first appear or become a stubborn problem in the genital area. Lesions may vary from discrete scaly papules to erythematous, fissured plaques with macerated, white scales in the flexures (inguinal, genitocrural, intergluteal). The differential diagnosis of discrete papulosquamous lesions includes lichen planus, secondary lues, flat warts, extramammary Paget's disease, and intraepithelial neoplasia. In the uncircumcised penis, lesions on the glans appear erosive. It is important to distinguish flexural psoriasis from diaper rash in infants and seborrheic dermatitis in adults because psoriasis takes longer to respond to therapy and is more likely to recur. Diagnosis is aided by finding typical lesions or markers of psoriasis elsewhere on the body. Rarely, a biopsy may be necessary. Therapy is as for intertrigo, although a medium-strength topical corticosteroid may be used initially. Recurrences may be prevented by regular use of topical imidazole creams and lotions.

Contact Dermatitis

Contact dermatitis may be acute or chronic and may be of an allergic or irritant nature. Irritant dermatitis may be caused by a chronic discharge, overcleansing, and therapeutic modalities such as trichloroacetic acid or 5-fluorouracil. Allergic contact dermatitis is pruritic, while irritant dermatitis causes burning. Both are often intermittent. Some of the more common allergens include preservatives (e.g., ethylenediamine, propylene glycol, formaldehyde releasers), medications (e.g., neomycin), fragrances, and latex (e.g., condoms). Chronic use of panty liners that are impregnated with fragrances and formaldehyde may cause low-grade, chronic, allergic dermatitis, resulting in a pattern similar to lichen simplex chronicus. A good history, including information regarding partners' use of topical medications and barrier contraceptives, is generally sufficient to establish the etiology of an acute problem. The presence of a spongiotic dermatitis with eosinophils on histologic evaluation favors an allergic etiology, and at that point patch testing

may be helpful. Therapy consists of discontinuing the offending agent followed by the use of topical steroids.

Lichen Simplex Chronicus

Lichen simplex chronicus refers to idiopathic, chronic pruritus resulting in thickened skin from constant rubbing. It is otherwise known as localized neurodermatitis, or pruritus vulvae, when localized to the vulva. The skin becomes hyperkeratotic, hyperpigmented, and resembles cobblestones, with broken-off hairs and prurigo nodules. The labia majora, mons, perineum, and scrotal sac are the areas most often involved. Histology is frequently necessary to differentiate this from other papulosquamous diseases mentioned in the previous section. The mainstay of therapy is topical steroids, and it is often necessary to start with a potent preparation for the first 3 to 4 weeks. Because itching is usually most intense as the patient is trying to fall asleep, sedating antihistamines taken before bedtime and the use of an icebag for immediate but temporary relief of pruritus are very helpful measures. Regular follow-up to monitor progress and provide encouragement is necessary for a good outcome.

Lichen Planus

Lichen planus can involve both the keratinized and mucosal surfaces of the genitalia. On keratinized skin, it looks like lichen planus elsewhere on the body. Annular lesions are frequently seen on the glans. On mucosal surfaces such as the uncircumcised glans, inner surface of the labia minora, vulva, and vagina there are prominent white, lacy patches bordering extensive erosions. Erosive lichen planus is one of the causes of desquamative vulvovaginitis.[80] In the vulva, the erosive lesions of lichen planus can cause agglutination of the clitoral hood, sclerosis, and/or absorption of the interlabial sulci and the labia minora. The process extends into the vagina, resulting in a serosanguineous to purulent discharge with eventual scarring and shortening of the vaginal canal. Pruritus may be present at the onset, but dyspareunia, burning pain, and spotting quickly supervene. Erosive lichen planus needs to be differentiated from lichen sclerosus, desquamative inflammatory vaginitis, and other erosive diseases that may affect the vulva (see Table 139–3).[81] Important differential diagnoses for hypertrophic lichen planus include lichen simplex chronicus, hypertrophic lichen sclerosus, and intraepithelial neoplasia. The diagnosis is aided by finding typical evidence of the disease elsewhere on the skin or oral cavity. The definitive diagnosis can be established on biopsy.

Therapy is a major problem in both hypertrophic and erosive lichen planus. Systemic steroids, dapsone, antimalarial agents, retinoids, immunosuppressive agents, and topical steroids have at best been only temporarily palliative. In my experience, superpotent topical steroids have resulted in rapid reepithelialization of the erosive form, although we do not yet know what side effects will occur from long-term use of these agents. Intralesional steroid injections are helpful for the hypertrophic variety. It is important to treat concomitant abnormal discharges resulting from chronic cervicitis, bacterial vaginosis, or candidal vulvitis. Prospective follow-up of these patients is necessary, not only to assess the efficacy of therapy but also to monitor for malignant change. Although there are no documented reports of squamous cell carcinoma arising from erosive lichen planus in the genitalia, there is a demonstrated increased risk in erosive oral lichen planus.[82]

Lichen Sclerosus

Lichen sclerosus is the currently accepted terminology (see Table 139–1) for a dermatosis that has been known as vulvar dystrophy, lichen sclerosus et atrophicus, kraurosis vulvae, and, in the male, balanitis xerotica obliterans. This dermatosis, which can affect any part of the body, occurs most often in the anogenital area of post-menopausal women, although it has been reported in all age groups of both sexes. Lichen sclerosus in prepubertal girls is rare, has a tendency to improve with increasing age,[83] but may persist to adulthood.[84] It is rare in males, and the glans and prepuce are often the only sites involved, with phimosis as the leading complication.[85] An autoimmune etiology for lichen sclerosus has been proposed based on the presence of autoantibodies in patients' sera, an association with other autoimmune diseases,[85, 86] and an association with HLA-A29 and B44, separately and together.[87] The role of *Borrelia burgdorferi* in the pathogenesis of lichen sclerosus continues to be unsettled. PCR studies from Europe show positive *Borrelia* antigen in lesions,[88] and spirochetes have been demonstrated by immunoperoxidase staining.[89]

Lichen sclerosus in the genitalia appears as ivory-colored atrophic or white, hyperkeratotic papules that coalesce into shiny, sclerotic plaques leading to phimosis in males. In females, the plaques may become sclerotic, bullous, ulcerated, or hemorrhagic (Fig. 139–7) and the epidermis may be thin and shiny or thick and white. End-stage vulvar lichen sclerosus shows total loss of identifiable structures, and the introitus can be reduced to a slit-like opening (Fig. 139–8). In women, the perianal area is frequently involved, giving rise to obstipation.

Early lichen sclerosus is generally very pruritic, but as it becomes chronic, symptoms secondary to erosions of stenotic orifices supervene. Depending on the stage of lichen sclerosus, the differential diagnosis may include lichen planus, lichen simplex chronicus, and the scarred end-stage of the different erosive conditions afflicting the genitalia. Multiple biopsy samples from noneroded lesions may be necessary to arrive at the correct diagnosis. Current therapy for lichen sclerosus relies on the use of superpotent topical steroids such as 0.05% clobetasol propionate. This results in rapid relief of symptoms with accompanying evidence of histologic improvement.[90] Whether persistent use of these agents will eventually reverse the disease process is still not known. Until the advent of the superpotent topical steroids, the mainstay

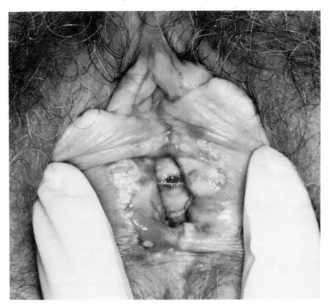

FIGURE 139–7. Lichen sclerosus showing small, yellow-white plaques, erosions, and hemorrhages. Note that the different parts of the vulva have not been obliterated.

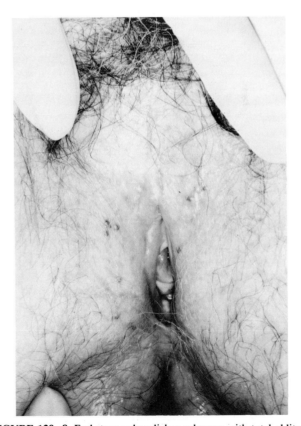

FIGURE 139–8. End-stage vulvar lichen sclerosus with total obliteration of its parts so that only a slit-like opening remains. Note small hemorrhagic vesicles.

of treatment was 2% testosterone propionate in white petrolatum, which resulted in clinical and histologic improvement.[91] For symptomatic children, progesterone, 100 mg/oz, was used. Vulvectomies are no longer indicated except in the presence of malignant change. However, excision of the diseased prepuce may be all that is necessary in males.

SYSTEMIC DISEASES

Diseases that give rise to erosions, aphthae, or ulcers on the genitalia are especially important in the evaluation of women with vulvodynia (see Table 139–3). In both sexes, recurrent ulcers on the genitalia should alert one to recurrent herpes simplex, aphthosis, Behçet's disease, and inflammatory bowel disease. Besides giving rise to aphthae, Crohn's disease may result in extraintestinal lesions that are suppurative granulomas. Pyoderma gangrenosum may present as "knife-cut" ulcers in the deep folds of the genital area.

NEOPLASMS

Benign Neoplasms

With a few exceptions, benign epidermal, dermal, and adnexal neoplasms occur on the genitalia as they would on the rest of the body.[92] Those with special predilection or importance in the genitalia are discussed here.

Angiokeratomas are common lesions in the genitalia of older men and women. When single, they are sometimes confused with melanomas. They are more frequently multiple (Fig. 139–9), dark red to purple papules, usually between 1 to 3 mm in diameter. When numerous on the scrotum of a young male, the possibility of Fabry's disease (angiokeratoma corporis diffusum)

might be considered. Angiokeratomas usually do not require therapy.

Bartholin's cyst is a cystic swelling in the posterolateral aspect of the vulvar vestibule caused by obstruction of Bartholin's duct. When sizable, it might cause pain. Because the obstruction tends to be recurrent, marsupialization is the treatment of choice.

Idiopathic calcinosis of the scrotum occurs as asymptomatic, grayish or yellowish white, firm nodules on scrotal skin. Its origin is not clear, and some believe that the calcifications are the residue of ancient epidermoid cysts. Draining lesions may be excised.

Pearly penile papules are small, smooth, dome-shaped or papillomatous papules occurring in the corona of the penis. They are a type of angiofibromas[93] and are asymptomatic and require no therapy (see Fig. 139–6).

Nonvenereal sclerosing lymphangitis of the penis presents as asymptomatic purplish cords around the coronal sulcus of the penis. Despite its name, it is most likely a post-traumatic phlebitis of superficial penile veins.[94] No therapy is needed.

Malignant Tumors

Intraepithelial Neoplasia

Equivalent classification and terminology apply to vaginal, cervical, penile, and anogenital intraepithelial neoplasia (see Table 139–2). Squamous intraepithelial neoplasia of the external genitalia comprise carcinoma in situ, Bowen's disease, bowenoid papulosis, and erythroplasia of Queyrat. The multifocal lesions (bowenoid papulosis) (Fig. 139–10) are more common in young persons and are associated with HPV (most commonly, types 16, 18, 31, and 33).[95, 96] These lesions appear as multiple, white, skin-colored or hyperpigmented flat papules of varying sizes. Although some of these lesions may progress to invasive squamous carcinoma,[97] most tend to follow a benign course (except possibly in immunosuppressed persons) so that the currently accepted

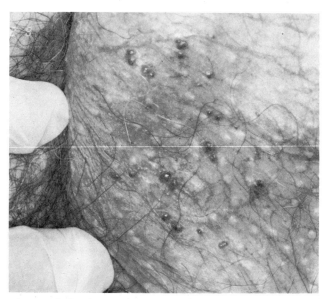

FIGURE 13–9. These angiokeratomas are 1- to 3-mm, dome-shaped, very superficial purple papules on the labia majora.

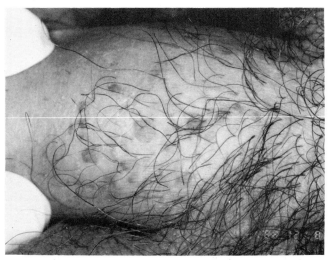

FIGURE 139–10. Penile flat warts are difficult to distinguish from the multifocal papular lesions of penile intraepithelial neoplasia III (bowenoid papulosis).

therapy is local destruction with careful longitudinal follow-up. Visualization is aided by application of acetic acid before colposcopy. Differential diagnosis of these multiple, discrete lesions includes flat warts, genital lentiginosis, and seborrheic keratoses. The solitary form of intraepithelial neoplasia, also known as Bowen's disease of the vulva or erythroplasia of Queyrat on the male genitalia, is more common in the older age group. This presents anywhere on the vulva of older women as a red or hyperpigmented, velvety to hyperkeratotic, pruritic plaque. In older men, it presents as a red, glazed patch, usually on the glans penis. These solitary lesions have a tendency to become invasive squamous cell carcinomas and are thus treated by excision, laser vaporization, or 5-fluorouracil. Follow-up is important.

Extramammary Paget's disease appears in the anogenital areas of older men and women as well-dermarcated, pruritic, erythematous, scaly, or eczematous plaques. This condition should be considered if a red, scaly eruption on or near genital skin does not resolve with topical therapy. Extramammary Paget's disease encompasses three entities: a primary intraepidermal carcinoma with apocrine differentiation, carcinoma of apocrine glands that colonizes the adjacent epidermis, and intraepithelial spread from nearby internal carcinomas, such as those of the rectum or bladder.[98] In all of these types, cells with abundant pale cytoplasm and atypical nuclei are scattered within the epidermis on biopsy. The cells of most cases stain with antisera to carcinoembryonic antigen.[99] Because the area of involvement is generally larger than what is superficially visible, margin control is necessary during the excision process.

Squamous Cell Carcinoma

Verrucous carcinoma, also known as giant condyloma of Buschke and Lowenstein, can reach enormous sizes in both men and women. These are now considered a type of squamous cell carcinoma despite their bland histologic appearance because of their tendency to recur after, and despite, extensive surgery. Radiation therapy can cause the tumor to become more aggressive.

Squamous cell carcinoma of the scrotum is associated with contact to tar and mineral oils.[100] Penile squamous cell carcinoma is almost never seen in circumcised males, suggesting that hygiene is important. There are indications that these cancers are also related to HPV[101] or to lichen sclerosus or may represent a progression of Bowen's disease. They may present as red or white plaques, verrucous lesions, or ulcers. Treatment is generally surgical, with amputation and node dissection depending on the stage of the cancer.

Squamous cell carcinoma, although rare, is the most frequent malignancy found in the vulva. Although other causes of chronic irritation may predispose to squamous cell carcinoma, most of the cases can likely be accounted for by progression of Bowen's disease (Fig. 139–11), HPV infection, and lichen sclerosus. In a review of slides of 107 patients with lichen sclerosus, 5% had concomitant invasive squamous cell carcinoma.[102] In evaluating histologic sections of vulvar squamous cell carcinoma, areas adjacent to the cancer showed evidence of lichen

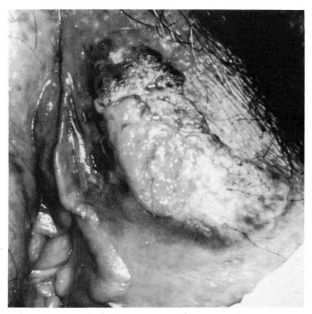

FIGURE 139–11. Squamous cell carcinoma on the vulva of a 20-year old woman who is on immunosuppressive chemotherapy for systemic lupus erythematous. She had evidence of human papillomavirus infection on other parts of the vulva.

sclerosus 30% of the time, squamous intraepithelial neoplasia 30% of the time, and a combination of lichen sclerosus and intraepithelial neoplasia in the rest.[99] Squamous cell carcinoma may appear as verrucous lesions, red or white plaques, and ulcers. Therapy is mostly surgical with total vulvectomy and node dissection depending on the stage.

Melanoma

Melanomas in the genitalia are rare. In a study of vulvar melanoma derived from data collected from a network of population-based cancer registries that includes about 10% of the U.S. population, Weinstock[103] found the incidence of vulvovaginal melanoma to be 1.6% of all melanomas in women and they were more common in older white women. In general, prognosis is poor and therapy is dependent on tumor thickness and whether metastases are present. Early diagnosis is the best treatment. Genital lentiginosis, in which the irregularly shaped pigmented patches are benign[104] needs to be differentiated from in situ melanoma. In genital lentiginosis, also known as vulvar or penile melanosis, there is abundant melanin in the basal layer of the epidermis with a discernible increase in the number of melanocytes.

VULVODYNIA

In 1983, a task force of the International Society for the Study of Vulvar Disease defined *vulvodynia* as chronic vulvar discomfort characterized by the patient's complaint of burning, irritation, or rawness.[3] This disorder was described as "excessive sensitiveness or hyperesthesia of the vulva" in *The Practical Home Physician* in 1886.[105] A hundred years later, this complaint of vulvar burning appears to have become more commonplace. One can speculate that there may be an environmental trigger (e.g., a virus, increased stress) or that women sense a certain freedom to discuss problems dealing with their genitalia. Systematic investigation of the possible causes and therapies for vulvodynia is just now beginning. As such, knowledge is nascent and much needs to be determined. For now, an algorithm for diagnosis is presented in Table 139–4. The first group of conditions that can give rise to chronic vulvar burning are those associated with ulcers and erosions of the mucocutaneous surfaces of the vulva. The second group of conditions have findings confined to the vulvar vestibule alone. The third group have in common unprovoked burning pain within and outside the vulvar vestibule. The clitoris, urethral orifice, anus, upper inner thighs and gluteal areas, and posterior leg may be involved in varying combinations.

Vulvar Vestibulitis Syndrome

In 1981, Friedrich defined the criteria for making a diagnosis of vulvar vestibulitis syndrome[106]: (1) pain on penile entry (introital dyspareunia), (2) findings confined to focal erythema within the vulvar vestibule, and (3) exquisite tenderness on light palpation of erythematous areas. Some of these cases had previously been reported as focal vulvitis,[107] infections of the minor vestibular gland,[108] and minor vestibular gland syndrome.[109] Numerous attempts to demonstrate an infectious or irritant etiology have not been fruitful. In a survey conducted in a private gynecologic practice, 15% of patients fulfilled the above criteria for the syndrome.[110] The typical patient complains of painful intercourse or inability to have intercourse. In those who are not sexually active, complaints range from pain on touching the vulvar vestibule, to pain on tampon insertion, on prolonged sitting, on riding a bicycle, on crossing the legs, or on wearing tight jeans. Except for these activities, patients are asymptomatic. Clinical findings are meager and confined to the vulvar vestibule. The mucosa may range from smooth to micropapillary. There is always erythema around the openings of Bartholin's ducts, at times accompanied by erythema around the openings of Skene's glands and around the ostia of minor vestibular glands at the base of the hymen (Fig. 139–12; see color plate). In long-standing and more severe cases, erythema and splitting at the fourchette are seen.

Histologic examination of these focal erythematous areas has revealed nonspecific submucosal and periglandular chronic inflammation with occasional metaplasia of the ostia of some vestibular glands.[111]

What are the candidate etiologies of this syndrome?

1. Trauma. We have encountered vulvar vestibulitis syndrome after 5-fluorouracil and CO_2 laser treatment of the vulva for condylomata acuminata.

2. HPV infection. With the use of molecular biologic techniques, HPV has been demonstrated in some samples,[111-113] but the yield of HPV is no higher than in an asymptomatic population.[56]

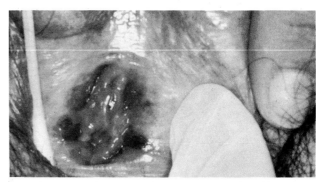

FIGURE 139–12. In this patient with vulvar vestibulitis syndrome there is marked erythema in the vulvar vestibule around the openings of Bartholin's ducts and Skene's ducts. Application of light pressure on these areas by an applicator tip elicits exquisite tenderness. (See color plate.)

3. Chronic candidiasis. In my experience, about 30% of patients with vulvar vestibulitis syndrome experience symptomatic, potassium hydroxide or culture positive candidiasis at some point.[114] However, 3- to 6-month courses of systemic anticandidal therapy have not produced lasting relief despite subsequent negative cultures.

4. Idiopathic. Most cases fall into this category. I believe idiopathic vulvar vestibulitis syndrome may just be an earlier stage of pudendal neuralgia.

The first rule of therapy is to discontinue everything the patient has been using or taking to get the patient to baseline levels. The next strategy is conservative management consisting of the application of bland barrier preparations such as white petrolatum or zinc oxide supplemented with topical anesthetics such as lidocaine ointment or EMLA (eutectic mixture of prilocaine and lidocaine). For those with demonstrable *Candida* on potassium hydroxide or culture, systemic anticandidal therapy may be initiated and continued for 3 to 6 months after cultures have turned negative. Although first reported as treatment for condylomatous vulvitis,[115] interferon alfa administered intradermally into the vestibule has provided temporary relief in women with idiopathic vulvar vestibulitis.[116] The long-term benefit of this modality is not known. For patients with long-standing (>2 years) entry dyspareunia of such severity as to almost totally prevent sexual intercourse, surgical excision of the vulvar vestibule with mobilization of the vaginal mucosa[106, 107, 113] offers about a 65% rate of success. Success is measured by increased ability to engage in pain-free intercourse. The long-term benefit from this procedure needs to be reported. In women presenting with vulvar vestibulitis after topical 5-fluorouracil or laser therapy, reassurance that their symptoms will most likely clear up with conservative therapy is important. Rare spontaneous remissions have also been encountered.

Zoon's Vulvitis

This entity[117] must be analogous to that which occurs on the penis, and it is possible that this represents the chronic form of vulvar vestibulitis syndrome in which the infiltrate is composed almost completely of plasma cells. Intralesional interferon alfa and local excision have both been reported to successfully clear the problem.

Pudendal Neuralgia

To facilitate the study and understanding of the chronic vulvar pain syndrome characterized by constant, burning pain and dyspareunia, Turner and Marinoff[118] suggested grouping these cases under the rubric of pudendal neuralgia. In contrast to vulvar vestibulitis syndrome, the burning pain is unprovoked and extends outside the vulvar vestibule. It is often accompanied by a deep aching component with occasional paroxysms of severe lancinating pain. The similarity of these symptoms to those described for post–herpes zoster neuralgia[119] and diabetic neuropathy suggested neuropathic pain in the area innervated by the pudendal nerve (S-2 to S-5). Pudendal neuralgia secondary to nerve injury is not new.[120, 121] It has been reported in males after straddle injuries in wartime.[122] In my practice, there are patients who date the onset of their problems to some form of injury, such as from falls, automobile accidents, bicycling accidents, and spinal laminectomies, or to having been maintained in a prolonged lithotomy position for a surgical procedure. In most cases, a clear traumatic incident cannot be recalled.

Affected patients vary in age from the late teens to the 70s, but most are in their mid 20s to mid 30s. Additional complaints include deep itching, formication, a painful burning sensation on light touch, discomfort or burning on movement of pubic hairs, entry to postcoital dyspareunia, and a sensation of labial swelling. Some patients experience dysuria and frequency, clitoral pain, "sciatica-like" pains, and radiation of pain to the perianal area. It is clear that these patients' complaints extend well outside the vulvar vestibule. In general, their discomfort is aggravated during the midcycle or just before the onset of their menstrual period, as well as by sitting and standing for long periods of time.

Visible changes are generally limited to mild erythema around the openings of the vestibular glands. The vulvar mucosa may be smooth or micropapillary. There are generally no visible changes on the surrounding skin except for the rare scar from trauma or surgical procedure and the equally rare acute lesion of genital HSV infection. Sensory testing of the area innervated by the pudendal nerve (Fig. 139–13) using a sharp-pointed stick and a cotton-tipped applicator reveals a multiplicity of responses. A sharp prick may be perceived as dull (hypalgesia) or extremely painful (hyperalgesia) or may evoke diffuse pain that lasts much longer than the inciting stimulus (hyperpathia). When a cotton-tipped applicator is used to put light pressure on the ostia of vestibular glands, severe sharp pain occurs. Lightly stroking the mucosal surfaces of the labia minora, of the vestibule and, sometimes, of the urethral orifice and the clitoris is generally perceived as burning pain (allodynia). These sensory findings may vary somewhat from day to day and are not defined by strict dermatomes, although they stay in the general area innervated by the pudendal nerve.

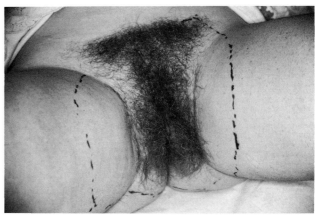

FIGURE 139–13. In pudendal neuralgia, abnormal sensory findings can be elicited within the rhomboidal area roughly corresponding to the field supplied by the pudendal nerve.

In the majority of cases, the cause is idiopathic. There are rare reports of pudendal neuralgia with recurrent HSV infection,[123, 124] and we have seen several such cases. Other reported causes include sacral meningeal cysts,[125] neurofibroma,[120] and trauma to the nerve as it traverses Alcock's canal.[121]

Drug therapy of the idiopathic cases relies on the use of tricyclic antidepressants (e.g., amitriptyline and imipramine) and topical anesthetics for milder cases and anticonvulsants for those with accompanying paroxysmal pain. Tricyclic antidepressants relieve the neuropathic pain of post–herpes zoster neuralgia[126] and diabetic neuropathy independent of their antidepressant effects.[127] This class of drugs blocks norepinephrine reuptake at synapses, thus increasing norepinephrine-mediated inhibition of spinal cord neurons involved in pain perception.[128] Additional actions such as decreasing α_2- and β-adrenergic receptor sensitivity and potentiating responses to α_1-adrenergic receptor antagonists[129] may also come into play. Before prescribing these medications, familiarize yourself with their pharmacokinetics and side effects, some of which are sommnolence, postural hypotension, anticholinergic effects, tachycardia, hypertension, weight gain, and photosensitivity. Individual patients vary in the type of side effects they experience and the dose they can tolerate. It is best to start with the lowest dose of 10 mg of amitriptyline or 25 mg of imipramine before bedtime and allow the patient's condition to stabilize before increasing the dose. It may take 2 to 3 weeks to tell if the medication is having any effect. These medications should also be discontinued in a stepwise fashion. Most often, the therapeutic dose for pain, generally not more than 75 mg per day of either medication, is much lower than the dose at which antidepressant effects are seen. Of the medications in this class, amitriptyline and imipramine have been the most studied.

Phenytoin and carbamazepine are the two most commonly used anticonvulsants for the treatment of neuralgic pain and have been helpful in the group of patients who experience paroxysmal stabbing or shooting pains in addition to the constant burning component. The anticonvulsants work by increasing the threshold at which nerve transmission occurs.[130] Besides monitoring for side effects (e.g., somnolence, hepatitis), blood levels of the medication should be checked to make sure that therapeutic levels are achieved. Regular blood cell counts and liver transaminase levels should also be monitored. Drug interactions are frequent with this class of drugs so that other medications that the patients are taking should be noted.

Acyclovir prophylaxis has limited use. It appears helpful in those exceptional patients in whom active recurrences of HSV can be documented.

There are anecdotal reports that topical anesthetics, topical steroids, and capsaicin offer temporary relief as do hydroxyzine, some muscle relaxants, and intermittent courses of systemic antibiotics.

Some patients experience some relief from cold applications to the area. When present, the etiology of irritating vaginal discharges needs to be determined and appropriate therapy initiated since the mere presence of a discharge at the introitus can irritate an already hypersensitive mucosa. Topical anesthetics offer some measure of relief once the patient gets over the initial irritation from the anesthetic vehicle.

Whether there is a role for total vestibulectomy for relief of the vestibular component of this problem remains to be studied carefully. The same applies to laser ablation of the vulvar vestibule, which in my experience has actually aggravated the problem.

There are anecdotal and case reports[131] documenting temporary relief from pudendal and epidural nerve blocks, with or without the addition of systemic corticosteroids. It is not uncommon to experience immediate relief from nerve blocks and nerve sections, but complicating neuritis frequently leads to more pain, which makes such procedures questionable for the management of chronic pain.[132] Some studies are underway to test the efficacy of sympathetic blocks.

Biofeedback, stress reduction techniques, acupuncture, transepidermal nerve stimulation, and muscle relaxation techniques are some of the alternative therapies that have been tried in other pain syndromes and need to be systematically evaluated with respect to this problem.

Most of the women suffering from vulvodynia have at one time or another been labeled as having a psychosomatic illness. At the moment, there are no data that show that these patients are innately depressed or have some other personality disorder or psychiatric diagnosis. However, it is known that while the majority of chronic pain patients do not suffer from major depression, the prevalence of major depression in this population is three to four times that in normal persons.[133] In addition to an understanding physician, support groups and psychological consultations are encouraged to help patients cope with the different ramifications of this problem.

Perineal Pain Syndromes

Other syndromes listed in Table 139–4 have been described with varying combinations of pain involving the structures located within the perineum. In several, such as levator syndrome and prostatodynia (in males),

dyspareunia is also a problem. However, in none of the descriptions of these entities has there been any mention of sensory abnormalities.

TOPICAL THERAPY FOR THE VULVA

Topical therapy is tailored to the stage of the disease. In general, harsh chemicals should be avoided.

Cleansing

Tepid tap water is best for regular cleansing. Soap is not necessary. When the area is so irritated that even plain water cannot be tolerated, pure mineral oil makes a good cleansing agent.

Wet Dressings and Baths

Open wet dressings or tub baths are useful for drying lesions that are weeping, eroded, or ulcerated. They are also effective for gentle debridement of adherent scales and crusts. Although plain water works well, the addition of colloidal oatmeal, cornstarch, sea salt, baking soda, or Epsom salt (magnesium sulfate) is said to result in more soothing solutions. The addition of Domeboro powder to tap water to make Burow's solution or of household vinegar to tap water results in solutions with both astringent and antiseptic properties.

Bases of Topical Therapeutic Agents

As a general rule, lotions and light creams work best in this warm, moist, and hairy environment. A pure petrolatum base is well tolerated where the mucosa is eroded.

For the treatment of weeping or denuded lesions it is sometimes necessary to compound "shake lotions" incorporating active therapeutic agents, since most commercially available lotions contain irritating alcohols in their bases. A modification of such a lotion base is 15 g zinc oxide, 15 g talc, 10 g glycerin, and water to make 100 mL. Such a lotion dries into a fine powder and, as the name implies, needs to be shaken before use. Once the acute stage passes, commercially available therapeutic lotions and light creams may be substituted, depending on the patient's tolerance. Generic formulations vary considerably with regard to bases and preservatives,[134] and this is an instance in which prescribing a specific preparation with known ingredients has merit.

Protective Agents

Pastes, which are combinations of white petrolatum and powders such as talc, bentonite, aluminum oxide, and zinc oxide, are useful in protecting surrounding tissues from irritating discharges or exudates. Besides providing a physical barrier, the powder content provides some absorptive capability. Readily available and inexpensive pastes include Lassar's paste and zinc oxide ointment.

Topical Steroids

The guiding principle is to choose the appropriate strength in the appropriate vehicle to achieve the shortest exposure possible. Acute dermatoses can be expected to show some response to a midpotency steroid after 48 hours and to clear within 2 weeks. Subacute to chronic dermatoses may be treated with a midpotent to potent topical steroid for 2 weeks and switched to a milder preparation for maintenance therapy. Similar to the experience with the use of fluorinated topical steroids on the face, some patients have the propensity to develop rosacea-like eruptions in the genital area after chronic use of topical steroids. Rebound erythema, epidermal atrophy, telangiectasia, milia, persistent erythema, and opportunistic yeast and fungal infections have also been seen with unrestricted use of potent topical steroids. The mucosal surfaces of the labia minora (Fig. 139–14) and the glans penis seem to be more vulnerable. Persistent purple discoloration of the glans penis has been noted after chronic application of fluorinated steroids.

Other Therapies

Topical cytotoxic agents, caustic solutions, cryotherapy, laser therapy, and other destructive modalities cause burn-like injuries, and healing depends on the modality used and the depth of destruction. Discomfort may persist for a while after reepithelialization has occurred.

Topical anesthetics such as 5% lidocaine ointment or EMLA cream are useful for pain relief when the mucosal surfaces are eroded.

Vaginal dilators may be helpful in keeping the canal patent during the reepithelialization of an erosive vulvitis.

Psychological support and reassurance are important aspects of the treatment of diseases affecting the genitalia. Fear of sexual transmission and the possibility or actuality of interference with normal sexual function are problems to be discussed openly and addressed.

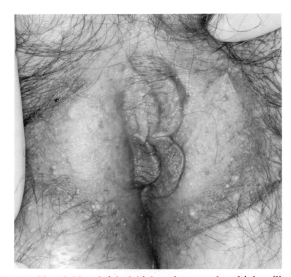

FIGURE 139–14. Note bright labial erythema and multiple milia after prolonged use of Lotrisone cream for mild vulvar irritation. At this point, the patient was complaining of burning.

References

1. Ridley CM, Frankman O, Jones ISC, et al. New nomenclature for vulvar disease. Am J Obstet Gynecol 1989;160:769–770.
2. Wilkinson EJ, Kneale B, Lynch PJ. Report of the ISSVD Terminology Committee. J Reprod Med 1986;31:973–974.
3. Burning vulva syndrome: Report of the ISSVD task force. J Reprod Med 1984;29:457.
4. McLean JM. Embryology and congenital anomalies of the vulval area. In: Ridley CM, ed. The Vulva, 2nd ed. London: Churchill Livingstone, 1988:1–38.
5. Wilson JD. Testosterone uptake by the urogenital tract of the rabbit embryo. Endocrinology 1973;92:1192–1197.
6. Smith HR, Hosker GL, Warrell GW. The role of partial denervation of the pelvic floor in the etiology of genitourinary prolapse and stress incontinence of urine: A neurophysiological study. Br J Obstet Gynaecol 1989;96:24–28.
7. Drake TE, Maibach HI. *Candida* and candidiasis: Cultural conditions, epidemiology, and pathogenesis. Postgrad Med 1973;53:83.
8. Christoph RA, Buchanan L, Begalia K, et al. Pain reduction in local anesthetic administration through pH buffering. Ann Emerg Med 1988;117:27–30.
9. Melish ME, Glasgow LA. The staphylococcal scalded skin syndrome: The expanded clinical syndrome. J Pediatr 1971;78:958.
10. Dhar V, Roker MLSO, Adami Z, et al. Streptococcal vulvovaginitis in girls. Pediatr Dermatol 1993;10:366–367.
11. Freeman RG, McBride ME, Knox JM. Pathogenesis of trichomycosis axillaris. Arch Dermatol 1969;100:90–95.
12. Holmes KK. The *Chlamydia* epidemic. JAMA 1981;245:1718–1723.
13. Wasserheit JN. Pelvic imflammatory disease and infertility. Md Med J 1987;36:58–63.
14. Tam MR, Stamm WE, Handsfield HH, et al. Culture-independent diagnosis of *Chlamydia trachomatis* using monoclonal antibodies. N Engl J Med 1984;310:1146–1150.
15. Westrom L, Evaldson G, Holmes KK, et al. Taxonomy of vaginosis; bacterial vaginosis—a definition. In: Mardh P-Am, Taylor-Robinson D, eds. Bacterial Vaginosis. Stockholm: Almquist and Wiksell, 1984:259–260.
16. Sobel JD. Bacterial vaginosis—an ecologic mystery. Ann Intern Med 1989;111:551–553.
17. Pheifer TA, Forsyth PS, Durfee MA, et al. Nonspecific vaginitis: Role of *Haemophilus vaginalis* and treatment with metronidazole. N Engl J Med 1978;298:1429.
18. Swedberg J, Steiner JF, Deiss F, et al. Comparison of single-dose vs one-week course of metronidazole for symptomatic bacterial vaginosis. JAMA 1985;254:1046.
19. Sobel JD. Vulvovaginitis. Dermatol Clin 1992;10:339–359.
20. Addison WA, Livengood CH III, Hill GB, et al. Necrotizing fasciitis of vulvar origin in diabetic patients. Obstet Gynecol 1984;63:473–479.
21. Bahlmann JCM, Fourie IJH, Arndt TCH. Fournier's gangrene; necrotizing fasciitis of the male genitalia. Br J Urol 1983;55:85–88.
22. Umbert IJ, Winkelmann RK, Oliver GF, et al. Necrotizing fasciitis: A clinical, microbiologic, and histopathologic study of 14 patients. J Am Acad Dermatol 1989;20:774–781.
23. Kalter DC, Tschen JA, Cernoch PL, et al. Genital white piedra: Epidemiology, microbiology and therapy. J Am Acad Dermatol 1986;14:982–993.
24. Odds FC. Genital candidiasis. Clin Exp Dermatol 1982;7:345–354.
25. Sobel JD. Candidal vulvovaginitis. Clin Obstet Gynecol 1993;36:153–165.
26. Sobel JD. Vulvovaginal candidiasis—what we do and do not know. Ann Intern Med 1984;101:390–392.
27. Robertson WH. A concentrated therapeutic regimen for vulvovaginal candidiasis. JAMA 1980;244:2549–2550.
28. Hilton E, Isenberg HD, Alperstein P, et al. Ingestion of yogurt containing *Lactobacillus acidophilus* as prophylaxis for candidal vaginitis. Ann Intern Med 1992;116:353–357.
29. Sobel JD. Recurrent vulvovaginal candidiasis: A prospective study of the efficacy of maintenance ketoconazole therapy. N Engl J Med 1986;315:1455–1458.
30. Sobel JD. Fluconazole maintenance therapy in recurrent vulvovaginal candidiasis. Int J Gynecol Obstet 1992;37(S1):17.

31. Becker TM, Blount JM, Douglas J, et al. Trends in molluscum contagiosum in the United States: 1966–1983. Sex Transm Dis 1986;13:18.
32. Johnson RE, Nahmias AJ, Madger LS, et al. A serial epidemiologic survey of the prevalence of herpes simplex virus type 2 infection in the United States. N Engl J Med 1989;321:7–12.
33. Sullivan-Bolyai J, Hall HF, Wilson C, et al. Neonatal herpes simplex virus infection in Kings County, Washington. JAMA 1983;250:3059–3062.
34. Langenberg A, Benedetti J, Jennifer-Jenkins BS, et al. Development of clinically recognizable genital lesions among women previously identified as having "asymptomatic" herpes simplex virus type 2 infection. Ann Intern Med 1989;110:882–887.
35. Koelle DM, Benedetti J, Langenberg A, et al. Asymptomatic reactivation of herpes simplex virus in women after the first episode of genital herpes. Ann Intern Med 1992;116:433–437.
36. Kalinyak JE, Fleagle G, Docherty J. Incidence and distribution of herpes simplex virus types 1 and 2 from genital lesions in college women. J Med Virol 1977;1:175–181.
37. Kaufman RH, Gardner HL, Rawls WE, et al. Clinical features of herpes genitalis. Cancer Res 1973;33:1446–1451.
38. Kaufman RH, Faro S. Herpes genitalis: Clinical features and treatment. Clin Obstet Gynecol 1985;28:152–163.
39. Corey L, Adams HG, Brown ZA, et al. Genital herpes simplex infection: Clinical manifestations, course and complications. Ann Intern Med 1983;98:958–972.
40. Mosley RC, Corey L, Benjamin D, et al. Comparison of viral isolation, direct immunofluorescence, and indirect imunoperoxidase techniques for determination of genital herpes simplex virus infection. J Clin Microbiol 1981;13:913–915.
41. Motyl MR, Bottone EJ, Janda MJ. Diagnosis of herpesvirus infections: Correlation of Tzanck preparations with viral isolation. Diagn Microbiol Infect Dis 1984;2:157–160.
42. Bryson YJ, Dillon M, Lovett M, et al. Treatment of first episodes of genital herpes simplex virus infection with oral acyclovir: A randomized double-blind controlled trial in normal subjects. N Engl J Med 1983;308:916–921.
43. Corey L, Fife KH, Benedetti J. Intravenous acyclovir for the treatment of primary genital herpes. Ann Intern Med 1983;98:914–921.
44. Reichman RC, Badger GJ, Mertz GJ, et al. Treatment of recurrent genital herpes simplex infections with oral acyclovir. JAMA 1984;251:2103–2107.
45. Kaplowits LG, Baker D, Gelb L. Prolonged continuous acyclovir treatment of normal adults with frequently recurrent genital herpes simplex virus infection. JAMA 1991;265:747–751.
46. Straus SE, Seidlin M, Takiff HE, et al. Effect of oral acyclovir on symptomatic and asymptomatic virus shedding in recurrent genital herpes. Sex Transm Dis 1989;16:107–113.
47. Erlich KS, Mills J, Chatis P, et al. Acyclovir-resistant herpes simplex virus infections in patients with the acquired immunodeficiency syndrome. N Engl J Med 1989;320:293–296.
48. Erlich KS, Jacobson MA, Koehler JE, et al. Foscarnet therapy for severe acyclovir resistant herpes simplex virus type 2 infections in patients with acquired immunodeficiency syndrome. Ann Intern Med 1989;110:710–713.
49. Wheatley RJ, Arvin A, Prober C, et al. Predictors of morbidity and mortality in neonates with herpes simplex virus infections. The National Institute of Allergy and Infectious Diseases Collaborative Antiviral Study Group. N Engl J Med 1991;324:450–454.
50. Brown ZA, Benedetti J, Ashley R. Neonatal herpes simplex virus infections in relation to asymptomatic matenal infection at the time of labor. N Engl J Med 1991;324:1247–1252.
51. Nahmias AJ, Roizman B. Infection with herpes simplex virus 1 and 2. N Engl J Med 1973;289:667–673.
52. Izuma AK, Edwards J. Herpes zoster and neurogenic bladder dysfunction. JAMA 1973;224:1748–1750.
53. Oriel JD. Natural history of genital warts. Br J Vener Dis 1971;47:1–13.
54. Condyloma acuminatum—United States 1966–1981. MMWR 1981;32:306–308.
55. Consultations for condyloma acuminata, United States, 1966–1983. MMWR 1983;33:81.
56. Bauer HM, Yiting MS, Gree CE, et al. Genital human papillomavirus infection in female university students as determined by PCR-based method. JAMA 1991;265:472–477.

57. Green J, Monteiro E, Bolton VN, et al. Detection of human papillomavirus DNA by PCR in semen from patients with and without penile warts. Genitourin Med 1991;67:207–210.
58. Chief Medical Office of the Department of Health and Social Security: Sexually transmitted diseases. Br J Vener Dis 1983; 59:134–137.
59. Carmichael JA, Clarice DH, Moher D, et al. Cervical carcinoma in women aged 34 and younger. Am J Obstet Gynecol 1986;154:264–269.
60. Crook T, Tidy JA, Vousden HK. Degradation of p53 can be targeted by HPV E6 sequences distinct from those required for p53 binding and trans-activation. Cell 1991;67:547–556.
61. Syrjanen KJ. Natural history of genital HPV infections. Papillomavirus Rep 1989;23:1–12.
62. Gissman L, zurHausen H: Partial characterization of viral DNA from human genital warts (condyloma acuminata). Int J Cancer 1980;25:605–609.
63. Ferenczy A, Mitae M, Nagai N, et al. Latent papillomavirus and recurrent genital warts. N Engl J Med 1985;313:784–788.
64. Moscicki AB, Palefsky JM, Gonzales J, et al. Colposcopic and histologic findings and human papillomavirus (HPV) DNA test variability in young women positive for HPV DNA. J Infect Dis 1992;166:951–957.
65. Koss LG, Durfee GR. Unusual patterns of squamous epithelium of the uterine cervix: Cytologic and pathologic study of koilocytotic atypia. Ann NY Acad Sci 1956;63:1245–1261.
66. Berth-Jones J, Hutchinson PE. Modern treatment of warts: Cure rates at 3 and 6 months. Br J Dermatol 1992;127:262–265.
67. Krebs HB. Treatment of vaginal condylomata acuminata by weekly topical application of 5-fluorouracil. Obstet Gynecol 1987;70:68–71.
68. Sillman FH, Sedlis A, Boyce JB. A review of lower genital intraepithelial neoplasia and the use of topical 5-fluorouracil. Obstet Gynecol Surv 1985;40:190–220.
69. Eron L, Judson F, Tucker S, et al. Interferon therapy for condylomata acuminata. N Engl J Med 1986;315:1059–1064.
70. Reichman RC, Oakes D, Bonnez W, et al. Treatment of condyloma acuminatum with three different interferons administered intralesionally. Ann Intern Med 1988;108:675–679.
71. Gross G, Ikenberg H, Roussaki A, et al. Systemic treatment of condylomata acuminata with recombinant interferon-alpha-2A: Low dose superior to the high-dose regimen. Chemotherapy 1986;32:537–541.
72. Kirby PK, Kiviat N, Beckman A, et al. Tolerance and efficacy of recombinant interferon gamma in the treatment of refractory genital warts. Am J Med 1988;85:183–188.
73. Gross G, Pfister H, Hagedorn M, et al. Effect of oral aromatic retinoid (Ro-109359) on human papillomavirus–induced common warts. Dermatologica 1983;166:48–53.
74. Lutzner MA, Blanchet-Bardon C. Oral retinoid treatment of human papillomavirus type 5–induced epidermodysplasia verruciformis. N Engl J Med 1980;302:1091.
75. Olsen EA, Kelly FF, Vollmer RT, et al. Comparative study of systemic interferon alfa-n1 and isotretinoin in the treatment of resistant condylomata acuminata. J Am Acad Dermatol 1989;20:1023–1030.
76. Lin YL, Borenstein LA, Selvakumar R, et al. Effective vaccination against papilloma development by immunization with L1 or L2 structural protein of cottontail rabbit papillomavirus. Virology 1992;187:612–619.
77. Campo MS. Vaccination against papillomavirus. Cancer Cells 1991;11:421–426.
78. Fisher LM. Isis drug approved for testing. New York Times, March 5, 1992, p D4.
79. Riva J, Sedlacek T, Cunnane M, et al. Extended carbon dioxide laser vaporization in the treatment of subclinical papillomavirus infection of the lower genital tract. Obstet Gynecol 1989; 73:25–30.
80. Edwards L, Friedrich EG Jr. Desquamative vaginitis: Lichen planus in disguise. Obstet Gynecol 1988;71:832–836.
81. Edwards L. Desquamative vulvitis. Dermatol Clin 1992; 10:325–337.
82. Sigurgeirsson B, Lindelof B. Lichen planus and malignancy: An epidemiologic study of 2071 patients and a review of the literature. Arch Dermatol 1991;127:1684–1688.
83. Berth-Jones J, Graham-Brown RA, Burns DA. Lichen sclerosus

et atrophicus—a review of 15 cases in young girls. Clin Exp Dermatol 1991;16:14–17.
84. Myerick TRH, Ridley CM, McGibbon DH, et al. Lichen sclerosus et atrophicus and autoimmunity—a study of 350 women. Br J Dermatol 1988;108:41.
85. Chalmers RJG, Burton PA, Bennett RF, et al. Lichen sclerosus et atrophicus: A common and distinctive cause of phimosis in boys. Arch Dermatol 1984;120:1025–1027.
86. Harrington CI, Dunsmore IR. An investigation into the incidence of autoimmune disorders in patients with lichen sclerosus et atrophicus. Br J Dermatol 1981;104:563–566.
87. Purcell KG, Spencer LV, Simpson PM, et al. HLA antigens in lichen sclerosus et atrophicus. Arch Dermatol 1990;126: 1043–1045.
88. Schempp C, Bocklage H, Lange R, et al. Further evidence for *Borrelia burgdorferi* infection in morphea and lichen sclerosus et atrophicus confirmed by DNA amplification. J Invest Dermatol 1993;100:717–720.
89. Aberer E, Stanek G. Histological evidence for spirochetal origin of morphea and lichen sclerosus et atrophicans. Am J Dermatopathol 1987;9:374–379.
90. Dalziel KL, Millard PR, Wojnarowska F. The treatment of vulval lichen sclerosus with a very potent topical steroid (clobetasol propionate 0.05%) cream. Br J Dermatol 1991;124:461–464.
91. Friedrich EG Jr. Vulvar dystrophy. Clin Obstet Gynecol 1985;28:178–187.
92. Hood AF, Lumadue J. Benign vulvar tumors. Dermatol Clin 1992;10:371–385.
93. Ackerman AB, Kornberg R. Pearly penile papules: Acral angiofibromas. Arch Dermatol 1973;108:673–675.
94. Findlay GH, Whiting DA. Mondor's phlebitis of the penis. Clin Exp Dermatol 1977;2:65–67.
95. Crum CP. Vulvar intraepithelial neoplasia: Histology and associated viral changes. In: Wilkinson EJ, ed. Pathology of the Vulva and Vagina. New York: Churchill Livingstone, 1987:79–101.
96. Barrasso R, De Brux J, Croissant O, et al. High prevalence of papillomavirus-associated penile intraepithelial neoplasia in sexual partners of women with cervical intraepithelial neoplasia. N Engl J Med 1987;317:916–923.
97. Pilotti S, Rilke F, Shah KV, et al. Immunohistochemical and ultrastructural evidence of papillomavirus infection associated with in situ and microinvasive squamous cell carcinoma of the vulva. Am J Surg Pathol 1984;8:751.
98. Jones RE, Austin C, Ackerman AB. Extramammary Paget's disease: A critical reexamination. Am J Dermatopathol 1979; 1:101–132.
99. Leibowitch M, Neill S, Pelisse M, et al. The epithelial changes associated with squamous cell carcinoma of the vulva: A review of the clinical, histological, and viral findings. Br J Obstet Gynaecol 190;12:1135–1139.
100. Lee WR, Alderson MR, Downes JE. Scrotal cancer in the northwest of England. Br J Indust Med 1972;29:188–195.
101. Martinez I. Relationship of squamous cell carcinoma of the cervix uteri to squamous cell carcinoma of the penis among Puerto Rican women married to men with penile carcinoma. Cancer 1969;24:777–780.
102. Hart WR, Norris HJ, Helwig EB. Relation of lichen sclerosus et atrophicus of the vulva to development of carcinoma. Obstet Gynecol 1975;45:369–376.
103. Weinstock MA. Malignant melanoma of the vulva and vagina in the United States: Patterns of incidence and population-based estimates of survival. (In press).
104. Barnhill RL, Albert LS, Shama SK, et al. Genital lentiginosis: A clinical and histopathologic study. J Am Acad Dermatol 1990;22:453–460.
105. Friedrich E. Vulvar Diseases, 2nd ed. Philadelphia: WB Saunders Co., 1983:238.
106. Friedrich EG. Vulvar vestibulitis syndrome. J Reprod Med 1987;32:110–114.
107. Peckham BM, Maki DG, Patterson JJ, et al. Focal vulvitis: A

characteristic syndrome and cause of dyspareunia: Features, natural history, and management. Am J Obstet Gynecol 1986; 154:855–864.
108. Woodruff JD, Parmley TH. Infection of the minor vestibular gland. Obstet Gynecol 1983;62:609–612.
109. Marinoff SC, Turner MLC. Hypersensitivity to vaginal candidiasis or treatment vehicles in the pathogenesis of minor vestibular gland syndrome. J Reprod Med 1986;31:796–799.
110. Goetsch MF. Vulvar vestibulitis: Prevalence and historic features in a general gynecologic practice population. Am J Obstet Gynecol 1991;164:1609–1614.
111. Pyka RE, Wilkinson EJ, Friedrich EG Jr, et al. The histopathology of vulvar vestibulitis syndrome. Int J Gynecol Pathol 1988;7:249–257.
112. Turner ML, Marinoff SC. Association of human papillomavirus with vulvodynia and the vulvar vestibulitis syndrome. J Reprod Med 1988;36:533–537.
113. Umpierre SA, Kaufman RH, Adam E, et al. Human papillomavirus DNA in tissue biopsy specimens of vulvar vestibulitis patients treated with interferon. Obstet Gynecol 1991;78:693–695.
114. Marinoff SC, Roe A, Turner ML. Total vestibulectomy and vaginal advancement in the treatment of vulvar vestibulitis syndrome. Presented at XII Congress of the ISSVD in Quebec, Canada, September 1993.
115. Horowitz BJ. Interferon therapy for condylomatous vulvitis. Obstet Gynecol 1989;73:446–448.
116. Marinoff SC, Turner ML, Hirsch RP, Richard G. Intralesional alpha interferon: Cost-effective therapy for vulvar vestibulitis syndrome. J Reprod Med 1993;38:19–24.
117. Davis J, Shapiro L, Baral J. Vulvitis circumscripta plasmacellularis. J Am Acad Dermatol 1983;8:413–416.
118. Turner MLC, Marinoff SC. Pudendal neuralgia. Am J Obstet Gynecol 1991;165:1233–1236.
119. Watson PN, Evans RJ. Postherpetic neuralgia. Arch Neurol 1986;43:836–840.
120. Tognetti F, Poppi M, Gaist G, et al. Pudendal neuralgia due to solitary neurofibroma. J Neurosurg 1982;56:732–733.
121. Amarenco G, Le Cocquen-Amarenco A, Kerdraon J, et al. Perineal neuralgia. Presse Med 1991;20:71–74.
122. Zuerler G. Reizung des Nervus pudendus (Neuralgie). Berl Klin Wochenschr 1915;52:1260–1261.
123. Layzer RB, Connant MA. Neuralgia in recurrent herpes simplex. Arch Neurol 1974;31:233–237.
124. Howard EJ. Postherpetic pudendal neuralgia. JAMA 1985; 253:2196.
125. Van de Kelft E, Van Vyve M. Chronic perineal pain related to sacral meningeal cysts. Neurosurgery 1991;29:223–226.
126. Watson CP, Evans RJ, Reed K, et al. Amitriptyline versus placebo in postherpetic neuralgia. Neurology 1982;32:671–673.
127. Max MB, Culnane M, Schafer RNC, et al. Amitriptyline relieves diabetic neuropathy pain in patients with normal or depressed mood. Neurology 1987;37:589–596.
128. Dubner R, Bennet GJ. Spinal and trigeminal mechanisms of nociception. Ann Rev Neurosci 1983;6:381–418.
129. Racagni G, Brunello N. Transsynaptic mechanisms in the action of antidepressant drugs. Trends Pharmacol Sci 1984;5:527–531.
130. Swerdlow M. Review: Anticonvulsant drugs and chronic pain. Clin Neuropharmacol 1984;7:51–82.
131. Bensigor-Le Henaff M, Labat JJ, Robert R, et al. Perineal neuralgia in connection with suffering pudendal nerves. Agressologie 1991;5:277–279.
132. Wood KM. Peripheral nerve and root chemical lesions. In Wall PD, Melzack R, eds. Textbook of Pain, 2nd ed. New York: Churchill Livingstone, 1989:768–771.
133. Sullivan MJL, Reesor K, Mikail S, et al. The treatment of depression in chronic low back pain: Review and recommendations. Pain 1992;50:5–13.
134. Fisher AA: Problems associated with "generic" topical medications. Cutis 1988;41:313–314.

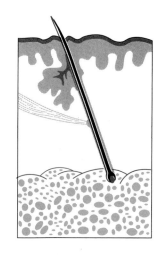

What Benign and Malignant Proliferations of Cells Affect the Skin, and How Are They Treated?

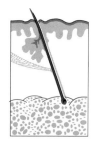

chapter 140

Molecular Mechanisms of Photocarcinogenesis: The Role of *ras* and *p53* Alterations

SAGARIKA KANJILAL
and HONNAVARA N. ANANTHASWAMY

Cells that proliferate in defiance of the normal restraints of the cell cycle give rise to tumors or neoplasms. As long as the neoplastic cells remain clustered together in a single group, the tumor is considered benign; however, if the cells invade surrounding tissues or spread to distant sites (metastasis), the tumor is considered to be malignant or cancerous. Cancers are categorized according to their origin, if it is known, or state of differentiation. Those arising from epithelial cells are termed carcinomas and in the skin they mainly consist of basal cell carcinomas (BCCs) and squamous cell carcinomas (SCCs). In the skin, in addition to epithelial neoplasms, melanomas arise from melanocytes and constitute the majority of metastatic neoplasms. More than 800,000 skin cancers are reported each year in the United States alone, and there is concern that the numbers will rise as a result of the depletion of the ozone layer.

Genetic changes that hyperactivate stimulatory genes (oncogenes) or inactivate inhibitory genes (tumor suppressor genes) are involved in the development of neoplasms. Such changes allow the abnormal cells to pass on their aberrant characteristics to their progeny (although epigenetic changes have been determined to play a part in some cases). The effect of activation of oncogenes is dominant, that is, only one of the two copies present in a cell need undergo the change. On the other hand, direct inactivation of tumor suppressor genes may have a recessive mode of action, that is, both copies of the gene have to be quiescent or absent in order to free the cell of their growth control properties. Aberrations in the cellular environment disrupt the delicate balance between the processes of growth, differentiation, and physiologic programmed cell death (apoptosis), and result in the formation of immortalized cells. Because cancers do not arise immediately after exposure to carcinogens, and because the chances for developing cancer increase with age, it is likely that multiple genetic alterations cooperate in the development of the neoplastic state.

Agents that cause genetic changes, or *mutagens* as they are termed, may present themselves to living organisms as chemicals, viruses, or as radiant energy. This chapter focuses on solar ultraviolet (UV) radiation, a naturally occurring environmental carcinogen associated with cancers of the skin. Lesions induced by UV radiation have unique characteristics that in effect, leave "signature" mutations on the affected genes. Thus far, mutations in the *ras* family of oncogenes and in the *p53* tumor suppressor gene have been characterized in skin carcinomas.

PHOTOBIOLOGY OF SOLAR ULTRAVIOLET RADIATION

Solar Ultraviolet in the Etiology of Skin Cancers

The importance of sunlight in the pathogenesis of skin cancer was recognized as early as 1894.[1] Basal and squamous cell carcinomas occur most frequently on sun-exposed regions of the body.[2] The incidence of these neoplasms correlates with the amount of accumulated sun exposure and is inversely related to the protective action of skin pigments. It has been demonstrated, in studies using laboratory animals, that most of the deleterious effects arise from exposure to the UV component of sunlight.[3, 4] As we shall see in the second half of this chapter, recent advances using molecular techniques have confirmed the role of UV radiation in the etiology of epidermal neoplasms.

Solar Ultraviolet Spectrum

The UV region of the solar spectrum is divided into three parts; UVA (320 to 400 nm), UVB (280 to 320 nm), and UVC (200 to 280 nm) (Fig. 140–1A). The shorter wavelengths of UV radiation reaching the earth's surface extend into the absorption spectra of nucleic acids (Fig. 140–1B) and proteins, and energy in this region of overlap is absorbed into the skin, producing erythema, burns, and eventually keratoses.[5] These biologic effects are brought about through damage at unsaturated chemical bonds such as those in the bases of DNA and RNA, and in the aromatic amino acids of proteins. Epidemiologic and clinical studies indicate that UVB is responsible for the induction of most skin cancers in humans.[6, 7] For a long time UVA was believed to be noncarcinogenic, but recent studies have demonstrated both the carcinogenicity of UVA,[8, 9] as well as its ability to enhance the development of UVB-induced skin cancers.[10]

Although UVC is a potent mutagen, it assumes a less significant role in the pathogenesis of human skin cancers because it does not pass through the stratospheric ozone layer.[11] Additionally, transmission of solar radiation through the skin drops off sharply below 300 nm, thereby providing a natural barrier to the most harmful fraction of UV rays.[12, 13] Much public and scientific attention is now focused on measuring alterations in the ozone layer and the resultant shift in the intensity and wavelength spectrum of solar UV radiation reaching the earth's surface.[11]

DNA Photoproducts Induced by Ultraviolet Radiation

DNA as the Target in Photodamage

Several lines of evidence implicate DNA as the primary target involved in most of the biologic effects of UV irradiation:

1. The action spectra for mutagenesis, cellular transformation, and cell death closely follow the absorption spectrum for DNA (see Fig. 140–1B).[5, 14, 15]
2. Removal of photolesions from irradiated DNA by enzymatic photoreactivation reduces the incidence of UV-induced cellular transformation and tumor formation in the Amazon molly (*Poecilia formosa*) and in the South American opossum (*Monodelphis domestica*).[16, 17]
3. Introduction of proto-oncogenes damaged in vitro by UV radiation into normal cells leads to tumorigenic transformation.[18, 19]
4. Individuals suffering from DNA repair deficiency disorders such as xeroderma pigmentosum (XP) are sunlight sensitive and highly cancer prone.[20, 21]

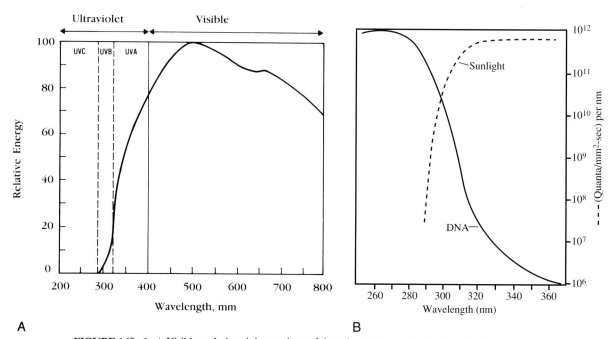

FIGURE 140–1. *A*, Visible and ultraviolet portions of the solar spectrum; *B*, Overlap of solar spectrum with the action spectrum of DNA. (*A* from Kripke ML. Sunlight and skin cancer. Reprinted from Texas Medicine, Cancer Update 1986;82:52–53; *B* from Setlow RB. The wavelengths in sunlight effective in producing skin cancer: A theoretical analysis. Proc Natl Acad Sci USA 1974;71:3363–3366.)

Major Components of Photodamage

UV radiation damages DNA by direct interaction and also via the involvement of endogenous cellular photosensitizers. The predominant UV-induced DNA photoproducts are (1) the cis-syn diastereoisomers of cyclobutane-type pyrimidine dimers (Py⬦Py) and (2) the pyrimidine (6-4) pyrimidone lesions and their alkali-labile Dewar valence isomers.[22-24] These two major groups of UV photoproducts result from the covalent association of adjacent pyrimidines (Fig. 140–2). The cyclobutane pyrimidine dimers (Fig. 140–2*C*) are formed when the double bonds between the C5 and C6 carbon atoms of two adjacent pyrimidines become saturated, producing a four-membered ring structure. As a result of this dimerization, the angle between the bases is reduced and the DNA helix is distorted.[25] In the (6-4) lesion the C6 position of a 5′ pyrimidine is covalently

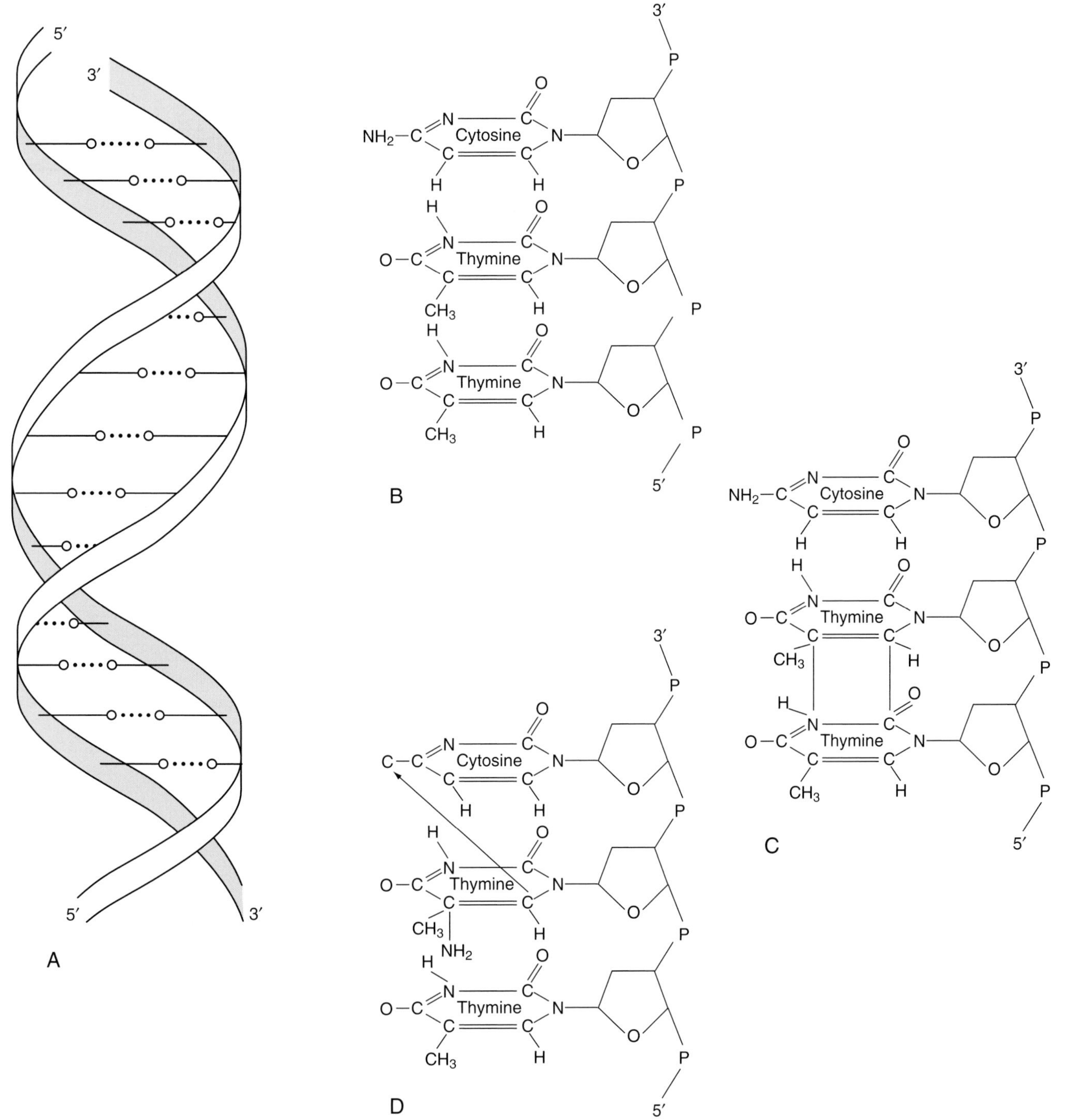

FIGURE 140–2. *A*, A DNA double helix; *B*, Adjacent pyrimidines; *C*, Adjacent pyrimidines showing a thymine⬦thymine cyclobutane dimer; and *D*, Adjacent pyrimidines showing a thymine-cytosine (6-4) lesion.

linked to the C4 position of its adjacent 3' pyrimidine (Fig. 140–2D). The relative yield or sequence specificity of either photolesion has been noted to be similar in double- or single-stranded naked DNA as well as in protein-bound DNA from UV-irradiated mammalian cells (there was a 50% decrease in the total number of lesions in this case due to cellular shielding).[23] While, on average, (6-4) lesions occur a third as often as the cyclobutane dimers,[26] the ratio varies considerably depending upon the nucleotides flanking the lesion site. The potential of photodimerization is enhanced by the presence of a 5' pyrimidine and lowered by a 5' purine, especially a guanine.[23, 27] Both photolesions appear to form preferentially in runs of tandemly located pyrimidine residues that are often "hot spots" of UV-induced mutations.[28]

The distribution of pyrimidine dimers between the four possible dipyrimidine sites is wavelength dependent, with dimer formation at cytosine-containing sites being augmented by UVB irradiation (the ratio of dimers at TT:CT:TC:CC is 68:13:16:3 for UVC and 52:19:21:7 for UVB.[23, 27] The relative proportion of the Dewar isomer of (6-4) lesions is also increased during UVB irradiation as compared with UVC irradiation due to simultaneous formation and photoisomerization in the presence of UVB.[29] These subtle wavelength dependent changes may have implications at the levels of DNA repair and mutagenesis.

Minor Components of Photodamage

UV radiation also induces other types of DNA lesions such as single-strand breaks, DNA-protein cross-links, and unstable pyrimidine photohydrates. The photohydrates are rare lesions (up to 100 times less frequent than pyrimidine dimers) formed by UVC and UVB in comparable amounts. In both instances cytosine photohydrates predominate over thymine photohydrates.[23, 30] UVA is also known to produce single-strand breaks[31] and alkalilabile sites through the action of reactive oxygen species such as superoxide anion, singlet oxygen, and hydrogen peroxide.[32] Occasional double-strand breaks have been observed in UV-irradiated DNA, but it is possible that they arise from lesions at closely opposed dipyrimidine sequences. Photoproducts involving purine bases in double-stranded DNA occur at a very low frequency and account for less than 1% of the total light-induced damage.[33] These photoproducts include modification reactions such as the photochemical addition of amino acids and photoalkylation by alcohols, amines, and other compounds.

Repair of DNA Photolesions

The DNA Repair Systems

Both cyclobutane dimers and (6-4) lesions, if left unrepaired, obstruct the progression of DNA and RNA synthesizing machineries and disrupt cellular processes. Thus, a number of repair pathways operate in human cells to overcome the harmful effects of DNA damaging agents.[34] In the versatile repair pathway known as excision repair,[34] a portion of the damaged strand is enzymatically excised and subsequently replaced using the intact opposite strand as template. The pathway consists of multiple steps,[35] and genes involved at a number of stages have been identified.[36] Proteins that bind preferentially to damaged DNA without any sequence specificity are thought to serve as markers that pinpoint the damage to the repair system. Such proteins may also function as "molecular matchmakers" that enhance the probability of interaction between other components of the repair complex and a damaged stretch of DNA in the absence of stabilizing effects arising from specific sequences.[37] The enzyme photolyase is present in many species and mediates reactivation of cyclobutane dimers in the presence of long wavelengths of light.[38] A recent study using a defined substrate containing a (T◇T) dimer has indicated the absence of the enzyme in human volunteers.[39] However, a new photoreactivating enzyme that specifically repairs (6-4) lesions has been reported in the fruit fly *Drosophila melanogaster*.[40] A UV-dose–dependent binding activity present in mammalian cells[41] recognizes (6-4) photoproducts and the trans-syn isomer of cyclobutane type dimers.[42] The activity is enhanced in cells that are resistant to the anticancer drug cisplatin[43] and absent in some XP patients assigned to the complementation group E.[44, 45]

The Hierarchy of DNA Repair

The local structure of DNA is important in determining the rate of repair (Table 140–1). Photolesions are preferentially excised from transcriptionally active chromatin,[46] with the transcribed strands of transcriptionally active genes being repaired at a faster rate than the nontranscribed strands.[47, 48] In addition, (6-4) lesions are removed more efficiently than are the cyclobutyl dimers.[49] It is the repair of (6-4) lesions that closely matches the overall rate of DNA repair[49, 50] and coincides with the recovery from a majority of biologic effects of UV light (including cell killing, sister-chromatid exchange, mutagenesis, and inhibition of DNA synthesis).

Human Genetic Repair Deficiency Diseases

A number of genetic disorders arise from defects in the cellular system responsible for processing DNA damage.[51] They are often associated with increased incidence of malignancies, mutagenesis, and chromosomal instability, with patients usually exhibiting radiation sensitivity from an early age. XP, Cockayne's syndrome, Bloom syndrome, and hereditary dysplastic nevus syndrome are examples of diseases in which the patients exhibit UV sensitivity.[52] As previously mentioned, malfunctions of

TABLE 140–1. The Hierarchy of DNA Repair

Transcriptionally active regions	>	Transcriptionally inactive regions
Transcribed strand	>	Nontranscribed strand
Pyrimidine (6–4) pyrimidone lesions	>	Pyrimidine dimers

the excision repair pathway lead to the various forms of XP, and a number of genes associated with the disease have been identified recently.[52-55] In Cockayne's syndrome, preferential repair of active genes is deficient, whereas DNA ligase I is thought to be involved in the defect in Bloom's syndrome.[56, 57] In dysplastic nevus syndrome, DNA excision repair appears to be normal but the cells exhibit hypermutability by UV radiation, and the incidence rate of melanomas in some of these patients is about 400-fold higher than average.[58] A study in which the rate of pyrimidine dimer removal was measured in skin biopsy specimens from basal cell nevus syndrome patients indicated that patients with BCC exhibited decreased excision repair compared with cancer-free subjects.[59] Reduced DNA repair capacity has been found to be a particularly important risk factor for young individuals with BCC and for those with a family history of skin cancer.[60] Patients with reduced repair capacities who have been overexposed to sunlight are at a fivefold greater estimated risk for developing BCC than control groups. The estimated risk seems to be related to the sex of the patient inasmuch as it was found to be increased by 10-fold for female subjects.[60]

Biologic Effects of Ultraviolet Radiation

Mutagenesis at DNA Photolesions

The genetic background of the individual is an important factor in determining the biologic consequences of UV radiation. For example, when exposed to UVB, persons with sun-sensitive (Type I) skin have a higher amount of pyrimidine dimer formation than do those with sun-insensitive (Type IV) skin.[61] Both cyclobutane dimers and (6-4) lesions cause mutations in human cells.[25] These mutations are predominantly C→T and CC→TT transitions at sequences containing adjacent pyrimidine nucleotides[62] and have become the *signature* of UV-induced mutagenesis.[25] It has been proposed that the C→T transitions arise during semiconservative replication of DNA due to misincorporation of A residues in the newly synthesized strand in accordance with the A rule (Fig. 140-3).[63] According to this hypothesis, when the DNA polymerase comes across lesions on the DNA template that it cannot interpret, it inserts A residues by default. Thus, according to this rule the (T◊T) cyclobutane dimer, which is the most frequent UV lesion in human cells, should be nonmutagenic (Fig. 140-3A) because the normal complimentary residue to T is A. The CC→TT tandem mutations predicted by the rule at (C◊C) cyclobutane dimers have actually been observed in human cells (Fig. 140-3B).[64] Such mutations have also been shown to arise from exposure to oxidizing agents.[65] Model building of (6-4) T-C and C-C photoproducts indicates that although the 5′ base pairs correctly, the 3′ base resembles a noninstructional apurinic/apyrimidinic site, and should result in a C→T mutation at only the 3′ nucleotide of (6-4) lesions (Fig. 140-3C). The applicability of the A rule to UV mutagenesis has been questioned[23] because the rule was originally conceived to explain misincorporations opposite basic sites.

Also, photoproducts at TT sequences are now thought to be misinstructive rather than noninstructive. In addition to single base substitutions, a number of deletions, insertions, and multiple base changes have also been observed, and their numbers are higher with UVB irradiation than with UVC.[23]

Photocarcinogenesis

Carcinogenesis is usually a multistep process involving initiation, promotion, and progression.[66] For instance, a subthreshold dose of a DNA-damaging agent may initiate the process of carcinogenesis by inducing mutations at one or more sites in the DNA. These mutations may lie dormant for several years until subsequent exposure to tumor-promoting agents (which need not be carcinogenic in themselves) leads to the appearance of tumors. UV radiation is a potentially complete carcinogen because it does not require additional extraneous effectors as initiators or promoters. Rodent skin cancers induced by repeated exposure to UV radiation have provided researchers with excellent model systems for investigating the harmful effects of UV radiation because the etiology of these tumors is well defined and other known risk factors are carefully controlled.[67] Other well-described systems include the South American opposum[17] and back-crossed hybirds of the southern platyfish, *Xiphophorus maculatus*, and the green swordtail, *Xiphophorus helleri*.[10] Either a single large dose,[68] or the accumulation of several small doses of UV radiation,[3, 4, 69] is sufficient to induce skin cancers in experimental animals. The effect of different wavelengths of UV radiation has been extensively studied both in experimental animals as well as in cells cultured in vitro, and the carcinogenic effects of UVA, UVB, and UVC are now well documented.[67-71] Skin cancer induction is usually associated with the appearance of precancerous lesions (actinic keratoses) at the site of UV exposure, indicating that the disease develops in multiple sequential stages that involve direct interaction between the carcinogen and the affected cells. There have been numerous studies examining the association of BCCs and SCCs with genetic make-up, age, and anatomic site of the animals. The rate of tumor development and antigenicity were found to vary in three inbred strains of mice although the tumor types and frequencies were comparable in all.[72] Albino mice (BALB/cAnN) developed tumors earlier than agouti (C3H/HeN) or black (C57BL/6N) mice. In all three cases, fibrosarcomas were the most common type of tumor followed by SCCs.

Photosuppression of Local and Systemic Immune Responses

Another rapidly emerging role of UV is at the level of interference with the immune mechanisms that protect against tumor development.[73, 74] The tumors induced in the above mentioned study, by chronic exposure to UV radiation, were highly antigenic and did not grow when transplanted to normal syngeneic recipients (Fig. 140-4).[72, 75] All tumors grew readily in immunosuppressed mice, indicating that the rejection seen in normal mice was immunologically mediated. This suggested that

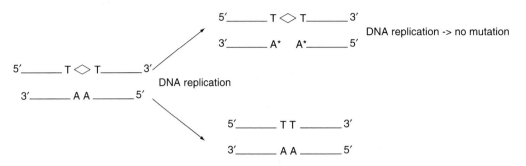

A, Replication past unrepaired T◇T lesion

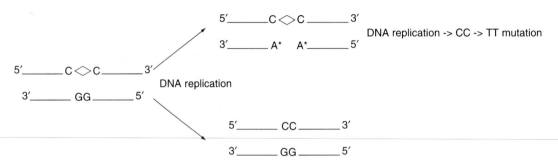

B, Replication past unrepaired C◇C lesion

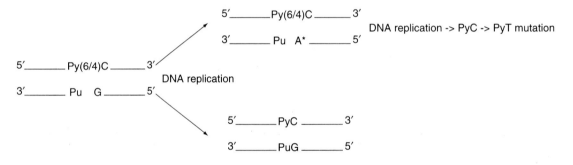

C, Replication past unrepaired Py(6-4)C lesion

'A*' Denotes insertion of A residues opposite noninstructional sites.

FIGURE 140–3. The A rule. *A,* Replication past unrepaired T◇T lesion; *B,* Replication past unrepaired C◇C lesion; and *C,* Replication past unrepaired Py(6-4)C lesion.

the original (autochthonous) tumor-bearing animals must have been immunocompromised in order for the tumors to have grown. Subsequent studies revealed that the UV-induced tumors from the agouti mice were immunogenic as well, bringing about a specific memory response during tumor regression,[75, 76] and that UV radiation suppresses specific immune responses, thereby allowing the growth of the tumors.

UV radiation exerts both local and systemic effects on the host's immune system. Local effects at the site of UVB exposure are mediated mainly via qualitative and quantitative changes in the Langerhans cells that reside in the epidermis.[77] The number of these cells is decreased in irradiated murine skin; those remaining are morphologically altered and unable to present antigens to the

Th2 subset of T helper cells.[78] Moreover, under the influence of cytokines released from surrounding UV-induced keratinocytes, the Langerhans cells become converted to antigen-presenting cells that induce T cell tolerance.[79] Yet another effect of exposure to UVB radiation is the recruitment of melanophages to the epidermis.[80] The melanophages present antigens to suppressor cells, further down-regulating the local immune response.

Systemic immune suppression is associated with the release of immunomodulatory cytokines and immunosuppressive substances by UV-irradiated epidermal cells.[74] The release of at least some of these factors seems to be wavelength dependent because UVB exposure suppresses delayed type hypersensitivity whereas UVA is

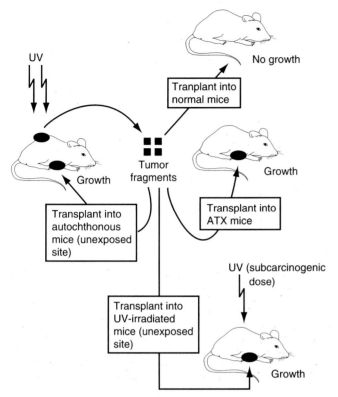

FIGURE 140-4. Antigenicity of UV-induced murine skin tumors and the immunosuppressive action of UV radiation ATX, adult thymectomy followed by 450 R whole-body x-irradiation. (Modified from Kripke ML, Fisher MS. Immunologic aspects of tumor induction by ultraviolet radiation. Natl Cancer Inst Monogr 1978;50:179–183.)

responsible for decreasing contact hypersensitivity.[81] Keratinocyte-derived interleukin-10[82] interacts with antigen presenting cells and impairs their function by down regulating major histocompatibility complex class II antigen expression and by blocking the production of monokines. Although this suppresses cellular immune reactions such as delayed type hypersensitivity, antibody production remains unaffected. Enhanced expression of interleukin-10 mRNA and secretion of interleukin-10 into the medium has been demonstrated in UV-irradiated in vitro keratinocyte cultures.[82] Recent advances indicate that suppression of contact hypersensitivity by UV may be mediated by the secretion of tumor necrosis factor-alfa.[79]

Photomodulation of Enzymes

A number of enzymes that are induced during chemical promotion of tumors are also activated by UV irradiation–induced DNA damage.[83, 84] Increase in membrane fluidity brought about by UVB irradiation[85] may be involved in some of the photomodulatory effects such as the activation of β-adrenergic adenylate cyclase which leads to accumulation of cyclic adenosine monophosphate.[86] Protein kinase C, another enzyme involved in chemical promotion, has been found to be enhanced in cultured mammalian cells by UVA alone.[87] This leads to the translation-independent activation of several general transcription factors including AP-1, NFκB, and the

serum response factor.[84] UVA also stimulates arachidonic acid release and cyclooxygenase activity, thus increasing the substrate as well as the enzyme required for the synthesis of prostaglandins.[88]

MOLECULAR MECHANISMS OF ULTRAVIOLET-INDUCED CARCINOGENESIS

Cooperation Between Genes During Carcinogenesis

A total of 10^{16} cell divisions, each with the probability of 10^{-6} spontaneous mutations per gene, takes place during the course of an average human lifetime. The probability of spontaneous mutagenesis is governed by the fidelity of DNA replication and repair processes, and for a normal individual it translates to 10^{10} mutations per gene in a single lifetime. If each mutational event was sufficient to convert a normal cell to a cancer cell, we would not be able to function as viable organisms. Epidemiologic studies indicate that the chances of developing cancer are not constant for each year; rather, the probability increases with age.[89] Also, because cancers do not arise immediately after exposure to the carcinogen, it follows that multiple hits at different loci are required for tumor growth and progression. It has been estimated statistically that, depending on the life span of the cell type, somewhere between three and seven mutational events are usually necessary to convert normal cells into cancer cells. Thus cancers originating in regions where the cells exhibit a rapid turnover, such as the epidermis, where the cells are continuously shed and replenished, require a large number of genetic alterations.[90]

Several investigators have shown that genetic alterations can cooperate to induce the neoplastic state.[91-93] For example, genes such as *myc* may function in the establishment or immortalization of cells whereas activation of *ras* or *ras*-like genes may confer the transformed phenotype.[93] Two genes that have been extensively investigated in skin cancers include *ras* and *p53*, and details of these studies will be discussed in the following sections (reviewed in references 94–96). Rearrangement of c-*myb*,[97] and appearance of polymorphic alleles of epidermal growth factor receptor and a protein kinase C,[98] have also been recorded in cases of skin cancer such as melanomas.

Role of Oncogenes and Tumor Suppressor Genes

The molecular mechanisms by which UV-induced mutations lead to the transformation of normal cells into cancer cells are just beginning to be elucidated.[94-96] The carcinogenic process begins when the cellular DNA is damaged either due to endogenous or exogenous causes (Table 140-2). Important endogenous mutagenic events include misincorporation of nucleotides by DNA polymerase, depurination of purine-containing nucleotides, deamination of 5-methylcytosine, and oxidative damage from free radicals generated by cellular processes.[99, 100]

TABLE 140-2. Sources of Mutations

Spontaneous endogeneous	Errors in DNA replication or repair, depurination, deamination, oxidative damage from free radicals generated by cellular processes
Superimposed exogeneous	Environmental carcinogens such as UV, chemical pollutants, biological toxins such as aflatoxin

TABLE 140-3. Cellular Organization of Proto-oncogenes

Biologic Function	Location	Proto-oncogene
Growth factor		(EGF), c-*sis* (PDGF)
Growth factor receptor with tyrosine-specific protein kinase activity	Transmembrane	*erb* B (EGF receptor), (PDGF receptor)
Tyrosine-specific protein kinase	Cell membrane/ cytoskeleton cytoplasm	c-*src* c-*fes*
Signal transduction via GTP binding	Cell membrane	H-*ras*, K-*ras*, N-*ras*
Serine/threonine-specific protein kinase	Cytoplasm	c-*raf*
Transcription/ replication regulation	Nucleus	c-*myc*, c-*jun*, c-*fos*

The contribution of environmental sources is often superimposed over internal lesions, leaving "signature" mutations that allow researchers to trace the path of tumorigenic transformation.[25, 99, 101] The genetic alterations including substitutions, insertions, deletions, and translocations occur mainly in two classes of interacting genes, proto-oncogenes and tumor suppressor genes.

Proto-oncogenes act as crucial growth regulators in normal cell division (during embryogenesis, wound healing, and regeneration of skin and liver), differentiation, and apoptosis.[102-107] They encode proteins that act as growth factors, receptor and nonreceptor tyrosine kinases, serine-threonine kinases, extranuclear proteins involved in signal transduction, and nuclear transcription-modulatory DNA-binding factors (Table 140–3). Activation of proto-oncogenes to cancer-causing onco-genes occurs via recombination with the genome of retroviruses or by point mutations and gross DNA rearrangements such as translocation or gene amplification. Production of the more potent mutant form of the gene product or simple overexpression leads to the transformed phenotype (Fig. 140–5A).[104]

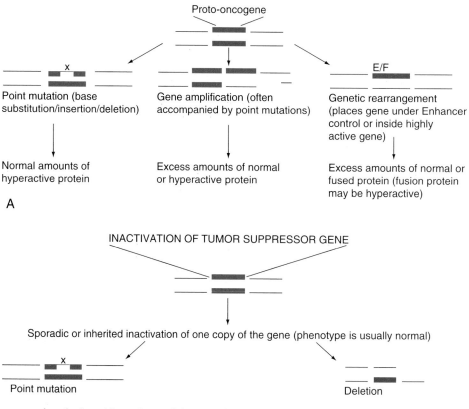

FIGURE 140-5. *A*, Activation of proto-oncogene to oncogene; *B*, Inactivation of tumor suppressor gene. The proto-oncogene or tumor suppressor gene is indicated by the heavy black bar.

Tumor suppressor genes act as negative growth regulators and mutations or deletions of such genes (Fig. 140-5*B*) have been documented for various types of cancers.[108-113] Aside from *p53*, other tumor suppressor genes associated with epidermal BCC or SCC may soon be identified. Linkage studies have indicated the association of Gorlin syndrome and Ferguson-Smith syndrome with genetic markers on chromosome 9q.[114, 115] Patients suffering from these diseases are predisposed to the development of nevoid BCCs and multiple SCC-like lesions respectively. Molecular studies on sporadic and familial cases of BCC and SCC have confirmed the involvement of chromosome 9,[116] and researchers are currently trying to further narrow down the location of the putative tumor suppressor gene(s).

ras Gene Mutations in Human Skin Cancers

The *ras* oncogene family has been implicated in the development of a variety of human cancers.[103, 117, 118] This family of guanosine triphosphate (GTP)-binding proteins consists of three members, H-*ras*, K-*ras* and N-*ras*, each coding for a 21-kd protein and sharing approximately 70% sequence homology.[117] The ras proteins are localized on the inner surface of the cell membrane, where they participate in growth control by helping in the transduction of signals (stimuli such as the binding of activator molecules to transmembrane receptor molecules) from the cell surface to the nucleus. A number of recent studies have elegantly elucidated parts of this pathway (Fig. 140-6; reviewed in references 119 and 120). When the epidermal growth factor receptor is stimulated, it undergoes autophosphorylation, which enables the intracellular portion of the molecule to recruit a complex containing two proteins called GRB2 and mSOS. The latter protein then activates ras-GDP (c-H-ras was mentioned in this model) to ras-GTP. Activated ras then binds to *raf*-1, which phosphorylates other kinases and thus activates a kinase cascade that ultimately activates transcription factors (such as *myc* and possibly the gene products of *jun* and *ets*) in the nucleus.

Most *ras* mutations detected in various forms of cancer have been localized to codons 12, 13, and 61 for all three members of the *ras* family.[118] Amino acid changes at these locations result in the continuous activation of ras. Inactivation of ras normally occurs via the hydrolysis of the bound GTP to GDP. The low intrinsic GTPase activity of ras is enhanced by at least a factor of 4 $\times$ 10^3 by a GTPase activating protein known as GAP. The transforming ras mutant, ras^{Val112} not only exhibits a 10-fold reduced intrinsic GTPase activity, but also has a 1 $\times$ 10^3-fold lower rate of GAP-induced GTP hydrolysis when compared with wild type ras.[121] Thus even though ras^{Val112} associates with 10 times less raf-1 than does normal ras,[122] the mutant form remains in the active signal transducing form much longer. A recent study indicates that mutation at codon 12 also dissolves an obstructive secondary structure that is normally present in the unmodified DNA sequence.[123] Because the normal secondary structure impedes the progress of DNA polymerase α,[124] it is possible that the same structure also

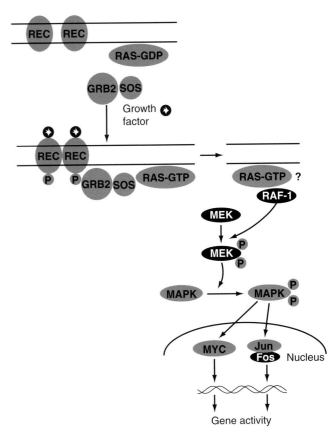

FIGURE 140-6. Major steps in the ras pathway for transmitting growth signals to the cell nucleus. Binding of growth factor to the extracellular portion of the receptor leads to autophosphorylation of the receptor, which then binds the GRB2-Sos complex. Sos activates ras, which may in turn lead to activation of Raf-1 and MEK, and ultimately to altered gene expression. (From Marx J. Forging a path to the nucleus. Science 1993;260:1588-1590. Copyright 1993 by the AAAS.)

hinders RNA polymerase and thereby controls ras production at the transcriptional level. A mutation at codon 12 may therefore enhance the transcription of the gene, although this hypothesis remains to be studied.

Single Base Substitutions

Our initial studies revealed that three of eight non-melanoma human skin cancers, occurring on sun-exposed sites, contained activated c-H-*ras* oncogenes that could induce transformation of NIH 3T3 cells.[125] Analysis of 40 skin tumors (24 SCCs and 16 BCCs) revealed that there was a G→T base change at the second position of codon 12 in the H-*ras* gene in 11 SCCs and 5 BCCs.[126] A twofold higher mutation frequency has been documented in skin tumors from XP patients as compared with those from people with no known genetic disorders.[127, 128] Other studies have shown a relatively lower frequency of *ras* activation in skin cancers from otherwise normal people.[129, 130] Corominas and associates found that only 13% of human SCCs contained mutations in H-*ras*.[129] In addition, van der Schroeff and colleagues detected only one BCC with a H-*ras* mutation (codon 61) and three with K-*ras* mutations (codon 12) out of the 30 cases that were examined.[130] These differences may be a reflection of the ethnic backgrounds of the groups studied. Activation of *ras* oncogenes has also been detected in melanomas[131, 132] and in benign self-regressing human and animal keratoacanthomas.[129] The latter observation leads to the conclusion that *ras* activation may play a role in the early stages of carcinogenesis.[129, 133] A 20% incidence rate of *ras*-activating mutations was also observed in UV-induced murine skin tumors.[134]

In vitro experiments have confirmed the role of UV radiation in *ras* activation and subsequent cellular transformation. Introduction of UVC-irradiated N-*ras* proto-oncogene DNA (but not unirradiated control DNA) led to the transformation of Rat-2 cells.[18] The mutations were found mainly at dipyrimidine sites in codons 12 and 61. In addition, treatment of the UV-irradiated transforming DNA with photoreactivating enzyme prior to transfection reduced the transformation frequency several-fold. More recently, we demonstrated the activation of human c-H-*ras* by in vitro UVB-irradiation followed by transfection into NIH 3T3 cells.[19] Analysis of the resulting *ras* mutations showed changes in codon 12 similar to those detected in sunlight-induced skin tumors.

Gene Amplification

Apart from point mutations, amplification of *ras* has been reported in human SCCs,[126] melanomas,[135] and in skin tumors from XP patients.[128] In most cases amplification was accompanied with point mutations or other rearrangements, but some cases exhibited simple amplification of the unmutated sequence.[126, 128]

Loss of Heterozygosity

The human c-H-*ras*-1 gene is located on the short arm of chromosome 11 and exhibits restriction fragment length polymorphism with the restriction enzyme *BamHI*.[136] The generation of such allelic restriction fragments at the locus is useful in the genetic analysis of cancer susceptibility. In fact, one of the c-H-*ras* alleles is deleted in several types of human cancers and such loss of heterozygosity is thought to unmask recessive mutations.[137] We examined 17 patients who were heterozygous for the c-H-*ras* gene in their normal skin DNA and found that 5 (4 BCCs and 1 SCC) showed a loss in one of the c-H-*ras* alleles in the tumor DNA.[138] These results suggest that loss of heterozygosity at the *ras* gene locus may also play a role in the pathogenesis of human skin cancers.

p53 Mutations in Human Skin Cancer

The *p53* tumor suppressor gene is located on the short arm of chromosome 17 and encodes a 53-kd phosphoprotein with oncosuppressive properties that help maintain the normalcy of cells by modulating DNA replication, or the transcription of growth inhibitory or stimulatory genes.[99, 110, 113, 139] The protein accumulates

in the cytoplasm during the G1 phase of the cell cycle and migrates to the nucleus at the beginning of the S phase.[140] Multiple phosphorylation of p53 is brought about by four protein kinases, including cdc2 kinase (an enzyme required for mitosis in mammalian cells), and the phosphorylated state of the protein is maximal during mitosis.[141] A variety of DNA-damaging agents bring about a dramatic increase in the intracellular levels of p53 that lead to G1 arrest, allowing the cellular repair pathways to remove DNA lesions before the onset of DNA synthesis and mitosis.[142, 143] This cell cycle arrest is mediated by the 21-kd protein product of the *Cip1/sid1/Waf1* gene, which blocks the Ckd enzymes (reviewed in reference 144). Equally erythemogenic doses of UVA, UVB, and UVC given to healthy volunteers are all capable of increasing p53 expression in a wavelength-specific pattern.[145] UVA induction of p53 is virtually confined to the basal layer, UVC induces p53 in the granular layer and upper stratum spinosum of the epidermis, and UVB induction is diffuse and equally intense throughout the epidermis.

Structural analyses have indicated that p53 is composed of three functional domains: an N-terminal domain that functions as a transcriptional activator; a central conformationally important region; and a positively charged C-terminal domain that is involved in DNA binding.[139, 146, 147] Two cellular proteins, Hsc 70 and mdm2, can interact with p53.[148, 149] The relationship between p53 and mdm2 seems to be functionally important because mdm2 is overexpressed (due to gene amplification) in many cancers and the protein-protein interaction inhibits p53-dependent transactivation.[149] The central region of p53 is conformationally flexible, and mutations of the type found in human cancers frequently alter this structure.[150] Such mutations also increase the half-life of the protein from 6 to 20 minutes up to 4 to 8 hours, allowing the intracellular accumulation of high levels of the mutant protein.[151] The C-terminal domain of native unmodified p53 exhibits very weak sequence-specific DNA-binding activity. However, conformational alteration, probably via interaction with other cellular proteins, dramatically enhances this activity.[147]

Sequence analysis of the *p53* gene in mammals, amphibians, birds, and fish has revealed five blocks of evolutionarily conserved amino acid sequence (Fig. 140-7).[152] A striking number of missense mutations detected in human cancer are at codons corresponding to conserved amino acids.[99] While the properties of p53 have been extensively investigated, many questions remain as to the mechanisms by which it participates in growth control. Of particular interest to those in the field of cancer research is the acquisition of oncogenic properties by some mutants whereas others simply lose their tumor suppressive properties.

Alterations in *p53* are the most frequently observed genetic lesions in human cancers and include allelic loss, point mutations, rearrangements, deletions, and insertions. In recent years, germ line transmission of mutant forms has been described in the cancer-prone patients suffering from Li-Fraumeni syndrome,[153, 154] and transgenic mice deficient in this gene are predisposed to the

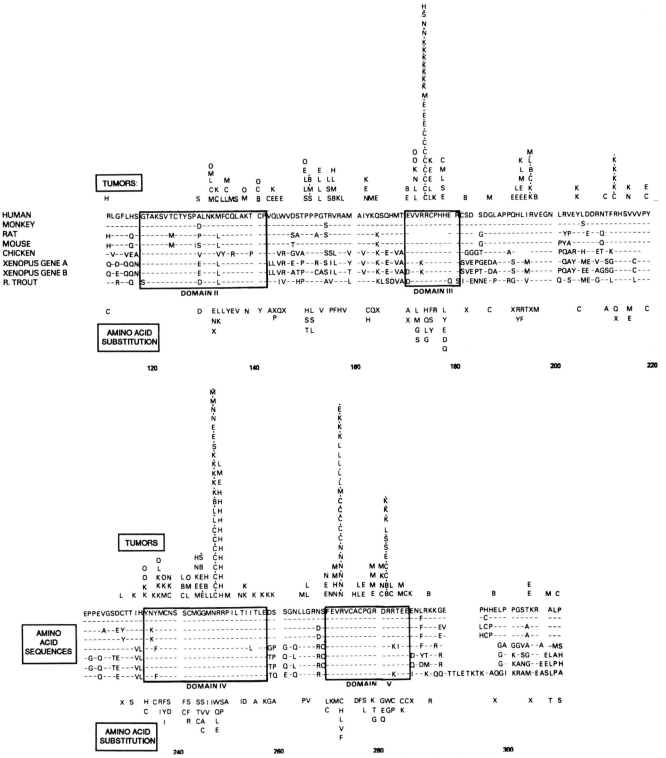

FIGURE 140-7. The domains of the *p53* gene and distribution of mutations found in various cancers. (From Hollstein M, Sidransky D, Vogelstein B, et al. *p53* mutations in human cancers. Science 1991;253:49-53. Copyright 1991 by the AAAS.)

development of tumors.[155] Also, although the normal allele of *p53* is functional in maintaining the normalcy of cells, some mutant alleles act to promote transformation.[99, 110, 113, 139] Although *p53* alterations have been defined in many cancers, its involvement in skin tumorigenesis had not been investigated until recently when an

examination of 10 SCCs indicated the presence of mutations in exon 7 in 2 cases.[156] One of the tumors had a mutation in codon 244, whereas the other had a mutation in codon 248. Interestingly, the mutations in both codons occurred at CC sequences. Similarly, Brash and colleagues[101] have reported that mutations in *p53* occur frequently (58%) in human skin cancers. Of the 24 invasive SCCs examined, 3 exhibited CC→TT double base changes and 5 had C→T transitions reinforcing the notion that UV-induced mutations play a direct role in the development of skin cancers. Our recent studies have shown that *p53* mutations occur at a much higher frequency (around 90%) in human skin cancers than previously reported (Kanjilal S, Ananthaswamy HN, unpublished data). *p53* mutations have also been detected in tumors occurring at sun-exposed sites on the skin of patients suffering from XP.[157] Rady and associates have found C→T transitions in 7 of 14 human BCCs,[158] and Shea and coworkers have detected the overexpression of a mutant p53 protein in 30 of 36 human BCCs of the head and neck regions.[159] Keratinocytes surrounding the BCC also had elevated levels of the p53 protein, in contrast to keratinocytes from the buttock, which had normal levels of the protein, indicating that *p53* alteration may be one of the early events of tumorigenesis in the epidermis. Ziegler and associates have reported that *p53* mutations occur in 56% of human basal cell skin cancers and that 45% of these tumors bear a second point mutation on the other *p53* allele.[160] The mutations were UV-induced, and two thirds were located at nine hot spots, of which seven were specific for skin cancer. Five patients with more than one actinic keratosis on sun-damaged areas of the arm were found to harbor distinct *p53* mutations, indicating that alteration of *p53* is an early event in UV radiation–induced skin carcinogenesis.[161]

Murine models have provided strong evidence for the involvement of *p53* mutations in the pathogenesis of UV-induced skin cancers.[162, 163] Analogous to human skin cancers, UV-induced murine skin cancers also contain C→T and CC→TT transitions at pyrimidine-rich sequences; interestingly, 100% of tumors analyzed contained mutations.[162] Based on comparative sequencing, the experiments showed that the gene was mutated in a strand-specific manner, with a pronounced bias for the nontranscribed strand. The strand specificity was most prominent for mutations at TC sequences, the primary site of (6-4) photoproduct formation. The tumors were also shown to consist of heterogeneous populations of cells carrying mutations at different regions of the *p53* gene.

However, *p53* mutations do not seem to be as important in the development of melanomas (a detailed discussion on melanomas is to be found in Chapter 151), where they occur at a much lower frequency.[164] Instead, inactivation of *nf-1* tumor suppressor activity on chromosome 17 may be involved in the process.[165] During the last five years, melanoma susceptibility genes (i.e., genes that are crucial in a large majority of melanomas, specially the hereditary cases) have been localized to chromosomes 1, 6, and 9 (reviewed in reference 164). Deletion mapping in melanomas and in a person carrying a germ line rearrangement of chromosome 9, as well as linkage analysis, has indicated a region in the middle of the short arm of chromosome 9 as the site of a melanoma susceptibility gene.[166–168] The region lies between two genetic markers, IFNA and D9S3, and is 2 to 3 million base-pairs in length, opening up the possibility that the susceptibility gene may be identified in the near future.

CONCLUSION

UV radiation present in sunlight is an ubiquitous environmental carcinogen that is involved in the pathogenesis of skin cancers. In addition to its mutagenic properties, UV radiation exerts local and systemic immunosuppressive effects on exposed individuals. Recently much attention has been focused on the mechanism by which UV radiation induces skin cancer. Molecular analysis of human skin cancers originating on sun-exposed body sites and mouse skin tumors induced by UV radiation has provided new information on the role of oncogenes and tumor suppressor genes in UV radiation carcinogenesis. In particular, mutations in *ras* and *p53* genes have been detected in both the human and murine skin cancers, suggesting that *ras* activation as well as *p53* inactivation plays a role in UV radiation carcinogenesis. Although the genes implicated in the pathogenesis of human and mouse skin cancers may be similar to those involved in other types of cancer, UV-induced skin cancers display unique UV-signature mutations (C→T and CC→TT) at dipyrimidine sequences that are not commonly found in other types of human or mouse cancers.

ACKNOWLEDGMENT

This work was supported by USPHS Grant RO1-CA-46523 from the National Cancer Institute.

References

1. Unna PG. Die Histopathologic der Hautkrankheiten. Berlin: Hirschwald A, 1894.
2. MacKie R. Links between exposure to ultraviolet radiation and skin cancer. J R Coll Phys London 1987;21:91–96.
3. Blum HF. Carcinogenesis by Ultraviolet Light. Princeton: Princeton University Press, 1959.
4. Urbach F. The Biologic Effects of Ultraviolet Radiation. New York: Pergamon Press, 1969.
5. Setlow RB. The wavelengths in sunlight effective in producing skin cancer: A theoretical analysis. Proc Natl Acad Sci USA 1974;71:3363–3366.
6. Urbach F. Evidence and epidemiology of ultraviolet-induced cancers in man. Natl Cancer Inst Monogr 1978;50:5–10.
7. Scotto J, Fears TR. Skin cancer epidemiology: Research needs. Natl Cancer Inst Monogr 1978;50:169–177.
8. Strickland P. Photocarcinogenesis by near-ultraviolet (UVA) radiation in Sencar mice. J Invest Dermatol 1986;87:272–275.
9. Setlow RB, Grist E, Thompson K, et al. Wavelengths effective in induction of malignant melanoma. Proc Natl Acad Sci USA 1993;90:6666–6670.
10. Matsui MS, DeLeo VA. Longwave ultraviolet radiation and promotion of skin cancer. Cancer Cells. 1991;3:8–12.
11. Frederick JE. Ultraviolet sunlight reaching the earth's surface; a review of recent research. Photochem Photobiol 1993;57:175–178.
12. Bruls WAG, van Weelden H, van der Leun JC. Transmission of UV-radiation through human epidermal layers as a factor influencing the minimal erythema dose. Photochem Photobiol 1984;39:63–67.
13. Freeman SE, Hacham RW, Gange DJ, et al. Wavelength dependence of pyrimidine dimer formation in DNA of human skin irradiated in situ with ultraviolet light. Proc Natl Acad Sci USA 1989;86:5605–5609.
14. Sutherland BM, Delihas NC, Oliver RP, et al. Action spectra for ultraviolet light–induced transformation of human cells to anchorage-independent growth. Cancer Res 1981;41:2211–2214.
15. Doniger J, Jacobson ED, Krell K, et al. Ultraviolet light spectra for neoplastic tranformation and lethality of Syrian hamster embryo cells correlate with spectrum for pyrimidine dimer forma-

tion in cellular DNA. Proc Natl Acad Sci USA 1981;78: 2378–2382.

16. Hart RW, Setlow RB, Woodhead AD. Evidence that pyrimidine dimers in DNA can give rise to tumors. Proc Natl Acad Sci USA 1977;75:5574–5578.

17. Ley RD, Applegate LA, Fry RJM, et al. Photoreactivation of ultraviolet radiation–induced skin and eye tumors of *Monodelphis domestica*. Cancer Res 1991;51:6539–6542.

18. van der Lubbe JLM, Rosdorff HJM, Bos JL, et al. Activation of N-*ras* induced by ultraviolet irradiation in vitro. Oncogene Res 1988;3:9–20.

19. Pierceall WE, Ananthaswamy HN. Transformation of NIH 3T3 cells by transfection with UV-irradiated human c-Ha-*ras*-1 proto-oncogene DNA. Oncogene 1991;6:2085–2091.

20. Cleaver JE. Defective repair replication of DNA in xeroderma pigmentosum. Nature 1968;218:652–656.

21. Cleaver JE, Bootsma D. Xeroderma pigmentosum: biochemical and genetic characteristics. Annu Rev Genet 1975;9:19–38.

22. Setlow RB, Carrier WL. Pyrimidine dimers in ultraviolet-irradiated DNA's. J Mol Biol 1966;17:237–254.

23. Sage E. Distribution and repair of photolesions in DNA: Genetic consequences and the role of sequence context. Photochem Photobiol 1993;57:163–174.

24. Mitchell DL, Nairn RS. The biology of the 6-4 photoproduct. Photochem Photobiol 1989;49:805–819.

25. Brash DE. UV Mutagenic photoproducts in *Escherichia coli* and human cells: A molecular genetics perspective on human skin cancer. Photochem Photobiol 1988;48:59–66.

26. Mitchell DL. The relative cytotoxicity of (6-4) photoproducts and cyclobutane dimers in mammalian cells. Photochem Photobiol 1988;48:51–57.

27. Mitchell DI, Jen J, Cleaver JE. Sequence specificity of cyclobutane pyrimidine dimers in DNA treated with solar (ultraviolet B) radiation. Nucleic Acids Res 1992;20:225–229.

28. Sage E, Cramb E, Glickman BU. The distribution of UV damage in the lac I gene of *Escherichia coli*: correlation with mutation spectrum. Mutat Res 1992;269:285–299.

29. Rosenstein BS, Mitchell DL. Action spectra for the induction of pyrimidine (6-4) pyrimidone photoproducts and cyclobutane dimers in normal human skin fibroblasts. Photochem Photobiol 1987;45:775–780.

30. Mitchell DL, Jen J, Cleaver JE. Relative induction of cyclobutane dimers and cytosine photohydrates in DNA irradiated *in vitro* and *in vivo* with ultraviolet-C and ultraviolet-B light. Photochem Photobiol 1991;54:741–746.

31. Peak MJ, Peak JG, Carnes BA. Induction of direct and indirect single-strand breaks in human cell DNA by far- and near-ultraviolet radiations: Action spectrum and mechanisms. Photochem Photobiol 1987;45:381–387.

32. Danpure HJ, Tyrrell RM. Oxygen dependence of near-UV (365 nm) lethality and the interaction of near-UV and x-rays in two mammalian cell lines. Photochem Photobiol 1976;23:171–177.

33. Duker NJ, Gallagher PE. Purine photoproducts. Photochem Photobiol 1988;48:35–39.

34. Rubin JS. The molecular genetics of the incision step in the DNA excision repair process. Int J Radiat Biol 1988;54:309–365.

35. Wood RD. Seven genes for three diseases. Nature 1991;350:190.

36. Lehmann AR, Hoeijmakers JHJ, van Zeeland AA, et al. Workshop on DNA repair. Mutat Res 1992;273:1–28.

37. Sancar A, Hearst JE. Molecular matchmakers. Science 1993; 259:1415–1420.

38. Friedberg EC. DNA damage and human disease. In: DNA Repair. New York: WH Freeman, 1985:505–574.

39. Li YF, Kim S-T, Sancar A. Evidence for lack of DNA photoreactivating enzyme in humans. Proc Natl Acad Sci USA 1993; 90:4389–4393.

40. Todo T, Takemori H. Ryo H, et al. A new photoreactivating enzyme that specifically repairs ultraviolet light-induced (6-4) photoproducts. Nature 1993;361:371–374.

41. Kanjilal S. Damage-specific DNA-binding proteins from human cells. Pennsylvania State University Ph.D. thesis, 1992.

42. Reardon JT, Nichols AF, Keeney S, et al. Comparative analysis of binding of human damaged DNA-binding protein (XPE) and Escherichia coli damage recognition protein (Uvr A) to the major ultraviolet photoproducts: T'c,s:T, T't,s:T, T'6-4:T, and T'Dewar:T. J Biol Chem 1993;268:1301–1306.

43. Chao CC-K, Huang S-L, Huang H, et al. Cross-resistance to UV radiation of a cisplatin-resistant human cell line: Overexpression of cellular factors that recognize UV-modified DNA. Mol Cell Biol 1991;11:2075–2080.

44. Chu G, Change E. Xeroderma pigmentosum group E cells lack a nuclear factor that binds to damaged DNA. Science 1988;242: 564–567.

45. Kataoka H, Fujiwara Y. UV damage-specific DNA-binding protein in xeroderma pigmentosum group E. Biochem Biophy Res Commun 1991;175:1139–1143.

46. Bohr VA, Smith CA, Okumuto DS, et al. DNA repair in an active gene: Removal of pyrimidine dimers from the DHFR gene of CHO cells is much more efficient than in the genome overall. Cell 1985;40:359–369.

47. Hanawalt PC, Mellon IM, Scicchitana D, et al. Relationships between DNA repair and transcription in defined DNA sequences in mammalian cells. In: Lambert MW, Laval J, eds. DNA Repair Mechanisms and Their Biological Implications in Mammalian Cells. New York: Plenum Press, 1989:325–337.

48. Mellon I, Spivak G, Hanawalt PC. Selective removal of transcription-blocking DNA damage from the transcribed strand of the mammalian DHFR gene. Cell 1987;51:241–249.

49. Thomas DC, Okumuto DS, Sancar et al. Preferential DNA repair of (6-4) photoproducts in the dihydrofolate reductase gene of chinese hamster ovary cells. J Biol Chem 1989;264: 18005–18010.

50. Ehmann UK, Cook KH, Friedberg EC. The kinetics of thymine dimer excision in ultraviolet-irradiated human cells. Biophys J 1978;22:249–264.

51. Lehmann AR, Norris PG. DNA repair and cancer: Speculations based on studies with xeroderma pigmentosum. Cockayne's syndrome and trichothiodystrophy. Carcinogenesis 1989;10: 1353–1356.

52. Hansson J. Inherited defects in DNA repair and susceptibility to DNA-damaging agents. Toxicol Let 1992;64/65:141–148.

53. Digweed M. Human genetic instability syndromes: Single gene defects with increased risk of cancer. Toxicol Let 1993;67: 259–281.

54. Miura N, Miyamoto I, Asahina H, et al. Identification and characterization of xpac protein, the gene product of XPAC (xeroderma pigmentosum group A complementing) gene. J Biol Chem 1991;266:19786–19789.

55. Weeda G, Ma LB, vanHam RC, et al. Structure and expression of the human XPBC/ERCC-3 gene involved in DNA repair disorders xeroderma pigmentosum and Cockayne's syndrome. Nucleic Acids Res 1991;19:6301–6308.

56. Venema J, Mullenders LHF, Natarajan AT, et al. The genetic defect in Cockayne syndrome is associated with a defect in repair of UV-induced DNA damage in transcriptionally active DNA. Proc Natl Acad Sci USA 1990;87:4707–4711.

57. Petrini JHJ, Huwiler KG, Weaver DT. A wild-type DNA ligase I gene is expressed in Bloom's syndrome cells. Proc Natl Acad Sci USA 1991;88:7615–7619.

58. Greene MH, Clark Jr WH, Tucker MA, et al. High risk of malignant melanoma in melanoma-prone families with dysplastic naevi. Ann Intern Med 1985;102:458–465.

59. Alcalay J, Freeman SE, Goldberg LH, et al. Decreased excision repair of pyrimidine dimers in skin of basal cell nevus syndrome patients by simulated solar radiation (abstract). J Invest Dermatol 1990;94:502.

60. Wei Q, Matanoski GM, Farmer ER, et al. DNA repair and aging in basal cell carcinoma: A molecular epidemiology study. Proc Natl Acad Sci USA 1993;90:1614–1618.

61. Freeman SE, Gange RW, Matzinger EA, et al. Higher pyrimidine dimer yields in skin of normal humans with higher UVB sensitivity. J Invest Dermatol 1986;86:34–36.

62. Hsia HC, Lebkowski JS, Leong PM, et al. Comparison of ultraviolet irradiation-induced mutagenesis of the *lacI* gene in *Escherichia coli* and in human 293 cells. J Mol Biol 1989;205:103–113.

63. Tessman I. A mechanism of UV-reactivation. In: Bukhari A, Ljungquist E, eds. Abstracts of the Bacteriophage Meeting. Cold Spring Harbor: Cold Spring Harbor Laboratory, 1976:87.

64. Bredberg A, Kraemer K, Seidman M. Restricted ultraviolet mutational spectrum in a shuttle vector propagated in xeroderma pigmentosum cells. Proc Natl Acad Sci USA 1986;83: 8273–8277.

65. Tkeshelashvili LK, Reid TM, McBride TJ. Leob LA. Nickel induces a signature mutation for oxygen free radical damage. Cancer Res 1993;53:4172–4174.

66. Hennings H, Glick AB, Greenhalg DA, et al. Critical aspects of initiation, promotion, and progression in multistage epidermal carcinogenesis. Proc Soc Exp Biol Med 1993;202:1–8.

67. Ananthaswamy HN, Kripke ML. Experimental skin carcinogenesis by ultraviolet radiation. In: Soter NA, Baden HP, eds. Pathophysiology of Dermatologic Diseases. New York: McGraw-Hill, 1991:483–505.

68. Strickland PT, Burns FJ, Albert RE. Induction of skin tumors in the rat by a single exposure to ultraviolet radiation. Photochem Photobiol 1979;30:683–688.

69. Forbes PD. Experimental ultraviolet light photocarcinogenesis: an overview. J Invest Dermatol 1981;77:139–143.

70. Ananthaswamy HN. Lethality and transformation of 10T1/2 mouse embryo fibroblast cell line by various wavelengths of ultraviolet radiation. Photodermatology 1984;1:265–269.

71. Ananthaswamy HN, Kripke ML. *In vitro* transformation of primary cultures of neonatal BALB/c mouse epidermal cells with ultraviolet-B radiation. Cancer Res 1981;41:2882–2890.

72. Kripke ML. Latency, histology, and antigenicity of tumors induced by ultraviolet light in three inbred mouse strains. Cancer Res 1977;37:1395–1400.

73. Kripke ML. Immunological mechanisms in ultraviolet radiation carcinogenesis. Adv Cancer Res 1981;34:69–106.

74. Rivas JM, Ullrich SE. Ultraviolet B radiation and skin immunology. In: Dean J, Luster M, Munson A, Kimber I, eds. Immunotoxicology and Immunopharmacology, 2nd edition. New York: Raven, 1993, in press.

75. Kripke ML. Antigenicity of murine skin tumors induced by ultraviolet light. J Natl Cancer Inst 1974;53:1333–1336.

76. Fisher MS, Kripke ML. Nature of a systemic alteration induced in mice by ultraviolet irradiation and its relationship to ultraviolet carcinogenesis. Proc Natl Acad Sci USA 1977;74:1688–1692.

77. Toews GB, Bergstresser PR, Steilein JW. Epidermal Langerhans cell density determines whether contact hypersensitivity or unresponsiveness follows skin painting with DNFB. J Immunol 1980;124:445–449.

78. Simon JC, Cruz PC, Bergstresser PR, et al. Low dose ultraviolet B-irradiated Langerhans cells preferentially activate CD4+ cells of the T helper 2 subset. J Immunol 1990;145:2087–2091.

79. Yoshikawa T, Streilein JW. Tumor necrosis factor-alpha and ultraviolet light have similar effects on contact hypersensitivity in mice. Regional Immunol 1990;3:139–144.

80. Baadsgaard O, Cooper KD, Lisby S, et al. UVB and UVC, but not UVA, induce the appearance of T6-DR+ antigen-presenting cells in human epidermis. J Invest Dermatol 1987;89:113–118.

81. Kim T-Y, Kripke ML, Ullrich SE. Immunosuppression by factors released from UV-irradiated epidermal cells: Selective effects on the generation of contact and delayed hypersensitivity after exposure to UVA or UVB radiation. J Invest Dermatol 1990;94:26–32.

82. Rivas JM, Ullrich SE. Systemic suppression of delayed-type hypersensitivity by supernatants from UV-irradiated keratinocytes: An essential role for keratinocyte-derived IL-10. J Immunol 1992;149:3865–3871.

83. Hug DH, Hunter JK. Photomodulation of enzymes. J Photochem Photobiol 1991;10:3–22.

84. Fornace Jr AJ. Mammalian genes induced by radiation. Annu Rev Genet 1992;26:507–526.

85. Hug DH. The activation of enzymes with light. In: Smith KC, ed. Photochemical and Photobiological Reviews, vol. III. New York: Plenum, 1978:1–33.

86. Iizuka H, Ishida-Yamamoto A, Kajita S, et al. Effects of UVB irradiation on epidermal adenylate cyclase response in vitro: Its relation to sunburn cell formation. Arch Dermatol Res 1988;280:163–167.

87. Matsui MS, DeLeo VA. Induction of protein kinase C by ultraviolet radiation. Carcinogenesis 1990;2:229–234.

88. Hanson DL, DeLeo VA. Long wave ultraviolet radiation stimulates arachidonic acid release and cyclooxygenase activity in mammalian cells in culture. Photochem Photobiol 1989;49:423–430.

89. Armitage P, Doll R. The age distribution of cancer and a multistage theory of carcinogenesis. Br J Cancer 1954;8:1–12.

90. Alberts B, Bray D, Lewis, J, et al. Cancer. In: Molecular Biology of the Cell, 2nd edition. Garland, 1989:1187–1218.

91. Fearon ER, Vogelstein B. A genetic model for colorectal tumorigenesis. Cell 1990;61:759–767.

92. Land H, Parada LF, Weinberg RA. Cellular oncogenes and multi-step carcinogenesis. Science 1983;222:771–778.

93. Spandidos DA, Lang JC. Immortalizaton by truncated *myc* or *ras* genes and synergism between *myc* and *ras* genes in cell transformation. Anticancer Res 1989;9:1149–1152.

94. Kanjilal S, Pierceall WP, Ananthaswamy HN. Ultraviolet radiation in the pathogenesis of skin cancers: Involvement of *ras* and *p53* genes. Cancer Bull 1993;45:205–211.

95. Ananthaswamy HN, Pierceall WE. Molecular mechanisms of ultraviolet radiation carcinogenesis. Photochem Photobiol 1990; 52:1119–1136.

96. Ananthaswamy HN, Pierceall WE. Molecular alterations in human skin tumors. In: Klein-Szanto AJP, Anderson MW, Barrett JC, Slaga TJ, eds. Comparative Molecular Carcinogenesis. New York: Wiley-Liss, 1992:61–84.

97. Linnenbach AJ, Huebner K, Reddy EP, et al. Structural alteration in the *myb* proto-oncogene and deletion within the gene encoding a-type protein kinase C in human melanoma cell lines. Proc Natl Acad Sci USA 1988;85:74–78.

98. Megidish T, Mazurek N. A mutant protein kinase C that can transform fibroblasts. Nature 1989;342:807–811.

99. Hollstein M, Sidransky D, Vogelstein B, et al. *p53* mutations in human cancers. Science 1991;253:49–53.

100. Kendric CS. Spontaneous mutagenesis: Experimental, genetic and other factors. Mutat Res 1990;277:139–162.

101. Brash DE, Rudolph JA, Simon JA, et al. A role for sunlight in skin cancer: UV-induced *p53* mutations in squamous cell carcinoma. Proc Natl Acad Sci USA 1991;88:10124–10128.

102. Anderson MW, Reynolds SH, You MH, et al. Role of protooncogene activation in carcinogenesis. Environ Health Perspect 1992;98:13–24.

103. Bishop JM. Cellular oncogenes and their retroviruses. Annu Rev Biochem 1983;52:301–354.

104. Hunter T. Cooperation between oncogenes. Cell 1991;64:249–270.

105. Cantlet LC, Auger KR, Carpenter C, et al. Oncogenes and signal transduction. Cell 1991;64:281–302.

106. Cross M, Dexter TM. Growth factors in development, transformation, and tumorigenesis. Cell 1991;64:271–280.

107. Hockenbery D, Nunez G, Milliman C, et al. Preventing cell suicide: A new role for oncogenes. Nature 1990;348:334.

108. Marshall CJ. Tumor suppressor genes. Cell 1991;64:313–326.

109. Lee WH, Brookstein R, Hong F, et al. Human retinoblastoma susceptibility gene: Cloning, identification, and sequence. Science 1987;235:394–1399.

110. Chen P-L, Chen Y, Bookstein R, Lee W-H. Genetic mechanisms of tumor suppression by the human *p53* gene. Science 1990;250:1576–1580.

111. Klein G. Genes that can antagonize tumor development. FASEB J 1993;7:821–825.

112. Anderson MJ Stanbridge EJ. Tumor suppressor genes studied by cell hybridization and chromosome transfer. FASEB J 1993;7:826–833.

113. Zambetti GP, Levine AJ. A comparison of the biological activities of wild-type and mutant p53. FASEB J 1993;7:855–865.

114. Gailini MR, Bale SL, Leffell DJ, et al. Developmental defects in Gorlin syndrome related to a putative tumor suppressor gene on chromosome 9. Cell 1992;69:111–117.

115. Goudie DR, Yuille MA, Leversha MA, et al. Multiple self-healing squamous epitheliomata (ESSI) mapped to chromosome 9q22-q31 in families with common ancestry. Nature Genet 1993;3:165–169.

116. Quinn AG, Campbell C, Healy E, et al. Chromosome 9 allele loss occurs in both basal and squamous cell carcinomas of the skin. J Invest Dermatol 1994;102:300–303.

117. Barbacid M. *Ras* genes. Annu Rev Biochem 1987;56:779–827.

118. Bos JL. *Ras* oncogenes in human cancer: review. Cancer Res 1989;49:4682–4689.

119. Marx J. Forging a path to the nucleus. Science 1993;260:1588–1590.

120. McCormick F. How receptors turn ras on. Nature 1993;363:15–16.

121. Vogel US, Dixon RA, Schaber MD, et al. Cloning of bovine GAP and its interaction with oncogenic ras p21. Nature 1988;335:90–93.
122. Moodie SA, Willumsen BM, Weber MJ, et al. Complexes of Ras. GTP with Raf-1 and mitogen-activated protein kinase kinase. Science 1993;260:1658–1661.
123. Daaka Y, Wickstorm E. Target dependence of antisense oligonucleotide inhibition of the c-Ha-ras p21 expression and focus formation in T24-tranformed NIH3T3 cells. Oncogene Res 1990;5:267–275.
124. Hoffmann J-S, Fry M, Ji J, et al. Codons 12 and 13 of H-*ras* protooncogene interrupt the progression of DNA synthesis catalyzed by DNA polymerase α. Cancer Res 1993;53:2895–2900.
125. Ananthaswamy HN, Price JE, Goldberg LH, Bales ES. Detection and identification of activated oncogenes in human skin cancers occurring on sun-exposed body sites. Cancer Res 1988;48:3341–3346.
126. Pierceall WE, Goldberg LH, Tainsky MA, et al. Ras gene mutation and amplification in human nonmelanoma skin cancers. Mol Carcinog 1991;4:196–202.
127. Daya-Grosjean L, Robert C, Drougard C, et al. High mutation frequency in *ras* genes of skin tumors isolated from DNA repair deficient xeroderma pigmentosum patients. Cancer Res 1993;53:1625–1629.
128. Suarez HG, Daya-Grosjean L, Schlaifer D, et al. Activated oncogenes in human skin tumors from a repair-deficient syndrome, xeroderma pigmentosum. Cancer Res 1989;49:1223–1228.
129. Corominas M, Kamino H, Leon J, et al. Oncogene activation in human benign tumors of the skin (keratoacanthomas): Is H-*ras* involved in differentiation as well as proliferation? Proc Natl Acad Sci USA 1989;86:6372–6376.
130. van der Schroeff JG, Evers LM, Boot AJM, et al. *Ras* oncogene point mutations in basal cell carcinomas and squamous cell carcinomas of the human skin. J Invest Dermatol 1990;94:423–425.
131. Shukla VK, Hughes DC, Hughes LE, et al. *Ras* mutations in human melanotic lesions: K-*ras* activation is a frequent and early event in melanoma development. Oncogene Res 1989;5:121–127.
132. van't Veer LJ, Burgering BMT, Versteeg R, et al. N-*ras* mutations in human cutaneous melanoma from sun-exposed body sites. Mol Cell Biol 1989;9:3114–3116.
133. Kumar R, Sukumar S, Barbacid M. Activation of *ras* oncogenes preceding the onset of neoplasia. Science 1990;248:1101–1104.
134. Pierceall WE, Kripke ML, Ananthaswamy HN. N-*ras* mutation in ultraviolet radiation-induced murine skin cancers. Cancer Res 1992;52:3946–3951.
135. Funato T, Take A, Ichikawa K, et al. Expression of p21 ras protein in human melanoma cell lines. Neoplasma 1989;36:513–518.
136. Goldfarb M, Shimizu K, Perucho M, et al. Isolation and preliminary characterization of a human transforming gene from T24 bladder carcinoma cells. Nature 1982;296:404–409.
137. Hansen MF, Cavenee WK. Genetics of cancer predisposition. Cancer Res 1987;47:5518–5527.
138. Ananthaswamy HN, Applegate LA, Goldberg LH, Bales ES. Deletion of the c-Ha-ras-1 allele in human skin cancers. Mol Carcinogen 1989;2:298–301.
139. Levine AJ, Momand J, Finlay CA. The *p53* tumor suppressor gene. Nature 1991;351:453–456.
140. Shaulsky G, Ben-Ze'ev A, Rotter V. Subcellular distribution of the p53 protein during the cell cycle of Balb/c 3T3 cells. Oncogene 1990;5:1707–1711.
141. Bischoff JR, Friedman PN, Marshak DR, et al. Human p53 is phosphorylated by p60-cdc2 and cyclin B-cdc2. Proc Natl Acad Sci USA 1990;87:4766–4770.
142. Zhan Q, Carrier F, Fornace Jr AJ. Induction of cellular p53 activity by DNA-damaging agents and growth arrest. Mol Cell biol 1993;13:4242–4250.
143. Kuerbitz SJ, Plunkett BS, Walsh WV, et al. Wild-type p53 is a cell cycle checkpoint determinant following irradiation. Proc Natl Acad Sci USA 1992;89:7491–7495.
144. Marx J. How *p53* suppresses cell growth. Science 1993;262:1644–1645.
145. Campbell C, Quinn AG, Angus B, et al. Wavelength specific patterns of p53 induction in human skin following exposure to UV radiation. Cancer Res 1993;53:2697–2699.
146. Frebourg T, Barbier N, Kassel J, et al. A functional screen for germ line *p53* mutations based on transcriptional activation. Cancer Res 1992;52:6976–6978.
147. Hupp TR, Meek DW, Midgley CA, et al. Regulation of the specific DNA binding function of p53. Cell 1992;71:875–886.
148. Pinhasi-Kimhi O, Michalovitz O, Ben-Ze'ev, et al. Specific interaction between the p53 cellular tumor antigen and major heat shock proteins. Nature 1986;320:182–185.
149. Momand J, Zambetti GP, Olson DC, et al. The *mdm*-2 oncogene product forms a complex with the p53 protein and inhibits p53-mediated transactivation. Cell 1992;69:1237–1245.
150. Stephen CW, Lane DP. Mutant conformation of *p53*: Precise epitope mapping using a filamentous phage epitope library. J Mol Biol 1992;225:577–583.
151. Hinds PW, Finlay CA, Quartin RS, et al. Mutant *p53* DNA clones from human colon carcinomas cooperate with ras in transforming primary rat cells: a comparison of the "hot spot" mutant phenotypes. Cell Growth Differentiation 1990;1:571–580.
152. Soussi T, Caron de Formentel C, May P. Structural aspects of the p53 protein in relation to gene evolution. Oncogene 1990;5:945–952.
153. Malkin D, Li FP, Strong LC, et al. Germ line *p53* mutations in a familial syndrome of breast cancer, sarcomas, and other neoplasms. Science 1990;250:1233–1238.
154. Srivastava S, Zou Z, Pirollo K, et al. Germ-line transmission of a *p53* gene in a cancer-prone family with Li-Fraumeni. Nature 1990;348:747–749.
155. Donehower LA, Harvey M, Slagle BL, et al. Mice deficient for *p53* are developmentally normal but susceptible to spontaneous tumours. Nature 1992;356:215–221.
156. Pierceall WE, Mukhopadhyay T, Goldberg LH, et al. Mutations in the *p53* tumor suppressor gene in human cutaneous squamous cell carcinomas. Mol Carcinog 1991;4:445–449.
157. Sato M, Nishigori C, Zghal M, et al. Ultraviolet-specific mutations in *p53* gene in skin tumors in xeroderma pigmentosum patients. Cancer Res 1993;53:2944–2946.
158. Rady P, Scinicariello F, Wagner RF Jr, et al. *p53* mutations in basal cell carcinomas. Cancer Res 1992;52:3804–3806.
159. Shea CR, McNutt NS, Volkenandt M, et al. Overexpression of p53 protein in BCC in human skin. Am J Pathol 1992;141:25–29.
160. Ziegler A, et al. Mutation hotspots due to sunlight in the *p53* gene of nonmelanoma skin cancers. Proc Natl Acad Sci USA 1993;90:4216–4220.
161. Ziegler A, Jonason AS, Leffell DJ, et al. Sunburn and p53 in the onset of skin cancer. Nature 1994;372:773–776.
162. Kanjilal S, Pierceall WP, Kripke ML, et al. High frequency of *p53* mutations in ultraviolet radiation-induced murine skin tumors: evidence for strand bias and tumor heterogeneity. Cancer Res 1993;53:2961–2964.
163. Kress S, Sutter C, Strickland PT, et al. Carcinogen-specific mutational pattern in the *p53* gene in ultraviolet B radiation–induced squamous cell carcinomas of mouse skin. Cancer Res 1992;52:6400–6403.
164. Lassam NJ, From L, Kahn HJ. Overexpression of p53 is a late event in the development of malignant melanoma. Cancer Res 1993;53:2235–2238.
165. Jhonson MR, Look AT, DeClue JE, et al. Inactivation of the *nf-1* gene in human melanoma and neuroblastoma cell lines without impaired regulation of GTP.Ras. Proc Natl Acad Sci USA 1993;90:5539–5543.
166. Travis J. Closing in on melanoma susceptibility gene(s). Science 1992;258:1080–1081.
167. Fountain JW, Karayiorgou M, Ernstoff MS, et al. Homozygous deletions within human chromosome band 9p21 in melanoma. Proc Natl Acad Sci USA 1992;89:10557–10561.
168. Cannon-Albright LA, Goldgar DE, Meyer LJ, et al. Assignment of a locus for familial melanoma, MLM, to chromosome 9p13-p22. Science 1992;258:1148–1152.

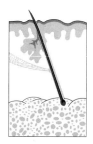

chapter 141

Malignant Neoplasms of Keratinocytes

Disease Description: Actinic (Solar) Keratosis, Bowen's Disease, Keratoacanthoma, Squamous Cell Carcinoma, Basal Cell Carcinoma, and Merkel Cell Carcinoma

Barry Leshin and Wain L. White

Actinic (Solar) Keratosis

DEFINITION

Actinic keratoses (AK), also referred to as solar keratoses, are one of the most common potentially serious manifestations of chronic ultraviolet radiation (UVR) exposure. The term *solar keratosis* is more precise than AK because the latter includes keratoses due to radiation, psoralens and ultraviolet light, and arsenic, which may have different features from those produced by sunlight. Solar keratoses can be conceived of as evolving lesions of squamous cell carcinoma in situ, but because so few of them progress to invasive neoplasia, they are not usually considered malignancies. AKs typically begin to appear in the fourth and fifth decades, and increase in number with advancing years. Individuals who are fair-skinned, with blue eyes and red or blond hair, are partic-

ularly susceptible. Similarly, individuals whose occupation or recreation takes them out of doors are regularly affected.

CLINICAL PRESENTATION

AKs are poorly circumscribed macules and papules, usually several millimeters to a centimeter in diameter, arising in a sun-exposed distribution. These lesions often have an adherent scale, and are variably rough depending on the degree of hyperkeratosis. Lesions arising on the dorsal hands and forearms tend to be much thicker than those on the face. AKs on the ears, too, may be thickened, and some protrude as a cutaneous horn. Occasionally, lesions are more easily palpated than seen. Some AKs are remarkably tender and readily pointed out by the patient. Others are inflamed and erythematous. Less commonly, AKs are hyperpigmented, and occasionally are difficult to distinguish from lentigo maligna and seborrheic keratoses. Lesions arising on the lip are referred to as actinic cheilitis, which typically is manifested by confluent scaliness, focal erosion, fissures and lack of definition of the vermilion border.

The natural history of AKs is controversial. Montgomery and Dorffel, in 1932, observed that up to 20% of untreated AKs will transform into squamous cell carcinoma (SCC).[1] More recently, Marks and associates[2] observed that in more than a third of 616 individuals, 25.9% of AKs remitted spontaneously within a year. This remission was more likely to occur in persons who were able to alter UVR exposure. Moreover, this study cited a malignant transformation rate of 0.24%. A subsequent study by Marks and colleagues[3] revealed that only 60% of SCCs developing in a population of 6416 patients arose from a preexisting AK. On the other hand, because 37 of 38 patients developing SCC had coexisting AKs, these authors felt that the presence of AKs was a significant marker for a population at risk for SCC.

PATHOLOGY

Common to all actinic keratoses is the presence of atypical keratinocytes along the basal cell layer, and usually in the lower third of the epidermis, and disordered cornification marked by singly dyskeratotic keratinocytes, a diminished granular layer, and parakeratosis. A hallmark of solar keratosis is alternating orthokeratosis and parakeratosis on the surface that results from the abnormal cornification of the epidermis between the preserved normal epithelial adnexa (acrotrichia, acrosyringia) (Fig. 141–1). Except for atropic lesions, actinic keratoses show budding of the atypical keratinocytes into the upper papillary dermis.

The evolution of a solar keratosis into an invasive SCC is a biologic continuum that is artificially divided histopathologically as a guide to therapy. The term *hyperplastic* or *acanthotic* solar keratosis applies to those lesions in which the atypical keratinocytes extend below half the thickness of the papillary dermis but not into the reticular dermis. Once the atypical keratinocytes bridge the superficial vascular plexus and extend into the reticular dermis, the lesion is better classified as a superficially invasive SCC.[4]

In addition to this vertical neoplastic progression, some solar keratoses evolve horizontally as the atypical keratinocytes begin to populate the epithelial structures of the follicular infundibula and lastly encroach on the acrosyringia. As this occurs, the keratin production of the infundibula becomes altered and the alternating ortho- and parakeratosis becomes more confluently parakeratotic.

There is confusion in the literature between the difference in a hypertrophic and a hyperplastic solar keratosis. Some use the terms interchangeably.[6] Others refer to the solar keratoses that occur on or near acral skin as hypertrophic because there is often a markedly thickened cornified layer in these lesions, possibly as a consequence of superimposed lichen simplex chronicus.[7]

Solar keratosis can be hyperpigmented as a consequence of increased melanin produced by associated melanocytes that is transferred to the keratinocytes, but there is no melanocytic neoplasm in these lesions. Some pigmented solar keratoses probably represent collision with a solar lentigo.[6, 8] They must be distinguished histologically from early malignant melanoma in situ on severely sun-damaged skin (lentigo maligna), which requires a demonstrable melanocytic proliferation.

Although only a very small number of solar keratoses ever eventuate into invasive SCC, we embrace the concept that solar keratoses are, in fact, the earliest manifestation of SCC in situ.[9] In some solar keratoses one can find complete full-thickness atypia of the epidermis (called the bowenoid type) between normal acrotrichia and acrosyringia. As these lesions evolve horizontally and the atypical changes encompass the epithelial adnexa, they become indistinguishable from Bowen's type of SCC in situ. As long as the alternating ortho- and parakeratosis is preserved, despite the fact that there are foci of full-thickness epidermal keratinocytic atypia and peripheral involvement of the epithelial adnexa by the atypical cells, the lesion is still classified as a solar keratosis and not as fully developed SCC in situ.

In all solar keratoses there are varying degrees of solar elastosis present in the dermis, often vascular telangiectasia, and a variable inflammatory cell infiltrate. A dense band of lymphocytes can fill the papillary dermis and abut the dermoepidermal junction forming a lichenoid pattern, and such lesions must be distinguished from lichenoid dermatoses and lichen planus–like keratoses. The key to the diagnosis of a lichenoid solar keratosis turns on the alternating ortho- and parakeratosis within the cornified layer, relative sparing of the adnexa by the atypical keratinocytes, and striking cytologic atypia in the basal layer, although in lichenoid dermatoses and lichen planus–like keratoses some basal layer cytologic atypia may be present as a consequence of the interface inflammation.[5] Attempts to distinguish these lesions by

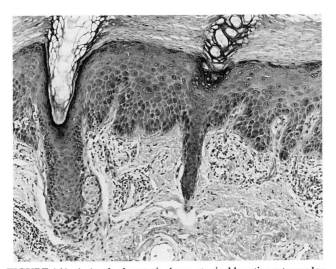

FIGURE 141–1. A solar keratosis shows atypical keratinocytes replacing the lower half of the epidermis, projecting into the papillary dermis, and sparing of the adjacent acrosyringium and acrotrichium. Although the granular layer is present, there is compact parakeratin that alternates with the normal basketweave cornified layer above the uninvolved actrotrichium and acrosyringium.

the number of epidermal Langerhans cells suggest a difference but not a diagnostic distinction.[10]

Actinic cheilitis is a manifestation of solar keratoses on the vermilion, usually of the lower lip. Because of the lack of epidermal adnexa, regularly alternation ortho- and parakeratosis is not evident, but disordered cornification and maturation and cytologic atypia are the same as solar keratoses elsewhere. Because the vermilion of the lip does not contain the same anatomic landmarks as skin it is more difficult to differentiate a hyperplastic actinic cheilitis from early invasive SCC. In this location, in part because of the higher incidence of metastases in squamous cell carcinomas arising on the lip, any prominent hyperplasia in actinic cheilitis extending around the superficial capillaries even suggesting invasive disease is best considered superficial SCC.[11]

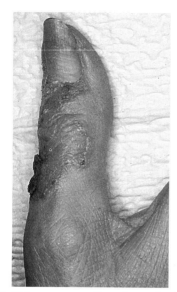

FIGURE 141–2. This squamous cell carcinoma in situ, Bowen's disease, of the thumb has a raised thread-like border around the crusting plaque. (Courtesy of June K. Robinson, M.D.)

Bowen's Disease

DEFINITION

Bowen's disease refers to SCC in situ and may arise anywhere on the skin; however, when it occurs on the mucous membrane of the glans penis it is termed erythroplasia of Queyrat. It has a protracted course that over many years may progress to invasive SCC. In the early small stage arising on actinically damaged skin, it may be called bowenoid actinic keratosis. In the anogenital area, it can be clinically distinguished from bowenoid papulosis, which occurs as multiple small lesions in young adults.

CLINICAL PRESENTATION

Lesions are characterized by macules or plaques of scaly erythema up to several centimeters in diameter, and may simulate an inflammatory dermatosis. Some lesions of Bowen's disease are pigmented. The variable degree of hyperkeratosis and margination give rise to the following basic clinical patterns: (1) nodular crusted or ulcerated plaques; (2) less nodular lesions with a raised thread-like border (Fig. 141–2); (3) scaly, keratotic plaques similar to large actinic keratosis; and (4) slightly elevated scaly flesh-colored plaques.

Bowen's disease most commonly arises on the head and neck, but is noted to arise on sun-protected skin as well.[12] It also can arise from the nail bed, palms and soles, and mucous membranes. Patients may have more than one lesion.

PATHOLOGY

Bowen's disease is SCC in situ in which atypical keratinocytes are arranged throughout the entire thickness of the epidermis. In contrast to solar keratosis, the atypical

cells in Bowen's disease often replace the acrotrichia and eventually acrosyringia but may spare the basal cell layer (Fig. 141–3). This full-thickness involvement of the epidermis in Bowen's disease eventually results in loss of the granular layer with the production of parakeratosis. At the periphery of some lesions, there may be atypical keratinocytes singly or in small nests involving adjacent normal epidermis. This so-called pagetoid or nesting variant must be recognized as one form of SCC in situ and is distinctly different from the pagetoid adenocarcinoma cells observed in extramammary Paget's disease and malignant melanoma in situ.[13] Careful inspection will demonstrate intercellular bridges between cells in pagetoid Bowen's disease, mucin producing and signet ring cells and sometimes small ductal structures in extramammary

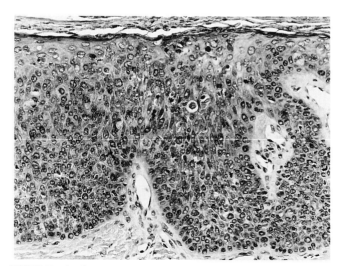

FIGURE 141–3. Bowen's disease is squamous cell carcinoma in situ that demonstrates markedly atypical keratinocytes throughout the epidermis that replace the granular layer and produce parakeratosis, but, in early lesions, spare the basal layer.

Paget's disease, and nests of atypical cells at the dermoepidermal junction and/or melanin production in most cases of melanoma in situ.

Bowen's disease may also show psoriasiform hyperplasia, hyperkeratosis, papillomatosis, and an extensive inflammatory cell infiltrate in the dermis. Some lesions, on the other hand, can be atrophic and others heavily pigmented.[13] As with solar keratoses, there is a somewhat arbitrary distinction between in situ and early invasive disease; however, once atypical cells, often showing signs of cornification, can be demonstrated within the reticular dermis, it is then considered invasive SCC.

PATHOGENESIS

Chronic solar exposure as well as other forms of radiation including ultraviolet light, psoralens and ultraviolet light, and inhalation of mustard gas are implicated in causing Bowen's disease.[14] This neoplasm may occur as a late sequela of chronic arsenic toxicity, especially in agriculture workers using arsenical powders in crop dusting of grapes, potatoes, and tobacco. Human papillomavirus types 12, 13, and 34 have been implicated in Bowen's disease.

DIFFERENTIAL DIAGNOSIS

Any persistent chronic scaling macule or plaque may suggest Bowen's disease. Biopsy is required to differentiate it from superficial basal cell carcinoma and actinic keratosis (Table 141–1).

Keratoacanthoma

DEFINITION

Keratoacanthoma (KA) is an unusual entity, difficult to classify nosologically in the spectrum of epidermal neoplasms as either benign or malignant. Classically considered a benign epithelial neoplasm, KA shares many clinical and histologic features with SCC, and indeed, some consider it to be a form of SCC that usually, but not invariably, involutes.

CLINICAL DESCRIPTION

KAs typically arise on sun-damaged, hair-bearing, light-colored skin in mid- to late life. Males are much more commonly affected than females by a ratio of 2:1. Lesions have been rarely noted to occur on mucous membranes and other non–hair-bearing skin such as the lips, intraorally, and subungually.[15] While usually painless, KAs in certain locations, such as subungual and intraoral, are painful. The typical solitary KA is a dis-

tinctive, well-circumscribed, dome-shaped papule or nodule with a central keratin-filled crater (Fig. 141–4). The lesion is rapidly progressive, reaching 1.0 to 2.5 cm over a 6- to 8-week period. After a stationary phase of 2 to 8 weeks, KAs typically spontaneously involute over a 2- to 8-week period, leaving an atrophic, crenelated scar in their wake. In many instances, KAs persist. Local invasiveness can be significant, and destruction of normal tissue may have cosmetic and functional impact. Although some authors state that KAs never metasta-

TABLE 141–1. Clinical Differential Diagnosis of Malignant Neoplasms of Keratinocytes

Actinic Keratosis (Solar Keratosis)

Seborrheic keratosis
Lentigo maligna
Superficial basal cell carcinoma
Lentigines

Bowen's Disease

Superficial basal cell carcinoma
Psoriasis or chronic eczema
Paget's disease
Actinic keratosis
Tertiary syphilis

Keratoacanthoma

Squamous cell carcinoma
Solar keratosis
Trichofolliculoma
Basal cell carcinoma
Verruca

Squamous Cell Carcinoma

Actinic keratosis
Disorders with pseudoepitheliomatous hyperplasia:
    Blastomycosis or bromoderma, giant seborrheic keratosis
Verruca and condyloma acuminata
Basal cell carcinoma
Keratoacanthoma
Bowen's disease
Eccrine poroma
Melanocytic nevus
Pyogenic granuloma

Basal Cell Carcinoma

Nodular Type
Nonpigmented melanocytic nevus
Squamous cell carcinoma
Pyogenic granuloma
Malignant melanoma
Seborrheic keratosis
Merkel cell carcinoma

Superficial Type
Actinic keratosis
Chronic cutaneous lupus erythematosus
Bowen's disease
Psoriasis and seborrheic dermatitis

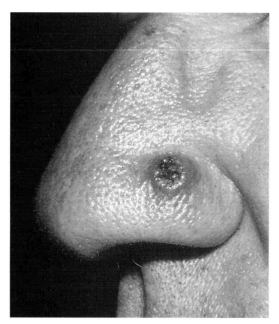

FIGURE 141–4. Keratoacanthoma. This rapidly enlarging lesion is slightly erythematous and demonstrates the characteristic central hyperkeratosis seen in these lesions.

because of its distinctive architecture (Fig. 141–5*A*). It is an exoendophytic proliferation of cornifying squamous epithelium having a central crater filled with orthokeratotic scale. The edges of the lesion show buttresses of well-differentiated squamous epithelium lipping the opening to the crater, and the base of the lesion consists of irregular lobules that usually extend deep into the reticular dermis. The overall lesion is symmetrical, but confusion often arises in tangentially sectioned specimens or incomplete biopsy specimens because the characteristic flask- or cup-shaped architecture cannot be recognized. The peripheral cells of the proliferation are more basaloid and in the center of the aggregations there is a distinct glassy eosinophilic hue to the cell cytoplasm that contains abundant glycogen. The lobules of epithelial cells demonstrate cornification with little to no intervening granular layer—a finding that is sometimes called "abrupt" cornification (Fig. 141–5*B*).[18] The abundant glycogenation and keratin formation without an intervening granular layer mimic changes of tricholemmal keratinization seen in the outer follicular sheath that has led to the histogenetic postulation that keratoacanthomas are primarily tumors with follicular differentiation. The presence of keratoacanthomas on mucous membranes and volar skin in some of the multiple KA

size,[16] others hold that occasional lesions, especially in immunosuppressed patients, are capable of distant spread.[17] Clinicopathologic correlation can at times be difficult. Lesions morphologically consistent with KA may be SCC when examined histologically. Lesions recalcitrant to treatment and otherwise simulating SCC may represent typical KA histologically.

Waiting for a KA to involute can have disastrous consequences. The metastasis of an invasive SCC that morphologically simulated a KA is a paradigm of a clinical paradox: If a presumptive benign diagnosis can be proven incorrect by subsequent biologic activity, should not all such lesions be treated as malignant? It is for this reason that most authorities treat KA as a well-differentiated SCC.

KA has several well-documented variants. *Giant keratoacanthoma* is a rapidly progressive lesion with growth up to 3 cm in diameter. The bulk of such neoplasms accounts for their significant local destructiveness. *Keratoacanthoma centrifugum marginatum* is characterized by rapidly enlarging plaque with central clearing, resulting in an annular configuration. Lesions greater than 20 cm have been described. *Multiple KA* has several forms. The Grysbowski type is characterized by eruptive lesions in a generalized distribution. Lesions occur by the hundreds, and do not usually spontaneously involute. The Ferguson-Smith type arises in early adulthood, and often occurs in kindreds. Also arising in a generalized distribution, lesions are fewer in number and have a greater tendency towards spontaneous involution.

PATHOLOGY

Keratoacanthoma is most readily diagnosed at scanning magnification of an optimally sectioned specimen

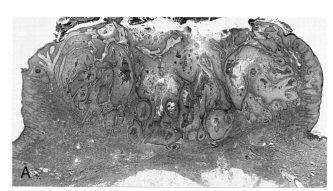

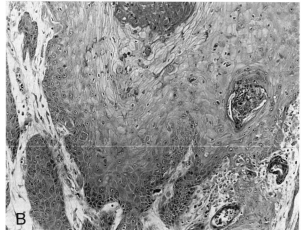

FIGURE 141–5. *A,* A scanning view of a keratoacanthoma demonstrates the characteristic architectural features of a relatively symmetrical exoendophytic proliferation of cornifying squamous cells. A central crater is framed by epithelial buttresses. *B,* Aggregations of squamous cells show abundant pale staining "glassy" cytoplasm producing keratin without an intervening granular layer. Cytologic atypia is confined to the periphery of the aggregations, and microabscesses are present.

settings, however, indicates that certainly this is not always the case.

There is a broad range of acceptance as to the degree of cytologic atypia, the number of atypical mitotic figures, and the amount of parakeratosis that can be accepted in KA. Certainly, when these are absent the diagnosis of KA can be accepted. When they are present the histologic picture merges with well-differentiated SCC and there is no single histologic feature that is generally agreed upon that can always separate these two entities.[19, 20]

The surrounding stroma, particularly in rapidly growing lesions, can have a dense infiltrate of mixed inflammatory cells including eosinophils, neutrophils, and tissue macrophages (histiocytes). Microabscesses are seen around the base of the lesion as well as within the epithelial islands. There is little fibroplasia surrounding keratoacanthomas until involution begins. In the late stages of regression fibroplasia with suppurative granulomatous inflammation is present at the base of the lesions with little in the way of residual squamous proliferation. Also, as keratoacanthomas regress, an increased number of apoptotic dyskeratotic keratinocytes are seen within the proliferated squamous islands, a feature that is regularly seen in subungual keratocanthomas, in which the apoptotic cells often calcify.[21]

At the periphery and base of some keratoacanthomas, intravascular and perineural involvement can be demonstrated. The presence of these features, however, does not necessarily affect the overall biologic behavior or prognosis of the KA.[22, 23] The presense of elastotic fibers and collagen bundles within the epithelial islands is also commonly seen in KA, and although this feature has been used by some to help to distinguish KA from SCC, it is not reliable.

In the final analysis, the diagnosis of KA can only be made based on a proper biopsy specimen in which the overall architecture can be assessed. Even in this setting the distinction from a well-differentiated SCC may be difficult because some lesions show features of both,[24, 25] a finding that has prompted the term *keratocarcinoma.*[26]

Because of the many cases with overlapping histology and clinical course, there remain many important and unanswered questions as to the true nature of the KA. Is its limited growth potential and ability to self-involute an intrinsic characteristic of the neoplasm or is it in fact a function of the host environment in which it arose? Simply dismissing KA as a type of well-differentiated SCC denies the potentially important information waiting to be discovered about the tumorigenesis and progression of this neoplasm. Because there are so many cases in which the histologic features are conflicting between KA and well-differentiated SCC, in the practical setting of determining treatment of a given lesion in an individual patient, treating these as a type of well-differentiated SCC, particularly in the inmmunocompromised patient, seems to be an appropriate approach at our current level of understanding.

Some authorities suggest that some types of multiple keratoacanthomas are distinctive histopathologically from the solitary type. This is particularly true of the multiple keratoacanthomas of the Ferguson-Smith type.[27, 28] There are certainly different clinicopathologic

settings in which these neoplasms evolve, but there is great confusion in the literature as to their distinct histopathology. Even though the lesions can be quite large and deeply invasive, they ultimately involute.[29] In a given neoplasm, particularly an early lesion, there seems to be little that is histologically reliably distinctive from the other types of KA.[30, 31]

Squamous Cell Carcinoma

DEFINITION

SCC is the second most common form of skin cancer, representing 20% of cutaneous malignancies.[32, 33] Over 100,000 cases of SCC are diagnosed annually in the United States, accounting for an incidence rate of 41.4 per 100,000 persons.[34] The incidence has been increasing at a rate of 4% to 8% since the 1960s.[35] This keratinocytic neoplasm most commonly affects individuals in mid- to late life, and most commonly arises in areas of chronic sun exposure. SCCs characteristically cause local tissue destruction and in advanced cases may cause considerable functional and cosmetic morbidity. Cutaneous SCC carries greater risk for metastases than does basal cell carcinoma (BCC), and in some instances has an explosive growth rate.

CLINICAL PRESENTATION

The typical SCC is a hyperkeratotic, skin-colored papule, nodule, or plaque arising on sun-damaged skin (Fig. 141–6). Associated erythema is variable, depending on the inflammatory response to the neoplasm. Larger lesions may have subcutaneous extension. When associated with pain, the clinician should be aware that this is an indication of perineural extension. Several parameters of SCC are significant in assessing its biologic behavior, that is, tendency for local recurrence and/or metastases.

Location

The central zone of the face is an area at high risk for local recurrence.[36–42] Tumors in this region may have significant subclinical extension, and therefore are frequently inadequately removed. Accounting for this subclinical extension are numerous resistance planes, such as the perichondrium of auricular and nasal cartilages and the tarsal plates of the eyelids, or embryonic fusion planes at the junction of the nasal ala and nasolabial fold, and along the nasal columella, or in the periauricular region.[43–45] Tumors will grow down to these planes, and rather than penetrate initially will "fan out." The resulting flask-shaped or eccentric configurations result in underestimation of tumor extent from surface topographic features (Fig. 141–7A and B).

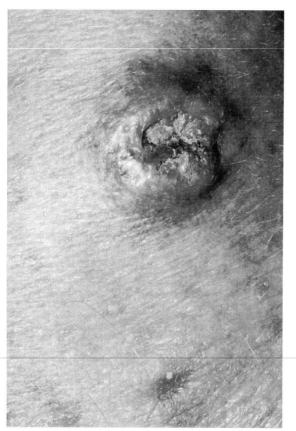

FIGURE 141-6. Squamous cell carcinoma. This ulcerated nodule is arising on the sun-damaged cheek of an elderly woman. Although present for less than 6 weeks, the tumor has significant subcutaneous extension.

SCC arising on the temple, dorsal hands, lips, ear, scalp, and penis is at significant risk for metastases.[46, 47] Zitelli observed that larger surgical margins are required to histologically clear SCC in these high-risk areas.[48] SCC arising in areas of chronic ulceration, sinus tracts, and chronic osteomyelitis also has increased risk of metastases.

Size

As would be expected, the larger the tumor, the more likely the chance for local recurrence.[46–49] Cure rates by Mohs micrographic surgery fall significantly as tumor size increases. Tumors less than 1 cm have a 99.5% cure rate by this technique, compared with 82.3% for tumors 2 to 3 cm, and 58.9% for tumors greater than 3 cm.[50] Rowe and coworkers describe a local recurrence rate of 7.4% for tumors under 2 cm in diameter, contrasted to 15.2% for tumors greater than 2 cm.[47] Margins of excision therefore are adjusted according to size, with a 4-mm margin recommended for tumors less than 2 cm, and 6 mm for tumors of 2 cm or greater.[48]

Depth of Invasion

As would be expected from the above discussion, more deeply invasive tumors have a much greater tendency for local recurrence and metastases.[46, 51–54] Of particular importance is penetration of tumor through the dermis to the subcutaneous adipose tissue, which may occur up to 30% of the time.[48] Such tumors have been noted to have a local or regional recurrence rate of 19.8%.[53] Rowe and coworkers observed a local recurrence rate of 5.3% for tumors less than 4 mm in depth, compared with a rate of 17.2% for tumors 4 mm or greater.[47] Tumors greater

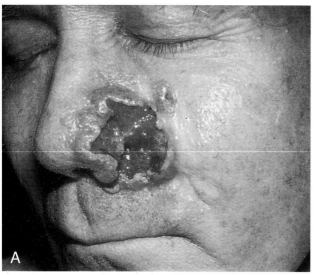

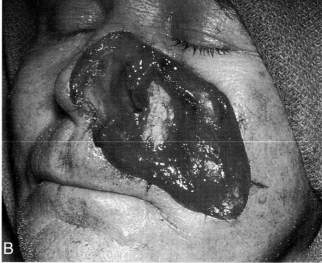

FIGURE 141-7. *A,* The epicenter of this ulcerated squamous cell carcinoma arises over the embryonic fusion planes of the nasolabial fold. Clinically, the white indurated area extends along the nasolabial fold toward the cheek. *B,* The postoperative surgical defect following Mohs micrographic excision demonstrates the substantial subclinical extent that frequently occurs in tumors arising in this region.

than 1 cm in diameter, or of histologic grade 2 or higher, are more likely to extend to the subcutaneous tissue.[48]

Degree of Histologic Differentiation

Histologic grade has significant impact on subclinical tumor extension. Less well differentiated SCC, Broder grades 2 or higher, generally requires larger resections, and therefore has greater likelihood of local recurrence.[48] Rowe and coworkers report an overall recurrence rate of 13.6% for well-differentiated tumors compared with 28.6% for poorly differentiated SCCs.[47]

Presence of Perineural Extension

A subset of SCC has a neurophilic growth pattern. These tumors invade the perineural space, which can serve as a conduit for significant subclinical extension. Tumors with perineural invasion are at greater risk for local recurrence following treatment.[55, 56] Rowe and coworkers note a 47.2% local recurrence rate for perineural tumors.[47]

Metastases and Death Rates

Actinically derived SCC has been traditionally regarded as having extremely low propensity for metastases.[57] Multiple studies have reported metastatic rates of 0.3% to 3.7% for such tumors. Rowe and coworkers attribute this low rate to short follow-up periods, and their meta-analyses noted a metastatic rate of 5.2% for previously untreated tumors.[47] SCCs arising at specific high-risk sites such as the lip, ear, penis, scrotum, and anus carry much greater risk.[47, 50, 58-60] Dinehart and Pollack have noted a metastatic rate of 7% in patients who have undergone Mohs excision of SCCs.[46]

Parameters of size, depth of penetration, histologic differentiation, and presence of perineural extension (as described above) carry much greater significance. Size greater than 2 cm,[46, 47, 60] depth of invasion to at least 4 mm,[47, 61] and Broder's histologic classification of 2 or greater[53, 54, 57, 60] are various factors defining a tumor at higher risk for metastases. Additionally, underlying immunosuppression may significantly impact on propensity for metastases.[47, 62] When SCC does metastasize, typically it is to regional lymph nodes. Hematogenous dissemination, though rare, has also been well documented. Five-year survival in patients with regional lymph node metastases is 26%, and 23% in patients with distant metastases.[63]

Verrucous Carcinoma

Verrucous carcinoma is often regarded as a clinicopathologic subtype of SCC. This low-grade, indolent neoplasm is usually exophytic with a wart-like appearance and may cause significant local tissue destruction, but carries a very low risk for metastases. Verrucous carcinoma characteristically arises on the foot (epithelioma cuniculatum), or on the glans penis (giant condyloma of Buschke and Lowenstein),[64] and clinically has marked wart-like hyperkeratosis. When seen in the mouth (oral florid papillomatosis), hyperkeratosis is manifested by diffuse leukokeratosis.[65-67]

PATHOLOGY

SCC most commonly consists of a proliferation of atypical squamous cells that originates in the epidermis and extends into the reticular dermis and below. The cells usually demonstrate rather abundant eosinophilic cytoplasm with large vesicular nuclei and prominent nucleoli. Mitotic figures are common, many being atypical. There are variable degrees of differentiation in these neoplasms with individual cell keratinization or more organized cornification in the form of squamous eddies and horn pearl formations. As indicated in the discussion on solar keratoses, there are no universally accepted criteria that separate the hyperplastic solar keratosis from the superficial SCC; however, involvement of the reticular dermis is one of the more reproducible features for the diagnosis of carcinoma (Fig. 141–8A).

Several histologic subtypes of SCC may be recognized morphologically, such as spindle and acantholytic, but have little relationship to biologic behavior. Spindle cell SCC must be distinguished from other poorly differentiated spindle cell malignancies such as malignant melanomas and superficial malignant fibrous histiocytoma (Fig. 141–8B). One can often identify focal cornification and intercellular bridges as a clue to squamous differentiation, but where none is demonstrable with sections stained by hematoxylin and eosin, the application of immunoperoxidase studies can usually distinguish these lesions; SCC is positive for cytokeratin and negative for S-100 antigen and macrophage markers.

Some squamous cell carcinomas show extensive acantholysis and present an adenoid or pseudoglandular appearance and must be distinguished from an adenocarcinoma. This acantholytic variety almost invariably arises from an acantholytic solar keratosis (Fig. 141–8C).[68, 69]

The degree of differentiation as determined by the amount of cornification has been used to grade SCC, but most cutaneous squamous carcinoma is moderately to well differentiated. SCC can invade and infiltrate nerves, blood vessels, lymphatics, and fascial planes, and a poorly differentiated tumor with a highly invasive appearance is certainly an indication that the lesion may be progressive biologically. On the other hand, well-differentiated lesions in immuncompromised patients may also be aggressive neoplasms.[7, 16] In contradistinction to spindle cell squamous carcinoma and acantholytic squamous carcinoma, verrucous carcinoma is a distinct clinicopathologic entity that is characterized by a large papillated exoendophytic proliferation that has hyperkeratosis and parakeratosis. It is difficult in some cases to distinguish a large condyloma from a verrucous carcinoma because the bulbous rete in verrucous carcinoma contain very well differentiated squamous cells with little to no

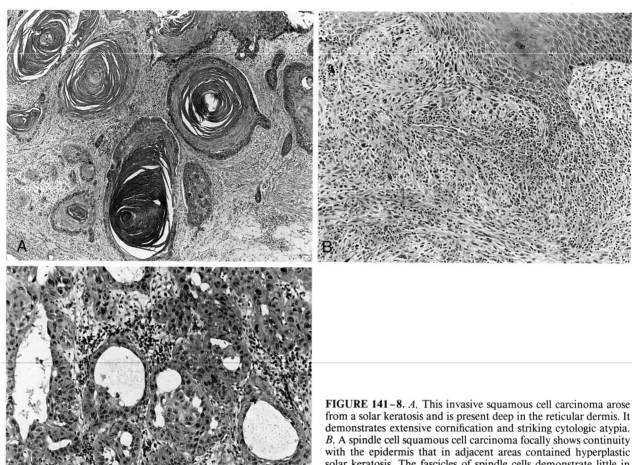

FIGURE 141–8. *A,* This invasive squamous cell carcinoma arose from a solar keratosis and is present deep in the reticular dermis. It demonstrates extensive cornification and striking cytologic atypia. *B,* A spindle cell squamous cell carcinoma focally shows continuity with the epidermis that in adjacent areas contained hyperplastic solar keratosis. The fascicles of spindle cells demonstrate little in the way of preserved squamous differentiation. *C,* An acantholytic squamous cell carcinoma demonstrates the pseudoglandular pattern that simulates adenocarcinoma. Keratinization is preserved in adjacent cells (upper right).

cytologic atypia. In fact, if a squamous proliferation shows any significant degree of squamous atypia above the basal cell layer, it should be classified as a well-differentiated squamous cell carcinoma, not a verrucous carcinoma.[70] In verrucous carcinoma the aggregations extend deep into the reticular dermis and have lobulated borders that give the appearance of a pushing margin (Fig. 141–9).

Intraepithelial abscesses can develop in long-standing lesions and keratin-filled cysts may develop within the tumor mass[71] Because of these features, some lesions may be difficult to distinguish from a pseudocarcinomatous hyperplasia associated with deep fungal or mycobacterial infections. The granulomatous inflammation seen in those infections, however, is usually not seen in verrucous carcinoma. The well-differentiated nature of these neoplasms sometimes requires multiple biopsies for diagnosis, and, as with keratoacanthoma, biopsies must be deep enough to include the base of the lesion and large enough to display the overall architecture of the lesion to establish a definitive diagnosis.

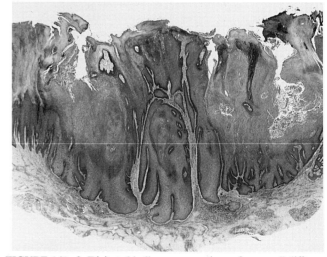

FIGURE 141–9. Digitated bulbous aggregations of very well differentiated keratinocytes characterize the typical features of verrucous carcinoma. The base of the neoplasm has a lobulated endophytic appearance. Cytologic atypia is confined to the basal cell layer and slightly above.

PATHOGENESIS

Many etiologic factors exist in the development of SCC. Recognition of occupational chemical exposure as a cause of SCC dates to Percivall Pott's account of scrotal tumors developing in chimney sweeps.[72] Since then, other hydrocarbons have been implicated.[73] Cutaneous SCC has also been linked to chronic arsenic exposure through well water, medicinals, herbicides, and insecticides.[74, 75] Exposure to x-radiation and other forms of radiation have also been established as etiologic.[76, 77] Substantial evidence supports a role of human papillomavirus in the development of some squamous cell carcinomas.[78] Patients with depressed host immunity, either iatrogenically as in the transplant population[79] or by virtue of an underlying disease (e.g., chronic lymphocytic leukemia) are at increased risk for SCC. Moreover, such neoplasms in this setting often display aggressive behavior. Various local changes may undergo malignant degeneration in the form of SCC, such as sites of thermal injury, chronic ulcerations and sinus tracts, hidradenitis suppurativa,[80] chronic cutaneous lupus erythematosus, and chronic osteomyelitis.[81] Finally, underlying genetic predisposition in the form of xeroderma pigmentosum,[82] epidermodysplasia verruciformis,[83] recessive dystrophic epidermolysis bullosa[84] and oculocutaneous albinism[85] may play a role in the development of SCC.

Despite this wide array of etiologies, the single most significant predisposing factor for the development of SCC is chronic ultraviolet light exposure. Several epidemiologic, clinical, and basic investigative data support this conclusion. The incidence of cutaneous SCC is greater among whites, as compared to blacks and Asians.[86, 87] Moreover, the incidence of SCC is also greater in non-Latino whites as compared to Latinos,[86] and correlates inversely with latitude.[84, 86] SCC also occurs more frequently in fair-skinned individuals who sunburn easily, and most frequently arises in sun-exposed skin. Solar radiation in the ultraviolet light B (290 to 320 nm) range generates SCC in experimental animals.[35, 89, 90] Occupational sun exposure may be an important risk factor for the development of SCC.[91]

Basal Cell Carcinoma

DEFINITION

BCC is a malignant neoplasm of epithelial cells that resemble the germinative cells of hair follicles more than they do the cells of the basal layer of the epidermis. It is the most frequently encountered cancer in man. Over half a million BCCs are diagnosed in the United States annually, outnumbering SCC 4 to 1.[86]

CLINICAL PRESENTATION

Basal cell carcinoma has multiple distinctive clinical forms, and in its most frequent presentations may be recognized and diagnosed by close inspection. Moreover, the clinical subtypes of BCC can often be correlated with histologic subtypes. This clinicopathologic correlation is so strong that several of the clinical subtypes are named by their histologic appearance. It should be emphasized, however, that BCC is protean in its manifestations, and clinical simulants abound. For this reason, biopsy for histologic evaluation is paramount. The various clinical forms of BCC include:

1. Nodular BCC. The most frequent form of BCC, nodular BCC presents as a waxy, opalescent or translucent papule or nodule associated with overlying fine telangiectasias (Fig. 141–10). Ulceration or erosion of the surface is a frequent finding. In larger ulcerated lesions, the tumor's surface appears to have been nibbled by a small animal, and hence the name of rodent ulcer.

Some nodular BCCs have an endophytic growth pattern, and surface topography belies its true extent. These tumors frequently have a plaque configuration, and actual tumor extent is best assessed clinically by palpation of tissue induration. Histologically, these lesions may have an infiltrative or micronodular pattern. Subclinical extent may be significant, which frequently accounts for inadequate treatment. For this reason, such tumors are more likely to recur after therapy, and therefore are categorized as aggressive BCC.

BCCs may occasionally be pigmented, with degree of pigmentation being quite variable. Depending on the degree of pigmentation, lesions may resemble nevi or melanoma.

2. Morpheaform or sclerosing BCC. This subtype of BCC has a scar-like appearance. A dermal plaque with overlying epidermal atrophy in a sun-exposed distribution and no history of antecedent trauma should heighten clinical suspicion for this tumor subtype. As with micronodular and infiltrative patterns of nodular BCC, subclinical extension is often great and treatment failures frequent.

3. Superficial BCC. This BCC subtype most commonly arises on the trunk and extremities, but may be

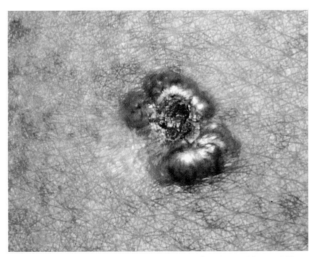

FIGURE 141–10. Nodular basal cell carcinoma. This umbilicated papule has a rolled, pearly rim with overlying fine telangiectasias.

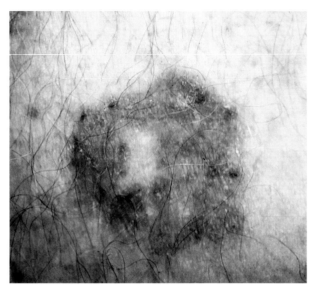

FIGURE 141-11. Superficial basal cell carcinoma. This form of basal cell carcinoma is characterized by scaly erythema. Focal erosion and central regression are evident.

seen anywhere on the body. The tumors are characterized by an erythematous macule or patch (Fig. 141–11). In lieu of erythema, lesions may be variably pigmented. There also may be an overlying fine scale, or lesions may be superficially eroded and with hemorrhagic scale crust. A fine thread-like ridge may be observed at the peripheral margin. Originally described as multicentric,[92, 93] Madsen and others[94-96] have substantiated the unicentric nature of this neoplasm. Clinically silent projections of this tumor account for difficulty in management. This type of BCC is the variant most frequently seen in chronic arsenism, and as a late sequelae of radiation therapy. Individuals may have broad areas of superficial BCC that are multiple and disconnected and are referred to as "field-fire" BCC. This true multicentricity is likely a field effect, with all affected tissue having similar local carcinogenic factors accounting for the tumor.

As with SCC, certain parameters define BCCs that pose greatest risk to affected individuals. Several of these correlate closely with those for SCC, namely location, histologic subtype, clinical characteristics, and size.

Location

The factors discussed for SCC are also wholly relevant for BCC. The typically more indolent growth pattern of BCC (as compared to SCC) accounts for the resistance and fusion planes of the central facial zone being a more significant determinant of subclinical extension.

Size

Size is also a good predictor of high risk BCCs. Mohs observed that cure rates with Mohs micrographic surgery (MMS) decreased as tumor size increased. He reported a cure rate of 99.8% for tumors less than 2 cm in diameter,

98.6% for tumors between 2 and 3 cm, and 90.5% for tumors greater than 3 cm.[50, 97] Robins similarly observed a cure rate of 98% for tumors less than 2 cm, and 92% for tumors greater than 5 cm.[98]

Histology

Unlike SCC, BCC is not histologically graded according to degree of differentiation. However, several histologic subtypes are notoriously difficult to manage. In particular, micronodular, infiltrative, and morpheiform BCCs have a much higher incidence of positive surgical margins after surgical excision (18.6% to 33.3%) as compared with tumors with a nodular or superficial histologic pattern.[99] Morpheiform BCC may have significant subclinical extent. Salasche and Amonette reported an average subclinical extension of morpheiform BCC of 7.2 mm in 51 patients undergoing MMS.[100] Similarly, Siegle and associates observe significant subclinical extension in infiltrative BCC.[101] BCC with marked squamous differentiation has been observed by some to be a more virulent tumor. Borel reported a local recurrence rate of 45.7% and metastatic incidence of 8.6% of 35 such tumors as compared to rates of 24.2%/0.09% for BCC, and 21.9%/7.9% for SCC.[102] Perineural extension of BCC may be especially problematic. As with SCC, the perineural space can serve as a conduit for significant subclinical tumor extension.[103]

PATHOLOGY

Numerous histopathologic subtypes of basal cell carcinomas have been described but there are only a few that are well-established clinicopathologic entities. These include nodular, morpheiform, superficial, fibroepitheliomatous, and infundibulocystic types. The others, such as keratotic, adenoid, infiltrating, micronodular, and pigmented, are variations of these basic clinicopathologic entities. Regardless of the morphologic variation of the lesion, all basal cell carcinomas have in common the presence of basaloid cells arranged in aggregations of various sizes and shapes, slightly elongated nuclei aligned at least focally in a palisade at the periphery of some aggregations, neoplastic cells with hyperchromatic nuclei with little or no definable cytoplasm, and varying numbers of mitotic figures accompanied by karyorrhexis and pyknosis. In almost all forms of BCC, clefts can be identified between the neoplastic cells and the adjacent stroma which may be altered by deposition of connective tissue mucin, edema, an infiltrate of inflammatory cells and fibroblasts, and neovascularization.[104] The vast majority of the neoplasms show some attachment to the undersurface of the epidermis and, with few exceptions such as the morpheiform variant, the epithelial component predominates over the stromal elements.

Nodular BCC is the most frequently encountered type and is composed of large, rounded aggregations of basaloid cells that usually have distinct peripheral palisading and prominent clefts around the aggregations that separate the neoplastic epithelium from the stroma, which is often myxoid and shows solar elastosis (Fig. 141–12*A*). These lesions are often cystic as a consequence of central tumor necrosis or mucin deposition within the epithelial aggregations.[105] The overlying epidermis may be ulcerated.

A micronodular variant is separated by some as being different biologically because of the high propensity for local recurrence, but others consider it a variant of nodular BCC.[6, 104] Likewise, an infiltrative BCC is a variant of nodular BCC in which the base of the lesion consists of infiltrative cords, strands and jagged aggregations of basaloid cells in a fibroblastic stroma (Fig. 141–12*B*). The amount of surrounding fibroplasia is variable but sclerosis is not well developed.[6]

Superficial basal cell carcinoma is composed of multiple buds of basaloid cells that project from the basal layer of the epidermis into the papillary dermis. There is usually distinct peripheral palisading around these nests with varying amounts of fibroplasia, inflammatory cell infiltrate and fibromyxoid change to the surrounding stroma (Fig. 141–12*C*). Although histologically these lesions appear to be multifocal, three-dimensional reconstruction studies both with and without computer enhancement have demonstrated that these in fact are unicentric in origin.[95, 96, 106] The histologic multifocal appearance of these neoplasms arises from the reticulated growth of a neoplasm that in horizontal pathologic sectioning demonstrates intervening uninvolved epidermis. Ulceration and varying amounts of melanin deposition may be present in superficial BCC.

Morpheiform BCC is also know as sclerosing, fibrosing, and desmoplastic types of BCC. The neoplasm is

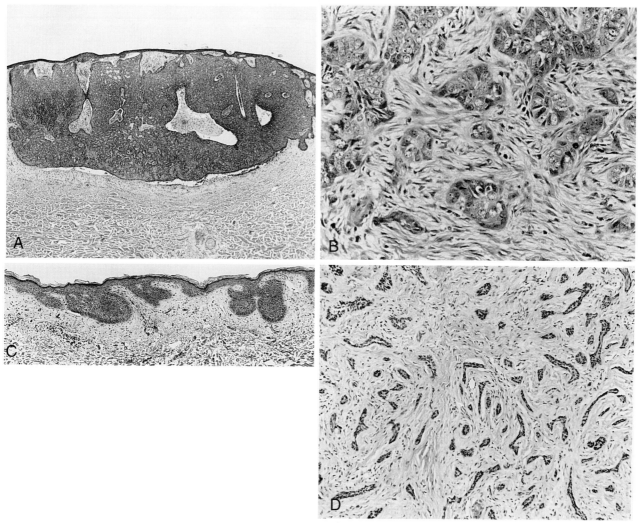

FIGURE 141–12. *A,* Nodular basal cell carcinoma shows large aggregations of cells with high nuclear/cytoplasmic ratios, like the cells of the basal layer of the epidermis, which are aligned in a palisade at the periphery of the proliferations that resemble a picket fence. These cells are separated from the adjacent altered myxoid stroma by an artifactual cleft. *B,* An infiltrating basal cell carcinoma demonstrates jagged nests of basaloid cells separated in a fibrotic stroma. This carcinoma has large vesicular nuclei with an open chromatin pattern that has been described as "metatypical" basal cell carcinoma. *C,* Buds of basaloid cells project in several foci from the base of the epidermis into the papillary dermis, which has an altered myxoid stroma. Clefts are focally present between the neoplastic epithelial cells and the stroma. *D,* Morpheiform basal cell carcinoma is composed of delicate cords and geometric aggregations of basaloid cells separated in a dense desmoplastic stroma.

Illustration continued on following page

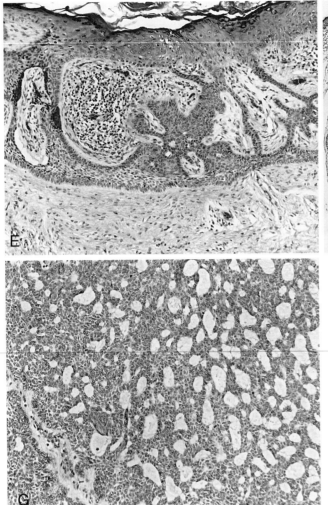

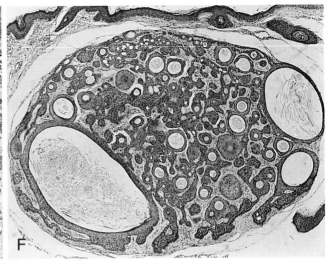

FIGURE 141–12. *Continued E,* Fibroepithelial basal cell carcinoma demonstrates a fenestrated pattern of cords of squamous cells with peripheral palisades of more basaloid cells with clefts separating them from the stroma at one periphery (left). The anastomosing epithelial cords are surrounded by a loose myxoid stroma. *F,* Infundibulocytic basal cell carcinoma shows anastomosing cords of squamous cells in somewhat of a radial array with keratin cysts and distal aggregations of basaloid cells that simulate follicular germs or the aggregations of superficial basal cell carcinoma. *G,* A reticulated basal cell carcinoma is composed of a lace-like arrangement of basaloid cells.

composed of narrow cords and even strings of single cells that are branched and separated in a dense fibrotic and sclerotic stoma. Attachment to the epidermis is often inconspicuous in these neoplasms and, in some foci, the stromal elements may predominate over the epithelial components. This pattern is distinct from the infiltrative variant of nodular BCC. Deep dermal invasion and subcutaneous involvement are not uncommon (Fig. 141–12D).[107]

This variant of BCC, first described by Pinkus as a premalignant fibroepithelioma,[108] is characterized by thin, trabeculated basaloid cells that extend from the epidermis as elongated cords forming a fenestrated pattern. They may also contain horn pseudocysts. These neoplasms, although often superficial, can extend deep into the dermis and even the subcutaneous tissue. Focally, at the periphery of the anastomosing cords, however, aggregations of small basaloid cells aligned in a palisade can usually be demonstrated; and in these foci clefts may separate them from the adjacent stroma. The mesenchymal proliferation is usually a loose myxoid stroma; but discrete clefts do not usually separate the elongated, reticulated epithelial cords from the adjacent stroma (Fig. 141–12E). Necrosis en masse is uncommon in the fibroepithelial variant.[5, 104]

Infundibulocystic BCC is the most recently described clinicopathologic type of basal cell carcinoma that consists of anastomosing cords of squamous epithelial cells often showing small keratin cysts.[104, 109] The cords end distally in small aggregations of basaloid cells that simulate follicular germs. These lesions often have an overall benign architectural pattern, being very small and well circumscribed (Fig. 141–12F). Clefts between the epithelial cells and surrounding stroma are not a constant feature. Melanin may be present in the epithelial cells and amyloid present in the surrounding stoma.

Ackerman and coworkers have classified infundibulocystic BCC as an indolent type of BCC that shows follicular differentiation.[104, 109] The true biologic potential of these lesions and their distinction from basaloid follicular hamartoma remain controversial.[110–112] They are often seen juxtaposed to a nodular BCC and are the common type of BCC arising in the basal cell nevus syndrome.[104]

Other morphologic variants of basal cell carcinomas are thought to be histologic subtypes of the major clinicopathologic entities, primarily nodular BCC. These include adenoid types that have abundant stromal mucin around a reticulated epithelial pattern (Fig. 141–12G); keratotic types that have prominent squamous differentiation with squamous eddy formation and keratinaceous cysts; and adamantinoid BCC that shows ameloblastic changes. Rarely true eccrine and apocrine differentiation have been reported in basal cell–like carcinoma.[113, 114] Likewise, sebaceous differentiation may be seen in some cases.[6]

Squamous differentiation is common in BCC, particularly near the dermoepidermal junction, and the surface of these lesions may be indistinguishable from a solar keratosis.[7] In persistent (recurrent) BCC, there is often a greater degree of squamous differentiation. Rarely indubitable SCC may be juxtaposed to BCC but the term *basosquamous carcinoma* is to be avoided unless both types are distinctly seen in a biphasic pattern.[115] Metatypical types of BCC are thought to be a variant with some squamous differentiation that has more nuclear anaplasia and an infiltrative pattern. Peripheral palisading is less obvious and the cells are large with more abundant pale-staining cytoplasm,[6, 107, 116] although the use of this type as a specific entity is to be discouraged (Fig. 141–12*B*).[7]

Rarely, BCC can be associated with a malignant mesenchymal component (carcinosarcoma) that in some cases may show chondroid and osteoid differentiation. These rare lesions can be highly aggressive and metastasize as poorly differentiated sarcomas.[107] Some basal cell carcinomas may be composed partially or entirely of cells having abundant clear cytoplasms. Although initially considered a function of tricholemmal differentiation, recent data suggest that these clear cell basal carcinomas are a result of lysosomal degeneration.[117]

PATHOGENESIS

Like SCC, BCC is related to chronic UVR exposure. More than 99% of individuals developing BCC are Caucasians, and 85% of these tumors arise on the head and neck. Of all sites, the nose is most commonly involved, accounting for 25% to 30% of all tumors. Men are slightly more commonly affected. Ninety-five per cent of individuals with BCC are between 40 and 79 years old.[118] Fair-skinned individuals who burn rather than tan are most susceptible. Other genetic factors also play a key role, with individuals of Scotch, Celtic, or Scandinavian ancestry especially prone. Affected persons usually have a history of significant occupational and/or recreational sun exposure.

There exist other significant risk factors for the development of BCC. Prior injury such as trauma, burns, or vaccinations at the tumor site is frequently noted by persons with BCC.[119, 120] As with SCC X-irradiation may be a risk factor for the subsequent development of BCC.[121] Carcinoma arising as a late sequela of radiation therapy most frequently takes the form of BCC on the head, neck, and trunk, and SCC on the hands.[122] As with SCC and Bowen's disease, prior exposure to inorganic arsenic can also lead to the formation of BCC.[123] In this setting, tumors are often multiple, truncal, and superficial lesions. Patients with certain genetic syndromes, such as xeroderma pigmentosum,[75] nevoid BCC syndrome,[124] albinism,[125] and Bazex syndrome,[126] are more

prone to the development of BCC. Nevus sebaceus[127] and linear unilateral basal cell nevus[128] are developmental hamartomas that may give rise to BCC. Finally, immunosuppressed individuals are prone to the development of BCC, although their risk is greater for SCC than for BCC.

Although BCC is rarely life threatening or health threatening, its capacity for local tissue destruction can result in significant functional or cosmetic morbidity. Untreated or inadequately treated BCCs have an insidious growth pattern and may result in death. Metastasis from BCC is a rare event, with estimates of metastatic incidence ranging from 0.0028% to 0.1%.[129-130a] Metastasis is associated with the metatypical (basosquamous) BCC and with duration and size of the lesion. The most frequent site of metastasis is lung, followed by bone, lymph nodes, and liver. For these reasons, great importance is attached to the early diagnosis and treatment of this malignancy.

Merkel Cell Carcinoma (see Chapter 148)

June K. Robinson

DEFINITION

Trabecular cell carcinoma or Merkel cell carcinoma is a primary neuroendocrine neoplasm of the skin that is commonly clinically diagnosed as a BCC. It may also mimic a BCC pathologically. Inasmuch as it is frequently mistaken for a BCC, Merkel cell carcinoma is included in this chapter despite the fact that it is not derived from epidermal keratinocytes.

CLINICAL PRESENTATION

This recently reported tumor[131-133] is slightly more prevalent in elderly females and occurs as a solitary lesion on the face,[134, 135] extremities, or buttocks.[136] Although the clinical behavior of MCC is difficult to predict, the aggressive nature of the tumor is illustrated by 39% of 229 cases having at least one local recurrence, one half having lymph node metastases, and 15% of patients dying of metastatic disease.[136, 137] The 5-year survival rate for patients with regional disease is 30%.

This slow-growing asymptomatic papule or nodule rarely ulcerates. It presents as a pink to red or violet firm, dome-shaped, usually solitary, lesion. Lymph node involvement is present in greater than 50% of patients.

PATHOLOGY

Most Merkel cell carcinomas are dermally based masses of small round cells with scant cytoplasm and hyperchromatic nuclei. The aggregations of cells vary from solid to loosely arranged, and some lesions show

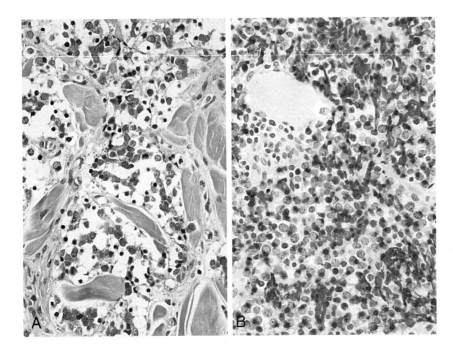

FIGURE 141–13. *A,* Merkel cell carcinoma can display a trabecular pattern, and typically has cells with scant cytoplasm, hyperchromatic nuclei, and small nucleoli. *B,* A Merkel cell carcinoma stained with antiserum to keratin filaments. Many cells have perinuclear globular staining, corresponding to balls of intermediate filaments seen by electron microscopy.

the trabecular pattern that led to its original name of trabecular carcinoma of the skin (Fig. 141–13*A*).[131] The nuclei of the cells of most Merkel cell carcinomas have small and sometimes multiple nucleoli, and in many cases nuclear detail is obscured by easily induced crush artifact. Mitotic figures, necrotic cells, and nuclear debris are frequent findings.

There are several variant appearances of Merkel cell carcinoma. In some cases, aggregations of neoplastic cells are present in the epidermis in a pagetoid pattern, either with or without dermal involvement.[138] There can be adjacent solar keratosis, Bowen's disease, or melanoma in situ, raising the possibility of divergent differentiation of the neoplastic cells. Sweat duct differentiation, small aggregations of squamous keratinocytes, and rosette-like groupings of cells are other unusual findings.[139]

The cells of Merkel cell carcinoma contain neurosecretory granules that can be seen by electron microscopy. These membrane-bound structures are 80- to 180-nm, round, and have an electron-dense core surrounded by a lucent space. These granules are best seen in glutaraldehyde fixed rather than routinely processed material. Another ultrastructural hallmark is the presence of perinuclear balls of intermediate filaments.

Although these ultrastructural findings are distinctive, immunohistochemistry can easily distinguish Merkel cell carcinoma from other small round cell neoplasms, such as lymphoma and leukemia. Staining with antisera to low-molecular-weight keratin reveals the perinuclear filament balls seen by electron microscopy (Fig. 141–13*B*). The cells of Merkel cell carcinoma also stain for neurofilaments and a variety of neuropeptides.[141–143] The claim has been made that neurofilament antigens are present in cutaneous Merkel cell carcinoma, but not in the cells of oat cell carcinoma of the lung metastatic to the skin, which can have a similar microscopic appearance.[140] The cells of Merkel cell carcinoma do not express S100 protein, unlike small cell variants of melanoma, nor CD45

(leukocyte common antigen) unlike those of most hematopoietic lymphoid neoplasms. High expression of CD44 may correlate with an increased risk of metastasis.[144]

The pathologic differential diagnosis of Merkel cell carcinoma is presented in Table 141–2.

PATHOGENESIS

Merkel cells function as specific slowly adapting sensory receptors of touch in the dermis and the basal layer of the epidermis. Normal Merkel cells share many ultrastructural and immunohistochemical features with those of Merkel cell carcinomas. Although most normal Merkel cells reside in the basal layer of the epidermis, most Merkel cell carcinomas are dermal neoplasms, with no epidermal connection, suggesting that epidermal Merkel cells are only the source of a minority of these neoplasms.

DIFFERENTIAL DIAGNOSIS

Clinically the firm solid tumor of Merkel cell carcinoma must be distinguished from SCC, desmoplastic

TABLE 141–2. Pathological Differential Diagnosis of Merkel Cell Carcinoma (by Light Microscopy)

Eccrine sweat gland carcinoma
Small cell bronchogenic carcinoma (oat cell)
Metastatic neuroendocrine carcinoma of many origins
Small cell lymphoma
Neuroblastoma
Malignant melanoma
Basal cell carcinoma

TABLE 141–3. Clinical Differential Diagnosis of Merkel Cell Carcinoma

Squamous cell carcinoma
Basal cell carcinoma
Adnexal tumors
Metastatic cancer
Desmoplastic and amelanotic melanoma

TABLE 141–4. Treatment of Merkel Cell Carcinoma

A. Wide local excision with margins 2.5–3.0 cm
B. Adjuvant
  Radiotherapy
  Chemotherapy

melanoma, amelanotic melanoma, metastatic carcinoma, BCC, and adnexal tumors (Table 141–3).

TREATMENT

Management of this tumor (Table 141–4) begins with wide local excision with margins of 2.5 to 3 cm followed by careful and frequent follow-up examinations including palpation of lymph nodes, liver, and spleen. Periodic liver function tests and chest radiographs should be obtained and compared with baseline studies.

Prophylactic lymph node dissection or irradiation are advocated by some because of the high incidence of regional metastasis;[145] however, this is not routinely recommended.

Radiotherapy and adjuvant chemotherapy have been used and may be palliative in the early stages of the disease but are unproven in advanced disease.[146] The most effective regimens include *cis*-platinum and are those used to treat small cell carcinoma of the lung, but responses are short lived.[147]

Treatment

Roy C. Grekin, John K. Geisse, Lawrence W. Margolis, and Jerome Potozkin

The ease of access to these tumors, combined with their perceived lack of aggressive behavior, has led to a wide variety of surgical and nonsurgical treatment methods. Success rates have been very high for the treatment of primary tumors with cure rates for BCC as a group reported at 90% or better (Table 141–5). SCC also has high cure rates with a variety of treatments (Table 141–6). As more is learned about these neoplasms, more specific information is available to allow the practitioner to better tailor treatment selections for more predictable outcomes. It is apparent that certain subtypes and presentations of BCC and SCC can result in a high percentage of treatment failures, leading to significant local morbidity and in some cases metastasis and death (see below). Histology, size, depth, location, recurrence, and prior treatment all play a role in determining appropriate treatments (Figs. 141–14 and 141–15). Physicians' knowledgeable about the nature of the specific tumor being treated use this information to choose the optimum therapy. Only with thoughtful, rational, case-by-case analysis can the therapeutic results be maximized. A reproducible algorithmic (Figs. 141–14 and 141–15) approach in the treatment of epidermal neoplasms can attain high cure rates with low morbidity for the patient.

TABLE 141–5. Five-year Recurrence Rates for Primary and Previously Treated Basal Cell Carcinoma

Treatment Method	Primary	Recurrent
Excision	10.1%	17.4%
Curettage and electrodesiccation	7.7%	40%
Cryotherapy	7.5%	13% (<5 yrs)
Radiation therapy	8.7%	9.8%
All non-Mohs micrographic surgery methods	8.7%	20%
Mohs micrographic surgery	1%	5.6%

Adapted by permission of the publisher from Rowe DE, Carroll RJ, Day CL Jr. Long term recurrence rates in previously untreated (primary) basal cell carcinoma: Implications for patient follow-up, J Dermatol Surg Oncol 1989;15:315–327; and Rowe DE, Carroll RJ, Day CL. Mohs surgery is the treatment of choice for recurrent (previously treated) basal cell carcinoma. J Dermatol Surg Oncol 1989;15:30. Copyright 1989 by Elsevier Science Inc.

TABLE 141–6. Five-year Recurrence Rates for Primary and Previously Treated Squamous Cell Carcinoma

Treatment Method	Primary	Recurrent
Excision	8.1%*	23.3%
Curettage and electrodesiccation	3.7%	N/A
Radiation therapy	10%	N/A
All non-Mohs micrographic surgery methods	7.9%	N/A
Mohs micrographic surgery	3.1%	10%

*Reported recurrence rates are higher for primary tumors of the lip (10.5%) and the ear (18.7%).

N/A, not available.

Adapted from Rowe DE, Carroll RJ, Day CL. Prognostic factors for local recurrence, metastasis, and survival rates in squamous cell carcinoma of the skin, ear, and lip, implications for treatment modality selection. J Am Acad Dermatol 1992;26:976–990.

TREATMENT OF BASAL CELL AND SQUAMOUS CELL CARCINOMA, BOWEN'S DISEASE, AND SOLAR KERATOSES

Basal Cell Carcinoma

BCC can be treated with multiple modalities providing 90% cure rates for primary disease in most instances (Table 141–5).[148–153, 171] These cure rates can be predicted by a number of easily measured variables, most importantly the histologic subtype or growth pattern of the tumor. The preoperative biopsy helps us determine the most appropriate treatment. Aggressive growth pattern tumors such as the morpheaform or sclerosing, micronodular, or infiltrative variants of BCC require excisional surgery with histologic margin control for adequate cure rates.[154–156] These aggressive tumors do not lend themselves well to superficial or ablative procedures such as curettage and electrodesiccation, cryotherapy, or shave excision.[154–157] Circumscribed growth pattern tumors, such as nodular and superficial BCC do quite well with a variety of treatments, and in some circumstances, superficial or ablative surgery can result in less morbidity than full-thickness excisional surgery.[158–161]

Cure rates for ablative surgery and excisional surgery vary with a number of factors including the clinical size of the tumor, the location, the histologic subtype, and whether or not it is recurrent (Table 141–5 and 141–6).[149–152, 157, 160, 161] Cure rates for ablative surgery are less than the 90% figure quoted above for BCC exceeding 0.5 cm in diameter on the face and over 2.0 cm in diameter on the trunk and extremities.[148–153, 171, 181] In these instances, consideration should be given for excisional surgery with adequate margin control.[149–152, 162.] Cure rates for BCC exceeding 0.5 mm in diameter of the central facial zone are less than acceptable for methods other than Mohs micrographic surgery (Table 141–5).[149–152, 157, 160–162, 171] Aggressive growth pattern tumors with sclerosing stromas create treatment dilemmas that result in unacceptable cure rates when routine modalities are employed.[154–156]

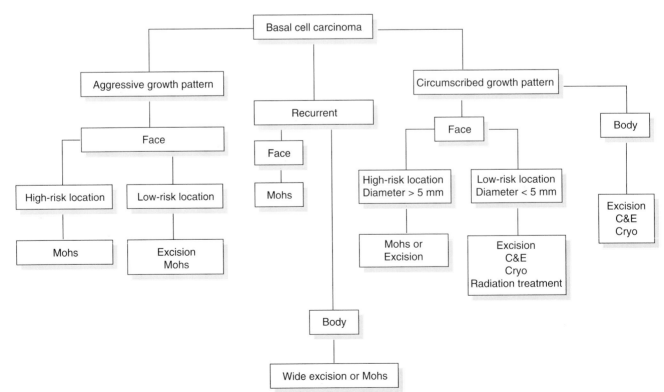

FIGURE 141–14. Flow chart for decision making in treatment of basal cell carcinoma. Cryo, cryosurgery; C&E, curettage and electrodesiccation; Mohs, Mohs micrographic surgery.

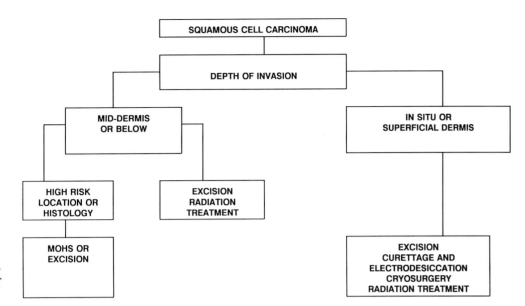

FIGURE 141–15. Flow chart for decision making in treatment of squamous cell carcinoma.

Squamous Cell Carcinoma

SCC can also be treated satisfactorily with different modalities (Table 141–6). The therapeutic choice for SCC varies with a number of the same parameters as BCC. However, histologic growth pattern is less important in SCC than clinical size and depth of invasion with the exception of rare histologic subtypes such as adenosquamous cell carcinoma.[163–167] Poorly differentiated SCC may behave aggressively but prognosis is often not affected by the degree of differentiation in a well-differentiated tumor.[163–167] SCC exceeding 1 cm in diameter and tumors that invade into the mid-dermis or deeper, particularly those involving cartilage and bone, are high-risk tumors. SCC of the lip, ear, temple, genitalia, and those associated with preexistent conditions such as radiation or burn scars are all higher risk tumors.[163, 164] In these instances, excisional surgery with careful margin control should be the treatment of choice.[163–165] Postoperative radiation therapy may also be considered for these aggressive high-risk tumors on a case-by-case basis.

Superficial or ablative procedures such as curettage and electrodesiccation, cryotherapy, and shave excision should be reserved for SCC in situ (Bowen's disease) or SCC that invades only the superficial dermis.[164, 166] The depth of invasion can be measured with an adequate preoperative biopsy. Because shave biopsies often demonstrate tumor transected at the deep margin, approximation of depth of invasion can be determined only by clinical inspection. Tumors that are indurated with an undermining infiltrative border are often deeply invasive and should be treated with excisional surgery.[164, 165]

Solar Keratoses

Solar keratoses are very common precursors to SCC and are a good predictor of patients at risk for developing non–melanoma skin cancer (NMSC).[163, 170, 173] Solar keratoses may require treatment to decrease pain, dis-comfort, pruritus, crusting, and progression to SCC.[168] The rate of malignant conversion has been said to be less than 1%, but even this low rate of transformation translates into a significant 10% lifetime risk of developing invasive SCC.[169, 170] Other authors report that up to 20% of solar or actinic keratoses will transform into SCC in 10 to 25 years.[163] Certainly the histogenesis of many SCCs can be associated with solar keratoses upon review of biopsy material.[163] These factors, when taken into consideration, warrant treatment of solar keratoses, particularly when patients are symptomatic.

Solar keratoses respond well to a variety of destructive modalities, especially liquid nitrogen, curettage, topical acids or caustics, 5-fluorouracil (5FU), and shave excision. Topical chemotherapy usually consists of 5FU for large areas of closely placed actinic keratosis with very diffuse borders (Fig. 141–16). Actinic cheilitis, erythroplasia of Queyrat, and other cutaneous dysplasias such as vulvar and intraoral leukoplakia have also been treated with topical 5FU. Such treatment is viewed as safe and efficacious with minimal systemic absorption; however, temporary unsightly inflammatory changes and crusting of the precancerous skin usually occur about 5 to 15 days after starting twice-daily topical application of 1% to 5% 5FU. The patient is advised to continue therapy for 3 weeks. Sunlight intensifies the cutaneous reaction during the treatment time. If a lower concentration of topical 5FU (0.1% to 1%) is used to try to limit the intensity of the erythematous response, the duration of treatment is extended over 10 to 12 weeks. The endpoint of treatment with any concentration of 5FU is disappearance of the last lesion. One may perform a biopsy on lesions that fail to disappear to confirm a suspected diagnosis other than actinic keratosis. At times topical steroids are given concurrently with 5FU to reduce the severity of the response. A schedule of weekly treatment on two sequential nights over a period of 10 weeks is also designed to limit the intensity of the response.

Cryosurgery may be performed with firm pressure and whitening of the surface of the lesion for 10 to 15 seconds

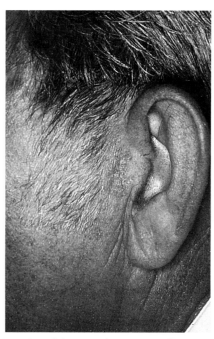

FIGURE 141-16. A 2.0-cm erythematous scaling patch in the left pre-auricular area was present for over 6 months. Biopsy showed an actinic keratosis. (Courtesy of June K. Robinson, M.D.)

twice at one sitting. Depigmentation usually results after applying topical liquid nitrogen to actinic keratosis. Bowen's disease of the skin requires two freeze-thaw cycles of 30 seconds each.

For hyperkeratotic lesions, shave biopsy followed by curettage provides a more expedient and effective treatment modality than others. In addition, this provides a pathology specimen for confirmation of the diagnosis. Shave biopsies must be carried into the dermis to avoid transecting the atypical keratinocytes, which can result in equivocal diagnoses.

Ablative Treatment Techniques

Long-term cure rates (over 5 years) for NMSC are critically important when reporting treatment outcomes.[148-153, 171] In evaluating outcome statistics for the treatment of NMSC, most studies report outcomes on a given group of patients monitored over time minus the patients lost to follow-up. These lost patients are usually excluded from the data used to compute cure rates. This leads to inaccurate statistics, often under- or over-reporting cure rates. Complicated formulas to take into account expected outcome in the patients lost to follow-up have been devised and used in the elegant series of articles by Silverman and associates.[149-152] Overall, we can expect close to 90% cure rates for primary tumors with these various techniques (Tables 141-5 and 141-6).[148-152]

Curettage and Electrodesiccation

Curettage and electrodesiccation (C&E) has been used successfully with cure rates that approach 90% for nonag-

gressive growth pattern BCC and superficial SCC.[158-160] Its limitations are based upon the experience of the surgeon, the carefulness and thoroughness of the curettage, and the depth and extent of the electrodesiccation as well as the number of cycles that are performed.[160, 161] Careful studies evaluating these parameters in different clinical settings have not been done, but inexperienced surgeons have poorer outcomes than experienced clinicians.[172] C&E should be done initially with a large curette to debulk the tumor followed by a 2-mm curette to feel small extensions of superficial and nodular BCC and superficial well-differentiated SCC.[160] The curette should be thoroughly used in every direction to eradicate all tumor extensions.[160] Electrodesiccation should be performed by fulgurating a margin of clinically normal appearing skin around the curettage site then carefully electrodesiccating the entire wound bed while maintaining a dry field to get a uniform depth of destruction.[160] This provides approximately 1 mm of margin of necrotic tissue with each desiccation cycle (Fig. 141-17). Most dermatologists utilize a Hyfrecator device that can produce a fairly uniform electrosurgical injury with each cycle. At least two, if not three, full cycles of curettage followed by electrodesiccation should be performed to obtain the documented 90% overall cure rate (see Atlas of Cutaneous Surgery, Chapter 6).[148, 150, 160, 161, 172]

Cure rates for the treatment of BCC with C&E vary depending upon the site and clinical size of the BCC (Table 141-5).[149-152, 157, 160, 161] BCCs of the trunk that approach 2 cm and above in diameter have much less satisfactory results with C&E than with other modalities.[149-152] No well-controlled studies have been done to evaluate the success of C&E for the treatment of superficially invasive SCC.[164, 166] C&E has been demonstrated to be less than adequate for some immunocompromised patients.[184] It seems prudent given the metastatic potential of SCC to suggest that all but the most superficial SCCs be removed by excision in order to obtain histologic confirmation of clear margins (Table 141-6).[163-166, 170]

C&E scars are often hypopigmented and slightly depressed. Hypertrophic scarring occurs with this technique, particularly over the dorsal hands, digits, shoulders, and chest. C&E of large superficial pattern BCC of the central trunk may heal with a more acceptable scar than excisional surgery, which by necessity would be three times as long as the curettage site is wide. Excisional scars on the trunk may spread over time, particularly in younger patients. On the other hand, C&E wounds usually require 3 to 4 weeks of wound care before complete re-epithelialization. Wound healing for such defects on the lower extremity can be prolonged, necessitating chronic wound care and causing discomfort over many weeks.

Tumors that recur after C&E often develop infiltrative growth patterns and grow underneath the scars. This leads to much greater subclinical extension than might be predicted by physical examination.[158, 161, 162] Recurrent tumors have an increased risk of perineural invasion and invasion of deeper structures, and are often poorly demarcated. All of these factors lead to an unacceptable 40% to 50% recurrence rate after repeat C&E to treat a

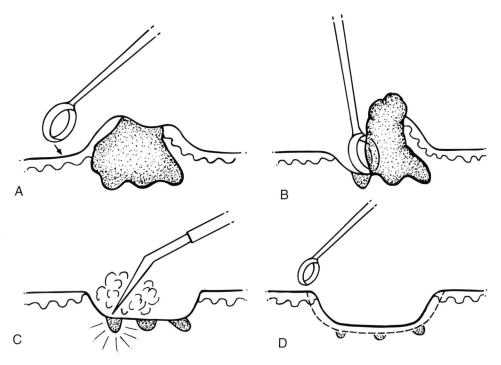

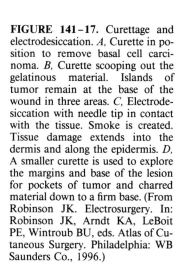

FIGURE 141-17. Curettage and electrodesiccation. *A,* Curette in position to remove basal cell carcinoma. *B,* Curette scooping out the gelatinous material. Islands of tumor remain at the base of the wound in three areas. *C,* Electrodesiccation with needle tip in contact with the tissue. Smoke is created. Tissue damage extends into the dermis and along the epidermis. *D,* A smaller curette is used to explore the margins and base of the lesion for pockets of tumor and charred material down to a firm base. (From Robinson JK. Electrosurgery. In: Robinson JK, Arndt KA, LeBoit PE, Wintroub BU, eds. Atlas of Cutaneous Surgery. Philadelphia: WB Saunders Co., 1996.)

recurrent lesion.[148, 157, 161, 162, 171] Therefore, NMSC recurrent after C&E and sclerosing or aggressive growth pattern should be treated with full-thickness excisional surgery with histologic margin control.[148, 157, 161, 162, 171]

In summary, C&E offers an efficient, and cost-effective means to eradicate primary nonaggressive growth pattern BCC and superficially invasive SCC. These wounds heal by second intention and can sometimes result in a better cosmetic outcome for large superficial tumors of the central trunk when compared with large elliptical excisions. Smaller lesions in selected facial areas can be treated with reasonable cure rates and fair cosmesis.

Cryosurgery

Cryosurgery is useful to eradicate superficial solar keratosis. With adequate control of the depth and intensity of the freeze, extensive necrosis can be obtained, extending utility of the procedure to malignant lesions.[135] Treatment of BCC requires two cycles of at least 60 seconds' thaw time for adequate clearance. The full thickness of the tumor must be frozen to −40° C to −70° C for complete necrosis.[135] In an ideal situation, thermocouples are used to measure the temperature reached and sustained at a given depth in the dermis or subcutis below the tumor.[135] Cryosurgery, like C&E, does not provide material for histologic margin control; thus an estimate of the depth of invasion of the tumor must be made clinically or, ideally, with preoperative biopsies measuring the extent of the tumor invasion. Tumor thickness varies with each case and is not necessarily consistent throughout a given tumor. Even with sophisticated techniques, an educated guess is used to evaluate the extent of tumor invasion and thus the depth of freeze required for adequate control. The same can be said for the lateral extent of tumors, which must be approxi-

mated by clinical exam prior to cryosurgery. This is probably less accurate than using the curette to determine the lateral extent of tumor for NMSC,[174] with the exception of sclerosing BCC. In fact, some cryosurgeons are now recommending curettage prior to freezing to help determine margins and to debulk the tumor.[186]

Cryosurgery for malignancies utilizes liquid nitrogen (−195.8° C) delivered in a number of different ways including cryogenic spray, cotton-tip applicators, and various cryoprobes. Although freeze depth is most accurately determined by thermocouple, many cryosurgeons feel comfortable estimating it, especially after prior experience with thermocouples. Each individual cryosurgeon has his or her own favored routine, and unfortunately studies reporting cure rates for NMSC treated with liquid nitrogen do not utilize a standardized technique.

Although cryosurgery is technically easy for the physician, it is not necessarily less invasive for the patient. Anesthesia is required due to the severe pain associated with the cold temperature and long freeze times. Appropriate treatment of malignancies results in an exudative, sometimes painful wound that heals over 3 to 4 weeks, depending upon the extent of the disease and the depth and duration of the freeze. These wounds usually heal with somewhat atrophic hypopigmented scars and are subject to postoperative complications similar to those of other surgical techniques (see *Atlas of Cutaneous Surgery*, Chapter 6).

Cryosurgery of NMSC can be an effective, efficient procedure.[144, 171, 185, 186] Clearly this is a valuable modality for well-trained, experienced dermatologists but has the same limitations as C&E in that adequate margin control cannot be confirmed and thus recurrence in or underneath the resultant scar can lead to increased morbidity.[157] The available literature reports high cure rates for BCC in experienced hands.[148, 171] These studies involve small numbers of patients, particularly when long-term cure rates are evaluated.[148, 171] No long-term data are available to evaluate the use of cryosurgery for SCC.

Carbon Dioxide Laser Ablation

Carbon dioxide (CO_2) laser ablation is occasionally used to treat superficially invasive or in situ SCC (Bowen's disease) with excellent results.[175] It can also be used in a similar fashion for superficial BCC.[176] The CO_2 laser offers some advantage over electrodesiccation because it can precisely de-epithelialize tissue when used in a defocused mode. Sophisticated superpulsed and ultra-pulsed CO_2 lasers can limit the depth of penetration of heat delivered to the tissue resulting in more superficial destruction than is possible with electrosurgery while still completely removing the epidermis.[172] This has some advantage when treating superficial tumors, although it is slight and may not warrant the purchase of, or routine use of, a more expensive device in place of other therapeutic modalities except in unusual circumstances. Also, the decreased depth of thermal damage might lead to higher recurrence rates.

Tumors that particularly lend themselves to CO_2 ablative surgery are in situ SCC of the digits and the periungual regions. Here the CO_2 laser can remove the nail plate and allow easy access to involved nail bed. Invasive SCC of the digit can be a relatively high-risk tumor, and consideration should be given for microscopically controlled excision of these tumors versus ablative surgery where no histologic margins are obtained.

In a similar fashion, SCC in situ of the penis and vulva can be adequately eradicated with CO_2 laser ablation with less risk of dysfunctional scarring than other modalities.[175] Extensive solar damage of the vermilion or actinic cheilitis, while not carcinoma in situ, is a premalignant field and can be effectively eradicated using defocused CO_2 laser light.[178, 180] The superpulsed CO_2 laser is particularly useful in these clinical scenarios due to its ability in the hands of an experienced operator to completely de-epithelialize tissue with minimal dispersion of heat to the underlying dermis. It results in far less morbidity than traditional vermilionectomy and repair.

The virtue of CO_2 laser therapy is its precise limitation of tissue injury. This is an advantage for subsequent wound healing and scar formation. Unfortunately, superficial BCC and SCC in situ can extend deeply down follicular structures. These extensions could be missed by CO_2 laser ablation as well as by other superficially ablative modalities.

In summary, the CO_2 laser can provide some advantages over standard modalities in selected cases. Sill, there are no absolute indications for CO_2 laser ablation over other standard modalities.

Excisional Techniques

Shave Excision

Superficial BCC, SCC in situ, and SCC invasive only to the superficial dermis can be extirpated with reasonable histologic margin control using tangential excision.

No good studies measuring outcome in large numbers of cases using this technique are available in the current literature. Potential outcome with shave excision can be compared to full-thickness excision because with adequate histologic processing, surgical margins can be evaluated in the same fashion as an ellipse. As with full-thickness excision, complete margin control does not always result in complete cure; despite negative margins, recurrences develop after excisional surgery (see below).

Shave or tangential excision is also technique dependent and is not done in a standardized fashion. Modalities vary from simple scalpel shave excision, as is done for diagnostic biopsies, straight razor excision using the Gillette blue blade or single-edged razors, sharp scissors excision, and large planar blade escision using blades such as those used to harvest split-thickness skin grafts. First, accurately delineate the cliniclal margins prior to the instillation of anesthesia. Then, debulk the tumor by curettage.[171, 187] A tangential excision is made around and under the curettage defect with a 2- to 5-mm margin of normal-appearing skin depending upon the preoperative size of the tumor.[181, 187] This disk or wafer of tissue should then be flattened and affixed to paper prior to placement in formalin. This prevents excessive curling of the lateral edges, allowing for appropriate histologic sectioning and examination of margins. The pathologist needs to be instructed, preferably in schematic or diagrammatic fashion, as to how to process the tissue. Breadloaf sectioning is the minimum standard for excisional specimens.

Shave excisions or tangential excisions heal by second intention and thus should be performed in areas of the body where the skin is thick such as the central trunk. These wounds often heal with excellent cosmesis, but atrophic hypopigmented or hypertrophic scars may result. Wound healing may be improved slightly by avoiding or limiting the use of electrosurgery, Monsel's solution, or aluminum chloride for hemostasis; these can cause damage to the tissue surrounding the surgical margins. This may be avoided by the use of simple pressure or gelatin-based hemostatic agents such as Gel Foam. Occlusive biosynthetic dressings may improve patient comfort, minimize wound care, and accelerate re-epithelialization in the initial weeks of healing. There may be some advantage to shave excision over ablative therapies because it offers the opportunity for histologic margin control. In some patients, the final result may be cosmetically more acceptable. As with C&E, these procedures should be done for superficial tumors where complete excision would result in a larger procedure and scar that may be less acceptable.

Excision

Excisional surgery has been the standard of care for NMSC against which other modalities have been measured. Excisional surgery offers similar to slightly better cure rates than C&E or cryosurgery for primary tumors.[148-153, 171] These cure rates approach and sometimes exceed 90% depending upon the characteristics of the tumor.[148, 151]

For recurrent disease, excision is superior to nonexcisional modalities.[171] Full-thickness excision and layered closure give excellent cosmetic results, particularly for the central face (Fig. 141–18). Excision offers the ability to completely extirpate even aggressive growth pattern BCC or invasive SCC with adequate histologic margin control. Cure rates do not approach those of Mohs micrographic surgery (see below) because of significant differences in pathology processing and examination which results in loss of margin control. Adequate preoperative

pathology with adjustment of surgical margins to take into account aggressive growth pattern BCC and deeply invasive SCC improves the likehood of complete excision. The standard surgical margin for BCC up to 1 cm in diameter has been reported to be 4 mm to obtain 90% cure rates.[148, 151, 171, 181, 182] By increasing the surgical margin to 6 to 9 mm for aggressive growth pattern BCC and for deeply invasive SCC, better control of margins and ultimately better cure rates can be ex-

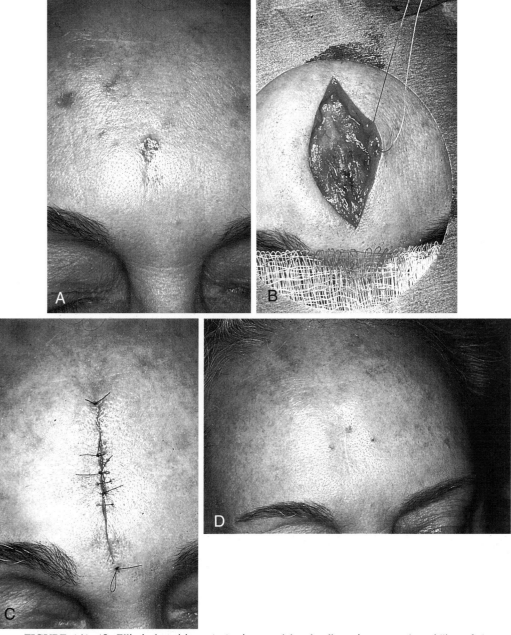

FIGURE 141–18. Elliptical excision. *A,* A pigmented basal cell carcinoma at the midline of the forehead is excised with 4-mm margins. *B,* The 3 : 1 dimensions of the excision allow 30-degree angles at the apices. The area is undermined readily in this area of relative laxity. The first suture placed is a buried subcutaneous suture in the middle of the incision. *C,* Wound edges are easily approximated with subcutaneous sutures. The running subcuticular suture has incorporated two crossover cutaneous loops. Slight adjustments of the wound edges to produce eversion are made with three interrupted sutures in the center of the incision. *D,* Appearance of forehead 1 year later. (From Robinson JK. Elliptical incisions and closures. In: Robinson JK, Arndt KA, LeBoit PE, Wintroub BU, eds. Atlas of Cutaneous Surgery. Philadelphia: WB Saunders Co., 1996.)

pected.[165, 181-183] Curettage prior to excision for non-sclerosing growth pattern BCC can better estimate the horizontal and vertical extent of tumor infiltration, thus allowing for more complete excision and better margin control as well as less loss of normal-appearing skin.[174] Curettage is best performed with a 2-mm curette using gentle-to-moderate pressure to find small tumor extensions and at the same time avoiding excessive or unintentional curettage of uninvolved surrounding skin. The latter issue can be particularly problematic in severely sun-damaged skin where the epidermis is thin, friable, and easily detached with minimal pressure. Signs of excessive curettage include extensive ecchymosis around the lateral margins of the treatment site occurring when the skin is stripped off rather than scooped out as is seen with nodular BCC (see *Atlas of Cutaneous Surgery*, Chapter 9).

When performing curettage followed by excision, pathologists must be informed of the procedure or at least be familiar with these types of specimens to know that the central ulceration is in fact part of a carcinoma that has been previously confirmed on biopsy. With preoperatively confirmed carcinoma, the curettings can be discarded although some instances and medical legal implications suggest that submitting the curettings as a separate specimen in addition to the excisional specimen may be warranted to reconfirm the proper site, diagnosis, and need for surgery.

Surgical ellipses are frequently the treatment of choice for primary NMSC, especially on the head and neck and for histologically infiltrative tumors. Curettage prior to excision has been shown to result in better control of the margins[174] and is therefore often a routine part of all NMSC excisions after preoperative biopsy confirmation of the diagnosis.

RADIATION

Inasmuch as most skin cancers can be treated with a variety of methods, it is important to select which form of treatment is most appropriate for each patient. After a complete evaluation of the tumor, the treatment options can be compared regarding cure rate and expected cosmetic and functional result.

Radiation is an excellent choice for skin cancer of the central face, including the eyelids, nose, and lips. It is also often the ablative treatment of choice in skin cancer of the ears or large areas of the forehead and scalp. Surgical literature suggests that radiation is contraindicated in large lesions involving cartilage because of the risk of radionecrosis and chondritis.[188, 189] However, current radiation literature clearly indicates that properly fractionated radiation can be used in these lesions, and in fact, is often the treatment of choice with high cure rates and preservation of function with minimal risk of complication.[190-192] Radiation has the advantage of being able to treat all visible tumor in addition to subclinical disease with a margin of uninvolved normal tissue without alteration of the anatomy. Therefore, in properly selected patients, the outcome is often an excellent cosmetic and functional result with high cure rates.

Prior to initiating radiation, one must carefully evaluate the lesion as to its margins and depth of invasion. If there is any suspicion of spread or invasion of tumor into underlying tissues or adjoining structures in evaluative studies, computed tomography or magnetic resonance imaging scans should be performed (Fig. 141–19).

The margin of normal appearing tissue included in the field of radiation is usually 5 mm in small tumors. However, sclerosing or morpheaform basal cell carcinomas tend to infiltrate widely, and the margins should be at least 10 mm in these tumors to avoid geographic misses.[193] Tumors with perineural invasion require special attention because they have a higher likelihood of nodal involvement, and can also spread great distances

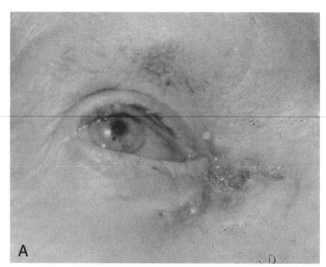

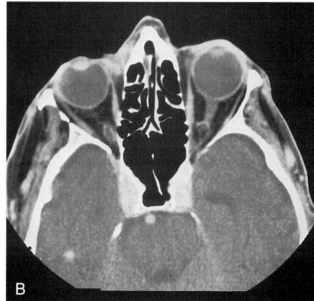

FIGURE 141–19. *A*, 85-year-old male with a 2 × 2 cm superficial appearing basal cell carcinoma in the right inner canthus area has pulled the lacrimal duct and the lower eyelid away from the globe. *B*, Computed tomographic scan showed the lesion actually extended 1.5 cm into the orbit. Therefore, the patient was treated with 9 meV electron with 0.5-cm bolus at 225 cGy per day to 6750. Superficial orthovoltage would have underdosed the lesion at depth—patient remains free of tumor 18 months after treatment.

along neural sheaths.[194-196] Well-differentiated squamous cell carcinomas are generally treated in the same fashion as basal cell carcinomas. However, poorly differentiated squamous cell tumors or those over 3 cm in size may spread to lymph nodes, and consideration should be given to the use of wider margins, or to even include regional lymph nodes, such as cervical and preauricular nodes in the radiation field.[197, 198] Tissue beyond the treated area should be protected with individually cut lead shields. In addition underlying tissue such as the lens, cornea, nasal septum, and teeth can be protected by shields placed under the eyelid, and in the nasal cavity, or under the lips. With the use of orthovoltage x-rays, lead-covered shielding with a layer of wax is utilized. The layer of wax absorbs scattered radiation off the lead and prevents mucosal reaction. With electron beam, the shielding under the eyelids is with stainless steel.

Types of Radiation

After evaluating the extent of the tumor, one selects the optimal energy of radiation. The choices range from low-energy x-ray machines to electron beams of various energies. On rare occasions, for particularly extensive tumors, high-energy photons or a combination of various beams is indicated.

The most commonly utilized x-ray energies range from 100 kV to 250 kV, and should be adequately filtered. Energies of 50 kV have been utilized, but have very rapid fall-off and may not provide adequate dose at depth. In recent years most radiation oncology departments have electron beams ranging from 6 to 18 meV. With the use of a wax bolus of varying thickness shaped to the contour of the area to be treated, the electron beam can deliver a very even dose throughout the entire depth of the tumor, and then rapidly fall off, sparing the underlying normal tissue. Table 141–7 compares various orthovoltage x-rays and electron energies for delivered doses at various depths.

The dermatology literature indicates that most basal cell carcinomas penetrate to a depth of 2 to 5 mm.[199, 200] Therefore, softer, less penetrating, radiation beams have been recommended.[201, 202] As seen in Table 141–7, a typical 50-kV beam with a half-value layer of 0.7 mm aluminum delivers 85% of surface dose at 2 mm, and

only 65% at 5 mm. Therefore, these low-energy soft x-ray beams should be utilized only on very small superficial lesions such as small eyelid tumors. Most radiation oncologists believe that a homogeneous dose of radiation should be delivered throughout the entire tumor, and therefore use a more penetrating filtered-beam x-ray.

Time and Dose Fractionation

The determination of the optimum time-dose relationship in skin cancer has been extensively studied. Strandquist examined skin reaction for various dose-fractionation schemes.[203] This work was further expanded by Von Essen, who applied iso-effect lines for a 99% tumor regression versus 3% skin necrosis and related this data not only to the dose per fraction, and total dose, but also to the size of the area to be treated.[204] His finding of different slopes for skin necrosis and tumor regression allows for development of favorable therapeutic ratios. He also demonstrated that larger areas do not tolerate radiation as well, and therefore require a more fractionated course of treatment using smaller daily doses taken to a higher overall total dose over a greater period of time. Further studies on cosmesis have demonstrated that delayed effects of radiation such as telangiectasia, fibrosis, and pigmentation can be minimized with the use of a more fractionated schema.[205] Turesson studied late radiation changes on normal skin in women with breast cancer treated to internal mammary nodes.[206] He found fewer late skin changes in patients treated daily versus once or twice weekly. Late cosmetic results in patients specifically treated for skin cancer have also been shown to be superior in patients treated with greater fractionation. Traenkle studied the incidence of late necrosis in 1751 patients treated with five different dose schedules.[207] The overall and time and total doses were consistent with widely used time-dose schedules. Patients treated with fewer large doses had a markedly higher rate of necrosis as compared with multiple smaller doses of radiation. Inasmuch as the choice of radiation over surgery in a specific patient is often based on the radiation advantage of giving a better cosmetic and functional result, it seems prudent to select that dose-fractionation schema that will give not only the highest chance for

TABLE 141-7. Comparison of Orthovoltage X-ray and Electron Beam Delivered Dose at Varying Depths

Energy HVL	50kV .7 mm Al	100kV 4 mm Al	150kV 5 mm Cu	6 meV Electron 1-cm Bolus	9 meV Electron 1-cm Bolus
			% of Depth Dose		
Surface	100	100	100	98	96
1 mm	92	98	99	99	96
2 mm	85	96	98	100	97
5 mm	65	91	97	99	99
1 cm	45	81	93	75	100
1.5 cm	36	71	87	30	95
2.0 cm	23	63	80	4	78

HVL, half-value layer.

TABLE 141-8. Orthovoltage X-ray Recommendations

Size of Lesion	Daily Dose	Fractions	Total Dose
Up to 2 cm	300	15-17	4500-5100 cGy*
Over 2 cm without cartilage involved	250	20-22	5000-5500 cGy
Large lesions with cartilage involved	200	30-33	6000-6600 cGy

*1 cGy is equivalent to 1 rad.

tumor control, but also the best cosmetic result (Table 141-8).

Larger, thicker lesions are often treated with electron beam, which allows a homogeneous dose throughout the entire tumor with minimum dose delivered to deep structures. When using the electron beam, a dose correction must be made to achieve equivalent doses to orthovoltage x-rays. The relative biologic effectiveness of electrons is 85% to 90% of 200 kilovolt peak (kVP).[208, 209] Therefore the daily dose and total dose are both 10% to 15% higher than the corresponding orthovoltage doses.

Results of Radiation

Rowe and colleagues compiled a comprehensive review of recurrence rates of all basal cell carcinomas reported in the literature from 1947 to 1988.[210] Patients treated with radiation revealed a recurrence rate of 5.3% (319/6072) for patients monitored less than 5 years, and 8.7% (485/5549) for patients monitored at least 5 years. This large retrospective study does not account for selection of modality by site, size, or extent of lesion, nor did it compare cosmetic and functional results. However, this exhaustive review of almost 40,000 basal cell carcinomas does provide approximate results of what might be expected with each modality.

Fitzpatrick reviewed 1166 eyelid tumors treated with radiation.[211] The control rate of 5 years was 93.3% for SCC, and 95% for BCC. The overall complication rate was 9.6%, but most felt it to be related to extensive tumor damage prior to treatment, and less than half of these were considered serious. The cosmetic results were generally considered excellent. Petrovich reviewed 646 patients with carcinoma of the eyelids, pinna, and nose.[212] The 464 basal cell carcinomas had a 5-year actuarial control rate of 99% compared with 94% control rate for the 115 squamous cell carcinomas and 95% of 67 patients with mixed basal cell and squamous cell features. The 5-year control rates were 99% for tumors under 2 cm in diameter, 92% for lesions 2 to 5 cm in diameter, and 60% for massive tumors. Cartilage and bone involvement were seen in 23 patients with a 5-year control rate of 80%. No cartilage, bone, or soft tissue necrosis was noted, and no serious complications were reported. The most common treatment schedule was 5100 cGy in 17 fractions over 21 to 23 days. Tumors with bone and cartilage involvement received 7000 cGy at 200-cGy daily fractions. The cosmetic result was considered excellent for those lesions treated with 300 cGy a day or less.

Petrovich also reviewed an additional 250 patients with lip carcinomas (247 squamous cell, 3 basal cell) with an overall control rate of 89%.[213] The failure rate was 6% for Stage 1 and Stage 2 (227 patients), 10% for Stage 3 (10 patients), and 53% for Stage 4 (19 patients). Nodal involvement was noted in 23 patients, 48% of whom failed. In 227 patients the failure rate was 7%. Five (2%) patients developed complications, all of whom had massive tumor involvement of the mandible prior to radiation.

Lovett reported on 339 skin carcinomas (242 basal and 97 squamous cell).[214] Control rate of the tumor correlated with size. Lesions under 1 cm had a 97% (86/89) control for BCC and 91% (21/23) for SCC. For lesions 1 to 5 cm, the control rate was 87% (116/133) and 76% (39/51) respectively for BCC and SCC. Lesions over 5 cm were controlled 87% (13/15—BCC) and 56% (9/16 SCC). The cosmesis was evaluated in 261 patients. It was scored good or excellent in 92%, fair in 3.1% and poor in 7.3%. This also related to tumor size with 98% good or excellent results in tumors under 1 cm in size, 83% in tumors 1.1 to 3 cm, and 69% in lesions greater than 3 cm.

Chemotherapy/Radiation

Thus far there have been only a few reports of systemic chemotherapy used for basal cell and squamous cell carcinomas of the skin. Because the overall results with radiation and surgery have been excellent with few metastases, systemic chemotherapy has been unnecessary in most patients. However, far advanced skin cancers have been shown to be responsive to a variety of combinations of 5FU, cisplatin, bleomycin, and adriamycin.[215-217] The chemotherapy was often combined with radiation or surgery. Response rates of 70% to 80% have been reported with complete responses in the range of 30%. These results are not surprising considering the excellent results obtained in squamous or basaloid carcinoma of the anal canal and anal verge using a combination of radiation and chemotherapy.[218, 219] In these patients, the chemotherapy has been 5FU and mitomycin or cisplatin given with concurrent radiation in the range of 4500 Gy. This multi-modality treatment has produced local control rates of 90% in several series. Therefore in advanced skin cancers or in the rare metastatic skin cancer, systemic chemotherapy in combination with surgery or radiation warrants further evaluation.

Summary

In summary, with careful attention to treatment planning, time-dose relationships, and appropriate selection beam quality, radiation can provide high cure rates with very good to excellent cosmetic and functional results and a low complication rate. In properly selected patients radiation remains the treatment of choice for many epithelial skin cancers (Fig. 141-20).

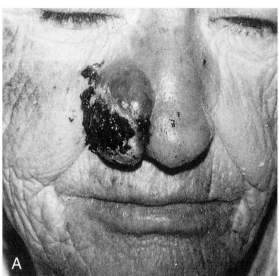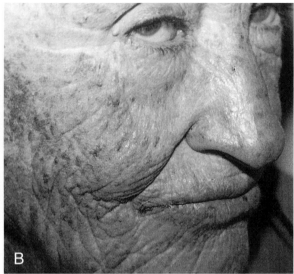

FIGURE 141–20. *A*, 72-year-old female with a 3.5 × 3.0 basal cell carcinoma on the right side of the nose—treated with 12-meV electrons with bolus at 225 cGy per day to 6975 cGy. *B*, 5 years after radiation treatment—no evidence of disease.

MOHS MICROGRAPHIC SURGERY

Historical Perspective

Mohs micrographic surgery (MMS) utilizes microscopically controlled excision in the extirpation of cutaneous malignancies. The technique was first described by Dr. Frederic Mohs in 1941.[220] He observed that application of a 20% zinc chloride paste to tumor-bearing tissue resulted in in situ fixation of the tumor with excellent preservation of microscopic detail. Combining this with horizontal rather than vertical sectioning allowed skin cancer excision with precise microscopic control. The combination of the fixative with the surgery spawned the term *chemosurgery*.

In the "fixed-tissue" technique, the gross tumor is debulked and zinc chloride paste is applied. Each stage required overnight fixation except when very small areas were involved. Wounds were required to heal by second intention due to residual sloughing of the fixed tissue. Cure rates utilizing this technique have been reported as 99% for primary basal cell carcinomas and 96% to 98% for recurrent basal cell carcinomas.[220–226] However, the procedure was slow due to fixation periods, the paste caused considerable pain, and slides were hard to read due to inflammatory infiltrates.

Theodore Tromovitch improved the applicability of the procedure with the description of the fresh tissue technique in 1970. The fresh tissue technique omits the zinc chloride paste, thereby decreasing the perioperative pain associated with in situ fixation, allowing for multiple stages in one day and permitting reconstruction to be performed immediately following extirpation of the tumor (Figs. 141–21*A* and *B*). Tromovitch and Stegman later reported their treatment results with the fresh tissue technique as similar to the fixed technique.[227] The fresh tissue technique has proven its benefits and now ac-

counts for the overwhelming majority of MMS procedures performed today.[228, 229]

Mohs micrographic surgery is the official nomenclature for the procedure: however, many synonyms exist including chemosurgery, Mohs surgery, Mohs histographic surgery, and perhaps the most descriptive, microscopically controlled excision. MMS is a precise technique that requires meticulous attention to detail and is learned during a one- or two-year fellowship.

Technique

MMS is almost always performed in the ambulatory setting. Initially, the gross tumor is delineated with a surgical marking pen. Local anesthesia is obtained. The gross tumor is then debulked with a curette (Fig. 141–21*C*). After debulking, the first stage is excised (Fig. 141–21*D*). In contrast to the technique for standard surgical excisions where the incision is made with the scalpel blade perpendicular to the skin, the Mohs surgeon incised the tissue with the scalpel blade angled at 30 to 45 degrees to the skin, slightly undercutting the tumor. The beveled edge created is essential to permit simultaneous microscopic examination of the entire undersurface and epidermal edge of the excised layer of tissue. Typically the excision is performed with 1- to 3-mm margins around the debulked tumor. Once the specimen is excised, hemostasis is obtained by electrodesiccation and a dressing is applied. The patient is escorted to the waiting area while the tissue is processed (usually 30 to 60 minutes). An anatomic map is created corresponding to the exact orientation of the excised tissue with respect to the patient. The excised specimen is divided into sections amenable to frozen sectioning and that will fit on a microscope slide. The nonepidermal edges of the specimens are color coded with tissue dye. The orientation of

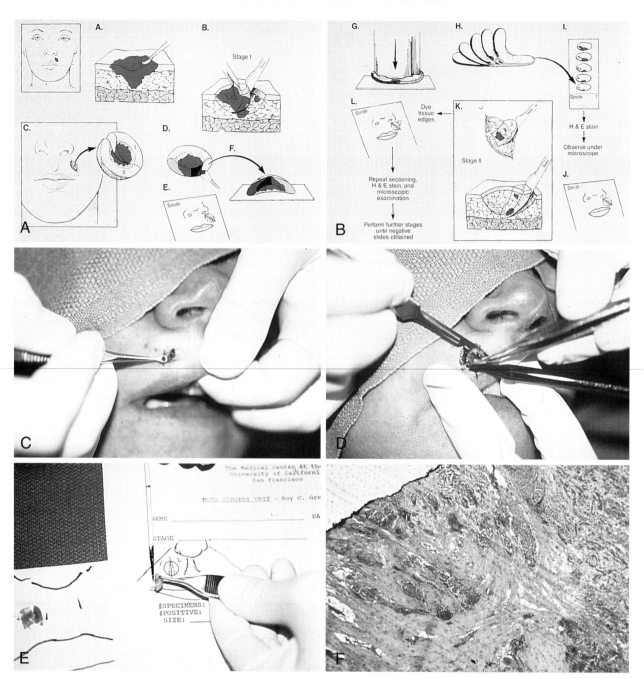

FIGURE 141–21. *A* and *B,* Schematic of Mohs micrographic surgery, fresh tissue technique. *A,* A, Tumor of upper lip has the edges delineated by curettage. B, A layer of tissue is removed from around and under the wound created by the curettage. Shaded areas indicate extent of tumor, which may not be clinically apparent. C, After excision of the specimen, it is subdivided, and D, dyes are applied to its surface to maintain its orientation. E, A map is created that corresponds to the orientation of the excised tissue. F, The surface of the specimen is inverted in preparation for mounting on the cryostat chude. *B,* G, The specimen is flattened on the chuck. H, Serial horizontal frozen sections are cut. I, The sections are stained and mounted on a glass slide. J, The slides are interpreted by the Mohs surgeon and remaining tumor marked on the anatomic map. K, The tumor remaining in the surgical field is excised in another layer, or a second stage of surgery. L, The specimen preparation mapping and interpretation are repeated. *C,* Curettage of right upper lip basal cell carcinoma. *D,* Excision of stage 1. Note angle of scalpel and rim of normal tissue. Glass eyedropper is attached to a suction device. *E,* Staining and mapping of stage I specimens. *F,* Frozen section with tumor present at the margin dyed with India ink.

the specimens and color coding is noted on the anatomic map (Fig. 141–21*A* and *E*). The surgeon then gives the tissue to a technician for processing. The tissue sections are placed inverted (deep margin up) on a cryostat chuck and flattened so that the epidermal margin is on the same level as the deep tissue plane (Fig. 141–21*A*). Horizontal frozen sections are then cut allowing for complete examination of the surgical margin. The slides are then stained with hematoxylin and eosin (or toluidine blue) and examined under a microscope by the surgeon, who serves

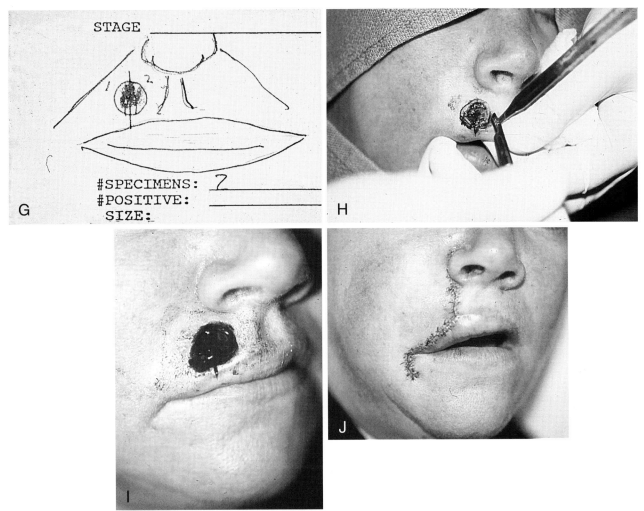

FIGURE 141–21. *Continued G,* Residual tumor precisely noted on map. *H,* Excision of stage II. *I,* Postoperative defect after three stages of Mohs micrographic surgery completed resection of the basal cell carcinoma. *J,* Immediate repair with advancement flap.

the dual roles of surgeon and pathologist. Tumor presence at any surgical margin is noted and precisely plotted on the anatomic map (Fig. 141–21*G*). The patient is returned to the operative suite, reanesthetized, and a tissue layer is excised only at the site of residual tumor as demarcated on the map and processed as above (Fig. 141–21*B* and *H*). The procedure is repeated until a tumor-free plane is reached (Fig. 141–21*B* and *J*). This precise method of microscopically controlled excision allows for minimal sacrifice of normal tissue as standard "safety margins" are not needed. The fresh tissue technique allows for repair of the surgical defect to be performed immediately after a tumor-free plane is obtained (Fig. 141–21*J*). Repair options include healing by secondary intent, side-to-side closure, skin grafting, and various skin flaps. On infrequent occasions, the surgery must be extended over a 2-day period because of a more extensive tumor. Multidisciplinary approaches to more complicated closures usually are performed one or more days after tumor excision.

Indications

The most common skin cancers treated with MMS are BCC and SCC. Cure rates stated below are for BCC unless otherwise noted. MMS affords the dermatologic surgeon two major advantages in treating cutaneous malignancies. The first is the highest possible cure rates (94%–99%).[222, 230-232] The second is tissue preservation, allowing high cure rates while removing the minimum amount of tissue. These advantages are due in large part to two important aspects of MMS not found in standard excisions or other cancer treatments. These are the careful mapping techniques and the horizontal sectioning. Routine histologic sectioning of surgical specimens is vertical in nature—frequently a "breadloaf" technique. This results in examination of 0.1% to 0.5% of the surgical margin.[233] This "sampling" of the margins has inherent error because nonvisualized margins may harbor cancer cells. To reduce the chance of sampling error or false-negative examination, an extra safety margin of tis-

TABLE 141-9. Recurrence Rate After Surgical Excision of Primary Basal Cell Carcinoma in High-Risk Areas of the Head and Neck

Anatomic Location	Recurrence Rate (5 Years)
Ear	42.9%
Nasal-labial groove	20.2%
Scalp	14.7%
Forehead	8.4%
Nose	5.5%
Periocular	5.3%
Malar cheek	4.0%
Neck	2.5%

Adapted by permission of the publisher from Silverman ML, Kopt AW, Bart RS, et al. Recurrence rates of treated basal cell carcinoma. J Dermatol Surg Oncol 1992;18:471–476. Copyright 1992 by Elsevier Science Inc.

sue is removed. This allows for excellent cure rates (90%–95%) for primary nodular and superficial basal cell carcinomas but may sacrifice tissue unnecessarily. This is not important in most areas but on the nose, eyelids, lips, or ears it becomes more important because functional and cosmetic repairs become difficult. For selected tumor types (e.g., recurrent, infiltrative, poorly defined clinical margins), the random safety margins may still be inadequate (Table 141–9). By examining 100% of the surgical margin there is no sampling error in MMS. This provides for high cure rates for all BCC and SCC despite their microscopic appearance or history. It also removes the need for a safety margin allowing the surgeon to spare as much tissue as possible while still obtaining the desired cure rate.

To take full advantage of the 100% marginal examination and reduce the risk of false-negative readings due to "skip areas" of tumor growth, the technique is most amenable to neoplasms that are characterized by contiguous growth and those that have a histologic appearance recognizable by frozen section examination. Therefore MMS is best suited in the management of BCC and SCC, the two most common neoplasms (Table 141–10). However, it has been applied to many other tumors (see below).

Even though MMS is the most efficacious modality in the treatment of cutaneous neoplasms,[234, 235] it is not always indicated (see Tables 141–5 and 141–6). Most primary skin cancers may be managed via standard less expensive surgical modalities with adequate cure rates. To maintain its place in our treatment regimen as a cost-effective procedure, MMS must be used for properly indicated tumors. One may divide the true value of the technique into two categories: (1) situations in which the cutaneous malignancy is more likely to recur due to its aggressive behavior, histologic appearance, or location; and (2) tumors that are anatomically located in areas in which tissue conservation is important (Fig. 141–22; see Table 141–10).[236-239]

Subclinical Tumor Spread

Subclinical tumor spread tends to increase as clinical tumor size enlarges beyond 2 cm.[285, 286] Perineural inva-

TABLE 141-10. Indications for Mohs Micrographic Surgery in Treatment of Basal Cell Carcinoma and Squamous Cell Carcinoma

I. Primary tumors with higher risks of recurrence
   A. Histologic variants
      1. Basal cell carcinoma
         a. Morpheaform
         b. Infiltrative
         c. Micronodular
      2. Squamous cell carcinoma
         a. Poorly differentiated
         b. Adenosquamous
         c. Sclerosing or desmoplastic
      3. Location
         Lower nose, ears, eyelids, perioral
      4. Perineural invasion
      5. Indistinct clinical margins
      6. Diameter greater than 2-cm basal cell carcinoma; 1-cm squamous cell carcinoma
      7. Deeply invasive or eroded tumors
II. Primary tumors in areas where tissue preservation is important
   A. Lower nose
   B. Periorbital
   C. Periauricular
   D. Lips
   E. Digits
   F. Genitalia
III. Recurrent basal cell carcinoma and squamous cell carcinoma
IV. Incompletely excised tumors

sion, associated with radiating pain, paresthesias, or numbness, is another situation well suited to MMS. Perineural invasion occurs with BCC; however, it is more likely and more threatening in squamous cell carcinoma.[287-289, 292] Perineural invasion correlates with

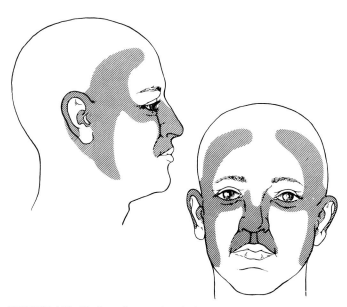

FIGURE 141-22. Locations on head where Mohs micrographic surgery is indicated for primary basal cell carcinoma. (From Swanson NA. Mohs surgery, technique, indications, applications, and future. Arch Dermatol 1983;119:761–773. Copyright 1983, American Medical Association.)

higher recurrence rates and places the patient at increased risk for metastatic disease.[290-293]

Standard histopathologic processing methods are inadequate in evaluating margins in tumors that display perineural invasion. MMS is ideal in this setting because it allows the Mohs surgeon to map out the involved nerve and continue excising tissue until the involved nerve is shown to be free of tumor. In addition the patient may require adjuvant radiation therapy in order to obtain the highest cure rate possible, particularly with SCC.

Incompletely Excised Tumors

Incompletely excised tumors are disconcerting to both patient and physician. Clinical observation can be a disservice to the patient because recurrence rates for incompletely excised tumors on the face may range from 33% to 82%.[255, 294] When the tumor recurs, re-excision may require a large disfiguring procedure. Because appropriate margins were not clinically discernible in the first surgical excision, there is the possibility of residual tumor again with immediate narrow re-excision, and wide re-excision may unnecessarily sacrifice normal tissues.

The Mohs technique is ideally suited to treating incompletely excised lesions. A conservative narrow re-excision is performed, the tissue is bisected along the long axis and processed in the usual fashion for MMS.[295] If residual tumor is found, it can be precisely localized and surgically traced and removed. This technique allows the physician to maximize the likelihood that the tumor has been adequately treated while minimizing tissue loss and the number of subsequent procedures.

Recurrent Tumors

Clinically recurrent tumors are the result of residual tumor cells left at the time of initial excision whether undetected histologically or detected histologically by a positive margin but not re-excised.[259] Often the tumors are clinically poorly circumscribed with indistinct margins. Histologically there is a greater stromal-to-tumor cell ratio allowing for "pseudo-skip areas" and increasing the possibility of false-negative microscopic examination. Scar from prior procedures tends to hide and obscure tumor, inhibiting the ability to assess the extent of tumor by curettage. MMS provides microscopic control in establishing excisional margins for recurrent lesions. In an extensive review of 5-year recurrence rates for recurrent BCC, Rowe and associates reported a 5.6% recurrence rate for MMS compared with significantly higher rates for other modalities (see Table 141–5) with much greater variability.[296] Based on these recurrence rates of previously recurrent tumors, they and other investigators have concluded that MMS is the treatment of choice for recurrent tumors.[297]

MMS is particularly suited to the treatment of BCCs that recur after radiation therapy. These tumors tend to be aggressively invasive, usually occur in cosmetically important areas (which prompted the original nonsurgical approach), and are particularly prone to recur again if retreated with radiation therapy or standard surgical excision.[298]

Squamous Cell Carcinoma

SCC is the second most common skin cancer, accounting for about 20% of lesions.[299, 300] Certain areas are more prone toward developing SCC then BCC, such as the ear, lower lip,[304-306] fingers, and genitals. SCC in these areas are well suited to treatment with MMS for both curative and tissue-conservative reasons (see Table 141–10).[276, 282, 283, 307-311] Cure rates may be slightly lower for SCC versus BCC when treated with MMS due to a more difficult histologic picture and the increased tendency for metastasis.

Although precise rates of metastasis of SCC are not known, locations at higher risk for metastasis are the lower lip, ear, penis, and digits. Perineural SCCs are at particularly high risk for metastasis as are tumors greater than 1 cm in diameter and also recurrent lesions.[301, 312-318] Management should include regional lymph node examination, with radiography and fine needle aspiration biopsy of suspicious adenopathy. For large primary SCC (>1 cm), lesions with perineural spread, or those with anaplastic histology, an extra margin of 3 to 5 mm beyond the clear MMS stage may help limit recurrence or metastasis. Adjunct radiation therapy may also be helpful in selected cases. Prospective studies are ongoing to determine metastatic rates, tumors and locations at most risk, and appropriate treatment combinations. Frequent follow-up at intervals of 1 to 2 months during the first postoperative year is recommended for SCC.

Application to Other Cutaneous Malignancies

MMS has been applied to tumors other than BCC and SCC with the same objectives of performing tissue-sparing surgery with high cure rates. However, tumors that exhibit skip areas or satellite lesions in their growth patterns are not fully amenable to MMS. MMS has been applied to a variety of skin cancers including microcystic adnexal carcinoma,[319-322] apocrine adenocarcinoma,[323] malignant cylindroma,[324] syringoid eccrine carcinoma,[325] adenoid cystic carcinoma,[326] malignant trichoepithelioma,[327] dermatofibrosarcoma protuberans,[328-331] extramammary Paget's disease,[332-334] leiomyosarcoma,[335] malignant fibrous histiocytoma and atypical fibroxanthoma,[336] eccrine porocarcinoma,[337] Merkel cell carcinoma,[338] angiosarcoma,[339] and sebaceous carcinoma.[340-343] Although MMS has been applied to this array of malignancies, there are currently no large-series reports of the use of MMS with these tumors.

Melanoma

The application of MMS in the treatment of melanoma is a controversial issue. Most Mohs surgeons (authors included) do not utilize MMS in the management of cutaneous melanoma. A minority of authors have held the fixed-tissue technique to be an effective therapeutic option in the management of melanoma.[222, 344-347] However, many practitioners believe that frozen-section evaluation of melanocytes is imprecise. This is further complicated by the inflammation associated with the use of zinc chloride paste in the fixed-tissue technique. One study evaluating the sensitivity and specificity of frozen sections as compared with paraffin sections for the same block found a sensitivity of 100% in detecting melanoma and a specificity of 90%.[348] Despite this study, few Mohs surgeons utilize MMS technique for the treatment of melanoma and those that do usually reserve this technique for superficial lesions.[349, 350] It remains unknown if MMS offers sufficient benefit to the patient in terms of melanoma recurrence or metastasis in order to warrant the time and expense of MMS versus primary excision.

Limitations of MMS

The limitations of MMS fall into three broad categories, which are tumor-related, patient-related, and technical errors. As MMS is predicated upon the interpretation of frozen sections, only those tumors that may be easily identified with frozen sections may be treated with MMS. As previously mentioned, MMS is more likely to fail in assessing tumors with discontiguous growth or those displaying satellitosis. At times tumors may be too large or deeply invasive to allow curative surgery.

Patient-related limitations may be poor health, surgical phobia, or intolerance to local anesthesia. Technical limitations include mapping errors, poor sectioning, poor staining, and slide interpretation error. The procedure should only be performed by those with advanced training in the technique.

Conclusion

MMS is a surgical procedure based upon the precise microscopically controlled excision of cutaneous malignancies. Neoplasms amenable to frozen-section evaluation and demonstrating contiguous growth patterns may be candidates for MMS. Due to horizontal tissue sectioning, which provides examination of 100% of the surgical margin, the technique offers tissue-sparing properties along with higher cure rates as compared with standard surgical excision. MMS requires meticulous attention to procedural detail, knowledge of superficial head and neck anatomy, and understanding of tumor biology and histology. It is a time-consuming, labor- and resource-intensive procedure; therefore, it is more expensive than other surgical destructive methods. To maintain its place in our armamentarium against cutaneous malignancy, its use must be reserved for those tumors that fulfill the indications discussed above. To further assure its most efficacious application, MMS is best performed by trained physicians doing sufficient volume commensurate with maintaining the necessary skills and knowledge base.

RECONSTRUCTION WITH FLAPS AND GRAFTS FOLLOWING EXCISION OF SKIN CANCER

Following skin cancer excision, the four general categories of management of the resulting defect are healing by second intention, side-to-side closure, skin grafting, and a variety of skin flaps. The decision to use a skin flap or graft to repair a wound should always be taken in the context of the local anatomy, tumor biology with likelihood of recurrence, and the desires and health of the patient. Healing by second intention or side-to-side closure is often the best option due to their relative simplicity. However, if these modalities are unable to close the particular defect, or if they will result in significant anatomic distortion or loss of function, flaps or grafts should be considered.

Although this text will go into some detail, the complexity of these advanced surgical techniques mandates far more in-depth reading, practical training, and proctored experience to fully prepare the surgeon to perform skin flaps and grafts. Knowledge of superficial anatomy, tumor biology, wound healing, wound dressings and recognition and management of complications are all important aspects of advanced surgery; however, they are beyond the scope of this chapter and must be gleaned from more directed surgical texts (see *Atlas of Cutaneous Surgery*).

Nomenclature for Cutaneous Flaps

A standardized nomenclature facilitates not only educational description of flap surgery but is important for concise and informative clinical documentation of procedures.[351, 352] In this text *primary defect* refers to the wound that requires closure. The *secondary defect* is created by movement of the flap. The object of flap repairs is to redirect the tension of the closure from the primary to the secondary defect. Location, size, and configuration of the secondary defect, therefore, become very important parameters. It does little good in most cases to close a primary defect but leave a secondary defect that cannot be closed or whose closure causes anatomic distortion.

Primary motion describes the movement of the flap into the primary defect. Flaps are either *advanced, rotated,* or *transposed* into place. The type of motion is generally how flaps are classified.

Secondary motion is one of the most difficult concepts in flap surgery and yet is one of the more important. The term defines the combined effects of the elastic forces attempting to return the skin of the flap to its original position and the reaction of surrounding tissue to both the primary motion of the flap and the closure of the secondary defect. The surgeon must understand and anticipate the secondary motion in a particular closure in order to properly choose and orient a flap.

The *pedicle* or *base* of a flap is its connection to surrounding tissue. It is the lifeline of the flap not only carrying blood flow in, but also blood and lymphatic fluid out. The size and location of the base are important determinants of flap survival. The location of the base in relation to the distal aspect of the flap is often used to describe the flap as being superiorly, inferiorly, medially, or laterally based.

The first stitch placed in flap surgery is termed the *tension-bearing suture,* and was formerly called the *key suture.*[353] This is an important stitch essentially doing most of the work of the closure by moving the flap into the primary defect and redirecting the closure tensions to the secondary defect. It is not inappropriate to set this stitch several times, varying each placement in an effort to arrive at the best combination of primary and secondary tension vectors. It is not uncommon at the completion of the procedure to replace the tension-bearing su-

ture with a more delicate, finely placed stitch (see Introduction to Tissue Movement in *Atlas of Cutaneous Surgery*).

Advancement Flaps

These flaps represent the most straightforward tissue movement. They are sliding flaps whose primary motion is linear as they are pulled into the primary defect. Classically they are rectangular in shape although in practice they can assume several geometric shapes to take advantage of skin tension lines and cosmetic borders for camouflage purposes (Fig. 141–23).[352, 354] In order to ensure

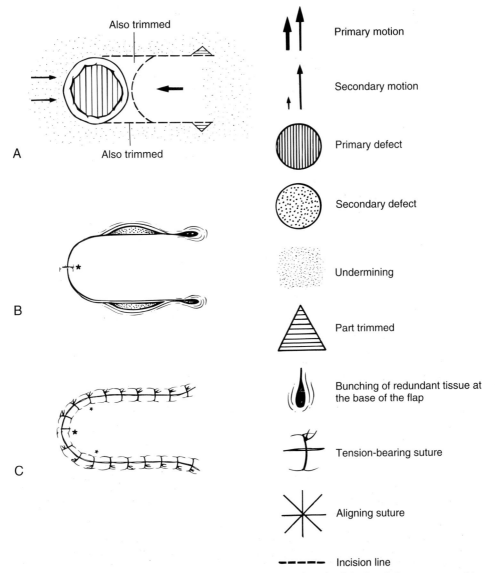

Primary motion

Secondary motion

Primary defect

Secondary defect

Undermining

Part trimmed

Bunching of redundant tissue at the base of the flap

Tension-bearing suture

Aligning suture

Incision line

FIGURE 141–23. *A–C,* There are instances when the cosmetic unit of the face is better preserved by rounding the tip of the single advancement flap, thus forming a U-shaped incision. As a general principle of planning advancement flaps, the length of a single advancement flap will be two to three times the length of the defect to be covered. If there is a lot of secondary motion about the flap, the flap's length may be planned shorter. The flap's dimensions in facial locations should not exceed a length-to-width ratio of 3:1. The right hand column shows the symbols used to illustrate the surgical concepts in the drawing in this section. (From Moy RK, Robinson JK. Advancement flap. In: Robinson JK, Arndt KA, LeBoit PE, Wintroub BU, eds. Atlas of Cutaneous Surgery. Philadelphia: WB Saunders Co., 1996.)

that the pedicle provides adequate blood flow, the design of these flaps should not exceed a length-to-width ratio of more than 3:1.[355, 356] Exceptions to this rule occur in quite vascular areas such as the nasal dorsum or helix of the ear, where longer lengths are supportable. In the less vascular areas of the trunk and extremities, shorter length-to-width ratios may be required.

The flap is designed as much as possible to take advantage of local skin tension lines and cosmetic borders.[352] The location of the pedicle should consider regional blood flow patterns and lymphatic drainage. Generally inferiorly or laterally based flaps are best, but the most important determinant is tissue availability and the relation of the defect and flap to surrounding anatomic structures. Because the secondary motion of advancement flaps is essentially equal and opposite in direction to the primary motion, it is unwise to move advancement flaps up toward free margins such as the lower lip or eyelid because this may cause eclabion or ectropion.[352] Movement across or parallel to free margins is recommended.

Following design and cutting of the flap, undermining is performed in a mid to high fat plane under and around the flap and primary defect.[351, 354] It is especially important to undermine well beyond the base of the flap to facilitate movement. The tension-bearing suture (Fig. 141–23B) is placed through the center of the advancing edge of the distal flap and pulls the flap across, thus closing the primary defect. This action creates two wounds of unequal length along both sides of the flap as the inner flap margins are shorter than the outer surrounding skin margins (Fig. 141–23B).[352, 356, 357] The redundant tissue can be excised as triangles of tissue generally from the base area or may be sewn out by halving the excess and sharing it along the entire length of the flap.[352, 356, 357]

There are several variations of advancement flaps. These include bilateral advancement flaps (H-plasty), single-arm advancement flaps (Burrow's wedge advancement flap), O to T or V to T advancement flaps, and island pedicle advancement flaps.[358] Each offers specific advantages relative to ease of tissue movement, limitations of the effects of primary and secondary motion, blood supply, and camouflage.[351, 352, 354–358]

The H-plasty is two classical advancement flaps moved towards each other across the primary defect (Fig. 141–24).[358] The equal and opposite motion of the two flaps cancels out the effects of secondary motion, minimizing the impact on surrounding structures. Also since each flap covers only half the defect they are smaller and move less, resulting in better relative blood flow to the flaps and less tension on the closure.

Single-arm advancement flaps are designed with only one incision emanating from an edge of the primary defect. This flap is characterized by removal of two cutaneous triangles hence the synonyn "Burow's wedge advancement flap."[359] The first triangle is removed from the base of the flap and both facilitates movement of the flap and removes redundant tissue created along the skin outside the flap incision. The second wedge excised triangulates the wound to create a favorable 30-degree closure angle.[359] These are widely based well-vascularized

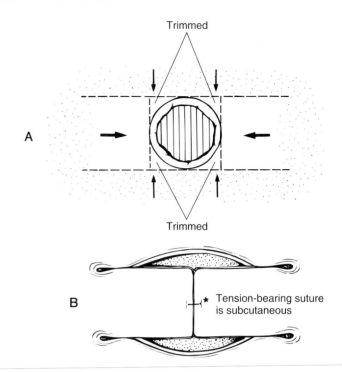

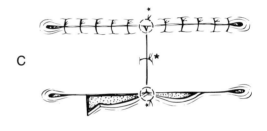

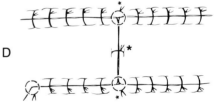

FIGURE 141–24. *A,* Diagram of the motion of the bilateral (double) advancement flap or H-plasty. The length of each flap may be 1.5 to 2 times the length of the defect. *B,* After the tension-bearing suture is placed, the gaping secondary defects appear superior and inferior to the flaps. Each secondary defect is an elliptical wound with unequal sides. Each secondary defect is closed using the rule of halves. *C,* The superior secondary defect is partially closed by a suture at its midpoint. This (*asterisk*) single-tip stitch also aligns the flaps through the tips of both flaps. The larger redundancy (bulging) is inferiorly and laterally placed. *D,* It is revised with a "hockey stick" repair. (From Moy RK, Robinson JK. Advancement flap. In: Robinson JK, Arndt KA, LeBoit PE, Wintroub BU, eds. Atlas of Cutaneous Surgery. Philadelphia: WB Saunders Co., 1996.)

flaps generally selected to take advantage of local anatomy for camouflage purposes.

Bilateral single-arm advancement flaps are termed O-T, V-T, or A-T advancement flaps.[358] Like the H-plasty they are generally selected to limit effects of both primary and secondary motion on anatomic structures and to utilize cosmetic units and skin tension lines to best hide incision lines (Fig. 141–25).[351, 352, 354–357]

The island pedicle flap is fundamentally different from most of the other flaps.[360] Depending on tissue laxity and elasticity a triangular flap 1.5 to 3 times the defect size is designed. The point of the triangle is a 30-degree angle and is opposite the advancing flap edge (Fig. 141–26). This triangle of skin is not undermined but rather the incision is carried straight down through fat to fascia. The surface skin is nourished by blood flow through this column or pedicle of fat. Because the pedicle is cut free from surrounding tissue, connected only at its base to fascia, it is able to swing or advance forward into the primary defect. Movement is facilitated by side-to-side closure of the secondary defect, which has the effect of pushing the triangular flap into the primary defect. Island pedicle flaps require a reasonably abundant layer of underlying fat to both nourish and allow movement of the flap. They are difficult to camouflage in some areas

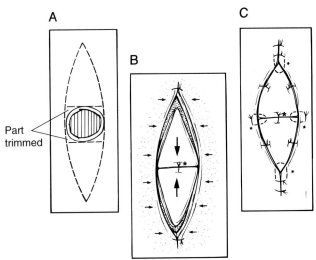

FIGURE 141–26. V-Y plasty or island advancement flap. *A,* The four rounded tips of the advancing flaps are trimmed, and the 3:1 dimensions of the total length of an ellipse are planned. *B,* The V-shaped island of tissue is raised on its narrow pedicle of subcutaneous fat and advanced forward. The entire flap is dissected from the base until a small central vertical line of tissue is formed from the center of the island. The ability to develop this pedicle depends on the availability of fat in the region. For instance, it is difficult to develop island advancement flaps on a pedicle in the forehead because of the relative dearth of fat but it is easier to develop them on the lip or cheek. The flap is advanced, and with a skin hook holding the flap in place, the tension-bearing sutures close the secondary defects. If in the process of suturing these flaps they turn white, they should be returned to their original position because the blood supply in the pedicle has been kinked or stretched too much and is impaired. The aligning suture is placed into the advancing edges of the two flaps, and tip stitches align the tails of the flaps. *C,* Then subcutaneous sutures are placed to close the remaining secondary defects. (From Moy RK, Robinson JK. Advancement flap. In: Robinson JK, Arndt KA, LeBoit PE, Wintroub BU, eds. Atlas of Cutaneous Surgery. Philadelphia: WB Saunders Co., 1996.)

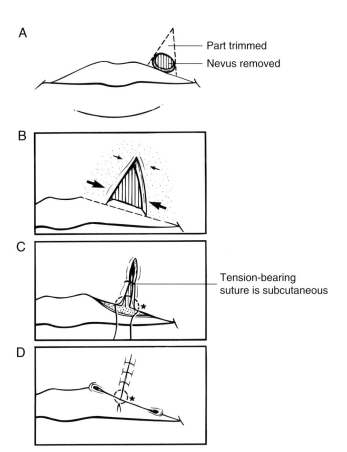

FIGURE 141–25. *A,* The circular nevus is converted to a triangular shape whose base lies on the vermilion border. *B,* The horizontal incisions are made along the vermilion, and all aspects of the flaps are undermined. The critical strategy is to mobilize the tissue under the flap by widely undermining (*stippled area*). The primary motion of the flaps is advancement, but there is a small element of rotation about the apex of the vertical limb of the A-T incision. *C,* The tension-bearing suture is a buried subcutaneous one that is placed first and creates the secondary defect. Then a tip stitch aligns the tips of the flaps. *D,* Bulging redundancies are created laterally. (From Moy RK, Robinson JK. Advancement flap. In: Robinson JK, Arndt KA, LeBoit, PE, Wintroub BU, eds. Atlas of Cutaneous Surgery. Philadelphia: WB Saunders Co., 1996.)

due to the triangular incision and often resemble a graft.[361]

Because advancement flaps are pulled into place they are most useful in areas of reasonable tissue elasticity. The linearity of the incision lines of advancement flaps also makes them appropriate for use in areas with straighter skin tension lines or cosmetic borders. Common anatomic locations for advancement flaps include the forehead and supra-brow areas, cheeks, lips, nasal sidewall, pre-auricular skin and helix of the ear (see *Atlas of Cutaneous Surgery*, Chapter 10).[351, 355]

Rotation Flaps

Like advancement flaps, rotation flaps are sliding flaps that are pulled into place across the primary defect. As the name implies, their vector of motion is arcuate.[362, 363] This rotational movement about an axis point provides advantages to and additional closure options over advancement flaps. The act of rotation results in less reliance on tissue elasticity for flap movement, allowing rotation flaps to be useful in areas of inelastic skin such as the scalp or nasal dorsum. The design characteristics create a broad-based flap with excellent blood flow and survival rates that can therefore be made considerably larger than most advancement flaps. The arcuate design of these flaps facilitates camouflage in curvilinear facial skin tension lines and cosmetic borders.[351, 352, 354–357]

The design of a rotation flap is dependent upon, among other things, the size of the primary defect, the extensibility of donor tissue, the proximity of free anatomic margins (e.g., eyelids, lips) and the tension that can be tolerated across the secondary defect.[351, 355, 356, 362, 363] In general the larger the flap-to-defect ratio the less the tension at either primary or secondary closure site. This is particularly important when working around free margins, which may be distorted by too much tension.[351, 355, 356, 362, 363] However, very extensible skin allows for smaller flaps to effect the closure, which are more efficient to do and create fewer incision lines and less risk of bleeding or infectious complication.

One may begin designing rotation flaps by considering the flap and primary defect as a half circle with a flap-to-defect size ratio of 3 or 4:1.[351, 355, 356, 362, 363] As experience is gained with flap movement and in judging tissue extensibility, variations on these design and size parameters can be made. Once the flap is cut and undermined, the tension-bearing suture is placed. As with the advancement flap, this suture is placed through the leading edge of the flap, pulling it over and anchoring it across the primary defect. This creates the secondary defect, which is crescentic in shape and located along the arc of the flap. This crescentic defect has margins of unequal length with a longer outer and shorter inner edge. The outer excess skin may be sewn out by employing the "rule of halves" and sharing it along the length of the inner edge. More commonly the outer edge is short-

ened by removing a triangle of tissue (dog-ear). This may be done anywhere along the margin but is usually placed at the distal-most point from the primary defect. This location of the dog-ear also helps with rotation of the flap by freeing up tissue surrounding the flap base which otherwise tethers the flap.[351, 355, 356, 362, 363]

A tissue protrusion is created by the flap motion around the axis of rotation near the primary defect. This also is called a dog-ear and must be removed both to facilitate flap movement and for aesthetic reasons. It is important to begin the excision of this dog-ear on the side opposite the flap base so as not to cut into and shorten the base in any way.[351, 355, 356, 362, 363]

One advantage of rotation flaps is the ability to make changes in their size and rotational characteristics after they are initially designed and cut. If the flap does not move as easily as it should or if there is too much tension at either the primary or secondary defect, the surgeon has options to remedy the problems. The first is to simply enlarge the flap by extending the arcuate incision beyond the existing base. Because of their broad base, rotation flaps can be very large and are not limited by length-to-width ratios as are advancement flaps. By increasing flap-to-defect size ratios, tension is decreased.[351, 355, 356, 358, 362, 363]

The other option is to perform a back cut (Fig. 141–27).[351, 352] This technique is accomplished by cutting into the base of the flap starting at the point most distant from the primary defect along the curvilinear incision line defining the arc of rotation. This has the effect of moving the tethering point that inhibits rotation closer to the defect, lengthening the inner arc of the flap, and there-

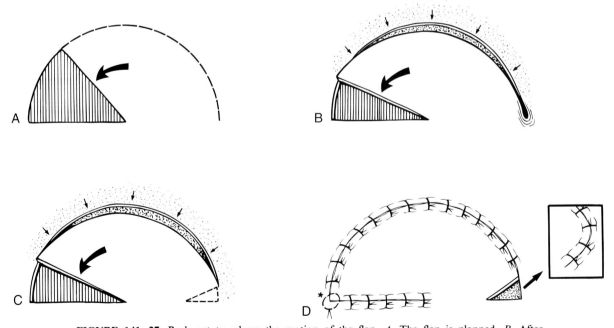

FIGURE 141–27. Back cut to release the motion of the flap. *A,* The flap is planned. *B,* After undermining the area around the flap, the flap is elevated but it is impossible to close the primary defect. *C,* A small back cut into the base of the flap allows the primary motion of the flap rotation to proceed. The primary defect is closed. *D,* The bunching of redundant tissue about the pivot point may be used to close the secondary defect by incorporating a Z-plasty or just closed using the principle of halves as shown here. (From Whitaker D. Rotation flap. In: Robinson JK, Arndt KA, LeBoit PE, Wintroub BU, eds. Atlas of Cutaneous Surgery. Philadelphia: WB Saunders Co., 1996.)

fore increasing the rotational capacity. This is a somewhat risky procedure because it narrows the base, limiting blood flow into the flap. Back cuts should start small and should rarely exceed one fourth of the base length.[351, 352]

Rotation flaps can be employed in most regions of the body because their broad-based design, rotational movement, and large size allow good movement in either extensible or nonextensible skin. They work very well in the inelastic skin of the scalp, where advancement flaps do not move well and the secondary defect of transposition flaps is hard to close.[351, 355, 356, 358, 362, 363] This is also true for the extremities and trunk, where the broad base is a further advantage in these less well vascularized areas. These are good regions to practice rotation flaps initially because of the high success rates and lack of cosmetic sensitivity.

Rotation flaps have great utility and versatility on the face, being especially useful where curvilinear skin tension lines and cosmetic borders exist.[352, 354] They are frequently employed in the pre-auricular and temple regions of the cheek, upper lip, and nose. In all these examples the accurate flap incision is carefully aligned within a cosmetic border or skin tension line, and flap-to-defect size ratios take into account local tissue extensibility and the proximity of free anatomic margins.[2, 3]

As with advancement flaps, double-rotation flaps are a design variation that aids in camouflage, decreases anatomic distortion, and facilitates wound closure when donor skin is limited or very extensible. Double rotations take two general forms.[351] The first is two flaps rotating in opposite directions toward each other along the same arc. This variation is similar to A-T or O-T bilateral advancement flaps except for the rotational vector of movement. Each flap closes half the wound and therefore is smaller than a single flap would be for the same size defect. Also, as with the O-T repairs, the opposing movement limits many of the effects of both primary and secondary motion on surrounding tissue and structures. They are therefore useful in midline locations such as the chin and nasal tip. The other double-rotation flap variation of note is called the O-Z repair due to the final appearance of the incisional lines (Fig. 141–28).[351] The two flaps are raised from opposite sides of the defect and rotate toward each other along opposite arcs of a theoretical circle. The Z-like scar configuration is difficult to camouflage, and so utility of this closure is limited to areas such as the scalp, dorsal hand, and lateral forehead/temple (see *Atlas of Cutaneous Surgery*, Chapter 11).[351]

Transposition Flaps

Transposition flaps also rotate from their donor area into the primary defect but they are different from classic rotation flaps in many ways. These flaps are named because after they are designed and cut, they are elevated up and transposed (rotated over) intervening tissue into the primary defect.[351, 352, 354–358, 364–367] Unlike the previous two flap types discussed, which are pulled into place, transposition flaps are pushed into the primary

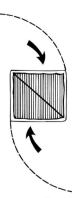

FIGURE 141–28. Double-rotation flap (O-Z). The square defect is subdivided into two triangular defects. Each triangular defect is closed with its own rotation flap. (From Whitaker D. Rotation flap. In: Robinson JK, Arndt KA, LeBoit PE, Wintroub BU, eds. Atlas of Cutaneous Surgery. Philadelphia: WB Saunders Co., 1996.)

defect by forces created by closure of the secondary defect. This is an important concept.[351, 352, 354–358, 364–367] These flaps tend to drape into place with very little tension around the primary defect, making them useful in many areas, particularly around free anatomic margins. All of the tension of these repairs is centered across closure of the secondary defect. Therefore placement of this defect, that is, the flap donor site, is extremely important to a successful procedure. In general, the direction of secondary defect closure vectors should parallel any local free margins to avoid pulling up or down on them.[351, 352, 354–358, 364–367]

Transposition flaps tend to be very economical in tissue use, which broadens their applicability, decreases scar length, and lowers complication risks. In most cases the size of a transposition flap is approximately the size of the primary defect. The design and orientation of these geometric flaps is critical, requiring very careful planning. Once they are cut and elevated they cannot be enlarged if they are too small. Transposition flaps carry several nominal designations based on their shape or location, but with a few modifications the principles behind the design and movement of them are the same.[351, 352, 354–358, 364–367]

The defect is measured and the flap drawn equal to or slightly larger in size and shape (Fig. 141–29). The flap will rotate between 45 and 90 degrees.[351, 352, 354–358, 364–367] It extends from the side of the defect and if that defect is not circular, it is best to initiate the flap off a shorter diameter. Designing the flap off a long axis results in a longer, more narrow flap with excessive rotation that may compromise blood flow. It is best to orient the secondary defect within or parallel to a cosmetic border or skin tension line.[352, 354] However, due to the 90-degree rotation, this is not always possible. The flap and skin surrounding the donor site is undermined. Some undermining around the primary defect may aid closure and help prevent thickening of the flap ("pin-cushion effect").[368] The tension-bearing suture in transposition flaps closes the secondary defect (Fig. 141–29).[351, 352, 354–358, 364–367] As mentioned, this pushes the flap into the primary defect. The next suture, the aligning suture, secures the flap in place and the rest of the procedure is essentially fine-tuning.

Two dog-ears are created (Fig. 141–29).[351, 352, 354–358, 364–367] The first is at the tip of the donor site and may be designed into the flap by creating a 30-degree angle there when excised (Fig. 141–29). Otherwise it is removed after closure of the secondary defect. The second results from transposition of the flap and occurs at the axis of rotation at the flap base closest to the primary defect. This is best excised after the flap is fixed in place so that the precise amount of tissue necessary is removed.

Examples of the banner-type of transposition flap include the glabella flap and the nasolabial-fold flap.[369–372] In both these examples the donor site incisions are well camouflaged in a glabellar frown line and along the melo-labial fold respectively.[370–372] The flaps drape into their primary defects with minimal or no tension, creating no distortion of the eyelids or nasal alar rim.[369–372] It is important to thin the fat on these flaps to minimize thickening ("pin-cushioning").[368] Other useful areas for this flap are the repair of superior helical defects with a pre-auricular flap and repair of lateral lower eyelid defects with a flap harvested from redundant upper eyelid skin.[372]

A commonly employed variation on the transposition flap is the rhombic flap [351, 352, 354–357, 365–367] (Fig. 141–30). This is a geometric flap with two 60-degree and two 120-degree angles in the shape of a rhombus. The defect is designed as this rhombic shape, the sides measured and the flap created with the identical (or 10%–20% larger) dimensions. It is wide based compared with its size and length, so it is a safe, well-vascularized flap. Its sharply defined angles facilitate camouflage within well-demarcated skin tension lines and cosmetic borders when compared with the banner-type flap. Rhombic flaps are quite useful for repair of nasal alar defects with a nasal sidewall donor site, mid and lateral cheek, upper lip, temple, and lower eyelid defects.[351, 352, 354–357, 365–367] Depending on the angularity of local skin tension lines and borders and the initial shape of the primary defect, the flap may be rounded to fit the defect or the defect extended to approximate the rhombic shape.

Another variation on the transposition flap is the 30-degree angle flap or Webster flap named for its originator.[374] This flap was designed to eliminate the 60-degree angles of the rhombic flap, which create significant closure dog-ears at the tip of the secondary defect and point of rotation of the flap. The 30-degree angle flap is predicated on the ability to close part of the primary defect with side-to-side motion.[374] Therefore it is not useful in

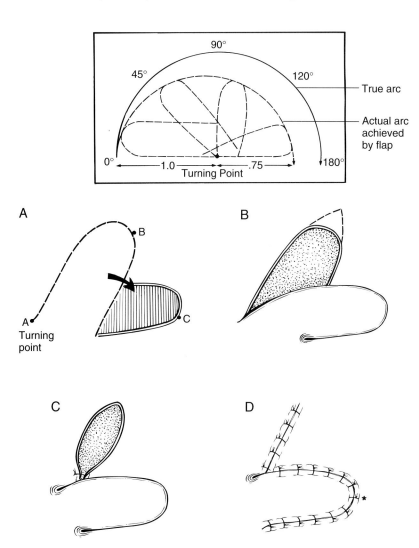

FIGURE 141–29. Transposition flap with 60-degree arc of motion. *A,* Planning the transposition flap requires the ability to predict the length of the flap necessary to cover the primary defect. By recognizing that the flap length depends on the motion about the turning point A; the distance AC is used to plot AB, the line of maximal tension. As the flap turns through an ever larger arc, the length of the flap shortens. *B,* The area around the secondary defect is undermined widely before placement of the first suture. *C,* The first suture closes the secondary defect and produces bunching at the base of the flap. This redundancy may be revised in a second procedure. The bunching may be somewhat corrected by suturing techniques using closure of wounds of unequal heights. *D,* The final closure results in a lengthy incision line. (From Robinson JK. Transposition flap. In: Robinson JK, Arndt KA, LeBoit PE, Wintroub BU, eds. Atlas of Cutaneous Surgery. Philadelphia: WB Saunders Co., 1996.)

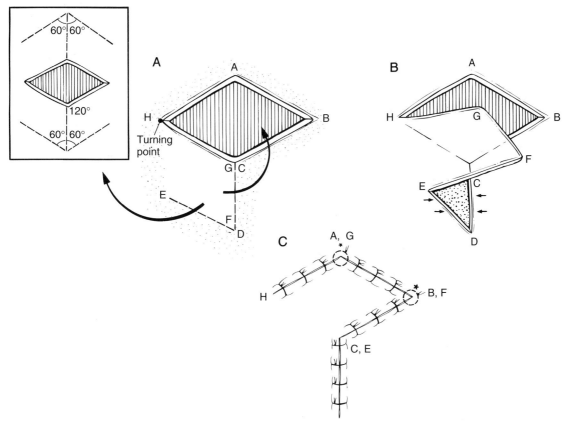

FIGURE 141–30. Rhombic flap. For any rhombus, there are four different possible flaps to construct off the 120-degree angle (short axis of the rhombus). To decrease the amount of "pincushioning" it is generally better to try to use an inferiorly based flap. *A,* The flap CDE is designed so that CD is the same length as AB and DE is the same as BC. The angle GFE is 60 degrees and fits into the angle ABC. *B,* As the flap is elevated, it collapses into the primary defect. The skin around the secondary defect is extensively undermined. *C,* The tension-bearing suture placed first closes the secondary defect (point CE). (From Robinson JK. Transposition flap. In: Robinson JK, Arndt AK, LeBoit PE, Wintroub BU, eds. Atlas of Cutaneous Surgery. Philadelphia: WB Saunders Co., 1996.)

areas of minimal tissue movement or near free margins such as the nasal tip and alae, the mid forehead, scalp, eyelids, and lips. The primary defect is defined as in the rhombic flap repair with a 60-degree angle at the tip and lateral 120-degree angles. Side-to-side closure will account for one half of the closure, creating a 30-degree angle at the tip. Therefore the flap is drawn with a 30-degree tip angle negating any dog-ear in this location. The flap base needs to be only half as wide as the primary defect diameter because it will need to fill only half of the defect. The flap must be harvested as close to 90 degrees from the long axis of the primary defect as possible.[374] If it is too close to paralleling the long axis, closure of the secondary defect will compete with available tissue extensibility for the side-to-side component of the repair. If a nearly vertically oriented 30-degree angle flap can be performed, this would indicate enough local tissue movement to allow side-to-side repair, thus obviating the need for a flap altogether. Care must be taken to avoid harvesting the flap so close to 90 degrees off the vertical axis that the base is compromised, risking necrosis.

The 30-degree angle flap is useful in areas with good tissue extensibility and with well defined skin tension lines to accommodate the sharp lines and angles of the repair. These include the cheeks, glabella, and nasal sidewall and dorsum.[351, 352, 354]

The bilobed flap is designed to allow for transposition flap repair in situations where donor skin is inadequate immediately adjacent to the primary defect.[351, 352, 354–358, 370, 375, 376] As the name implies, two separate lobes are designed in this flap (Fig. 141–31). The first lobe is designed the size and shape of the primary defect. The lack of donor skin extensibility would prevent primary closure of the secondary defect created by the first lobe of the flap. Therefore a second lobe is designed, generally one half to two thirds the size of the first, to transpose into and close the secondary defect. The tertiary defect created by the second lobe is closed side to side, the first stitch representing the tension-bearing suture in this repair. Following placement of the tension-bearing suture, the first lobe of the flap is anchored in place across the primary defect. A dog-ear is removed from the point of rotation at the base of the flap and then the second lobe sutured in place (Fig. 141–31). As can be seen from the figure, the flap resembles a broken-up rotation flap in its motion. Its advantages over a rotation flap include less undermining and tissue movement and the transposition flap characteristics of

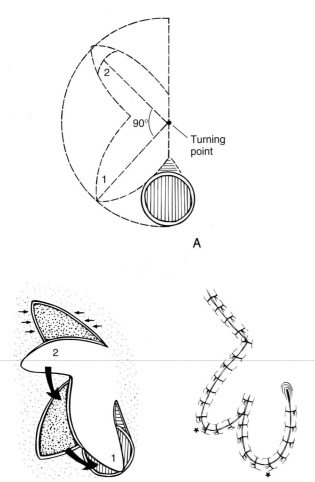

FIGURE 141-31. *A,* The first lobe forms a 45-degree angle with the defect and is planned to be the same width as the defect. The second lobe is at a 90-degree angle with the first and incorporates the potentially discarded tip that forms the ideal 30-degree angle for closure at the apex. Both flaps move about the turning point, forming an arc. This arc includes the rim of the defect and forms a circle of the motion of the flaps into the defect. The radius of the circle is the length of the lobe of each flap. The second lobe is shorter than the first because the secondary motion about the secondary defect will allow closure. A triangle of skin is excised between the defect and the pivot point of the flap before it is moved. The pivot point generally lies about one radius of the defect away from the defect. *B,* As the flaps are elevated, both move together. *C,* The tension-bearing suture placed first closes the secondary defect and pushes the flaps in place. (From Robinson JK. Transposition flap. In: Robinson JK, Arndt KA, LeBoit PE, Wintroub BU, eds. Atlas of Cutaneous Surgery. Philadelphia: WB Saunders Co., 1996.)

draping across the wound without pulling on free margins. The multiple zig-zagging lines of the flap make camouflage difficult in many areas. The bilobed flap is most useful on the nasal tip and alae, where donor skin is scarce.[351, 352, 354-358, 370, 375, 376] Frequently a dermabrasion 6 to 10 weeks postoperatively improves camouflage.

There are instances in which a flap repair is indicated but adequate donor skin is not available within the same or the adjacent cosmetic unit. In these situations skin may be harvested from a greater distance and transposed over intervening cosmetic units into the recipient site on a long pedicle.[351, 352, 354-357, 370, 377-379] The distal flap is

sutured in place, but the pedicle remains attached at the donor site and is temporarily left free over the intervening tissue. These staged or interpolation flaps require at least two and often three stages to complete.[351, 352, 354-357, 370, 377-379] After placement of the distal flap in stage one, a 3- to 4-week delay must ensue to allow the development of a local blood supply to nourish the distal skin and replace the need for the pedicle. At that point the pedicle is severed and replaced to the donor area or discarded. A touch-up procedure may be required several weeks later. These flaps have utility in repair of the nasal tip with a midline forehead flap or melo-labial fold flap or in repair of the mid-helix with a retro-auricular flap (see *Atlas of Cutaneous Surgery,* Chapter 12).[351, 352, 354-357, 370, 377-379]

Flap Selection

There are often several flaps capable of repairing a particular defect. Mastering the thought processes behind appropriate flap selection is as important as learning how to do the flaps themselves. Knowledge of anatomy, cosmetic units and skin tension lines, tissue movement vectors and resulting effects, and tissue survival characteristics as a result of these flap dynamics forms the basis of good judgment in flap surgery.[351, 352, 354-357]

In designing a flap repair, one must first determine where available donor skin is located and whether enough is present to reach and fill the primary defect. Certain classic areas exist for various cosmetic unit defects, but they vary from patient to patient as far as amount and extensibility and must therefore be examined before each repair. This can be accomplished by gently moving the tissue from side to side or pinching it between thumb and forefinger. Examples of donor areas include the glabella, nasal sidewall, and medial cheek for nasal defects; the temple and glabella for forehead defects; and melo-labial fold cheek skin for the upper lip.[351, 352, 354-357]

Next it is important to assess the effects on surrounding tissue of moving the flap and closing the secondary defect, that is, primary and secondary motion.[351, 352, 354-357] It does little good to close a defect with such tension as to cause severe distortion to surrounding anatomic structures. To ensure (as much as possible) flap survival, closure design needs to take into account an adequate pedicle, appropriately placed to provide sufficient blood flow in and blood and lymphatic flow out. Because most flaps in dermatologic surgery are of random pattern blood flow, length-to-width ratios are important.[351, 352, 354-357] Excessive tension can limit blood flow even in widely based flaps.

Appreciation of skin tension lines and cosmetic units is important in order to take advantage of them for flap movement and camouflage. A well-executed flap whose incision lines cross rather than parallel skin tension lines and cosmetic borders will result in a poor aesthetic outcome.[351, 352, 354-357]

Lastly, danger zones must be noted to avoid damage to important nerves, vessels, and Stinson's duct and to limit effects on free margins.[354] Flap surgery plays an important but complex role in treatment of skin cancers. The result of the repair is as important to the patient as the removal of the neoplasm.

Skin Grafting

There are three main types of skin grafting relevant to skin cancer excision repair. These include split-thickness, full-thickness, and composite grafts. They are each quite different in their structure, indications, metabolic requirements, cosmetic outcome, and technique.

Split-Thickness Skin Grafts

Split-thickness skin grafts (STSGs) consist of the epidermis and a portion of the dermis (Fig. 141–32). The amount of dermis included determines whether the graft is a thin, medium, or thick STSG. The thicker the graft, the more adnexal structures persist, including hairs. This has an effect on the final texture and appearance of the graft. However, as the thickness of the grafts increases, so do their metabolic needs. Graft thickness generally varies between 0.01 to 0.03 inches.[358, 380-384]

Harvesting of STSGs is usually done with either a power-driven device with a rapidly oscillating knife blade or a hand-operated blade with a special sheath to control thickness.[380-384] The former allows the surgeon to very rapidly harvest large-sized very uniform grafts, but are expensive and bulky. A Weck blade is a sheathed manually operated knife that with practice can produce adequate STSGs (see *Atlas of Cutaneous Surgery*, Chapter 13).

An advantage of STSGs is that they may be harvested quite quickly, they produce coverage for large areas, and the donor sites do not require repair.[380] The most common donor regions are in noncosmetically sensitive areas and include the anterior and lateral thighs, hip, buttock, and upper inner arm (Fig. 141–33).[358, 380, 381, 383, 384] Disadvantages related to the donor sites include a large, albeit superficial wound that is often painful, takes 2 to 3 weeks for initial healing, and leaves a frequently hypopigmented or hypertrophic scar.

The decision to repair a defect with a STSG is based on several considerations. These include the size, depth, vascularity, and location of the defect, the cosmetic and functional requirements of the patient, tumor biology, and relative morbidity of other repair options.[380, 384]

Because the donor site heals by second intention, STSGs can be harvested to cover far larger areas than a full-thickness skin graft (FTSG) and most random blood flow pattern flaps used in dermatologic surgery. They are therefore considered for large defects of the forehead, scalp, lateral cheeks, ears, and extremities when adequate donor skin does not exist for flap repair and the defect size would not allow for closure of a FTSG donor site.[358, 380, 384]

The thinness of STSGs results in lower metabolic requirements for the graft versus thicker grafts, allowing for better survival in wounds with poor vascularity. STSGs are therefore useful to cover wounds down to periosteum, perichondrium, muscle fascia, and over fat on extremities.[380, 384]

However, the thinness of STSGs is also problematic for a number of reasons. First, they cannot be expected to fill the depth of most defects as can flaps or thicker grafts. In some regions the wound-healing process will eventually elevate the graft and fill the defect, but this may take months to years and cannot always be predicted. The lack of depth of the grafts results in a loss of adnexal structures, particularly hair follicles. This, combined with the distant donor site, produces a repair that

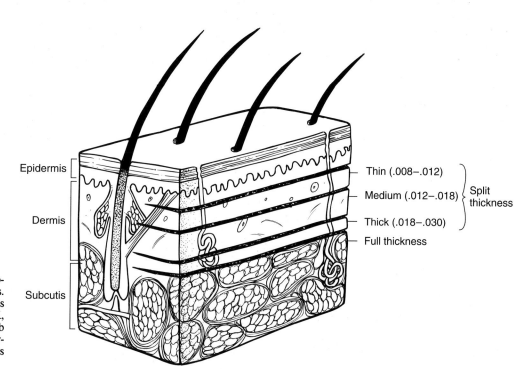

FIGURE 141–32. Schematic representation of skin graft thickness. (From Leffell DJ. Split-thickness skin grafts. In: Robinson JK, Arndt KA, LeBoit PE, Wintroub BU, eds. Atlas of Cutaneous Surgery. Philadelphia: WB Saunders Co., 1996.)

Epidermis

Dermis

Subcutis

Thin (.008–.012)
Medium (.012–.018) Split thickness
Thick (.018–.030)
Full thickness

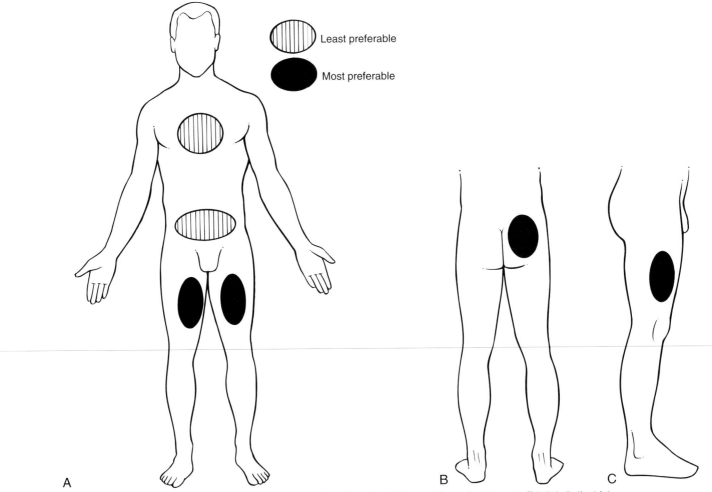

FIGURE 141–33. Useful donor locations for split-thickness skin grafts (From Leffell DJ. Split-thickness skin grafts. In: Robinson JK, Arndt KA, LeBoit PE, Wintroub BU, eds. Atlas of Cutaneous Surgery. Philadelphia: WB Saunders Co., 1996.)

rarely matches surrounding skin in color, texture, or hair-bearing characteristics (Fig. 141–34).[380, 382, 384, 385] Lastly, the thinner the graft, the greater the wound contraction that will occur.[358, 383] Therefore STSGs at free margins or cosmetic borders are likely to result in significant anatomic distortion as well as textural and pigmentary changes.

These problems notwithstanding, STSGs are still often likely to produce less morbidity in some patients when compared with large flaps, staged flaps, or free flaps. Patient and defect selection is critical when deciding upon choosing a STSG. Older patients with large defects benefit from the speed of the procedure and the lack of tissue undermining and movement. In paler complected patients, the tissue match is better. For large wounds of the forehead, alopecic scalp, posterior auricle, trunk, and extremities where donor tissue for flaps is scant, STSGs are particularly useful.

Another important use for STSGs is as temporary coverage following removal of particularly invasive tumors or those whose excisional margins are suspect. In these cases the STSG provides a "skin window" over the wound, possibly allowing earlier detection of recurrences

than would be possible through a flap or FTSG.[380] If there is no recurrence one or two years post-operatively then the STSG can be excised and more elegantly repaired.

The technique for split-thickness skin grafting is uncomplicated and quick but does require expensive equipment for larger defects.[380-384] Both the donor and recipient sites are anesthetized and prepped. The desired graft thickness is selected on the dermatome. Harvesting a graft of greater than 3×3 cm will usually require at least two and sometimes three people. One person operates the dermatome and stabilizes one side of the donor site, which must be kept firm and as flat as possible. Another person (or two) stabilizes the opposite side of the donor site and guides the graft away from the blade as it is harvested to prevent bunching and tearing of the graft (Fig. 141–35). The actual harvesting takes a matter of seconds with a power-driven dermatome. A Weck blade is slower but still rapid by "flap" standards.

A partial-thickness wound is created that can be covered in many ways. Use of any of a number of synthetic occlusive dressings such as Opsite, Omiderm, or Allevyn provides simple coverage, decreases pain, requires infre-

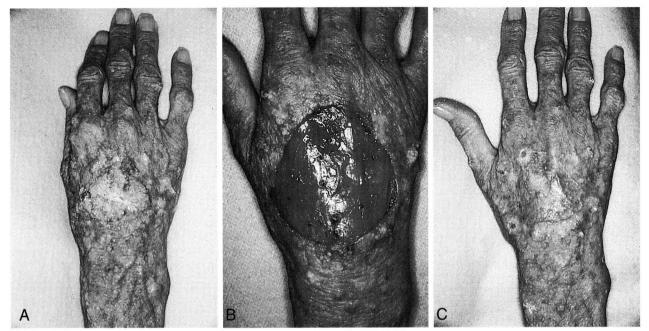

FIGURE 141–34. Squamous cell carcinoma of the hand with graft. *A,* A large well-differentiated squamous cell carcinoma covers the dorsum of the right hand of this immunosuppressed renal transplant patient. *B,* Following resection with Mohs micrographic surgery, there is sparing of the tendon sheaths; however, skin adjacent to the wound contains other primary lesions. The defect was repaired with a split-thickness skin graft from the anterior thigh donor site. *C,* Six months after the resection and repair, the patient has full function of the hand. The three other primary lesions adjacent to the graft edges were treated with excisional surgery. (Courtesy of June K. Robinson, M.D.)

quent wound care, and may speed healing.[380, 384] Daily wound care with ointment and nonstick dressings is also efficacious. Interestingly, the donor site is almost universally more painful than the primary defect in the postoperative period.

The harvested graft may be placed in sterile saline until applied or immediately sutured in place. No further preparation usually is needed except to cut it to precisely

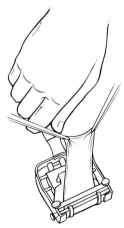

FIGURE 141–35. Split-thickness skin graft being harvested with power-driven Brown dermatome. One person guides the graft away from the blade as it is harvested. (From Leffell DJ. Split-thickness skin grafts. In: Robinson JK, Arndt KA, LeBoit PE, Wintroub BU, eds. Atlas of Cutaneous Surgery. Philadelphia: WB Saunders Co., 1996).

fit the recipient site and this is done as it is sewed into place. One modification may be to mesh the graft by cutting slits in the STSG. Meshing allows the graft to expand and cover a larger area. Also, the slits permit serous or bloody exudates to pass through and be absorbed by the dressing rather than elevate the graft off its bed preventing reattachment of capillaries, that is, graft death.[384] This process is most often used for larger truncal or extremity wounds, those overlying muscle or when covering defects when hemostasis is a problem.

The graft is anchored in place with four to eight or more paired 4-0 to 6-0 nylon or polypropylene sutures depending on the graft size. Many physicians prefer to leave one arm of each suture quite long to be used with its paired counterpart to tie a bolstering or stent dressing in place. The remaining graft margins are sutured with a simple running stitch. Use of a rapidly absorbable material such as 6-0 gut obviates the need for removal in the future. Staples may be used for larger grafts in less cosmetically sensitive areas. For larger grafts or those in concave areas, central "basting" sutures help stabilize the graft to the wound.[386] These are best placed early in the repair before the margins of the graft are secured so that any bleeding stimulated by suture placement into the graft bed may be controlled.

There are several ways to dress and secure a STSG depending on the surgeon's particular experience, preference, and graft location.[358, 381, 384, 386] The author prefers to apply a thin layer of antibiotic ointment and cover this with a nonstick permeable first layer (e.g., N-Terface).

Over this, saline-moistened sterile cotton balls are molded into place one at a time to match the contour of the defect. The first postoperative night this is secured in place with Steri-Strips. The patient returns in one day and the dressing is removed and the wound examined for hemorrhage, hematoma, or seroma formation. With hemostasis assured, the same N-Terface and moist cotton dressing is applied but this time the long sutures are used to tie the bolster in place and it is left for 5 to 7 days (Fig. 141–36). Daily wound care is discouraged so as not to disturb the graft and prevent capillary reattachment.

Typically by the end of 1 week, the graft will exhibit either complete or partial "take," that is, blood flow to the transplanted skin has been re-established and the graft will appear pink. If this does not occur within 1 or 2 weeks it is unlikely the graft will survive. Although a black, escharotic graft does not always signify failure of the graft to take, it is not a good sign and implies at least partial graft loss.[358] Factors leading to this include a poorly vascularized graft bed, hematoma, or seroma, infection, or shearing forces due to graft movement that inhibit vascular reattachment.[380, 384]

When the graft fails to survive, causative factors should be identified and rectified. The area should be cleaned, monitored frequently, and gently debrided as necrotic tissue undergoes autolysis and separates. The wound can then heal by second intention with subsequent scar revision or be regrafted (see *Atlas of Cutaneous Surgery*, Chapter 13).

Full-Thickness Skin Grafts

FTSGs are comprised of epidermis and the entire dermis without subcutaneous fat.[358, 381–384] They are still thin compared with flaps or composite grafts and are therefore useful for coverage of shallow defects, particularly of the nose, ears, eyelids, and digits. They are advantageous for the patient in that they provide rapid repair of the defect without additional tissue movement and incision lines in the area of the primary defect. In some regions, such as digits, ears, and nasal tip, there simply isn't a good tissue reservoir to effect a flap repair, making grafting the only reasonable option. FTSGs provide advantages over STSGs in many cases. Because they are thicker, there is much less retraction or shrinkage of the graft, particularly in areas over a rigid superstructure such as the ears, nose, and digits.[358, 382, 384] The added thickness also includes more adnexal structures allowing for a more normal texture postoperatively. This can be a problem as one does not wish to transfer hair-bearing skin to non–hair-bearing areas. Also, the added thickness causes increased metabolic needs for the graft, and they require more vascular recipient beds.[383, 384, 387, 388] FTSGs are usually harvested nearer to the recipient site allowing for better pigment, textural, and thickness match.

Because FTSGs include the entire dermis down to the fat they must be excised when harvested. The donor defect must then be sutured closed. This limits the size of the graft to a width that can be sutured shut and also one in which the donor site can be camouflaged. Common donor areas for facial wound include the pre-auricular crease, retro-auricular skin and sulcus, supraclavicular neck, and the melo-labial fold (Fig. 141–37).[358, 381, 384] For extremity defects, the inguinal crease provides a good tissue reservoir. Although there is little shrinkage of FTSGs, it is a good idea to harvest them with 10% to 20% greater dimensions than measured in the primary defect to ensure adequate material for coverage.[387]

A FTSG can be harvested in a number of

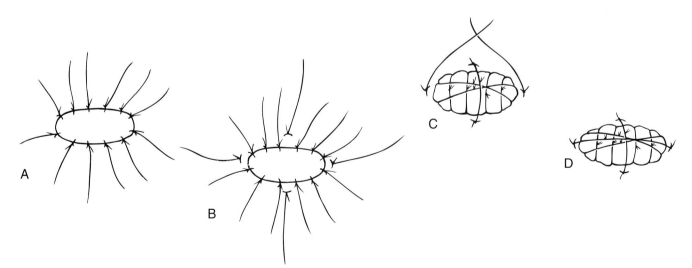

FIGURE 141–36. *A,* Sutures for the bolster are placed into the graft and wound margin like a regular interrupted suture, but one tail is left long enough to tie over the dressing. A hemostat should be available to temporarily hold all ends together so they do not get in the way of placing the next suture. *B,* Some surgeons also place four sutures into the skin away from the graft. *C,* At least four pairs (eight sutures total) should be used, and each should be tied to its corresponding suture on the other side of the bolster. Always tie the sutures that are 180 degrees away from each other rather than going in sequence around the bolster. *D,* If the surgeon chooses to use tie-over sutures distant from the graft, these sutures are tied last. (From Leffell DJ: Split-thickness skin grafts. In: Robinson JK, Arndt KA, LeBoit PE, Wintroub BU, eds. Atlas of Cutaneous Surgery. Philadelphia: WB Saunders Co., 1996.)

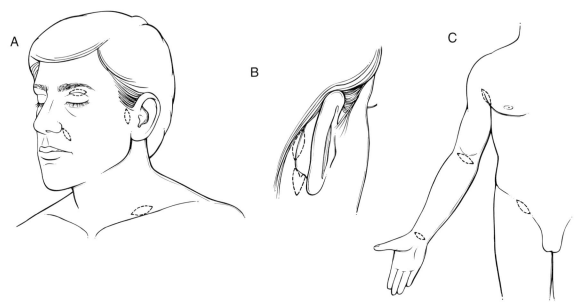

FIGURE 141–37. Donor sites commonly used to produce compatible tissue for full-thickness skin grafts of the head and neck. (From Roenigk RK, Zalla MJ. Full-thickness skin grafts. In: Robinson JK, Arndt KA, LeBoit PE, Wintroub BU, eds. Atlas of Cutaneous Surgery. Philadelphia: WB Saunders Co., 1996.)

ways.[358, 381, 384, 387] One technique is to make a template of the defect and use this to design the graft in the donor area. Because most grafts are round to ovoid, dog-ears must be cut out to close the donor site. A second method is to measure the primary defect diameter and use this as the width measurement for a standard ellipse with a 3 : 1 length-width ratio. This obviates the need to separately remove the dog-ears and helps ensure that adequate skin will be harvested. A third technique is to turn the circular primary defect into an ellipse or partial ellipse by cutting out triangular dog-ears and closing as much of the defect side to side as possible. The dog-ears removed can then be inserted as FTSGs into the remaining defect. This gives the best tissue match due to the donor site proximity, but increases incision lines in the area.[389]

Once the graft is harvested, it must be completely defatted (Fig. 141–38). Any fat left will interfere with revascularization of the graft. This is generally achieved by draping the graft fat side up over a moistened gauze pad on the second or third finger of the nondominant hand. A curved iris or blepharoplasty scissor (one blade serrated) is then used to carefully defat the graft.[381, 384, 387]

The graft is sutured in place much like the STSGs discussed above.[381, 384, 387] It is more imperative with FTSGs to ensure that the borders are meticulously sutured to avoid gaps, step-offs, or hypertrophic margins. Occasionally, one to three thin fenestrations may be cut to aid serous or hemorrhagic drainage from under the graft, but they may alter the final cosmetic appearance. Four to eight paired anchoring sutures are placed with one arm left long for use in a tie-over dressing. The graft is then trimmed to precisely fit the primary defect (Fig. 141–39). Central basting sutures may be placed for added graft security and attachment to the base.[384] These may be set in either a visualized or nonvisualized manner

(the author prefers the former). Final wound approximation may be achieved with a fine simple running suture such as 6-0 gut. The same N-Terface and moist cotton dressing technique described for STSGs above may be used for FTSGs. Either a tie-over bolster or firm taping to secure the graft for 1 week is generally employed. As with STSGs, graft survival is usually evident by 5 to 7 days postoperatively although in some instances it may take longer.[384] Cosmetic appearance can frequently be improved at 6 to 10 weeks by dermabrasion (see *Atlas of Cutaneous Surgery*, Chapter 14).[383, 390]

Composite Grafts

Composite grafts contain skin and at least one additional tissue layer including fat, muscle, cartilage, or bone.[358, 381, 383, 384, 391, 392] They are employed to reconstruct deep defects involving multiple tissue planes and when full-thickness structural loss occurs such as through-and-through defects of the nasal ala or helix of the ear. Hair transplantation represents a type of composite grafting, skin plus fat, and is applicable to cancer reconstruction for repair of eyebrow defects.[381, 393]

Repair of full-thickness alar defects is the most common use of these grafts in dermatologic cancer surgery. The structure of the nose and surrounding facial anatomy does not provide an abundant tissue reservoir for local alar repair. Side-to-side closure results in collapse and narrowing of the nasal passage. Forehead flaps are often used but are bulky and may not reproduce the fine curve of the alar rim. They require at least two stages and often more to fine-tune the repair. They cause a significant forehead scar as well. Large nasal-labial fold flaps folded under to recreate the alar rim are also bulky and may distort important cosmetic structures and borders of

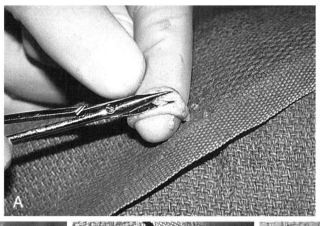

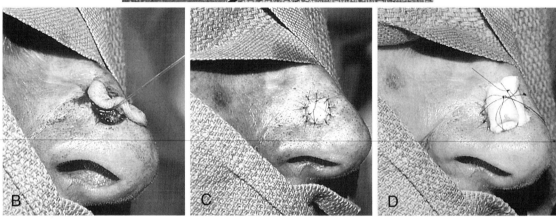

FIGURE 141–38. *A,* Defatting the graft with Gradle scissors. White dermal tissue remains on the graft, which is draped over the surgeon's left index finger. *B,* Placement of a central absorbable tacking suture. *C,* Graft sutured in place. *D,* Dental roll bolster dressing suture in place. (From Roenigk RK, Zalla MJ. Full-thickness skin grafts. In: Robinson JK, Arndt KA, LeBoit PE, Wintroub BU, eds. Atlas of Cutaneous Surgery. Philadelphia: WB Saunders Co., 1996.)

the central face. Both of these flaps may require cartilage implants from the ear to establish alar integrity and prevent collapse during respiration.

A skin-cartilage-skin composite graft from the ear can obviate many of the drawbacks to flap repair of full-thickness alar defects. Harvested from the superior crus or mid-helix (Fig. 141–40) the graft provides an excellent contour match for the nasal ala, structural rigidity, and minimal wound contraction.[381, 383, 384] The donor site is easily sutured primarily with good camouflage. The procedure is quite rapid compared with the flap procedures, is one stage, and results in less morbidity to surrounding structures.

However, there are several drawbacks to the use of composite grafts in some situations.[383, 392] The recipient bed is much smaller in relation to the graft size because it is in contact only with the graft edges, unlike STSGs and FTSGs, where the entire undersurface is in contact with the bed.[384] This increases the failure rate for composite grafts and decreases their maximum size. In general, composite grafts cannot exceed 1 to 2 cm in maximum diameter, with smaller grafts more likely to survive.[381, 383, 384] With these parameters, no portion of the graft is more than 5 to 10 mm from its nutrient source. In less vascular ares (e.g., radiation dermatitis, scar), in smokers, or in patients with compromised oxygenation

for any reason, success rates of these grafts diminish significantly. Improved success rates are dependent on choosing appropriate patients and defects and using the smallest graft possible to achieve reconstructive goals. Meticulous technique is imperative in delicately harvesting and handling the graft and in preparing the recipient site.[351, 381, 383]

The recipient site area can be maximized by beveling the edges or by using hinged flaps turned down from above the defect or up from the nasal septum.[394] This provides a richer recipient bed as well as an inner lining for the graft. Hemostasis is critical but should be done with fine pinpoint electrodesiccation or pressure to minimize char tissue.

The graft must be delicately sutured in place with a minimum of sutures utilizing small tissue bites.[394] The inner mucosal surface is secured first with an absorbable 6-0 suture.[384] The outer margin is next sutured, carefully aligning the skin and alar rim margins without tension. The cartilage does not require suturing (Fig. 141–41). Postoperative dressings need to stabilize and secure the graft in place without great pressure or bulkiness. An intranasal stent of Vaseline gauze or Xeroform gauze is required. The outer surface may be dressed with Steri-Strips and a light bandage to protect from trauma.[381, 384, 394]

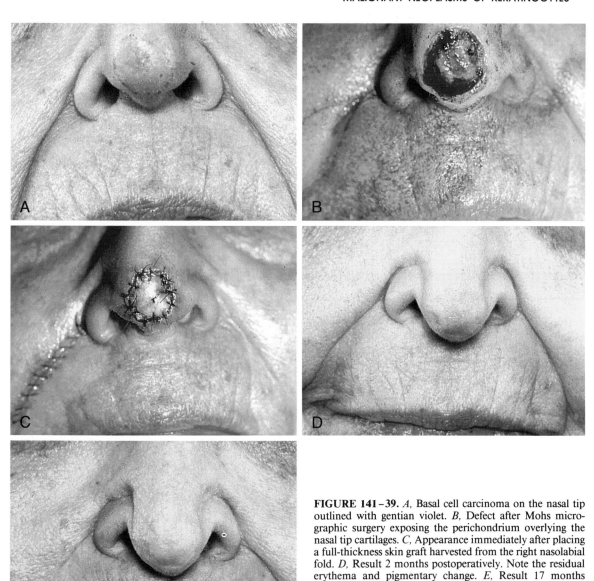

FIGURE 141–39. *A*, Basal cell carcinoma on the nasal tip outlined with gentian violet. *B*, Defect after Mohs micrographic surgery exposing the perichondrium overlying the nasal tip cartilages. *C*, Appearance immediately after placing a full-thickness skin graft harvested from the right nasolabial fold. *D*, Result 2 months postoperatively. Note the residual erythema and pigmentary change. *E*, Result 17 months postoperatively. Note that erythema and pigmentary change have resolved. The graft is cosmetically acceptable, and the donor site is imperceptible. This is an excellent result. (From Roenigk RK, Zalla MJ. Full-thickness skin grafts. In: Robinson JK, Arndt KA, LeBoit PE, Wintroub BU, eds. Atlas of Cutaneous Surgery. Philadelphia: WB Saunders Co., 1996.)

Some authors suggest frequent ice packs to chill the graft and theoretically lower its metabolic requirements for the first several days until the recipient vessels have attached to the graft.[384] Systemic steroids have also been employed to lessen inflammation around the graft. Because nasal mucosa has been breached, it is prudent to give prophylactic antibiotics.[381] This is accomplished with one dose of dicloxacillin, 2 g 1 hour preoperatively, and a second dose of 1 g 6 hours later.

Graft survival should be evident by 5 to 7 days. Success rates are reported by various authors at from 50% to 90% depending on the patient, defect, size, and technique.

EMERGING TECHNIQUES FOR TREATMENT OF MALIGNANT NEOPLASMS OF KERATINOCYTES

Photodynamic Therapy: Mechanism of Action, Technique, and Applications in the Treatment of Cutaneous Malignancy

Raab first employed photodynamic therapy (PDT) by delivering light to acridine-dye treated paramecium cultures with lethal results in 1900.[395] Jesionek and Tappenier attempted the first PDT of skin cancer in 1903.[396] They applied eosin dye to lip cancer followed by light

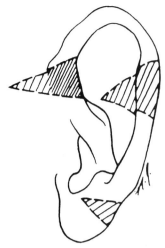

FIGURE 141-40. Composite graft donor sites of the left ear.

tizer and opened the door to the modern era of PDT.[399] But it was Thomas Dougherty and his colleagues in the 1970s and 1980s who first presented multiple ongoing studies on the use of HPD in PDT in animals and humans. Their work contributed much to the knowledge we now possess on the mechanisms of PDT, its clinical efficacy, and its current status in our armamentarium against cutaneous malignancy.[400-402]

PDT is a unique therapy requiring three essential elements to be present simultaneously. These are the *sensitizer, light,* and *oxygen*.[403] Each of these alone is without effect. However, when combined in the right concentration with the appropriate wavelength and energy of light, the light-activated sensitizer causes a photo-oxidative reaction toxic to cells. Concentration of the sensitizer in the tumor results in a highly localized tumor-specific reaction. PDT has promise as a possible anticancer therapy due to its selectivity, safety, and potential efficacy.

Technique

The technique of PDT involves two steps (Fig. 141-42).[404] The first is administration of the photosensitizer. This is generally done by intravenous injection, although experiments with topical and intralesional application have been done. During the next 24 to 72 hours, depending on the agent and protocol, the sensitizer is either selectively concentrated or preferentially retained by neoplastic tissue. This sets up a gradient of sensitizer concentration between tumor and surrounding tissue that is important in producing selective tumor destruc-

exposure. Although they were not successful, interest in the technique prevailed and numerous chemicals were investigated as photosensitizers. In 1911 Hausman first experimented with hematoporphyrin, and since then the porphyrin-based derivatives have been the major focus of interest in developing PDT.[397] Figge and coworkers in the 1940s demonstrated an affinity for neoplastic tissues by hematoporphyrin either due to selective uptake or preferential retention.[398] The synthesis of hematoporphyrin derivative (HPD) by Lipson and associates in the 1960s improved the tumor specificity of the photosensi-

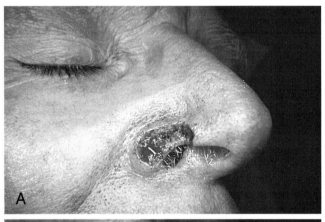

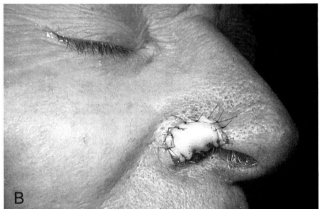

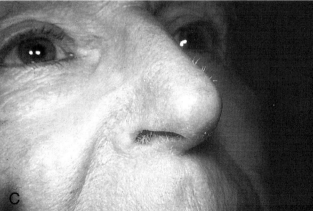

FIGURE 141-41. *A,* Loss of alar rim after resection of a basal cell carcinoma. The defect is a full-thickness loss approximately 1.8 cm in length. *B,* After placement of a skin-fat composite graft from a supraclavicular donor site, the graft is blanched white. The alar rim contour has been restored by the bulk of the skin-fat "sandwich." *C,* The final result shows restoration of the contour of the alar rim without retraction of the alar. (From Haas AF, Glogau RD. Composite graft. In: Robinson JK, Arndt KA, LeBoit PE, Wintroub BU, eds. Atlas of Cutaneous Surgery. Philadelphia: WB Saunders Co., 1995.)

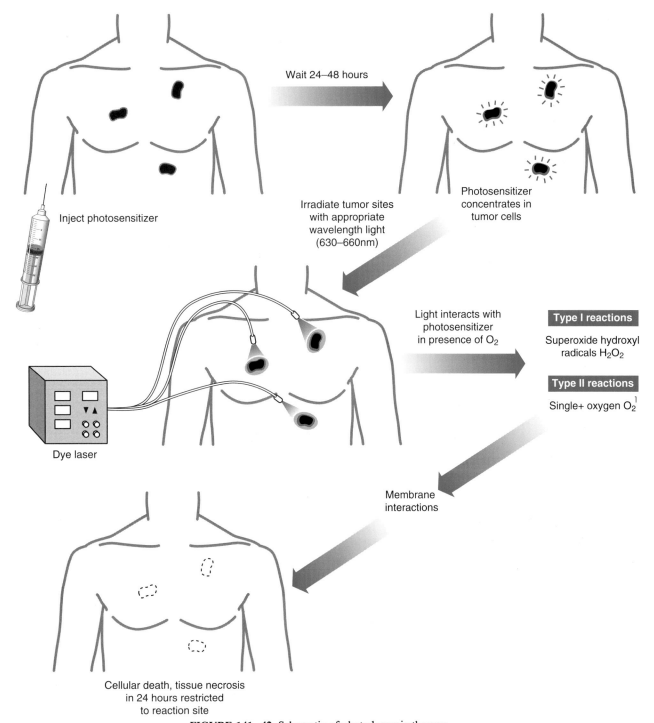

Wait 24–48 hours

Inject photosensitizer

Photosensitizer concentrates in tumor cells

Irradiate tumor sites with appropriate wavelength light (630–660nm)

Dye laser

Light interacts with photosensitizer in presence of O_2

Type I reactions

Superoxide hydroxyl radicals H_2O_2

Type II reactions

Single+ oxygen O_2^1

Membrane interactions

Cellular death, tissue necrosis in 24 hours restricted to reaction site

FIGURE 141–42. Schematic of photodynamic therapy.

tion. Light of appropriate wavelength is then delivered to activate the sensitizer within the tumor. This light, generally long-wavelength visible light, is low energy and has no effect on normal, nonsensitized skin. The light-activated sensitizer is lethal to cells (the putative mechanisms of action will be discussed below), equally so to normal or neoplastic. Three factors contribute to the selectivity of destruction. The first is a focused delivery of the light via fiber-optic cable. The second is the concen-

tration gradient of photosensitizer from tumor to surrounding normal tissue. This gradient is typically 2 : 1 to 8 : 1, depending on the agent. The third is a phenomenon known as photobleaching.[403] This defines the destruction of the sensitizer by the incident light. The threshold of light delivery for photobleaching is below that necessary for the photodestructive effect of PDT. Therefore, in areas of low sensitizer concentration the agent may be substantially destroyed prior to causing significant cellular damage. In areas of high sensitizer concentration enough agent survives photobleaching to allow for the photodynamic effect and cellular damage.

The molecular damage in PDT occurs instantly during the light-sensitizer reaction.[404] Effects appear clinically within hours as edema and erythema. They progress to frank necrosis as early as 24 hours after treatment and usually within 2 to 3 days. Eschar formation ensues, with sloughing in 2 to 3 weeks. Re-epithelialization and healing occurs over 4 to 8 weeks depending on the size and depth of the lesion. Healing is generally cosmetically quite good due to the selectivity of destruction and sparing of stromal tissues (Fig. 141–43).[405]

Short-term side effects include pain, burning, and eschar formation at the treatment site. The only long-term reactions are occasional hypertrophic scarring and prolonged photosensitivity with currently used agents (Photofrin I and II) lasting 3 to 8 weeks.[404] This photosensitivity is due to visible light and occurs in all patients. It cannot be prevented with sunscreens, and sun avoidance must be practiced until the agent is cleared sufficiently from the skin. Newer sensitizers with more rapid clearing rates will lessen this problem.

PDT does not directly involve DNA damage.[403] Mutagenesis testing has been negative, further supporting the safety of the technique.[406, 407]

Mechanism of Action

To produce the photodynamic effect all three components, the photosensitizer, light, and oxygen, must simultaneously be present. The cytotoxity in PDT is most likely due to a photo-oxidation reaction. When oxygen drops below levels of 2% in the system, no cytotoxic reaction takes place.[408] Two main types of photo-oxidative reactions occur.[403, 404] In *type I* photo-oxidation, the excited sensitizer reacts with a substrate by way of hydrogen ion or electron transfer to form radicals that react with molecular oxygen to form reactive oxygenated products. In *type II* reactions, energy from the excited sensitizer is transferred directly to oxygen, generating singlet oxygen, a highly reactive species.

The site of damage appears to be in cellular membranes including the plasma membrane, mitochondria, endoplasmic reticulum, nuclear membranes, and lysosomes.[409] The effect is rapid with loss of cellular viability noted in vitro to occur within 4 hours.[410]

Besides the direct cellular effect of PDT, there is a marked vascular effect. The vascular reactions may be due to both direct endothelial cell damage and the release of vasoactive substances[404] (eiconsanoids, histamine, factor VIII, tumor necrosis factor). Platelet clumping is seen within seconds of treatment followed eventually by stasis, hemorrhage, and coagulation necrosis.[404] Interestingly this may have a self-limiting effect on the photodynamic reaction because oxygen is such a necessary component. The vascular effects alone can result in tumor necrosis, and may in fact explain tumor death at depths below that which the delivered light can actually reach.

Photosensitizers

The ideal sensitizer is selectively absorbed or retained in tumor tissue such that concentrations are severalfold higher than in surrounding normal tissue. The sensitizer should be nontoxic without activation and rapidly cleared to avoid prolonged photosensitivity.

Most work has been done with either hematoporphyrin derivative (HPD) or the more refined dihematoporphyrin ether (DHE). Why these agents are retained in tumor cells is unknown. Selective retention may be related to a lower pH in tumor cells altering the charge status of the sensitizer and increasing binding to cellular molecules. Sensitizers are found to bind to low-density lipoproteins, and neoplastic cells exhibit increased

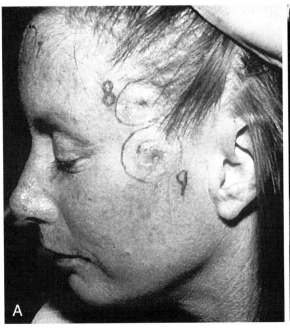
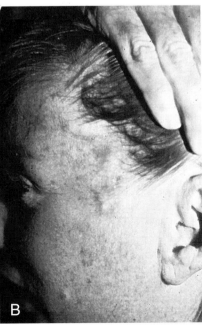

FIGURE 141–43. *A,* Two basal cell carcinomas before treatment with photodynamic therapy. *B,* Three months after treatment there is slight erythema and hypopigmentation at the site.

low-density lipoprotein receptor-mediated endocytosis. There may be pooling of sensitizer in tumors due to poor lymphatic development or leaky vessels. Finally, it is known that the sensitizers have an affinity for cells of the reticulo-endothelial system, and tumor-associated macrophages and monocytes may locally trap the agents.[403, 404]

HPD and DHE[403, 404] are rapidly cleared from circulation with only 1% of the injected dose remaining after 24 hours. The agents concentrate in tissue with liver, spleen, and kidney having the highest concentrations. For DHE, tumor-to-skin ratios in rodents are less than 2:1. DHE has five absorption bands from 400 nm (highest) to 630 nm (lowest). Despite giving the least absorption, 630 nm is used for treatment because it penetrates more deeply. Slow complete tissue elimination accounts for the prolonged photosensitivity. For these reasons, many other agents are under investigation to improve tumor-to-normal tissue ratios and allow more rapid elimination.

Chlorins are porphyrins derived from chlorophyll.[411] Chlorin-e6, (NPe6, mono-L-aspartyl chlorine e6 [MACE]) is a short-acting agent. It is rapidly taken up by tumor, and light treatment gives maximal results when given 2 hours after injection. By 12 hours after injection no effect is seen. Vascular effects seem to predominate, indicating that high plasma concentrations are important. Very little skin sensitization is reported and the rapid clearing would negate long-term photosensitivity.

Purpurins[412] are intermediate acting agents. The metallo-derivative (tin ethyletiopurpurin [SnET2]) absorbs in the 630- to 715-nm range. Response is best when light is delivered 24 hours after injection. Rapid clearing occurs, with minimal photosensitivity noted after about 1 week.[413] Benzo-porphyrin derivative is a short-acting chlorine absorbing at 690 nm. Peak activity is 3 hours after injection with 50% to 60% clearing in 48 hours.[414]

5-Aminolevulinic acid is a precursor of protoporphyrin IX in the hemoglobin synthesis pathway. In aqueous solution it passes through abnormal keratin. Complete responses in PDT of basal cell carcinoma have been reported when 5-aminolevulonic acid is applied topically.[415]

Clinical Experience with Cutaneous Malignancy

Although newer agents are being worked with in Phase I and II trials, the majority of experience in treating cutaneous malignancy is with the use of Photofrin I and II (HPD and DHE). These sensitizers are in Phase III clinical studies. As experience with dosing regimens, light energy, and time delay has been gained, efficacy and management of side effects are improving.

Most cutaneous experience is with BCC, SCC, metastatic adenocarcinoma, and Kaposi's sarcoma.

Early studies met with disappointing success, with control rates for BCC and SCC being in the 50% to 80% range.[416, 417] Compared with existing surgical modalities, this was deemed unacceptable, leading Pennington and coworkers[417] to state "that this modality has no place in the treatment of these tumors at the present time." How-

ever, alterations in dosing and light delivery have produced marked improvements in response rates. In general, by decreasing the sensitizer dose to 1 mg/kg and increasing the light dose at 630 nm to 150 to 250 joules/cm^2, response rates have improved while photosensitivity has lessened in intensity and duration.

Precise comparisons with existing surgical modalities are hampered by lack of long-term follow-up and histologic evidence of cure. In 1987 Waldow and colleagues[418] obtained complete response rates of six BCCs and three SCCs when evaluated at 3 months. In 1989 Keller and associates[419] reported complete responses in six infiltrating facial BCCs and two facial SCCs with greater than 4 years of follow-up. Two nasal alar BCCs required three and four treatments respectively to obtain a complete response. It has been noted by this group and others that infiltrating, morpheaform, and nasal tumors respond less well than nodular and superficial tumors or those in other locations.

Wilson and coworkers[420] from the Roswell Park Cancer Institute in Buffalo, NY, have probably the greatest clinical experience in treating cutaneous malignancy. They reported in 1992 on 37 patients on whom they treated 151 primary or recurrent BCC. They achieved an 88% (133/151) complete response rate with one application of PDT. Eleven of the 18 partial responses were retreated with a complete response at 14 to 29 months' follow-up. There were 24 recurrences (15.9%). Nineteen of these were retreated with a complete response clinically; however 5 of these recurred between 5 and 9 months after treatment and were referred for surgical removal.

PDT has not been found successful in treating melanomas.[421]

Summary

PDT is a promising therapy for cutaneous cancers. It may offer distinct advantages for patients with multiple tumors, poor surgical candidates, tumors in functionally or cosmetically sensitive areas, or those with surgical phobias. It may be of adjunctive help in shrinking large or inoperable tumors. Unlike radiation therapy, multiple PDT treatments to a single region are safe.

Development of new rapidly acting photosensitizers with a shorter duration of solar sensitivity and refinement of light delivery techniques will significantly improve PDT applicability and solidify its utility in treatment of cutaneous cancers.

Interferons

The interferons are a class of proteins that possess a myriad of biologic properties including antiviral, antiproliferative, antineoplastic, and immune enhancing activities. Isaacs and Lindenmann first described interferon in 1957 when they reported that virally infected cells liberate a protein that offered a protective effect upon noninfected cells. This agent was referred to as interferon to represent viral "interference."[421] Interferon is also important in other host defense activity. Currently, the interferons are Food and Drug Administration–approved for the treatment of Kaposi's sarcoma, chronic hepatitis B, hepatitis C, hairy-cell leukemia, chronic granulomatous disease, and condylomata acuminata.[422] Intense investigation is under way to define a potential role for interferons in cutaneous oncology.

The interferons are comprised of three families designated alpha (α), beta (β), and gamma (γ). Recombinant DNA technology has resulted in the ability to isolate human interferon genes, and clone them. This has permitted large-scale production of recombinant interferons.[423–425].

The interferons exert their effects upon cells via their interactions with cell surface receptors. The alpha and beta interferons utilize the same receptor, whereas gamma interferon has a unique receptor.[426] The interferons exert specific antitumor effects through a variety of mechanisms including direct antiproliferative effects, regulation of oncogenes, and depletion of cellular metabolites.[427–430] In addition, the interferons serve in an immunostimulatory fashion via their ability to enhance antitumor activity of effector cells.[431–435]

Within the realm of cutaneous oncology, the interferons have been most widely investigated in the treatment of BCC. In one large multicenter, double-blind, placebo-controlled study, intralesional recombinant interferon alfa-2b was found to yield an 80% cure rate at 1 year follow-up in patients with superficial or noduloulcerative BCCs (Fig. 141–44).[436] Injections were given three times per week over 3 weeks with a cumulative dose of 13.5 million IU. A similar study with a sustained-release formulation of interferon alfa-2b requiring only once-weekly injections over 3 weeks demonstrated an 80% cure rate with a 16-week follow-up period.[437] Interferon gamma has not been effective in the treatment of BCCs.[439]

Stenquist and colleagues evaluated the efficacy of interferon alfa-2b in BCCs with more aggressive clinical and histologic subtypes.[440] Fifteen patients with morpheaform or recurrent BCCs were referred for Mohs surgery. Prior to surgery patients received 13.5 million IU of interferon alfa-2b over 3 weeks. At the time of surgery complete resolution of tumor was found in only four subjects (27%).

In the above studies side effects associated with intralesional interferon was most frequently reported as erythema at the treatment sites and dose-dependent flu-like symptoms. With respect to the high cure rates obtained with standard surgical modalities, and their relatively low cost, intralesional interferon is not considered to be standard therapy in the management of BCC. However, it may be indicated in a select group of patients with nodular or superficial BCC who are averse to or unable to undergo surgery.

The therapeutic effect of interferon alpha has been evaluated in the treatment of cutaneous SCC. The combined results of two uncontrolled studies with varied doses of interferon alpha reveal a cure rate of 62%.[441, 442] Both of these studies lack long-term follow-up and defined their cure rates at less than 3 months. A recent study evaluated the efficacy and cosmesis with intralesional alfa-2b in the treatment of actinically induced, primary cutaneous SCCs.[443] Eighteen weeks following therapy with intralesional interferon alfa-2b (1.5 million IU injected three times per week for 3 weeks), treatment sites were excised and examined for histologic evidence of residual tumor. A complete response was demonstrated in 30/34 (88.2%), with investigators and patients reporting very good to excellent cosmetic results in 93.9% of the cases. The lack of marginal control is problematic with this potentially metastatic tumor. Therefore, the authors feel longer follow-up periods and treatment numbers are required before adding this modality to our therapeutic options for SCC. The effectiveness of intralesional interferon in the treatment of keratoacanthoma has been limited to case reports, with no controlled studies to date.[444, 445]

Intralesional interferon alpha has been proven to be

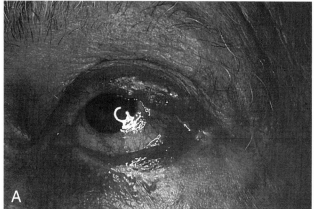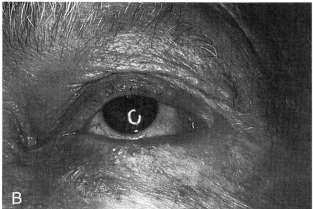

FIGURE 141–44. *A,* Prior to treatment, the primary nodular basal cell carcinoma involves the upper eyelid, lateral canthus, and lower eyelid. Reconstruction techniques are limited by prior surgical procedures in the region and the chronic radiodermatitis sustained after treatment for acne as a teenager. *B,* Response to a course of intralesional interferon alfa-2b given as nine injections over 3 weeks with a total of 13.5 million IU (1.5 million IU/injection). This patient is now 18 months after treatment. (Courtesy of June K. Robinson, M.D.)

efficacious in treating actinic keratoses when injected on multiple occasions.[446] However, in the context of effective standard treatments the cost and necessity for multiple injections renders intralesional interferon impractical in the management of actinic keratoses.

The interferons are biologic response modifiers with multiple activities. They show initial promise in the treatment of select populations of patients with cutaneous malignancies. However, their full potential in treating cutaneous malignancies will not be realized until long-term studies demonstrate their efficacy, fiscal benefits, and patient convenience.

Retinoids

The retinoids are a class of pharmacologic agents comprised of vitamin A (retinol) and its synthetic analogues, which include tretinoin, isotretinoin, etretinate, and acitretin. These agents are efficacious in the treatment of acne, psoriasis, pityriasis rubra pilaris, Darier's disease, and other disorders of keratinization. Other indications for these agents are currently under intense investigation.

The potential role for vitamin A as a therapeutic agent in the treatment of malignancies was first described by Fujimaki, who noted the development of gastric carcinomas in rats fed vitamin A–deficient diets.[447] More recent animal studies have demonstrated the efficacy of vitamin A in the inhibition of neoplastic cell growth and reversal of metaplasia.[448, 449] Vitamin A attenuates DNA synthesis, cellular growth, and decreases the number of squamous cell carcinomas in Swiss male albino mice with chemically induced SCCs by 3-methylcholanthrene.[449]

The investigation of vitamin A as a potential agent in the treatment of cutaneous malignancies in humans has been limited by its relatively low therapeutic index and high side effect profile. Hypervitaminosis A in the adult is characterized by dry scaly skin, brittle hair, cheilitis, bone and joint pain, nosebleeds, headache, fatigue, anorexia, weight loss, and rarely pseudotumor cerebri.[450] Vitamin A is also teratogenic.

The Agents

The most widely used retinoids include tretinoin, isotretinoin, etretinate, and recently introduced acitretin.

Tretinoin (all-trans retinoic acid) is a topically applied metabolite of vitamin A. It is widely used as a standard therapy in acne vulgaris. It has been demonstrated to alter the effects of photoaging on both a clinical and histopathologic basis. Decreased facial wrinkling and reversal of ultraviolet-induced dermal and epidermal structural changes are proven effects of topically applied tretinoin.[451–454]

Isotretinoin (Ro 4-3780) was the first vitamin A derivative available for systemic use in the United States. It has gained widespread use because of its dramatic therapeutic effect upon severe cystic acne. It is also efficacious in the management of the disorders of keratinization.

Etretinate and its metabolite acitretin represent the third-generation retinoids. Etretinate has been used in the treatment of psoriasis and pityriasis rubra pilaris. Acitretin is currently in use for investigational treatment of disorders of keratinization.

Mechanisms of Action

Tumorigenesis has been described in terms of initiation and promotion. Initiation refers to the permanent genotypic changes which occur in a population of cells following exposure to a carcinogen. Tumor promotion causes the genotypic changes to be phenotypically manifest. Utilizing the mouse skin model Yuspa et. al. were able to show that retinoids effect tumorigenesis by inhibiting promotion.[455] Others have demonstrated retinoid potential as an anti-carcinogen by inhibiting free radical-generating compounds.[456] Some have suggested that the retinoids may exert their antineoplastic effect by enhancing intercellular communication by increasing the number of gap junctions present on cell membranes.[457–459]

The retinoids have demonstrated the ability to inhibit the proliferation of a variety of cultured tumor lines.[460–464] They induce a dose-dependent antiproliferative effect in HL-60 (acute promyelocytic leukemia), MCF7 (mammary carcinoma), SCC4, SCC15, A431 (squamous cell carcinomas), and melanoma cell lines.[465–467] In addition to eliciting a dose-dependent growth inhibition of squamous cell carcinoma lines, retinoic acid inhibits markers of squamous differentiation including type 1 transglutaminase, cholesterol sulfate, involucrin expression, and keratin expression.[468, 469]

The retinoids may exert their effect upon cellular proliferation via the enhanced expression of epidermal growth factor receptors. Epidermal growth factor binding capacity correlates with growth inhibition.[470–472] Retinoic acid induces the expression of transforming growth factor–β, a potent inhibitor of epithelial cell growth.[473] Many tumor cell lines manifest sensitivity to the antiproliferative qualities of transforming growth factor–β.[475]

In addition to their direct antiproliferative effect, the retinoids' antineoplastic characteristics may be a function of their ability to induce and maintain normal epithelial differentiation. The retinoids exert their activity at the nuclear level. Retinoic acid receptors are members of the steroid-thyroid family of nuclear receptors. These nuclear receptors influence cellular metabolism by their interaction at specific DNA sequences known as retinoic acid response elements.[475, 476] It has been postulated that the mRNA induced by the retinoic acid response elements directs protein synthesis that eventuates in cellular differentiation and growth inhibition.[477] In vitro studies have elucidated the ability of the retinoids to induce cellular differentiation in a variety of neoplastic cell lines.[478–483]

With their ability to interfere with tumor promotion and their direct effects upon cellular growth and differentiation, the retinoids' potential role as antineoplastic agents has been and is currently under intense investigation. The retinoids have been explored in their ability to function as both chemopreventive and chemotherapeutic agents.

Actinic Keratosis

The first report of the use of tretinoin in the treatment of facial AK was by Stuttgen.[484] Since then Bollag and Ott have reported a partial response of 45% and complete regression of 40% of AK treated with topically applied tretinoin.[485] Others have reported similar results.[486]

A recent double-blind study compared the efficacy of Ro 14-9707 (an arotinoid methyl sulfone) with tretinoin in the treatment of actinic keratosis. This study revealed a 37.8% decrease in the number of actinic keratoses with Ro 14-9707 and a 30.3% response rate for those treated with tretinoin.[487] Topical tretinoin has been used in combination with topical 5-fluorouracil, yielding a higher response than either used as monotherapy.[488, 489]

Several studies have investigated the efficacy of systemic retinoids in treating actinic keratosis. The first double-blind crossover study was reported by Moriarty and coworkers.[490] This group evaluated 50 patients with actinic keratoses during a 4-month period. Subjects were randomly assigned to receive etretinate (75 mg/day) or placebo for 2-month intervals. Of the patients completing treatment with etretinate, 37/44 (84%) had a complete or partial response whereas only 2/42 (5%) subjects receiving placebo had any response. In a similar study, Watson found etretinate to be efficacious in the treatment and prevention of actinic keratosis.[491, 492]

Limited by their side effect profile, the systemic retinoids may prove most useful in the management of high-risk patients prone to develop multiple actinic keratoses. Topical retinoids for the treatment of AK lessen the toxicities of systemic retinoids, but they are not nearly as effective as existing treatments. They may function best to slowly reverse existing mild disease, as a chemopreventive agent, or in combination with other topical therapies.

Keratoacanthoma

Surgical modalities are highly efficacious in the treatment of keratoacanthomas (KAs), and lesions are known to regress spontaneously, both contributing to the limited investigation of retinoid therapy in the management of these tumors.

Although preliminary studies are encouraging, further investigation is needed to delineate the role of retinoids in the treatment and prevention of KAs. Haydey and colleagues reported the ability of oral isotretinoin, 6 mg/kg for 13 to 16 weeks, to prevent the development of new KAs in a patient with multiple KAs. New lesions developed 8 weeks following the treatment, implying the need for continuous therapy.[493] Other case reports have found isotretinoin useful in the treatment and prevention of KAs with excellent cosmetic results and limited scarring.[494–496] Longer remission rates were reported with etretinate than with isotretinoin with follow-up periods up to 24 months.[497] This may be related to the much longer elimination period for etretinate from the body.

Basal Cell Carcinoma

Because local measures are extremely efficacious in the treatment of BCCs, there is little utility in using retinoids in their treatment. Peck and associates found an 8% response of patients with multiple BCCs treated with high-dose isotretinoin (3.1 mg/kg/day).[498] An additional study by Hughes and colleagues found no effect of etretinate upon untreated BCCs.[499]

Cristofolini and coworkers suggest that etretinate may be an adjuvant therapy in patients with the nevoid BCC syndrome. They found an 83% regression rate of the tumors for a period of 1 year.[500] These limited studies have led to the investigation of retinoids as chemoprophylactic agents. In patients with the nevoid BCC syndrome, isotretinoin has been shown to attenuate the formation of new BCCs.[498, 500]

In a 3-year prospective controlled study, isotretinoin was demonstrated to prevent tumorigenesis in high-risk patients.[501] Kraemer and associates studied five patients with xeroderma pigmentosum and found that isotretinoin (2 mg/kg/day) resulted in a 65% decrease in tumor formation when compared with the 2 years preceding therapy.[501] These high doses were accompanied by toxicities (cutaneous, elevated triglycerides, hepatotoxicity, and skeletal abnormalities). This chemopreventive effect diminished over the 1-year post-treatment follow-up period.

Although there are multiple reports of high-dose retinoid therapy as effective chemoprophylactic agents in the management of BCC, the practical widespread use of chronic high-dose retinoid therapy is limited by significant toxicity. This led to a large multicenter clinical trial to test the effectiveness of chronic low-dose isotretinoin (10 mg daily) in preventing the formation of new BCCs in patients with previously treated BCCs.[502] Tangrea and associates report the results of eight centers with a total of 981 patients. After 36 months of treatment, there was no difference in the rate of occurrence of BCCs in patients treated with isotretinoin versus placebo.

Squamous Cell Carcinoma

As surgical modalities are proven to be highly effective in the treatment of localized primary SCCs, the retinoids have been evaluated in the role they may play in patients with advanced disease, those with multiple lesions, and as chemopreventive agents in high-risk groups for developing multiple cutaneous malignancies. Recent work has focused upon utilizing retinoids with other pharmacologic agents in the management of advanced squamous cell carcinoma.

Lippman and coworkers treated patients with advanced SCC for whom standard surgical or radiation therapy was unsuccessful with isotretinoin (1 mg/kg for at least 4 weeks) and found major disease regression in 4/4 patients.[503] Other studies utilizing isotretinoin or etretinate, with an additional 10 patients with advanced cutaneous SCCs, show an overall response rate of approximately 70%.[504–506]

In high-risk populations the chemopreventive effects of the retinoids in SCCs have been explored. Etretinate has been effective in chemoprevention of SCCs in renal transplant patients with no evidence of induction of kidney rejection.[507] In patients with xeroderma pigmentosum, isotretinoin was found to result in a 79% decrease in the number of cutaneous malignancies during a 2-year treatment period.[501] This chemopreventive effect was not sustained following discontinuation of isotretinoin. In patients treated for SCC of the head and neck at risk for developing second primary tumors, isotretinoin was found effective in preventing second primary tumors, however, it did not prevent recurrence of the original tumor.[508]

Current research has expanded into the potential for the retinoids to be used in conjunction with other agents with non-overlapping side effect profiles. In cultured tumor cell lines (including SCC), retinoids and interferons show additive and synergistic antiproliferative effects.[509-511] In one prospective, phase II study, the combined systemic therapy of isotretinoin and interferon alfa-2a proved highly effective in the treatment of advanced squamous cell carcinoma of the skin.[512]

Future Directions

The retinoids hold promise in the treatment and prevention of cutaneous malignancy. A plethora of laboratory evidence supports the potential for retinoids to attenuate neoplasia. Although preliminary clinical studies demonstrate retinoid activity against cutaneous neoplasia, to date there is a lack of large clinical trials supporting the efficacy of these agents in the management of cutaneous malignancies. The presence of retinoid-associated toxicities further limit their utility. They may be most beneficial as chemopreventive agents, to shrink large tumors prior to surgery or radiation or in palliation of inoperable malignancies. Future investigation is needed to develop retinoids with higher therapeutic ratios and to explore the potential for the retinoids to behave in an additive or synergistic fashion with other agents.

References

1. Montgomery H, Dorffel J. Verruca senilis und keratoma senilis. Arch Dermatol Syphilol Berlin 1932;166:286–287.
2. Marks R, Foley P, Goodman G, et al. Spontaneous remission of solar keratoses: The cause for conservative management. Br J Dermatol 1986;115:649–655.
3. Marks R, Rennie G, Selwood TS. Malignant transformation of solar keratoses to squamous cell carcinoma. Lancet 1988;1: 795–797.
4. Jones RE Jr, ed. What is the boundary that separates a thick solar keratosis and a thin squamous cell carcinoma? Am J Dermatopathol 1984;6:301–306.
5. Ackerman AB, White WL, Guo Y, et al. Differential Diagnosis in Dermatopathology IV. Philadelphia: Lea and Febiger, 1994.
6. Weedon D. Tumours of the epidermis. In Weedon D, ed. The Skin. Edinburgh: Churchill Livingstone, 1992:729–776.
7. Murphy GF, Elder DE. Atlas of tumor pathology: Non-melanocyte tumors of the skin. Washington, DC: Armed Forces Institute of Pathology, 1991:32–38.
8. Subrt P, Jorizzo JL, Apisarnthanarax P, et al. Spreading pigmented actinic keratosis. J Am Acad Dermatol 1983;8:63–67.
9. Lever WF, Schaumberg-Lever G. Histopathology of the skin, 7th edition. Philadelphia: JB Lippincott, 1990:542–546.
10. Prieto VG, Casal M, McNutt NS. Immunohistochemistry detects differences between lichen planus-like keratosis, lichen planus and lichenoid actinic keratosis. J Cutan Pathol 1993;20: 143–147.
11. Mollar R. Reymann F, Hou-Jensen K. Metastases in dermatological patients with squamous cell carcinoma. Arch Dermatol 1979;115:703–705.
12. Kossard S, Rosen R. Cutaneous Bowen's disease. J Am Acad Dermatol 1992;27:406–410.
13. Strayer DS, Sana Cruz DJ. Carcinoma in situ of the skin: A review of the histopathology. J Cutan Pathol 1980;7:244–259.
14. Klehr NW: Late manifestations in former mustard gas workers with special reference to cutaneous findings. Z Hautkr 1984;59: 1161–1164.
15. Ghadially FN, Barton BW, Kerridge DF. The etiology of keratoacanthoma. Cancer 1963;16:603–611.
16. Kern WH, McCray MK. The histopathologic differentiation of keratoacanthoma and squamous cell carcinoma of the skin. J Cutan Pathol 1980;7:318–325.
17. Piscioli F, Zumiani G, Boi S, Christofolini MA: A gigantic metastasizing keratoacanthoma. Report of a case and discussion of classification. Am J Dermatopathol 1984;6:123–129.
18. Murphy GF, Elder DE. Non-melanocytic tumors of the skin. Atlas of Tumor Pathology. Washington, DC: Armed Forces Institute of Pathology. 1991:21–27.
19. Lawrence N, Reed RJ. Actinic keratoacanthoma: Speculating on the nature of the lesion and the role of cellular immunity in its evolution. Am J Dermatopathol 1990;12:517–533.
20. Ackerman AB, Mendonca AMN, Guo Y. Differential Diagnosis in Dermatopathology I, 2nd edition. Philadelphia: Lea and Febiger, 1992:122–125.
21. Stoll DM, Ackerman AB. Subungual keratoacanthoma. Am J Dermatopathol 1980;2:265–271.
22. Cooper PH, Wolfe JT III. Perioral keratoacanthomas with extensive perineural invasion and intravenous growth. Arch Dermatol 1988;124:1397–1401.
23. Calonje E, Jones WL. Intravascular spread of keratoacanthoma: An alarming but benign phenomenon. Am J Dermatopathol 1992;14:414–417.
24. Hodak E. Jones RE, Ackerman AB. Solitary keratoacanthoma is a squamous cell carcinoma: Three examples with metastases. Am J Dermatopathol 1993;15:332–342.
25. Reed RJ. Response to Drs. Hodak et al. Am J Dermatopathol 1993;15:347–351.
26. Kwittken J. A histologic chronology of the clinical course of the keratocarcinoma (so-called keratoacanthoma). Mt Sinai J Med (NY) 1975;42:127–135.
27. Burgdorf WHC, Koester G. Multiple cutaneous tumors: What do they mean? J Cutan Pathol 1992;19:449–457.
28. Mackie RM. Epidermal skin tumours. In: Champion RH, Barton JL, Ebling FJG, eds. Textbook of Dermatology. London: Blackwell Scientific, 1992:1459–1504.
29. Witten VH, Zak FG. Multiple primary self-healing prickle cell epithelioma of the skin. Cancer 1952;5:539–550.
30. Rook A, Moffatt JL. Multiple self-healing epithelioma of Ferguson-Smith type: Report of a case of unilateral distribution. Arch Dermatol 1956;74:525–532.
31. Winklemann RK, Brown J. Generalized eruptive keratoacanthoma: Report of cases. Arch Dermatol 1968;97:615–623.
32. Shiffman NJ. Squamous cell carcinoma of the skin of the pinna. Can J Surg 1975;18:279–283.
33. Ames FC, Hickey RC. Metastasis from squamous cell carcinoma of the extremities. South Med J 1982;75:920–923.
34. Scotto J, Fearst R, Fraumeni JF. Incidence of nonmelanoma skin cancer in the United States. NIH Publication No. 83-2433. Washington, DC: US Department of Health and Human Services, 1983.
35. Glass AF, Hoover RN. The emerging epidemic of melanoma and squamous cell skin cancer. JAMA 1989;262:2097–2100.
36. Cottell WI, Proper S. Mohs' surgery, fresh tissue technique: Our technique with a review. J Dermatol Surg Oncol 1982; 8:576–587.
37. Levine H, Bailin P, Wood B, et al. Tissue conservation in treatment of cutaneous neoplasms of the head and neck: Combined use of Mohs' chemosurgical and conventional surgical techniques. Arch Otolaryngol 1979;105:140–144.
38. Levine JL, Bailin PL. Basal cell carcinoma of the head and neck: Identification of the high-risk patient. Laryngoscope 1980;90:955–961.

39. Mora CG, Robins P. Basal-cell carcinoma in the center of the face: Special diagnostic, prognostic and therapeutic considerations. J Dermatol Surg Oncol 1978;4:315–321.
40. Robins P. Chemosurgery: My 15 years of experience. J Dermatol Surg Oncol 1981;7:779–789.
41. Swanson NA. Mohs surgery: Technique, indications, applications, and the future. Arch Dermatol 1983;119:761–773.
42. Tromovitch TA, Stegman SJ. Microscopic-controlled excision of cutaneous tumors: Chemosurgery, fresh tissue technique. Cancer 1978;41:653–658.
43. Granstrom G, Aldenberg F, Jeppsson P-H. Influence of embryonal fusion lines for recurrence of basal cell carcinomas in the head and neck. Otolaryngol Head Neck Surg 1986; 95:76–82.
44. Mohs FE, Lathrop TG. Modes of spread of skin cancer. Arch Dermatol Syph 1952;66:427–439.
45. Panje WR, Ceilley RI. The influence of embryology of the mid-face on the spread of epithelial malignancies. Laryngoscope 1979;89:1914–1920.
46. Dinehart SM, Pollack SV. Metastases from squamous cell carcinoma of the skin and lip. J Am Acad Dermatol 1989; 21:241–248.
47. Rowe DE, Carroll RJ, Day CL. Prognostic factors for local recurrence, metastasis, and survival rates in squamous cell carcinoma of the skin, ear, and lip. J Am Acad Dermatol 1992;26:976–990.
48. Brodland DG, Zitelli JA: Surgical margins for excision of primary cutaneous squamous cell carcinoma. J Am Acad Dermatol 1992;27:241–248.
49. Mohs FE, Snow SN. Microscopically controlled surgical treatment for squamous cell carcinoma of the lower lip. Surg Gynecol Obstet 1985;160:37–41.
50. Mohs FE. Chemosurgery: Microscopically Controlled Surgery for Skin Cancer. Springfield, IL: Charles C. Thomas, 1978.
51. Albright SD III. Treatment of skin cancer using multiple modalities. J Am Acad Dermatol 1982;7:143–171.
52. Johnson TM, Rowe DE, Nelson BR, et al. Squamous cell carcinoma of the skin (excluding lip and oral mucosa). J Am Acad Dermatol 1992;26:467–484.
53. Immerman SC, Scanlon EF, Christ M, et al. Recurrent squamous cell carcinoma of the skin. Cancer 1983;51:1537–1540.
54. Shiu MH, Chu F, Fortner JG. Treatment of regionally advanced epidermoid carcinoma of the extremity and trunk. Surg Gynecol Obstst 180;150:558–562.
55. Weimar VM, Ceilley RI, Babin RW. Squamous-cell carcinoma with invasion of the facial nerve and underlying bone and muscle: Report of a case. J Dermatol Surg Oncol 1979; 5:526–531.
56. Cottell WI. Perineural invasion by squamous-cell carcinoma. J Dermatol Surg Oncol 1982;8:589–599.
57. Lund HZ. How often does squamous cell carcinoma metastasize? Arch Dermatol 1965;92:635–637.
58. Frierson HF, Cooper PH. Prognostic factors in squamous cell carcinoma of the lower lip. Hum Pathol 1986;17:346–354.
59. Moller R, Reymann F, Hou-Jensen K. Metastases in dermatological patients with squamous cell carcinoma. Arch Dermatol 1979;115:703–705.
60. Breuninger H, Black G, Rassner G. Microstaging of squamous cell carcinomas. Am J Clin Pathol 1990;94:624–627.
61. Friedman H, Friedman HI, Cooper PH, et al. Prognostic and therapeutic use of microstaging of cutaneous squamous cell carcinoma of the trunk and extremities. Cancer 1985;56: 1099–1105.
62. Dinehart SM, Chu DZJ, Maners AW, et al. Immunosuppression in patients with metastatic squamous cell carcinoma from the skin. J Dermatol Surg Oncol 1990;16:271–274.
63. Epstein E, Epstein NN, Bragg K, et al. Metastases from squamous cell carcinoma of the skin. Arch Dermatol 1968; 97:245–249.
64. Schwartz RA. Buschke-Loewenstein tumor: Verrucous carcinoma of the penis. J Am Acad Dermatol 1990;23:723–727.
65. Headington JT. Verrucous carcinoma. Cutis 1978;21:207–211.
66. Mohs FE, Sahl WJ. Chemosurgery for verrucous carcinoma. J Dermatol Surg Oncol 1979;5:302–306.
67. Swanson NA, Taylor WB. Plantar verrucous carcinoma: Literature review and treatment by Mohs' chemosurgery. Arch Dermatol 1980;116:794–797.
68. Johnson WC, Helwig EB. Adenoid squamous cell carcinoma (adenocanthoma). A clinocopathologic study of 155 patients. Cancer 1966;19:1639–1650.
69. Nappi O, Pettinato G, Wick MR. Adenoid (acantholytic) squamous cell carcinoma of the skin. J Cutan Pathol 1989; 16:114–121.
70. Cubilla AL, Barreto J, Caballero C, et al. Pathologic features of epidermoid carcinoma of the penis. A prospective study of 66 cases. Am J Surg Pathol 1993;17:753–763.
71. McKee PH, Wilkinson JD, Black MM, et al. Carcinoma (epithelioma) cuniculatum: A clinicopathological study of nineteen cases and review of the literature. Histopathology 1981; 5:425–436.
72. Potter M. Percivall Pott's contribution to cancer research. NCI Monogr 1963;10:1–6.
73. Hueper WC. Chemically induced skin cancer in man. NCI Monogr 1963;10:377–391.
74. Tseng WP. Effects and dose-response relationships of skin cancer and blackfoot disease with arsenic. Environ Health Perspect 1977;19:109–119.
75. Neubauer O. Arsenical cancer: A review. Br J Cancer 1947;1:192–251.
76. Sadamori N, Mine M, Hori M. Skin cancer among atom bomb survivors. Lancet 1989;1:1267.
77. Traenkle H. X-ray induced skin cancer in man. NCI Monogr 1963;10:423–432.
78. Moy RL, Eliezri YD, Nuovo GJ, et al. Human papillomavirus type 16 DNA in periungual squamous cell carcinomas. JAMA 1989;261:2669–2673.
79. Gupta AK, Cardella CJ, Haberman HF. Cutaneous malignant neoplasms in patients with renal transplants. Arch Dermatol 1986;122:1288–1293.
80. Mendonca H. Squamous cell carcinoma arising in hidradenitis suppurativa. J Dermatol Surg Oncol 1991;17:830–832.
81. Goldberg DJ, Arbesfeld D. Squamous cell carcinoma arising in a site of chronic osteomyelitis: Treatment with Mohs micrographic surgery. J Dermatol Surg Oncol 1991;17:788–790.
82. Robbins JH, Kraemer KH, Lutzner MA, et al. Xeroderma pigmentosum: An inherited disorder with sun sensitivity, multiple cutaneous neoplasms, and abnormal DNA repair. Ann Intern Med 1974;80:221–248.
83. Kaspar TA, Wagner RF, Jablonska S, et al. Prognosis and treatment of advanced squamous cell carcinoma secondary to epidermodysplasia verruciformis: A worldwide analysis of 11 patients. J Dermatol Surg Oncol 1991;17:237–240.
84. Newman C, et al. Squamous cell carcinoma secondary to recessive dystrophic epidermolysis bullosa: A report of 4 patients with 17 primary cutaneous malignancies. J Dermatol Surg Oncol 1992;18:301–305.
85. Keeler CE. Albinism, xeroderma pigmentosum, and skin cancer. Natl Cancer Inst Monogr 1963;10:349–359.
86. Scotto J, Fears TR, Fraumeni JF, et al. Incidence of Nonmelanoma Skin Cancer in the United States. Washington, DC: Public Health Service, 1983. National Institutes of Health publication 1983;83–2433.
87. Stone JL, Elpern DJ, Reizner G, et al. Incidence on non-melanoma skin cancer in Kawai during 1983. Hawaii Med J 1986;45:281–286.
88. Giles G, Marks R. Foley P. Incidence of non-melanocytic skin cancer treated in Australia. Br Med J 1988;296:13–17.
89. Freeman RG. Data on the action spectrum for ultraviolet carcinogenesis. J Natl Cancer Inst 1975;55:1119–1121.
90. Winkleman RK, Zollman PE, Baldes EJ. Squamous cell carcinoma produced by ultraviolet light in hairless mice. J Invest Dermatol 1963;40:217–224.
91. Vitasa BC, Taylor HR, Strickland PT, et al. Association of nonmelanoma skin cancer and actinic keratosis with cumulative solar ultraviolet exposure in Maryland watermen. Cancer 1990;65:2811–2817.
92. Zackheim HS. Origin of the human basal cell epithelioma. J Invest Dermatol 1963;40:283–297.

93. Sanderson KV. The architecture of basal cell carcinoma. Br J Dermatol 1961;73:455–474.
94. Madsen A. The histogenesis of superficial basal cell epitheliomas. Unicentric or multicentric origin. Arch Dermatol Syphil 1955;72:29–30.
95. Madsen A. The theory of the multicentric origin of basal cell epithelioma lacks evidence. Act Dermatovener 1956;36:102–111.
96. Lang PG Jr, McKelvey AC, Nicholson JH. Three-dimensional reconstruction of the superficial multicentric basal cell carcinoma using serial sections and a computer. Am J Dermatopathol 1987;9:198–203.
97. Mohs FE. Micrographic surgery for the microscopically controlled excision of eyelid cancer: History and development. Adv Ophthal Plast Reconstr Surg 1986;5:381–408.
98. Robins P. Chemosurgery: My 15 years of experience. J Dermatol Surg Oncol 1981;7:779–789.
99. Sexton M, Jones DB, Maloney ME. Histologic pattern analysis of basal cell carcinoma. J Am Acad Dermatol 1990;23:1118–1126.
100. Salasche SJ, Amonette R. Morpheaform basal-cell epitheliomas: A study of subclinical extensions in a series of 51 cases. J Dermatol Surg Oncol 1981;7:387–392.
101. Siegle RJ, MacMillan J, Pollack SV. Infiltrative basal cell carcinoma: A nonsclerosing subtype. J Dermatol Surg Oncol 1986;12:830–836.
102. Borel DM. Cutaneous basosquamous carcinoma: A review of the literature and report of 35 cases. Arch Pathol Lab Med 1973;95:293–297.
103. Hanke CW, et al. Perineural spread of basal-cell carcinoma. J Dermatol Surg Oncol 1983;9:742–747.
104. Ackerman AB, DeViragh PA, Chongchitnant N. Neoplasms with follicular differentiation. Philadelphia: Lea & Febiger, 1993:605–658.
105. Schwartz RA, Hansen RC, Maize JC. The blue-grey cystic basal cell epithelioma. J Am Acad Dermatol 1980;2:155–160.
106. Madsen A. De L'epithelioma baso-cellulaire superficiel. Acta Dermatovener 1941;7(Suppl.):1–161.
107. Farmer ER, Helwig EB. Metastatic basal cell carcinoma: A clinicopathologic study of seventeen cases. Cancer 1980;46:748–757.
108. Pinkus H. Premalignant fibroepithelial tumors of skin. Arch Dermatol 1953;67:598–615.
109. Walsh N, Ackerman AB. Infundibulocystic basal cell carcinoma: A newly discussed variant. Modern Pathol 3:599–608, 1990.
110. Walsh N, Ackerman AB. Basaloid follicular hamartoma: Solitary and multiple types (letter). J Am Acad Dermatol 1993;29:125–127.
111. Brownstein MH. Reply to Drs Walsh and Ackerman (letter). J Am Acad Dermatol 1993;29:127–129.
112. White WL, Abernethy JL. Other questions on basaloid follicular hamartoma. Arch Dermatol 1994;130:254–255.
113. Sakamoto F, Ito M, Sato S, et al. Apocrine epithelioma. J Am Acad Dermatol 1985;13:355–363.
114. Sanchez NP, Winkelmann RK. Basal cell tumor with eccrine differentiation (eccrine epithelioma). J Am Acad Dermatol 1982;6:514–518.
115. Lopes de Faria J. Basal cell carcinoma of the skin with areas of squamous cell carcinoma: A basosquamous cell carcinoma? J Clin Pathol 1985;38:1273–1277.
116. McGibbon DH. Malignant epidermal tumours. J Cutan Pathol 1985;12:224–238.
117. Barr RJ, Alpern KS, Santa Cruz DJ, et al. Clear cell basal cell carcinoma: An unusual degenerative variant. J Cutan Pathol 1993;20:308–316.
118. Miller SJ. Biology of basal cell carcinoma (Part I). J Am Acad Dermatol 1991;24:1–13.
119. Dix CR. Occupational trauma and skin cancer. Plast Reconstr Surg 1960;26:546–554.
120. Noodleman RF, Pollack SV. Trauma as a possible etiologic factor in basal cell carcinoma. J Dermatol Surg Oncol 1986;12:841–846.
121. Allison JR. Radiation-induced basal-cell carcinoma. J Dermatol Surg Oncol 1984;10:200–203.
122. Everall JD, Dowd PM: Influence of environmental factor excluding ultraviolet radiation on the incidence of skin cancer. Bull Cancer 1978;65:241–247.
123. Schoolmaster WL, White DR. Arsenic poisoning. South Med J 1980;73:198–207.
124. Milstone EB, Helwig EB. Basal cell carcinoma in children. Arch Dermatol 1973;108:523–527.
125. Ademiluyi SA, Ijaduola GT. Occurrence and recurrence of basal cell carcinoma of the head and neck in Negroid and albinoid Africans. J Laryngol Otol 1987;101:1324–1328.
126. Plosila M, Kiistala R, Niemi KM. The Bazex syndrome: follicular atrophoderma with multiple basal cell carcinomas, hypotrichosis and hypohidrosis. Clin Exp Dermatol 1981;6:31–41.
127. Goldstein GD, Whitaker DC, Argenyi ZB, et al. Basal cell carcinoma arising in a sebaceous nevus during childhood. J Am Acad Dermatol 1988;18:429–430.
128. Anderson TE, Best PV. Linear basal cell neavus. Br J Dermatol 1962;74:20–23.
129. Mikhail GR, Nims LP, Kelly AP Jr, et al. Metastatic basal cell carcinoma. Review, pathogenesis and report of two cases. Arch Dermatol 1977;113:1261–1269.
130. von Domarus H, Steven PJ. Metastatic basal cell carcinoma. Report of five cases and review of 170 cases in the literature. J Am Acad Dermatol 1984;10:1043–1060.
130a. Lo JS, Snow SN, Reizner GT, et al. Metastatic basal cell carcinoma: Report of twelve cases with a review of the literature. J Am Acad Dermatol 1991;24:715–719.
131. Toker C. Trabecular carcinoma of the skin. Arch Dermatol 1972;105:107–110.
132. Tang CK, Toker C. Trabecular carcinoma of the skin: An ultrastructural study. Cancer 1978;42:2311–2321.
133. Tang CK, Toker C. Trabecular carcinoma of the skin: Further clinicopathologic and ultrastructural study. Mt Sinai J Med NY 1979;46:516–523.
134. Figerio B, Capella C, Eusebi V, et al. Merkel cell carcinoma of the skin: The structure and origin of normal Merkel cells. Histopathology 1983;7(2):229–249.
135. Pilotti S, Rilke F, Lombardi L. Neuroendocrine (Merkel cell) carcinoma of the skin. Am J Surg Pathol 1982;6(3):243–254.
136. Wide MR. Goellner JR, Scheithauer BW, et al. Primary neuroendocrine carcinomas of the skin (Merkel cell tumors): A clinical, histologic, and ultrastructural study of 13 cases. Am J Clin Pathol 1983;79:6–13.
137. Shaw JHF, Rumball E. Merkel cell tumor: Clinical behavior and treatment. Br J Surg 1991;78:138–143.
138. LeBoit PE, Crutcher W, Shapiro PE. Pagetoid epidermal spread in cutaneous neuroendocrine (Merkel cell) carcinoma. Am J Surg Pathol 1992;16:584–592.
139. Gould E, Albores-Saavedra J, Dubner B, et al. Eccrine and squamous differentiation in Merkel cell carcinoma. An immunohistochemical study. Am J Surg Pathol 1988;12:768–772.
140. Shah IA, Netto D, Schlageter MO, et al. Neurofilament immunoreactivity in Merkel cell tumor. A differentiating feature from small cell carcinoma. Mod Pathol 1993;6:3–9.
141. Saurat JH, Chavez P, Carraux P, et al. A human monoclonal antibody reaction with Merkel cells: Immunofluorescence, immunoperoxidase and immunoelectron microscopy. J Invest Dermatol 1983;81:249–253.
142. Gu J, Polak JM, Topia FJ, et al. Neuron-specific enolase in the Merkel cells of mammalian skin. Am J Pathol 1981;104:63–68.
143. Merot T, Margolis RJ, Dahl D, et al. Coexpression of neurofilament and keratin proteins in cutaneous neuroendocrine carcinoma cells. J Invest Dermato 1986;86:74–77.
144. Penneys NS, Shapiro S: CD44 expression in Merkel cell carcinoma may correlate with risk of metastasis. J Cutan Pathol 1994;21:22–25.
145. Taxy JB, Ettinger DS, Wharom MD. Primary small cell carcinoma of the skin. Cancer 1980;46:2308–2311.
146. Hitchcock CL, Bland KI, Laney RG, et al. Neuroendocrine (Merkel cell) carcinoma of the skin: Its natural history, diagnosis, and treatment. Ann Surg 1988;207:201–207.
147. George TK, Di Saint 'Agnese PA, Bennett JM: Chemotherapy for metastatic Merkel cell carcinoma. Cancer 1985;56:1034–1038.
148. Rowe DE, Carroll RJ, Day CL Jr. Long term recurrence rates in

previously untreated (primary) basal cell carcinoma: Implications for patient follow-up. J Dermatol Surg Oncol 1989;15:315–327.

149. Silverman MK, Kopf AW, Grin CM, et al. Recurrence rates of treated basal cell carcinoma, part 1: Overview. J Dermatol Surg Oncol 1991;17:L713–718.

150. Silverman MK, Kopf AW, Grin MC, et al. Recurrence rates of treated basal cell carcinoma, part 2: Curettage-electrodesiccation. J Dermatol Surg Oncol 1991;17:720–726.

151. Silverman MK, Kopf AW, Grin CM, et al. Recurrence rates of treated basal cell carcinoma, part 3: Surgical excision. J Dermatol Surg Oncol 1992;18:471–476.

152. Silverman MK, Kopf AW, Gladstein AH, et al. Recurrence rates of treated basal cell carcinoma, part 4: X-ray therapy. J Dermatol Surg Oncol 1992;18:549–554.

153. Reymann F. Basal cell carcinoma of the skin: Recurrence rate after different types of treatment. Dermatologica 1980; 161:217–226.

154. Melcalf JS, Maize JC. Histopathologic considerations in the management of basal cell carcinoma. Semin Dermatol 1989; 8(4):259–265.

155. Lang PG, Maize JC. The histologic evolution of the recurrent basal cell carcinoma and treatment implications. J Am Acad Dermatol 1986;14:186–196.

156. Sexton MF, Jones DB, Maloney M. Histologic pattern analysis of basal cell carcinoma. A study of 1,039 consecutive neoplasms. J Am Acad Dermatol 1990;23:1118–1126.

157. Suhge d'Aubermont PC, Bennett RG. Failure of C&E for removal of basal cell carcinoma. Arch Dermatol 1984; 120:1456–1460.

158. Popkin GL. C&E. NY State J Med 1968;68:866.

159. Popkin GL, Bart RS. Excision versus C&E as office procedures for the treatment of basal cell carcinomas. J Dermatol Surg Oncol 1975;1:33–35.

160. Salasche SJ. C&E in the treatment of mid-face basal cell carcinoma. J Am Acad Dermatol 1983;8:496.

161. Salasche SJ. Status of curettage and desiccation in the treatment of primary basal cell carcinoma. J Am Acad Dermatol 1984;10:285.

162. Wagner RF, Cottel WI. Multifocal recurrent basal cell carcinoma following primary tumor treatment by electrodesiccation and curettage. J Am Acad Dermatol Surg 1987;17(6): 1047–1049.

163. Johnson TM, Rowe DE, Nelson BR, Swanson NA. Squamous cell carcinoma of the skin (excluding lip and oral mucosa). J Am Acad Dermatol 1992;26:467–484.

164. Rowe DE, Carroll RJ, Day CL. Prognostic factors for local recurrence, metastasis, and survival rates in squamous cell carcinoma of the skin, ear, and lip, implications for treatment modality selection. J Am Acad Dermatol 1992;26:976–990.

165. Brodland DG, Zitelli JA. Surgical margins for excision of primary cutaneous squamous cell carcinoma. J Am Acad Dermatol 1992;27:241–248.

166. Dzubow LM, Rigel DS, Robbins P. Risk factors for local recurrence of primary cutaneous squamous cell carcinomas, Treatment by microsurgically controlled excision. Arch Dermatol 1982;118:900–992.

167. Banks ER, Cooper PH. Adenosquamous cell carcinoma of the skin: A report of 10 cases. J Cutan Pathol 1991;18:227–234.

168. Marks R, Foley P, Goodman G, et al. Spontaneous remission of solar keratoses. Br J Dermatol 1986;115:649–655.

169. Marks R, Kennie G, Selwood TS. Malignant transformation of solar keratoses to squamous cell carcinoma. Lancet 1988;1:795–797.

170. Kwa RE, Campana K, Moy RL. Biology of cutaneous squamous cell carcinoma. J Am Acad Dermatol 1992;26:1–26.

171. Rowe DE, Carroll RJ, Day CL. Mohs surgery is the treatment of choice for recurrent (previously treated) basal cell carcinoma. J Dermatol Surg Oncol 1989;15:4.

172. Kopf AW, Bart RS, Schrager D, et al. Curettage-electrodesiccation-treatment of basal cell carcinomas. Arch Dermatol 1977;113:439–443.

173. Marks R, Rennie G, Selwood T. The relationship of basal cell carcinoma and squamous cell carcinoma to solar keratoses. Arch Dermatol 1988;124:1034–1042.

174. Johnson TM, Tromovitch TA. Combined C&E (C&E) treatment for basal cell carcinoma. J Am Acad Dermatol 1991;24:613–617.

175. Greenbaum SS, Glogau RG. CO_2 laser treatment of erythroplasia of Queyrat. J Dermatol Surg Oncol 1989;15:747–750.

176. Adams EL, Price NM. Treatment of the basal cell carcinomas with the CO_2 laser. J Dermatol Surg Oncol 1979;5:803–806.

177. Hobbs ER, Bailin PL, Wheeland RG. Superpulsed lasers: Minimizing thermal damage with short duration, high irradiance pulses. J Dermatol Surg Oncol 1987;13:955–964.

178. Dufresne RG, Garrett AB. CO_2 laser treatment of chronic actinic cheilitis. J Am Acad Dermatol 1988;19:976–878.

179. Johnson TM, Sebastien TS, Nelson BR. CO_2 laser treatment of actinic cheilitis. J Am Acad Dermatol, 1992;27:737–740.

180. Zelickson BD, Roenigk RK. Actinic cheilitis treated with the CO_2 laser. Cancer 1990;65:1307–1311.

181. Wolf DJ, Zitelli JA. Surgical margins for basal cell carcinoma. Arch Dermatol, 1987;123:340–344.

182. Robinson JK. What are adequate treatment and follow-up care for nonmelanoma cutaneous cancer? Arch Dermatol 1987; 123:331–333.

183. Salasche SJ, Amonette RA. Morpheaform basal cell epitheliomas: A study of subclinical extensions in a series of 51 cases. J Dermatol Surg Oncol 1981;7:387–393.

184. Lobo DV, Chu P, Grekin RC, Berger TG. Non-melanoma skin cancers and infection with the human immuno-deficiency virus. Arch Dermatol 1992;128:623–627.

185. Roenigk RK, Roenigk HH. Current surgical management. J Dermatol Surg Oncol 1990;16(2):136–151.

186. Torre D. Cryosurgery instrumentation and depth dose monitoring. In: Clinics in Dermatology: Advances in Cryosurgery, vol. 8. New York: Elsevier, 1990:48.

187. Brooks NA. Curettage and shave excision. J Am Acad Dermatol 1984;10:279–284.

Radiation of Skin Cancer

188. Metcalf PB. Carcinoma of the pinna. N Engl J Med 1954;251:991–995.

189. Schewe EJ, Pappalardo C. Carcinoma of the external ear. Am J Surg 1962;104:753–755.

190. Parker RG, Wildermuth O. Radiation therapy of lesions overlying cartilage; carcinoma of the pinna. Cancer 1962;15:57–62.

191. Mendenhal WM, Parson JT, Mendenhall NP, et al. T2-T4 carcinoma of the skin of the head and neck, treated with radical irradiation. Int J Radiation Oncol Biol Phys 1987;13:975–981.

192. Petrovich Z, Kuisk H, LangHolz B, et al. Treatment of carcinoma of the skin with bone and/or cartilage involvement. Am J Clin Oncol 1988;11:10–12.

193. Bart RS, Kopk AW, Gladstein AH. Treatment of morphea-type basal cell carcinomas with radiation therapy. Arch Dermatol 1977;113:783–786.

194. Mendenhall WM, Parson JT, Mendenhall NP, et al. Carcinoma of the skin of the head and neck with perineural invasion. Head and Neck 1989;11:301–308.

195. Goepfert H, Dichtel WJ, Medina JE, et al. Perineural invasion in squamous cell skin cancer of the head and neck. Head Neck 1989;11:301–308.

196. Ballantyne A, McCarten AB et al. The extension of cancer of the head and neck through peripheral nerves. Am J Surg 1963;106:651–667.

197. Cassissi NJ, Dickerson DR, Million R. Squamous cell carcinoma of the skin metastatic to parotid nodes. Arch Otolaryngol 1987;104:336–339.

198. Mendenhall NP, Million R, Cassissi N. Parotid area lymph node metastases from cancer of this skin. Int J Radiat Oncol Biol Phys 1985;11:707–714.

199. Zacarian SA. Cryosurgery of skin cancer: Fundamentals of technique and application. Cutis 1975;16:449–460.

200. Atkinson HR. Skin carcinoma depth and dose homegeneity in dermatological x-ray therapy. Aust J Dermatol 1962; 6:208–212.

201. Goldschmidt H, Sherwin WK. Office radiotherapy of cutaneous carcinomas, radiation techniques, dose schedules, and radiation protection. J Dermatol Surg Oncol 1983;9:31–46.

202. Farina AT, Leider M, Newall J, et al. Modern radiotherapy for malignant epitheliomas. Arch Dermatol 1977;113:650–654.
203. Strandquist M. Studien Uber Die Kumulative Urkung Der Roetgenstrahlen Bei Fractionerung. Acta Radiol 1944; 55(Suppl.):1–292.
204. Von Essen CF. A spatial model of time-dose area relationships in radiation therapy. Radiology 1963;81:881–883.
205. Hliniak A, Maciejewski B. The influence of the number of fractions, overall treatment time and field size on the local control of cancer of the skin. Br J Radiol 1983;56:596–598.
206. Turesson I, Notter G. The influence of fraction size in radiotherapy on the late normal tissue reaction—II: Comparison of the effects of daily and twice a week fractionation on human skin. Int J Radiat Oncol Biol Phys 1984;10:599–606.
207. Traenkle HL, Mulay D. Further observations of the late radiation necrosis following therapy of skin cancer. Arch Dermatol 1960;81:908–913.
208. Williams PC; Hendry JH. The RBE of megavoltage photons and electron beams. Br J Radiol 1978;51:220.
209. Sinclair WK, Kohn HI. The relative biological effectiveness of high energy photons and electrons. Radiology 1964; 82:800–814.
210. Rowe EE, Carroll RJ, Day CL Jr. Long term recurrence rates in previously untreated (primary) basal cell carcinoma; implications for patient follow-up. J Dermatol Surg Oncol 1989; 15:315–325.
211. Fitzpatrick PJ, Thompson GA, Easterbrook WM, et al. Basal and squamous cell carcinoma of the eyelids and their treatment by radiotherapy. Int J Radiat Oncol Biol Phys 1984; 10:449–454.
212. Petrovich Z, Kuisk H, LangHolz B et al. Treatment results and patterns of failure in 646 patients with carcinoma of the eyelids, pinna and nose. Am J Surg 1987;154:447–450.
213. Petrovich Z, Parker RG, Luxton G, et al. Carcinoma of the lip and selected site of head and skin. A clinical study of 896 patients. Radiother Oncol 1987;8:11–17.
214. Lovett Rd, Perez CA, Shapiro SJ, et al. External irradiation of epithelial skin cancer. Int J Radiat Oncol Biol Phys 1990; 19:235–242.
215. Guthrie TH, Porubsky ES, Luxenberg MN, et al. Cisplatinum based chemotherapy in advanced basal and squamous cell carcinomas of the skin. Results in 28 patients including 13 patients receiving multimodality therapy. J Clin Oncol 1990;8:342–346.
216. Khansur T, Kennedy A. Cisplatin and 5-fluorouracil for advanced locoregional and metastatic squamous cell carcinoma of the skin. Cancer 1991;67:2030–2032.
217. Sadek H, Azli, Wendling JL, Curthosovic. Treatment of advanced squamous cell carcinoma of the skin with cisplatinum, 5 Fluorouracil and Bleomycin. Cancer 1990;66:1692–1696.
218. Nigro N, Vaitkevicius VK, Buroker T, et al. Combined therapy for cancer of the anal canal. Dis Colon Rectum 1981;24:73–75.
219. Cummings BJ, Keane TJ, O'Sullivan CN. Epidermoid anal cancer: Treatment by radiation alone or by radiation and 5-Fluorouracil with and without Mitomycin C. Int J Radiat Oncol Biol Phys 1991;21:1115–1125.

Mohs Micrographic Surgery

220. Mohs RE, Chemosurgery. A microscopically controlled method of cancer excision. Arch Surg 1941;42:279–295.
221. Bart R, Schrager D, Kopf A, et al. Scalpel excision of basal cell carcinoma. Arch Dermatol 1978;114:739–742.
222. Mohs FE. Chemosurgery: Microscopically controlled surgery for skin cancer. Springfield, IL: Charles C. Thomas, 1978.
223. Tromovitch TA, Beirne GA, Beirne CG. Cancer chemosurgery. Cutis 1965;1:523–529.
224. Phelan JT, Milgrom H. The use of Mohs chemosurgery technique of the treatment of skin cancers. Surg Gynecol Obstet 1967;125:549–560.
225. Robins P. Chemosurgery: A surer method to treat basal cell epithelioma. Consultant 1974;14:137–142.
226. Robins P, Menn H. Chemosurgery in the treatment of skin cancer. Hosp Pract 1970;5:40–50.
227. Tromovitch TA, Stegman SJ. Microscopic-controlled excision. Dermatol Digest 1976;15:12–19.
228. Tromovitch TA, Stegman SJ. Microscopically controlled excision of skin tumors. Arch Dermatol 1974;110:231–232.
229. Mohs FE. Chemosurgery for skin cancer: Fixed tissue and fresh tissue techniques. Arch Dermatol 1976;112:211–215.
230. Tromovitch TA, Stegman SJ. Microscopic controlled excision of cutaneous tumors: Chemosurgery, fresh tissue technique. Cancer 1978;41:653–658.
231. Robins P. Chemosurgery: My 15 years of experience. J Dermatol Surg Oncol 1981;7:779–789.
232. Roenigk RK, Ratz JL, Bailin PL, Wheeland RG. Trends in the presentation and treatment of basal cell carcinomas. J Dermatol Surg Oncol 1986;12:860–865.
233. Davidson TM, Nahum AM, Astarita RW. Microscopic controlled excisions for epidermoid carcinoma of the head and neck. Otolaryngol Head Neck Surg 1981;89:244–251.
234. Rowe DE, Carrol RJ, Day CL Jr. Long-term recurrence rates in previously untreated (primary) basal cell carcinoma: Implications for patient follow-up. J Dermatol Surg Oncol 1989;15:315–328.
235. Silverman ML, Kopt, AW, Bart RS, et al. Recurrence rates of treated basal cell carcinomas. J Dermatol Surg Oncol 1992;18:471–476.
236. Bailin PL, Levine HL, Wood HL, Tucker H. Tissue conservation in treatment of cutaneous neoplasms of the head and neck. Arch Otolaryngol 1979;105:140–144.
237. Levine JL, Bailin PL. Basal cell carcinoma of the head and neck: Identification of the high-risk patient. Laryngoscope 1980;90:955–961.
238. Mora CG, Robins P. Basal cell carcinoma in the center of the face: Special diagnostic, prognostic and therapeutic considerations. J Dermatol Surg Oncol 1978;4:315–321.
239. Robins P, Albom MJ. Recurrent basal cell carcinomas in young women. J Dermatol Surg Oncol 1975;1:49–52.
240. Albright SD III. Treatment of skin cancer using multiple modalities. J Am Acad Dermatol 1982;7:143–171.
241. Roenigk R, Roenigk H. Current surgical management of skin cancer in dermatology. J Dermatol Surg Oncol 1990; 16:136–151.
242. Swanson N. Mohs surgery technique, indications, applications, and the future. Arch Dermatol 1983;119:761–773.
243. Silverman M, Kopt A, Grin C, Bart R, Levenstein M. Recurrence rates of treated basal cell carcinomas: part 2: Curettage and electrodesiccation. J Dermatol Surg Oncol 1991;17:720–726.
244. Spiller W, Spiller R. Treatment of nasal cell epithelioma by curettage and electrodesiccation. J Am Acad Dermatol 1984; 11:808–814.
245. Whelan C, Deckers P. Electrocoagulation for skin cancer: An old oncologic tool revisited. Cancer 1981;47:2280–2287.
246. Freeman R, Knox J, Heaton C. The treatment of skin cancer: A statistical study of 1,341 stain tumors conparing results with irradiation, surgery, and curettage followed by electrodesiccation. Cancer 1964;17:535–538.
247. Reymann F, Kopp H. Treatment of basal cell carcinoma of the skin with ultrasoft X-rays. Dermatologica 1978;156:40–47.
248. Bart R, Kopt A, Petratos M. X-ray therapy of skin cancer: Evaluation of a "standardized" method of treating basal cell epitheliomas. In: Proceedings of the Sixth National Cancer Conference in 1968. Philadelphia: JB Lippincott, 1970: 559–569.
249. Fitzpatrick P, Jamieson D, Thompson G, Alt W. Tumors of the eyelids and their treatment by radiotherapy. Radiology 1972;104:661–665.
250. Silverman M, Kopt A, Bart R, et al. Recurrence rates of treated basal cell carcinomas: part 4: X-ray therapy. J Dermatol Surg Oncol 1992;18:549–554.
251. Zacarian SA. Cryosurgery of skin cancer in proper perspective. J Dermatol Surg Oncol 1975;1:33–38.
252. Biro L, Price E. Basal cell carcinoma on eyelids: Experience with cryosurgery. J Dermatol Surg Oncol 1979;5:397–401.
253. Graham G. Statistical data on malignant tumors in cryosurgery: 1982. J Dermatol Surg Oncol 1983;9:238–239.
254. Ceilley RI, Blumsted RM, Smith WH. Malignancies on the external ear: Methods of ablation and reconstruction of defects. J Dermatol Surg Oncol 1979;5:762–767.

255. Thomas P. Treatment of basal cell carcinomas of the head and neck. Rev Surg 1970;27:293–294.

256. Freeman RH. Histopathologic considerations in the management of skin cancer. J Dermatol Surg Oncol 1976;2:215–219.

257. Sloane JT. The value of typing basal cell carcinomas and predicting recurrence after surgical excision. Br J Dermatol 1977;96:127–131.

258. Salasche SJ, Amonette RA. Morpheaform basal cell epitheliomas. A study of subclinical extensions in a series of 51 cases. J Dermatol Surg Oncol 1981;7:387–399.

259. Lang PG, Maize JC. Histologic evaluation of recurrent basal cell carcinoma and treatment implications. J Am Acad Dermatol 1986;14:186–196.

260. Metcalf JS, Maize JC. Histopathologic considerations in the management of basal cell carcinoma. Semin Dermatol 1989; 8:259–265.

261. Weimar MW, Ceilley RI. Basal cell carcinoma of a medial canthus with invasion of supraorbital and supratrochlear nerves: Report of a case treated by Mohs technique. J Dermatol Surg Oncol 1979;5:279–282.

262. Monheit GD, Callahan MA, Callahan A. Mohs micrographic surgery for periorbital skin cancer. Dermatol Clinics 1989; 7:677–697.

263. Koplin L, Zaren HA. Recurrent basal cell carcinoma. Plast Reconstr Surg 1980;65:656–663.

264. Dubin N, Kopf AW. Multivariate risk score for recurrence of cutaneous basal cell carcinomas. Arch Dermatol 1983; 119:373–377.

265. Barton FE. Principles of nasal reconstruction. J Dermatol Surg Oncol 1982;8:568–574.

266. Beard C. Management of malignancy of the eyelids. Am J Ophthalmol 1981;92:1–6.

267. Mohs FE. Micrographic surgery for the microscopically controlled excision of eyelid cancers. Arch Ophthalmol 1986; 104:901–909.

268. Robins P, Rodriguez-Sains R, Rabinovitz H, Rigel D. Mohs surgery for periocular basal cell carcinomas. J Dermatol Surg Oncol 1985;11:1203–1207.

269. Anderson RL, Cielly RI. Multispecialty approach to excision and reconstruction of eyelid tumors. Ophthalmology 1978; 85:1150–1163.

270. Baylis HI, Cies WA. Indications of Mohs chemosurgical excision of eyelid and canthal tumors. Am J Ophthalmol 1975;80:116–122.

271. Downes RN, Walker NPJ, Collin JRO. Micrographic (Mohs) surgery in the management of periocular basal cell epitheliomas. Eye 1990;4:160–168.

272. Rosen HM. Periorbital basal cell carcinoma requiring ablative craniofacial surgery. Arch Dermatol 1987;123:376–378.

273. Pless J. Carcinoma on the external ear. Scand J Plast Reconstr Surg 1976;10:147–151.

274. Niparko JK, Swanson NA, Baker SR, et al. Local control of auricular, periauricular, and external canal cutaneous malignancies with Mohs surgery. Laryngoscope 1990;100:1047–1051.

275. Robins P, Nix M. Analysis of persistent disease on the ear following Mohs surgery. Head and Neck Surgery 1984;6:998–1006.

276. Mohs FE, Snow SN, Messing EM, Kuglitsch ME. Microscopically controlled surgery in the treatment of carcinoma of the penis. J Urol 1985;133:961–966.

277. Brown MD, Zachary CB, Grekin RC, Swanson NA. Genital tumors: Their management by micrographic surgery. J Am Acad Dermatol 1988;18:115–122.

278. Nahass GT, Blauvelt A, Leonardi CL, Penneys NS. Basal cell carcinoma of the scrotum. Report of three cases and review of the literature. J Am Acad Dermatol 1992;26:576–578.

279. Moritz DL, Lynch WS. Extensive Bowen's disease of the penile shaft treated with fresh tissue Mohs micrographic surgery in two separate operations. J Dermatol Surg Oncol 1991;17:374–378.

280. Stiller M, Klein W, Dorman R, Albom M. Bilateral vulvar basal cell carcinomata. J Am Acad Dermatol 1993;28:836–838.

281. Sober AJ. Diagnosis and management of skin cancer. Cancer 1983;51:2448–2452.

282. Tomsick RS, Menn H. Squamous cell carcinoma of the fingers treated with chemosurgery. South Med J 1984;77:1124–1126.

283. Albom MJ. Squamous cell carcinoma of the finger and nail bed. A review of the literature and treatment by the Mohs surgical technique. J Dermatol Surg 1975;1:476–477.

284. Mikhail GR. Subungual basal cell carcinoma. J Dermatol Surg Oncol 1985;11:1222–1223.

285. Burg G, Hirsch RD, Konez B, et al. Histographic surgery: Accuracy of visual assessment of the margins of basal-cell epithelioma. J Dermatol Surg Oncol 1975;1:21–24.

286. Wolf DJ, Zitelli JA. Surgical margins for basal cell carcinoma. Arch Dermatol 1987;123:340–344.

287. Ballantyne AJ, McCarter AB, Ibanez ML. The extension of cancer of the head and neck through peripheral nerves. Am J Surg 1963;106:651–667.

288. Geopfert H, Dichtel WJ, Medina JE, et al. Perineural invasion in squamous cell skin carcinoma of the head and neck. Am J Surg 1984;148:542–547.

289. Mark GJ. Basal cell carcinomas with intraneural invasion. Cancer 1977;40:2181–2187.

290. Dandy DJ, Munro DD. Squamous cell carcinoma of the skin involving the median nerve. Br J Dermatol 1973;89:527–531.

291. Hanke CW, Wolf RL, Hochman SA, et al. Perineural spread of basal cell carcinoma. J Dermatol Surg Oncol 1983;9:742–747.

292. Morris JGL, Joffe R. Perineural spread of cutaneous basal and squamous cell carcinomas. The clinical appearance of spread into the trigeminal and facial nerves. Arch Neurol 1983;40:424–429.

293. Weimer VM, Ceilly RI, Babin RW, et al. Chemosurgical reports. Squamous cell carcinoma with invasion of the facial nerve and underlying bone and muscle. Report of a case. J Dermatol Surg Oncol 1979;5:526–530.

294. Bieley HC, Kirsner RS, Reyes BA, Garland LD. The use of Mohs micrographic surgery for determination of residual tumor in incompletely excised basal cell carcinoma. J Am Acad Dermatol 1992;26:754–756.

295. Swanson NA, Tromovitch TA, Stegman SJ, Glogau RG. A novel method of re-excising incompletely excised basal carcinomas. J Dermatol Surg Oncol 1980;6:438–439.

296. Rowe DE, Carroll RJ, Day CL Jr. Mohs surgery is the treatment of choice for recurrent (previously treated) basal cell carcinoma. J Dermatol Surg Oncol 1989;15:424–431.

297. Menn H, Robins P, Kopf AW, Bart RS. The recurrent basal cell epithelioma: A study of recurrent, re-treated basal cell epitheliomas. Arch Dermatol 1971;103:628–631.

298. Smith SP, Grande DJ. Basal cell carcinoma recurring after radiotherapy: A unique, difficult treatment subclass of recurrent basal cell carcinoma. J Dermatol Surg Oncol 1991;17:26–30.

299. Giles GG, Marks R, Foley P. Incidence of non-melanocytic skin cancer treated in Australia. Br Med J 1988;296:13–17.

300. Scotto J, Feurs TR, Fraumeni JF Jr. Incidence of non-melanoma skin cancer in the United States. Publication #83-2433. Bethesda, MD: National Institutes of Health, 1983.

301. Cottel WI. Perineural invasion by squamous cell carcinoma. J Dermatol Surg Oncol 1982;8:589–600.

302. Rank BK, Wakefield AR. Surgery of basal cell carcinoma. Br J Surg 1958;45:531–547.

303. Dzubow LM, Rigel DS, Robins P. Risk factors for local recurrence of primary cutaneous squamous cell carcinomas. Arch Dermatol 1982;118:900–902.

304. Jorgensen K, Elbrond O, Anderson AP. Carcinoma of the lip. A series of 1869 patients. Acta Otolaryngol 1973;75:302–313.

305. Baker SR. Cancer of the lip. In: Myers EN, Suen JY, eds. Cancer of the Head and Neck. New York: Churchill Livingstone, 1989:363–415.

306. Ju DMC. On the etiology of cancer of lower lip. Plast Reconst Surg 1973;52:151–154.

307. Robins P, Dzubow LM, Rigel DS. Squamous cell carcinoma treated by Mohs surgery. An experience with 414 cases in a period of 15 years. J Dermatol Surg Oncol 1981;7:800–801.

308. Knabel MR, Koranda FC, Panje WR, et al. Squamous cell carcinoma of the upper lip. J Dermatol Surg Oncol 1982;8:487–491.

309. Mohs FE, Snow SN, Microscopically controlled surgical treatment for squamous cell carcinoma of the lower lip. Surg Gynecol Obstet 1985;160:37–41.

310. Mehregan DA, Roenigk RK. Management of superficial squa-

mous cell carcinoma of the lip with Mohs micrographic surgery. Cancer 1990;66:462–468.

311. Brown MC, Zachary CB, Grekin RC, Swanson NA. Penile tumors: Their management by Mohs micrographic surgery. J Dermatol Surg Oncol 1987;13:1163–1167.

312. Byers RM, Obrien J, Waxler J. The therapeutic and prognostic implications of nerve invasion in cancer of the lower lip. Int J Radiat Oncol Biol Phys 1978;4:215–217.

313. Sack JG, Ford CN. Metastatic squamous cell carcinoma of the lip. Arch Otolaryngol 1979;105:187–191.

314. Mendenhall NP, Million RR, Cassisi NJ. Parotid area lymph node metastases from carcinoma of the skin. Int J Radiat Oncol Biol Phys 1985;11:707–714.

315. Blake GB, Wilson JSP. Malignant tumours of the ear and their treatment. Tumours of the auricle. Br J Plast Surg 1974;27:67–76.

316. Modulin JJ. Cancer of the skin: Surgical treatment. Mo Med 1954;51:364–367.

317. Shiffman NJ. Squamous cell carcinoma of the skin of the pinna. Can J Surg 1975;18:279–283.

318. Levine H. Cutaneous carcinoma of the head and neck: Management of massive and previously uncontrolled lesions. Laryngoscope 1983;93:87–105.

319. Fleischmann HE, Roth RJ, Wood CC, Nickoloff BJ. Microcystic adnexal carcinoma treated by microscopically controlled excision. J Dermatol Surg Oncol 1984;10:873–875.

320. Cooper PH. Sclerosing carcinomas of sweat ducts (microcystic adnexal carcinoma). Arch Dermatol 1986;122:261–264.

321. Chow WC, Cockerell CJ, Geronemus RG. Microcystic adnexal carcinoma of the scalp. J Dermatol Surg Oncol 1989;15:768–771.

322. Wallace RD, Bernstein PE. Microcystic adnexal carcinoma. Ear Nose Throat J 1991;70:789–793.

323. Dhawann SS, Nanda VS, Grekin S, Rabinovitz HS. Apocrine adenocarcinoma: Case report and review of the literature. J Dermatol Surg Oncol 1990;16:468–470.

324. Lo JS, Peschen M, Snow SN, et al. Malignant cylindroma of the scalp. J Dermatol Surg Oncol 1991;17:897–901.

325. Moy RL, Rivkin JE, Lee H, et al. Syringoid eccrine carcinoma. J Am Acad Dermatol 1991;24:857–860.

326. Chesser RS, Bertler DE, Fitzpatrick JE, Mellette JR. Primary cutaneous adenoid cystic carcinoma treated with Mohs micrographic surgery toluidine blue technique. J Dermatol Surg Oncol 1992;18:175–176.

327. Hunt SJ, Abell E. Malignant hair matrix tumor ("malignant trichoepithelioma") arising in the setting of multiple hereditary trichoepithelioma. Am J Dermatopathology 1991;13:272–281.

328. Goldberg DJ, Maso M. Dermatofibrosarcoma protuberans in a 9-year-old child: Treatment by Mohs micrographic surgery. Pediatr Dermatol 1990;7:57–59.

329. Schuller DE, Snyderman CH, Quivey JM. Dermatofibrosarcoma protuberans (clinical conference). Head Neck 1990;12:178–181.

330. Mikhail GR, Lynn BH. Dermatofibrosarcoma protuberans. J Dermatol Surg Oncol 1978;4:81–84.

331. Robinson JK. Dermatofibrosarcoma protuberans resected by Mohs surgery (chemosurgery). J Am Acad Dermatol 1985;12:1093–1098.

332. Coldiron BM, Goldsmith BA, Robinson JK. Surgical treatment of extramammary Paget's disease. A report of six cases and a reexamination of Mohs micrographic surgery compared with conventional surgical excision. Cancer 1991;67:933–938.

333. Wagner RF, Cotell WI. Treatment of extensive extramammary Paget disease of male genitalia with Mohs micrographic surgery. Urology 1988;16:415–418.

334. Mohs FE, Blanchard L. Microscopically controlled surgery for extramammary Paget's disease. Arch Dermatol 1979;115:706–708.

335. Davidson LL, Frost ML, Hanke CW, Epinette WW. Primary leiomyosarcoma of the skin. Case report and review of the literature. J Am Acad Dermatol 1989;21:1156–1160.

336. Brown MD, Swanson NA. Treatment of malignant fibrous histiocytoma and atypical fibrous xanthomas with micrographic surgery. J Dermatol Surg Oncol 1989;15:1287–1292.

337. Snow SN, Reizner GT. Eccrine porocarcinoma of the face. J Am Acad Dermatol 1992;27:306–311.

338. Roenigk RK, Goltz RW. Merkel cell carcinoma—a problem with microscopically controlled surgery. J Dermatol Surg Oncol 1986;12:332–336.

339. Goldberg DJ, Kim YA. Angiosarcoma of the scalp treated with Mohs micrographic surgery. J Dermatol Surg Oncol 1993;19:156–158.

340. Dixon RS, Mikhail GR, Slater HC. Sebaceous carcinoma of the eyelid. J Am Acad Dermatol 1980;3:241–243.

341. Ratz JL, Luu-Duong S, Kulwin DR. Sebaceous carcinoma of the eyelid treated with Mohs surgery. J Am Acad Dermatol 1986;14:668–673.

342. Dzubow LM. Sebaceous carcinoma of the eyelid: Treatment with Mohs surgery. J Dermatol Surg Oncol 1985;11:40–44.

343. Folberg R, Whitaker DC, Tse DT, Nerad JA. Recurrent and residual sebaceous carcinoma after Mohs excision of the primary lesion. Am J Ophthalmol 1987;103:817–823.

344. Mohs FE. Chemosurgery for the microscopically controlled excision of cutaneous cancer. Head Neck Surg 1978;1:150–163.

345. Mohs FE. Chemosurgical treatment of melanoma. Arch Dermatol 1950;62:269–279.

346. Mohs FE. Chemosurgery for melanoma. Arch Dermatol 1977;113:285–291.

347. Brooks NA. Fixed-tissue micrographic surgery in the treatment of cutaneous melanoma. An overlooked cancer treatment strategy. J Dermatol Surg Oncol 1992;18:999–1000.

348. Zitelli JA, Moy RL, Abell E. The reliability of frozen sections in the evaluation of surgical margins for melanoma. J Am Acad Dermatol 1991;24:102–106.

349. Zitelli JA. Mohs surgery for lentigo maligna. Arch Dermatol 1991;127:1729–1730.

350. Kaspar TA, Wagner RF Jr. Mohs micrographic surgery for thin stage 1 malignant melanoma: Rationale for a modern management strategy. Cutis 1992;50:350–351.

351. Tromovich TA, Stegmen SJ, Glogau RG. Flaps and grafts in dermatologic surgery. Chicago: Year Book, 1989:1–5.

352. Summers BK, Siegle RJ: Facial cutaneous reconstructive surgery: General anesthetic principles. J Am Acad Dermatol 1993;29:669–681.

353. Robinson JK. Tissue Movement. In: Robinson JK, Arndt K, LeBoit P, Wintroub R, eds. Atlas of Cutaneous Surgery. Philadelphia: WB Saunders Co., 1995.

354. Salache SJ, Bernstein G, Senkarik M. Surgical Anatomy of the Skin. Norwalk, CT: Appleton & Lange, 1988:25–35.

355. Whitaker DE: Rotation pattern flaps. In: Wheeland RG, ed. Cutaneous Surgery. Philadelphia: WB Saunders Co., 1994:329–352.

356. Dzubow LM: Flap dynamics. J Dermatol Surg Oncol 1991;17:116–128.

357. Summers BK, Siegle RJ. Facial cutaneous reconstructive surgery: Facial flaps. J Am Acad Dermatol 1993;29:917–941.

358. Swanson NA. Atlas of Cutaneous Surgery. Boston: Little, Brown, 1987:1–177.

359. Gormley DE. A brief analysis of the Burow's wedge/triangular principle. J Dermatol Surg Oncol 1985;11:121–123.

360. Dzubow L. Subcutaneous pedicle island flaps. J Dermatol Surg Oncol 1986;12:591–596.

361. Zitelli JA, Brodland DG. Regional approach to reconstruction of the upper lip. J Dermatol Surg Oncol 1991;17:143–148.

362. Winton GB, Salasche SJ. The rotation flap. J Assoc Military Dermatol 1989;15:3–7.

363. Bennett RG. Local skin flaps on the cheeks. J Dermatol Surg Oncol 1991;17:161–165.

364. Monheit GD. The rhomboid flap. In: Dermatologic Surgery. St. Louis: Mosby, 1988.

365. Dzubow LM. Design of an appropriate rhombic flap for a circular defect created by Mohs microscopically controlled surgery. J Dermatol Surg Oncol 1988;14:126–128.

366. Larrabee WFJ, Trachy R, Sutton D, Cox K. Rhomboid flap dynamics. Arch Otolaryngol 1981;107:755–757.

367. Borges AF. The rhombic flap. Plast Reconstr Surg 1981;67:458–466.

368. Kaufman JA, Kiene KL, Moy RL. Role of tissue undermining in the trap-door effect of transposition flaps. J Dermatol Surg Oncol 1993;19:128–132.

369. Masson JK, Mendelsohn BC. The banner flap. Am J Surg 1977;134:419–423.

370. Salasche SJ, Grabski WJ. Flaps for the central face. In: Grekin RC, ed. New York: Churchill Livingstone, 1990:1–93.
371. Field LM: Design concepts for the nasolabial fold flap. Plast Reconstr Surg. 1983;71:283–285.
372. Zitelli JA. The nasolabial fold flap as a single-stage procedure. Arch Dermatol 1990;126:1445–1448.
373. Wiggs EO. Periocular flaps. J Dermatol Surg Oncol 1992; 18:1069–1073.
374. Webster RC, Davidson TM, Smith RC. The thirty degree transposition flap. Laryngoscope 1978;88:85–94.
375. McGregor JC, Soutar DS. A critical assessment of the bilobed flap. Br J Plast Surg 1981;34:197–205.
376. Zitelli JA: The bilobed flap for nasal reconstruction. Arch Dermatol 1989;125:957–959.
377. Jackson IT. Local Flaps in Head and Neck Reconstruction. St. Louis: CV Mosby, 1985.
378. Mellette JR. Ear reconstruction with local flaps. J Dermatol Surg Oncol 1991;17:176–182.
379. Zitelli JA, Fazio MJ: Reconstruction of the nose with local flaps. J Dermatol Surg Oncol 1991;17:184–189.
380. Skouge JW. Techniques for split-thickness skin grafting. J Dermatol Surg Oncol 1987;13:841–849.
381. Skouge JW. Skin grafting. In: Grekin RC, ed. New York: Churchill Livingstone, 1991.
382. Wheeland RG. Skin grafts: In: Roenigk RK, Roenigk HH, eds. Dermatologic Surgery, 1st edition. New York: Marcel Dekker, 1989:323–345.
383. Hill TG. Skin grafts. In: Wheeland RG, ed. Cutaneous Surgery, 1st edition. Philadelphia: WB Saunders Co., 1994:318–328.
384. Johnson TM, Ratner D, Nelson. Soft tissue reconstruction with skin grafting. J Am Acad Dermatol 1992;27:151–165.
385. Mir Y, Mir L: The problem of pigmentation in the cutaneous graft. Br J Plast Surg 1961;14:303–307.
386. Glogau RG, Stegman SJ, Tromovitch TA. Refinements in split-thickness grafting technique. J Dermatol Surg Oncol 1987; 13:853–858.
387. Salasche SJ, Feldman BD. Skin grafting: Perioperative technique and management. J Dermatol Surg Oncol 1987; 13:863–869.
388. Hirokawa RH, Stark TW, Prevet CW, et al. Skin grafts. Otolaryngol Clin North Am 1982;15:133–145.
389. Chester E. Closure of surgical defect in a nose using island grafts from the nose. J Dermatol Surg Oncol 1982;8:790–791.
390. Robinson JK. Improvement of the appearance of full-thickness skin grafts with dermabrasion. Arch Dermatol 1987;123:1340–1345.
391. Avelar JM, Psillakis JM, Viterbo F. Use of large composite grafts in the reconstruction of deformities of the nose and ear. Br J Plast Surg 1984;37:55.
392. Tromovitch TA, Stegman SJ, Glogau RG. Flaps and Grafts in Dermatologic Surgery. Chicago: Yearbook, 1989.
393. English FP, Forester TCG. The eyebrow graft. Ophthalmic Surg 1979;10:39–41.
394. Mares MD, Yessenow RS: The use of composite auricular grafts in nasal reconstruction. J Dermatol Surg Oncol 1988; 14:994–999.
395. Rabb O. Uber die Wirkung Fluoreszierenden Stoffen. Infusoria Z Biol 1900;39:524.
396. Jesionek A, Tappeiner VH. Zur Behandlung der Hautcarcinomit mit fluorescierenden Stoffen. Muench Med Wochneshr 1903;47:2042.
397. Hausman W. Die sensibilisierende Wirkung des Hematoporphyrins. Biochem Z 1911;30:267.
398. Figge FHJ, Weiland GS, Manganiello LOJ. Cancer detection and therapy. Affinity of neoplastic embryonic and traumatized tissue for porphyrins and metalloporphyrins. Proc Soc Exp Biol Med 1948;68:640.
399. Lipson RL, Baldes EJ. The photodynamic properties of a particular hematoporphyrin derivative. Arch Dermatol 1960;82:508.
400. Dougherty TJ, Grindey GE, Field R, et al. Photoradiation therapy. Cure of animal tumors with hematoporphyrin and light. J Natl Cancer Inst 1975;55:115–121.
401. Dougherty TJ, Kaufman JE, Goldfarb A, et al. Photoradiation therapy for the treatment of malignant tumors. Cancer Res 1978;38:2628–2635.

402. Dougherty TJ. Photosensitizers: Therapy and detection of malignant tumors. Photochem Photobiol 1987;45:874–889.
403. Pass HI. Photodynamic therapy in oncology: Mechanisms and clinical use. J Natl Cancer Inst 1993;85:443–456.
404. Henderson BW, Dougherty TJ. How does photodynamic therapy work? Photochem Photobiol 1992;55:145–157.
405. Barr H, MacRobert AJ, Tralau CJ, et al. The significance of the nature of the photosensitiser for photodynamic therapy: Quantitative and biological studies in the colon. Br J Cancer 1990;62:730–735.
406. Gomer CJ, Rucker N, Banerjee A, Benedict WF. Comparison of mutagenicity and induction of sister chromatid exchange in Chinese hamster cells exposed to hematoporphyrin derivative photoradiation, ionising radiation, or ultraviolet radiation. Cancer Res 1983;43:2622–2627.
407. Ben-Hur E, Fujihara T, Suzuki F, Elkind MM. Genetic toxicology of the photosensitization of Chinese hamster cells by phthalocyanines. Photochem Photobiol 1987;45:227–230.
408. Mitchel JB, McPherson S, DeGraff W, et al. Oxygen dependence of hematoporphyrin derivative-induced photoinactivation of Chinese hamster cells. Cancer Res 1985;45:2008–2011.
409. Moan J, Berg K, Kvam E, et al. Intracellular localization of photosensitizers. In: Photosensitizing Compounds. Their Chemistry, Biology and Clinical Use. Chichester, UK: Wiley, 1989:95–107.
410. Bellnier DA, Dougherty TJ. Membrane lysis in Chinese hamster ovary cells treated with hematoporphyrin derivative plus light. Photochem Photobiol 1982;36:43–47.
411. Spikes JD. Chlorins as photosensitizers in biology and medicine. J Photochem Photobiol B 1990;6:259–274.
412. Morgan AR, Rampersauld A, Garbo GM. New sensitizers for photodynamic therapy: Controlled synthesis of purpurins and their effect on normal tissue. J Med Chem 1989;32:904–908.
413. Morgan AR, Garbo GM, Keck RW, et al. Metallopurpurins and light: Effect on transplantable rat bladder tumors and murine skin. Photochem Photobiol 1990;51:589–592.
414. Richter AM, Waterfield E, Jain AK, et al. Photosensitizing potency of structural analogues of benzoporphyrin derivative (BPD) in a mouse tumor model. Br J Cancer 1991;63:87–93.
415. Kennedy JC, Pottier RH, Pross DC. Photodynamic therapy with endogenous protoporphyrin IX: Basic principles and present clinical experience. J Photochem Photobiol B 1990; 6:143–148.
416. Carruth JAS, McKenzie AL. Pilot study on photoradiation therapy in the treatment of superficial tumors of the skin and head and neck. Clin Oncol 1985;11:47–50.
417. Pennington DG, Waner M, Knox A. Photodynamic therapy for multiple skin cancers. Plast Recon Surg 1988;82:1067–1071.
418. Waldow SM, Lobraico RV, Kohler IK, et al. Photodynamic Therapy for Treatment of Malignant Cutaneous Lesions. Lasers Surg Med 1987;7:451–456.
419. Keller GS, Razum NJ, Doiron DR. Photodynamic therapy for nonmelanoma skin cancer. Fac Plas Surg 1989;6:180–184.
420. Wilson BD, Mang TS, Stoll H, et al. Photodynamic therapy for the treatment of basal cell carcinoma. Arch Dermatol.

Interferons

421. Isaacs A, Lindenmann J. Virus interference. I. The Interferon. Proc R Soc Lon [Biol] 1957;147:258–273.
422. Baron S. Mechanism of recovery from viral infection. In: Smith DM, Laufferr MA, eds. Advances in Virus Research. New York: Academic Press, 1963:39–60.
423. Pestka S. The human interferons—from protein purification and sequence to cloning and expression in bacteria: Before, between, and beyond. Arch Biochem Biophys 1983;221:1–37.
424. Wagner WH. Interferons. Pharm Ind 1983;45:1141–1149.
425. Wagner WH. Interferson. Pharm Ind 1983;45:1283–1290.
426. Stiem ER, Kronenberg LH, Rosenblatt HM, et al. Interferon: Immunobiology and clinical significance. Ann Intern Med 1982;96:80–93.
427. Fleischmann WR Jr, Newton RC, Fleischmann CM, et al. Discrimination between nonmalignant and malignant cells by combinations by IFNgamma and IFNalpha/beta. J Biol Response Mod 1984;3:397–405.

428. Wells V, Mallucci L. Expression of the 2-5A system during the cell cycle. Exp Cell Res 1985;159:27–36.
429. Sekar V, Atmar VJ, Joshi SR, et al. Inhibition of ornithine decarboxylase in human fibroblast cells by type I and type II interferons. Biochem Biophys Res Commun 1983;114: 950–954.
430. Yasui H, Takai K, Yoshida R, Hayaishi O. Interferon enchances tryptophan metabolism by inducing pulmonary indolamine 2,3-dioxygenase: Its possible occurrence in cancer patients. Proc Natl Acad Sci USA 1986;83:6622–6626.
431. Nathan CF, Murray HW, Wiebe ME, Rubin BY. Identification of interferon gamma as the lymphokine that activates human macrophage oxidative metabolism and antimicrobial activity. J Exp Med 1983;158:670–689.
432. Weigert DA, Stanton GJ, Johnson HM, Recombinant gamma interferon enhances natural killer cell activity similar to natural gamma interferon. Biochem Biophys Res Commun 1983; 111:525–529.
433. Chen L, Tourvieille B, Burns GF, et al. Interferon: A cytotoxic T lymphocyte differentiation signal. Eur J Immunol 1986; 16:767–770.
434. Houghton AN, Thomson TM, Gross D, et al. Surface antigens of melanoma and melanocytes: specificity of induction of Ia antigens by human gamma—interferon. J Exp Med 1984; 160:255–269.
435. Schwartz R, Momburg F, Moldenhauer G, et al. Induction of HLA class-II antigen expression of human carcinoma cell lines by IFN-gamma. Int J Cancer 1985;35:245–250.
436. Cornell RC, Greenway HT, Tucker SB, et al. Intralesional interferon therapy for basal cell carcinoma. J Am Acad Dermatol 1990;23:694–700.
437. Edwards L, Tucker SB, Perednia D, et al. The effect of an intralesional sustained release formulation of interferon alfa-2b on basal cell carcinomas. Arch Dermatol 1990;126:1029–1032.
438. Buechner SA. Intralesional interferon alpha-2b in the treatment of basal cell carcinoma. Immunohistochemical study on cellular immune reaction leading to tumor regression. J Am Acad Dermatol 1991;24:731–734.
439. Edwards L, Whiting D, Rogers D, et al. The effect of intralesional gamma on basal cell carcinomas. J Am Acad Dermatol 1990;22:496–500.
440. Steinquist B, Wennberg AM, Gisslen H, Larko O. Treatment of aggressive basal cell carcinomas with intralesional interferon: Evaluation of efficacy by Mohs surgery. J Am Acad Dermatol 1992;27:65–69.
441. Ikic D, Padovan I, Pipic N, et al. Treatment of squamous cell carcinoma with interferon. Int J Dermatol 1991;30:58–61.
442. Wickramasinghe L, Hindson TC, Wacks H. Treatment of neoplastic skin lesions with intralesional interferon. J Am Acad Dermatol 1989;20:71–74.
443. Edwards L, Berman B, Rapini RP, et al. Treatment of cutaneous squamous cell carcinoma by intralesional interferon alpha-2b therapy. Arch Dermatol 1992;128:1486–1489.
444. Grob JJ. Suzini F, Richard MA, et al. Large keratoacanthomas treated with intralesional interferon alfa-2a. J Am Acad Dermatol 1993;29:237–241.
445. Wickramasinghe L, Hindson TC, Wacks H. Treatment of neoplastic skin lesions with intralesional interferon. J Am Acad Dermatol 1989;20:71–74.
446. Edwards L, Levine N, Weidner M, et al. Effect of a2-Interferon on actinic keratoses. Arch Dermatol 1986;122:779–782.

Retinoids

447. Fujimaki Y. Formation of carcinoma in albino rats fed on deficient diets. J Cancer Res 1926;10:469–470.
448. Chopra DP. Retinoid reversal of squamous metaplasia in organ cultures of tracheas derived from hamsters fed on Vitamin A-deficient diets. Europ J Cancer Clin Oncol 1983;9:847–857.
449. Lupulesca A. Inhibition of DNA synthesis and neoplastic cell growth by Vitamin A (retinol). J Natl Cancer Inst 1986; 77:149–156.
450. Dicken CH. Retinoids: A review. J Am Acad Dermatol 1984; 11:541–552.
451. Kligman AM, Grove GL, Hirose R, Leyden JJ. Topical tretinoin for photoaged skin. J Am Acad Dermatol 1988; 15:836–859.
452. Weiss JS, Ellis CN, Headington JT, et al. Topical tretinoin improves photoaged skin: A double-blind vehicle controlled study. JAMA 1988;259:527–532.
453. Kligman AM, Dogadkina D, Lauker RM. Effects of topical tretinoin on non-sun-exposed protected skin of the elderly. J Am Acad Dermatol 1993;29:25–33.
454. Griffiths CEM, Russman AN, Majmudar G, et al. Restoration of collagen formation in photodamaged human skin by tretinoin (retinoic acid). N Engl J Med 1993;329:530–535.
455. Yuspa SH, Lichti V. Retinoids and skin carcinogenesis. In Saurat, ed. Retinoids: New Trends in Research and Therapy. Retinoid Symposium, Geneva 1984. Basel: Karger, 1985: 56–65.
456. Athar M, Agarwal R, Wang ZY, et al. All-trans retinoic acid protects against conversion of chemically induced and ultraviolet B radiation induced skin papillomas to carcinomas. Carcinogenesis 1991;12:2325–2329.
457. Prutkin L. Mucous metaplasia and gap junctions in the vitamin A acid-treated skin tumor, keratoacanthoma. Cancer Res 1975; 35:364–369.
458. Elias PM, Grayson S, Gross EG, et al. Influence of topical and systemic retinoids on basal cell carcinoma cell membranes. Cancer 1981;48:932–938.
459. Lowenstein WR. Junctional intercellular communication and the control of growth. Biochem Biophys Acta 1979;560:1–65.
460. Lotan R. Effects of vitamin A and its analogs (retinoids) on normal and neoplastic cells. Biochem Biophys Acta 1980; 605:33–91.
461. Lotan R, Nicolson GL. Inhibitory effects of retinoic acid or retinyl acetate on the growth of untransformed, transformed and tumor cells in-vitro. J Natl Cancer Inst 1977; 59:1717–1722.
462. Jetten AM, Kim JS, Sacks PG, et al. Inhibition of growth and squamous cell differentiation markers in cultured human head and neck squamous carcinoma cells by B-all-trans retinoic acid. Int J Cancer 1990;45:195–202.
463. Lacroix A, Lippman ME. Binding of retinoids to human breast cancer cell lines and their effect on cell growth. J Clin Invest 1980;656:586–591.
464. Sidell N. Retinoic acid induced growth inhibition and morphological differentiation of human neuroblastoma cells in vitro. J Natl Cancer Inst 68:589–593.
465. Frey JR, Peck R, Bolag W. Antiproliferative activity of retinoids, interferons alpha and their combination in five human transformed cell lines. Cancer Letters 1991;57:223–227.
466. Meyskens F, Fuller B. Characterization of the effects of different retinoids on the growth and differentiation of human melanoma cell lines and selected subclones. Cancer Res 1980; 40:2194–2196.
467. Ponec M, Weerheim A, Kempenaar J, Boonstra J. Proliferation and differentiation of squamous cell carcinoma cell lines and normal keratinocytes: Effects of epidermal growth factor, retinoids, and hydrocortisone. In Vitro Cell Dev Biol 1988; 24:764–770.
468. Jetten AM, Kim JS, Sacks PG, et al. Inhibition of growth and squamous cell differentiation markers in cultured human head and neck squamous cell carcinoma cells by B-all-trans retinoic acid. Int J Cancer 1990;45:195–202.
469. Sacks PG, Oke V, Amos B, et al. Modulation of growth differentiation and glycoprotein synthesis by B-all-trans retinoic acid in a multicenter tumor spheroid model for squamous cell carcinoma of the head and neck. Int J Cancer 1989;44:926–933.
470. Sidell N. Retinoic acid-induced growth inhibition and morphologic differentiation of human neuroblastoma cells in vitro. J Natl Cancer Inst 1982;68:589–593.
471. Behzadian MD, Shimuzu N. Variant of A431 cell isolated by ricin A-conjugated monoclonal antibody directed to EGF receptor: Phosphorylation of EGF receptor and phosphatidylinositol. Somatic Cell Mol Genet 1985;11:579–591.
472. Huang CC. Effect of retinoids on the growth of squamous cell carcinoma of the palate in rats. Am J Otolaryngol 1986;7:55–57.
473. Glick A, McCune B, Abdulkaren N, et al. Complex regulation

of TGFb expression by retinoic acid in the vitamin A deficient rat. Development 1991;111:1081–1086.

474. Smith MA. Parkinson DR, Cheson BD, Friedman MA. Retinoids in cancer therapy. J Clin Oncol 1992;10:839–864.

475. Evans R. The steroid and thyroid hormone receptor superfamily. Science 1988;240:889–895.

476. Petkovich M, Brand N, Krust A, et al. A human retinoic acid receptor which belongs to the family of nuclear receptors. Nature 1987;330:440–450.

477. Umesono K, Giguere V, Glass C, et al. Retinoic acid and thyroid hormone induce gene expression through a common responsive element. Nature 1988;336:262–265.

478. Smith MA, Parkinson DR, Cheson BD, Friedman MA. Retinoids in cancer therapy. J Clin Oncol 10:839–864.

479. Strickland S, Mahdavi V. The induction of differentiation in teratocarcinoma stem cells by retinoic acid. Cell 1978; 15:393–403.

480. Huang ME, Ye YC, Chai JR. Use of all-trans retinoic acid in the treatment of acute promyelocytic leukemia. Blood 1988;72:567–575.

481. Collins S. The HI-60 promyelocytic leukemia cell line: Proliferation, differentiation, and cellular oncogene expression. Blood 1987;70:1233–1244.

482. Imaizumi M, Breitman T. Retinoic acid-induced differentiation of the human promyelocytic leukemia cell lines, HI-60, and fresh human leukemia cells in primary culture: A model for differentiation inducing therapy of leukemia. Eur J Haematol 1887;38:289–302.

483. Bollag W, Holdener EE. Retinoids in cancer prevention and therapy. Annals of Oncology 1992;3:513–526.

484. Stuttgen G. Zur lokalbehandlung von keratosen mit vitamin-A-saure. Dermatologica 1962;124:65–80.

485. Bollag W, Ott F, Vitamin A acid in benign and malignant epithelial tumors of the skin. Acta Dermatol Venereol (Stockh) 1975;74:163–166.

486. Belisario JC. Recent advances in topical cytotoxic therapy of skin cancer and pre-cancer. In: Melanoma and Skin Cancer: Proceedings of the International Cancer Conference, Sydney, 1972:349–365.

487. Misiewicz J, Sendagorata E, Golebiowska A, et al. Topical treatment of multiple actinic keratoses of the face with arotinoid methyl sulfone (Ro 14-9706) cream versus tretinoin cream: A double-blind comparative study. J Am Acad Dermatol 1991;24:448–451.

488. Robinson TA, Kligman A. Treatment of solar keratoses of the extremities with retinoic acid and 5-fluorouracil. Br J Dermatol 1975;92:703–706.

489. Bercovitch L. Topical chemotherapy of actinic keratosis of the upper extremity with tretinoin and 5-fluorouracil: A double-blind controlled study. Br J Dermatol 1987;116:549–552.

490. Moriarty M, Dunn J, Darragh A, et al. Etretinate in treatment of actinic keratosis: A double blind crossover study. Lancet 1982;1:364–365.

491. Watson AB. Preventative effect of etretinate therapy on multiple actinic keratosis. Cancer Detect Prev 1986;9:161–165.

492. Hughes BR, Marks R, Pearse AD, Gaskell SA. Clinical response and tissue effects of etretinate treatment of patients with solar keratosis and basal cell carcinoma. J Am Acad Dermatol 1988;18:522–9.

493. Haydey RP, Reed ML, Dzubow LM, Shupack JL. Treatment of keratoacanthomas with oral 13-cis-retinoic acid. N Engl J Med 1980;303:560–562.

494. Shaw JC, White CR. Treatment of multiple keratoacanthomas with oral isotretinoin. J Am Acad Dermatol 1986;15:1079–1082.

495. Goldberg LH, Rosen T, Becker J, Knauss A. Treatment of solitary keratoacanthomas with oral isotretinoin. J Am Acad Dermatol 1990;23:934–936.

496. Gupper C, Berretti B. Cutaneous neoplasia and etretinate. In: Spitzy KH, Karrer K, eds. Proceedings of the 13th International Congress of Chemotherapy. Vienna: VH Egermann, 1983:201.

497. Cristofolini M, Piscioli F, Zumiani G, Scappini P. The role of etretinate (Tegison, Tigason) in the management of keratoacanthoma. J Am Acad Dermatol 1985;12:633–638.

498. Peck GL, DiGiovanna JJ, Sarnoff DS, et al. Treatment and prevention of basal cell carcinoma with oral isotretinoin. J Am Acad Dermatol 1988;19:176–185.

499. Hughes BR, Marks R, Pearse AD, Gaskell SA. Clinical response and tissue effects of etretinate treatment of patients with solar keratosis and basal cell carcinomas. J Am Acad Dermatol 1988;18:522–529.

500. Cristofolini M, Zumiani G, Scappini P, Piscioli F. Aromatic retinoid in the chemoprevention of the progression of nevoid basal-cell carcinoma syndrome. J Dermatol Surg Oncol 1984;10:778–781.

501. Kraemer KH, DiGiovanna JJ, Moshell AN, et al. Prevention of skin cancer in xeroderma pigmentosum with use of oral isotretinoin. N Engl J Med 1988;318:1633–1637.

502. Tangrea JA, Edwards BK, Taylor PR, et al. Long-term therapy with low-dose isotretinoin for prevention of basal cell carcinoma: A multicenter trial. J Natl Cancer Inst 1992;84:328–332.

503. Lippman SM, Meyskens FL. Treatment of advanced squamous cell carcinomas of the skin with isotretinoin. Ann Intern Med 1987;107:499–502.

504. Grupper CH, Berretti B. Cutaneous neoplasia and etretinate. In: Proceedings of the 13th International Congress of Chemotherapy (Spitzy KH, Karrer K, eds.). Vienna, VH Egermann, 1983:201, 224–227.

505. Meyskens FL, Gilmartin E, Alberts DS, et al. Activity of isotretinoin against squamous cell cancers and preneoplastic lesions. Cancer Treat Rep 1982;66:1315–1319.

506. Levine N, Miller RC, Meyskens FL. Oral isotretinoin therapy: Use in patient with multiple cutaneous squamous cell carcinomas and keratoacanthomas. Arch Dermatol 1984;120:1215–1217.

507. Kelly JW, Sabto J, Gurr FW, Bruce F. Retinoids to prevent skin cancer in organ transplant recipients. Lancet 1991;338:1407.

508. Hong WK, Lippman SL, Itri LM, et al. Prevention of secondary primary tumors with isotretinoin in squamous-cell carcinoma of the head and neck. N Engl J Med 1990;323:795–801.

509. Frey JR, Peck R, Bollag W. Antiproliferative activity of retinoids, interferon-alpha and their combination in five human transformed cell lines. Cancer Lett 1991;57:223–227.

510. Higuchi T, Hannigan GE, Malkin D, et al. Enhancement by retinoic acid and dibutyryl cyclic adenosine 3′:5′-monophosphate of the differentiation and gene expression of human neuroblastoma cells induced by interferon. Cancer Res 1991;51:3958–3964.

511. Marth C, Kirchebner P, Daxenbichler G. The role of polyamines in interferon and retinoic acid mediated synergistic antiproliferative action. Cancer Lett 1989;44:55–59.

512. Lippman SM, Parkinson DR, Itri LM, et al. 13-cis-Retinoic acid and interferon alpha-2a: Effective combination therapy for advanced squamous cell carcinoma of the skin. J Natl Cancer Inst 1992;84:235–241.

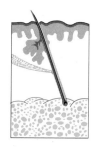

chapter 142

Benign Neoplasms of the Epidermis

BRUCE R. SMOLLER and GLORIA GRAHAM

Dermatosis Papulosa Nigra

CLINICAL DESCRIPTION

Dermatosis papulosa nigra is a condition that occurs almost exclusively in the black population. It has been estimated that lesions of dermatosis papulosa nigra occur in about 50% of blacks.[1] It is also seen occasionally in other non-Caucasian patients. It usually appears in early adulthood as multiple asymptomatic, hyperpigmented papules on the face and neck, and progresses with age (Fig. 142–1). Lesions are about 1 to 5 mm in diameter. Some authors suggest a female predominance of 2:1,[1] but others believe the lesions occur with equal frequency in men and women.[2] Lesions of dermatosis papulosa nigra do not spontaneously regress. There have been no reports of malignant degeneration, and the lesions are not associated with any systemic diseases or syndromes.

PATHOLOGY

Lesions of dermatosis papulosa nigra are rarely biopsied, given their small size and classic clinical appearance. However, histologically, they do have a characteristic, if not completely specific, appearance. There is a slightly hyperkeratotic stratum corneum with an underlying acanthotic epidermis. The epidermis occasionally has a gently lobulated configuration, similar to that seen in a fibroepithelial polyp. The keratinocytes are basaloid, somewhat resembling those seen in a seborrheic keratosis, and rare horned pseudocysts may be present. No mitoses or cytologic atypia are seen. There is fibrosis present within the most superficial portion of the papil-lary dermis, and the remainder of the dermis is unremarkable.

PATHOGENESIS

Some authors believe dermatosis papulosa nigra to be a variant of seborrheic keratosis. Other dermatologists view seborrheic keratoses and dermatosis papulosa nigra as variants of epidermal nevus with delayed onset (Table 142–1). Others regard dermatosis papulosa nigra as a variant of fibroepithelial papilloma (acrochordon).

DIAGNOSIS AND DIFFERENTIAL DIAGNOSIS

The clinical differential diagnosis of dermatosis papulosa nigra is relatively small, as these lesions have a classic appearance (Table 142–2). Lesions that might be considered would include multiple seborrheic keratoses or verrucae; fibroepithelial polyps; and, less likely, small, benign appendage tumors such as syringomas or trichoepitheliomas. Multiple pigmented melanocytic nevi might rarely be mistaken for dermatosis papulosa nigra.

Histologically, the differential diagnosis is also relatively small (Table 142–2). Any individual lesion could be histologically mistaken for a small seborrheic keratosis or a fibroepithelial polyp. However, the clinical appearance of multiple lesions concentrated on the face and neck would strongly suggest a diagnosis of dermatosis papulosa nigra.

TREATMENT

While often no treatment is needed or desired by the patient, these small papules may be removed by curet-

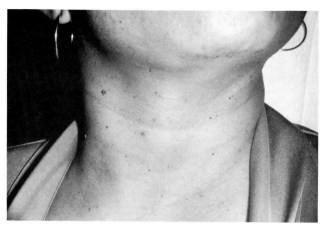

FIGURE 142–1. Dermatosis papulosa nigra shows hyperpigmented papules on the neck. (Courtesy of June K. Robinson, M.D.)

TABLE 142–2. Differential Diagnosis of Dermatosis Papulosa Nigra

Clinical
Verruca plana
Seborrheic keratosis
Fibroepithelial polyp
Syringoma
Trichoepithelioma
Melanocytic nevi

Histologic
Seborrheic keratosis
Verruca plana
Fibroepithelial polyp

tage or scissors excision. Chemical peeling using alpha hydroxy acids will soften and flatten these lesions and does seem to prevent some new lesions. Light electrodesiccation is successful but may result in hyperpigmentation. Cryosurgery using a probe results in variable pigmentation and is not the treatment of choice for dermatosis papulosa nigra. Daily use of lactic acid or other alpha hydroxy acids containing lotions or creams is useful. Kauh[3] reported on the use of curettage with a small, sharp curette without anesthesia. There was little bleeding and no postoperative complications in several hundred patients, mostly African-Americans, who were followed for 10 years.

TABLE 142–1. Differential Diagnosis of Epidermal Nevus

Clinical
Seborrheic keratosis
Nevus sebaceus of Jadassohn
Lichen striatus
Linear psoriasis
Compound melanocytic nevus
Verruca vulgaris

Histologic
Seborrheic keratosis
Acrokeratosis verruciformis of Hopf
Acanthosis nigricans
Confluent and reticulated papillomatosis of Gougerot and Carteaud
Lichen simplex chronicus
Verruca vulgaris
Nevus sebaceus of Jadassohn
Dermatosis papulosa nigra

Pale Cell Acanthoma

CLINICAL DESCRIPTION

Pale cell (or clear cell) acanthoma most commonly presents on the lower extremities, especially the thighs. More than 80% of patients with clear cell acanthoma are over 50 years of age. While most lesions are solitary, multiple lesions can occur simultaneously. It can occur in patients of any age, though it is infrequent in children, and affects men and women equally. These tumors present as nontender, erythematous papules or nodules that can be up to 1 cm in diameter (Fig. 142–2). Ulceration is infrequent. There can be a slight overlying scale. These tumors are believed to be entirely benign, with no reports of malignant transformation.

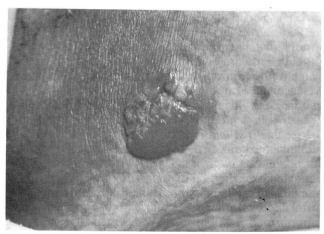

FIGURE 142–2. Pale cell acanthoma presents as a nontender erythematous nodule on the extremity. (From Callen JP, Greer KE, Hood AF, et al. Color Atlas of Dermatology. Philadelphia: WB Saunders Co., 1993:141.)

PATHOLOGY

Pale cell acanthomas have a very characteristic histologic pattern (Fig. 142–3). The low-power appearance is very reminiscent of psoriasis, but keratinocytes within the lesional skin show an abrupt and marked cytoplasmic pallor when compared with adjacent nonlesional skin. There is elongation of the rete ridges, with suprapapillary thinning. Neutrophils can be identified within the pale-staining epidermis, and in small microabscesses within the overlying parakeratotic keratin layer. The granular layer is diminished to absent. Occasional mitotic figures can be observed within the keratinocytes, but no atypical mitoses are seen. Cytologic atypia is not a feature of these tumors. A periodic acid–Schiff (PAS) stain demonstrates strong positivity in the cytoplasm of the lesional cells, and predigestion with diastase reveals extreme sensitivity, suggesting the intracytoplasmic material to be glycogen. This pallor is not present within cells in the acrosyringia and acrotrichia. At either edge of the lesion, the surrounding keratinocytes form a collarette, helping to demarcate the borders of the lesion.

PATHOGENESIS

Pale cell acanthomas have been postulated to arise as a result of a focal lack of cytoplasmic phosphorylase within a small clone of keratinocytes. This enzyme deficiency permits the excessive accumulation of glycogen within the cytoplasm of keratinocytes within pale cell acanthomas. Cells within these lesions have also been shown to lack cytochrome oxidase and succinic dehydrogenase.[4]

DIAGNOSIS AND DIFFERENTIAL DIAGNOSIS

The main clinical differential diagnoses include other erythematous nodules such as pyogenic granuloma, Ka-

TABLE 142–3. Differential Diagnosis of Pale Cell Acanthoma
Clinical
Hemangioma
Kaposi's sarcoma
Xanthogranuloma
Spitz's nevus
Pyogenic granuloma
Dermatofibroma
Basal cell carcinoma
Squamous cell carcinoma in situ
Psoriasis
Nummular dermatitis
Histologic
Psoriasis
Dermatophyte infection
Eccrine poroma

posi's sarcoma and other vascular neoplasms, Spitz's nevi, and xanthogranulomas (Table 142–3). Other lesions that can clinically be mistaken for clear cell acanthoma include dermatofibroma, basal cell carcinoma, and squamous cell carcinoma in situ. In some cases, the epidermal scales are more marked and papulosquamous lesions such as nummular dermatitis and psoriasis enter the clinical differential diagnosis.

While pale cell acanthosis is an epithelial reaction pattern that can occur in many conditions, the histologic differential diagnosis of pale cell acanthoma is quite limited (Table 142–3). The low-power appearance is quite similar to that of psoriasis, but the sharply demarcated staining characteristics of the keratinocytes in pale cell acanthomas are not a feature of psoriasis. The psoriasiform epidermal hyperplasia and neutrophilic infiltrate also raise the possibility of a dermatophyte infection. However, no fungi are demonstrated within this lesion. The cytoplasmic pallor can sometimes be seen in appendageal neoplasms such as eccrine poroma. However, in poromas, ductular differentiation is readily apparent, and the keratinocytes appear more basaloid than in pale cell acanthomas.

TREATMENT

The pale cell or clear cell acanthomas are often solitary tumors. A shave or excisional biopsy with suture closure is effective therapy. For multiple lesions, cryosurgery has proven effective. Williams et al.[5] treated multiple lesions with liquid nitrogen, using a cotton-wool swab with a diameter smaller than the lesion. Freezing was continued until a 1-mm ring of normal tissue was frozen around the nodule. A repeat freeze-thaw cycle was used. Multiple lesions were treated on the lower leg, thigh, and back. Fernandez-Obregon[6] treated a solitary lesion with open spray technique.

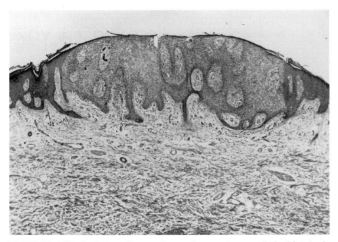

FIGURE 142–3. Pale cell acanthoma has a characteristic histologic pathogen reminiscent of psoriasis, but keratinocytes show an abrupt and marked cytoplasmic pallor. Note elongation of the rete ridges with suprapapillary thinning.

Seborrheic Keratosis

CLINICAL DESCRIPTION

Seborrheic keratoses are macular or papular lesions that vary in color from waxy yellow to dark brown. They most commonly have a velvety or verrucous surface but may also be flat. A greasy, hyperkeratotic scale is frequently seen overlying the lesions and is a helpful diagnostic clue in differentiating these lesions from other pigmented neoplasms (see later discussion). Seborrheic keratoses may occur in any anatomic location and vary in size from 1 mm to several centimeters (Fig. 142–4). Stucco keratosis, a variant of seborrheic keratosis, occurs almost exclusively in acral locations (described below).

Seborrheic keratoses are the most common cutaneous neoplasms. They occur in the majority of elderly Caucasian patients but are not limited to this population. There is no predilection for either sex, with approximately equal incidences in men and women. Seborrheic keratoses are unusual in childhood and increase in number and size with progressive age. They are most commonly asymptomatic, though occasional lesions are pruritic. The major concern is one of cosmesis, and occasional confusion with more worrisome pigmented lesions such as malignant melanoma. The heavily pigmented variant of seborrheic keratosis, melanoacanthoma, is easily confused with melanoma (see later). These lesions are invariably benign, and there are no reports of malignant degeneration; however, sometimes basal cell carcinoma can exist within the same pathologic specimen as a seborrheic keratosis. Spontaneous regression of these lesions has not been reported.

Seborrheic keratoses are a component of the Leser-Trélat syndrome.[7] In this condition, the rapid onset of multiple, pruritic seborrheic keratoses has been associated with the development of gastrointestinal malignancy, leukemias, and lymphomas.[8, 9] Many authors believe this association to be fortuitous and not a real syndrome.[10,11] A study by Lindelof and associates[10] evaluated 1752 cases of seborrheic keratoses. In 62 patients, a malignancy was diagnosed within 1 year before or after the diagnosis of seborrheic keratosis. Of these 62 patients, 6 were believed to have presented with the sign of Leser-Trélat. If one considered squamous cell carcinoma of the skin, there was a slightly increased risk of cancer in the study population. There were also 5 cases of Leser-Trélat in the control group, and these investigators concluded that there was no evidence to support the contention that eruptive seborrheic keratoses are related to internal cancer risk. Smith and colleagues[17] have reported one occurrence of melanoma arising in a seborrheic keratosis. Kitagawa[13] reported on a tricholemmal tumor arising in a seborrheic keratosis. DNA replicating cells were located in the basal and parabasal cell layers, suggesting that this tumor might have had a malignant tendency.

PATHOLOGY

Seborrheic keratoses have several characteristic histologic appearances. Common to all forms is a proliferation of basaloid keratinocytes that have ovoid nuclei, without prominent nucleoli, small amounts of cytoplasm, and variable amounts of melanin. There is no cytologic atypia seen, and mitoses are usually seen only in inflamed or irritated lesions. One characteristic histologic feature of seborrheic keratosis is the "horn pseudocyst." These are crypts lined by keratinocytes containing keratohyaline granules. As these invaginations have irregular shapes, cross-sectioning renders a cystic appearance to their profiles. Pseudocysts contain laminated or basketweave keratin and are most prevalent in the acanthotic type of seborrheic keratoses, but can be seen in any subtype (Fig. 142–5). Reticulated seborrheic keratoses show less epidermal thickening. Rather than growing as a flat-bottomed, acanthotic plaque, reticulated seborrheic keratoses grow with a pattern of progressive elongation and interanastamosis of adjacent rete ridges. The proliferating keratinocytes are identical in appearance to those seen in the acanthotic types of lesions, but the growth pattern is somewhat different. Reticulated seborrheic keratoses have fewer pseudo-horn cysts.

When seborrheic keratoses become irritated, there is a characteristic pattern of squamous eddies that form within the keratinocytic proliferation. These whorls of keratinocytes may show mild cytologic atypia and occasional mitotic figures, and care should be taken to avoid overdiagnosis as squamous cell carcinoma.

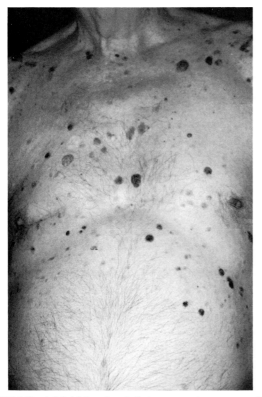

FIGURE 142–4. Multiple seborrheic keratoses show waxy yellow to dark brown keratotic papules varying in size from 1 mm to several cm.

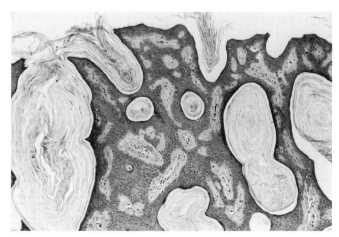

FIGURE 142–5. Pseudocysts are noted in this acanthotic form of seborrheic keratosis.

TABLE 142–4. Differential Diagnosis of Seborrheic Keratosis
Clinical
Epidermal nevus
Verruca vulgaris
Condyloma accuminatum
Fibroepithelial polyp
Actinic keratosis
Melanocytic nevus
Melanoma
Histologic
Verruca vulgaris
Fibroepithelial polyp
Condyloma accuminatum
Acanthosis nigricans
Epidermal nevus
Confluent and reticulated papillomatosis of Gougerot and Carteaud
Acrokeratosis verruciformis of Hopf
Lentigo senilis
Tumor of the follicular infundibulum

PATHOGENESIS

The pathogenesis of these very common cutaneous lesions remains largely unknown. Some workers have classified them as epidermal nevi with delayed onset, based largely upon the clinical and histologic similarities. Others regard them as proliferations of follicular infundibular keratinocytes.

In treating seborrheic keratoses in the genital area (43 cases), it was found by Zhu and coworkers[14] that 53% of these cases contained human papillomavirus (HPV) DNA sequences. Only 3% of nongenital seborrheic keratoses contained HPV DNA sequences. Zhao and colleagues[15] studied 89 seborrheic keratoses and found HPV only in 4 of these cases.

DIAGNOSIS AND DIFFERENTIAL DIAGNOSIS

The clinical differential diagnosis of a seborrheic keratosis depends somewhat on the clinical appearance of the lesion (Table 142–4). Hyperkeratotic and papillomatous seborrheic keratoses may resemble verruca vulgaris or epidermal nevi. Smaller, macular lesions may resemble solar lentigines, but these lesions are seldom hyperkeratotic, as are most seborrheic keratoses. Pigmented seborrheic keratoses may be confused with melanocytic neoplasms.[16, 17] When in doubt, biopsy is required to exclude a malignant lesion.

Stern, Boudreaux, and Arndt[18] assessed physician performance in treating 527 seborrheic keratoses. These lesions were removed by 133 clinicians associated with four different institutions. A correct preoperative diagnosis was given in 49% of cases. Dermatologists demonstrated the highest rate of accuracy: 61% versus 35% for all other physicians. A suitable procedure for the actual preoperative diagnosis was used in only 50% of cases. If the preoperative diagnosis was correct, the lesion was eight times more likely to receive appropriate treatment. Many lesions were excised and sutured, especially by non-dermatologists. However, surgical excision requires more resources and tends to have more adverse conse-

quences, such as wound dehiscence and infection, and generally yields less acceptable cosmetic results than cryosurgery, electrosurgery, curettage, or shave excision. Therefore, it was felt that the latter procedures are more satisfactory forms of treatment for seborrheic keratoses.

Entry into this study required a pathologic diagnosis of seborrheic keratosis. The study did not look at how often the diagnosis of seborrheic keratosis may be made clinically and is not confirmed by histopathologic evaluation. Teaching all physicians to diagnose these very common lesions with accuracy would be most appropriate.

Pigmented tumors of the eyelids may be difficult to identify. D'Hermies and colleagues[19] point out the importance of precise diagnosis of these pigmented tumors in which the differential diagnosis may include sweat gland cysts, pigmented basal cell carcinoma, nevus, and malignant melanoma. Epiluminescence microscopy, a technique that permits closer visual inspection of pigmented lesions, shows multiple comedo-like openings in seborrheic keratoses. This finding is also intensified with freezing, wherein the cryopattern that develops helps to differentiate the seborrheic keratoses from nevi and other pigmented lesions.

In an evaluation of a more elderly population, a study by McFadden and Hande[20] showed that in patients greater than 70 years of age (257 patients), 15.6% had seborrheic keratosis, 13.6% had basal cell carcinoma, and 13.2% had solar keratosis. A skin biopsy was required in 27% of this group and surgical treatment required in 31%, compared with 12% and 16%, respectively, of all new patients during the same time period. It is true that in dealing with patients with multiple skin tumors, this age group is more likely to require surgical intervention with follow-up visits. Patients' concerns about these lesions vary considerably, requiring that some patients be seen more often for reassurance than others.

Sloan and Jaworsky[21] have shown that 1.4% of clinically diagnosed seborrheic keratoses had evidence of squamous cell carcinoma in situ. These lesions were more common in elderly patients and more likely to occur on the head and neck. This suggests that sun damage plays a role in the development of cancer in these cases.

The histologic differential diagnosis of a seborrheic keratosis is quite limited (Table 142–4). Acanthotic lesions may be confused with eccrine poromas, but no ductular differentiation is observed in seborrheic keratoses. More papillomatous lesions may be mistaken for epidermal nevi, as described earlier. Verruca vulgaris is often frequently in the histologic differential diagnosis, but these lesions display features of papillomavirus not seen in seborrheic keratosis, such as keratohyalin granule clumping and perinuclear vacuolization. Ectatic vessels within the papillary dermal tips are also more suggestive of verruca vulgaris than of seborrheic keratosis. Reticulated seborrheic keratoses may be mistaken for solar lentigines. It has been suggested by some authors that these lesions represent a spectrum of the same condition.[22] Solar lentigines are not usually hyperkeratotic. Fortunately, the distinction is of academic importance only, and of no clinical significance.

TREATMENT

In an era of nonreimbursement for treatment of these lesions, many patients are agreeing to conservative management using lactic acid or other alpha hydroxy acid creams or lotions. Chemical peeling with alpha hydroxy acid compounds or trichloroacetic acid (TCA) may result in flattening and lightening of the lesions, especially on the face. Cryosurgery combined with a TCA chemical peel results in removal of seborrheic keratosis, actinic keratosis, and lentigines on the face and scalp in a one-time procedure.[23]

Seborrheic keratosis may be treated with liquid nitrogen applied with a cotton-tipped applicator, with one of the cryosurgical spray or probe units, or with a newly described unit—the Frigipoint.[24] The latter is a dipstick type of cryoprobe that has a thermal conductive housing chamber or reservoir tapered to tips with diameters of 2 to 10 mm. There is a cryogen-absorbent material within the housing chamber, and there is a low thermal conductivity handle. While liquid nitrogen spray will produce a greater depth of destruction than the Frigipoint, this can be used for actinic keratosis, molluscum, various types of verruca, lentigines, and seborrheic keratoses.

Multiple flat to mildly elevated seborrheic keratoses on the trunk or extremities may be treated, especially if they are pruritic, burn, sting, or become inflamed. Cryosurgery using a spray or cotton-tipped applicator until a 1- to 2-mm rim of normal skin is frozen around the lesion results in eradication of many of the lesions in one treatment session. Thicker lesions may respond best to a few seconds of freezing until the lesions are moderately firm and then removed by quick curettage. Aluminum chloride or Monsel's solution is used for hemostasis. Simple aftercare with soap and water is usually sufficient. This is similar to the technique for removal of seborrheic kera-

toses by curettage followed by application of oxidized cellulose.[25] Electrodesiccation of multiple small lesions on the face followed by wiping the area with gauze results in an excellent cosmetic appearance. Laser carbon dioxide vaporization may be used, especially for lesions in cosmetically sensitive areas. Dermabrasion for giant seborrheic keratosis has been used.[26]

Patients with POEMS syndrome, which is associated with cryoglobulinemia, lymphoma, multiple seborrheic keratoses, and ichthyosis, have a cryoprecipitant showing monoclonal IgM with kappa light chains.[27] Cryosurgery in this group of patients might prove to cause greater destruction or delay in healing; therefore, an alternative therapy should be used.

Stucco Keratosis

CLINICAL DESCRIPTION

Stucco keratosis, a clinically distinct variant of seborrheic keratosis, presents almost exclusively in acral locations as hyperkeratotic, white-gray, verrucous, exophytic growths.[28] The lesions are usually less than 1 cm, but they can rarely grow to several centimeters. Occasionally, the lesions may appear pigmented. They are most commonly seen in elderly patients, and there is no sex predominance. Clinically, these lesions can easily be scraped off with the use of a fingernail, with bleeding points from the papillary dermal capillaries. These tumors are invariably benign, with no incidence of malignant transformation. Stucco keratoses are not known to be associated with any syndromes.

PATHOLOGY

Histologically, stucco keratoses demonstrate marked orthokeratotic hyperkeratosis. Underlying the thickened stratum corneum, there is a verrucous proliferation of the epidermis. Each projection has a spike-like surface. The keratinocytes are basaloid, with lack of progressive maturation. However, the most superficial cells do have keratohyaline granules and the granular layer is often slightly thickened. Pseudo-horn cysts, such as those seen in seborrheic keratoses, are not observed. There is no cytologic atypia seen, and mitoses are infrequent. There may be some increase in basal keratinocyte melanin, but there is no increase in numbers of melanocytes. The occasional pigment seen clinically within these lesions is a result of the thickened stratum corneum.

PATHOGENESIS AND ETIOLOGY

Stucco keratoses are a distinct variant of seborrheic keratosis with a marked propensity to develop on the extremities. There may be a relation with chronic solar exposure.

DIAGNOSIS AND DIFFERENTIAL DIAGNOSIS

The clinical differential diagnosis of a stucco keratosis includes congenital lesions such as acrokeratosis verruciformis of Hopf; lesions that occur early in life, such as epidermal nevi; lesions that may occur at any time during life, such as verruca vulgaris; and lesions that occur later in life, such as actinic keratoses (Table 142–5). Also to be considered in the clinical differential diagnosis are solar lentigines and large cell acanthomas. Stucco keratoses can be distinguished from acrokeratosis verruciformis based upon age at onset and family history. Similarly, epidermal nevi can be distinguished by history, as well as by the usual linear pattern of these lesions, not ordinarily seen in stucco keratoses. In verruca vulgaris, one can sometimes see the ectatic vessels present in the papillary dermis, clinically. This feature is not seen in stucco keratoses. Solar lentigines are, as a rule, more pigmented than the stucco keratoses and are not ordinarily hyperkeratotic. Large cell acanthomas are not ordinarily markedly hyperkeratotic and do not have a verrucous appearance. Actinic keratoses are frequently difficult to distinguish clinically.

Histologically, the differential diagnosis would include the same list of entities, but several lesions that are not at all clinically similar enter the list (Table 142–5). Acanthosis nigricans and Dowling-Degos disease and confluent and reticulated papillomatosis of Gougerot and Carteaud may demonstrate very similar histologic appearances. Parakeratosis is a frequent feature of actinic keratoses and verruca vulgaris and helps to distinguish these lesions from stucco keratoses, which are covered by orthokeratotic keratin. Further, cytologic atypia required for the diagnosis of actinic keratosis is not seen in stucco keratoses. Solar lentigines and large cell acanthomas do not have the papillomatous architecture of stucco keratoses. The number and prominence of melanocytes in solar lentigines are also increased compared with stucco keratoses, and the keratinocytes in large cell acanthomas are significantly larger than those seen in stucco keratoses. Acanthosis nigricans sometimes is characterized by papillomatous projections that have blunted surfaces as opposed to the spike-like surfaces of stucco keratoses.

However, this is a very inconstant finding. Confluent and reticulated papillomatosis may be histologically identical to stucco keratosis, but frequently fungi can be demonstrated in the small foci of parakeratosis seen. The lesions of Dowling-Degos disease, acrokeratosis verruciformis of Hopf, and epidermal nevi may be histologically identical to stucco keratoses and can only be distinguished based upon clinical history and presentation.

TREATMENT

Many patients are happy just to be told that the lesions are benign and request no therapy. Lotions containing lactic acid or alpha hydroxy acid are effective in softening and flattening these lesions and also in preventing the appearance of new lesions. Applications of 35% TCA may remove small lesions. Electrodesiccation or instrument curettage is effective, and cryosurgery using 5 to 10 seconds of spray or 5 seconds with a cryoprobe will often result in cure. Freezing is continued until there is a 1- to 2-mm halo (lateral spread of freeze) beyond the lesion. Soap and water cleansing of the treatment site is sufficient.

Melanoacanthoma

CLINICAL DESCRIPTION

Melanoacanthoma is a heavily pigmented variant of a seborrheic keratosis.[29] Hyperkeratosis often overlies these papular or, rarely, macular lesions, which are sharply demarcated from the surrounding normal skin (Fig. 142–6). Much like other seborrheic keratoses, they have a "stuck-on" appearance, which helps to differentiate these benign keratinocytic neoplasms from melanocytic proliferations. There have been no reports of malignant degeneration of melanoacanthoma, and the significance of these lesions lies only in distinguishing

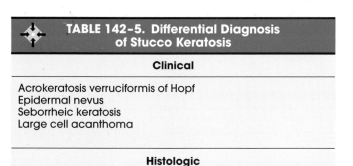

TABLE 142–5. Differential Diagnosis of Stucco Keratosis
Clinical
Acrokeratosis verruciformis of Hopf
Epidermal nevus
Seborrheic keratosis
Large cell acanthoma
Histologic
Acrokeratosis verruciformis of Hopf
Dowling-Degos disease
Epidermal nevus
Seborrheic keratosis
Large cell acanthoma
Acanthosis nigricans

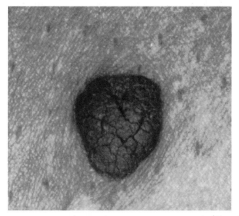

FIGURE 142–6. Melanoacanthoma presents as a darkly pigmented keratotic papule with a "stuck-on" appearance.

them from other, potentially malignant pigmented neoplasms.

PATHOLOGY

The histologic features of a melanoacanthoma are very similar to those of a seborrheic keratosis. There is a proliferation of banal-appearing keratinocytes that resemble normal basal keratinocytes. These cells are frequently densely pigmented. There is a concomitant increase in benign-appearing melanocytes throughout the lesion (Fig. 142–7). These cells are readily identifiable by their paler and more abundant cytoplasm than the surrounding keratinocytes. The proliferating melanocytes comprise only a minority of cells contained within the lesion. There is no cytologic atypia seen in these lesions, and mitoses are not ordinarily observed.

DIAGNOSIS AND DIFFERENTIAL DIAGNOSIS

The clinical differential diagnosis of melanoacanthoma consists of other pigmented cutaneous lesions (Table 142–6). Melanocytic nevi and melanomas do not have the hyperkeratosis displayed by most melanoacanthomas. In addition, melanomas are usually more variegated in pigmentation and less sharply demarcated from the surrounding nonlesional skin. Solar lentigines may also be confused clinically with melanoacanthoma, but these lesions are not usually hyperkeratotic and are invariably macular.

Histologically, the differential diagnosis is quite similar to that described earlier for seborrheic keratosis (Table 142–6). The only significant additional entities to be considered are proliferations of melanocytes such as melanocytic nevi and melanoma. In these cases, unlike in melanoacanthoma, there is a nesting of the proliferating melanocytes. In addition, the proliferation of melano-

TABLE 142–6. Differential Diagnosis of Melanoacanthoma
Clinical
Melanoma
Pigmented basal cell carcinoma
Seborrheic keratosis
Histologic
Seborrheic keratosis
Melanoma
Paget's disease
Squamous cell carcinoma in situ

cytes is confined to the dermoepidermal junction in melanocytic nevi, with upwardly migrating, pagetoid cells not frequently seen. In melanomas, single melanocytes can be seen at all levels of the epidermis, as in melanoacanthoma. However, melanocytes with melanomas are cytologically atypical.

TREATMENT

Once the diagnosis is determined, this lesion may be eradicated by electrodesiccation with or without curettage, depending on the thickness of the lesion, or cryosurgery using a spray or spray and cone. The spray time is usually 10 to 15 seconds using an intermittent spray. If the lesion is 0.6 cm or less in size, cryoprobe or liquid nitrogen on cotton swab may be used. Since this is a benign lesion, no treatment at all is acceptable.

References

1. Grimes PE, Arora S, Minus HR. Dermatosis papulosa nigra. Cutis 1983;32:385–392.
2. Hairston MA, Reed RJ, Derbes VJ. Dermatosis papulosa nigra. Arch Dermatol 1964;89:655–658.
3. Kauh YC, Young C. Lecture to Seventh International Zagazig Conference on Dermatology and Venereology. Dermatol Times 1992;13(8):40.
4. Wellas GC, Wilson Jones E. Degos' acanthoma (acanthome a cellules claires). A report of five cases with particular reference to the histochemistry. Br J Dermatol 1967;79:249–358.
5. Williams REA, Lever R, Seywright M. Multiple clear cell acanthomas: Treatment by cryotherapy. Clin Exp Dermatol 1989;14:300–301.
6. Fernandez-Obregon AC. Residents' corner: Cryosurgery of clear cell acanthoma. J Dermatol Surg Oncol 1986;12(7):689–692.
7. Gitlin MC, Pirozzi DJ. The sign of Leser-Trélat. Arch Dermatol 1975;111:792–793.
8. Liddell K, White JE, Cladville JW. Seborrheic keratoses and carcinoma of the large bowel. Br J Dermatol 1975;92:449–452.
9. Greer KC, Haukurs H, Hess C. Leser-Trélat associated with acute leukemia. Arch Dermatol 1978;114:1552.
10. Lindelof B, Sigurgeirsson B, Melander S. Seborrheic keratoses and cancer. J Am Acad Dermatol 1992;26(6):947–950.
11. Rampen FHJ, Schwengle LEM. The sign of Leser-Trélat: Does it exist? J Am Acad Dermatol 1989;21:50–55.
12. Smith KJ, Skelton HG III, Lupton GP, et al. Adenocarcinoma arising in a seborrheic keratosis. Arch Dermatol 1991;127(11):1738–1739.

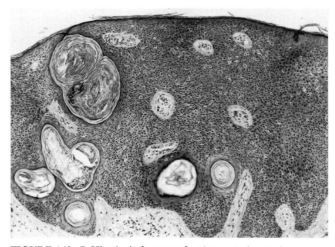

FIGURE 142–7. Histologic features of melanoacanthoma show a proliferation of banal appearing keratinocytes resembling normal basal keratinocytes. The cells are densely pigmented with a concomitant increase in melanocytes throughout the lesion. There is no cytologic atypia.

13. Kitagawa K, Amagai M, Miyakawa S, et al. Trichilemmal tumor arising in a seborrheic keratosis: Analysis of cell kinetics by BrdU staining. J Dermatol 1991;18(6):334–339.

14. Zhu WY, Leonardi C, Penneys NS. Detection of human papillomavirus DNA in seborrheic keratosis by polymerase chain reaction. J Dermatol Sci 1992;4(3):166–171.

15. Zhao YK, Lin YX, Luo RY, et al. Human papillomavirus (HPV) infection in seborrheic keratosis. Am J Dermatopathol 1989;11(3):209–212.

16. Hodge SJ, John MD, Newell GB. Malignant skin tumors presenting as seborrheic keratosis. J Kentucky Med Assoc 1984;82(5):221–223.

17. Yakar JB, Sagi A, Mahler D, et al. Malignant melanoma appearing in seborrheic keratosis. J Dermatol Surg Oncol 1984;10(5):382–383.

18. Stern RS, Boudreaux C, Arndt KA. Diagnostic accuracy and appropriateness of care for seborrheic keratoses: A pilot study of an approach to quality assurance for cutaneous surgery. JAMA 1991;265:74–77.

19. D'Hermies F, Elmaleh C, Gemin Y, et al. Pigmented seborrheic wart on the skin of the eyelid. J Francais D Ophtalmologie 1992;15(11):633–635.

20. McFadden N, Hande KO. A survey of elderly new patients at a dermatology outpatient clinic. Acta Derm Venereol 1989;69(3):260–262.

21. Sloan JB, Jaworsky C. Clinical misdiagnosis of squamous cell carcinoma in situ as seborrheic keratosis: A prospective study. J Dermatol Surg Oncol 1993;19(5):413–416.

22. Mehregan AH. Lentigo senilis and its evolution. J Invest Dermatol 1975;65:429–433.

23. Chiarello SE. Cryopeeling. J Dermatol Surg Oncol 1992;18:329–332.

24. Karakashian GV, Sweren RJ. Frigipoint: A new cryosurgical instrument. J Dermatol Surg Oncol 1989;15(5):514–517.

25. Mohs FE. Seborrheic keratoses, scarless removal by curettage and oxidized cellulose. JAMA 1970;212:1956–1958.

26. Pepper E. Dermabrasion for the treatment of a giant seborrheic keratosis. J Dermatol Surg Oncol 1985;11(6):646–647.

27. Fishel B, Brenner S, Weiss S, et al. POEMS syndrome associated with cryoglobulinemia, lymphoma, multiple seborrheic keratosis, and ichthyosis. J Am Acad Dermatol 1988;19:979–982.

28. Kocsard E, Ofner F. Keratoelastoidosis verrucosa of the extremities (stucco keratoses of the extremities). Dermatologica 1966;133:225–235.

29. Mishima Y, Pinkus H. Benign mixed tumor of melanocytes and malpighian class. Arch Dermatol 1960;81:539–550.

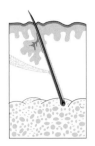

chapter 143

Cysts of Epithelial Adnexal Origin

JAG BHAWAN and S. TERI MCGILLIS

Cysts are among the most common benign lesions encountered by the dermatologist and dermatologic surgeon. To the clinician, "cyst" describes any round to dome-shaped mobile lesion that contains expressible material. Many different lesions, therefore, are grouped into this general category when first evaluated. Their true nature may not be established until pathologic evaluation is done. Cysts may then be classified by a wide variety of factors, including histologic similarities, common origins, as well as the nature of the cystic contents. One histologic classification scheme groups cysts into those that are keratinizing or nonkeratinizing (Table 143–1). This chapter does not include cysts seen in the skin that are not of epithelial or adnexal origin.[1] The expressed contents of a cyst may also help in characterizing a cyst (Table 143–2).

CYSTS LINED BY SQUAMOUS EPITHELIUM

Cysts lined by squamous epithelium represent approximately 80% of all cysts and thus are frequently encountered. The appearance of cyst lining and contents of the cyst on histologic evaluation will determine the true origin of the cyst (see Table 143–1).

Infundibular Cysts

The majority of keratinizing cysts are infundibular, meaning they arise from the infundibular portion of the pilosebaceous unit. Although many use the term *epidermal incision cyst* as a synonym, its use should be restricted to those cysts produced by implantation of epidermis into the dermis or subcutis. These cysts occur primarily on the neck, chest, and face and have a predilection for periauricular areas. Not unexpectedly, this distribution pattern closely mimics that of acne vulgaris. In fact, persons with a history of acne may be more susceptible to developing infundibular cysts (Fig. 143–1). The genitalia are also a frequent site for development of infundibular cysts, and in such instances the cysts have a propensity to calcify.[2, 3] The male-to-female ratio is approximately 2:1 and not unexpectedly reflects the severity of acne in the population. Similarly, cysts are rare in childhood. Infundibular cysts may be solitary or multiple and can range from 3 mm to several centimeters in diameter. Many contain a small punctum that marks the connection of the cyst to the overlying epidermis either by the pilar canal of a follicle or by a sinus tract (Fig. 143–2). These cysts are lined by stratified squamous epithelium resembling the interfollicular epidermis and the follicular infundibulum. A prominent granular layer is seen. The cysts contain laminated keratin (Fig. 143–3). Often these cysts rupture, resulting in suppuration (Fig. 143–4), foreign body granulomatous reaction, and/or granulation tissue with chronic inflammation. At times the subcutis may be involved, resulting in lobular panniculitis (Fig. 143–5). An interesting Koebner phenomenon of psoriasis has been reported in an epidermal inclusion cyst.[4] Histogenetically, these cysts commonly arise in the follicular infundibulum from occlusion of the pilar canal or from traumatically implanted epidermis. Regardless of the histogenesis, the histologic features are indistinguishable. Furthermore, cysts having features of both epidermal and trichilemmal keratinization can also be seen. The presence of a punctum aids greatly in the diagnosis of a cyst. Treatment of cysts is sought not only for cosmetic reasons but also because of discomfort that can result when cysts become inflamed or infected. When inflammation or infection occurs, cysts may resemble an abscess or foreign body granuloma (Fig. 143–6). Dark cysts may occur in dark-skinned patients as well as in patients with hemochromatosis.[5, 6] Multiple infun-

**TABLE 143-1. Cysts of Epithelial
Adnexal Origin**

Cysts Lined by Squamous Epithelium

Infundibular cysts (epidermoid, epidermal inclusion,
   follicular)
Trichilemmal cyst (isthmus-catagen, sebaceous, pilar)
Eruptive vellus hair cyst
Milium
Steatocystoma

Cysts Lined by Nonsquamous Epithelium

Apocrine hidrocystoma
Eccrine hidrocystoma

dibular cysts can be seen in patients with basal cell nevus syndrome and Gardner's syndrome. Cysts in patients with basal cell nevus syndrome can have features that overlap with steatocystoma,[7] and those in patients with Gardner's syndrome have foci similar to pilomatricoma.[8] In such cases the distribution is not typically in acne-prone areas. Viruses such as molluscum contagiosum and human papillomavirus can be associated with infundibular cysts.[9, 10] This is likely due to localization of the virus in the cells of the follicular ostia that then later give rise to the cyst. Epidermal inclusion cysts have also been known to arise after surgical procedures such as rhinoplasty.[11] Infundibular cysts can also arise after treatment of other diseases, such as cutaneous T-cell lymphoma, although their etiology in such cases has not been fully elucidated.[12, 13] A multitude of lesions or multiple recurring cysts should alert the clinician to the possibility of an underlying condition.

Eruptive Vellus Hair Cysts

Eruptive vellus hair cysts are multiple and clinically appear as a hyperpigmented papular eruption on the chest, abdomen, and flexural aspects of the extremities. The lesions are usually smooth but may be crusted, umbilicated, or keratotic. They tend to occur with greater frequency in children and adolescents.[14, 15] Although less common, congenital and familial cases have been described.[16, 17] Esterly and associates[18] described the condition in 1977 and have suggested that the condition represents a developmental anomaly of the vellus hair follicle. Microscopically, the cysts can easily be misdiagnosed as

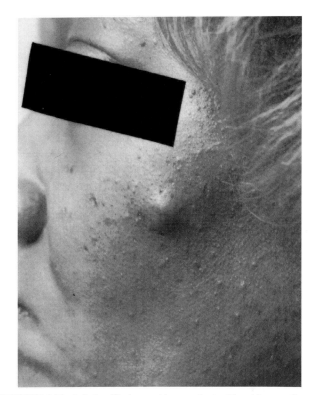

FIGURE 143-1. Infundibular cyst in a patient with a history of acne vulgaris.

follicular or epidermal inclusion cysts since they are lined by squamous epithelium. They contain several cross-sections of vellus hair shafts (Fig. 143-7). These cysts may be difficult to histologically distinguish from a comedone or milium, which may also rarely show vellus hair. However, the clinical features of eruptive vellus hair cysts are quite characteristic.[17, 18]

Many lesions will regress spontaneously once the vellus hair has been shed through transepidermal elimination. The carbon dioxide laser has been used to treat this condition without recurrence of lesions.[19]

Milia

Milia appear clinically as miniature epidermal inclusion cysts. They range from 0.5 to 2.0 mm. They are white to yellow and may be singular or multiple. Milia occur primarily on the face with a predilection for the

Problem	Lesion Contents	Probable Etiology	Classification
Cystic lesion	Oily, yellow, clear gray, mucoid	Steatocystoma Apocrine hidrocystoma Eccrine hidrocystoma Mucous cyst	Nonkeratinization
	Cheesy, whitish yellow, foul smelling	Milia Trichilemmal cyst Infundibular cyst	Keratinizing

TABLE 143-2. Differential Diagnosis of Epithelial and Adnexal Cysts

Note: Lesion location, number, size, and history also help in establishing a differential diagnosis.

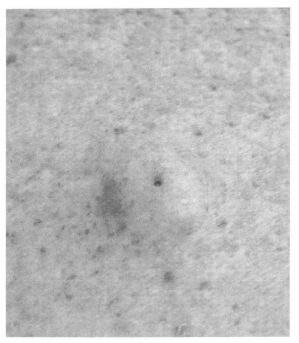

FIGURE 143-2. The presence of a punctum indicates a superficially located cyst. The punctum is not always centrally located.

thin skin of the periorbital region. Primary and secondary forms have been described.[20] Primary milia occur de novo in adults as well as in children. On questioning, many patients give a history of using powder cosmetics or cleansing granules. Either of these products may be abrasive enough to invaginate portions of the vellus follicular ostia, leading to milia formation.

Secondary milia occur as a consequence of healing of denuded areas of skin. They occasionally develop after trauma, such as dermabrasion, burns, or chemical peels. Any disease, in fact, that results in de-epithelialization may be predisposed to milia. Blistering conditions such as porphyria cutanea tarda, epidermolysis bullosa, and bullous pemphigoid and some inflammatory conditions that fibrose the superficial dermis such as lichen sclerosus et atrophicus have resulted in milia formation.[21] Microscopically, milia are tiny epidermoid cysts (Fig. 143-8). They are lined by stratified squamous epithelium containing keratin. Histogenetically these lesions may be derived from follicular infundibular epithelium and arise in the upper portion of eccrine ducts or by epidermal inclusion after trauma as a consequence of an inflammatory process. Histologic differentiation between these types is not possible.

Milia are easily expressed after lancing the overlying skin with a No. 27 needle or a microsharp blade. It is helpful to express milia by compressing the lesion between two cotton-tipped swabs. Retinoic acid cream may be a useful adjuvant treatment to prevent further milia formation.

Trichilemmal Cysts

Trichilemmal cysts are the second most frequently encountered of the keratinizing cysts, representing approximately 15% of excised lesions.[22] They mainly occur on the scalp, where they present as smooth, firm, mobile nodules (Fig. 143-9). Overlying hair growth is normal unless the cysts exceed several centimeters in size. They are seen more frequently in women, which may reflect a more detailed attention to hair styling practices that may identify the cyst. Unlike infundibular cysts, a punctum is not typically seen and inflammation is relatively uncommon. Trichilemmal cysts have thick walls and are more easily enucleated intact, compared with infundibular cysts, which tend to rupture easily. They can be solitary or multiple. When multiple, cysts are likely inherited as an autosomal dominant trait.[23] In such predisposed persons many cysts develop at a remarkably early age.

This cyst has several names. They were initially mistakenly called sebaceous cysts or wens. The term *pilar*

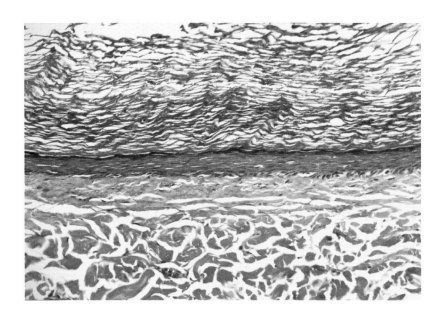

FIGURE 143-3. Part of epidermal inclusion cyst containing laminated layers of keratin. The cyst is lined by squamous epithelium similar to the epidermis including the granular layer.

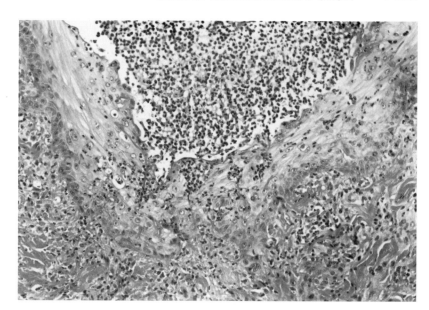

FIGURE 143–4. Ruptured epidermal inclusion cyst with abundant intracystic and pericystic neutrophilic infiltrate.

cyst is often used and was first suggested by McGavran, who recognized their close association with hair follicles.[22] The term *trichilemmal cyst* was later used by Pinkus because their walls are similar to that of the outer root sheath (trichilemma) at the level of the follicular isthmus.[24] It is now thought that the term *trichilemmal cyst* most accurately describes this lesion. These cysts differ from infundibular cysts in having the squamous epithelial lining without the granular layer. Because of the resemblance of its lining to the isthmus of hair follicle or a catagen hair, these have also been called isthmus-catagen cysts. The epithelial cells on the luminal side have pale cytoplasm and appear swollen (Fig. 143–10). Keratinization is abrupt, and the contents of the cyst appear compact, frequently with focal calcification and cholesterol clefts.[21] Various histologic features resulting from rupture of these cysts are similar to those seen with ruptured infundibular cysts.

Proliferating Trichilemmal Cysts (Pilar Tumor of the Scalp)

Proliferating trichilemmal cysts are large, multilobulated nodules or exophytic lesions most commonly occurring on the scalp. In many cases they may cause overlying areas of alopecia. They occur predominantly in women and most often are noted after the age of 60.[25] Proliferating trichilemmal cysts may also be found in persons with multiple hereditary trichilemmal cysts. This suggests a common histogenesis of these two cysts.[26] Proliferating pilar cysts can grow to large sizes if neglected; a lesion as large as 25 cm has been reported.[27] Proliferating trichilemmal cysts are particularly important since they can be easily confused microscopically with squamous cell carcinoma.[28] These lesions are characterized by a well-circumscribed multicystic structure containing keratin with proliferating lobules of squamous epithelium.

There is abrupt trichilemmal type of keratinization in the squamous epithelial islands (Fig. 143–11). The stroma is usually fibrous with variable inflammatory reaction including foreign body giant cells. Because of variable de-

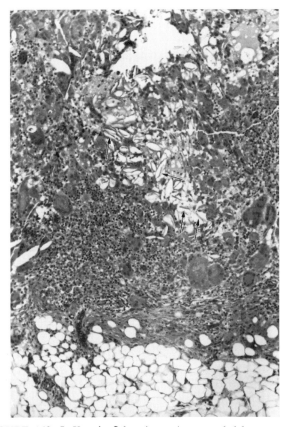

FIGURE 143–5. Keratin flakes *(arrows)* surrounded by acute and chronic inflammatory infiltrate, including foreign body giant cells extending into the subcutaneous fat.

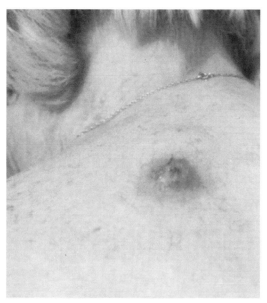

FIGURE 143-6. Infected cyst with erythema that extends beyond lesion margins.

gree of atypia, confusion with squamous cell carcinoma is easy. Abrupt keratinization, low miotic activity, minimal pleomorphism, and sharp demarcation between stroma and the adjacent dermis are helpful in differentiating these lesions from squamous cell carcinoma. A malignant proliferating pilar cyst with metastasis has also been reported.[29, 30]

Like trichilemmal cysts, adequate treatment involves complete surgical excision. Malignant transformation is often preceded by a sudden change in the preexisting nodule.[27] These cysts should be treated aggressively with immediate excision.

CYSTS LINED BY NONSQUAMOUS EPITHELIUM

Steatocystoma Multiplex

Despite common misuse of the term *sebaceous cyst,* the steatocystoma is the only cyst that actually contains sebaceous cells or lobules in its lining. The steatocystoma can occur singularly (simplex) but most often occurs as a multiple lesion complex known as steatocystoma multiplex.[31, 32] It is inherited as an autosomal dominant condition (Fig. 143-12).

Steatocystomas are usually small, ranging in size from 0.5 to 3.0 cm. They are first noted around the time of puberty, although a case of onset at birth has been described.[33] Approximately 25% of cases occur on the face; however, the chest, back, axilla, and groin areas can be affected. Most patients seek advise sometime around puberty when they are most concerned about a diagnosis. When many lesions are present, they become a cosmetic concern. Lesions rarely become inflamed or infected.

Histologic features of both steatocystoma multiplex and simplex are similar.[32] These cysts are lined by few to several layers of squamous epithelial cells without a granular layer. A thick, wavy homogeneous eosinophilic cuticular layer is characteristic of these lesions and lines the luminal side of the epithelium (Fig. 143-13). Frequently, sebaceous glands and/or abortive hair follicles can be seen in the cyst wall. Vellus hair may be seen within the cystic cavity at times.

Histogenetically, these cysts are pilosebaceous. The presence of sebaceous glands in its wall and a cuticle similar to that of the sebaceous duct has supported a sebaceous origin.[32, 33]

It is important to differentiate this condition from eruptive vellus hair cysts, which can also present in young persons. Some investigators suggest that the two disorders may, in fact, be related.[34] Steatocystomas will discharge a yellowish oily material when gently lanced

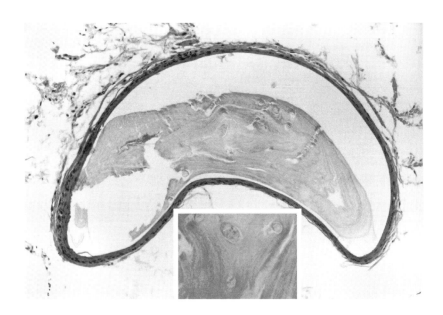

FIGURE 143-7. Eruptive vellus hair cyst lined by squamous epithelium contains numerous vellus hair. Inset shows vellus hair in higher magnification.

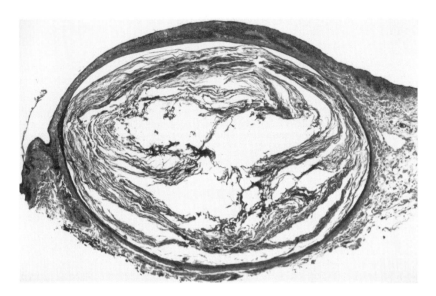

FIGURE 143–8. This tiny milium cyst shares histologic features with an infundibular or epidermal inclusion cyst.

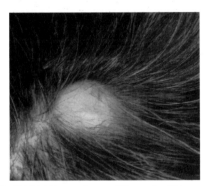

FIGURE 143–9. Trichilemmal cyst of the scalp. Note overlying alopecia typically seen with larger cysts.

with a No. 11 blade, and this greatly aids in differentiating these two conditions.

Surgical excision of cysts is reasonable when they are few. Patients with a plethora of lesions should be ap-

proached more cautiously. The carbon dioxide laser has been reported to treat multiple lesions of steatocystoma multiplex.[35] Incision and drainage, cryosurgery, and electrocautery have all been successful; however, the surgeon should weigh the consequences of having either the lesions or multiple small scars. Sato and associates[36] have successfully treated lesions with aspiration therapy alone with good cosmesis. Although medical management has little to offer, suppurative cases of steatocystoma multiplex may respond to therapy with isotretinoin.[37]

Hydrocystomas

Apocrine hydrocystomas are solitary cystic lesions that occur primarily on the face. They present as a translucent nodule with a bluish gray hue (Fig. 143–14). The lesions clinically may be confused with blue nevus and melanoma.[38] Lancing these lesions gives rise to a gela-

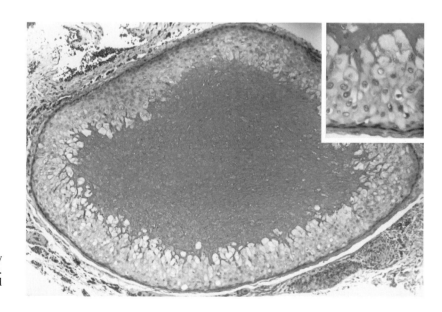

FIGURE 143–10. A trichilemmal cyst is lined by squamous epithelium and lacks a granular layer. Note the swollen, pale, epithelial cells on the luminal side seen clearly in inset.

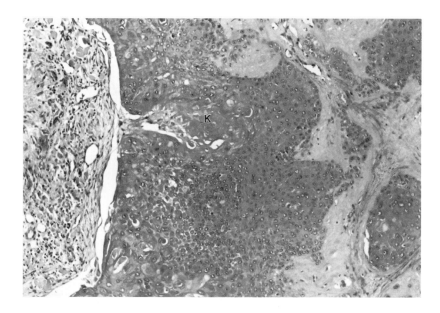

FIGURE 143-11. Proliferating masses of squamous epithelium with abrupt keratinization (K). Note the sharp demarcation of the stroma and lack of atypica.

tinous material. These cysts are characterized by one or many cystic spaces lined by columnar cells. The lumen may be folded and have papillary projections. The lining epithelium shows "decapitation" characteristic of apocrine secretion (Fig. 143-15). These cells are periodic acid–Schiff positive and diastase resistant. Elongated myoepithelial cells can be seen around the epithelial lin-

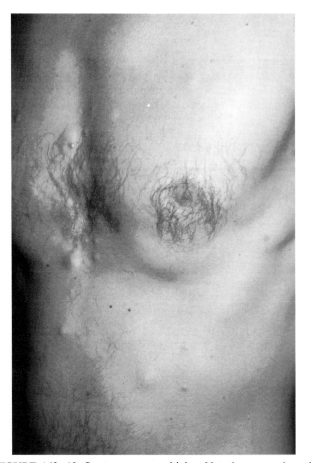

FIGURE 143-12. Steatocystoma multiplex. Note larger number of lesions of varying sizes, predominantly in the presternal area.

ing. The cause of the bluish color often seen clinically is not clearly known. The Tyndall phenomenon,[39] lipofuscin,[40] and extravasation of red blood cells[41] have been postulated as possible causes. The presence of melanin and melanocytes has also been reported in one case.[38]

Eccrine hydrocystomas are often solitary. They range in size from 1 to 3 mm and are yellowish to slightly blue. They tend to be tense or firm to the touch. Differentiation of apocrine from eccrine hydrocystomas can be difficult clinically and, at times, histologically. A solitary cystic space usually lined by two layers of cuboidal epithelial cells characterizes the eccrine hidrocystoma (Fig. 143-16). Only one layer of cells may be seen in some areas. Eccrine ducts may be seen close by or entering the cyst.[42] Intraluminal papillary projections are rarely observed.

Since many hydrocystomas are solitary facial lesions, it is important to rule out conditions that they can mimic, such as basal cell carcinomas, sebaceous carcinoma, nevi, melanoma, and hemangiomas. Although lancing a lesion may confirm its cystic nature, it is important to keep in mind that basal cell carcinomas may also form cystic areas. If there is any doubt as to the diagnosis, cysts should be removed completely by simple excision or punch biopsy.

SURGICAL MANAGEMENT OF KERATINIZING CYSTS

The most frequently noted reasons for treating cysts includes painful inflammation, infection, desire for diagnosis, or cosmetic concerns. Inflamed and infected cysts should be identified since treatment differs from that of cysts that are quiescent (Table 143-3).

Inflamed Cysts

Inflamed cysts present as erythematous, dome-shaped lesions that are tender to the touch. Inflammation occurs

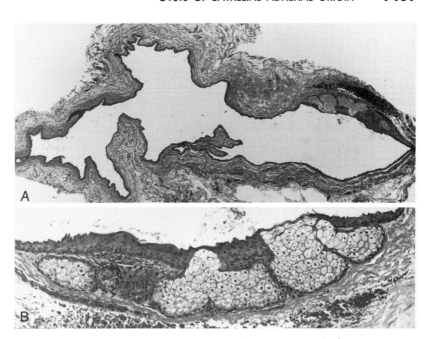

FIGURE 143–13. *A,* Irregular cyst lined by squamous epithelium. *B,* Sebaceous glands in the cyst wall and the thick homogeneous eosinophilic cuticle are easily seen in higher magnification.

when a cyst ruptures and spills its contents into the dermis. Such cysts are commonly found in patients with acne who have squeezed or manipulated their lesions. Initial treatment should be conservative and include warm compresses along with an injection of triamcinolone acetonide (usually 2.5 to 5.0 mg/mL). These measures often hasten and encourage resolution. At the least, inflammation subsides and the cyst can then be treated as a quiescent cyst.

Infected Cysts

Infection tends to occur in large cysts that have been present for many years. Infected cysts are extremely tender, with erythema that extends well beyond the cyst

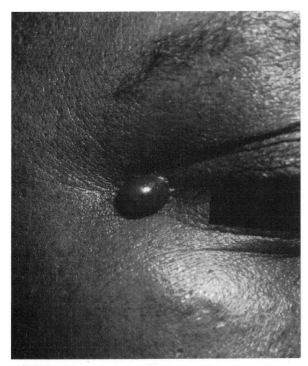

FIGURE 143–14. Apocrine hydrocystoma. Dark nodule at the corner of the eye.

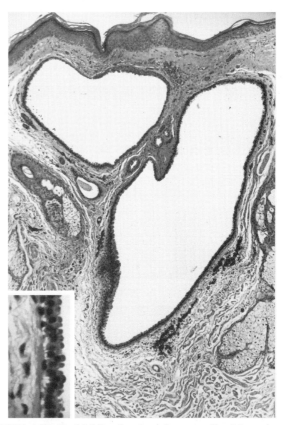

FIGURE 143–15. Multiloculated cystic spaces lined by columnar epithelium. Characteristic apocrine ("decapitation") secretion is seen on higher magnification in inset.

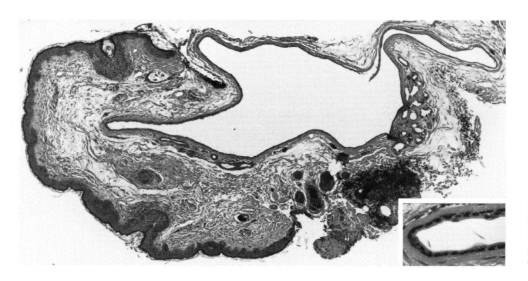

FIGURE 143–16. Irregular cystic space lined by flattened epithelium. Several eccrine ducts are seen in close association. The eccrine nature of epithelium is evident in inset.

margins (see Fig. 143–6). This is in contrast to inflamed cysts in which the erythema localizes to the lesion site. Inflamed cysts may be fluctuant and spontaneously drain purulent material.

Complete excision of infected lesions should be postponed until infection is under control. This will avoid potential seeding of the infection. Instead, proper management includes incision and drainage, systemic antibiotics, or a combination approach. Infected lesions should not be treated with intralesional steroids, since steroids may weaken the stromal collagen. This, in turn, leads to delayed healing and increases the incidence of wound dehiscence. Proper incision and drainage technique will not only provide immediate relief but will also lead to the most optimal cosmetic results.

Some form of an anesthetic should be used. In very fluctuant lesions, a topically applied refrigerant such as ethylchloride or anesthetic such as eutectic mixture of local anesthetics (EMLA), prilocaine and lidocaine (Astra, Westborough, MA), may suffice. Local anesthesia can be used, but the low pH of infected tissues can render the anesthetic less effective.[43] Care should be taken to avoid injection into the cyst since the excess pressure can cause premature rupture.

Once the area is anesthetized, drainage of the cyst is initiated by using a large-gauge needle, such as a No. 14 or 16, or a No. 11 scalpel blade. The smallest drainage port possible should be attempted first. Enough drainage to reduce pressure and provide comfort may be facilitated with a syringe attached to a large-bore needle. However, if drainage is not possible, the lesion should be incised.

When possible, incisions should be made along resting skin tension lines. Gentle pressure with the blade causes easy entry into the infected cavity, resulting in oozing of purulent material from the wound. Further compression with gauze will facilitate additional drainage. Purulent drainage, which should be cultured, is frequently followed by the typical cheesy foul-smelling keratinous debris characteristic of most cysts. Because many cysts contain *Staphyloccocus aureus,* an antibiotic such as erythromycin should be started empirically until culture results are final.[44] Once the cyst is drained, saline lavage of the infected cavity may further loosen and remove any remaining cyst wall fragments. Such fragments often serve as a nidus for inflammation. If the cavity is large, as is often the case on the trunk, iodoform-impregnated gauze or other packing material can be placed into the cavity to facilitate further drainage (Fig. 143–17).

Infected wounds should not be sutured. It is customary to allow infected sites to heal by second intention. Patients should be told that unacceptable scars may require revision at some later date. Delayed primary closure at 5 to 7 days after incision and drainage has been done with

TABLE 143-3. Treatment of Epithelial and Adnexal Cysts		
Cyst Type	**Treatment**	**Concerns**
Inflamed cyst	Warm compresses, intralesional steroids	Distinguish from infected cyst
Infected cyst	Incision and drainage	Culture and sensitivity studies
	Antibiotics	May require excision at later date
	Wound packing	
Quiescent cyst	Removal of cyst wall lining imperative for all methods	Assess anatomy, size, and mobility before surgery
Freely mobile	Punch or incise and evacuate contents of cyst; then remove lining. Dissect or excise.	Local anesthesia should not be injected into cyst cavity. Be aware of risk of rupture. Excision results in a longer scar than dissection.
Slightly mobile	Dissect or excise.	
Firm/nonmobile	Dissect or excise.	

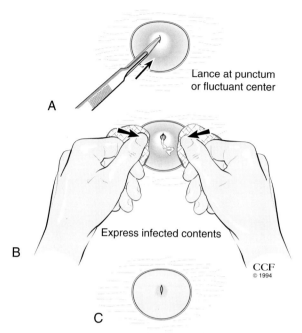

FIGURE 143–17. Diagrammatic representation of approach to infected cysts. *A*, Lance at punctum or fluctuant center of cyst. *B*, Manually express contents. *C*, Packing of cavity may be necessary.

good results.[45] If there is any evidence of ongoing infection or inflammation, surgical therapy should be deferred.

Treatment of Quiescent Cysts

Cysts that are neither inflamed nor infected are amenable to a wide variety of treatments, including excision,[46] piezosurgery[47] (pressure extraction), and electric current.[48] Any approach should have as its goal complete removal or destruction of the cyst wall. Recurrence is to be expected if only the cyst contents are expressed, leaving the lining behind to re-form the cyst. Anatomic location, size, and mobility of the cyst should be considered before initiating surgery. These factors help in selecting the best treatment.

Anatomic Location

Keratinizing cysts for the most part are easily identified. If a punctum is visible, the diagnosis is rarely questioned. On occasion, however, there may be some concern as to the true origin of the cystic lesion. The parotid gland can produce cystic lesions that mimic infundibular cysts of the cheek; and, not infrequently, inflamed lymph nodes may be mistaken for benign cysts. It is always important, therefore, to look for the presence of a punctum and palpate or ballotte the lesion for cystic mobility. Deep palpation and/or immobility may signal a subcutaneous nodule other than a cyst. Lesions on the scalp that appear dome shaped may actually be nodules of obscure origin such as hemangiomas, cephaloceles, or dermoid

tumors. Baldwin and coworkers[49] emphasize that lesions of the scalp may require careful preoperative studies such as radiographic or tomographic evaluation to distinguish rarer intracranial and intraosseous lesions that may mimic benign cysts. Developmental anomalies may present as midline lesions. Thymic cysts and thyroglossal duct cysts present on the neck as asymptomatic masses and can resemble benign subcutaneous cysts.[50, 51] If suspected, these cysts require more complete evaluation by an otolaryngologist. Cutaneous bronchogenic cysts are rare developmental abnormalities that occur in the lower part of the neck, the shoulders, and the chin. They often present as solitary lesions and may drain a mucoid material, similar to that seen in nonkeratinizing cysts. Branchial abnormalities may also appear as cysts, sinuses, fistulae, and skin polyps containing cartilage. Branchial cleft cysts are most commonly noted during the second and third decades of life and may be associated with sudden swelling and discomfort at that time. Erythema that typically accompanies inflamed or infected follicular cysts is usually not seen and helps determine the diagnosis. If there is any doubt as to the location or nature of the "cyst," further evaluation may be warranted before attempting surgical removal.

Size

Size of the cystic lesion can provide information regarding the most optimal method for removal. Pilar cysts of the scalp, for example, are often large and can produce areas of overlying alopecia. The cyst in essence acts as a natural tissue expander by stretching the surrounding tissues. In such cases, the surgeon should plan in advance to remove redundant tissue to more accurately correct the resultant defect. This effectively eliminates the alopecia.

Mobility

The mobility of a cyst on palpation may indicate how bound down it may be to surrounding tissues. Bennett[52] has classified cysts into three categories based on their mobility. Freely mobile cysts usually indicate that the cyst wall is thin and not well connected to surrounding stroma. They also tend to have a visible punctum. These cysts are much more easily evacuated, giving an option for removal other than excision. Slightly movable cysts generally occur in areas of thicker dermis such as the back. Firm to nonmobile cysts often have much scar tissue tethering them into place. Neither of these latter cyst types typically has a punctum and therefore should not simply be evacuated. In such cases, the cyst as well as surrounding fibrotic tissue must be removed.

Steps to Removing Quiescent Cysts

Ballottement

It is important to gently manipulate the cystic lesion before excision. Is the cyst freely mobile, slightly mobile, or firm and bound down? The periphery of the cyst should be marked since the cyst generally feels larger than it is when removed. This is because of a tethering effect of surrounding tissues. In most circumstances, the incision or excision should not extend beyond the palpable boundaries of the cyst. The anticipated incision line should be along skin tension lines and should include the punctum if one is present.

Anesthesia

Local anesthesia is used according to area. A solution of lidocaine with 1:100,000 epinephrine is adequate for most areas. It is best to infiltrate the area peripheral to the perceived outline of the cyst. By infiltrating with the bevel of the needle facing up and injecting the anesthetic slowly, it is possible to achieve circumferential blanching. This avoids injecting directly into the cyst itself, which would place it under undue pressure and encourage it to rupture prematurely.

Removal

The surgeon is presented with several options for cyst removal. Cysts that appear superficial and are freely mobile or with a well-visualized punctum can simply be incised with a No. 15 blade or punched with a routine trephine device at the punctum site. The punctum site represents attachment of the cyst to overlying epidermis and is not always at the center of the lesion. By manually squeezing the incised area, the cystic contents will be extruded, followed by portions of or the entire cyst lining or sac. The sac is well recognized by its bluish gray shiny texture. To extract the remainder of the cyst sac, a fine forceps such as a mosquito forceps can be inserted through the incision or punch site and gently manipulated and pulled (Fig. 143–18). Krull[53] has reported that a curette may then be helpful in scraping away any re-

maining wall portions. In some cases it is also helpful to gently cauterize this cavity. The heat may serve to further destroy any remaining cyst wall fragments. The cyst wall and not the keratinous debris should be sent for pathologic evaluation. Benign-appearing cysts have on occasion been found to be associated with squamous cell carcinomas or other neoplasms.[54-56]

For slightly mobile and firmer cysts or those without a visual punctum, the approach is to excise the cyst in such a manner that the wall is completely removed. This can be done by dissecting the cyst from surrounding tissues and delivering it through a small ellipse or by totally excising the cyst. The advantage of dissection is that a smaller wound site and therefore a smaller scar result. Dissection, however, requires greater skill since the risk of cystic rupture is higher. These cysts are very difficult to express through an incision or punch wound. In any case, be it by dissecting or by excising, removal of the entire cyst and its lining is ensured (Fig. 143–19). To dissect the cyst, a curved or elliptical incision is made within the palpable cyst boundaries. This should extend to just below the skin. The cyst wall should then become visible as a shiny layer. By using skin hooks and curved dissecting scissors, the cyst wall is separated from surrounding tissue by gentle undermining at a level between the cyst and the subcutaneous tissues surrounding it. The curve of the scissors tip should parallel the curve of the cyst wall. Complete separation of the cyst wall is possible if it is not bound down by fibrosis. In most cases, once the subcutaneous fat is reached, the cyst is easily freed up and can be gently "rolled" out of the excisional site. A cotton-tipped applicator or the blunt end of a scalpel handle may assist in this maneuver. To help stabilize the specimen and to facilitate dissection, the overlying skin can be left attached to the cyst and gently held with forceps (Fig. 143–20). (For further information, see Robinson et al., *Atlas of Cutaneous Surgery*, Chapter 9.)

At times, it is impossible to avoid rupturing the cyst or

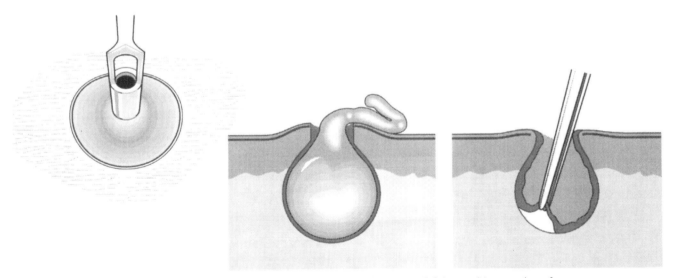

FIGURE 143–18. Diagrammatic representation of removing a superficial cyst with extraction of cyst lining.

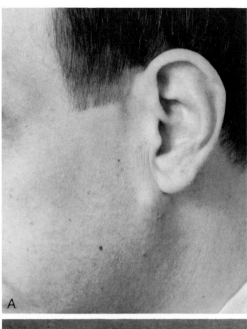

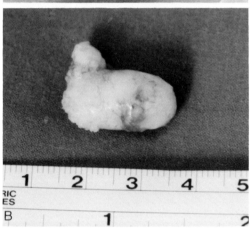

FIGURE 143–19. *A,* Preoperative photograph of a slightly mobile cyst below the earlobe. *B,* Complete specimen with cyst wall intact after dissection.

spilling its foul-smelling debris into the surgical field. Debris should be completely removed since it serves as a source of inflammation. This is accomplished by using gauze or a cotton-tipped applicator and wiping it free of the wound. The remainder of the sac and its contents may then be removed by further dissection without further spillage. The sac can also be evacuated completely, and the wall then dissected from surrounding tissue. The disadvantage in this case is that the entire sac is more difficult to visualize once spillage occurs. The remaining dead space should be rinsed with normal saline to remove any residual debris before closure. Cauterization of the wound site usually suffices for hemostasis (Fig. 143–21).

Closing the wound begins with assessing the defect for the amount of dead space and any redundant tissue that previously overlaid the cyst. Dead space can be closed by placing interrupted buried absorbable sutures similarly

to closing a routine excision site. If the wound is deep, as it often is on the back, the dead space can be closed with a single five-point suture (Fig. 143–22). This "purse strings" the base and side walls together and eliminates excess space. Redundant skin edge tissue can be trimmed away and the fresh edges sutured together, being careful to avoid removing too much skin since this may put added tension on the wound. Redundant skin that is not trimmed will eventually settle into place, so this is always an option, especially if the surgeon is uncertain as to how much should be removed. Firm cysts can be dissected in the manner described earlier or excised in total as an ellipse with the cyst at the center. This method removes all fibrotic tissue and avoids potential rupture of the cyst sac. The only drawback is that the final scar line is longer and, therefore, is less desirable for removing large cysts where an extensive scar may result. In such cases, dissection can be attempted first with the option for excision left open should the surgeon run into difficulty.

At the close of the procedure, the patient should have assurance that the cyst has been completely removed. The decision to prescribe antibiotics should be left to the discretion of the surgeon.

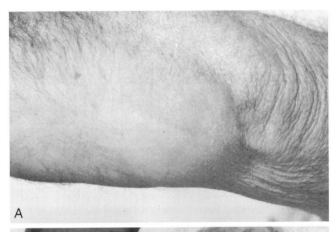

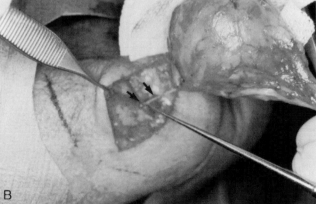

FIGURE 143–20. *A,* Preoperative photograph of large slightly mobile cyst of the elbow. *B,* Intraoperative photograph showing "rolling" of the complete specimen out of the wound site. Skin hook and arrows identify the ulnar nerve. (Courtesy of Allison Vidimos, M.D.)

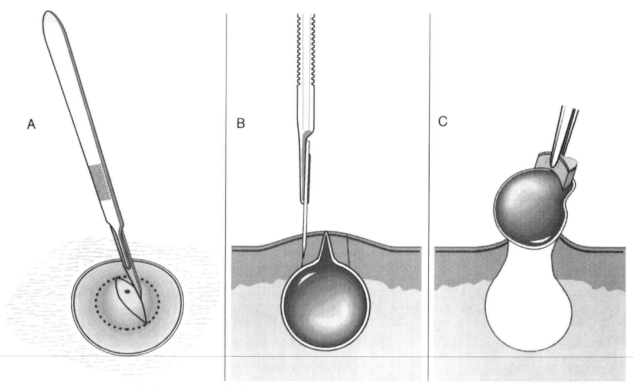

FIGURE 143-21. *A* through *C*, Diagrammatic representation of removing a slightly mobile cyst by dissecting it from surrounding tissues.

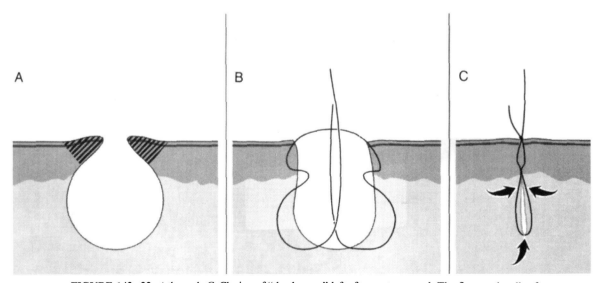

FIGURE 143-22. *A* through *C*, Closing of "dead space" left after cyst removal. The floor and walls of the cavity are brought together. Note that excess redundant tissue was excised before closure.

References

1. Kurban RS, Bhawan J. Cutaneous cysts lined by nonsquamous epithelium. Am J Dermatopathol 1991;13:509–517.
2. Swinehart JM, Golitz LE. Scrotal calcinosis: Dystrophic calcification at epidermoid cysts. Arch Dermatol 1982;118:985–988.
3. Malhotra R, Franks S, Bhawan J. Idiopathic calcinosis of the scrotum. Cutis 1981;27:396–398.
4. Bhawan J, Malhotra RL, Bernhard J. Psoriasis in epidermal cyst: An inside and outside Koebner phenomenon. Am J Dermatopathol 1988;10:142–143.
5. Fieselman DE, Reed RJ, Ichinose H. Pigmented epidermal cyst. J Cutan Pathol 1985;2:163–165.
6. Leyden JJ, Lockshin NA, Kriebel S. The black keratinous cyst: A sign of hemochromatosis. Arch Dermatol 1972;106:379–381.
7. Barr RJ, Headley JL, Jensen JL, Howell JB. Cutaneous keratocysts of nevoid basal cell carcinoma syndrome. J Am Acad Dermatol 1986;14:572–576.
8. Cooper PH, Fechner RE. Pilomatricoma-like changes in the epidermal cysts of Gardner's syndrome. J Am Acad Dermatol 1983;8:639–644.
9. Egawa K, Iraba Y, Honda Y, et al. Cystic papilloma: Human papillomavirus in a palmar epidermoid cyst. Arch Dermatol 1992;128:1658–1659.
10. Kato N, Veno H. Two cases of plantar epidermal cyst associated with human papillomavirus. Clin Exp Dermatol 1992;17:252–256.
11. Grocutt M, Fatah MF. Recurrent multiple epidermoid inclusion of cysts following rhinoplasty: An unusual complication. J Laryngol Otol 1989;103:1214–1216.
12. Smith SP, Konnikov N. Eruptive epidermal cysts and multiple squamous cell carcinomas after therapy for cutaneous T-cell lymphoma. J Am Acad Dermatol 1991;25:940–943.
13. Oliwiecki S, Ashworth J. Mycosis fungoides with a widespread follicular eruption, comedones and cysts. Br J Dermatol 1992;127:54–56.
14. Burns DA, Calnan CD. Eruptive vellus hair cysts. Clin Exp Dermatol 1981;6:209–213.
15. Watson A. Eruptive vellus hair cysts. Int J Dermatol 1982;21:273–275.
16. Steifler RE, Bergfeld WF. Eruptive vellus hair cysts: An inherited disorder. J Am Acad Dermatol 1980;3:425–429.
17. Piepkorn MW, Clark L, Lombardi DL. A kindred with congenital vellus hair cysts. J Am Acad Dermatol 1981;5:661–665.
18. Esterly NB, Actzin DF, Pinkus H. Eruptive vellus hair cysts. Arch Dermatol 1977;113:500–503.
19. Huerter CJ, Wheeland RG. Multiple eruptive vellus hair cysts treated with carbon dioxide laser vaporization. J Dermatol Surg Oncol 1987;23:260–263.
20. Epstein W, Kligman AM. The pathogenesis of milia and benign tumors of the skin. J Invest Dermatol 1956;26:1–11.
21. Leepard B, Sneddon IB. Milia occurring in lichen sclerosis et atrophicus. Br J Dermatol 1975;92:711–714.
22. McGavran MN, Binnington B. Keratinous cysts of the skin: Identification and differentiation of pilar cysts from epidermal cysts. Arch Dermatol 1966;94:499–508.
23. Leppard BJ, Sanderson KV, Wells RS. Hereditary trichilemmal cysts: Hereditary pilar cysts. Clin Exp Dermatol 1977;2:23–32.
24. Pinkus H. "Sebaceous cysts" are trichilemmal cysts. Arch Dermatol 1969;99:544–555.
25. Baptista AP, Silva LGE, Born MC. Proliferating trichilemmal cysts. J Cutan Pathol 1983;10:178–187.
26. Hendricks DL, Liang MO, Borochovitz D, et al. A case of multiple pilar tumors and cysts involving the scalp and back. Plast Reconstr Surg 1991;87:763–767.
27. Casas Jg, Woscoff A. Giant pilar tumor of the scalp. Arch Dermatol 1980;116:1395–1398.
28. Brownstein MH, Arluk DJ. Proliferating trichilemmal cyst: A simulant of squamous cell carcinoma. Cancer 1981;48:1207–1214.
29. Saida T, Oohara K, Hori Y, Tsuchiya S. Development of a malignant proliferating trichilemmal cyst in a patient with multiple trichilemmal cysts. Dermatologica 1983;166:203–208.
30. Mehrgan AH, Lee KC. Malignant proliferating trichilemmal tumors: Report of three cases. J Dermatol Surg Oncol 1987;13:1339.
31. Noojin RO, Reynolds JP. Familial steatocystoma multiplex: Twelve cases in three generations. Arch Dermatol Syph 1948;57:1013–1018.
32. Brownstein MH. Steatocystoma simplex: A solitary steatocystoma. Arch Dermatol 1982;118:409–411.
33. Sachs W. Steatocystoma multiplex congenitale: Ten cases in three generations. Arch Dermatol Syph 1938;38:877–880.
34. Ohtake N, Kubota Y, Takayama O, et al. Relationship between steatocystoma multiplex and eruptive vellus hair cysts. J Am Acad Dermatol 1992;26:876–878.
35. Krahenbuhl A, Eichmann A, Pfaltz M. CO$_2$ laser therapy for steatocystoma multiplex. Dermatologica 1991;183:294–296.
36. Sato K, Shibuya K, Taguchi H, et al. Aspiration therapy in steatocystoma multiplex. Arch Dermatol 1993;129:35–37.
37. Statham BN, Cunliffe WJ. The treatment of steatocystoma multiplex suppurativum with isotretinoin. Br J Dermatol 1984;111:246.
38. Malhotra R, Bhawan J. The nature of pigment in pigmented apocrine hidrocystoma. J Cutan Pathol 1985;12:106–109.
39. Smith JD, Chernosky ME. Apocrine hidrocystoma (cystadenoma). Arch Dermatol 1974;109:700–702.
40. Cramer HJ. Das schwarze Hidrocystom (Monfort). Dermatol Monatsschr 1980;166:114–118.
41. Hashimoto K, Lever WF. In: Appendage Tumors of the Skin. Eccrine hidrocystoma. Springfield, IL: Charles C Thomas, 1968:52–54.
42. Hashimoto K, Lever WF. In: Appendage Tumors of the Skin. Apocrine hidrocystoma. Springfield, IL: Charles C Thomas, 1968:19–25.
43. Bieter RN. Applied pharmacology of local anesthetics. Am J Surg 1936;34:500–508.
44. Brook I. Microbiology of infected epidermal cysts. Arch Dermatol 1989;125:1658–1661.
45. Miyata T, Torisu M. A new surgical approach for treating infected epidermoid cysts using delayed primary closure. Jpn J Surg 1989;19:532–534.
46. Thaller SR, Bauer BS. Cysts and cyst-like lesions of the skin and subcutaneous tissue. Clin Plast Surg 1987;14:327–340.
47. Shelley ED, Shelley WV. Piezosurgery: A conservative approach to encapsulated skin lesions. Cutis 1986;38:123–126.
48. Davis WE, Templer JW, Renner GJ. Postauricular epidermoid cysts: Treatment with electric current. Laryngoscope 1984;94:124.
49. Baldwin HE, Berck CM, Lynfield YL. Subcutaneous nodules of the scalp: Preoperative management. J Am Acad Dermatol 1991;25:819–830.
50. Berger RC, McAdams AJ. Thymic cysts. Arch Pathol 1966;82:535–541.
51. Sanusi ID, Carrington PR, Adams DN. Cervical thymic cyst. Arch Dermatol 1982;118:122–124.
52. Bennett RG. Fundamentals of Cutaneous Surgery. St. Louis: CV Mosby, 1988:734–739.
53. Krull EA. The "Little" curet (surgical gems). J Dermatol Surg Oncol 1978;4:656.
54. Yaffe HS. Squamous cell carcinoma arising in an epidermal cyst (letter). Arch Dermatol 1982;118:961.
55. Iked I, Ono T. Basal cell carcinoma originating from an epidermoid cyst. J Dermatol 1990;17:643–646.
56. Shah LK, Rane SS, Holla VV. A case of squamous cell carcinoma arising in an epidermal cyst. Indian J Pathol Microbiol 1989;32:138–140.

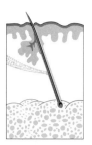

chapter 144

Neoplasms of the Pilosebaceous Unit

BRETT COLDIRON and BRUCE R. SMOLLER

Introduction

Pilosebaceous neoplasms are best classified by their suspected cells of origin or differentiation. Pilosebaceous tumors can differentiate toward the hair bulb, inner and outer root sheath, sebaceous gland, and lining epithelium.[1-5] The majority of pilosebaceous tumors are rare and benign. Some might question the need for exact categorization. The recognition of these tumors is informative to the astute clinician. For example, there is a genetic syndrome of multiple trichoepitheliomas, which can become disfiguring and may be associated with adjacent, but discrete, basal cell carcinoma.[6] There are also syndromes of multiple cylindromas, tricholemmomas, and sebaceous adenomas. Multiple tricholemmomas are associated with Cowden's syndrome (in which carcinomas of the breast and thyroid can occur),[7-10] and sebaceous adenomas are associated with Muir-Torre syndrome and possible gastrointestinal malignancy.[11] Nevus sebaceus can give rise to a variety of low-grade, and rarely high-grade malignancies (discussed in Chapter 174). Finally, certain pilosebaceous tumors may mimic metastatic malignancies, so being able to identify these neoplasms, clinically and histologically, assumes some importance. Some of these tumors are so rare, and of little clinical significance[1-4] (Table 144-1).

Immunohistochemistry is of less use in differentiating pilosebaceous tumors than those of sweat gland origin.[3] Pilosebaceous tumors differentiate toward various follicular structures, for which there are few available markers.

Pilar differentiation, in its most primitive form, is represented by small buds of basaloid epithelium that resemble embryonic hair germ. Advanced pilar differentiation is manifested by the formation of structures resembling those of the hair matrix, papilla, inner or outer root sheath, or hair shaft, alone or in combination. The overall architecture of the tumor also aids in defining it.

Basal cell carcinoma (see Chapter 141) can be conceived of as the prototypical pilar carcinoma, with differentiation toward the germinative cells of the developing follicles. Other malignant follicular neoplasms are rare. Only a few have been well characterized.[12] The inciting factor for growth of these tumors, benign or malignant, is unknown.

Many of these tumors are clinically impossible to identify, remaining anonymous dermal or subcutaneous nodules until removed and examined histologically. A clinical differential diagnosis for each of these would be needlessly redundant and is discussed only if the specific tumor has unique clinical features (Tables 144-2 and 144-3).

Dilated Pore of Winer

CLINICAL DESCRIPTION AND EPIDEMIOLOGY

Dilated pore of Winer is a benign proliferation of epithelium, which forms a characteristic cone-shaped, giant follicular orifice. It is found on the trunk, head, and neck, in all age groups.[13] Occasionally multiple lesions are present. Lesions appear as small to large dermal nodules with a central, usually oxidized and black, keratin plug. They resemble a giant open comedone but are more complex histologically.

TABLE 144-1. Rare Tumors of the Pilosebaceous Unit

Follicular hamartoma
Tumor of follicular infundibulum
Trichodiscoma
Trichoblastic fibroma
Trichogerminoma
Perifollicular fibroma
Fibrofolliculoma
Trichoadenoma

TABLE 144-3. Differential Diagnosis of Subcutaneous Nodules

Pilomatricoma
Lipoma
Angiolipoma
Sarcoid nodule
Foreign body granuloma
Eosinophilic granuloma
Panniculitis
Dermatofibrosarcoma protuberans

PATHOLOGY

Dilated pore of Winer is typified by a follicle with a characteristic cone-shaped infundibulum whose orifice is wide and distended with keratin, and which tapers as it extends into the deep dermis and occasionally subcutis. The tumor may be multilobular, connecting to a central ostium. Finger-like projections of squamous follicular epithelium radiate from the outer wall of the pore. There is no proliferation of basaloid buds around the periphery of the central opening as is seen in the histologically similar trichofolliculoma.[13]

PATHOGENESIS AND ETIOLOGY

The mode of keratinization in the dilated pore of Winer is epidermal or infundibular, with a granular layer and laminated keratin, suggesting that the lesion arises from the infundibulum.[3,4]

DIAGNOSIS AND DIFFERENTIAL DIAGNOSIS

Dilated pore of Winer is usually clinically distinct but can be confused with pilar sheath acanthoma, seborrheic keratosis, keratoacanthoma, giant comedo, and epidermal cyst.

TREATMENT

These tumors do not undergo malignant degeneration, so that observation and reassurance may suffice for some patients. Excision is curative.

TABLE 144-2. Differential Diagnosis of Dermal Nodules

Pilomatricoma
Sebaceous cyst
Sarcoid nodule
Foreign body granuloma
Eosinophilic granuloma
Atypical fibroxanthoma
Squamous cell carcinoma
Metastatic carcinoma
Dermatofibroma
Dermatofibrosarcoma protuberans
Glomus tumor
Hidradenoma
Hidradenoma papilliferum

Pilar Sheath Acanthoma

CLINICAL DESCRIPTION AND EPIDEMIOLOGY

Pilar sheath acanthoma is a pore-like tumor that usually occurs on the upper lip of older adults.[5] These tumors are solitary and measure 5 to 10 mm in diameter. The papule may have a central keratin plug.

PATHOLOGY

The histologic appearance is similar to that of a dilated pore of Winer. A centrally dilated follicular orifice is distended with keratin. There are bulbous aggregates of squamous epithelium lining the sides of the opening, but cytologic atypia and increased mitoses are not seen. Scattered dyskeratotic cells and a peripheral palisade of keratinocytes with tiny nuclei are often present, as are hints of sebaceous ductular differentiation. Epithelial proliferation is typically more elaborate than in the dilated pore of Winer.

PATHOGENESIS AND ETIOLOGY

The lobules of pilar sheath acanthoma show differentiation toward the follicular isthmus, as evidenced by dyskeratotic cells and a palisade of cells with small nuclei.

DIAGNOSIS AND DIFFERENTIAL DIAGNOSIS

Pilar sheath acanthoma can be differentiated from dilated pore of Winer by its location (upper lip), and histopathologically by the more extensive projections of its epithelial wall.

TREATMENT

Assurance may be adequate; excision is curative.

Trichofolliculoma and Sebaceous Trichofolliculoma

CLINICAL DESCRIPTION AND EPIDEMIOLOGY

Trichofolliculomas are solitary skin-colored nodules 3 to 5 mm in diameter.[4, 14] They usually have a central pore from which a woolly tuft of white hairs may project[15] (Fig. 144–1). This tuft of hairs is highly diagnostic.

PATHOLOGY

The tumors are characterized by a central pore that opens to the overlying surface, and around which are aggregated clusters of basal keratinocytes. These small islands of cells recapitulate the bulbar portions of follicles and frequently contain small vellus hairs. The islands of basaloid cells bear some resemblance to basal cell carcinoma, but the overall configuration of the neoplasm is well circumscribed, and it fails to show epithelial stromal clefts, myxoid stroma, palisading, necrosis en masse, or mitotic activity such as that seen in basal cell carcinoma.[18]

PATHOGENESIS AND ETIOLOGY

The trichofolliculoma is derived from the bulbar portion of the hair follicle. This epithelium becomes highly differentiated, reflecting all portions of the pilosebaceous complex.

DIAGNOSIS AND DIFFERENTIAL DIAGNOSIS

The diagnosis can often be made clinically because of the tuft of hairs emerging from the tumor. If this is absent, trichofolliculoma could be confused with basal cell carcinoma, closed comedone, epidermal cyst, sebaceous adenoma, and pilar sheath acanthoma.

TREATMENT

Assurance of benignity is often adequate. Biopsy may be indicated to obtain a definitive diagnosis. Elliptical excision including full thickness of dermis is curative.

Trichoepithelioma

CLINICAL DESCRIPTION AND EPIDEMIOLOGY

Two forms of trichoepithelioma exist: the common, solitary (sporadic) and the rare, multiple (autosomal dominant) form[6] (Fig. 144–2A). These entities are discrete: that is, patients with solitary trichoepitheliomas do not later develop multiple ones. There is an association between multiple trichoepitheliomas and multiple cylindromas.

Solitary lesions are pale or skin-colored papules and nodules that may reach 2 cm in diameter (Fig. 144–2B). The face of adults is the usual site. Clinically these lesions are easily confused with basal cell carcinoma. In the multiple form, many papules develop in childhood and are scattered on the face, neck, scalp, and upper trunk. The papules are skin colored to slightly pink. Papules are concentrated in the nasolabial fold, preauricular cheek, and forehead (Fig. 144–2A).

PATHOLOGY

Trichoepitheliomas share many features with basal cell carcinoma and can be difficult to distinguish from it. Both conditions feature proliferations of basaloid cells within the dermis, but unlike basal cell carcinomas, trichoepitheliomas usually do not have a connection to the overlying epidermis, and the neoplasm is usually well circumscribed. The tumor cells are arranged in rounded cribiform structures and may be indented by "papillary mesenchymal bodies," which are indentations filled by cells resembling follicular papillae. These structures are only rarely seen in basal cell carcinoma.[16] There is extensive keratinization, with the formation of small horn cysts. These can rupture, leading to a granulomatous response and sometimes calcification in the surrounding dermis. The stroma is collagenous with many fibroblasts, with none of the mucinous change often seen in basal cell carcinoma. Other features of basal cell carcinoma such as clefts between the epithelial and mesenchymal components of the tumor, mitotic figures, and apoptotic cells are not common features in trichoepithelioma[17, 18] (Figs. 144–3 and 144–4).

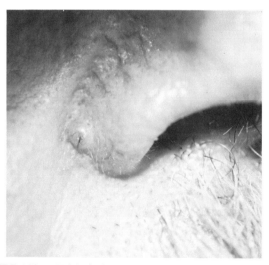

FIGURE 144–1. Trichofolliculoma. The tuft of hairs in this example is black, not white, an exception to the rule.

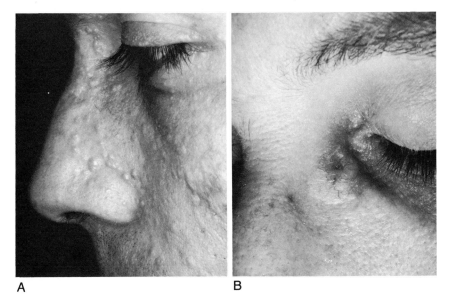

FIGURE 144–2. *A,* Hereditary multiple trichoepithelioma over the nasal sidewall and nasolabial fold area. *B,* Solitary trichoepithelioma–basal cell carcinoma. This tumor was originally diagnosed as trichoepithelioma. It slowly continued to enlarge, and a repeat, larger biopsy showed basal cell carcinoma. (*A* courtesy of June K. Robinson, M.D.)

A   B

PATHOGENESIS AND ETIOLOGY

These tumors are derived from trichogenic epithelium and differentiate toward hair germ, bulb, and infundibulum.

DIAGNOSIS AND DIFFERENTIAL DIAGNOSIS

Trichoepithelioma can be confused with basal cell carcinoma, sebaceous hyperplasia, syringoma, and hidrocystoma. The "adenoma sebaceum" of tuberous sclerosis, lesions of which are truly angiofibromas, can also present with many skin-colored papules on the central part of the face.

Biopsy is usually required in order to distinguish trichoepithelioma from basal cell carcinoma. History of a long-standing lesion with little change may be suggestive, but this same history is often obtained with basal cell carcinoma.

TREATMENT

The well-circumscribed nature of the benign process of this lesion makes it possible to excise it with narrow clinical margins.

A "malignant trichoepithelioma" occurring in the setting of multiple hereditary trichoepitheliomas has been reported, but this is a very rare event.[19] Basal cell carcinoma has also been reported among multiple trichoepitheliomas. The tumors were excised, while sparing the benign trichoepitheliomatous tissue, with Mohs' surgery.[20]

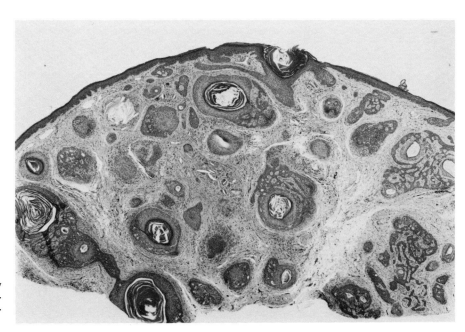

FIGURE 144–3. Trichoepithelioma, low power, hematoxylin and eosin. Note proliferation of basal cells in dermis without connection to epidermis.

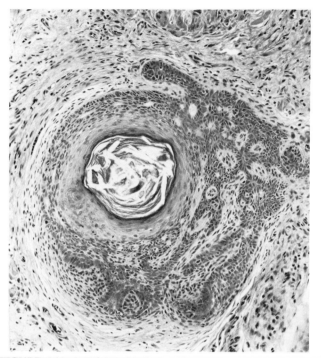

FIGURE 144-4. Trichoepithelioma, high power, hematoxylin and eosin. Note formation of basaloid cells into follicular structures and lack of retraction artifact. There are several papillary mesenchymal bodies indenting the basaloid proliferation.

Some "trichoepitheliomas" continue to enlarge and cause local destruction, making the distinction from basal cell carcinoma a moot point. These tumors should be treated as basal cell carcinoma. There are also instances in which keratotic basal cell carcinoma is identified on a more adequate re-biopsy of trichoepithelioma (see Fig. 144-2).

Desmoplastic Trichoepithelioma

CLINICAL DESCRIPTION AND EPIDEMIOLOGY

Desmoplastic trichoepithelioma is usually a small, sclerotic, depressed plaque found on the face of a young woman.[5, 21] These lesions are usually solitary, although a familial pattern of multiple desmoplastic trichoepitheliomas has been reported.[6] Trichoepithelioma and desmoplastic trichoepithelioma have little in common, clinically or histologically. Patients with one of these lesions typically do not develop the other, and trichoepitheliomas do not evolve into desmoplastic trichoepitheliomas.

PATHOLOGY

The desmoplastic variant of trichoepithelioma shows marked similarity to morpheaform basal cell carcinoma,

with scant strands of epithelium coursing between densely sclerotic stroma. However, as mentioned earlier, many other features of basal cell carcinoma are not seen in desmoplastic trichoepithelioma,[28] and many features can distinguish these entities. Perhaps the most useful are the sharp circumscription of fibrotic stroma from the adjacent dermis in desmoplastic trichoepithelioma, and the presence of thick rims of collagen around strands of cytologically bland cells within it (Fig. 144-5).

PATHOGENESIS AND ETIOLOGY

Desmoplastic trichoepithelioma is derived from trichogenic epithelium and can differentiate to form structures that range from bulbar to infundibular.

DIAGNOSIS AND DIFFERENTIAL DIAGNOSIS

Desmoplastic trichoepithelioma may be confused with morpheaform basal cell carcinoma, granuloma annulare, eccrine carcinoma, and syringoma.

Pilomatricoma

CLINICAL DESCRIPTION AND EPIDEMIOLOGY

Pilomatricoma, also known as calcifying epithelioma of Malherbe, presents as a deep dermal or subcutaneous

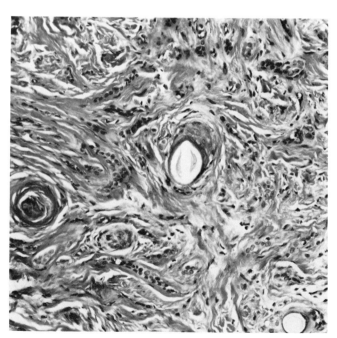

FIGURE 144-5. Desmoplastic trichoepithelioma features strands of cytologically bland epithelial cells and small keratinizing cysts embedded in sclerotic stroma.

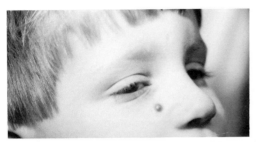

FIGURE 144-6. Pilomatricoma on right cheek of 8-year-old male. This tumor was successfully removed with curettage and light electrodesiccation.

nodule. Lesions are very firm and painless. Size is variable, ranging from 5 mm to 3 or 4 cm in diameter. The clinical presentation can range from an erythematous epidermal nodule, as seen in children (Fig. 144-6), to a hard nodule that is flesh colored to blue-black in coloration.

Children are frequently affected, and tumors are frequently found on the face or upper extremity.[22] Multiple lesions and familial patterns have been reported. There is a hereditary variant that is associated with myotonic dystrophy.[23]

PATHOLOGY

Pilomatricoma grows as a cystic structure that is usually present within the deep reticular dermis (Fig. 144-7). While in most sections it does not connect with the overlying epidermis, fortuitous sections show contiguity with follicular epithelium. These tumors are characterized by a proliferation of small, basaloid cells, with dark nuclei, small nucleoli, and virtually no visible cytoplasm lining the cystic structure. Scattered mitoses may be present within these cells, but atypical mitoses are not seen. More centrally located, larger eosinophilic "shadow" cells with clear, nonstaining nuclei are apparent (Fig. 144-8). These represent dying and dead keratinocytes derived from the lining wall. Earlier lesions show a predominance of the basaloid cells; in older nodules, the eosinophilic cells become more apparent. The mode of cornification resembles that of the hair matrix, which forms, among other structures, the cortex of the hair shaft through a similar dissolution of nuclei. Rupture, or the exposure of shadow cells to the dermis by keratinization of the entire matrical cell population, results in a foreign body granulomatous reaction and fibrosis. In these cases, calcification is present and bone formation is not uncommon.[24]

PATHOGENESIS AND ETIOLOGY

Pilomatricoma is a cystic neoplasm whose principal routes of differentiation are toward hair.

DIAGNOSIS AND DIFFERENTIAL DIAGNOSIS

The clinical differential diagnosis of pilomatricoma includes many deep dermal or subcutaneous benign tumors, cysts, and lipomas. Pilomatricoma does not have an epidermal pore as does an epidermoid cyst and is much firmer than a lipoma. The diagnosis is most often made on biopsy but can be suspected if there is a dermal

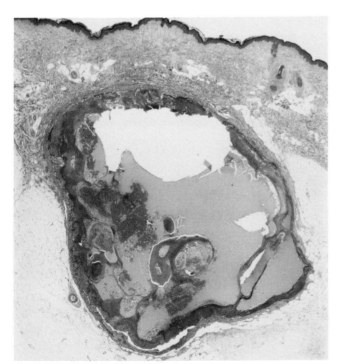

FIGURE 144-7. Pilomatricoma presents as a cystic dermal or subcutaneous nodule.

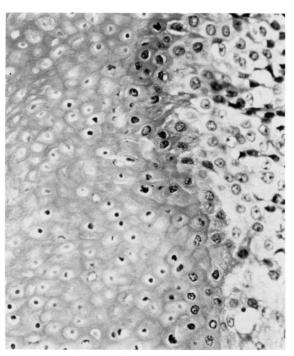

FIGURE 144-8. Shadow cells in a pilomatricoma recapitulate the keratinization that the hair matrix undergoes to become a hair shaft.

or subcutaneous nodule that has a bluish hue, given an appropriate clinical setting.

Histologically, pilomatricoma can be confused with a ruptured, calcified, tricholemmal cyst, but examination with high magnification will reveal shadow cells.

TREATMENT

Complete excision is usually curative. Recurrence after supposed complete excision has been reported in up to 3% of cases.[3]

Tricholemmoma and Cowden's Syndrome

CLINICAL DESCRIPTION AND EPIDEMIOLOGY

Tricholemmomas are relatively common, benign tumors.

Solitary tricholemmoma presents as a verrucous, hyperkeratotic, or smooth papule. These lesions range in size from a few millimeters to over 1 cm in size. The face is usually affected.

The autosomal dominantly inherited form (Cowden's syndrome) is associated with internal malignancy. Cowden's syndrome consists of multiple tricholemmomas on the face that appear in the third or fourth decade.[8] Patients also have benign keratoses of the distal extremities, and fibromas and papillomas of the oral mucosa. These growths may appear as "cobblestones" on the lip. There is a propensity to develop multiple benign and malignant tumors. The most prominent of these is carcinoma of the breast. Up to 29% of women with Cowden's syndrome eventually develop breast cancer.[7] The thyroid gland, gastrointestinal tract, ovaries, and uterus can also develop benign and malignant tumors.[9]

PATHOLOGY

Histologically, there is a proliferation of keratinocytes extending down from the overlying surface in an endophytic manner. In some lesions, there is a centrally located follicle. Tricholemmoma features large keratinocytes with abundant, eosinophilic to clear cytoplasm. The surface can be papillated with enlargement and clumping of keratohyalin granules, similar to that seen in human papillomavirus infection of the skin. However, most authors do not believe this lesion to be papillomavirus induced and no studies have yet shown the virus or its antigens in tricholemmoma.[25] Mitoses are not uncommon, but atypical ones and mitoses are unusual. Surrounding the lesion, there is a markedly thickened, periodic acid–Schiff positive basement membrane, simu-

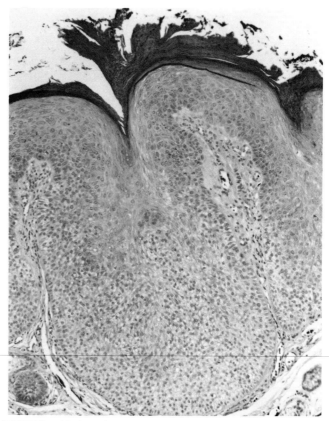

FIGURE 144–9. Tricholemmoma, high power, hematoxylin and eosin. Note large keratinocytes and thickened basement membrane.

lating the vitreous membrane of the outer root sheath of the hair follicle[10] (Fig. 144–9).

PATHOGENESIS AND ETIOLOGY

Tricholemmomas may arise from the follicular infundibulum, but their principal route of differentiation is toward the outer root sheath.

DIAGNOSIS AND DIFFERENTIAL DIAGNOSIS

The solitary tricholemmoma is a small keratotic papule. Multiple tricholemmomas, as seen in Cowden's syndrome, are warty clusters around the mouth, ears, and nose and can be confused with verrucae.

Histologically, tricholemmomas must be distinguished from verrucae.

TREATMENT

The solitary tumor is usually diagnosed and treated with the biopsy. Multiple lesions may be excised, electrodesiccated, or removed with the carbon dioxide laser. More importantly, patients with multiple lesions must be evaluated, and followed closely, for the development of internal malignancies.

Pilomatrix Carcinoma

CLINICAL DESCRIPTION AND EPIDEMIOLOGY

Pilomatrix carcinoma is a locally aggressive variant of benign pilomatricoma. This is a rare malignancy, and most reports involve nodules on the face 1 to 1.5 cm in diameter. Most often the diagnosis is made histologically, since the malignant variety cannot be reliably distinguished clinically.[27,28]

PATHOLOGY

The histologic appearance is similar to that of benign pilomatricoma except that there is local infiltration, more cellular necrosis, many mitotic and atypical mitotic figures, and cellular atypia.

PATHOGENESIS AND ETIOLOGY

Pilomatrix carcinoma presumably arises from the hair matrix as pilomatricoma. It is not known if this malignancy arises spontaneously or degenerates from a benign pilomatricoma.

DIAGNOSIS AND DIFFERENTIAL DIAGNOSIS

Diagnosis and differential diagnosis is the same as for benign pilomatricoma. Histopathologically, basal cell carcinoma with matrical differentiation also needs to be considered.[29]

TREATMENT

Complete local excision is usually curative. Margins should be checked for complete excision. Two cases of metastases have been reported.[30,31]

Sebaceous Hyperplasia

CLINICAL DESCRIPTION AND EPIDEMIOLOGY

Sebaceous hyperplasia is perhaps the most common of all pilosebaceous tumors and probably of the least significance.

It is a disproportionate enlargement of sebaceous glands found on the forehead and cheeks of middle-aged or older individuals. These areas of hyperplasia consist of

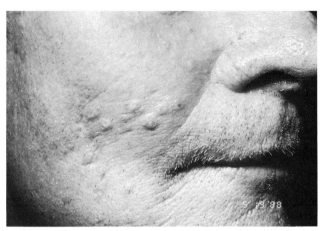

FIGURE 144–10. Sebaceous hyperplasia of the cheek consists of umbilicated papules with a yellowish hue.

one or more 2- to 4-mm umbilicated papules that have a yellowish hue (Fig. 144–10).

PATHOLOGY

Histologically, sebaceous hyperplasia is characterized by an increased number of mature sebocytes aggregated into large nodules that cluster around a central duct. The sebaceous lobules show a proper maturation sequence of the sebocytes, with only a single rim of basaloid cells at the periphery, and mature sebocytes within the central portions of the lobules.

PATHOGENESIS AND ETIOLOGY

Sebaceous hyperplasia is thought to be due to chronic ultraviolet exposure because it is frequently found in association with other signs of solar damage. Sebaceous hyperplasia is also a common sequela to radiation treatment. Labeling studies with tritiated thymidine have shown that the sebocyte migration time from basal cell to center of sebaceous lobule is distinctly prolonged.[32] This probably accounts for the sebaceous gland enlargement. Only one or a few glands are enlarged, in contrast to rhinophyma.

DIAGNOSIS AND DIFFERENTIAL DIAGNOSIS

It is very important to learn to recognize sebaceous hyperplasia in order to avoid many unnecessary biopsies to rule out basal cell carcinoma. Sebaceous hyperplasia must be distinguished from rhinophyma, basal cell carcinoma, nevus sebaceus, and dermal nevus. This can usually be determined clinically, based on the yellowish coloration and central dell that is usually present in sebaceous hyperplasia.

TREATMENT

Many treatments are satisfactory for sebaceous hyperplasia. Often a tangential biopsy will provide diagnostic material as well as remove the lesion. Any destructive method, including curettage, cryotherapy, mild electrodesiccation, CO_2 laser surgery, or topical application of acids, is effective.

Sebaceous Adenoma and the Muir-Torre Syndrome

CLINICAL DESCRIPTION AND EPIDEMIOLOGY

Sebaceous adenoma varies from a small nodule to an ill-defined plaque, usually yellow or tan-yellow in color, located on the face or scalp. Sebaceous adenomas can arise within a nevus sebaceus.[12] They usually arise on older patients. Sebaceous adenoma (epithelioma or sebaceoma) is benign tumor and may be a marker for an autosomal dominant, genetic syndrome: the Muir-Torre syndrome.

The Muir-Torre syndrome consists of multiple facial sebaceous adenomas, sebaceous epitheliomas, sebaceous carcinomas, keratoacanthomas, and gastrointestinal carcinomas, particularly adenocarcinoma of the colon.[33] Carcinomas of the tracheobronchial tree, genitourinary tract, and endometrium have also been documented. Solitary sebaceous adenomas have been associated with the Muir-Torre syndrome.[11] The skin lesions usually appear in childhood. The exact mode of inheritance is not known.

PATHOLOGY

Sebaceous adenomas have a lobular configuration with a connection to the epidermis (Fig. 144–11). The tumors are located in the papillary and superficial reticular dermis. The relative amount of basaloid peripheral sebocytes is increased in comparison with mature, lipid-containing sebocytes. There is a predominance of mature sebocytes over basaloid cells. The distinction between sebaceous adenomas and sebaceous hyperplasia is made based upon loss of the clustering architecture and increased numbers of basaloid cells in the adenomas. Distinction from sebaceous epithelioma is often difficult, but there is an increase in the number of basaloid cells in the epithelioma.

PATHOGENESIS AND ETIOLOGY

These tumors are derived from sebaceous epithelium and usually occur on sun-damaged skin.

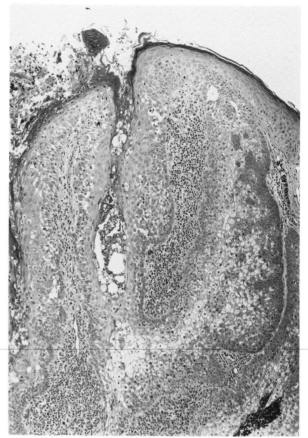

FIGURE 144–11. Sebaceous adenoma features an endophytic lobular proliferation in which basaloid cells are present at the periphery and sebocytes are found centrally.

DIAGNOSIS AND DIFFERENTIAL DIAGNOSIS

Biopsy is usually required to obtain the diagnosis. Clinical and histologic differential diagnosis includes sebaceous hyperplasia, basal cell carcinoma, and sebaceous epithelioma.

TREATMENT

Excision is curative. Family history should be sought and evaluation for Muir-Torre syndrome performed when indicated.

Sebaceous Epithelioma

CLINICAL DESCRIPTION AND EPIDEMIOLOGY

Sebaceous epithelioma is usually found on the face or scalp as a small pearly to yellow nodule that may be ulcerated. It can arise in nevus sebaceus[34] and can be found in the Muir-Torre syndrome. Troy and Ackerman proposed that the concept of sebaceous epithelioma is flawed and proposed that these benign neoplasms are composed of dermal lobules of sebocytes and basaloid cells without connection to the epidermis.[35] These authors distinguish sebaceoma from the rare basal cell carcinoma with sebaceous differentiation.

PATHOLOGY

Sebaceous epithelioma is less differentiated than sebaceous adenoma. It demonstrates peripheral palisading of basaloid cells with irregular masses of sebocytes. Some cases are indistinguishable from, and in fact are, basal cell carcinoma with sebaceous differentiation.

PATHOGENESIS AND ETIOLOGY

Sebaceous epithelioma is thought to be derived from a primitive cell destined for sebaceous differentiation.

DIAGNOSIS AND DIFFERENTIAL DIAGNOSIS

Clinically and histologically, sebaceous epithelioma is easily confused with basal cell carcinoma, sebaceous hyperplasia, and sebaceous adenoma.

TREATMENT

Excision is curative.

Sebaceous Carcinoma

CLINICAL DESCRIPTION AND EPIDEMIOLOGY

Sebaceous carcinoma is quite rare and is usually found on the eyelids, although rare cases arise at other sites. Sebaceous carcinoma accounts for 1% to 3% of eyelid malignancies. It is an aggressive neoplasm, metastasizing first to regional nodes and later to the liver, lung, and brain. Approximately 33% of patients may develop metastases, although this is based on a series of only 44 patients.[36] The 5-year mortality rate is thought to be about 20%.[37] Lesions appear as asymptomatic, firm, nonencapsulated nodules, usually on the upper eyelid (Fig. 144–12). The eyelid malignancies frequently have pagetoid spread of neoplastic cells widely in the epidermis.

Some lesions are associated with previous radiation treatment to the area for unrelated conditions.[38] Sebaceous carcinoma is also seen in association with the Muir-Torre syndrome.

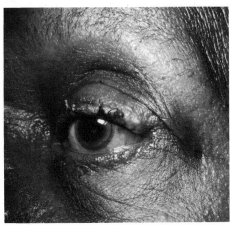

FIGURE 144–12. Sebaceous carcinoma. Note thickening of lid and yellowish nodule involving the upper lid. This tumor was removed with Mohs' surgery, sparing the eye. There is no recurrence at 4 years follow-up.

PATHOLOGY

Sebaceous carcinomas are often poorly differentiated carcinomas present mainly within the dermis. Multiple lobules of basaloid, undifferentiated cells are present in the dermis. In the central portions of the lobules, more mature sebocytes are present (Fig. 144–13). There is marked nuclear atypia and pleomorphism, and mitoses are common. Keratinization may be present within some of the tumor lobules and may be predominant in some tumors.

Histologically, sebaceous carcinoma can be confused with squamous cell carcinoma, particularly if lipidization of the tumor is not prominent. Fat stains, on frozen sections, can help with this distinction, as can a microvascular pattern with immunoperoxidase staining for epithelial membrane antigen.

In about half of cases, there is pagetoid spread of tumor cells throughout all levels of the epidermis.[38] It had long been thought that pagetoid spread heralded a worse prognosis, though this has been refuted.[37] These pagetoid cells have abundant, clear, foamy cytoplasm and nuclear atypia. In this situation, sebaceous carcinoma can be confused with Bowen's disease, extramammary Paget's disease, Merkel cell carcinoma, and amelanotic melanoma.

PATHOGENESIS AND ETIOLOGY

Sebaceous carcinoma is thought to be derived from the sebaceous glands of structures near the eye, most commonly the meibomian glands, followed, in descending frequency, by the glands of Zeis, the caruncle, and the eyebrows.[39, 40]

DIAGNOSIS AND DIFFERENTIAL DIAGNOSIS

The clinical presentation of sebaceous carcinoma is subtle, and diagnosis can be difficult. The lesion can

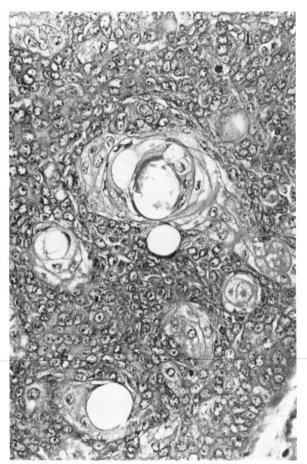

FIGURE 144-13. Sebaceous carcinoma, hematoxylin and eosin. There are atypical cells with many mitoses, among which are foci of sebaceous ductal differentiation and clusters of sebocytes.

mimic ruptured cysts, blepharitis, conjunctivitis, chalazion, and later basal cell carcinoma, or other adnexal tumors. Diagnosis is usually a late one, and this contributes to the poor outcome of some patients.[41]

TREATMENT

Treatment is surgical, with complete excision verified by negative margins. The Mohs technique has been used with some success for sebaceous carcinoma, although recurrences have been reported.[42] It has been suggested that this malignancy may be multifocal, although why this would be is uncertain. This author (BC) believes there may be skip areas as a result of previous treatment or spontaneous regression.

A particularly difficult situation to treat with the Mohs or any other technique is the pagetoid spread of tumor onto the conjunctiva of the eye. It is almost impossible to cut frozen sections of conjunctiva. In this circumstance, it may be better to use widespread cryosurgery on the conjunctiva and follow up with frequent conjunctival biopsies. If the conjunctival disease recurs, orbital exenteration may be the only option to prevent eventual metastatic disease.

Oil red O fat stains are of great help in tracking this tumor with Mohs' surgery. The fat in a sebaceous carcinoma stains in a unique microglobular pattern, allowing ready distinction from surrounding meibomian gland or other fatty tissue.

Metastatic disease to the lymph nodes of the neck occurs most commonly. Neck dissection, superficial parotidectomy, and radiation therapy are indicated in this circumstance.

References

1. Smith KJ, Skelton HG, Holland TT. Recent advances and controversies concerning adnexal neoplasms. New Dev Dermpath 1992;10:117–160.
2. Marrogi AJ, Wick MR, Dehner LP. Benign cutaneous adnexal tumors in childhood and young adults, excluding pilomatrixoma: Review of 28 cases and literature. J Cutan Pathol 1991;18:20–27.
3. Cotton D. Troublesome tumors 1: Adnexal tumours of the skin. J Clin Pathol 1991;44:543–548.
4. Mehregan AH. Infundibular tumors of the skin. J Cutan Pathol 1984;11:387–395.
5. Mehregan H, Brownstein MH. Pilar sheath acanthoma. Arch Dermatol 1978;114:1495–1497.
6. Shapiro PE, Kopf AW. Familial multiple desmoplastic trichoepitheliomas. Arch Dermatol 1991;127:83–87.
7. Brownstein H, Mehregan AH, Bikowski JB, et al. The dermatopathology of Cowden's syndrome. Br J Dermatol 1979;100:667–673.
8. Brownstein MH, Mehregan AH, Bikowski JB. Trichilemmomas in Cowden's disease. JAMA 1977;238:26.
9. Gentry WC, Eskritt NR, Gorlin RJ. Multiple hamartoma syndrome (Cowden's disease). Arch Dermatol 1972;106:682.
10. Shaprio SD, Lambert CW, Schwartz RA. Cowden's disease. A marker for malignancy. Int J Dermatol 1988;27:232–237.
11. Rothenberg J, Lambert WC, Vail JT, et al. The Muir-Torre (Torre's) syndrome: The significance of a solitary sebaceous tumor. J Am Acad Dermatol 1990;23:638–640.
12. Wick MR, Coffin CM. Sweat gland and pilar carcinomas. In: Wick MR, ed. Pathology of Unusual Malignant Cutaneous Tumors. New York: Marcel Dekker, 1985.
13. Winer LH. The dilated pore, a trichoepithelioma. J Invest Dermatol 1954;23:181–188.
14. Gray FHR, Helwig EB. Trichofolliculoma. Arch Dermatol 1962;86:619–625.
15. Pinkus H, Sutton RL. Trichofolliculoma. Arch Dermatol 1965;91:46–49.
16. Brooke JD, Fitzpatrick JE, Golitz LE. Papillary mesenchymal bodies: A histologic finding useful in differentiating trichoepitheliomas from basal cell carcinomas. J Am Acad Dermatol 1989;21:523–528.
17. Brownstein MH. The genodermatology of adnexal tumors. J Cutan Pathol 1984;11:457–465.
18. MacDonald DM, Wilson-Jones E, Marks R. Sclerosing epithelial hamartoma. Clin Exp Dermatol 1977;2:153–160.
19. Hunt SJ, Abell E. Malignant hair matrix tumor ("malignant trichoepithelioma") arising in the setting of multiple hereditary trichoepitheliomas. Am J Dermatopathol 1991;13:275–281.
20. Johnson CJ, Bennett RG. Occurrence of basal cell carcinoma among multiple trichoepitheliomas. J Am Acad Dermatol 1993;28:322–326.
21. Kalloinen M, Twomi ML, Dammer K et al. Desmoplastic trichoepithelioma: Clinicopathologic features and immunohistochemical study of basement membrane proteins, laminin and type IV collagen. Br J Dermatol 1984;111:571–577.
22. Moehlenbeck F. Pilomatrixoma (calcifying epithelioma). Arch Dermatol 1973;108:532–536.
23. Chiaramonti A, Gilgor RS. Pilomatrixomas associated with myotonic dystrophy. Arch Dermatol 1978;114:1363–1365.
24. Booth JC, Kramer H, Taylor KB. Pilomatrixoma: Calcifying epithelioma (Malherbe). Pathology 1969;1:119–127.
25. Leonardi CL, Zhu WY, Kinsey WH, Penneys NS. Trichilemmo-

mas are not associated with human papilloma virus DNA. J Cutan Pathol 1991;18:193–197.

26. Lever WF, Schaumberg-Lever G. Histopathology of the Skin, 7th ed. Philadelphia: JB Lippincott, 1990:593.

27. Lopansri S, Mihm MC. Pilomatrix carcinoma or calcifying epithelioma of Malherbe: A case report and review of literature. Cancer 1980;45:2368–2373.

28. Tateyama H, Eimoto T, Tada T, Niwa T. Malignant pilomatrixoma. An immunohistochemical study with anti–hair keratin antibodies. Cancer 1992;69:127–132.

29. Aloi FG, Molinero A, Pippione M. Basal cell carcinoma with matrical differentiation. Matrical carcinoma. Am J Dermatopathol 1088;10:509–513.

30. Gould E, Kurzon R, Kowalczyk P, et al. Pilomatrix carcinoma with pulmonary metastases. Cancer 1984;54:370–272.

31. Mir R, Cortes E, Papantoniou PA, et al. Metastatic trichomatrical carcinoma. Arch Pathol 1986;110:660–663.

32. Luderschmidt C, Plewig G. Circumscribed sebaceous hyperplasia: Autoradiographic and histoplanometric studies. J Invest Dermatol 1978;70:207–209.

33. Lynch HT, Lynch PM, Pester J, Fusaro RM. The cancer family syndrome. Rare cutaneous phenotypic linkage of Torre's syndrome. Arch Intern Med 1981;141:607–611.

34. Zackheim HS. The sebaceous epithelioma: A clinical and histologic study. Arch Dermatol 1964;89:107.

35. Troy JL, Ackerman AB. Sebaceoma. A distinctive benign neoplasm of adnexal epithelium differentiating toward sebaceous cells. Am J Dermatopathol 1984;6:7–13.

36. Wick MR, Goellner JR, Wolfe JT, et al. Adnexal carcinomas of the skin II. Extraocular sebaceous carcinomas. Cancer 1985;56:1163–1172.

37. Margo CE, Lessner A, Stern GA. Intraepithelial sebaceous carcinoma of the conjunctiva and skin of the eyelid. Ophthalmology 1992;99:227–231.

38. Russell WG, Page DL, Hough AJ, et al. Sebaceous carcinoma of meibomian gland origin: The diagnostic importance of pagetoid spread of neoplastic cells. Am J Clin Pathol 1980;73:504–511.

39. Lemos LB, Santa Cruz DJ, Baba N. Sebaceous carcinoma of the eyelid following radiation therapy. Am J Surg Pathol 1978;2:305–311.

40. Loeber CW, Fenske NA. Basal cell, squamous cell, and sebaceous gland carcinomas of the periorbital region. J Am Acad Dermatol 1991;25:685–690.

41. Gurin DM, Rapini RP. Aggressive sebaceous carcinoma of the eyelid: An elusive diagnosis. Cutis 1993;52:40–42.

42. Folberg R, Whitaker DC, Tse DT, et al. Recurrent and residual sebaceous carcinoma after Mohs' excision of the primary lesion. Am J Ophthalmol 1987;103:817–823.

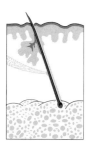

Neoplasms with Eccrine or Apocrine Differentiation

BRUCE R. SMOLLER and BRETT COLDIRON

Tumors that differentiate toward the eccrine sweat coil or duct make up 1% of all cutaneous neoplasms. Most are benign and can often be controlled with simple excision. The traditional classification and nomenclature are based on differentiation and histopathologic pattern. Immunophenotypic data have also played a role in their classification (Fig. 145–1).[1-3]

Apocrine tumors can differentiate toward either the secretory coil, the duct, or both. Because apocrine and eccrine ducts are indistinguishable, and the apocrine duct is not divided into distinct portions, the precise differentiation of apocrine neoplasms cannot be as easily pinpointed as that of eccrine tumors. The more common tumors are discussed in this chapter. Those tumors that are less common are listed in Table 145–1. The reader is referred to monographs and textbooks of dermatopathology for detailed descriptions of these entities.

ECCRINE NEOPLASMS

Cylindroma

Clinical Description

Cylindromas occur sporadically as single lesions or as multiple lesions, usually in patients with a family history of similar lesions. An autosomal dominant inheritance pattern has been postulated in these familial cases. Single lesions are more frequent. Cylindromas are asymptomatic, firm, dermal or subcutaneous nodules that usually arise during early adulthood. Ulceration is rare. Cylindromas are usually smaller than 1 cm, except in patients with multiple lesions, in whom individual lesions can

grow to be many centimeters in diameter (Fig. 145–2). The head and neck are frequent sites. Malignant transformation is extremely rare and is more often seen in patients with multiple cylindromas.[4, 5]

Pathology

Cylindromas are situated in the reticular dermis or subcutis and are not connected to the epidermis. They are usually unifocal and grow as sharply circumscribed, expansile nodules. Sheets of relatively small, hyperchromatic cells are arranged in angulated, interlocking nests, surrounded by densely eosinophilic basement membrane material, in a pattern described as "jigsaw puzzle–like" (Fig. 145–3). The two types of cells that ordinarily comprise the normal eccrine duct are also seen in cylindromas: cells with slightly vesicular nuclei and small amounts of cytoplasm admixed with cells with darker nuclei and virtually no identifiable cytoplasm. Duct formation is often difficult to find. Abundant mitotic activity and cytologic atypia are not found. The material surrounding the nests of keratinocytes has been shown to be predominantly reduplicated type IV collagen.

Pathogenesis and Etiology

The histogenesis of cylindroma is still controversial. Most authors now believe cylindromas display eccrine differentiation.[6, 7] However, some histochemical and ultrastructural properties of the cells in this neoplasm are suggestive of apocrine glandular epithelium. The reports of tumors with features of both eccrine spiradenoma and cylindroma favor eccrine differentiation.[8]

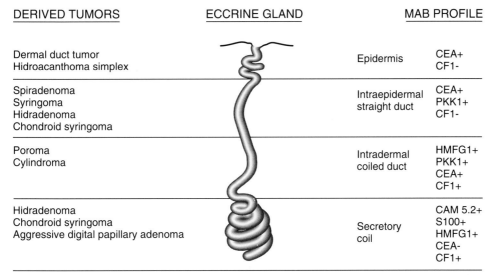

DERIVED TUMORS	ECCRINE GLAND	MAB PROFILE
Dermal duct tumor Hidroacanthoma simplex	Epidermis	CEA+ CF1-
Spiradenoma Syringoma Hidradenoma Chondroid syringoma	Intraepidermal straight duct	CEA+ PKK1+ CF1-
Poroma Cylindroma	Intradermal coiled duct	HMFG1+ PKK1+ CEA+ CF1+
Hidradenoma Chondroid syringoma Aggressive digital papillary adenoma	Secretory coil	CAM 5.2+ S100+ HMFG1+ CEA- CF1+

FIGURE 145–1. Origin and monoclonal antibody profile of eccrine appendage tumors. CEA, carcinoembryonic antigen; PKK1, cytokeratins 8, 18, 19; HMFG1, human milk fat globulin; CAM 5.2, cytokeratins 8, 18; CF1, cystic fluid protein. (Data from references 1, 3, 28, and 61.)

Diagnosis and Differential Diagnosis

The clinical differential diagnosis is that of a dermal or subcutaneous nodule. Because there are no distinguishing clinical characteristics, diagnosis is made on biopsy. The diagnosis of cylindroma can be made solely on clinical observations when multiple large lesions are present, especially on the head and neck.

The histologic differential diagnosis is limited. In some cases, differentiation from eccrine spiradenoma can be difficult, and some lesions are composites of both neoplasms.

Treatment

Excision is curative. The rare cases with malignant transformation require wider excision to prevent local recurrence.

Syringoma

Clinical Description

Syringomas are benign, flesh colored to slightly yellow, soft, papules, usually found scattered on the lower eyelids. There is a female predilection, with onset at puberty.[9] They can be found where apocrine glands are found, including axillae, umbilicus, groin, and vulva,

**TABLE 145–1. Rare Eccrine
and Apocrine Tumors**

Eccrine nevus
Syringofibroadenoma
Papillary eccrine adenoma
Dermal duct tumor
Apocrine nevus
Tubular apocrine adenoma

despite the fact that they are thought to be of eccrine sweat duct origin.[10] Rare presentations include eruptive and linear lesions.[11]

Pathology

There is a well-circumscribed proliferation of small ductal structures embedded in a dense fibrous stroma in the papillary and superficial reticular dermis, without epidermal connections. The ductal structures often appear tadpole-like (Fig. 145–4). Surrounding a central duct are several layers of cuboidal cells. The innermost layer(s) is composed of keratinocytes, and the outermost, if present, of myoepithelial cells. Small cornifying cysts can be present.

In the rare, clear cell variant the ductular lining cells have excessive glycogen. These lesions may be a marker for diabetes mellitus.[12, 13]

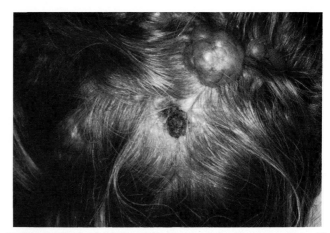

FIGURE 145–2. Multiple cylindromas on scalp. (Courtesy of June K. Robinson, M.D.)

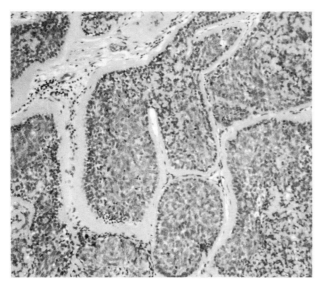

FIGURE 145-3. Cylindroma, low-power view. Note angulated epithelial islands surrounded by hyalinized basement membrane material (H&E, ×160).

TABLE 145-2. Histologic Differential Diagnosis of Syringoma
Desmoplastic trichoepithelioma
Morpheaform basal cell carcinoma
Sclerosing sweat duct carcinoma
Microcystic adnexal carcinoma
Chondroid syringoma
Adenosquamous carcinoma

Treatment

Reassurance is often the best therapy. If the patient desires treatment, syringomas can be unroofed with fine scissors and chemically cauterized, removed with a punch biopsy, or flattened to the contour of the surrounding skin by treating gently with electrodesiccation, or with the defocused beam of the carbon dioxide laser.

Chondroid Syringoma and Malignant Chondroid Syringoma

Clinical Description

This tumor is also called mixed tumor of the skin.[14] It appears as a firm dermal or subcutaneous nodule, 0.5 to 3 cm in diameter, usually on the head or neck of elderly men. The overlying skin may be fixed to the nodule but is otherwise unaltered (Fig. 145-5). Malignant chondroid syringoma has a similar clinical presentation except that this tumor is more often found on the extremities.

Pathology

Chondroid syringomas are sharply circumscribed dermal or subcutaneous proliferations with no connection to the overlying epidermis. They are composed of a proliferation of ductular elements lined by two layers of cells. These epithelial elements grow in two patterns, the

Pathogenesis and Etiology

Syringoma is thought to differentiate toward the eccrine sweat duct. Its cells do not react with monoclonal antisera that identify determinants found only in eccrine secretory structures (see Fig. 145-1).

Diagnosis and Differential Diagnosis

Clinically, syringoma can be confused with sebaceous hyperplasia, eruptive xanthoma, hidrocystoma, and acne vulgaris. Table 145-2 is a list of the entities that cause the most difficulty in the histologic differential diagnosis of syringoma. Its differentiation from microcystic adnexal carcinoma is the most difficult of these, but the carcinoma is poorly circumscribed and extends much deeper.

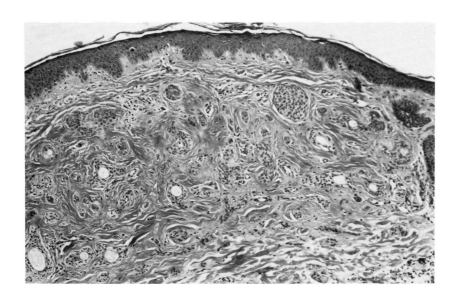

FIGURE 145-4. Syringoma, low-power view. Note tadpole-like ducts (H&E).

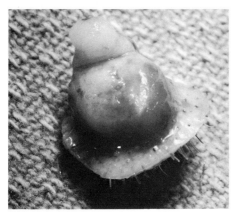

FIGURE 145–5. Chondroid syringoma. Note mucoid appearance of gross specimen removed from the upper lip of a middle-aged man.

more common one suggesting apocrine differentiation and the less frequently encountered pattern being more suggestive of eccrine differentiation. Branching tubules lined by cells showing decapitation secretion occur in the apocrine type, and small round tubules are the hallmark of the eccrine type of mixed tumor (Fig. 145–6).[14]

The epithelial elements are embedded within a basophilic stroma that is rich in acidic mucin and often contains chrondrocytes. Large polygonal cells with eosinophilic cytoplasm (myoepithelial cells) are often embedded in this stroma, which can comprise up to half of the neoplasm. Cytologic atypia is not seen, and mitoses are rare.[15]

Malignant chondroid syringoma shares many features with its benign counterpart with the addition of large cysts due to necrosis, nuclear atypia, many mitotic figures, vascular invasion, and infiltration of adjacent structures. These features need not be present, however, and metastatic disease has been reported from a primary lesion that seemed histologically benign.[16]

Pathogenesis and Etiology

Chondroid syringoma can show either eccrine or apocrine differentiation. Both ductal and secretory structures can be found on electron microscopy.[17]

Diagnosis and Differential Diagnosis

Biopsy is usually needed for diagnosis. Clinically, because they are so firm, chondroid syringoma can be confused with pilomatricoma or a calcified trichilemmal cyst. Histologically, small chondroid syringomas with eccrine differentiation can be confused with syringoma. Large lesions with abundant epithelial components could be confused with a mucinous basal cell carcinoma.

Malignant chondroid syringoma can be confused with its benign counterpart and with extraskeletal myxoid chondrosarcoma.

Treatment

Excision of the benign chondroid syringoma is usually curative. Malignant chondroid syringoma can recur locally or metastasize.[16, 18] It should be excised with margin control and patients observed for recurrent or metastatic disease.

Poroma and Porocarcinoma

Clinical Description

Poromas are benign neoplasms that differentiate toward the poroid and cuticular cells of the acrosyringium. They make up about 10% of all sweat gland tumors.[19, 20] They present as solitary, slowly growing, flesh-colored to erythematous dome-shaped papules or nodules in older adults.[21] Most are found on the sides or the sole of the foot where the density of sweat glands is high (620/cm²). Poromas have also been reported on

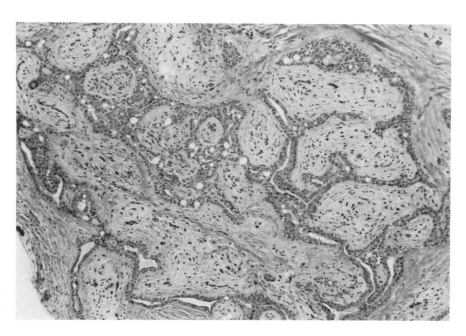

FIGURE 145–6. Chondroid syringoma, apocrine type. Note tubules embedded in mucinous stroma (H&E).

extremities, chest, back, and scalp. Poromas are usually painless, unless they are on the sole of the foot.

Porocarcinoma is the rare malignant counterpart to poroma. It occurs as a solitary nodule or plaque, usually on the extremities or head of an elderly person. These tumors can arise from within benign poromas and are often diagnosed after a rapid increase in size in a previously indolent lesion.[22, 23]

Pathology

Eccrine poroma is a sharply demarcated tumor that extends downward from the overlying epidermis, growing as a broad plate-like extension. The tumor cells are pale, small, cuboidal keratinocytes with monomorphous nuclei. Their pink cytoplasm is due to increased glycogen (Fig. 145–7). This glycogen is accentuated with a periodic acid–Schiff stain, which also highlights the occasional ductular lumina.[24] Variants of poroma include a form in which nests are present within the epidermis (hidroacanthoma simplex) and one in which only dermal nests occur (dermal duct tumor).

Porocarcinoma is poorly circumscribed and shows larger atypical cells and numerous mitoses. Lymphatic invasion is often present. Metastatic poromas often spread to the skin and are frequently epidermotropic.[25]

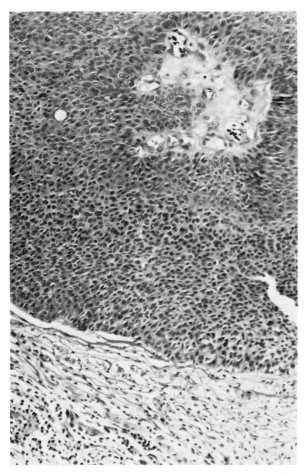

FIGURE 145–7. Eccrine poroma, low-power view. Note broad plate-like extension into the dermis (H&E).

Pathogenesis and Etiology

Poromas differentiate toward the poroid cells and cuticular cells of the acrosyringium.[3]

Diagnosis and Differential Diagnosis

Clinically, poromas are unique but can be confused with neurofibroma, a large callus, or squamous cell carcinoma. Other lesions that should be included in the clinical differential diagnosis are listed in Table 145–3. Histologically, poromas superficially resemble psoriasis, seborrheic keratoses, and occasionally basal cell carcinoma.

Porocarcinoma can be confused with squamous and basal cell carcinoma. The differential diagnosis of cutaneous metastases of porocarcinoma includes extramammary Paget's disease, mammary Paget's disease, Bowen's disease, and amelanotic melanoma.

Treatment

Complete excision of benign poroma is curative. Porocarcinoma is aggressive, with local extension as well as metastatic disease being reported.[26, 27] Recurrent benign poroma and malignant porocarcinoma should be considered for microscopically controlled excision. Porocarcinoma must be observed for the possibility of metastatic disease.

Clear Cell Hidradenoma and Hidradenocarcinoma

Clinical Description

Clear cell hidradenoma is also known as nodular hidradenoma, eccrine acrospiroma, eccrine sweat gland adenoma, clear cell sweat gland adenoma, clear cell myoepithelioma, and solid-cystic hidradenoma.

Clear cell hidradenomas are solitary, dermal nodules, measuring from 0.5 to 2 cm in diameter (Fig. 145–8). There is no particular distribution and no way to determine the diagnosis from clinical appearance. The skin covering these lesions is usually normal in appearance, although red to blue coloration, and occasional ulceration, has been described.[28]

Hidradenocarcinoma usually appears as a solitary, 1- to 5-cm ulcerated nodule, most commonly on the hands and feet. It can also occur on the scalp and face. It usually

TABLE 145-3. Clinical Differential Diagnosis of Eccrine Poroma
Pyogenic granuloma
Fibroma
Hemangioma
Amelanotic melanoma
Basal cell carcinoma
Squamous cell carcinoma
Dermatofibroma
Epidermal nevus

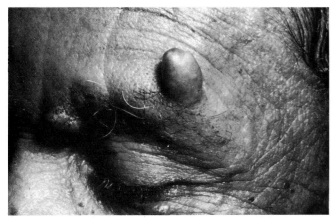

FIGURE 145–8. Hidradenoma on eyebrow of elderly male. Diagnosis was made pathologically.

TABLE 145–4. Histologic Differential Diagnosis of Clear Cell Hidradenoma
Metastatic adenocarcinoma (especially renal cell carcinoma)
Balloon cell melanoma
Squamous cell carcinoma
Chondroid syringoma
Glomus tumor

occurs in older individuals, and metastatic disease is common.[29-31]

Pathology

Clear cell hidradenoma most commonly grows in a nodular, expansile pattern. The lobules of the tumor are surrounded by condensed collagen. Clear cell change is helpful when prominent. The lobules are composed of well-circumscribed masses of ductal and secretory cells and occasional tubules. There are solid and cystic areas. In solid areas there are two distinct cell populations. These consist of cuboidal ductal cells and columnar secretory cells. The columnar cells may have cytoplasms that contain mucin. Cells showing decapitation secretion can also be seen. Usually there is no connection to the overlying epidermis.[30] An eosinophilic, hyalinized stroma on the edges of the tumor sends slender projections into the tumor. Mitotic activity, without atypical mitoses, is usually seen. Multiple separate foci of growth, atypical mitoses, zonal necrosis, and invasion into vascular spaces or along perineurial sheaths are features that raise the possibility of clear cell hidradenocarcinoma.[31]

Pathogenesis and Etiology

Hidradenomas are primitive adnexal tumors that show differentiation spanning the entire eccrine and apocrine apparatus. Although some histochemical and ultrastructural studies support an eccrine origin, unequivocal evidence of apocrine differentiation can be present in the form of decapitation secretion in some cases.

Hidradenocarcinoma is thought to arise independently from clear cell hidradenoma and may be of eccrine origin. However, some lesions have been initially diagnosed as clear cell hidradenoma, only to be redefined as hidradenocarcinoma after several local recurrences.[32]

Diagnosis and Differential Diagnosis

Clinically, clear cell hidradenoma resembles many of the other dermal nodules (see Table 144–2). Histologically, when clear cell change is prominent these tumors can be confused with metastatic renal cell carcinoma or balloon cell melanoma. Other entities in the histologic differential diagnosis are seen in Table 145–4. The presence of cytokeratin in a clear cell neoplasm suggests renal cell carcinoma, as well as clear cell hidradenoma, and the absence of cytokeratin suggests melanoma. Since eccrine tumors can express S-100 protein, the expression of this antigen is not helpful in distinguishing clear cell hidradenoma from melanoma.

Treatment

Excision is curative. When occasional lesions recur, reexcision with margin control is indicated. Hidradenocarcinomas must be approached aggressively. Generous biopsy of a suspected hidradenocarcinoma is required because malignant change may be present only focally. Good margin control is needed on excision. Local recurrence rates of up to 50% and metastatic rates of up to 60% have been reported.[28]

Aggressive Digital Papillary Adenoma and Adenocarcinoma

Clinical Description

These are rare tumors that occur under the nail bed, most commonly in white men, and usually involving fingers.[33] The toes, palms, and soles can also be involved. Clinical history usually reveals a single, painless, enlarging mass. Ulceration is uncommon, and tumors rarely compromise digital function.

The variant termed *adenocarcinoma* has a similar presentation, and the diagnosis is made on biopsy. Some regard both variants as malignant—the "adenoma" as a low-grade and the "adenocarcinoma" as a high-grade malignant neoplasm.

Pathology

Aggressive digital papillary adenoma is characterized by one or several nodules with glandular differentiation situated in the reticular dermis. In most cases, no connection to the overlying epidermis can be identified. The glands are lined by one to two layers of mildly atypical cells. Myoepithelial cells are also seen lining the glandular spaces. Nonsulfated acid mucopolysaccharides can be demonstrated within the glandular spaces. Immunoperoxidase reveals that most cases stain with antisera to carcinoembryonic antigen, cytokeratins, and S-100 protein, as do normal eccrine glands. Greater atypia, pleomorphism, and necrosis are seen in the adenocarcinoma, with less glandular differentiation. Invasion of bone and vasculature is seen only with the adenocarcinoma.

Pathogenesis and Etiology

The tumors are believed to demonstrate eccrine glandular differentiation.

Diagnosis and Differential Diagnosis

Histologically, the tumor could be mistaken for papillary eccrine adenoma. Aggressive digital papillary adenocarcinoma resembles many metastatic adenocarcinomas, especially ductal adenocarcinoma of the breast.

Treatment

These tumors are difficult to remove and have a recurrence rate of up to 50%. The adenoma must be excised with margin control. The most reasonable treatment for the adenocarcinoma seems to be excision with margin control or simple amputation at the distal interphalangeal joint. The adenocarcinoma may metastasize many years after removal of the primary tumor.[33]

Eccrine Spiradenoma

Clinical Description

Eccrine spiradenoma is usually a solitary dermal nodule that can be found in all age groups. They are often present on the trunk and extremities and range from 1 to 2 cm in diameter. Nodules are dome shaped and skin colored. They are often painful.[34] Malignant eccrine spiradenoma does occur and arises from within benign eccrine spiradenoma but is quite rare.[35-37]

Pathology

Eccrine spiradenoma is a tumor of the middle to deep reticular dermis or subcutis with no connection to the epidermis. It grows as small well-circumscribed nodules, which are surrounded by compressed collagen (Fig. 145–9). There are two populations of epithelial cells. The larger cells have vesicular nuclei and scant cytoplasm and are admixed with smaller, darker-staining cells with almost no visible cytoplasm. Lymphocytes are almost always scattered within the interlacing cords of epithelial cells.[38] Ductular differentiation may be obvious. In other cases it is possible to find ductular structures only with the use of special stains. Surrounding the nests of epithelial tumor cells, hyalinized, densely eosinophilic basement membrane material (predominantly type IV collagen) is present in variable amounts. Infrequently, areas that are histologically indistinguishable from cylindroma are seen.[7]

Pathogenesis and Etiology

Eccrine spiradenoma does not display definitive signs of differentiation from any specific part of the eccrine apparatus. Some authors believe that they are derived from the outer cells of the intradermal straight duct.[3]

Diagnosis and Differential Diagnosis

Clinically, a diagnostic clue is pain on palpation. Otherwise, the differential diagnosis of dermal nodules is applicable (see Table 144–2, Chapter 144).

The histologic differential diagnosis is seen in Table 145–5. There may be initial confusion with basal cell carcinoma; however, two distinct types of epithelial cells and thickened basement membrane are not features of that neoplasm. Rounded lobules occur in spiradenoma, while closely packed angulated nests are found in cylin-

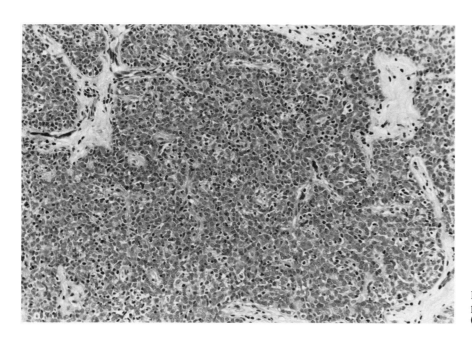

FIGURE 145–9. Eccrine spiradenoma, high-power view. Note the two cell populations (H&E, ×160).

TABLE 145-5. Histologic Differential Diagnosis of Eccrine Spiradenoma
Basal cell carcinoma
Glomus tumor
Lymphoma
Lymphocytoma cutis
Merkel cell carcinoma
Cylindroma
Metastatic carcinoma

droma. Spiradenomas with large cystic or dilated vascular spaces can be confused with glomangiomas.

Treatment

Excision is curative.

Eccrine Carcinoma and its Variants

The classification of eccrine carcinomas is difficult, but several well-defined subtypes have been described.[1] These include microcystic adnexal carcinoma, syringoid eccrine carcinoma, and mucinous eccrine carcinoma. Sweat gland carcinoma is rare, with about 200 cases reported in the literature.

All of these tumors are difficult to cure with conventional excision, and microscopically controlled excision is probably preferable.[39] These tumors infiltrate deeply and widely. Metastatic disease has been reported.[40-43]

Lesions have few distinctive features and are difficult to diagnose clinically and histologically. Metastatic adenocarcinoma should always be ruled out since it can mimic primary sweat gland carcinoma.

Microcystic Adnexal Carcinoma

Clinical Description

This slow-growing, deeply invasive malignancy usually presents as a sclerotic plaque on the face of older women. (Fig. 145-10).[44-46] When stretched under good illumination these plaques have a yellowish hue. These tumors can invade deeply, even into bone, and extend along the sheaths of nerves.

Pathology

Small nests of bland-appearing keratinocytes are seen coursing throughout the papillary and reticular dermis and often into the subcutaneous fat. There is sclerotic stroma (Fig. 145-11). Mucin is scant. In some areas, the keratinocytes form ductular structures that are similar to those seen in syringoma. In other areas there are small keratinizing cysts suggesting differentiation toward the follicular infundibulum. Other features of follicular differentiation such as sebocytes and trichohyaline granules can be present. Marked cytologic atypia is not a feature of microcystic adnexal carcinoma, and necrosis is not present. The mitotic rate is very low. Diagnostic features

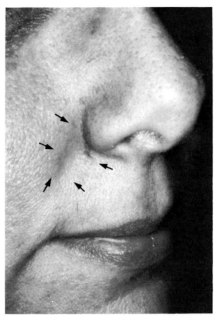

FIGURE 145-10. Microcystic adnexal carcinoma of the junction of the lip and the alar base (*outlined with arrows*) of a middle-aged woman. This firm plaque has a yellowish hue. (Courtesy of June K. Robinson, M.D.)

include poor circumscription, deep extension of tumor, perineural invasion, and both follicular and ductal differentiation.[46-48]

Pathogenesis and Etiology

These tumors stain positively for hair-specific cytokeratin (AE13) and carcinoembryonic antigen, lending support to both pilar and eccrine origin.[1] Others have suggested that the ductular differentiation is apocrine.[49]

Diagnosis and Differential Diagnosis

The diagnosis is typically delayed for many years as the sclerotic plaque slowly enlarges. The clinical and histologic differential includes morpheaform basal cell carcinoma, desmoplastic trichoepithelioma, syringoma, and other sweat gland tumors (see Table 145-2).

Treatment

This tumor extends deeply and diffusely through the dermis and fat far beyond the visible tumor. Recurrences are frequent even following seemingly complete excision, and margin control is essential. Mohs' micrographic surgery is generally regarded as a good approach to these tumors.[50] This tumor may extend for long distances perineurally.

Syringoid (Sclerosing) Sweat Duct Carcinoma

Clinical Description

Syringoid sweat duct carcinoma is usually a solitary tumor or plaque found on the face or scalp of the elderly.

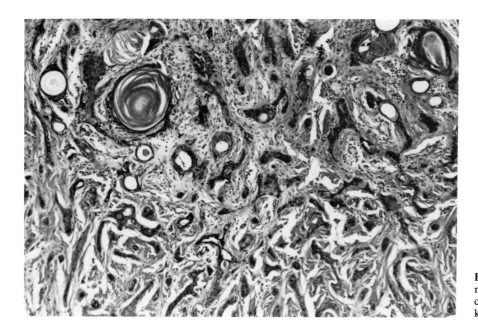

FIGURE 145–11. Microcystic adnexal carcinoma, high-power view. Note nests of keratinocytes coursing through fibrotic matrix. A small keratinizing cyst is at upper left (H&E).

On the scalp, it causes local alopecia. The surface of the lesion may be verrucous and secrete fluid. This tumor is slow growing and locally invasive. Several reports of metastases have been reported.[39] The clinical appearance and behavior of this tumor are similar to those of microcystic adnexal carcinoma.[39, 47]

Pathology

Histologically, a poorly circumscribed neoplasm with sclerotic stroma and slender tubules, some having a tadpole-like appearance, is found in the dermis. There is nuclear atypia and hyperchromatism that can vary from slight to marked deep dermal invasion and crowding of tubules. This is the only sweat gland malignancy aside from porocarcinoma with a characteristic epidermal change, consisting of acanthosis and papillomatosis.

Pathogenesis and Etiology

These tumors are of eccrine origin, but their precise differentiation has not yet been determined.

Diagnosis and Differential Diagnosis

Syringoid carcinomas may appear as verrucous hyperkeratotic plaques. In these cases, the clinical differential diagnosis would include the lesions listed in Table 145–6. In other cases, the clinical appearance may be nondescript. Histologically, there may be marked similarity to syringoma if only small, partial biopsy specimens are available for examination. However, unlike syringoma, there may be deep infiltration, cells may be anaplastic, and numerous mitoses may be present.[39] Microcystic adnexal carcinoma can also be confused with syringoid carcinoma. However, syringoid carcinomas do not display follicular differentiation, cysts, or prominent perineural invasion. As is the case with all eccrine carcinomas, metastatic adenocarcinoma also needs to be

excluded. These tumors are usually more anaplastic and mitotically active than are syringoid carcinomas. Organ-specific differentiation, when present, is also helpful in differentiating metastatic lesions from primary syringoid carcinomas.

Treatment

Syringoid carcinomas extend far beyond their visible borders. Excision with good margin control is essential. Most of these tumors occur on the head and neck where the tissue-sparing features of Mohs' micrographic surgery may be helpful.

Mucinous Carcinoma

Clinical Description

This tumor most frequently arises in the major and minor salivary glands.[51] Approximately 60 cases have been reported. It can also occur in the skin and presents as a solitary nodule, usually on the eyelid or scalp.[52] The appearance of the tumor ranges from bluish to pink or red to simply a skin-colored dermal nodule.[53] The surface can be smooth, bumpy, or crusted. These tumors are locally invasive but rarely metastasize.

TABLE 145–6. Differential Diagnosis of Verrucous Plaques
Nevus sebaceus of Jadassohn
Hidradenoma papilliferum
Lichen simplex chronicus
Epidermal nevus
Nevus comedonicus
Sweat gland carcinoma
Lichen amyloidosis

Pathology

Nests of small cuboidal epithelial cells with slight nuclear atypia, forming duct-like structures, are arranged in cribriform patterns within the dermis. The nests float in pools of acid mucin, restrained by fibrocollagenous septa. Invasion of nerves, blood vessels, and muscle have all been reported.[53]

Pathogenesis and Etiology

Mucinous carcinoma is believed to originate from the sweat gland or a primary germ cell of the sweat gland.

Diagnosis and Differential Diagnosis

Care must be taken to exclude a salivary gland origin of this tumor, which can extend directly or perineurally to the skin. Clinical diagnosis is difficult, and a generous biopsy is needed for definitive diagnosis.

This tumor histologically is quite similar to mucinous carcinomas arising from the breast, bowel, or other sites,[54, 55] Almost all visceral mucinous carcinomas that metastasize are large enough to declare themselves clinically, so that an isolated cutaneous mucinous carcinoma of more than a few weeks' duration is likely to be primary. Histologically, the basaloid proliferation can be confused with the adenoid pattern of basal cell carcinoma and eccrine epithelioma. The basaloid proliferation does not show palisading, and there is no connection to the epidermis as is usually seen in the other two neoplasms.

Treatment

Mucinous carcinoma is locally aggressive with a high recurrence rate.[56] Perineural invasion is frequent. Local lymph node metastases occur, and rarely there is widespread metastatic disease.[57] Excision with good margin control is essential. Mohs' micrographic surgery has been used successfully for this tumor.[58, 59] Patients with primary mucinous carcinoma of the skin should be evaluated for the possibility of metastatic disease, particularly from the breast and gastrointestinal tract.

APOCRINE NEOPLASMS

Syringocystadenoma Papilliferum

Clinical Description

Most of these tumors occur on the face and scalp as verrucous, skin-colored papules merging into plaques. Up to 30% of cases arise within a nevus sebaceus of Jadassohn and may show a linear or zosteriform distribution.[60] Lesions may enlarge or spontaneously develop at puberty.

Pathology

A cystic structure in the mid dermis is filled with numerous papillary infoldings. The epidermis is hyperkeratotic and verrucous. An opening to the surface may be seen. There are two cell layers in the papillary projections: the inner layer is columnar epithelium demonstrating decapitation secretion, and the outer is a basaloid to cuboidal layer. Small lumina can be seen (Fig. 145–12). The stroma is heavily infiltrated with plasma cells.

Pathogenesis and Etiology

The origin of this tumor is debated. Syringocystadenoma papilliferum shows positive immunoreactivity for gross cystic disease fluid protein, indicating apocrine origin.[61] The many plasma cells bear IgA, similar to those of the secretory immune system.

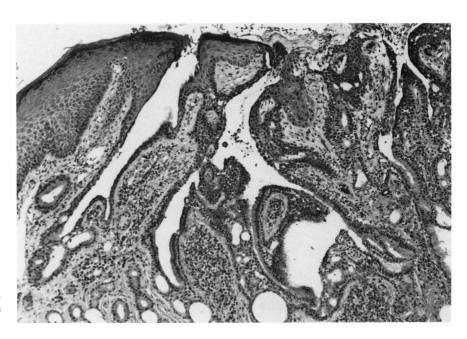

FIGURE 145–12. Syringocystadenoma papilliferum, high-power view. Note two cell layers in papillary projections (H&E).

TABLE 145-7. Histologic Differential Diagnosis of Syringocystadenoma Papilliferum

Hidradenoma papilliferum
Tubular apocrine adenoma
Erosive adenomatosis of the nipple
Adenocarcinoma
Cutaneous endometriosis

Diagnosis and Differential Diagnosis

Clinical diagnosis is difficult. Table 145–6 displays a partial differential diagnosis of verrucous plaques.

The histologic differential diagnosis is seen in Table 145–7. This tumor can readily be distinguished from hidradenoma papilliferum by the intense infiltration of plasma cells into the stroma of the tumor.

Treatment

Excision is curative. Rare malignant change has been reported.[62]

Hidradenoma Papilliferum

Clinical Description

These are usually solitary, skin-colored, pink or red dermal nodules that range in size from a few millimeters to several centimeters. There is no overlying epidermal change. Location is a clue to diagnosis. They occur almost exclusively in white women older than 30 years of age. The major site of involvement is the anogenital area, but lesions have also been reported on the nipple, supernumerary nipple, eyelid, and external ear.[63]

Pathology

Within the reticular dermis is a well-circumscribed proliferation of cells that grow along papillomatous fibrovascular fronds. Tubules and glands are lined by cells with abundant eosinophilic cytoplasm and small, central nuclei. Decapitation secretion is prominent. Beneath this layer of cells, there is a second layer of small cuboidal-appearing myoepithelial cells. (Fig. 145–13).

Pathogenesis and Etiology

This tumor recapitulates the apocrine secretory coil.

Diagnosis and Differential Diagnosis

The clinical differential diagnosis is difficult because a variety of other dermal nodules occur in the anogenital area of women. Histologically, this tumor can be confused with syringocystadenoma papilliferum, but it does not have the plasma cell infiltrate seen with syringocystadenoma papilliferum and does not ordinarily open to the skin surface. There could also be confusion with tubular apocrine adenoma and erosive adenomatosis of the nipple (see Table 145–7).

Treatment

Excision is curative.

Apocrine Carcinoma

Clinical Description

These rare tumors present as red to purple, often ulcerated, solitary, or multiple cystic masses 1 to 5 cm in size. They are found in areas where apocrine gland density is highest, namely, the axilla, anogenital skin ear

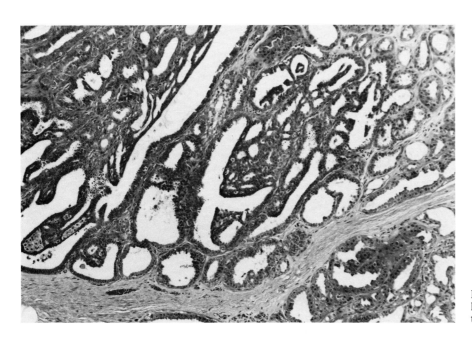

FIGURE 145–13. Hidradenoma papilliferum, high-power view. Note areas of tubule formation and two cell layers (H&E).

canal, and eyelid. Apocrine carcinomas are the most commonly fully malignant neoplasms arising in nevus sebaceus of Jadassohn. They have also been reported in the ear canal and eyelid. Men are affected about twice as often as women, and patients are usually older than age 40.[64]

Pathology

Apocrine carcinomas are usually poorly circumscribed neoplasms with solid, tubular, or papillary patterns. Their hallmark is the presence of cells with voluminous eosinophilic cytoplasm and decapitation secretion.[64]

Pathogenesis and Etiology

These malignancies are believed to arise from normal apocrine glands.

Diagnosis and Differential Diagnosis

Clinically, apocrine carcinoma could be confused with angiosarcoma. The diagnosis is made by biopsy. Histologically, metastatic adenocarcinoma to the skin, particularly from the breast, must be excluded.

Treatment

Treatment is aggressive, with margin control essential.[65]

Extramammary Paget's Disease

Clinical Description

Extramammary Paget's disease is a rare adenocarcinoma usually restricted to the epidermis. It is an indolent disorder of the elderly that eventually can become invasive, metastasize, and cause death.[66-69]

Extramammary Paget's disease presents as a well-circumscribed reddish brown plaque, usually in the anogenital region, although cases have been reported on the chest, axilla, posterior knee, and ear canal. The plaque may be eroded, moist, or velvety (Fig. 145–14). Patients commonly complain of itching, and occasionally pain, at the site.

There are cases that are due to direct extension of an internal adenocarcinoma, especially those of the rectum, bladder, or prostate.[67, 70-73] Internal malignancy must be ruled out before planning therapy (Fig. 145–15).

Pathology

Extramammary Paget's disease is histologically similar to mammary Paget's disease. There is a proliferation of large, atypical cells with abundant, frequently pale-staining cytoplasm usually restricted to the otherwise unremarkable epidermis. Aggregations of cells appear to compress nonneoplastic basal keratinocytes in some cases. Other intraepidermal tumors, which can have similar-appearing large cells, do not ordinarily spare the basal layer as is sometimes seen in Paget's disease and

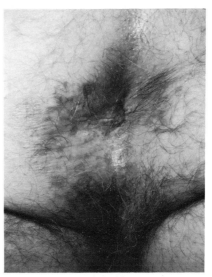

FIGURE 145–14. Extramammary Paget's disease of the rectum. This came to attention after a long history of pruritus ani. Note this tumor was recurrent after CO$_2$ laser ablation. No internal malignancy was present, although the disease did extend into the rectal mucosa.

extramammary Paget's disease. Immunohistochemical stains are helpful in making the diagnosis but do not reliably distinguish Paget's disease of the nipple from extramammary Paget's disease.[74, 75] The cells of extramammary Paget's disease tend to produce acidic mucins rather than the neutral ones produced by those of mammary Paget's disease.

Pathogenesis and Etiology

The cause of extramammary Paget's disease is unknown. It is thought to be of apocrine gland origin, although this is debated. Many believe that it originates from pluripotential epidermal keratinocytes or from rare intraepidermal cells that are committed to sudoriferous differentiation. In 10% or less of cases, extramammary Paget's disease is a direct extension to the epidermis from an underlying adenocarcinoma of the gastrointestinal or urogenital tract. In the majority of cases there is no underlying malignancy and it is apparently an adenocarcinoma of the epidermis that arises de novo. Human papillomavirus DNA has been sought in extramammary Paget's disease and not found.[76]

Diagnosis and Differential Diagnosis

It may take 5 to 10 years before a correct diagnosis is reached, because of confusion with other, more common, maladies (Table 145–8). The histologic differential diagnosis is identical to that of mammary Paget's disease.

Treatment

Extramammary Paget's disease eventually becomes invasive, and it is generally agreed that it should be excised if possible. The disorder always extends beyond the margin of obviously affected tissue and may be multifocal.[77]

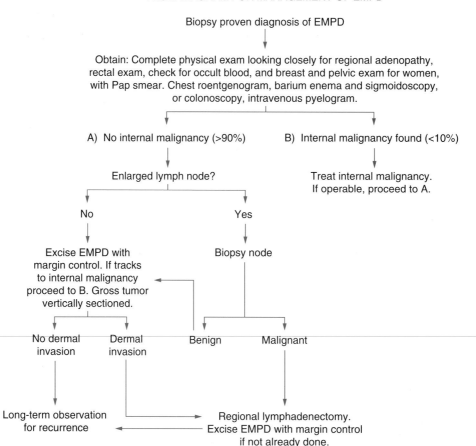

FIGURE 145–15. Flow diagram for the evaluation and treatment of extramammary Paget's disease. (From Coldiron BM, Goldsmith BA, Robinson JK. Surgical treatment of extramammary Paget's disease. Cancer 1991;67:933–938.)

The use of 5-fluorouracil cream to delineate more of the truly affected area has been reported to be helpful.[78]

Extramammary Paget's disease should be excised with careful margin control, or recurrences are notoriously common. The cure rates obtained with Mohs' micrographic surgery versus conventional excision are not significantly different if careful margin control is used in the conventional surgery.[79] However, Mohs' micrographic surgery usually offers the more accurate margin control and can be performed with the use of local anesthesia as an outpatient procedure.[80, 81] This greatly reduces the morbidity, and mortality, of fragile elderly patients who cannot tolerate long periods of general anesthesia. Most Mohs' micrographic surgeons prefer to let the wounds created after resection of the lesions heal by secondary intention because of the high recurrence rate and possibly multifocal nature of this tumor. Radiation therapy and chemotherapy may help with palliation in the rare patient with metastatic disease or whose tumor is inoperable, even under local anesthesia.[82]

Mammary Paget's Disease

Clinical Description

Paget's disease of the breast appears as a solitary, unilateral, erythematous plaque that originates from the nipple. The lesion is sharply defined, and the vast majority of patients are women. The plaque is often crusted, oozing, or scaly and sometimes ulcerated.

This cutaneous lesion is almost always associated with an underlying carcinoma of the breast, from which it may be a direct extension. There is often metastatic disease to the axillary lymph nodes.[83]

Pathology

Paget's disease is characterized by a proliferation of large cells with abundant pale-staining cytoplasm

TABLE 145-8. Differential Diagnosis of Extramammary Paget's Disease	
Clinical	**Histologic**
Dermatophytosis	Mammary Paget's disease
Contact dermatitis	Squamous cell carcinoma
Seborrheic dermatitis	in situ (Bowen's disease)
Psoriasis	Melanoma
Squamous cell carcinoma	Eccrine porocarcinoma
in situ (Bowen's disease)	Sebaceous carcinoma

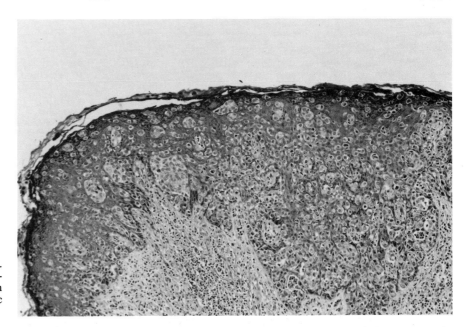

FIGURE 145–16. Mammary Paget's disease. Large nests of atypical Paget's cells fill epidermis. This can be very difficult to distinguish from extramammary disease on histologic sections.

throughout the epidermis. Interspersed between unremarkable keratinocytes, these large cells are present at all layers within the epidermis (Fig. 145–16). A pattern of suprabasilar proliferation, with sparing and compression of the basal keratinocytes, is a very helpful diagnostic feature when present. In some cases there is striking nuclear hyperchromatism and atypia. There may be prominent cytoplasmic vacuolization, with the nuclei pushed to the side of the cell in a signet-ring pattern. In other cases, mucinous change is readily apparent within the cytoplasm of individuals cells. The cells can be highlighted with a periodic acid–Schiff with diastase stain, and stain less strongly for acid mucin with colloidal iron or alcian blue. In addition, it has been shown that a high percentage of cells in Paget's disease stain with antibodies directed against epithelial membrane antigen and carcinoembryonic antigen and against antikeratin monoclonal antibody Cam 5.2.[74]

Pathogenesis and Etiology

Mammary Paget's disease is an adenocarcinoma that has been thought to be due to a direct extension to the epidermis from the underlying ductal carcinoma. In rare cases, no such carcinoma is evident. Studies suggest that the cells of mammary Paget's disease may be of an origin that is different from that of the underlying carcinoma.[84]

Diagnosis and Differential Diagnosis

Other clinical entities that could be confused with mammary Paget's disease are erosive adenomatosis of the nipple, nummular dermatitis, seborrheic dermatitis, psoriasis, and dermatophyte infection. Histologically, mammary Paget's disease can be confused with extramammary Paget's disease, Bowen's disease, and superficial malignant melanoma.

Treatment

The patient needs an evaluation for breast carcinoma and appropriate treatment.

References

1. Smith KJ, Skelton HG, Holland TT. Recent advances and controversies concerning adnexal neoplasms. New Dev Dermopathol 1992;10:117–160.
2. Marrogi AJ, Wick MR, Dehner LP. Benign cutaneous adnexal tumors in childhood and young adults, excluding pilomatrixoma: Review of 28 cases and literature. J Cutan Pathol 1991;18:20–27.
3. Cotton D. Troublesome tumors: I. adnexal tumours of the skin. J Clin Pathol 1991;44:543–548.
4. Lotum M, Trattner A, Kahanovich S, et al. Multiple dermal cylindroma undergoing a malignant transformation. Int J Dermatol 1992;81:642–644.
5. Gerretson AL, van der Putte SCJ, Deenstra W, van Vloten WA. Cutaneous cylindroma with malignant transformation. Cancer 1993;72:1618–1623.
6. Crain RC, Helwig EB. Dermal cylindroma (dermal eccrine cylindroma). Am J Clin Pathol 1961;35:504–515.
7. Abenoza P, Ackerman AB, eds. Neoplasms with Eccrine Differentiation: Cylindromas. Philadelphia: Lea & Febiger, 1990: 251–272.
8. Goette DK, McConnell MA, Fowler VR. Cylindroma and eccrine spiradenoma coexistent in the same lesion. Arch Dermatol 1982;118:273–274.
9. Friedman SJ, Butler DF. Syringoma presenting as milia. J Am Acad Dermatol 1987;16:410–414.
10. Thomas J, Majmudar B, Gorelkin L. Syringoma localized to the vulva. Arch Dermatol 1979;115:95–96.
11. Hashimoto K, Dibella A, Borsuk GM, et al. Eruptive hidradenomas and syringoma. Arch Dermatol 1967;96:500–519.
12. Fiebelman CE, Maize JC. Clear syringoma: A study by conventional and electron microscopy. Am J Dermatopathol 1984; 6:139–150.
13. Saitoh A, Ohtake N, Fukuda S, Tamaki K. Clear cells of eccrine glands in a patient with clear cell syringoma associated with diabetes mellitus. Am J Dermatopathol 1993;15:166–168.
14. Headington JT. Mixed tumors of the skin: Eccrine and apocrine types. Arch Dermatol 1961;84:989–996.
15. Inglesias DF, Forcelledo FF, Sanchez ST, et al. Chondroid syrin-

goma: A histological and immunohistochemical study of 15 cases. Histopathology 1990;17:311–317.

16. Harrist TJ, Aretz TH, Mihm MC, et al. Cutaneous malignant mixed tumor. Dermatologica 1981;117:719–724.

17. Varela-Duran J, et al. Ultrastructure of chondroid syringoma. Cancer 1979;44:148–156.

18. Hirsh P, Helwig EB. Chondroid syringoma. Arch Dermatol 1961;84:835–847.

19. Pylyser K, Wolf-Peters C, Marien K. Histology of eccrine poromas: Study of 14 cases. Dermatologica 1983;167:243–249.

20. Pinkus H, Rogin J, Goldman P. Eccrine poroma: Tumors exhibiting features of the epidermal sweat duct unit. Arch Dermatol 1956;74:511–521.

21. Johnson RC, Rosenmeier GJ, Keeling JH. A painful step: Eccrine poroma. Arch Dermatol 1992;128:1530–1533.

22. Bottles K, Sagebiel R, McNutt NS, et al. Malignant eccrine poroma: Case report and literature review. Cancer 1984;53:1579–1585.

23. Matloub H, Cunningham M, Yousif N, et al. Eccrine porocarcinoma. Ann Plast Surg 1988;20:351–355.

24. Pinkus H. The discovery of eccrine poroma. Dermatology 1979;2:26–38.

25. Landa NG, Winkelmann RK. Epidermotropic eccrine porocarcinoma. J Am Acad Dermatol 1991;24:27–31.

26. Dummer R, Becker JC, Boser B, et al. Successful therapy of metastatic eccrine poroma using perilesional interferon α and interleukin 2. Arch Dermatol 1992;128:1127–1128.

27. Pinkus H, Mehregan AH. Epidermotrophic eccrine carcinoma. Arch Dermatol 1963;88:597–606.

28. Murphy GF, Elder DE. Cutaneous appendage tumors. In: Rosai J, Sobin LH, eds. Atlas of Tumor Pathology: Non-Melanocytic Tumors of the Skin, 3rd series, fascicle 1. Bethesda, MD: Armed Forces Institute of Pathology, 1991:61–152.

29. Headington JT, Niederhuber JE, Beals TF. Malignant clear cell acrospiroma. Cancer 1978;41:641–647.

30. Hernandez-Perez E, Cestoni-Parducci R. Nodular hidradenoma and hidradenocarcinoma. J Am Acad Dermatol 1985;12:15–20.

31. Hernandez-Perez E, Cruz FA. Clear cell hidradenocarcinoma: Report of an unusual case. Dermatologica 1976;153:249–252.

32. Keasbey LE, Hadley GG. Clear cell hidradenoma. Report of three cases with widespread metastases. Cancer 1954;7:934–952.

33. Kao GF, Helwig EB, Grahm JH. Aggressive digital papillary adenoma and adenocarcinoma: A clinicopathological study of 57 patients, with histochemical, immunopathological, and ultrastructural observations. J Cutan Pathol 1987;14:129–146.

34. Kersting DW, Helwig EG. Eccrine spiradenoma. Arch Dermatol 1956;73:199–205.

35. Engel J, Meads GE, Joseph NG, Stavraky W. Eccrine spiradenoma: A report of malignant transformation. Can J Surg 1991;34:477–480.

36. Argenyi ZS, Nguyen AV, Balogh K, et al. Malignant eccrine spiradenoma: A clinicopathologic study. Am J Dermatopathol 1992;14:381–390.

37. Cooper PH, Frierson HF, Morrison AG. Malignant transformation of eccrine spiradenoma. Arch Dermatol 1985;121:1445–1448.

38. Al-Nafussi A, Blessing K, Rahilly M. Non-epithelial cellular components in eccrine spiradenoma: A histological and immunohistochemical study of 20 cases. Histopathology 1991;18:155–160.

39. Moy RL, Rivkin JE, Lee H, et al. Syringoid eccrine carcinoma. J Am Acad Dermatol 1991;24:864–867.

40. Okada N, Junko O, Sato K, Kitano Y. Metastasizing eccrine sweat gland carcinoma. Arch Dermatol 1984;120:768–769.

41. Dzubow LM, Grossman DJ, Johnson B. Chemosurgical report: Eccrine adenocarcinoma: Report of a case, treatment with Mohs surgery. J Dermatol Surg Oncol 1986;12:1049–1053.

42. Hirsch LF, Enterline HT, Rosato EF, Rosato FE. Sweat gland carcinoma. Ann Surg 1971;174:283–287.

43. Morris DM, Sanusi ID, Lanehart WH. Carcinoma of eccrine sweat glands: Experience with chemotherapy, autopsy findings in a patient with metastatic eccrine carcinoma and a review of the literature. J Surg Oncol 1986;31:26–30.

44. Yuh WT, Engelken JD, Whitaker DC, Dolan KD. Bone marrow invasion of microcystic adnexal carcinoma. Ann Otol Rhinol Laryngol 1991;100:601–603.

45. Borenstein A, Seidman DS, Trau H, Tsur H. Case report: Micro-

cystic adnexal carcinoma following radiotherapy in childhood. Am J Med Sci 1991;301:259–261.

46. Birkby CS, Argenyi AB, Whitaker DC. Microcystic adnexal carcinoma with mandibular invasion and bone marrow replacement. J Dermatol Surg Oncol 1989;15:308–312.

47. Nickoloff BJ, Fleischmann HE, Carmel J. Microcystic adnexal carcinoma. Arch Dermatol 1986;122:290–294.

48. Cooper PH, Mills SE. Microcystic adnexal carcinoma. J Am Acad Dermatol 1984;10:908–914.

49. LeBoit PE, Sexton M. Microcystic adnexal carcinoma of the skin: A reappraisal of the differentiation and differential diagnosis of an underrecognized neoplasm. J Am Acad Dermatol 1993;29:609–618.

50. Fleischmann HE, Roth RJ, Wood C, Nickoloff BJ. Microcystic adnexal carcinoma treated by microscopically controlled excision. J Dermatol Surg Oncol 1984;10:873–875.

51. Salzman MJ, Eades E. Primary cutaneous adenoid cystic carcinoma: A case report and review of the literature. Plast Reconstr Surg 1991;88:140–144.

52. Mehregan AH, Hashimoto K, Rahbari H. Eccrine adenocarcinoma: A clinicopathologic study of 35 cases. Arch Dermatol 1983;119:104–115.

53. Fukamizu H, Tomita K, Inque K, Takigawa M. Primary mucinous carcinoma of the skin. J Dermatol Surg Oncol 1993;625–628.

54. Cooper PH, Adelson GL, Holthaus WH. Primary cutaneous adenoid cystic carcinoma. Arch Dermatol 1984;120:774–777.

55. Headington JT. Primary mucinous carcinoma of the skin. Cancer 1977;39:1055–1063.

56. Serab JA, Grahm JH. Primary cutaneous adenoid cystic carcinoma. J Am Acad Dermatol 1987;17:113–118.

57. Wright JD, Font RL. Mucinous sweat gland adenocarcinoma of eyelid: A clinicopathologic study of 21 cases with histochemical and electron microscopic observations. Cancer 1979;44:1757–1768.

58. Yeung KY, Stinson JC. Mucinous (adenocystic) carcinoma of sweat glands with widespread metastases. Cancer 1977;39:2556–2562.

59. Lang PG, Metcalf JS, Maize JC. Recurrent adenoid cystic carcinoma of the skin managed by microscopically controlled surgery (Mohs' surgery). J Dermatol Surg Oncol 1986;12:395–396.

60. Permalatha S, Rao NR, Yesudian P, et al. Segmental syringocystadenoma papilliferum in an unusual location. Int J Dermatol 1985;24:520–521.

61. Mazoujian G, Margolis R. Immunohistochemistry of gross cystic fluid protein (GCDFP-15) in 65 benign sweat gland tumors of the skin. Am J Dermatopathol 1988;10:28–35.

62. Dissanayake RV, Salm R. Sweat-gland carcinomas: Prognosis related to histological type. Histopathology 1980;4:445–466.

63. Santa Cruz DJ, Prioleau PG, Smith ME. Hidradenoma papilliferum of the eyelid. Arch Dermatol 1981;117:55–56.

64. Warkel RL, Helwig EB: Apocrine gland adenoma and adenocarcinoma of the axilla. Arch Dermatol 1978;198–203.

65. Paties C, Taccagni GL, Papotti M, et al. Apocrine carcinoma of the skin: A clinicopathologic, immunocytochemical, and ultrastructural study. Cancer 1991;71:375–381.

66. Chaudhuri SPR, Smoller BR. Extramammary Paget's disease: Diagnosis and disease pattern. Cutis 1992;50:195–196.

67. Saida T, Iwata M. Ectopic extramammary Paget's disease affecting the lower anterior aspect of the chest. J Am Acad Dermatol 1987;17:910–913.

68. Gibson JR, Baker H, Pegum JS, Pollack DJ. Multifocal extramammary Paget's disease. J R Soc Med 1983;76:426–427.

69. deBlois GG, Patterson JW, Hunter SB. Extramammary Paget's disease: Arising in knee region in association with sweat gland carcinoma. Arch Pathol Lab Med 1984;108:713–716.

70. Turner AG. Pagetoid lesions associated with carcinoma of the bladder. J Urol 1980;123:124–126.

71. Ojeda VJ, Heenan PJ, Watson SH. Paget's disease of the groin associated with adenocarcinoma of the urinary bladder. J Cutan Pathol 1987;14:227–231.

72. Fukutani K, Kawabe K, Niijima T, Oohara K. Transitional cell carcinoma of the urinary tract associated with extramammary Paget's disease: A report of two cases. Urol Int 1987;42:71–73.

73. Chandra JJ. Extramammary Paget's disease: Prognosis and rela-

tionship to internal malignancy. J Am Acad Dermatol 1985; 13:1053–1055.

74. Helm KF, Goellner JR, Peters MS. Immunohistochemical stains in extramammary Paget's disease. Am J Dermatopathol 1992; 14:402–407.

75. Jones RE, Austin C, Ackerman AB. Extramammary Paget's disease: A critical reexamination. Am J Dermatopathol 1979; 1:101–132.

76. Snow SN, Desouky S, Lo JS, Kurtycz D. Failure to detect human papillomavirus DNA in extramammary Paget's disease. Cancer 1992;69:249–251.

77. Gunn RA, Gallager HS. Vulvar Paget's disease: A topographic study. Cancer 1980;46:590–594.

78. Eliezri YD, Silvers DN, Horan DB. Role of preoperative topical 5-fluorouracil in preparation for Mohs microscopic surgery of extramammary Paget's disease. J Am Acad Dermatol 1987; 17:497–505.

79. Coldiron BM, Goldsmith BA, Robinson JK. Surgical treatment of extramammary Paget's disease. Cancer 1991;67:933–938.

80. Mohs FE, Blanchard L. Microscopically controlled surgery for extramammary Paget's disease. Arch Dermatol 1979;115:706.

81. Wagner RF, Cottel WI. Treatment of extensive extramammary Paget disease of male genitalia with Mohs micrographic surgery. Urology 1988;31:415–418.

82. Voigt H, Basserman R, Nathrath W. Cytoreductive combination chemotherapy for regionally advanced unresectable extramammary Paget carcinoma. Cancer 1992;70:704–708.

83. Ashikari R, Park K, Huvos AG, et al. Paget's disease of the breast. Cancer 1979;26:680–685.

84. Meissner K, Riviere A, Haupt G, Loning T. Study of Neu-protein expression in mammary Paget's disease with and without underlying breast carcinoma and in extramammary Paget's disease. Am J Pathol 1990;137:1305–1309.

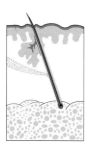

Angiogenesis, Vascular Malformations and Proliferations

JAMES NIGRO, ROBERT A. SWERLICK, NORBERT T. SEPP, ROY G. GERONEMUS, PHILIP E. LEBOIT, and ILONA J. FRIEDEN

ANGIOGENESIS

Angiogenesis is the process by which new blood vessels are formed. It is a critical process in embryologic development and normal wound healing. Additionally, pathologic angiogenesis is a key feature of many disorders, including tumor growth and spread, and is associated with a variety of ocular disorders, inflammatory arthritis, and hyperproliferative skin disease. The exact sequence of events that results in the formation of new blood vessels is not fully understood, but the formation of new blood vessels appears to be regulated by a complex interplay of soluble growth, inflammatory, and chemotactic factors, and the influence of the extracellular matrix.

Embryologic Angiogenesis

The embryologic development of the vascular system initially differs from the formation of blood vessels in mature organisms. Development of the vascular system has been most intensively studied in the chicken egg, in which primitive mesenchymal cells differentiate into precursors of endothelial cells termed *angioblasts,* from which all endothelial cells are subsequently derived.[1]

The formation of a mature vascular system within the developing embryo and the formation of blood vessels within the adult share many common mechanisms. Endothelial cells needed to form new blood vessels in the adult must be recruited from preexisting blood vessels.[2-4] Increases in vascular permeability and vasodilatation often result in signals that induce angiogenesis. Subsequently, endothelial cells enlarge, form pseudopods, migrate, and form vascular sprouts.

Endothelial cells recruited for angiogenesis are usually derived from the microvasculature and most commonly from tortuous venular segments.[2-4] They may produce a variety of proteases capable of degrading basement membrane proteins prior to migration; angiogenic substances such as basic fibroblast growth factor (bFGF) are also potent modulators of endothelial cell protease activity.[5, 6]

The initial phase of angiogenesis strictly depends on migration of endothelial cells; migration of endothelial cells from preexisting vessels alone is sufficient to form vascular sprouts early in angiogenesis.[7] As the angiogenic process continues, proliferation of endothelial cells becomes necessary. Mitotic foci are found not at the leading edge of endothelial cells, but away from areas of most active migration. Endothelial cells then migrate following paths of least resistance along fibrin strands. Lumens may form by endothelial cells covering preexisting fluid-filled cavities or may form by coalescence of intracytoplasmic lumens in adjacent endothelial cells, a process that is recapitulated in several vascular neoplasms in which similar vacuoles are present, such as angiolymphoid hyperplasia with eosinophilia and spindle cell hemangioendothelioma.[3]

Pathologic Angiogenesis

Although angiogenesis is necessary for normal homeostasis, pathologic angiogenesis is also central to the growth of neoplasms and to destructive processes that affect the skin, joints, bone, and eyes. The growth of many solid tumors depends on their ability to induce an adequate vascular supply.[8, 9] Tumor cells grown in avascular tissues (such as the anterior chamber of the eye) or in vitro in soft agar form nodules that grow to only 2 to 3 mm in diameter. However, tumor cell nodules subsequently transplanted into vascular sites resume their rapid growth.[10] Additional studies have shown that incorporation of genes coding for angiogenic growth factors increases tumor cell aggressiveness in vivo.[11]

Chronic inflammation almost invariably accompanies neovascularization and, until recently, it has been virtually impossible to determine whether angiogenesis may occur independently of inflammation. Tissue damage in inflammatory conditions is often directly attributable to associated vascular proliferation. For example, much of the joint destruction in rheumatoid arthritis is due to new blood vessel growth that invades the joint and destroys cartilage. Ocular neovascularization, the most common cause of blindness, is characteristic of a variety of eye disorders. The pathophysiology of psoriasis may also depend on angiogenesis.[12] An improved understanding of factors that induce angiogenesis or the identification of agents that can inhibit angiogenesis is central to developing strategies for therapeutic intervention in neoplastic and inflammatory disorders.

Models of Angiogenesis

The formation of blood vessels and regulation of angiogenesis in vivo is complex and controlled by a variety of soluble factors and extracellular matrix proteins, as well as by differences in endothelial cell phenotype and function. Current understanding of the complex cascade of events that lead to angiogenesis is the result of studies that use both in vivo and in vitro models.[10] Prior to the development of techniques to culture endothelial cells, particularly those derived from capillaries, angiogenesis

was largely studied in vivo, using two models: the chorioallantoic membrane of chick embryo and the corneal pocket of the rabbit. These models were valuable in defining the range of angiogenic substances, particularly soluble ones, but they were limited. They did not reflect the angiogenic potential of certain mediators, particularly pro-inflammatory cytokines, that induce vascular proliferation in association by causing inflammation, rather than having a direct effect on endothelial cells.

Cultured endothelial cells, particularly those derived from capillaries, allow for more direct examination of the mechanisms that regulate angiogenesis.[13–15] Placement of these cells on various substrates can induce the formation of capillary-like structures in vitro,[14] which occurs rapidly if endothelial cells are plated on basement membrane gels or if they are overlaid with type I collagen gels.[16] Soluble growth factors such as bFGF can also induce changes in endothelial cell behavior in vitro, resembling those seen in early angiogenesis.[17] Basic fibroblast growth factor induces endothelial cell migration and invasion of collagen gels to form capillary-like structures in vitro.

Angiogenic Factors (Table 146–1)

Fibroblast Growth Factors

The fibroblast growth factors (FGFs) are a family of mitogenic polypeptides.[18] The most widely studied FGF members are two closely related proteins, acidic FGF (aFGF) and basic FGF (bFGF), closely related proteins of about 18,000 kd that share 53% amino acid homology. The product of the int-2 and K-FGF oncogenes code for FGF-like proteins and have been implicated in the pathophysiology of tumors such as Kaposi's sarcoma.[19] Oncogenes coding for other FGF-like polypeptides have been isolated from gastric and bladder cancers.[20]

FGF is produced by a variety of cells, including endothelial cells in vivo and in vitro.[21–23] Neither aFGF or bFGF has an appropriate signal sequence necessary for

TABLE 146–1. Angiogenic Factors

	MW	Source	Mitogen	Chemotactic	Comments
bFGF	18,000	Tumor cells, endothelial cells, macrophages	Yes	Yes	Induces endothelial cell tube formation in collagen gels in vitro
aFGF	16,400				
VPF/VEGF	45,000	Keratinocytes, tumor cells	Yes	?	Induces tube formation—synergistic with FGF
PD-ECGF	45,000	Platelets	No	?	Works independent of heparin
TGF-α	5,500		Yes	?	Causes angiogenesis when injected subcutaneously
Angiogenin	14,100	Human plasma, normal human cells		?	Homologous to pancreatic ribonuclease
TGF-β	25,000	Many cells and tissues	No	?	Inhibits cell proliferation but increases matrix synthesis
IL-8	8,000	Endothelial cells, leukocytes, keratinocytes	Yes	Yes	Leukocyte activator. Related to a number of small chemotactic cytokines, some of which are angiostatic
TNF-α	17,000	Leukocytes, keratinocytes	No	No	Proinflammatory polypeptide when exposed to vascular lumens. Induces vascular sprouting when introduced in extravascular location
Angiotropin	4,500	Monocytes	No	Yes	Cu^{2+}-containing polyribonucleotide. Induces vasodilation and angiogenesis

secretion.[24] Basic FGF is both associated with endothelial cells and bound to their basement membranes. Treatment of endothelial cell basement membranes with heparin or proteases liberates bFGF, suggesting that basement membrane serves as a reservoir of FGF. This finding also suggests that heparin and related polysaccharides play a key role in mediating and modulating the effects of FGF.[25, 26]

Both acidic and basic FGF have been shown to induce angiogenesis in vivo in both the chick chorioallantoic membrane (CAM) and the rabbit cornea model.[18] The mechanisms by which FGF induces angiogenesis have been intensively studied in vitro. Basic FGF is 30 to 100 times more effective a mediator of angiogenesis than aFGF. FGF is a potent mitogen for endothelial cells, particularly capillary endothelial cells at doses less than 5 ng/mL. It has other effects, which are probably important, particularly in the early phases of angiogenesis. It is a potent stimulator of chemotaxis in microvascular endothelial cells.[27, 28] FGF stimulation of endothelial cells induces invasion of collagen gels and amniotic membrane and the formation of vascular-like structures.[16, 29] These responses also induce protease production and secretion as well as changes in cell surface integrin expression.[30, 31] Each of these effects is likely to be critical in the migration of endothelial cells from preexisting blood vessels across the matrix of granulation tissue in healing wounds. Similar effects on endothelial cells can be induced by the protein kinase C agonist PMA.[30, 32] Both PMA and FGF cause endothelial cells to invade collagen gels and form capillary-like structures in vitro.[17]

Vascular Endothelial Cell Growth Factor

Vascular endothelial cell growth factor (VEGF) (also known as *vascular permeability factor,* VPF) is a 45- to 46-kd protein secreted by a variety of tissues that induces angiogenesis and enhances vascular permeability. It is a highly glycosylated cationic dimer of 23- to 24-kd subunits.[33-36] Like FGF, VEGF is also a heparin-binding growth factor, but it appears to be structurally related to the family of platelet-derived growth factors (PDGFs). Unlike PDGF, which is mitogenic for smooth muscle cells, VEGF is a potent endothelial cell mitogen and induces a brisk angiogenic response in rabbit corneal and CAM assays.

Recent in situ hybridization studies have demonstrated expression of VEGF mRNA by keratinocytes adjacent to wounded skin. This production is probably particularly important in cutaneous wound healing because small breaks in the epidermis are generally accompanied by locally increased vascular permeability followed by tufts of new capillary growth. VEGF affects cultured endothelial cells in a manner similar to bFGF,[16] but VEGF alone appears to be about half as potent as bFGF in inducing angiogenesis in vitro. VEGF and bFGF together may act synergistically to induce angiogenesis in vitro.[16]

Platelet-Derived Endothelial Cell Growth Factor

Platelet-derived endothelial cell growth factor (PD-ECGF) is a 45-kd growth factor synthesized by platelets, fibroblasts, and selected carcinoma cells.[37, 38] PD-ECGF is a specific mitogen for endothelial cells and also potentiates the mitogenic effects of bFGF. Additionally, it is chemotactic for endothelial cells and induces angiogenesis in vivo.

Other Mediators of Angiogenesis

Angiogenin. Angiogenin is a 14-kd cationic single-chain polypeptide that stimulates angiogenesis in the CAM and rabbit cornea.[39] It is structurally related to pancreatic RNAase A, but shares little functional activity. Although it has been found in cell culture supernatants from the human adenocarcinoma HT-29 and normal lymphocytes, the liver appears to be the major source of angiogenin synthesis in vivo.

Angiogenin does not directly induce endothelial cell proliferation or migration in vitro,[39] but it does bind to specific cell surface receptors on endothelial cells and induces a transient rise in intracellular diacylglycerol. In vivo, angiogenin is a potent inducer of angiogenesis in the CAM assay. Because angiogenin does not directly induce endothelial cell proliferation or migration, it has been suggested that it might stimulate angiogenesis indirectly via an intermediary molecule.

Angiotropin. Angiotropin is a small (4.5-kd) copper-containing polyribonucleopolypeptide that has been characterized from the supernatants from concanavalin-A–activated peripheral porcine monocytes.[40, 41] It is a potent stimulator of endothelial cell migration and, when added to cultures of microvascular endothelial cells, induces them to rapidly reorganize into capillary-like structures. Angiotropin is also a potent inducer of angiogenesis in the CAM assay. Unlike FGF, angiotropin is not mitogenic for endothelial cells in vitro.

Transforming Growth Factor (TGF)-α. TGF-α is a 5.5-kd polypeptide that is closely related to and utilizes the same receptor as epidermal growth factor. TGF-α is mitogenic for endothelial cells and induces angiogenesis in vivo,[42] but does not induce endothelial cell migration. It is produced by macrophages and selected tumor cells.

Transforming Growth Factor (TGF)-β. TGF-β may function as both an inducer and inhibitor of angiogenesis. When injected into the skin of mice, TGF-β rapidly stimulates the formation of highly vascularized granulation tissue.[43] Paradoxically, TFG-β is not mitogenic in vivo for endothelial cells and actually inhibits endothelial cell proliferation.[44, 45] It also inhibits FGF-induced induction of proteases as well as FGF-stimulated collagen gel invasion.[6] Its effects on angiogenesis in vivo may be because of its potent chemotactic effects on monocytes, which release angiogenic factors.[46, 47] It may also act as a differentiating factor after the proliferative phase of angiogenesis, promoting connective tissue synthesis and endothelial cell differentiation.

Tumor Necrosis Factor (TNF)-α. TNF-α has overlapping activities with interleukin (IL)-1 in that stimulation of endothelial cells with TNF also results in adhesion molecule induction and leukocyte binding. TNF is not mitogenic for endothelial cells in vitro but, like TFG-β, is capable of inducing neovascularization in vivo.[48, 49] Injection of as little as 3.5 ng into the rabbit cornea results in angiogenesis.

Interleukin (IL)-8. IL-8 is angiogenic when implanted in the rat or rabbit cornea and induces proliferation and chemotaxis of human umbilical vein endothelial cells.[50, 51] In these studies, repeat examination 6 weeks after placing angiogenic doses of IL-8 demonstrated significant regression of corneal vascularity, suggesting that IL-8–induced angiogenesis is dynamic and modulated as might normally be seen in wound healing.

Anti-angiogenic Factors

Experimental and clinical observations demonstrating the clear association between angiogenesis and pathology in inflammatory and neoplastic disorders spurred investigations into the development of therapeutic approaches to inhibit angiogenesis. A variety of agents have been shown to demonstrate anti-angiogenic activity; however, their mechanisms of action are only poorly understood (Table 146–2). Selected corticosteroid drugs are potent angiostatic agents that can be administered in conjunction with heparin or heparin fragments.[52] The anticoagulant activity of heparin does not necessarily mediate this effect. Although corticosteroids are used alone to treat hemangiomas, they appear to have no effect alone in vitro, and their clinical efficacy may be due to endogenous levels of heparin.

Endothelial cell migration through basement membranes depends on secretion of collagenase and other proteases. For example, bFGF-induced angiogenesis appears to be at least in part dependent on induction of plasminogen activator activity. A number of unrelated collagenase inhibitors have been shown to inhibit angiogenesis. Minocycline inhibits collagenase activity in rheumatoid synovium and is as effective as angiostatic steroid-heparin combinations in inhibiting corneal angiogenesis.[53, 54] Methoxyprogesterone inhibits both collagenase and plasminogen activator activity, and also inhibits corneal vascularization. Modified chitin, a polysaccharide characteristic of insect exoskeleton, is also a potent inhibitor of collagenase, heparinase, and of angiogenesis and tumor growth.

Platelet factor 4 (PF4) is a small polypeptide derived from platelet granules that is a potent inhibitor of angiogenesis. PF4 specifically inhibits endothelial cell proliferation and migration in vitro.[55] Interestingly, PF4 is very closely related to IL-8, a factor that has been shown to induce angiogenesis, endothelial cell proliferation, and endothelial cell migration. Another platelet-derived protein, *thrombospondin* also inhibits angiogenesis. Like PF4, thrombospondin also binds to heparin and inhibits endothelial cell proliferation.[56]

Consumption of a plant-based diet can prevent the development and progression of chronic diseases that are associated with extensive neovascularization; however, little is known about the mechanisms. High concentrations of antiangiogenic isoflavonoids are found in the urine of healthy human vegetarians. The isoflavonoid genistein is the most potent and inhibits endothelial cell proliferation and in vitro angiogenesis.[57] Inhibitors of angiogenesis have also been isolated from bacteria and fungal sources.[58] These agents not only inhibit angiogenesis in the CAM assay but also inhibit tumor growth in vivo, presumably in inhibiting tumor-induced angiogenesis.

Interferon (IFN) alfa inhibits endothelial cell migration and proliferation in vitro and inhibits lymphocyte-induced angiogenesis in vivo, and is currently being used as a treatment of hemangiomas of infancy. However, tumor-associated neovascularization has not responded to similar therapy.

Anti-inflammatory agents also inhibit angiogenesis, and this effect may be partially responsible for their therapeutic effects. D-penicillamine and gold thiomalate, agents used in the treatment of arthritis, and methotrexate have been shown to inhibit angiogenesis.[59-61] D-penicillamine and methotrexate inhibit endothelial cell proliferation in vitro and angiogenesis in vivo in the rabbit corneal assay. Gold thiomalate also inhibits endothelial cell proliferation in vitro as well as the release of angiogenic factors by macrophages in vivo.

TABLE 146-2. Anti-angiogenic Factors

	Source/Examples	
Anti-angiogenic steroids	Cortisone and hydrocortisone	Activity induced in the presence of heparin
Genistein	Dietary sources	Isoflavonoids. High concentrations found in urine of vegetarians.
Interferon alfa	Primarily leukocytes	Family of >20 closely related proteins. Inhibits endothelial cell proliferation and migration.
Collagenase inhibitors	Minocycline, cartilage-derived factors, medroxyprogesterone, chemically modified chitin	Diverse mechanisms involved
Platelet factor 4	Platelets	Closely related to IL-8, which induces angiogenesis. Heparin binding-factor, which inhibits endothelial cell migration and proliferation
Bacterial and fungal derived angiostatic agents	1. *Arthrobacter* species 2. *Aspergillus fumigatus*	1. Sulfated-polysaccharide-petidoglycan complex 2. Analogues of fumagillin (angioinhibins), antibiotics secreted by *Aspergillus fumigatus*. Both inhibit tumor growth in vitro
D-penicillamine		Copper chelator. Inhibits endothelial cell proliferation in vitro
Thrombospondin	Platelets	450-kd protein with diverse biologic effects
Gold analogues		Inhibits endothelial cell proliferation and macrophage release of angiogenic factors

VASCULAR BIRTHMARKS

Until recently, the nomenclature and classification of vascular birthmarks have been confusing. Terms such as *strawberry birthmark, nevus flammeus,* and *cavernous hemangioma* are purely descriptive and fail to take into account histopathology, pathogenesis, and natural history. The work of Mulliken and Glowacki[62] has utilized the histology and natural history of vascular birthmarks to simplify their classification. The result is an understandable and useful approach to the evaluation and management of vascular lesions in infants and children (Table 146–3). The vast majority of vascular birthmarks can be classified as either *hemangiomas* or *vascular mal-*

formations based on their presentation, natural history, and histologic features. The term *hemangiomas of infancy* will be applied to these lesions in this section because there are many other types of hemangiomas that occur later in life as described in the last part of this chapter.

Hemangiomas are benign vascular neoplasms characterized by the rapid proliferation and slow involution of the endothelial lining of capillary walls. Although they are the most common tumors of infancy, these lesions have virtually no risk of malignant transformation. Hemangiomas in children can be present at birth, but most lesions are first noted during early infancy. They typically undergo a phase of rapid growth in the first year of

TABLE 146–3. Vascular Birthmarks

Condition	Age of Onset	Location	Clinical Description	Systemic Manifestations	Associated Syndromes	Natural History
Hemangioma of infancy	Birth to 6 wks	Variable	Raised, red, tense tumors; subcutaneous lesions with overlying bluish discoloration	Obstruction of vital structures; cardiac failure with extensive internal lesions	Kasabach-Merritt Sternal clefting Coarctation of Aorta Dandy-Walker malformations	>90% involute completely by age 9 years
Nevus simplex	Birth	Eyelids Forehead Nape of neck	Pink, irregular macules and patches	None	None	Facial lesions resolve by age 2 yrs; nuchal lesions persist
Capillary malformations (port-wine stain)	Birth	Anywhere; facial lesions may follow cutaneous innervation of trigeminal nerve	Red-violaceous patches, color deepens with age	Limb overgrowth	Sturge-Weber Cobb Phakomatosis-pigmento-vascularis Klippel-Trenaunay	Persist throughout life; may develop nodules within port-wine stain
Venous malformation	Birth	Variable	Bluish-purple subcutaneous masses; can be solitary, localized, or diffuse	Hemorrhage of visceral lesions	Gorham's Maffucci's Blue rubber bleb nevus Cutis marmorata telangiectasia congenita	Lesions are persistent; may not be clinically evident until adulthood
Arteriovenous malformation	Birth	Variable	Pink to blue discoloration overlying a pulsatile mass	Potentially fatal hemorrhage, pain	See Combined malformations	Lesions are persistent; may not be clinically evident until adulthood
Lymphatic malformation	Birth	Anywhere	Single or multicystic lesions; subcutaneous lesions may resemble venous malformations or deep hemangiomas	None	See Combined malformations	Lesions are persistent, some cystic lesions may spontaneously collapse
Combined malformation	Birth	Variable	Variable	Variable	Klippel-Trenaunay Parkes-Weber Wyburn-Mason Riley-Smith Bannayan-Zonana Proteus	Persistent

life followed by slow involution, and they generally resolve completely during childhood.[63]

In contrast, vascular malformations are developmental anomalies of blood vessels that occur in utero. These lesions consist of ectatic vessels in which endothelial cell proliferation is normal. Vascular malformations may be composed of abnormal capillaries, veins, arteries, lymphatics, or combinations thereof. Capillary malformations, also known as port-wine stains, are the most common cutaneous vascular malformation. By definition, these lesions are present at birth, although some may not be clinically evident until later in life. The growth of vascular malformations is commensurate with the growth of the child, and, unlike hemangiomas, they are not capable of spontaneous resolution.[62]

Certain older terms such as *cavernous hemangioma* are confusing because many lesions carrying this diagnosis are actually venous malformations. Other outmoded terms include juvenile, cellular, and/or hypertrophic hemangioma, as well as benign hemangioendothelioma. Vascular malformations can be classified according to the type or types of vessels present. Although this schema applies nicely to vascular birthmarks, it cannot be used for acquired vascular lesions, those beginning in older children or adults. In this setting, the term *hemangioma* or *angioma* is still used, both clinically and histopathologically to describe many vascular neoplasms.

Hemangiomas of Infancy

Hemangiomas of infancy are benign neoplasms largely composed of capillaries and venules. They usually are present or develop during the first few weeks of life. They are characterized by a period of rapid growth followed by a period of slow involution leading to complete resolution in the majority of cases.

Clinical Description

Hemangiomas of infancy occur in 1.1% to 2.6% of newborns and are present in 10% to 12% of 1-year-old infants. The incidence of hemangiomas in the general population varies according to sex, race, and gestational age. By a ratio of 3:1, females are more likely than males to be affected.[64] Whites are more commonly affected than either Asian or black infants.[65, 66] Premature infants have an increased incidence of hemangiomas; very low birth-weight infants (500 to 1000 g) are especially at risk, with an incidence as high as 22.9%.[67]

Hemangiomas are noted at birth in approximately 25% of cases and by 4 weeks in 88%.[68] Deeper lesions are sometimes inapparent until several months of age because they can proliferate with minimal change in the overlying skin.[64] Hemangiomas most commonly occur on the head and neck (50% to 59%) and trunk (22% to 25%). Less common sites include the extremities (17%) and the genitalia (1% to 4%).[63, 64, 69] Although hemangiomas usually occur singly, multiple lesions have been noted in 16% to 30% of affected individuals.[64, 69]

Hemangioma precursors may appear as pale patches (Fig. 146–1*A*), thread-like telangiectasia with or without a pale halo, macular erythema, bluish discolorations, or small areas of skin ulceration, and can initially be confused with nevus anemicus, a port-wine stain, or a bruise.[66, 70]

The appearance of hemangiomas of infancy depends on whether the proliferation of endothelial cells occurs in the dermal or subcutaneous vasculature. Dermal lesions are bright red, raised, and are usually well-demarcated with a firm texture (Fig. 146–1*B*). Subcutaneous hemangiomas usually present as soft, enlarging masses with a bluish discoloration of the overlying skin. Lesions involving both the dermis and subcutis may share both appearances (Fig. 146–2). Hemangiomas of infancy vary in size from a few millimeters to rare cases involving the entire face, the majority of a limb, or a significant portion of the torso.

Proliferation is most rapid in early infancy between 3 and 6 months, but growth may continue until 12 months of age, and occasionally into the second year of life. After the proliferative phase, the lesion tends to plateau for months to several years, followed by a phase of slow involution. Lesions change in color from a bright crimson to a dull, faded red. Graying is first noted in the

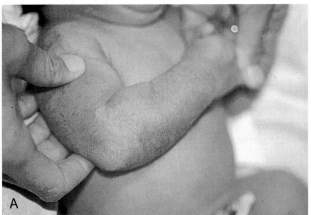
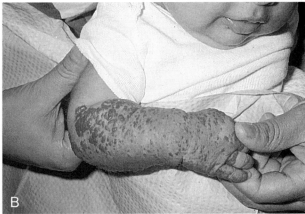

FIGURE 146–1. *A*, Hemangioma precursor: An area of blanching on the arm of a 1-day-old infant. *B*, By 1 month of age, a superficial hemangioma has developed in this area.

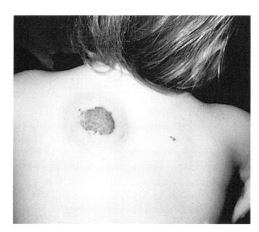

FIGURE 146-2. Superficial and deep hemangioma.

center and progresses centrifugally. The hemangioma gradually softens and the overall texture becomes flabby. Areas of normal skin slowly appear and increase in size until the lesion fully involutes. Complete resolution occurs in 50% to 60% of patients by 5 years of age, in 75% by age 7, and 90% by age 9. In some cases, hemangiomas improve well into adolescence.[71] Although the rate of involution and the degree of resolution are not usually influenced by the sex or race of the patient, the size of the lesion, site, or the duration of the proliferative phase, anecdotal data suggest that hemangiomas involving the lip or nose may have poor outcomes after involution.[63, 71]

Complications

Although most hemangiomas of infancy resolve without consequence, approximately 40% of patients are left with some residual abnormality of the skin, including telangiectasia, atrophy, hypopigmentation, or scarring. Complications develop in about 20% of patients. These range from minor ulceration and bleeding to severe sequelae such as respiratory compromise, cardiac failure, consumptive coagulopathy, and irreversible cutaneous distortion.[72]

Ulceration, the most common complication, usually occurs in large, rapidly growing, tense, superficial hemangiomas. Lip and perianal lesions are more likely to be affected. Once ulceration occurs, scarring is inevitable and can be quite disfiguring in extensive cases.[64, 68] Minor bleeding and superficial infections occur less frequently and are generally self-limited events.[73]

Proliferating hemangiomas can lead to obstruction of critical anatomic structures. Patients with lesions involving the eyelids and orbit are at risk for developing permanent ophthalmologic sequelae such as amblyopia, astigmatism, strabismus, ptosis, proptosis, and optic nerve atrophy. The severity of amblyopia depends on how long the eyelid is closed, but permanent damage can occur even if it is closed for a few days.[74, 75] Upper eyelid lesions are more common and are associated with more complications, especially astigmatism, but any hemangioma that increases orbital pressure or causes even partial closure of the eyelids is of great concern.[76]

Hemangiomas of infancy that obstruct the nasal passages or the oropharynx can cause respiratory failure.[70] Potentially life-threatening subglottic hemangiomas may lead to severe constriction of the trachea. Patients usually present with stridor, often at a few weeks of age, and may be initially misdiagnosed as having tracheomalacia, viral croup, or asthma.[77, 78] Hemangiomas involving the maxillary and mandibular regions can cause dental malocclusion, whereas lesions in the parotid area can obstruct the external auditory canal and cause conductive hearing loss.[79]

Infants with *diffuse neonatal hemangiomatosis* have multiple cutaneous hemangiomas in association with visceral hemangiomas, most often in the liver and gastrointestinal tract. Skin lesions, usually 1 to 10 mm in size, develop during the first few weeks of life, varying in number from a few to hundreds. Visceral lesions may also be present in the central nervous system (CNS), lungs, and other organs. Associated systemic complications include high-output cardiac failure, obstructive jaundice, gastrointestinal hemorrhage, respiratory failure, consumptive coagulopathy, and central nervous system bleeding resulting in a mortality rate of 80% in untreated patients.[80] The presence of multiple cutaneous hemangiomas without systemic involvement has been called *benign neonatal hemangiomatosis.* In general, spontaneous and uneventful involution of the hemangiomas occurs by 2 years of age. Infants with multiple cutaneous hemangiomas (especially with 10 or more) are best regarded as part of a continuum with variable degrees of cutaneous and visceral involvement.

The *Kasabach-Merritt syndrome* is a coagulopathy characterized by platelet trapping within a hemangioma. It usually presents at birth or within the first few months of life. The typical presentation is that of a large, rapidly enlarging hemangioma that develops a tense, woody consistency with taut overlying skin covered with petechiae and purpura, which gradually spread to adjacent areas. Other findings include epistaxis, melena, and hematuria.[81] Although any site can be affected, the syndrome is most commonly seen in subcutaneous lesions of the torso or extremities. Rarely, it can be seen in association with small multiple lesions or visceral hemangiomas.[80] Although symptoms usually resolve with involution and treatment can reduce morbidity, death rates may still approach 20% to 30%.[81-83]

Associated Syndromes

Hemangiomas of infancy are rarely associated with underlying structural malformations, but a few well-defined exceptions have been described. Infants with lumbosacral hemangiomas may have associated spinal and genitourinary anomalies.[84, 85] Early evaluation of the spinal cord with either high-resolution ultrasonography or magnetic resonance imagery (MRI) is recommended.[86] Large facial hemangiomas can occur in the Dandy-Walker malformation and other posterior fossa abnormalities.[87] Facial hemangiomas can also be seen in association with coarctation of the right-sided aortic arch, supraumbilical abdominal raphe, and sternal clefting.[88-90]

Pathology

Hemangiomas of infancy begin as densely cellular dermal or subcutaneous proliferations, and evolve to form distinct vessels. Early lesions demonstrate solid masses and strands of cells with few if any discernible lumina.[91] Endothelial cells comprise only a minority of the lesion at this stage because they are outnumbered by cuboidal interstitial cells, which are a mixture of pericytes, and dermal dendrocytes. It can be difficult to discern vascular lumina. Later on, small vascular channels lined by plump endothelial cells gradually increase in number. Most mitotic figures are within interstitial rather than endothelial cells. Endothelial cell nuclei are generally uniform in appearance.[92] A 30- to 40-fold increase in the number of mast cells as compared with normal tissues may indicate a role for these cells in the pathogenesis of hemangiomas of infancy.[93] Electron microscopy reveals a thickened, multilaminated basement membrane that may result from cyclic endothelial proliferation and death. Additional findings on electron microscopy suggestive of intracellular activity include convoluted nuclear membranes, swollen mitochondria, rough endoplasmic reticulum, and clusters of free ribosomes.[92]

The involutional phase is characterized by a tendency for vessels to be arranged in distinct lobules, with interspersed bands of fibrous connective tissue. Vascular channels are fewer in number, tend to be widely dilated, and have a flattened endothelium. As regression continues, the number of mast cells returns to normal.[93] The basement membrane remains multilaminated; however, it is thinned and disordered.[92]

Pathogenesis and Etiology

Although the pathogenesis of hemangiomas is not fully understood, angiogenic factors are probably central to their development. Mast cells release heparin, which binds to endothelial cells resulting in the release of FGFs. Paradoxically, however, heparin can be an inhibitor of angiogenesis in the presence of steroids.[94] The growth of hemangiomas may also be influenced by hormones, particularly estrogen, which, in one study, was four times higher in infants with hemangiomas than in normal infants.[95]

Diagnosis and Differential Diagnosis

The diagnosis of superficial hemangiomas rarely requires more than a complete history and physical examination. The characteristic rapid proliferation and slow involution of these lesions are unique findings that do not occur in other pediatric vascular processes. However, an occasional deep hemangioma may be slow to involute and may be confused with a static vascular malformation. Conversely, hemangiomas presenting as a high-flow mass at birth may be mistaken for an arteriovenous malformation (AVM). Occasionally, pyogenic granulomas may also be confused with hemangiomas.

Although repetitive examinations over time usually establish the proper diagnosis, the correct identification of subcutaneous as well as intramuscular and visceral hemangiomas may require further investigation. MRI is the most reliable noninvasive technique for distinguishing hemangiomas from vascular malformations, meningoceles, dermoid cysts, and other neoplastic processes. Ultrasonography with color flow imaging is the most cost-effective technique, but proliferating hemangiomas may be difficult to distinguish from AVMs because both are high-flow lesions.[72] Biopsy is rarely needed to establish the diagnosis of hemangioma of infancy, except to rule out other, rapidly growing soft-tissue tumors such as rhabdomyosarcoma, adrenocortical carcinoma, and Langerhans cell histiocytosis.[96, 97] A rare vascular proliferation termed *kaposiform hemangioendothelioma* can also induce the Kasabach-Merritt syndrome. This condition mostly affects infants but can also occur in children and young adults. The name derives from its histologic resemblance to Kaposi's sarcoma.[98]

Treatment of Hemangiomas

The vast majority of hemangiomas eventually involute without complications and require no treatment, but approximately 20% cause complications such as ulceration, irreversible cutaneous expansion and/or obstruction of vital structures (eyes, nose, airway), which require intervention.[72] Even in cases requiring no treatment, the concerns of parents regarding the natural history and prognosis should be addressed. The lesions(s) should be carefully monitored on a regular basis during the proliferative phase and the possible need for medical intervention acknowledged should the hemangioma grow too rapidly, ulcerate, or develop other complications. Serial photographs of prior patients with involuting and resolved hemangiomas can help to reassure parents that their infants will also likely have good outcomes.

Newer laser treatments, such as pulsed dye laser, have caused a resurgence of interest in the possibility of early treatment of hemangiomas to prevent ensuing proliferation, irreversible cutaneous changes, and disfigurement. The ability of laser treatment to affect the course of hemangiomas depends on the growth phase of the hemangioma, its thickness, and the characteristics of the laser that is used. The flashlamp-pumped pulsed-dye laser (585-nm wavelength, 450-microsecond pulse width) can selectively destroy vascular tissue with little risk to surrounding skin. Limited uncontrolled studies show this laser's efficacy in the treatment of hemangiomas during the involutional phase of growth and of superficial hemangiomas (less than 3-mm thickness) during the proliferative phase (Fig. 146-3*A* and *B*).[99] During the proliferative phase, repeated treatments at short intervals (e.g., every 2 to 4 weeks) are often required to prevent progression. Moreover, growth of a deeper component may not be inhibited by this method, and hemangiomas with a significant deep component are not likely to benefit from pulsed-dye laser therapy alone. The best results with the use of the pulsed-dye laser occur with the treatment of resolving superficial hemangiomas, particularly the telangiectatic component.[99, 101, 102] Decreased pain and increased healing have also been reported with pulsed-dye laser treatment of ulcerated hemangiomas (Fig. 146-4*A* and *B*).[100]

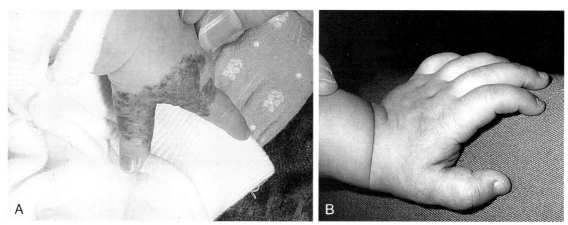

FIGURE 146-3. *A,* Hemangioma of the hand prior to treatment with pulsed-dye laser. *B,* Virtual complete resolution of hemangioma after multiple treatments with pulsed-dye laser.

Continuous-wave lasers, including the argon (488–514 nm), continuous-wave dye (488–620 nm), carbon dioxide (10,600 nm), krypton (548, 570 nm); Nd:YAG (1064 nm), and KTP (532, 1064 nm), as well as the quasi-continuous-wave lasers, including the copper vapor (510, 578 nm), have been used to treat hemangiomas, but these lasers do not specifically injure vessels, thus increasing the possibility of scarring and pigmentary loss.[101, 102] The Nd:YAG penetrates further and has been used in the treatment of deep hemangiomas. Its use is limited however, because it can induce a high degree of nonspecific thermal damage, which can lead to significant scarring. Several studies, however, have reported good results in the treatment of carefully selected patients.

Medical therapies, such as corticosteroids and interferon alfa, are usually necessary if functional impairment, involvement of vital structures (such as the airway, liver, or gastrointestinal tract), coagulopathy, or irreversible cutaneous changes ensue. Systemic and intralesional corticosteroids both induce early regression of hemangiomas and reduce their morbidity and mortality. Prednisone or prednisolone, 2 to 4 mg/kg per day, is usually given orally and, depending on the age of the patient, generally must be continued for one to several months before tapering gradually.[70, 103] A response is usually evident within a few days to weeks. Approximately one third of hemangiomas shrink dramatically, one third stop growing but do not shrink significantly, and one third do not respond.[103] Infants treated with systemic corticosteroids must be closely monitored for potentially severe side effects, such as growth suppression and hypertension. Parents must be made aware of the potential for severe complications of seemingly innocuous infections such as varicella, as well as the need for tapering the medication and giving stress doses of corticosteroids in medical or surgical emergencies to avoid adrenal insufficiency. Live viral vaccine administration should be deferred until therapy is discontinued.

Intralesional corticosteroids are often used by ophthalmologists in the treatment of orbital hemangiomas, and are occasionally used in other superficial well-localized lesions. Although complications associated with intralesional therapy of periorbital hemangiomas are uncommon, the consequences are potentially severe and include soft tissue atrophy, eyelid necrosis, and perforation

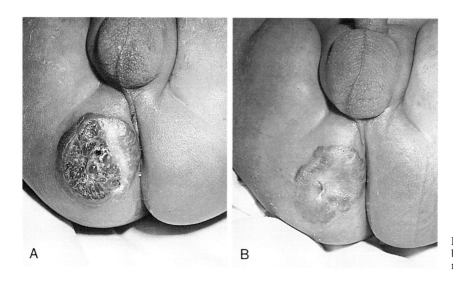

FIGURE 147-4. *A,* Ulcerated hemangioma on the buttock. *B,* Nearly complete healing after one treatment with pulsed-dye laser.

of the globe.[74, 75] When the hemangioma involves the retrobulbar region, intralesional steroids are not recommended because there is a high risk of central retinal artery occlusion, optic nerve damage, and retrobulbar hematoma.[104]

Interferon alfa 2α and β have been used successfully in cases of life-threatening hemangiomas that are unresponsive to systemic corticosteroids. The usual dose is 3 million units/m² per day injected subcutaneously. Although treatment usually accelerates regression of lesions, 6 to 12 months of continuous therapy may be required.[105] Side effects include mild fever, flu-like symptoms, and neutropenia. Occasionally, significant hemodynamic changes will occur during the first 48 to 72 hours of therapy, especially in patients with massive hemangiomas who already have significant circulatory compromise. Such patients should be monitored in an intensive care unit while treatment with interferon is initiated.[106]

Port-Wine Stains

Definition

Port-wine stains (nevus flammeus) are vascular malformations usually localized to the papillary and superficial reticular dermal vessels. They always occur at birth and, unlike hemangiomas, they are permanent and do not resolve. Lesions are usually isolated but may be associated with other vascular malformations or occur as a component of a variety of congenital syndromes.

Clinical Description

Port-wine stains occur in approximately 0.3% of neonates,[107] with equal frequency in males and females. Although lesions occur in all races, they are more common in whites.[108] The size of the lesions varies from several millimeters in diameter to more than 50% of the body surface area.[109] Although the face and neck are most commonly involved, any site may be affected. About one half of facial port-wine stains are restricted to one of the three trigeminal sensory areas, whereas the remainder involve more than one sensory region, cross the midline, or occur bilaterally.[110] The mucous membranes are often involved contiguously with the dermal capillary malformation. Extensive facial port-wine stains are more likely than small isolated lesions to be associated with truncal and extremity lesions as well as with neurologic, ophthalmologic, and other congenital abnormalities.[111, 112]

Although most newborns with port-wine stains have pink, well-circumscribed macular lesions, the generalized erythema commonly seen in newborns and its similarity to hemangioma precursors may prevent accurate diagnosis for several weeks. The size of the lesion increases proportionately with the growth of the child and the color generally deepens from light pink to red to dark purple with age. In rare instances, the port-wine stain may appear to lighten, especially during infancy and early childhood.[70] Progressive darkening and cutaneous hypertrophy of initially macular lesions occurs in approximately two thirds of patients by age 45. Lesions may develop a "cobblestone" texture and can become studded with angiomatous nodules, including pyogenic granulomas.[113]

Pathology

Port-wine stains are characterized by ectasia of capillaries located in the papillary and superficial reticular dermis. The abnormalities are generally limited to the upper 0.8 mm of the dermis with a mean vessel depth of 0.46 mm. Early lightly colored lesions may be virtually identical histologically to normal skin. However, as the patient ages, the vessels in the port-wine stain progressively dilate and there is stasis of erythrocytes. Clinically this correlates with gradual darkening of the lesion, whereas the "cobblestone" pattern seen in older patients is associated with localized exaggeration of the ectatic process and prominent stasis of erythrocytes throughout the entire malformation.[114] Although an increased number of vessels may be present, this finding does not correlate with the age or clinical appearance of the lesion.[111] Components of the vessel wall, including collagenous basement membrane protein (type IV collagen), factor VII, and fibronectin, have been shown to have equivalent distributions in port-wine stains and normal skin. These findings suggest that the structural abnormality in these lesions is in the supporting dermal elements rather than an abnormality of the vessel wall.[114] The number of cutaneous nerves, especially those in perivascular regions of port-wine stains, are significantly reduced. The resultant alteration in neural modulation of vascular tone could lead to the characteristic ectasia of vessels of these lesions.[115]

Pathogenesis and Etiology

The pathogenesis of vascular malformations including port-wine stains is not completely understood. It is believed that these lesions are a result of errors in the morphogenic processes that shape the vascular system between the fourth and tenth week of embryonic life. These anomalies are sporadic, nonfamilial developmental errors. A number of unproven etiologies have been postulated, including a defect in processes of thrombosis and fibrinolysis, aberrations of the autonomic nervous system, and abnormal dynamics in the developing vascular system.[116]

Diagnosis and Differential Diagnosis

A complete history and physical examination are usually sufficient to correctly diagnose a port-wine stain. Occasionally, a nevus simplex (salmon patch) or hemangioma precursor may be mistaken for a port-wine stain. Nevus simplex is usually located in the midline whereas port-wine stains generally do not cross the midline. Early hemangiomas and their precursor lesions are often red and macular in appearance, and the early proliferation of these lesions helps distinguish them from port-wine stains. In darkly pigmented infants, mongolian spots and the nevi of Ota and Ito can resemble vascular malformations. Close inspection will usually establish the proper diagnosis; biopsy is rarely necessary.

Management of Capillary Malformations

Patients with port-wine stains corresponding to the first branch of the trigeminal nerve (V1) are at risk for Sturge-Weber syndrome (see Sturge-Weber syndrome, in Syndromes Associated with Cutaneous Vascular Malformations). Similarly, those with involvement of the upper or lower eyelid (or both) may have associated glaucoma and should be evaluated regularly by an ophthalmologist. Those with port-wine stains of the lower extremity need periodic leg-length measurements during early childhood (see Klippel-Trenaunay syndrome, in Complex and Combined Vascular Malformations). In the past decade, the use of lasers, particularly the pulsed-dye laser, has dramatically improved the treatment of port-wine stains. Other therapeutic options, including surgical excision, skin grafting, radiation treatment, tattooing, and cosmetic camouflage have generally been ineffective. The use of continuous-wave lasers often resulted in textural change of the skin and, at times, permanent depigmentation. The pulsed-dye laser has been demonstrated to have a very low incidence of side effects in the treatment of port-wine stains in infants, children, and adults.[117–119] Most studies have indicated an incidence of atrophic scarring of 1% or less with virtually no hypertrophic scarring when the laser is used in the appropriate therapeutic energy fluence range.

In addition to efficacy and safety, a major advantage of pulsed-dye laser treatment has been a decreased need for anesthesia. Many adults can tolerate the procedure without local anesthesia. Most younger children, however, require sedation as well as the use of local, topical, regional, or general anesthesia in the treatment of medium to large lesions. Multiple treatments are required to obtain the maximum benefit. It is rare to see complete clearing in one or two sessions, as may be noted with a continuous-wave laser source. Although one study reported complete clearing of all patients after six treatment sessions,[117] other studies have noted significant but incomplete clearing after multiple treatments.[118–120] The

degree of clearing is, in large part, related to the anatomic location of a port-wine stain.[121] Facial port-wine stains usually respond most quickly, except those distributed over the central portion of the face, in particular, the second branch of the trigeminal nerve, which respond more slowly (Fig. 146–5*A* and *B*).

Although the use of the continuous-wave lasers, such as the argon and continuous-wave tunable dye lasers, became less frequent in the treatment of many vascular lesions, they continue to play a significant role in the treatment of the hypertrophic component of port-wine stains, despite their higher incidence of scarring and pigmentary alteration.[122] Modification of the delivery method of the laser light has led to renewed interest in the use of continuous-wave lasers. Robotized scanning devices that can be attached to any continuous-wave or copper vapor laser light source have been developed, and preliminary studies comparing test areas in port-wine stains irradiated with the continuous-wave dye laser with the pulsed-dye laser show little clinically significant difference between the two.[117, 118] Greater patient acceptance has been noted, at least in part due to the absence of the post-treatment darkening that occurs with the pulsed dye laser.[123]

The psychological trauma associated with facial port-wine stains has been well documented. Patients frequently experience feelings of stigmatization, difficulties in interpersonal relationships, and feelings of guilt, embarrassment, anxiety, and depression. In addition, many people believe that they are at significant personal, professional, and social disadvantage due to their port-wine stain. Psychological evaluation followed by treatment of either the birthmark itself or the resultant emotional issues can be beneficial for the patient.[124, 125]

Nevus Simplex (Salmon Patch)

Nevus simplex is an extremely common vascular birthmark seen in 25% to 40% of all newborns. The lesions are composed of ectatic dermal capillaries that are presumed to be the result of persistent fetal circulation. The nevus simplex or salmon patch has also been termed

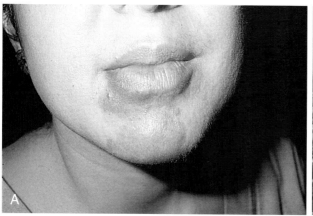
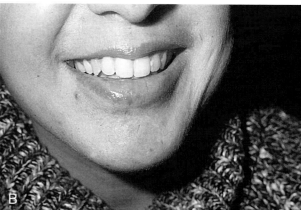

FIGURE 146–5. *A,* Port-wine stain of the chin. *B,* Nearly complete resolution after five treatments with pulsed-dye laser.

angel's kiss or *stork bite,* depending on the location of the lesion. Sites of predilection include the glabella, eyelids, and most commonly, the nape of the neck. The lesions are light pink to scarlet, flat, easily blanched, and usually deepen in color with vigorous activity, fever, crying or increases in ambient temperature.[126] Salmon patches are more common in white than Asian and black infants; however, there is no sex predilection.[127, 128] These lesions must be distinguished from port-wine stains because salmon patches tend to fade over time with complete resolution occurring by age 3 in the vast majority of cases. The exception is nevus simplex of the nape of the neck and some glabellar lesions, which may persist into adulthood. Some authors have referred to persistent lesions as *medial telangiectatic nevus.*[129] Lesions usually respond to pulsed-dye laser within two or three treatments, but therapy is not usually indicated unless the lesions persist beyond 3 years of age.[126]

Other Malformations (Venous, Arteriovenous, Lymphatic, and Combined)

Definition

Like port-wine stains, vascular malformations of veins, arteries, and lymphatic vessels are anomalies that occur during embryogenesis. Although they are almost always present at birth, significant signs and symptoms leading to the correct diagnosis may not be apparent until later in life. Vascular malformations may occur singly or as combined lesions and may affect cutaneous, subcutaneous, and visceral structures.

Venous Malformations

These low-flow vascular lesions are the second most common vascular malformation. They usually present as a faint blue patch or soft blue mass, often with ill-defined borders (Fig. 146–6). Lesions are usually present at birth but may occasionally become evident later in life. Venous malformations (VMs) are generally soft and compressible and have no increased skin temperature, thrill or bruit, such as would be evident in a higher-flow

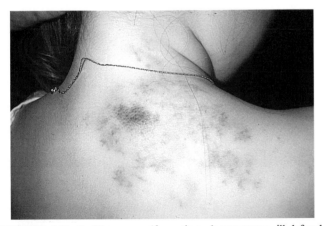

FIGURE 146–6. Venous malformation demonstrates ill-defined borders with blue and purple discoloration.

malformation. Over time, they may slowly enlarge, due to increasing ectasia. Firm areas may become evident due to phleboliths, thrombosis, or hemorrhage. Swelling and/or pain may be episodic, due to thrombosis or hemorrhage. A chronic consumption coagulopathy with prolonged prothrombin time, partial thromboplastin time, and decreased fibrinogen and clotting factors may occur in large VMs.

Craniofacial VMs may require treatment due to expansion and compression of adjacent structures or distortion of facial features. MRI can be used to delineate the extent of the lesions. Limb VMs may also involve deeper structures, including the muscle, joints, and even bone. Lower extremity lesions should be evaluated with MRI because knee joint involvement requires synovectomy and surgical removal of the VM to prevent recurrent hemarthrosis and loss of function of the joint. Doppler flow studies can also be used to document deeper venous anomalies and to assure that arteriovenous shunting (e.g., Parkes Weber syndrome) is not present.[72]

Percutaneous sclerotherapy with agents such as alcohol or sotradecol may decrease extensive VMs where surgical removal is not possible. These treatments are generally done with fluoroscopic guidance (usually under general anesthesia) to ensure that the injected material stays in the intended vasculature. Marked swelling for several weeks after therapy is usually followed by significant shrinkage of the VM. Limb VMs are more difficult to treat than craniofacial lesions. Custom-made elastic stockings are an important part of the management of VMs, usually necessary on a life-long basis.

Cutis marmorata telangiectatica congenita (congenital phlebectasia) is characterized by reticulated mottling of the superficial vasculature with some areas of apparent decreased perfusion and other areas with dilated venules and capillaries. When the distribution is localized, it tends to be sharply demarcated with strict observation of the midline. The condition is present at birth and tends to improve with age, although some patients have lesions that remain relatively fixed throughout life. Associated cutaneous findings include port-wine stain, atrophy of the skin overlying the dilated vessels, and superficial ulceration with scarring. Other associated anomalies include hyperplasia or hypoplasia of an affected limb, skeletal abnormalities, mental retardation, and glaucoma in cases with periorbital involvement.[130, 131]

Arteriovenous Malformations

Arteriovenous malformations (AVMs) are high-flow vascular malformations that can involve any structure including the skin, subcutaneous tissues, musculoskeletal system, and the viscera. Arteriovenous anomalies occur less frequently than other forms of vascular malformations, but have more severe sequelae, including tissue ischemia and ulcerations, pain, hemorrhage, and cardiac failure.

In contrast to other malformations, AVMs often go undiagnosed until adulthood. Their expression can be precipitated by puberty, pregnancy, trauma, or surgery. Skin findings, which vary from faint pink or bluish macules to a pulsating mass, are frequently the first indication of an underlying AVM. Specific symptoms include a sensation of heaviness, especially when in a dependent position, throbbing or stabbing pain, pulsation or thrill, hyperhidrosis or hypertrichosis overlying the lesion, and hyperthermia.[132]

Lesions are usually solitary but may involve much larger areas of vasculature than are evident at the outset. Lesions have a remarkable ability to recruit new vessels, particularly after trauma or surgery, behaving much like a malignancy. With time, draining veins become more evident with increased tortuosity. Careful physical examination of the skin and surrounding structures, including auscultation for bruits, may help differentiate AVMs from hemangiomas and other vascular malformations. Duplex Doppler studies can confirm the presence of arteriovenous shunting. MRI can help delineate the extent of lesions and demonstrate areas of flow void corresponding to the fast-flowing arteries and veins. Angiography is always required prior to therapy.

If AVMs remain quiescent during childhood, no treatment may be necessary until after puberty. Intervention is usually undertaken if complications develop, and should be performed by a multidisciplinary team, including interventional radiologists and surgeons familiar with the difficult treatment decisions involved. Although superselective arterial embolization may be palliative, reducing shunting and local vascular output, embolization followed by complete surgical excision may actually be curative in well-localized AVM. Partial embolization or resection can result in severe and even uncontrollable recurrences.[72]

Lymphatic Malformations

Lymphatic malformations present as localized or diffuse malformations of the lymphatic vessels. Solitary lymphatic cysts, so-called cystic hygromas, are most common on the neck. They are fluid filled and frequently communicate with adjacent lymphatic structures. Localized multicystic lymphatic malformations of the skin and mucosa, so-called lymphangioma circumscriptum, present as clusters of clear, fluid-filled vesicles that often become discolored by bleeding from surrounding capillaries. These lesions often have deeper components not initially evident, but that become apparent if the lesion recurs after a "complete excision." Extensive lymphatic malformations usually present with lymphedema of the affected area, often in association with more superficial vesicular skin lesions. In some cases, deeper connective tissues and viscera may be affected. Severe complications, including recurrent leakage of lymph, recurrent cellulitis, and cosmetic disfigurement, can occur.

Lymphatic malformations feature dilated, thin-walled vessels whose lumens contain frothy appearing proteinaceous material, and are devoid of erythrocytes unless the lesion has been traumatized. These vessels are dispersed throughout the superficial and deep dermis, and subcutis. Delicate valves are present in some vessels. Collections of small lymphocytes are sometimes seen in the adjacent dermis. Deep vessels can be partially sur-

rounded by fascicles of smooth muscle. In lymphangioma circumsciptum, round, dilated lymphatic vessels are present just beneath a hyperplastic and hyperkeratotic epidermis.

Some superficial lymphangiomas (lymphangioma circumscriptum) and the cutaneous component of deeper lymphangiomas may benefit from laser therapy. Carbon dioxide laser vaporization of individual and grouped lymphangiomas may be helpful in obliterating these lesions. Vaporization in the defocused mode often controls lymphorrhea, which may be quite symptomatic for some patients.[133] Because of deeper components, lesions may recur following any surgical technique, including laser ablation, electrosurgery, cryotherapy, and superficial excision. Many of these techniques may lead to scarring, which may be hypertrophic. Some lymphatic malformations with a capillary or venous component may be susceptible to continuous-wave light sources that are absorbed well by vascular tissue. Under these circumstances, the argon, copper vapor, continuous-wave dye, krypton, and KTP lasers may be of benefit. In cases with diffuse lymphatic malformations, support garments may be very helpful in avoiding progressive lymphangiectasia. Prophylactic antibiotics may also help if recurrent infection becomes a problem.

Complex and Combined Vascular Malformations

Virtually any vessel type may combine with another to cause combined malformations (Fig. 146–7). The most well recognized of these malformations is the *Klippel-Trenaunay syndrome,* characterized by soft tissue hypertrophy, and bony overgrowth of an extremity in association with an overlying port-wine stain. In the vast

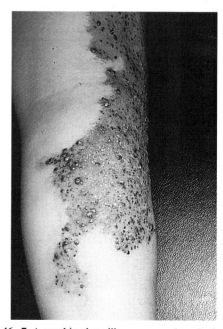

FIGURE 146–7. A combined capillary, venous, lymphatic malformation: Multiple venous and lymphatic ectasias developing in a port-wine stain.

majority of cases, a single lower extremity is affected. However, patients with upper extremity, multiple extremity, and extensive truncal involvement have all been described. The port-wine stain is invariably present at birth, but the limb overgrowth and venous anomalies may not be evident in infancy. The capillary malformation can vary greatly in color from light pink to dark purple and almost always has an associated venous or lymphatic malformation.

Limb overgrowth is generally secondary to variable combinations of increased adipose tissue, lymphedema, muscle hypertrophy, and dilated venous vasculature. Bony hypertrophy may also contribute to increased girth of the affected extremity. The enlargement of the limb is often disproportionate, with hypertrophy of the toes and feet being more prominent. Limb length discrepancy may be mild, but does not progress in a predictable fashion; close follow-up together with orthopedic consultation and x-ray "scanograms" can be used to determine if clinically significant disproportionate growth is occurring in the legs. If the discrepancy is significant, compensatory shoes and ultimately premature epiphyseal closure of the longer leg may be necessary.[134] Deep venous aplasia or hypoplasia may also be present, and may lead to disastrous consequences if sclerotherapy or vein stripping is undertaken without adequate evaluation of the underlying venous vasculature.[135] Lymphoscintigraphy may also help evaluate the lymphatic system.

In the *Parkes Weber syndrome,* limb hypertrophy is seen in association with multiple arteriovenous fistulas and an overlying port-wine stain. Venous anomalies are not usually present and extremity overgrowth is proportionate without accentuation of the feet or toes. The limb length discrepancy is often considerable. Other complications associated with the high-flow malformation, such as congestive heart failure, result in a poor prognosis for many of these patients.[134]

Syndromes Associated with Cutaneous Vascular Malformations

The *Sturge-Weber syndrome* (SWS) is characterized by the presence of a facial port-wine stain and leptomeningeal and choroidal angiomatosis, but partial SWS can occur with only skin and CNS or eye involvement as well. The location and extent of the port-wine stain determines the risk for the development of SWS. Only patients with V1 port-wine stains can develop SWS, but because of overlap in the distribution of V1 and V2 enervation, patients with infraorbital port-wine stains may be affected.[72] Those with complete involvement of V1, 2, and 3 or bilateral port-wine stains are at highest risk (approximately 25%) for developing the syndrome.[112] Those with involvement of cheek but not eyelids (V2) or the V3 dermatome alone have essentially no risk of SWS.[110, 136]

The most common neurologic findings are seizures, usually beginning in the first year of life, and mental retardation, which occurs in 30% to 55% of patients with CNS involvement, usually those with extensive CNS involvement and epilepsy. Less common neurologic findings include hemiplegia, hemiatrophy, microcephaly,

cortical blindness, increased intracranial pressure, and intracranial hemorrhage.[137, 138]

The most common ophthalmologic finding is ipsilateral choroidal angiomatosis. The increased vasculature rarely causes retinal dysfunction in childhood, but undetected anterior displacement of the retina may lead to amblyopia. Adults are at risk for retinal detachment, ectopic bone formation, and retinal degeneration.[139, 140] Glaucoma is the most significant ophthalmologic sequela, occurring in 30% to 71% of patients.[136, 141] Nearly all cases are associated with ipsilateral port-wine stains of both the upper and lower eyelids, but in rare instances, only the upper or lower eyelid is affected.[112, 136, 142] Because eye problems can occur later in life, all patients with eyelid lesions should have periodic ophthalmologic examinations even if the results of the initial examination were normal.

Skull roentgenograms may demonstrate characteristic railroad track–like calcifications of the brain parenchyma but are rarely seen before 1 year of age. Computed tomography is more sensitive in detecting small calcifications; MRI may demonstrate abnormalities such as parenchymal atrophy and choroid plexus enlargement even earlier.[143] Electroencephalography can be used to define the location and type of seizure activity that may be present.

Phakomatosis pigmentovascularis is the association of port-wine stains with pigmented lesions, either nevus spilus, dermal melanocytosis (such as nevus of Ota or Ito), or linear or whorled epidermal hyperpigmentation. Associated epidermal nevus and nevus anemicus have also been described. It has been described most commonly in Asians. The port-wine stains are usually extensive. Some patients also have ocular melanosis as well as systemic abnormalities, including seizures, hemiplegia, limb hypertrophy, and malignant colon polyposis.[144, 145]

The blue rubber bleb nevus syndrome is the association of multiple cutaneous venous malformations of the skin and gastrointestinal tract. The syndrome is rare; less than 100 cases have been reported in the literature. The skin lesions may be present at birth but are usually noted during childhood and tend to increase in size and number over time. The venous malformations are generally located on the trunk and upper extremities, are compressible, and range in size from a few millimeters to several centimeters in diameter; they may be spontaneously painful and occasionally have associated hyperhidrosis.[146, 147] Cutaneous blue rubber bleb nevi often are muscular vessels with an ovoid profile, a thick-walled inferior portion, and a thin-walled superficial one.

The gastrointestinal tract, especially the small bowel, is the most frequent site of extracutaneous involvement, although venous malformations have also been reported in the respiratory tract, central nervous system, eye, liver, spleen, and genitourinary tract.[148] Gastrointestinal and other visceral lesions are frequently injured and may bleed profusely, requiring transfusion and surgical intervention. Many patients continue to develop new lesions with advancing age, and surgical excision is often followed by recurrence of the malformation. Acute massive gastrointestinal hemorrhage is the most common cause of death.[146, 147]

Gorham's syndrome is the association of venous and lymphatic malformations of the skin and skeleton with osteolytic bone disease. Clinical presentation usually occurs during adolescence but has been reported in infancy as well as in the elderly.[149] The presence of intraosseous vascular lesions leads to gradual osteolysis of the affected bone until the entire area is replaced with fibrous connective tissue. Typically bones of the shoulder and pelvic girdles are involved, but any region may be affected.[150] Usually one bone or group of bones is affected although a multicentric form has also been described.[151] Deformity of the involved area, pathologic fractures, and muscular weakness occur secondary to the osteolysis and usually result in permanent sequelae. The disease is self-limited and tends to undergo spontaneous arrest after several years.[152]

Maffucci's syndrome is characterized by the presence of dyschondroplasia and multiple subcutaneous venous malformations. The disease is believed to be a congenital, nonhereditary disorder of mesodermal dysplasia. Onset is usually during childhood and there is an equal sex predilection.[153] The skeletal changes result from a defect in endochondral ossification that leads to irregular growth (dyschondroplasia), cartilage proliferation, and the eventual formation of endochondromas. The lesions most commonly involve the distal extremities, although tumors have been reported to involve the spine, thorax, pelvis, and skull.[154]

Mucosal and visceral VMs may also occur and cutaneous lymphatic malformations have also been described. Phlebolith formation may complicate any site of venous anomaly; intraoral and hand lesions are at a particular risk for hemorrhage.[70]

A predisposition to neoplasia during adulthood has been well documented. Malignant transformation of endochondromas to chondrosarcomas has been noted in 15% to 20% of patients. Similarly, vascular lesions are also at risk for sarcomatous degeneration. Other associated tumors include fibrosarcomas, gliomas, ovarian neoplasms, pituitary adenoma, and pancreatic adenocarcinoma.[155]

Proteus syndrome is an overgrowth syndrome characterized by the variable presence of port-wine stains, epidermal nevi, limb asymmetry, and partial gigantism of one or more body segments. Many patients with the syndrome have previously been diagnosed as having Klippel-Trenaunay syndrome. Other features include macrocephaly, skull exostoses, lipomas, and cerebriform thickening of the skin of an extremity, which is highly characteristic.[156]

The *Wyburn-Mason syndrome* is a very rare disorder characterized by a unilateral retinal AVM and an ipsilateral mid-brain AVM; ipsilateral cutaneous vascular malformations are occasionally present. The skin lesions are usually port-wine stains in a trigeminal distribution. Vascular malformations of the mandible, maxilla, palate, and oral mucosa have also been described.[157]

The *Riley-Smith syndrome* is an autosomal dominant condition described in five members of the same family. It consists of macrocephaly without hydrocephalus or neurologic impairment, pseudopapilledema, and cutaneous capillary, venous, and lymphatic malformations.[158]

Bannayan-Zonana syndrome is a rare autosomal dominant disorder characterized by benign macrocephaly, lipomas, and subcutaneous or visceral mixed vascular malformations. Some lesions may have histologic features of both adipose and vascular tissue. Visceral involvement can be extensive, resulting in life-threatening obstruction of vital organs, including the gastrointestinal tract and the central nervous system.[159]

Cobb syndrome or cutaneomeningospinal angiomatosis is a rare condition characterized by the presence of a truncal port-wine stain or mixed malformation (previously referred to as *angiokeratoma*) in association with a vascular malformation of the spinal cord. The cutaneous lesion is located in a dermatomal distribution approximately corresponding to the segments of the spinal cord that are involved.[160] Size can vary from a few centimeters to a large linear unilateral band overlying the cervical, thoracic, or lumbar spine. The sacral area is rarely involved. Neurologic findings depend on the level of the spinal angioma and can include back or leg pain, leg weakness, sensory disturbances, and loss of sphincter control. Although the onset of symptoms is usually gradual, occasionally a patient will present with severe pain followed by complete paralysis within hours or days. Other findings include scoliosis or kyphoscoliosis occurring in one fourth of patients, as well as rare instances of congenital heart disease, spina bifida occulta, café-au-lait spots, and ipsilateral hypertrophy of the extremities.[161–163]

ACQUIRED VASCULAR PROLIFERATIONS

There are a bewildering array of acquired vascular proliferations (Table 146–4). Some are clearly hamartomatous, hyperplastic, or neoplastic, whereas others are difficult to classify along traditional lines. The differentiation of many of these lesions—capillary, venular, arteriolar, and so forth—has not been precisely defined. Only one neoplasm, angiosarcoma, is universally accepted as malignant; some regard Kaposi's sarcoma to be a hyperplasia or angiomatosis (see Chapter 125).

Hyperplasias of Blood Vessels

A hyperplasia is a proliferation of cells that is initiated by a stimulus, but stabilizes or regresses when that stimulus ceases. Several important cutaneous vascular proliferations meet these conditions. The most common by far is due to venous stasis, and usually results in swelling of the skin of the lower legs accompanied by mottled red-brown discoloration. Microscopic examination shows tortuous capillaries and venules within a thickened papillary dermis, often accompanied by extravasated erythrocytes and siderophages. Venous stasis is covered in detail in Chapter 65, but acroangiodermatitis, an exaggerated form of venous stasis, is discussed below. Vascular hyperplasias can also result from bacterial infections, as in bacillary angiomatosis due to *Rochalimaea*, and verruga peruana due to *Bartonella bacilliformis* (see Chapter 115). The rare entity angioendotheliomatosis clearly

TABLE 146-4. Acquired Vascular Growths

Condition	Age of Onset	Location	Clinical Description	Systemic Manifestations	Associated Syndromes	Natural History
Acroangiodermatitis	Variable	Lower extremities	Coalescent red-purple papules overlying a deeper vascular abnormality	None	None	Persistent
Reactive angioendotheliomatosis	Adults	Variable	Red, blue, or purple papules	None	Disseminated intravascular coagulation Endocarditis Vasculitis Cryoglobulinemia	Slow resolution
Pyogenic granuloma	Variable	Face, lips, periungual	Rapidly growing, red, glistening, pedunculated papules	None	May arise within port-wine stain	Hemorrhage and ulceration if left untreated
Acquired tufted hemangioma	Children Young adults	Neck, back	Pink patch developing small pink or red papules within patch	None	None	Persistent
Acral arteriovenous hemangioma	Adults	Digits, face	Small, superficial, dermal, bluish papules	None	None	Persistent
Epithelioid hemangioma	Adults	Ears, scalp	Multiple pink, red, or brown smooth papulonodules	Hypertension Eosinophilia	None	Persistent
Glomus tumor	Adults	Digits	Solitary red-purple painful nodules	None	None	Persistent
Angiokeratoma	Variable	Genitalia, trunks, legs	Solitary or multiple dark red scaly papules and plaques	None	Fabry's disease Fucosidosis β-galactosidase deficiency	Persistent
Cherry hemangioma	Elderly	Trunk	Very small round, smooth, red papules	None	None	Persistent
Targetoid hemosiderotic hemangioma	Adults	Trunk	Solitary, red-purple papule surrounded by targetoid zones of pallor and purplish discoloration	None	None	Persistent

consists of two conditions: one is an intravascular lymphoma (malignant angioendotheliomatosis); and the other, a reactive condition described herein. Intravascular papillary endothelial hyperplasia, or Masson's lesion, is not a primary process but a hyperplasia of fibroblasts and endothelial cells recruited into an organizing thrombus. Canalization of the thrombus results in a papillary pattern in which branching struts of collagen are lined by protuberant endothelial cells. It is generally confined to the dilated lumina of preexistent vascular neoplasms such as those of angiokeratoma.[164]

Acroangiodermatitis

Definition. Acroangiodermatitis is a superficial localized form of vascular hyperplasia due to abnormal blood flow. It is also known as pseudo–Kaposi's sarcoma. Cases due to venous hypertension alone have been termed acroangiodermatitis of Mali, whereas those in

which an arteriovenous shunt is present have been termed the *Bluefarb-Stewart syndrome.*

Clinical Description. Acroangiodermatitis presents with coalescent red to purple papules over a circumscribed area of skin, usually on the legs or feet (Fig. 146–8). Underlying the cutaneous findings are a variety of vascular problems, including chronic venous insufficiency, paralysis of the affected limb, a congenital or acquired arteriovenous shunt, or damage to vessels from amputation or intravenous drug abuse.[165]

Pathology. Biopsies of acroangiodermatitis show an exaggeration of the findings seen in venous stasis, and are described above. The papillary dermis is often packed with small, round, thick-walled vessels arranged back to back. Sometimes dermal dendrocytes that have ingested hemosiderin appear spindled, and there can be increased numbers of spindled fibroblasts, resulting in a superficial resemblance to Kaposi's sarcoma (Fig. 146–9).

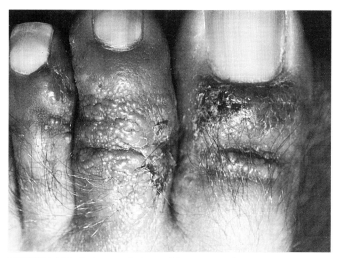

FIGURE 146–8. Acroangiodermatitis presents with closely set purple papules. The dorsal toes are a favored location.

Pathogenesis and Etiology. The mechanism at work in acroangiodermatitis is clearly vascular proliferation driven by venous hypertension.

Diagnosis and Differential Diagnosis. The diagnosis of acroangiodermatitis should be considered if purplish papules or nodules arise on the skin of the toes, either unilaterally or bilaterally, or on an amputation stump. A triangular distribution over the dorsal first and second toes is characteristic. Studies of blood flow may help detect an underlying anomaly. Biopsy is useful to rule

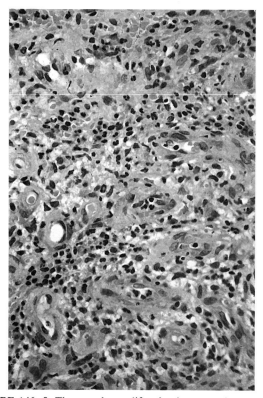

FIGURE 146–9. The vascular proliferation in acroangiodermatitis is composed of small round thick-walled vessels in the papillary dermis, in contrast to Kaposi's sarcoma, in which slit-like or jagged vessels with thin walls are present, generally sparing the papillary dermis.

out Kaposi's sarcoma or angiosarcoma. Acroangiodermatitis is not usually difficult for expert dermatopathologists to distinguish from Kaposi's sarcoma, despite its designation of *pseudo-Kaposi's sarcoma*. In acroangiodermatitis, the pathologic changes are centered in the papillary dermis, whereas those of Kaposi's sarcoma usually spare that site and instead revolve around preexistent vessels and adnexa, at least early on. The vessels of acroangiodermatitis, in contrast to those of Kaposi's sarcoma, are thick walled and invested by pericytes.

Treatment. Correction of arteriovenous shunting or other underlying condition, if possible, may improve the condition or help prevent its progression. Treatment of venous hypertension with pressure garments may also be helpful. Some individual lesions may respond to laser ablation, with either continuous-wave or pulsed-dye laser.

Reactive Angioendotheliomatosis

Definition. Reactive angioendotheliomatosis is a rare condition in which endothelial cells and pericytes proliferate due to several different stimuli that have in common the occlusion of vascular lumina.

Clinical Description. Reactive angioendotheliomatosis generally occurs in patients with systemic diseases, including endocarditis, vasculitis, disseminated intravascular coagulation, and cryoglobulinemia. Its lesions are erythematous, purple or blue papules that are usually on the limbs, face, or trunk, and, in cases due to cryoglobulinemia, on the acra.[166, 167] The condition is limited to the skin and resolves over time.

Pathology. Reactive angioendotheliomatosis features small clusters or tufts of vessels with rounded shapes that are invested by pericytes and sometimes by myxoid connective tissue. In cases due to disseminated intravascular coagulation, thrombi can be present in vessel lumina, and in those due to cryoproteins, their precipitates can be similarly identified. Inflammatory infiltrates can also be present; these may be a reaction to ischemia from luminal occlusion in some cases and may be the residuum of a small vessel leukocytoclastic vasculitis in others.

Pathogenesis and Etiology. Reactive angioendotheliomatosis appears to be mediated by the blockage of the lumina of small vessels, either by cryoproteins or fibrin in cases arising from small vessel vasculitis. Although microscopic foci of vascular proliferation due to such occlusion are common, clinically evident lesions are exotically rare. The reason for some patients' inability to shut off this reaction is unknown.

Diagnosis and Differential Diagnosis. The diagnosis of reactive angioendotheliomatosis is a histologic one. Among its differential diagnoses is malignant angioendotheliomatosis, also known as intravascular or angiotropic lymphoma. The latter is typified by bruise-like skin lesions accompanied by a variety of unusual symptoms due to involvement of vessels in other organs. Lymph nodes are generally not involved. In contrast to the proliferation of well-formed small, round vessels surrounded by pericytes in reactive angioendotheliomatosis, angiotropic lymphoma features the plugging of vessels by cells with scant cytoplasm and atypical nuclei. A B-cell immunophenotype is usually present, although occasional patients have T-cell neoplasms.

Treatment. The treatment of reactive angioendotheliomatosis is generally that which is appropriate for the underlying systemic condition. Once the vaso-occlusive stimulus is removed, cutaneous lesions slowly involute.

Telangiectases

Telangiectases are due to ectasia of preexistent blood vessels with little proliferation of endothelial cells, pericytes, or smooth muscle, unlike the case in benign vascular neoplasms. Telangiectases affecting large areas of skin such as port-wine stains are considered earlier in this chapter. Some of the conditions listed below feature slight proliferation of vessels in addition to ectasia. In *angioma serpiginosum,* small pinhead-sized erythematous puncta are arranged in circinate or serpentine patterns. Nearly any part of the skin can be affected. Dilated capillaries are present in enlarged dermal papillae. *Spider angioma* or nevus araneus is found on the upper trunk and face and has a central punctum from which fine vessels radiate. Spider angiomas are sensitive to estrogen, and enlarge during pregnancy and are often found in patients with cirrhosis of the liver. *Venous lakes* are blue papules that occur on the face of older patients, favoring the lips and ears. Elastosis of the walls of vessels due to actinic damage appears to cause weakening of the vessel wall and its subsequent dilatation. Lesions whose lumina house thrombi have been termed *thrombosed capillary aneurysms.* In *generalized essential telangiectasia* there are small lesions that resemble spider angiomas over much of the cutaneous surface. The condition is transmitted as an autosomal dominant trait. It usually has its onset in the fourth decade, and mostly affects women. The process is fortunately limited to the skin. In unilateral nevoid telangiectasia the dermatomes innervated by either the trigeminal or third or fourth cervical nerves are the sites of telangiectases, which can either present at birth or in later life, when they can blossom under the influence of estrogens. Secondary telangiectases can be due to collagen vascular diseases, actinic damage, and other causes. *Caliber persistent arteries* are due to vessels that do not diminish in size as they approach the surface of the lip, resulting in an erosive area.

Treatment of Telangiectasia. Treatment depends on the location and extent of lesions. Small well-localized lesions may be treated with electrocautery using an epilating needle, or copper vapor or pulsed-dye laser using a yellow light source. Larger areas of telangiectasia on the upper body are best treated with either pulsed-dye or copper vapor laser; those on the legs are usually treated with injection of sclerosing agents such as saline or sotradecol. Treatment of venous lakes is best done with lasers.

Benign Vascular Lesions

Benign vascular neoplasms of the skin include proliferations with capillary, venular, smooth muscle, arteriolar, and venous composition and varying components of en-

dothelial cells, pericytes, smooth muscle, and glomus cells. Some of these lesions may truly be hamartomatous, such as acral arteriovenous hemangioma, and others may have a hamartomatous element alongside a proliferative one, such as angiolymphoid hyperplasia with eosinophilia, in which AVMs frequently underlie nodules of large cuboidal or epithelioid endothelial cells. There is debate as to whether the proliferations in such lesions as pyogenic granuloma are reactive or neoplastic.

Pyogenic Granuloma (Lobular Capillary Hemangioma)

Definition. Pyogenic granulomas are neither pyogenic in origin nor do they feature granulomatous inflammation. Instead they are lobular proliferations of capillaries and venules that present as exophytic lesions, and are often related to minor trauma by the patient. The concept of lobular capillary hemangioma links the classic exophytic pyogenic granuloma with other dermal, intravascular, and subcutaneous lesions that have similar microscopic appearances.[168] However, similar lobular structures can be present in unrelated lesions, such as regressing infantile hemangiomas and in florid stasis vascular changes.[169]

Clinical Features. Pyogenic granulomas are typically glistening red or pink excrescences, which rapidly evolve into polypoid or pedunculated papules or nodules with eroded surfaces that eventually reepithelialize. Common sites are the lips, periungual skin, and face. They often bleed, at times profusely, a characteristic that has led some authors to refer to them as the "Band-Aid disease" (Fig. 146–10). Pyogenic granulomas can arise within preexistent vascular malformations such as nevus flammeus or in acquired ones such as spider angiomas. The concept of lobular capillary hemangioma links conventional pyogenic granulomas with epulis gravidarum, which are oral lesions that appear during pregnancy, and with dermal, intravascular, or subcutaneous lesions that present as pink to skin-colored papules and nodules. Some also consider tufted angioma to be part of this spectrum.[170]

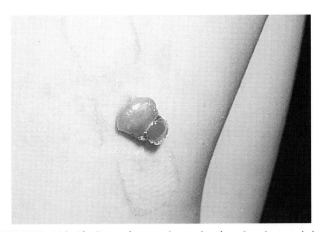

FIGURE 146–10. Pyogenic granuloma showing the characteristic "Band-Aid" sign.

Pathology. Early pyogenic granulomas appear as volcanic protrusions of ulcerated granulation tissue that project through a rent in the epidermis. As lesions mature, a lobular pattern of well-formed small, round vessels is formed grouped around ectatic, irregularly shaped spaces that contain many erythrocytes (Fig. 146–11). The vessels are surrounded by concentrically arranged spindle-shaped pericytes that impart much of the cellularity of these lesions. Lobules are divided by bands of connective tissue, which are initially myxoid and later become fibrotic. Over time, the ulcerated surfaces of pyogenic granulomas re-epithelialize. At the bases of many pyogenic granulomas are paired arterioles and veins, which some believe represent an underlying AVM.

In dermal, subcutaneous, and intravascular lesions, similar lobules of vessels divided by connective tissue septa are present as they are in the submucosa of oral epulis gravidarum.

Pathogenesis and Etiology. The supposition that pyogenic granulomas and related lesions are hyperplasias rather than true neoplasms is supported by their occurrence following minor trauma or hormonal or pharmacologic stimulation. They can be found in scars of acne patients who have been treated with retinoids, in pregnant women as well as in women taking birth control pills, in skin affected by chronic graft versus host disease, and in satellite array around the site of attempted ablation of a single larger lesion. To others, the repeatable lobular pattern and the failure of lesions to involute indicate that they are neoplasms.

Diagnosis and Differential Diagnosis. The diagnosis of pyogenic granuloma can be made clinically if a rounded red, glistening papule with a history of rapid growth over a few weeks is found at a characteristic site or setting. It can be difficult to exclude melanotic melanoma or, in an immunocompromised patient, Kaposi's sarcoma and bacillary angiomatosis. These latter conditions can so mimic pyogenic granuloma that expert clinicians with extensive experience with these entities cannot tell them apart without a biopsy. Histologically, all three conditions can feature a polypoid contour, ulcerated surface, and collarettes of adnexal epithelium. Histologic criteria for their separation are enumerated in Table 115–2.

Treatment. Treatment depends on the size and location of the lesion. Often curettage and electrodesiccation is sufficient in eradicating solitary lesions. Other treatment options include pulsed-dye and carbon dioxide laser, cryotherapy, and surgical exision. Recurrences and the development of multiple satellite lesions following therapy have been reported.[170a, 170b]

Acquired Tufted Angioma

Definition. Acquired tufted angioma is a benign vascular proliferation in which lobules similar to those of pyogenic granuloma are scattered widely in the dermis, causing faint pink to red papules within a pink patch of skin.[170] The condition is termed *angioblastoma* in the Japanese literature.

Clinical Appearance. Acquired tufted angioma begins as a pink patch, generally over the dorsal neck and upper back of children or teenagers (Fig. 146–12). As the vascular lobules become more defined, they become palpable. Some lesions harbor exophytic papules similar to those of conventional pyogenic granuloma. Papules with the histologic features of a tufted angioma occurred in the skin of a liver allograft recipient, but regressed with modulation of immunosuppressive therapy. The lesions of acquired tufted angioma are stable over time.

Pathology. In acquired tufted angioma, vascular lobules similar to those seen in pyogenic granuloma and other lobular vascular proliferations stud the superficial and deep dermis and subcutis; lobules are separated by areas of normal dermis or fat (Fig. 146–13). Narrow semilunar spaces are present at the peripheries of many lobules (Fig. 146–14).

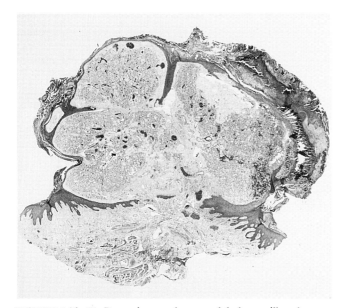

FIGURE 146–11. Pyogenic granuloma, or lobular capillary hemangioma in its fully developed form, is a polypoid proliferation composed of lobules of capillaries and venules separated by bands of connective tissue.

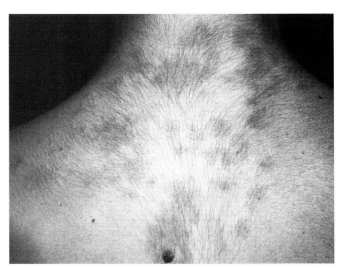

FIGURE 146–12. Tufted angioma often presents as a pink patch within which are slightly elevated or flat but palpable erythematous foci.

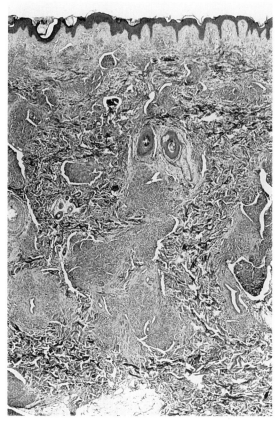

FIGURE 146-13. There are scattered lobules of capillaries and venules similar to those of pyogenic granuloma throughout the dermis of tufted angioma.

Pathogenesis and Etiology. The pink patches in which acquired tufted angiomas arise could represent an underlying vascular malformation. This supposition is buttressed by the reported occurrence of one lesion in a nevus flammeus in an adult and by reports of pyogenic granuloma arising in another nevus flammeus.

Diagnosis and Differential Diagnosis. A pink patch of tufted angioma contains slightly elevated papules and has a lumpy consistency, unlike a nevus flammeus, which is flat. Tufted angioma can be distinguished on biopsy from other vascular proliferations that present as large pink patches.

Treatment. Small lesions can be excised, but the extent of large ones makes resection problematic. Pulsed-dye laser, soft x-ray therapy, and electrocautery have been used in some cases.[170, 170c, 171]

Acral Arteriovenous Hemangioma

Definition. Acral arteriovenous hemangiomas are small, superficial dermal clusters of arterioles, veins, and vessels with features intermediate between them.[172] The traditional name for these lesions was cirsoid aneurysm.

Clinical Description. These superficial arteriovenous shunts present as small, asymptomatic red papules on the digits or periorificial facial skin of adults.

Pathology. The vessels of these hemangiomas are found as clusters of thick-walled, muscular vessels in a well-circumscribed area of the dermis (Fig. 146-15). With stains for elastic tissue, some have the internal and external elastic laminae seen in arteries, whereas in others, the elastica resembles that of veins, with only external fibers in the adventitia.

Diagnosis and Differential Diagnosis. The color and distribution of acral arteriovenous hemangiomas raise the possibilities of perniosis and cryoglobulinemia, which are temperature sensitive, whereas arteriovenous hemangiomas are not. Definitive diagnosis is made on biopsy.

Treatment. Local excision is usually curative.

Angiolymphoid Hyperplasia with Eosinophilia (Epithelioid Hemangioma)

Definition. Angiolymphoid hyperplasia with eosinophilia (ALHE) is a benign proliferation of large, protuberant (hence, epithelioid or histiocytoid endothelial cells) that is often accompanied by dense lymphoid infiltrates and frequently by peripheral or lesional eosinophilia. It is unknown whether the condition is hyperplastic or neoplastic.

Clinical Description. Lesions of ALHE are smooth-surfaced tan, pink, red, or brown papules or nodules often found on the skin of the head, with a predilection for the area around the ears (Fig. 146-16). Although usually asymptomatic, they can be painful, and because some of them are associated with an underlying AVM, they may be pulsatile. Multiple lesions are common, and

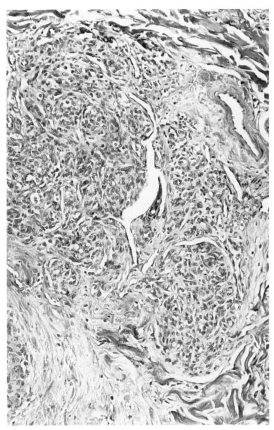

FIGURE 146-14. Semilunar clefts surround a lobule in tufted angioma.

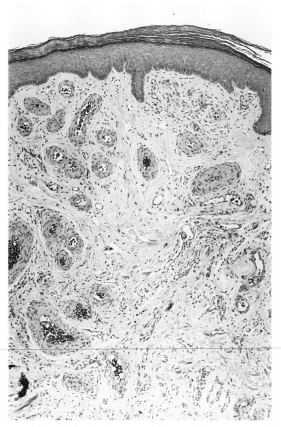

FIGURE 146–15. Redundant muscular vessels are present in the dermis in an acral arteriovenous hemangioma.

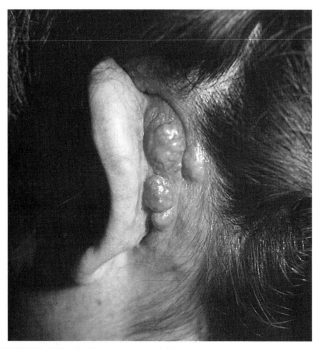

FIGURE 146–16. The area around the ears is a characteristic location of angiolymphoid hyperplasia with eosinophilia. (From Callen JP, Greer KE, Hood AF, et al. Color Atlas of Dermatology. Philadelphia: WB Saunders Co., 1993:143.)

eruptive presentation occasional.[173] The condition described as papular angioplasia of the face appears to represent multiple facial papules of ALHE.[174] A few patients with ALHE had hypertension that responded to surgical removal of the lesions.[175]

Pathology. The vascular proliferation of ALHE is generally based in the dermis, but it can extend into the subcutis. It is usually well circumscribed, except in the case of rapidly growing eruptive lesions. There can be discrete vessels with thick walls, or nodules of so-called epithelioid endothelial cells. These so-called hobnail cells bulge into vascular spaces and have plump ovoid shapes, abundant eosinophilic cytoplasm, and large vesicular nuclei contained in their bulbous adluminal ends. Large, malformed arteriolar and venous segments are often present at the base of the proliferation. Lymphocytic infiltration varies from scant to dense with many lymphoid follicles. Eosinophils can likewise range from none to many (Fig. 146–17).

Pathogenesis and Etiology. Because some examples of ALHE have tortuous arterioles and veins at their bases, it has been conjectured that arteriovenous shunting causes ALHE. A clinical history of trauma and histologic evidence of vascular damage is present in some patients and may cause the shunt. The inverse is also possible; cytokines produced by the vascular proliferation could

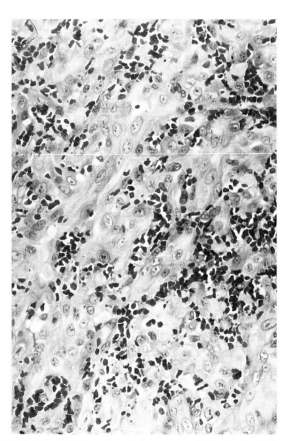

FIGURE 146–17. There is a broad range of histologic findings in angiolymphoid hyperplasia with eosinophilia, but the constituents include vessels with large plump ovoid endothelial cells, lymphoid follicles or dense lymphocytic infiltrates, numerous eosinophils, and redundant arterioles and veins. In this field there are vessels that contain erythrocytes bounded by large, protuberant endothelial cells.

induce arterioles and veins to elongate and become tortuous. Renin has been immunohistochemically identified in the endothelial cells of ALHE, and its product, angiotensin II, may be responsible for some of the vascular proliferation and for the hypertension that rare patients develop as a consequence of ALHE.[175] Both pregnancy and oral contraceptive use have been linked to ALHE, and its endothelial cells contain estrogen receptor protein.[176]

Diagnosis and Differential Diagnosis. The diagnosis of ALHE is made on biopsy, although the characteristic location of lesions around the ears may alert the clinician. ALHE shares a number of features with Kimura's disease, and indeed the two conditions have been confused and many have used these terms synonymously. Kimura's disease is a lymphoid proliferation of the subcutis of the head and neck that usually affects young Asian adults. Like ALHE, there is peripheral blood eosinophilia. Unlike ALHE, its lesions are bulky subcutaneous masses rather than dermally based papules or nodules. While nodules of epithelioid endothelial cells are a hallmark of ALHE, the vessels of Kimura's disease feature far less proturberant endothelial cells that are similar to those found in the high endothelial venules of lymph nodes.[177] On biopsy, the differential diagnosis includes bacillary angiomatosis, bartonellosis, and a low-grade variant of angiosarcoma known as epithelioid hemangioendothelioma. The latter features cords of epithelioid endothelial cells set in a myxoid stroma without well-differentiated vessels, unlike the case in ALHE.[178] To date, no eosinophils have been demonstrated in epithelioid hemangioendothelioma.

Treatment. Individual lesions of ALHE can be removed surgically. Care should be taken to adequately excise the arteriolar and venous segments at their bases. Intralesional corticosteroid therapy is sometimes successful. In one case, extensive widespread lesions of ALHE were successfully treated with intravenous vinblastine (15 mg/week).[179] A compelling reason for drastic treatment of these benign lesions should be present, however, because there is no recorded case of ALHE evolving into angiosarcoma, even though the lesions persist indefinitely.

Glomus Tumors

Definition. Glomus tumors are benign neoplasms characterized by vascular spaces surrounded by a proliferation of modified smooth muscle cells resembling the arrangement seen in the arteriovenous glomus—a cuff that surrounds the shunt between arterioles and veins on the skin of the digits and elsewhere. Both normal and neoplastic glomus cells are small and cuboidal and have round monomorphous nuclei. Glomus tumors are relatively solid while glomangiomas have fewer glomus cells arranged around ectatic vessels. This distinction may depend more on the location of lesions than on a real biologic difference, however. The dermis of acral skin is less distensible, hence, the solidity of glomus tumors; however, many patients will have lesions at other sites where their growth is not compressed.[180] Glomangiomyomas resemble glomangiomas, but also contain con-

ventional smooth muscle cells. Glomangiosarcomas, malignant neoplasms of glomus cells, are extraordinarily rare.

Clinical Description. Glomus tumors are solitary red or purple nodules found on the skin of the fingers or toes, sites rich in normal glomus apparatus. Subungual papules can erode underlying bone and cause nail dystrophy. Glomus tumors generally occur in adults, and are included in the spectrum of painful cutaneous tumors along with angioleiomyoma, neurilemoma, eccrine spiradenoma, and leiomyoma. Lancinating pain can follow a gentle touch, or exposure to cold.

Multiple lesions (glomangiomas) affecting other sites can have a similar appearance but are less often painful (Fig. 146–18). Glomangiomas are not clinically distinctive. Rare cases have been associated with thrombocytopenia as part of the Kasabach-Merritt syndrome.

Pathology. Glomus tumors of the acra are well-circumscribed dermal nodules in which masses of glomus cells surround inconspicuous venules. Myxoid stroma is often present (Fig. 146–19). In glomangiomyomas, ectatic venules are surrounded by concentric ribbons of glomus cells. Glomangiomyomas feature spindled smooth muscle cells with abundant eosinophilic cytoplasm and blunt-ended nuclei, as well as cells with features intermediate between glomus cells and fully differentiated myocytes.

Pathogenesis and Etiology. Glomus tumors are presumed to derive from the cells that line the canal of Sucquet-Hoyer. In the case of multiple glomangiomas, the derivation is obscure either because the cells of an arteriovenous anastomosis in a nonacral site could give rise to these lesions, or because they could derive from pluripotential cells in the walls of arterioles.

Diagnosis and Differential Diagnosis. A solitary painful red acral papule is likely to be a glomus tumor. Inasmuch as an excisional biopsy is curative, the diagnosis is almost always confirmed histologically. Eccrine spiradenoma shares a composition of small cuboidal cells with glomus tumors and is also painful. It features duc-

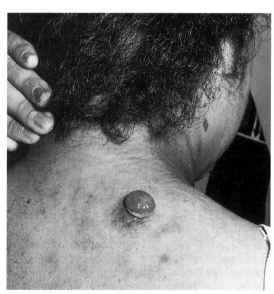

FIGURE 146–18. A glomangioma presenting as a glistening nodule.

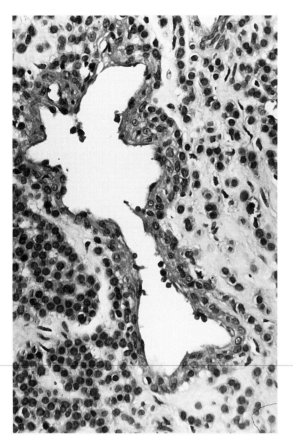

FIGURE 146–19. Glomus tumors feature compact aggregations of cells with small monomorphous round nuclei surrounding venules.

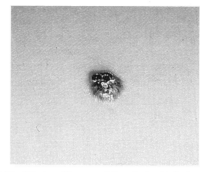

FIGURE 146–20. A solitary angiokeratoma is dark red and scaly.

tular differentiation, as well as pale and dark epithelial cells and infiltrates of lymphocytes.

Treatment. Excisional biopsy is usually curative. Multiple glomus tumors can also be surgically excised, but depending on the location, the resultant scars may be more disfiguring than the lesions themselves.

Angiokeratoma

Definition. The angiokeratomas are a group of benign vascular neoplasms in which marked dilated, thin-walled vessels are situated beneath a hyperplastic and hyperkeratotic epidermis.

Clinical Presentation. Each type of angiokeratoma has a characteristic clinical setting. In solitary angiokeratoma, there is a well-circumscribed dark red, scaly papule of at least 0.5 mm diameter, which is often found on the leg (Fig. 146–20).[181] Multiple lesions of similar appearance can sometimes occur. Thrombosis of the superficial vessels of an angiokeratoma cause the lesion to appear black, simulating melanoma. Angiokeratoma of Mibelli largely occurs as small multiple lesions on the skin of the dorsal toes (and sometimes fingers) in patients with cold intolerance and, sometimes, perniosis. Angiokeratoma of Fordyce affects scrotal or vulvar skin and, sometimes, that of the adjacent abdomen or thigh. This also features multiple lesions. Angiokeratoma corporis diffusum is a component of several metabolic diseases, including Fabry's disease (X-linked recessive α-galactosidase A de-

ficiency disease that results in ceramide trihexidose accumulation in several organs). Other storage diseases in which angiokeratoma corporis diffusum occurs are fucosidosis and β-galactosidase deficiency. In angiokeratoma corporis diffusum, many small papular angiokeratomas occur around the waist and at other sites. Angiokeratoma circumscriptum is a rare condition in which a solitary plaque composed of contiguous papular angiokeratomas occupies a large area of skin.

Pathology. Sections of all of the various angiokeratomas show a combination of thin-walled, ectatic vascular spaces that contain erythrocytes and epidermal hyperplasia with compact hyperkeratosis (Fig. 146–21). The vessels are often enclosed by pointed rete ridges, and such scant collagen bundles intervene between their walls that they sometimes appear to touch the undersurface of the epidermis. In the angiokeratomas of Mibelli and Fordyce, there are only a few vessels, so that a profile similar to that of a telangiectasis is present beneath a hyperkeratotic epidermis.

In addition to the features seen in other types of angiokeratomas, those associated with Fabry's disease have periodic acid–Schiff inclusions in endothelial cells. On frozen section, the granules are Sudan black positive and anisotropic when examined under polarized light. Elec-

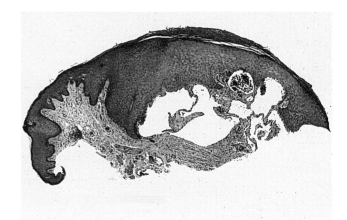

FIGURE 146–21. In all of the angiokeratomas, dilated thin-walled vessels with rounded shapes abut an irregularly hyperplastic and hyperkeratotic epidermis. In this solitary lesion, there are many vascular spaces; in the angiokeratomas of Mibelli and Fordyce, only a few telangiectatic spaces are present.

tron microscopy reveals that the inclusions have a lamellar internal structure.

Pathogenesis and Etiology. Angiokeratomas could conceivably result from elevated venular pressure in some settings. Angiokeratoma of Fordyce sometimes occurs above a varicocele, and correction of the aberrant vessel can lead to resolution of the lesion. In angiokeratoma corporis diffusum, metabolic deposits could cause vessel walls to weaken and dilate. The epidermal hyperplasia and hyperkeratosis common to angiokeratomas is likely a reaction to the growth of vessels near the epidermis; similar epidermal changes occur in verrucous hemangiomas, verrucous lesions of Cobb's syndrome, and in the central papular areas of targetoid hemosiderotic hemangiomas.

Diagnosis and Differential Diagnosis. The diagnosis of solitary angiokeratoma is usually made clinically, but confirmed by biopsy. Thrombosed angiokeratomas are often so dark in color that they are suspected of being melanoma. Angiokeratoma of Mibelli can sometimes be difficult to distinguish from cryoglobulinemia or perniosis, but its lesions are more sharply circumscribed. The epidermal changes of angiokeratoma histologically resemble those of verrucous hemangioma, a congenital lesion in which vessels are present throughout the thickness of the dermis.[182]

Treatment. Solitary angiokeratomas are cured by simple excision. Multiple angiokeratomas can be excised, frozen, electrodesiccated, or treated with lasers.

Cherry Hemangioma

Definition. Cherry hemangiomas are small bright red papules composed of ectatic vessels. They arise in middle age, are nearly always present in the elderly, and are also known as senile hemangiomas.

Clinical Presentation. Cherry hemangiomas are only a few millimeters in diameter, are bright red and smooth surfaced. They are most commonly found on the skin of the abdomen.

Pathology. A gently domed proliferation of vessels is present in the papillary dermis. Dilated, thin-walled vessels containing erythrocytes are present beneath thinning epidermis. These vessels have round contours and sometimes a hint of an epithelial collarette defining the lateral borders. The walls of some vessels in older lesions are surrounded by rims of sclerosis.

Diagnosis and Differential Diagnosis. Cherry hemangiomas are easily diagnosed clinically by their small size and distribution. Minute lesions can be confused with petechiae. Very few people have not seen such a lesion on the skin of another, usually a parent. Histologic examination is usually a consequence of their removal by shave technique rather than of a diagnostic biopsy.

Treatment. Lesions can be treated with shave excision, light electrocautery, cryotherapy, copper vapor laser, or pulsed-dye laser.

Targetoid Hemosiderotic Hemangioma

Definition. Targetoid hemosiderotic hemangiomas are solitary benign vascular neoplasms that feature a central papular component and a macular periphery.[183]

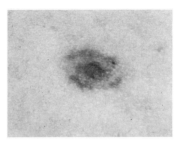

FIGURE 146-22. Targetoid hemosiderotic hemangioma is so called because an erythematous halo surrounds a central papule.

Clinical Presentation. These lesions are generally found on the skin of the trunk, sometimes at sites of trauma. The central papular area is often ringed by a zone of pallor, peripheral to which is another annulus that is purplish in hue. This ring expands and then fades, leaving the central papule (Fig. 146-22).

Pathology. The central papular areas of targetoid hemosiderotic hemangioma resemble angiokeratoma in many respects. There is often a small area of irregular epidermal hyperplasia and hyperkeratosis with closely apposed, dilated, thin-walled vessels. Protuberant endothelial cells bulge into the ectatic vascular spaces in a hobnail pattern. The periphery of targetoid hemosiderotic hemangiomas is flat, with angulated, thin-walled vessels interposed between reticular dermal collagen bundles. Siderophages and sparse lymphoid infiltrates are common constituents (Fig. 146-23).

Pathogenesis and Etiology. Although most consider this lesion a form of hemangioma, others believe that they are traumatized hemangiomas, which could explain the presence of hemosiderin. Venular pressure, either due to the structure of the lesion or its traumatic disruption might account for the angiokeratoma-like central papular area.

Diagnosis and Differential Diagnosis. Although the diagnosis can be made clinically, so few clinicians are familiar with the condition that it is usually only diagnosed on biopsy. The presence of angulated thin-walled vessels between collagen bundles, siderophages, and di-

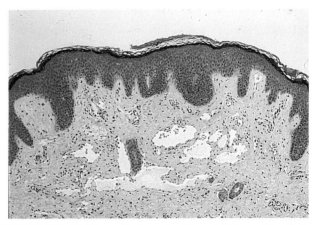

FIGURE 146-23. The central papule of targetoid hemosiderotic hemangioma resembles an angiokeratoma because ectatic vessels nearly abut the epidermis. Thin-walled angulated vessels are present between dermal collagen bundles at the periphery of the lesion.

lated vascular spaces that surround preexistent structures (the promontory sign) raises the possibility of Kaposi's sarcoma. Unlike Kaposi's sarcoma, however, targetoid hemosiderotic hemangioma does not follow the courses of preexistent vessels and almost always lacks plasma cells.

Treatment. The diagnosis is almost always made on biopsy. If the central portion of the lesion is removed, the procedure is curative.

Miscellaneous Hemangiomas

Other distinctive hemangiomas include *microvenular hemangioma,* in which short, straight vessels invested by pericytes form a meshwork between collagen bundles. Because of this infiltrative pattern, the proliferation can be mistaken for Kaposi's sarcoma.[184] In *glomeruloid hemangioma,* small round knots of vessels cause red papules in patients with the POEMS syndrome (polyneuropathy, organomegaly, endocrinopathy, monoclonal paraproteinemia, and skin findings, including sclerodermoid areas) as well as glomeruloid and other types of hemangiomas. Droplets of protein within the cytoplasms of the endothelial cells of the "glomerulus" are a hallmark of the condition.[185] *Sinusoidal hemangioma* causes small red papules and consists of a well-circumscribed collagenous mass containing markedly ectatic thin-walled vessels. Many such lesions have incorrectly been termed *cavernous hemangiomas* by pathologists.[186] True cavernous hemangiomas are far larger and deeper than sinusoidal hemangiomas. *Multinucleate cell angiohistiocytoma* causes tan to red papules on the dorsal hands and feet. Small thin-walled vessels are present in both the superficial and deep dermis, and multinucleated stellate mesenchymal cells are present between the intervening collagen bundles.[187]

Angiosarcoma and Its Variants

Definition. Angiosarcoma is a malignant neoplasm whose cells differentiate toward blood, vascular, or lymphatic endothelium. The traditionally recognized forms of angiosarcoma are highly malignant. The recently recognized conditions termed *epithelioid hemangioendothelioma, retiform hemangioendothelioma,* and the *Dabska tumor* appear to be low-grade forms of angiosarcoma. As indicated above, some also believe that spindle cell hemangioendothelioma belongs in this group.

Clinical Presentation. Classic angiosarcoma of the skin occurs in only a few settings, such as the scalp and face of elderly patients, lymphedematous limbs, and skin that has been irradiated. Angiosarcoma of the head of elderly patients presents as an ill-defined bruise-like patch, usually involving the central or upper face, the scalp, or both.[188] Over time, plaques develop, and blue or purplish nodules emerge (Fig. 146–24). In some angiosarcomas, vesicular areas that can contain blood develop. The best known presentation of angiosarcoma due to lymphedema is the Stewart-Treves syndrome, in which the disease develops in the arm of a patient who has undergone a mastectomy and axillary lymph node dis-

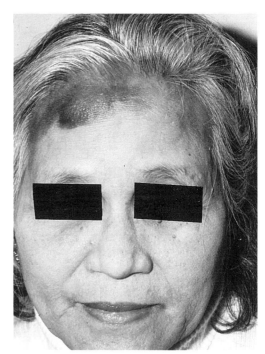

FIGURE 146–24. The face and scalp are frequently involved areas of angiosarcoma in elderly patients.

section for breast carcinoma.[189] Oddly, angiosarcoma can also occur following mastectomy in patients who did not have a node dissection, and in some patients who underwent lymph node dissection but did not have lymphedema. Lymphedema due to other causes such as Milroy's disease, venous stasis, or obesity can also predispose to angiosarcoma. Post-radiation angiosarcoma is rare, and generally follows irradiation by a decade or more.[190] The lower abdomen has been a common site. Far less common antecedents of angiosarcoma are benign vascular proliferations and ulcers.[191]

The classic forms of angiosarcoma grow relentlessly and almost always recur following resection because of their vague circumscription. They metastasize both to lymph nodes and to the lungs.

Several conditions are designated with the curious and misleading term *hemangioendothelioma.* Some of these appear to be low-grade angiosarcomas, whereas the status of others is controversial. *Epithelioid hemangioendothelioma* can be a primary cutaneous neoplasm or can spread to the skin from a source in the deep soft tissue or viscera.[178] The few reported primary cases have been deep dermal nodules with no particular localization. Whether this condition overlaps with epithelioid angiosarcoma has been debated.[192] The *Dabska tumor,* also termed *endovascular papillary angioendothelioma of childhood* or *Dabskoid angiosarcoma,* can present at birth or in the first decade of life as diffuse swelling or as a dermal mass.[193] Similar lesions in older patients have recently been described as *retiform hemangioendothelioma.*[194] *Spindle cell hemangioendothelioma* causes large, deep, well-circumscribed masses in the soft tissue and skin of the distal extremities. Some of the affected patients have had vascular anomalies such as congenital lymphedema, Maffucci's syndrome or the Klippel-Trenaunay syndrome. The advent of new lesions has implied metastasis to those who consider the condition a lowgrade form of angiosarcoma, but others believe that additional lesions are a consequence of multicentric disease.[195, 196]

Pathology. The classic forms of angiosarcoma have similar histologic features. In patches of angiosarcoma, jagged vessels lined by endothelial cells with large and often protuberant hyperchromatic nuclei infiltrate between reticular dermal collagen bundles. The lining of those vessels often forms small papillations that project into their lumina. Tangential sections of those papillations often create the illusion that the angiosarcoma cells are floating within the lumen (Fig. 146–25). Nodular lymphocytic infiltrates are often present both at the periphery of the neoplasm and within it. These can persist in later lesions.

Nodules or plaques of angiosarcoma have a more solid growth pattern. Either spindled or epithelioid cells can predominate. Erythrocytes are usually present in the slitlike interstices between these cells. Epithelioid areas often have cells with intracytoplasmic vacuoles, recapitulating the mode of luminal formation within solid cords of endothelial cells in embryonic vessels.

Epithelioid hemangioendothelioma features cords and strands of large polygonal or plump ovoid cells with copious cytoplasm and prominent intracytoplasmic vacuoles. The cords are disposed between thickened collagen bundles and myxoid stroma. Epithelioid angiosarcoma has similar cells without the distinctive stromal findings.

Dabska's tumor and retiform hemangioendothelioma both contain large angulated vascular spaces into which hobnail-shaped endothelial cells project. Spindled cells are present in between these spaces. Lymphocytes are intimately mixed with papillary structures that project into lumina in Dabska's tumor.

Spindle cell hemangioendotheliomas are marked by large cavernous vascular spaces, within which thrombi and phleboliths can occur. Septations that contain spindled endothelial cells and are lined by protuberant or epithelioid endothelial cells impart an alveolar appearance microscopically. Large intracytoplasmic vacuoles are often present within the bulging endothelial cells, which have been termed *blister cells* as a consequence.

Pathogenesis and Etiology. The cause of angiosarcoma in areas of lymphedematous skin may be impaired local immunity. Radiation clearly damages endothelial cells, which, along with fibroblasts, can have an abnormal cytologic appearance. The causes of other forms of cutaneous angiosarcoma are obscure.

Diagnosis and Differential Diagnosis. The diagnosis of angiosarcoma is often made clinically if the presentation is of one of its classic forms, and is confirmed by biopsy. The clinical differential diagnosis of a flat red patch on the face or scalp of an adult is broad, but if the lesion is of recent onset, angiosarcoma becomes more likely.

Histologic findings in patches of angiosarcoma can be difficult to distinguish from those of Kaposi's sarcoma because both feature small angulated vessels that infiltrate between collagen bundles. The degree of nuclear atypia is far greater in angiosarcoma than in Kaposi's sarcoma, and the cells of Kaposi's sarcoma practically never form intraluminal papillations. Early patches of Kaposi's sarcoma display increased cellularity around preexistent structures, whereas those of angiosarcoma do not. Kaposi's sarcoma is also the differential diagnosis of the spindled solid areas of angiosarcoma seen in nodules and plaques. Spindled nodules of Kaposi's sarcoma are often well circumscribed compared with those of angiosarcoma. Although sparse infiltrates of lymphocytes and plasma cells are frequent in Kaposi's sarcoma, lymphoid follicles are rare. Solid areas of epithelioid endothelial cells in angiosarcoma can be difficult to distinguish from melanoma, carcinoma, and other malignancies. Immunohistochemistry and electron microscopy can both be of help in this setting. The cells of angiosarcoma express a variety of endothelial antigens such as CD31, CD34, and factor VIII related antigen, and also express the L-fucose moiety present in all blood groups and recognized by Ulex europaeus lectin. Ultrastructural examination can reveal Weibel-Palade bodies, which contain factor VIII. In poorly differentiated lesions, there can be loss of one or more of these antigens. The broad immunophenotypic spectrum of angiosarcoma has blurred the traditional distinction between lesions with blood vascular and lymphatic differentiation.

Treatment. Early diagnosis and complete excision with wide and deep margins is the best approach to classic angiosarcoma, but unfortunately misdiagnoses and temporizing surgical measures prevent the salvage of many

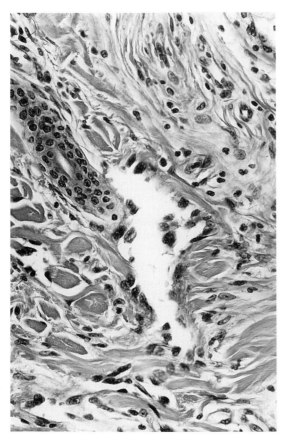

FIGURE 146–25. Papillations lined by endothelial cells with hyperchromatic nuclei are present in angiosarcoma.

patients. Locally recurrent disease has a grim prognosis, and ultimately, many face and scalp lesions become unresectable. Radiation therapy can be useful for extensive lesions.[188] The low-grade forms of angiosarcoma (or those reputed to be) are usually cured by complete excision, although metastases (or the emergence of multicentric lesions) can sometimes occur.

References

1. Sabin FR. On the origin of the cells of the blood. Physiol Rev 1922;2:38–69.
2. Phillips GD, Whitehead RA, Knighton DR. Initiation and pattern of angiogenesis in wound healing in the rat. Am J Anat 1991;192:257–262.
3. Barnhill RL, Wolf JE. Angiogenesis and the skin. J Am Acad Dermatol 1987;16:1226–1242.
4. Clark ER, Clark EL. Microscopic observations on the growth of blood capillaries in the living mammal. Am J Anat 1939;64:251–301.
5. Sato Y, Rifkin DB. Autocrine activities of basic fibroblast growth factor: Regulation of endothelial cell movement, plasminogen activator synthesis, and DNA synthesis. J Cell Biol 1988;107:1199–1205.
6. Saksela O, Moscatelli D, Rifkin DB. The opposing effects of basic fibroblast growth factor and transforming growth factor beta on the regulation of plasminogen activator activity in capillary endothelial cells. J Cell Biol 1987;105:957–963.
7. Sholley MM, Ferguson GP, Seibel HR, et al. Mechanisms of neovascularization: Vascular sprouting can occur without proliferation of endothelial cells. Lab Invest 1984;51:624.
8. Folkman J. The role of angiogenesis in tumor growth. Semin Cancer Biol 1992;3:65–71.
9. Folkman J, Shing Y. Angiogenesis. J Biol Chem 1992;267:10931–10934.
10. Folkman J. Angiogenesis: Initiation and control. In: Fishman AP, ed. Endothelium. New York: New York Academy of Sciences, 1982:212–227.
11. Ferrara NJ, Winer T, Burtin A, et al. Expression of vascular endothelial growth factor does not promote transformation but confers a growth advantage in vivo to Chinese hamster ovary cells. J Clin Invest 1993;91:160–170.
12. Malhotra R, Stenn KS, Fernandez LA, et al. Angiogenic properties of normal and psoriatic skin associated with epidermis, not dermis. Lab Invest 1989;61:162–165.
13. Ono M, Okamura K, Nakayama Y, et al. Induction of human microvascular endothelial tubular morphogenesis by human keratinocytes: Involvement of transforming growth factor-alpha. Biochem Biophys Res Commun 1992;189:601–609.
14. Kubota Y, Kleinman H, Marin GR, et al. Role of laminin and basement membrane in the differentiation of human endothelial cells into capillary-like structures. J Cell Biol 1988;107:1589.
15. Vernon RB, Angello JC, Arispe MLI, et al. Reorganization of basement membrane matrices by cellular traction promotes the formation of cellular networks in vitro. Lab Invest 1992;66:536–547.
16. Montesano R. 1992 Mack Forster Award Lecture. Review. Regulation of angiogenesis in vitro. Eur J Clin Invest 1992;22:504–515.
17. Montesano R, Vassalli JD, Baird A, et al. Basic fibroblast growth factor induces angiogenesis in vitro. Proc Natl Acad Sci USA 1986;83:7297–7301.
18. Gospodarowicz D, Neufeld G, Schweigerer L. Molecular and biological characterization of fibroblast growth factor, an angiogenetic factor which also controls proliferation and differentiation of mesoderm and neuroectoderm derived cells. Cell Diff 1986;19:1–17.
19. Bovi PD, Basilico C. Isolation of a rearranged human transforming gene following transfection of Kaposi sarcoma DNA. Proc Nat Acad Sci USA 1987;84:5660–5664.
20. Dickson C, Peters G. Potential oncogene product related to growth factors. Nature 1987;326:833.
21. McNeil PL, Muthukrishnan L, Warder E, et al. Growth factors are released by mechanically wounded endothelial cells. J Cell Biol 1989;109:811–822.
22. Hannan RL, Kourembanas S, Flanders KC, et al. Endothelial cells synthesize basic fibroblast growth factor and transforming growth factor beta. Growth Factors 1988;1:7–17.
23. Tsuboi R, Sato Y, Rifkin DB. Correlation of cell migration, cell invasion, receptor number, proteinase production, and basic fibroblast growth factor levels in endothelial cells. J Cell Biol 1990;110:511–517.
24. Mignatti P, Rifkin DB. Release of basic fibroblast growth factor, an angiogenic factor devoid of secretory signal sequence: A trivial phenomenon or a novel secretion mechanism? J Cell Biochem 1991;47:201–207.
25. Klagsbrun M. Mediators of angiogenesis: The biological significance of basic fibroblast growth factor (bFGF)-heparin and heparan sulfate interactions. Semin Cancer Biol 1992;3:81–87.
26. Folkman J. Shing Y. Control of angiogenesis by heparin and other sulfated polysaccharides. Adv Exp Med Biol 1992;313:355–364.
27. Daviet I, Herbert JM, Maffrand JP. Involvement of protein kinase C in the mitogenic and chemotaxis effects of basic fibroblast growth factor on bovine cerebral cortex capillary endothelial cells. FEBS Lett 1990;259:315–317.
28. Stokes CL, Rupnick MA, Williams SK, et al. Chemotaxis of human microvessel endothelial cells in response to acidic fibroblast growth factor. Lab Invest 1990;63:657–668.
29. Mignatti P, Tsuboi R, Robbins E, et al. In vitro angiogenesis on the human amniotic membrane: Requirements for basic fibroblast growth factor-induced proteinases. J Cell Biol 1989;108:671–682.
30. Swerlick RA, Brown EJ, Xu Y, et al. Expression and modulation of the vitronectin receptor on human dermal microvascular endothelial cells. J Invest Dermatol 1993;99:715–722.
31. Enenstein J, Waleh NS, Kramer RH. Basic FGF and TGF-beta differentially module integrin expression of human microvascular endothelial cells. Exp Cell Res 1992;203:499–503.
32. Montesano R, Orci L. Tumor promoting phorbol esters induce angiogenesis in vitro. Cell 1985;40:469–477.
33. Ferrara N, Houck KA, Jakeman LB, et al. The vascular endothelial growth factor family of polypeptides. J Cell Biochem 1991;47:211–218.
34. Brown LF, Yeo KT, Berse B, et al. Expression of vascular permeability factor (vascular endothelial growth factor) by epidermal keratinocytes during wound healing. J Exp Med 1992;176:1375–1379.
35. Keck PJ, Hauser SD, Krivi G, et al. Vascular permeability factor, an endothelial cell mitogen related to PDGF. Science 1989;246:1309–1312.
36. Dvorak HF, Sioussat TM, Brown LF, et al. Distribution of vascular permeability factor (vascular endothelial growth factor) in tumors: Concentration in tumor blood vessels. J Exp Med 1991;174:1275–1278.
37. Heldin CH, Usuki K, Miyazono K. Platelet-derived endothelial cell growth factor. J Cell Biochem 1991;47:208–210.
38. Miyazono K, Usuki K, Heldin CH. Platelet-derived endothelial cell growth factor. Prog Growth Factor Res 1991;3:207–217.
39. Lee FS, Vallee BL. Structure and action of mammalian ribonuclease (angiogenin) inhibitor. Prog Nucleic Acid Res Mol Biol 1993;44:1–30.
40. Hockel M, Jung W, Vaupel P, et al. Purified monocyte-derived angiogenic substance (angiotropin) induces controlled angiogenesis associated with regulated tissue proliferation in rabbit skin. J Clin Invest 1988;82:1075–1090.
41. Hockel M. Sasse J, Wissler HJ. Purified monocyte-derived antiogenic substance (angiotropin) stimulates migration, phenotypic changes, and "tube formation" but not proliferation of capillary endothelial cells in vitro. J Cell Physiol 1987;133:1–13.
42. Schreiber AB, Winkler ME, Dernyck R. Transforming growth factor alpha: A more potent angiogenic factor than epidermal growth factor. Science 1986;232:1250–1253.
43. Roberts AB, Sporn MB, Assoian RK, et al. Transforming growth factor type beta: Rapid induction of fibrosis and angiogenesis in vivo and stimulation of collagen formation in vivo. Proc Natl Acad Sci USA 1986;83:4167–4171.

44. Baird A, Durkin T. Inhibition of endothelial cell proliferation by type beta-transforming growth factor: Interactions with acidic and basic fibroblast growth factors. Biochem Biophys Res Commun 1986;138:476–482.

45. Muller G, Behrens J. Nussbaumer U, et al. Inhibitory action of transforming growth factor beta on endothelial cells. Proc Natl Acad Sci USA 1987;84:5600–5604.

46. Falcone DJ, McCaffrey TA, Friedman AH, et al. Transforming growth factor-beta 1 stimulates macrophage urokinase expression and release of matrix-bound basic fibroblast growth factor. J Cell Physiol 1993;155:595–605.

47. Pepper MS, Vassalli JD, Orci L, et al. Biphasic effect of transforming growth factor-beta 1 on in vitro angiogenesis. Exp Cell Res 1993;204:356–363.

48. Fajardo LF, Kwan HH, Kowalski J, et al. Dual role of tumor necrosis factor-alpha in angiogenesis. Am J Pathol 1992; 140:539–544.

49. Frater-Schroder M, Risau W, Hallman R, et al. Tumor necrosis factor alpha, a potent inhibitor of endothelial cell growth in vitro, is angiogenic in vivo. Proc Natl Acad Sci USA 1987;84:5277–5281.

50. Strieter RM, Kunkel SL, Elner VM, et al. Interleukin-8. A corneal factor that induces neovascularization. Am J Pathol 1992;141:1279–1284.

51. Koch AE, Polverini PJ, Kunkel SL, et al. Interleukin-8 as macrophage-derived mediator of angiogenesis. Science 1992;258: 1798–1801.

52. Folkman J, Brem H. Angiogenesis and inflammation. In: Gallin JI, Goldstein IM, Snyderman R, eds. Inflammation: Basic Principles and Clinical Correlates. New York: Raven Press, 1992:821–839.

53. Tamrgo RJ, Bok RA, Brem H. Angiogenesis inhibition by minocycline. Cancer Res 1991;51:672–675.

54. Greenwald RA, Golub LM, Lavietes B, et al. Tetracyclines inhibit human synovial collagenase in vivo and in vitro. J Rheumatol 1987;14:28–32.

55. Maione TE, Gray GS, Petro J, et al. Inhibition of angiogenesis by recombinant platelet factor 4 and related peptides. Science 1990;247:77–79.

56. Mosher DF. Physiology of thrombospondin. Annu Rev Med 1990;41:85–97.

57. Fotsis TM, Peper H, Adlercreutz G, et al. Genistein, a dietary-derived inhibitor of in vitro angiogenesis. Proc Natl Acad Sci USA 1993;90:2690–2694.

58. Ingber D, Fujita T, Kishimoto S, et al. Synthetic analogues of fumagillin that inhibit angiogenesis and suppress tumour growth. Nature 1990;348:555–557.

59. Matsubara T, Saura R, Hirohata K, et al. Inhibition of human endothelial cell proliferation in vitro and neovascularization in vivo by D-penicillamine. J Clin Invest 1989;83:158–167.

60. Hirata S, Matsubara T, Saura R, et al. Inhibition of in vitro vascular endothelial cell proliferation and in vivo neovascularization by low-dose methotrexate. Arthritis Rheum 1989;32: 1065–1073.

61. Koch AE, Burrows JC, Polverini PJ, et al. Thiol-containing compounds inhibit the production of monocyte/macrophage-derived angiogenic activity. Agents Actions 1991;34:350–357.

62. Mulliken JB, Glowacki J. Hemangiomas and vascular malformations in infants and children: A classification based on endothelial characteristics. Plast Reconstr Surg 1982;69:412–420.

63. Finn MC, Glowacki J, Mulliken JB. Congenital vascular lesions: Clinical application of a new classification. J Pediatr Surg 1983;18:894–900.

64. Moroz B. Long-term follow-up of hemangiomas in children. In: Williams HB, ed. Symposium on Vascular Malformations and Melanotic Lesions. St. Louis: CV Mosby, 1983:162–171.

65. Grabb WC, Dingman R, Oneal RM, et al. Facial hamartomas in children: Neurofibroma, lymphangioma, and hemangioma. Plast Reconst Surg 1980;66:509–527.

66. Hidano A, Nakajima S. Earliest features of the strawberry mark in the newborn. Br J Dermatol 1972;87:138–144.

67. Amir J, Metsker A, Krikler R, et al. Strawberry hemangioma in preterm infants. Pediatr Dermatol 1986;3:331–332.

68. Simpson JR. Natural history of cavernous haemangiomata. Lancet 1959;2:1057–1059.

69. Nakayama H. Clinical and histological studies of the classification and the natural course of the strawberry mark. J Dermatol 1981;8:277–291.

70. Esterly NB. Cutaneous hemangiomas, vascular stains, and associated syndromes. Curr Probl Pediatr 1987;17:1–69.

71. Bowers RE, Graham EA, Tomlinson KM. The natural history of the strawberry nevus. Arch Dermatol 1960;82:667–679.

72. Enjolras O, Mulliken JB. The current management of vascular birthmarks. Pediatr Dermatol 1993;10:311–333.

73. Margileth AM, Museles M. Current concepts in diagnosis and management of congenital cutaneous hemangiomas. Pediatrics 1965;36:410–416.

74. Bilyk JR, Adamis AP, Mulliken JB. Treatment options for periorbital hemangioma of infancy. Int Ophthalmol Clin 1992; 32:95–109.

75. Goldberg NS, Rosanova MA. Periorbital hemangiomas. Dermatologic Clinics 1992;10:653–661.

76. Stigmar G, Crawford JS, Ward CM, et al. Ophthalmic sequelae of infantile hemangiomas of the eyelids and orbit. Am J Ophthalmol 1978;85:805–813.

77. Riding K. Subglottic hemangioma: A practical approach. J Otolaryngol 1992;21:419–421.

78. Rodriguez LR, DiMaio M, Kidron D, et al. Late presentation of a subglottic hemangioma masquerading as asthma. Clin Pediatr 1992;31:753–775.

79. Mulliken JB. Capillary (port-wine) and other telangiectatic stains. In: Mulliken JB, Young AE, et al, eds. Vascular Birthmarks—Hemangiomas and Malformations. Philadelphia: WB Saunders—Co., 1988:170–195.

80. Margileth AM. The management of disseminated eruptive hemangiomata in infants. Pediatr Dermatol 1984;1:312–317.

81. Martins AG. Hemangioma and thrombocytopenia. J Pediatr Surg 1970;5:641–648.

82. Lang PG, Dubin HV. Hemangioma-thrombocytopenia syndrome. Arch Dermatol 1975;111:105–107.

83. Shin WKT. Hemangiomas of infancy complicated by thrombocytopenia. Am J Surg 1968;116:896–906.

84. Goldberg NS, Hebert AA, Esterly NB. Sacral hemangiomas and multiple congenital abnormalities. Arch Dermatol 1986; 122:6847.

85. Burns AJ, Kaplan LC, Mulliken JB. Is there an association between hemangioma and syndromes with dysmorphic features? Pediatrics 1991;88:1257–1267.

86. Esterly NB. Hemangiomas in infants and children: Clinical observations. Pediatr Dermatol 1992;9:353–355.

87. Reese V, Frieden IJ, Ferriero D, et al. The association of facial hemangiomas with Dandy-Walker and other posterior fossa malformations. Pediatr Dermatol 1992;9:190.

88. Igarashi M, Uchida H, Kajii T. Supraumbilical midabdominal raphe and facial cavernous hemangiomas. Clin Genet 1985; 27:196–198.

89. Vaillant L, Lorette G, Chantepie A, et al. Multiple cutaneous hemangiomas and coarctation of the aorta with right aortic arch. Pediatrics 1988;81:707–709.

90. Hersh JH, Waterfill D, Rutledge J, et al. Sternal malformation/vascular dysplasia association. Am J Med Genet 1985; 21:177–186.

91. Lever WF. Tumors of vascular tissue. In: Lever WF, Schaumburg-Lever G, eds. Histopathology of the Skin, 7th edition. Philadelphia: JB Lippincott, 1990:689–721.

92. Mulliken JB. Pathogenesis of hemangiomas. In: Mulliken JB, Young AE, eds. Vascular Birthmarks—Hemangiomas and Malformations. Philadelphia: WB Saunders Co., 1988:63–76.

93. Glowacki J, Mulliken JB. Mast cells in hemangiomas and vascular malformations. Pediatrics 1982;70:48–51.

94. Folkman J, Langer R, Linhardt RJ, et al. Angiogenesis inhibition and tumor regression caused by heparin or a heparin fragment in the presence of cortisone. Science 1983;221: 719–725.

95. Sasaki GH, Pang CY, Wittliff JL. Pathogenesis and treatment of infant skin strawberry hemangiomas: Clinical and in vitro studies of hormonal effects. Plast Reconstr Surg 1984;73:359–370.

96. Saracco S, Abramowsky C, Taylor S, et al. Spontaneously regressing adrenocortical carcinoma in a newborn: A case report with DNA ploidy analysis. Cancer 1988;62:507–511.

97. Messenger GG, Kamei R, Honig PJ. Histiocytosis X resembling cherry angiomas. Pediatr Dermatol 1985;3:75–78.

98. Zukerberg LR, Nickoloff BJ, Weiss SW. Kaposiform hemangioendothelioma of infancy and childhood. An aggressive neoplasm associated with Kasabach-Merritt syndrome. Am J Surg Pathol 1993;17:321–328.

99. Garden JM, Bakus AD, Paller AS. Treatment of cutaneous hemangiomas by the flashlamp-pumped pulsed dye laser: Prospective analysis. J Pediatr 1992;120:550–560.

100. Morelli J. Tan OT, West WL. Treatment of ulcerated hemangiomas with pulsed tunable dye laser. Am J Dis Child 1991;145:1062–1064.

101. Ashinoff R, Geronemus RG. Capillary hemangiomas and treatment with the flashlamp-pumped dye laser. Arch Dermatol 1991;127:202–205.

102. Sherwood KA, Tan OT. The treatment of capillary hemangioma with the flashlamp-pumped dye laser. J Am Acad Dermatol 1990;22:136–137.

103. Enjolras O, Riche MC, Merland JJ, et al. Management of alarming hemangiomas in infancy: A review of 25 cases. Pediatrics 1990;85:491–498.

104. Kushner BJ. The treatment of periorbital infantile hemangioma with intralesional corticosteroid. Plast Reconstr Surg 1985;76:517–524.

105. Ezekowitz RAB, Mulliken JB, Folkman J. Interferon alfa-2a therapy for life-threatening hemangiomas. N Engl J Med 1992;326:1456–1463.

106. White CW. Treatment of hemangiomatosis with recombinant interferon alfa. Semin Hematol 1990;27:15–22.

107. Jacobs AH, Walton RG. The incidence of birthmarks in the neonate. Pediatrics 1976;58:218–222.

108. Pratt AG. Birthmarks in infants. Arch Dermatol 1953;67:302–305.

109. Williams HB. Hemangiomas and lymphangiomas. Adv Surg 1981;13:317–349.

110. Enjolras O, Riche MC, Merland JJ. Facial port-wine stains and Sturge-Weber syndrome. Pediatrics 1985;76:48–51.

111. Barsky SH, Rosen S, Geer D, et al. The nature and evolution of port wine stains: A computer assisted study. J Invest Dermatol 1980;74:1543–1575.

112. Tallman B, Tan OT, Morelli JG, et al. Location of port-wine stains and the likelihood of ophthalmic and/or central nervous system complications. Pediatrics 1991;87:323–327.

113. Swerlick RA, Cooper PH. Pyogenic granuloma (lobular capillary hemangioma) within port-wine stains. J Am Acad Dermatol 1983;8:627–630.

114. Finley JL, Noe JM, Arndt KA, et al. Port-wine stains—morphologic variations and developmental lesions. Arch Dermatol 1984;120:1453–1455.

115. Smoller BR, Rosen S. Port-wine stains—a disease of altered neural modulation of blood vessels? Arch Dermatol 1986;122:177–179.

116. Young AE. Pathogenesis of vascular malformations. In: Mulliken JB, Young AE, eds. Vascular Birthmarks—Hemangiomas and Malformations. Philadelphia: WB Saunders Co., 1988:107–113.

117. McDaniel DH, Mordon S. Hexascan: A new robotic scanning laser handpiece. Cutis 1990;45:300–305.

118. Tan O, Stafford TJ, Murray S, et al. Histologic comparison of the pulsed dye laser and copper vapor laser effects on pig skin. Lasers Surg Med 1990;10:551–558.

119. Neumann RA, Knobler RM, Leonhartsberger H, et al. Comparative histochemistry of port-wine stains after copper vapor laser (578 nm) and argon laser treatment. J Invest Dermatol 1992;99:160–167.

120. Pickering JW, Walker RHB, Halewy CN. Copper vapor laser treatment of port-wine stains and other vascular malformations. Br J Plast Surg 1990;43:273–282.

121. Waner M, Dinehart SM. Comparison of the copper vapor and flashlamp-pumped pulsed dye laser in the treatment of facial telangiectases. J Dermatol Surg Oncol 1993;19:370–376.

122. Scheibner A, Wheeland RG. Argon-pumped tunable dye laser therapy for facial port-wine stain hemangiomas in adults—a new technique using small spot size and minimal power. J Dermatol Surg Oncol 1989;15:277–289.

123. Riche MC, Merland JJ. Embolization of vascular birthmarks. In: Mulliken JB, Young AE, eds. Vascular Birthmarks—Hemangiomas and Malformations. Philadelphia: WB Saunders Co., 1988:436–453.

124. Lanigan SW, Cotterill JA. Psychological disabilities amongst patients with port-wine stains. Br J Dermatol 1989;121:209–215.

125. Silverman RA. Hemangiomas and vascular malformations. Pediatr Clin North Am 1991;38:811–833.

126. Leung AKC, Telmesani AMA. Salmon patches in Caucasian children. Pediatr Dermatol 1989;6:185–187.

127. Smith MA, Manfield PA. The natural history of salmon patches in the first year of life. Br J Dermatol 1962;73:31–33.

128. Tan KL. Nevus flammeus of the nape, glabella and eyelids—a clinical study of frequency, racial distribution, and association with congenital anomalies. Clin Pediatr 1972;11:112–118.

129. Pasyk KA, Wlodarczyk SR, Jakobczak MM, et al. Familial medial telangiectatic nevus: Variant of nevus flammeus—port-wine stain. Plast Reconstr Surg 1993;91:1032–1041.

130. Picascia DD, Esterly NB. Cutis marmorata telangiectatica congenita: Report of 22 cases. J Am Acad Dermatol 1989;20:1098–1104.

131. Rogers M, Poyzer KG, Shenkman L. Cutis marmorata telangiectatica congenita. Arch Dermatol 1982;118:895–899.

132. Young AE. Arteriovenous malformations. In: Mulliken JB, Young AE, eds. Vascular Birthmarks—Hemangiomas and Malformations. Philadelphia: WB Saunders Co., 1988:228–245.

133. Wheeland RG, Bailin PL, Kronberg E. Carbon dioxide (CO_2) laser vaporization for the treatment of multiple trichoepithelioma. J Dermatol Surg Oncol 1984;10:470–475.

134. Young AE. Combined vascular lesions. In: Mulliken JB, Young AE, eds. Vascular Birthmarks—Hemangiomas and Malformations. Philadelphia: WB Saunders Co., 1988:246–274.

135. Gloviczki P, Hollier LH, Telander RL, et al. Surgical implications of Klippel-Trenaunay syndrome. Ann Surg 1983;197:353–362.

136. Sullivan TJ, Clarke MP, Morin JD. The ocular manifestations of the Sturge-Weber syndrome. J Pediatr Ophthalmol Strabismus 1992;29:349–356.

137. Gomez MR, Bebin EM. Sturge-Weber syndrome. In: Gomez MR, ed. Neurocutaneous Diseases: A Practical Approach. Boston: Butterworths, 1987:356–367.

138. Bein EM, Gomez MR. Prognosis in Sturge-Weber disease: Comparison of unihemispheric and bihemispheric involvement. J Child Neurol 1988;3:181–184.

139. Font RL, Ferry AP. The phakomatoses. Int Ophthalmol Clin 1972;12:1–50.

140. Witschel H, Font RL. Hemangioma of the choroid: A clinicopathologic study of 71 cases and a review of the literature. Surv Ophthalmol 1976;20:415–431.

141. Miller SJH. Ophthalmic aspects of the Sturge-Weber syndrome. Proc R Soc Med 1963;56:419–421.

142. Greenwald MJ, Weiss A. Ocular manifestations of the neurocutaneous syndromes. Pediatr Dermatol 1984;2:98–117.

143. Chamberlain MC, Press GA, Hesselink JR. MR imaging and CT in three cases of Sturge-Weber syndrome: Prospective comparison. AJNR 1989;10:491–496.

144. Hasegawa Y, Yasuhara M. Phakomatosis pigmentovascularis type IVa. Arch Dermatol 1985;121:651–655.

145. Horio T, Ogawa M. Pigmentovascular nevus. Arch Dermatol 1973;107:463–464.

146. Gallo SH, McClave SA. Blue rubber bleb nevus syndrome: Gastrointestinal involvement and its endoscopic presentation. Gastrointestinal Endoscopy 1992;38:72–76.

147. Morris L, Lynch PM, Gleason WA, et al. Blue rubber bleb nevus syndrome: Laser photocoagulation of colonic hemangiomas in a child with microcytic anemia. Pediatr Dermatol 1992;9:91–94.

148. Rice JS, Fischer DS. Blue rubber-bleb nevus syndrome. Arch Dermatol 1962;86:503–511.

149. Ross J, Schinella R. Massive osteolysis. Am J Med 1978;65:367–372.

150. Pedicelli G, Mattia P, Zorzoli AA, et al. Gorham's syndrome. JAMA 1984;252:1449–1451.

151. Fornasier VL. Hemangiomatosis with massive osteolysis. J Bone Joint Surg 1970;52:444–451.

152. Mendez AA, Keret D, Robertson W, et al. Massive osteolysis of the femur (Gorham's disease): A case report and review of the literature. J Pediatr Orthop 1989;9:604–608.

153. Lewis RJ, Ketcham A. Maffucci's syndrome, functional and neoplastic significance, case report and review of the literature. J Bone Joint Surg 1973;55:1465–1479.

154. Elmore SM, Cantrell WC. Maffucci's syndrome: Case report with a normal karyotype. J Bone Joint Surg 1966;48:1607–1613.

155. Johnson TE, Nasr AM, Nalbandian RM, et al. Enchondromatosis and hemangioma (Maffucci's syndrome) with orbital involvement. Am J Ophthalmol 1990;110:153–159.

156. Clark RD, Donnai D, Rogers J, et al. Proteus syndrome: An expanded phenotype. Am J Med Genet 1987;27:99–117.

157. Berg BO. Unusual neurocutaneous syndromes. Neurol Clin 1985;3:165–178.

158. Riley HD, Smith WR. Macrocephaly, pseudopapilloedema and multiple hemangiomata: A previously undescribed heredofamilial syndrome. Pediatrics 1960;26:293–300.

159. Klein JA, Barr RJ. Bannayan-Zonana syndrome associated with lymphangiomyomatous lesions. Pediatr Dermatol 1990;7:48–53.

160. Jessen RT, Thompson S, Smith EB. Cobb syndrome. Arch Dermatol 1977;113:1587–1590.

161. Kissel P, Dureux JB. Cobb syndrome: Cutaneomeningospinal angiomatosis. In: Bruyn GW, Vinken PJ, eds. Handbook of Clinical Neurology, vol. 14. New York: North Holland, 1972:429–445.

162. Gordon-Firing S, Purriel JA, Pereyra D, et al. Aporte de un neuvo caso de sindrome de Cobb: Angiomatosis cutaneomeningoespinal. Acta Neurol Latinoam 1981;27:99–111.

163. Doppman JL, Wirth FP, DiChiro G, et al. Value of cutaneous angiomas in the arteriographic localization of spinal-cord arteriovenous malformations. N Engl J Med 1969;281:1440–1446.

164. Hashimoto H, Daimaru Y, Enjoji E. Intravascular papillary endothelial hyperplasia. A clinicopathologic study of 91 cases. Am J Surg Pathol 1983;5:539–546.

165. Strutton G, Weedon D. Acro-angiodermatitis. A simulant of Kaposi's sarcoma. Am J Dermatopathol 1987;9:85–89.

166. Wick MR, Rocamora A. Reactive and malignant "angioendotheliomatosis." A discriminant clinicopathologic study. J Cutan Pathol 1988;15:260–271.

167. LeBoit PE, Solomon AR, Santa Cruz DJ, Wick MR. Angiomatosis with luminal cryoprotein deposition. J Am Acad Dermatol 1992;27:969–973.

168. Mills SE, Cooper PH, Fechner RE. Lobular capillary hemangioma. The underlying lesion of pyogenic granuloma. A study of 73 cases from the oral and nasal mucous membranes. Am J Surg Pathol 1980;4:471–479.

169. LeBoit PE. Lobular capillary proliferation. The underlying process in diverse benign cutaneous vascular neoplasms and reactive conditions. Semin Dermatol 1989;8:298:310.

170. Wilson Jones E, Orkin M. Tufted angioma (angioblastoma). A benign progressive angioma, not to be confused with Kaposi's sarcoma or low-grade angiosarcoma. J Am Acad Dermatol 1989;20:214–225.

170a. Warner J, Jones EW. Pyogenic granuloma recurring with multiple satellites: A report of 11 cases. Br J Dermatol 1968;80:218–227.

170b. Patrice SJ, Wiss K, Mulliken JB. Pyogenic granuloma (lobular capillary hemangioma): A clinicopathologic study of 178 cases. Pediatr Dermatol 1991;8:267–276.

170c. Bernstein EF, Kantor G, Howe N, et al. Tufted angioma of the thigh. J Am Acad Dermatol 1994;31:307–311.

171. Kimura S. Ultrastructure of so-called angioblastoma of the skin before and after soft x-ray therapy. Jpn J Dermatol 1981;8:235–243.

172. Conelly MG, Winkelmann RK. Acral arteriovenous tumor. A clinicopathologic review. Am J Surg Pathol 1985;9:15–21.

173. Olsen TG, Helwig EB. Angiolymphoid hyperplasia of the skin. A clinicopathologic study of 116 cases. J Am Acad Dermatol 1985;12:781–796.

174. Wilson Jones E, Marks R. Papular angioplasia. Vascular papules of the face and scalp simulating malignant vascular tumors. Arch Dermatol 1970;102:422–427.

175. Fernandez LA, Olsen TG, Barwick KW, et al. Renin in angiolymphoid hyperplasia with eosinophilia. Its possible effect on vascular proliferation. Arch Pathol Lab Med 1986;110:1131–1135.

176. Moy RL, Luftman DB, Nguyen QH, Amenta JS. Estrogen receptors and the response to sex hormones in angiolymphoid hyperplasia with eosinophilia. Arch Dermatol 1992;128:825–828.

177. Kuo T-T, Shih L-H, Chan H-L. Kimura's disease. Involvement of regional lymph nodes and distinction from angiolymphoid hyperplasia with eosinophilia. Am J Surg Pathol 1988;12:843–854.

178. Resnik KS, Kantor GR, Spielvogel RL, Ryan E. Cutaneous epithelioid hemangioendothelioma without systemic involvement. Am J Dermatopathol 1993;15:272–276.

179. Massa MC, Fretzin DF, Chowdhury L, Sweet DL. Angiolymphoid hyperplasia demonstrating extensive skin and mucosal lesions controlled after vinblastine therapy. J Am Acad Dermatol 1984;11:333–339.

180. Cooper PH. Vascular tumors. In: Farmer ER, Hood AF, ed. Pathology of the skin, 1st edition. East Norwalk, CT: Appleton & Lange, 1990:827–829.

181. Imperial R, Helwig EB. Angiokeratoma. A clinicopathological study. Arch Dermatol 1967;95:166–175.

182. Rossi A, Bozzi M, Barra E. Verrucous hemangioma and angiokeratoma circumscriptum. Clinical and histopathologic differential characteristics. J Dermat Surg Oncol 1989;15:88–91.

183. Santa Cruz DJ, Aronberg J. Targetoid hemosiderotic hemangioma. J Am Acad Dermatol 1988;19:550–558.

184. Hunt SJ, Santa Cruz DJ, Barr RJ. Microvenular hemangioma. J Cutan Pathol 1991;18:235–240.

185. Chan JKC, Fletcher CDM, Hicklin GA, Rosai J. Glomeruloid hemangioma. A distinctive cutaneous lesion of multicentric Castleman's disease associated with POEMS syndrome. Am J Surg Pathol 1990;14:1036–1046.

186. Calonje E, Fletcher CDM. Sinusoidal hemangioma. A distinctive benign vascular neoplasm within the group of cavernous hemangiomas. Am J Surg Pathol 1991;15:1130–1135.

187. Wilson Jones E, Cerio R, Smith NP. Multinucleate cell angiohistiocytoma. An acquired vascular anomaly to be distinguished from Kaposi's sarcoma. Br J Dermatol 1990;122:651–663.

188. Holden CA, Spittle MF, Wilson Jones E. Angiosarcoma of the face and scalp, prognosis and treatment. Cancer 1987;59:1046–1057.

189. Cooper PH. Angiosarcomas of the skin. Semin Diagn Pathol 1987;4:2–17.

190. Goette DK, Detlefs RL. Postirradiation angiosarcoma. J Am Acad Dermatol 1985;12:922–926.

191. Cooper PH. Angiosarcomas of the skin. Semin Diagn Pathol 1987;4:2–17.

192. Marrogi AJ, Hunt SJ, Santa Cruz DJ. Cutaneous epithelioid angiosarcoma. Am J Dermatopathol 1990;12:350–356.

193. Manivel JC, Wick MR, Swanson PE, et al. Endovascular papillary angioendothelioma of childhood. A vascular leison characterized by "high" endothelial cell differentiation. Hum Pathol 1986;177:1240–1244.

194. Calonje E, Fletcher CDM, Wilson Jones E, Rosai J. Retiform hemangioendothelioma. A distinctive form of low-grade angiosarcoma delineated in a series of 15 cases. Am J Surg Pathol 1994;18:115–125.

195. Scott GA, Rosai J. Spindle cell hemangioendothelioma. Report of seven additional cases of a recently described vascular neoplasm. Am J Dermatopathol 1988;10:281–288.

196. Calonje E, Fletcher CDM. Sinusoidal hemangioma. A distinctive benign vascular neoplasm within the group of cavernous hemangiomas. Am J Surg Pathol 1991;15:1130–1135.

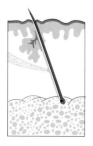

Neoplasms of Muscle and Fat, Liposuction Surgery of Fat Hypertrophy

JAMES E. FITZPATRICK and WILLIAM P. COLEMAN, III

The usually solitary, subcutaneous, well-circumscribed nodular lesions of this group of tumors may be difficult to clinically distinguish from one another and from scars or keloids. Most smooth and striated muscle tumors require biopsy to identify the muscular or fat origin.

TUMORS OF MUSCLE

Leiomyoma

Clinical Description. Cutaneous leiomyoma may present in a group of pinhead to pea-sized firm nodules that are relatively superficial in the skin of the back, face, or extensor surfaces of the extremities. These grouped lesions may aggregate in linear or arciform patterns or coalesce into plaques. Solitary subcutaneous leiomyomas vary in size from pea sized to walnut sized and are especially prevalent on the extensor surfaces of the lower extremities, scrotum, labia majora, and nipples. Pain may be a prominent symptom in patients with larger lesions.

Pathology. Scanning magnification of pilar leiomyomas demonstrates a reticular dermal tumor associated with a normal or attenuated epidermis (Fig. 147–1). In some cases, the tumor may be adjacent to or surround a hair follicle. The tumor fascicles are distinct from the surrounding connective tissue, but the tumor is not encapsulated and individual fascicles may be separated from the main body of the tumor by collagen. Fascicles that have been cut on end will characteristically demonstrate round nuclei with perinuclear vacuoles. At high power, longitudinally oriented fascicles are composed of rather straight spindle-shaped cells that demonstrate fusiform, rounded, or blunt ends (Fig. 147–1, *inset*). Nuclei with blunt ends are the most distinctive and have been described as being "eel-like" or "cigar-shaped." Another characteristic feature is the presence of perinuclear vacuoles at the tips of some nuclei. Genital leiomyomas are histologically identical except that they are often more cellular.[1]

Angioleiomyomas differ from pilar leiomyomas in that they are sharply delineated from the surrounding tissue by a true capsule and are deeper, usually in the deep reticular dermis or subcutaneous tissue (Fig. 147–2). The tumor demonstrates several to many endothelial-lined vascular spaces that are often slit-like or stellate in shape. These vascular spaces are surrounded by concentric smooth muscle coats arranged in fascicles that may be ill defined in some areas. At high power, the tumor cells are indistinguishable from the smooth muscle cells found in pilar leiomyomas. Some angioleiomyomas may demonstrate focal hemorrhage, vascular thrombosis, myxoid stroma, or fat cells.[2] Those cases with abundant lipocytes have been termed angiomyolipomas or angiolipoleiomyomas.[3]

Pathogenesis. The pathogenesis of cutaneous leiomyomas has not been elucidated, but it appears that they

The opinions or assertions contained herein are the views of the authors and are not to be considered as reflecting the views of the Department of the Army or the Department of Defense. This is a US government work and is in the public domain.

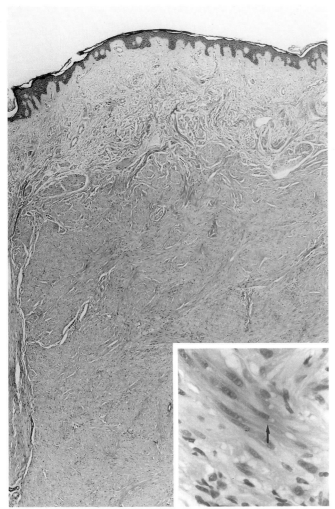

FIGURE 147-1. Scanning view of pilar leiomyoma demonstrating a dermal tumor composed of intersecting fascicles of spindle cells (hematoxylin-eosin [H&E], ×20). *Inset,* High-power appearance of pilar leiomyoma showing characteristic straight spindle-shaped cells with blunt tips and perinuclear vacuoles *(arrow)* (H&E, ×400).

arise from any type of normal smooth muscle. The superficial tumors arise from the pilar arrector muscles, dartos muscle, or mamillary muscle. Angioleiomyomas arise from the muscular wall of blood vessels. The consistent lack of internal elastic lamina suggests that most of these tumors arise from veins, although rare tumors may demonstrate internal elastic laminae and probably arise from arteries. Multiple leiomyomas are often familial, suggesting that their formation is under genetic control.

Differential Diagnosis. Clinically, pilar leiomyomas may be difficult to differentiate from other tumors such as dermatofibromas and other spindle cell neoplasms, although the presence of pain particularly on cold stimulation is highly suggestive. Pilar leiomyomas are histologically distinctive but may be confused with dermatofibromas, dermatomyofibromas, and neurofibromas. The diagnosis of leiomyoma can usually be established by identifying the characteristic blunt-tipped nuclei associated with perinuclear vacuoles, a feature that is absent

in fibrous and neural spindle cell tumors. The diagnosis can be confirmed by performing a trichrome stain, which will demonstrate diffuse red staining of the abundant cytoplasm of the smooth muscle cells. Since dermatofibromas, dermatomyofibromas, and neurofibromas are composed of fusiform cells with minimal cytoplasm, the nuclei will be surrounded by blue or green connective tissue depending on the counterstain used. Rare ambiguous cases may require immunoperoxidase confirmation with smooth muscle–specific actin that will decorate smooth muscle. Angioleiomyomas are histologically distinctive but may still be confused with other encapsulated spindle cell tumors such as neurilemmomas. Angioleiomyomas stain positive with trichrome, while neurilemmomas will demonstrate minimal positivity.

Treatment. The degree of symptoms and extent of involvement determine the therapy. Solitary lesions and smaller plaques can be excised with a layered closure. Radiation therapy has not proven effective.

If there is a family history, genetic counseling should be considered. In women affected with multiple cutaneous leiomyomatosis, the uterus should be examined for involvement.[4]

Leiomyosarcoma

Clinical Description. This solitary malignant tumor of smooth muscle is rare in either the cutaneous or subcutaneous tissue forms, with only 230 reported cases.[5] The cutaneous variant arises from the arrectores pilorum or genital smooth muscle, while subcutaneous leiomyosarcomas arise from vascular smooth muscle. This is an important distinction, since the prognosis of these two tumors is vastly different. The dermal tumors only rarely

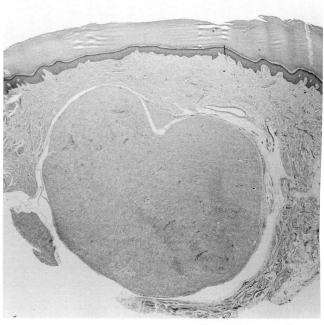

FIGURE 147-2. Low-power appearance of angioleiomyoma demonstrating characteristic circumscription (H&E, ×10).

metastasize, but the subcutaneous ones do so in 30% to 40% of cases. The most common site of metastasis is the lung.

These poorly circumscribed tumors do not have a distinctive clinical appearance and usually become clinically suspicious because of rapid enlargement or ulceration. While seen in any location, they are frequently present on the extremities.

Pathology. At scanning magnification, the cutaneous leiomyosarcomas are composed of interlacing fascicles of atypical spindle-shaped cells. The overlying epidermis may be normal, attenuated, or ulcerated. The spindle cells vary from benign-appearing smooth muscle cells to highly anaplastic multinucleated giant cells (Fig. 147–3). In general, the cells are larger, plumper, and more hyperchromatic than their benign counterparts. Even within some tumors, different fields may demonstrate varying degrees of differentiation. The number of mitotic figures varies from rare to more than one per high-power field. Subcutaneous leiomyosarcomas differ from cutaneous leiomyosarcomas by their location, sharp circumscription, and frequent presence of irregular vascular spaces within the tumor.[6]

Pathogenesis. The pathogenesis of leiomyosarcomas is unknown, but a significant number of patients report a prior history of trauma, suggesting that local factors may be important. Less commonly reported factors have included ionizing radiation and lupus vulgaris.

Differential Diagnosis. Histologically, leiomyosarcomas must be differentiated from other spindle cell neoplasms. In both variants of leiomyosarcomas, the histologic diagnosis hinges on recognizing the smooth muscle origin of the tumor cells. Even in anaplastic tumors, a careful search will often demonstrate a fascicular growth pattern associated with at least some straight spindle-shaped cells with blunt tips and perinuclear vacuoles (Fig. 147–3). The diagnosis can be confirmed by the demonstration of abundant red-staining cytoplasm by a trichrome stain. Immunoperoxidase stains, particularly smooth muscle–specific actin and desmin, are useful because smooth muscle cells are typically decorated by these monoclonal antibodies. Negative immunoperoxidase markers do not exclude leiomyosarcoma, since up to 10% of cases may lack smooth muscle–specific actin reactivity and up to 50% may lack desmin reactivity.[7] Rare cases may also require electron microscopy to exclude other spindle cell neoplasms.

Treatment. Survival improves with early detection and adequate excision. While the tumor may appear encapsulated at the time of surgical resection, this is a false capsule of compressed stoma. Enucleation of the mass that leaves this apparent capsule will result in recurrence of the tumor. Wide local excision offers as good a chance at survival as an amputation. Postoperative radiation therapy may provide effective adjuvant therapy.[8] Adjuvant chemotherapy does not offer a significant survival advantage.[9]

Rhabdomyoma

This benign nodule of striated muscle may represent a hamartoma and is usually a well-circumscribed cutaneous mass. Rhabdomyomas can be seen in adults or fetuses. Fetal rhabdomyomas usually appear in young boys as subcutaneous tumors near the ear. In women, rhabdomyomas may appear as genital polyps in the vaginal or vulvar areas. In adult men, these tumors localize in the muscles of the head and neck region.

Pathology. Rhabdomyomas are well-defined tumors

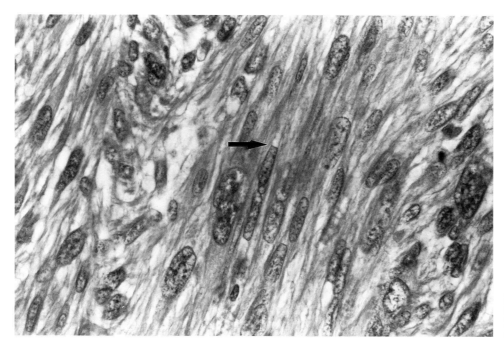

FIGURE 147–3. High-power appearance of leiomyosarcoma showing blunt-tipped nuclei with apical vacuole *(arrow)* (H&E, ×400).

that are usually surrounded by compressed connective tissue. The tumor is composed of large, round to polygonal cells that are separated from each other by a thin layer of fibrovascular tissue. The individual cells demonstrate intensely eosinophilic cytoplasm with one or more vesicular nuclei that are peripherally located. The cytoplasm may be variably granular or vacuolated. Cross-striations are present in some but not all cells.[10] A distinctive feature is the presence of rod-like crystalline structures of the cytoplasm that are thought to represent Z-band material.

Pathogenesis. The pathogenesis of rhabdomyomas has been debated, with some authorities favoring a true neoplasm and others favoring abnormal tissue development. The association of certain types of rhabdomyomas with tuberous sclerosis suggests that at least some cases are the result of a hamartomatous process.

Differential Diagnosis. Rhabdomyomas can be histologically confused with granular cell tumors and hibernomas. In contrast to granular cell tumors, rhabdomyomas demonstrate increased glycogen, cross-striations, and cytoplasmic rod-like crystals and lack pustulo-ovoid bodies of Milian. Hibernomas lack these structures and also demonstrate varying numbers of characteristic "mulberry" cells.

Treatment. Local excision is curative.

Rhabdomyosarcoma

Rhabdomyosarcomas are seen primarily in children. These appear as soft tissue masses or arise in congenital nevi. They may present as surface nodules singly or as multiple small lesions.

Pathology. Cutaneous rhabdomyosarcomas that are likely to be encountered by dermatologists include embryonal rhabdomyosarcoma and alveolar rhabdomyosarcoma. Embryonal rhabdomyosarcoma may demonstrate one or more different histologic patterns depending on the degree of differentiation. The least differentiated tumors are composed of cells that are small, round to oval basophilic nuclei without discernible cytoplasm or other distinctive features. Mitotic figures are frequently present in high numbers. More differentiated cells demonstrate larger nuclei that may be more vesicular associated with intensely eosinophilic cytoplasm. Highly differentiated embryonal rhabdomyosarcomas are composed of spindle-shaped or strap-shaped cells with some cells demonstrating abundant eosinophilic cytoplasm and cross-striations (Fig. 147–4). Alveolar rhabdomyosarcomas are composed of poorly differentiated round to oval basophilic cells with minimal cytoplasm that are poorly cohesive in the center of the tumor aggregates, producing an alveolar pattern.

Pathogenesis. Although rhabdomyosarcomas are generally classified as malignant tumors of striated muscle, it has also been proposed that these tumors arise from primitive mesenchymal cells that merely demonstrate striated muscle differentiation. Extrinsic factors appear to be of minimal importance, although rare cases have occurred following trauma and ionizing radiation.[11]

Poorly differentiated rhabdomyosarcomas that are composed of hyperchromatic undifferentiated round cells are difficult to separate from other small round cell tumors (Table 147–1). Even undifferentiated tumors will often demonstrate cells with eosinophilic filamentous material (myofilaments) in the cytoplasm that surrounds the nucleus. If this feature is lacking, the diagnosis can be established by electron microscopy or the demonstration of myoglobin by immunoperoxidase technique. Myoglobin reactivity is specific for striated muscle differentiation but may be absent in a minority of

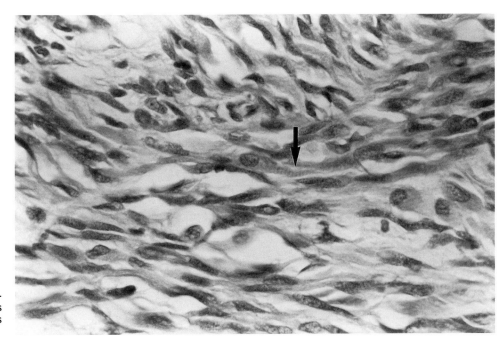

FIGURE 147–4. Rhabdomyosarcoma demonstrating strap-like cells with diagnostic cross-striations *(arrow)* (H&E, ×200).

TABLE 147-1. Differential Diagnosis of Cutaneous Small Cell Malignancies

Carcinoid
Extraskeletal Ewing's sarcoma
Malignant lymphoma
Merkel cell carcinoma
Neuroepithelioma
Oat cell carcinoma
Rhabdomyosarcoma
Small cell squamous cell carcinoma
Small cell sweat gland carcinoma

tumors. In tumors that are more differentiated, the diagnosis can be established by the demonstration of strap cells with cross-striations. If the cross-striations are difficult to visualize by routine hematoxylin and eosin stains, phosphotungstic acid hematoxylin may enhance visualization.

Treatment. Treatment is by complete surgical excision followed by chemotherapy or radiation therapy.

TUMORS OF FAT

Nevus Lipomatosus Superficialis

Clinical Description. Nevus lipomatosus superficialis is a rare lesion that is usually asymptomatic. It appears as a circumscribed group of soft nodules that often have a folded surface. Lesions are skin colored or pale yellow. They appear chiefly in the pelvic or gluteal areas and are usually present at birth.

Pathology. Nevus lipomatosus superficialis is a benign malformation that is grossly both exophytic and endophytic. Microscopically, it demonstrates a normal or slightly attenuated epidermis associated with a dermal proliferation of mature lipocytes in the reticular dermis that may extend to the papillary dermis. The lipocytes may demonstrate connections to the underlying normal fat or be separated from the subcutis by collagen. The lipocytes are most commonly formed as small aggregates around blood vessels but may be present as solitary lipocytes between collagen bundles.[12] Less commonly, spindle cells representing immature fat cells are present.

Pathogenesis. The pathogenesis of nevus lipomatosus superficialis is not certain. Since this tumor is often congenital, it is most likely that the tumor arises from lipocytes or primitive lipoblasts that are abnormally sequestered in the dermis. It has been also proposed that the tumor is due to degenerative changes of connective tissue with secondary fatty replacement or the displacement of subcutaneous fat into the dermis.

Differential Diagnosis. Nevus lipomatosus superficialis is clinically difficult to differentiate from other tumors that are soft and polypoid such as soft fibromas and neurofibromas. Histologically, the tumor can be difficult to distinguish from large soft fibromas that can also demonstrate lipocytes in the dermis. Clinical information that favors a diagnosis of nevus lipomatosus superficialis includes presence at birth, large tumor or plaque, and presence of linear lesions. Microscopically, a pedunculated architecture favors a soft fibroma.

Lipoma

Clinical Description. Lipomas are found quite commonly in the adult population. They are primarily seen on the trunk but may appear on an part of the body. Although they are usually solitary, they may be multiple and range in size from a few millimeters to 20 or more centimeters. Most lipomas are painful when compressed.

A familial form of lipoma, *multiple familial lipomatosis,* is autosomal dominant. Hundreds of lesions may be seen over the entire body. *Madelung's disease,* or benign symmetrical lipomatosis, is a form of multiple lipomatosis in which the lesions are poorly circumscribed and congregate especially around the neck and occiput. This causes a classic "horse collar" appearance.

Pathology. Lipomas resemble normal adipose tissue both grossly and microscopically. Grossly, they typically demonstrate one or more yellow to yellow-orange lobules that are delineated from the surrounding tissue by a thin fibrous pseudocapsule. Less commonly, they may demonstrate an infiltrative growth pattern into surrounding normal tissue such as muscle.[13]

At low power, the appearance of lipomas is indistinguishable from that of normal adipose tissue except that the normal lobular architecture is lost and the fat lobules appear larger than normal. Since lipomas are often surgically removed by shelling out the tumor, the edges of the tumor are rounded with a thin fibrous capsule (Fig. 147-5). High-power examination of the tumor demonstrates rather uniform mature fat cells that are round, oval, or polygonal in shape. The fat cells of lipomas are indistinguishable from normal fat cells, although they are generally more variable in size and may be larger. An intensely basophilic crescent-shaped nucleus is present at the rim of the cell where it is compressed by a large unilocular space that represents lipid that has been removed in tissue processing (Fig. 147-5, *inset*). Small nuclear lipid invagination may be present in some nuclei. Secondary changes as a result of trauma or impaired vascularization include focal cystic fat necrosis, lipid-laden macrophages, and microhemorrhages. It is likely that the so-called mobile encapsulated lipoma (nodulocystic fat necrosis) is not a tumor but is the result of trauma to normal subcutaneous fat that has resulted in vascular insufficiency of fat and fibrous capsule formation around the necrotic tissue.[14] The lipomas of adiposis dolorosa (Dercum's disease), benign symmetrical lipomatosis (Madelung's disease), and familial multiple lipomatosis, which is autosomal dominant, are indistinguishable from ordinary lipomas.

Histologic variations of lipomas include fibrolipomas, myxolipomas, and fibromyxolipomas. Fibrolipomas are most commonly encountered in the posterior neck and

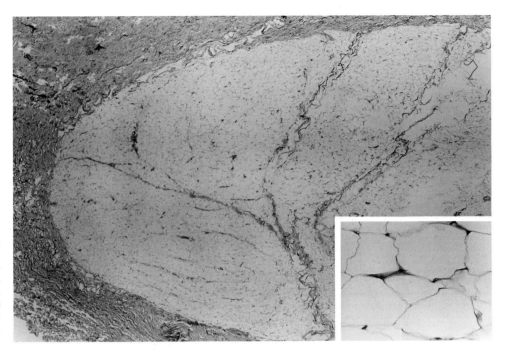

FIGURE 147–5. Scanning magnification of lipoma demonstrating characteristic lobular architecture and compression of surrounding normal collagen (H&E, ×20). *Inset,* Typical appearance of lipoma cells showing round to polygonal unilocular lipocytes with compressed nuclei (H&E, ×200).

upper back and demonstrate thickened fibrous septa with interspersed mature adipocytes. Fibrolipomas often lack the delicate fibrous pseudocapsule of routine lipomas. Myxolipomas are lipomas that demonstrate focal or diffuse accumulation of mucin between the lipocytes. This mucin stains readily with colloidal iron or other acid mucopolysaccharide stains. Mast cells are frequently present in lipomas associated with increased mucin. Fibromyxolipomas demonstrate a combination of mature fat, increased collagen, and stromal mucin.

Pathogenesis. The pathogenesis of lipomas has not been elucidated, but the observation that some cases are familial suggest that their development is under genetic control. This is further supported by studies reporting that one half of lipomas demonstrate structural rearrangement of chromosome 12.[15] Rarely, proliferation of fatty tissue indistinguishable from lipomas can be found at sites of trauma or surgery, suggesting that local factors may also induce adipose proliferation.

Differential Diagnosis. Clinically, lipomas may be confused with epidermoid cysts, other benign fatty tumors, and liposarcomas. Needle aspiration may help to determine cystic lesions. The histologic differential diagnosis of classic lipomas would include normal adipose tissue and well-differentiated liposarcoma. Normal adipose tissue can usually be excluded by the loss of normal lobular architecture and smooth edges of the neoplasm associated with a delicate fibrous capsule. Well-differentiated liposarcomas can be difficult to distinguish from lipomas but can usually be differentiated clinicopathologically. Clinically, liposarcomas are usually larger, demonstrate insidious growth, and are more likely to infiltrate normal structures. Microscopically, some areas may be indistinguishable from lipomas. Other areas demonstrate features of liposarcomas, including variation in the

size and shape of lipocytes, hyperchromatic nuclei, and multivacuolar lipoblasts.

Treatment. Excision or liposuction surgery is employed for lipomas. For further discussion of liposuction surgery, see the end of this chapter.

Angiolipoma

Clinical Description. Although confused with lipomas in their clinical presentation, these lesions are smaller and more mobile than lipomas. Angiolipomas may also be painful. They are primarily located on the arms and the trunk.

Pathology. Angiolipomas grossly demonstrate one or more sharply circumscribed lobules that resemble normal adipose tissue except for a reddish tint secondary to increased vascularization. Like lipomas, angiolipomas may lack a pseudocapsule and demonstrate an infiltrative growth pattern into normal tissue such as striated muscle.

Microscopically, at low power the tumor is delineated from the surrounding normal tissue by a thin fibrous pseudocapsule (Fig. 147–6). At higher powers, the tumor is composed of mature lipocytes interspersed with variable numbers of thin, branching vascular spaces (Fig. 147–6, *inset*). The proportion of these two components varies from area to area such that some areas may appear indistinguishable from routine lipomas while other areas may be highly vascular. A characteristic feature of angiolipomas is the presence of microthrombi within the vessels. Additional histologic findings include variable fibrosis between the fat cells and vasculature. Vascular channels and spindle-shaped fibroblasts may totally replace the lipocytes in some areas.[16]

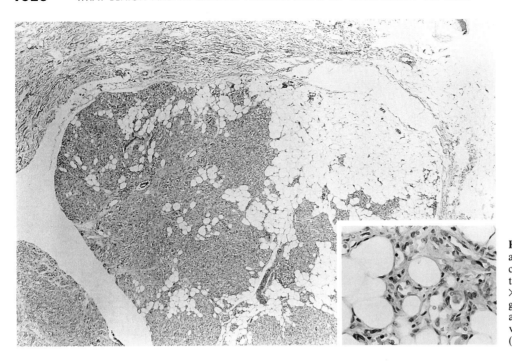

FIGURE 147-6. Scanning view of angiolipoma demonstrating sharp circumscription and admixture of mature fat and vascular elements (H&E, ×20). *Inset,* High-power view of angiolipoma showing mature lipocytes admixed with vascular spaces. Some vessels demonstrate thrombosis (H&E, ×100).

Pathogenesis. The pathogenesis of angiolipomas is not known, but as in the case of lipomas, the presence of familial cases suggests that the development of this tumor is probably under genetic control in some patients.

Differential Diagnosis. Clinically, angiolipomas are difficult to differentiate from routine lipomas and other fatty tumors; however, the presence of pain favors the former. The histologic differential diagnosis of angiolipoma includes routine lipoma, capillary hemangioma, Kaposi's sarcoma, and angiomyolipoma. The degree of vascularization needed to differentiate lipoma from angiolipoma has not been established, but conspicuous vessels and microthrombi indicate angiolipoma. Capillary hemangiomas may form subcutaneous lobules resembling angiolipomas but can usually be excluded because they lack adipocytes and microthrombi. Angiolipomas with fibrosis may demonstrate some resemblance to subcutaneous Kaposi's sarcoma, but the sharp circumscription, presence of true vascular channels, absence of mitotic figures, and presence of microthrombi are features that favor the former. Angiomyolipomas are distinguished by the demonstration of significant smooth muscle.

Treatment. Surgical excision is called for.

Spindle Cell Lipoma

Clinical Description. Clinically, these usually appear as painless solitary, firm subcutaneous masses that are small and slow growing. They are seen primarily on the upper back and neck.

Spindle cell lipomas are grossly well-circumscribed fatty tumors composed of one or more lobules that vary in color from yellow to gray associated with a thin compressed fibrous pseudocapsule. Less commonly, the tumor may demonstrate infiltrative margins.

Pathology. Microscopically, the tumor is a lobular tumor with sharply delineated borders composed of an admixture of mature lipocytes and uniform-appearing spindle cells. In some areas the lipocytes predominate, and other areas demonstrate almost complete replacement of the fat by the spindle cells. The stroma varies from myxoid to collagenous with myxoid areas often demonstrating moderate numbers of mast cells.[17]

Pathogenesis. The pathogenesis of spindle cell lipomas is not clear. The nature of the spindle cells has not been established, although it is most likely that they represent either fibroblasts or prelipoblasts; the former is more likely because these cells produce abundant collagen.

Differential Diagnosis. Clinically, spindle cell lipomas are impossible to differentiate from other benign and malignant fatty tumors, and the diagnosis is established histologically. The differential diagnosis of spindle cell lipoma includes liposarcoma and fibrosarcoma. Liposarcomas may demonstrate sclerotic areas, but the smaller size, circumscription, uniform bland spindle cell component, presence of thick collagen bundles, absence of lipoblasts, and lack of atypia are features that favor spindle cell lipoma. Fibrosarcoma with infiltration into fat can be excluded by the small size of the tumor, presence of circumscription, and lack of cytologic atypia.

Pleomorphic Lipoma

Pleomorphic lipomas, clinically and grossly resembling routine lipomas, are composed of one or more yellowish to yellowish-orange lobules that demonstrate sharp circumscription from surrounding normal tissue. Microscopically, the tumor is sharply circumscribed and demonstrates a thin fibrous pseudocapsule at the edge of the tumor. Examination under high power demonstrates numerous mature lipocytes associated with variable numbers of bizarre hyperchromatic mononuclear or multinuclear cells (Fig. 147-7). These cells are markedly

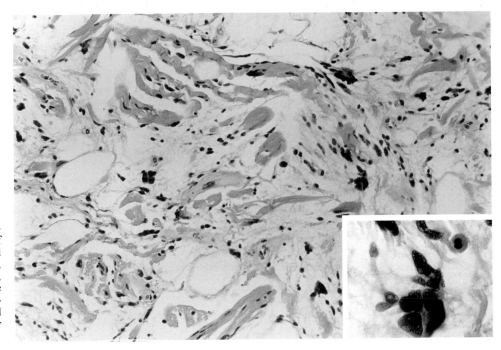

FIGURE 147-7. Pleomorphic lipoma demonstrating an admixture of mature fat, spindle cells, atypical floret-like multinucleated giant cells, and fibromyxoid stroma (H&E, ×100). *Inset*, Characteristic floret-like multinucleated giant cell demonstrating hyperchromatic nuclei arranged in a pattern reminiscent of a flower (H&E, ×400).

pleomorphic in shape and size and vary from spindle shaped to stellate. A characteristic feature is the presence of "floret-like" giant cells in which the nuclei are arranged in a circular, often overlapping configuration around eosinophilic cytoplasm reminiscent of the petals of a flower (Fig. 147-7, *inset*). These cells are usually associated with fibromyxoid stroma. The number of these floret-like giant cells varies from numerous to rare. In some tumors the pleomorphic component may be present focally, while in other cases the entire tumor may demonstrate this pattern. Thick collagen bundles may also be present.[18]

Pathogenesis. The pathogenesis of this rare neoplasm is unknown, but it is probably closely related to spindle cell lipoma because up to 25% will demonstrate areas resembling spindle cell lipoma. Despite the alarming histologic appearance, this is felt to be a benign tumor.

Differential Diagnosis. Clinically, pleomorphic lipomas cannot be differentiated from other benign and malignant adipose tumors. Histologically, pleomorphic lipoma is most commonly confused with pleomorphic liposarcoma. Features that favor pleomorphic lipoma over liposarcoma include smaller size, well-circumscribed margins, floret-like giant cells, absence of mitotic figures, paucity of lipoblasts, and presence of thick collagen bundles.

Hibernoma

Hibernomas are well-circumscribed rare benign tumors that clinically resemble lipomas. They are usually solitary and are found on the back, neck, or axilla. They may be reddish brown in color and tend to be mobile and symptomatic. They have a lobular architecture and a distinct tan to brownish color—hence the name "brown fat." At low power, the tumor cells are arranged in distinct lobules separated by interlobular septa that are often highly vascular. At high power, the lobules are composed of distinctive lipocytes that may entirely fill the lobules or be intermixed with white fat cells. The fat cells may either be round or oval and separated from adjacent cells by loose stroma or assume a polygonal outline if the hibernoma cells impinge on one another. The distinctive hibernoma or "mulberry" cell demonstrates a centrally placed nucleus that may be hyperchromatic or demonstrate a solitary nucleolus. The cytoplasm may be either eosinophilic and granular or multivacuolated.[19]

Hibernomas are the only known benign tumors of brown fat. Brown fat is more common and metabolically important in several other species of animal, especially species that hibernate, but not in humans. In humans, brown fat is seldom found past infancy.[20]

Differential Diagnosis. Hibernomas demonstrate such a distinctive histologic appearance that confusion with other tumors is unlikely. Hibernomas with prominent eosinophilic granular cytoplasm may be confused with other tumors such as granular cell tumors; however, the presence of multivacuolated cytoplasm in at least some of the cells will exclude these possibilities. Liposarcomas with variable eosinophilic granular cytoplasm or multivacuolated cytoplasm may resemble hibernoma but can be excluded on the basis of increased cellularity and presence of cytologic atypia.

Treatment. Treatment with surgical excision is curative of this benign process.

Lipoblastoma

Lipoblastoma is a rare benign tumor that occurs in young children.

Clinical Description. Lipoblastomas grossly demonstrate either a well-circumscribed lobular appearance or a diffuse growth pattern that may infiltrate into normal structures such as muscle. Lipoblastomas are distinctly less yellow-orange than normal fat or routine lipomas and may demonstrate a gelatinous appearance in some cases.

Pathology. Microscopically, lipoblastomas resemble fetal fat. They demonstrate very distinct lobules separated by highly vascularized septa with a variably myxoid stroma. The composition of different lobules is highly variable, with some lobules demonstrating marked uniformity of the cells while other lobules demonstrate an admixture of mature and immature fat cells. The immature fat cells may vary from undifferentiated spindle- or stellate-shaped cells associated with myxoid stroma to lipoblasts. The more mature areas usually demonstrate less myxoid stroma. Lipoblasts are smaller than mature lipocytes and are characterized by one or more cytoplasmic lipid droplets. Those with a single cytoplasmic lipid droplet demonstrate a characteristic "signet ring" appearance.[21]

Pathogenesis. Lipoblastomas are generally considered to be tumors of immature white fat. That this tumor is found almost exclusively in infancy and childhood suggests the possibility that at least some cases merely represent residual areas of fat that have not yet fully matured.

Differential Diagnosis. Clinically, lipoblastomas cannot be differentiated from other fatty tumors, although the young age at the time of presentation is suggestive. Histologically, lipoblastomas may be confused with some variants of liposarcoma. At low power, lipoblastomas demonstrate a distinctive lobular architecture that is typically absent in liposarcomas. At high power, lipoblastomas do not demonstrate mitotic figures, nuclear hyperchromatism, or multinucleated giant cells. Clinicopathologic correlation is also helpful, since liposarcomas occur in adults and lipoblastomas are usually discovered in childhood.

Treatment. Treatment is by surgical excision.

Liposarcoma

Clinical Description. Liposarcoma occurs most frequently in adults 40 to 60 years old and is rare in children. There is a predilection for the lower leg. The tumors are often large lobulated masses greater than 10 cm in diameter with poorly defined margins. Some are firm and yellow; others are soft and gray. Hemorrhage and necrosis within the mass frequently occur. The tumor enlarges rapidly and is painful and nonmobile.

Pathology. Microscopically, liposarcomas have been divided into four main subtypes. This division is somewhat artificial, since tumors with a mixed pattern may occur. Myxoid liposarcomas are the most common subtype and are characterized by an admixture of lipoblasts, signet ring cells, and mature lipocytes associated with a myxoid stroma and prominent vascularity. Myxoid liposarcomas may demonstrate hyperchromatic cells and multinucleated giant cells, but these are uncommon. Mitotic figures may be rare or absent. Round cell liposarcomas are closely related to myxoid liposarcomas but are

characterized by more cellularity and cytologically atypical round cells that often demonstrate a signet ring appearance. Mitotic activity is typically much higher than in myxoid liposarcomas. Well-differentiated liposarcomas are composed primarily of seemly mature lipocytes that demonstrate an infiltrative growth pattern and more variation in size than typically observed in either normal fat or lipomas. Interspersed throughout the tumor are hyperchromatic, often somewhat pleomorphic cells that may be multinucleated. The atypical cells may be associated with a fibrous or myxoid stroma and may be more common in septa. Mitotic figures are usually rare or absent. Pleomorphic liposarcomas demonstrate large hyperchromatic nuclei that often demonstrate irregular nuclear contours as a result of one or more lipid vacuoles (Fig. 147–8). Multinucleated giant cells and atypical mitotic figures are commonly present.[22]

Pathogenesis. The pathogenesis of liposarcomas is unknown, but most cases appear to arise from normal fat with only rare cases arising from preexisting lipomas. Studies on two tumors reported that liposarcomas demonstrate clonal abnormalities of chromosome 12.[15] Liposarcomas have been reported to occur in sites of previous trauma, but this is rare.

Differential Diagnosis. Liposarcomas may be difficult to differentiate from other benign fatty tumors and sarcomas. In general, liposarcomas can be differentiated from benign fatty tumors by clinicopathologic correlation because liposarcomas tend to be painful, arise deep, and demonstrate an infiltrative growth pattern. Microscopically, most liposarcomas demonstrate varying combinations of cytologic atypia and evidence of immature fat formation in the form of lipoblasts or signet ring cells. Large lesions may need to be sampled in multiple areas, since diagnostic features may be focal.

Treatment. Treatment is with excision. Metastasis to lungs can occur.

TREATMENT OF BENIGN TUMORS AND HYPERTROPHY OF FAT

In recent years, liposuction surgery has been adapted for the treatment of lipomas.[23-25] Liposuction removes fat by using a cannula attached to a source of negative pressure. The fat is suctioned out in a tunneling fashion rather then en bloc to prevent large dead spaces, seromas, and hematomas. Instead of sharply removing the entire lipoma, the tumor is extensively suctioned, leaving multiple tunnels throughout the lesion. Healing and contraction of these tunnels shrink the size of the tumor. The advantage of liposuction over standard surgical excision is the small incision (3 to 4 mm) (Fig. 147–9). It also allows better recontouring of the area as opposed to sharp excision, which may result in a depression. Another compromise approach is to make a small surface incision (1 to 2 cm) and with blunt dissection or curettage remove the lipoma in fragments.

Liposuction and curettage of a lipoma are both time-consuming procedures that may take twice as long as excision. Lipomas are often very firm and encapsulated, making blunt dissection of the tumor quite difficult. Be-

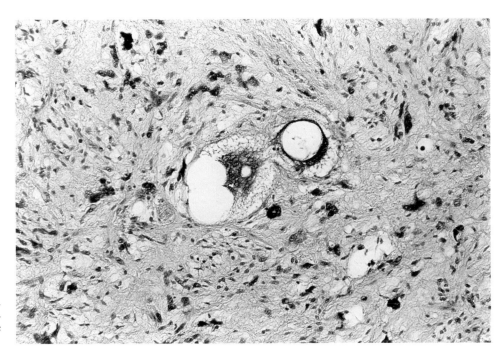

FIGURE 147–8. Pleomorphic liposarcoma showing bizarre hyperchromatic lipoblasts with intracytoplasmic lipid droplets (H&E, ×100).

cause the tumor is not under direct visualization, palpation allows the liposuction surgeon to determine the extent of tumor removal. Postoperatively, compression tape must be applied over the surgical site to effectively eliminate dead space. This reduces the risk of postoperative hematomas or seromas.

Fat Hypertrophies

Many individuals develop localized adiposities that apparently respond to weight gain or loss differently than fat stores elsewhere in the body. Metabolically, these fat cells have been shown to be more active in storing triglycerides and resistant to releasing free fatty acids.[26] With weight gain, these fat cells disproportionately enlarge while remaining more resistant to weight loss than other adipocytes. In spite of exercise and dieting, many individuals are prone to development of these adipose hypertrophies. These bulges are fancifully termed "love handles," "saddlebags," "turkey gobblers," etc.

In 1974, Dr. Giorgio Fischer used blunt suction-assisted cannula dissection to reduce the adiposity.[27] Tunneling through the fat was preferred over creation of large dead spaces because of early problems with hematomas and seromas and occasionally infection.

The chief areas where liposuction is performed are the upper thighs, abdomen, and flanks (Fig. 147–10). The neck, arms, knees, and ankles are also amenable to liposuction in many individuals. Facial liposuction may be

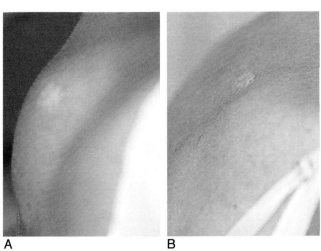

A   B

FIGURE 147–9. *A,* Recurrent lipoma of the upper back has a hypopigmented scar from a prior attempted removal. The area is prepared for liposuction surgery. *B,* Two months after liposuction surgery, the contours are excellent with only the preoperative scar remaining. (Courtesy of William P. Coleman, III, M.D.)

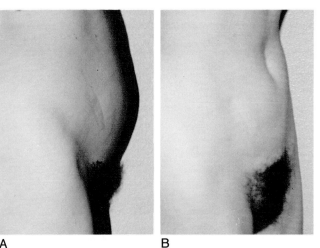

A   B

FIGURE 147–10. *A,* Preoperative excessive fat of the lower abdomen in a woman who does not have other significant areas of fat deposition. *B,* At 1-year follow-up, there are excellent contour changes. The dimple of the lower right quadrant is the top of the appendectomy incision that was present preoperatively. (Courtesy of William P. Coleman, III, M.D.)

performed with or without simultaneous facelifting. The male breast can be recontoured by removal of excess fat in patients with pseudogynecomastia and gynecomastia. Likewise, liposuction may be performed in conjunction with formal breast reduction for females with mammary hypertrophy.

The worst potential complication of any procedure is death. A few patients have died as a result of this procedure because of an anesthetic mishap in cases performed under general anesthesia.[28, 29] There are no known liposuction deaths resulting from procedures performed under local anesthesia.[30] Another important pattern is the association of deaths in liposuction patients who underwent simultaneous abdominoplasty.[31] These patients developed fat or pulmonary thromboemboli, a complication associated with abdominoplasty alone. There is some question whether the liposuction had any effect on these fatal outcomes, but the association of these two procedures is a clear risk factor. Death from infection after liposuction occurred under the care of two physicians who had multiple postoperative liposuction infections during a short period of time. Evidence points to a lack of sterile technique. There have been no deaths in patients upon whom liposuction was performed under local anesthesia as a solo procedure with proper attention to sterile technique. Necrotizing fasciitis has been reported as a rare complication of liposuction. This may also be due to overaggressive liposuction. Excessive blood loss was the most feared complication of liposuction during the early days of its evolution. Before the development of local tumescent anesthesia, it was quite typical for the liposuction aspirate to contain 40% or more of blood.[30] Consequently, removal of 2000 cc or more of fat and fluid necessitated blood replacement in some patients. This problem led to extensive use of autologous blood transfusions with its attendant complications.

In 1987, Jeffrey Klein introduced tumescent local anesthesia, which involves the infiltration of large volumes of dilute lidocaine and epinephrine throughout the adiposity.[32] This resulted in excellent regional anesthesia as well as reduced blood loss. Klein has shown that proper use of this technique yields an aspirate that is approximately 1% blood, completely eliminating the need for transfusions.[33] This has allowed larger volumes of fat to be removed safely under local anesthesia.[34]

Inadvertent penetration of adjacent viscera with the liposuction cannula has been reported in a few individuals. This has chiefly occurred in the abdominal area where cannulas were forced through hernias or other defects in the muscle wall. This has not been reported in patients who had liposuction surgery under local anesthesia. The tumescent method also has the advantages of providing a firm fatty layer upon which to operate, which eliminates the need for aggressive thrusts of the cannula as may occur under general anesthesia without proper infiltration of the fatty layers. In fact, using the tumescent method, liposuction is a very delicate and precise procedure in which the location of the cannula is carefully controlled at all times.

In addition to these serious complications of liposuction, a number of sequelae occur occasionally after this procedure (e.g., contour abnormalities, hematomas, and seromas). These are presumed to be due to variations between individual patients. Although these occur occasionally, most subside with no long-term ill effects. If the patient is prepared for the possibility of such sequelae, their occurrence postoperatively can be handled more gracefully by the operating surgeon.[35, 36]

Various contour abnormalities may occur on the surface skin after liposuction. This is far more likely if large cannulas are used, especially in the superficial fatty layers. These large tunnels may collapse, leaving visible dents or waffling on the skin surface. Although superficial liposuction was discouraged in the early years of this procedure, it has become common to use small cannulas in the superficial fat in order to encourage redraping of the overlying skin. As long as cannulas smaller than 3 mm are used in the upper layers of subcutaneous tissue, waffling or dents usually should not occur. Larger cannulas should be restricted to use below a 1-cm buffer of the superficial fat. Patients must also recognize that preoperatively most individuals already have various dimples and waffling of their skin and fatty layer. Often liposuction will improve the appearance of these, but there is also some risk of new ones occurring.

Hematomas and seromas, although common in the early days of liposuction, are now quite rare. The tumescent anesthetic approach decreases the potential for these. If a hematoma or seroma were to occur, needle drainage is usually sufficient to ablate it, especially if followed by several days of compression. If left untreated, a hematoma or seroma may result in infection.

Some patients complain of cutaneous loss of sensation after liposuction. This is usually temporary, although there have been a few permanent cases. All patients must be warned of this possibility.

Some patients take much longer than others to complete healing from liposuction. Persistent edema in the area of treatment may last for several months postoperatively and be very frustrating to physician and patient alike. All patients should be warned that the final results of the contouring may not be apparent for up to 6 months postoperatively. Some patients continue to improve even after this long period of time.

Liposuction, like any procedure, produces a great variety of results ranging from no appreciable improvement to near perfection. Even when the same technique is used on similar patients, different results can be anticipated. All patients must be informed of the possibility that they will not be satisfied with the final results of their contouring. Many patients achieve the best results after a second or third touch-up liposuction.

Preparing for Liposuction

The physician must be certain that the patient is in good physical health prior to undergoing liposuction. In particular, bleeding disorders must be ruled out. Severe cardiovascular disease is incompatible with injection of large volumes of epinephrine and must be ruled out as well. Patients with wound healing problems or metabolic abnormalities such as diabetes should be approached carefully.

A panel of preoperative blood tests including a complete blood count with platelets, a general chemistry, a prothrombin time, and a partial thromboplastin time should be performed on every liposuction patient. Some physicians also perform hepatitis screens or HIV studies. If there is any doubt as to the general health of the patient, clearance for surgery should be sought from an internist.

The patient must be instructed to avoid taking any medications that could increase bleeding. This includes discontinuing aspirin, nonsteroidal antiinflammatory agents, vitamin E, and other anticoagulants at least 10 days prior to the procedure. Furthermore, alcohol is contraindicated for at least 48 hours prior to liposuction. The patient should be thoroughly prepared for the details of the procedure as well as his or her expected postoperative behavior. All patients who receive any form of sedation should have a responsible driver take them home and stay with them until they are fully capable of caring for themselves. Many patients assume they should fast prior to all surgery. However, with liposuction performed under local anesthesia with sedation, a normal breakfast is allowed. Many patients who fast become hypoglycemic and dizzy preoperatively or at the sight of needles.

All patients should have their operative consents signed prior to administration of any sedatives.[35] For physicians who prefer preoperative sedation either the morning or the night before surgery, consents must be signed at an earlier preoperative appointment. Such preoperative visits afford an ideal time to discuss last-minute details, sign consents, and pay fees. This often avoids last-minute misunderstandings and allows the patient a final chance to decline surgery if he or she is uncertain about proceeding.

Once the surgical sites have been marked with the patient standing, the patient can then recline on the operating table. If the operating suite contains a shower, this is the ideal place to wash the entire body with a surgical scrub. If a shower is not available, the assistant performs this scrub with the assistance of the patient.

The surgeon begins initial anesthetic infiltration at the sites of cannula insertion using 1% lidocaine with epinephrine and using a No. 11 blade to incise the skin. A 12- to 14-gauge injection cannula is to be inserted through these incisions into the fat compartment. These injection cannulas are then attached directly with IV lines to 1-L bags containing the tumescent anesthetic solution. This maintains a closed sterile system for delivery of the anesthetic.[37] Although the force of gravity will aid in delivery of the anesthetic from the intravenous bag through the cannula, some sort of pressure around the bags helps to accelerate this process. Mechanical blood pumps are ideal for this purpose. These can be placed around the intravenous bag and inflated, forcing the fluid into the fatty space. Electronic pumps have also been developed, which accelerate this process. Using these devices, over 1 L of anesthetic fluid can be injected in 5 minutes.

Once enough anesthetic has been instilled into the operative area, the overlying skin becomes firm and vasoconstriction of the subcutaneous and cutaneous vessels is apparent from the pallor of the overlying skin. The surgeon waits approximately 15 minutes after instillation of the anesthetic before proceeding with the liposuction, and there is usually no significant bleeding during the procedure.

Instrumentation

Liposuction requires a blunt cannula and a source of suction. Although this seems simple, several variations have been introduced. The source of suction can be a syringe or a mechanical pump. It is possible to efficiently perform liposuction using a 50-cc syringe attached directly to a cannula.[38] This allows liposuction to be performed with totally disposable equipment; however, it does require that the surgeon maintain constant pressure on the syringe plunger. This necessitates delays during the procedure when the syringe becomes filled with fat.

Most liposuction surgeons employ an electric suction pump that is attached to the cannula via clear plastic tubing. These pumps develop approximately one atmosphere of pressure. The mechanical pumps allow continuous liposuction without delay. Also, the amount of pressure developed can be modulated as necessary. However, these pumps are expensive and require maintenance and clean-up after the procedure.

Cannulas are available in many shapes and sizes. The most crucial dimension is the diameter of the instrument. Originally, liposuction was performed with 8-mm or larger cannulas, which sometimes resulted in "cave-in," as the tunnel collapsed resulting in surface dimpling and waviness. Currently, most liposuction surgeons use cannulas of 6 mm or smaller. The large cannulas are used for debulking, whereas smaller cannulas (2 to 3 mm) are used for superficial liposuction, feathering, and pretunneling.

The length of the cannula is also important. When the insertion site is a great distance from the periphery of the adiposity, longer instruments are required. It is possible, for instance, to suction the entire posterior thigh through a small incision behind the knee. This requires a cannula 45 cm in length or more. Shorter cannulas are more efficient and are used whenever permitted.

The aperture or hole in the tip of the cannula determines how aggressive and efficient the instrument is. Cannulas designed with apertures near the tip perform more like a curette and tear at the fat. These are more aggressive and are used when the fat is quite firm or fibrotic (male love handles). When the aperture is placed further down the shaft of the instrument, the blunt tip is more gentle to the tissues. Cannulas have been designed in a multitude of patterns with holes placed in various configurations. Experience with various instruments allows the surgeon to become comfortable with a few configurations. It is not necessary to purchase all of the different variations.

Liposuction Technique

Liposuction begins with insertion of a small cannula into the subcutaneous layer. The location of this cannula must be known at all times. The nondominant hand acts as a constant sentinel to be certain that the tip is in the right location. Suctioning is a smooth process wherein the dominant hand acts as a piston. Strokes should be continued through a tunnel approximately 8 to 10 times or until there is no resistance. This process may need to be repeated several times throughout the length of the tunnel. Meanwhile, the nondominant hand holds the fatty layer firm and can be used to squeeze the fat cells around the tip of the cannula. This tunneling process should be continued throughout the fatty layer with each tunnel separated from the next by the diameter of the cannula. Several layers of tunnels can be developed from deep to superficial. However, the surgeon must be careful not to create large dead spaces by suctioning in a windshield wiper fashion. The smallest cannulas can be used close to the overlying dermis. Superficial suctioning using small (2 to 3 mm) cannulas may help to tighten the overlying skin.

After the entire adiposity has been suctioned adequately using the small cannula, a larger instrument can then be employed. This larger cannula should be used only in the deeper fat, sparing the most superior 1 cm. Pretunneling with the smaller cannula allows easier introduction of the larger instrument. Fat will flow more rapidly through the tubing when using larger cannulas. Using small cannulas in the superficial fat and progressively larger instruments as the liposuction proceeds down to the deeper layer will achieve the best results. This approach helps to tighten the overlying skin postoperatively.

As the liposuction proceeds, the surgeon should automatically "feather" the procedure by doing less suctioning at the periphery of the adiposity. This allows a smoother transition zone between the suctioned and nonsuctioned areas. Some surgeons prefer to perform a final tunneling around the periphery of the adiposity without suction. This "peripheral mesh dissection" is an alternative to feathering during the procedure.[39]

Postoperative Care

Once the liposuction is complete, the operative areas should be massaged to milk out any excess tumescent fluid. Often this fluid will drip from the incisions for up to 24 hours. Patients must be advised of this so that they will not become frightened and assume that they are bleeding. The incisions are closed with a single suture. Sometimes, the edges of the incision need to be excised if they have been excessively traumatized during the procedure. These wounds are dressed with a bland antibiotic ointment, nonstick pads, and gauze squares secured with tape. Over this, a compression garment is applied.

Various compression garments are now manufactured for liposuction. These are available in a number of shapes and sizes to conform to various anatomic sites. Although originally tape compression was used for liposuction, it has largely been abandoned because of discomfort. Compression garments can be removed and the patient allowed to shower postoperatively. The patient should be advised to wear the compression garments continuously for 14 days after the liposuction. When the patient has an active lifestyle, it is also useful to wear these garments an additional 2 weeks. This provides additional compression and support of tissue that may feel sensitive or bruised. Patients can usually exercise lightly after 3 days and without restriction by 3 weeks.

The most successful liposuction is performed in patients who follow a regular pattern of exercise and dieting. Part of the postoperative follow-up should include reinforcement of these concepts. Patients who engage in any form of regular exercise should be encouraged to do so. A sensible diet must be maintained in order to realize maximum benefits from the procedure. Patients who gain excessive amounts of weight after liposuction may be disappointed to see accumulation of excess fat around the periphery of the liposuction site, which merely causes a new deformity. The liposuctioned areas are usually resistant to future excessive fat storage.

The surgeon should plan to see the patient at regular intervals throughout the healing stage to be certain that no complications are developing. The main reason for these follow-ups is to provide the patient some emotional support during the recovery. Many patients are enthusiastic during the first week or two after liposuction and then gradually become more discouraged as they do not see visible results from their procedure. Many individuals do not show any dramatic change from their liposuction for 3 or more months after the procedure. Although patients are advised of this preoperatively, it is important for patients to be continuously reminded during the healing stages.

It is also important to remind patients that secondary or touch-up procedures may be required. This is particularly important if the anticipated results are not present after 3 to 6 months following liposuction. As with any procedure, there is a great variation in individual response. Some patients achieve dramatic benefits from liposuction, whereas others may notice only slight improvement. (For additional information, see Robinson et al., *Atlas of Cutaneous Surgery,* Chapter 28.)

References

1. Orellana-Díaz O, Hernández-Pérez E. Leiomyoma cutis and leiomyosarcoma: A 10-year study and a short review. J Dermatol Surg Oncol 1983;9:283–287.
2. Hachisuga T, Hashimota H, Enjaji M. Angioleiomyoma: A clinicopathologic reappraisal of 562 cases. Cancer 1984;54:126–130.
3. Fitzpatrick JE, Mellette JR Jr, Hwang RJ, et al. Cutaneous angiolipoleiomyoma. J Am Acad Dermatol 1990;23:1093–1098.
4. Reed WB, Walker R, Horowitz R. Cutaneous leiomyomata with uterine leiomyomata. Acta Derm Venereol 1973;53:409–416.
5. Landry MM, Sarna DP, Boucree TB. Leiomyosarcoma of the buttock. J Am Acad Dermatol 1991;24:618–620.
6. Fields JP, Helwig EB. Leiomyosarcoma of the skin and subcutaneous tissue. Cancer 1981;47:156–159.
7. Azumi N, et al. Immunophenotypic diagnosis of leiomyosarcomas and rhabdomyosarcomas with monoclonal antibodies to muscle-specific actin and desmin in formalin-fixed tissue. Mod Pathol 1988;1:469–474.
8. Sim FH, Pritchard DJ, Reiman HM, et al. Soft tissue sarcomas: Mayo Clinic experience. Semin Surg Oncol 1988;4:38–44.
9. Elias AD, Artman KH. Adjuvant chemotherapy for soft tissue sarcoma: A critical appraisal. Semin Surg Oncol 1988;4:59–65.
10. Sangueza O, Sangueza P, Jordan J, et al. Rhabdomyoma of the tongue. Am J Dermatopathol 1990;12:492–495.
11. Enzinger FM, Weiss SW. Soft Tissue Tumors, 2nd edition. St. Louis: CV Mosby, 1988:448–488.
12. Chanoki M, Sugamoto I, Suzuki S, et al. Nevus lipomatosus superficialis of the scalp. Cutis 1989;43:143–144.

13. Harrington AC, Adnot J, Chesser RS. Infiltrating lipomas of the upper extremities. J Dermatol Surg Oncol 1990;16:834–837.
14. Hurt MA, Santa Cruz DJ. Nodular-cystic fat necrosis. A reevaluation of the so-called mobile encapsulated lipoma. J Am Acad Dermatol 1989;21:493–498.
15. Mrozek K, Karakousis CP, Bloomfield CD. Chromosome 12 breakpoints are cytogenetically different in benign and malignant lipogenic tumors: Localization of breakpoints in lipoma to 12q15 and in myxoid liposarcoma to 12q13.3. Cancer Res 1993; 53:1670–1675.
16. Howard WR, Helwig EB. Angiolipoma. Arch Dermatol 1960; 82:924–931.
17. Enzinger FM, Harvey DA. Spindle cell lipoma. Cancer 1975; 36:1852–1859.
18. Digregorio F, Barr RJ, Fretzin DF. Pleomorphic lipoma: Case reports and review of the literature. J Dermatol Surg Oncol 1992;18:197–202.
19. Novy EG Jr, Wilson JW. Hibernomas, brown fat tumors. Arch Dermatol 1956;73:149–157.
20. Dardick I. Hibernoma: A possible model of brown fat histogenesis. Hum Pathol 1978;9:321–329.
21. Chung EB, Enzinger FM. Benign lipoblastomatosis. An analysis of 35 cases. Cancer 1973;32:482–492.
22. Enzinger FM, Weiss SW. Soft Tissue Tumors, 2nd edition. St. Louis: CV Mosby, 1988:346–382.
23. Coleman WP III. Non-cosmetic applications of liposuction. J Dermatol Surg Oncol 1988;14:1085–1090.
24. Field L, Skouge J, Anhalt T, et al. Blunt liposuction cannula dissection with and without suction assisted lipectomy in reconstructive surgery. J Dermatol Surg Oncol 1988;14:1116–1122.
25. Pinski K, Roenigk H. Liposuction for lipomas. Dermatol Clin 1990;8:483–492.
26. Brownell K, Steen S. Modern methods for weight control: The physiology and psychology of dieting. Phys Sports Med 1987;15:12:122–137.
27. Fischer A, Fischer G. First surgical treatment for molding body's cellulite with three 5-mm incisions. Bull Int Acad Cosmet Surg 1976;3:35.
28. Teimourian B. Complications associated with suction lipectomy. Clin Plast Surg 1989;16:385–394.
29. Teimourin B, Rogers WB. A national survey of complications associated with the suction lipectomy: A comparative study. Plast Reconstr Surg 1989;84:628–631.
30. Chrisman B, Coleman WP III. Determining safe limits for untransfused outpatient liposuction: Personal experience and review of the literature. J Dermatol Surg Oncol 1988;14:1095–1102.
31. Chrisman K. Death following suction lipectomy and abdominoplasty (letter). Plast Reconstr Surg 1986:78:428.
32. Klein JA. The tumescent technique for liposuction surgery. Am J Cosmet Surg 1987:4:263.
33. Klein JA. Tumescent technique for regional anesthesia permits lidocaine doses of 35 mg/kg for liposuction: Peak plasma lidocaine levels are diminished and delayed 12 hours. J Dermatol Surg Oncol 1990;16:248–263.
34. Lillis PJ. The tumescent technique for liposuction surgery. Dermatol Clin 1990;8:439–450.
35. Coleman WP III, Coleman J. Liposuction and the law. Dermatol Clin 1990;5:569–580.
36. Guidelines of care for liposuction. American Academy of Dermatology, 1990.
37. Coleman WP III, Badame A, Phillips H. A new technique for injection of tumescent anesthetic mixtures. J Dermatol Surg Oncol 1991;17:535–537.
38. Fournier P. Why the syringe and not the suction machine? J Dermatol Surg Oncol 1988;14:1062–1069.
39. Fournier P. Reduction syringe undermining. Dermatol Clin 1990;8:539–551.

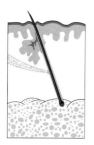

chapter 148

Neural Tumors (Other than Tuberous Sclerosis and Neurofibromatosis)

ZSOLT B. ARGENYI

Cutaneous neural tumors are a small, but important part of clinical dermatology. For decades, these tumors were often misdiagnosed histopathologically because of confusing classifications; consequently, their clinical relevance was poorly understood. Indeed, cutaneous neural tumors clinically often look alike and most of them are benign. However, their correct diagnosis can be helpful in recognizing important clinical syndromes and can contribute to better patient management. Moreover, with the advancement of immunohistochemistry, new variants of cutaneous neural neoplasms have been described.[1]

This chapter should provide a practical clinicopathologic guide for the dermatologist to establish the correct diagnosis of the most important cutaneous neural tumors so that proper treatment can be initiated. For a detailed discussion of rare or controversial entities the reader is referred to several papers and textbooks.[2-8]

Classification, Terminology, and Histogenesis

Cutaneous neural tumors can be classified into two major groups: those derived from peripheral nerves and those from ectopic or heterotopic neural tissue (Table 148–1). The former group is often subdivided into true nerve sheath neoplasms and hamartomatous tumors, although this classification may not be accepted without reservation.[2, 3]

Cutaneous neural tumors either arise from or differentiate toward one or more elements of the nervous system.[9] During their differentiation neural neoplasms often recapitulate to varying degrees the morphogenesis of normal peripheral nerves.[10] Therefore, the knowledge of the organization of the normal peripheral nerve is crucial to understanding the histogenesis of tumors arising from it. The peripheral nerve can be compared to a conventional telephone cable, in which each axon and its surrounding Schwann cell layer correspond with the telephone wires with their insulation. The basic units of a peripheral nerve are nerve fibers, composed of axons and the surrounding Schwann cells. These fibers form nerve fascicles and are held together by a sheath of specialized cells, which is called the perineurium. The space between the individual nerve fibers is called the endoneurium. As in a telephone cable system where the smaller cable units are separated, protected, and held together by an outer wrapping, bundles of nerve fascicles are also encased in a supportive fibrous sheath that is called the epineurium.[10] This architectural arrangement is recognizable in many cutaneous neural neoplasms. The most important constituent cells are the Schwann cell, the perineurial cell, and the various nonspecific mesenchymal cells, such as fibroblasts and mast cells. These cells are capable of proliferation and, therefore, malignant transformation. Other elements of the peripheral nerve, which are cell parts or products (i.e., axons and myelin), cannot duplicate. Schwann cells are derived from the neural crest,[11] and there is good evidence that perineurial cells are modified fibroblasts of mesodermal origin.[5, 12] This difference in histogenesis is also reflected by the distinct antigenic expression of these cells. Schwann cells contain S-100 protein[13, 14] but not epithelial membrane anti-

TABLE 148-1. Classification of Cutaneous Neural Neoplasms

Tumors of the Peripheral Nerves	Tumors of Ectopic or Heterotopic Neural Tissue
True neuromas	Nasal glioma
Traumatic type	Extracranial meningioma
Palisaded, encapsulated type	Neuroectodermal tumors
True nerve sheath tumors	Peripheral neuroepithelioma (neuroblastoma)
Schwannoma	
Neurofibroma	
Nerve sheath myxoma	
Granular cell tumor	
Malignant nerve sheath neoplasms	

gen,[15] whereas perineurial cells stain for epithelial membrane antigen but not for S-100 protein. Axons contain a specific type of intermediate filament called neurofilaments, and myelinated axons contain myelin basic protein, both of which can be detected by immunohistochemistry.[16] These and other immunohistochemical markers often help to establish the correct diagnosis.[17]

Clinically Important Cutaneous Neural Tumors

TRUE NEUROMAS

Traumatic or Amputation Neuroma

Definition. Neuromas are proliferations of neural tissue in which Schwann cells and axons are present in roughly equal numbers. Traumatic or amputation neuromas are complex regenerative proliferations of nerve fibers secondary to injury.

Clinical Description. Traumatic neuromas are relatively uncommon, but they can occur at any age and in either sex.[18] Traumatic neuromas are usually solitary, skin-colored or reddish purple, firm papules or nodules at sites of wounds, surgical scars, and amputations.[19] On the lower extremities they tend to be multiple. Early lesions are asymptomatic, but after a few months they gradually become sensitive and painful, frequently with a lancinating character. Variable tingling and itching can be associated with the pain.[18, 19]

In neonates and small infants, the lesions may be located at the lateral-volar aspects of the hand, in which case they represent amputation neuromas secondary to amputation in utero of supernumerary digits.[20] These tumors are occasionally referred to as "rudimentary supernumerary digits"; however, on histologic examination they do not contain either normal or rudimentary elements of a digit.

The clinical differential diagnosis of traumatic neuroma includes hypertrophic scar, dermatofibroma, angiomyoma, and granuloma.

Pathology. Traumatic or amputation neuromas are usually well-circumscribed nodular lesions located at any level of the dermis or the subcutis. They are encased by a fibrous sheath, although the distal end can be poorly defined. The proliferation is composed of a chaotic, poorly organized tangle of fascicles of various sizes and shapes (Fig. 148–1A).[2, 3] Between the fibers are variable amounts of fibrous tissue with or without inflammatory cells or mucin.[5, 21] The constituent cells are Schwann cells and perineurial cells with spindle-shaped nuclei and cytoplasm. Special stains show many axons in an irregular pattern (Fig. 148–1B).[2, 3, 21]

Pathogenesis and Etiology. Any extrinsic damage to nerve fibers can cause a neuroma. Amputation neuroma is considered the most common form and represents an attempted, but failed regeneration of the nerve fibers after transection.[2, 3, 5] After transection, the distal segments of the nerve fibers degenerate, whereas the proximal segments regenerate in an attempt to reunite with the distal portion of the transected nerve fibers.[22] In case of severe trauma, this regenerative process is unsuccessful and the growing nerve fibers form a tangle of fascicles within fibrotic tissue.[1] Despite marked variations in arrangement, size, and shape of the regenerating fascicles, in traumatic neuromas the constituent fibers have a Schwann cell to axon ratio close to a normal 1:1, which helps to distinguish true neuromas from nerve sheath neoplasms.[18–21, 23]

Diagnosis and Differential Diagnosis. The diagnosis of traumatic neuroma is usually suspected by the history of a painful or symptomatic small mass at a site of injury and is confirmed by pathologic examination after biopsy.

Treatment. Simple surgical excision suffices in most cases.

Palisaded Encapsulated Neuroma

Definition. Palisaded encapsulated or solitary circumscribed neuromas are complex hamartomatous proliferations of nerve fibers without apparent previous tissue injury.[24]

Clinical Description. Palisaded encapsulated neuromas develop spontaneously and gradually, without evidence of obvious previous trauma.[24] They manifest in adults (mean age, 45.5 years) with about equal occurrence in males and females. The individual lesions are asymptomatic, rubbery, firm, skin-colored or pink papules and nodules in a size range of 0.2 to 0.6 cm. Approximately 90% of them are located on the face, mostly around the nose, but they also occur on the cheek, chin, and lips.[25–27] The remaining 10% occur elsewhere, including the trunk and extremities. The most common clinical diagnoses include intradermal nevi, basal cell carcinoma, adnexal tumors, and neurofibroma.[25]

The other less common, but important setting with which the dermatologist should be familiar is the multiple mucosal neuromata syndrome.[28, 29] In this syndrome there are numerous, soft, skin- or mucosa-colored papules and nodules around the lips, on the tongue, and eyelids, and in the oral cavity. Histologically, these lesions are also true neuromas but are multiple and often

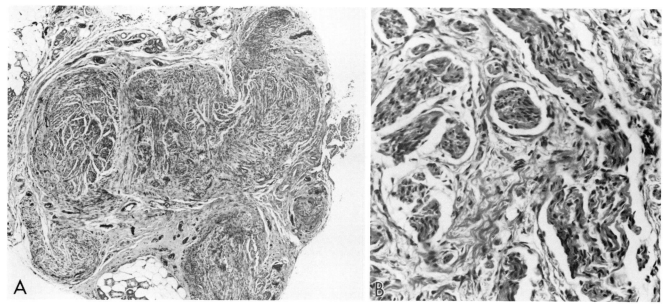

FIGURE 148-1. *A,* Traumatic neuroma. The chaotic proliferation of nerve fascicles is embedded in a fibrous stroma (H&E, ×10). *B,* The individually proliferating fascicles retain their resemblance to normal nerves, but their shape and size markedly vary (H&E, ×50).

not encapsulated. This syndrome is usually part of the multiple endocrine neoplasia syndrome (type 2b), in which pheochromocytoma and medullary carcinoma of the thyroid also occur; therefore, its early recognition can be lifesaving.[29, 30]

Pathology. Palisaded encapsulated neuroma is a well-circumscribed, ovoid or round tumor located in the mid dermis, although some lesions may extend to the subcutis.[24] The lesions appear encapsulated by a thick condensation of collagen fibers around the tumor, and there is often some clefting from the adjacent dermis (Fig. 148-2A). This encapsulation is not always evident.[25-27, 31] The parenchyma is composed of interwoven

fascicles of spindled cells. The fascicles are compactly and relatively uniformly arranged, separated only by clefts (see Fig. 148-2B). There is no evidence of extensive fibrosis, inflammation, granulation tissue, degenerative changes, or foreign bodies, in contradistinction to traumatic neuromas. Increased vasculature is rare.[32] The spindled cells have eosinophilic cytoplasm with indistinct cell membranes. The nuclei are elongated, are wavy with tapered ends, and have an evenly basophilic chromatin pattern. Occasionally, a parallel arrangement of the nuclei is present, but, despite its name, distinct palisading or Verocay body formation is rare. There is no appreciable nuclear pleomorphism, and mitotic figures

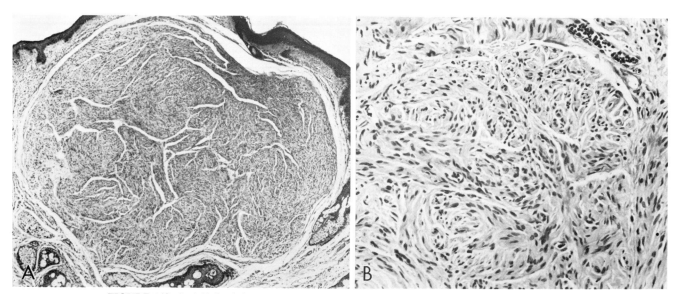

FIGURE 148-2. *A,* Palisaded encapsulated neuroma. The well-circumscribed dermal nodule appears encapsulated (H&E, ×10). *B,* The fascicles are tightly arranged with occasional palisading of nuclei (H&E, ×50). (*A* and *B,* from Argenyi ZB. Newly recognized neural neoplasms relevant to the dermatopathologist. Dermatol Clin 1992;10:219-234.)

are scant or absent. Special stains show abundant axons in a variable pattern.[21, 31, 32] A histologic variant of this tumor can be seen in the multiple mucosal neuromata syndrome.[28] In this variant, the tumors are cytologically and to some extent architecturally similar to palisaded encapsulated neuromas but are not encapsulated and are multiple.[29, 30]

Pathogenesis and Etiology. Palisaded encapsulated neuroma was described by Reed and coworkers,[24] who proposed that it was due to hyperplasia of nerve fibers. There is an overgrowth of axons and their sheath cells within the confinement of the perineurium.[25-27, 31] The tumor most likely represents a hamartomatous growth in which there is a close reduplication of the normal axon to Schwann cell ratio (Fig. 148-3). The cause of the overgrowth of neurites is not known; and although minor tissue injury such as inflammation induced by acne was suggested,[25] a definite traumatic origin cannot be established in the majority of cases.[21, 31, 32]

Diagnosis and Differential Diagnosis. The diagnosis is made on histologic examination. Most palisaded encapsulated neuromas are facial papules, clinically thought to be intradermal nevi, basal cell carcinoma, or small cysts.

Treatment. This tumor is benign, and no cases of malignant transformation or metastasis have been reported. The treatment is usually simple excision or, in case of superficial location, the lesion can be shelled out (i.e., "enucleated") from the surrounding dermis.

TRUE NERVE SHEATH NEOPLASMS

In contrast to neuromas, true nerve sheath neoplasms are proliferations of the endoneurial or perineurial nerve sheath elements of the cutaneous nerves.[4, 5] Axons do not duplicate in these lesions.[33]

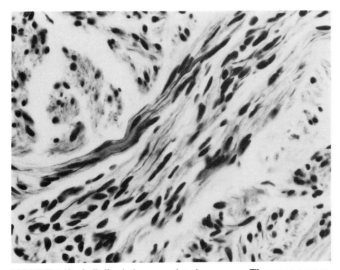

FIGURE 148-3. Palisaded encapsulated neuroma. There are numerous axons present, seen as thin dark lines parallel with the long axis of the fascicles (Bielschowsky's silver impregnation, ×100).

Common Schwannoma (Neurilemmoma)

Definition. Schwannomas are benign neoplasms of Schwann cells, with only minor populations of other types of neural cells.

Clinical Description. Schwannomas are relatively uncommon tumors that can occur at any age but are most often evident in adults and are slightly more frequent in females than in males.[34, 35] They present as solitary, soft, pink to yellow smooth-surfaced dermal or subcutaneous nodules or tumors. Their size ranges between 0.5 and 3.0 cm, but extreme exceptions do occur. They are most commonly found on the flexor aspects of the extremities along the larger nerve trunks, followed by head and neck areas.[36, 37] The tumors are usually asymptomatic, but rarely pain and tenderness occur, especially if the tumor is forcefully moved and the attached nerve is being placed under tension. Motor disturbances and paresthesias are extremely rare.[35]

The solitary schwannoma can be part of von Recklinghausen's disease and can be associated with various central nervous system tumors. Rare cases of multiple schwannomas have also been described under the term *neurolemmomatosis* but are not consistently associated with von Recklinghausen's disease.[38, 39]

Pathology. Schwannomas are well-circumscribed, nodular or ovoid tumors located in the deep dermis or subcutis (Fig. 148-4A). They are almost invariably encapsulated.[31, 40, 41] The tumors are composed of hypercellular (also called Antoni-A type of tissue) and hypocellular (Antoni-B type of tissue) areas. The hypercellular areas show proliferation of spindle cells with indistinct cytoplasmic membranes and uniform nuclei. Nuclear palisading and arrangement of palisaded nuclei in double rows, so-called Verocay bodies, are characteristic features of these tumors (Fig. 148-4B).[40, 41] Mitotic figures are absent or rare. The hypocellular areas show variable degrees of degeneration, including cystic, edematous, mucinous, fibrotic, and vascular changes. Degenerative changes are often associated with some degree of cytologic atypia. These so-called ancient schwannomas should not be confused with the more specific entity of cellular schwannomas, which may display similar degenerative changes but rarely occur in the skin.[42, 43] As a general rule, schwannomas are devoid of axons or they can be detected only at the site at which they are attached to a nerve.

Pathogenesis and Etiology. Schwannomas exclusively derive from the proliferation of periaxonal or endoneurial Schwann cells.[3, 4] As a result of the Schwann cell proliferation, the remaining normal nerve fibers are displaced to the periphery of the tumor, creating a virtual lack of the other components of a peripheral nerve. Indeed, only after careful dissection can the attached nerve trunk be demonstrated.[2, 40, 41] Since only the Schwann cells proliferate, the neoplasm will remain within the confinement of the perineurium, forming an encapsulated tumor. The cause of the exclusive Schwann cell proliferation is unknown.

Diagnosis and Differential Diagnosis. The clinical differential diagnosis includes lipoma, angiolipoma, adnexal tumors, dermoid cysts, leiomyoma, nevi, and

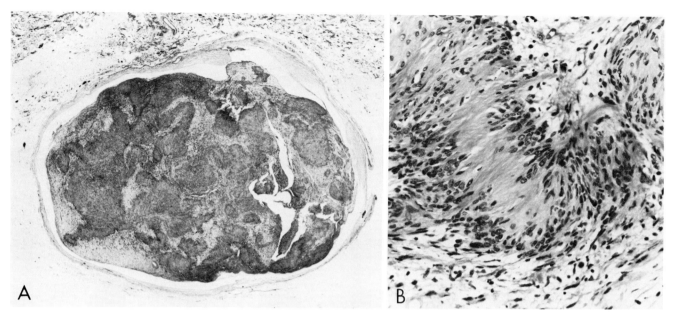

FIGURE 148-4. *A*, Solitary cutaneous schwannoma. Encapsulated nodule in the deep dermis composed of hypercellular and hypocellular areas (H&E, ×5). *B*, Hypercellular areas often show nuclear palisading and Verocay bodies (H&E, ×66).

ganglions. The diagnosis is made by histopathologic examination (see Tables 148-2 and 148-3).

Treatment. The tumor is benign, and a simple excision is almost invariably curative. If the clinical diagnosis is reasonably firm, the lesion can be removed by careful enucleation, which preserves normal nerve function.

Neurofibroma

Definition. A neurofibroma is a tumor composed of a complex proliferation of neuromesenchymal tissue (Schwann cells, perineurial cells, fibroblasts, and mast cells and their products).[2, 3]

Clinical Description. The ordinary, solitary forms of cutaneous neurofibromas are relatively common in adults and equally present in both sexes. They are usually solitary, skin-colored, soft or rubbery papules or nodules; and with time they may become pedunculated.[4, 44] They grow slowly and are asymptomatic. A "buttonhole sign" is often present. There are several clinical and pathologic subtypes of neurofibroma, such as the diffuse, pigmented, and plexiform variants.[4] Plexiform neurofibroma is especially important because it has a characteristic clinical appearance and it is considered pathognomonic of von Recklinghausen's disease.[4, 45] Typically, these tumors are baggy or pedunculated rope-like dermal and subcutaneous masses that on occasion are covered by hyperpigmented skin.[45-47] Recognition and correct patient management is crucial in these cases, especially in forme fruste cases of von Recklinghausen's disease, when the other cutaneous stigmata are not obvious[45] (see Chapter 166). About 10% of patients with common types of neurofibromas have multiple lesions, and some of these patients may have neurofibromatosis.

Pathology. Neurofibromas are poorly to well circum-

scribed, unencapsulated nodular or oblong lesions that can be located anywhere in the dermis and subcutis (Fig. 148-5*A*). The common solitary variant is usually present in the superficial dermis and is frequently pedunculated.[2-4] The tumor is composed of a fine fibrillary lattice of haphazardly arranged slender spindle cells (see Fig. 148-5*B*). The stroma can be variably vascular, fibrotic, edematous, or myxomatous.[2-4] Besides the Schwann cells and perineurial cells, plump fibroblasts and mast cells are present. Palisading of nuclei can occur, but true Verocay body formation is extremely rare. As opposed to the superficial forms, neurofibromas, which are seated in the deep dermis, subcutis, and other deep, soft tissues, are usually encapsulated by the perineurium or the epineurium and may show a plexiform growth pattern (Fig. 148-6).[2-4] By special stains rare scattered axons can be demonstrated in both the superficial and the deep variants.[4]

Pathogenesis and Etiology. Neurofibromas differ from schwannomas in that several cell types are involved in their histogenesis. Regardless of the various histologic subtypes of neurofibromas (e.g., solitary, diffuse, combined, plexiform), the basic process is proliferation of the entire "neuromesenchyme," which includes the Schwann cells, endoneurial fibroblasts, perineurial cells, mast cells, and so on.[2, 3] Since the extent of proliferation of each cell line is often different, the resulting histologic composition and architecture are variable. As stated earlier, the axons do not duplicate; therefore their relative ratio to the Schwann cells will be less than 1:1. Although the basic process of multiple cell type proliferation is common in all types of neurofibroma, the cause of the individual growth patterns, such as solitary, diffuse, and plexiform, is not known.

Diagnosis and Differential Diagnosis. The clinical differential diagnosis includes dermal nevi, neuromas, soft

TABLE 148–2. Clinical Features of Benign Neural Neoplasms

	Traumatic Neuroma	Palisaded Encapsulated Neuroma	Neurofibroma (Common, Solitary Type)	Schwannoma (Neurilemmoma)	Nerve Sheath Myxoma	Cellular Neurothekeoma	Granular Cell Tumor
Incidence Age	Uncommon; Any	Rare; Adults (mean age, 45.5 years)	Very common; Adults (20–60 years)	Uncommon; Adults (20–50 years)	Rare; Adults (mean age, 48 years)	Rare; Early adulthood (mean age, 24 years)	Rare; Adults (30–50 years)
Gender	Any	1:1 = M:F	1:1 = M:F	F > M	1:2 = M:F	F > M	1:3 = M:F
Number	Usually solitary	Usually solitary	Usually solitary	Usually solitary	Usually solitary	Usually solitary	Usually solitary
Location	At sites of trauma, surgical scars, amputations	90% face, 10% elsewhere	Trunk, head	Flexor aspects of extremities, head	Head and upper extremities	Predominantly on head, but also anywhere	30% tongue, 70% elsewhere, mainly head and neck
Size	0.5–2 cm	0.2–0.6 cm	0.2–2.0 cm	0.3–3.0 cm	0.5–1 cm	0.5–3 cm	0.5–3.0 cm
Clinical appearance	Skin-colored, firm papules or nodules	Skin-colored or pink, rubbery, firm papules or nodules	Skin-colored, soft or rubbery papules or nodules, sometimes pedunculated	Soft, pink, yellow smooth-surfaced nodules or tumors	Soft, skin-colored papules and nodules	Pink, red, brown firm papules and nodules	Skin-colored, brownish red raised, firm nodules; may have ulceration and verrucous surface
Symptoms	Variable, tingling, itching, lancinating pain	Asymptomatic	Asymptomatic; "buttonhole" sign may be present	Asymptomatic; rarely painful, tender or paresthetic; occasionally freely movable	Asymptomatic	Usually asymptomatic, rarely sore or itchy	Asymptomatic or occasionally tender or pruritic
Association	NA	A variant is part of multiple mucosal neuromata syndrome, marfanoid habitus, neuroendocrine neoplasms	If multiple, may be part of von Recklinghausen's disease (10%)	Rarely with von Recklinghausen's disease or central nervous system tumors	NA	NA	10% multiple; predilection for blacks; rare in children
Clinical differential diagnosis	Hypertrophic scar, dermatofibroma, granuloma	Dermal nevi, basal cell carcinoma, neurofibroma	Dermal nevi, dermatofibroma, neuroma, soft fibroma	Lipoma, angiolipoma, adnexal tumors, dermoid or pilar cysts, leiomyoma, ganglion	Myxoid cysts, ganglions, dermal nevi, fibrolipoma	Dermatofibroma, keloid, hemangioma, dermal nevi	Dermatofibroma, neurofibroma, adnexal tumor, dermal nevi
Other	"Rudimentary supernumerary digit" is considered as variant	May be induced by minor trauma	Plexiform variant is pathognomonic for von Recklinghausen's disease	May be multiple; syndrome of "schwannomatosis"			Visceral forms occur; malignant transformation may occur (3%)

NA, not applicable.

TABLE 148–3. Histologic Differential Diagnostic Features of Common Cutaneous Neural Neoplasms

Feature	Traumatic Neuroma	Palisaded Encapsulated Neuroma	Neurofibroma	Schwannoma
Location in the skin	Any level of dermis or subcutis	Upper or mid dermis	Any location in the dermis	Deep dermis or subcutis
Growth pattern	Usually well circumscribed but may be irregular at the distal end	Well circumscribed, nodular, rarely plexiform	Poorly to well circumscribed	Well circumscribed, nodular or ovoid
Encapsulation	Usually encased by fibrous sheath	Yes, by perineurium	Not encapsulated in the dermis	Yes, by perineurium
Architecture	Chaotic, poorly organized tangle of fascicles of various sizes and shapes	Compactly arranged fascicles; frequent clefts between fascicles	Fine fibrillary lattice of haphazardly arranged spindle cells in variably dense matrix	Hypercellular areas (Antoni-A), fascicles in various patterns, hypocellular areas (Antoni-B), edematous, myxoid
Constituent cell types	Schwann cells, fibroblasts, perineurial cells, inflammatory cells, macrophages	Schwann cells (99%), perineurial cells (in capsule only)	Schwann cells, perineurial cells, fibroblasts, mast cells	Schwann cells (99%), perineurial cells (in capsule only)
Cytologic features	Spindle cells with indistinct cytoplasmic membrane and tapered slender nuclei	Spindle cells with indistinct cytoplasmic membrane and tapered slender nuclei	Spindle cells with slender nuclei, plump fibroblasts	Spindle cells with indistinct cytoplasmic membrane and slender nuclei
Nuclear palisading	None	Usually present, but indistinct	Rarely	Yes, prominent in Antoni-A areas
Verocay bodies	None	None	None	Often
Nerve fibers (axons)	Yes, abundant irregular pattern	Yes, abundant often in parallel arrangement	Yes, rare, scattered	None or only at the site of the connecting nerve
Other important features	Nerve of origin frequently present, extensive fibrosis	Nerve of origin frequently present, no fibrosis	Variable fibrosis and myxoid changes, occasional blood vessels, mast cells	Mast cells; may have extensive degenerative changes (hyalinization, hemorrhage, etc.) in Antoni-B areas ("ancient changes")
Histopathologic differential diagnosis	Hypertrophic scar, neurofibroma, schwannoma	Traumatic neuroma, schwannoma, angioleiomyoma, myofibroma	Dermatofibroma, hypertrophic scar, dermatofibrosarcoma protuberance, traumatic neuroma, neural nevus	Palisaded, encapsulated neuroma, angiomyoma, fibrous histiocytoma

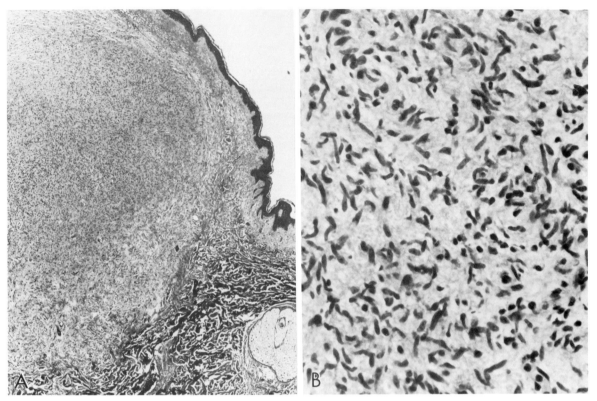

FIGURE 148–5. *A,* Cutaneous neurofibroma. A well-circumscribed but not encapsulated nodular mass in the upper dermis (H&E, ×10). *B,* The tumor contains diffuse proliferation of spindle cells with slender, ovoid nuclei in a fibrillary matrix (H&E, ×100).

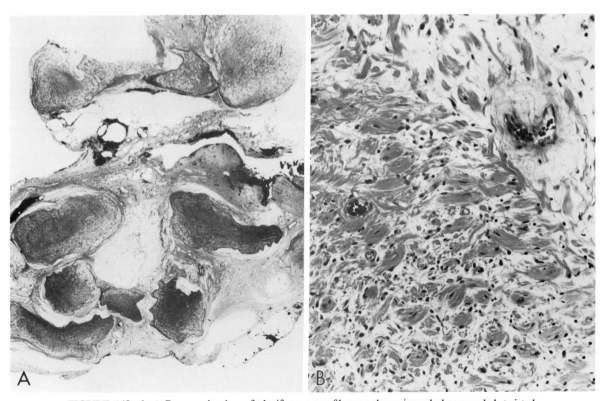

FIGURE 148–6. *A,* Panoramic view of plexiform neurofibroma shows irregularly expanded, twisted nerve fascicles (H&E, ×25). *B,* Diffuse proliferation of spindle cells in a fibrotic and myxoid stroma (H&E, ×50).

fibromas, and dermatofibroma. The diagnosis is confirmed by histopathologic examination (see Tables 148–2 and 148–3).

Treatment. Neurofibromas are usually treated by simple excision. The treatment of plexiform neurofibromas and multiple cutaneous neurofibromas is discussed in detail in Chapter 166.

Nerve Sheath Myxoma and Cellular Neurothekeoma

Definition. Nerve sheath myxoma, which is also often designated as neurothekeoma, is a recently described tumor composed of nerve sheath cells and mucinous stroma arranged in a lobular pattern.[48–53] Nerve sheath myxoma can be subclassified into classic, myxoid type and cellular types.[54–58]

The neural origin of the cellular variant still awaits confirmation.

Classic Nerve Sheath Myxoma

Clinical Description. The classic or myxoid type of neural sheath myxoma occurs commonly in middle-aged adults (mean age, 48 years) with an approximate 1:2 male-to-female ratio. The lesions are soft, skin-colored papules and nodules, are generally 0.5 to 1.0 cm in diameter, and are typically located on the head and upper extremities.

Pathology. Microscopically, the classic myxoid type of nerve sheath myxoma is a well-defined, lobular or plexiform neoplasm that is usually located in the reticular dermis (Fig. 148–7*A*). It often appears encapsulated by compression of the surrounding fibrous tissue.[56, 58] There is hypocellular myxoid stroma with rare, scattered, spindled, stellate, or dendritic cells (see Fig. 148–7*B*). The

cells usually have scant, pale cytoplasm with indistinct cytoplasmic contours and hyperchromatic, ovoid, or angulated nuclei. Nucleoli are small, and mitotic figures are rare or absent. On occasion, multinucleated giant cells with eosinophilic cytoplasm can be identified. Histochemically, the myxoid stroma stains strongly positively for acidic mucopolysaccharides.[48, 58] While entrapped nerves in and around the tumor can be identified, the presence of scattered axons or direct continuity of axons with tumor cells has not been established.[58] The histopathologic differential diagnosis of classic nerve sheath myxoma includes the myxoid plexiform neurofibroma, pacinian neurofibroma, myxoid cysts, "ganglions," and variants of focal cutaneous mucinosis.

Cellular Neurothekeoma

Clinical Description. The cellular form of nerve sheath myxoma, or as originally proposed, the cellular neurothekeoma,[54, 55] is also a tumor of adulthood, but it usually affects younger adults (mean age, 24 years). As in the classic form, this variant is more common in women and occurs predominantly on the head.[55] However, cases from essentially all body sites have been reported. Unlike the classic type of nerve sheath myxoma, cellular neurothekeoma is characterized by firm, pink, red, brown papules or nodules ranging from 0.5 to 3.0 cm.[56] Clinical symptoms are mild or nonspecific and seem to relate to the size and firmness of the tumor.

Pathology. On histologic sections, cellular neurothekeoma is composed of ill-defined multilobular masses or fascicles in the reticular dermis (Fig. 148–8*A*).[54–58] In some cases, the growth pattern can be frankly infiltrative or dissecting without any hint of a residual capsule and there may be involvement of superficial subcutis. Cytologically, the predominant cell types are epithelioid or polygonal cells with usually ample eosinophilic cyto-

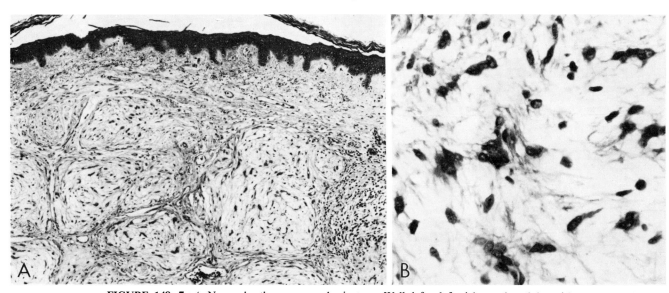

FIGURE 148–7. *A,* Nerve sheath myxoma, classic type. Well-defined fascicles and nodules with myxoid stroma (H&E, ×10). *B,* Spindle and stellate cells embedded in mucinous material (H&E, ×100). (*A,* from Argenyi ZB. Newly recognized neural neoplasms relevant to the dermatopathologist. Dermatol Clin 1992;10:219–234.)

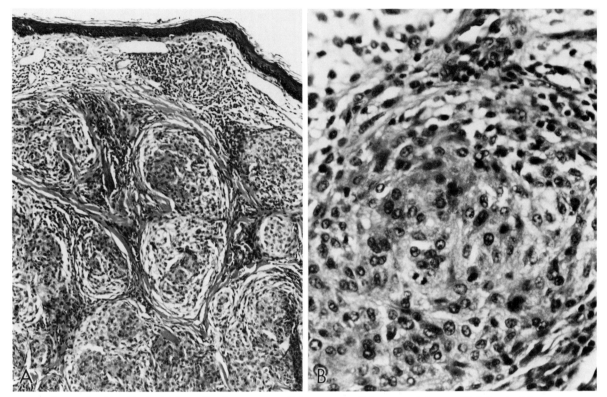

FIGURE 148-8. *A,* Nerve sheath myxoma, cellular type or cellular neurothekeoma: Ill-defined epithelioid nests are dispersed in a hyalinized stroma (H&E, ×10). *B,* Whorl-like arrangement of epithelioid cells showing nuclear pleomorphism and rare mitotic figures (H&E, ×100).

plasm and round nuclei with an "open" chromatin pattern (see Fig. 148-8*B*).[56-58] Many cells have prominent nucleoli.

Less often, the constituent cells are spindled or plump with hyperchromatic nuclei as seen in the classic form of nerve sheath myxoma.[58] Mitotic figures are often present but are normal. The stroma can be markedly fibrotic or even hyalinized. An obvious direct connection with peripheral nerves has not been established, but branches of preexisting nerve fibers can be demonstrated by special stains. Microscopically, the differential diagnosis of cellular neurothekeoma includes epithelioid Spitz nevus, deep penetrating nevus, plexiform spindle cell nevus, the fascicular variant of cellular blue nevus, and, to a lesser extent, spindle cell malignant melanoma.[56]

Pathogenesis and Etiology. Nerve sheath myxoma has a controversial histogenesis that is reflected in a plethora of terms (e.g., cutaneous lobular neuromyxoma, myxomatous perineurioma, myxoma of the nerve sheath). Both Schwann cells and perineurial cells are present in classic neural sheath myxoma.[49-53, 58] The reason for extreme mucin production is unknown, although mucin is part of the normal endoneurium. Some authors speculated that nerve sheath myxoma could represent a variant of neurofibroma with extreme myxoid degeneration.[53] This degeneration may explain the virtual lack of axons in these tumors. Although the available immunohistochemical and ultrastructural data support the nerve sheath differentiation in the classic, myxoid variant, there is no uniformly accepted view regarding the histo-

genesis of the cellular variant.[58] Although cellular neurothekeomas have some features suggesting neural differentiation, they usually do not express S-100 protein (as do Schwann cells) or epithelial membrane antigen (as perineurial cells do) but can be partially positive for smooth muscle specific antigen and for a melanocyte marker, NKI/C3 antigen. Some lesions have features of both the classic and cellular variants, but the exact route of differentiation in cellular neurothekeoma is unknown.[55, 56]

Diagnosis and Differential Diagnosis. Neural sheath myxomas are usually asymptomatic and clinically are mistaken for myxoid cysts, ganglions, dermal nevi, fibrolipomas, and adnexal neoplasms.[49-53, 56] The clinical impression of cellular neurothekeoma is usually of a dermatofibroma, keloid, hemangioma, dermal nevus, or even pyogenic granuloma.[58] The diagnosis is made histopathologically (see Tables 148-2 and 148-3).

Treatment. Both variants of nerve sheath myxoma are benign. They are usually treated by simple excision; however, in case of incomplete removal, nerve sheath myxoma may recur.

Granular Cell Tumor

Definition. Granular cell tumor is a descriptive term for a heterogeneous group of neoplasms composed of cells with granular cytoplasm due to the accumulation of lysosomal granules. Most cutaneous granular cell neoplasms are of neural origin, but granular cell change occurs in a variety of neoplasms.[59]

Clinical Description. Granular cell tumor is a relatively rare tumor that occurs mainly in adults (age 30–50 years) with a 1:3 male-to-female ratio. The tumor is characteristically solitary, and 70% of them are located on the head and neck areas with 30% of these confined to the tongue.[60, 61] In approximately 10% of the cases, the lesions are multiple, with a predilection for blacks.[62] The tumor presents as asymptomatic or occasionally tender or pruritic, skin-colored, brownish red, firm dermal or subcutaneous papules or nodules ranging in size from 0.5 to 3.0 cm. Occasionally the surface can show ulceration or verrucous changes.

Pathology. The dermis contains a poorly circumscribed nodule or infiltrative collection of polygonal, pale-staining cells. The cells have abundant, granular, faintly eosinophilic cytoplasm with round, dark nuclei (Fig. 148–9).[61] With periodic acid–Schiff reaction the granules are positive but diastase resistant. Rare mitotic figures are occasionally encountered.[61] The tumor is devoid of axons. Increased numbers of mast cells are present in some lesions. The overlying epidermis is frequently acanthotic.

Pathogenesis and Etiology. The neural origin of this tumor is debatable and is primarily based on the observation that granular cells sometimes are intimately associated with nerves and other neural tumors.[61-64] In addition, granular cells contain S-100 protein and Leu-7 antigen, as do Schwann cell tumors.[65, 66] However, the classic form of this tumor does not resemble any other types of peripheral nerve sheath tumor. Recent immunohistochemical studies suggest a neural crest–derived peripheral nerve–related cell differentiation.[67] Despite the controversy about its histogenesis, the tumor is histologically distinct and rarely presents a diagnostic problem.

Diagnosis and Differential Diagnosis. The clinical differential diagnosis includes dermatofibroma, adnexal tumors, dermal nevi, and verrucous keratoses.[61] The

diagnosis is made microscopically. Granular cell tumors can evoke pseudocarcinomatous hyperplasia of overlying epithelium, and superficial biopsy samples have been mistaken for squamous cell carcinoma, especially on the tongue. A variety of epithelial and mesenchymal neoplasms can show granular cell change, including basal cell carcinoma, leiomyoma, and leiomyosarcoma.[59]

Treatment. Granular cell tumors are slowly growing lesions with usually benign behavior. However, in approximately 3% of the cases, malignant behavior was reported, mainly in visceral or deep locations. The general treatment is simple, complete excision.

Malignant Peripheral Nerve Sheath Tumor

The term *malignant peripheral nerve sheath tumor* is preferable to the widely used but confusing terminology of neurosarcoma, neurofibrosarcoma, and malignant schwannoma.[68-70] This term implies that any cellular component of the peripheral nerve could give rise to these tumors, although their relative participation can be extremely variable. Interestingly, in the majority of the cases, the perineurial or endoneurial fibroblasts rather than Schwann cells form the bulk of the tumor (Fig. 148–10).[68] Malignant peripheral nerve sheath tumor is a tumor of deep soft tissues and rarely involves the skin.[71] However, it is of great clinical importance because in approximately 50% of the cases it is associated with neurofibromatosis, especially with plexiform neurofibromas.[72-74] These features are discussed in more detail in Chapter 166 under neurofibromatosis.

TUMORS AND TUMOR-LIKE CONDITIONS OF ECTOPIC AND HETEROTOPIC NEURAL TISSUE OF THE SKIN

These lesions develop from embryologically misplaced neural tissue within the skin. They range from benign

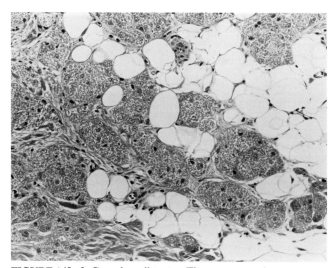

FIGURE 148–9. Granular cell tumor. The tumor may show a nodular or infiltrative growth pattern. The large polygonal cells have finely granular cytoplasm and round nuclei (H&E, ×50).

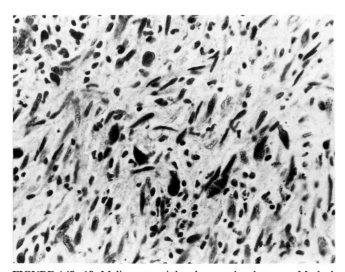

FIGURE 148–10. Malignant peripheral nerve sheath tumor. Marked cellular pleomorphism with cytologic atypia and mitotic activity (H&E, ×100).

malformations to cellular proliferations with potential for metastasis.

The clinicopathologic features of the cutaneous heterotopic neural tissues are much more variable than those of the tumors of the peripheral nerves. Although these tumors in general are extremely rare, the dermatologist should be familiar with their cardinal features. For this reason, only a concise discussion is provided here. A more comprehensive overview of the differential diagnostic features of cutaneous ectopic and heterotopic neural tumors is summarized in Table 148–4.

Nasal Glioma

The term *nasal glioma* is misleading because the tumor is due to embryologic displacement of brain tissue and is not a true neoplasm.[75] Ectopic brain tissue can be found along cranial closure lines, most commonly around the nasal bones.[76, 77] The lesion contains predominantly glial tissue, and the neurons are often absent or degenerated (Fig. 148–11).[77]

Cutaneous Meningioma

There are three distinct pathways by which these tumors develop.[78] In type I, nests of ectopic arachnoid lining cells are misplaced during embryogenesis. This type is usually located on the scalp, on the forehead, and in the paravertebral area. In some cases the cells are part of a rudimentary cystic channel and such lesions are more appropriately designated as rudimentary meningoceles.[79, 80] Type II variants develop along the course of the cranial nerves and therefore are mostly located on the head. It is postulated that these cells are derived from

the dura mater extending along the channels of the cranial nerves.[78] Type III lesions are cutaneous metastasis or direct extensions of central nervous system meningiomas.[78] With the exception of the rudimentary meningocele, the main histopathologic features of meningiomas are similar in all three types (Fig. 148–12).

Cutaneous Neuroblastoma and Peripheral Neuroepithelioma

Cutaneous tumors with features of neuroblastoma are either metastases of classic neuroblastoma of adrenal or ganglionic origin or, exceedingly rarely, derived from peripheral heterotopic primitive neuroectodermal tissue.[81, 82] The former is relatively common in childhood, whereas the latter variant has paradoxically been described mainly in adults.[83, 84] Irrespectively of the histogenesis, the two types are histologically indistinguishable, because both are composed of small, round blue tumor cells (Fig. 148–13).[83]

Metastatic cutaneous neuroblastomas in children often manifest multiple, reddish, violaceous, or bluish papules or nodules, mimicking the "blueberry sign" due to extramedullary hematopoiesis seen in various severe congenital infections in infants, such as toxoplasmosis and cytomegalovirus infection.[85–87]

Treatment

Although most cutaneous neural malformation can be effectively treated by simple excision, the surgery should be preceded by radiologic and neurosurgical consultations. This is especially important if nasal glioma, cutaneous meningioma or meningocele is suspected.[75–80] Ex-

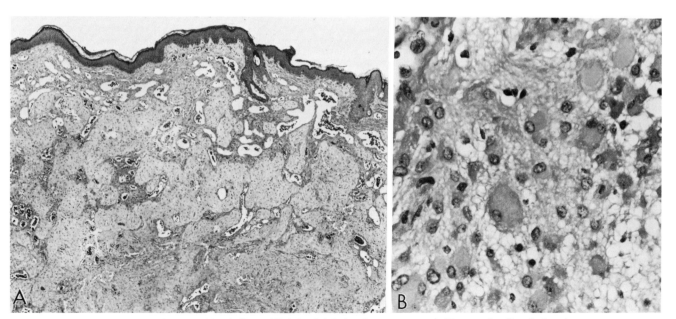

FIGURE 148–11. *A,* Nasal glioma. Ill-defined, lobulated mass surrounded by vascular fibrotic dermis (H&E, ×10). *B,* Round and ovoid glial cells admixed with large oligodendrocytes embedded in neuropile-type tissue (H&E, ×100).

TABLE 148–4. Tumors and Tumor-like Conditions of Ectopic and Heterotopic Neural Tissue of the Skin

	Nasal Glioma	Cutaneous Meningioma	Rudimentary Meningocele	Peripheral Neuroblastoma
Incidence	Rare	Extremely rare	Rare	Extremely rare
Age	Neonates	Neonates or infants	Neonates, young adults	Late adulthood
Location	Most common near the root of the nose but can be intranasal	Scalp, forehead, paravertebral areas	Scalp, forehead, paravertebral areas	Head and trunk
Size	0.5–3.0 cm	0.5–4.0 cm	0.5–3.0 cm	0.5–5.0 cm
Clinical appearance	Firm, smooth, red-purple nodules or tumors	Soft to firm nodules often with alopecia	Soft to firm nodules, often with alopecia	Soft, skin-colored or red, often ulcerated nodules
Clinical differential diagnosis	Hemangioma, nasal polyp, xanthoma, dermoid cysts	Skin tag, fibroma, cyst, nevi	Skin tag, fibroma, cyst, nevi	Lipoma, dermatofibroma, metastatic tumor
Associations	Encephalocele (20%) with intracranial connections	May be associated with von Recklinghausen's disease and acoustic neuromas	May be associated with other developmental abnormalities (encephalocele)	NA
Other	NA	Metastasis of central nervous system meningioma must be excluded	NA	Metastasis of ganglionic or adrenal neuroblastoma and extension of olfactory neuroblastoma must be excluded, especially in children
Histopathologic features	Lobulated neural tissue (glial cells, astrocytes, rarely true neurons)	Solid nests and strands, whorls of epithelioid or spindle cells, psammoma bodies	Cystic or cavernous spaces, scattered meningothelial cells, pseudovascular pattern, psammoma bodies	Rosette-like (Homer Wright type) structures of small, round, blue cells, extensive infiltration and necrosis
Biologic course	Benign	Locally aggressive and destructive	Benign	Extremely malignant with widespread metastases

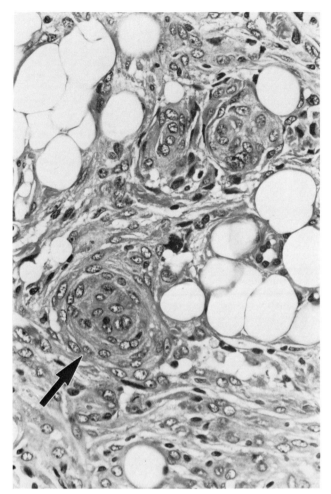

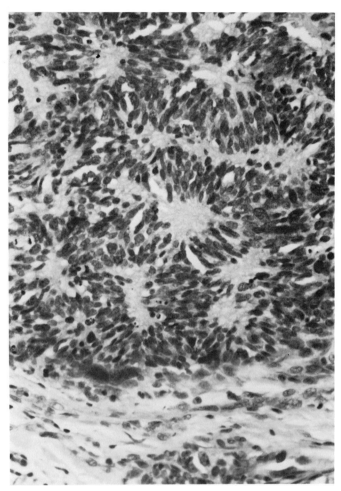

FIGURE 148-12. Cutaneous meningioma. Diffuse and nested pattern of epithelioid cells infiltrating the subcutaneous fat. Note the whorl-like arrangement of the cells *(arrow)* (H&E, ×100).

FIGURE 148-13. Cutaneous neuroblastoma. The tumor is composed of small cells with small, round to ovoid nuclei that can be arranged in rosettes. The fibrillary material in the center of Homer Wright type rosettes is characteristic (H&E, ×100).

treme caution and cranial imaging are required before these lesions are sampled or removed because they can communicate with the brain, and cerebrospinal fluid leakage and subsequent meningoencephalitis and other neurologic damage may occur.[75-80] Metastatic meningiomas and peripheral neuroblastomas often require aggressive surgery and adjuvant oncologic therapy.[64, 78, 82, 83]

Acknowledgments

The author wishes to thank Joel Carl for preparation of the photographs and Susan Lee for administrative assistance.

References

1. Argenyi ZB. Recent developments in cutaneous neural neoplasms. J Cutan Pathol 1993;20:97–108.
2. Harkin JC, Reed RJ. Tumors of the peripheral nervous system. In: Atlas of Tumor Pathology, 2nd series, fascicle 3, vol 10. Washington, DC: Armed Forces Institute of Pathology, 1969:19–168.
3. Reed RJ, Harkin JC. Tumors of the peripheral nervous system. In: Atlas of Tumor Pathology, 2nd series, fascicle 3 (supplement). Washington, DC: Armed Forces Institute of Pathology, 1983; S1–S52.
4. Enzinger FM, Weiss SW: Benign tumors of peripheral nerves. In: Soft Tissue Tumors, 2nd ed. St. Louis: CV Mosby, 1988:906–929.
5. Reed ML, Jacoby RA. Cutaneous neuroanatomy and neuropathology: Normal nerves, neural-crest derivates, and benign neural neoplasms in the skin. Am J Dermatopathol 1983;5:335–362.
6. Lassmann H, Jurecka W, Lassmann G, et al. Different types of benign nerve sheath tumors: Light microscopy, electron microscopy and autoradiography. Virchows Arch [A] 1977;375:197–210.
7. Erlandson RA, Woodruff JM. Peripheral nerve sheath tumors: An electron microscopic study of 43 cases. Cancer 1982;49:273–287.
8. Argenyi ZB. Newly recognized neural neoplasms relevant to the dermatopathologist. Dermatol Clin 1992;10:219–234.
9. Weedon D. Neural and neuroendocrine tumours. In: Symmers WSTC, ed. Systemic Pathology, 3rd ed, vol IX. New York: Churchill Livingstone, 1992:923–942.
10. Ortiz-Hidalgo C, Weller RO. Peripheral nervous system. In: Sternberg SS, ed. Histology for Pathologists. New York: Raven Press, 1992;169–193.
11. Le Douarin NM, Smith J. Development of peripheral nervous system from the neural crest. Annu Rev Cell Biol 1988;4:375–404.
12. Bunge MB, Wood PM, Tynan LB, et al. Perineurium originates from fibroblasts: Demonstration in vitro with a retroviral marker. Science 1989;243:229–231.
13. Takahashi K, Isobe I, Ohtsuki Y, et al. Immunohistochemical study on the distribution of α and β subunits of S-100 protein in human neoplasm and normal tissue. Virchows Arch [B] 1984; 45:385–396.
14. Weiss SW, Lageloss JM, Enzinger FM. Value of S-100 protein in the diagnosis of soft tissue tumors with particular reference to benign and malignant Schwann cell tumors. Lab Invest 1983; 49:299–308.

15. Perentes E, Nakagawa Y, Ross G, et al. Expression of epithelial membrane antigen in perineurial cells and their derivatives: An immunohistochemical study with multiple markers. Acta Neuropathol 1987;75:160–165.

16. Kawahara E, Yoshio O, Akishi O, et al. Expression of glial fibrillary acidic protein (GFAP) in peripheral nerve sheath tumors: A comparative study of immunoreactivity of GFAP, vimentin, S-100 protein, and neurofilament in 38 schwannomas and 18 neurofibromas. Am J Surg Pathol 1988;12:115–120.

17. Perentes E, Rubinstein LJ. Recent applications of immunoperoxidase histochemistry in human neurooncology: An update. Arch Pathol Lab Med 1987;111:796–812.

18. Matthews GJ, Osterholm JL. Painful traumatic neuromas. Surg Clin North Am 1972;51:1313–1324.

19. Burtner DD, Goodman M. Traumatic neuroma of the nose. Arch Otolaryngol 1972;103:108–109.

20. Shapiro L, Juklin EA, Brownstein HM. Rudimentary polydactyly. Arch Dermatol 1973;108:223–225.

21. Argenyi ZB, Santa Cruz D, Bromley C. Comparative light-microscopic and immunohistochemical study of traumatic and palisaded, encapsulated neuromas of the skin. Am J Dermatopathol 1992;14:504–510.

22. Lundborg G. Nerve regeneration and repair: A review. Acta Orthop Scand 1987;58:145–169.

23. Lassmann H, Ammerer HP. Schwann cells and perineurium in neuroma: Some morphological aspects. Virchows Arch [B] 1974;15:313–321.

24. Reed RJ, Fine RM, Meltzer HD. Palisaded, encapsulated neuromas of the skin. Arch Dermatol 1972;106:865–870.

25. Dover JS, From L, Lewis A. Palisaded encapsulated neuromas: A clinicopathologic study. Arch Dermatol 1989;125:386–389.

26. Albrecht S, Kahn HJ, From L. Palisaded encapsulated neuroma: An immunohistochemical study. Mod Pathol 1989;2:403–406.

27. Fletcher CDM. Solitary circumscribed neuroma of the skin (so-called palisaded, encapsulated neuroma): A clinicopathologic and immunohistochemical study. Am J Surg Pathol 1989;13:574–580.

28. Williams ED, Pollock DJ. Multiple mucosal neuromata with endocrine tumors: A syndrome allied to von Recklinghausen's disease. J Pathol Bacteriol 1966;91:71–80.

29. Gorlin RJ, Sedano HO, Vicers RA, et al. Multiple mucosal neuromas, pheochromocytomas and medullary carcinoma of the thyroid: A syndrome. Cancer 1968;22:293–299.

30. Ayala F, Derosa G, Scippa L, et al. Multiple endocrine neoplasia, type IIb. Dermatologica 1981;162:292–299.

31. Argenyi ZB. Immunohistochemical characterization of palisaded encapsulated neuroma. J Cutan Pathol 1990;17:329–335.

32. Argenyi ZB, Cooper PH, Santa Cruz D. Plexiform and other unusual variants of palisaded encapsulated neuroma. J Cutan Pathol 1993;20:34–39.

33. Feigin I. Skin tumors of neural origin. Am J Dermatopathol 1983;5:397–399.

34. Das Gupta TK, Brasfield RD, Strong EW, et al. Benign solitary schwannomas (neurilemomas). Cancer 1969;24:355–366.

35. Whitaker WG, Droulias C. Benign encapsulated neurilemoma: A report of 76 cases. Am Surg 1976;42:675–678.

36. White NB. Neurilemomas of the extremities. J Bone Joint Surg [Am] 1967;49:1605–1610.

37. Jacobs RL, Barmada R. Neurilemoma: A review of the literature with six case reports. Arch Surg 1971;102:181–186.

38. Shishiba T, Niimura M, Ohtsuka F, et al. Multiple cutaneous neurilemomas as a skin manifestation of neurilemmomatosis. J Am Acad Dermatol 1984;10:744–754.

39. Izumi AK, Rosato FE, Wood MG. Von Recklinghausen's disease associated with multiple neurilemomas. Arch Dermatol 1971;104:172–176.

40. Vilanova JR, Burgos-Bretones JJ, Alvarez JA, et al. Benign schwannomas: A histopathological and morphometric study. Pathology 1982;137:281–286.

41. Dahl I, Hagmar B, Idvall I. Benign solitary neurilemoma (schwannoma): A correlative cytological and histological study of 28 cases. Acta Pathol Microbiol Immunol Scand 1984;92:91–101.

42. Argenyi ZB, Balogh K, Abraham AA. Degenerative ("ancient") changes in benign cutaneous schwannoma: A light microscopic, histochemical and immunohistochemical study. J Cutan Pathol 1993;20:148–153.

43. Woodruff JM, Susin M, Godwin TA, et al. Cellular schwannoma: A variety of schwannoma sometimes mistaken for a malignant tumor. Am J Surg Pathol 1981;5:733–744.

44. Oshman RG, Phelps RG, Kantor I. A solitary neurofibroma on the finger. Arch Dermatol 1988;124:1185–1186.

45. Riccardi VM. Neurofibromatosis: The importance of localized or otherwise atypical forms. Arch Dermatol 1987;123:882–883.

46. Jurecka W. Plexiform neurofibroma of the skin. Am J Dermatopathol 1988;10:209–217.

47. Riccardi VM. Von Recklinghausen neurofibromatosis (review). N Engl J Med 1981;305:1617–1627.

48. Harkin JC, Reed RJ. Myxoma of nerve sheath. In: Tumors of the Peripheral Nervous System, 2nd series, fascicle 3. Washington, DC: Armed Forces Institute of Pathology, 1969:60–65.

49. Gallager RL, Helwig EB. Neurothekeoma: A benign cutaneous tumor of neural origin. Am J Clin Pathol 1980;74:759–764.

50. Angervall L, Kindblom L-G, Haglid K. Dermal nerve sheath myxoma: A light and electron microscopic, histochemical and immunohistochemical study. Cancer 1984;53:1752–1759.

51. Aronson PJ, Fretzin DF, Potter BS. Neurothekeoma of Gallager and Helwig (dermal nerve sheath myxoma variant): Report of a case with electron microscopic and immunohistochemical studies. J Cutan Pathol 1985;12:506–519.

52. Fletcher CDM, Chan JK-C, McKee PH. Dermal nerve sheath myxoma: A study of three cases. Histopathology 1986;10:135–145.

53. Holden CA, Wilson-Jones E, MacDonald DM. Cutaneous lobular neuromyxoma. Br J Dermatol 1982;106:211–215.

54. Rosati LA, Fratamico FCM, Eusebi V. Cellular neurothekeoma. Appl Pathol 1986;4:186–191.

55. Barnhill RL, Mihm MC. Cellular neurothekeoma: A distinctive variant of neurothekeoma mimicking nevomelanocytic tumors. Am J Surg Pathol 1990;14:113–120.

56. Barnhill RL, Dickerson GR, Nickeleit V, et al. Studies on cellular origin of neurothekeoma: Clinical, light microscopic, immunohistochemical, and ultrastructural observations. J Am Acad Dermatol 1991;25:80–88.

57. Calonje E, Wilson-Jones E, Smith NP, et al. Cellular "neurothekeoma": An epithelioid variant of pilar leiomyoma? Morphological and immunohistochemical analysis of a series. Histopathology 1992;20:397–404.

58. Argenyi ZB, LeBoit PE, Santa Cruz D, et al. Nerve sheath myxoma (neurothekeoma) of the skin: Light microscopic and immunohistochemical reappraisal of the cellular variant. J Cutan Pathol 1993;20:294–303.

59. LeBoit PE, Barr RJ, Burrall S, et al. Primitive polypoid granular cell tumor and other cutaneous granular cell neoplasms of nonneural origin. Am J Surg Pathol 1991;15:48–58.

60. Apisarnthanarax P. Granular cell tumor: An analysis of 16 cases and review of the literature. J Am Acad Dermatol 1981;5:171–182.

61. Lack EE, Wosham GF, Callihan MD, et al. Granular cell tumor: A clinicopathologic study of 110 patients. J Surg Oncol 1980;13:301–316.

62. Goette DK, Olson EG. Multiple cutaneous granular cell tumors. Int J Dermatol 1982;21:271–272.

63. Khansur T, Balducci L, Tavassoli M. Granular cell tumor: Clinical spectrum of the benign and malignant entity. Cancer 1987;60:220–222.

64. Cadotte M. Malignant granular-cell myoblastoma. Cancer 1974;33:1417–1422.

65. Armin A, Connelly EM, Rowden G. An immunoperoxidase investigation of S-100 protein in granular cell myoblastomas: Evidence for Schwann cell derivation. Am J Clin Pathol 1983;79:37–44.

66. Raju GC, O'Reilly AP. Immunohistochemical study of granular cell tumour. Pathology 1987;19:402–406.

67. Buley ID, Gatter KC, Kelly PMA, et al. Granular cell tumours revisisted: An immunohistological and ultrastructural study. Histopathology 1988;12:263–274.

68. Enzinger FM, Weiss SW. Malignant tumors of peripheral nerves. In: Soft Tissue Tumors, 2nd ed. St. Louis: CV Mosby, 1988:781–815.

69. Trojanowski JQ, Kleinman GM, Proppe KH. Malignant tumors of nerve sheath origin. Cancer 1980;46:1202–1212.

70. Storm FK, Eilber FR, Mirra J, et al. Neurofibrosarcoma. Cancer 1980;45:126–129.
71. George E, Swanson PE, Wick MR. Malignant peripheral nerve sheath tumors of the skin. Am J Dermatopathol 1989;11:213–221.
72. D'Agostino AN, Soule EH, Miller RH: Sarcomas of the peripheral nerves and somatic soft tissues associated with multiple neurofibromatosis (von Recklinghausen's disease). Cancer 1963; 16:1015–1027.
73. Guccion JG, Enzinger FM. Malignant schwannoma associated with von Recklinghausen's neurofibromatosis. Virchows Arch [A] 1979;383:43–57.
74. Herrera GA, deMoraes HP. Neurogenic sarcomas in patients with neurofibromatosis (von Recklinghausen's disease). Virchows Arch [A] 1984;403:361–376.
75. Kopf AW, Bart RS. Nasal glioma. J Dermatol Surg Oncol 1978;4:128–130.
76. Gebhart W, Hohlbrugger H, Lassmann H, et al. Nasal glioma. Int J Dermatol 1982;21:212–215.
77. Fletcher CDM, Carpenter G, McKee PH. Nasal glioma: A rarity. Am J Dermatopathol 1986;8:341–346.
78. Lopez DA, Silveirs DN, Helwig EB. Cutaneous meningiomas: A clinicopathologic study. Cancer 1974;34:728–744.
79. Sibley DA, Cooper PH. Rudimentary meningocele: A variant of "primary cutaneous meningioma." J Cutan Pathol 1989;16: 72–80.
80. Marrogi AJ, Swanson PE, Kyriakos M, et al. Rudimentary meningocele of the skin: Clinicopathologic features and differential diagnosis. J Cutan Pathol 1991;18:178–188.
81. Argenyi ZB, Bergeld WF, McMahon JT, et al. Primitive neuroectodermal tumor in the skin with features of neuroblastoma in an adult patient. J Cutan Pathol 1986;13:420–430.
82. Van Nguyen A, Argenyi ZB. Cutaneous neuroblastoma: Peripheral neuroblastoma. Am J Dermatopathol 1993;15:7–14.
83. Enzinger FM, Weiss SW. Tumors of the sympathetic nervous system. In: Soft Tissue Tumors, 2nd ed. St. Louis: CV Mosby, 1988;816–836.
84. Klapman MH, Chun DC. Cutaneous and subcutaneous neuroblastoma in children and adults: Case report and population study. J Am Acad Dermatol 1991;24:1025–1027.
85. Van Erp, Gronigen IFR. Cutaneous metastases in neuroblastoma. Dermatologica 1968;136:265–269.
86. Shown TE, Durfee MF. Blueberry muffin baby: Neonatal neuroblastoma with subcutaneous metastases. J Urol 1970;104: 193–195.
87. Lucky AW, McGuire J, Komp D. Infantile neuroblastoma presenting with cutaneous blanching nodules. J Am Acad Dermatol 1982;6:389–391.

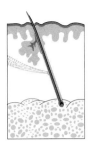

chapter 149

Fibrous Neoplasms

FREDERICK S. FISH and HIDEKO KAMINO

Dermatofibroma

CLINICAL DESCRIPTION

Dermatofibroma is a common fibrohistiocytic tumor that has been called by a number of names, including fibrohistiocytoma, nodular subepidermal fibrosis, histiocytoma cutis, and sclerosing hemangioma. Dermatofibromas occur as papules or nodules on the extremities in approximately 80% of cases. The legs of women are a common location, possibly as a result of shaving or other minor trauma, and there are reports of cases involving the palms and soles.[1] Although they have been reported to occur at any age, dermatofibromas most frequently affect individuals in early to middle adult life. There is no racial predilection. Although usually solitary, in about 20% of patients multiple lesions will be found,[2] and there are reports of generalized dermatofibromas,[3] especially in immunosuppressed patients.[4] Multiple dermatofibromas have been reported in systemic lupus erythematosus unrelated to immunosuppressant therapy.[4, 5] Rare cases have been reported with basal cell carcinoma occurring in conjunction with a dermatofibroma,[6] but more commonly follicular induction occurs.

The typical dermatofibroma presents as a slow-growing, round to oval, firm nodule with a dermal component that is attached to the overlying skin. It ranges in size from a few millimeters to several centimeters. Some lesions are dome shaped, while others appear depressed. The color can range from red-brown to a dusky brown color (Fig. 149 – 1). Rarely they may appear dark brown or black, and if there is a significant vascular component, they are reddish. The surface of the lesions may be smooth or rough. They are usually asymptomatic but occasionally may be slightly pruritic or painful on pressure. The clinical differential diagnosis includes scar, atypical nevus, and melanoma (Table 149 – 1). A simple

maneuver to help confirm the diagnosis can be done by applying lateral compression, which causes the central portion of the dermatofibroma to "dimple."[7] Larger lesions that extend into the fat and are several centimeters in diameter may be confused with dermatofibrosarcoma protuberans.

PATHOLOGY

Dermatofibromas are usually well circumscribed nodules confined to the dermis, measuring 1 to 2 cm in diameter and composed of plump fibroblasts arranged as intersecting fascicles (Fig. 149 – 2). The likely cell of origin is the dermal dendrocyte. There are variable proportions of mononucleated and multinucleated foamy histiocytes, with hemosiderin deposits in their cytoplasm (Fig. 149 – 3).[8-11] Scattered between the cells, and predominantly at the periphery of the lesion, are thick "keloidal" collagen bundles that are birefringent when examined with polarizing lenses (Fig. 149 – 4).[12] Additional features are epidermal hyperplasia and a perivascular lymphoplasmacytic infiltrate at the periphery of the nodule. Although most dermatofibromas are easy to diagnose histologically, there are some variants that may be more difficult to diagnose, such as dermatofibroma with atypical cells,[13-16] atrophic dermatofibroma,[17] dermatofibroma with extension into the subcutaneous tissue,[18] palisading dermatofibroma,[19] dermatofibroma with osteoclast-like giant cells,[20] dermatofibroma with granular cells,[21] dermatofibroma with follicular and sebaceous induction in the overlying epidermis,[6, 22] and dermatofibroma with lymphoid follicles.[23] Two variants of dermatofibroma that could pose a dilemma in the differential diagnosis with malignant lesions are described.

Dermatofibroma with Atypical Cells

The presence of cytologic atypia in some dermatofibromas could be a problem in distinguishing them from

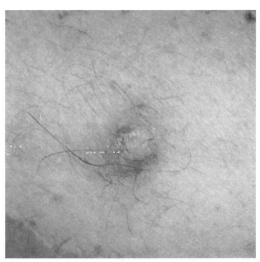

FIGURE 149–1. Typical clinical presentation of dermatofibroma.

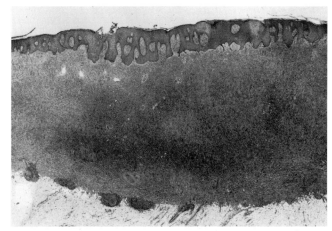

FIGURE 149–2. Dermatofibroma. Well-circumscribed nodule associated with epidermal hyperplasia and a peripheral inflammatory infiltrate.

atypical fibroxanthoma (superficial malignant fibrous histiocytoma). In 1963, Levan and associates[13] described two cases of dermatofibromas with atypical cells and used the name "pseudosarcomatous dermatofibroma." More recently, similar cases have been reported under the following names: atypical ("pseudosarcomatous") cutaneous histiocytoma,[14] atypical cutaneous fibrous histiocytoma,[15] and dermatofibroma with monster cells.[16]

In addition to the histologic features described earlier for the common type of dermatofibroma, dermatofibromas with atypical cells have mononucleated and multinucleated cells with large pleomorphic and hyperchromatic nuclei, some of which have prominent nucleoli (Fig. 149–5). The nuclear atypia is most commonly seen in the large cells with "histiocytic" differentiation rather than in the fibroblastic cells. The atypical "histiocytic" cells have abundant foamy cytoplasm, frequently with hemosiderin deposits. Despite the striking nuclear atypia, these lesions are characterized by rare mitotic figures. If mitoses are present, they are not atypical. This latter feature distinguishes dermatofibroma with atypical cells from atypical fibroxanthoma, in which typical and atypical mitotic figures are common.[24]

TABLE 149-1. Differential Diagnosis of Fibrous Neoplasms
Dermatofibroma
Lightly pigmented
Scar
Keloid
Xanthoma
Neurofibroma
Darkly pigmented
Atypical nevus
Kaposi's sarcoma
Melanoma
Larger lesions
Dermatofibrosarcoma protuberans
Dermatofibrosarcoma Protuberans
Early phase
Scar
Morphea
Intermediate phase
Dermatofibroma
Keloid
Advance phase
Malignant fibrous histiocytoma
Fibrosarcoma
Atypical Fibroxanthoma
Squamous cell carcinoma
Basal cell carcinoma
Epidermoid cyst
Ulcerated pyogenic granuloma

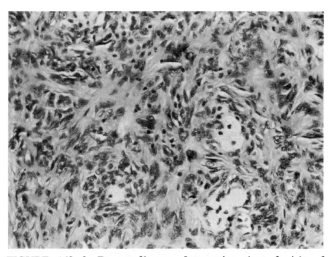

FIGURE 149–3. Dermatofibroma. Intersecting short fascicle of plump fibroblasts and foamy histiocytes.

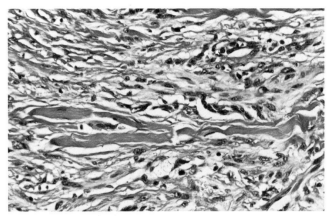

FIGURE 149–4. Thick "keloidal" collagen bundles typical of dermatofibroma.

Dermatofibroma Extending into the Subcutaneous Tissue

Dermatofibromas are usually confined to the dermis and, in most instances, do not pose a diagnostic problem. However, when they are composed predominantly of fibroblasts and extend to the subcutaneous tissue it can be difficult to distinguish them from an early lesion of dermatofibrosarcoma protuberans.[18] Differentiation between these two entities could be especially difficult if the lesions are incompletely excised and the biopsy specimens are small or fragmented.

The dermatofibroma extending into the subcutaneous tissue has the same histologic components as the more common dermal type of dermatofibroma described earlier. There are two main patterns of extension of dermatofibroma into the subcutaneous tissue.[18] The most frequent pattern consists of irregular extensions into the subcutaneous tissue in a vertical or radial fashion, predominantly along the septa, which acquire a wedge-shaped appearance (Fig. 149–6). The second pattern is well circumscribed with a deep smooth margin that bulges into the subcutaneous tissue (Fig. 149–7). In both

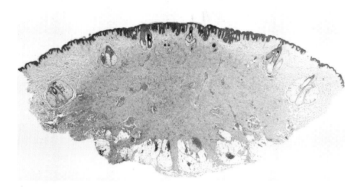

FIGURE 149–6. Dermatofibroma extending into the subcutaneous tissue in a radial pattern.

patterns, fat cells are admixed with fibroblasts, collagen bundles, and a lymphoplasmacytic infiltrate only at the interface between the lesion and the subcutaneous tissue or in areas of preexisting fat cells around the base of hair follicles or eccrine glands.

Immunostains for factor XIIIa, KP1 (CD68), lysozyme, MAC387, and HAM56 are positive in variable degrees in dermatofibroma. CD34 is a helpful marker to distinguish between dermatofibroma, whose cells are mostly negative, and dermatofibrosarcoma protuberans, in which most cells are positive.

TREATMENT

Dermatofibromas that require treatment may be treated in several ways. For smaller lesions that protrude above the skin surface, tangential shave excision is often an excellent treatment. This will contour the lesion to the skin surface. There will still be a firm area left within the dermis, but the protuberant portion will be removed and can be sent for histologic analysis. Smaller lesions may also respond to cryosurgery, which may eliminate the discoloration as well as flattening out the raised portion of the nodule.[25] In larger symptomatic lesions, simple

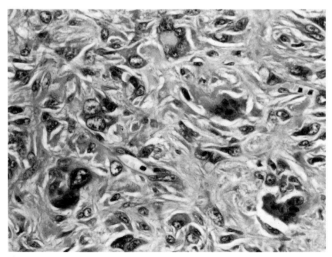

FIGURE 149–5. Dermatofibroma with mononucleated and multinucleated cells with atypical nuclei.

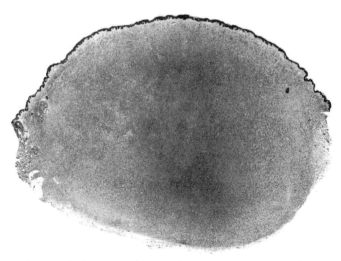

FIGURE 149–7. Dermatofibroma with a smooth base bulging into the subcutaneous tissue.

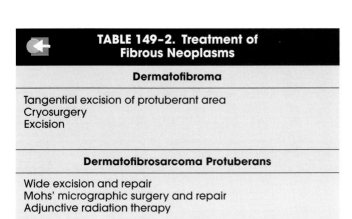

TABLE 149-2. Treatment of Fibrous Neoplasms
Dermatofibroma
Tangential excision of protuberant area
Cryosurgery
Excision
Dermatofibrosarcoma Protuberans
Wide excision and repair
Mohs' micrographic surgery and repair
Adjunctive radiation therapy
Atypical Fibroxanthoma
Excision with 1.0-cm clinical margin
Mohs' micrographic surgery

excision is the treatment of choice (Table 149-2). The excision should be carried down to the level of the fat plane. In one study there was a reported recurrence rate of approximately 4%,[26] and lesions that extend deeper into the subcutis have a greater chance of recurrence.

Dermatofibrosarcoma Protuberans

CLINICAL DESCRIPTION

Dermatofibrosarcoma protuberans is a soft tissue neoplasm of intermediate malignancy and should be separated from both benign and malignant fibrohistiocytoma. It is considered a low-grade sarcoma of the skin. The incidence of dermatofibrosarcoma protuberans has been estimated at 0.8 cases per 1 million persons per year.[27] However, a population study in Rochester, Minnesota, disclosed a significantly higher incidence of 5 cases per million.[28] Dermatofibrosarcoma protuberans has a pronounced tendency to recur but is of low metastatic potential.

The tumor typically presents during early or middle adult life (from ages 20 to 50 years) and has been reported in all races. Men are affected slightly more frequently than women. The most common site of occurrence is the trunk and proximal extremities, followed by the head and neck area and distal extremities.[29] In up to 20% of cases, antecedent trauma is reported.[30] The trauma has ranged from 2 months to 20 years before tumor recognition, making a true association uncertain. However, several cases have been reported describing dermatofibrosarcoma protuberans arising in a surgical scar, vaccination site, and burn scar.[31, 32]

Dermatofibrosarcoma protuberans appears initially as a dusky, indurated plaque that often escapes recognition for an extended period of time. The color can range from brown to bluish red, and there is often a blue or reddish discoloration of the surrounding skin (Fig. 149-8).[29] Ini-

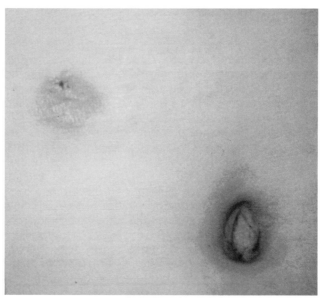

FIGURE 149-8. Early plaque stage of dermatofibrosarcoma protuberans on the anterior chest near the umbilicus.

tial lesions are usually flat, or in some cases even depressed, and may resemble morphea.[33, 34] Over time the plaque areas become larger and gradually nodules develop within the sclerotic area. These may be flesh colored, dusky red, or red-brown. The nodules may become quite large in advanced tumors (Fig. 149-9). They usually exhibit steady growth and are frequently asymptomatic. In one study, 25% of the patients experienced some pain or tenderness associated with the tumor.[29]

The clinical differential diagnosis of early dermatofibrosarcoma protuberans includes scar tissue and mor-

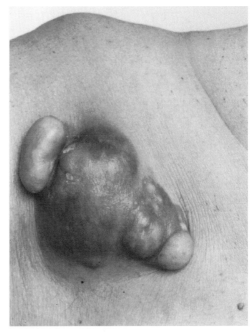

FIGURE 149-9. Multinodular stage of a large dermatofibrosarcoma protuberans.

phea. Once nodules begin to develop, intermediate lesions can be confused with larger dermatofibromas. The advanced lesions must be differentiated from malignant fibrous histiocytoma and fibrosarcoma (see Table 149–1).

A rare variant of dermatofibrosarcoma protuberans, found in less than 5% of cases is termed the *Bednar tumor.* It is a pigmented form that occurs predominantly in blacks and contains melanin.[35]

PATHOLOGY

The classic descriptions of dermatofibrosarcoma protuberans have been based on the fully developed large nodular lesions.[29, 30] However, dermatofibrosarcoma protuberans similar to other malignant neoplasms has an earlier plaque or nonprotuberans stage that may be more difficult to diagnose.[33, 34, 36] This earlier stage could be confused with benign lesions such as dermatofibroma, dermatomyofibroma, or diffuse neurofibroma.

The plaque lesions of dermatofibrosarcoma protuberans are characterized by a flat surface, lower cellularity, lack of a storiform pattern, and slender spindle-shaped neoplastic cells arranged in long horizontal fascicles parallel to the skin surface. When the subcutaneous tissue is infiltrated, it has a multilayered appearance with cells and fascicles also in a horizontal, parallel arrangement (Fig. 149–10).[18, 36] The slender, neoplastic

cells have uniform nuclei with no evidence of cytologic atypia. Mitotic figures are rare and range from 0 to 1 per 10 high-power fields. The preexisting collagen bundles are infiltrated by the neoplastic cells and appear cellular and wavy at the periphery of the plaques. Toward the center of the plaques, instead of thick collagen bundles, there are thin collagen fibers identified between the slender neoplastic cells that are not refractile when examined with polarized light. Compared with the adjacent uninvolved skin the dermis appears thinner and the eccrine coils and subcutaneous tissue are closer to the skin surface in the plaque areas. An inflammatory infiltrate of lymphocytes is minimal or absent. The adnexal structures are infiltrated in variable degrees or become completely obliterated. The overlying epidermis is of normal thickness or slightly thinned.[36]

The nodular stage of dermatofibrosarcoma protuberans usually develops within a plaque, but there are lesions that are nodular from an early stage with no evidence of a preexisting plaque lesion. The nodular stage of dermatofibrosarcoma protuberans is characterized by higher cellularity and slender to oval cells arranged as short intersecting fascicles in the typical "storiform" pattern (Fig. 149–11).[30, 37–39] The cells have slender to oval nuclei with a variable degree of hyperchromatism. Mitoses are frequent and range from 3 to 5 per 10 high-power fields. In addition, in some cases there are myxomatous areas with plump neoplastic cells and increased vascularity.[40] In other cases, fibrosarcoma-

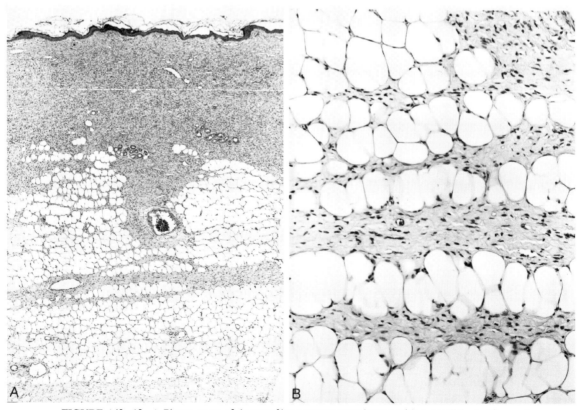

FIGURE 149–10. *A,* Plaque stage of dermatofibrosarcoma protuberans with a parallel, multilayered pattern of infiltration into the subcutaneous tissue. *B,* Closer view reveals bundles of slender cells in a horizontal, parallel arrangement.

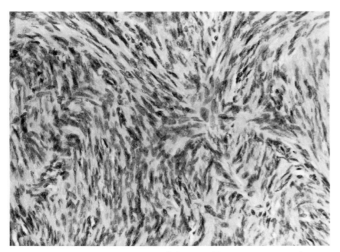

FIGURE 149–11. Nodular area of dermatofibrosarcoma protuberans with cellular bundles intersecting in a storiform pattern.

tous areas are also present with fascicles of cells arranged in a characteristic "herringbone" pattern.[41] In these areas nuclear atypia is more prominent and there is an increased mitotic rate ranging from 10 to 15 mitoses per 10 high-power fields. In the nodular areas, dermatofibrosarcoma protuberans infiltrates the subcutaneous tissue between fat cells in a "honeycomb" or "lace-like" pattern. Fully developed nodular areas replace and obliterate the subcutaneous tissue in a solid pattern of growth. Adnexal structures are mostly absent. The overlying epidermis is usually thinned. In the variant of pigmented dermatofibrosarcoma protuberans known as Bednar tumor, pigmented dendritic melanocytes are scattered between the neoplastic spindle-shaped cells.[35]

Most dermatofibrosarcoma protuberans neoplasms have a combination of plaque and nodular areas. The plaque areas can be seen at the sides of the nodules, above subcutaneous nodules, and less frequently underneath the nodules. Deep-seated plaques surround and infiltrate the fascia and skeletal muscle in a parallel fashion. Because plaques extend beyond the nodules and infiltrate the surrounding tissues as thin layers of slender, spindle-shaped cells that blend with the normal connective tissue cells, the surgical margins of excision may be very difficult to evaluate.[36]

Immunostaining for CD34 is strongly positive in the plaque areas and weak to moderately positive in the nodular areas. A positive immunostain with CD34 is helpful in the differential diagnosis of dermatofibrosarcoma protuberans, which is mostly positive, from dermatofibroma, which is negative.[42–44] Because plaque areas are strongly positive for CD34, this antibody is very helpful in evaluating the infiltrating margins of this tumor in the surgical excisions including specimens taken by Mohs' micrographic surgery.

TREATMENT

Dermatofibrosarcoma protuberans grows by direct extension spreading outward and downward with irregular tracts of tumor following along paths of least resistance. The tumor can invade to involve deeper structures, including muscle and even bone. Recurrences are common because the infiltrating growth pattern extends well beyond the clinical margins. Dermatofibrosarcoma protuberans metastasizes in less than 4% of cases.[30] The metastatic potential of this tumor is probably overestimated because tumors in the older literature that were defined as deeply penetrating dermatofibrosarcoma protuberans would now be categorized as malignant fibrous histiocytomas.[29, 37, 45] Cases that metastasize are almost always recurrent tumors with a considerable time interval between diagnosis and metastasis. When metastases do occur, the lung is the most common target organ, followed by the regional lymph nodes.[30]

Dermatofibrosarcoma protuberans has a strong propensity to recur even after wide excision. Taylor and Helwig[29] reported a 49% recurrence rate in 98 cases; Pack and Tabah,[38] a 24% recurrence rate in 17 patients; and Hajdu,[39] a 54% recurrence rate after wide excision in a series of 119 cases. Roses[46] evaluated the surgical margins and reported a 41% recurrence rate with clinical margins less than 2 cm and a 20% recurrence rate with clinical margins of at least 3 cm. Being even more aggressive in resection, McPeak and Cruz[31] reported a 11% recurrence rate in 27 patients treated with a 3-cm margin that was taken beyond clinically involved skin down to and including fascia.

Recurrences of dermatofibrosarcoma protuberans typically occur within 3 years. In Hadju's series,[39] most recurrences were noted within the first year, and in Taylor and Helwig's series[29] nearly 40% of recurrences were noted in the first year, and 75% within the first 3 years. Occasional late recurrences have been reported.[38] Recurrences are mainly due to incomplete excision. Because this tumor grows with very irregular projections that extend far beyond the clinical borders, it is difficult to determine adequate surgical margins.

Treatment of dermatofibrosarcoma protuberans is primarily surgical. Radiation has a limited role that has been used as a primary treatment in some cases when the tumor could not be resected. It has also been used in selected cases as an adjunct to surgery.[47] Radiation should be used with caution since cases of fibrosarcomatous change within dermatofibrosarcoma protuberans have been reported after radiation therapy.[48] Chemotherapy has no role at present (see Table 149–2).

Current recommendations for the surgical treatment of dermatofibrosarcoma protuberans call for wide excision with a 3 cm or greater margin down to and including fascia. There is no evidence to indicate that prophylactic lymph node dissection is warranted. Three-centimeter margins especially in the head and neck region are often difficult to obtain without significant functional and cosmetic problems. Mohs' micrographic surgery has shown great promise in treating this tumor. Mohs reported seven cases of dermatofibrosarcoma protuberans treated with the Mohs' technique in which there was no recurrence after 5 years. In five of these cases the fixed tissue technique was used, which is seldom used today,[49] and in two cases the fresh tissue technique was used. Robinson[50] reported four cases that were followed for 5 years with no recurrences. Mikhail and Lynn[51] used Mohs' surgery in two cases and had no recurrence after 5 years. Hobbs and coworkers[52] reported 10 cases that were treated at the Cleveland Clinic by the Mohs' method between 1979 and 1986. All of these patients had undergone previous surgery before Mohs' excision and subsequently underwent reconstructive surgery with no recurrences being reported thus far.

Atypical Fibroxanthoma

CLINICAL DESCRIPTION

Atypical fibroxanthoma most commonly presents on the nose, cheek, and ear regions of elderly patients. Some cases have been reported on the trunk and limbs of younger individuals. Atypical fibroxanthoma usually appears as an asymptomatic solitary nodule or nodular ulcer (Fig. 149–12). Typically, the tumor is less than 2 cm and as it enlarges it may erode and ulcerate. Lesions that are present on the extremities are often larger, are less well demarcated, and extend deeper.[53]

The clinical differential diagnosis includes squamous cell carcinoma, basal cell carcinoma, epidermoid cyst, and ulcerated pyogenic granuloma (see Table 149–1). The etiology of atypical fibroxanthoma is uncertain, but ultraviolet light probably plays a role since these tumors are most commonly seen on severely actinically damaged facial skin in elderly patients. Several cases have been reported where previous radiation therapy was

thought to be an etiologic factor, although this is not well documented.[54] Atypical fibroxanthoma is best thought of as a superficial form of malignant fibrous histiocytoma. Because of its superficial location and small size, atypical fibroxanthoma usually pursues a relatively benign course.[53] In rare cases, the tumor has metastasized to regional lymph nodes.[55, 56]

PATHOLOGY

Atypical fibroxanthoma is characterized histopathologically by a predominantly dermal expansile nodular growth on chronically sun-damaged skin of elderly patients that may extend into the upper portion of the subcutaneous fat. The lesions usually measure from 1 to 2 cm in diameter. The neoplasm is composed of atypical cells with fibroblastic and histiocytic differentiation. The fibroblastic cells are spindle shaped and arranged as long fascicles and admixed with larger cells with histiocytic differentiation that have abundant foamy cytoplasm (Fig. 149–13). In both types of cells, the nuclei are large, pleomorphic, and hyperchromatic and the cells are frequently multinucleated. There are many typical and atypical mitotic figures.[24, 30, 57, 58] Between the cells there are variable amounts of collagen fibers. The neoplasm usually has a dome-shaped appearance and abuts at the dermoepidermal junction with thinning of the overlying epidermis, with frequent crusting and secondary erosion or ulceration. Because of the proximity of the neoplasm to the epidermis, the differential diagnosis includes spindle cell squamous cell carcinoma and spindle cell amelanotic malignant melanoma. Atypical fibroxanthoma shares similar histologic features with the pleomorphic variant of malignant fibrous histiocytoma and some authors consider atypical fibroxanthoma to be the superficial variant of malignant fibrous histiocytoma.[30] The histologic differential diagnosis includes dermatofibroma with atypical cells, which is described earlier. The main distinguishing feature for dermatofibroma with atypical cells is the lack of atypical mitoses. Pleomorphic fibroma

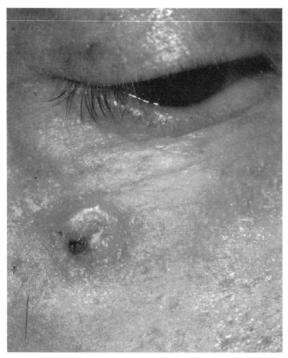

FIGURE 149–12. Atypical fibroxanthoma presenting as a crusted nodule on sun-damaged skin.

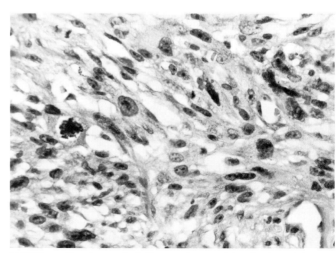

FIGURE 149–13. Atypical fibroxanthoma with spindle and irregularly shaped cells with foamy cytoplasm and pleomorphic nuclei. One atypical mitosis is present.

shares with atypical fibroxanthoma the presence of atypical spindle-shaped and multinucleated cells. However, pleomorphic fibroma is a high-domed to polypoid hypocellular lesion and mitotic figures are rarely present.[59]

Immunohistochemical stains are usually needed for a definitive diagnosis of atypical fibroxanthoma. Positive reactivity for α_1-antitrypsin, α_1-antichymotrypsin, and actin; and negative reactivity for S-100 protein, HMB-45, and cytokeratins would support the diagnosis of atypical fibroxanthoma.

TREATMENT

Surgical excision is the recommended treatment of atypical fiboxanthoma. Because these tumors can extend into the superficial subcutaneous tissue, excision with margin control is recommended. Electrodesiccation and curettage is not recommended because it does not allow for removal of the subcutaneous portion of the tumor. If frozen section margin control is not available, excision with a 1-cm margin is probably reasonable. The excision should be carried well into the subcutaneous tissue to ensure complete tumor removal.[60] Mohs' micrographic surgery has been used to treat a limited number of cases and has shown excellent results.[61] Mohs' surgery offers the advantage of tissue conservation, especially in cosmetically important areas of the face. If an atypical fibroxanthoma does recur and involves deeper subcutaneous tissues, the possibility of transformation to a malignant fibrous histiocytoma should be considered and aggressive therapy is indicated.

References

1. Bedi TR, Pandhi RK, Bhutani LK. Multiple palmoplantar histiocytomas. Arch Dermatol 1976;112:1001–1003.
2. Rentiers PL, Montgomery H. Nodular subepidermal fibrosis (dermatofibroma vs histiocytoma). Arch Dermatol Syph 1949;59:568–583.
3. Baraf CS, Shapiro L. Multiple histiocytomas: Report of a case. Arch Dermatol 1970;101:588–590.
4. Newman DM, Walter JB. Multiple dermatofibromas in patients with systemic lupus erythematosus on immunosuppressive therapy. N Engl J Med 1973;289:842–843.
5. Lin RY, et al. Multiple dermatofibromas and systemic lupus erythematosus. Cutis 1986;37:45–49.
6. Goette DK, Helwig EB. Basal cell carcinomas and basal cell carcinoma–like changes overlying dermatofibromas. Arch Dermatol 1975;111:589–592.
7. Fitzpatrick TB, Gilchrist BA. Dimple sign to differentiate benign from malignant pigmented cutaneous lesions. N Engl J Med 1977;296:1518.
8. Ackerman AB. Histologic Diagnosis of Inflammatory Skin Diseases. Philadelphia: Lea & Febiger, 1978:735–745.
9. Ackerman AB, Niven J, Grant Kels J. Dermatofibroma vs. dermatofibrosarcoma protuberans. In: Differential Diagnosis in Dermatopathology. Philadelphia: Lea & Febiger, 1982.
10. Lever WF, Schaumburg-Lever G. Histopathology of the Skin, 7th ed. Philadelphia: JB Lippincott, 1990.
11. Vilanova JR, Flint A. The morphological variations of fibrous histiocytomas. J Cutan Pathol 1974;1:155–164.
12. Barr RJ, Young EM, King DF. Non-polarizable collagen in dermatofibrosarcoma protuberans: A useful diagnostic aid. J Cutan Pathol 1986;13:339–346.
13. Levan NE, Hirsch P, Kwong MC. Pseudosarcomatous dermatofibroma. Arch Dermatol 1963;88:276–280.
14. Fukamizu H, Oku T, Inoue K, et al. Atypical ("pseudosarcomatous") cutaneous histiocytoma. J Cutan Pathol 1983;10:327–333.
15. Leyva WH, Santa Cruz DJ. Atypical cutaneous fibrous histiocytoma. Am J Dermatopathol 1986;8:467–471.
16. Tamada S, Ackerman AB: Dermatofibroma with monster cells. Am J Dermatopathol 1987;95:380–387.
17. Beer M, Eckert F, Schmoeckel C. The atrophic dermatofibroma. J Am Acad Dermatol 1991;25:1081–1082.
18. Kamino H, Jacobson M. Dermatofibroma extending into the subcutaneous tissue: Differential diagnosis from dermatofibrosarcoma protuberans. Am J Surg Pathol 1990;14:1156–1164.
19. Schwob VS, Santa Cruz DJ. Palisading cutaneous fibrous histiocytoma. J Cutan Pathol 1986;13:403–407.
20. Kutchemeshgi M, Barr RJ, Henderson CD. Dermatofibroma with osteoclast-like giant cells. Am J Dermatopathol 1992;14:397–401.
21. LeBoit PE, Barr RJ. Unusual mesenchymal proliferations associated with dermatofibromas (abstract). J Cutan Pathol 1991;18:376.
22. Requena L, Roo E, Yus ES. Plate-like sebaceous hyperplasia overlying dermatofibroma. J Cutan Pathol 1992;19:253–255.
23. Barker SM, Winkelmann RK: Inflammatory lymphadenoid reactions with dermatofibroma/histiocytoma. J Cutan Pathol 1986;13:222–226.
24. Fretzin DF, Helwig EB. Atypical fibroxanthoma of the skin: A clinicopathologic study of 140 cases. Cancer 1973;31:1541–1552.
25. Lanigan SW, Robinson TWE. Cryotherapy for dermatofibromas. Clin Exp Dermatol 1987;12:121–123.
26. Niemi KM. The benign fibrohistiocytic tumours of the skin. Acta Derm Venereol 1970;50(Suppl 63):1–66.
27. Bendix-Hansen K, Myhre-Jensen O, Kaae S. Dermatofibrosarcoma protuberans: A clinico-pathological study of nineteen cases and review of world literature. Scand J Plast Reconstr Surg 1983;17:247–252.
28. Chuang TY, Su WP, Muller SA. Incidence of cutaneous T cell lymphoma and other rare skin cancers in a defined population. J Am Acad Dermatol 1990;23:254–256.
29. Taylor HB, Helwig EB. Dermatofibrosarcoma protuberans: A study of 115 cases. Cancer 1962;15:717–725.
30. Enziger FM, Weiss SW. Soft Tissue Tumors, 2nd ed. St. Louis: CV Mosby, 1988.
31. McPeak CJ, Cruz T, Nicastri AD. Dermatofibrosarcoma protuberans: An analysis of 86 cases—5 with metastasis. Ann Surg 1967;166:803–816.
32. McLelland J, Chu T. Dermatofibrosarcoma protuberans arising in a BCG vaccination scar. Arch Dermatol 1988;124:496.
33. Page EH, Asaad DM. Atrophic dermatofibroma and dermatofibrosarcoma protuberans. J Am Acad Dermatol 1987;17:947–950.
34. Lambert WC, Abramovits W, Gonzalez-Serva A, et al. Dermatofibrosarcoma non-protuberans: Description and report of five cases of a morpheaform variant of dermatofibrosarcoma. J Surg Oncol 1985;28:7–11.
35. Dupree WB, Langloss J, Weiss SW. Pigmented dermatofibrosarcoma protuberans (Bednar tumor): A pathologic, ultrastructural, and immunohistochemical study. Am J Surg Pathol 1985;9:630–639.
36. Kamino H, Garcia JA, Clark RE. Histopathologic characterization of plaque areas of dermatofibrosarcoma protuberans (abstract). Lab Invest 1992;66:32A.
37. Fletcher CDM, Evans BJ, MacArtney JC, et al. Dermatofibrosarcoma protuberans: A clinicopathological and immunohistochemical study with a review of the literature. Histopathology 1985;9:921–938.
38. Pack GT, Tabah EJ. Dermatofibrosarcoma protuberans: A report of thirty-nine cases. Arch Surg 1951;63:391–411.
39. Hajdu SI. Pathology of Soft Tissue Tumors. Philadelphia: Lea & Febiger, 1979:60–83.
40. Frierson HF, Cooper PH. Myxoid variant of dermatofibrosarcoma protuberans. Am J Surg Pathol 1983;7:445–450.
41. Ding J, Hashimoto H, Enjoji M. Dermatofibrosarcoma protuberans with fibrosarcomatous areas. Cancer 1989;64:721–729.
42. Anthony PP, Ramani P. Endothelial markers in malignant vascular tumours of the liver: Superiority of QB-END/10 over von Willebrand factor and Ulex europaeus agglutinin. J Clin Pathol 1991;44:29–32.
43. Aiba S, Tabata N, Ishii H, et al. Dermatofibrosarcoma protuberans

is a unique fibrohistiocytic tumor expressing CD34. Br J Dermatol 1992;127:79–94.

44. Kamino H, Burchette JL, Garcia JD. Immunostaining for CD34 in plaque and nodular areas of dermatofibrosarcoma protuberans (abstract). J Cutan Pathol 1992;19:530.

45. Weiss SW. Proliferative fibroblastic lesions: From hyperplasia to neoplasia. Am J Surg Pathol 1986;10(Suppl 1):14–25.

46. Roses DF, Valensi Q, LaTrenta G, et al. Surgical treatment of dermatofibrosarcoma protuberans. Surg Gynecol Obstet 1986; 162:449–452.

47. Marks LB, Suit HD, Rosenberg AE, et al. Dermatofibrosarcoma protuberans treated with radiation therapy. Int J Radiat Oncol Biol Phys 1989;17:379–384.

48. Wrotnowski U, Cooper PH, Shmookler BM. Fibrosarcomatous change in dermatofibrosarcoma protuberans. Am J Surg Pathol 1988;12:287–293.

49. Mohs FE. Chemosurgery: Microscopically Controlled Surgery for Skin Cancer. Springfield, IL: Charles C Thomas, 1978:251.

50. Robinson JK. Dermatofibrosarcoma protuberans resected by Mohs surgery (chemosurgery): A 5-year prospective study. J Am Acad Dermatol 1985;12:1093–1098.

51. Mikhail GR, Lynn BH. Dermatofibrosarcoma protuberans. J Dermatol Surg Oncol 1978;4:81–84.

52. Hobbs ER, Wheeland RG, Bailin PL, et al. Treatment of dermatofibrosarcoma protuberans with Mohs micrographic surgery. Ann Surg 1988;207:102–107.

53. Fretzin DF, Helwig EB. Atypical fibroxanthoma of the skin: A clinicopathologic study of 140 cases. Cancer 1973;31:1541–1552.

54. Hudson AW, Winkelmann RK. Atypical fibroxanthomas of the skin. Cancer 1972;29:413.

55. Jacobs DS, Edwards WD, Ye RC. Metastatic atypical fibroxanthoma of the skin. Cancer 1975;35:457.

56. Helwig ED, May D. Atypical fibroxanthoma of the skin with metastases. Cancer 1986;57:368.

57. Weiss SW, Enzinger FM. Malignant fibrous histiocytoma: An analysis of 200 cases. Cancer 1978;41:2250–2266.

58. Harris M. The ultrastructural study of benign and malignant fibrous histiocytoma. Histopathology 1980;4:29–44.

59. Kamino H, Lee JY, Berke A. Pleomorphic fibroma of the skin: A benign neoplasm with cytologic atypia: A clinicopathologic study of eight cases. Am J Surg Pathol 1989;13;107–113.

60. Roenigk RK, Roenigk HH. Surgical dermatology: Advances in current practice. St. Louis: CV Mosby, 1993:201–210.

61. Brown MD, Swanson NA. Treatment of malignant fibrous histiocytoma and atypical fibrous xanthomas with micrographic surgery. J Dermatol Surg Oncol 1989;15:1287–1292.

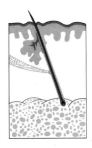

chapter 150

Melanocytic Nevi

Benign Melanocytic Neoplasms: Congenital and Acquired Nevi

Clay J. Cockerell, Timothy M. Johnson, and Neil A. Swanson

DEFINITION

A melanocytic neoplasm refers to a "new growth" composed of cells with differentiation toward melanocytes. These may be benign (i.e., melanocytic nevi) or malignant (i.e., melanoma). Melanocytes are cells derived from the neural crest and are demonstrable in the epidermis by the eighth week of gestation.[1] They may assume a number of different shapes and forms. Some of the morphologic variants of melanocytes include cells that are small and round, large and round, pagetoid (abundant pale-staining cytoplasm and enlarged nuclei), balloon (extensive clear cytoplasm with small nuclei), oval, spindle, cuboidal, epithelioid, multinucleated, and dendritic.[2] Any of these cell types may be present in greatest number in a given melanocytic nevus, which explains the large number of variants that have been described (Table 150–1).

CLINICAL DESCRIPTION AND PATHOLOGY

Intraepidermal Melanocytic Proliferations

Intraepidermal melanocytic proliferation refers to an increase in the number of melanocytes confined to the epidermis usually associated with epidermal hyperpigmentation. Many of these represent early stages in the development of more fully developed lesions, whereas others represent end-stage processes. *Ephelides,* also known as freckles, are small, tan, uniformly pigmented macules that are usually 1 to 3 mm in diameter. They are induced by ultraviolet irradiation and are seen most commonly in persons with Fitzpatrick skin type 1 or 2. They darken with exposure to ultraviolet irradiation and fade when light exposure diminishes. Histologically, there is a slight increase in the amount of melanin in the basal cell layer with a normal number of melanocytes. This correlates with the fact that these lesions are due to an overproduction of melanin by a normal number of melanocytes.[3] Ephelides develop as a protective measure against the harmful effects of ultraviolet irradiation in persons who do not tan well.

Lentigo is a Latin word that means "lentil shaped" and has come to mean any lentil-shaped spot on the skin like a freckle. For this reason, lentigo should not be used in an unmodified fashion since the term may be applied to a number of different lesions, ranging from lentigo maligna, a variant of melanoma in situ, to genetic disorders in which myriad small, benign, pigmented lesions are present. The simple lentigo (*lentigo simplex*) is a very common lesion the precise incidence of which is unknown. Clinically, these are macular or slightly raised areas of brown or brownish black pigmentation that are usually round or oval and usually less than 5 mm in diameter (Fig. 150–1; see color plate). There may be slight scaling on the surface, but skin surface markings are unaltered. Pigmentation is usually uniform, although there may be slight irregularities at the margin especially near follicular ostia.[4] These lesions usually arise in childhood and are generally few in number, although they may be present in great numbers in patients with certain syndromic disorders such as the Peutz-Jeghers syndrome and central facial lentiginosis associated with cardiac dis-

TABLE 150-1. Classification of Melanocytic Nevi

Intraepidermal Melanocytic Proliferation

Ephelis (freckle)
Lentigo simplex (simple lentigo)
PUVA lentigo
Mucosal lentigo
Solar-induced melanocytic proliferation
Idiopathic intraepidermal melanocytic proliferation
Café-au-lait macule

Melanocytic Nevi

Junctional nevus
Compound nevus
Intradermal nevus
 "Neural" nevus
Congenital melanocytic nevus
Nevus spilus
Blue nevus
 Mongolian spot, nevus of Ota, nevus of Ito
 Combined blue nevus

Variants of Melanocytic Nevi

Spitz nevus
Desmoplastic nevus
Deep penetrating nevus
Genital nevus
Persistent (recurrent) nevus
Nevi on volar skin
Desmoplastic nevus
Cockade nevus
"Dysplastic" or atypical nevus
Growing nevus in children

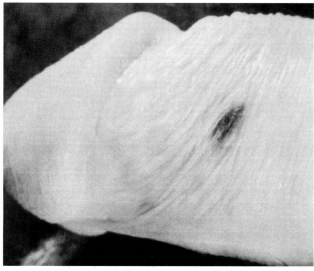

FIGURE 150-1. Lentigo simplex (simple lentigo). (See color plate.)

the dermoepidermal junction with an increase in the amount of melanin in the epidermis and cornified layer (Fig. 150-2). Melanocytes may be dendritic in lentigines on mucosal surfaces, on volar skin, and in the nail unit. In addition, there may be slight elongation of the epidermal retia with melanophages in the papillary dermis. Although lentigines are generally readily diagnosed both clinically and histologically, they may be confused with melanoma in situ and other intraepidermal melanocytic proliferations associated with sun exposure. Clinical correlation should be helpful in distinguishing these proliferations since evolving melanoma is generally much broader, is composed of atypical-appearing melanocytes, and is generally present on sun-damaged skin. No histologic difference can be appreciated between lentigines associated with genetic syndromes and those that are isolated.

ease.[5, 6] In many cases, lentigines develop into junctional and compound nevi, although others may remain stable throughout life. Histopathologically, there is an increase in the number of small typical-appearing melanocytes at

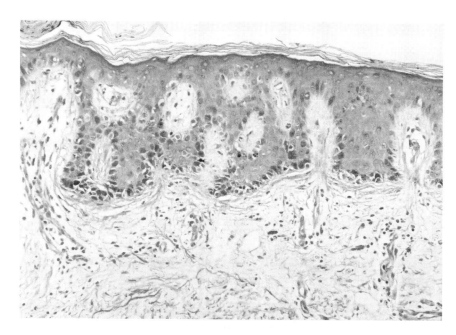

FIGURE 150-2. Lentigo simplex, histology. There is elongation of epidermal retia with hyperpigmentation and a slight increase in the number of normal-appearing melanocytes (H&E, original magnification × 200).

A number of intraepidermal melanocytic proliferations may arise as a consequence of ultraviolet irradiation. The *PUVA lentigo* is a macular pigmented lesion that develops on the skin of patients receiving photochemotherapy that is characterized histologically by the presence of an increased number of large, somewhat atypical melanocytes confined primarily to the basal cell layer and associated with hyperpigmentation.[7] In spite of the atypical cytologic features, no increase in the incidence of melanoma has been demonstrated. The primary significance of these lesions is that histologically they may simulate melanoma in situ. The fact that they are generally smaller and have minimal numbers of melanocytes situated in suprabasilar locations assists in histopathologically distinguishing these two disorders.

Solar lentigines are macular tan-brown pigmented areas in the skin that vary from 0.1 to 1 cm or greater in diameter and usually develop as a consequence of long-standing sun exposure. These are not truly melanocytic neoplasms but are keratinocytic proliferations that feature increased production of melanin by a normal complement of melanocytes. Histologically, there are epithelial changes characterized by rounded buds of keratinocytes at the tips of epidermal retia. These are distinct from the thinner, more delicate elongated epidermal retia seen in simple lentigines. Solar lentigines may remain stable or can evolve into reticulated seborrheic keratoses. When dense infiltrates of lymphocytes arise within these lesions and assault the basal layer, the term *benign lichenoid keratosis* or *lichen planus–like keratosis* is applied.

Mucosal lentigines develop on the oral or genital mucosa and are characterized by diffuse tannish to dark brown macular pigmentation that may range from less than 0.5 cm to several centimeters in diameter.[8, 9] Histologically, there is an increase in melanin in the basal keratinocytes with an increase in the number of dendritic melanocytes in the epithelium without cytologic atypia. The terms *melanosis vulvae* and *melanosis peni* refer to variants of this same process in which there may be slight epithelial hyperplasia.

Other conditions may be associated with histologic findings of slight melanocytic proliferation without clinical evidence of a melanocytic neoplasm. Long-standing sun damage may produce a slight increase in the number of melanocytes confined to the dermoepidermal junction and in some cases, with involvement of adnexal structures. This process is a histologic finding only and is not associated with clinical evidence of a melanocytic neoplasm. It is important to distinguish this from melanoma in situ in which there is more prominent pagetoid spread of atypical melanocytes and formation of nests of melanocytes at the dermoepidermal junction. Clinical correlation is an important element in making the diagnosis. Some have referred to this phenomenon as "atypical junctional melanocytic hyperplasia," but this confusing term, which does not connote any specific melanocytic lesion either clinically or histologically, is probably best avoided. In addition to solar-induced melanocytic hyperplasia, melanocytes may be slightly increased in number in the epidermis overlying angiofibromas as well as in normal skin of the eyelid.

Café-au-lait macules are well circumscribed tan macules that range from 1 to 20 cm in diameter. These lesions are characterized by an increase in the numbers of melanocytes at the basal cell layer of the epidermis as well as an increase in the amount of melanin. Histologically, there are features that are similar to those seen in ephelides, although enlarged melanosomes are often visualized on routine histologic examination.

Melanocytic Nevi

The word "nevus" refers to an abnormal or faulty growth in the skin that is generally synonymous with the term *hamartoma*. *Melanocytic nevus* refers to an abnormal but benign proliferation of melanocytes in the skin that is generally associated with the formation of nests of cells. Although there may be many different varieties of nevi, the most common are those in which melanocytes are situated mostly at the dermoepidermal junction, known as *junctional melanocytic nevi, compound melanocytic nevi* in which there are nests of melanocytes at the dermoepidermal junction as well as in the dermis, and *intradermal melanocytic nevi* in which melanocytes are situated predominantly within the papillary and reticular dermis. There are many distinct variants of nevi in the skin each with different histopathologic findings. Nevi may be present at the time of birth or may be acquired. They are relatively rare in infancy, increase in frequency during childhood and adolescence, reach a plateau in middle age, and undergo slow resolution with advancing age.[10] It has been estimated that the average number of nevi in whites is 20 by the time the individual has reached 20 years of age.

Simple lentigines, junctional nevi, compound nevi, and *intradermal nevi* lie on a continuum of evolution.[11] In childhood, most acquired melanocytic nevi are composed of melanocytes that proliferate at the dermoepidermal junction forming *junctional nevi*. It is thought that over the course of time, nests of melanocytes migrate into the upper papillary dermis to form *compound melanocytic nevi*. Eventually, the junctional component diminishes and virtually all the melanocytes are situated in the papillary and reticular dermis. In long-standing lesions, nests of melanocytes may exhibit neural differentiation, forming structures with features similar to Meissner's corpuscles. Clinically, junctional nevi are usually small, round, flat, or slightly raised, light brown to dark brown or black macules on the skin that range from 1 mm to 1 cm in greatest diameter (Fig. 150–3; see color plate). They are usually round with no distortion of skin markings. These lesions tend to be short-lived and are found most commonly in children, except when they occur on the palms and soles. Compound nevi are raised, often papillomatous lesions that are usually circular (Fig. 150–4; see color plate). They may assume colors that range from skin colored and light tan to brownish black. Although many are papular, some may be oriented horizontally, having features of a plaque. Intradermal nevi are usually brownish to skin-colored papules characterized by a smooth or papillary surface and a soft rubbery texture (Fig. 150–5; see color plate).

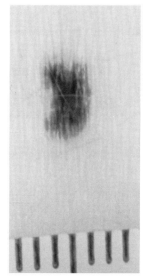

FIGURE 150-3. Junctional nevus. (See color plate.)

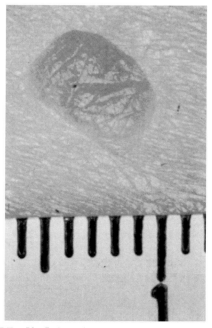

FIGURE 150-5. Intradermal nevus. (See color plate.)

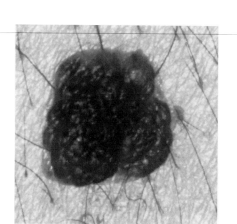

FIGURE 150-4. Compound nevus. (See color plate.)

Histologically, *junctional melanocytic nevi* are characterized by proliferations of melanocytes that are dendritic or spindle shaped and confined to the dermoepidermal junction (Fig. 150-6). There is usually abundant melanin in melanocytes and often in keratinocytes overlying the junctional nests. Melanin may be present in the granular and cornified layers in small columns, especially in lesions from volar skin. Lesions are small, well circumscribed, and symmetrical with regular distribution of pigment across the lesion. *Compound melanocytic nevi* have a similar proliferation of melanocytes at the dermoepidermal junction with the added feature of having small nests of round cells in the papillary and often the reticular dermis (Fig. 150-7). Melanocytes may vary in

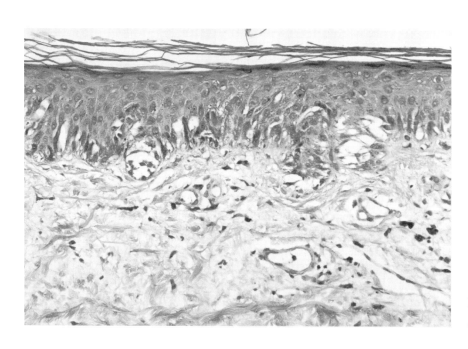

FIGURE 150-6. Junctional nevus. There is a proliferation of melanocytes arranged in small nests at the dermoepidermal junction (H&E, original magnification × 200).

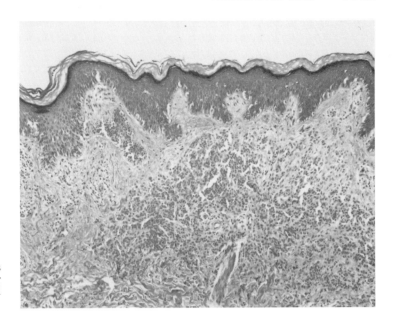

FIGURE 150–7. Compound nevus. There are nests of nevus cells at the dermoepidermal junction accompanied by similar cells in the papillary and upper reticular dermis (H&E, original magnification × 200).

shape, some appearing spindled while others appear distinctly neural. Melanin is usually present superficially rather than at the depth of the lesion. *Intradermal melanocytic nevi* are characterized by nests of cells similar to those seen in the dermal component of compound nevi with minimal junctional melanocytic proliferation (Fig. 150–8). As mentioned previously, late lesions may exhibit neural differentiation with differentiation toward Meissner's corpuscles.

PATHOGENESIS

The factors that initiate the development of nevi are unknown. Heredity may play a role since excessive numbers of nevi can be a family trait. Lesions may undergo eruptive growth in adolescence, in pregnancy, and after

the administration of corticosteroids[12] or human growth hormone.[13] Melanocyte-stimulating hormone causes lesions to increase in pigmentation.

DIFFERENTIAL DIAGNOSIS

The clinical differential diagnosis of nevi may include a number of different entities. Junctional nevi, especially those on the volar skin of acral surfaces, may be confused with hemorrhage into the cornified layer that develops after trauma, traumatic tattoos, thrombosed hemangiomas, as well as evolving melanoma (Table 150–2). Of the aforementioned conditions, evolving melanoma is the most important to be distinguished. In general, evolving melanomas are broader, are asymmetrical, and have a poorly circumscribed border in contrast to junc-

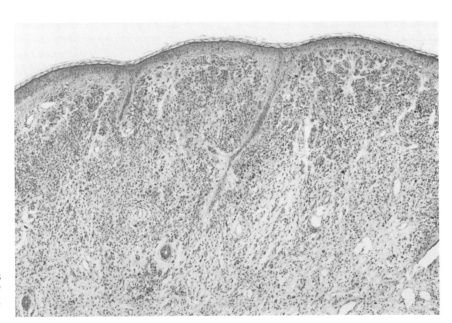

FIGURE 150–8. Intradermal nevus. Melanocytes are arranged in nests and aggregations entirely within the papillary and reticular dermis (H&E, original magnification × 200).

TABLE 150-2. Differential Diagnosis of Benign Melanocytic Neoplasms

Acquired Nevi
Junctional nevus
Traumatic tattoo
Thrombosed hemangioma
Talon noir or other hemorrhage into the cornified layer
Melanoma
Lentigo
Compound nevus and intradermal nevus
Basal cell carcinoma
Molluscum contagiosum
Verruca
Sebaceous gland hyperplasia
Achrochordon
Melanoma
Dermatofibroma
Neurofibroma
Spitz nevus
Pyogenic granuloma
Dermatofibroma
Juvenile xanthogranuloma
Melanoma
Deep penetrating nevus (blue nevus)
Melanoma
Desmoplastic nevus
Dermatofibroma
Spitz nevus

Congenital Nevi
Melanoma
Nevus spilus

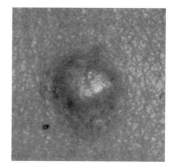

FIGURE 150-9. Spitz nevus (spindle and epithelioid cell nevus). (See color plate.)

though they are usually solitary, they may be numerous and widespread or grouped (agminated Spitz nevi). The most important element of Spitz nevus is that histologically there may be features similar to melanoma. This is because the cells that make up the lesions are large with abundant eosinophilic-staining cytoplasm that may be either spindle shaped or cuboidal (Fig. 150-10). Cells may be in mitosis, and there may be abundant single melanocytes at all levels of the epidermis. Other histologic features allowing distinction between this benign process and melanoma are the small, well-circumscribed, symmetrical distribution of the melanocytes and the fact that the melanocytes are smaller at the bases of lesions than at the surface. There is also epithelial hyperplasia and hyperkeratosis as well as a sparse infiltrate of lymphocytes scattered throughout the lesion. Some lesions may be heavily pigmented, and one variant of Spitz nevus known as *pigmented spindle cell tumor* may be very dark.[15] Clinically, Spitz nevi are usually thought to be benign but they are often confused with other nonmelanocytic lesions, such as pyogenic granuloma, dermatofibroma, or juvenile xanthogranuloma. Although melanoma is the most important histologic differential diagnostic consideration, occasionally these nevi may be confused with xanthogranulomas.

Desmoplastic nevus occurs on the extremities of young adults, and although it is clinically recognized as a nevus, it may simulate a dermatofibroma.[16] Histologically, there is a relatively small number of nevus cells embedded in thick, collagenous stroma often with overlying epidermal hyperplasia. Nevus cells are usually present singly rather than in nests and may be large and bizarre with copious cytoplasm. Mitotic figures are rare, however. Some consider these to be variants of Spitz nevi.

Balloon cell nevi clinically appear similar to other types of acquired melanocytic nevi.[17] Histologically, there is a predominant population of cells with extensive vacuolization of their cytoplasm. *Halo nevus* refers to a melanocytic nevus surrounded by a depigmented halo of otherwise normal skin.[18] It is seen most commonly in older children and young teenagers. Patients can develop depigmented halos around several nevi simultaneously. Histologically, there is a striking lymphocytic infiltrate admixed with nevus cells in the dermis and at the dermoepidermal junction. A loss of epidermal melanocytes can be demonstrated in the depigmented halo area,

tional nevi, which are small, symmetrical, and well circumscribed. Furthermore, melanocytes in evolving melanoma are cytologically atypical and involve epithelial structures of adnexa. Compound nevi may be confused clinically with basal cell carcinoma, molluscum contagiosum, verrucae, sebaceous gland hyperplasia, and other benign skin-colored to brownish papules on the skin. Intradermal nevi may be confused with skin tags and other benign epithelial lesions. Histologically, these are usually distinct, although some cases of unusual-appearing compound nevi may be difficult to distinguish from melanoma. In such cases, criteria used to diagnose each must be carefully applied.

Variants of Melanocytic Nevi

There are a number of distinct variants of melanocytic nevi that are important to recognize. *Spitz nevus,* also known as the nevus of spindle and/or epithelioid cells, was first described by Sophie Spitz in 1948 as benign juvenile melanoma.[14] Spitz nevi generally have features of compound or intradermal nevi clinically but often have a somewhat yellowish or orange color (Fig. 150-9; see color plate). They most often occur in children but may be seen in any age group and are quite common in young adults. They occur on any part of the body but are usually present on the face, trunk, or extremity. Al-

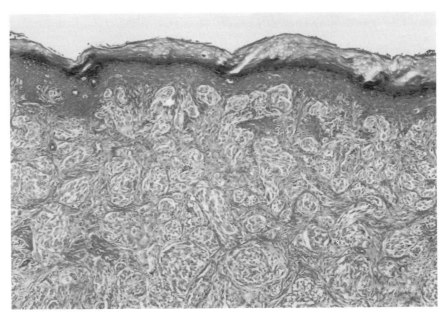

FIGURE 150-10. Spitz nevus. There is a proliferation of spindle and cuboidal "epithelioid" melanocytes at the dermoepidermal junction and focally above it as well as in the dermis beneath. Note the epidermal hyperplasia, hypergranulosis, and hyperkeratosis (H&E, original magnification × 200).

which may be a consequence of antimelanocyte antibodies that have been found in some patients with these lesions, a cytotoxic T-cell reaction, or both.

Nevus spilus, also known as speckled and lentiginous nevus, is clinically characterized by a flat, macular area that is usually darker than the surrounding skin, containing dark central lentigo-like lesions.[19] These lesions are relatively uncommon, although in one study they were shown to be present coincidentally in 1% of persons. Histologically, there is an admixture of areas with features similar to simple lentigo, whereas in other areas, features suggestive of either compound or congenital nevi are noted.

There are several variants of melanocytic nevi that are important because they may simulate melanoma histologically. Nevi on the genitalia may be associated with large pagetoid-appearing melanocytes as well as scattered melanocytes above the dermoepidermal junction.[2] These lesions exhibit the architectural features of benignancy and clinically are characterized by small brown to brownish black lesions. Congenital nevi biopsied shortly after birth may show a proliferation of nests of nevus cells that vary in size and shape at all levels of the epidermis as well as single melanocytes in a pagetoid distribution.[21] Some cells may be large, hyperchromatic, and slightly atypical. Mitotic figures are absent, and the dermal component usually shows features of a characteristic congenital nevus. Persistent (recurrent) nevi also may be associated with pagetoid spread of melanocytes with

atypical cytologic features.[22] In general, these features are present only at the site overlying the scar from the previous procedure (Figs. 150-11 and 150-12). Many persistent nevi develop as a consequence of incomplete removal of congenital nevi or compound nevi containing a

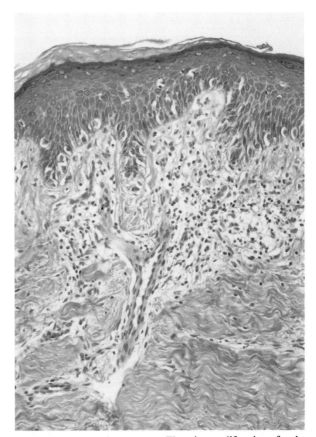

FIGURE 150-12. Persistent nevus. There is a proliferation of melanocytes arranged singly and in small nests at the dermoepidermal junction and slightly above it. These changes were confined to zones above the scar in the dermis visible at the bottom of the photomicrograph (H&E, original magnification × 200).

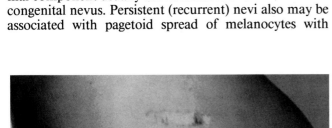

FIGURE 150-11. Persistent ("recurrent") nevus.

deep dermal component so that residual preexisting nevus cells are often visible microscopically.

Many benign melanocytic nevi are characterized by proliferations of melanocytes that are situated wholly in the dermis. These are thought to arise from dermal melanocytes that became arrested in the dermis before birth and never reached the basal cell layer, the normal location of melanocytes in the skin. These are generally referred to as "blue nevi" and its variants. *Mongolian spot, nevus of Ota,* and the *nevus of Ito* all are characterized by proliferations of dendritic melanocytes in the dermis.[23] Mongolian spot clinically appears most commonly as a macular blue-gray pigmentation at birth on the sacral area. The lesion is quite common in dark-skinned persons, being present in over 90% of Asian infants, although it is less common in whites, being seen in only 1% of infants. The nevus of Ota, also known as nevus fuscoceruleus ophthalmomaxillaris, and the nevus of Ito, known as nevus fuscoceruleus acromioclavicularis, are characterized by diffuse grayish blue patches involving the face and sclera and the acromioclavicular region, respectively. Both have histologic features that are identical to those of mongolian spot, namely, diffuse proliferations of dendritic melanocytes scattered throughout the dermis. Small "nevus of Ota–like macules" sometimes occur on the skin of the cheeks of Asians.

The *blue nevus* is an area of bluish gray or blue-black dermal pigmentation produced by heavily pigmented melanocytes in the deep papillary and reticular dermis (Fig. 150–13; see color plate). The "blue" color is a result of the transmission of black from melanin in the dermis through the dermis in association with the surrounding contrast of the normal skin color. Classically, two forms have been described: the cellular blue nevus and the common blue nevus.[24] These are oversimplifications, as there are a number of different variants depending on the numbers of melanocytes and the stromal changes surrounding them. In the "common" type, den-

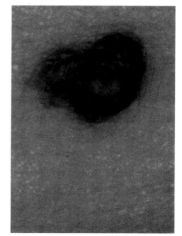

FIGURE 150–13. Blue nevus. (See color plate.)

dritic melanocytes are found singly or in small aggregations usually in the reticular dermis often centered around appendages, vessels, and nerves (Fig. 150–14). There may be associated melanophages as well. Cellular blue nevi possess both spindle and dendritic melanocytes, although larger cells with neural differentiation may also be present. Minimal cytologic atypia or mitotic activity is seen. Features of blue nevi may be observed in combination with other types of benign melanocytes (i.e., those of "ordinary" or Spitz nevus type). In such cases, the term *combined nevus* is appended to these lesions. Blue nevi must be distinguished from heavily pigmented nodular melanoma and are usually easily done so on the basis of architectural features of benignancy as well as a lack of atypical cytologic features.

Deep penetrating nevus is thought by many to be a subset of a blue nevus.[25] It occurs most commonly on the face, upper trunk, or proximal extremities of young persons and is a heavily pigmented, dome-shaped lesion that

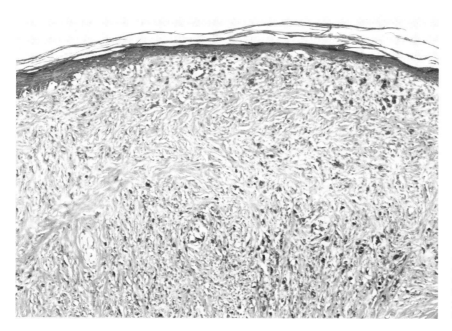

FIGURE 150–14. Blue nevus. There is a proliferation of dendritic melanocytes in the dermis that are heavily pigmented. Occasionally, there may be a component of melanocytes at the dermoepidermal junction as in this case (H&E, original magnification × 200).

ranges from 2 to 9 mm. Histologically, the lesion has the overall pattern of a benign lesion with a wedge shape with the apex extending to the subcutaneous fat. There are nests and fascicles of heavily pigmented nevus cells, many of which are somewhat large, with granular cytoplasm and prominent eosinophilic nucleoli. Mitotic figures are rare, but there may be slight pleomorphism of cells. The importance of the lesion is that it may histologically simulate malignant melanoma because of its deep extension.

Congenital Melanocytic Nevi

A congenital melanocytic nevus refers to a melanocytic nevus that is present at the time of birth. These lesions are present in 1% of all newborns and have been divided into three sizes: small lesions less than 1.5 cm in diameter, intermediate-sized lesions 1.5 to 20 cm in greatest diameter, and giant lesions with a diameter of greater than 20 cm.[26] At birth, these may be pale macules that over the course of time become darker and may develop outgrowths of terminal hair. Both pigment and hair growth increase at puberty. Histologically, there may be junctional, compound, and intradermal variants. Generally, there is an increase in the number of melanocytes at the epidermal basal cell layer with minimal cells in the papillary dermis and numerous melanocytes involving the upper reticular dermis, sometimes in a band-like configuration. Nevus cells are also present between the collagen bundles in the reticular dermis and may be present prominently around blood vessels and adnexal structures. Some forms tend to be situated more superficially and have lesser density of melanocytes than those situated more deeply in which diffuse replacement of the dermis and extension into the subcutaneous fat by nevus cells are often noted.

One of the most important elements of the diagnosis of a congenital nevus concerns the likelihood for the development of melanoma in association with these lesions, which appears to be proportionate to the size of the lesion. There is a well-documented risk for malignant degeneration in giant congenital nevi. The risk for the development of melanoma for small and intermediate-sized congenital nevi is extremely low, although the phenomenon has been documented.

Differentiation Between Benign and Malignant Melanocytic Lesions

"Suspicious" pigmented lesions are those in which there is clinical concern about the possible diagnoses of melanoma and are defined as those with the clinical features of asymmetry, irregular borders, jet-black or variegated colors (especially with shades of red, white, and blue-gray), or diameter greater than 6 mm. Additionally, any pigmented lesion with a history of recent growth, color change, tenderness, pruritus, or bleeding is suspicious. A family or personal history of melanoma or atypical nevi is also important.[26] A biopsy to rule out melanoma is indicated for suspicious pigmented lesions.

Any biopsy of a suspicious pigmented lesion should extend to the underlying adipose tissue to enable accurate measurement of thickness if the lesion proves to be melanoma.[28, 29] This is imperative, because while several factors are used to determine the overall prognostic index, the Breslow depth of invasion measured in millimeters is the major factor that most accurately determines the treatment and prognosis for malignant melanoma.[30]

Communication between the clinician and the dermatopathologist is essential. Accurate clinical impressions should be conveyed to the dermatopathologist to maximize correlation. For example, if the clinician strongly favors a malignant lesion and the initial sections show features of benignancy, the pathologist may need to section deeper into the block to exclude the possibility of a malignant lesion arising in a benign one. Similarly, describing the clinical history of recurrence is important because a recurrent benign melanocytic nevus may easily be misinterpreted histologically as a dysplastic nevus or melanoma.

BIOPSY TECHNIQUES (Table 150–3)

Excisional Biopsy

Complete excision of a pigmented lesion suspicious for melanoma is desired (Fig. 150–15). This is the first stage

TABLE 150-3. Treatment of Benign Melanocytic Neoplasms

Acquired Nevi

1. Biopsy to rule out melanoma when clinically suspicious
2. Cosmetically disfiguring lesions:
   a. Saucerization (tangential, shave) excision
   b. Excision with primary closure, graft or flap repair
   c. Serial excision
   d. Tissue expansion and excision with repair
   e. Some dermal variants as nevus of Ota and Ito may be improved by laser surgery:
      Epidermal and dermal pigmented process:
         694 nm Q-switched ruby laser (pulsed)
         755 nm Q-switched alexandrite (pulsed)
         1064 nm Q-switched Nd:YAG (pulsed)
   f. Some epidermal variants, i.e., lentigines, may be improved by treatment with
      Laser surgery:

510 nm	Flashlamp-pumped dye (short-pulsed)
511 nm	Copper vapor (quasi-continuous)
514 nm	Argon (continuous)
521, 531 nm	Krypton (continuous)
532 nm	KTP (continuous)
532 nm	Frequency-doubled Q-switched Nd:YAG (pulsed)

Chemical peeling
Dermabrasion

Congenital Nevi

1. Excision with primary closure, graft, or flap repair
2. Serial excision
3. Tissue expansion and excision with repair
4. Observation

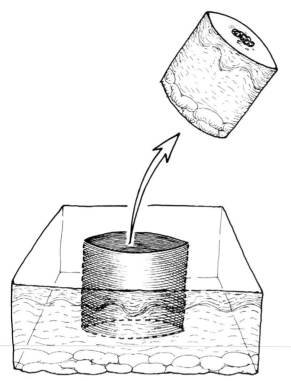

FIGURE 150–15. Elliptical excisional biopsy. The entire lesion is completely removed with a 2- to 3-mm margin of surface skin. The excision is carried into the subcutaneous adipose tissue.

chemical cautery (aluminum chloride, Monsel's solution), or fibrin foam. The wound is allowed to heal by second intention, which usually occurs over 3 to 6 weeks, depending on the size of the wound. A shave biopsy through the dermis is never recommended for any suspicious pigmented lesion, owing to the risk of transection of the lesion. (For further information, see Robinson et al., *Atlas of Cutaneous Surgery*, Chapters 4 and 9.)

Incisional Biopsy

Three types of incisional biopsies are acceptable for a biopsy of a suspicious lesion: punch biopsy, elliptical incisional biopsy, and saucerization. Removal of the most elevated and/or clinically suspicious area of the lesion to the adipose tissue is indicated during any incisional biopsy. The elliptical incision (wedge) and the incisional saucerization biopsies are useful for relatively large lesions when complete excision is difficult. The surgical techniques are similar to the elliptical excision and the saucerization excision described previously.[30] Incisional biopsy does not increase the risk of metastasis of a melanoma.[27, 28]

The use of local skin flaps and skin grafts are discussed elsewhere in the text. Conventional tissue expansion is discussed briefly for excision of large congenital nevi.[32, 33] The management of large congenital nevi should be approached on an individual basis. Due to the risk of progression to melanoma, excision is often recommended.[34] This can be accomplished by the use of serial excisions or tissue expansion. Tissue expansion is performed by gradual inflation of a balloon-type device placed beneath the skin. Once the desired degree of tissue expansion has been achieved after a period of about 6 weeks, the tissue expansion device is removed. The adjacent lesion is then excised, and the expanded tissue is used to reconstruct the surgical defect.

Advantages of tissue expansion over conventional reconstructive techniques include the ability to biologically greatly increase the amount of skin available for soft tissue reconstruction (Figs. 150–16 and 150–17). In most cases the expanded tissue will cover both the donor and recipient sites resulting in an easily manageable secondary defect. Tissue expansion provides excess adjacent donor tissue with good to excellent tissue match in terms of color, texture, and hair-bearing properties. This is particularly important for maximal cosmesis on the face and scalp. The expansion process produces angiogenesis in the expanded tissue, resulting in a highly vascular flap with good survival potential. Sensation is also usually preserved in the expanded tissue. Finally, tissue expansion can usually be performed, if desired, in children younger than 1 year of age. Disadvantages include the need for two operations—one to place the expander and another to remove it and complete the excision and reconstruction. Multiple office visits are required to infuse saline into the expander during the expansion process over a period of several weeks. Disfigurement usually occurs as the expansion process proceeds. This is temporary, and most patients tolerate this transient deformity without great difficulty. For most areas of the

of a two-stage procedure if the lesion is, in fact, a melanoma. The second stage consists of a wide local excision to the fascia with margins ranging from 0.5 to 3 cm, dependent on the Breslow depth of invasion.[29, 30] Before the excisional biopsy, the lesion may be examined with a Wood lamp to help delineate subclinical pigment extension. The planned excisional lines can then be marked with ink with 2- to 3-mm margins. The excision is designed with the long axis corresponding to the relaxed skin tension lines. The length-to-width ratio may range from 2:1 to 4:1, depending on anatomic location and skin elasticity. The optimal angle at the tip of the ellipse is 20 degrees. M-plasties may be used at the tips of the ellipse to shorten the length of the excision. After perpendicular incision of the skin, the tissue is removed with scissors or scalpel at a uniform depth and placed in 10% formalin solution. Failure to remove the tissue at a uniform depth, with a deeper excision in the center and more superficial excision at the apices, will result in pseudo dog-ears. If necessary, undermining may be achieved to provide greater skin mobility. After meticulous hemostasis with spot electrocoagulation, the wound is closed in a standard two-layer closure with absorbable and nonabsorbable sutures or with a simple cutaneous closure with nonabsorbable sutures.[31]

The excisional saucerization represents a modification of the excision technique. No sutures are used, and the wound heals by second intention (granulation). The scalpel is placed on the skin at a 45- to 60-degree angle. The skin is cut with the scalpel or scissors through the dermis to the underlying adipose tissue and removed. Meticulous hemostasis is achieved with spot electrocoagulation,

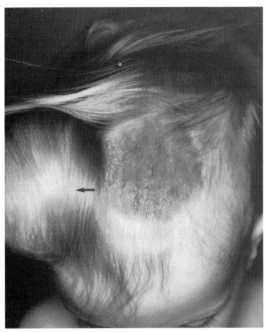

FIGURE 150–16. Congenital nevus located on the scalp in an infant. A tissue expander was placed and inflated adjacent to the lesion (*arrow*). (Courtesy of Shan Baker, M.D.).

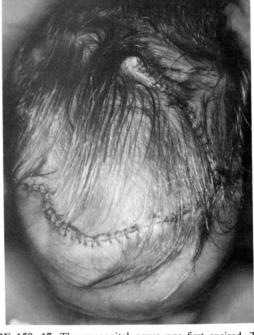

FIGURE 150–17. The congenital nevus was first excised. The expanded adjacent tissue was then used to close the defect with hair-bearing tissue and a rotation flap. (Courtesy of Shan Baker, M.D.)

body, complications are infrequent and usually minor. These include infection, hematoma, seroma, pain, mechanical device failure, exposure or extrusion of the expander, tissue necrosis, and bone resorption. Tissue expansion is an extraordinary procedure based on the skin's ability to stretch and increase in surface area in response to a mechanical force.

Atypical Melanocytic Nevi

Clay J. Cockerell

DEFINITION

Atypical melanocytic nevus, formerly termed "dysplastic nevus," refers to a benign melanocytic neoplasm that displays a characteristic constellation of clinical and histologic findings that in some forms has been associated with the development of malignant melanoma. Because the term *dysplastic nevus* is controversial, it has been recommended by a National Institutes of Health Consensus Conference that the term *dysplastic nevus* no longer be used to describe the clinical presentation.[35] Although it has been recommended that *nevus with architectural disorder* or *Clark's nevus* be substituted for the pathologic description, because the phrase "dysplastic nevus" is firmly entrenched in clinical practice and in the literature it is likely to be used for some time to come. Although *atypical nevus* is used synonymously with *dysplastic nevus* in this chapter, the terms are in transition. Regardless of terminology it is important that the criteria used to diagnose this lesion on both clinical and histologic grounds be understood and that it be recognized that there is concern and controversy regarding the potential for development of melanoma in association with these lesions.

CLINICAL DESCRIPTION

Clinical criteria that are characteristic of atypical nevi include melanocytic lesions with variegated colors of tan,

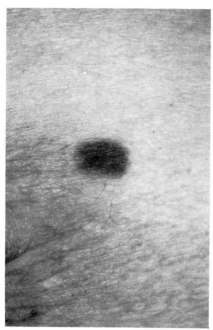

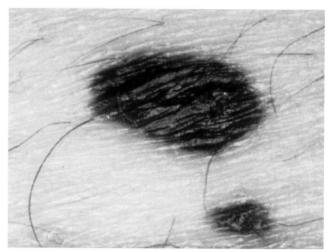

FIGURE 150–19. Junctional type of atypical melanocytic nevus. Two lesions are located very close to each other. (See color plate.)

FIGURE 150–18. Compound type of atypical melanocytic nevus. Note the peripheral spread of pigment. Lesion is located at the junction of the areola in a young woman. (See color plate.) (Courtesy of June K. Robinson, M.D.)

brown, and, frequently, areas of dyspigmentation; irregular angulated outlines; and size 5 to 10 mm or larger with location predominantly on the back, chest, abdomen, and arms.[36] They may be solitary or present in multiplicity. Individual lesions may have a central papular component surrounded by a "halo" of brown, or they may appear as mamillated plaques (Figs. 150–18 and 150–19; see color plate).

PATHOLOGY

The histologic features of atypical nevi, while not entirely specific, consist of nests of melanocytes at the

dermoepidermal junction at the bases and sides of epidermal retia, elongation of epidermal retia, slight coalescence of nests of junctional melanocytes ("bridging"), fibrosis surrounding epidermal retia, and a sparse infiltrate of lymphocytes in the papillary dermis (Fig. 150–20).[37–40] Although the melanocytes may be large and somewhat pleomorphic, they do not demonstrate cytologic atypia to the degree observed in melanoma. Lesions are generally larger than 5 to 6 mm in greatest diameter when they are sampled, although the histologic features noted earlier may be seen when they are much smaller. In compound lesions, there is a central component of intradermal nests of typical-appearing melanocytes associated with a proliferation of melanocytes arranged singly and in nests at the dermoepidermal junction extending beyond the intradermal component. Four histologic features defined by Clark and others are generally found. These include "basilar melanocytic hyperplasia" (increase in the number of melanocytes at the dermoepidermal junction arranged in solitary units and in nests),

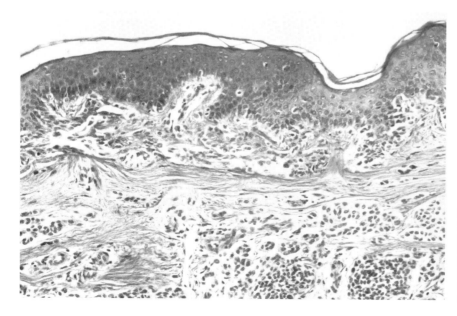

FIGURE 150–20. Compound type of atypical ("dysplastic") melanocytic nevus. There is a component of dermal nevus cells with melanocytes at the dermoepidermal junction that have coalesced focally ("bridging") around which there is fibroplasia. There is also a sparse infiltrate of lymphocytes in the dermis. Note the absence of significant cytologic atypia.

"random" cytologic atypia (scattered melanocytes within the nevus component having enlarged nuclei and slight pleomorphism), a sparse lymphocytic infiltrate in the dermis, and lamellar fibrosis and/or concentric eosinophilic fibroplasia (thickened collagen bundles arranged in "plates" beneath retia or surrounding them, respectively).[37, 38]

Although criteria for clinical and histologic diagnosis of atypical nevi are discussed extensively in the literature, it should be noted that the specificity of these criteria is in question and has remained controversial.[41] Many atypical nevi display features clinically similar to those of evolving melanoma, namely, asymmetry, border irregularity, color irregularity, and diameter greater than 6 mm.[42] In addition, the histologic features that have been described as being specific for atypical nevi have been demonstrated in other lesions such as growing nevi in children and nevi in pregnancy.[43, 44] Thus, for a diagnosis of atypical nevus to be rendered with certainty, it is becoming increasingly recognized that clinicopathologic correlation is required.

PATHOGENESIS AND ETIOLOGY

The pathogenesis of the familial atypical nevus syndrome remains unclear, although some studies have suggested that it is transmitted in autosomal dominant fashion associated with linkage to the short arm of chromosome 1 (1P36).[46] This, too, is controversial since several studies have refuted this finding and have suggested that heritability is polygenic.[47-49] The risk of melanoma is more likely related to nevus density and total number of nevi than their morphologic features. Whether there is a circulating stimulatory growth factor that leads to the expression of numerous pigmented lesions in these patients has yet to be defined.

DIAGNOSIS AND DIFFERENTIAL DIAGNOSIS

The most important feature of atypical nevi is that their presence has been correlated with melanoma risk. In the original paper published in 1978 by Clark and coworkers, it was established that families existed in which there were many individuals with large numbers of unusual-appearing nevi who developed melanoma with greater frequency than those in the general population (Fig. 150–21; see color plate).[45] Melanoma arising in association with a preexisting atypical nevus was documented. Since that original paper, it has become well-accepted that a familial melanoma syndrome associated with multiple unusual-appearing nevi exists. However, significant controversy still exists with regard to precisely what is required to establish that diagnosis. As mentioned earlier, the method used to diagnose atypical nevi is controversial and varies among persons. Some workers have stated that the diagnosis can be made by the evaluation of histologic features alone, whereas others have averred that such nevi may be diagnosed using either histologic or clinical criteria.[37, 50]

Once a diagnosis has been made, the question arises as to how many lesions are necessary for the diagnosis of the atypical nevus syndrome. According to some experts, a patient with even a solitary atypical nevus should be defined as having the syndrome.[37] A less strict definition has been proposed such that the presence of two to three or more clinically and histologically characteristic lesions in a given individual is diagnostic.[51]

A number of different clinical subsets have been created depending on the presence or absence of atypical nevi and melanoma in family members. The sporadic subtypes are only weakly correlated with melanoma risk if at all. On the other hand, persons with multiple atypical nevi and a strong family history of melanoma in first-degree relatives are at risk for the development of melanoma that may reach 100% over the course of a lifetime.[52] Thus, it is essential that a distinction be made between these subtypes. Studies of atypical nevus syndrome families have demonstrated approximately 32,000 affected persons in the United States, an incidence that is slightly higher but similar to that of other familial cancer syndromes such as Gardner's syndrome.[53] The prevalence of sporadic atypical nevi has been estimated to range from 5% to 53% of populations in different studies.[54, 55] Thus, if a loose definition for the atypical nevus syndrome is used, namely, the presence of one lesion being sufficient for the diagnosis, over 50% of white individuals in the United States could be said to be affected with a familial syndrome associated with malignancy. As mentioned previously, studies have shown that melanoma risk correlates more with the total nevus density or nevus number than morphologic features of individual lesions.[55, 56] Therefore, the most reasonable conclusion is that patients with atypical nevi and a personal or family history of melanoma are those afflicted with the familial form of the disorder and are at greatest risk for the development of melanoma. Those with many nevi, regardless of clinical or histologic features, are also at increased risk for development of melanoma albeit less than patients with the familial atypical nevus syndrome.

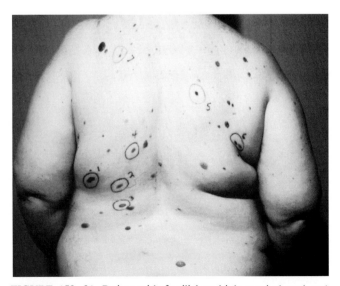

FIGURE 150–21. Patient with familial multiple atypical nevi and melanoma. Lesion 1 was shown to represent melanoma following excision. (See color plate.)

Another important point that has remained controversial is whether atypical nevi are truly precursors of melanoma or whether they serve primarily as markers for an increased risk of melanoma development. Most patients with familial atypical nevus syndrome who develop melanoma most commonly develop them on normal skin where there is no preexisting melanocytic nevus.[52] Nevertheless, the existence of atypical nevi seen histologically in association with melanoma has been estimated to range from less than 1% to 83%.[57, 58] The reason for this marked disparity is, in all likelihood, a consequence of overinterpretation of melanocytic proliferation at the edge of melanoma as representing residual atypical nevus. Unless an incontrovertible atypical ("dysplastic") nevus can be demonstrated histologically, it is generally considered unreasonable by most experts to render the diagnosis of melanoma arising in association with an atypical ("dysplastic") nevus.

Although the atypical nevus syndrome remains a controversial topic, it is important nonetheless that a rational approach to managing patients with this disorder be followed.[59] Since the clinical criteria for the diagnosis of atypical nevi and melanoma overlap significantly, the most important aspect of the diagnosis lies in distinguishing these two. All experts agree that atypical nevi are "stable" lesions and do not tend to increase rapidly in size or change appreciably in color; therefore, careful observation should enable clinicians to distinguish between these since evolving melanoma tends to become darker and change in size and shape over time. Special attention should be given to the development of zones of black within a lesion because this finding has been correlated with evolving melanoma.[53]

TREATMENT

In that many patients with atypical nevi have numerous lesions, wholesale biopsy, excision, and removal is not feasible. One alternative that has been proposed is that a series of regional photographs be taken for baseline documentation of the clinical morphology of lesions followed by periodic observation and comparison.[60] In patients with only a few lesions, follow-up at 12-month intervals is generally considered sufficient. In patients with a personal or family history of melanoma, careful observation at up to 4-month intervals is necessary. Any lesions documented to have changed should be subjected to biopsy. Furthermore, family members of index cases should be examined. All affected patients should be advised to avoid potential carcinogens such as ultraviolet irradiation that could lead to a synergistic effect with regard to the development of melanoma.[61]

Since the histologic criteria for the diagnosis of atypical ("dysplastic") nevi are not specific, it is essential that patients not be overdiagnosed as having atypical ("dysplastic") nevi to avoid their being labeled as having a syndrome associated with malignancy. Histologic features seen in atypical ("dysplastic") nevi may be observed in recurrent nevi, growing nevi, and junctional nevi in children among others so that it is essential that the diagnosis not be rendered unless there is clinical correlation.[59] It is recommended that lesions having histologic features suggestive of nevi with architectural disorder be interpreted simply as compound or junctional nevi with commentary made that there are histologic features similar to those observed in lesions taken from patients with familial melanoma. Whether such findings are of importance depends on whether there is a personal or family history of melanoma. It has been suggested by others that nevi be "graded" with respect to the degree of "dysplasia" within individual lesions. Nevertheless, until further studies demonstrate conclusively that melanoma risk correlates with histologic features, such a practice does not seem warranted.

Because it has been recommended by the National Institutes of Health that the term *dysplastic nevus* no longer be used,[35] some experts have proposed that the term *Clark's nevus* be used as a name for this lesion in that Wallace H. Clark, Jr. and colleagues were the first to scientifically study and define this syndrome.[62] Whether this eponym is accepted will in all likelihood depend on usage and, possibly, discussion at future consensus conferences.

References

1. Sagebiel RW, Odland GF. In: Riley V, ed. Pigmentation: Its Genesis and Biologic Control. New York: Appleton-Century-Crofts, 1972:43.
2. Maize JC, Ackerman AB. Pigmented Lesions of the Skin. Philadelphia: Lea & Febiger, 1987.
3. Breathnach AS, Wyllie LM. Electron microscopy of melanocytes and melanosomes in freckled human epidermis. J Invest Dermatol 1964;42:389–394.
4. Bolognia JL, Shapiro PE, Perifollicular hypopigmentation: A cause of variegate pigmentation and irregular border in melanocytic nevi. Arch Dermatol 1992;128:514–517.
5. Giardiello RM, Welsh SB, Hamilton SR, et al. Increased risk of cancer in the Peutz-Jeghers syndrome. N Engl J Med 1987; 316:1511–1514.
6. Atherton DJ, Pitcher DW, Wells RS, et al. A syndrome of various cutaneous pigmented lesions, myxoid neurofibromata and atrial myxoma: The NAME syndrome. Br J Dermatol 1980;103: 421–429.
7. Haensler T, Christophers E, Honigman H, et al. Skin tumours in the European PUVA study. J Am Acad Dermatol 1987; 16:108–116.
8. Spann CR, Owen LG, Hodge SJ. The labial melanotic macule. Arch Dermatol 1987;123:1029–1031.
9. Barnhill RL, Albert LS, Shama SK, et al. Genital lentiginosis. J Am Acad Dermatol 1990;22:453–460.
10. Maize JC, Foster G. Age-related changes in melanocytic nevi. Clin Exp Dermatol 1979;4:49–58.
11. Lund HZ, Stobbe GD. The natural history of the pigmented nevus: Factors of age and anatomic location. Am J Pathol 1949; 25:1117–1145.
12. Goldman L, Richfield DF. Effect of corticotropin and cortisone on development and progress of pigmented nevi. JAMA 1951; 147:941–943.
13. Bourguignon J-P, Pierard GE, Emould C, et al. Effects of human growth hormone therapy on melanocytic naevi. Lancet 1993; 341:1505–1506.
14. Spitz S. Melanomas of childhood. Am J Pathol 1948;24:591–609.
15. Sagebiel RW, Chinn EK, Egbert BM. Pigmented spindle cell nevus: Clinical and histologic review of 90 cases. Am J Surg Pathol 1981;8:645–653.
16. Barr RJ, Morales RV, Graham JH. Desmoplastic nevus: A distinct histologic variant of mixed spindle cell and epithelioid cell nevus. Cancer 1980;46:557–564.
17. Schrader WA, Helwig EB. Balloon cell nevi. Cancer 1967; 20:1502–1514.

18. Frank SB, Cohen HJ. The halo nevus. Arch Dermatol 1964; 89:367–373.
19. Stewart DM, Altman J, Mehregan AH. Speckled lentiginous nevus. Arch Dermatol 1978;114:895–896.
20. Osburn K, Schosser RH, Everett MA. Congenital pigmented and vascular lesions in newborn infants. J Am Acad Dermatol 1987;16:788–792.
21. Silvers DN, Helwig EB. Melanocytic nevi in neonates. J Am Acad Dermatol 1981;41:166–175.
22. Park HK, Leonard DD, Arrington JH, Lund HZ. Recurrent melanocytic nevi: Clinical and histologic review of 175 cases. J Am Acad Dermatol 1987;17:285–292.
23. Sun CC, Lu YC, Lee EF, et al. Naevus fuso-caeruleus zygomaticus. Br J Dermatol 1987;117:545–553.
24. Leopold JG, Richardson DB. The interrelationship of blue and common nevi. J Pathol 1968;95:37–43.
25. Seab JA Jr, Graham JH, Helwig EB. Deep penetrating nevus. Am J Surg Pathol 1989;13:39–44.
26. Rhodes AR, Weinstock MA, Fitzpatrick TB, et al. Risk factors for cutaneous melanoma: A practical method of recognizing predisposed individuals. JAMA 1987;258:3146–3154.
27. Sober AJ, Fitzpatrick TB, Mihm MC Jr. Primary melanoma of the skin. J Am Acad Dermatol 1980;2:179–197.
28. Lederman JS, Sober AJ. Does biopsy type influence survival in clinical Stage I cutaneous melanoma? J Am Acad Dermatol 1985;13:983–987.
29. Ho VC, Sober AJ. Therapy for cutaneous melanoma: An update. J Am Acad Dermatol 1990;22:159–176.
30. Early Melanoma NIH Consensus Conference. Diagnosis and treatment of early melanoma. JAMA 1992;268:1314–1319.
31. Swanson NA. Basic techniques. In: Swanson NA, ed. Atlas of Cutaneous Surgery, vol. 1. Boston: Little, Brown & Co, 1987: 14–62.
32. Argenta LC, Marks MW, Pasyk KA. Advances in tissue expansion. Clin Plast Surg 1988;12:159–171.
33. Baker S, Swanson NA. Clinical applications of tissue expansion in head and neck surgery. Laryngoscope 1990;10:313–319.
34. Kang S, Milton GW, Sober AJ. Childhood melanoma. In: Balch CM, Houghton AN, Milton GW, et al., eds. Cutaneous Melanoma, 2nd ed, vol 1. Philadelphia: JB Lippincott, 1992:312–315.
35. National Institutes of Health Consensus Development Conference. Diagnosis and treatment of early melanoma. JAMA 1992;268: 1314–1319.
36. Greene MH, Clark WH Jr, Tucker MA, et al. Acquired precursors of cutaneous malignant melanoma: The familial dysplastic nevus syndrome. N Engl J Med 1985;312:91–97.
37. Elder DE, Kraemer KH, Greene MH, et al. The dysplastic nevus syndrome: Our definition. Am J Dermatopathol 1982;4:455–460.
38. Elder DE, Goldman LI, Goldman SC, et al. Dysplastic nevus syndrome: A phenotypic association of sporadic cutaneous melanoma. Cancer 1980;46:1787–1794.
39. Clark WH Jr. The dysplastic nevus syndrome. Arch Dermatol 1988;124:1207–1210.
40. Consensus conference: Precursors to malignant melanoma. JAMA 1984;251:1864–1866.
41. Grob JJ, Andrac L, Romano MH, et al. Dysplastic nevus in nonfamilial melanoma: A clinicopathological study of 101 cases. Br J Dermatol 1988;118:745–752.

42. Friedman RJ, Rigel DS, Kopf AW. Early detection of malignant melanoma: The role of physician examination and self examination of the skin. Ca 1985;35:130–151.
43. Eng AM. Solitary small active junctional nevi in juvenile patients. Arch Dermatol 1983;119:35–38.
44. Klein LJ, Barr RJ. Histologic atypia in clinically benign nevi: A prospective study. J Am Acad Dermatol 1990;22:275–282.
45. Clark WH Jr, Reimer RR, Greene MH, et al. Origin of familial malignant melanomas from heritable melanocytic lesions: The B-K mole syndrome. Arch Dermatol 1978;114:732–738.
46. Bale SJ, Tucker MA, et al: Mapping the gene for hereditary cutaneous malignant melanoma-dysplastic nevus to chromosome 1p. N Engl J Med 1989;320:1367–1372.
47. Van Haeringen A, Bergman W, Nelen MR, et al. Exclusion of the dysplastic nevus syndrome (DNS) locus from the short arm of chromosome 1 by linkage studies in Dutch families. Genomics 1989;5:61–64.
48. Cannon-Albright LA, Goldgar DE, Wright EC, et al. Evidence against the reported linkage of the cutaneous melanoma-dysplastic nevus syndrome locus to chromosome 1p36. Am J Hum Genet 1990;46:912–918.
49. Happle R, Traupe H, Vakilzadeh F, et al. Arguments in favor of a polygenic inheritance of precursor nevi. J Am Acad Dermatol 1982;6:540–543.
50. Cooke KR, Spears GFS, Elder DE, et al. Dysplastic nevi in a population-based study. Cancer 1989;63:1240–1244.
51. Clark WH Jr, Elder DE, Guerry D IV, et al. A study of tumor progression: The precursor lesions of superficial spreading and nodular melanoma. Hum Pathol 1984;15:1147–1165.
52. Rigel DS, Rivers JK, Kopf AW, et al. Dysplastic nevi: Markers for increased risk of melanoma. Cancer 1989;63:386–389.
53. Kraemer KH, Greene MH. Dysplastic nevus syndrome, familial and sporadic precursors of cutaneous melanoma. Dermatol Clin 1985;3:225–237.
54. Crutcher WA, Sagebiel RW. Prevalence of dysplastic naevi in a community practice (letter). Lancet 1984;1:729.
55. Piepkorn M, Meyer LJ, Goldgar DE, et al. The dysplastic melanocytic nevus: A prevalent lesion that correlates poorly with clinical phenotype. J Am Acad Dermatol 1989;20:407–415.
56. Holly EA, Kelly FW, Shpall SN, Chiu SH. Number of melanocytic nevi as a major risk factor for malignant melanoma. J Am Acad Dermatol 1987;17:459–468.
57. Rigel DS, Friedman RJ, Kopf AW, et al. Precursors of malignant melanoma: Problems in computing the risk of malignant melanoma arising in dysplastic and congenital nevocytic nevi. Dermatol Clin 1985;3:361–365.
58. Lopansri S, Mihm MC Jr. Clinical and pathological correlation of malignant melanoma. J Cutan Pathol 1979;6:180–194.
59. Cockerell CJ. A rational approach to the understanding and management of the dysplastic nevus syndrome concept. Pathol Annu 1993;28:121–144.
60. Slue W, Kopf AW, Rivers JK. Total-body photographs of dysplastic nevi. Arch Dermatol 1988;124:1239–1243.
61. MacKie RM, Freudenberger T, Aitchison TC. Personal risk factor chart for cutaneous melanoma. Lancet 1989;2:487–490.
62. Ackerman AB. What naevus is dysplastic, a syndrome, and the commonest precursor of malignant melanoma? A riddle and an answer. Histopathology 1988;13:241–256.

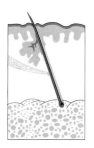

chapter 151

Melanoma

HOWARD K. KOH, RAYMOND L. BARNHILL,
and GARY S. ROGERS

DEFINITION

Cutaneous melanoma arises from malignant melanocytes located in the skin.[1] Noncutaneous primary sites of melanocytes also include mucosal epithelia, retina, and leptomeninges.

Treatment and control of this increasingly common cancer requires a multidisciplinary approach including dermatologists, surgeons, oncologists, immunologists, primary care physicians, pathologists, epidemiologists, health educators, environmentalists, and public health professionals, among others. We will review the current state of knowledge of melanoma and outline approaches for treatment and control.

CLINICAL DESCRIPTION

Epidemiology

Decades of steady increases in the incidence of cutaneous melanoma throughout the industrialized world have made it a common cancer.[1-7] The rise in the melanoma incidence and mortality rate is second only to lung cancer in women (Fig. 151-1).

In the United States, the incidence of melanoma has almost tripled in the past four decades, faster than that of any other cancer.[4, 6, 8] This rise is not explained by any temporal change in diagnostic criteria,[9] although early detection efforts may be contributing to some degree. Approximately 32,000 Americans will be found to have melanoma in 1994, and 6900 will die from the disease.[10] Projections suggest that by the year 2000, one in 90 Americans will develop melanoma.[8] Melanoma affects all adult age groups, with the median age at diagnosis being 53.[1, 5]

While the current 5-year survival rate of 83% represents a vast improvement over the 49% rate in 1950,[5] the mortality rate has increased almost 150% in the United States in the past 40 years. In addition, deaths from melanoma in young adults contribute to many years of potential life lost.[11]

Inasmuch as the precise etiology of melanoma is unknown, ongoing research has focused on risk factors, genetic factors, exposure to ultraviolet (UV) light, and environmental exposures. Of the major risk factors for melanoma (Table 151-1),[12-21] the importance of genetic factors is reflected in that about 6% of persons with melanoma have a family history of this cancer; also, those with a family history of melanoma in parents or offspring have an estimated eightfold increased risk of developing the disease themselves.[12-16]

Epidemiologic and case control studies suggest a role for sunlight in the pathogenesis of melanoma (Table 151-1).[20-26] Although radiation in the ultraviolet B (UVB) range (290-320 nm) may be causative, the precise action spectrum for human melanoma remains unknown.[22, 23] A growing body of evidence supports the hypothesis that the risk of melanoma depends more on intermittent recreational sun exposure, especially early in life, than on simple cumulative sun exposure.[20-26] Worldwide, the incidence of melanoma generally correlates inversely with latitude, with rates higher in locations closest to the equator and progressively lower in areas closer to the poles.[20-23] Whites, especially those with a tendency to burn rather than (or instead of) tan when exposed to sunlight (type 1 or 2 skin) have much higher rates of melanoma than nonwhites.[20-23] Furthermore, investigators have linked blistering sunburns in childhood or adolescence with increased rates of melanoma later in life.[20-26] Migration studies suggest that childhood or adolescence represents a "critical period" for UV burn.[20, 22-23] Furthermore, in xeroderma pigmentosum, a rare autosomal recessive disorder characterized by deficient repair of UVB-damaged DNA, there is a 1000-fold increased rate of skin cancer, including melanoma.[27]

TRENDS IN SEER INCIDENCE AND U.S. MORTALITY RATES
BY PRIMARY CANCER SITE
1973–1990

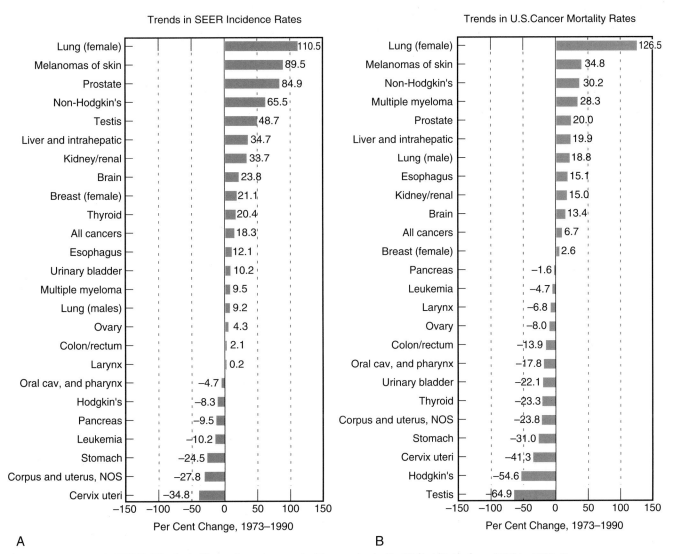

FIGURE 151–1. *A,* Change in melanoma incidence rates in the United States from 1973 to 1990. *B,* Change in melanoma mortality rates in the United States from 1973 to 1990. SEER, surveillance, epidemiology, and end-results.

However, not all evidence readily links UV light with melanoma.[20-23, 25] Melanoma rates are relatively low in persons with outdoor occupations.[17, 22-23, 25] Except for the lentigo maligna melanoma subtype, melanoma does not regularly occur on maximally sun exposed skin, such as the face (a notable exception to this is seen in Australia, where high rates of melanoma on the face are being described).[28] The linkage of blistering sunburns to increased melanoma risk may be confounded by phenotype (easy burning) as a risk factor. Also, aside from one recent report,[29] studies have failed to induce melanoma regularly in animals using UV light alone.

Many speculate that increased recreational sun exposure has contributed to the rising incidence of melanoma.[5, 25] In addition, the depletion of the earth's stratospheric ozone layer, induced and exacerbated by man-made chlorofluorocarbons,[30, 31] may increase the amount of UV light reaching the earth and contribute to the rising incidence in the coming decades.[21] A recent report from Canada has documented increased UVB reaching the earth, due to ozone depletion.[32] Similarly, some preliminary evidence has linked melanoma to sun beds and tanning parlors.[33, 34]

Clinical Presentation

Because cutaneous melanoma is a uniquely visible tumor, the early detection and recognition of melanoma is the key to possible cure.[35] An ABCD guideline helps the observer to suspect the diagnosis of melanoma in any pigmented lesion: A—asymmetry, B—border irregularity, C—color variegation or dark black color, and D—diameter greater than 0.6 cm (the size of a pencil eraser).

TABLE 151-1. Summary of Risk Factors for the Development of Cutaneous Melanoma

Risk Factor	Relative Risk*
Adulthood (≥15 yr)	88
Pigmented lesions:	
Dysplastic mole(s) (and familial melanoma)	148
Dysplastic mole(s) (but no familial melanoma)	7-70
Lentigo maligna	10
Higher than average number of benign melanocytic nevi	2-64
Congenital mole	17-21
White race (vs. black)	12
Previous cutaneous melanoma	5-9
Cutaneous melanoma in parents, children, or siblings	2-8
Immunosuppression	2-8
Excessive sun exposure	3-5
Sun sensitivity	2-3

*Degree of increased risk for persons with the risk factor compared with persons without the risk factor. Relative risk of 1.0 implies no increased risk.

Modified with permission from the New England Journal of Medicine, 1991;325:171-182.

The possibility of melanoma should be considered when a patient reports a new pigmented lesion, or a change in a preexisting mole, such as a change in the color, size, shape, or surface. The typical patient with melanoma usually experiences no skin discomfort whatsoever (such as itching or burning)—pain is uncommon and usually associated with late presentation.[36] Hence, the visual examination remains the most reliable means of identification.[35]

Evaluation of the visual examination as a screening tool should determine its sensitivity, specificity, and predictive value. A number of reports have documented dermatologists' accuracy in the diagnosis of melanoma in the clinical setting. Kopf and associates noted an overall accuracy of 64%; in a later report, Grin and colleagues noted improvement in clinical diagnosis of melanoma from 1955 through 1982 with a sensitivity of 84.5% and a specificity of 72.4% in the most recent period (1974 to 1982).[37, 38] Perednia and coworkers found significant differences between dermatologists in assessment of skin images when measures of diagnostic sensitivity, reproducibility, and reliability were assessed.[39] Preliminary evaluation of screening data from the American Academy of Dermatology programs finds the predictive value positive of a visual examination by a dermatologist is 27% to 31% in Massachusetts and 10% to 16% in national American Academy of Dermatology screenings.[40, 41] Recent research has used epiluminescence microscopy (dermoscopy) to aid in clinical recognition of melanoma; however, its use currently remains restricted to specialized centers.[42]

Melanoma can occur anywhere on the skin surface, but not infrequently occurs on the back and other areas that are difficult for persons to inspect themselves (Fig. 151-2). Because patients with melanoma on such areas may be unaware of the existence of these lesions, early detection by physicians, nurses, spouses, family members, and others can be exceedingly important.[35]

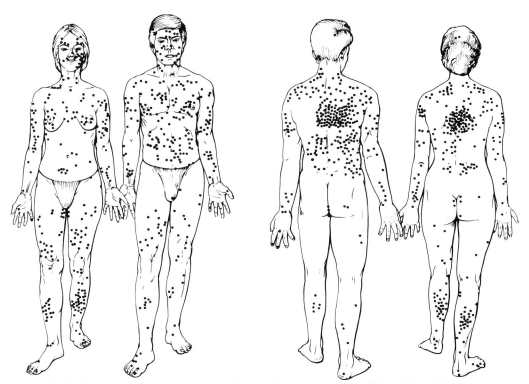

FIGURE 151-2. Body site distribution of melanoma. (Reprinted from Koh HK, Geller AC, Miller DR, et al. Skin Cancer: Prevention and control. In: Greenwold P, Kramer BS, Weel DL (eds.). Cancer Prevention and Control. By courtesy of Marcel Dekker Inc., 1995:611-640.)

The four classic histogenetic types of melanoma are defined by their clinical and histologic characteristics and by the history of progression of the lesion. Although prognostic differences among the various types can largely be accounted for by the tumor thickness at the time of diagnosis, anatomic site, and sex of the patient, there is still reason to believe that these types are distinctive processes reflecting different pathophysiologies.[43]

Regardless of type, nearly all cutaneous melanomas begin as proliferations of neoplastic melanocytes within the epidermis (Fig. 151–3; see color plate) and sometimes its epithelial adnexal structures—eccrine ducts and hair follicles, a stage termed *melanoma in situ.* Lentigo maligna and the intraepidermal forms of superficial spreading and acral lentiginous melanoma all have histologically distinctive growth patterns. By definition, nodular melanomas lack an in situ component, presumably present early on but overrun by the rapid proliferation of melanoma cells in the dermis.

Lentigo maligna is most commonly seen in atrophic sun-damaged skin of the head and neck in patients in the fifth decade or older. It begins as an irregularly bordered tan or brown macule, and typically enlarges over many years to become an irregularly shaped patch (Fig. 151–4; see color plate).[43] In time, one or more papules or nodules can develop within the patch. The raised areas can be the same color as the patch, or any shade of pink, red, and brown. Palpable areas within a lentigo maligna herald the presence of invasion, and the lesion is then termed *lentigo maligna* melanoma. Rarely, lentigo maligna or lentigo maligna melanoma (LMM) can be amelanotic, appearing as a reddish, scaly area. The actual size of a lentigo maligna or LMM is often underestimated clinically. Examination under Wood's light can sometimes reveal the true size of the lesion.

Superficial spreading melanoma can occur anywhere on the skin. It rarely arises before the fourth decade of life and appears to evolve more rapidly than LMM.[43] By the time that most lesions are recognized, they are over 2.5 cm in diameter and may be palpable (Fig. 151–5; see color plate). They often have angulated or notched borders. There is great variability in the color of these lesions, and shades of pink, red, tan, brown, and black are often haphazardly arranged. Papular or nodular areas

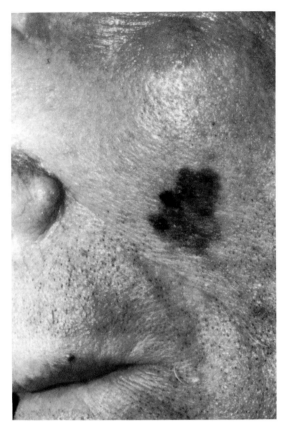

FIGURE 151–4. Lentigo maligna melanoma on the face. (See color plate.)

signify invasion of the dermis and can be ulcerated. Often, superficial spreading melanomas begin in a long-standing nevus, noted as a change by the patient.

Nodular melanoma appears clinically as a papule or nodule of melanoma. A common misconception is that nodular melanoma is any melanoma in which a nodule is present; nodules occur in superficial spreading, lentigo maligna, and acral lentiginous melanomas. Nodular melanoma is most common on the trunk in men and on the

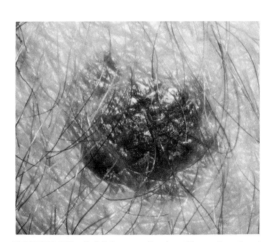

FIGURE 151–3. Melanoma in situ. (See color plate.)

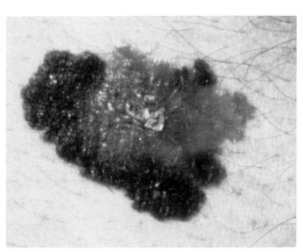

FIGURE 151–5. Superficial spreading melanoma. (See color plate.)

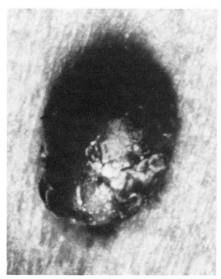

FIGURE 151-6. Nodular melanoma. (See color plate.)

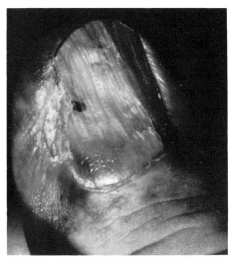

FIGURE 151-7. Acral lentiginous melanoma demonstrates Hutchinson's sign, the spreading of pigmentation onto the proximal nail fold. (See color plate.) (Reprinted with permission from the New England Journal of Medicine, 1991;325:171-182.)

legs of women. It evolves rapidly, seemingly within months, and is elevated when first encountered. Most nodular melanomas are 1 to 2 cm at the time that they are diagnosed, which is most often in the fifth decade of life. Their color ranges from pink in amelanotic lesions to black, or "thundercloud gray" (Fig. 151-6; see color plate).

Acral lentiginous melanoma is found on the palms, soles, and nail beds.[1] Not all melanomas on these sites are of this type. Acral lentiginous melanoma is defined in part by its histologic appearance and some acral melanomas are of the superficial spreading or nodular varieties. Acral lentiginous melanoma appears to be equally common in all races, and is the only form of melanoma consistently found in dark-skinned individuals. Its peak incidence is in persons of 65 years of age or older. It presents as a dark brown patch with irregular borders, within which papules, nodules, or plaques can supervene. Subungual melanoma may extend onto the skin of the proximal nail fold, a finding known as Hutchinson's sign (Fig. 151-7; see color plate).

In addition to the classic forms of melanoma, some unusual ones can be suspected clinically.

Melanoma arising in a congenital nevus presents as an area of change within the lesions. In small congenital nevi, the picture resembles that seen when superficial spreading melanoma arises in an acquired nevus. In large or giant congenital nevi, melanoma can be heralded by a palpable nodule within the dermal substance of a nevus. Melanoma can develop in congenital nevi in neonates or children, in whom other forms of melanoma are rare. Not all papules or nodules that arise in congenital nevi are melanoma; several unusual proliferations behave in a benign fashion. Nonetheless, significant change within a congenital nevus merits a biopsy.

Melanoma arising in a blue nevus (malignant blue nevus) presents as an area of change in a long-standing dark brown or blue lesion. Malignant blue nevi are often situated on the scalp, where it is difficult for patients to monitor lesions.

Mucosal melanoma can present to the dermatologist as a dark patch that spills over onto the cutaneous surface of the lip, genitalia, or anus. Mucosal melanomas are histogenetically similar to acral lentiginous melanomas, and occur with similar frequency in all races. Because the prognosis of invasive mucosal melanoma is poor, early recognition and treatment is paramount.

Regression of melanoma is a cell-mediated immune process whereby lymphocytes destroy the cells of a melanoma, in whole or in part. Regression of a flat area of melanoma results in a white or gray area within it (or sometimes engulfing the entire lesion). In some melanomas in which most of the lesion has regressed, the pigmented, residual areas may be small and separated by broad white or gray zones. Regression of melanoma in situ can accompany persistence of the invasive component, so that a flat depigmented area can be present next to a pigmented or amelanotic raised one (Fig. 151-8; see color plate). Regression can also occur in papules or nodules of melanoma. Complete regression of melanoma can account for the inability to find a primary lesion on examination of a patient with metastatic melanoma.

Halo reactions or even patches of vitiligo can also occur around melanomas and around benign nevi.

Invasive melanomas in which spindled cells predominate can induce desmoplasia. Desmoplastic melanoma presents as a firm plaque that is often amelanotic. Areas of desmoplastic melanoma occur more frequently in the lentigo maligna and acral lentiginous variants. Desmoplastic melanoma can also be found without any evident flat area of melanoma, and if amelanotic, this form is particularly difficult to diagnose. A lesion suspected to be a scar or fibroma that recurs following its incomplete removal should raise suspicion of desmoplastic melanoma. Desmoplastic melanoma, often neurotropic (i.e., it can invade along nerves), can produce neurologic changes.

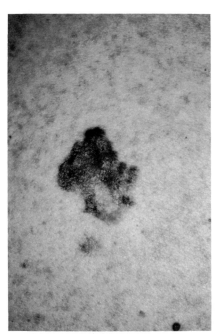

FIGURE 151–8. Regression of melanoma results in flat white or gray areas within a melanoma. (See color plate.) (Courtesy of June K. Robinson, M.D.)

TABLE 151-2. Histopathologic Criteria for the Diagnosis of Melanoma

Radial Growth Phase

Architecture

Asymmetry of general architecture
Poorly defined margins
Loss of nevus architecture
Variation in size, shape, placement of nests
Confluence or fusion of nests
Diminished cohesion of cells in nests
Upward migration of cells (pagetoid spread)
Lack of maturation of melanocytes with descent into the dermis

Cytology

Uniformly atypical (continuous as opposed to variable) population of cells exhibiting cellular enlargement, nuclear enlargement, nuclear pleomorphism, nuclear hyperchromatism, prominent nucleoli

Vertical Growth Phase

Architecture

Expansile nodule or plaque in papillary dermis larger than intraepidermal nests; also, diffuse infiltration of the reticular dermis and subcutaneous fat

Cytology

Usually greater atypicality, frequent loss of pigment synthesis

Satellite metastases of melanoma appear as papules adjacent to a primary melanoma or near the scar of an excised melanoma. Both satellite and distant cutaneous metastases present as symmetrical domed papules. Their colors vary just as those of papules or nodules of primary melanoma do. Rapid growth, or the swift appearance of new lesions often signifies the nature of the process.

A rare form of metastatic melanoma is characterized by diffuse darkening, or melanosis of the skin and often of the sclerae. Patients with generalized melanosis have a dismal prognosis, reflecting widespread metastatic disease, permeation of cutaneous vessels by melanoma cells, increased epidermal melanin, and permeation of the dermis by melanophages. These patients can even have melanuria.

PATHOLOGY

Most cutaneous melanomas begin as an intraepidermal proliferation of melanocytes, designated melanoma in situ when they meet the following criteria: (1) increased frequency of predominantly basilar melanocytes, or melanocytes dispersed at all levels of the epidermis (pagetoid spread); (2) a relatively monomorphous population of markedly atypical melanocytes; (3) both of the above present for a minimum breadth, such as one high-power field, or 0.5 to 1 mm.[44, 45]

One theory proposes that tumor progression in melanoma can be divided into so-called radial and vertical growth phases, linked to the biologic properties of the neoplastic cells (Table 151–2). In radial growth phase, neoplastic melanocytes spread centrifugally within the epidermis, and sometimes appear to infiltrate the papillary dermis as small nests or single cells. In the vertical growth phase, neoplastic melanocytes acquire the ability to form larger nodules. Criteria have been proposed to enable pathologists to distinguish melanoma in radial growth phase from those in which vertical growth has supervened.[44, 45] Accumulating evidence suggests that the radial and vertical growth phases have distinctive biologic properties that explain why some melanomas remain entirely intraepidermal for prolonged periods of time (corresponding to relatively macular pigmented lesions), whereas other lesions display rapid invasion of the dermis to form an expansile nodule or plaque (Table 151–2).[46-48] The radial growth phase appears to lack metastatic potential.[46-48] The vertical growth phase signifies a focal qualitative change resulting in a population or clone of cells that have a growth advantage over the surrounding population.[45-48] This property of forming compact aggregates of cells seems to correlate with the lesion's capacity for metastasis.[46-48] The vertical growth phase differs from that of the radial growth phase cytologically as well as architecturally, displaying more cellular enlargement and greater nuclear atypicality. Cells that enter vertical growth may have a concomitant reduction in, or complete loss of, pigment synthesis, causing the nodule or papule to, at times, appear amelanotic.[46-48]

Classification of Growth Phases: Radial and Vertical

Although no particular type of radial growth phase significantly affects prognosis,[49] recognizing radial growth phase patterns can help the clinician understand the pathogenesis and developmental biology of melanoma. However, of note, some radial growth phases are difficult to categorize. Any radial growth phase pattern may occur in any anatomic location; possibly the particular anatomic site may have more to do with the actual pathogenesis of melanoma than the histologic pattern of the radial growth phase. Also, although melanoma thickness has much greater prognostic significance than the radial growth phase pattern, anatomic site may influence biologic behavior more than actual histopathologic pattern of the radial growth phase.[50] For example, lentigo maligna melanoma seems more directly linked to cumulative sun exposure than any of the other types of melanoma, whereas acral lentiginous melanoma seems least related to the influence of ultraviolet light.[51, 52] Superficial spreading melanoma most often arises in melanocytic nevi.[47, 53, 54] In all likelihood, the rapidity of progression to vertical growth phase from an intraepidermal component varies among tumor types, being the most rapid in nodular melanoma and the most indolent in lentigo maligna melanoma.[54]

Superficial Spreading Melanoma

Superficial spreading melanoma, the most common type of melanoma (about 70% of all melanomas), histologically presents with a prominent intraepidermal proliferation of malignant melanocytes that are at least focally scattered in single-cell array throughout the epidermis.[44, 46, 47, 54] Because the distribution of these cells resembles that of the cells of Paget's disease, the pattern is often called pagetoid. The pagetoid cells may spread up to and include the granular cell layer or may be confined to the lower portions of the epidermis (Fig. 151–9). The cells have abundant cytoplasm, are round or ovoid (also called epithelioid), and contain round nuclei. The nuclei are large, have irregularly dispersed heterochromatin, especially around their margins, and possess nucleoli that usually stain pink. The nuclei vary in size, and multinucleate forms may be present. The cytoplasm has a finely granular texture and usually stains pink-tan. The epi-

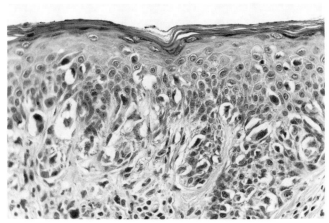

FIGURE 151–10. Superficial spreading melanoma, radial growth phase. Higher magnification shows intraepidermal melanoma and extension of single melanoma cells into the papillary dermis (H & E, × 313).

dermis itself is frequently hyperplastic, but may be of normal thickness or even atrophic.[44]

The radial growth phase of superficial spreading melanoma may be entirely intraepidermal (melanoma in situ or level I).[43, 44, 53, 55] More often, however, single cells or small clusters of cells similar in character to those in the intraepidermal component fill the dermis (level II) (Fig. 151–10). The papillary dermis may contain fibroplasia, a patchy or band-like lymphocytic infiltrate, occasional melanophages, and increased vascularity, especially in inflamed lesions. Mitoses are sometimes noted among the invasive dermal cells. If the papillary dermis contains nests larger than those in the epidermis or the constituent cells have a different appearance, early vertical growth has probably supervened, and the potential for metastasis has developed.[46, 47]

The fully evolved vertical growth phase is defined by expansile nodule formation in the papillary dermis, with widening of the papillary dermis and compression of the papillary reticular dermal junction.[44, 46–48, 56] Single cells may infiltrate the reticular dermis or the subcutaneous fat. Some vertical growth phases do not form expansile nodules but instead extend directly into the deep portions of the skin.[54] Vertical growth phase cells in superficial spreading melanoma usually are large epithelioid cells that commonly aggregate in nests.[44, 46, 47, 53, 54] However, spindle-shaped cells (or a mixture of spindle-shaped, epithelioid, and small epithelioid cells) may be present.

Expansile-nodule formation (level III disease) represents the fully evolved vertical growth phase, which may extend into the reticular dermis (Clark level IV) and infiltrate the subcutaneous fat (Clark level V).[46, 47, 55]

Lentigo Maligna Melanoma

LMM comprises about 5% of all melanomas, and occurs most commonly on the maximally sun exposed skin of the head and neck.[43, 44, 47, 53–55, 57, 58] The radial growth phase, lentigo maligna, is characterized by a mainly basilar or lentiginous proliferation of atypical

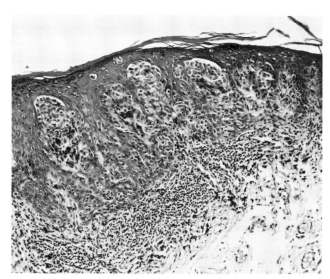

FIGURE 151–9. Superficial spreading melanoma, radial growth phase. Note pagetoid spread of melanoma cells within epidermis (H & E, × 160).

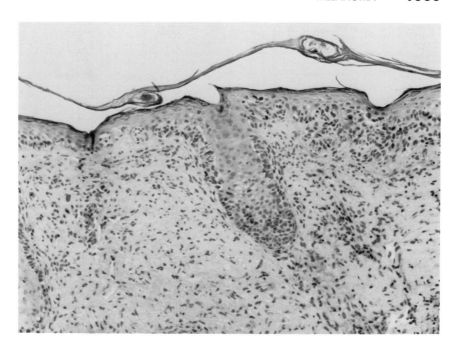

FIGURE 151–11. Lentigo maligna melanoma, radial growth phase. There is a predominantly basilar proliferation of atypical melanocytes along the dermoepidermal junction and also involving the hair follicle epithelium in the center of the field (H & E, × 125).

melanocytes that is associated with an atrophic epidermis, extension of this cellular proliferation along the dermoepidermal junction of appendages (in many instances), and prominent solar elastosis of the dermis (Fig. 151–11).[43, 44, 53, 54, 56] The cells comprising this proliferation often exhibit scant cytoplasm and pleomorphic, hyperchromatic nuclei.[44] With progression, many of these cells often are spindle shaped and form dyscohesive nests along the dermoepidermal junction. This pattern of nesting may also prominently involve the skin appendages. With further progression, the cells often take on an epithelioid cell appearance, resembling the cells of superficial spreading melanoma.[44] Pagetoid spread may also develop in more advanced lesions.

The initial invasion of the papillary dermis may be difficult to recognize because of increased numbers of fibroblasts, dendrocytes, and melanophages.[44] Another problem is that cross sections of junctional nests associated with adnexal structures may simulate dermal invasion.

The invasive component of LMM is most commonly composed of spindle cells, with epithelioid cells and small round melanoma cells occasionally observed.[43, 44, 53–55, 57] Invasion of the dermis may develop from adnexal nests of melanoma cells. The vertical growth phase of LMM may also be desmoplastic or neurotropic.[47] The desmoplastic pattern is characterized by a fibrotic stroma entrapping spindle cells with hyperchromatic nuclei, singly, and in fascicles.

Acral Lentiginous Melanoma

Acral lentiginous melanoma, about 2% to 10% of all melanoma, is a pattern of melanoma involving the palms, soles, and nail apparatus.[47, 54, 59–64] A somewhat similar histologic pattern sometimes occurs in the mucosa.[54] The histologic changes that occur in the radial growth phase of acral lentiginous melanoma involve a predominant proliferation of large, highly atypical cells along the dermoepidermal junction in a hyperplastic epidermis. The cells are frequently associated with prominent melanin production; this allows for easy recognition of their dendritic processes, some of which reach the granular cell layer (Fig. 151–12). In this tumor, the nuclei of the malignant melanocytes are usually round or spindled, often hyperchromatic, and often contain condensed chromatin around the nuclear margin and small nucleoli. The cytoplasm is usually filled with fine melanin granules that are visible in its dendritic portions. Necessary for the diagnosis are contiguous, uniformly atypical cells along the basilar region of the epidermis. These cells sometimes aggregate in nests along the dermoepidermal junction, but this feature is not usual. Single-cell infiltration of the papillary dermis is associated with a fibrotic and lymphocytic host response, and melanophages are usually present. The radial growth phase of acral lentiginous melanoma may occasionally show pagetoid spread.[44] Such a change is more common after tumor cells have infiltrated the papillary dermis or once the vertical growth phase has begun.[47, 54, 59–64] The vertical growth phase of acral lentiginous melanoma may consist of spindle cells, epithelioid cells, or small melanoma cells.[54] When the cells are spindle shaped, the vertical growth phase is often associated with a desmoplastic or fibrotic response and neurotropism (see the discussion on desmoplastic melanoma). The fibrotic response in the desmoplastic/neurotropic vertical growth phase may be so intense that, clinically, the lesion is mistaken for a type of fibroma or fibromatosis.

Nodular Melanoma

Nodular melanoma (NM), about 15% to 30% of all melanoma, conceptually represents direct tumor progression to the vertical growth phase.[46, 47, 54, 65] If this tumor arises from a de novo proliferation of basilar mel-

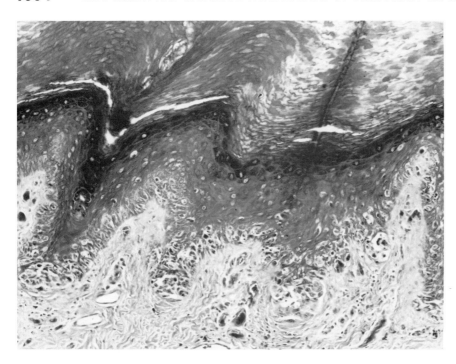

FIGURE 151–12. Acral lentiginous melanoma, radial growth phase. There is a contiguous proliferation of highly pleomorphic melanocytes in a lentiginous pattern along the dermoepidermal junction (H & E, × 125).

anocytes or a radial growth component, the vertical growth phase rapidly follows. In most instances, little or no intraepidermal remnant is adjacent to the expansile nodule that forms in the papillary dermis. A useful standard suggests that intraepidermal melanoma extending three rete ridges beyond the dermal component differentiates radial growth phase subtypes from nodular melanoma. NM may represent rapid tumor development of any type of intraepidermal or intraepithelial precursor.[65] The nodular proliferation itself is most commonly composed of epithelioid cells, but spindle cells, small epithelioid (nevoid or nevus-like) cells, and mixtures of cells may be present (Fig. 151–13). Most cases of NM are at least level III lesions when first recognized.

Polypoid and amelanotic variants of NM deserve special mention; however, these variants may also arise with other subtypes of melanoma in the vertical growth phase. In some instances, distinguishing NM from metastatic melanoma is difficult, if not impossible, without clinical information.[66, 67]

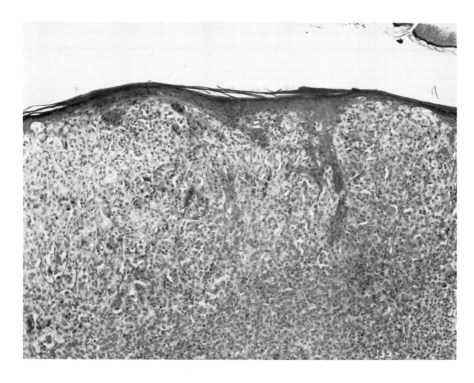

FIGURE 151–13. Nodular melanoma (vertical growth phase). There is a cohesive nodule of epithelioid melanoma cells filling the dermis. The vertical growth phase of any subtype of melanoma may have this appearance (H & E, × 79).

Other Forms of Melanoma

Other forms of melanoma include desmoplastic and neurotropic melanomas. Desmoplastic melanoma involves substantial deposition of collagen. The cells of desmoplastic melanoma have a propensity to infiltrate the perineurium and endoneurium of the cutaneous nerves (neurotropism).[68, 69] The collagenization of cells, elongated shape, and occasional lack of pigment can make these cells resemble fibroblasts (Fig. 151–14). In addition to infiltrating nerves, these tumors may form patterns that resemble nerves or neuroidal structures.[69] Desmoplastic melanoma usually occurs in lentigo maligna or acral lentiginous melanoma but can also occur without an overlying radial growth phase.

Malignant blue nevus is an extremely rare form of melanoma originating from or associated with a preexisting benign blue nevus and characterized by a dense nodular or multinodular proliferation of variably pigmented spindle cells without involvement of the epidermis.[70-77] Because there are no specific histologic features that distinguish the cells of malignant blue nevi from those of other melanomas, a contiguous remnant of benign blue nevus must be present.[77] Malignant blue nevus has a dismal prognosis, perhaps because lesions are often thick with the propensity to involve the scalp, a vascular site.

Metastatic melanoma frequently enters into the differential diagnosis of anaplastic epithelial metastatic tumors and maintains properties that suggest the diagnosis in many instances.[66] These include the presence of melanin in at least part of the tumor, a nested growth pattern, and the presence of epithelioid cells or a combination of epithelioid and spindle cells in the lesion. Cytologically, the presence of cells with melanin in their cytoplasm is characteristic of metastatic melanoma. In addition to epithelioid and spindle cells, metastatic melanomas may contain nevoid cells, largely undifferentiated blastic cells, and anaplastic giant forms, as seen in undifferentiated malignant tumors. All pigment synthesis is frequently lost. In epidermotropic metastatic melanoma, the epidermis is focally colonized by atypical melanocytes.

Special Pathology Studies in Melanoma

Diagnosis of melanoma is based on clinical findings, detection of the above characteristics, and, when necessary, results from ancillary tests. These procedures might include silver stains (such as the Fontana-Masson stain) for the detection of melanin, immunohistochemical analyses using panels of antibodies (including, for example, those reactive to S-100 protein, HMB-45, and vimentin), and electron microscopy to determine whether melanosomes are present.[66]

Immunohistochemical analysis can determine whether melanoma is present in primary or metastatic poorly differentiated malignant neoplasms that have little or no pigment, in spindle-cell tumors, in tumors that exhibit pagetoid epidermal patterns but that are not obvious melanoma (for instance, in extramammary Paget's disease), and in small cell malignant tumors suggesting melanoma, lymphoma, or neuroendocrine carcinoma.[49, 78-80]

The markers used most often for the routine evaluation of paraffin-embedded specimens include S-100 protein and HMB-45.[79, 80] S-100 protein is expressed by virtually all melanomas and melanocytic nevi but unfortunately also by a variety of other tumors. HMB-45 is a more specific marker of melanocytic lineage, but does not discriminate between benign and malignant neoplasms. HMB-45 usually fails to mark desmoplastic melanoma but these tumors usually express S-100 protein.[80] In general, these two reagents should be used in concert

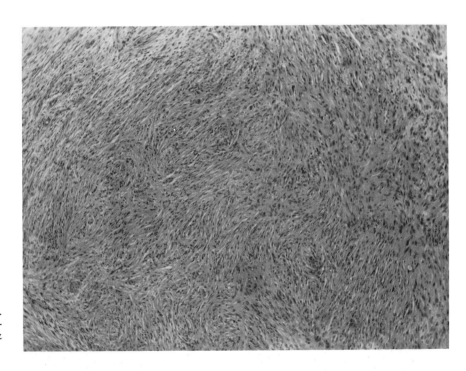

FIGURE 151–14. Desmoplastic melanoma. Fascicles of spindle cells are disposed in a fibrous matrix, forming a fibrotic nodule (H & E, × 79).

with a panel of antibodies against other tumor markers, such as cytokeratins, vimentin, and leukocyte common antigen.

Host Response in Melanoma

Lymphoid response and regression are common in the radial growth phase of melanoma.[44] This lymphoid reaction is presumed to be an indication of antigenic alteration in melanocytic cells. With the onset of vertical growth phase, lymphoid response is more variable but may still be present both at the base and within the expansile nodule (tumor-infiltrating lymphocytes). Some authors have reported decreasing density of the basal lymphoid reaction with increasing tumor thickness.[81]

Regression encompasses a broad spectrum of histopathologic changes, ranging from degenerating melanoma cells accompanied by dense lymphoid infiltrates (active or early inflammatory regression) to a constellation of findings that apparently result from partial or, rarely, complete destruction of a melanocytic lesion by the host response (end-stage regression).[82] The latter changes generally consist of variable degrees of fibrosis, prominent vascularity (and angiogenesis), melanophages, and lymphocytic infiltrates that affect and frequently thicken the papillary dermis.[83] These alterations are accompanied by variable obliteration of the melanocytic tumor in both the epidermis and dermis and by effacement of the epidermal rete pattern. These changes may involve any part or proportion of a lesion, but the process is most often focal or segmental. The interior zones or the periphery may be affected. The end stage of regression frequently occurs in the radial growth phase but is less common during vertical melanoma growth.

Regression of melanoma presents a number of dilemmas to the pathologist.[84] Some halo nevi may suggest melanoma because of the presence of cytologic atypia. Further, lymphoid infiltrates may obscure cytologic detail in melanocytes. Also difficult is the diagnosis of partially regressed melanoma.[85] Attention to asymmetry and to marked cytologic atypia of residual melanocytes, along with increased vigilance for the other characteristics of melanoma, is helpful in making the diagnosis.

The presentation of metastatic melanoma from an unknown primary tumor usually prompts a careful examination for evidence of a regressed lesion.[66] The fact that metastases are occasionally associated with thin melanomas (usually under 1 mm) with regressive change raises questions about the prognostic significance of regression.[85-87] A number of investigators have in fact found that regression per se does affect survival or risk of metastasis.[85-87] However, at present, the question has not been totally resolved, principally because of differences in definitions of regression and varying thresholds for recording regression in different study populations.[82]

PATHOGENESIS AND ETIOLOGY

Melanocytes arise from neural crest tissue during early fetal development before migrating to the skin and several other peripheral sites. While primarily residing in the basal layer of the epidermis, melanocytes use the enzyme tyrosinase to synthesize melanin pigment, which in turn serves to protect cells against UV damage.[88]

At least six growth factors and their receptor systems (including nerve growth factor, epidermal growth factor/alpha-transforming growth factor, and fibroblast growth factor) are active in the human melanocyte system.[89-91] Major antigens identified on melanocytes of all stages of tumor progression include high-molecular-weight oncofetal proteins (chondroitin sulfate proteoglycan), growth factor receptors, cation transport and binding proteins (e.g., transferrin-related p97 or melanotransferrin), class II HLA antigens, and gangliosides (e.g., GD2, GD3).[88, 92-94] Investigators propose that a range of differentiation stages, defined by morphologic features and differing antigen expression in cultured cells, could describe and delineate the pathway of tumor progression from benign to malignant melanocytes.[92]

Recent work has described karyotypic abnormalities in melanoma, particularly nonrandom alterations involving chromosomes 1p, 6, 7, 9, and 11.[95-97] Research in oncogene activation and regulation in melanoma[98, 99] has focused specifically on mutations of the ras oncogene family, but these mutations have not been directly implicated in melanoma initiation.[99] Alteration of the tumor suppressor gene p53 appears, at this time, to play only a minor role in melanoma progression.

The relationship between melanocytic nevi and melanoma is complex. Different reports suggest that the proportion of melanomas that arises from melanocytic nevi ranges from 18% to 85%.[100] Hence, some melanomas arise in conjunction with ordinary melanocytic nevi, while others appear to develop de novo.

DIAGNOSIS AND DIFFERENTIAL DIAGNOSIS

A number of melanocytic and nonmelanocytic lesions mimic melanoma (Figs. 151–15 and 151–16; see color plate).[101-103] In addition, the fact that the average white adult may have a dozen or more pigmented lesions (including melanocytic nevi) further complicates the early recognition of melanoma.[13, 102-104] Ordinary melanocytic nevi enlarge, darken, or increase in number at certain times in life, such as during puberty or pregnancy. However, as a rule, most melanocytic nevi change together, whereas the changes of melanoma may stand out in a distinctive way. Melanocytic nevi arise in childhood, adolescence, or young adulthood and are characterized by regular borders and even pigmentation (sometimes with a regular stippled pattern). The common type of blue nevus, a smooth nodule that is "gun metal" or blue-black in color, is generally less than 1 cm in diameter, has a well-defined, regular border, and usually occurs on the buttocks, presacral area, or dorsa of the hands or feet. Lentigo simplex is usually less than 5 mm in diameter and is a sharply defined, oval, uniformly pigmented (or regularly stippled) tan-brown or black macule; it may have a reticulated (net-like) pigmentation pattern. Solar lentigines, commonly called "freckles" or "liver spots," appear as lightly pigmented, tan macules or patches in sun-exposed areas.[101-104]

Nonmelanocytic pigmented lesions that may resemble

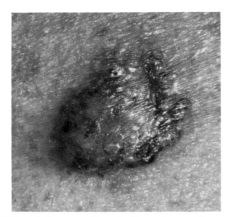

FIGURE 151–15. Pigmented basal cell carcinoma. (See color plate.)

melanoma include seborrheic keratosis, pigmented basal cell carcinoma (Fig. 151–15), appendage tumors, and vascular lesions.[35, 101] Seborrheic keratoses are brown or black, well-demarcated plaques with a "stuck-on" or occasionally greasy appearance. Close examination shows a warty texture. Basal cell carcinoma, classically a pearly, translucent facial papule with telangiectases, can resemble melanoma when it contains melanin, which gives the lesion a blue or black color.[1] Solar lentigines, which are pigmented keratinocytic proliferations, can resemble lentigo maligna.

Several vascular lesions may look like melanoma.[35, 101] An ulcerated pyogenic granuloma can resemble amelanotic melanoma. A hemangioma may also appear as a red or blue-purple lesion. Angiokeratoma in particular may resemble melanoma in its appearance when thrombosis of its superficial vessels occurs. Kaposi's sarcoma (Fig. 151–16), increasingly seen in patients with acquired immunodeficiency syndrome, presents as a red, blue, or violaceous macule, papule, nodule, or plaque, which may be confused with melanoma. Hemorrhage beneath a nail plate can simulate subungual melanoma.

The major class of precursor lesions, dysplastic nevi (atypical moles), was first described in 1978. These nevi are both markers for increased melanoma risk (when large or present in abnormal numbers) and potential precursor lesions from which melanoma may develop.[104–111] Initially described in family pedigree studies, these nevi are more commonly seen in the nonfamilial setting as so-called sporadic dysplastic nevi. Disagreements on precise, reproducible definitions and clinicopathologic correlations of dysplastic nevi have hindered efforts to determine their prevalence and proper management.[112] A recent National Institutes of Health Conference on Early Melanoma recommended dropping the term *dysplastic nevi*, using the term *atypical moles* instead.[113] At the present time both terms are used in the literature. In general, dysplastic nevi (atypical moles) are larger than common melanocytic nevi and have clinical features (such as haphazard pigmentation and irregular borders) that are qualitatively similar to but quantitatively not as extreme as those seen in melanoma. Histologically, they differ from common melanocytic nevi in their atypical architectural, cytologic, and stromal features.[114] Some hold that dysplastic nevi are exceedingly common and that their histopathologic features are not specific. Regardless, numbers of melanocytic nevi clearly mark patients as being at an increasing risk of developing melanoma. Further information on dysplastic nevi is in Chapter 150.

Other melanoma precursor lesions include the rare giant congenital melanocytic nevi, which carry at least a 6% to 7% lifetime risk of malignant transformation.[115] Small- to medium-sized congenital melanocytic nevi appear also to be precursor lesions, although the lack of definitive histologic criteria distinguishing these lesions from acquired nevi of similar size complicates proper analysis of this issue.[104, 116, 117]

Histologic Differential Diagnosis of Melanoma

Spitz nevus, pigmented spindle-cell nevus, dysplastic nevus, halo nevus, combined nevus, recurrent nevus, and cellular blue nevus are commonly mistaken for melanoma (Table 151–3).[44] Spitz nevi and their atypical variants are frequently misdiagnosed as melanoma because the former contain large cells, occasionally have marked cellular pleomorphism, can have foci with an upward migration of melanocytes (a pagetoid pattern), and occasionally lateral extension of their intraepidermal components beyond the bulk of dermal neoplasm.[118] Nonetheless, Spitz nevi generally can be distinguished from melanoma by their symmetry and orderly maturation, by the upward migration of groups of cells rather than single cells, by their lack of fully evolved cellular atypia, and by the absence of atypical mitotic figures.[118]

Pigmented spindle-cell nevi and particularly their atypical variants mimic melanoma because of their striking fascicles of heavily pigmented spindle cells and, usually, some upward migration of cells. In atypical variants, lateral basilar single-cell proliferation and nuclear atypia may be present. In general, these lesions can be distinguished from melanoma by their overall symmetry, the limitation of pagetoid spread to the lower epidermis, their fairly regular fascicles (both vertically and horizontally disposed), and uniformity of cell type. Fully evolved cellular atypia is not present.[119]

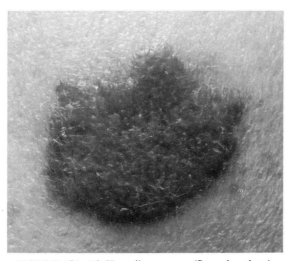

FIGURE 151–16. Kaposi's sarcoma. (See color plate.)

TABLE 151–3. Histopathologic Differential Diagnosis of Melanoma

Superficial Spreading Melanoma

Spindle- and epithelioid-cell (Spitz) nevus
Pigmented spindle-cell nevus
Dysplastic nevus
Halo nevus
Recurrent nevus
Epidermotropic metastatic melanoma
Mycosis fungoides
Paget's disease (including extramammary Paget's disease)
Bowen's disease
Sebaceous carcinoma

Lentigo Maligna Melanoma

Dysplastic nevus
Pigmented spindle-cell nevus
Atypical fibroxanthoma
Pigmented actinic keratosis
Lentiginous junctional or compound nevus
Spindle-cell squamous cell carcinoma

Acral Lentiginous Melanoma

Lentiginous melanocytic proliferations
Acral nevus
Fibrous histiocytoma

Nodular Melanoma

Spitz nevus
Metastatic melanoma
Histiocytoid hemangioma
Kaposi's sarcoma (tumor stage)
Fibrous histiocytoma

Desmoplastic/Neurotropic Melanoma

Desmoplastic (Spitz) nevus
Blue nevus
Cellular neurothekeoma (nerve sheath myxoma)
Malignant peripheral nerve sheath tumor
Fibrous histiocytoma

Malignant Blue Nevus

Cellular blue nevus
Metastatic melanoma
Malignant peripheral nerve sheath tumor

The atypical nevus, particularly when it has significant cytologic atypia, may mimic melanoma.[120–121] Dysplastic or atypical nevi can usually be distinguished from melanoma by their retention of nevoid or lentiginous architectural patterns. Upward migration of cells, if present, is usually not pronounced. Cytologic atypia is present in a minority of cells and is not fully evolved. Distinguishing between severely atypical dysplastic nevi and melanoma in situ can be difficult. In general, however, in melanoma in situ the normal epidermal rete ridge pattern is lost, basilar melanocytes are distributed without regard for rete ridges, single melanocytes pre-

dominate in some areas and are distributed throughout the upper layers of the epidermis (pagetoid spread), and fully evolved, consistent cytologic atypia is present.

Halo nevi, lesions that often undergo spontaneous clinical regression, often contain evidence of cytologic atypia, which atypia has led some authors to interpret the lesion as a type of melanocytic dysplasia. Therefore, these lesions must be carefully evaluated to rule out melanoma. Halo nevi generally are distinguished from melanoma by their architectural symmetry, maturation, and lesser degree of cytologic atypia. Mitotic figures are occasionally present in the deeper areas of the dermal portion of halo nevi.[121]

Combined nevus refers to a nevus composed of two juxtaposed populations of melanocytic cells that have different characteristics.[122, 123] Originally introduced to describe ordinary acquired compound or dermal nevi associated with a blue nevus component, the term now encompasses a much broader spectrum of nevi, including two distinct cell populations. Most commonly, the pathologist encounters either common acquired or congenital nevi that have been removed because they appeared almost completely blue-black or because of focal darkening within them. These nevi usually contain compound or dermal elements and discrete focal aggregates of pigmented epithelioid or plump spindle cells in the dermis. These cells frequently show low-grade cytologic atypia, hence the concern about melanoma. The significance of these features is unclear, but they may mark the inception of aberrant proliferation or of a form of dysplasia. Distinction of these nevi from melanoma is based on their symmetry and lower degree of cytologic atypia.[122, 123]

The recurrent nevus phenomenon is heralded by the development of pigmentation at the site of a previously removed nevus.[124, 125] Histologically, a junctional or compound proliferation of nevus cells usually appears along a flattened epidermis and is above a dermal scar. Changes of concern are an irregular disposition of the intraepidermal melanocytes and frequent epithelioid cytologic changes accompanied by occasional nuclear atypia. Recurrent nevi can be distinguished from melanoma by their usually low grade of nuclear atypia and by their confinement of the process to the area above the scar. However, it is important that the original biopsy specimen be reevaluated to rule out melanoma.

Histopathologic Reporting of Melanoma

The pathology report should include at the very least the diagnosis, that is, melanoma, in situ or invasive; depth of tumor invasion in millimeters measured vertically from the granular layer of the epidermis; and the adequacy of surgical margins. Other information that may be important in prognostic modeling should be recorded if possible (Table 151–4).[56]

TREATMENT

The treatment of melanoma includes surgery of the primary lesion, prognostic factors and staging, considera-

TABLE 151-4. Example of Reporting of Melanoma

Diagnosis:	Melanoma
Subtype:	Nodular
Measured depth:	1.00
Anatomic level:	III
Ulceration:	Absent
Regression:	Absent
Vertical growth phase:	Present, consisting of epithelioid cells
Mitotic rate:	4/mm^2
Tumor-infiltrating lymphocytes:	None
Microscopic satellites:	None
Associated nevus/precursor:	None
Completely excised:	

tion of adjuvant therapy, and treatment of metastatic disease (Tables 151–5 and 151–6).

Biopsy Technique for Suspected Melanoma

Many lesions can simulate melanoma on clinical examination.[35, 42, 101] Histologic interpretation of the biopsy specimen[53, 126] can confirm the diagnosis of mela-

TABLE 151-5. Staging Systems for Melanoma

Traditional Three-Stage System

Stage	Criteria	5-Year Survival Rate
I (thickness categories)	Skin	80%
≤0.75 mm		96%
0.76–1.49 mm		87%
1.50–2.49 mm		75%
2.50–3.99 mm		66%
≥4.00 mm		47%
II	Nodal Involvement	36%
III	Distant metastases	5%

American Joint Committee on Cancer Staging System*

Stage	Criteria
IA	Localized melanoma, ≤0.75 mm, or Clark level II (T1,N0,M0)
IB	Localized melanoma, 0.76–1.5 mm, or Clark level III (T2,N0,M0)
IIA	Localized melanoma, 1.5–4 mm, or Clark level IV (T3,N0,M0)
IIB	Localized melanoma, >4 mm, Clark level V (T4,N0,M0)
III	Limited nodal metastases involving only one regional lymph node basin, or <5 in-transit metastases but without nodal metastases (any T,N1,M0)
IV	Advanced regional metastases (any T,N2,M0) or any distant metastases (any T,any N,M1 or M2)

*When the thickness and level of invasion criteria do not coincide within a T classification, thickness should take precedence.

Adapted from Balch C, Milton G, eds. Cutaneous Melanoma. Philadelphia: JB Lippincott, 1985; Friedman RJ, Rigel DS, et al., eds. Cancer of the Skin. Philadelphia: WB Saunders Co., 1991:201.

TABLE 151-6. Recommended Margins of Surgical Resection for Primary Cutaneous Melanoma

Thickness	Surgical Margin
In situ	0.5-cm border of clinically normal skin and layer of subcutaneous tissue
≤2 mm thick	1-cm margin of clinically normal skin and layer of subcutaneous tissue down to fascia
>2 mm thick	2- to 3-cm margin

noma and, by enabling measurement of the thickness of the neoplasm, help determine the patient's prognosis, appropriate surgical management, and potential need for other therapy.[53, 126, 127]

Before performing the diagnostic biopsy, the physician should palpate the regional draining lymph nodes and record the presence or absence of adenopathy. Because subtle palpable adenopathy can develop and persist for several weeks as a consequence of the biopsy procedure itself, delaying lymph node examination until after the biopsy could potentially result in inaccurate clinical staging of the patient.[128]

For the cutaneous lesion suspected of being a melanoma, the diagnostic procedure of choice is a biopsy that conservatively excises the entire lesion. This is generally a simple office procedure. Removal in toto permits the pathologist to evaluate the full breadth and depth of the lesion and also prevents sampling error. Exceptions to the rule of biopsy in toto fall into three categories: (1) lesions so large that complete conservative excision would require significant surgery such as a skin flap or graft; (2) lesions located in anatomic sites where complete removal would cause an unacceptable cosmetic deformity (should the diagnosis prove to be benign); and (3) fragile patient health status. Only under these three circumstances should biopsy in parte be performed.[1] Sampling by shave, curettage, or needle biopsy technique may compromise the histologic interpretation, provide insufficient material for an accurate histologic diagnosis, and preclude accurate determination of the thickness of the lesion.[128, 129]

The margins of the excision should be outlined with a sterile marker before infiltration of the local anesthetic solution. The margin of the excision need be no more than 1 mm outside the visible edge of the lesion. The orientation of the ellipse should be located parallel to the lymphatic drainage (rather than along the relaxed skin tension lines) to facilitate future definitive surgery, should the biopsy reveal the lesion to be melanoma. The depth of the incision should extend into the subcutaneous fat but need not be carried down to the underlying muscular fascia. The physician should handle the specimen gently and take great care not to crush the biopsy specimen with tissue forceps, which could render accurate histologic interpretation impossible.[130]

The remainder of the procedure follows conventional excisional skin surgery. There is no contraindication to tissue undermining at the level of the subcutaneous fat, if necessary, to facilitate wound closure without skin tension. Likewise, there is no contraindication to the use of electrocautery. Once hemostasis is obtained, the physician can close the defect in successive layers, first burying some absorbable suture to close the subcutaneous fat and deep dermis (dead space) and then opposing the epidermis with simple interrupted nylon or running Prolene sutures.[130]

If the anatomic location or size of the lesion prevents simple biopsy in toto (see earlier discussion), an incisional biopsy can minimize the risk of sampling error by using a relatively narrow ellipse that spans the entire breadth of the lesion to include the most raised or most deeply pigmented portion of the tumor.[130]

An incisional biopsy does not compromise survival of the patient, and there is no evidence that "seeding" of tumor occurs with biopsy in parte.[130] Diagnosis by the punch biopsy technique is less desirable than by incisional biopsy, because it is more likely to result in sampling error; however, if a biopsy in parte by punch technique is necessary, the same principles of incisional biopsy should be observed. The biopsy should include the most elevated or darkest portion of the lesion and some of the underlying subcutaneous fat (Fig. 151–17). If a punch biopsy of a raised area is performed, the

dermatologist should be confident that the specimen will contain normal tissue beneath the neoplasm so that the ascertainment of thickness is not compromised, that is, the punch should extend deeply into the subcutis. The pathologist should always be informed that such a biopsy is a sampling of a much larger lesion. Several punch biopsies in various areas of the tumor reduce the risk of sampling error.[131]

Prognostic Factors and Staging

Multiple clinical and pathology studies have defined prognostic factors for melanoma. The 5-year survival rates for melanoma decline steadily with increasing clinical stage. Traditionally, melanoma was staged according to whether disease was confined to skin (stage I), nodes (stage II), or was metastatic (stage III). The American Joint Commission on Cancer (AJC) has proposed a revised four-stage system, dividing traditional stage I lesions into two categories at the 1.50-mm mark. In addition, the prognosis depends on a number of other factors. For melanoma confined to the skin, Clark and colleagues[53] first proposed that poorer prognosis correlated with increasing levels of microinvasion into the dermis or subcutaneous tissue (describing five Clark levels of invasion). Soon thereafter, Breslow[126, 132] found that vertical tumor thickness (as measured by an ocular micrometer from the top of the granular cell layer to the deepest point of tumor penetration) was a better predictor. Since then, many studies have confirmed the dominance of vertical tumor thickness (in millimeters) as the best prognostic indicator for melanoma confined to the skin.[133–138] For localized melanoma, discrete thickness categories mark where survival rates decline most rapidly. For example, most patients with thin stage I lesions (lesions ≤ 0.75 mm thick) can expect prolonged disease-free survival and even cure after treatment, whereas those with thicker lesions (> 4.0 mm) have much higher likelihood of dying of metastatic disease. The limited data available suggest that melanoma in situ is associated with relative 5-year survival rates approaching 100%.[139–141]

In addition to tumor thickness, a number of other clinical and histologic factors affect prognosis for localized melanoma. Anatomic site of the melanoma is one important factor[133, 138, 142]; with equivalent thickness, lesions on the scalp, hands, and feet appear to carry a poorer prognosis.[133–138, 143] Older patients and men have poorer prognosis than younger patients and women, but these differences largely reflect variations in thickness and site.[132–138]

Histologic features associated with an unfavorable prognosis include high mitotic activity, the presence of microscopic satellites of tumor (defined as discrete nests of tumor cells > 0.05 mm in diameter located in reticular dermis or subcutaneous fat and separated from the bulk of the tumor by normal tissue), the presence of a vertical growth phase, ulceration, high prognostic index (derived by multiplying the thickness in millimeters by the number of mitoses per square millimeter) and increased tumor volume.[144–147] DNA aneuploidy measure-

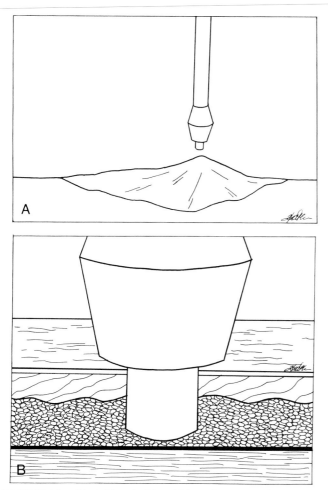

FIGURE 151–17. *A,* If an incisional biopsy is to be performed, the most raised or darkest portion of the pigmented lesion should be sampled in order to plan the surgical resection. This sampling may be performed with a punch biopsy. *B,* The depth of the incisional biopsy should extend into the subcutaneous fat, but need not reach the underlying fascia.

ments by flow-cytometry techniques may also have prognostic value.[148]

As noted earlier, multivariate analyses do not show the histopathologic subtype to be of major prognostic significance.[149] The 5-year survival rates for stage I (AJC stages I and II) melanoma differ by subtype: lentigo maligna melanoma and superficial spreading melanoma have better 5-year survival rates (about 90%) than do acral lentiginous melanoma (about 75% to 80%) and nodular melanoma (about 60%).[7] These differences tend to reflect varying tumor thickness at the time of presentation. In addition, the long-held contention that lentigo maligna melanoma has an inherently better prognosis than other subtypes has now been challenged.[131]

The overall 5-year survival in stage II (AJC stage III) disease is about 30% to 35% but varies according to the clinical status of the nodes (macroscopic versus occult metastases) and the number of nodes involved with the tumor.[7, 150, 151] Stage III (AJC stage IV) disease is generally incurable and has a median survival of 6 months.[152, 153] Common sites for the dissemination of melanoma include the skin, lymph nodes, bone, lungs, liver, spleen, and especially the central nervous system.[1, 7, 152, 153] Like lung cancer and breast cancer, melanoma commonly metastasizes to the brain.[7, 154]

Once the diagnosis of melanoma has been confirmed by careful histologic examination of the biopsy specimen, the melanoma must be staged to determine prognosis and treatment plan. In evaluating the newly diagnosed melanoma patient, the clinician should perform a thorough history that searches for signs and symptoms of metastatic disease, including symptoms of malaise, decreased exercise tolerance, weight loss, headaches, and bone or abdominal pain. The physical examination should then focus special attention to the skin, regional draining lymph node basin(s), lungs, central nervous system, liver, and spleen. In the absence of signs or symptoms of metastasis, laboratory or radiologic tests, aside from baseline chest radiography and possibly serum transaminase and alkaline phosphatase, are not routinely necessary for staging purposes.[155] In particular, routine liver-spleen scans, magnetic resonance imaging and computed tomography have not been shown to be cost effective for evaluating patients with thin tumors.[156] In such tests, for patients with stage I tumors less than 0.76 mm in thickness (AJC stage I), the false-positive rate will far exceed the true detection of metastases.[1, 155] The risks of iatrogenic complications and increased costs associated with some radiographic and nuclear medicine studies suggest that, in patients with thin tumors who are clinically free of disease, extensive testing is unnecessary.

Experts debate whether patients with thicker tumors need more extensive laboratory staging evaluation, including computed tomography or magnetic resonance imaging of the head, chest, abdomen, and pelvis.[155] Some argue that at the very least, these studies can serve as a baseline for future reference in these high-risk patients.

Once signs or symptoms of metastasis exist, that is, the patient has progressed to clinical stage II or III (AJC stages III and IV) disease, a full metastatic work-up includes an evaluation of liver, lungs, bone, and brain.[155]

Surgical Excision of Stage I Melanoma

Although wide surgical excision has been the accepted treatment for stage I (AJC stages I and II) melanoma, newer data suggest that narrower margins may suffice. First, a prospective trial of patients with primary melanomas with thickness 2 mm or less showed similar disease-free (and overall) survival rates in those randomized to either narrow excision (1-cm margins) or wide excision (at least 3-cm margins).[157] This randomized multicenter trial of over 600 patients led by the National Cancer Institute, Milan, Italy, assessed the efficacy of narrow excision for thin primary melanomas.[157] The authors found somewhat increased rates of local recurrence but no difference in rates of metastatic disease in the two groups of patients. Another prospective multi-institutional trial of 486 patients with melanoma 1.0 to 4.0 mm thick (trunk or proximal lesions) randomized patients to 2- or 4-cm surgical margins. There was no difference in 5-year survival rate or overall recurrence.[158] Other studies have noted that increased local recurrence rate (i.e., persistence of tumor in contiguity with the operative site) in the narrow-margin group did not adversely affect survival.[159] Clinicians should distinguish between local recurrence, defined as persistence of the tumor in contiguity with the surgical scar (incomplete excision of the primary lesion), and satellitosis, which is a local metastasis occurring within 5 cm of the surgical site and associated with a poor prognosis.

Thus, the newest recommendation for definitive therapeutic melanoma surgery for lesions up to 1 mm in thickness is a 1-cm margin of normal skin surrounding the tumor or biopsy area,[157, 160] a conclusion also supported by the National Institutes of Health Consensus Conference on Early Melanoma.[113] In situ lesions can safely be removed with 0.5-cm margins.[113] The recommendation for lesions greater than 1 mm in thickness continues to be a 2-cm (or 3-cm) margin of healthy surrounding skin (see Table 151–6).

It is important to note that the Milan study excluded melanomas occurring on the head and neck.[157] The recurrence rate (tumor persistence in the margin of excision) is high for melanomas arising on these anatomic sites.[159, 161] This may, in part, be caused by the "field effect" of sun-damaged melanocytes surrounding melanoma on the face, particularly at the periphery of lentigo maligna melanomas.

The 1-cm resection margin for thin lesions not located on critical anatomic sites greatly simplifies melanoma surgery. The procedure can often be performed entirely under local anesthesia. Simple primary closure or a local skin flap can repair the defect, avoiding the need for myocutaneous flaps, extensive skin grafting, general anesthesia, and costly inpatient stays.[158]

The surgeon can minimize the risk of local recurrences (tumor persistence) by marking the 1-cm margin with a sterile ruler and skin-marking pen prior to infiltration of the local anesthetic solution.[130, 160] This will avoid the tissue distortion caused by the injection of the solution. If the prior diagnostic biopsy did not remove the entire tumor, use of a Wood's lamp can help determine the clinical border of the tumor.[162] Then, with use of surgical

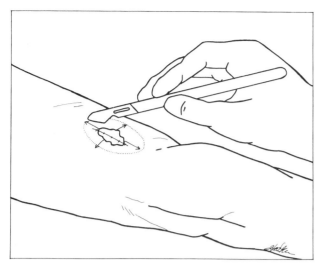

FIGURE 151–18. If a lymph node dissection is planned on the extremities, the excisional biopsy and the definitive surgery should be oriented parallel to the lymphatic drainage, not the relaxed skin tension lines. The margin of excision should be measured from the clinical border (Wood's light–assisted) of the tumor.

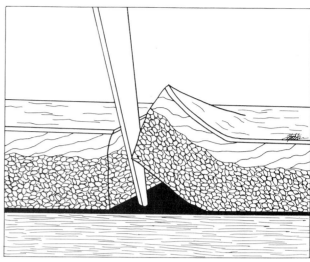

FIGURE 151–19. On the trunk and extremities, the depth of the excision should extend to the underlying muscular fascia but the fascia should not be removed. Scalp melanomas should be excised in depth to the periosteum. Facial tumors may require dissection at the level of the superficial muscular aponeurosis or muscular fascia.

lighting, the surgeon can map the 1-cm margin around the Wood's lamp–assisted clinical border.

If a lymph node dissection is planned, the long axis of the excision should be oriented toward the regional draining lymph node group (Fig. 151–18). This tenet of surgical oncology takes precedence over orientation parallel to relaxed skin tension lines. The surgery is simplified when the diagnostic biopsy is oriented similarly (see above).[130] In certain anatomic locations, especially on the extremities, the long axis of the excision will be perpendicular to the relaxed skin tension lines. Thus, extensive undermining may be necessary to close the defect. In contrast to earlier opinions on the subject, there is no contraindication to tissue undermining after en bloc removal of the tumor.[130] On the head and neck and extremities, the surgeon should anticipate the possible need for a local flap to achieve wound closure without undue skin tension.

The depth of the excision should extend to but not include the underlying muscular fascia because there is no difference in disease-free and overall survival in patients with the fascia removed compared with patients where the fascia was left intact (Fig. 151–19). Removing the fascia may delay healing, increase postoperative morbidity without improving survival, and perhaps increase the rate of lymph node metastases. The fascial dissection plane can, in most instances, be easily defined on the trunk and extremities. On the scalp, a high-risk anatomic site independent of tumor thickness, dissection should proceed in the subgaleal plane.[130, 163] There is no universally accepted approach governing the depth of excision for melanomas on the face. Depth of dissection can be performed along the superficial muscular aponeurotic system or the muscular fascia. Great care should be exercised to preserve branches of the facial nerve, especially on the temple, zygomatic arch and mandibular notch, where these branches course superficial to the muscular

fascia. If the tumor is located near a free margin, that is, ear, nasal ala, eyelid, or lip, a wedge resection is often used. The high recurrence rate and decreased survival[163, 164] associated with melanomas arising on these sites may, in part, be due to inadequate resection margins taken on these critical locations.

No guidelines exist for depth of excision for in situ melanoma. Conservative resection appears prudent. Depth of resection should include at least the full thickness of the dermis and a portion of the subcutis to assure that the basal portions of hair follicles are removed. This superficial resection facilitates healing by granulation if deemed appropriate by the surgeon. Ablative modalities such as CO_2 and argon laser have resulted in high recurrence rates, possibly due to the partial-thickness nature of the wounds created, which do not destroy melanoma cells in the lower portions of hair epithelium.[130]

Mohs Micrographic Surgery

In theory, the Mohs micrographic surgery technique should provide the same high cure rate and tissue sparing for melanoma as it does for patients with basal or squamous cell carcinoma.[165] Although skin surgeons have used both the fixed and fresh tissue techniques of Mohs micrographic surgery to treat melanoma,[165, 166] insufficient data as yet exist to assess the long-term efficacy of this treatment modality. Notably, several potential pitfalls exist for the use of Mohs surgery to treat melanoma.[167, 168] It is often difficult for a dermatopathologist to distinguish single melanoma cells at the periphery of the tumor from the enlarged but non-neoplastic melanocytes ubiquitously present in photodamaged skin. Freeze artifact, an unavoidable consequence of performing frozen section analysis, produces vacuolated keratinocytes and alters melanocyte morphology, further complicating the interpretation of histologic sections processed by the

Mohs fresh tissue technique. Also, foci of regression, which can occur both within and at the periphery of melanomas, produce histologic "skip" areas rendering the tumor discontiguous and further complicating Mohs surgery.[168]

Melanomas arising on critical anatomic sites such as the central face and distal extremities pose special problems for achieving appropriate margins without precipitating excess surgical morbidity in terms of functional or cosmetic outcome. No guidelines exist for margin reduction when treating melanomas arising on these sites. In fact, the distal extremities, ears, and certain areas of the face are associated (thickness for thickness) with a poorer prognosis than other anatomic sites.[142, 169] Thus, arbitrary reduction in surgical margins on these critical anatomic sites may not be appropriate. For tumors arising on these high-risk sites, a randomized, prospective trial of Mohs surgery versus conventional surgery would be helpful.

Lymph Node Dissection

Patients with melanoma and palpable lymph nodes require therapeutic lymph node dissection for diagnostic and therapeutic purposes. Controversy focuses on the value of elective (prophylactic) dissection of regional draining lymph nodes in patients who are clinically and radiographically free of regional and distant disease.[170-172] A subset of patients with stage I (AJC stages I and II) disease will have microscopic metastatic disease in nonpalpable lymph nodes.[173, 174] Hence, elective regional node dissection (for otherwise healthy patients with primary tumors associated with clearly defined lymphatic drainage) might improve the prognosis.[175-180] The theory supporting elective regional lymph node dissection (ELND) contends that melanoma may, in some cases, spread in a sequential manner from the primary tumor site along lymphatics to the regional nodes and then to distant sites. Removal of the draining nodes containing microscopic disease could then possibly prevent distant dissemination.

However, there is no clear consensus regarding the efficacy of ELND. Although nonrandomized studies do suggest a benefit for patients with intermediate-thickness primary lesions, neither of the two prospective randomized node dissection studies performed to date demonstrated improved survival for patients treated with immediate prophylactic (versus delayed therapeutic) node dissection.[172, 181, 182] In a study of more than 300 patients with clinically negative nodes, Davis and coworkers[183] found only 15 (5%) to harbor occult metastases in the regional draining lymph nodes. Thus, only a small subset of patients may benefit from ELND. With the advent of improved prognostication of survival and risk of tumor recurrence, two factors are preeminent in evaluating the potential utility of ELND. These factors are (1) depth of primary tumor invasion, determined by either Breslow thickness or Clark level, and (2) anatomic location of the primary melanoma.[170, 183-185]

Patients with thin lesions, less than 1.5 mm in thickness or Clark level I or II, have such a low risk of regional node metastasis that ELND is not justified given the risk of surgical complication from the dissection, and the long-term sequelae of the lymphadenectomy. In a study of 151 patients with unambiguous drainage (extremity lesions), Wanebo and colleagues[184] determined that there was only a 4% risk of metastases for Clark level II lesions. In contrast, patients with deeply invasive tumors, that is, greater than 4 mm in thickness or Clark level V, are also poor candidates for ELND because of the high probability (> 40%) of disease being present beyond the regional draining lymph nodes.[184]

Patients with tumors located on the midline of the trunk or head and neck are believed to be poor candidates for ELND because of the pattern of lymphatic drainage to two or more nodal basins. Thus, ELND for tumors located on sites of ambiguous drainage would entail extensive surgery, involving multiple lymphadenectomies, with the morbidity and complication rate exceeding therapeutic benefit.[171, 185, 187]

Lymphoscintigraphy can help define the primary pattern of lymphatic drainage from the tumors located in an area of ambiguous drainage. Although this radiographic technique can, in some instances, inform the surgeon of the primary draining nodal group, survival data have not shown an advantage for ELND on the head and neck and trunk.[170, 171, 183, 185] A study of 289 patients with head and neck primary melanomas (followed in some cases over 21 years) did not find improved survival for those who had undergone ELND.[171] Others have found a similar lack of efficacy of ELND in patients in whom the trunk or head and neck is the primary site of the melanoma.[170, 185]

Thus, ELND does not appear to improve survival for patients with primary lesions on the head and trunk, or for thin (<1.50 mm) or thick (>4.00 mm) melanomas on an extremity. The most heated debate now centers on the remaining group of patients, those with intermediate-thickness lesions located on an extremity. Review of the literature suggests that the rate of micrometastases, that is, clinically negative, histologically positive lymph nodes, in this select group ranges from 9.6% to 27%.[184, 187-189] At best, patients with intermediate-thickness extremity melanomas may theoretically derive a modest benefit from ELND.[170, 183, 184, 187] Prospective randomized studies are currently in progress to assess efficacy versus cost and morbidity of the procedure in stage I intermediate-thickness extremity melanomas.

Adjuvant Therapy

After surgery, patients require regular follow-up because of the risk of metastasis and increased risk of a second primary cutaneous melanoma.[164, 192] Patients with nodal disease or thick primary lesions who are at high risk for recurrence of distant metastasis need effective adjuvant therapy to prolong the disease-free survival. Many adjuvant strategies have been employed, including chemotherapy, nonspecific immunotherapy (e.g., bacillus Calmette-Guérin, Corynebacterium parvum, levamisole, and transfer factor), active specific immunotherapy, chemoimmunotherapy, adjuvant isolated regional perfusion for extremity melanoma, and radiation therapy. However, none of these strategies have definitively improved survival.[193-199] Specifically, newer investigations disagree about the possible benefit of levamisole.[198, 199] Recent investigations are testing several melanoma vaccines and interferon in the adjuvant setting.[200, 201]

Although limb perfusion has been available for years as a treatment in the adjuvant or metastatic setting, its proper role is still a matter of debate. For melanoma located on an arm or leg, regional perfusion of the tumor-bearing extremity with otherwise lethal doses of chemotherapeutic agents can be performed with minimal systemic absorption. The technique involves canalizing the major vessels of the affected extremity, cutting off blood and lymphatic flow to and from the limb using a tourniquet, and then perfusing the limb via an extracorporeal circuit through the arterial and venous cannulae. The chemotherapy can be administered through this extracorporeal circuit, avoiding systemic exposure to the agent. However, the technique has been associated with severe, permanent, and occasionally life-threatening complications in as many as 10% of patients treated. Some retrospective studies suggest a survival benefit in the adjuvant setting.[1, 7, 202] One prospective study has indicated some benefit from this adjuvant modality.[203] Other prospective trials are currently under way to evaluate the utility of limb perfusion in the adjuvant treatment of patients with thick primary lesions or nodal metastases.

Investigators have explored whether radiotherapy can play a role as an adjuvant treatment in patients with high-risk primary tumors.[204, 205] Following excision of high-risk primary melanomas on the head and neck, Ang and associates[205] gave patients a total of 2400 cGy to 3000 cGy to the area in four to five divided doses of 600 cGy. A total of 83 patients (with thick primary tumors, nodal disease, or recurrences in the regional nodes at various times after surgery) had high 3-year disease-free survival rates. A prospective, controlled clinical trial to evaluate these preliminary findings is needed. Preliminary data from cooperative trials suggest a role for adjuvant interferon given intravenously or in a subcutaneous fashion for nodal disease or thick primary disease—we await the publication of the full reports of these studies. An interesting report of high-dose chemotherapy with autologous bone marrow transplant as adjuvant therapy for multi-node positive melanoma requires confirmation by other groups.[206]

Treatment of Metastatic Disease

Because widespread metastatic melanoma is generally incurable, the goal of treatment should be palliation. In deciding from among the treatment options, the clinician must consider the site and extent of metastases, the tempo of the clinical course, and the overall performance status of the patient.[207] Traditionally, chemotherapy, radiation, and surgery have been the first approaches. Of the chemotherapeutic agents, the most commonly used single agent is dacarbazine, which has an aggregate re-

sponse rate of approximately 15% to 25%.[208, 209] These responses are usually partial, of short duration (3 to 6 months), and more likely to occur in skin, soft tissue, node, and lung metastases than other sites.[207, 208] Other commonly used single agents include the nitrosoureas, and cisplatin.[207] Compared with single agents, combination chemotherapy has not appreciably improved remission and survival rates.[1, 207, 208] Some investigators suggest that the addition of tamoxifen with chemotherapy improves response rates. Isolated limb perfusion, used principally with melphalan and hyperthermia, clearly palliates locally advanced melanoma of the extremity, but its impact on overall survival is still a matter of debate.[1, 209-212]

At one time considered a radioresistant tumor, metastatic melanoma can respond to radiation therapy. The complete response rate is roughly 25%,[213-217] and the partial response rate of treating metastatic nodules is approximately 35%.[205] Larger dose-per-fraction radiotherapy may be more effective than conventional for primary and metastatic melanoma.[205, 217, 218] Some investigators find the combination of chemotherapy or hyperthermia with external beam radiation significantly improves disease-free survival in patients with metastatic melanoma.[219-221] Several clinical trials are studying new and innovative modalities for the radiotherapy of metastatic melanoma. One such experimental therapy is boron neutron capture therapy,[222-227] a binary therapy that entails ingestion of a stable isotope of boron (^{10}B) followed by exposure to a thermal (low energy) or epithermal neutron beam. Future large-scale trials must determine the future role of boron neutron capture therapy and other radiotherapy modalities for treatment purposes.

Complete surgical excision of accessible, limited metastases may be associated with prolonged survival[228]; more often, however, widespread metastases will preclude the possibility of surgery.

The unsatisfactory response to traditional treatments for metastatic melanoma has stimulated many experimental trials with innovative therapies. High-dose chemotherapy, using either single or combination agents followed by autologous bone marrow rescue, can produce high response rates but is complicated by considerable toxicity, including fatalities.[229, 230] Whether newer support with growth factors (e.g., recombinant human GM-CSF) can accelerate bone marrow recovery in this setting and reduce future toxicity remains to be seen.[231] Interferon (administered in various doses and treatment schedules) produces about an overall 20% response rate in metastatic melanoma, although a small proportion of patients have had prolonged remissions.[232-234] Preliminary studies have reported some remissions with the use of monoclonal antibodies (against p97 and the gangliosides GD2 and GD3), autologous or allogeneic vaccines against metastatic melanoma, targeted toxin therapy, anti-idiotypic antibody, and other agents.[235-246] At present, none of these innovative therapies can be recommended outside of a study setting. Future studies must evaluate the efficacy of these approaches in properly controlled studies.

Of the investigational therapies, much attention has

focused on adoptive immunotherapy.[247] This therapy has particular relevance, because the immune system may have a critical role in the well-described phenomenon of spontaneous regression in melanoma.[248] The process of adoptive immunotherapy employs three steps—leukapheresis to obtain lymphocytes from patients, incubation of the collected cells ex vivo with interleukin 2 (IL-2) to generate and expand lymphokine-activated killer cells, and then reinfusion of the lymphokine-activated killer cells in conjunction with IL-2 into the patient.[249] To date, the clinical trials using IL-2 and lymphokine-activated killer cells in metastatic melanoma have shown an overall response rate of about 15% to 20%.[247, 249–252] Most of the remissions have been partial and seen primarily in patients with skin, nodal, or lung metastases. Some responses are durable and take place in otherwise nonresponsive sites. Unfortunately, the toxicity of IL-2 due primarily to a capillary-leak syndrome includes pressor-dependent hypotension, severe respiratory compromise, and liver and renal dysfunction.[247, 249–252] The goal of current research is to improve the remission rate of adoptive immunotherapy while limiting its toxicity. Trials are testing IL-2 alone using various dosages and routes of administration (bolus versus continuous infusion), or in combination with lymphokine-activated killer cells.[247, 249, 252] In addition, these trials are combining IL-2 with other agents, such as chemotherapeutic drugs or other biologic response modifiers (such as alpha interferon and tumor necrosis factor), in the hopes of obtaining an additive or synergistic effect.[247, 249, 253–259] Another generation of immunotherapy studies use even more potent tumor-infiltrating lymphocytes with IL-2; techniques using retroviral gene transduction to alter these lymphocytes may further heighten their antitumor potency.[256–259] However, tumor-infiltrating lymphocytes cannot be successfully obtained or generated in many patients and may require a substantial commitment of time and resources. Finally, new reports suggest a role for immunotherapy by direct in vivo gene transfer into tumors, but this method also requires broader confirmation.[260]

Early Detection and Prevention

The contrast between near-certain death from metastatic disease and possible cure of thin melanoma underscores the potential of prevention and early detection.[261, 262] The theoretical appeal of the early detection of melanoma and other skin cancer lies in the fact that these conditions are increasingly common, early disease has a high survival rate, and the screening examination (a visual examination by a qualified observer) is noninvasive, takes several minutes, and is regarded as reliable in diagnostic settings.[261–264] However, formal screening for melanoma is in its infancy, and few data are available on its yield and efficacy. No randomized prospective trial of skin cancer screening currently exists. Short of this, in 1985, the American Academy of Dermatology launched an annual, free, national melanoma/skin cancer screening effort that has so far reached more than 700,000 Americans and supplied education to millions

more.[265] This volunteer program has heightened public awareness, but a rigorous evaluation of this effort has only just begun. More data are needed to demonstrate whether screening for melanoma can reduce mortality rates.[261–267] In the meantime, whether skin cancer screening should be general public health policy is commonly a matter of debate.[267–269] Several organizations do currently advocate screening for persons at high risk.[268–270] There may be potential benefit from a screening examination of the skin during a routine physical examination (casefinding), but general physicians need more training to develop the proper expertise to recognize melanoma.[271]

At the present time, recommendations are for high-risk persons to minimize sun exposure, use sunscreens when possible, and until more data emerge, be encouraged to perform regular self-examination of the skin.[272] The management of patients with small- to medium-sized congenital nevi is controversial[273]; for now, patients should consider excision of the lesion at puberty, when surgery under local (not general) anesthesia is feasible.[12, 104]

While we await a better understanding of the etiology of melanoma, it is appropriate to initiate education and primary prevention strategies that can complement secondary prevention. Education should be of particular value in this uniquely visible and recognizable tumor. Public education can alert persons to recognize and seek prompt care for suspicious pigmented lesions. Such efforts in the United Kingdom and Australia have resulted in higher percentages of persons presenting with thin melanomas.[274–276] In addition, a United Kingdom study utilizing education and special pigmented lesion clinics in Scotland found a drop in mortality rates (in women only).[276] Other efforts must intensify to preserve the ozone layer, decrease the production of chlorofluorocarbons, consider regulation of tanning parlors, and instill habits of regular sunscreen use and sun protection, especially in children and adolescents.[277]

Proper monitoring of patients with atypical moles should help prevent melanoma-related deaths.[278] Although the optimal interval for monitoring is unknown, most authorities recommend at least once or twice yearly skin examinations (with selective excision of the most atypical or changing pigmented lesions) for persons with atypical nevi.[279] Serial photography may help the physician evaluate changes in pigmented lesions during follow-up.[280]

The rising incidence and mortality rates of cutaneous melanoma around the world have stimulated an interest in better management and control strategies. Future efforts for melanoma control will likely come from increased public and professional education,[281] rigorous evaluation of the proper role of screening, a better understanding of tumor biology, further refinements of surgical treatments, adjuvant therapies, and new therapies for advanced and metastatic disease.

References

1. Koh HK. Cutaneous melanoma. N Engl J Med 1991;325:171–182.

2. Feldman AR, Kessler L, Myers MH, Naughton MD. The prevalence of cancer: Estimates based on the Connecticut Tumor Registry. N Engl J Med 1986;315:1394–1397.
3. Cancer Incidence in Five Continents. Vol. 1, Berlin, Germany: Springer-Verlag, 1966; vol 5, Lyon, France: International Agency for Research on Cancer, 1987.
4. Davis DL, Hoel D, Fox J, Lopez A. International trends in cancer mortality in France, West Germany, Italy, Japan, England and Wales, and the USA. Lancet 1990;336:474–481.
5. National Cancer Institute. Cancer statistics review 1973–1989. Bethesda, MD: Department of Health and Human Services, 1992. (NIH publication number 92-2789.)
6. Glass AG, Hoover RN. The emerging epidemic of melanoma and squamous cell skin cancer. JAMA 1989;262:2097–2100.
7. Balch CM, Houghton AN, Milton GW, et al. Cutaneous Melanoma, 2nd ed. Philadelphia: JB Lippincott, 1992.
8. Rigel DS, Kopf AW, Friedman RJ. The rate of malignant melanoma in the United States: Are we making an impact? J Am Acad Dermatol 1987;17:1050–1053.
9. Van Der Esch EP, Muir CS, Nectoux J, et al. Temporal change in diagnostic criteria as a cause of the increase of malignant melanoma over time is unlikely. Int J Cancer 1991;47:483–490.
10. Boring CC, Squires TS, Tong T. Cancer Statistics, 1993. A Cancer Journal for Clinicians 1993;43:7–26.
11. Albert VA, Koh HK, Geller AC, et al. Years of potential life lost: Another indicator of the impact of cutaneous malignant melanoma on society. J Am Acad Dermatol 1990;23:308–310.
12. Rhodes AR, Weinstock MA, Fitzpatrick TB, et al. Risk factors for cutaneous melanoma. JAMA 1987;258:3146–3154.
13. MacKie RM, Freudenberger T, Aitchison TC. Personal risk-factor chart for cutaneous melanoma. Lancet 1989;2:487–490.
14. Evans RD, Kopf AW, Lew RA, et al. Risk factors for the development of malignant melanoma—I: Review of case control studies. J Dermatol Surg Oncol 1988;14:393–408.
15. Duggleby WF, Stoll H, Priore RL, et al. A genetic analysis of melanoma—polygenic inheritance as a threshold trait. Am J Epidemiol 1981;114:63–72.
16. Kopf AW, Hellman LJ, Rogers GS, et al. Familial malignant melanoma. JAMA 1986;256:1915–1919.
17. Gellin GA, Kopf AW, Garfinkel L. Malignant melanoma: A controlled study of possibly associated factors. Arch Dermatol 1969;99:43–48.
18. Lee JAH, Strickland D. Malignant melanoma: Social status and outdoor work. Br J Cancer 1980;41:757–763.
19. Swerdlow AJ, English J, MacKie RM, et al. Benign melanocytic nevi as a risk factor for malignant melanoma. Br Med J 1986;292:1555–1559.
20. Elwood JM, Gallagher RP, Hill GB, et al. Pigmentation and skin reaction to sun as risk factors for cutaneous melanoma: Western Canada Melanoma Study. Br Med J 1984;288:99–102.
21. Longstreth J, ed. Ultra-violet radiation and melanoma. With a special focus on assessing the risks of stratospheric ozone depletion. Environmental Protection Agency, Office of Air and Radiation, December 1987.
22. Koh HK, Kligler BE, Lew RA. Sunlight and cutaneous malignant melanoma: Evidence for and against causation. Photochem Photobiol 1990;51:765–779.
23. Sober AJ. Solar exposure in the etiology of cutaneous melanoma. Photodermatology 1987;4:23–31.
24. Lew RA, Sober AJ, Cook N, et al. Sun exposure habits in patients with cutaneous melanoma: A case-control study. J Dermatol Surg Oncol 1983;9:981–986.
25. Armstrong BK. Epidemiology of malignant melanoma: Intermittent or total accumulated exposure to the sun? J Dermatol Surg Oncol 1988;14:835–849.
26. Holman CDJ, Armstrong BK, Heenan PJ. Relationship of cutaneous malignant melanoma to individual sunlight-exposure habits. J Natl Cancer Inst 1986;76:403–414.
27. Kraemer KH, Lee MM, Scotto J. Xeroderma pigmentosum: Cutaneous, ocular and neurologic abnormalities in 830 published cases. Arch Dermatol 1987;123:241–250.
28. Green A, MacLennan R, Youl P, Martin N. Site distribution of cutaneous melanoma in Queensland. Int J Cancer 1993;53:232–236.
29. Ley RD, Applegate LA, Padilla RS, et al. Ultraviolet radiation-induced malignant melanoma in Monodelphis domestica. Photochem Photobiol 1989;50:1–5.
30. Molina MJ, Rowland FS. Stratospheric sink for chlorofluoromethanes: Chlorine atom-catalyzed destruction of ozone. Nature 1974;249:810–812.
31. Bowman KP. Global trends in total ozone. Science 1988;239:48–50.
32. Kerr JB, McElroy CT. Evidence for large upward trends of ultraviolet-B radiation linked to ozone depletion. Science 1993;262:1032–1034.
33. Swerdlow AJ, English JS, MacKie RM. Fluorescent lights, UV lamps, and risk of cutaneous melanoma. Br Med J 1988;297:647–649.
34. Walter SD, Marrett LD, From L. The association of cutaneous malignant melanoma with the use of sunbeds and sunlamps. Am J Epidemiol 1990;131:232–243.
35. Sober AJ, Fitzpatrick TB, Mihm MC, et al. Early recognition of cutaneous melanoma. JAMA 1979;242:2795–2799.
36. Fitzpatrick T, Milton G, Balch CW, et al. Clinial characteristics. In: Balch CM, Houghton AN, Milton GW, et al, eds. Cutaneous Melanoma, 2nd ed. Philadelphia: JB Lippincott, 1992:223–233.
37. Kopf AW, Mintzis M, Bart RS. Diagnostic accuracy in malignant melanoma. Arch Dermatol 1975;111:1291–1292.
38. Grin CM, Kopf AW, Welkovich B, et al. Accuracy in the clinical diagnosis of malignant melanoma. Arch Dermatol 1990;126:763–766.
39. Perednia DA, Gaines J, Rossum AC. Variability in physician assessment of lesions in cutaneous images and its implications for skin screening and computer-assisted diagnosis. Arch Dermatol 1992;128:357–364.
40. Koh HK, Geller AC, Miller DR, et al. Evaluation of melanoma/skin cancer screening in Massachusetts 1986–1989 (abstract). New York: American Public Health Association, 1990.
41. Koh HK, Norton LA, Geller AC, et al. Confirmed melanomas found in national skin cancer screening. Cancer, 1995, submitted for publication.
42. Pehamberger H, Binder M, Steiner A, Wolff K. In vitro epiluminescence microscopy: Improvement of early diagnosis of melanoma. J Invest Dermatol 1993;100:356S–362S.
43. Clark WH Jr. A classification of malignant melanoma in man correlated with histogenesis and biological behavior: In: Montagna W, Hu F, eds. Advances in Biology of the Skin, vol. VIII. Oxford: Pergamon Press, 1967:621–647.
44. Barnhill RL, Mihm MC Jr. The histopathology of cutaneous malignant melanoma. Diagn Pathol 1993;10(1):47–75.
45. Barnhill RL. Melanocytic nevi and tumor progression: Perspectives concerning histomorphology, melanoma risk and molecular genetics. Dermatology 1993;187:86–90.
46. Clark WH, Elder DE, Guerry D IV, et al. A study of tumor progression: The precursor lesion of superficial spreading and nodular melanoma. Hum Pathol 1984;15:1147–1165.
47. Clark WH Jr, Elder DE, Van Horn M. The biologic forms of malignant melanoma. Hum Pathol 1987;17:433–450.
48. Clark WH. Tumor progression and the nature of cancer. Br J Cancer 1991;64:631–644.
49. Schmitt FC, Bacchi CE. S-100 protein: Is it useful as a marker in diagnostic immunocytochemistry? Histopathology 1989;15:281.
50. Vollmer R. Pathology of melanoma. In: Seigler H, ed. Clinical Management of Melanoma. The Hague: Martinus Nijhoff, 1982:9–40.
51. Heenan PJ, Armstrong BK, English DR, et al. Pathological and epidemiological variants of cutaneous malignant melanoma. In: Elder DE, ed. Pathobiology of Malignant Melanoma, Pigment Cell, vol. VIII. Basel, Switzerland: Karger, 1987:107–146.
52. Holman CDJ, Armstrong BK. Cutaneous malignant melanoma and indicators of total accumulated exposure to the sun: An analysis separating histogenetic types. J Natl Cancer Inst 1984;73:75–82.
53. Clark WH Jr, From L, Bernardino EA, et al. The histogenesis and biologic behavior of primary human malignant melanoma of the skin. Cancer Res 1969;29:705–727.
54. Reed RJ. The pathology of human cutaneous melanoma. In: Costanzi JJ (ed). Malignant Melanoma, vol. I. The Hague: Martinus Nijhoff, 1983:85–116.
55. Elder DE, Ainsworth AM, Clark WH Jr. The surgical pathology

of primary cutaneous malignant melanoma. In: Clark WH Jr, Goldman LI, Mastrangelo MJ, eds. Human Malignant Melanoma. New York: Grune & Stratton, 1979:55–108.

56. Clark WH Jr, Elder DE, Guerry D IV, et al. Model predicting survival in Stage I melanoma based on tumor progression. J Natl Cancer Inst 1989;81:1893–1904.

57. Clark WH Jr, Mihm MC Jr. Lentigo maligna and lentigo-maligna melanoma. Am J Pathol 1969;55:39–67.

58. Heenan PJ, Matz LR, Blackwell JB, et al. Inter-observer variation between pathologists in the classification of cutaneous malignant melanoma in western Australia. Histopathol 1984;8:717–729.

59. Reed RJ. Acral lentiginous melanoma. In: New Concepts in Surgical Pathology of the Skin. New York: Wiley & Sons, 1976:89–90.

60. Arrington JH III, Reed RJ, Ichinose H, et al. Plantar lentiginous melanoma: A distinctive variant of human cutaneous malignant melanoma. Am J Surg Pathol 1977;1:131–143.

61. Coleman W, Loria PR, Reed RJ, et al. Acral lentiginous melanoma. Arch Dermatol 1980;116:773–776.

62. Patterson RH, Helwig EB. Subungual malignant melanoma: A clinical-pathologic study. Cancer 1980;46:2074–2087.

63. Blessing K, Kernohan NM, Park KGM. Subungual malignant melanoma: Clinicopathological features of 100 cases. Histopathology 1992;19:425–429.

64. Rigby HS, Briggs JC. Subungual melanoma: A clinicopathological study of 24 cases. Br J Plast Surg 1992;45:275–278.

65. Heenan PJ, Holman CDJ. Nodular malignant melanoma: A distinct entity or a common end stage? Am J Dermatopathol 1982;4:477–478.

66. Elder DE. Metastatic melanoma. In: Elder DE, ed. Pathobiology of Malignant Melanoma, Pigment Cell, vol. VIII. Basel, Switzerland: Karger, 1987:182–204.

67. Komberg R, Harris M, Ackerman AB. Epidermotropically metastatic malignant melanoma. Am J Surg Pathol 1979;3:301–311.

68. Bruijn JA, Mihm MC Jr, Barnhill RL. Desmoplastic melanoma. Histopathology 1992;20:197–205.

69. Reed RJ, Leonard D. Neurotropic melanoma. A variant of desmoplastic melanoma. Am J Surg Pathol 1979;3:301–311.

70. Kwittken J, Negri L. Malignant blue nevus: Case report of a Negro woman. Arch Dermatol 1966;94:64–69.

71. Merkow LP, Burt RC, Hayeslip DW, et al. A cellular and malignant blue nevus. A light and electron microscopic study. Cancer 1969;24:888–896.

72. Hernandez JF. Malignant blue nevus: A light and electron microscopic study. Arch Dermatol 1973;107:741–744.

73. Rubinstein N, Kopolovic J, Wexler MR, et al. Malignant blue nevus. J Dermatol Surg Oncol 1985;11:921–923.

74. Wetherington GM, Norin AL, Sadove AM. Locally invasive cellular blue nevus of the scalp. Plast Reconstr Surg 1987;79:114–117.

75. Temple-Camp CRE, Saxe N, King H. Benign and malignant cellular blue nevus: A clinicopathologic study of 30 cases. Am J Dermatopathol 1988;10:289–296.

76. Goldenhersh MA, Savin RC, Barnhill RL, et al. Malignant blue nevus: Case report and literature review. J Am Acad Dermatol 1988;19:712–722.

77. Connelly J, Smith JL Jr. Malignant blue nevus. Cancer 1991;67:2653–2657.

78. Cochran AJ, Wen D-R. S-100 protein as a marker for melanocytic and other tumours. Pathology 1985;17:340–345.

79. Gown AM, Vogel AM, Hoak D, et al. Monoclonal antibodies specific for melanocytic tumors distinguish subpopulations of melanocytes. Am J Pathol 1986;123:195–239.

80. Wick MR, Swanson PE, Rocamora A. Recognition of malignant melanoma by monoclonal antibody HMB-45. An immunohistochemical study of 200 paraffin-embedded cutaneous tumors. J Cutan Pathol 1988;15:201.

81. McGovern VJ, Shaw HM, Milton GW, et al. Lymphatic infiltration and survival in malignant melanoma. In: Ackerman AB, ed. Pathology of Malignant Melanoma. New York: Masson, 1981:341.

82. Kang S, Barnhill RL, Mihm MC Jr, et al. Histologic regression in malignant melanoma: An interobserver concordance study. J Cutan Pathol 1993;20:126–129.

83. Barnhill RL, Levy MA. Regressing thin cutaneous malignant

84. McGovern VJ. Spontaneous regression of melanoma. Pathology 1975;7:91–99.

85. Sondergaard K, Hou-Jensen K. Partial regression in thin primary cutaneous malignant melanomas clinical stage I: A study of 486 cases. Virchows Arch 1985;408:241–247.

86. Ronan SG, Eng AM, Briele HA, et al. Thin malignant melanomas with regression and metastases. Arch Dermatol 1987;123:1326–1330.

87. Slingluff CL, Vollmer RT, Reintgen DS, et al. Lethal "thin" malignant melanoma: Identifying patients at risk. Ann Surg 1988;208:150–161.

88. Fitzpatrick TB, Szabo G. The melanocyte: Cytology and cytochemistry. J Invest Dermatol 1959;32:197–209.

89. Herlyn M, Clark WH, Rodeck U, et al Biology of disease: Biology of tumor progression in human melanocytes. Lab Invest 1987;56:461–474.

90. Ellis DL, Kafka SP, Chow JC, et al. Melanoma, growth factors, acanthosis nigracans, the sign of Leser-Trelat, and the multiple acrochordons. N Engl J Med 1987;317:1582–1587.

91. Halaban R, Ghosh S, Baird A. bFGF is the putative natural growth factor for human melanocytes. In Vitro Cell Dev Biol 1987;23:47–52.

92. Houghton AN, Eisinger M, Albino AP, et al. Surface antigens of melanocytes and melanomas: Markers of melanocyte differentiation and melanoma subsets. J Exp Med 1982;156:1755–1766.

93. Thomson TM, Real FX, Murakami S, et al. Differentiation antigens of melanocytes and melanoma: Analysis of melanosome and cell surface markers of human pigmented cells with monoclonal antibodies. J Invest Dermatol 1988;90:459–466.

94. Herlyn M, Koprowski H. Melanoma antigens: Immunological and biological characterization and clinical significance. Ann Rev Immunol 1988;6:283–308.

95. Balaban G, Herlyn M, Guerry D IV, et al. Cytogenetics of human malignant melanoma and premalignant lesions. Cancer Genet Cytogenet 1984;11:429–439.

96. Bale SJ, Dracopoli NC, Tucker MA, et al. Mapping the gene for heredity cutaneous malignant melanoma-dysplastic nevus to chromosome 1p. N Engl J Med 1989;320:1367–1372.

97. Trent JM, Meyskens FL, Salmon SE, et al. Relation of cytogenetic abnormalities and clinical outcome in metastatic melanoma. N Engl J Med 1990;322:1508–1511.

98. Wittbrodt J, Adam J, Malitschek B, et al. Novel putative receptor tyrosine kinase encoded by the melanoma inducing Tu locus in Xiphophorus. Nature 1989;341:415–421.

99. Albino AP, Nanus DM, Mentle IR, et al. Analysis of ras oncogenes in malignant melanoma and precursor lesions: Correlation of point mutations with differentiation phenotype. Oncogene 1989;4:1363–1374.

100. Elder DE, Greene MH, Bondi EE, et al. Acquired melanocytic nevi and melanoma: The dysplastic nevus syndrome. In: Ackerman AB, ed. Pathology of Malignant Melanoma. New York: Masson, 1981:185–215.

101. Koh HK. When to refer the patient with a pigmented lesion. Hosp Pract 1986;21:47–54.

102. Nicholls EM. Development and elimination of pigmented moles, and the anatomical distribution of primary malignant melanoma. Cancer 1973;32:191–195.

103. Pack G, Lenson N, Gerber D. Regional distribution of moles and melanoma. Arch Surg 1952;65:862–869.

104. Rhodes AR. Melanocytic precursors of cutaneous melanoma. Med Clin North Am 1986;70:3–37.

105. Clark WH, Reimer RR, Greene M, et al. Origin of familial malignant melanomas from heritable melanocytic lesions. The B-K mole syndrome. Arch Dermatol 1978;114:732–738.

106. Greene MH, Clark WH, Tucker MA, et al. Acquired precursors of cutaneous malignant melanoma. The familial dysplastic nevus syndrome. N Engl J Med 1985;312:91–97.

107. Lynch HT, Frichot BC, Lynch JF. Familial atypical multiple mole–melanoma syndrome. J Med Genet 1978;15:352–356.

108. Greene MH, Clark WH, Tucker MA, et al. High risk of malignant melanoma in melanoma-prone families with dysplastic nevi. Ann Int Med 1985;102:458–465.

109. Kraemer K, Greene M, Tarone R, et al. Dysplastic naevi and cutaneous melanoma risk. Lancet 1983;2:1076–1077.

110. Rigel DS, Rivers JK, Kopf AW, et al. Dysplastic nevi: Markers for increased risk for melanoma. Cancer 1989;63:386–389.

111. Piepkorn M, Meyer LJ, Goldgar D, et al. The dysplastic melanocytic nevus: A prevalent lesion that correlates poorly with clinical phenotype. J Am Acad Dermatol 1989;20:407–415.

112. Ackerman AB. Pathobabel: Confusing terminology in the language of melanocytic neoplasia. In: Cascinelli N, Santinami M, Veronesi U, eds. Cutaneous Melanoma: Biology and Management. Milan: Masson: 1990:127–132.

113. NIH Consensus Development Panel on Early Melanoma. Diagnosis and treatment of early melanoma. JAMA 1992;168:1314–1319.

114. Clemente C, Cochran AJ, Elder DE, et al. Histopathologic diagnosis of dysplastic nevi: Concordance among pathologists convened by the World Health Organization Melanoma Programme. Hum Pathol 1991;22:313–319.

115. Lorentzen M, Pers M, Bretteville-Jensen G. The incidence of malignant transformation in giant pigmented nevi. Scand J Plast Reconstr Surg 1977;11:163–167.

116. Rhodes AR, Melski JW. Small congenital nevocellular nevi and the risk of cutaneous melanoma. J Pediatr 1982;100:219–224.

117. Rhodes AR, Silverman RA, Harrist TJ, et al. A histologic comparison of congenital and acquired nevomelanocytic nevi. Arch Dermatol 1985;121:1266–1273.

118. Reed RJ, Ichinose H, Clark WH Jr, et al. Common and uncommon melanocytic nevi and borderline melanomas. Semin Oncol 1975;2:119–147.

119. Barnhill RL, Barnhill MA, Berwick M, et al. The histological spectrum of pigmented spindle cell nevus: A review of 120 cases with emphasis on atypical variants. Human Pathol 1991;22:52–58.

120. Barnhill RL, Hurwitz S, Duray PH, et al. The dysplastic nevus: Recognition and management. Plast Reconstr Surg 1988;81:280–289.

121. Barnhill RL, Roush GC, Duray PH. Correlation of histologic architectural and cytoplastic features with nuclear atypia in atypical (dysplastic) nevomelanocytic nevi. Hum Pathol 1990;21:773–780.

122. Fletcher V, Sagebiel RW. The combined nevus. In: Ackerman AB, ed. Pathology of Malignant Melanoma. New York: Masson, 1981:273–283.

123. Pulitzer DR, Martin PC, Cohen AP, et al. Histologic classification of the combined nevus. Am J Surg Pathol 1991;15:1111–1122.

124. Kornberg R, Ackerman AB. Pseudomelanoma: Recurrent melanocytic nevus following partial surgical removal. Arch Dermatol 1975;111:1588.

125. Park HK, Leonard DD, Arrington JH, et al. Recurrent melanocytic nevi. Clinical and histologic review of 175 cases. J Am Acad Dermatol 1987;17:285–292.

126. Breslow A. Thickness, cross-sectional areas and depth of invasion in the prognosis of cutaneous melanoma. Ann Surg 1970;172:902–908.

127. Ackerman AB. Association of malignant melanomas with melanocytic nevi. In: Roses DF, Harris MN, Ackerman AB, eds. Diagnosis and Management of Cutaneous Malignant Melanoma. Philadelphia: WB Saunders Co., 1982:51–53.

128. Macy-Roberts E, Ackerman AB. A critique of techniques of biopsy of clinically suspected malignant melanomas. Am J Dermatopathol 1982;4:391–395.

129. Roses DF, Ackerman AB, Harris MN: Assessments of biopsy techniques and histopathologic interpretations of primary cutaneous melanomas. Ann Surg 1979;189:294.

130. Rogers, GS: Surgical management of stage I malignant melanoma. Dermatol Clin 1989;9:649–655.

131. Koh HK, Michalik E, Sober AJ, et al. Lentigo maligna melanoma has no better prognosis than other types of melanoma. J Clin Oncol 1984;2:994–1001.

132. Breslow A: Tumor thickness, level of invasion and node dissection in stage I cutaneous melanoma. Ann Surg 1975;182:572–575.

133. Day CL, Mihn MC, Lew RA, et al. Cutaneous malignant melanoma: Prognostic guidelines for physicians and patients. CA 1982;32:113–122.

134. Vollmer RT. Malignant melanoma: A multivariate analysis of prognostic factors. Path Ann 1989;24:383–407.

135. Balch CM, Soong SJ, Milton GW, et al. A comparison of prognostic factors and surgical results in 1,786 patients with localized (stage 1) melanoma treated in Alabama, USA, and New South Wales, Australia. Ann Surg 1982;196:677–683.

136. Cascinelli N, Morabito A, Bufalino R, et al. Prognosis of stage 1 melanoma of the skin: WHO collaborating centres for evaluation of methods of diagnosis and treatment of melanoma. Int J Cancer 1980;26:733–739.

137. Schmoeckel C, Bockelbrink A, Bockelbrink H, et al. Low- and high-risk malignant melanoma—1. Evaluation of clinical and histological prognosticators in 585 cases. Eur J Cancer Clin Oncol 1983;19(2):227–235.

138. Thorn M, Adami HO, Ringborg U, et al. The association between anatomic site and survival in malignant melanoma. An analysis of 12,353 cases from the Swedish Cancer Registry. Eur J Cancer Clin Oncol 1989;25:483–491.

139. Lemish WM, Heenan PJ, Holman CDJ, et al. Survival from preinvasive and invasive malignant melanoma in Western Australia. Cancer 1983;52:580–585.

140. Elder DE, Clark WH Jr. Tumor progression and prognosis in malignant melanoma. Pigment Cell 1987;8:51–80.

141. Sagebiel RW. The dysplastic melanocytic nevus. J Am Acad Dermatol 1989;20:496–501.

142. Rogers GS, Kopf AW, Rigel DS, et al. Effect of anatomical location on prognosis in patients with clinical stage 1 melanoma. Arch Dermatol 1983;119:644–649.

143. Day CL, Sober AJ, Kopf AW, et al. A prognostic model for clinical stage 1 melanoma of the upper extremity: The importance of anatomic subsites in predicting recurrent disease. Ann Surg 1981;193:436–440.

144. Harrist TJ, Rigel DS, Day CL, et al. "Microscopic satellites" are more highly associated with regional lymph node metastases than is primary melanoma thickness. Cancer 1984;53:2183–2187.

145. Kopf AW, Gross DF, Rogers GS, et al. Prognostic index for malignant melanoma. Cancer 1987;59:1236–1241.

146. Sorenson FB. Objective histopathologic grading of cutaneous malignant melanomas by stereologic estimation of nuclear volume. Cancer 1989;63:1784–1798.

147. Clark WH, Elder DE, Guerry D IV, et al. Model predicting survival in stage I melanoma based on tumor progression. J Natl Cancer Inst 1989;81:1893–1904.

148. Kheir SM, Bines SD, VonRoenn JM, et al. Prognostic significance of DNA aneuploidy in stage I cutaneous melanoma. Ann Surg 1988;207:455–461.

149. Ackerman AB. Malignant melanoma: A unifying concept. Am J Dermatopathol 1980;2:309–313.

150. Cascinelli N, Vaglini M, Nava M, et al. Prognosis of skin melanoma with regional node metastases (stage 2). J Surg Oncol 1984;25:240–247.

151. Balch CW, Soong SJ, Murad TM, et al. A multifactorial analysis of melanoma. 3. Prognostic factors in melanoma patients with lymph node metastases (stage 2). Ann Surg 1981;193:377–388.

152. Balch CM, Soong S, Murad TM, et al. A multifactorial analysis of melanoma. IV. Prognostic factors in 200 melanoma patients with distant metastases (stage III). J Clin Onc 1983;1:126–134.

153. Presant CA, Bartolucci AA, Southeastern Cancer Study Group. Prognostic factors in metastatic malignant melanoma: The Southeastern Cancer Study Group experience. Cancer 1982;49:2192–2196.

154. Choi KN, Withers HR, Rotman M: Intracranial metastases from melanoma: Clinical features and treatment by accelerated fractionation. Cancer 1985;56:1–9.

155. Rogers GS: Melanoma update: Advances in diagnostic technique. J Dermatol Surg Oncol 1989;15:605–607.

156. Buzaid AC, Sandler AB, Mani S, et al. Role of computed tomography in the staging of primary melanoma. J Clin Oncol 1993;11:638–643.

157. Veronesi U, Cascinelli N, Adamus J, et al. Thin stage 1 primary cutaneous malignant melanoma: Comparison of excision with margins of 1 or 3 centimeters. N Engl J Med 1988;318:1159–1162.

158. Balch CM, Urist MM, Karakousis CP, et al. Efficacy of 2-cm surgical margins for intermediate-thickness melanomas (1 to 4

mm): Results of a multi-institutional randomized surgical trial. Ann Surg 1993;218:262–269.

159. Kelly J, Sagebiel RW, Calderon W, et al. The frequency of local recurrence and microsatellites as a guide to reexcision margins for cutaneous malignant melanoma. Ann Surg 1984;200:759–763.

160. Rogers GS. Narrow versus wide margins in malignant melanoma. J Dermatol Surg Oncol 1989;15:33–34.

161. Roses DF, Harris MN, Ackerman AB: Diagnosis and Management of Cutaneous Melanoma. Philadelphia: WB Saunders Co., 1983:121–123.

162. Reyes BA, Robbins P. Use of Wood's light to determine the edge of a malignant melanoma. J Dermatol Surg Oncol 1988;1:22–23.

163. Urist MM, Balch CM, Soong SJ, et al. The influence of surgical margins and prognostic factors predicting the risk of local recurrence in 3445 patients with primary cutaneous melanoma. Cancer 1985;55:1398–1402.

164. Rogers GS, Kopf AW, Rigel D, et al. Hazard analysis for stage I cutaneous malignant melanoma. Arch Dermatol 1986; 5:999–1102.

165. Mohs FE. Fixed tissue micrographic surgery for melanoma of the ear. Arch Otolaryngol 1988;114:625–631.

166. Mohs FE. Micrographic surgery for satellite metastases of malignant melanoma. J Dermatol Surg Oncol 1986;12:471–476.

167. Dhawan SS, Woolf DJ, Robinowitz HS, et al. Lentigo maligna: The use of rush permanent sections in therapy. Arch Dermatol 1990;126:928–931.

168. Headington JT: A dermatopathologist looks at Mohs micrographic surgery. Arch Dermatol 1990;126:950–951.

169. Balch CM, Murad TM, Soong SJ, et al. A multifactorial analysis of melanoma: I. Prognostic histopathological features comparing Clark's and Breslow's staging methods. Ann Surg 1978; 188:732–742.

170. Coit DG, Brennan MF. Extent of lymph node dissection in melanoma of the trunk and lower extremity. Arch Surg 1989; 124:162–166.

171. Loree TR, Spiro RH: Cutaneous melanoma of the head and neck. Am J Surg 1989;158:388–391.

172. Veronesi U, Adamus J, Bandeira DC, et al. Inefficacy of immediate node dissection in stage 1 melanoma of the limbs. N Engl J Med 1977;297:627–630.

173. Day CL, Sober AJ, Lew RA, et al. Malignant melanoma patients with positive nodes and relatively good prognoses: Microstaging retains prognostic significance in clinical stage 1 melanoma patients with metastases to regional nodes. Cancer 1981; 47:955–962.

174. Koh HK, Sober AJ, Day CL, et al. Prognosis of clinical stage 1 melanoma patients with positive elective regional node dissection. J Clin Oncol 1986;4:1238–1244.

175. McCarthy WH, Shaw HM, Milton GW. Efficacy of elective lymph node dissection in 2,347 patients with clinical stage I malignant melanoma. Surg Gynecol Obstet 1985;161:575–580.

176. Goldsmith HS, Shah JP, Kim DH. Prognostic significance of lymph node dissection in the treatment of malignant melanoma. Cancer 1970;26:606–609.

177. Balch CM: The role of elective lymph node dissection in melanoma: Rationale, results, and controversies. J Clin Oncol 1988;6:163–172.

178. Roses DF, Provet JA, Harris MN, et al. Prognosis of patients with pathologic stage 2 cutaneous malignant melanoma. Ann Surg 1985;201:103–107.

179. Cohen MH, Ketcham AS, Felix EL, et al. Prognostic factors in patients undergoing lymphadenectomy for malignant melanoma. Ann Surg 1977;186:635–642.

180. Roses DF, Harris MN, Gumport SL, et al. Regional lymph node dissection for malignant melanoma of the extremities. Surgery 1981;89:654–659.

181. Sim FH, Taylor WF, Pritchard DJ, et al. Lymphadenectomy in the management of stage 1 malignant melanoma: A prospective randomized study. Mayo Clin Proc 1986;61:697–705.

182. Veronesi U, Adamus J, Bandeira DC, et al. Delayed regional lymph node dissection in stage 1 melanoma of the skin of the lower extremities. Cancer 1982;49:2420–2430.

183. Davis NC, McLeod GR, Beardmore GL. Primary cutaneous melanoma: A report from the Queensland Melanoma Project. CA 1976;2:80–107.

184. Wanebo HJ, Fortner JG, Woodruff J, et al. Selection of the optimum surgical treatment of stage I melanoma by depth of microinvasion. Ann Surg 1975;182:302–309.

185. Pritchard DJ, Sim FH. Surgical management of malignant melanoma of the trunk and extremities. Mayo Clin Proc 1989; 64:846–851.

186. Hiyama DT. Malignant melanoma: Current management. Ohio Med 1990;86:360–365.

187. Silberman AW. Malignant melanoma: Practical consideration concerning prophylactic lymph node dissection. Ann Surg 1987;206:206–209.

188. Sim FH, Taylor WF, Pritchard DJ, et al. Lymphadenectomy in the management of stage 1 malignant melanoma: A prospective randomized study. Mayo Clin Proc 1986;61:697–705.

189. Roses DF, Harris MN, Hidalgo D, et al. Correlation of the thickness of melanoma and regional lymph node metastases. Arch Surg 1982;198:921–927.

190. Davis NC: Cutaneous melanoma: The Queensland experience. Curr Probl Surg 1976;13:1–6.

191. Day CL, Lew RA. Malignant melanoma prognostic factors 7: Elective lymph node dissection. J Dermatol Surg Oncol 1985; 11:233–239.

192. Cascinelli N, Fontana V, Cataldo I, et al. Multiple primary melanoma. Tumori 1975;61:481–486.

193. Koh HK, Sober AJ, Harmon DC, et al. Adjuvant therapy of cutaneous malignant melanoma: A critical review. Med Pediatr Oncol 1985;13:244–260.

194. Eilber FR, Morton DL, Holmes EC, et al. Adjuvant immunotherapy with BCG in treatment of regional-lymph-node metastases from malignant melanoma. N Engl J Med 1976;294:237–240.

195. Veronesi U, Adamus J, Aubert C, et al. A randomized trial of adjuvant chemotherapy and immunotherapy in cutaneous melanoma. N Engl J Med 1982;307:913–916.

196. Franklin HR, Koops HS, Oldhoff J, et al. To perfuse or not to perfuse? A retrospective comparative study to evaluate the effect of adjuvant isolated regional perfusion in patients with stage 1 extremity melanoma with a thickness of 1.5 mm or greater. J Clin Oncol 1988;6:701–708.

197. Cumberlin R, DeMoss E, Lassus M, et al. Isolation perfusion for malignant melanoma of the extremity: A review. J Clin Oncol 1985;3:1022–1030.

198. Spitler LE. A randomized trial of levamisole versus placebo as adjuvant therapy in malignant melanoma. J Clin Oncol 1991;9:736–740.

199. Quirt IC, Shelley WE, Pater JL, et al. Improved survival in patients with poor-prognosis malignant melanoma treated with adjuvant levamisole: A phase III study by the National Cancer Institute of Canada Clinical Trials Group. J Clin Oncol 1991;9:729–735.

200. Wallack MC, Bash J, Bartolucci A. Improvement in disease-free survival of melanoma patients in conjunction with serologic response in a phase Ia/Ib Southeastern Cancer Study Group trial of vaccinia melanoma oncolysate. Am Surg 1989;55:243–247.

201. Bystryn JC, Oratz R, Harris MN, et al. Immunogenicity of a polyvalent melanoma antigen vaccine in humans. Cancer 1988;61:1065–1070.

202. Rege VB, Leone LN, Soderberg CH Jr. Hyperthermic adjuvant chemotherapy for stage I malignant melanoma of the extremities. Cancer 1983;52:2033–2041.

203. Ghussen F, Kruger I, Smalley RV, et al. Hyperthermic perfusion with chemotherapy for melanoma of the extremities. World J Surg 1989;13:598–602.

204. Cooper JS. Radiation therapy for cancers of the skin. Dermatol Clin 1991;9:683–687.

205. Ang KK, Byers RM, Peters LJ, et al. Regional radiotherapy as adjuvant treatment for head and neck malignant melanoma: Preliminary results. Arch Otolaryngol Head Neck Surg 1990; 16:169–172.

206. Meisenberg BR, Ross M, Vredenburgh JJ, et al. Randomized trial of high dose chemotherapy with autologous bone marrow support as adjuvant therapy for high-risk, multi-node-positive malignant melanoma. J Natl Cancer Inst 1993;85:1080–1085.

207. Creagan ET. Regional and systemic strategies for metastatic malignant melanoma. Mayo Clin Prac 1989;64:852–860.

208. Hill GJ, Krementz ET, Hill HZ. Dimethyl triazeno imidazole

carboxamide and combination therapy for melanoma. Cancer 1984;53:1299–1305.

209. Ghussen F, Nagel K, Groth W, et al. A prospective randomized study of regional extremity perfusion in patients with malignant melanoma. Ann Surg 1984;200:764–768.

210. Ghussen F, Kruger I, Groth W, et al. The role of regional hyperthermic cytostatic perfusion in the treatment of extremity melanoma. Cancer 1988;61:654–659.

211. Krementz ET, Carder RD, Sutherland CM, et al. The use of regional chemotherapy in the management of malignant melanoma. World J Surg 1979;3:289.

212. Stehlin JS, Giovanella BC, Ipolyi PD, et al. Seven years' experience with hyperthermic perfusion for melanoma of the extremities. World J Surg 1979;3:305.

213. Barranco SC, Romsdahl MM, Humphrey RM. The radiation response of human malignant melanoma cells grown in vitro. Cancer Res 1971;31:830–833.

214. Dewey DL. The radiosensitivity of melanoma cells in culture. Br J Radiol 1971;44:816.

215. Orton CG, Ellis F. A simplification in the use of the NSD concept in practical radiotherapy. Br J Radiol 1973;46:529–537.

216. Sause WT, Cooper JS, Rush S, et al. R.T.O.G. 83-05: A randomized trial evaluating fraction size in external beam radiation therapy. Proceedings of the American Society of Clinical Oncology 1989;8:283.

217. Overgaard J. The role of radiotherapy in recurrent and metastatic malignant melanoma: A clinical radiobiological study. Int J Rad Oncol Biol Phys 1986;12:867–872.

218. Ziegler JC, Cooper JS. Brain metastases from malignant melanoma: Conventional vs. high-dose-per-fraction radiotherapy. Int J Rad Oncol Biol Phys 1986;12:1839–1842.

219. Klausner JM, Gutman M, Rozin RR, et al. Conventional fractionation radiotherapy combined with 5-fluorouracil for metastatic malignant melanoma. Am J Clin Oncol. 1987;10:448–450.

220. Hidalgo V, Dy C, Fernandez-Hidalgo O, et al. Simultaneous radiotherapy and cis-platinum for the treatment of brain metastases. A pilot study. Am J Clin Oncol 1987;10:205–209.

221. Overgaard J, Overgaard M. Hyperthermia as an adjuvant to radiotherapy in the treatment of malignant melanoma. Int J Hyperthermia 1987;3:483–501.

222. Matalka KZ, Bailey MQ, Barth RF, et al. Boron neutron capture therapy of intracerebral melanoma using boronophenylalanine as a capture agent. Cancer Res 1993;53:3308–3313.

223. Coderre JA, Glass JD, Packer S, et al. Experimental boron neutron capture therapy for melanoma: Systemic delivery of boron to melanotic and amelanotic melanoma. Pigment Cell Res 1990;3:310–318.

224. Allen BJ. The potential of neutron capture therapy in the management of uncontrollable localised tumours. Australas Radiol 1990;34:297–305.

225. Kobayashi T, Kanda K, Ujeno Y, et al. Biomedical irradiation system for boron neutron capture therapy at the Kyoto University Reactor. Basic Life Sci 1990;54:321–339.

226. Fairchild RG, Slatkin DN, Coderre JA, et al. Optimization of boron and neutron delivery for neutron capture therapy. Pigment Cell Res 1989;2:309–318.

227. Mishima Y, Ichihashi M, Tsuji M, et al. Treatment of malignant melanoma by selective thermal neutron capture therapy using melanoma seeking compound. J Invest Dermatol 1989;92(5 Suppl.):321S–325S.

228. Overett TK, Shiu MH. Surgical treatment of distant metastatic melanoma. Cancer 1985;56:1222–1230.

229. Shea TC, Antman KH, Eder JP, et al. Malignant melanoma: Treatment with high-dose combination alkylating agent chemotherapy and autologous bone marrow support. Arch Dermatol 1988;124:878–884.

230. Wolff SN, Herzig RH, Fay JW, et al. High-dose thiotepa with autologous bone marrow transplantation for metastatic melanoma: Results of phase I-II studies of the North American Bone Marrow Transplantation Group. J Clin Oncol 1989;7:245–249.

231. Brandt SJ, Peters WP, Atwater SK, et al. Effect of recombinant human granulocyte-macrophage colony-stimulating factor on hematopoietic reconstitution after high-dose chemotherapy and autologous bone marrow transplantation. N Engl J Med 1988;318:869–876.

232. Creagan ET, Ahmann DL, Frytak S, et al: Recombinant leukocyte A interferon (rIFN-alpha A) in the treatment of disseminated malignant melanoma. Analysis of complete and long-term responding patients. Cancer 1986;58:2576–2578.

233. Legha SS, Papadopoulos NEJ, Plager C, et al. Clinical evaluation of recombinant interferon alfa-2A (Roferon-A) in metastatic melanoma using two different schedules. J Clin Oncol 1987;5:1240–1246.

234. Kirkwood JM, Ernstoff MS, Davis CA, et al. Comparison of intramuscular and intravenous recombinant alpha-2 interferon in melanoma and other cancers. Ann Int Med 1985;103:32–36.

235. Ferrone S, Chen ZJ, Liu CC, et al. Human high molecular weight-melanoma associated antigen mimicry by mouse antiidiotypic monoclonal antibodies MK2-23. Experimental studies and clinical trials in patients with malignant melanoma. Pharmacol Ther 1993;57:259–290.

236. Vadhan-Raj S, Cordon-Cardo C, Caarswell E, et al. Phase 1 trial of a mouse monoclonal antibody against GD3 ganglioside in patients with melanoma: Induction of inflammatory responses at tumor sites. J Clin Oncol 1988;6:1636–1648.

237. Mitchell MS, Harel W, Kempf RA, et al. Active-specific immunotherapy for melanoma. J Clin Oncol 1990;8:856–869.

238. Berd D, Maguire HC, McCue P, et al. Treatment of metastatic melanoma with an autologous tumor-cell vaccine: Clinical and immunologic results in 64 patients. J Clin Oncol 1990;8:1858–1867.

239. Spitler LE, del Rio M, Khentigan A, et al. Therapy of patients with malignant melanoma using a monoclonal antimelanoma antibody-Ricin A chain immunotoxin. Cancer Res 1987;47:1717–1723.

240. Murphy JR, Bishai W, Borowski M, et al. Genetic construction, expression, and melanoma-selective cytotoxicity of a diphtheria toxin-related alpha-melanocyte-stimulating hormone fusion protein. Proc Natl Acad Sci USA 1986;83:8258–8262.

241. Jacquillat C, Khayat D, Banzet P, et al. Final report of the French multicenter phase II study of the nitrosourea fotemustine in 153 evaluable patients with disseminated malignant melanoma including patients with cerebral metastases. Cancer 1990;66:1873–1878.

242. Wick MM. Therapeutic effect of dopamine infusion on human malignant melanoma. Cancer Treat Rep 1982;66:1657–1659.

243. Creagan ET, Long HJ, Ahmann DL, et al. Phase 2 evaluation of L-alanosine (NSC-153353) for patients with disseminated malignant melanoma. Am J Clin Oncol 1984;7:543–544.

244. Croghan MK, Booth A, Meyskens FL. A phase 1 trial of recombinant interferon-alpha and alpha-difluoromethylornithine in metastatic melanoma. J Biol Response Mod 1988;7:409–415.

245. Goodman GE, Beaumier P, Hellstrom I, et al. Pilot trial of murine monoclonal antibodies in patients with advanced melanoma. J Clin Oncol 1985;3(3):340–352.

246. Levine N, Meyskens FL Jr. Topical vitamin A acid therapy for cutaneous metastatic melanoma. Lancet 1980;2:224–226.

247. Rosenberg SA, Lotze MT, Yang JC, et al. Experience with the use of high-dose interleukin-2 in the treatment of 652 cancer patients. Ann Surg 1989;210:474–485.

248. Nathanson L. Spontaneous regression of malignant melanoma: A review of the literature on incidence, clinical features, and possible mechanisms. Nat Cancer Inst Monogr 1976;44:67–76.

249. Rosenberg SA, Lotze MT, Muul LM, et al. A progress report on the treatment of 157 patients with advanced cancer using lymphokine-activated killer cells and interleukin-2 or high-dose interleukin-2 alone. N Engl J Med 1987;316:889–897.

250. Cascinelli N, Belli F, Marchini S, et al. A phase 2 study of the administration of recombinant interleukin 2 (rIL-2) plus lymphokine activated killer (LAK) cells in stage 4 melanoma patients. Tumori 1989;75:233–244.

251. Parkinson DR, Abrams JS, Wiernik PH, et al. Interleukin-2 therapy in patients with metastatic malignant melanoma: A phase 2 study. J Clin Oncol 1990;8:1650–1656.

252. West WH, Tauer KW, Yannelli JR, et al. Constant-infusion recombinant interleukin-2 in adoptive immunotherapy of advanced cancer. N Engl J Med 1987;316:898–905.

253. Rosenberg SA, Lotze MT, Yang JC, et al. Combination therapy with interleukin-2 and alpha-interferon for the treatment of patients with advanced cancer. J Clin Oncol 1989;7:1863–1874.

254. Mitchell MS, Kempf RA, Harel W, et al. Effectiveness and tolerability of low-dose cyclophosphamide and low-dose intravenous interleukin-2 disseminated melanoma. J Clin Oncol 1988; 6:409–424.

255. Dillman RO, Oldham RK, Barth NM, et al. Recombinant interleukin-2 and adoptive immunotherapy alternated with Dacarbazine therapy in melanoma: A National Biotherapy Study Group Trial. J Natl Cancer Inst 1990;82(16):1345–1349.

256. Rosenberg SA, Packard BS, Aebersold PM, et al. Use of tumor-infiltrating lymphocytes and interleukin-2 in the immunotherapy of patients with metastatic melanoma. A preliminary report. N Engl J Med 1988;319:1676–1680.

257. Kradin RL, Lazarus DS, Dubinett SM, et al. Tumour-infiltrating lymphocytes and interleukin-2 in treatment of advanced cancer. Lancet 1989;1:577–580.

258. Topalian SL, Solomon D, Avis FP, et al. Immunotherapy of patients with advanced cancer using tumor-infiltrating lymphocytes and recombinant interleukin-2: A pilot study. J Clin Oncol 1988;6:839–853.

259. Rosenberg SA, Aebersold P, Cornetta K, et al. Gene transfer into humans—immunotherapy of patients with advanced melanoma, using tumor-infiltrating lymphocytes modified by retroviral gene transduction. N Engl J Med 1990;323:570–578.

260. Plautz GE, Yang ZY, Wu BY, et al. Immunotherapy of malignancy by in vitro gene transfer into tumors. Proc Natl Acad Sci USA 1993;90:4645–4649.

261. Koh HK, Lew RA, Prout MN. Screening for melanoma/skin cancer: Theoretic and practical considerations. J Am Acad Dermatol 1989;20:159–172.

262. Weary PE: A two-year experience with a series of rural skin and oral cancer detection clinics. JAMA 1971;217:1862–1863.

263. Koh HK, Geller AC, Miller DR, et al. Can screening for melanoma/skin cancer save lives? In: Rigel D, ed. Dermatologic Clinics. Philadelphia: WB Saunders, 1991:795–804.

264. Koh HK, Caruso A, Gage I, et al. Evaluation of melanoma/skin cancer screening in Massachusetts: Preliminary results. Cancer 1990;65:375–379.

265. Koh HK, Geller AC, Miller DR, et al. Early detection of melanoma: An ounce of prevention may be a ton of work. J Am Acad Dermatol 1993;28:645–647.

266. Rigel DS, Friedman RJ, Kopf AW, et al. Importance of complete cutaneous examination for the detection of malignant melanoma. J Am Acad Dermatol 1986;14:857–860.

267. Miller AB, Chamberlain J, Day NE, et al. Report on a workshop of the UICC project on evaluation of screening for cancer. Int J Cancer 1990;46:761–769.

268. Hayward RS, Steinberg EP, Ford DE, et al. Preventive care guidelines: 1991. Ann Int Med 1991;114:758–783.

269. Fisher M, Eckhart C, eds: Screening for skin cancer. In: Guide to Clinical Preventive Services. An Assessment of the Effectiveness of 169 Interventions. Report of the U.S. Preventive Services Task Force. Baltimore: Williams & Wilkins, 1989:71–76.

270. American Cancer Society: Report on cancer-related health checkup. Cancer 30:194–240, 1980.

271. Cassileth BR, Clark WH, Lusk EJ, et al. How well do physicians recognize melanoma and other problem lesions? J Am Acad Dermatol 1986;14:555–560.

272. Friedman RJ, Rigel DS, Kopf AW. Early detection of malignant melanoma: The role of physician examination and self-examination of the skin. CA 1985;35:4–25.

273. Alper J. Congenital nevi: The controversy rages on. Arch Derm 1985;121:734–735.

274. Bonett A, Roder D, Esterman A. Epidemiologic features of melanoma in South Australia: Implications for cancer control. Med J Aust 189;151:502–509.

275. Theobald T, Marks R, Hill D, et al. Goodbye Sunshine: Effects of a television program about melanoma on beliefs, behavior, and melanoma thickness. J Am Acad Dermatol 1991;25:717–723.

276. MacKie RM, Hole D. Audit of public education campaign to encourage earlier detection of malignant melanoma. Br Med J 1992;304:1012–1015.

277. Marks R, Hill D. Behavioural change in adolescence: A major challenge for skin-cancer control in Australia. Med J Aust 1988;149:514–515.

278. Vasen HFA, Bergman W, Van Haeringen A, et al. The familial dysplastic nevus syndrome. Natural history and the impact of screening on prognosis. A study of nine families in the Netherlands. Eur J Cancer 1989;25:337–341.

279. Kopf A, Rivers J, Friedman R. Dysplastic nevi. In: Friedman R, Rigel D, Kopf A, et al, eds. Cancer of the Skin. Philadelphia: WB Saunders Co., 1991;125–141.

280. Slue W, Kopf AW, Rivers JK. Total-body photographs. Arch Dermatol 1988;124:1239–1243.

281. Grossman DJ. Public and professional materials on skin cancer. J Am Acad Dermatol 1989;21:1012–1018.

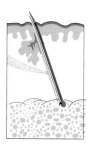

chapter 152

Mastocytosis

JACK LONGLEY

DEFINITION

Mastocytosis, also known as mast cell disease, is a heterogeneous group of disorders characterized by increased numbers of mast cells in a variety of tissues, most often the skin. The localization of mast cells to different organs and the release of their mediators locally and into the systemic circulation result in a number of symptom-complexes that vary from one individual to another.[1-3]

CLINICAL DESCRIPTION

Mast cell disease occurs in all races and affects both sexes equally.[1-6] Most cases of cutaneous mastocytosis are self-limited and unreported, so the true incidence and prevalence of this condition are unknown, but an estimated 1 in 1000 to 1 in 8000 individuals visiting a general dermatology clinic has some form of mastocytosis.[5, 7] The peak incidence of mastocytosis is in children; in over half of all patients the disease is diagnosed before the age of 6 months.[1, 5] There is a second peak of incidence in young adults.[1, 3, 5, 6] Mastocytosis tends to be transient in children and chronic in adults.[1]

Mastocytosis may be limited to one organ or may be classified as systemic if more than one organ system is involved. The disease may be further classified prognostically as indolent, aggressive, or associated with mast cell leukemia or other hematologic abnormalities.[2, 8]

General Features of Cutaneous Mastocytosis

Although there is overlap in the morphology of the individual lesions and clinical presentation, patients with cutaneous mastocytosis can be generally classified into those with solitary mastocytoma, urticaria pigmentosa, diffuse or erythrodermic mastocytosis, and telangiectasia macularis eruptiva perstans. The number of mast cells infiltrating the dermis in cutaneous mastocytosis varies from a relatively small number that is undetectable on physical examination to larger aggregations forming papules, nodules, or diffuse thickening of the skin. Papular or nodular lesions with dense dermal infiltrates may have a yellowish hue that is accentuated by diascopy.[9] Darier's sign, which is the development of urtication and a delayed, axonally mediated erythematous flare, can usually be elicited by rubbing or other minor trauma to a lesion (Fig. 152–1). Such physical stimulus causes mast cell degranulation with the release of mast cell mediators and local tissue effects of vasodilatation, increased vascular permeability, and edema. In addition, any of the forms of cutaneous mastocytosis may show hyperpigmentation, which is caused by increased epidermal melanin pigment.[10] Patients may have prolonged dermographism or flushing as well as localized or generalized pruritus, occasionally without visible skin lesions.[11, 12] Lesions in infants occasionally form tense blisters that may rarely be hemorrhagic and that usually heal without scarring unless secondary infection occurs. Unusual severe complications in infancy include hypotension and shock, severe diarrhea and dehydration, and, very rarely, a bleeding diathesis.[3, 6, 13]

Mastocytoma

The term *mastocytoma* has been used to describe nodular infiltrates of mast cells occurring as a single or one of several isolated lesions (solitary mastocytoma) and to refer to lesions that are a component of more generalized cutaneous mastocytosis. Solitary mastocytomas occur almost exclusively in the first 2 years of life and are often present at birth (see Fig. 152–1).[1, 6, 14, 15] These solitary nodules typically are found on the trunk and extremities and range in size from 5 to 60 mm in diameter.[1] Darier's sign, epidermal pigmentation, the formation of vesicles or bullae, and localized flushing are common; generalized flushing has rarely been reported.[1, 5, 6, 16] Although lesions with these clinical characteristics may occasionally be the first of many lesions, extensive involvement is

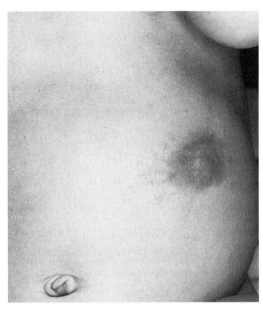

FIGURE 152–1. A solitary mastocytoma in an infant showing a wheal and flare following minor physical irritation (Darier's sign).

usually manifest within 1 or 2 months.[1] Lesions that are truly solitary usually regress completely or become asymptomatic and rarely persist into adulthood.[1]

Urticaria Pigmentosa

The term *urticaria pigmentosa* refers to the clinical characteristics of the lesions in the most common form of cutaneous mastocytosis; they urticate and they are pigmented. Several to several thousand individual lesions may be present, and they are typically round or oval, reddish brown macules or papules on the trunk and extremities (Fig. 152–2). There may be occasional individual nodular lesions, or there may be clustering of papules to form plaques or a generalized cobblestone appearance with exaggeration of normal skin markings.[3, 6] The individual lesions tend to be larger in very young children and smaller, macular, and relatively stable in older children and adults.[3, 6, 9] Pruritus, dermo-

graphism, flushing, telangiectasia, and petechiae or ecchymoses can occur in lesions or in clinically normal skin as a result of mast cell mediator release.[6, 9] Most patients, particularly children, have an extremely good prognosis. Over half will experience complete clearance by adolescence, and most of the remainder have only residual, lightly pigmented asymptomatic macules.[1] When onset occurs in adolescence or adulthood, the lesions are more likely to persist or progress slowly and remain symptomatic. Perhaps 25% of patients with adult-onset urticaria pigmentosa develop systemic mastocytosis.[1]

Diffuse and Erythrodermic Mastocytosis

Diffuse infiltration of the skin is rare and occurs almost exclusively in infants, although it may persist into adult life.[3, 17–19] Blisters occurring in the neonatal period may be the first indication of diffuse involvement, with later development of a "doughy" thickening of the skin. Involvement may be limited to large plaques or may include the entire skin surface (Fig. 152–3; see color plate). The skin surface may be smooth or covered with minute papules causing a resemblance to grain leather (peau chagriné). Scattered nodules and larger papules are not uncommon.[20] The color of the skin may appear normal, focally or diffusely hyperpigmented, or bright red. Tan or brown, freckle-like macules typical of urticaria pigmentosa may coexist.[3] When the dermal mast cell infiltrate is dense, the skin may have a yellowish hue similar to that seen in pseudoxanthoma elasticum.[9] Although diffuse cutaneous mastocytosis often resolves spontaneously, these patients are at higher risk of systemic involvement, severe complications, and persistence of mastocytosis into adulthood.[3, 6]

Telangiectasia Macularis Eruptiva Perstans

Telangiectasia macularis eruptiva perstans is a rare form of cutaneous mastocytosis that occurs almost exclusively in adults. The lesions tend to be widespread and may involve the face. As the descriptive name suggests, individual lesions consist of telangiectases on an erythematous or hyperpigmented macular background. Darier's sign may be evident. Pigmentation ranges from light tan to brown.[3, 6] Rarely, there may also be scattered

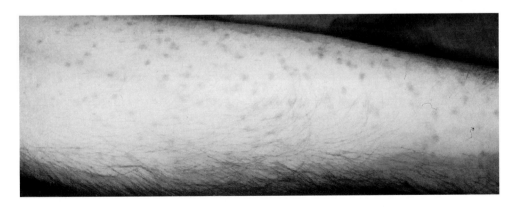

FIGURE 152–2. Extensive macular and papular lesions of urticaria pigmentosa in an adult.

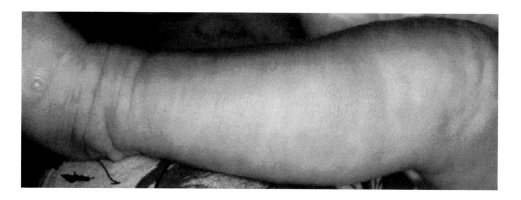

FIGURE 152-3. Hyperpigmented and thickened skin in an infant with diffuse cutaneous mastocytosis. Subepidermal bulla (*far left, dorsal ankle*) is caused by edema of the superficial dermis, secondary to mast cell mediator release. (See color plate.)

papules or individual lesions more typical of urticaria pigmentosa.[21]

Systemic Mastocytosis

The vast majority of patients with cutaneous mastocytosis do not have systemic involvement, although evidence of bone involvement may be detected in as many as 10% of patients with urticaria pigmentosa undergoing radiologic survey.[22, 23] Many patients with systemic mastocytosis have indolent disease that has a good prognosis and that can be controlled pharmacologically. After the skin, the skeletal and hematopoietic systems are the systems next most commonly involved, followed by the reticuloendothelial system, including the liver, the gastrointestinal system, and the cardiovascular and central nervous systems.[2] Patients with mastocytosis may present with complaints of nausea, vomiting, diarrhea, episodic abdominal pain, weight loss, headache, fatigue, episodic flushing, chest pain, tachycardia, hypotension, syncope, or dizziness.[2, 3, 24] Any of these symptoms may be caused by chemical mediators released from mast cells into the systemic circulation from one organ, or by local, high concentrations of mediators released in the affected organ. Malabsorption, gastritis, and peptic ulcer disease with hemorrhage or perforation are associated with hyperchlorhydria caused by high levels of histamine. Steatorrhea, asymptomatic hepatosplenomegaly, anemia, myelodysplastic and myeloproliferative syndromes, lymphoma, and leukemia may occur, especially in adults with systemic mastocytosis. In cases of mastocytosis associated with serious hematologic abnormality or malignancy, the overall prognosis is determined by the response of these associated conditions to therapy. True mast cell leukemia is very rare and has a dismal prognosis.

PATHOLOGY

Lesions of mastocytosis are characterized by increased numbers of mast cells in various tissues. Generally, there is an accentuation of normal mast cell distribution; that is, there is a tendency for the infiltrating mast cells to be perivascular, perineural, and near epithelial surfaces. The degree of infiltration varies widely from the subtle superficial perivascular mast cell infiltrates of telangiectasia

macularis eruptiva perstans that are problematic to diagnose histologically, to the massive superficial and deep infiltrates that may extend into the subcutaneous fat and that are more commonly seen in mastocytomas or other nodular lesions.[15] However, there is considerable overlap in the histologic features of various forms of mastocytosis so that a specific lesion usually cannot be ascribed to one of the clinical forms of mastocytosis on the basis of histopathology alone.

The infiltrating mast cells are usually monotonous and have round or oval, darkly staining, bland nuclei and a moderate amount of finely granular cytoplasm that gives the cells a distinctive appearance like a fried egg (Fig. 152-4; see color plate).[25] They may be larger than normal mast cells and are occasionally irregular or dendritic, or show spindling of their cytoplasm and nuclei. Spindled mast cells are sometimes associated with fibrosis of the papillary dermis. Sometimes nuclear irregularities and hyperchromasia are present, but these changes do not necessarily indicate malignancy. The cytoplasms of mast cells contain tiny amphophilic granules that show metachromasia in Giemsa- or toluidine blue-stained sections (see Fig. 152-4, *inset*).

Any lesions of mastocytosis may show the effects of mast cell degranulation, such as edema and the recruitment of eosinophils, superimposed on the basic pattern of mast cell infiltration. Additional histologic features include hyperpigmentation caused by increased melanin that is found exclusively in the basal layer of the epidermis, telangiectases in lesions of telangiectasia macularis eruptiva perstans, and massive edema with subepidermal blister formation in bullous lesions.

PATHOGENESIS AND ETIOLOGY

Most of the symptoms of mast cell disease are caused by mast cell mediators that can be released by a number of factors, including specific immunologic triggers such as the occupation of mast cell surface Fcε receptors by antigen-IgE complexes. Less specific factors such as complement and nonimmunologic stimuli including physical trauma and changes in temperature, venoms from snakes and insects, polypeptides found in shellfish, and a number of drugs are also capable of triggering mediator release. The most commonly implicated drugs are aspirin, alcohol, and narcotics. Radiographic contrast

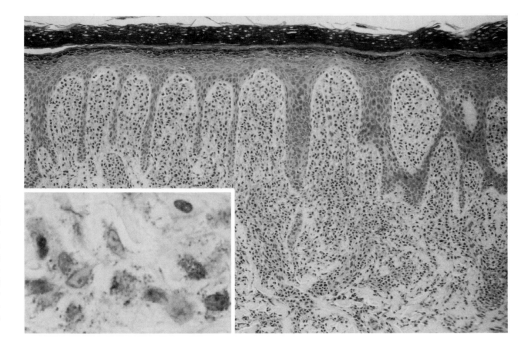

FIGURE 152–4. Infiltrating mast cells in cutaneous mastocytosis are larger than normal mast cells and resemble fried eggs. Highly charged, sulfated acid mucopolysaccharides cause metachromatic (purple) staining of mast cell granules in Giemsa-stained sections (*inset*), in contrast to the eosinophilic (pink) granules of eosinophils recruited by mast cell degranulation. (See color plate.)

dyes and various drugs associated with anesthesia may also cause mast cell degranulation and release of mediators.[4]

The mediators released from stimulated mast cells include histamine, arachidonic acid and its metabolites, cytokines, and neutral proteases. The effects of these mediators may be seen locally in the skin as urtication, vasodilatation, and pruritus; systemically they contribute to anaphylaxis or gastrointestinal and central nervous system disturbances.

More specifically, histamine causes pruritus and a wheal and flare locally, and its release into the general circulation may result in widespread vasodilatation, bronchospasm, increased gastric acid secretion, and spasmodic contractions of the gastrointestinal tract.[26] Arachidonic acid metabolites include the prostaglandins and leukotrienes.[27] Prostaglandins induce sensations of pruritus and pain in the skin and rhinorrhea, bronchorrhea, and hypotension systemically. A group of leukotrienes released from activated mast cells have been identified as the slow-reacting substances of anaphylaxis (SRS-A). These leukotrienes have been shown to alter vascular tone and permeability and promote constriction of coronary arteries and bronchial tissues, thereby contributing to hypotension, chest pain, and decreased expiratory flow rate.[28-34] A cytokine, tumor necrosis factor–α, has been identified as a product of human mast cells and is a proinflammatory peptide that stimulates the recruitment of inflammatory cells and the release of a cascade of other mediators.[35-41] The neutral proteases have local anticoagulant effects. Another product of human mast cells, platelet activating factor, may contribute to systemic anaphylaxis as well as having anticoagulant effects locally.[42, 43]

The transient clinical course of most cases of mastocytosis and the histologic finding of increased numbers of mast cells in an accentuation of their normal distribution have suggested that mastocytosis may represent a hyperplastic response to abnormal stimuli rather than a true neoplasm.[15, 44, 45] Additional support for this concept has come from the finding that the injection of a cytokine called mast cell growth factor (also known as stem cell factor or c-*kit* ligand) induces mast cell hyperplasia in the skin of experimental animals.[46, 47] Although elevations of circulating mast cell growth factor have not been identified in patients with systemic mastocytosis, mast cell growth factor can be produced locally in the skin by keratinocytes and fibroblasts, and increased local concentrations of soluble mast cell growth factor have been identified in lesions of human cutaneous mastocytosis.[47, 48] Mast cell growth factor not only causes mast cell proliferation but also stimulates melanocyte proliferation and melanin pigment production.[49] Thus, alterations in the local metabolism of mast cell growth factor in the skin of patients with cutaneous mastocytosis may explain both the characteristic mast cell proliferation and the hyperpigmentation of these lesions.

DIAGNOSIS AND DIFFERENTIAL DIAGNOSIS

The diagnosis of cutaneous mastocytosis can be established when lesions of classic morphology are identified and a positive Darier's sign is elicited.[1] No further diagnostic investigation is needed in young children with limited disease. Skin biopsy is the most common and most effective confirmatory test. The infiltration of local anesthetics adjacent to the lesion rather than directly into it and the use of anesthetics without epinephrine have been recommended to avoid mast cell degranulation, which can make histologic identification of mast cells more difficult. Lesions of mastocytosis may bleed excessively when biopsied, perhaps because of the anticoagulant effects of heparin and other mast cell mediators.

In adolescent patients and in adults with extensive, persistent, or progressive cutaneous disease, a baseline radiologic survey may be considered. Identification and knowledge of focal involvement of the skeletal system may prevent undue expense and concern if such changes were to be discovered incidentally at a later date and confused with a manifestation of malignancy. A radiologic survey and bone scan are indicated in any patients with symptoms referable to the skeletal system. Bone marrow biopsy is indicated in individuals with hematologic abnormalities.

In patients with atypical presentations or unusual symptom-complexes, biochemical determination of mast cell mediators can support a diagnosis of suspected mast cell disease. Determination of urinary Nτ-methylhistamine, a metabolite of histamine that is elevated in patients with mastocytosis, can be obtained through the Department of Laboratory Medicine at Vanderbilt University School of Medicine.[50, 51] Levels of this metabolite and other mast cell products may be elevated with anaphylaxis as well as in mast cell disease, so the results must be interpreted in the clinical context; identification of chronically elevated levels of mast cell products is the most useful finding. Although not yet generally available, determination of urinary prostaglandin D_2 metabolites may be even more specific for mastocytosis.

In the differential diagnosis of the lesions of cutaneous mastocytosis one must consider pigmented, telangiectatic, and nodular lesions as well as pruritus, dermographism, and flushing (Table 152–1). The presence of Darier's sign, urtication of a hyperpigmented skin lesion on stroking it, allows easy differentiation of individual lesions in most cases, but biopsy may be necessary, particularly in older patients in whom Darier's sign may be absent. Papular lesions of mastocytosis having a yellowish hue may resemble eruptive xanthomas, but these lesions may be differentiated by the presence of a brown halo in the former and a red halo in the latter. Crusting vesicular lesions of cutaneous mastocytosis in infants may resemble impetigo. Langerhans cell histiocytosis can be differentiated from mastocytosis clinically by the distribution of lesions and histopathologically. Both the carcinoid syndrome and mastocytosis may present as episodic flushing and nonspecific gastrointestinal and cardiovascular symptoms. In the absence of characteristic skin lesions of mastocytosis, these syndromes may be differentiated by noting that the flushing associated with carcinoid syndrome is evanescent, typically lasting 10 minutes or less while that of mastocytosis typically lasts 30 minutes or more.[9] These two syndromes can be further differentiated by examining urine for 5-hydroxyindoleacetic acid or Nτ-methylhistamine. The former is usually elevated in the carcinoid syndrome, and the latter is elevated in mastocytosis.[52]

Although most patients with mastocytosis have cutaneous involvement, occasional patients may present with few or no skin lesions and pruritus or a constellation of vague complaints (inability to concentrate, headache, fatigue, dizziness, syncope, nausea, vomiting, diarrhea, abdominal pain, weight loss, epiuodic flushing, tachycardia, or chest pain).[3, 4, 11, 24] Any of these symptoms may be the presenting complaint and may be due to episodic release of mast cell mediators. In such eases, a careful

TABLE 152–1. Differential Diagnosis of Cutaneous Mastocytosis*

Mastocytoma(s)

Melanocytic nevus
Lentigo
Impetigo (crusted vesicular lesion)
Xanthogranuloma (juvenile xanthogranuloma)
Connective tissue nevus
Leiomyoma (may show pseudo-Darier's sign)

Urticaria Pigmentosa

Melanocytic nevi or lentigines
Café-au-lait spots
Leiomyomas
Neurofibromas
Xanthogranulomas (multiple juvenile xanthogranulomas)
Eruptive xanthomas

Diffuse/Erythrodermic Mastocytosis

Blistering diseases of the newborn
  Impetigo
  Toxic epidermal necrolysis
  Staphylococcal scalded skin syndrome
  Epidermolysis bullosa
  Congenital bullous ichthyosiform erythroderma
Infiltrative process
  Langerhans' cell histiocytosis
  Pseudoxanthoma elasticum (rarely)

Telangiectasia Macularis Eruptiva Perstans

Telangiectasia
  Essential
  Dermatoheliosis
  Acne rosacea
  Liver disease
  Poikiloderma
Nevoid telangiectasia

*This table was prepared with help from Dr. Jean Bolognia.

history for other symptoms of mastocytosis including the identification of known triggers of mast cell degranulation, a thorough physical examination for hepatosplenomegaly, a radiologic survey, bone marrow biopsy, or determination of urinary Nτ-methylhistamine may ultimately allow a diagnosis of mastocytosis. A therapeutic trial of antihistamines or sodium cromoglycate may confirm the diagnosis.

TREATMENT

Since most cases are self-limited and not life-threatening, reassurance of the usual benign course of this disease and avoidance of specific factors known to trigger mast cell degranulation may be sufficient (Table 152–2). Therapeutic intervention is generally directed at amelioration of symptoms; however, in certain situations, therapy may be directed against specific cutaneous lesions. Acceptable temporary cosmetic results may be ob-

TABLE 152–2. Treatment of Cutaneous Mastocytosis

A. Reassure patient of usually benign course, when appropriate
B. Avoid known triggers of mast cell degranulation*
  1. Immunologic (allergens)
  2. Physical (heat, cold, sunlight, trauma)
  3. Biologic toxins (snake and insect venoms; biologic peptides associated with *Ascaris*, jellyfish, and shellfish)
  4. Drugs (aspirin, alcohol, narcotics, polymyxin B, amphotericin B, thiamine, D-tubocurarine, quinine, radiographic dyes, scopolamine, gallamine, decamethonium)
C. Symptomatic therapy
  1. Treatment of anaphylaxis (epinephrine, fluids)
  2. Antihistamines
     a. H_1 blockers (chlorpheniramine, hydroxyzine, doxepin)
     b. H_2 blockers (cimetidine, ranitidine)
     c. H_3 blockers (no reports yet)
  3. Antiprostaglandins (aspirin)
  4. Disodium cromoglycate (Gastrocrom)
  5. Photochemotherapy (PUVA)
D. Treatment of lesions
  1. Excision of solitary mastocytomas
  2. Topical corticosteroids (betamethasone dipropionate under occlusion)
  3. Local corticosteroid injection (triamcinolone acetonide)
  4. Systemic corticosteroids (severe cases)

*Section B was modified from DiBacco RS, DeLeo VA. Mastocytosis and the mast cell. J Am Acad Dermatol 1982; 7:709–722.

tained for individual lesions by treatment with potent topical corticosteroids (0.05% betamethasone dipropionate ointment, applied as a thin film and occluded for 8 hours daily, for 6 weeks), or with the injection of corticosteroids.[53] Excision of symptomatic solitary mastocytomas may rarely be indicated, for instance, if severe cardiovascular or respiratory symptoms are being produced.[1]

Patients or the parents of children with extensive involvement or prominent cardiovascular symptoms should be taught to recognize developing shock and the emergency management of anaphylactic reactions. These patients should wear Medical Alert bracelets and have epinephrine available for injection.[3, 54, 55] Patients with mastocytosis should be cautioned that they may be at increased risk for adverse reactions when undergoing general anesthesia.[56, 57]

Histamine receptor antagonists are the primary therapy for mastocytosis and may be used to control symptoms related to the skin, the gastrointestinal tract, and the cardiovascular system. Therapy may be begun with a single type 1 histamine (H_1) receptor antagonist. After maximum tolerated levels are achieved, other H_1-receptor blockers may be added. H_2-receptor blockers may be necessary, particularly for the control of gastrointestinal effects associated with hyperchlorhydria.[3, 58–60] Oral disodium cromoglycate may prevent release of histamine and other mediators and thus be effective in controlling diarrhea. Dosages are 20 to 40 mg/kg in four divided doses in patients younger than the age of 2 years, 100 mg

four times a day from ages 2–12, and 200 mg four times a day for adults.[61] Two or 3 weeks of treatment may be required before a maximum clinical response is achieved. Although it is poorly absorbed, oral disodium cromoglycate also appears to have beneficial effects on cutaneous and central nervous system symptoms.[62]

Symptoms of mastocytosis may be caused by other circulating mediators besides histamines. Symptoms associated with high levels of circulating prostaglandins may be controlled using aspirin, 975 mg given orally four times a day in adults. The use of aspirin to treat mastocytosis in the pediatric age group has not been reported. Because of aspirin's ability to cause mast cell degranulation, which could precipitate severe respiratory and cardiovascular symptoms in patients with mastocytosis, aspirin therapy must be initiated slowly in a hospital setting in which maximum levels of blockade with antihistamines has been achieved.[3, 63, 64] The use of enteric-coated tablets has been advised but may not be as effective as regular aspirin owing to lower peak blood levels.[3, 63, 64]

Photochemotherapy using psoralens and ultraviolet A radiation (PUVA) may decrease itching and provide cosmetic benefits.[65–67] The benefits from PUVA, however, are temporary, and this modality should be administered only by those experienced in its use because of potential side effects, such as the development of cutaneous carcinomas.[3, 4]

Systemic corticosteroids may be beneficial in patients with severe cutaneous involvement, malabsorption, or ascites that is otherwise uncontrollable.[60] Interferon alfa 2b may also be effective in patients with several forms of mastocytosis.[68] In patients with aggressive systemic mastocytosis and in those with associated hematologic malignancies, death usually results from bleeding caused by severe thrombocytopenia. Splenectomy is controversial but may have a beneficial effect in a selected group of patients.[69] In patients with an associated hematologic malignancy, the prognosis is limited by the ability to control that malignancy.

References

1. Caplan RM. The natural course of urticaria pigmentosa. Arch Dermatol 1963;87:146–157.
2. Travis WD, Li C-Y, Bergstrahl EJ, et al. Systemic mast cell disease: Analysis of 58 cases and literature review. Medicine 1988;67:345–368.
3. Stein DH. Mastocytosis: A review. Pediatr Dermatol 1986;3:365–375.
4. DiBacco RS, DeLeo VA. Mastocytosis and the mast cell. J Am Acad Dermatol 1982;7:709–722.
5. Fine J. Mastocytosis. Int J Dermatol 1980;19:117–123.
6. Soter NA. The skin in mastocytosis. J Invest Dermatol 1991;96(Suppl):32S–39S.
7. Sagher F, Even-Paz Z. Mastocytosis and the Mast Cell. Chicago: Year Book Medical Publishers, 1967.
8. Metcalfe DD. Conclusions: Clinical advances in mastocytosis: An interdisciplinary round table discussion. J Invest Dermatol 1991;96(Suppl):64S–65S.
9. Selyne H. The Mast Cells. London: Butterworth, 1965:264.
10. Lever W, Schaumberg-Lever G. Histopathology of the Skin, 7th ed. Philadelphia: JB Lippincott, 1990.

11. Kendall ME, Fields JP, King LE Jr. Cutaneous mastocytosis without clinically obvious skin lesions. J Am Acad Dermatol 1984; 10:903–905.

12. Brownstein MH, Rabinowitz AD. The invisible dermatoses. J Am Acad Dermatol 1983;8:579–588.

13. Campbell EW Jr, Hector D, Gossain V. Heparin activity in systemic mastocytosis. Ann Intern Med 1979;90:940–941.

14. Johnson WC, Helwig EB. Solitary mastocytosis (urticaria pigmentosa). Arch Dermatol 1961;84:806–815.

15. Mihm MC, Clark WH, Reed RJ, et al. Mast cell infiltrates of the skin and the mastocytosis syndrome. Hum Pathol 1973; 4:231–239.

16. Birt AR, Nickerson M. Generalized flushing of the skin with urticaria pigmentosa. Arch Dermatol 1959;80:311–317.

17. Atherton DJ, Wells RS. Diffuse mastocytosis. Br J Dermatol 1981;105:84–85.

18. Golitz LE, Weston WL, Lane AT. Bullous mastocytosis: Diffuse cutaneous mastocytosis with extensive blisters mimicking scalded skin syndrome or erythema multiforme. Pediatr Dermatol 1984;1: 288–294.

19. Sahihi T, Esterly NB. Atypical diffuse cutaneous mastocytosis. Am J Dis Child 1972;124:133–135.

20. Meneghini CL, Angelini G. Systemic mastocytosis with diffuse crocodile-like pachydermic skin, pedunculated pseudofibromas and comedones. Br J Dermatol 1980;102:601–607.

21. Parkes Weber F, Rast H. Telangiectasia macularis eruptiva perstans: A telangiectatic and relatively pigmentless variety of urticaria pigmentosa of adults. Acta Derm Venereol 1935; 16:216–224.

22. Bendel WL, Race GH. Urticaria pigmentosa with bone involvement. J Bone Joint Surg [Am] 1963;45:1043–1056.

23. Lucaya J, Perez-Candela V, Aso C, et al. Mastocytosis with skeletal and gastrointestinal involvement in infancy. Radiology 1979; 131:363–366.

24. Duffy TJ. Clinical problem solving: Getting the story right. N Engl J Med 1993;328:1333–1336.

25. Ackerman AB. Histologic Diagnosis of Inflammatory Skin Diseases: A Method by Pattern Analysis. Philadelphia: Lea & Febiger, 1978.

26. Cavanah DK, Casale DB. Histamine. In: Kaliner MA, Metcalfe DD, eds. The Mast Cell in Health and Disease. New York: Marcel Dekker, 1992:321–342.

27. Schwartz LB, Austen KF. Structure and function of the chemical mediators of mast cells. Prog Allergy 1984;34:271–321.

28. Corey EJ, Clark DA, Goto G, et al. Stereospecific total synthesis of a slow reacting substance of anaphylaxis, leukotriene C-1. J Am Chem Soc 1980;108:1436–1439.

29. Hanna CJ, Bach MK, Pare PD, et al. Slow-reacting substance (leukotrienes) contract human airway and pulmonary vascular smooth muscle in vitro. Nature 1981;290:343–344.

30. Lewis RA, Austen KF, Drazen JM, et al. Slow reacting substances of anaphylaxis: Identification of leukotrienes C-1 and D from human and rat sources. Proc Natl Acad Sci USA 1984;77: 3710–3714.

31. Murphy RC, Hammarström S, Samuelsson B. Leukotriene C: A slow reacting substance from murine mastocytoma cells. Proc Natl Acad Sci USA 1979;76:4275–4279.

32. Pfeffer MA, Pfeffer JM, Lewis RA, et al. Cardiovascular responses to leukotriene C_4 (LTC_4) in the intact rat. Clin Res 1982; 30:484A.

33. Weiss JW, Drazen JM, Coles N, et al. Bronchoconstrictor effects of leukotriene C in human subjects. Science 1982;216:196–197.

34. Weiss JW, Drazen JM, McFadden ER Jr, et al. Comparative bronchoconstrictor effects of histamine and leukotrienes C and D (LTC and LTD) in normal human volunteers. Clin Res 1982;30:571A.

35. Burd PR, Rogers HW, Gordon JR, et al. Interleukin-3–dependent and –independent mast cells stimulated with IgE and antigen expressed multiple cytokines. J Exp Med 1989;170:245–257.

36. Gordon JR, Galli SJ. Mast cells as a source of both preformed and immunologically inducible TNF-α/cachectin. Nature 1990; 346:274–276.

37. Galli SJ. New insights into "the riddle of the mast cells": Microenvironmental regulation of mast cell development and phenotypic heterogeneity. Lab Invest 1990;62:5–33.

38. Gordon JR, Burd PR, Galli SJ. Mast cells as a source of multifunctional cytokines. Immunol Today 1990;11:458–464.

39. Leung DYM, Pober JS, Cotran RS. Expression of endothelial-leukocyte adhesion molecule-1 in elicited late phase allergic reactions. J Clin Invest 1991;87:1805–1809.

40. Plaut M, Pierce JH, Watson CJ, et al. Mast cell lines produce lymphokines in response to cross-linkage of FcεRI or to calcium ionophores. Nature 1989;339:64–67.

41. Walsh LJ, Trinchiere G, Waldorf HA, et al. Human dermal mast cells contain and release tumor necrosis factor, which induces endothelial leukocyte adhesion molecule 1. Proc Natl Acad Sci USA 1991;88:4220–4224.

42. Halonen M, Fisher HK, Blair C, et al. IgE-induced respiratory and circulatory changes during systemic anaphylaxis in the rabbit. Am Rev Respir Dis 1976;114:961–969.

43. Pinckard RN, Halonen M, Palmer JD, et al. Intravascular aggregation and pulmonary sequestration of platelets during IgE-induced systemic anaphylaxis in the rabbit: Abrogation of lethal anaphylactic shock by platelet depletion. J Immunol 1977;119:2185–2193.

44. Galli SJ. New concepts about the mast cell. N Engl J Med 1993;328(4):257–265.

45. Metcalfe DD. Classification and diagnosis of mastocytosis: Current status. J Invest Dermatol 1991;96(Suppl):2S–4S.

46. Tsai M, Shih LS, Newlands GFJ, et al. The rat c-kit ligand, stem cell factor, induces the development of connective tissue-type and mucosal mast cells in vivo: Analysis by anatomical distribution, histochemistry, and protease phenotype. J Exp Med 1991; 174:125–131.

47. Galli SJ, Iemura A, Garlick DS, et al. Reversible expansion of primate mast cell populations in vivo by stem cell factor. J Clin Invest 1993;91:148–152.

48. Longley BJ, Morganroth GS, Tyrrell L, et al. Altered metabolism of mast-cell growth factor (c-kit ligand) in cutaneous mastocytosis. N Engl J Med 1993;328:1302–1307.

49. Halaban R, Tyrrell L, Longley J, et al. Pigmentation and proliferation of human melanocytes and the effects of melanocyte-stimulating hormone and ultraviolet B light. Ann NY Acad Sci 1993;680:290–301.

50. Granerus G, Roupe G, Swanbeck G. Decreased urinary histamine metabolite after successful PUVA treatment of urticaria pigmentosa. J Invest Dermatol 1981;76:1–3.

51. Keyzer JJ, De Monchy JGR, Van Doormaal JJ, et al. Improved diagnosis of mastocytosis by measurement of urinary histamine metabolites. N Engl J Med 1983;309:1603–1605.

52. Engelman K. The carcinoid syndrome. In: Beeson PB, et al., eds. Textbook of Medicine. Philadelphia: WB Saunders Co., 1979:2207–2213.

53. Burton JB, Lavker RM, Schechter NM, et al. Treatment of urticaria pigmentosa with corticosteroids. Arch Dermatol 1985; 121:1516–1523.

54. Muller UR, Horat W, Wuthrich B, et al. Anaphylaxis after Hymenoptera stings in three patients with urticaria pigmentosa. J Allergy Clin Immunol 1983;72:685–689.

55. Turk J, Oates JA, Roberts LJ. Intervention with epinephrine in hypotension associated with mastocytosis. J Allergy Clin Immunol 1983;71:189–192.

56. James PD, Krafchik BR, Johnston AE. Cutaneous mastocytosis in children: Anesthetic conditions. Can J Anaesth 1987;34:522–524.

57. Scott HW Jr, Parriss WC, Sandidge PC, et al. Hazards in operative management of patients with systemic mastocytosis. Ann Surg 1983;197:507–514.

58. Hirschowitz BI, Groarke MB. Effect of cimetidine on gastric hypersecretion and diarrhea in systemic mastocytosis. Ann Intern Med 1979;90:769–771.

59. Gerrard JW. Urticaria pigmentosa: Treatment with cimetidine and chlorpheniramine. J Pediatr 1979;94:843–844.

60. Metcalfe DD. The treatment of mastocytosis: An overview. J Invest Dermatol 1991;96(Suppl):55S–59S.

61. Hurwitz S. Clinical Pediatric Dermatology: A Textbook of Skin Disorders of Childhood and Adolescence, 2nd ed. Philadelphia: WB Saunders Co., 1993.

62. Soter NA, Austen KF, Wasserman SI. Oral disodium cromoglycate in the treatment of systemic mastocytosis. N Engl J Med 1979;301:465–469.

63. Roberts LJ II, Sweetman BJ, Lewis RA, et al. Increased production of prostaglandin D_2 in patients with systemic mastocytosis. N Engl J Med 1980;303:1400–1404.

64. Roberts LJ. Personal communication, March 1993.

65. Christophers E, Honigsmann H, Wolf K, et al. PUVA treatment of urticaria pigmentosa. Br J Dermatol 1978;98:701–702.

66. Granerus G, Olafsson JH, Roupe G. Studies on histamine metabolism in mastocytosis. J Invest Dermatol 1983;80:410–416.

67. Vella Briffa D, Eady RAJ, James MP, et al. Photochemotherapy (PUVA) in the treatment of urticaria pigmentosa. Br J Dermatol 1983;109:67–75.

68. Kluin-Nelemans HC, Jansen JH, Breukelman H, et al. Response to interferon alfa-2b in a patient with systemic mastocytosis. N Engl J Med 1992;326:619–623.

69. Friedman B, Darling G, Norton J, et al. Splenectomy in the management of systemic mast cell disease. Surgery 1990;107:94–100.

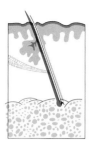

chapter 153

Langerhans Cell Histiocytosis

CHRISTOPHER R. SHEA and N. SCOTT MCNUTT

DEFINITION

Langerhans cells are cutaneous dendritic cells derived from bone marrow precursors; they are the major antigen-presenting cells of the skin and are only weakly phagocytic. These cells are normally present in the epidermis, have a characteristic immunophenotype (CD1a+, S-100+), and contain unique Birbeck granules, demonstrated by electron microscopy. Langerhans cells are related to so-called indeterminate dendritic cells in the dermis, which share the CD1a-positive, S-100–positive phenotype but lack Birbeck granules.

Langerhans cell histiocytosis comprises a broad spectrum of clinical diseases having proliferation of Langerhans cells in common. The most limited form includes skin lesions of congenital self-healing reticulohistiocytosis and solitary, indolent lesions (eosinophilic granulomas) of bone or other organs. Multifocal Langerhans cell histiocytosis lesions of the head classically produce diabetes insipidus, proptosis, and lytic bone lesions (Hand-Schüller-Christian disease) or, more commonly, an incomplete form of this triad. Disseminated, often fatal involvement of viscera and skin (Letterer-Siwe disease) constitutes the acute, fulminant end of the Langerhans cell histiocytosis spectrum. Because of this clinical heterogeneity, only gradually did a unified pathologic concept of Langerhans cell histiocytosis evolve.[1, 2] The term Langerhans cell histiocytosis is now preferred to histiocytosis X.[3]

CLINICAL DESCRIPTION

Langerhans cell histiocytosis can occur at any age but onset is most common between 1 and 15 years of age. In general the Letterer-Siwe form occurs in infants, Hand-Schüller-Christian disease in older children, and solitary eosinophilic granuloma in young adults; exceptionally, Letterer-Siwe disease may occur as late as the eighth decade of life.[4, 5] Langerhans cell histiocytosis is reported more often in whites than blacks. Males and females are equally affected, but the pattern of organ involvement may vary between the sexes; for instance, pulmonary involvement is much more common in males.[6]

Skin lesions[7] may be the sole manifestation of Langerhans cell histiocytosis; they occur in almost all patients with Letterer-Siwe disease and up to half of patients with Hand-Schüller-Christian disease. Lesions include erythematous, brown, or yellow papules, plaques, nodules, vesicles, pustules, ulcers, and purpura. The typical distribution is in flexural and seborrheic regions such as the scalp, hairline, retroauricular areas, axillae, groin, and perineum (Figs. 153–1 and 153–2). Skin lesions are often hemorrhagic in patients with Letterer-Siwe disease.

Congenital self-healing reticulohistiocytosis[8] is a limited form of Langerhans cell histiocytosis not yet described when the unified concept of the histiocytosis X spectrum was first proposed.[1] It is present at birth or shortly thereafter and involutes spontaneously within the first year of life. Affected infants have multiple or, rarely, solitary red-brown or purple-blue nodules on the torso and extremities. The nodules ulcerate and heal with hyperpigmentation and atrophic scarring. Systemic involvement is absent, except for occasional hepatomegaly or hematologic abnormalities.

Eosinophilic granulomas are the most common manifestation of Langerhans cell histiocytosis.[9] They may occur in any organ, including skin and lung, but have a predilection for flat bones, particularly of the calvaria; rib, mandible, femur, ilium, and scapula are also commonly involved, but small bones such as phalanges are generally spared. Lesions are asymptomatic or painful; infiltration of vertebral bodies can lead to collapse and

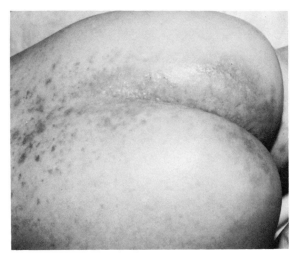

FIGURE 153–1. Langerhans cell histiocytosis in a 6-month-old girl with purpuric papules and superficial erosions mimicking a persistent candidal diaper dermatitis. Similar lesions were present on the scalp and postauricular areas. (Courtesy of Sharon Raimer, M.D.)

spinal cord compression. Radiographs show well-demarcated radiolucencies.

Neurologic signs and symptoms in Langerhans cell histiocytosis result from widespread dissemination or direct extension of calvarial lesions and include headache, vertigo, ataxia, seizures, and sometimes cognitive defects. Involvement of the hypothalamus and pituitary in children may cause diabetes insipidus[10] or growth hormone deficiency. Otolaryngologic and oral manifestations of Langerhans cell histiocytosis are common and can be the presenting complaint. They include external otitis, chronic otitis media, aural discharge, retroauricular swelling, conductive hearing loss, gingival bleeding, loosening of teeth, and buccal ulceration.[11, 12]

Pulmonary lesions[6] may be isolated in adults but in children are usually associated with disseminated disease. Signs and symptoms include failure to thrive, chest pain, dyspnea, and hemoptysis. Pneumothorax may follow

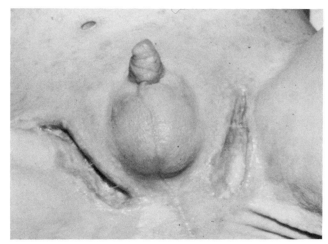

FIGURE 153–2. Ulcerated infiltrated plaques in a 2-year-old with Langerhans cell histiocytosis with multiorgan involvement. (Courtesy of Sharon Raimer, M.D.)

rupture of subpleural cysts. Oxygen diffusion and lung compliance are reduced.

Hepatic involvement is common in disseminated Langerhans cell histiocytosis, presenting as hepatomegaly with elevation of liver enzymes and conjugated bilirubin. Prolonged cholestasis secondary to sclerosing cholangitis is associated with progression to chronic hepatic failure, portal hypertension, and bleeding esophageal varices. Diarrhea in Langerhans cell histiocytosis may be secondary to abnormal bile salt metabolism or to intestinal infiltration.

Hematologic manifestations are associated with disseminated disease and include pancytopenia and bleeding diathesis due to hypersplenism or bone marrow infiltration; hemolytic anemia and peripheral eosinophilia may also occur. Severe hematopoietic involvement predisposes to fatal sepsis.

Functional abnormalities due to involvement of several organs are associated with a worse prognosis.[13, 14] In addition to a complete history and physical examination, recommended laboratory evaluation[15] includes assessment of the complete and differential blood cell count, reticulocyte count, erythrocyte sedimentation rate, direct and indirect Coombs' test, liver function tests, serum amylase level, prothrombin and partial thromboplastin times, serum protein electrophoresis, urinalysis, urinary specific gravity after water deprivation, chest films, and skeletal survey. Additional studies, such as pulmonary function testing, arterial blood gases, and bone marrow biopsy, should be based on clinical suspicion or abnormal findings from screening tests. Tests of immunologic function are indicated in disseminated cases.

PATHOLOGY

Pathologic findings are similar in all organs; this discussion emphasizes cutaneous pathology. On routine histopathology the dermis has a diffuse, nodular, or occasionally perivascular infiltrate of mononuclear Langerhans cells, each 15 to 25 μm in diameter, having a moderate amount of homogeneous, eosinophilic or pale cytoplasm, a lobular nucleus with a central, longitudinal groove ("coffee bean" appearance) or hilar indentation ("kidney" appearance), and a small nucleolus (Fig. 153–3; see color plate). There is not significant nuclear cytologic atypia.[16] Epidermotropism of the Langerhans cells is common, and ulceration may occur. The infiltrate may be composed almost entirely of Langerhans cells, particularly in cases of Letterer-Siwe disease, or may be admixed with eosinophils, lymphocytes, and phagocytic macrophages. Hemorrhage is common in Letterer-Siwe lesions. Chronic lesions of Langerhans cell histiocytosis may be xanthomatous, with vacuolated cells and Touton giant cells; late lesions are fibrotic and contain relatively few Langerhans cells. In congenital self-healing reticulohistiocytosis the infiltrate contains many giant cells with ground-glass cytoplasm and periodic acid–Schiff-positive, diastase-resistant cytoplasmic inclusions.[8]

Immunohistochemistry helps to identify the pathognomonic Langerhans cells in the infiltrate[17] and has virtually replaced enzyme histochemistry. In formalin-

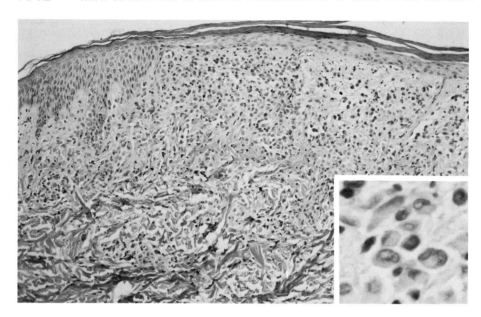

FIGURE 153-3. Biopsy specimen has a nodular infiltrate of Langerhans cells in the dermis, with focal hemorrhage, epidermal atrophy, and parakeratosis (hematoxylin-eosin, × 200). *Inset*, Demonstrates lobular nuclei and eosinophilic cytoplasm of the dermal Langerhans cells infiltrate (× 1300). (See color plate.)

fixed, paraffin-embedded tissue the most useful positive marker is S-100 protein, which Langerhans cells strongly express in the cytoplasm and, frequently, the nucleus. Peanut agglutinin reacts in a characteristic halo pattern around the plasma membrane, with a perinuclear dot, unlike the diffuse, cytoplasmic reactivity of non–Langerhans cell histiocytes. The cells of Langerhans cell histiocytosis also express HLA-DR (detected with LN3).[18] Non–Langerhans cell macrophage markers such as MAC387, lysozyme, and α_1-antitrypsin are usually negative. CD1a (using OKT6) and CD4 (using OKT4 or Leu-3) are detected on unfixed, frozen specimens. CD1a immunoreactivity may not be completely diagnostic of Langerhans cell histiocytosis, however, having also been reported in unusual cases of juvenile xanthogranuloma[19] and indeterminate cell histiocytoma.[20, 21] Cells of Lan-

gerhans cell histiocytosis express interferon gamma[22] and heterogeneous surface markers resembling various states of Langerhans cell activation and differentiation.[23]

Electron microscopy is still the diagnostic standard. The cytognomonic Birbeck granules of Langerhans cells are intracytoplasmic and measure 33 nm in width and 190 to 360 nm in length. In two dimensions they appear rod shaped, with a central, crystalline striation and a terminal, vesicular dilatation giving a "tennis racquet" appearance; three-dimensional reconstructions show that Birbeck granules are disc or cup shaped in most cases.[24] Cells of Langerhans cell histiocytosis may have more Birbeck granules than do normal, epidermal Langerhans cells. Birbeck granules are formed by invagination of the plasma membrane and have fuzzy surfaces similar to those lining clathrin-coated pits (Fig. 153–4). Besides

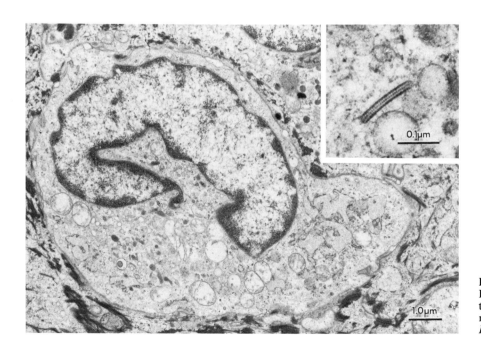

FIGURE 153-4. Electron microscopy of a Langerhans cell in Langerhans cell histiocytosis demonstrates indented nucleus and numerous intracytoplasmic Birbeck granules. *Inset* shows a typical Birbeck granule.

Birbeck granules, other ultrastructural features of Langerhans cells are characteristic but not diagnostic, including trilaminar membranous loops and laminated substructures of lysosomes.

PATHOGENESIS AND ETIOLOGY

A genetic basis for Langerhans cell histiocytosis has not been established. Family history is usually negative, but there have been several occurrences in monozygotic twins.[25] The incidence of associated congenital anomalies may be increased.[26]

A fundamental question is whether Langerhans cell histiocytosis is neoplastic or reactive. Clinical thinking on this matter has been influenced by the attempts to stage Langerhans cell histiocytosis by organ involvement, analogously to lymphoma, and by the use of treatment modalities (radiation and cytotoxic chemotherapy) generally reserved for malignant neoplasms. Indeed, some cases of Langerhans cell histiocytosis are considered malignant, on the basis of cytologic atypia, aggressive clinical course, and infiltration of unusual organs.[27] Despite one early report of aneuploidy, however, two series comprising 42 patients showed euploidy in all cases.[28, 29] The Langerhans cells constituting the infiltrate are usually monomorphous and cytologically banal. Furthermore, Langerhans cell histiocytosis often remains indolent and may even involve spontaneously,[30, 31] suggesting that autonomous cellular division, the sine qua non of neoplasia, is not a constant feature of Langerhans cell histiocytosis. On the other hand, recent studies demonstrating clonality of the infiltrate provide strong evidence for the neoplastic, if not necessarily malignant, nature of Langerhans cell histiocytosis.[32, 33]

Immunologic derangements may be important in pathogenesis. Abnormalities of suppressor T-cell number and function have been documented.[34] Abnormal regulation and expression of cytokines, including macrophage colony-stimulating factor and platelet-derived growth factor, may contribute to Langerhans cell proliferation.[35] Pulmonary lesions of Langerhans cell histiocytosis are much more common in cigarette smokers, suggesting a possible role for chronic irritation or antigenic stimulation.[6] Human herpesvirus-6 DNA has been detected in some lesions of Langerhans cell histiocytosis.[36]

DIFFERENTIAL DIAGNOSIS

The clinical differential diagnosis (Table 153–1) of cutaneous lesions of Langerhans cell histiocytosis is broad. The scaly plaques resemble seborrheic dermatitis; ulcerative, nodular, or mucosal lesions, however, should alert the clinician. In boys, Wiskott-Aldrich syndrome, like Letterer-Siwe disease, presents as hemorrhagic, persistent, eczematoid lesions that respond poorly to conservative topical care. The possibility of acrodermatitis enteropathica may be entertained when Langerhans cell histiocytosis presents as crusted, perineal papules and pustules in a child with diarrhea and failure to thrive;

TABLE 153–1. Differential Diagnosis of Langerhans Cell Histiocytosis
Clinical
Seborrheic dermatitis
Wiscott-Aldrich syndrome
Acrodermatitis enteropathica
Intertrigo
Candidiasis
Mastocytosis
Lymphoma
Xanthoma disseminatum
Infectious ulcer
Extramammary Paget's disease
Pathologic
CD30-positive T-cell lymphoma
Allergic contact dermatitis
Dermal hypersensitivity reaction
Sinus histiocytosis with massive lymphadenopathy
Malignant melanoma
Hairy cell leukemia

however, acral distribution is not typical of Letterer-Siwe disease. Simple intertrigo and candidiasis are also diagnostic considerations. Red-brown papules and nodules of Langerhans cell histiocytosis may resemble mastocytomas; the absence of urtication on stroking (Darier's sign) is helpful. Infiltrated plaques of Langerhans cell histiocytosis may mimic cutaneous lymphoma. Other histiocytic syndromes, such as xanthoma disseminatum, may closely resemble Langerhans cell histiocytosis clinically and histologically, and differentiation may require immunohistochemistry.[18] Isolated eosinophilic granulomas of the skin, particularly those on the perineum or vulva, may suggest infectious ulcers or extramammary Paget's disease.

The histopathologic differential diagnosis (see Table 153–1) includes CD30-positive T-cell lymphoma with a population of reactive Langerhans cells. Resolving lesions of allergic contact dermatitis or dermal hypersensitivity reactions may contain prominent infiltrates of Langerhans cells with accompanying eosinophils, resembling Langerhans cell histiocytosis. Sinus histiocytosis with massive lymphadenopathy (Rosai-Dorfman disease) may occur as dermal infiltrates of S-100–positive histiocytes; the presence of plasma cells and lymphophagocytosis in sinus histiocytosis with massive lymphadenopathy and the absence of eosinophils help to distinguish it from Langerhans cell histiocytosis.[37] Malignant melanoma, like Langerhans cell histiocytosis, presents as infiltrates of S-100–positive cells with pagetoid epidermal spread; banal cytology and absence of melanin pigment favor Langerhans cell histiocytosis. Hairy cell leukemia cutis causes dermal infiltrates of S-100–positive mononuclear cells, but they are usually smaller and have less cytoplasm than cells of Langerhans cell histiocytosis and are separated from one another by a pericellular space. In summary, the other disorders in the pathologic differential diagnosis can often be separated from Lan-

TABLE 153-2. Treatment of Langerhans Cell Histiocytosis

Excision
Intralesional corticosteroid injection
Local radiation therapy
Hormone replacement
Psoralen photochemotherapy
Topical nitrogen mustard
Systemic chemotherapy
Immunotherapy

gerhans cell histiocytosis on the basis of the relative monomorphism of the Langerhans cell histiocytosis infiltrates, their epidermotropism, their lack of phagocytosis, and their immunophenotype in frozen (CD1a-positive) and paraffin (S-100–positive) sections. Electron microscopy to demonstrate Birbeck granules may be necessary in some cases.

TREATMENT

Therapeutic decisions (Table 153–2) depend on symptoms and extent of disease. For limited disease, such as solitary eosinophilic granuloma, simple excision may be curative. Spontaneous regression is also possible. Intralesional corticosteroid injection (50 to 150 mg methylprednisolone for bone lesions) or local radiation therapy (6 to 10 Gy) is often effective for local disease. Antidiuretic hormone and growth hormone are given for the respective endocrine deficiency syndromes.

Patients with extensive cutaneous disease may respond to psoralen photochemotherapy[4] (two to four times per week for several months) or topical nitrogen mustard[5] (10 mg in 50 ml normal saline applied daily). Patients with disseminated disease may require prednisone, alone or in combination with cytotoxic agents such as vinblastine, methotrexate, and 6-mercaptopurine[38]; at present, etoposide (150 mg per day for 3 days intravenously, repeated in three to six cycles) seems to be the most active chemotherapeutic agent.[39] Immunotherapy with thymic extracts, thymopentin, and suppressin (a thymus-derived peptide that stimulates CD8-positive lymphocytes) has been tried and largely abandoned. Interferon has given mixed results. Cyclosporine and biologic response modifiers have not been adequately studied.

References

1. Lichtenstein L. Histiocytosis X: Integration of eosinophilic granuloma of bone, "Letterer-Siwe disease," and "Schüller-Christian disease" as related manifestations of a single nosologic entity. Arch Pathol 1953;56:84–102.
2. Komp DM. Historical perspectives of Langerhans cell histiocytosis. Hematol Oncol Clin North Am 1987;1:9–21.
3. Broadbent V, Gadner H, Komp DM, et al (Clinical writing group of the Histiocyte Society). Histiocytosis syndromes in children: II. Approach to the clinical and laboratory evaluation of children with Langerhans cell histiocytosis. Med Pediatr Oncol 1989;17:492–495.
4. Neumann C, Kolde G, Bonsmann G. Histiocytosis X in an elderly patient: Ultrastructure and immunocytochemistry after PUVA photochemotherapy. Br J Dermatol 1988;119:385–391.
5. Novice FM, Collison DW, Kleinsmith DM, et al. Letterer-Siwe disease in adults. Cancer 1989;63:166–174.
6. Soler P, Kambouchner M, Valeyre D, et al. Pulmonary Langerhans cell granulomatosis (histiocytosis X). Annu Rev Med 1992;43:105–115.
7. Winkelmann RK. The skin in histiocytosis X. Mayo Clin Proc 1969;44:535–549.
8. Hashimoto K, Bale GF, Hawkins MS, et al. Congenital self-healing reticulohistiocytosis (Hashimoto-Pritzker type). Int J Dermatol 1986;25:516–523.
9. Bollini G, Jouve JL, Gentet JC, et al. Bone lesions in histiocytosis X. J Pediatr Orthop 1991;11:469–477.
10. Dunger DB, Broadbent V, Yeoman E, et al. The frequency and natural history of diabetes insipidus in children with Langerhans cell histiocytosis. N Engl J Med 1989;321:1157–1162.
11. Cunningham MJ, Curtin HD, Jaffe R, et al. Otologic manifestations of Langerhans cell histiocytosis. Arch Otolaryngol Head Neck Surg 1989;115:807–813.
12. DiNardo LJ, Wetmore RF. Head and neck manifestations of histiocytosis-X in children. Laryngoscope 1989;99:721–724.
13. Rivera-Luna R, Martinez-Guerra G, Altamirano-Alvarez E, et al. Langerhans cell histiocytosis: Clinical experience with 124 patients. Pediatr Dermatol 1988;5:145–150.
14. Raney RB Jr, D'Angio GJ. Langerhans cell histiocytosis (histiocytosis X): Experience at the Children's Hospital of Philadelphia, 1970–1984. Med Pediatr Oncol 1989;17:20–28.
15. Lavin PT, Osband ME. Evaluating the role of therapy in histiocytosis-X. Hematol Oncol Clin North Am 1987;1:35–47.
16. Risdall RJ, Dehner LP, Duray P, et al. Histiocytosis X (Langerhans cell histiocytosis): Prognostic role of histopathology. Arch Pathol Lab Med 1983;107:59–63.
17. Fartasch M, Vigneswaran N, Diepgen TL, et al. Immunohistochemical and ultrastructural study of histiocytosis X and non-X histiocytoses. J Am Acad Dermatol 1990;23:885–892.
18. Zelger B, Cerio R, Orchard G, et al. Histologic and immunohistochemical study comparing xanthoma disseminatum and histiocytosis X. Arch Dermatol 1992;128:1207–1212.
19. Andersen WK, Knowles DM, Silvers DN. CD1 (OKT6)-positive juvenile xanthogranuloma; OKT6 is not specific for Langerhans cell histiocytosis (histiocytosis X). J Am Acad Dermatol 1992;26:850–854.
20. Levisohn D, Seidel D, Phelps A, et al. Solitary congenital indeterminate cell histiocytoma. Arch Dermatol 1993;129:81–85.
21. Wood GS, Haber RS. Novel histiocytoses considered in the context of histiocyte subset differentiation. Arch Dermatol 1993;129:210–214.
22. Neumann C, Schaumburg-Lever G, Döpfer R, et al. Interferon gamma is a marker for histiocytosis X cells in the skin. J Invest Dermatol 1988;91:280–282.
23. Groh V, Gadner H, Radaszkiewicz T, et al. The phenotypic spectrum of histiocytosis X cells. J Invest Dermatol 1988;90:441–447.
24. Sagebiel RW, Reed TH. Serial reconstruction of the characteristic granule of the Langerhans cell. J Cell Biol 1968;36:595–602.
25. Katz AM, Rosenthal D, Jakubovic HR, et al. Langerhans cell histiocytosis in monozygotic twins. J Am Acad Dermatol 1991;24:32–37.
26. Sheils C, Dover GJ. Frequency of congenital anomalies in patients with histiocytosis X. Am J Hematol 1989;31:91–95.
27. Ben-Ezra J, Bailey A, Azumi N, et al. Malignant histiocytosis X: A distinct clinicopathologic entity. Cancer 1991;68:1050–1060.
28. Rabkin MS, Wittwer CT, Kjeldsberg CR, et al. Flow-cytometric DNA content of histiocytosis X (Langerhans cell histiocytosis). Am J Pathol 1988;131:283–289.
29. McLelland J, Newton J, Camplejohn RS, et al. A flow cytometric study of Langerhans cell histiocytosis. Br J Dermatol 1989;120:485–491.
30. Corbeel L, Eggermont E, Desmyter J, et al. Spontaneous healing of Langerhans cell histiocytosis (histiocytosis X). Eur J Pediatr 1988;148:32–33.
31. Iwafuchi M, Watanabe H, Shiratsuka M. Primary benign histiocytosis X of the stomach: A report of a case showing spontaneous remission after 5½ years. Am J Surg Pathol 1991;15:489–496.

32. Yu RC, Chu C, Buluwela L, et al. Clonal proliferation of Langerhans cells in Langerhans cell histiocytosis. Lancet 1994; 343:767–768.
33. William CL, Busque L, Griffith BB, et al. Langerhans'-cell histiocytosis (histiocytosis X)—a clonal proliferative disease. N Engl J Med 1994;331:154–160.
34. Leitkin SL. Immunobiology of histiocytosis X. Hematol Oncol Clin North Amer 1987;1:49–61.
35. Barth J, Kreipe H, Radzun HJ, et al. Increased expression of growth factor genes for macrophages and fibroblasts in bronchoalveolar lavage cells of a patient with pulmonary histiocytosis X. Thorax 1991;46:835–838.
36. Leahy MA, Krecji M, Friednash M, et al. Human herpesvirus-6 is present in lesions of Langerhans cell histiocytosis. J Invest Dermatol 1993;100:642–645.
37. Thawerani H, Sanchez RL, Rosai J, et al. The cutaneous manifestations of sinus histiocytosis with massive lymphadenopathy. Arch Dermatol 1978;114:191–197.
38. McLelland J, Pritchard J, Chu AC. Current controversies. Hematol Oncol Clin North Am 1987;1:147–159.
39. Viana MB, Oliveira BM, Silva CM, et al. Etoposide in the treatment of six children with Langerhans cell histiocytosis (histiocytosis X). Med Pediatr Oncol 1991;19:289–294.

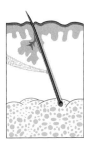

chapter 154

Multicentric Reticulohistiocytosis and Sinus Histiocytosis

PAUL CHU

Multicentric Reticulohistiocytosis

DEFINITION

Multicentric reticulohistiocytosis is a rare, systemic, histiocytic disorder that involves primarily the skin, mucosa, and joints. Skin lesions may precede, accompany, or follow development of polyarthritis, and nearly half of the patients develop lifelong disabling arthritis. Solitary papules with identical histopathologic features have been termed *reticulohistiocytic granuloma*.

CLINICAL DESCRIPTION

The age at onset of multicentric reticulohistiocytosis is most frequently in the fourth decade, but the disorder can occur at any age. Females are more likely to develop multicentric reticulohistiocytosis than males by a ratio of 3:1, and whites are affected more often.[1] Cutaneous eruptions of papules and nodules have a cephalocaudal distribution, with the face, scalp, neck, hands, and forearms most often involved. Approximately 50% of the cases of lesions occurring on the hands will have papules resembling beads arranged around the nail fold. Oral involvement occurs in half of the cases, with lips, buccal mucosa, tongue, and nasal septum being the most common sites.[1] Perianal and genital lesions have not been described. Lesions are pruritic in one third of the cases. Repeated regression and reappearance of cutaneous lesions has been noted. Patients often present with pain and swelling of the joints, and typically the arthritis and joint damage is very rapid. Destruction of the distal and proximal interphalangeal joints often results in an opera-glass-shaped deformity of the hands. Other joints such as shoulders, knees, wrists, hips, feet, ankles, elbows, and spine can also be involved.[2] Arthritic symptoms, like the skin eruption, will wax and wane; and as a general rule, multicentric reticulohistiocytosis will spontaneously disappear in about 8 years.

PATHOLOGY

Microscopically, sections stained with hematoxylin-eosin reveal a circumscribed, but unencapsulated proliferation of histiocytes, which may involve the entire thickness of the dermis. The epidermis is spared. The majority of the infiltrate is composed of multinucleated giant cells with abundant eosinophilic, finely granular, ground-glass cytoplasm (Fig. 154–1) that is periodic acid–Schiff positive and diastase resistant. Vesicular nuclei with distinct nuclear membranes and prominent nucleoli can appear haphazardly arranged within the cytoplasm, or they may be aligned along the periphery or cluster in the center of the cell. Thin, compressed collagen bundles as well as occasional mononuclear histiocytes, lymphocytes, and fibroblasts lie between the giant cells. Numerous electron-dense cytoplasmic granules, ranging from 50 to 250 nm in diameter, with a surrounding halo located adjacent to Golgi areas can be seen with electron microscopy.[3] These granules have many similarities to lysosomes. Identical pathologic features are evident in solitary reticulohistiocytic granuloma.

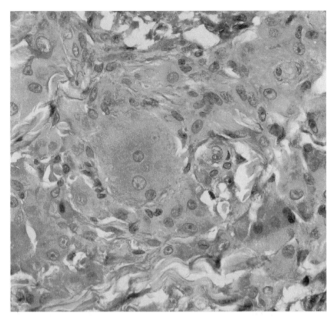

FIGURE 154-1. Multicentric reticulohistiocytosis. Numerous histiocytes and multinucleated forms are present in a background of finely granular, ground-glass cytoplasm.

PATHOGENESIS AND ETIOLOGY

The etiology of multicentric reticulohistiocytosis remains unknown. It was originally thought to be a storage disease because several patients had concomitant hypercholesterolemia and xanthelasma; but as more cases were reported, this finding can be regarded as an incidental occurrence.[1] Approximately one fourth of patients with multicentric reticulohistiocytosis have been found to have cancer of the colon, stomach, or ovary;[4] however, the occurrence of the disorder can predate detection of the neoplasm by a considerable period and thus a paraneoplastic disease etiology remains speculative at this time. Nevertheless, a search for an underlying neoplasm seems plausible.

DIAGNOSIS AND DIFFERENTIAL DIAGNOSIS

The diagnosis of multicentric reticulohistiocytosis is straightforward given the clinical and histologic findings, although other entities should be considered in the differential diagnosis (Table 154-1). Rheumatoid arthritis

 TABLE 154-1. Differential Diagnosis of Multicentric Reticulohistiocytosis

Rheumatoid arthritis
Xanthogranuloma
Reticulohistiocytoma
Benign cephalic histiocytosis
Congenital self-healing reticulohistiocytosis
Xanthoma disseminatum
Lepromatous leprosy

can show similar clinical findings, but cutaneous lesions will show palisaded granulomatous dermatitis. Solitary reticulohistiocytoma can have an identical histologic picture, but patients with this disorder do not have arthritis. Xanthogranulomas display macrophages with foamy cytoplasm, and even in the form of juvenile xanthogranulomas with disseminated small papules, arthritis is rare. Benign cephalic histiocytosis can easily be distinguished from multicentric reticulohistiocytosis on clinical and histologic grounds.

TREATMENT

In general, therapy for multicentric reticulohistiocytosis has been unrewarding. Anti-inflammatory agents such as aspirin, indomethacin, and corticosteroids may provide some relief to arthritic symptoms, but they do not alter the course of the disease. Chemotherapeutic agents such as azathioprine,[5] cyclophosphamide,[6] topical nitrogen mustard,[7] chlorambucil,[8] and methotrexate[9] have all been tried with some success.

Sinus Histiocytosis

DEFINITION

Sinus histiocytosis with massive lymphadenopathy, or Rosai-Dorfman disease, was first comprehensively described by Rosai and Dorfman in 1969.[10] The original patients presented with striking lymphadenopathy, which often affected cervical lymph nodes; and biopsy specimens revealed pale-staining mononuclear cells that distended the sinusoids.

CLINICAL DESCRIPTION

Since 1969, there have been over 400 documented cases of Rosai-Dorfman disease listed in the Sinus Histiocytosis Registry.[11] The clinical course is usually benign, characterized by recurrent episodes of exacerbations and remissions; however, fatalities have been reported.[11] The mean patient age is about 20 years, but neonates and the elderly can also be affected. Blacks are more frequently afflicted than whites, and 60% of the cases involve males. More than 40% of patients have extranodal disease, with respiratory tract, eyes, soft tissue, bones, and genitourinary tract being the most common sites. Skin lesions comprise 27% of extranodal disease and occur in 11% of all patients with Rosai-Dorfman disease.[12] Cutaneous lesions consist of solitary or multiple papules or nodules with a xanthomatous or erythematous hue (Fig. 154-2), ranging in size up to 4 cm. There is no predilection for a particular site. In rare cases, only cutaneous lesions have been found.[13]

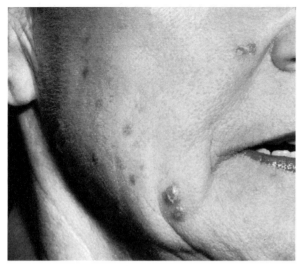

FIGURE 154-2. Several orange-red papules on the face of a 58-year-old woman with cutaneous Rosai-Dorfman disease.

PATHOLOGY

Cutaneous lesions, as well as lesions involving lymph nodes and other systemic organs, have similar histologic features.[13] The salient feature of cutaneous lesions is a dense, nodular infiltrate of histiocytes with abundant cytoplasm and medium to large, round, vesicular nuclei with small nucleoli. Lymphocytes, plasma cells, and neutrophils are present within the cytoplasm of the histiocytes and are surrounded by small "halos," signifying engulfment without digestion, a feature known as emperipolesis (Fig. 154-3). Thick-walled venules surrounded by cuffs of plasma cells at the periphery of the lesions, lymphoid aggregates and germinal centers, and histiocytes within lymphatic spaces can also be seen. Immunoperoxidase staining for S-100 protein marks the cytoplasm of the histiocytes and accentuates the emperipolesis.

PATHOGENESIS AND ETIOLOGY

The origin of the histiocytes in Rosai-Dorfman disease remains unknown. They share some immunophenotypic features with Langerhans cells and interdigitating reticulum cells in that they demonstrate strong positivity for S-100 protein; however, the cells of Rosai-Dorfman disease are negative for OKT6 (CD1) and OKM5. Additionally, these histiocytes label with antimacrophage antibodies such as CD11c, CD14, CD33, CD68, LN5, MAC387, and lysozyme.[14]

The etiology of Rosai-Dorfman disease is unknown, but it has been considered a disease characterized by abnormal immunologic response. Epstein-Barr virus has been implicated, but not all patients have positive titers to this virus.[12] Recently, human herpesvirus 6 genome was isolated in tissue from seven of nine patients with Rosai-Dorfman disease by in situ hybridization[15]; however, whether this represents a true infectious etiology or a secondary infection remains unclear.

DIAGNOSIS AND DIFFERENTIAL DIAGNOSIS

Cutaneous lesions of Rosai-Dorfman disease have similar histology to lesions seen in lymph nodes and can be recognized by those familiar with the diagnostic criteria. Emperipolesis and strong cytoplasmic staining of histiocytes with S-100 protein are hallmarks of this disease and can be used to differentiate it from histiocytosis X, xanthogranuloma, congenital self-healing reticulohistiocytosis, reticulohistiocytic granuloma, xanthoma disseminatum, and necrobiotic xanthogranuloma (Table 154-2).[13]

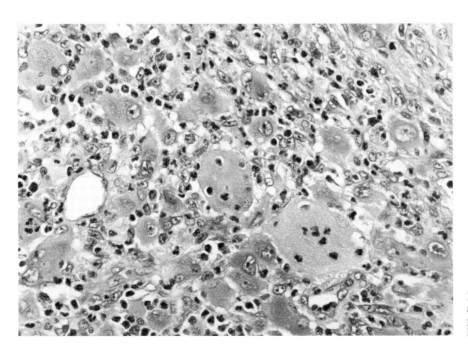

FIGURE 154-3. Sinus histiocytosis. Neutrophils and lymphocytes with surrounding halos (emperipolesis) are present within the cytoplasm of histiocytes.

TABLE 154-2. Differential Diagnosis of Rosai-Dorfman Disease

Histiocytosis X
Congenital self-healing reticulohistiocytosis
Necrobiotic xanthogranuloma
Xanthogranuloma
Xanthoma disseminatum
Eruptive xanthoma
Reticulohistiocytoma

TREATMENT

Treatment does not appear to be necessary for the majority of patients with this disease. Therapy other than surgery for Rosai-Dorfman disease has had dismal success. Patients with systemic disease with compromised visceral functions have received single or combination chemotherapeutic agents with variable responses.[16]

References

1. Barrow MV, Holubar K. Multicentric reticulohistiocytosis: A review of 33 patients. Medicine 1969;48:287–305.
2. Lesher JL Jr, Allen BS. Multicentric reticulohistiocytosis. J Am Acad Dermatol 1984;11:713–723.
3. Tani M, Keiichiro H, Takafumi N, et al. Multicentric reticulohistiocytosis: Electron microscopy and ultracytochemical studies. Arch Dermatol 1981;117:495–499.
4. Catterall MD, White JE. Multicentric reticulohistiocytosis and malignant disease. Br J Dermatol 1978;98:221–224.
5. Ehrlich GE, Young I, Nosheny SZ. Multicentric reticulohistiocytosis (lipoid dermatoarthritis): A multisystem disorder. Am J Med 1972;52:830–840.
6. Hanauer LB. Reticulohistiocytosis: Remission after cyclophosphamide therapy. Arthritis Rheum 1972;15:636–640.
7. Brandt F, Lipman M, Taylor JR. Topical nitrogen mustard therapy in multicentric reticulohistiocytosis. J Am Acad Dermatol 1982;6:260–262.
8. Ginsburg WW, O'Duffy JD, Morris JL. Multicentric reticulohistiocytosis: Response to alkylating agents in six patients. Ann Intern Med 1989;111:384–388.
9. Gourmelen O, LeLoët X, Fortier-Beaulieu M, et al. Methotrexate treatment of multicentric reticulohistiocytosis. J Rheumatol 1991;18:627–628.
10. Rosai J, Dorfman RF. Sinus histiocytosis with massive lymphadenopathy. Arch Pathol 1969;87:63–70.
11. Foucar E, Rosai J, Dorfman RF. Sinus histiocytosis with massive lymphadenopathy: An analysis of 14 deaths occurring in a patient registry. Cancer 1984;54:1834–1840.
12. Foucar E, Rosai J, Dorfman RF. Sinus histiocytosis with massive lymphadenopathy (Rosai-Dorfman disease): Review of the entity. Semin Diagn Pathol 1990;7:19–73.
13. Chu P, LeBoit PE. Histologic features of cutaneous sinus histiocytosis (Rosai-Dorfman disease): Study of cases both with and without systemic involvement. J Cutan Pathol 1992;19:201–206.
14. Paulli M, Rosso R, Kindl S. Immunophenotypic characterization of the cell infiltrate in five cases of sinus histiocytosis with massive lymphadenopathy (Rosai-Dorfman disease). Hum Pathol 1992; 23:647–654.
15. Levine PH, Jahan N, Murari P. Detection of human herpesvirus 6 in tissues involved by sinus histiocytosis with massive lymphadenopathy (Rosai-Dorfman disease). J Infect Dis 1992;166:291–295.
16. Komp DM. The treatment of sinus histiocytosis with massive lymphadenopathy (Rosai-Dorfman disease). Semin Diagn Pathol 1990;7:83–86.

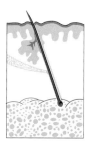

chapter 155

Other Histiocytoses of Childhood

SHARON S. RAIMER and RAMON L. SANCHEZ

The histiocytoses of childhood are a group of diseases with localized or generalized proliferations of cells of the monocyte-macrophage and/or dendritic cell systems.[1] The cells of both systems are derived from monocytes, which in turn originate from a bone marrow stem cell. Apart from the rare true malignant histiocytosis, the histiocytoses of childhood do not fulfill the criteria for malignancy but rather appear to result from abnormal or altered regulation of histiocyte activity.

Understanding of the histiocytoses has been hampered by the lack of a universally accepted classification of these diseases and the widespread use of eponyms to describe them. In 1987, the Histiocyte Society published their classification of histiocytoses based on immunophenotype and ultrastructural findings.[2] This classification is widely accepted, and a modification of it is used in this chapter (Table 155–1). Langerhans cell histiocytosis is discussed in Chapter 153. Only those other entities that are seen principally in children are discussed in detail here.

toplasm, vesicular nuclei that are frequently grooved, and small nucleoli.[6] Mitotic figures, if present, are few; and lymphocytes, giant cells, and foam cells are occasionally present. The cells are S-100 positive and CD1 positive, but no Birbeck granules are demonstrable on ultrastructural examination.[5] Because Birbeck granules may be present in as few as 5% of cells in Langerhans cell histiocytosis,[7] many cells must be examined before Langerhans cell histiocytosis can be excluded. Conversely, some cases previously diagnosed without ultrastructural examination of the histiocytic cells (as self-healing Langerhans cell histiocytosis) may represent this entity. It is unclear at present, but the indeterminant cell may actually represent a stage in the life cycle of the Langerhans cell.[5] It has been postulated to be a precursor or, conversely, because cultured Langerhans cells lose their Birbeck granules to be more "mature" than Langerhans cells. Indeterminant cells may reside in the dermis and help to repopulate epidermal Langerhans cells.

Indeterminant Cell Histiocytoma

Indeterminant cell histiocytomas are rare and have been reported most commonly in adults; however, two adolescents[3, 4] and one neonate have been described with this entity.[5] Clinically the disease may present as a solitary nodule, which was eroded in the neonate reported,[5] or more commonly as widespread papules or papulonodules.[6] In most patients the lesions have exhibited complete or partial spontaneous regression.

Histologically, the dermis is infiltrated diffusely with cytologically bland histiocytes with pale eosinophilic cy-

Juvenile Xanthogranuloma

Juvenile xanthogranuloma is a benign histiocytic tumor that occurs most commonly in infancy and early childhood and tends to be self-healing. Identical lesions can occur in adults. The pathogenesis of this tumor is unclear.

CLINICAL DESCRIPTION

The lesions of juvenile xanthogranuloma generally erupt as one or several small erythematous papules that

1620

TABLE 155-1. The Histiocytoses of Childhood

Class I: Dendritic Cell Histiocytoses

Langerhans cell histiocytosis
Indeterminant cell histiocytoma

Class II: Histiocytoses of Mononuclear Phagocytes Other than Langerhans Cells

Juvenile xanthogranuloma
Benign cephalic histiocytosis
Generalized eruptive histiocytoma
Xanthoma disseminatum
Hemophagocytic lymphohistiocytosis
Sinus histiocytosis with massive lymphadenopathy
Multicentric reticulohistiocytosis

Class III: Malignant Histiocytic Disorders

Monocytic leukemia
Malignant histiocytosis
True histiocytic lymphoma
Malignant Langerhans cell histiocytosis

develop into 2- to 20-mm (most commonly, 5–10 mm) yellowish-red nodules that frequently have telangiectases or may appear somewhat hyperpigmented particularly in dark-skinned individuals (Fig. 155–1). Lesions tend to slowly flatten as they resolve and frequently heal with small atrophic scars. Large exophytic or endophytic lesions measuring several centimeters in diameter have been reported but are rare.[8]

Lesions of juvenile xanthogranuloma occur most commonly on the upper part of the body.[9] Ocular involvement[10] is the most common extracutaneous manifestation, and lesions affecting the iris can lead to anterior chamber hemorrhage and glaucoma. Mucous membranes are occasionally involved,[11] and lesions have been reported in skeletal muscle,[12] lungs, liver, spleen,

testes, ovaries, colon, kidneys, heart, and bones.[13] Associations of juvenile xanthogranuloma with neurofibromatosis[14] or myelogenous leukemia[15] have been reported.

PATHOLOGY

Early lesions show a diffuse infiltration of spindle-shaped fibrohistiocytic cells (Fig. 155–2). Lipidization of the histiocytic cells can be subtle. As the lesion matures, a mixed cellular infiltrate with histiocytes, lymphocytes, eosinophils, and occasional neutrophils and plasma cells is seen. Touton giant cells, characterized by the wreath-like arrangement of multiple nuclei, are typically present (Fig. 155–3). In older lesions, foamy, lipid-laden histiocytes are more abundant, and resolution is marked by gradual fibrosis. The infiltrates commonly extend from just below the epidermis into the subcutaneous fat.

Shapiro and coworkers[16] described 17 cases of juvenile xanthogranuloma in infants and small children that showed a sheet-like or infiltrative arrangement of epithelioid and spindle-shaped cells with near absence of foamy cells and Touton giant cells. An important histologic feature was the presence of numerous mitoses, particularly in the superficial portion of the lesions. All the

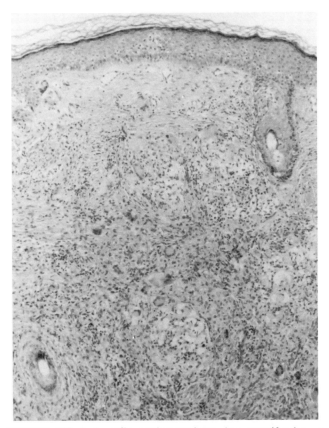

FIGURE 155-2. Juvenile xanthogranuloma, low magnification. A cellular infiltrate extends from the upper to the deep dermis. The epidermis is not altered. The infiltrate surrounds cutaneous adnexa and contains multiple giant cells as well as histiocytes and lymphocytes (hematoxylin-eosin, ×100).

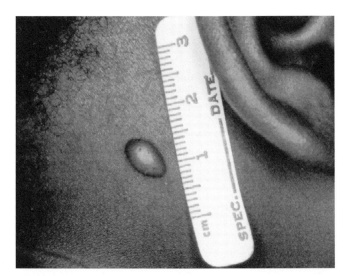

FIGURE 155-1. Solitary juvenile xanthogranuloma in a 6-month-old infant.

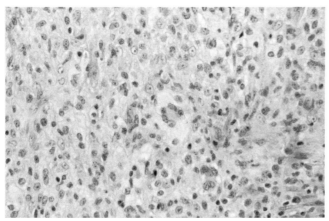

FIGURE 155-3. Juvenile xanthogranuloma, higher magnification. The giant cells can be recognized as Touton giant cells. The histiocytes have abundant cytoplasm and are admixed with lymphocytes (hematoxylin-eosin, ×280).

children with follow-up did well in spite of the worrisome histologic features.

Immunohistochemical studies have demonstrated that the histiocytic cells in the infiltrate of juvenile xanthogranuloma express macrophage markers[1] and are negative for peanut agglutinin and S-100 protein except for an occasional S-100–positive dendritic cell at the periphery of the lesion.[17] Ultrastructurally, lesional histiocytes have complex interdigitations of the cytoplasmic membrane[18] but no Birbeck granules.

DIAGNOSIS AND DIFFERENTIAL DIAGNOSIS

The diagnosis of juvenile xanthogranuloma is usually suspected on the basis of clinical morphology. A nodule of juvenile xanthogranuloma can be differentiated from a mastocytoma by failure of the lesion to urticate when stroked. Multiple lesions can be differentiated from benign cephalic histiocytosis, eruptive histiocytomas, and xanthoma disseminatum by clinical and/or histopathologic differences. Histologic examination is desirable to rule out Langerhans cell histiocytosis (Table 155–2).

TREATMENT

Surgical excision is usually curative, but treatment is generally unnecessary in children unless the lesions are symptomatic since cutaneous lesions tend to resolve

TABLE 155-2. Differential Diagnosis of Juvenile Xanthogranuloma
Mastocytoma
Dermatofibroma
Benign cephalic histiocytosis
Generalized eruptive histiocytoma
Xanthoma disseminatum
Langerhans cell histiocytosis

spontaneously. Adults may desire removal of lesions because juvenile xanthogranuloma arising in adulthood is frequently persistent.[9] An ophthalmologic examination is recommended for children with skin lesions of juvenile xanthogranuloma to rule out ocular involvement. Surgery or radiation therapy may be indicated for ocular lesions.[19]

Benign Cephalic Histiocytosis

The lesions of benign cephalic histiocytosis most commonly appear in the second half of the first year of life as yellow-red, 2- to 5-mm papules on the cheeks that spread to involve the forehead, ears, neck, and occasionally the upper body and buttocks. In reported cases, findings have been limited to the skin. The lesions generally do not increase in size and heal after several years, leaving flat or atrophic pigmented scars.[20]

The histology of early lesions shows a well-circumscribed infiltrate in the superficial and mid dermis composed primarily of histiocytes with some pleomorphism and scattered lymphocytes and eosinophils.[21] Older lesions may contain a few multinucleated giant cells, but the histiocytes contain no lipids. The cells are S-100 negative.[22] Ultrastructurally, approximately 20% of the histiocytes contain clusters of comma-shaped bodies,[23] but fatty droplets and Birbeck granules are absent. Since the condition is self-limiting, therapy is not indicated.

Generalized Eruptive Histiocytoma

Generalized eruptive histiocytoma is rare and has been reported more frequently in adults, but it also occurs in children.[18] The skin lesions consist of fine papules that are yellow to bluish red and range from 3 to 10 mm in size. The lesions tend to be symmetrically distributed on the face, trunk, and proximal limbs, and old lesions tend to fade as new ones appear. Mucous membrane involvement is rare and has not been reported in children,[23] and visceral lesions have not been observed. The disease lasts for a few years and then spontaneously resolves, usually without scarring.[23]

Histologic examination of the papular lesions reveals a monomorphous histiocytic infiltrate in the upper and mid dermis.[24] A few lymphocytes can be seen, but no lipid-laden cells or giant cells are observed, which differentiates the lesions from juvenile xanthogranulomas. Stains for S-100 protein are negative. Ultrastructural studies have shown that the histiocytic cells lack Birbeck granules but have cytoplasmic laminated bodies.[24]

Xanthoma Disseminatum

Xanthoma disseminatum is a rare sporadic histiocytic disease that occurs in both children (predominately older boys) and adults. Skin lesions are typically red-brown to yellow and tend to be most prominent on flexural surfaces, where they develop in clusters and may become confluent. The eyelids and conjunctiva may be involved, and the lips, pharynx, and larynx characteristically become infiltrated, occasionally resulting in respiratory difficulty. Diabetes insipidus, which occurs in up to 50% of patients, is the only characteristic sign of systemic disease.[25]

Histopathologically, lesions are similar to those of juvenile xanthogranuloma,[26] showing the presence of foamy histiocytes, inflammatory cells, and Touton giant cells. Lesional histiocytes do not bind S-100 or anti-CD1 (OKT6) antibodies and are negative for Birbeck granules by electron microscopy.

The skin lesions tend to be self-healing, with spontaneous resolution occurring over a 2- to 40-year period. Diabetes insipidus, when present, tends to be mild and may also resolve spontaneously. Troublesome cutaneous, mucosal, and ocular lesions have been managed successfully with conservative surgical excision and electrocauterization.[26] Xanthoma disseminatum responds poorly to chemotherapy and radiation.

Hemophagocytic Lymphohistiocytosis (Hemophagocytic Syndrome)

Hemophagocytic lymphohistiocytosis is a rare reactive histiocytosis in which there is widespread infiltration of multiple organs with lymphocytes and mature histiocytes that exhibit prominent erythrophagocytosis and cytophagocytosis.[27] This disease is frequently rapidly fatal and is therefore the most clinically significant of the class II histiocytoses. Early recognition is vital to patient survival. Many of the cases reported in the past as histiocytic medullary reticulosis fit well into this entity.

CLINICAL DESCRIPTION

The disease occurs most commonly in immunocompromised patients and is usually associated with either an infectious organism (most often a virus[28]) or a neoplastic lymphoid proliferation. The neoplastic lymphoid proliferations are usually of T-cell origin and occur as a familial syndrome in young children, 60% of whom are younger than 6 months of age.[29]

Clinical manifestations include fever and severe constitutional symptoms, hepatosplenomegaly, lymphadenopathy, coagulopathies, and pancytopenia. Skin mani-

festations occur in approximately 20% of patients, most commonly as panniculitis or purpura.[27]

PATHOLOGY

Skin biopsy specimens show erythrophagocytosis and frequently cytophagocytosis of other bone marrow–derived elements by cytologically benign histiocytes.[27] Infiltration of vessel walls and fat necrosis are generally present. Focal dermal necrosis associated with benign and malignant lymphoid infiltrates is common. Erythrophagocytotic histiocytes stain positively with antiserum to KP-1 (CD68) and are negative for S-100 protein.[27]

PATHOGENESIS AND ETIOLOGY

Hemophagocytic lymphohistiocytosis may result from cytokine production by reactive or malignant T cells.[27] Lymphocyte-derived cytokines appear to stimulate stem cells to undergo differentiation to histiocytes. Epstein-Barr virus, cytomegalovirus, and adenovirus appear to be the most common triggers of a reactive proliferation of T cells in immunocompromised individuals, but bacterial, fungal, and parasitic infections have also been reported to trigger the disease.[27]

DIAGNOSIS AND DIFFERENTIAL DIAGNOSIS

The diagnosis of hemophagocytic lymphohistiocytosis is based on the histopathologic finding of erythrophagocytosis by benign histiocytes. A few true malignancies such as histiocytic lymphomas and malignant histiocytosis, some T-cell lymphomas, acute myoblastic leukemia, and myelomas have been reported to exhibit erythrophagocytosis, but erythrophagocytosis is usually not a prominent finding and the cells in these conditions are cytologically malignant.[27]

TREATMENT

If immunosuppression is iatrogenic, then discontinuation of immunosuppressive therapy may result in clearing of the hemophagocytic lymphohistiocytosis.[28] Specific therapy for a known infectious agent should be given if available. If the patient is found to have a lymphoma, then cytotoxic therapy is generally indicated despite the immunosuppression induced by such therapy.[27]

Malignant Histiocytoses

Acute monocytic leukemia, malignant histiocytosis, and histiocytic lymphoma are malignancies of the monocyte–macrophage system of cells. Although they have been separated on clinical grounds, they form a spectrum of related entities and it is not always possible to differentiate them.[1]

Monocytic leukemia is a malignancy that primarily affects the bone marrow and blood, but extramedullary involvement is common. Darbyshire and associates[30] reviewed eight children with monocytic leukemia, all aged 12 months or younger at presentation. Skin involvement was present in six children, including single or multiple skin nodules in four and rash in two others. The skin involvement was the presenting manifestation in three children and preceded peripheral blood abnormalities by 1 to 3 months. Histologically, the skin biopsy specimens showed a dermal and subcutaneous infiltrate of closely packed, uniform, round cells with oval or slightly indented nuclei and moderate nongranular cytoplasm. Frequent mitoses were seen, but hemophagocytosis was not observed. Five patients were treated with a combination of etoposide and cyclophosphamide and of them three were surviving at the time of the publication.

Malignant histiocytosis and true histiocytic lymphoma originate theoretically from tissue macrophages. Malignant histiocytosis predominantly involves the sinuses of lymph nodes, while true histiocytic lymphoma effaces the lymph node architecture, similar to other non-Hodgkin's lymphomas.[31] Most clinicopathologic reports on these entities date to the availability of monoclonal antibodies and molecular diagnostic techniques. Most of the childhood malignancies classified in the past as histiocytic are examples of anaplastic large cell Ki-1 (CD30)-positive lymphomas of the T-cell type.[32] Presently, cases accepted as malignant histiocytosis and true histiocytic lymphoma should have phenotypic studies supporting a histiocytic lineage, with absence of T- and B-cell lineage markers and with a germline configuration for the T-cell receptor and immunoglobulin genes. Using these strict criteria, Ralfkiaer and colleagues[33] found four cases of true histiocytic lymphoma after reviewing 925 non-Hodgkin's lymphomas. Three of the four patients presented with skin tumors, and all four patients were adults.

Soria and colleagues[34] described two cases of true histiocytic lymphoma, one of them in a 7-month-old infant who presented with fever, cough, vomiting, and multiple red-violet–colored nodules 0.2 to 1 cm in diameter. After initial response to chemotherapy the patient experienced relapse with skin and multiorgan involvement, including bone marrow; and therefore a diagnosis of monocytic leukemia must be entertained.

Malignant Langerhans Cell Histiocytosis

Malignant Langerhans cell histiocytosis or malignant histiocytosis X has been reported to be a distinct clinicopathologic entity.[35] The disease occurs predominantly in men. Multisystem organ involvement is typically present, while skin lesions have been reported in less than half of the patients. The findings in two patients in whom the skin lesions were described (a 71-year-old man[36] and a 9-year-old girl[37]) were remarkably similar. The disease began with the rapid development of widespread papules, many of which progressed to nodules 1 to 3 cm in size. These lesions frequently developed central necrosis and ulceration as the disease progressed.

Infiltrating cells in this disease are cytologically atypical with nuclear pleomorphism and enlarged nucleoli, and cells tend to occur singly rather than in syncytium-like sheets.[35] The infiltrate is S-100 and CD1 positive,[6] and Birbeck granules are demonstrable ultrastructurally. All reported cases of malignant Langerhans cell histiocytosis have been rapidly fatal despite aggressive therapy with surgery, chemotherapy, and radiation therapy.

References

1. Malone M. The histiocytosis of childhood. Histopathology 1991;19:105–119.
2. Chu A, D'Angio GJ, Favara B, et al. Histiocytosis syndromes in children. Lancet 1987;1:208–209.
3. Miracco C, Raffaelli M, De Santi MM, et al. Solitary cutaneous reticulum cell tumor: Enzyme-histiochemical and electron-microscopic analogies with IDRC sarcoma. Am J Dermatopathol 1988;10:47–53.
4. Saijo S, Hara M, Kuramoto Y, et al. Generalized eruptive histiocytoma: A report of a variant case showing the presence of dermal indeterminant cells. J Cutan Pathol 1991;18:134–136.
5. Levisohn D, Seidel D, Phelps A, Burgdorf W. Solitary congenital indeterminant cell histiocytoma. Arch Dermatol 1993;129:81–85.
6. Wood GS, Haber RS. Novel histiocytoses considered in the context of histiocyte subset differentiation. Arch Dermatol 1993;129:210–214.
7. Divaris DXG, Ling FCK, Prentice RSA. Congenital self-healing histiocytosis: Report of two cases with histochemical and ultrastructural studies. Am J Dermatopathol 1991;13:481–487.
8. Resnick SD, Woosley J, Azizkhan RG. Giant juvenile xanthogranuloma: Exophytic and endophytic variants. Pediatr Dermatol 1990;7:185–188.
9. Cohen BA, Hood A. Xanthogranuloma: Report on clinical and histologic findings in 64 patients. Pediatr Dermatol 1989;6:262–266.
10. Zimmerman E. Ocular lesions of juvenile xanthogranuloma. Am J Ophthalmol 1965;60:1011–1016.
11. Ossoff RH, Esterly NB, Levine DK, et al. Intraoral and cutaneous xanthogranuloma. Ann Otol Rhinol Laryngol 1980:89:268–270.
12. Janney CG, Hurt MA, Santa Cruz DJ. Deep juvenile xanthogranuloma: Subcutaneous and intramuscular forms. Am J Surg Pathol 1991;15:150–159.
13. Webster SB, Reister HC, Harman LE. Juvenile xanthogranuloma with extracutaneous lesions. Arch Dermatol 1966;93:71–76.
14. Ackerman CD, Cohen BA. Juvenile xanthogranuloma and neurofibromatosis. Pediatr Dermatol 1991;8:339–340.
15. Cooper PH, Frierson HF, Kayne AL, Sabio H. Association of juvenile xanthogranuloma with juvenile myeloid leukemia. Arch Dermatol 1984;120:371–375.
16. Shapiro PE, Silvers DN, Treiber RK, et al. Juvenile xanthogranuloma with inconspicuous or absent foam cells and giant cells. J Am Acad Dermatol 1991;24:1005–1009.
17. Tahan SR, Pastel-Levy C, Bhan AK, Mihm MC Jr. Juvenile xanthogranuloma: Clinical and pathological characterization. Arch Pathol Lab Med 1989;113:1057–1061.
18. Seifert HW. Membrane activity in juvenile xanthogranuloma. J Cutan Pathol 1981;8:24–33.
19. MacLeod PM. Juvenile xanthogranuloma in the iris managed with superficial radiotherapy. Clin Radiol 1986;37:295–296.
20. Gianotti F, Caputo R, Ermacora E, et al. Benign cephalic histiocytosis. Arch Dermatol 1986;122:1038–1043.
21. Barsky BL, Lao I, Barsky S, Rhee HL. Benign cephalic histiocytosis. Arch Dermatol 1984;120:650–655.

22. de Luna ML, Geikin I, Golberg J, et al. Benign cephalic histiocytosis: Report of four cases. Pediatr Dermatol 1989;6:198–201.
23. Caputo R, Ermacora E, Gilmetti C, et al. Generalized eruptive histiocytoma in children. J Am Acad Dermatol 1987;17:449–454.
24. Caputo R, Alessi E, Allegra F. Generalized eruptive histiocytoma: A clinical, histologic, and ultrastructural study. Arch Dermatol 1981;117:216–221.
25. Kalty F, Hoffman MM, Lafrance A: Xanthoma disseminatum: Clinical and laboratory observations over a ten-year period. Dermatologia 1970;140:129–141.
26. Giller RH, Folberg R, Keech RV, et al. Xanthoma disseminatum: An unusual histiocytosis syndrome. Am J Pediatr Hematol Oncol 1988;10:252–257.
27. Smith KJ, Skeleton HG, Yeager J, et al. Cutaneous histopathologic, immunohistochemical, and clinical manifestations in patients with hemophagocytic syndrome. Arch Dermatol 1992;128:193–200.
28. Risdall RJ, McKenna RW, Nesbit ME, et al. Virus-associated hemophagocytic syndrome: A benign histiocytic proliferation distinct from malignant histiocytosis. Cancer 1979;44:993–1002.
29. Janka G. Familial haemophagocytic lymphohistiocytosis. Eur J Pediatr 1983;140:221–230.
30. Darbyshire PJ, Smith JHF, Oakhill A, et al. Monocytic leukemia in infancy: A review of eight children. Cancer 1985;56:1584–1589.
31. Weiss LM. Histiocytic and dendritic cell proliferation. In: Knowles DM, ed. Neoplastic Hematopathology. Baltimore: Williams & Wilkins, 1992:1459–1484.
32. Ornvold K, Carstensen H, Jinge J, et al. Tumors classified as "malignant histiocytosis" in children are T-cell neoplasms. Apmis 1992;100:558–566.
33. Ralfkiaer E, Delsol G, O'Connor NTJ, et al. Malignant lymphoma of true histiocytic origin: A clinical, histological, immunophenotypic and genotypic study. J Pathol 1990;160:9–17.
34. Soria C, Orradre JL, Garcia-Almagro D, et al. True histiocytic lymphoma (monocytic sarcoma). Am J Dermatopathol 1992;14:511–517.
35. Ben-Ezra J, Bailey A, Azumi N, et al. Malignant histiocytosis X: A distinct clinicopathologic entity. Cancer 1991;68:1050–1060.
36. Wood C, Wood GS, Deneau DG, et al. Malignant histiocytosis X. Cancer 1984;54:347–352.
37. Imamura M, Sakamoto S, Hanazono H. Malignant histiocytosis: A case of generalized histiocytosis with infiltration of Langerhans granule–containing histiocytes. Cancer 1971;28:467–475.

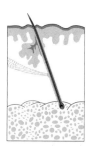

chapter 156

Cutaneous Lymphoid Hyperplasia

GARY S. WOOD

DEFINITION

Cutaneous lymphoid hyperplasia is a clinically benign, usually localized dermatosis characterized by dense lymphoid infiltration of the skin that may be idiopathic or secondary to a recognized foreign antigen. Several names have been used to refer to this disease in the past, including lymphocytoma cutis, pseudolymphoma, Spiegler-Fendt sarcoid, and lymphadenosis benigna cutis.[1, 2] Cutaneous lymphoid hyperplasia is the preferred term because it describes the basic underlying process that gives rise to the lesion and is unlikely to be confused with terms that refer to cutaneous lymphomas. In addition, the designation cutaneous lymphoid hyperplasia emphasizes the fact that this disorder is one special case of extranodal lymphoid hyperplasia that can occur in a wide variety of other organs besides the skin.[3]

The term *cutaneous pseudolymphoma* should be avoided because it is ambiguous. Some authors use it synonymously with cutaneous lymphoid hyperplasia, while others use it as an umbrella term to refer to any disease producing a dense or atypical cutaneous lymphoid infiltrate. These other diseases include T-cell disorders, such as lymphomatoid papulosis, pseudo-Hodgkin's disease, actinic reticuloid, angioimmunoblastic lymphadenopathy with dysproteinemia, lymphomatoid granulomatosis, Jessner's lymphocytic infiltrate, and drug-induced cutaneous T-cell lymphoma–like skin lesions.[3-6] Cutaneous lymphoid hyperplasia is typically a mixed B- and T-cell infiltrate that is nodular or diffuse but relatively dense. Jessner's lymphocytic infiltrate is typically a superficial and deep perivascular infiltrate composed of T cells. These other diseases also include disorders with prominent plasma cell infiltrates as seen in plasmacytoma, lues, and some cases of multicentric Castleman's disease.[3] None of these entities constitutes cutaneous lymphoid hyperplasia as defined in this chap-

ter. In addition to being the principal lesion, cutaneous lymphoid hyperplasia may occur as part of a distinct disease such as Kimura's disease, angiolymphoid hyperplasia with eosinophilia, cutaneous inflammatory pseudotumor, or systemic drug-induced lymphoid hyperplasia (e.g., secondary to phenytoin).[1, 2, 7-10]

CLINICAL DESCRIPTION

Cutaneous lymphoid hyperplasia occurs in adults of both sexes and also affects the pediatric age group. The male-to-female ratio is 1:2 to 1:3. Cutaneous lymphoid hyperplasia can involve any area of the skin but is most common on the face.[1, 11] The majority of cases present as a solitary or localized cluster of asymptomatic, erythematous to violaceous, papules or nodules that can coalesce into a plaque (Fig. 156–1). Uncommonly, the lesions may be widespread over a body region or even generalized in their cutaneous distribution. In cutaneous lymphoid hyperplasia that is not part of some other systemic lymphoid hyperplasia syndrome, constitutional symptoms are absent. There are no associated extracutaneous physical findings or laboratory abnormalities.

PATHOLOGY

The typical case of cutaneous lymphoid hyperplasia exhibits a patchy or confluent dense lymphoid infiltrate throughout the dermis that spares the epidermis and is separated from it by a narrow, so-called grenz zone (Fig. 156–2).[1, 2, 11-22] The infiltrate may extend into the subcutis but usually has a top-heavy distribution with attenuation in the deeper portions of the specimen. In occasional cases composed predominantly of T cells, there may also be epidermal infiltration by lymphoid cells. If

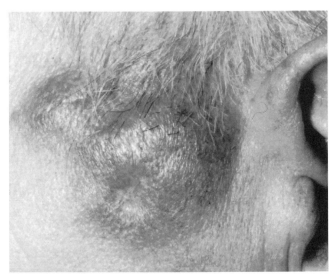

FIGURE 156–1. This patient exhibits a plaque typical of the localized form of cutaneous lymphoid hyperplasia.

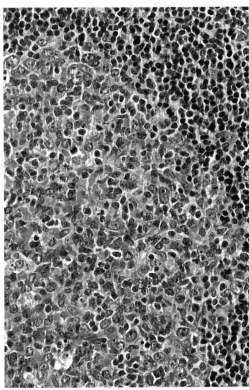

FIGURE 156–3. Cutaneous lymphoid hyperplasia. Higher-power view of a secondary lymphoid follicle shows a germinal center surrounded by a mantle zone of small mature lymphocytes *(top)*. Tingible body macrophages are also present within the germinal center. These features of secondary lymphoid follicles are similar whether the follicles occur in lymphoid tissues, skin, or other sites. They help to distinguish reactive follicular lymphoid hyperplasia from follicular B-cell lymphoma.

the B cells within the infiltrate are organized into primary and secondary lymphoid follicles, these may be apparent as nodular aggregates at low power. Otherwise, the infiltrate has a diffuse histologic appearance.

The cytologic features of the infiltrate vary from case to case.[1, 2, 11-22] There is generally a heterogeneous mixture of large and small lymphoid cells and histiocytes (macrophages, Langerhans cells, other dendritic cells). In many cases, plasma cells and eosinophils are also present. If B-cell nodules are present and have formed secondary lymphoid follicles, these will consist of a germinal center containing large, mitotically active lymphoid cells and tingible body macrophages surrounded by a mantle zone or cuff of small lymphocytes (Fig. 156–3).

The same range of cells that can occur in reactive follicles in lymph nodes is found in the follicles of cutaneous lymphoid hyperplasia. The T cells in the interfollicular areas of the dermis are usually small and round but may sometimes show mild enlargement and mild nuclear irregularities.

PATHOGENESIS AND ETIOLOGY

Cutaneous lymphoid hyperplasia may be idiopathic or arise in response to a wide variety of foreign antigens, including arthropod bites, stings, and infestations; tattoos; vaccinations; trauma; injection of foreign substances; pierced ear jewelry; and drugs.[1-5, 23-25] Some cases have been attributed to infection with *Borrelia burgdorferi.*[26] These associations suggest that cutaneous lymphoid hyperplasia begins as a reactive response to newly encountered antigens.

Immunophenotypic studies have shown that most cases of cutaneous lymphoid hyperplasia consist of a mixture of reactive polytypic B cells, T cells, macrophages, and dendritic cells.[2, 3, 11, 22, 27, 28] The B cells are often organized into primary and secondary lymphoid follicles analogous to those occurring in reactive lymphoid tissues. These are frequently present regardless of

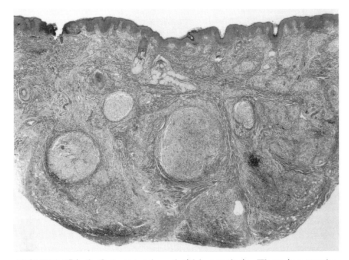

FIGURE 156–2. Cutaneous lymphoid hyperplasia. There is a patchy superficial and deep dermal lymphoid infiltrate containing several secondary lymphoid follicles with pale germinal centers. Lymphoid follicles are not detectable in all cases of cutaneous lymphoid hyperplasia. The infiltrate spares the epidermis and is separated from it by a narrow "grenz zone" of uninvolved dermis.

whether they can be recognized by routine histopathology.[11] Occasionally, B cells are rare or absent and the infiltrate is composed predominantly of T cells.[3, 11, 29-31] Molecular biologic analysis of immunoglobulin or T-cell receptor gene rearrangements indicates that in some cases there is a progression from polyclonal lymphoid hyperplasia to the emergence of a dominant monoclonal B-cell or T-cell population.[30-34] These cases of monoclonal cutaneous lymphoid hyperplasia are recognizable only by immunogenotypic analysis and are of clinical significance because they appear to constitute a subset of patients with cutaneous lymphoid hyperplasia who are at increased risk for the development of overt lymphoma. Thus, rather than being regarded as a completely benign condition, cutaneous lymphoid hyperplasia appears to be part of a spectrum of lymphoproliferative disease that includes polyclonal cutaneous lymphoid hyperplasia, monoclonal cutaneous lymphoid hyperplasia, and overt cutaneous lymphoma. Fortunately, most patients who present with cutaneous lymphoid hyperplasia do not progress to clinically malignant disease. The existence of a monoclonal, prelymphomatous process is not unique to cutaneous lymphoid hyperplasia but also occurs in the context of lymphoid hyperplasia in other tissues, lymphomatoid papulosis, angioimmunoblastic lymphadenopathy with dysproteinemia, and the so-called benign monoclonal gammopathies (now generally referred to as monoclonal gammopathies of uncertain significance).[3]

DIAGNOSIS AND DIFFERENTIAL DIAGNOSIS

Diseases that produce localized red or purple cutaneous papules, nodules, or plaques are the main disorders that should be considered in the clinical differential diagnosis of cutaneous lymphoid hyperplasia (Table 156–1). Various forms of lymphoma and leukemia are the major diseases involved in the histopathologic differential diagnosis. Leukemias and low-grade lymphomas often exhibit an extremely monomorphous cellular infiltrate that contrasts to the more heterogeneous cellular composition characteristic of cutaneous lymphoid hyperplasia. The lymphoid infiltrate in cutaneous lymphoid hyperplasia is often top heavy and diminishes in the deep dermis or subcutis. In contrast, lymphomas often exhibit a bottom-heavy infiltrate. In fact, it is crucial to obtain a deep biopsy when lymphoma is in the differential diagnosis because the most diagnostic areas are often in the deepest portions of the lymphomatous infiltrate.[35] Incisional biopsy using a scalpel is preferable, and care should be taken not to crush the specimen, since lymphoid cells are particularly fragile. Follicular lymphomas may be primary in the skin.[29, 35] The B-cell nodules in these tumors differ from the secondary lymphoid follicles observed in cutaneous lymphoid hyperplasia because the former characteristically lack the zonation into follicular areas and mantle zones and tingible body macrophages present in germinal centers. Infiltration of appendages, vascular walls, and peripheral collagen can be seen in cutaneous lymphoid hyperplasia as well as lymphoma.[11] Occasionally, reactive skin lesions histologically similar to cutaneous T-cell lymphoma may arise in patients taking carba-

TABLE 156-1. Differential Diagnosis of Cutaneous Lymphoid Hyperplasia

Clinical
Rosacea
Adnexal tumor
Granuloma faciale
Leukemia
Lupus erythematosus
Lymphoma
Metastatic neoplasm
Nodular granulomatous lesion (e.g., deep fungal)
Nodular infiltrative lesion (e.g., nodular amyloidosis)
Soft tissue tumor

Histopathologic
Actinic reticuloid
Angioimmunoblastic lymphadenopathy with dysproteinemia
Angiolymphoid hyperplasia with eosinophilia
Jessner's lymphocytic infiltrate
Kimura's disease
Leukemia
Lues
Lupus erythematosus
Lymphoma
Lymphomatoid contact dermatitis
Lymphomatoid papulosis
Merkel cell carcinoma
Metastatic small cell (oat cell) carcinoma
Multicentric Castleman's disease
Polymorphous light eruption

mazepine, phenytoin, or other drugs.[4-6] In addition to lymphomas and leukemias, other dense infiltrations of lymphoid cells or small round cells sometimes need to be considered in the differential diagnosis of cutaneous lymphoid hyperplasia (see Table 156–1). Usually, the overall clinicopathologic features of these diseases allow their distinction from cutaneous lymphoid hyperplasia. Occasionally, electron microscopy or immunohistologic studies to demonstrate lineage-specific markers are needed to reach a correct diagnosis.

In many cases of cutaneous lymphoid hyperplasia, the clinical and histopathologic features are classic and the diagnosis can be made with confidence on these grounds alone. In many other cases, however, the clinicopathologic features are atypical and the distinction between cutaneous lymphoid hyperplasia and lymphoma cannot be reached without additional evaluation. In these instances, two lines of investigation warrant pursuit.

First, lesional skin should be subjected to immunophenotypic and immunogenotypic analysis to search for evidence of monoclonal B-cell or T-cell populations. Immunophenotypic evidence of monoclonal B cells includes monotypic immunoglobulin light-chain restriction (abnormal κ/λ ratio) or immunoglobulin-negative B cells.[2, 3, 11, 22, 27, 28] Immunophenotypic evidence of monoclonal T cells includes lack of expression of one or more pan–T-cell antigens (CD2, CD3, CD5).[2, 3, 11, 22, 27, 28] Immunogenotypic evidence of B-cell or T-cell lymphoma includes monoclonal rearrangements of immunoglobulin or T-cell receptor genes.[3, 30-34] If immunophenotyping is positive in this regard, then the lesion should be classified as lymphoma. Otherwise, the lesion should be classified as polyclonal or monoclonal cutaneous lymphoid hyperplasia based on the results of immunogenotyping.

The second important aspect of patient evaluation involves a workup for evidence of lymphoid malignancy outside the skin. Conservative workup should include physical examination of peripheral lymph nodes, liver, and spleen; the complete blood cell count with differential review; and chest radiography. A more aggressive workup might also include bone marrow aspiration or biopsy and computed tomographic scans of the chest, abdomen, and pelvis. Suspected lymphoma or leukemia detected with these tests should then be confirmed and classified by histopathologic examination and, if necessary, immunophenotypic and immunogenotypic analysis.

TREATMENT

Lesions of cutaneous lymphoid hyperplasia that are not cosmetically or functionally problematic for the patient can be followed without specific therapy. Some lesions may eventually undergo regression, either spontaneously or in response to biopsy. Given the relatively high prevalence of monoclonality among cases of cutaneous lymphoid hyperplasia and reports of progression to overt lymphoma in some cases, long-term follow-up of patients is warranted regardless of therapy.

The major therapies that have shown benefit in cutaneous lymphoid hyperplasia are listed in Table 156–3. Because of the association with *Borrelia burgdorferi* in some cases, a therapeutic trial of appropriate antibiotics is often undertaken if there is no other apparent cause of the cutaneous lymphoid hyperplasia.[26] Localized lesions

are often amenable to surgical resection, and smaller lesions are often diagnosed and treated simultaneously by excisional biopsy. Cryotherapy has also been reported to be an effective surgical modality.[36] Lesions generally improve with intralesional corticosteroid therapy,[1] although repeated treatments may be required to achieve complete resolution of a lesion. Topical and systemic corticosteroids have also been used with success. Antimalarial agents have been used to treat the generalized variant of cutaneous lymphoid hyperplasia.[1] As a last resort, this disease can be treated with various forms of radiation therapy and usually exhibits rapid resolution. Relapse within the original or new sites may sometimes occur with any of these treatments.

Those cases of atypical cutaneous lymphoid hyperplasia in which an unequivocal distinction between localized cutaneous lymphoid hyperplasia and localized lymphoma cannot be made do not present an insurmountable therapeutic problem because they can be treated as localized cutaneous lymphoma (stage IEA in the Ann Arbor classification). This generally involves local radiation therapy with or without prior surgical excision of any lesional tissue remaining after adequate biopsy specimens have been obtained.

References

1. Brodell RT, Santa Cruz DJ. Cutaneous pseudolymphomas. Dermatol Clin 1985;3:719–734.
2. Wirt DP, Grogan TM, Jolley CS, et al. The immunoarchitecture of cutaneous pseudolymphoma. Hum Pathol 1985;16:492–510.
3. Neoplastic Hematopathology. Knowles DM, ed. Baltimore: Williams & Wilkins, 1992.
4. D'Incan M, Souteyrand P, Bignon YJ, et al. Hydantoin-induced cutaneous pseudolymphoma with clinical, pathologic, and immunologic aspects of Sézary syndrome. Arch Dermatol 1992; 128:1371–1374.
5. Welykyj S, Gradini R, Nakao J, et al. Carbamazepine-induced eruption histologically mimicking mycosis fungoides. J Cutan Pathol 1990;17:111–116.
6. Rijlaarsdam JU, Scheffer E, Meijer CJ, et al. Mycosis fungoides–like lesions associated with phenytoin and carbamazepine therapy. J Am Acad Dermatol 1991;24:216–220.
7. Urabe A, Tsuneyoshi M, Enjoji M. Epithelioid hemangioma versus Kimura's disease. Am J Surg Pathol 1987;11:758–766.
8. Googe PB, Harris NL, Mihm MC Jr. Kimura's diseases and angiolymphoid hyperplasia with eosinophilia: Two distinct histopathological entities. J Cutan Pathol 1987;14:263–271.
9. Hurt MA, Santa Cruz DJ. Cutaneous inflammatory pseudotumor. Am J Surg Pathol 1990;14:764–773.
10. Braddock SW, Harrington D, Vose J. Generalized nodular cutaneous pseudolymphoma associated with phenytoin therapy: Use of T-cell receptor gene rearrangement in diagnosis and clinical review of cutaneous reactions to phenytoin. J Am Acad Dermatol 1992;27:337–340.
11. Medeiros LJ, Picker LJ, Abel EA, et al. Cutaneous lymphoid hyperplasia: Immunologic characteristics and assessment of criteria recently proposed as diagnostic of malignant lymphoma. J Am Acad Dermatol 1989;21:929–942.
12. Caro WA, Helwig EB. Cutaneous lymphoid hyperplasia. Cancer 1969;24:487–502.
13. Evans HL, Winkelmann RK, Banks PM. Differential diagnosis of malignant and benign cutaneous lymphoid infiltrates: A study of 57 cases in which malignant lymphoma had been diagnosed or suspected in the skin. Cancer 1979;44:699–717.
14. Fisher ER, Park EJ, Wechsler HL. Histologic identification of malignant lymphoma cutis. Am J Clin Pathol 1976;65:149–158.
15. Lange Wantzin G, Hou-Jensen K, Nielsen M, et al. Cutaneous lymphocytomas: Clinical and histological aspects. Acta Derm Venereol 1982;62:119–124.

TABLE 156-2. Treatment of Cutaneous Lymphoid Hyperplasia

Antibiotics
Penicillin
Tetracycline

Anti-inflammatory
Antimalarials
Corticosteroids

Radiation
Localized electron-beam therapy
Orthovoltage therapy

Surgical
Cryosurgery
Excision

16. Mach KW, Wilgram GH. Characteristic histopathology of cutaneous lymphoplasia (lymphocytoma). Arch Dermatol 1966;94:26–32.
17. Burke JS, Hoppe RT, Cibull ML, et al. Cutaneous malignant lymphoma: A pathologic study of 50 cases with clinical analysis of 37. Cancer 1981;47:300–310.
18. Long JC, Mihm MC, Quazi R. Malignant lymphoma of the skin: A clinicopathologic study of lymphoma other than mycosis fungoides diagnosed by skin biopsy. Cancer 1976;38:1282–1296.
19. MacDonald DM. Histopathological differentiation of benign and malignant cutaneous lymphocytic infiltrates. Br J Dermatol 1982;107:715–718.
20. Saxe N, Kahn LB, King H. Lymphoma of the skin: A comparative clinico-pathologic study of 50 cases including mycosis fungoides and primary and secondary cutaneous lymphoma. J Cutan Pathol 1977;4:111–122.
21. Van Hale HM, Winkelmann RK. Nodular lymphoid disease of the head and neck: Lymphoma cutis, benign lymphocytic infiltrate of Jessner, and their distinction from malignant lymphoma. J Am Acad Dermatol 1985;12:455–461.
22. Rijlaarsdam JU, Meijer CJ, Willemze R. Differentiation between lymphadenosis benigna cutis and primary cutaneous follicular center cell lymphomas: A comparative clinicopathologic study of 57 patients. Cancer 1990;65:2301–2306.
23. Kobayashi Y, Nanko H, Nakamura J, et al. Lymphocytoma cutis induced by gold pierced earrings. J Am Acad Dermatol 1992;27:457–458.
24. Bernstein H, Shupack J, Ackerman AB. Cutaneous pseudolymphoma resulting from antigen injections. Arch Dermatol 1974;110:756–757.
25. Zinberg M, Heilman E, Glickman F. Cutaneous pseudolymphoma resulting from a tattoo. J Dermatol Surg Oncol 1982;8:955–958.
26. Abele DC, Anders KH. The many faces and phases of borreliosis: II. J Am Acad Dermatol 1990;23:401–410.
27. Ralfkiaer E, Lange Wantzin G, Mason DY, et al. Characterization of benign cutaneous lymphocytic infiltrates by monoclonal antibodies. Br J Dermatol 1984;111:635–645.
28. Smolle J, Torne R, Soyer HP, et al. Immunohistochemical classification of cutaneous pseudolymphomas: Delineation of distinct patterns. J Cutan Pathol 1990;17:149–159.
29. Rijlaarsdam JU, Scheffer E, Meijer CJ, et al. Cutaneous pseudo–T-cell lymphomas: A clinicopathologic study of 20 patients. Cancer 1992;69:717–724.
30. Griesser H, Feller AC, Sterry W. T-cell receptor and immunoglobulin gene rearrangements in cutaneous T-cell–rich pseudolymphomas. J Invest Dermatol 1990;95:292–295.
31. Bendelac A, Lesavre P, Boitard C, et al. Cutaneous pleomorphic T-cell lymphoma. J Am Acad Dermatol 1986;15:657–664.
32. Wood GS, Ngan B-Y, Tung R, et al. Clonal rearrangements of immunoglobulin genes and progression to B-cell lymphoma in cutaneous lymphoid hyperplasia. Am J Pathol 1989;135:13–19.
33. Rijlaarsdam JU, Bakels V, van Oostveen JW, et al. Demonstration of clonal immunoglobulin gene rearrangements in cutaneous B-cell lymphomas and pseudo-B-cell lymphomas: Differential diagnostic and pathogenetic aspects. J Invest Dermatol 1992;99:749–754.
34. Hammer E, Sangueza O, Suwanjinder P, et al. Immunophenotypic and genotypic analysis in cutaneous lymphoid hyperplasias. J Am Acad Dermatol 1993;28:426–433.
35. Garcia CF, Weiss LM, Warnke RA, et al. Cutaneous follicular lymphoma. Am J Surg Pathol 1986;10:454–463.
36. Graham GR, Stewart R. Cryosurgery for unusual cutaneous neoplasms. J Dermatol Surg Oncol 1977;3:437–442.

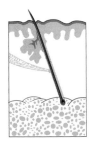

chapter 157

Lymphomatoid Papulosis

MARSHALL E. KADIN

DEFINITION

Lymphomatoid papulosis is a continuing self-healing eruption whose lesions are clinically benign but histologically contain malignant-appearing cells.[1] Despite the alarming histologic resemblance to lymphoma, individual lesions usually regress spontaneously within a few weeks. It is important to recognize lymphomatoid papulosis to avoid overtreatment of this clinically benign disease and to follow patients carefully because of their significant risk of developing lymphoma.

CLINICAL DESCRIPTION

Lesions first appear as red, painless, nonpruritic papules that undergo central necrosis, sometimes with scale, and heal with scarring, often leaving a depigmented or hyperpigmented area. Individual lesions may reach up to 2 cm but usually are smaller than 1 cm. There may be few to more than 100 lesions. Individual lesions regress spontaneously in 4 to 6 weeks. Some lesions develop while others regress (Fig. 157–1). Distribution of lesions is usually random but occasionally symmetrical, clustered, or disseminated. The buttocks, trunk, legs, and arms are most often involved. Hands and feet, including palms, soles, digits, face, scalp, and genitalia can be affected. Mucous membranes are spared. Papules sometimes coalesce to form nodules, plaques, or ulcers. The latter lesions can be difficult or impossible to distinguish from cutaneous lymphoma, and the distinction indeed may be arbitrary (Fig. 157–2).

Incidence and Prevalence

All ages are affected, with a range of onset from infancy to the eighth decade.[2] The median age at onset is in the fourth[2] or fifth decade.[3] There is a nearly equal distribution between males and females. This is in contrast to most lymphomas in Western countries, which have a clear male patient predominance. This difference may be explained by the fact that lymphomatoid papulosis is primarily a T-cell disorder whereas most non-Hodgkin's lymphomas in Western countries are derived from B cells. The overall prevalence of lymphomatoid papulosis is difficult to estimate owing to variable reporting, but the condition appears to be rare. In one study, the period prevalence rate of lymphomatoid papulosis was estimated to be 1.9 per 1 million per year population for Massachusetts and 1.2 per 1 million population per year for Pennsylvania.[2] Cases have been found in all regions of the United States, in Europe, and in Asia. All races are affected, but there appears to be a lower prevalence of lymphomatoid papulosis in blacks than has been reported for mycosis fungoides or adult T-cell leukemia.[4, 5]

Association with Lymphoma

Lymphomatoid papulosis is preceded by, coexistent with, or followed by a malignant lymphoma in an estimated 10% to 20% of cases.[6-8] The time to develop lymphoma is highly variable, but a median of 13 years has been observed.[3] Although the risk to develop lymphoma appears low, one recent report indicates that the risk may be higher, approaching 80%, when patients are followed for 15 years or longer.[3] The most common types of lymphoma to develop in patients with lymphomatoid papulosis are mycosis fungoides, Hodgkin's disease, and CD30-positive large cell lymphoma.[6]

Supported by NIH grant CA54062.

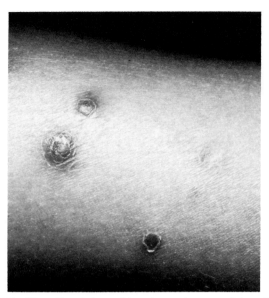

FIGURE 157–1. Four lesions of lymphomatoid papulosis in different stages of spontaneous regression.

Interestingly, the prognosis for lymphomas associated with lymphomatoid papulosis appears to be better than for the same lymphomas arising de novo.[6] In particular, patients with lymphomatoid papulosis who have mycosis fungoides or CD30-positive large cell lymphoma confined to the skin have a very good prognosis, whereas patients with systemic or extracutaneous CD30-positive large cell lymphoma have a poor prognosis.[6, 9] In a summary of the literature, the risk of developing lymphoma was much higher for male than female patients with lymphomatoid papulosis, with males accounting for 32 of 35 patients with associated lymphoma.[6] The risk to develop lymphoma also appears to be lower for patients who have lymphomatoid papulosis lesions of type B histology and highest for patients with diffuse large cell type

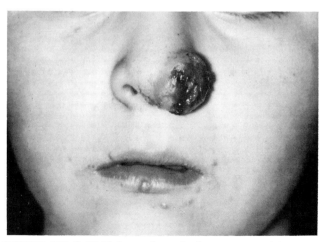

FIGURE 157–2. Multiple papules and a large tumor nodule on the face of a child with lymphomatoid papulosis.

lesions (see Pathology), although the number of cases is too small to be conclusive.[6]

PATHOLOGY

Histology

The histology of lymphomatoid papulosis depends on the stage of development of the lesion at the time of biopsy. Early lesions may have only a nonspecific perivascular lymphocytic infiltrate. Mid-stage lesions have a wedge shape (Fig. 157–3). Late-stage lesions have superficially dilated blood vessels and numerous inflammatory cells. Neutrophils can be seen infiltrating the epidermis, which can ulcerate. Large atypical mononuclear cells appear soon after the onset of lesions. Some of these have bilobed or multilobed nuclei and prominent eosinophilic nucleoli and thereby resemble Reed-Sternberg cells of Hodgkin's disease (Fig. 157–4). Mitoses, some of which appear multipolar or otherwise atypical, are common. Neutrophils, eosinophils, and small, normal-appearing lymphocytes are frequently present. Lesions composed predominantly of large atypical mononuclear cells and inflammatory cells are termed type A.[18] These are the most common type of lesion. The less frequent type B lesions resemble mycosis fungoides histologically. Type B lesions contain mononuclear cells with convoluted or cerebriform nuclei (Fig. 157–5). Infiltrates of type B lesions are often perivascular and focally epidermotropic. However, typical Pautrier abscesses, characteristic of mycosis fungoides, are seldom if ever encountered in lymphomatoid papulosis. Some lesions have an appearance intermediate between types A and B and are referred to as type A and B lesions. A third major type of lesion of lymphomatoid papulosis contains clusters of large atypical mononuclear cells as are found in type A lesions and may be difficult to distinguish histologically from CD30-positive large cell anaplastic lymphoma. However, the clusters of large atypical mononuclear cells in regressing lesions of lymphomatoid papulosis are usually confined to the upper dermis and do not infiltrate the subcutis as seen in CD30-positive lymphomas. Nevertheless, the distinction between lymphomatoid papulosis and CD30-positive lymphoma sometimes cannot be made by histology alone and such examples have been termed *borderline lesions*. Borderline lesions are associated with a favorable prognosis, similar to lymphomatoid papulosis in a multivariate Cox regression model of survival.[9]

Immunopathology

Lymphomatoid papulosis is, in most cases, a proliferation of activated CD4-positive helper T-lymphocytes that co-express Hodgkin's disease–associated antigens CD30, CD25, CD71, and HLA-DR but usually not CD15.[10] The T lymphocytes have an aberrant phenotype, lacking CD7 and one or more other common T-cell antigens, CD3, CD2, and CD5. In 20 to 25% of cases, no T-cell antigens are detected.

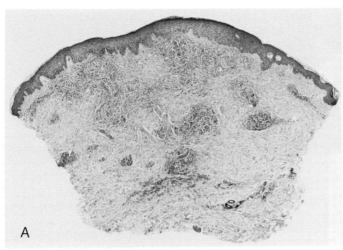

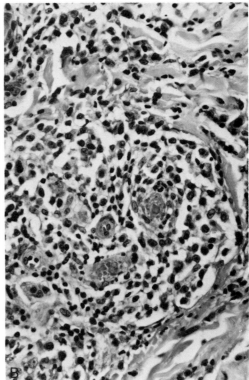

FIGURE 157–3. *A*, Type A lesions of lymphomatoid papulosis often have infiltrates with a wedge-shaped pattern. *B*, Large atypical cells with vesicular nuclei surround the walls of venules.

PATHOGENESIS AND ETIOLOGY

Lymphomatoid papulosis is a benign clonal proliferation of T lymphocytes in most cases.[11–13] Individual lesions contain one or more dominant T-cell populations detected as rearranged bands when Southern blots are probed for T-cell receptor beta or gamma genes.[11–13] Some lesions contain only polyclonal T cells, with no rearranged band.[12, 13] In one study, a lack of T-cell receptor gene rearrangements was associated particularly with type A histology, leading investigators to conclude that type A lesions arise from non-T, non-B lineage cells.[13]

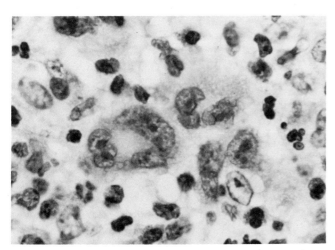

FIGURE 157–4. Reed-Sternberg–like cells in a type A lesion of lymphomatoid papulosis.

Separate lesions may be derived from the same[12–14] or different[11] T-cell clones. In one patient, three different lesions had different T-cell receptor rearrangement patterns, indicating that the lesions were not clonally related.[11] However, identical T-cell clones have also been observed and confirmed by DNA sequencing in spatially and temporally separate type A lesions.[14] The same T-cell receptor gene rearrangement has been found most often in multiple type B lesions.[12, 13] A clonal relationship between lymphomatoid papulosis and malignant CD30-positive anaplastic large cell lymphoma[15] or Hodgkin's disease[16] has been demonstrated in several cases.

DNA densitometry studies have shown that lesions of lymphomatoid papulosis often contained aneuploid cells.[17, 18] Aneuploid and polyploid cells (4n, 6n, 8n) were most frequent in type A lesions, whereas type B lesions contained predominantly 2n and few 4n cells.[18] Cytogenetics of a single lesion of lymphomatoid papulosis demonstrated the presence of aneuploidy and abnormal marker chromosomes.[19] By using modern banding methods the presence of clonal aneuploid cells in the regressing stage of lymphomatoid papulosis has been confirmed in our laboratory. We found more abnormal chromosomes in a CD30-positive anaplastic lymphoma that arose from lymphomatoid papulosis. These observations suggest that, like other neoplasms, lymphomatoid papulosis can progress from a polyclonal to an indolent monoclonal disorder that requires additional mutations, detectable as chromosome abnormalities, to confer a fully malignant phenotype.

The etiology of lymphomatoid papulosis is an

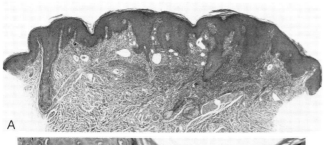

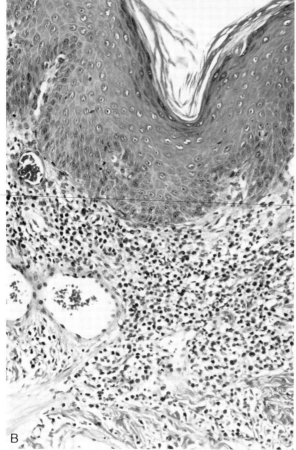

FIGURE 157–5. *A*, Type B lesions of lymphomatoid papulosis resemble mycosis fungoides in that there are lichenoid infiltrates accompanied by psoriasiform epidermal hyperplasia. *B*, Lymphocytes with slightly enlarged nuclei only tentatively infiltrate the epidermis in most lesions, in contrast to mycosis fungoides.

enigma. A viral etiology has been suggested but not confirmed.[20–23] No Epstein-Barr viral RNA was detected in a study of skin lesions and lymph nodes from nine patients with lymphomatoid papulosis.[24] Human T-cell lymphotropic virus type I (HTLV-I) proviral sequences have been detected in CD30-positive large cell anaplastic cutaneous T-cell lymphomas[25] but have not yet been reported in lymphomatoid papulosis.

A case-controlled study of 57 patients with lymphomatoid papulosis failed to uncover a significant risk factor for development of the condition. Patients with lymphomatoid papulosis, however, had a significantly increased frequency of prior or coexisting lymphoproliferative disorders, an increased frequency of nonlymphoid malignant lesions, and exposure to radiation ther-

apy.[2] Patients with lymphomatoid papulosis also reported more frequent exaggerated reactions to mosquito bites. Hypersensitivity to mosquito bites has been reported to induce a condition interpreted as malignant histiocytosis in some patients.[26] Most cases previously interpreted as malignant histiocytosis subsequently have been demonstrated to be T-cell lymphomas. A possible hypothesis is that lymphomatoid papulosis is a clonal proliferation of activated T cells initiated by an abnormal immune response to a common stimulus, such as a mosquito bite.

DIAGNOSIS AND DIFFERENTIAL DIAGNOSIS

Lymphomatoid papulosis is a combined clinical and pathologic diagnosis (Table 157–1). The essential clinical feature is spontaneous regression or self-healing of papulonodular lesions that appear in crops without a history of exposure to drug, toxin, or allergen. The distinctive pathology is the presence of large atypical cells, sometimes resembling Reed-Sternberg cells, surrounded by inflammatory cells. The distinctive immunopathology reveals Ki-1(CD30)-positive cells with aberrant expression (deletion) of T-cell antigens. Together, these features are diagnostic of lymphomatoid papulosis.

In the absence of an appropriate history, arthropod bite reactions can be histologically confused with lymphomatoid papulosis. However, the CD30-positive cells characteristic of lymphomatoid papulosis are absent in inflammatory infiltrates responding to arthropod bites.[27]

Lymphomatoid papulosis can be difficult to distinguish clinically from pityriasis lichenoides et varioliformis acuta (PLEVA). Patients with lymphomatoid papulosis are usually older, and their lesions may coexist with or follow lymphoma. The lymphocytes of PLEVA do not show the degree of atypia observed in lymphomatoid papulosis. The interface dermatitis, basal vacuolation, and dyskeratosis characteristic of PLEVA are generally absent in lymphomatoid papulosis. In pityriasis lichenoides, there are few or no CD30-positive cells and the predominant cell is usually CD8-positive instead of CD4-positive as in lymphomatoid papulosis.[28]

Lymphomatoid papulosis, especially type B, can closely resemble mycosis fungoides and may be a variant of that disorder. However, the lesions of lymphomatoid papulosis appear as discrete papules with central necrosis that is not typical of mycosis fungoides. Lesions of lymphomatoid papulosis do not have dense band-like infiltrates beneath the epidermis, show less epidermotropism, and lack Pautrier microabscesses characteristic of mycosis fungoides. Mycosis fungoides has few or no CD30-positive cells, and the aberrant expression of T-cell antigens characteristic of lymphomatoid papulosis is found only in plaques or tumors of mycosis fungoides.

Lymphomatoid papulosis comprises the benign end of a spectrum of lesions that ends in Ki-1(CD30)-positive malignant lymphoma.[29, 30] Type A and regressing lesions with clusters of large atypical cells (diffuse large cell type)[30] closely resemble CD30–positive cutaneous lymphomas. However, individual lesions of CD30–positive lymphomas are larger than 2 cm and show delayed, in-

TABLE 157-1. Differential Diagnosis of Lymphomatoid Papulosis

Disorder	Clinical Features	Histology	Immunophenotype
Lymphoid papulosis	Recurrent papulonodular eruption with spontaneous regression; 10%–20% develop systemic lymphoma	Perivascular or wedge-shaped infiltrate with Reed-Sternberg–like cells and many inflammatory cells; type A: Hodgkin's-like; type B: mycosis fungoides-like	Aberrant T-cell phenotype; CD30-positive, CD15-negative, LCA (CD45)-positive
Pityriasis lichenoides et varioliformis acuta	Maculopapular scaling; necrotic and often hemorrhagic lesions; self-healing; median age of patients younger than those with lymphomatoid papulosis; rare association with lymphoma	Small lymphocytes with minimal atypia; exocytosis; interface dermatitis; basal vacuolar and dyskeratotic changes in epidermis; papillary dermal hemorrhage	Numerous CD8-positive cells, especially at the dermal-epidermal junction; CD30-positive cells usually not present; HLA-DR-positive epidermis
Arthropod bite	Usual history of arthropod bite; rapid resolution of eruption	Superficial and deep lymphohistiocytic infiltrate with eosinophils; reactive germinal centers; scattered atypical lymphocytes	Mixed T- and B-cell infiltrate; CD30-positive cells rare or absent
Ki-1 (CD30)-positive anaplastic large cell lymphoma	One to several large ulcerating tumors; may show partial regression; can progress to involve regional lymph nodes and viscera; excellent prognosis when confined to skin	Sheets of large anaplastic cells; usually not epidermotropic; few small lymphocytes; occasionally numerous neutrophils	Sheets of CD30-positive cells; aberrant T-cell phenotypic in most cases; no lineage specific markers in some cases
Primary cutaneous Hodgkin's disease	One to several large deep-seated nodules; indolent course but some patients develop systemic Hodgkin's disease	Classic Reed-Sternberg cells surrounded by small lymphocytes; eosinophils, and other inflammatory cells	Reed-Sternberg cells; CD30-positive, CD15-positive, CD45-negative

TABLE 157-2. Treatment of Lymphomatoid Papulosis

Treatment	Dose/Frequency	Advantages	Disadvantages
Observation	Not applicable	Useful for minimal lesions; no risk of mutagenesis or toxicity	Recurrent lesions; possible progression to lymphoma
Methotrexate	10–20 mg orally weekly or biweekly	Excellent control of lesions; convenient	Cumulative hepatic toxicity possible; bone marrow suppression
PUVA	50–480 J/cm twice weekly	No systemic toxicity; useful when coexisting mycosis fungoides	Requires specialized facility; potential for eye injury
Topical carmustine	10 mg in dilute ethanol daily to total body surface for 1 to 4 months; maintenance therapy with 2 to 4 mg/mL 95% ethanol to individual papules	Useful when coexisting mycosis fungoides	Requires familiarity with treatment; skin irritation common; systemic bone marrow suppression possible
Topical mechlorethamine	10 mg in 45 mL of water to skin surface once daily	Safe, useful when coexisting mycosis fungoides	Allergic contact dermatitis common; cutaneous carcinogenesis
Oral antibiotics		Simple to administer	Inadequate control in most patients

complete, or no clinical regression. Extension of atypical cells into the subcutis, characteristic of CD30 lymphoma, seldom occurs in lymphomatoid papulosis. The many small lymphocytes and other inflammatory cells that surround large atypical mononuclear cells in lymphomatoid papulosis are, except for neutrophils, confined to the perimeter of CD30–positive cutaneous lymphomas.

Primary cutaneous Hodgkin's disease is a rare disorder that presents as large dermal and subcutaneous nodules that can regress spontaneously. The abnormal infiltrate of Hodgkin's disease is often in a nodular configuration with diagnostic, often multinucleated Reed-Sternberg cells containing huge inclusion–like eosinophilic nucleoli. The Reed-Sternberg cells are usually positive for Leu-M1(CD15) antigen and negative for leukocyte common antigen (LCA, CD45R0) whereas lymphomatoid papulosis cells are usually CD45R0 positive and CD15 negative.[31]

TREATMENT

Lymphomatoid papulosis is seldom cured by therapy. Therefore, the objective of treatment is to suppress the formation of new lesions and maintain the skin in an improved state. Various treatments have been reported to have some effectiveness in this regard, but the response rate is variable and unpredictable (Table 157–2).

In a minority of patients with mild lymphomatoid papulosis, systemic antibiotics such as tetracycline or erythromycin or conventional ultraviolet phototherapy (UVB) may be effective. Papules may continue to appear during treatment but are often smaller and less numerous than before treatment. The combination of UVB and erythromycin has been an effective combination in some cases.

For most patients who fail to respond to these simple measures, control of lymphomatoid papulosis may be achieved with photochemotherapy or topical mechlorethamine or carmustine (BCNU). Thomsen and Lange Wantzin[22] noted complete clearing or improvement of lesions with psoralens and ultraviolet A therapy (PUVA) at dosages ranging from 50 to 480 J/cm but virtually all patients relapse on cessation of therapy.[22] Vonderheid and colleagues[32] obtained remissions in four of seven patients with daily topical applications of mechlorethamine. Zackheim and coworkers[33] achieved clearing of lesions of lymphomatoid papulosis without side effects by daily application of 10 mg of carmustine in dilute ethanol. These treatments are well tolerated but require special expertise for administration.

For severe lymphomatoid papulosis or disease refractory to other therapies, excellent control can be achieved in more than 90% of cases with low doses of methotrexate.[22, 34] Weekly oral doses (10–20 mg) of methotrexate usually result in complete clearing within several weeks. The doses can then be spaced to maintain an adequate level of control. Some patients respond better to parenteral methotrexate, including those with disease that has become refractory to oral therapy. Thus, most patients can be kept clear or nearly clear of lesions with small oral doses of methotrexate at 10- to 14-day intervals or even

longer.[35] Blood cell counts and liver function tests must be monitored, and liver biopsy is recommended if the results are abnormal or if the cumulative methotrexate dose exceeds 2 g.

Other treatments have been tried in small numbers of patients with lymphomatoid papulosis with equivocal results. Two patients have been treated with oral isotretinoin, 0.5 mg/kg, with partial remission in one and no response in the other.[22] Acyclovir has been administered intravenously to a patient with lymphomatoid papulosis following Hodgkin's disease.[36] Complete clearing of the cutaneous lesions of lymphomatoid papulosis was observed immediately after intravenous injection of acyclovir. The patient had numerous relapses of his skin eruption with complete responses after each course of intravenous acyclovir. Interferon alfa 2b was given to another patient with lymphomatoid papulosis with good results.[37] When 1 mU of interferon alfa 2b was given three times weekly, 0.5-cm lesions disappeared, whereas larger lesions required up to 10 injections. Maintenance therapy of subcutaneous injections of 3 mU given in the abdomen three times a week reduced the number of lesions, which continued to respond to local injection of interferon alfa 2b.

It is important to avoid overtreatment of lymphomatoid papulosis with multiagent chemotherapy, which may result in unwarranted toxicity.[3,38] A transient but only temporary remission of lesions is commonly observed during multiagent chemotherapy or ionizing radiation therapy for lymphoma in patients with lymphomatoid papulosis.[37] Since cytotoxic therapies are immunosuppressive and potentially carcinogenic, they may not be appropriate for the management of uncomplicated disease.[38]

References

1. Macaulay W. Lymphomatoid papulosis: A continuing, self-healing eruption, clinically benign-histologically malignant. Arch Dermatol 1968;97:23–30.
2. Wang H, Lach L, Kadin M. Epidemiology of lymphomatoid papulosis. Cancer 1992;70:2951–2957.
3. Cabanillas F, Armitage J, Pugh W, et al. Lymphomatoid papulosis: A commonly unrecognized benign skin disorder, often misdiagnosed and treated as malignant lymphoma. Submitted for publication.
4. Greene M, Dalager N, Lamberg S, et al. Mycosis fungoides: Epidemiologic observations. Cancer Treat Rep 1979;63:597–606.
5. Blayney D, Blattner W, Robert-Guroff M, et al. The human T-cell leukemia-lymphoma virus in the southeastern United States. JAMA 1983;250:1048–1052.
6. Beljaards R, Willemze R. The prognosis of patients with lymphomatoid papulosis associated with malignant lymphoma. Br J Dermatol 1992;126:596–602.
7. Sanchez N, Pittelkow M, Muller S, et al. The clinicopathologic spectrum of lymphomatoid papulosis: Study of 31 cases. J Am Acad Dermatol 1983;8:81–94.
8. Weinman V, Ackerman A. Lymphomatoid papulosis: A critical review and new findings. Am J Dermatopathol 1981;3:129–163.
9. Paulli M, Berti E, Rosso R, et al. Ki-1/CD30 positive lymphoproliferative disorders of the skin: Clinicopathologic correlation and statistical analysis of 86 cases (abstract). Lab Invest 1994;70:118A.
10. Kadin M, Nasu K, Sako D, et al. Lymphomatoid papulosis: A cutaneous proliferation of activated helper T-cells expressing Hodgkin's disease-associated antigens. Am J Pathol 1985;119:315–325.

11. Weiss L, Wood G, Trela M, et al. Clonal T-cell population in lymphomatoid papulosis: Evidence of a lymphoproliferative origin for a clinically benign disease. N Engl J Med 1986;315:475–479.
12. Kadin M, Vonderheid E, Sako D, et al. Clonal composition of T-cells in lymphomatoid papulosis. Am J Pathol 1987;126:13–17.
13. Whittaker S, Smith N, Jones R, et al. Analysis of B, γ, and T-cell receptor genes in lymphomatoid papulosis: Cellular basis of two distinct histologic subsets. J Invest Dermatol 1991;96:786–791.
14. Chott A, Yockey C, Balk S, et al. The clonality of lymphomatoid papulosis as assessed by cloning and sequencing of TCRγ-chain genes (abstract). Lab Invest 1994;70:105A.
15. Volkenandt M, Bertino J, Shenoy B, et al. Molecular evidence for a clonal relationship between lymphomatoid papulosis and Ki-1 positive anaplastic large cell lymphoma. J Dermatol Sci 1993;6:121–126.
16. Davis T, Morton C, Miller-Cassman R, et al. Hodgkin's disease, lymphomatoid papulosis and cutaneous T-cell lymphoma derived from a common T-cell clone. N Engl J Med 1992;326:1115–1122.
17. Verallo V, Fand S. DNA measurements in lymphomatoid papulosis: Evidence for this new entity. J Invest Dermatol 1969;53:51–57.
18. Willemze R, Meijer C, Van Vloten W, et al. The clinical and histologic spectrum of lymphomatoid papulosis. Br J Dermatol 1982;107:131–144.
19. Espinoza C, Erkman-Balis B, Fenske N. Lymphomatoid papulosis: A premalignant T cell disorder. J Am Acad Dermatol 1985;13:736–743.
20. Sandbank M, Feuerman E. Lymphomatoid papulosis: An electron microscopic study of the acute and healing stages with demonstration of paramyxovirus-like particles. Acta Derm Venereol 1972;52:337–345.
21. Shamsuddin A, Nedwich A, Toker C. Lymphomatoid papulosis: Ultrastructural study with demonstration of intranuclear and intracytoplasmic virus-like particles. Dermatologica 1980;160:238–242.
22. Thomsen K, Lange Wantzin G. Lymphomatoid papulosis: A follow-up of 30 patients. J Am Acad Dermatol 1987;17:632–636.
23. Kadin M. Common activated helper T-cell origin for lymphomatoid papulosis, mycosis fungoides and some types of Hodgkin's disease. Lancet 1985;2:864–865.
24. Kadin M, Vonderheid E, Weiss L. Absence of Epstein-Barr viral RNA in lymphomatoid papulosis. J Pathol 1993;170:145–148.
25. Anagnostopoulos I, Hummel M, Kaudewitz P, et al. Detection of HTLV-1 proviral sequences in CD30-positive large cell cutaneous T-cell lymphomas. Am J Pathol 1990;137:1317–1322.
26. Hidano A, Kawakami M, Yago A. Hypersensitivity to mosquito bite and malignant histiocytosis. Jpn J Exp Med 1982;52:303–306.
27. Smoller B, Longacre T, Warnke R. Ki-1 (CD30) expression in differentiation of lymphomatoid papulosis from arthropod bite reactions. Mod Pathol 1992;5:492–496.
28. Varga F, Vonderheid E, Olbricht S, et al. Immunohistochemical distinction of lymphomatoid papulosis and pityriasis lichenoides et varioliformis acuta. Am J Pathol 1990;136:979–987.
29. Kadin M. Spectrum of Ki-1+ lymphomas. Curr Probl Dermatol 1990;19:132–143.
30. Willemze R, Beljaards R. Spectrum of primary cutaneous CD30 (Ki-1)-positive lymphoproliferative disorders: A proposal for classification and guidelines for management and treatment. J Am Acad Dermatol 1993;28:973–980.
31. Sioutos N, Kerl H, Murphy S, et al. Primary cutaneous Hodgkin's disease: Unique clinical, morphologic, and immunophenotypic findings. Am J Dermatopathol 1994;16:2–8.
32. Vonderheid E, Tan E, Kantor A, et al. Long-term efficacy, curative potential and carcinogenicity of topical mechlorethamine chemotherapy in cutaneous T-cell lymphoma. J Am Acad Dermatol 1989;20:416–428.
33. Zackheim H, Epstein EJ, Crain W. Topical carmustine therapy for lymphomatoid papulosis. Arch Dermatol 1985;121:1410–1414.
34. Lange Wantzin G, Thomsen K. Methotrexate in lymphomatoid papulosis. Br J Dermatol 1984;111:93–95.
35. Vonderheid EC, Sajjadian A, Kadin ME. Methotrexate for lymphomatoid papulosis and other primary cutaneous CD30-positive lymphoproliferative disorders. Submitted for publication.
36. Baumgartner G, Duschet P, Schwarz T, et al. Lymphomatoid papulosis: Remission following intravenously administered acyclovir. Dermatologica 1986;172:305–309.
37. Proctor S, Jackson G, Lemmard J. Lymphomatoid papulosis: Response to treatment with recombinant interferon-α 2b. J Clin Oncol 1992;10:170.
38. Zackheim H, LeBoit P, Gordon R, et al. Lymphomatoid papulosis followed by Hodgkin's lymphoma: Differential response to therapy. Arch Dermatol 1993;129:86–91.

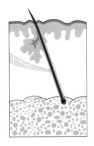

chapter 158

Cutaneous T-Cell Lymphoma

PETER W. HEALD, PHILIP E. SHAPIRO,
JENNIFER F. MADISON, PHILIP E. LEBOIT,
and RICHARD L. EDELSON

DEFINITION

Cutaneous T-cell lymphoma (CTCL) comprises a group of clinicopathologic entities that are neoplastic proliferations of T lymphocytes that home to the skin. Most of these begin as epidermotropic proliferations, but eventually the cells may lose their dependence on an epidermal environment for growth, and spread to the dermis, lymph nodes, blood, and viscera. Included in the spectrum of CTCL are such classically described conditions as mycosis fungoides, in which lesions evolve from patches to plaques and tumors, and Sézary's syndrome, in which the cells of CTCL circulate in the peripheral blood in large numbers and cause erythroderma. The concept of CTCL accounts for patients who evolve from mycosis fungoides to Sézary's syndrome, or vice versa.

In the last few years, it has become apparent that some normal T lymphocytes bear antigens on their cell membranes that enable them to migrate to the skin via specific binding to cutaneous endothelial cells. This realization has furthered the concept of "cutaneous T cells" and their malignant counterparts.

CLINICAL DESCRIPTION

Lymphomas of cutaneous T cells produce a wide variety of clinical and pathologic changes. Various clinicopathologic entities have been described, largely without reference to the overall spectrum of disease. Thus, one finds names of French clinicians, German cities, Greek letters, obscure antibodies, clinical findings, histologic terms, and immunopathologic terms in the names of CTCL syndromes. The following classification is based primarily on clinical morphology but also correlates with

pathobiology, inasmuch as the progression from patches and plaques to tumors and erythroderma is associated with loss of epidermotropism, greater cytologic atypia, immunophenotypic alterations, and a poorer prognosis.

Patches and Plaques

CTCL in which lesions evolve from patches into plaques and ultimately into tumors is termed *mycosis fungoides* and was initially described by Alibert.[1] Early lesions are typically dry, slightly scaly, pink lesions that can exhibit telangiectasia and atrophy. They tend to be broad, usually measuring at least several centimeters across, and distributed somewhat asymmetrically. There is a predilection for areas of skin that are protected by two layers of clothing such as the buttocks and breasts, but lesions can occur anywhere. The eruption may be intensely pruritic or asymptomatic and occasionally may be transitory, disappearing spontaneously without scarring. Often a patient will recall a preceding "chronic dermatitis" for 10 to 20 years that may have been considered as "therapeutically resistant" chronic contact dermatitis, atopic dermatitis, psoriasis, eczema, or neurodermatitis. Of 211 patients studied by the Mycosis Fungoides Cooperative Study Group, 77% were reported to have had antecedent, noninfectious skin conditions, 32% of which were diagnosed as "dermatitis, not otherwise specified."[2] Some patients with patch-stage lesions have traditionally been said to have *large plaque parapsoriasis* or *parapsoriasis en plaques*, terms that have been used to avoid labeling the patient with the diagnosis of a lymphoma, either because of uncertainty or because patch-stage disease is indolent and does not always progress to the plaque or tumor stage. As criteria for the histologic diagnosis of early patch-stage mycosis fungoides have become more precise, it is preferable to use the term CTCL where appropriate, and to simply express uncertainty as to the diagnosis if changes are not clear-cut.

The patch stage may last for months or years before progressing to the plaque stage, or plaques may appear to arise de novo. Plaques of CTCL appear as elevated, scaly, indurated lesions that may be sharply demarcated and are often discoid in shape (Fig. 158–1). In each patient, the lesions tend to be of uniform color, ranging from an erythematous to a violaceous hue. Occasionally, the plaques are quite scaly, simulating psoriasis, or are associated with crusts or papules. Plaques may spontaneously regress or may coalesce to form large plaques with annular, arcuate, or serpiginous borders, and may clear centrally with disease activity remaining at the periphery of the lesion, producing a geographic appearance (Fig. 158–2).

Erythroderma

Erythrodermic CTCL was first described by Besnier and Hallopeau in 1892.[3] In 1938, Sézary and Bouvrain described patients with generalized exfoliating erythroderma, intense pruritus, peripheral lymphadenopathy, and abnormal hyperchromatic mononuclear cells in the skin and peripheral blood.[4] These atypical circulating lymphocytes, termed *cellules monstreuses* (monster cells) by Sézary, are now referred to as Sézary cells. The term *Sézary syndrome* is best applied to patients with leukocytosis and Sézary cells. Erythrodermic CTCL is a broader term that encompasses all stages of erythrodermic and leukemic disease, whether or not Sézary cells are identified in the blood. When erythrodermic CTCL begins, there is widespread skin involvement and there is peripheral blood involvement, although the latter may not be apparent on a complete blood count. This is because the malignant lymphocytes may appear morphologically normal, and because they tend to replace normal lymphocytes, resulting in a total lymphocyte count that is not elevated. As the disease progresses and

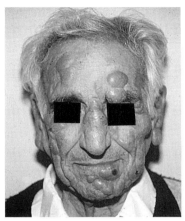

FIGURE 158–2. Plaques and nodules of cutaneous T-cell lymphoma (CTCL) on the face of a patient with the mycosis fungoides variant.

full-blown Sézary syndrome appears, there may be markedly depressed levels of normal circulation T cells and very little normal immunity left.[5] Indeed, Sézary's patients died of infection rather than of progressive disease.

Clinically, erythrodermic CTCL may start de novo, or appear after established plaque or tumor stage disease (Fig. 158–3). The erythroderma is usually generalized, but isolated areas of normal skin may be present. Pruritus is often intense, resulting in excoriation and exudation. The patient may have fever, chills, weight loss, malaise, and overwhelming pruritus. There may be scaling and fissuring of palms and soles, alopecia, ectropion, nail dystrophy, and ankle edema. These result in pain on walking and poor manual dexterity. Such patients become cutaneous cripples, being severely debilitated by the skin manifestations of this fatal disease. After a variable time, some patients with the erythrodermic form of CTCL develop tumors.

Tumors

Tumors generally arise at sites of previous skin involvement by CTCL but may occur in clinically normal skin. Nodules or tumors of CTCL are usually reddish

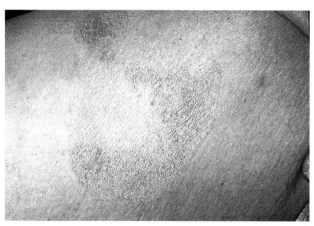

FIGURE 158–1. Patch-plaque lesion with discoid shape and arciform configuration.

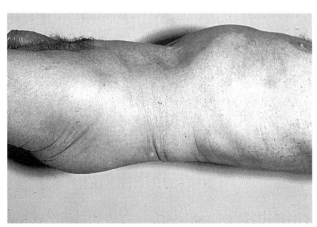

FIGURE 158–3. Erythrodermic CTCL.

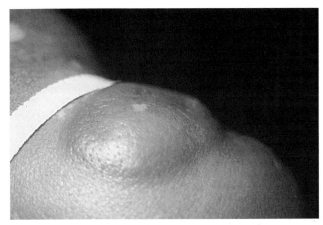

FIGURE 158-4. A tumor of CTCL with a smooth surface. The overlying epidermis shows only a hint of involvement, with hypopigmentation.

brown or purplish red. They may be smooth-surfaced (Fig. 158-4) but can become ulcerated with or without superinfection. Tumors may occur anywhere but have a predilection for the face and body folds—axillae, groin, antecubital fossae, neck, and in women, the inframammary area. Spontaneous resolution of tumors is observed but is quite rare. Their appearance in areas of long-standing plaques suggests local evolution of more aggressive subclones of malignant cells resulting in a "vertical growth phase" analogous to that described in melanoma. The occurrence of tumors de novo suggests spread by cells of an aggressive malignant T-cell clone.

Variations

In some examples of patch-stage CTCL, the clinical picture is dominated by a poikilodermatous appearance, in which there are atrophy and telangiectasis, often with hypo- or hyperpigmentation. This poikilodermatous form of CTCL is also known as poikiloderma vasculare atrophicans. It has been hypothesized to represent partial regression of the lymphoma due to an active host response.[6] Poikiloderma is not specific for CTCL, occurring in conditions such as dermatomyositis and radiation dermatitis, but its presence should raise the possibility of CTCL if it is distributed primarily on the trunk and pelvic girdle.

Alopecia mucinosa is a term applied to plaques that are clinically associated with alopecia and histologically associated with collections of mucin in follicular epithelium. Because these plaques occur on sites other than the scalp and alopecia may not be apparent, the term follicular mucinosis is often used. Follicular mucinosis manifests clinically as indurated plaques with superimposed follicular papules from which a gelatinous material can occasionally be expressed. The plaques may be solitary or multiple. Such lesions may be the presenting sign of CTCL, or they may develop in a patient with an established diagnosis of CTCL. Follicular mucinosis also occurs outside the setting of CTCL, as an idiopathic benign condition. CTCL-associated follicular mucinosis

can be distinguished from the benign idiopathic variety only if the patient has other changes that are diagnostic of CTCL, either in the lesion or in concurrent lesions. In the absence of such findings, especially in children or if the lesions begin on the head and neck, follicular mucinosis is usually the benign, idiopathic variety, but follow-up may be required to make that distinction with certainty.[7, 8]

Pagetoid reticulosis or Woringer-Kolopp disease most often presents as a solitary verrucous plaque on acral skin. The long duration, and slow growth of the disease are characteristic.[9-14] The term *pagetoid reticulosis* derives from the characteristic pattern of epidermal involvement, with many lymphocytes in the epidermis, producing a picture reminiscent of Paget's disease. There is a disseminated (Ketron-Goodman) form of pagetoid reticulosis that has many of the pathologic features of the classic form but has a less favorable prognosis.[9, 15, 16]

Granulomatous slack skin is a form of CTCL in which the lymphocytic infiltrate is associated with a granulomatous component and destruction of cutaneous elastic tissue. Patients with this condition develop large regions of lax skin, especially in the axillae and groins. Female patients have shown a tendency for breast destruction by the disease. Many patients with granulomatous slack skin are said to develop Hodgkin's disease, although detailed studies to ensure that they have not simply developed anaplastic T-cell lymphoma have not been published.[17-19]

Hypopigmented mycosis fungoides is a variant of patch or early plaque-stage mycosis fungoides that is seen in dark-skinned patients. Individual lesions have been confused with vitiligo on clinical grounds, although the distribution of lesions provides a clue to the correct diagnosis. In areas such as the Malaysian peninsula, this may be the most common presentation of patch-stage mycosis fungoides. Patients respond to therapy by repigmenting, and relapse is often heralded by a return of the hypopigmentation.[20-26]

Some patients with CTCL have lesions resembling those of a pigmented purpuric eruption.[27] In fact, the first patient in the North American literature that was reported to have lichen aureus[28] was later reported to have CTCL.[29] Patients with such lesions tend to have their disease distributed in a fashion similar to other types of patch-stage CTCL.

There are rare examples of CTCL with blisters[30, 31] or pustules.[32, 33] There are also a few reports of verrucous plaques,[34] some of which could also be categorized as examples of pagetoid reticulosis. Ulceration of plaques due to vasculitis has also been described.[35, 36]

Some examples of papuloerythroderma (Ofuji) may represent a variant of CTCL.[37-39] Papuloerythroderma was first described in 1984 and is characterized by eosinophilia, papules that coalesce, and erythroderma that spares skin folds, producing the "deck chair" sign (Fig. 158-5).[40-42]

The variations of CTCL mentioned above were described primarily as a result of their morphologic appearance. Variations of CTCL have also been described as a result of immunophenotypic analysis. The vast majority of CTCLs are malignancies of cells with immunologic

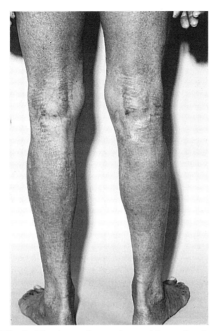

FIGURE 158–5. The legs of a patient with erythrodermic CTCL demonstrating the "deck chair sign" or "folded luggage sign." These terms refer to the creases of normal skin in natural skin folds, as shown here about the popliteal fossae.

Finally, a variant of CTCL described in just a few patients is gamma-delta T-cell lymphoma. These lymphomas were discovered as a result of investigation of "double negative" CTCL patients, that is, patients with malignant T cells that lacked both the CD4 and CD8 antigens. The CD4 and CD8 antigens are associated with the alpha-beta T-cell receptor complex, which is expressed on most mature T cells. By contrast, most mature human T cells do not express the gamma-delta receptor, although some such cells, whose function is unknown, have been found in normal human skin. Various morphologic features have been described in patients with cutaneous lymphomas of gamma-delta T cells,[46, 47] including spontaneously regressing subcutaneous and dermal tumors,[48] and patches and plaques with ulcerated plaques or nodules.[49, 50]

PATHOLOGY

There is a wide spectrum of histologic findings in cutaneous T-cell lymphoma, and the features in a particular biopsy are partially dependent on the type of clinical

and phenotypic characteristics of helper T cells (CD4+). There are some examples, however, where the malignant cells express the suppressor phenotype (CD8+). One form is very similar to that often seen with CD4+ CTCL, with a chronic course of patches and plaques and expression of the pan T-cell antigen CD2 but not CD7.[43] Other patients with CD8+ CTCL have been reported to have an aggressive, therapy-resistant disease characterized by papulonodular lesions, ulcers, and involvement of the palms and soles (Fig. 158–6).[43, 44] The immunophenotype of the cells in this variant is characteristically CD2 negative and CD7 positive.[43] A patient with this type of CD8+ CTCL and angiodestructive lesions has been described.[45]

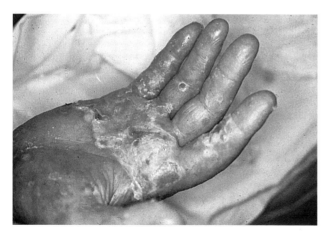

FIGURE 158–6. Nodular ulcerative lesions of CD8-positive CTCL. Lesions on the palms and soles are characteristically found in this variant.

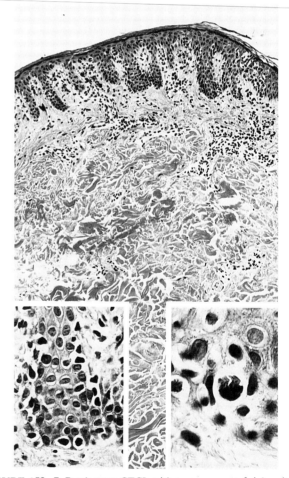

FIGURE 158–7. Patch-stage CTCL with a sparse, superficial perivascular lymphocytic infiltrate and slight epidermotropism without spongiosis. Left inset shows lymphocytes along the basal layer. Right inset shows a highly convoluted, "cerebriform" lymphocyte. (From Shapiro PE, Pinto F. The histologic spectrum of mycosis fungoides/Sézary syndrome (cutaneous T-cell lymphoma). Am J Surg Pathol 1994; 18:645–667.)

lesion from which the biopsy was taken.[6, 34, 51] Patches of CTCL typically show a sparse or moderately dense, perivascular or slightly lichenoid lymphocytic infiltrate most prominent around the superficial plexus (Fig. 158–7). There is usually epidermotropism, with little or no spongiosis, and a tendency of lymphocytes to be located along the basal layer. Cytologic atypia is not striking, but lymphocytes may be slightly enlarged, hyperconvoluted, and/or hyperchromatic, particularly those in the epidermis.[6, 51, 52] Pautrier's microabscesses, which are composed of a tightly packed cluster of lymphocytes surrounded by a clear space, are a fairly specific finding, although not present in the majority of biopsies.

Plaques of CTCL show similar changes to those in patch-stage lesions, but the infiltrates are more likely to be lichenoid, denser, and containing eosinophils and/or plasma cells (Fig. 158–8). The papillary dermis is expanded and contains collagen bundles that are coarse, due to the chronicity of the disease. Hyperkeratosis is more apparent, usually laminated and/or compact with subtle parakeratosis. Psoriasiform epidermal hyperplasia may be present.

The histologic features of the erythrodermic stage are varied. Sometimes the histopathologic picture resembles that seen in patch- or plaque-stage disease, but with less epidermotropism and, occasionally, with more spongiosis. In such cases, the diagnosis is more easily made by study of lymphocytes in peripheral blood (see Diagnosis and Differential Diagnosis).

Tumors of CTCL feature dense diffuse or nodular infiltrates (Fig. 158–9). In some patients, a polymorphous infiltrate is present, similar to that seen in the plaque stage but denser and deeper. In other patients, the

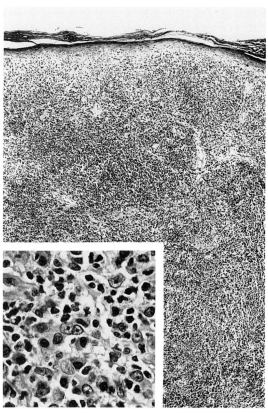

FIGURE 158–9. A tumor of CTCL with a dense diffuse infiltrate of atypical lymphocytes. Inset shows small as well as medium-sized to large atypical lymphocytes. Some large cells resemble immunoblasts, with large nucleoli and somewhat clear nuclei.

infiltrates are monomorphous, composed almost exclusively of neoplastic cells. Epidermotropism may be present in tumors, but it is found less frequently than in patch- or plaque-stage lesions, suggesting that the malignant T cells in tumors are less dependent on the epidermal microenvironment for growth. Transitions between these histologic variants and evolution from epidermotropic to nonepidermotropic variants in the same patient have been observed.

The cells of tumor-stage CTCL nearly always have striking nuclear atypia. Some biopsy specimens contain moderately enlarged, hyperconvoluted nuclei with diffuse nuclear hyperchromasia, whereas other biopsy specimens feature large vesicular nuclei and prominent nucleoli, a finding termed *blastic transformation*.[53] The cells of tumor-stage CTCL can resemble those of a variety of T-cell lymphomas that affect lymph nodes—including medium and large cell pleomorphic, and large cell anaplastic lymphoma using the classification of Suchi and Lennert.[54] Whether classification along these lines provides prognostic information awaits further study. Immunophenotypically, cells in these "transformed" lesions may show loss of some T-cell antigens, and acquisition of new antigens, such as CD15 (Leu M1) and CD30 (Ki-1), on the majority of cells, which may correlate with a poor prognosis.[55, 56] Despite the evolution of bizarre appearing cells in tumor-stage lesions, studies of clonality reveal that they represent the same

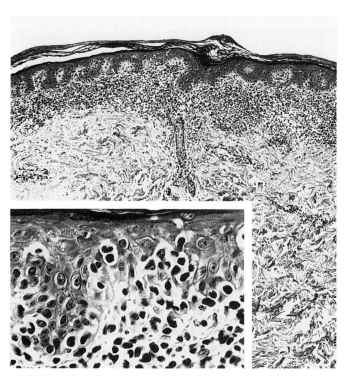

FIGURE 158–8. Plaque-stage CTCL with a band-like infiltrate unassociated with vacuolar alteration. Inset shows epidermotropism without spongiosis.

lineage as the smaller cells in patches and plaques from the same patient.[57]

Some clinical variants of CTCL show specific histologic features. In poikilodermatous CTCL, atrophy is associated with telangiectases, pigment incontinence, fibrosis, and sometimes subtle vacuolar alteration (Fig. 158–10). Epidermotropism and cytologic atypia may be present but tend not to be extensive, sometimes precluding a specific diagnosis on histologic grounds alone.

In follicular mucinosis, mucin and lymphocytes are present in follicular epithelium; associated features of CTCL (e.g., epidermotropism without spongiosis, lymphocytic atypia) may or may not be present. CTCL can show involvement not only of hair follicles and sebaceous glands, but of eccrine glands as well.[58, 59]

In pagetoid reticulosis there is verrucous epidermal hyperplasia coupled with even more striking epidermotropism than is usually found in CTCL. The lower half of the epidermis is permeated by lymphocytes with large irregular nuclei, and retraction of the cytoplasm of lymphocytes from neighboring keratinocytes often gives the impression that the lymphocytes are surrounded by halos.[9] Few eosinophils or plasma cells are present in the dermal infiltrates of pagetoid reticulosis, and in some cases it seems as if all of the atypical lymphocytes are contained within the epidermis. Pagetoid reticulosis also has distinctive immunohistochemical features—its cells express very low levels of CD45, or leukocyte common antigen and its related epitopes, CD45RA and CD45RO.[60] This can lead to its misdiagnosis if a page-

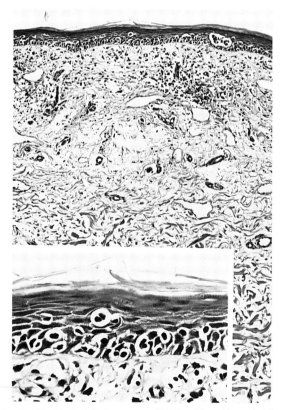

FIGURE 158–10. Poikilodermatous CTCL with epidermal thinning and flattening, telangiectases, papillary dermal fibrosis, and lymphocytes along the basal layer.

toid neoplasm is evaluated by a pathologist using a panel of antisera that does not contain the pan–T-cell antigen CD3, which is indeed present on these cells.

Granulomatous slack skin is characterized histologically by dense lichenoid or diffuse infiltrates of lymphocytes associated with collections of epithelioid histiocytes.[19] The histiocytes may contain huge numbers of nuclei, and may dominate the histologic picture, resulting in misdiagnosis as sarcoidosis or an infectious granuloma. Elastic tissue stain reveals marked diminution or absence of elastic fibers, which allows for the slack skin appearance noted clinically. Although Hodgkin's disease is said to eventuate in some patients with granulomatous slack skin, Reed-Sternberg and Hodgkin's cells are not found in its cutaneous infiltrates. Although granulomatous slack skin represents a striking clinical and histologic appearance, it is rare. A more common finding in biopsies of CTCL is the presence of a less obvious granulomatous component, consisting of a few scattered or clustered multinucleated histiocytes, or an interstitial pattern of histiocytes as can be seen in granuloma annulare.

Biopsy specimens of hypopigmented CTCL resemble those of patch-stage lesions that are not hypopigmented, but with diminished pigment in keratinocytes, presumably as a consequence of degenerative changes in melanocytes caused by lymphocytes.[21]

The variant of CTCL that clinically resembles a pigmented purpuric eruption is characterized histologically by a perivascular and interstitial, often lichenoid infiltrate of lymphocytes, with many extravasated erythrocytes. This is an exaggeration of the slight purpura seen in almost a third of biopsies of patch-plaque CTCL.[51] Distinction between this variant of CTCL and a true pigmented purpuric eruption can be facilitated by the presence of lymphocytes in the epidermis, especially if atypical or lining the basal layer. However, epidermotropism can occur in true pigmented purpuric eruptions, and clinicopathologic correlation is usually required to make certain distinctions.

Bullous CTCL is usually associated histologically with a subepidermal blister, although subcorneal and intraepidermal blisters have been reported. Usually there are other histologically typical features of CTCL in the biopsies, and the bullae may arise simply due to epidermal damage in areas of prominent epidermotropism. However, some lesions have been "cell poor," with negative immunofluorescent studies, and thus the etiology of bullae in CTCL is not entirely clear.[30, 31]

Very uncommonly, pustules are encountered in biopsies of patients with CTCL.[32, 33] Sometimes, this is due to coexistence of another disease, such as psoriasis, but rarely, it appears to be an intrinsic part of the disease. Biopsies show pustules at a subcorneal or slightly lower level, superimposed on changes of CTCL.

Verrucous lesions of CTCL show some overlap with examples of pagetoid reticulosis, and the epidermal hyperplasia and epidermotropism may be pathogenetically related. The epidermal hyperplasia can be so extensive that it produces a pseudocarcinomatous appearance.[34]

Biopsies of plaques of CTCL with ulceration due to necrotizing vasculitis, which occurred in patients with

CD4+ CTCL, showed epidermotropism and a perivascular or lichenoid lymphocytic infiltrate with fibrinoid necrosis of small blood vessels associated with neutrophils and nuclear dust or infiltration by atypical cells.[35, 36] Necrosis of a small artery due to occlusion by neoplastic lymphocytes has also been described.[51]

Biopsies of lesions of CD8+ CTCL have been associated with prominent epidermotropism.[43, 44] Biopsies from patients with the more aggressive form of the disease tend to show more acanthosis, including pseudocarcinomatous hyperplasia, more dermal involvement, and greater cytologic atypia, but these findings may be more reflective of the progress of the disease rather than the "type" of CD8+ CTCL, and there is no evidence that different forms of CD8+ CTCL can be distinguished from one another or from CD4+ CTCL on the basis of routine histologic examination.[43] The patient with angioinvasive and angiodestructive CD8+ CTCL showed a typical biopsy of plaque stage CTCL with the additional finding of occlusion of blood vessels in the upper and mid-dermis by atypical lymphocytes, with fibrinoid necrosis.[45]

In patients with gamma-delta T-cell lymphoma and primarily subcutaneous disease, biopsies have shown infiltrates of medium-sized or large atypical lymphocytes in the subcutis and dermis in a nodular or perivascular pattern, without epidermotropism.[46-48] By contrast, patients with gamma-delta T-cell lymphoma that manifested clinically as plaques had biopsies with prominent epidermotropism,[50] in one case associated with pronounced epidermal necrosis that suggested that the malignant cells were cytotoxic,[49] which is consistent with the observation that double negative T cells can lyse target cells with natural killer-like cytotoxicity.[61]

PATHOGENESIS AND ETIOLOGY

The clinical phenotype of cutaneous lymphoma can be viewed as the pathologic exaggeration of a physiologic process. An understanding of relevant aspects of T-cell and cutaneous immunology is important in the study of this disease.

The thymus is the primary site of T-cell differentiation. T cells are principally responsible for cell-mediated immunity and can be characterized by functional assays and by their surface proteins. Well-defined T-cell–associated antigens are summarized in Table 158–1. After a lymphocyte differentiates to become a T cell in the thymic medulla, it typically expresses the "pan–T-cell" antigens CD2+, CD3+, and co-expresses CD4 and CD8. In the thymic cortex it differentiates to become either a CD4+ helper cell or a CD8+ suppressor cell. The T-cell then circulates primarily in the vascular system that perfuses lymph nodes. Antigen-presenting cells home to lymph nodes draining inflammatory sites. In the lymph node, antigen presentation occurs via the T-cell receptor–mediated activation of previously naive (or virgin) T cells. At this point T cells change their expression of CD45 to the isoform known as CD45RO. CD45RO+CD4+ lymphocytes are thus referred to as "memory" helper T cells because they have already been specifically activated.

Memory T cells travel through the extravascular lymph system and traverse regions of the lymph nodes that are devoid of virgin cells. Reserve (naive) cells are thus largely in the recruitable circulation and the more valuable memory cells are on patrol.[62]

The tertiary sites of T-cell differentiation are in specialized environments such as the skin. The skin has a reserve of cytokines that can act on T cells and adhesion molecules that facilitate their differentiation. Only those lymphocytes with homing receptors for the cutaneous vascular adhesion molecules known as adressins have access to the skin. Lymphocytes that home to the skin differ from lymphocytes found in other organs in that they express the epitope known as cutaneous lymphoid antigen (CLA).[63] In CTCL, the cells of the epidermotropic stage express CLA whereas those of the nonepidermotropic tumor stage do not.

The CLA epitope on the membranes of T cells binds to endothelial lymphocyte adhesion molecule-1 (ELAM-1),[64] which is expressed on venules and undoubtedly plays a role in facilitating the passage of lymphocytes from the circulation to the skin. This surface protein also appears after specific T-cell receptor–mediated activation of a specific skin-homing lymphocyte. CLA-expressing cells in the circulation are memory cells readily recruitable to sites of cutaneous inflammation.

The following scenario illustrates some of the cellular aspects of cutaneous immunity. The immune response to an insult consists of a rapid nonspecific response fol-

TABLE 158–1. Antigens Commonly Associated with T Cells

Marker	Cells	Description
CD2	T cells	Adhesion molecule, present on most mature T cells, often lost in transformation
CD3	T cells	Transduces the activation signal from the antigen receptor
CD4	Helper T cell monocytes	Binds to Class II major histocompatability complex
CD8	Suppressor T cells	Binds to Class I major histocompatability complex
CD25	Activated T cells	IL-2 receptor (Tac), induced by HTLV-1
CD30	Activated T cells	Ki-1 marker, found in anaplastic T-cell lymphomas, lymphomatoid papulosis
CD45	Leukocyte common	Isoforms of CD45 appear with T-cell antigen activation
CD45RO	Memory cells	Irreversibly formed after T cell activation
CLA-1	Skin associated lymphocytes	Homing receptor that binds ELAM-1
TCR	T cells	Two varieties: alpha-beta and gamma-delta. These are proteins that bind specific antigens
V-beta	T cells	Variable region specific antibodies (approx. 45 different regions)

TCR, T-cell receptor.

lowed by the amplification of a specific immune response. Nonspecific responses rely on cytokines, endothelial cells, neutrophils, and monocyte-macrophages. Presumably, cytokines induce adhesion molecules and set up diffusion gradients to bring in the cells of the nonspecific response. But there are also adhesion molecules on cutaneous endothelial cells that are up-regulated to induce the egress of cutaneous lymphocytes. When appropriately presented with antigens, they become activated. Antigen-presenting cells also migrate to lymph nodes, draining the sites of inflammation to allow recruitment of lymphocytes. These recruited cells can then be directed back to the cutaneous site of inflammation by way of their skin-homing receptors. Cutaneous sites of inflammation are characterized by up-regulation of endothelial adressins, proteins that are specific for the cutaneous lymphocytes, recognized by the homing proteins on T cells.

These considerations have led to the concept of a cutaneous T cell. Clone-specific antibodies are available for identifying malignant cells in a few patients with CTCL (see below). Using these antibodies in patients with the leukemic CTCL, investigators have been able to clearly show that the circulating malignant cells are CD45RO+CLA+.[65] The diverse clinical entities that comprise CTCL can be grouped together because they are lymphomas of cutaneous T cells.

T-cell surface protein expression is not the only way to define subsets of T cells. A functional division of T cells can be based on the cytokines that they produce. The helper T-cell-1(Th1) type refers to a T cell that makes gamma-delta interferon and interleukin-2. A helper T cell -2(Th2) type produces interleukins 4, 6, and 10. Both resting and stimulated cells from the blood of patients with leukemic CTCL make cytokines of the Th2 type.[66] Although profiles of cytokine production have been obtained from only a few patients, the findings to date are consistent with the hypergammaglobulinemia (interleukins 4 and 6) and eosinophilia (interleukin 5, also made by Th2 cells) typical of patients with CTCL. Thus, the most commonly encountered malignant cutaneous T cell is a Th2 CD45RO+CLA+ T cell.

CTCL progresses from early lesions in which inflammatory cells can outnumber neoplastic ones, to late monomorphous collections of cytologically atypical lymphocyte cells or to the leukemic death of a patient. The dynamic interplay of the malignant cells, the skin, and the nonmalignant portions of the immune system contributes to the clinical picture of progressive disease.[67]

Early in the evolution of CTCL, the inflammatory response associated with lesions often obscures the diagnosis. The cause of this inflammation is twofold because it is produced by the pro-inflammatory nature of the CTCL cells and by the inflammatory aspects of the antitumor response. The patient's response may even be successful in completely destroying the lesion, leading to spontaneous remission of the individual lesion. Over time the immune response may weaken and the disease is allowed to grow unchecked. The importance of the antitumor response is emphasized by the previous discussion of the association between immunosuppression,

whether from cyclosporine or human immunodeficiency virus, and advanced CTCL.

CTCL may also progress by spreading from the skin to the peripheral blood. Serial studies of the keratinocyte membrane proteins of a patient who progressed from primary skin involvement to a leukemic picture provide insight into this process. During this transition, the keratinocyte surface protein intercellular adhesion molecule-1 (ICAM-1), which may attract lymphocytes to the epidermis, became undetectable. Thus, with decreasing affinity of the epidermis for the lymphocytes, leukemia may ensue.[68] The reticuloendothelial system involved in monitoring circulating cells fails in patients with Sézary syndrome. This failure could result from more aggressive subclones expressing lower amounts of surface proteins as has been observed with tumor progression.[55, 69] Another possibility is that the tumor-related immunosuppression (discussed later) reduces the ability of the host to respond to circulating cells.

CTCL is characterized by the evolution of a polymorphous infiltrate of several types of T cells to a monomorphous infiltrate. One way of observing this is to assess the CD4/CD8 ratio in skin. As the CTCL progresses, the proportion of CD4+ cells climbs to over 90%. Nonneoplastic cells, including reactive CD8+ cells, disappear from the skin.[70]

A similar phenomenon occurs in the peripheral blood. This can be demonstrated with beta-chain variable region antibodies. T cells that have rearranged their alpha and beta T-cell receptor genes express a single variable region beta-chain protein. Normally, none of the variable region antibodies reacts with more than 5% of circulating peripheral blood lymphocytes. A clonal expansion in the peripheral blood can easily be detected if an existing variable region antibody reacts with that clone. At the moment, antisera are only available to less than 25% of the variable regions, limiting the diagnostic utility of this technique. Similar to the skin, the peripheral blood shows a gradual replacement of normal lymphocytes by CTCL cells.[5] This phenomenon can lead to several surprising findings.

Results in six patients (whose clones were reactive with a variable-region antibody) are shown in Table 158–2. The alarming finding is that even with normal range white blood counts, these patients have markedly decreased numbers of circulating nonmalignant cells. For example, in a patient who had 64% CTCL cells, only 13% of the circulating lymphocytes were nonneoplastic, giving that patient a pathologically low number of normal T cells.[5] Does this nonmalignant lymphopenia explain the T-cell immunodeficiencies that clinically occur? CTCL patients have an increased rate of second malignancies;[71] Kaposi's varicelliform eruption;[72] tinea infection; pneumocystis carinii;[73] and cryptococcosis.[74] The loss of normal cells, schematized in Figure 158–11, may also play an accelerating role in the progression of CTCL. Because normal CD8 (and CD4) bearing cells are pivotal to the antitumor response, their depletion weakens this defense. The assessment of nonmalignant lymphopenia is discussed later in the section on staging and prognosis. This CTCL-induced immunodeficiency (as shown in Table

TABLE 158-2. Loss of Normal T Cells in Patients with Normal Range TLC

Patient	TLC c/mm³	CD4/CD8	Sézary cell (%)	V-Beta (%)	CD3 (%)	Normal T cell (c/mm³)
1	7184	50	32	67	92	1796
2	794	10	10	82	75	0
3	684	13	7	74	88	95
4	3276	17	9	78	82	131
5	5160	90	13	87	90	155
6	3650	14	5	59	91	1131
Range of normals	1500– 3000	.53– 3.77	0	0–5	54–81	800–2000

TLC, total lymphocyte count.

158–2 and Fig. 158–11) results in a loss of the T-cell reserve of patients. Immunophenotyping can demonstrate this occurrence earlier in skin lesions than in the peripheral blood. Thus, the tumor removes the host ability to sustain an antitumor response. Immunosuppression becomes an accelerating factor in the progression of the disease. Being aware of the T-cell deficiency helps clinicians in the differential diagnosis of findings encountered in the staging of patients.

Bacterial skin colonization and infections can exacerbate CTCL. The skin of patients with CTCL is often heavily colonized and antibiotics often improve many symptoms. In Japan, infestation with strongyloides is recognized to accelerate the course of retrovirus-associated adult T-cell lymphoma/leukemia. With an abundance of clonally expanded T cells in their skin, CTCL patients are vulnerable to anything that might activate and stimulate these T cells, such as a bacterial superantigen. Recently, a series of immunologically active bacterial proteins has been designated as superantigens. Superantigen stimulation of human and mouse T cells is restricted to particular T-cell receptor beta-chain variable gene segments. Superantigens bind to major histocompatibility class II molecules to mimic antigen presentation to the T cell by way of the T-cell receptor. It is likely

that some pathologic effects of these toxins are caused by their ability to activate T cells. CTCL cells have been shown to be selectively stimulated by specific bacterial superantigens.[75] Inasmuch as many of these proteins are found in skin-colonizing bacteria, it is possible they play a role in disease progression.

A retrovirus has been suggested as a cause of CTCL because of the similarities to adult T-cell lymphoma, and epidermotropic lymphoma that arises from a retroviral infection. The incubation period of the HTLV-1 virus extends into the fifth decade of life. The lure of finding tumor-associated virus in CTCL has attracted retroviral researchers to the field. The identification (by isolation and partial sequencing) of the putative HTLV-V was briefly in the limelight, and electron micrographs have purported the existence of a mycosis fungoides virus.[76] Leukemic CTCL cells from erythrodermic CTCL patients were found to contain viral transactivators.[77] Partially deleted HTLV-1 provirus was found in a cell line established from a patient with CTCL.[78] However, the relative lack of clustering of mycosis fungoides is a feature distinguishing that disease from HTLV-1–induced adult T-cell lymphoma.

Immunosuppression is associated with the development of CTCL, suggesting that active immunity against the development of cutaneous T-cell clones in the skin is a vital defense that, when compromised, leads to fatal outcomes. Patients infected with human immunodeficiency virus can develop CTCL.[79] Clinical observation has also shown that immunosuppression plays an accelerating role. Cyclosporine is an immunosuppressive medication that has not been successful with CTCL. When used, there has been rapid acceleration of disease.[80] Now that immunosuppressive regimens have been successful in prolonging organ transplants, there are patients reported with post-transplant T-cell lymphomas of skin.[81]

Karyotyping studies have been performed in CTCL in order to determine if a reproducible alteration that might account for its pathogenesis is present, as occurs with some malignancies. Although clonal chromosomal abnormalities have been described[82] and an association has been suggested between CTCL and rearrangements involving chromosome 10, which bears the gene for the interleukin-2 receptor, a consistently present alteration that accounts for the pathogeneis has not been found.[83]

The possibility that occupation or contact with chemi-

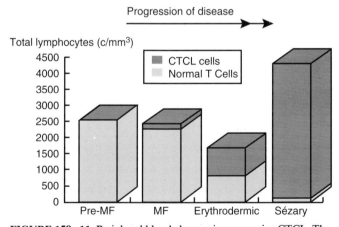

FIGURE 158–11. Peripheral blood changes in progressive CTCL. The progression of erythrodermic CTCL is depicted as inferred from the data in Table 158–2. The y-axis is the total lymphocyte count, which does not increase until significant amounts of the normal T cells are destroyed while the malignant clone expands. (MF, mycosis fungoides.)

cal is involved in the causation of CTCL has been explored in several epidemiologic studies. These studies have largely included patients specifically referred to tertiary centers, and as a result, there are conflicting findings regarding risk factors. Occupational exposure to hazardous chemicals was recorded in 30% of patients of the Mycosis Fungoides Cooperative Study Group.[84] A smaller survey found an increased relative risk for those in manufacturing or construction,[85] as did a retrospective survey of one country's 20-year experience with CTCL.[86] However, a telephone survey of several tertiary centers could find no correlation with occupation, although the data were weakened by a high drop-out rate.[87] An example of the difficulty of such surveys is exemplified by the latter, which showed that being in the paper industry had a protective effect. The sporadic reportings of clustered cases often suggest certain settings are involved in the disease. For example, several workers at a solid-fuel propellant plant developed mycosis fungoides.[88]

Aging contributes to the development of CTCL. Age-related increases of CTCL have been reported along with an increase in the incidence of CTCL overall. In a review of several cancer registries over an 11-year period an increase in incidence was clearly shown without an increase in survival probability. The latter finding is consistent with the increase not being due to improved detection methods. The incidence of the disease is age related, from a low of .05 cases/100,000/year for under age 40 to 1.28/100,000/year for patients 70 to 79 years old.[89]

Familial clusterings of CTCL are rare. Those reported to date are: father-daughter,[90] mother-daughter,[91] and brother-sister.[92] Hearsay examples have been passed along,[90] but not documented. A relative lack of familial or geographic clustering argues against a single causative agent of CTCL.

DIAGNOSIS AND DIFFERENTIAL DIAGNOSIS

The differential diagnosis of CTCL depends on the clinical presentation. Patch-stage lesions can be difficult to distinguish from chronic allergic contact or nummular dermatitis, and rarely from drug eruptions. Erythrodermic CTCL needs to be distinguished from idiopathic erythroderma (l'homme rouge), and that due to pityriasis rubra pilaris, atopic dermatitis, psoriasis, and drug eruptions. Tumor-stage lesions can be confused with pseudolymphomas and with lymphomas of other types. The following sections describe how evaluation of skin, lymph nodes, or blood can assist in making a diagnosis of CTCL.

Skin Lesions

Diagnosis of CTCL in patients with patch/plaque-stage disease is usually accomplished by combining clinical features with findings in routine skin biopsy. Diagnosis at an early stage is often difficult; an average of 6 years between onset of skin disease and diagnosis has been reported.[93] Part of the reason for this delay in diag-

nosis is the subtlety of changes found in biopsies of early disease and the difficulty in distinguishing those changes from inflammatory skin diseases. This has produced some interobserver variation in the diagnosis of biopsies thought to possibly represent CTCL.[94] However, recent advances in our understanding of early histologic changes in CTCL[6, 51] and adherence to definable criteria enable reliable diagnosis of CTCL if specimens are examined by experienced dermatopathologists with appropriate clinicopathologic correlation. Compared with spongiotic processes, patches or plaques of CTCL are more likely to show lymphocytes in the epidermis without epidermotropism, lymphocytes lining the basal layer, Pautrier's microabscesses, atypical lymphocytes, or a lichenoid infiltrate. Occasionally, spongiotic processes such as contact dermatitis may show striking resemblance to CTCL, as may some drug eruptions, particularly those caused by antiseizure medications.[95-97] Thus, the importance of clinicopathologic correlation in evaluating patients with suspected CTCL, as well as obtaining multiple or serial biopsies in questionable cases, cannot be overstated.

Because the changes of patch-stage mycosis fungoides are often subtle, there has been great interest in developing adjunctive techniques that would enable its objective diagnosis. Immunohistochemistry, the study of nuclear contour index by electron microscopy, flow and image cytometry seeking increased nuclear DNA content, and conventional light microscopy of thin plastic embedded sections have all been touted as methods to supplement routine histopathology. All of these techniques have limitations, but the most effort has gone into development of immunohistochemical methods for confirming the diagnosis in patch-stage lesions. Early interest in immunohistochemistry focused on the predominance of T-helper cells in the infiltrates of most cases of CTCL, but many inflammatory diseases with similar histologic patterns also are largely composed of CD4+ cells. Aberrant T-cell phenotypes, with loss of one or more of the antigens normally present on the membranes of mature peripheral blood T cells, is indeed a feature of CTCL but is more common in advanced lesions.[98] Inasmuch as T-cell antigens appear to be lost in a hierarchical manner, interest has focused on CD7, which is more frequently absent than CD2, CD3, or CD4, but studies conflict as to whether diminished CD7 expression is useful in distinguishing CTCL from inflammatory skin disease.[99] More recently, immunohistochemistry using antibodies that recognize the T-cell receptor beta-chain variable regions has been studied.[99, 100] As antibodies to the multitude of such variable regions become available, screening to detect clonality through immunohistochemistry may become practicable. In the meantime, immunophenotypic analysis of lymphocytic infiltrates in skin biopsy specimens is of most practical usefulness in biopsies of tumors, in which the findings on routine biopsy are sufficient for establishing a diagnosis of lymphoma, but not its type (e.g., B-cell vs T-cell).

More recently, techniques of molecular genetics, such as Southern blotting, have been used in the diagnosis of lymphomas. In CTCL, a malignant clone is present, with each neoplastic cell bearing the same unique, rearranged

DNA sequence that codes for its T-cell antigen receptor. If a malignant clone is present, the unique rearrangement of genes for this T-cell antigen receptor can be detected by a Southern blot if it is present in as little as 1% to 5% of a population of lymphocytes under study.[101, 102] The Southern blot can be performed on fresh tissue such as skin, but it is not yet in routine diagnostic use in most medical centers and, unfortunately, patches of CTCL are too sparsely infiltrated by malignant cells for a negative result to be considered reliable.[101, 103] Thus, these techniques are more useful for ruling out other types of lymphoma or pseudolymphomas from biopsy specimens with nodular or diffuse infiltrates. More recently, polymerase chain reaction, which can amplify minute quantities of DNA, has been used for detecting clonal T-cell receptor gene rearrangements,[104-107] even from patch-stage lesions. Furthermore, technical advances have allowed this technique to be used not only on fresh tissue, but on specimens that have already been fixed in formalin and embedded in paraffin. Although not yet established as a method of diagnosing early CTCL, given the sensitivity afforded by gene amplification through polymerase chain reaction, it seems likely that in the not too distant future, the gold standard for diagnosis of early CTCL may move beyond clinicopathologic correlation to molecular analysis.[99]

Lymph Nodes

A lymph node biopsy is usually not used for establishing an initial diagnosis of CTCL because in early stages of disease, when nodes are not clinically enlarged, the findings are noncontributory. By the time a diagnosis of CTCL can be established in a lymph node biopsy, there is usually sufficient evidence in the skin or blood to establish a diagnosis. Biopsy is usually recommended if lymph nodes are enlarged, especially for staging and prognosis. In advanced disease, one may see effacement of nodes by atypical cells.[108] In earlier stages, abnormalities are less striking and often interpreted with the nonspecific designation *dermatopathic lymphadenopathy*. Application of more sophisticated diagnostic techniques, however, is beginning to permit earlier detection of lymph node involvement. For example, clonal rearrangement of the T-cell receptor was detected by Southern blot analysis in lymph nodes that only showed dermatopathic changes histologically.[109, 110]

Peripheral Blood

Morphology and enumeration of circulating CTCL cells by light microscopy alone are difficult unless there is marked lymphocytosis. The resemblance of CTCL cells to reactive lymphocytes makes examination of peripheral blood smears useful only in experienced hands.[111] In addition, light microscopy blood smear morphology generally underestimates the level of circulating malignant cells.[5] Conventional electron microscopy to evaluate the degree of nuclear convolution is too time consuming to be of general value in the routine diagnosis of CTCL. It is also recognized that Sézary cells and reactive lymphocytes can have similar degrees of hyperconvolution.[112]

Flow cytometry has improved the reliability and reproducibility of detecting CTCL in the peripheral blood.[113] CD4/CD8 ratios can detect disease in the peripheral blood. There are two contributing features. In part, the elevated ratio is due to the malignant CD4+ cells entering the peripheral blood. Complementing this is a decrease in CD8+ lymphocytes. A question remains regarding the appropriate cutoff for defining blood involvement. In the laboratory at Yale University, normal patients have a CD4/CD8 ratio of 1.91 with a standard deviation of 0.93. Thus, 2.5% of the normal population would have CD4/CD8 ratios greater than 3.77 and 1% will have ratios greater than 4.04. For this reason, values over 4 are interpreted as pathologic in patients suspected of having CTCL. In one study, CD4/CD8 ratios were compared with T-cell gene rearrangement studies and it was shown that of 11 CTCL patients with positive T-cell gene rearrangement studies, 10 had CD4/CD8 ratios over 10.[114] There was one case in which a ratio lower than 2 occurred while the T-cell gene rearrangement study indicated a clonal population. This reflects that 1% to 5% involvement of the peripheral lymphocyte population by the malignant clone can be recognized by gene rearrangement studies, a level that is beneath detection by flow cytometry. In fact, genetic methods, such as Southern blotting and the polymerase chain reaction, that can assist in detecting clonal rearrangements of T-cell receptor genes, are the most sensitive methods currently available for identifying the presence of malignant cells in the peripheral blood.[103, 114-116] As these techniques become more available and as more data on their specificity are obtained, they may assume a wider role in the routine evaluation of peripheral blood of patients suspected of having CTCL.

STAGING AND PROGNOSIS

Staging

In any patient in whom a diagnosis of CTCL is established, there should be documentation of the extent of cutaneous involvement as well as an assessment for the presence of extracutaneous involvement and its severity. An approach to staging patients is shown in Table 158–3. The TNM scoring system (Table 158–4) is useful to assist staging but is in need of updating with current laboratory methods. Documentation of cutaneous disease can be assisted by total-body photography. In practice, biopsies of lymph nodes are not always performed if they are not clinically enlarged. Computerized axial tomography scan provides precise measurements of axillary and inguinal nodes along with surveillance pictures of viscera, pelvic, periaortic, and thoracic lymph nodes.

A practical approach for evaluating the peripheral blood is outlined in Figure 158–12. A complete blood count is checked for total lymphocyte count abnormalities, eosinophil count, and for overt lymphocyte nuclear abnormalities. We recommend a flow cytometry panel

TABLE 158-3. An Approach to Staging CTCL Patients

1. Complete history and physical examination, including whole body mapping of skin lesions
2. CBC with absolute lymphocyte count, eosinophil count
3. Flow cytometry for CD4, CD8, CD3, CD25, CD45RO, CLA, BE2
4. Immunophenotyping of fresh tissue with all lymphoid antigens
5. HTLV-I antibody
6. Liver and renal chemistries, antinuclear antibody
7. Biopsy or aspirate of enlarged lymph nodes
8. Chest x-ray
9. Computerized axial tomography of abdomen and pelvis
10. Cancer screening as per American Cancer Society: stool guaiac, mammograms

CTCL, cutaneous T-cell lymphoma; CBC, complete blood count.

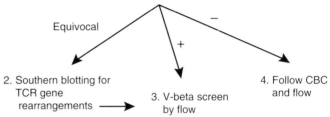

1. Complete blood count with flow cytometry for CD3, CD4, CD8, CD45RO, CLA.
- Look for lymphocytosis, elevated CD4/CD8, elevated levels of cutaneous T cells

Equivocal   −   +

2. Southern blotting for TCR gene rearrangements ⟶   3. V-beta screen by flow   4. Follow CBC and flow

FIGURE 158-12. An algorithm to guide the peripheral blood evaluation of CTCL patients utilizing flow cytometry and molecular studies. (CBC, complete blood count; TCR, T-cell receptor.)

TABLE 158-4. TNM Classification of CTCL

Classification	Description
T: skin*	
T_0	Clinically and/or histopathologically suspicious lesions
T_1	Limited plaques, papules, or eczematoid patches covering 10% or more of the skin surface
T_2	Generalized plaques, papules, or erythematous patches covering 10% or more of the skin surface
T_3	Tumors, one or more
T_4	Generalized erythroderma
N: lymph nodes†	
N_0	No clinically or palpably abnormal peripheral lymph nodes, pathology negative for CTCL
N_1	Clinically abnormal peripheral lymph nodes, pathology negative for CTCL
N_2	No clinically abnormal peripheral lymph nodes, pathology positive for CTCL
N_3	Clinically abnormal peripheral lymph nodes, pathology positive for CTCL
B: peripheral blood	
B_0	Atypical circulating cells not present or less than 5%
B_1	Atypical circulating cells present in 5% or more of total blood lymphocytes; record total white blood cell count and total lymphocyte counts and number of atypical cells/100 lymphocytes
M: visceral organs	
M_0	No involvement of visceral organs
M_1	Visceral involvement (must have confirmation of pathology and organ involved should be specified)

*Pathology of T_{1-4} is diagnostic of a CTCL. When characteristics of more than one T classification exist, both are recorded and the highest is used for staging, e.g., $T_4(3)$.

†The number of sites of abnormal nodes is recorded, e.g., cervical (left + right), axillary (left + right), axillary (left + right), inguinal (left + right), epitrochlear, submandibular, submaxillary, etc.

that initially includes CD4, CD8 and CD45RO, all of which are readily available. Any elevation of the CD4/CD8 ratio or elevation of CD45RO% or any clinical suspicion of occult leukemia (widespread skin involvement) should be followed by gene rearrangement studies that could confirm leukemic disease. The advantage of flow cytometry over the slightly more sensitive gene rearrangement study is that the latter answers the question "Is there peripheral blood involvement?" with a yes or no. Flow cytometry answers this question with a measure of how much CTCL is present and a measure of where the patient is on the progression of disease shown in Figure 158-11.

Flow cytometry can also be used for monitoring the blood of patients with CTCL. For example, patients in remission have normal values of CD45RO and CLA. Likewise, antibodies against the variable region of the T-cell receptor can be used in the follow-up of patients with CTCL who have clones that react with the available antibodies (see Table 158-2). Because antibodies to less than a quarter of the possible variable regions are available, they are more useful for monitoring selected patients than for establishing a diagnosis of CTCL.

Prognosis

Several factors allow the clinician to assess the prognosis of CTCL. Predicting the outcome of CTCL is a risky business, but in general there is a worse prognosis for greater degrees of skin involvement, depth of infiltrate, blastic transformation, loss of normal T cells, leukemia, lymph node and viscera involvement.[117-119] There are rough guidelines on what to expect in patients with CTCL. In general, the degree of skin involvement inversely correlates with prognosis. Involvement of 10% or less of the skin surface by patch-stage disease correlates with median survival of 12 years. Patients with patch-stage disease in general seem to have a median survival range of 7 to 12 years. Patients with limited plaque lesions (less than 10% surface area) have a better prognosis than patients with generalized plaque lesions (T2, greater than 10% surface). Prognosis is poorer in patients with tumors (T3) than in those with plaque lesions and is poorer still in those with erythroderma

(T4). Differences in prognosis in these groups may be related to the increase in the incidence of extracutaneous involvement with progressive stages of skin disease.[93, 120-122] Lymphadenopathy, whether due to dermatopathic change (N1) or infiltration by CTCL (N2, N3), is a sign of poor prognosis.[117, 118] The development of tumors, erythroderma, or node involvement signals a drop to 2 to 3 years' median survival.[93, 122-125] Patients with tumors or lymph node involvement have almost the same survival rate, suggesting that an involved node is biologically similar to a cutaneous tumor. Nearly all of the survival data compiled to date reflect studies performed before the availability of methods to assess antigen loss by phenotyping,[55, 69, 126] nonmalignant lymphopenia by flow cytometry,[5, 118] clonality, leukemia, or lymph node involvement by molecular techniques.[109, 115, 127] Because some of these techniques, as well as advances in routine histopathology, are permitting earlier diagnosis of CTCL, the prognostic figures cited above may underestimate survival. Furthermore, therapy may have an impact on outcome that can confound such survival estimates. As will be discussed in the next section, the side effects of some treatments can also accelerate the demise of the patient, in part by exacerbating the immunosuppression inherent in CTCL itself.

THERAPY

In this section, the therapeutic approach to CTCL will be discussed from two different perspectives that must be covered separately. For each modality there is a discussion of how to administer the treatment and what to watch for. The second part of this section will present strategies for using these modalities. Matching the clinical activity of the disease with the appropriate treatment option is the science of CTCL management. Fortunately, the tools used to help the clinician have improved to make this more of a science and less of an art.

The treatments listed in Table 158-5 are those that are used in the successful management of cutaneous lymphomas. The successful management also depends on a knowledge of the nature of CTCL, as discussed in the previous section. Many of the treatments to be discussed exploit the unique biology of cutaneous lympho-

TABLE 158-5. CTCL Treatments

Spot radiotherapy
Nitrogen mustard
Topical BCNU
PUVA, rePUVA, iPUVA
Total skin radiotherapy
ECP therapy
DAB-IL2 toxin
Chlorambucil/prednisone
Methotrexate
Etoposide
Fludarabine
Interferon
Polychemotherapy

PUVA, photochemotherapy with ultraviolet A light.

TABLE 158-6. Therapies Appropriate for Different Stages of CTCL

Stage	Therapy
Patch-stage CTCL	PUVA, NM, TSEB, BCNU
Plaque-stage CTCL	PUVA, NM, TSEB, BCNU
Erythrodermic CTCL	ECP, TSEB, DAB-IL2, CHL/PRED, MTX
Tumor-stage CTCL	TSEB + NM, PUVA, IFN, ECP, CHEMO, FAMP-IFN, DAB-IL2, MTX
Lymph node CTCL	RT, MTX, FAMP-IFN, CHEMO
Leukemic CTCL	ECP, MTX, CHL/PRED, VP16, FAMP-IFN, DAB-IL2
Visceral CTCL	MTX, FAMP-IFN, CHEMO

PUVA, photochemotherapy with ultraviolet A light; NM, nitrogen mustard; TSEB, total skin electron beam radiotherapy; BCNU, carmustine; ECP, extracorporeal photochemotherapy; DAB-IL2, diphtheria A toxin-interleukin-2 gene fusion product; CHL/PRED, chorambucil/prednisone; MTX, methotrexate; IFN, interferon; CHEMO, chemotherapy; FAMP, fludarabine monophosphate; RT, radiotherapy; VP16, etoposide.

cytes. After discussing practical and theoretical aspects of each modality, this section will cover the clinical applications of these treatments in different stages of CTCL (Table 158-6).

Spot Radiotherapy

The radiosensitivity of cutaneous lymphomas[12] has been exploited in a variety of regimens. The use of localized ("spot") radiotherapy depends on having a limited number of lesions that will allow the radiotherapist to practically administer 2000 to 3000 rads in 400- to 600-rad fractions over 5 to 10 treatment sessions. Small-field or "spot" radiotherapy will adequately eliminate localized lesions of cutaneous lymphoma.[128, 129]

Orthovoltage radiotherapy can be utilized but the less penetrating electron beam radiotherapy (discussed in detail later in this section) produces fewer side effects. Given the wide availability of spot radiotherapy, there usually are no geographic constraints on the use of this modality.

Topical Nitrogen Mustard Therapy

Topical nitrogen mustard (NM) therapy derives its success from delivering a lymphocyte-toxic mustard chemotherapy agent to the entire skin—the domain of the cutaneous lymphocyte. NM therapy is administered chronically and the ability of this chemotherapy agent to be tolerated over long periods of time undoubtedly plays a role in its success.[130-132] Cutaneous T cells are recirculating through the skin. The proliferative rates of the malignant cells are low enough to require long-term cutaneous-directed chemotherapy to therapeutically reduce their numbers.

NM is typically made up fresh daily as an aqueous solution of 10 mg of mechlorethamine hydrochloride dissolved in approximately 50 mL of tap water. The entire volume is then applied to the whole body surface by the patient. Paintbrushes can be used to facilitate the application. The patient should wear protective plastic gloves while applying the solution. A delayed hypersensitivity reaction may complicate treatment. This hypersensitivity has been circumvented by induction of tolerance to NM by topical desensitization or by concomitant use of photochemotherapy with ultraviolet A light (PUVA). Another alternative is to use 10 mg % NM in Aquaphor,[133] which avoids the problems of patients diluting their own chemotherapeutic agent and is potentially less sensitizing. After patients achieve a remission, NM is continued nightly for at least a month, then the frequency of application can be decreased to every other night for 3 to 6 months before tapering to a once or twice weekly application schedule that should be maintained for 1 to 2 years. Following cessation of therapy there can be relapse, which would most likely respond to subsequent courses of NM.

The prime advantage of NM is that patients can do the treatments at home without the inconveniences that can arise with other modalities such as electron beam or PUVA. However, there can be hypersensitivity and primary irritant reactions that may dampen the enthusiasm that is needed for compliance to this home-based regimen. The long-term effects of the development of second cutaneous malignancies are real and require periodic cancer screening exams.[134] In addition there can be cosmetic discomfort with hypo- and hyperpigmentation.

Topical Carmustine (BCNU) Therapy

Another topical chemotherapeutic regimen utilizes a solution of 25 to 50 mg of BCNU in dilute alcohol (100 to 200 cc) given on a daily or alternate-day schedule until a total dose of 200 to 600 mg is used. The BCNU is stable for at least 3 months in 95% alcohol when refrigerated. Patients can make up the stock solution and keep it in the refrigerator. Total skin applications of the BCNU are done in a manner similar to the NM described above.[135, 136] For spot therapy, an ointment preparation of 5 mg per mL BCNU in Aquaphor is stable at room temperature.

The advantages of BCNU therapy are similar to those of NM. The patient can perform treatments at home. The entire treatment course is more abbreviated. In general one achieves a remission within a few weeks and because of this and some irritant reaction that inevitably occurs, the treatment is stopped. Application is continued until that irritant reaction develops or for a maximum of 6 to 8 weeks. During therapy with BCNU, complete blood counts must be monitored but marrow suppression is usually avoided with total doses less than 600 mg. When significant relapses occur, subsequent cycles of therapy can be repeated. One advantage of the BCNU schedule over the NM schedule is that by being shorter, less frequent, and more intense, the BCNU schedule can often be carried out with the assistance of a visiting nurse with those patients who may not have the compliance level required for NM.

The disadvantages of BCNU are cutaneous with contact hypersensitivity (10%), severe erythema (33%), post-treatment telangiectasia (35%), and hematologic with mild bone marrow depression (30%).[135, 136]

Photochemotherapy with Ultraviolet A Light (PUVA)

PUVA must be regarded as both a remittive and a maintenance therapy. For inducing a remission, treatments should begin at three times per week frequency. A treatment session consists of the ingestion of 8-methoxypsoralen at .4 to .5 mg/kg. One and one-half hours later, the patient stands in an ultraviolet-A light box to activate the psoralen in the skin (see PUVA in Chapter 27). For PUVA therapy to be successful, patients have to be near a competent PUVA center so that the initial thrice-weekly schedule does not get excessively interrupted by travel problems. Because PUVA therapy results in many years of infrequent treatment sessions, it is important that patients identify PUVA as a friend worth visiting every couple of weeks. This bonding is impossible if a center is not accessible.

After most of the lesions have cleared, the frequency can be decreased to twice weekly until the patient has achieved a complete remission.[137-140] It is important to maintain the multiple treatment per week schedule for a minimum of 3 and a maximum of 6 months. If the patient's CTCL is not cleared by PUVA monotherapy, there are several options to boost the therapeutic response. Two of the more traditional choices at this point are retinoid therapy or interferon therapy. Both are proven in the role of PUVA boosters (discussed later).

As a maintenance therapy, PUVA is initially administered at once-weekly frequencies until 1 year has passed. At this point, 1 week can be added between treatments and a total of 25 sessions over a year will be needed. Should the patient still be in remission at this point, the same addition is carried out over 2 more years so that eventually patients are receiving 12 sessions per year, which is continued for at least 2 years. At this point, the patient should have been in remission for 5 years. Consideration should be given to stopping therapy at this point. There are no reports of patients experiencing relapse after 5 years of remission off all treatments. This would imply that a malignant cutaneous T cell could survive asymptomatically for 5 years. With 5 years of intermittent PUVA, it is less likely that one of these cells survived but it is still possible. Patients should not be considered cured unless they stay clear 5 years after stopping therapy.

Long-term side effects include atrophy and dryness of the skin. Patients with psoriasis treated with photochemotherapy have a 2% to 3% incidence of cutaneous epitheliomas, particularly those who have had previous x-ray irradiation of the skin or who sunburn easily.

Total-Skin Electron Beam Radiotherapy

Because electrons penetrate only to the dermis, electron beam therapy may be used without systemic effect.

The total dose of irradiation is important, and a dose of 3000 rads or more gives better complete remission rates and disease-free survival than do lower doses.[124, 141, 142] The major disadvantages are that this type of therapy is expensive, requires a specialized center, and takes up to 3 months for complete treatment. Local side effects include alopecia, atrophy of sweat glands and skin generally, radiodermatitis, and edema. When the total dose is highly fractionated, these complications are minimized and often avoided. The maximum radiation tolerance of the skin then becomes the limiting factor with treatment. Using the highly fractionated approach, patients can receive a second course of 3600 rads electron beam to re-induce a remission. As the total radiation dose increases, so does the risk of squamous cell carcinoma and radiodermatitis.

Only those portions of the skin that are directly exposed to the beam are radiated. Therefore, palms, soles, scalp, axillae, and perineum may need separate exposure to ensure total-body treatment. The eyelids are routinely covered with lead eye shields to protect the cornea and lens from the effects of radiation. If the eyelids are involved, 5-mm-thick contact lenses are worn between the lid and cornea within the conjunctival sac. Nail shields may also be used to prevent anonychia.

Extracorporeal Photochemotherapy

An extracorporeal photochemotherapy (ECP) therapy session begins when a patient ingests 8-methoxypsoralen at doses comparable to those used for PUVA. One to two hours later the patient has an intravenous line placed in an arm to allow a portion of the peripheral blood to course through the treatment device. The device separates the leukocytes from the ultraviolet-A shielding erythrocytes and it provides ultraviolet-A irradiation of the leukocytes. Lymphocytes treated with ECP achieve a "photoinactivated" state by which they are viable and intact but unable to respond in stimulation assays. This unique state may underlie the ability of the body to develop a response against the malignant cells. Cells removed from the treatment cassette can survive several days, with 90% dying off over 3 to 5 days. Thus, intact but inactivated cells circulate in the treated patient, and undoubtedly the cells encounter the reticuloendothelial system and other components of the immune system over several days after a treatment. After photoinactivation, the treated leukocytes are returned to the patient.

Treatments are performed for two consecutive days, typically at 4-week intervals. This strategy has been found to be effective therapeutically with minimal side effects. The total fraction of lymphocytes treated is less than 5%.

A mild febrile reaction has occurred in less than 10% of patients within 6 hours after re-infusion of their own treated leukocytes. In addition, erythematous lesions may become more intensely red and slightly edematous. This immediate reaction diminishes with subsequent treatments as the disease regresses. The treatment is non-immunosuppressive as judged by the lack of leukopenia,

opportunistic infections, and the preservation of delayed hypersensitivity skin testing.[143-145]

Diphtheria A Toxin–Interleukin-2 Gene Fusion Product (DAB-IL2)

DAB-IL2 is a recombinant protein produced by expression of a fusion of the gene for interleukin-2 with the gene for diphtheria toxin in genetically engineered *Escherichia coli*. It is an interleukin-2 (IL-2) receptor–specific cytotoxin by its killing of activated lymphocytes at drug concentrations of 10^{-11} M to 10^{-9} M, and such killing is blocked by the addition of excess IL-2 or monoclonal antibody to the IL-2 receptor. Doses of 750 kU/kg/per day for 5 days every 21 days, as long as improvement persists, are given for up to eight courses, or two courses beyond complete response.

One adverse effect is mild nausea following infusion. This can be relieved by administration of promethazine (Phenergan) or prochlorperazine (Compazine). The incidences of nausea are comparable to or less than effects associated with combination chemotherapy. Hair loss and mucositis do not occur. A macular papular eruption may occur following an initial course in 30% of patients, clearing within 10 days, often not recurring with subsequent courses. Effects on laboratory parameters include elevation of hepatic transaminases (up to five times normal) in 40% of patients, resolving within 14 days and typically decreasing with subsequent courses.[146, 147]

Chlorambucil-Prednisone

Chlorambucil combined with prednisone has been used as a low-dose chronic chemotherapy regimen for CTCL.[148, 149] Typically a patient would begin on 40 mg prednisone and 4 mg chlorambucil per day. If no hematologic toxicity is noted, the chlorambucil can be increased in 2-mg increments. Once the maximum response is achieved, the prednisone is tapered to a long-term tolerable dose of 20 mg every other day. The side effects of prednisone are well known, but at an alternating dose of 20 mg every other day, they are not severe. Chlorambucil, however, can produce bone marrow suppression and pose a threat for the later development of myelogenous leukemia.

Fludarabine Monophosphate

Fludarabine monophosphate (FAMP) is a chemotherapeutic agent that is very well tolerated and active against a wide range of lymphoid malignancies.[150] The regimen typically used with CTCL is a 5-day course of 50 to 100 mg/M² administered over 30 minutes intravenously. This is repeated monthly. Alopecia and mucositis are minimal. Rare neurologic sequelae have been noted with FAMP but otherwise it is very well tolerated. Typically FAMP is used in conjunction with interferon.

Interferon

Two types (alpha and gamma) of interferons have been found to have therapeutic effects in patients with CTCL. The most commonly used one is alpha, which has a distinct role as an adjunct therapy with PUVA and with FAMP. Dose ranging studies demonstrated that the best tolerated dose is 3 million units three times a week, and this is a good starting dose. The initial week of interferon (IFN) is complicated by a flu-like illness that may be accompanied by fever, myalgia, fatigue, and listlessness. As this wears off, with coaching and acetaminophen, patients are often left with a slight feeling of chronic fatigue. The long-term toxicity that causes most concern is neurologic—depression, neuropathy, dementia, and myelopathy. Autoimmune phenomena such as proteinuria, thrombocytopenia, and anemia may occur. With monitoring, the patient's ideal dose can safely be established. Should there be no problem with the 9 million units per week as outlined above, the dose can be increased up to a maximum of 36 million units per week.[151, 152]

Methotrexate

Two regimens for methotrexate have been implemented in the treatment of CTCL. One is a low-dose weekly regimen using doses from 20 to 60 mg per week.[53] The toxicities encountered are similar to those encountered with psoriasis patients undergoing methotrexate treatment: liver toxicity and bone marrow suppression. Typically the patient is told to avoid alcohol, after which a test dose of 20 mg intramuscular, intravenous, or oral methotrexate is given. If no toxicity appears, the dose can be gradually escalated as tolerated. A second regimen is one that must be carried out weekly at a chemotherapy center. Methotrexate is given intravenously at doses of 60 to 240 mg/M^2. This is followed by leucovorin rescue.[154] Side effects of the high-dose regimen included skin ulcerations, mucositis, anemia, and leukopenia.

Etoposide

Etoposide (VP16) is administered at low oral doses (50 mg/M^2) daily for 3 weeks followed by a rest week. The regimen does produce hair loss, and because of the risk for bone marrow toxicity it is necessary to monitor blood counts at least monthly. Even patients who have been heavily pretreated with chemotherapy are candidates for etoposide.[155, 156]

Polychemotherapy

Systemic high-dose chemotherapy does have a role as a palliative agent in advanced disease. Most patients with advanced disease will exhibit some degree of steroid sensitivity that makes the glucocorticoids a frequent component of therapy.[157-160] Adriamycin is very effective as a single-agent palliative regimen.[161] The combination regimen of cyclophosphamide, adriamycin, vincristine, and prednisone (CHOP) is one of the safer, better tolerated regimens for advanced CTCL, as it is for other non-Hodgkin's lymphomas.[162]

Treatment in Different Stages of Disease

Patch- and Plaque-Stage Disease

Patch- and plaque-stage disease respond to any of three commonly used approaches: topical chemotherapy, photochemotherapy, and total-skin electron beam radiotherapy. Cutaneous directed therapy of CTCL has several principles and guidelines. In early stages of CTCL, photochemotherapy, topical chemotherapy, and electron beam radiotherapy can induce remissions. In the earliest stages, there can be cures. However, the curative potential is not as dependent on the modality as it is dependent on having therapy matched to the clinical setting and administered with appropriate follow-up. The selection of cutaneous directed therapy should involve an assessment of geographic constraints, time commitments, compliance, and local expertise to help the proper decision making.

1. **Geographic constraints.** Only a few centers in the United States offer total-skin electron beam radiotherapy in a highly fractionated schedule with the Stanford technique. Some of these centers are New Haven, Philadelphia, San Francisco, Buffalo, Hanover, Detroit, Durham, Nashville, Chicago, St. Louis, Houston, and Stanford. With three to four sessions per week over 9 to 12 weeks, patients need to consider temporary residence near one of these centers. For PUVA therapy, as discussed, patients have to be near a competent PUVA center. Topical chemotherapy, on the other hand, can be done in the home.

2. **Time commitments.** Patients undergoing electron beam radiotherapy need to take a 9- to 12-week block of time to devote themselves to this therapy. Once this is completed, patients only need periodic check-ups. PUVA patients start out at thrice-weekly treatments that last 5 minutes or so. However, the pills may cause nausea and the treatment restricts outdoor activity so that many patients tend to "lay low" on treatment days. PUVA is continued at once-weekly, then biweekly, then monthly schedules for years. Topical chemotherapy requires a nightly commitment of 20 to 30 minutes along with restrictions on exposure of the treated skin to close contacts.

3. **Compliance.** With electron beam and PUVA, compliance is not only enforced but assiduously recorded in a treatment record. These therapies are certainly preferable when there is any reason to doubt the compliance of a patient with topical chemotherapy. In settings where poor compliance with topical chemotherapy is anticipated, local visiting nurse agencies can be particularly invaluable in inducing a remission.

All three approaches to patch-plaque disease (topical chemotherapy, photochemotherapy, electron beam) can induce remissions at rates of 80% to 90%.[124, 132, 136, 138] Because it was one of the first regimens of skin-directed therapy for CTCL, there is excellent long-term follow-up of NM-treated patients. Ninety per cent of patients with limited CTCL were treated with topical NM therapy and were in remission; 67% were maintained in a disease-free state for a short follow-up period. In a large series, disease-free intervals of more than 3 years have been achieved in 13%. Following cessation of therapy, some of these individuals experienced relapse.[124] Thus, the use of more long-term maintenance regimens seems prudent. One difference between BCNU and NM is that the former is typically given for a several-week course and then the patient goes off therapy until relapses require subsequent courses. Should a patient fail with any of the three skin-directed approaches, consideration should be given to utilizing one of the others.

PUVA is administered for CTCL as outlined earlier. Should patients not achieve clearing with PUVA, there are two proven PUVA boosters that can lead the patient into remission with PUVA. IFN at doses previously discussed can help PUVA clear refractory disease.[163] The side effects of IFN can often produce more disability and discomfort than the disease. Other patients may show no toxicity at all. For those who cannot tolerate IFN or for those who prefer an alternative, retinoid-PUVA therapy can also be successful. Isotretinoin (Accutane) or etretinate (Tegison) can be used at doses of 20 to 80 mg per day to boost a response to PUVA.[164] With retinoid or IFN PUVA boosters, the PUVA can usually be used successfully as maintenance therapy once the remission has been attained.

Whole-body electron beam irradiation brings about complete remission in 84% of patients, with a median survival time of 9 years.[131] Patients with limited plaque disease had the best survival rate (69% at 9 years) and the best relapse-free rate (42% at 10 years). The median disease-free interval was greater than 3 years in the limited plaque group, approximately 1 year for patients with generalized plaque-stage disease. Maintenance therapy for patch-plaque patients completing electron beam radiotherapy can be done with either PUVA or NM.[165]

Erythrodermic Disease

In the erythrodermic stage, patients can have varying degrees of circulating malignant cells, normal T cells, and variable levels of leukemia. This clinical heterogeneity makes a uniform treatment plan difficult; however, the earlier treatment is started in the course of the disease, the better the response to therapy.[166] The first-line treatment for erythrodermic CTCL is extracorporeal photochemotherapy (ECP), which can be used as monotherapy in patients that are not markedly leukemic and immunosuppressed. There are now 107 CTCL patients reported with ECP treatments and the results from all centers show about a 15% to 30% complete response rate.[145] Clearly, even a partial response can improve the quality of life of one of these cutaneous cripples. The onset of improvement may begin as early as 6 weeks into therapy and yet some patients do not completely clear until 12 months after starting therapy. Those patients who demonstrate marked clinical improvement are maintained on the every-4-week treatment schedule.

Once stable for an additional 6 months, patients are then gradually tapered by adding 1 week per cycle every three cycles. After this has been extended to one cycle of therapy every 8 weeks for three times, the therapy is stopped.

Patients with marked leukemia and immunosuppression need adjunctive therapy with ECP. Electron beam, IFN, methotrexate, and etoposide have all been used as adjuncts with varying degrees of success. The prolongation of electron beam–induced remissions with ECP has been noted in preliminary reports.[167] Markedly leukemic patients or patients refractory to the therapies above are candidates for DAB-IL2 or cytotoxic therapy with a polychemotherapy regimen.

Tumor-Stage Disease

Radiotherapy for tumor-stage disease is an effective modality for inducing a remission, and this modality remains the mainstay for tumor-stage treatment. The frontier in tumor-stage CTCL therapy is in the prolongation of survival. It appears that conventional therapy does not improve on survival, although remissions can be induced.

Patients with cutaneous tumors treated with electron beam alone have a guarded prognosis, with a 10-year survival rate of 28% and a median survival time of 2.7 years. Most of the relapses occurred within the first year after completion of therapy and were very rare after 3 years.[124, 141, 142] A protocol to study ECP therapy in conjunction with total-skin electron beam radiotherapy was begun after the first patient maintained a remission over 3 years on this regimen.[166] The initial results of this combined regimen are encouraging with 75% of ECP/electron beam patients alive at 5 years compared with 30% of those treated with electron beam alone.[167] The low toxicity of ECP therapy makes it an attractive candidate for maintenance therapy of patients with tumor-stage CTCL. NM therapy has also been successfully used as a maintenance therapy.

Lymph Node Disease

Involvement of lymph nodes with CTCL carries a prognostic impact similar to the development of tumor-stage disease. Many of the same modalities used in tumor stage apply here. Radiotherapy is a reliable way to ablate lymph node disease. Localized node involvement is amenable to spot orthovoltage therapy. However, total-nodal irradiation, which has been used in CTCL, does have significant bone marrow toxicity.[168] The bone marrow suppression can even manifest itself when the nodal irradiation port for limited disease includes significant portions of the iliac bones (pelvic or inguinal nodes), or spinal column (thoracic, neck, and axillary nodes). Patients need to be monitored with weekly complete blood counts. Superior vena cava syndrome is an emergency and should be treated with combined radiotherapy and intravenous steroids.[169] For patients who do not respond or cannot tolerate radiotherapy, polychemotherapy with a regimen that includes corticosteroids will provide a palliative respite from lymph node involvement.

Leukemic Disease

Hyperleukocytic disease is usually encountered in the evolution of erythrodermic disease, and parts of the treatment strategy are discussed above in that section. However, there are patients who can have pronounced leukemic involvement with only minimal plaque- or tumor-stage disease. In addition to therapy being directed at the latter components, it is necessary to therapeutically address the leukemia. Single-agent therapy with DAB-IL2, methotrexate, chlorambucil, or etoposide can often improve the hematologic picture. FAMP-IFN is a regimen that tends to be successful and tolerated better than polychemotherapy regimens.

Visceral Disease

Splenic enlargement is one of the most symptomatic visceral manifestations of CTCL. Patients that cannot be controlled with daily oral doses of corticosteroids may require splenic irradiation and possibly splenectomy. Similarly, involvement of other organs can be addressed with localized radiotherapy and (preferably) targeted chemotherapy. For example, lung lesions have been treated successfully with radiotherapy[170] whereas intrathecal chemotherapy has been useful for central nervous system involvement.[171] Because of the guarded prognosis that accompanies visceral CTCL, palliation is the goal.

References

1. Alibert JLM. Monographie des Dermatoses. Bailliere G, ed. Paris, 1835:413.
2. Lamberg SI, Bunn PA. Proceeding of the workshop on cutaneous T-cell lymphomas (mycosis fungoides and Sézary syndrome). Cancer Treat Rep 1979;63:561–572.
3. Besnier E, Hallopeau H. On the erythrodermia of mycosis fungoides. J Cutan Genito Urin Dis 1892;10:453.
4. Sézary A, Bouvrain Y. Erythrodermie avec presence de cellules monstreuses dans le derme et le sang circulant. Bull Soc Fr Dermatol Syphil 1938;45:254.
5. Heald P, Yan SL, Latkowski J, et al. Profound deficiency in normal circulating T-cells in erythrodermic cutaneous T-cell lymphoma. Arch Dermatol 1994;130:198–204.
6. Sanchez JL, Ackerman AB. The patch stage of mycosis fungoides. Am J Dermatopathol 1979;1:5–26.
7. Gibson LE, Muller SA, Leiferman KM, Peters MS. Follicular mucinosis: Clinical and histopathologic study. J Am Acad Dermatol 1989;20:441–447.
8. Mehregan D, Gibson L, Muller S. Follicular mucinosis: Histopathologic review of 33 cases. Mayo Clin Proc 1991;66:387–390.
9. Mandojana RM, Helwig EB. Localized epidermotropic reticulosis (Woringer-Kolopp disease): A clinicopathologic study of 15 new cases. J Am Acad Dermatol 1983;8:813–829.
10. Wood GS, Weiss LM, Hu Ch, et al. T-cell antigen deficiencies and clonal rearrangement of T-cell receptor genes in pagetoid reticulosis (Woringer-Kolopp Disease). N Engl J Med 1988;318:164–168.
11. Braun-Falco O, Schmoeckel C, Burg G, et al. Pagetoid reticulosis: A further case report with a review of the literature. Acta Dermatovener 1979;59(Suppl. 85):11–21.
12. Lever WF. Localized mycosis fungoides with prominent epidermotropism: Woringer-Kolopp disease. Arch Dermatol 1977;113:1254–1256.
13. Medencia M, Lorincz AL. Pagetoid reticulosis (Woringer-Kolopp Disease). Arch Dermatol 1978;114:262–268.
14. Tan RS-H, Macleod TIF, Dean SG. Pagetoid reticulosis, epidermotropic mycosis fungoides and mycosis fungoides: A disease spectrum. Br J Dermatol 1987;116:67–77.
15. Lacour JP, Juhlin L, El Baze P, et al. Disseminated pagetoid reticulosis associated with mycosis fungoides: Immunomorphologic study. J Am Acad Dermatol 1986;14:898–901.
16. Ketron LW, Goodman MH. Multiple lesions of the skin apparently of epithelial origin resembling clinically mycosis fungoides. Arch Dermatol Syph 1931;24:758–777.
17. Balus L, Bassetti F, Gentili G. Granulomatous slack skin. Arch Dermatol 1985;121:250–253.
18. LeBoit P, Beckstead JH, Bond B, et al. Granulomatous slack skin: Clonal rearrangement of the T-cell receptor beta gene is evidence for the lymphoproliferative nature of a cutaneous elastolytic disorder. J Invest Dermatol 1987;89:183–188.
19. LeBoit P, Zackheim H, White C. Granulomatous variants of cutaneous T-cell lymphoma. Am J Surg Pathol 1988;12:83–92.
20. Smith NP, Samman PD. Mycosis fungoides presenting with areas of cutaneous hypopigmentation. Clin Exp Dermatol 1978; 3:213–216.
21. Breathnach SM, McKee PH, Smith NP. Hypopigmented mycosis fungoides: Report of five cases with ultrastructural observations. Br J Dermatol 1982;106:643–649.
22. Zackheim HS, Epstein EH, Grekin DA, et al. Mycosis fungoides presenting as areas of hypopigmentation. J Am Acad Dermatol 1982;6:340–345.
23. Goldberg DJ, Schinella RS, Kechijian P. Hypopigmented mycosis fungoides. Am J Dermatopathol 1986;8:326–330.
24. Sigal M, Grossin M, Laroche L, et al. Hypopigmented mycosis fungoides. Clin Exp Dermatol 1987;12:53–55.
25. Misch KJ, McCleannan KA, Marsden RA, et al. Immunopathology of hypopigmented mycosis fungoides. Clin Exp Dermatol 1986;11:332–339.
26. Whitemore SE, Simmons-O'Brien E, Rotter FS. Hypopigmented mycosis fungoides. Arch Dermatol 1994;130:476–480.
27. Barnhill RL, Braverman IM. Progression of pigmented purpuralike eruptions to mycosis fungoides: Report of three cases. J Am Acad Dermatol 1988;19:25–31.
28. Farrington J. Lichen aureus. Cutis 1970;6:1251.
29. Waisman M, Waisman M. Lichen aureus. Arch Dermatol 1976;112:696–697.
30. Zina G, Bernengo MG, Zina AM. Bullous Sézary syndrome. Dermatologica 1981;163:25–33.
31. Kartsonis J, Brettschneider F, Weissmann A, Rosen L. Mycosis fungoides bullosa. Am J Dermatopathol 1990;12:76–80.
32. Ackerman AB, Miller RC, Shapiro L. Pustular mycosis fungoides. Arch Dermatol 1966;93:221–225.
33. Moreno JC, Ortega M, Conejo-Mir JS, Sanchez-Pedreno P. Palmoplantar pustulosis as a manifestation of cutaneous T-cell lymphomas (mycosis fungoides). J Am Acad Dermatol 1990;23:759.
34. LeBoit P. Variants of mycosis fungoides and related cutaneous T-cell lymphomas. Semin Diag Pathol 1991;8(2):73–81.
35. Granstein RD, Soter NA, Haynes HA. Necrotizing vasculitis within cutaneous lesions of mycosis fungoides. J Am Acad Dermatol 1983;9:128–133.
36. Nevin M, Armus S, Wolff M, Bisaccia E. Cutaneous T-cell lymphoma in association with leukocytoclastic vasculitis. Int J Dermatol 1991;30:443–444.
37. Nakajima M, Hashikawa Y, Komatsu Y, et al. Leukemic T-cell lymphoma with lichen ruber-like erythroderma. Rinsho Derm (Tokyo) 1988;30:1523–1527.
38. Grob JJ, Collet Villette AM, Horchowski N, et al. Ofuji papuloerythroderma. Report of a case with T-cell skin lymphoma and discussion of the nature of this disease. J Am Acad Dermatol 1989;20:927–931.
39. Ofuji S. Papuloerythroderma. J Am Acad Dermatol 1990;22:697.
40. Farthing CF, Staughton RCD, Harper JI, et al. Papuloerythroderma: A further case with the "deck chair sign." Dermatologica 1986;172:65–66.
41. Ofuji JS, Furukawa F, Miyachi Y, et al. Papuloerythroderma. Dermatologica 1984;169:125–130.
42. Nazzari G, Crorato F, Nigro A. Papuloerythroderma (Ofuji); two additional cases and review of the literature. J Am Acad Dermatol 1992;26:499–501.
43. Agnarsson BA, Vonderheid EC, Kadin ME. Cutaneous T-cell lymphoma with suppressor/cytotoxic (CD8) phenotype: Identification of rapidly progressive and chronic subtypes. J Am Acad Dermatol 1990;22:569–577.

44. Ohkohchi K, Aiba S, Tagami H. OKT8-reactive mycosis fungoides. Arch Dermatol 1986;122:20–22.
45. Fujiwara Y, Abe Y, Kuyama M, et al. CD8+ cutaneous T-cell lympoma with pagetoid epidermotropism and angiocentric and angiodestructive infiltration. Arch Dermatol 1990;126:801–804.
46. Fujita M, Miyachi Y, Furukawa F, et al. A case of cutaneous T-cell lymphoma expressing gamma-delta T-cell receptors. J Am Acad Dermatol 1993;28:355–360.
47. Avinoach I, Halevy S, Argov S, Sacks M. Gamma-delta T-cell lymphoma involving the subcutaneous tissue and associated with a hemophagocytic syndrome. Am J Dermatopath 1994; 16:426–433.
48. Burg G, Dummer R, Wilhelm M, et al. A subcutaneous delta positive T-cell lymphoma that produces interferon gamma. N Engl J Med 1991;325:1078–1081.
49. Heald P, Buckley P, Kacinski B, et al. Unique clinical and immunophenotypic correlations of cutaneous gamma-delta T-cell lymphoma. J Am Acad Dermatol 1992;26:865–870.
50. Berti E, Cerri A, Caviccini, et al. Primary cutaneous gamma-delta lymphoma presenting as disseminated pagetoid reticulosis. J Invest Dermatol 1991;96:718–722.
51. Shapiro PE, Pinto F. The histologic spectrum of mycosis fungoides/Sézary syndrome (cutaneous T-cell lymphoma): A review of 222 biopsies, including newly-described patterns and the earliest pathologic changes. Am J Surg Pathol 1994;18:654–667.
52. Nickoloff BJ. Light microscopic assessment of 100 patients with patch/plaque stage mycosis fungoides. Am J Dermatopathol 1988;10:469–478.
53. Braverman IM. Transformation in cutaneous T-cell lymphoma. J Invest Dermatol 1993;101:249–250.
54. Suchi T, Lennert K, Tu LY, et al. Histopathology and immunohistochemistry of peripheral T-cell lymphomas: A proposal for their classification. J Clin Pathol 1987;40:995–1015.
55. Salhany KE, Cousar JB, Greer JP. Transformation of cutaneous T-cell lymphoma to large cell lymphoma. Am J Pathol 1988;132:265–273.
56. Greer JP, Salhany KE, Sousar JB, et al. Clinical features associated with transformation of cerebriform T-cell lymphoma to a large cell process. Hematol Oncol 1990;8:215–227.
57. Wood GS, Bahler DW, Hoppe RT. Transformation of mycosis fungoides: T-cell receptor beta gene analysis demonstrates a common clonal origin for plaque-type mycosis fungoides and CD 30 large cell lymphoma. J Am Acad Dermatol 1987;17:40–52.
58. Aloi F, Tomasini C, Pippion M. Mycosis fungoides and eruptive epidermoid cysts: A unique response of follicular and eccrine structures. Dermatology 1993;187:273–277.
59. Zelger B, Sepp N, Weyrer K, et al. Syringotropic cutaneous T-cell lymphoma: A variant of mycosis fungoides? Br J Dermatol 1994;130:765–769.
60. Sterry W, Hauschild A. Loss of leukocyte common antigen (CD45) on atypical lymphocytes in the localized but not disseminated type of pagetoid reticulosis. Br J Dermatol 1991; 125:238–242.
61. Van de Griend R, Tax W, Van Krimpen B, et al. Lysis of tumor cells by CD3+4−8−16+ T-cell receptor clones, regulated via CD3 and CD16 activation sites, recombinant interleukin 2 and interferon beta. J Immunol 1987;138:1627–1633.
62. Mackay CR, Marston WL, Dudler L. Naive and memory T cells show distinct pathways of lymphocyte recirculation. J Exp Med 1990;171:801–817.
63. Picker LJ, Michie SA, Rott LS, et al. A unique phenotype of skin associated lymphocytes in humans. Preferential expression of the HECA-452 epitope by benign and malignant T cells at cutaneous sites. Am J Pathol 1990;136:1053–1068.
64. Picker LJ, Kishimoto TK, Smith CW, et al. ELAM-1 is an adhesion molecule for skin-homing T cells. Nature 1991;349:796–799.
65. Heald P, Yan SL, Edelson RL, et al. Skin selective lymphocyte homing mechanisms in the pathogenesis of leukemic cutaneous T-cell lymphoma. J Invest Dermatol 1993;101(2):222–226.
66. Vowels BR, Cassin M, Vonderheid EC, et al. Aberrant cytokine production by Sézary syndrome patients: Cytokine secretion pattern resembles murine Th2 cells. J Invest Dermatol 1992; 99:90–94.
67. Heald P, Edelson R. The immunobiology of cutaneous T-cell lymphoma. J Natl Cancer Inst 1991;83:400–404.
68. Nickoloff BJ, Griffiths CE, Baadsgaard O, et al. Markedly diminished epidermal keratinocyte expressions of intercellular adhesion molecule-1 (ICAM-1) in Sézary syndrome. JAMA 1989; 261:2217–2222.
69. Cerroni L, Rieger E, Hodl S, et al. Clinicopathologic and immunologic features associated with transformation of mycosis fungoides to large-cell lymphomas. Am J Pathol 1992;16:543–552.
70. Vonderheid EC, Tan E, Sobel EL, et al. Clinical implications of immunologic phenotyping in cutaneous T-cell lymphoma. J Am Acad Dermatol 1987;17:40–52.
71. Olsen EA, Deizell E, Jegasothy BV. Second malignancies in cutaneous T-cell lymphoma. J Am Acad Dermatol 1984;10:197–203.
72. Massessa JM, Grossman ME, Knobler EH, et al. Kaposi's varicelliform eruption in cutaneous T-cell lymphoma. J Am Acad Dermatol 1989;21:133–135.
73. Cohen ML, Weiss EB. Pneumocystis carinii pneumonia: Percutaneous lung biopsy and review of literature. Chest 1971; 60:195–199.
74. Frieden TR, Bia F, Heald P, Patterson T, Edelson R. Cryptococcosis in a patient with cutaneous T-cell lymphoma undergoing therapy with photopheresis and methotrexate. Clin Infect Dis 1993;17:77–78.
75. Tokura Y, Heald P, Yan SL, et al. Stimulation of cutaneous T-cell lymphoma cells with superantigenic staphylococcal toxins. J Invest Dermatol 1992;98:33–37.
76. Zucker-Franklin D, Coutavas E, Rush M, et al. Detection of human T-lymphotropic virus-like particles in cultures of peripheral blood lymphocytes from patients with mycosis fungoides. Proc Natl Acad Sci USA 1991;88:7630–7634.
77. Strair RK, Towle M, Heald PW, et al. Retroviral mediated transfer and expression of exogenous genes in primary lymphoid cells: Assaying for a viral transactivator activity in normal and malignant cells. Blood 1990;76:1201–1209.
78. Hall WW, Liu CR, Schneewind O, et al. Deleted HTLV-1 provirus in blood and cutaneous lesions of patients with mycosis fungoides. Science 1991;253:317–320.
79. Nahass GT, Draffert CG, Penneys NS. Cutaneous T-cell lymphoma associated with the acquired immunodeficiency syndrome. Arch Dermatol 1991;127:1020–1022.
80. Catteral MD, Addis BJ, Smith JL, et al. Sézary syndrome: Transformation to a high grade T-cell lymphoma after treatment with cyclosporin A. Clin Exp Dermatol 1983;8:159–169.
81. Iraftery MJ, Tidman MJ, Koffman G, et al. Post-transplantation T-cell lymphoma of the skin. Transplantation 1988;46:475–477.
82. Shapiro PE, Warburton D, Berger CL, Edelson RL. Clonal chromosomal abnormalities in cutaneous T-cell lymphoma. Cancer Genet Cytogenet 1987;28:267–276.
83. Kaltoft K, Hansen BH, Thestrup-Pedersen KT. Cytogenetic findings in cell lines from cutaneous T-cell lymphoma. Derm Clin 1994;12:295–304.
84. Fischman AB, Bunn PA, Guccion JG, et al. Exposure to chemicals, physical agents, and biologic agents in mycosis fungoides and the Sézary syndrome. Cancer Treat Rep 1979;63:591–596.
85. Cohen SR, Stenn KS, Braverman IM, et al. Mycosis fungoides: Clinicopathologic relationship, survival and therapy in 59 patients. Cancer 1980;46:2654–2666.
86. McFadden N, Nyfors A, Tanum G, et al. Mycosis fungoides in Norway 1960–1980. A retrospective study. Acta Derm Venereol 1983;109(Suppl.):1–13.
87. Whittemore AS, Holley E, Lee I, et al. Mycosis fungoides in relation to environmental exposure and immune responses: a case control study. J Natl Cancer Inst 1989;81:1560–1564.
88. Conrad ME, Omura GA, et al. Mycosis fungoides: Carcinogens and cerebral involvement. Am J Med Sci 1987;293:122–124.
89. Weinstock MA, Horm JW. Mycosis fungoides in the United States. Increasing incidence and descriptive epidemiology. JAMA 1988;260:42–46.
90. Shelley WB. Familial mycosis fungoides revisited. Arch Dermatol 1980;116:1177–1178.
91. Cameron OJ. Mycosis fungoides in mother and in daughter. Arch Dermatol Syphilol 1933;27:232–236.
92. Sandbank M, Katzenellenbogen I. Mycosis fungoides of prolonged duration in siblings. Arch Dermatol 1968;98:620–627.

93. Epstein EH Jr, Levin DL, Croft JD Jr, et al. Mycosis fungoides. Survival, prognostic features, response to therapy and autopsy findings. Medicine 1972;51:61–79.
94. Olerud JE, Kulin PA, Chew DE, et al. Cutaneous T-cell lymphoma: Evaluation of pretreatment; skin biopsy specimens by a panel of pathologists. Arch Dermatol 1992;128:501–507.
95. Ackerman AB, Breza TS, Capland L. Spongiotic simulants of mycosis fursoides. Arch Dermatol 1974;109:218–220.
96. Orbaneja JG, Diez LI, Lozano JLS, Salazar LL, Lymphomatoid contact dermatitis: A syndrome produced by epicutaneous hypersensitivity with clinical features and a histopathologic picutre similar to that of mycosis fungoides. Contact Derm 1976;2:139–143.
97. Rijlaarsdom JV, Schaffer E, Meijer CJLM, Willemze R. Cutaneous pseudo-T-cell lymphomas. Cancer 1992;69:717–724.
98. Ralfkiaer E. Immunohistochemical markers for the diagnosis of cutaneous lymphomas. Semin Diag Pathol 1991;8:62–72.
99. Fivenson DP, Nickoloff BJ. Immunodiagnosis in cutaneous T-cell lymphoma: How does gene expression of the variable region of the T-cell receptor fit into the diagnostic and pathophysiologic picutre of T-cell neoplasia. J Cutan Pathol 1992;19:1–5.
100. Bagot M, Wechsler J, Lescs M, Revuz J, et al. Intraepidermal localization of the clone in cutaneous T-cell lymphoma. J Am Acad Dermatol 1992;27:589–593.
101. Terhune MH, Cooper KD. Gene rearrangements and T-cell lymphomas. Arch Dermatol 1993;129:1484–1490.
102. Knowles DM. Immunophenotypic and antigen receptor gene rearrangement analysis in T-cell neoplasia. Am J Pathol 1989;134:761–785.
103. Weinberg JM, Rook AH, Lessin SR. Molecular diagnosis of lymphocytic infiltrates of the skin. Arch Dermatol 1993;129:1491–1500.
104. Lessin SR, Rook AH, Rovera G. Molecular diagnosis of cutaneous T-cell lymphoma: Polymerase chain reaction amplification of T-cell antigen receptor beta-chain gene rearrangements. J Invest Dermatol 1991;96:299–302.
105. McCarthy KP, Sloane JP, Kabarowski JHS, et al. The rapid detection of clonal T-cell proliferations in patients with lymphoid disorders. Am J Pathol 1991;138:821–828.
106. Bahler DW, Berry G, Oksenbery J, et al. Diversity of T-cell antigen receptor variable genes used by mycosis fungoides cells. Am J Pathol 1992;140:1–8.
107. Wood GS, Tung RM, Haeffner AC, et al. Detection of clonal T-cell receptor gamma gene rearrangements in early mycosis fungoides/Sézary syndrome by polymerase chain reaction and denaturing gradient gel electrophoresis (PCR/DGGE). J Invest Dermatol 1994;103:34–41.
108. Vonderheid EC, Diamond LW, Sue-Min L, et al. Lymph node histopathologic findings in cutaneous T-cell lymphoma: A prognostic classification system based on morphologic assessment. Am J Clin Path 1992;97:121–129.
109. Weiss LM, Hu E, Wood GS, et al. Clonal rearrangements of T-cell receptor genes in mycosis fungoides and dermatopathic lymphadenopathy. N Engl J Med 1985;313:539–544.
110. Bakels V, Van Oostveen JW, Geerts ML, et al. Diagnostic and prognostic significance of clonal T-cell receptor beta gene rearrangements in lymph nodes of patients with mycosis fungoides. J Pathol 1993;170:249–255.
111. Heaphy MR, Winkelmann RK. Variations in peripheral Sézary cell count. Arch Dermatol 176;112:594.
112. Bendelac A, O'Connor N, Daniel MT, et al. Non-neoplastic circulating Sézary-like cells in cutaneous T-cell lymphoma. Cancer 1987;60:980–986.
113. Yan SL, Heald PW. Flow cytometry in the evaluation of dermatology patients. Clinics in Dermatology 1991;9:31–40.
114. Bakels V, Van Oostveen JW, Gorkijn RL, et al. Diagnostic value of T-cell receptor beta gene rearrangement analysis in peripheral blood lymphocytes of patients with erythroderma. J Invest Dermatol 1991;97:782–786.
115. Weiss LM, Wood GS, Hu E, et al. Detection of clonal T-cell receptor gene rearrangements in the peripheral blood of patients with mycosis fungoides/Sézary syndrome. J Invest Dermatol 1989;92:601–604.
116. Ralfkiaer E, O'Connor NTJ, Crick J, et al. Genotypic analysis of cutaneous T-cell lymphomas. J Invest Dermatol 1987;88:762–765.
117. Bunn PA, Huberman MS, Whang-Peng J, et al. Prospective staging evaluation of patients with cutaneous T-cell lymphomas. Ann Intern Med 1980;93:223–230.
118. Sausville EA, Worsham GF, Matthews JM, et al. Histologic assessment of lymph nodes in mycosis fungoides/Sézary syndrome (cutaneous T-cell lymphoma): Clinical correlations and prognostic import of a new classification system. Hum Pathol 1985;16:1098–1109.
119. Marti RM, Estrach T, Reverter JC, et al. Prognostic clinicopathologic factors in cutaneous T-cell lymphoma. Arch Dermatol 1991;127:1511–1516.
120. Lamberg SI, Green SB, Byar DP, et al. Status report of 376 mycosis fungoides patients at 4 years: Mycosis fungoides cooperative group. Cancer Treat Rep 1979;63:701–711.
121. Green SB, Byar DP, Lamberg SI. Prognostic variables in mycosis fungoides. Cancer 1981;47:2671–2677.
122. Sausville EA, Eddy JL, Makuch RW, et al. Histopathologic staging at initial diagnosis of mycosis fungoides and the Sézary syndrome. Definition of three distinctive prognostic groups. Ann Intern Med 1988;109:372–382.
123. Oliver GF, Winkelmann RK. Unilesional mycosis fungoides: A distinct entity. J Am Acad Dermatol 1989;20:63–67.
124. Kaye FJ, Bunn PA, Steinberg SM, et al. A randomized trial comparing combination electron-beam radiation and chemotherapy with topical therapy in the initial treatment of mycosis fungoides. N Engl J Med 1989;321:1784–1790.
125. Weinstock MA, Horm JW. Mycosis fungoides in the United States. Increasing incidence and descriptive epidemiology. JAMA 1988;260:42–46.
126. Holden CA, Staughton R, Campbell M, et al. Differential loss of T lymphocyte markers in advanced cutaneous T-cell lymphoma. J Am Acad Dermatol 1982;6:507–510.
127. Kono D, Baccula R, Balderas R, et al. Application of a multiprobe RNAse protection assay and functional sequences to define VB gene diversity in Sézary syndrome. Am J Pathol 1992;140:823–830.
128. Levin OL, Behrman HT. Roentgen ray therapy of mycosis fungoides. Arch Dermatol Syphilol 1945;51:307–312.
129. Lo T. Electron beam irradiation for cutaneous lymphoma. Curr Probl Dermatol 1990;19:238–251.
130. Van Scott E, Wingers PL. Responses of mycosis fungoides to intensive external treatment with nitrogen mustard. Arch Dermatol 1970;102:507–515.
131. Vonderheid EC, Van Scott EJ, Wallner PE, et al. A 10 year experience with topical mechlorethamine for mycosis fungoides: Comparison with patients treated by total-skin electron-beam radiation therapy. Cancer Treat Rep 1979;63:681–687.
132. Vonderheid EC, Tan ET, Cantor AF, et al. Long term efficacy, curative potential, and carcinogenicity of topical mechlorethamine chemotherapy and cutaneous T-celll lymphoma. J Am Acad Dermatol 1989;20:416–425.
133. Price NM, Hoppe RT, Deneau G. Ointment based mechlorethamine treatment for mycosis fungoides. Cancer 1983;52:2214–2222.
134. Lee LA, Fritz KA, Golitz L, et al. Second cutaneous malignancies in patients with mycosis fungoides treated with topical nitrogen mustard. J Am Acad Dermatol 1982;7:590–598.
135. Zackheim HS, Epstein E, McNutt NA, et al. Topical carmustine for mycosis fungoides and related disorders: A 10 year experience. J Am Acad Dermatol 1983;9:363–372.
136. Zackheim HS, Epstein EH, Crain WR. Topical carmustine (BCNU) for cutaneous T cell lymphoma: A 15-year experience in 143 patients. J Am Acad Dermatol 1990;22:802–810.
137. Gilchrest BA. Methoxsalen photochemotherapy for mycosis fungoides. Cancer Treat Rep 1979;63:663–668.
138. Honigsmann H, Brenner W, Rauschmeier W, et al. Photochemotherapy for cutaneous T cell lymphoma. J Am Acad Dermatol 1984;10:238–245.
139. Powell F, Spiegel G, Muller S. Treatment of parapsoriasis and mycosis fungoides: The role of psoralen and long-wave ultraviolet light A (PUVA). Mayo Clin Proc 1984;59:538–546.
140. Rosenbaum MM, Roenigk HH, Caro WA, et al. Photochemo-

therapy in cutaneous T cell lymphoma and parapsoriasis en plaques. J Am Acad Dermatol 1985;13:613–622.

141. Hoppe RT, Cox RS, Fuks Z, et al. Electron-beam therapy for mycosis fungoides: The Stanford University experience. Cancer Treat Rep 1979;63:691–702.

142. Braverman IM, Yager NB, Chen M, et al. Combined total body electron beam irradiation and chemotherapy for mycosis fungoides. J Am Acad Dermatol 1989;16:45–60.

143. Edelson RL, Berger CL, Gasparro FP, et al. Treatment of cutaneous T cell lymphoma by extracorporeal photochemotherapy. N Engl J Med 1987;316:297–303.

144. Heald PW, Rook A, Perez M, et al. Treatment of erythrodermic cutaneous T-cell lymphoma patients with photopheresis. J Am Acad Dermatol 1992;27:427–433.

145. Heald P, Laroche L, Knobler R. Photoinactivated lymphocyte therapy of cutaneous T-cell lymphoma. Dermatol Clinic 1994; 12:443–449.

146. Meneghetti CM, LeMaistre CF. Initial clinical experiences with an interleukin-2 fusion toxin. Targeted Diagn Ther 1992; 7:395–401.

147. LeMaistre CF, Meneghetti C, Rosenblum M, et al. Phase I trial of an interleukin-2 fusion toxin in hematologic malignancies expressing the IL-2 receptor. Blood 1992;79:2547–2554.

148. Lorent A, Feermans W, Blondeel A, et al. Sézary syndrome: Treatment with a prednisolone chlorambucil combination. Dermatologica 1982;165:464–465.

149. Winkelmann RK, Diaz-Perez JL, Buechner SA. The treatment of Sézary syndrome. J Am Acad Dermatol 1984;10:1000–1004.

150. Von Hoff DD, Dahlberg S, Hartstock RJ, et al. Activity of fludarabine monophosphate in patients with advanced mycosis fungoides: A Southwest Oncology Group study. J Natl Cancer Inst 1990;82:1353–1355.

151. Bunn PA, Foon KA, Ihde DC, et al. Recombinant leukocyte A interferon: An active agent in advanced cutaneous T-cell lymphomas. Ann Intern Med 1984;101:484–487.

152. Olsen EA, Rosen ST, Vollmer RT, et al. Interferon alfa-2A in the treatment of cutaneous T-cell lymphomas. J Am Acad Dermatol 1989;203:395–407.

153. Zackheim HS, Epstein EH. Low dose methotrexate for Sézary syndrome. J Am Acad Dermatol 1989;21:757–762.

154. McDonald CJ, Bertino JR. Treatment of mycosis fungoides lymphoma: Effectiveness of infusions of methotrexate followed by oral citrovorum factor. Cancer Treat Rep 1978;62:1009–1014.

155. Rijlaarsdam JU, Huijgens PC, Beljaards RC, et al. Oral etoposide in the treatment of cutaneous large-cell lymphomas. Br J Dermatol 1992;127(5):524–528.

156. Einhorn LH. Daily oral etoposide in the therapy of cancer. Semin Oncol 1991;18:43–49.

157. Doberauer C, Ohl S. Advanced mycosis fungoides: Chemotherapy with etoposide, methotrexate, bleomycin, and prednimustine. Acta Derm Venereol (Stockh) 1989;69:538–540.

158. Zakem MH, Davis BR, Adelstein DJ, Hines JD. Treatment of advanced stage mycosis fungoides with bleomycin, doxorubicin, and methotrexate with topical nitrogen mustard (BAM-M). Cancer 1986;58:2622–2626.

159. Winkler CF, Sausville EA, Ihde DC, et al. Combined modality treatment of cutaneous T cell lymphomas. Results of a 6 year follow-up. J Clin Oncol 1986;4:1094–1103.

160. Hallahan DE, Griem M, Griem S, et al. Combined modality therapy for tumor stage mycosis fungoides: Results of a 10 year follow-up. J Clin Oncol 1988;6:1177–1183.

161. Levi JA, Diggs CH, Wiernik PH. Adriamycin therapy in advanced mycosis fungoides. Cancer 1977;39:1967–1975.

162. Longo DL, deVita VT, Young RC. CHOP versus intensive regimens in non-Hodgkin's lymphoma. N Engl J Med 1993; 329:580–582.

163. Mostow EN, Neckel SL, Oberhelman L, et al. Complete remissions in psoralen and UV-A (PUVA)-refractory mycosis fungoides-type cutaneous T-cell lymphoma with combined interferon alfa and PUVA. Arch Dermatol 1993;129:747–762.

164. Thomsen K, Hammar H, Molin L, et al. Retinoids plus PUVA (RePUVA) and PUVA in mycosis fungoides, plaque stage. Acta Derm Venereol (Stockh) 1989;69:536–538.

165. Price MN, Hoppe RT, Constantine VS, et al. The treatment of mycosis fungoides: Adjuvant topical mechlorethamine after electron beam therapy. Cancer 1977;40:2851–2853.

166. Heald PW, Perez MI, Christensen I, et al. Photopheresis therapy of cutaneous T-cell lymphoma: The Yale-New Haven Hospital experience. Yale J of Bio Med 1989; 62:629–638.

167. Kacinski BM, Wilson L, Goodrich A, et al. Adjuvant extracorporeal photoimmunotherapy or adjuvant adriamycin/cytoxan chemotherapy both prolong survival for cutaneous T-cell lymphoma patients treated with total skin electron beam therapy. Int J Rad Oncol:in press.

168. Micaily B, Campbell O, Moser C, et al. Total skin electron beam and total nodal irradiation of cutaneous T-cell lymphoma. Int J Radiat Oncol Biol Phys 1991;20:809–813.

169. Escalante CP. Causes and management of superior vena cava syndrome. Oncology 1993;7:61–68.

170. Stokar LM. Clinical manifestations of intrathoracic cutaneous T cell lymphoma. Cancer 1985;56:2694–2702.

171. Zackheim HS, Lebo CF, Wasserstein P, et al. Mycosis fungoides of the mastoid, middle ear and CNS. Arch Dermatol 1983b; 119:311.

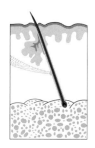

chapter 159

Other Cutaneous Lymphomas: B-Cell Lymphoma, Non– Mycosis Fungoides T-Cell Lymphoma, and Adult T-Cell Lymphoma/Leukemia

GÜNTER BURG, REINHARD DUMMER, and STEFAN DOMMANN

Whereas most nodal lymphomas are neoplasias of B lymphocytes, cutaneous lymphomas were thought to originate exclusively from T lymphocytes and usually were referred to as mycosis fungoides (MF) or as cutaneous T-cell lymphomas (CTCL).[1] However, besides these common types there were some cutaneous lymphomas exhibiting distinct clinical and histologic features, which in the European literature usually were referred to as "reticuloses."[2-4] Today, due to our knowledge on lymphocyte ontogeny and to the availability of modern techniques for differentiation, lineage-specific cell proliferations can be subdivided into various nosologic groups, including cutaneous B-cell lymphomas (CBCL) and non–MF-CTCL.

Table 159–1 is an overview of lymphoma classification, elaborated primarily for nodal lymphomas, which basically can also be used for cutaneous lymphomas. Almost 25% of cutaneous lymphomas are CBCL and 5% to 10% of CTCL are non–MF-CTCL.

Cutaneous B-Cell Lymphomas

DEFINITION

Cutaneous B-cell lymphomas (CBCL) are extranodal non-Hodgkin's lymphomas that occur primarily in the skin and are usually confined to the skin for many years. Nevertheless they are also systemic diseases of the lymphoid system and can spread into extracutaneous sites, such as lymph nodes, peripheral blood, bone marrow, and viscera. As in nodal lymphomas and leukemias, the cells that comprise the proliferating clone of tumor cells correspond to a counterpart whose differentiation stopped somewhere on the pathway between a stem cell and a fully differentiated peripheral B lymphocyte. Figure 159–1 shows the ontogeny of B lymphocytes and the

TABLE 159-1. Non-Hodgkin's Lymphomas Occurring in the Skin

Type of Lymphoma	Working Formulation
T-Cell Lymphomas	
Lymphomas of precursor T cells	ML, lymphoblastic (I)
T-lymphoblastic lymphoma/leukemia	
Lymphomas of peripheral T cells	
T-chronic lymphocytic leukemia	ML, small lymphocytic, consistent with CLL (A)
Mycosis fungoides (MF)	Mycosis fungoides (A)
Sézary's syndrome	Sézary's syndrome (A)
Pagetoid reticulosis, circumscribed, disseminated	
Pleomorphic T-cell lymphoma, HTLV-I±, small, medium, large	ML, polymorphous (H)
Immunoblastic lymphoma, T-cell type (Ki-1 +)	ML, large cell, immunoblastic (H)
Large cell anaplastic lymphoma, T-cell type (Ki-1+)	
B-Cell Lymphomas	
B-chronic lymphocytic leukemia	ML, small lymphocytic, consistent with CLL (A)
Lymphoplasmocytoid immunocytoma	ML, small lymphocytic plasmacytoid (A)
Plasmacytoma	Extramedullary plasmacytoma
Centroblastic/centrocytic lymphoma	ML, mixed small cleaved and large (B–G)
Skin-associated lymphoid tissue (SALT) lymphoma (?)	
Centrocytic (mantle cell) lymphoma	ML, small cleaved (E, G)
Immunoblastic lymphoma	ML, large cell, immunoblastic (H)
Burkitt's lymphoma	ML, small non-cleaved, Burkitt (J)

ML, malignant lymphoma; CLL, chronic lymphocytic leukemia; HTLV-I, human T-cell lymphotropic virus–I.

respective malignant B-cell lymphomas arising from the various stages of differentiation.

B lymphocytes are produced throughout life by primary B-cell production from hematopoietic cells in the marrow and through antigen-driven proliferation in secondary lymphoid tissue; only a small proportion of these cells survive and differentiate to become part of the rela-tively stable pools of peripheral B cells,[5] which need to receive regular signals to become long-lived cells. This stable pool consists of recirculating B cells and nonrecir-culating cells.

The most frequent type of CBCL originates from fol-licular cells. The recirculating follicular cells migrate to and from the follicles through T zones, which are impor-

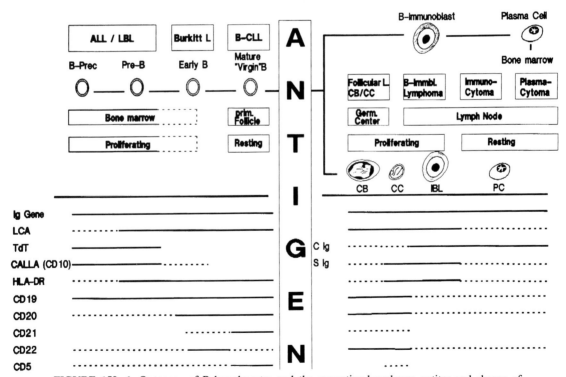

FIGURE 159-1. Ontogeny of B lymphocytes and the respective lymphoma entites and change of phenotype during B-cell maturation. ALL, acute lymphoblastic leukemia; LBL, lymphoblastic leuke-mia/lymphoma; L, lymphoma; CLL, chronic lymphocytic leukemia; B-Prec, B-precursor; CB/CC, centroblastic/centrocytic; Germ. Center, germinal center; CB, centroblast; CC, centrocyte; IBL, im-munoblast; PC, plasma cell; CIg, cytoplasmatic immunoglobulins; SIg, surface immunoglobulins.

tant for B-cell activation and the production of virgin B cells, most of which die after a short time but some of which receive signals that rescue them from apoptosis and recruit them into the recirculating follicular B-cell pool through the various layers of secondary follicles.[6]

CLINICAL DESCRIPTION

Clinically, CBCL can usually be differentiated from CTCL, owing to the monomorphous appearance of nodules and/or tumors, which may be solitary, grouped in a circumscribed area, or disseminated and which develop in a relatively short period of time from normal-looking skin.[7]

The head and neck area seems to be preferentially involved by infiltrates and tumors (Fig. 159–2A) for some unknown reason. Diffuse infiltration of facial skin may lead to leonine facies. The color of nodules and tumors of CBCL is deep red, and the surface is smooth without scaling or ulceration. The consistency of tumors is relatively firm compared with the soft consistency in CTCL.[8]

As opposed to CTCL, in which the clinical features may help in the discrimination of subtypes, the subtypes of CBCL cannot be differentiated on the basis of the clinical appearance of the skin lesions. The so-called reticulohistiocytosis of the back (Crosti's disease) is usually a follicular center cell lymphoma.[7, 9] Enlargement of peripheral lymph nodes, if at all, occurs early in the course of the disease and indicates neoplastic infiltration rather than dermatopathic lymphadenopathy as frequently seen in CTCL.

There is no current clinical staging classification for CBCL that can accurately predict the clinical course and prognosis of the disease. Attempts have been made with a modified TNM staging,[7, 8] but its prognostic reliability has not been sufficiently demonstrated.

The curve depicting survival in patients with cutaneous lymphoma shows significant flattening after about 7 years for CBCL, which crosses the CTCL curve at that time (Fig. 159–3). This indicates that there is a proportion of at least 50% of CBCL that has an exceptionally good prognosis. This is probably due to the special types of CBCL, which are true clonal malignant B-cell lymphomas but that biologically show features of pseudolymphomas and are referred to as pseudolymphomatous or "semimalignant" B-cell lymphomas (see later discussion).

PATHOLOGY

Histologically, CBCL show a typical architecture referred to as a B-cell pattern[7] that is different from the band-like subepidermal infiltrate seen in CTCL. In CBCL, the infiltrate is characterized by a sharply demarcated nodular, mostly bottom-heavy infiltrate in the middle or deep dermis, sparing a subepidermal border zone. These features are typical for small cell type, well-

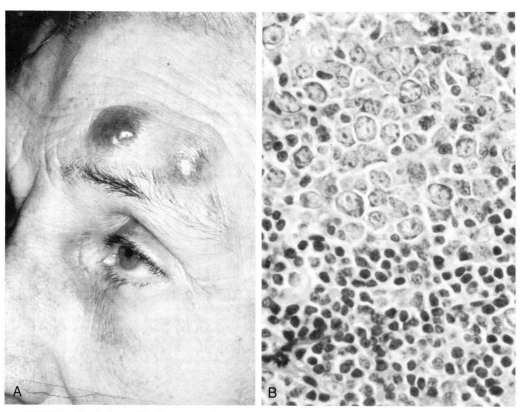

FIGURE 159–2. Centroblastic/centrocytic lymphoma (mixed small cleaved and large) of the skin. *A,* multiple nodules in the head and neck area. *B,* small cleaved and large uncleaved cells (Giemsa, ×400).

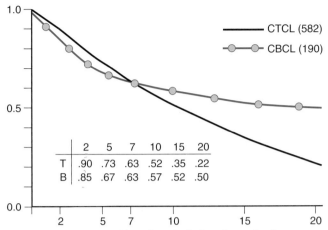

FIGURE 159–3. Probability of survival after diagnosis of cutaneous B-cell and cutaneous T-cell lymphoma. (Data from EORTC Cutaneous Lymphoma Study, 1993; N = 772.)

differentiated CBCL and may be lost in large cell CBCL with high-grade malignancy. Phenotyping of the infiltrate in CBCL reveals pan–B-cell antigen expression (HLA-DR, CD19, CD20, CD22) in addition to special differentiation antigens of the cell surface or intracytoplasmic immunoglobulins.[10]

Malignant B-Cell Lymphomas of Low-Grade Malignancy

Lymphocytic Lymphoma

Small lymphocytic lymphoma, B-cell type (SLL; category A in the Working Formulation) differs from chronic lymphocytic leukemia (CLL) by the lack of a leukemic blood picture. Histologically, SLL in the skin displays the typical B-cell pattern (well-circumscribed nodules in the dermis and subcutis without epidermotropism) commonly seen in all CBCL of low-grade malignancy. The small lymphocytes have a small round or oval nucleus with dense chromatin showing homogeneous dark staining; the small rim of cytoplasm cannot be seen. There is no formation of germinal centers. Eosinophils and plasma cells are usually absent. Surface immunoglobulins, κ and λ light chains, and B-cell differentiation antigens can be demonstrated by immunoenzymatic techniques using the respective pan–B-cell monoclonal antibodies (HLA-DR, CD19, CD20); the pan–T-cell antibody for CD5 is also positive in SLL and CLL.

Immunocytoma

This lymphoma is known as malignant lymphoma small lymphocytic or plasmacytoid in the Working Formulation (categories A and F, respectively). It represents the second most frequent clinicopathologic form of lymphoma occurring in the skin after follicular (centroblastic/centrocytic) lymphoma. Primary cutaneous immunocytoma generally has a favorable prognosis.

Histologically, cutaneous infiltrates in immunocytoma show a typical B-cell pattern with well-circumscribed

nodules in the dermis. Small well-differentiated cells showing morphologic features of both small lymphocytes and plasma cells predominate. A valuable diagnostic hallmark is the presence of intranuclear, periodic acid–Schiff-positive globular inclusions of immunoglobulins (Dutcher bodies). The proliferating cells are monoclonal and usually produce IgMκ.[11] In contrast to medullary plasmacytoma or macroglobulinemia, in immunocytoma the immunoglobulins are not secreted but are stored within the tumor cells; thus, no monoclonal gammopathy can be detected in the peripheral blood.

Follicular Center Cell Lymphomas (Centroblastic (CB)/Centrocytic (CC) and Centrocytic Lymphoma)

Reactive follicular centers mainly contain two types of B-lymphoid cells in addition to a network of dendritic cells and a few T lymphocytes. Centroblasts are medium- to large-sized cells with a vesicular, somewhat round nucleus and a few distinct nucleoli attached to the nuclear membrane. The cytoplasm is basophilic on Giemsa staining. Centrocytes are small- or medium-sized cells with irregular nuclei showing linear clefts.

Centroblastic/centrocytic (CBCC) lymphoma, also known as malignant lymphoma, intermediate grade, and mixed small and large cell in the Working Formulation, is the most frequent form, accounting for about 12% of cutaneous lymphomas and about 40% of CBCL. They are composed of centroblasts (at least 20%) and centrocytes (see Fig. 159–2B) and usually lack the sharp border between these two major cellular components, which is typically seen in follicular pseudolymphomas of the skin. In contrast to pseudolymphomas, in CBCL there are almost no tingible body macrophages and no eosinophils and the structure of the network of CD21+ dendritic reticulum cells, if present, is irregular. Special subtypes of CBCL may show immunoglobulin production or are cytogenetically related to lymphocytes arising from the mantle zone of lymph follicles (intermediate cell lymphoma), which show membrane-bound alkaline phosphatase.[12]

Centrocytic lymphoma (CC) is designated as malignant lymphoma of small or large cleaved cells in the Working Formulation and comprises about 1% cutaneous lymphomas and about 4% CBCL. Due to the clefted nuclei and the lack of follicular structures in this type of lymphoma, the histologic features may be misinterpreted as nonepidermotropic T-cell lymphoma. Therefore, immunophenotyping is mandatory in these cases. However, eosinophils or plasma cells, often present in CTCL, are usually absent in CC.

Malignant B-Cell Lymphomas of High-Grade Malignancy

Centroblastic Lymphoma

Centroblastic lymphoma (CB), which was called reticulum cell sarcoma 20 years ago, in the Working Formulation is referred to as malignant lymphoma, large-cell, noncleaved. It comprises about 1.5% of cutaneous lymphomas and about 6% of CBCL and may arise secondary from centroblastic/centrocytic lymphoma (see earlier discussion).

Histologically, typical features of B-cell or T-cell pattern are lacking in the skin. Epidermotropism may be present or absent. There may be remnants of large follicle-like structures. The predominant proliferating cell type resembles the large noncleaved basophilic follicular center cell (centroblast) and contains several medium-sized nucleoli situated predominantly at the nuclear membrane.

The differential diagnosis includes immunoblastic lymphoma, lymphoblastic lymphoma, and true histiocytic lymphoma. The histomorphologic and cytomorphologic border between centroblastic and immunoblastic lymphoma is not sharp.

Immunoblastic Lymphoma (IBL), B-Cell Type

This lymphoma, designated as malignant lymphoma, large-cell immunoblastic in the Working Formulation, was formerly referred to as reticulum cell sarcoma or histiocytic lymphoma and represents about 3% of cutaneous lymphoma and about 12% of CBCL.

Histologically, a diffuse pattern is commonly found. The infiltrate usually involves all levels of the dermis and subcutis. The immunoblast is a large round-to-oval cell with broad basophilic cytoplasm, a large vesicular nucleus, and a centrally placed nucleolus; the cytomorphologic features of T and B immunoblasts are both very similar, so that distinction must be based on immunophenotyping.

Lymphoblastic Lymphoma (LBL), Burkitt Type

The categorization of this lymphoma is not yet completely clear. It is thought to arise from early B cells by some and to be related to follicular center cell lymphoma by others. Usually, as in the Epstein-Barr virus (EBV)–associated Burkitt lymphoma, the EBV-unrelated type shows primary involvement of lymph nodes and internal organs. However, primary Burkitt-type lymphoma of the skin may occur, as seen in one of our cases without any extracutaneous involvement over a follow-up period of 5 years (Fig. 159–4A). The histological hallmark is the starry-sky appearance due to large macrophages within a relatively monomorphous infiltrate of small- to medium-sized lymphoid cells (see Fig. 159–4B).

Other and Rare Forms of Large B-Cell Lymphomas

Extramedullary plasmacytomas of the skin are extremely rare.[7] Histologically, a dense monomorphous infiltrate of plasma cells is seen.

Angiotropic (intravascular) lymphoma, formerly referred to as systemic or malignant angioendotheliomatosis,[13, 14] is characterized by dense accumulation of small to large mononuclear cells within the lumina of blood vessels, probably due to dysregulation of homing factors.[18]

Reticulohistiocytoma of the back in adults (Crosti's disease) in most of the cases is a follicular centroblastic/centrocytic lymphoma. It has little tendency to spread systemically.[9]

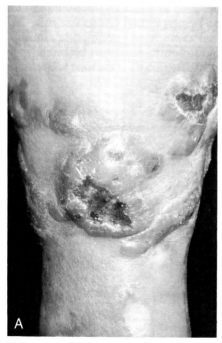
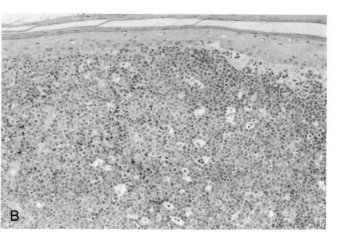

FIGURE 159–4. Cutaneous B-cell lymphoma, Burkitt type. *A,* Ulcerating tumors in a circumscribed area of one leg. *B,* Dense mononuclear cell infiltrate with macrophages in a starry-sky pattern (Burkitt-type fashion) (hematoxylin-eosin, × 100).

Anaplastic Ki-1 (CD30)-positive lymphomas usually express T-cell phenotype; however, B-cell types also exist.

Multilobated large B-cell lymphomas of the skin with flower-like multilobated nuclei and several nuclear protrusions have been reported.[15-17]

T-cell–rich large B-cell lymphoma is also very rare, especially when primarily occurring in the skin.

Semimalignant (Pseudolymphomatous) B-Cell Lymphomas of the Skin

This type of CBCL shares features of centroblastic-centrocytic lymphoma and of pseudolymphoma (Table 159–2).[19, 20] Clinically it is compatible with other low-grade malignant B-cell lymphomas of the skin, presenting as multiple nodules or tumors that do not regress spontaneously but may be controlled by nonaggressive therapeutic modalities such as topical or systemic glucocorticosteroids.

Histologically it differs from pseudolymphoma by covering the whole dermis, infiltrating into the subcutaneous fat, and showing monoclonal immunoglobulin-bearing or immunoglobulin-producing cells. Differentiation of this peculiar form of CBCL, also referred to as large cell lymphocytoma,[21, 22] is reasonable, since the prognosis of the disorder mandates control by nonaggressive rather than aggressive treatment modalities.

TREATMENT

B-cell lymphomas with exclusively cutaneous manifestations should be treated with locally aggressive modalities like x-rays or surgical excision. However, in cases showing disseminated spread of skin lesions, systemic therapy may be indicated, using glucocorticosteroids, (poly-)chemotherapy, interferons, or retinoids.

Non–Mycosis Fungoides Cutaneous T-Cell Lymphomas

DEFINITION

Mycosis fungoides (MF) is the prototypical peripheral CTCL of small cerebriform cell type. One of the distinctive features is development of the disease from an "eczematous" stage to a tumor stage, whose diagnosis can be difficult. Non–MF-CTCL display specific clinical, histologic, cytologic, or phenotypic features and therefore can be regarded as distinct nosologic subentities within the group of CTCL.

TABLE 159–2. Preferential Clinical, Histologic, and Phenotypical Criteria in Cutaneous B-Cell Lymphomas (CBCL), Semimalignant (SM) "Pseudolymphomatous" CBCL, and Pseudolymphomas (PSL)

Criteria	CBCL (%)	SM-CBCL (%)	PSL (%)
Clinical			
Number, distribution, and localization of skin lesions	Multiple generalized (100%)	Multiple confined to one region (70%)	Solitary, head (80%)
Extracutaneous involvement	Present (100%)	Absent (100%)	Absent (100%)
Type of and response to therapy	Aggressive, TR	Nonaggressive, TR	Nonaggressive, CR
Fatal outcome	Likely	No or late	No
Recurrences	Always	Mostly (>90%)	Rare (<10%)
Cure	Not possible	Not possible	Possible
Survival time	Affected	Usually nonaffected	Normal
Histologic			
Infiltrate extending into all levels of the dermis	Mostly (>70%)	Mostly (>60%)	Rarely (<5%)
Pattern of infiltrate	Diffuse or nodular Bottom > top heavy	Diffuse or nodular Bottom > top heavy	Nodular (>90%) Top > bottom heavy
Follicular center formation (hematoxylin-eosin)	Usually absent	Usually present	Usually present
Transformation into blast form (centroblastic, immunoblastic)	May occur	Never occurs	Never occurs
Eosinophilic granulocytes	Usually absent	Usually absent	Always present
Phenotypic			
Monotypic κ or λ light chain reaction of surface immunoglobulin	Present (100%)	Present (100%)	Absent (100%)
Percentage of cells expressing			
B-cell markers (CD20, MB2, CD45R)	High	High	Medium
T-cell markers (CD43, CD45RA, CD45 RO)	Low	Low	Medium
Network of CD21-positive dendritic reticulum cells	Mostly absent	Mostly present, bizarre	Mostly present, regular

TR, temporary response; CR, complete response.

CLINICAL DESCRIPTION AND PATHOLOGY

Pleomorphic and Large Cell Lymphomas

Pleomorphic T-cell lymphoma has an inconspicuous clinical appearance showing papules, plaques, tumors, or erythroderma with a male-to-female ratio of 5:1.[23] The neoplastic cells, which may be small, medium sized, or large, are pleomorphic; that is, they have a multishaped bizarre nucleus, usually with dense chromatin structure and abundant eosinophilic cytoplasm (Fig. 159–5). Adult T-cell leukemia/lymphoma (ATLL) is a human T-cell lymphotropic virus type I (HTLV-I)–positive variant of this subgroup. The clinical course of these lymphomas may be prolonged in the small cell variant or rapid in the medium and large cell variants.

Primary cutaneous CD30 (Ki-1)–positive anaplastic large cell lymphoma is a morphologic and phenotypic variant of large cell lymphomas, formerly referred to as histiocytic lymphoma or misdiagnosed as true malignant histiocytosis.[24-26] Characteristic clinical features are solitary or localized skin lesions in almost 90% of the cases, frequent spontaneous remission of skin lesions, rare secondary involvement of extracutaneous sites (25%), and a good prognosis.[27]

Histologically, there is a diffuse cohesive growth pattern with or without epidermotropism, often reaching into the subcutaneous tissue. The neoplastic cells are large with round or oval nuclei and abundant, often clear cytoplasm, simulating undifferentiated carcinoma, melanoma, or histiocytic disorders. Immunophenotypically, the hallmark is CD30 (Ki-1) positivity. In addition, most cells express a T-helper cell phenotype. However, there also exist CD30-positive large cell lymphomas of B-cell type, primarily occurring in the skin.

Immunoblastic lymphoma of T-cell type and multilobated T-cell lymphoma represent variants of large cell, non-MF peripheral T-cell lymphomas with high-grade malignancy showing distinct cytologic features with round or oval vesicular nuclei and central large nucleoli (immunoblasts) or irregular nuclei with lobulations (multilobated).[28]

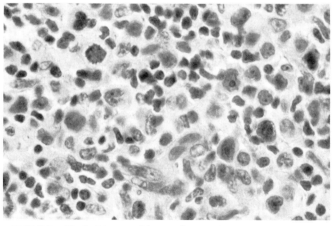

FIGURE 159–5. Pleomorphic (medium to large) T-cell lymphoma arising from mycosis fungoides (hematoxylin-eosin, × 400).

Non–MF-CTCL Showing Features of Distinct Tissue Tropism

Angiotropic lymphomas (intravascular lymphomatosis), formerly referred to as systemic angioendotheliomatosis,[16] are intravascular lymphomas that usually express the B-cell phenotype[29]; however, T-cell variants have been reported.[30] Clinically, multiple reddish violet cutaneous patches, plaques, or nodules are seen. In the final stage of the usually treatment-refractory and rapidly fatal disease, extracutaneous involvement (lung, liver) occurs. A skin biopsy specimen shows lymphoid cells confined to the lumina of dermal vessels. Immunohistologic studies revealed the lymphoid nature of the intravascularly proliferating tumor cells,[31] which subsequently has been confirmed in several studies by gene rearrangement assays. Speculations on the vascular confinement of angiotropic lymphoma focus on the role of cytokines and adhesion molecules in homing behaviors.

Subcutaneous ("lipotropic") lymphomas clinically often present as erythema nodosum or panniculitis.[32, 33] Histologically, they show dense infiltrates in the subcutaneous fat tissue, but without features of hemophagocytosis as seen in hemophagocytic panniculitis.[34] Rare variants may show clonal rearrangement of the δ chain of the T-cell receptor and produce high amounts of interferon gamma, resulting in progressing leukopenia and fever.[33]

Epidermolytic (T8-positive) CTCL within the spectrum of phenotypically distinct CTCL showing pronounced tropism to distinct tissue structures clinically appears with widespread erosions and ulcerations with rapid dissemination. Histologically, the epidermis is destroyed by a cytotoxic CD8-positive lymphoid infiltrate, which in the beginning is superficial but becomes tumorous in the final stage of the disease.

Granulomatous and Other Non–MF-CTCL

Granulomatous slack skin, originally described as progressive, atrophying, chronic granulomatous dermohypodermitis,[35] represents a rare condition with plaque-like lesions showing a wrinkled surface and large pendulous folds of skin in the axillae and in the groins. Histologically, sarcoid and tuberculoid granulomas are found with multinucleated giant cells, almost complete loss of elastic fibers, and remnants of elastic material in giant cells. Analysis of the T-cell receptor by Southern blot analysis has demonstrated a clonal population of cells.[36] There seems to be a close relationship of these variants to granulomatous forms of mycosis fungoides[37] or to sarcoid skin reactions, seen in association with Hodgkin's disease and CTCL.

Angioimmunoblastic lymphadenopathy, formerly termed lymphogranulomatosis X, is a lymphoproliferative disorder that can give rise to T-cell lymphoma. Skin involvement is usually seen secondarily in 40% of the patients[7] after manifestations of the disease in the lung, brain, and other organs. Histology of skin lesions reveals polymorphous cellular infiltrates and vessel changes that are not diagnostic.

Lymphomatoid granulomatosis[38] is primarily an extracutaneous disease involving skin (plaques, papules, ulcers) in almost 50% of the cases.[7] There are clinical similarities to Wegener's granulomatosis or to lethal midline granuloma. Histology shows characteristic angiocentric and angiodestructive infiltrates that range from cytologically bland to frankly malignant.

Lymphoepithelioid lymphoma (so-called Lennert's lymphoma) has also been reported in the skin.[39] It is histologically characterized by proliferation of CD4-positive lymphocytes with small clusters of epithelioid macrophages. Originally, the disorder was thought to be a variant of Hodgkin's disease. However, typical Sternberg-Reed cells are usually lacking and the reaction of CD30 is negative.[40]

In 1984, Ofuji and associates described a chronic dermatosis characterized by erythroderma-like changes, sparing the skinfolds with widespread red-brown flat pruritic papules with many eosinophils, which they termed "papuloerythroderma."[41] Additional cases have been reported since then[42]; however, the etiology and pathogenesis remain obscure, and it is not clear if the process is reactive or neoplastic.

TREATMENT

Non–MF cutaneous T-cell lymphomas are treated according to the same guidelines as MF in order to control rather than to cure the disease.

Pathogenesis and Etiology of Cutaneous Lymphomas

As in solid tumors, the development of lymphoma is probably a multistep process, starting with initiation by changes or damage of the cellular DNA and promotion due to a variety of factors. Eventually a malignant cell succeeds in escaping immunologic surveillance and leads to tumor formation[43] by clonal expansion.

Whereas in adult T-cell lymphoma in Japan and the Caribbean HTLV-I plays an important etiologic role, retroviral DNA cannot be detected in other non-MF lymphomas; however, integration of certain retroviral genomic information, such as the pX-region, into the lymphoid cells can code for uncontrolled production of promoter proteins, including interleukin-2 or other cytokines, in a minority of patients.

Translocation (t14,18) of the bcl-2 suppressor gene, which blocks programmed cell death (apoptosis), is a crucial event in follicular center cell–derived neoplasia of the lymph node. Similar cytogenetic changes may be important in cutaneous lymphomas but have not yet been demonstrated except in secondary skin involvement of primary nodal B-cell lymphomas.[44]

Diagnosis and Differential Diagnosis

Most CBCL can be diagnosed as such owing to their typical morphologic features of circumscribed, firm, dome-shaped nodules and tumors arising on normal-looking skin. However, in contrast to CTCL, differentiation of the various nosologic subtypes is not possible clinically. More information is provided by histomorphology showing a typical nodular B-cell pattern of the infiltrate, consisting of lymphoid cells, that can be differentiated according to their typical cytomorphology as large and small follicular center cells, immunoblasts, and multilobated and other cell types. In doubtful cases confirmation of the B-cell nature of the infiltrate can be achieved by demonstration of κ or λ light chain restriction on cryostat or on microwave-exposed paraffin sections, respectively, or by proving heavy chain restriction in the Southern blot analysis.

The differential diagnosis of CBCL primarily includes nodular pseudolymphomas and semimalignant (pseudolymphomatous) B-cell lymphomas of the skin with germinal center formation (see Table 159–2). Pseudolymphomas can be defined as reactive processes regressing either spontaneously or by nonaggressive treatment modalities without recurrences. In some cases the clinical course of the disease allows the conclusive diagnosis.

Adult T-Cell Lymphoma/Leukemia

DEFINITION

Adult T-cell lymphoma/leukemia (ATL) is a lymphoproliferative disorder etiologically associated with HTLV-I most frequently seen in endemic areas such as southern Japan and the Caribbean. The skin is involved in more than 50% of cases.[45, 46]

CLINICAL DESCRIPTION

Based on clinical features and laboratory findings the following subtypes of ATL have been differentiated[47]: smoldering, chronic lymphoma, and acute. In general, the disease starts between the fourth to sixth decades and most commonly affects men. Generalized lymphadenopathy is the most consistent finding. However, hepatosplenomegaly, bone marrow involvement, and a leukemic blood picture are also present in more than 50% of the cases.

Skin involvement occurs almost regularly during the course of the disease, presenting as papules, nodules, or tumors, as erythema, as lupus erythematosus-like lesions, or as erythroderma.

Typical laboratory findings are a leukemic blood picture, sometimes in conjunction with anemia, hypoalbuminemia, hypergammaglobulinemia, and hypercalcemia. A distinctive finding is the presence of peripheral blood lymphocytes with cloverleaf-shaped nuclei. The mean survival time is less than 3 years.

PATHOLOGY

The histopathologic findings in the skin usually show a diffuse infiltrate of medium to large pleomorphic (multi-shaped nuclei) cells with or without epidermotropism. However, there are great variations of cytomorphologic features. There may even be differences between the histomorphologic findings in the lymph node compared with skin infiltrates. No correlation exists between subtypes of ATL and histomorphologic classification according to the Working Formulation.[46] There is also pronounced heterogeneity of the phenotype of neoplastic cells from patients with ATL. Usually they show a helper/inducer T-cell phenotype (CD4 +, CD8 −), but other phenotypic profiles may be seen in some of the cases (CD4 −, CD8 + or CD4 −, CD8 −). Surface antigens of neoplastic cells from the skin (CD29 −, CD45RO +, CD45RA −; memory cell phenotype) may be different from those in the peripheral blood (CD45RA +, CD29 −, CD45RO −; naive cell phenotype) or lymph nodes,[46] constituting different maturational stages rather than distinct lineages.

PATHOGENESIS AND ETIOLOGY

Despite the existence of pleomorphic T-cell lymphomas without serologic evidence of HTLV-I infection, in the endemic variants clonal integration of retroviral DNA into the host cell genome plays an important role in pathogenesis. In clonal integration, retroviral DNA is present at the same point in each malignant cell. Clonal integration can be detected by Southern blot analysis and distinguishes ATL from other T-cell lymphomas in seropositive patients. It is speculated that activation of genes coding for the production of proteins that exhibit activating and proliferating capacities leads to proliferation of T cells.

DIAGNOSIS AND DIFFERENTIAL DIAGNOSIS

The diagnosis is based on clinical findings described earlier and on the demonstration of HTLV-I antibodies in the serum. Skin manifestations showing erythema, papules, tumors, or erythroderma fall in the category of skin lesions mostly seen in CTCL; however, confirmation of the diagnosis has to be achieved by histopathology and immunophenotyping.

The differential diagnosis, from a clinical point of view, includes the broad spectrum of peripheral CTCL and, from a pathologic point of view, other forms of HTLV-I–negative pleomorphic or anaplastic T-cell lymphomas.

TREATMENT

Like in other forms of noncurable T-cell lymphomas, the strategy of management of ATL should be control of the disease using treatment modalities that are appropriate according to the spread of the neoplastic process and its biologic aggressiveness. Disease confined to a few skin sites is often amenable to local modalities such as excision or local radiation therapy. In cases with widespread lesions, the whole spectrum from watchful waiting to nonaggressive chemotherapy (e.g., low-dose chlorambucil) to highly aggressive polychemotherapy or electron beam radiation therapy may be considered. Like in other CTCL, "experimental" treatment modalities may include the use of interferons and of new drugs (purine analogues).

References

1. Edelson RL (NHI Conference). Cutaneous T-cell lymphomas: Perspective. Ann Intern Med 1975;83:548–552.
2. Degos R, Ossipowski B, Civatte J, Touraine R. Reticuloses cutanées (reticuloses histiomonocytaires). Ann Dermatol Syphiligr 1957;84:125–152.
3. Gottron HA. Retikulosen der Haut. In: Gottron HA, Schönfeld W, eds. Dermatologie und Venerologie, vol IV. Stuttgart: Thieme, 1960:501–590.
4. Burg G, Braun-Falco O. Classification and differentiation of cutaneous lymphomas. Br J Dermatol 1975;93:597–599.
5. MacLennan I, Chan E. The dynamic relationship between B-cell populations in adults. Immunol Today 1993;14:29–37.
6. Liu YJ, Johnson GD, Gordon J, MacLennan ICM. Germinal centers in T-cell–dependent antibody responses. Immunol Today 1992;13:17–21.
7. Burg G, Braun-Falco O. Cutaneous Lymphomas, Pseudolymphomas, and Related Disorders. New York: Springer, 1983.
8. Burg G, Kaudewitz P, Klepzig K, et al. Cutaneous B-cell lymphoma. Dermatol Clin 1985;3:689–704.
9. Berti E, Alessi E, Caputo R, et al. Reticulohistiocytoma of the dorsum. J Am Acad Dermatol 1988;19:259–272.
10. Faure P, Chittal S, Gorguet B, et al. Immunohistochemical profile of cutaneous B-cell lymphoma on cryostat and paraffin sections. Am J Dermatopathol 1990;12:122–133.
11. Burg G, Kaudewitz P, Braun-Falco O, Mason DY. Immunoenzymatic typing of lymphoplasmacytoid skin infiltrates. J Dermatol Surg Oncol 1984;10:284–290.
12. Geerts ML, Burg G, Schmoeckel CH, Braun-Falco O. Alkaline phosphatase activity in non-Hodgkin's lymphomas and pseudolymphomas of the skin. J Dermatol Surg Oncol 1984;10:306–312.
13. Pfleger L, Tappeiner J. Zur Kenntnis der systemischen Endotheliomatose der kutanen Blutgefässe. Hautarzt 1959;10:359.
14. Tappeiner J, Pfleger L. Angioendotheliomatosis proliferans systematisata: Ein klinisch und pathologisch neues Krankheitsbild. Hautarzt 1963;14:67.
15. Putte van der SCJ, Toonstra T, De Weger RA, Unniv van JAM. Cutaneous T-cell lymphoma, multilobated type. Histopathology 1982;6:35–54.
16. Giannotti B, Gattorossi A, Moretti S, et al. Cytochemical and immunological findings in cutaneous multilobated cell lymphoma. In: MacDonald MD, ed. Immunodermatology. London: Butterworth, 1984;125–127.
17. O'hara J, Said J, Pinkus GS. Non-Hodgkin's lymphoma, multilobated B-cell type: Report of nine cases with immunoultrastructural evidence for a follicular center cell derivation. Hum Pathol 1986;17:593–599.
18. Ferry JA, Harris NL, Picker LJ, et al. Intravascular lymphomatosis (malignant angioendotheliomatosis): A B-cell neoplasm expressing surface homing receptors. Mod Pathol 1988;1:444–452.
19. Torne R, Roura M, Umbert P. Generalized cutaneous B-cell pseudolymphoma. Am J Dermatopathol 1989;11:544–548.
20. Burg G, Hess Schmid M, Küng E, et al. Semimalignant ("pseudo-

lymphomatous") cutaneous B-cell lymphomas. Dermatol Clin 1994;12:399–407.

21. Duncan SC, Evans HL, Winkelman RK. Large cell lymphocytoma. Arch Dermatol 1980;116:1142–1146.

22. Winkelman RK, Dabski K. Large cell lymphocytoma: Follow up, immunopathology studies and comparison to cutaneous follicular and Crosti lymphoma. Arch Dermatol Res 1987;279:81–87.

23. Sterry W, Siebel A, Mielke V. HTLV-1–negative pleomorphic T-cell lymphoma of the skin: The clinicopathological correlations and natural history of 15 patients. Br J Dermatol 1992;126:456–462.

24. Stein H, Mason DY, Gerdes J, et al. The expression of Hodgkin's disease associated antigen Ki-1 in reactive and neoplastic lymphoid tissue: Evidence that Reed-Sternberg cells and histiocytic malignancies are derived from activated lymphoid tissue. Blood 1985;66:848–858.

25. Agnarsson BA, Kadin ME. Ki-1 positive large cell lymphoma: A morphologic and immunological study of 19 cases. Am J Pathol 1988;12:264–274.

26. Kaudewitz P, Burg G, Stein H, Ki-1 (CD 30) positive cutaneous anaplastic large cell lymphomas. Curr Probl Dermatol 1990;19:150–156.

27. Beljaards RC, Kaudewitz P, Berti E, et al. Primary cutaneous CD 30-positive large cell lymphoma: Definition of a new type of cutaneous lymphoma with a favorable prognosis: A European multicenter study of 47 patients. Cancer 1993;71:2097–2104.

28. Kerl H, Cerroni L, Burg G. The morphologic spectrum of T-cell lymphomas of the skin: A proposal for a new classification. Semin Diagn Pathol 1991;8:55–61.

29. Wick MR, Mills SE. Intravascular lymphomatosis: Clinicopathologic features and differential diagnosis. Semin Diagn Pathol 1991;8:91–101.

30. Sepp N, Schuler G, Romani N, et al. Intravascular lymphomatosis (angioendotheliomatosis): Evidence for a T-cell origin in two cases. Hum Pathol 1990;21;1051–1058.

31. Bhawan J, Wolff SM, Ucci A, et al. Malignant lymphoma and malignant angioendotheliomatosis: One disease. Cancer 1985;55:570–576.

32. Gonzalez CL, Medeiros LJ, Braziel RM, Jaffe ES. T-cell lymphoma involving subcutaneous tissue: A clinicopathologic entity commonly associated with hemophagocytic syndrome. Am J Surg Pathol 1991;15:17–27.

33. Burg G, Dummer R, Wilhelm M, et al. A subcutaneous delta-positive T-cell lymphoma that produces interferon gamma. N Engl J Med 1991;325:1078–1081.

34. Winkelman RK. Pannikulitis mit Zellphagozytose, Fieber, Panzytopenie, Polyserositis und letaler hämorrhagischer Diathese. Hautarzt 1980;31:588–594.

35. Convit J, Kerdel F, Goihman M, et al. Progressive, atrophing, chronic granulomatous dermohypodermitis: Autoimmune disorder? Arch Dermatol 1973;107:271–274.

36. LeBoit PE, Beckstead JH, Bond B, et al. Granulomatous slack skin: Clonal rearrangement of the T-cell receptor gene is evidence for the lymphoproliferative nature of a cutaneous elastolytic disorder. J Invest Dermatol 1987;89:183–186.

37. Ackerman AB. Granulomatous mycosis fungoides. J Dermatol 1970;82:397–401.

38. Liebow AA, Carrington CRB, Friedman PJ. Lymphomatoid granulomatosis. Hum Pathol 1972;3:457–558.

39. Kiesewetter F, Haneke E, Lennert K, et al. Cutaneous lymphoepitheloid lymphoma (Lennert's lymphoma): Combined immunohistological, ultrastructural, and DNA-flow cytometric analysis. Am J Dermatopathol 1989;11:549–554.

40. Lennert K, Feller AC. Histopathology of Non-Hodgkin's Lymphomas. New York: Springer, 1992:167–186.

41. Ofuji S, Furukawa F, Miyachi Y, et al. Papuloerythroderma. Dermatologica 1984;169:125–130.

42. Lacour JP, Perrin C, Ortonne JP. Ofuji papuloerythroderma: A new European case. Dermatology 1993;186:190–192.

43. Dummer R, Posseckert G, Nestle F, et al. Soluble interleukin-2 receptors inhibit interleukin-2–dependent proliferation and cytotoxicity: Explanation for diminished natural killer cell activity in cutaneous T-cell lymphomas in vivo. J Invest Dermatol 1991;98:50–54.

44. Cerroni L, Volkenandt M, Rieger E, et al. bcl-2 protein expression and correlation with the interchromosomal 14;18 translocation in cutaneous lymphomas and pseudolymphomas. J Invest Dermatol 1994;102:231–235.

45. Ushiyama T, Yodoi J, Sagawa K, et al. Adult T-cell leukemia: Clinical and hematologic features of 16 cases. Blood 1977;50:481–492.

46. Nagatani T, Miyazawa M, Matsuzaki T, et al. Adult T-cell leukemia/lymphoma (ATL): Clinical, histological and immunohistochemical characteristics. Exp Dermatol 1992;1:248–252.

47. Shimoyama MI. Members of the Lymphoma Study Group (1984–1987). Diagnostic criteria and classification of clinical subtypes of adult T-cell leukemia-lymphoma: A report from the Lymphoma Study Group (1984–1987). Br J Haematol 1991;79:428–437.

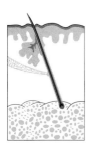

chapter 160

Leukemia Cutis

STANISLAW A. BUECHNER and W. P. DANIEL SU

DEFINITION

Cutaneous manifestations in leukemias present an important diagnostic challenge to dermatologists. The skin lesions can be classified as either specific or nonspecific. Lesions that are the direct result of infiltration and proliferation of leukemic cells in the skin are known as "specific lesions" or "leukemia cutis." Leukemic infiltration of the skin occurs in 3% to 11% of patients with adult leukemia.[1-4] Nonspecific lesions (leukemids) are common, occurring in approximately 30% of patients with leukemia.[5, 6] They may be related to anemia, thrombocytopenia, infection, and drugs or result from immunologic responses to tumor antigens. Histologically, there is no evidence of leukemic infiltration of the skin.

CLINICAL DESCRIPTION OF SPECIFIC LESIONS

Lymphocytic Leukemia

In chronic lymphocytic leukemia (CLL), specific lesions occur in 4% to 45% of patients but are uncommon in lymphocytic leukemia of the acute type.[5, 7] Clinically, the patients present with papules (Fig. 160–1), plaques, and nodules (Fig. 160–2).[4, 7-9] In a review of 289 cases of lymphocytic leukemia with skin lesions collected from the literature, tumors and large nodules were found in 50% of patients.[10] Although leukemic skin lesions can occur anywhere, the head, neck, trunk, and especially the face appear to the most common locations.[4] Rarely, the clinical features of the lesions may be atypical, and the initial appearance of cutaneous infiltrates of CLL has been reported in individual cases as chronic paronychia, subungual tumors involving several fingers, plaques on the volar surface of the hands and fingers, finger clubbing with periosteal bone destruction of the distal digits, papulovesicular eruption of the face, and exfoliative erythroderma.[7, 11, 12]

Hairy-Cell Leukemia

Specific skin lesions in hairy cell leukemia (HCL) are uncommon. Of the 600 cases with HCL reported in the literature, 48 (8%) were described as having specific skin lesions, of which 8 were proven by biopsy.[13] In another report of 113 cases of HCL from the Mayo Clinic, only one patient had skin infiltration by leukemic cells.[14] Specific cutaneous lesions were usually described as erythematous macules and papules.

Adult T-Cell Leukemia

Adult T-cell leukemia (ATL) is a disseminated malignancy of T lymphocytes infected by the human T-lymphotropic virus type I.[15] The cutaneous manifestations of ATL may vary from maculopapular rash, multiple nodular tumors, and bullous lesions to generalized erythroderma.[16] Skin involvement has been reported to occur in 40% to 70% of cases.[15] The diagnosis of ATL is based on detailed examination of blood and bone marrow, although the clinicopathologic differentiation of ATL from Sézary's syndrome may be difficult.

Granular Lymphocytic Leukemia

Lymphoproliferative disease of granular lymphocytes (LDGL) represents a heterogeneous family of diseases with an atypical lymphocytosis characterized by an expansion of lymphocytes with cytoplasmic azurophilic granules, usually referred to as "granular lymphocytes."[17] Phenotypically, the lymphocytes in LDGL have characteristics of either cytotoxic T cells (CD3+, CD8+) or natural killer cells (CD3+, CD16+).[18] LDGL shows less predilection for skin involvement than other T-cell malignancies do. In a large multicenter study, skin infiltration was observed in 5 of 151 patients and was a poor prognostic finding.[17]

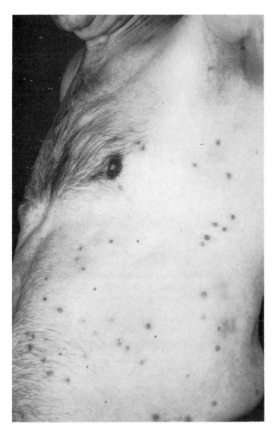

FIGURE 160-1. Chronic lymphocytic leukemia. Purplish macules and papules on trunk.

Myelogenous and Monocytic Leukemia

Involvement of the skin by acute myelogenous leukemia (AML) has been reported to occur in 13% of patients.[2] Patients with acute monocytic leukemia (AMOL, FAB-M5) and acute myelomonocytic leukemia (AMML, FAB-M4) have the highest incidence of both specific and nonspecific skin lesions. Documented mucocutaneous leukemic infiltrations range from 10% to 33% in AMOL and from 13% to 27% in AMML.[1, 3, 5] The cutaneous manifestations are quite varied and consist of multiple papules, nodules, and infiltrative plaques ranging in size from a few millimeters to several centimeters (Fig. 160-3).[1, 2, 4-6, 8] In a series of 877 patients with AML, leukemia cutis presented as multiple small skin lesions in 13 patients and as single skin lesions in 5 others.[19] Bullous lesions have also been described in AMOL and AMML.[20] The most common areas of involvement are the scalp, face, trunk, and extremities.[2, 4-6] Congenital monoblastic leukemia with papular and nodular skin lesions or nodules with blueberry-muffin appearance has rarely been described.[21] The finding of infiltrated, hyperplastic gingival lesions strongly favors the diagnosis of AMOL or AMML.

Leukemic gingival infiltrations were present in 67% of patients with AMOL and in 18% of those with AMML.[1] Hyperplasia, swelling, bleeding, and inflammation of the gingiva are characteristic findings. Usually skin involvement occurs during the course of disease or may be concomitant with or precede the diagnosis of systemic leukemia.[4] As late as 1990, nine cases of aleukemic leu-

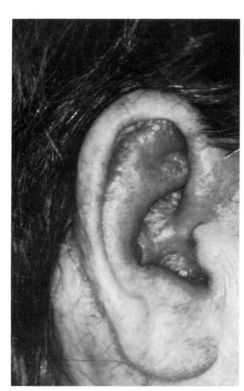

FIGURE 160-2. Chronic lymphocytic leukemia. Infiltrated plaque on ear.

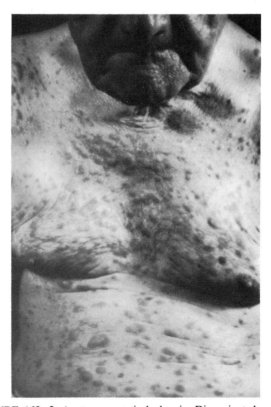

FIGURE 160-3. Acute monocytic leukemia. Disseminated papules and nodules on trunk.

kemia cutis of monocyte origin had been reported.[22] The skin lesions developed 2 to 18 months before systemic leukemia was diagnosed.

Cutaneous infiltration is an uncommon event during the course of acute granulocytic leukemia (AGL). Skin lesions include papules, plaques, and nodules without any particular distribution.[2, 5, 6, 8] Chloroma, or granulocytic sarcoma, is another rare condition that may occur in patients who have AGL or chronic granulocytic leukemia (CGL) in blast crisis.[4, 23] The term *chloroma* may be used when the tumor of myeloblast cells in the skin has a diagnostic greenish coloration due to the presence of myeloperoxidase. Granulocytic sarcomas develop in less than 3% of patients with AGL and may precede by months to years the development of systemic leukemia.

Specific skin lesions in CGL are uncommon. The incidence of skin lesions varies from 0% to 4%.[24] The lesions begin as erythematous papules, nodules, or plaques that may become purpuric and ulcerated.[4, 8] Skin involvement in chronic myelomonocytic leukemia (CMML), which almost exclusively affects elderly persons, is much less frequent, and only a few cases have been reported.

PATHOLOGY

Problems in histologic diagnosis of leukemia cutis arise because of variable patterns of infiltrations and cytomorphologic features that depend on cell differentiation and the origin of the neoplastic cells.[25] The diagnosis of leukemia cutis is based on the recognition of the predominant cell type, on the pattern of infiltration and on correlation with distinctive clinical and hematologic findings. Histochemical and immunohistochemical studies with monoclonal antibodies may be helpful in confirming the diagnosis. They are also important in distinguishing nonspecific from specific infiltrates.[26]

Lymphocytic Leukemia

In most cases of B-cell CLL there is a perivascular and periadnexal infiltrate of small- to medium-sized lymphocytes with dense nuclear chromatin. The infiltrate is usually present in the upper and lower dermis and may extend to the subcutaneous tissue. In the majority of cases, a grenz zone of uninvolved dermis separates the epidermis from the underlying dermal infiltrates.[7-9, 25] With regard to phenotype, there is considerable heterogeneity among the infiltrating cells in CLL. The majority of lymphocytes are negative for the T-cell marker (CD45Ro) and positive or negative for the B-cell marker (CD20).[26] CD20-positive B cells that inappropriately coexpress Leu-22 (CD43), a T-cell marker, can be demonstrated in routinely processed sections of B-cell CLL.[26] Monoclonality of SIg (light-chain restriction) is pathognomonic of B-cell malignancy. The predominant heavy-chain type in typical CLL is IgM or IgM and IgD.

The distinctive pathologic feature of HCL is a dense, diffuse, or patchy infiltrate of small uniform mononuclear cells with indented nuclei in the dermis surrounding and invading the blood vessels and skin ad-

nexa.[8, 13, 14] Histochemically, the majority of infiltrating hairy cells show diffuse cytoplasmic positivity by tartrate-resistant acid phosphatase staining.[14]

The histologic picture of ATL is that of a dense infiltrate of a variety of small, medium-sized, large, or pleomorphic lymphoid cells with convoluted nuclei that are present around the blood vessels or extend through the full thickness of the dermis.[16] Frequent mitotic figures were observed. The infiltrate can exhibit epidermotropism with or without Pautrier's microabscesses. Marker studies confirm that the majority of these cells are activated T-helper cells with a high level of expression of CD3, CD4, CD5, and CD25 antigens.[15]

Myelogenous and Monocytic Leukemia

In AGL and CGL, dense infiltrates involve all levels of the dermis. The epidermis is spared and separated from the infiltrates by distinct grenz zones. The infiltrate may overrun and destroy the blood vessels and adnexa. Typically, the leukemic cells spread contiguously, infiltrating the collagen bundles and subcutaneous fibrous septa. The neoplastic infiltrates in AGL are composed predominantly of large cells with round or oval vesicular nuclei and immature atypical myeloid cells with bizarre, clefted nuclei. Mitotic figures are a consistent finding in AGL.[1, 8, 23, 25] Granulocytes in various stages of differentiation, including mature neutrophilic granulocytes and metamyelocytes, are present in CGL.[24] Most of the leukemic cells in AGL and CGL stain strongly for intracytoplasmic lysozyme, and a smaller proportion of neoplastic cells has been found to contain chloroacetate esterase (using the Leder stain) or to react with antiserum to α_1-antitrypsin. CD43 (Leu-22) is strongly positive in most cases of AGL and CGL.[19, 25, 26]

The infiltrates in AMOL are principally monomorphous and composed mainly of atypical cells of various size and with a slightly basophilic and vacuolated cytoplasm and a large, often indented or kidney-shaped nucleus. In AMML, the infiltrates contain a mixture of immature monocytes with irregular nuclei, atypical myeloblasts, myelocytes, and occasional neutrophils.[1, 8, 25] Phenotypically, leukemic infiltrates are consistently positive for lysozyme, CD43 (Leu 22), CD45 (LCA), and CD15 (Leu-M1) in almost all AMOL and in the majority of AMML cases.[19, 26] Chloroacetate esterase is detected in only a minority of the leukemic cells in AMML and is absent in AMOL.[25, 26]

DIFFERENTIAL DIAGNOSIS

Some of the more common disorders in the differential diagnosis of leukemia are summarized in Table 160–1.

TREATMENT

Treatment of leukemia cutis is the same as that of the underlying systemic leukemia and consists of local radio-

TABLE 160-1. Differential Diagnosis of Leukemia Cutis

Cutaneous lymphomas
  Mycosis fungoides
  Sézary's syndrome
Hodgkin's disease
Histiocytosis X
Lymphomatoid papulosis
Angioimmunoblastic lymphadenopathy
Lymphomatoid granulomatosis
Lymphocytic infiltrate of Jessner
Actinic reticuloid
Lymphadenosis benigna cutis
Drug-induced pseudolymphoma
Arthropod bite reactions
Kaposi's sarcoma
Sarcoidosis
Mastocytosis
Vasculitis

therapy and chemotherapy. Chemotherapy has been used in all types of leukemia with skin involvement with varying degrees of success. The chemotherapy varies with the type of acute leukemia and includes various combinations of vincristine, L-asparaginase, daunorubicin, cytarabine, thioguanine, and prednisone. Administration of cytarabine, usually in conjunction with an anthracycline antibiotic, is considered the treatment of choice in AML. Bone marrow transplantation appears to be superior to chemotherapy alone. Busulfan is the agent of choice for patients with chronic myeloid leukemia.[27]

Because systemic chemotherapy adequate to induce and to maintain bone marrow remission does not necessarily control specific skin lesions in AML, the optimal management of leukemia cutis should consist of electron-beam irradiation in conjunction with systemic chemotherapy.[19] Patients with widespread leukemia cutis present at diagnosis of AML in the bone marrow may be treated successfully with whole-body electron beam radiation followed by chemotherapy. Total skin irradiation is superior to chemotherapy for treating the skin lesions.[22] The skin lesions in HCL respond well to systemic interferon alpha therapy, which is the treatment of choice.[13] Favorable results have been obtained with treating leukemia cutis with topical nitrogen mustard.[24]

References

1. Dreizen S, McCredie KB, Keating MJ, et al. Malignant gingival and skin "infiltrates" in adult leukemia. Oral Surg Oral Med Oral Pathol 1983;55:572-579.
2. Boggs DR, Wintrobe MM, Cartwright GE. The acute leukemias: Analysis of 322 cases and review of the literature. Medicine 1962; 41:163-225.
3. Ricevuti G, Mazzone A, Rossini S, et al. Skin involvement in hemopathies: Specific cutaneous manifestations of acute nonlymphoid leukemias and non-Hodgkin lymphomas. Dermatologica 1985;171:250-254.
4. Su WPD, Buechner SA, Li C-Y. Clinicopathologic correlations in leukemia cutis. J Am Acad Dermatol 1984;11:121-128.
5. Stawiski MA. Skin manifestations of leukemias and lymphomas. Cutis 1978;21:814-818.
6. Bluefarb SM, ed. Leukemia Cutis. Springfield, IL: Charles C Thomas, 1960.
7. Bonvalet D, Foldes C, Civatte J. Cutaneous manifestations in chronic lymphocytic leukemia. J Dermatol Surg Oncol 1984; 10:278-282.
8. Burg G, Braun-Falco O. Cutaneous Lymphomas, Pseudolymphomas, and Related Disorders. Berlin: Springer-Verlag, 1983; 341-374.
9. Greenwood R, Barker DJ, Tring FC, et al. Clinical and immunohistological characterization of cutaneous lesions in chronic lymphocytic leukemia. Br J Dermatol 1985;113:447-453.
10. Beek CH. Skin manifestations associated with lymphatic-leucaemia. Dermatologica 1948;96:350-356.
11. High DA, Luscombe HA, Kauh YC. Leukemia cutis masquerading as chronic paronychia. Int J Dermatol 1985;24:595-597.
12. Simon CA, Su WPD, Li C-Y. Subungual leukemia cutis. Int J Dermatol 1990;29:636-639.
13. Arai E, Ikeda S, Itoh S, et al. Specific skin lesions as the presenting symptom of hairy cell leukemia. Am J Clin Pathol 1988; 90:459-464.
14. Finan MC, Su WPD, Li C-Y. Cutaneous findings in hairy cell leukemia. J Am Acad Dermatol 1984;11:788-797.
15. Davey FR, Hutchison RE. Pathology and immunology of adult T-cell leukemia/lymphoma. Curr Opin Oncol 1991;3:13-20.
16. Chan H-L, Su IJ, Kuo T, et al. Cutaneous manifestations of adult T cell leukemia/lymphoma: Report of three different forms. J Am Acad Dermatol 1985;13:213-219.
17. Pandolfi F, Loughran TP Jr, Starkebaum G, et al. Clinical course and prognosis of the lymphoproliferative disease of granular lymphocytes: A multicenter study. Cancer 1990;65:341-348
18. McKenna RW. Lymphoproliferative disorder of granular lymphocytes: More questions than answers (editorial). Arch Pathol Lab Med 1992;116:235-237.
19. Baer MR, Barcos M, Farrell H, et al. Acute myelogenous leukemia with leukemia cutis: Eighteen cases seen between 1969 and 1986. Cancer 1989;63:2192-2200.
20. Eubanks SW, Patterson JW. Subacute myelomonocytic leukemia—an unusual skin manifestation. J Am Acad Dermatol 1983;9:581-584.
21. Gottesfeld E, Silverman RA, Coccia PF, et al. Transient blueberry muffin appearance of a newborn with congenital monoblastic leukemia. J Am Acad Dermatol 1989;21:347-351.
22. Ohno S, Yokoo T, Ohta M, et al. Aleukemic leukemia cutis. J Am Acad Dermatol 1990;22:374-377.
23. Sun NCJ, Ellis R. Granulocytic sarcoma of the skin. Arch Dermatol 1980;116:800-802.
24. Murphy WG, Fotheringham GH, Busuttil A, et al. Skin lesions in chronic granulocytic leukemia: Treatment of a patient with topical nitrogen mustard. Cancer 1985;55:2630-2633.
25. Buechner SA, Li C-Y, Su WPD. Leukemia cutis: A histopathologic study of 42 cases. Am J Dermatophathol 1985;7:109-119.
26. Ratnam KV, Su WPD, Ziesmer SC, et al. Value of immunohistochemistry in the diagnosis of leukemia cutis: Study of 54 cases using paraffin-section markers. J Cutan Pathol 1992;19:193-200.
27. Lee GR, Bithell TC, Foerster J, et al. Wintrobe's Clinical Hematology, 9th ed, vols 1 and 2. Philadelphia: Lea & Febiger, 1993.

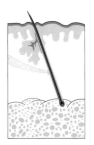

chapter 161

Cutaneous Metastases

GEORGE P. LUPTON and J. MICHAEL GAGNIER

DEFINITION

Cutaneous metastases represent spread of a preexisting malignancy to the skin. They are of diagnostic importance because, in addition to signifying a generally poor prognosis, they may be the first manifestation of an undiscovered malignancy or the first indication of metastasis of a presumably cured malignancy.

CLINICAL DESCRIPTION

In one study of nearly 2300 patients who died of internal carcinoma, only 2.7% had metastases to skin.[1] More recent studies have shown a significantly higher percentage of skin metastases. In a study of autopsies on more than 7500 patients with internal malignancy, 9% had metastases to skin.[2] Another study found cutaneous metastases in 10% of 4020 patients with metastatic cancer.[3]

The incidence of cutaneous metastasis depends on both the incidence and site of the primary neoplasm. The incidence varies as well by sex (Table 161–1).[3, 4] Despite the high frequency of prostate cancer (28% of all malignant neoplasms in men) and the significant mortality associated with this tumor (13% of cancer deaths in men),[5] cutaneous metastases from this malignancy are uncommon (less than 3%). Metastasis to skin from carcinoma of the thyroid gland, pancreas, liver, bladder, endometrium, and testis is rare, probably because of the relative infrequency of these primary carcinomas. In one study, melanoma was the most frequent source of cutaneous metastases in men, responsible for 32% of cases.[3] In a review of the files (1945–1993) at the Armed Forces Institute of Pathology (AFIP), melanoma accounted for 39% of all skin metastases in men and 20% of those in women. Although these figures may be somewhat skewed because of the selected case material received for consultation at the AFIP, melanoma is well known for its propensity to cutaneous metastasis.[2, 6] The origin and

All material in this chapter is in the public domain, with the exception of any borrowed figures or tables.

frequency of other cutaneous metastases were similar to those cited in Table 161–1.

The clinical appearance of skin metastases is usually not distinctive (Figs. 161–1 through 161–4). They may resemble the primary tumor in color and consistency and vary in size up to several centimeters. Most skin metastases are freely movable cutaneous or subcutaneous nodules that may be discrete, firm, and indolent. Plaque-like lesions also occur. Lesions may appear skin colored, erythematous, violaceous, or pigmented.

PATHOLOGY

Metastases to skin generally show histologic features bearing some resemblance to those of the primary tumor. Metastatic adenocarcinoma from the gastrointestinal tract usually reveals glands with intracytoplasmic and luminal mucin (Fig. 161–5). In a metastatic adenocarcinoma to the skin of the umbilicus in a woman (Fig. 161–6), the presence of psammoma bodies suggested an ovarian primary tumor. A cutaneous tumor consisting of clear cells may suggest a clear cell hidradenoma, but if a

TABLE 161–1. Origins of Malignancies Most Commonly Metastatic to Skin

Primary Site in Men	Range of Percentage of Cutaneous Metastases	Primary Site in Women	Range of Percentage of Cutaneous Metastases
Melanoma	13–39	Breast	69–71
Lung	12–24	Melanoma	5–20
Colon	11–19	Ovary	3–4
Oral cavity	9–12	Lung	2–4
Kidney	5–6	Oral cavity	1–2
Stomach	1–6	Colon	1–9

*Data from references 3 and 4 and Armed Forces Institute of Pathology.

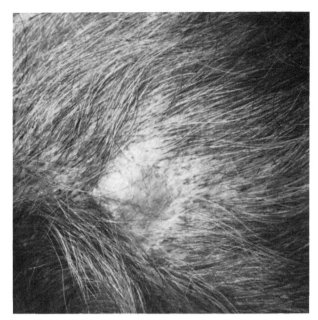

FIGURE 161-1. Alopecia neoplastica in metastatic breast carcinoma.

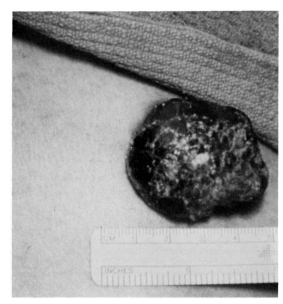

FIGURE 161-3. Exophytic cutaneous metastasis from lung carcinoma.

prominent vascular component is present (Fig. 161-7), metastatic renal cell carcinoma is likely. The absence of an epidermal component in a squamous cell carcinoma suggests the possibility of metastasis. Metastatic breast carcinoma often reveals a desmoplastic stroma infiltrated by anaplastic cells with an "Indian filing" pattern, as well as small aggregates of similar cells suggesting glandular differentiation (Fig. 161-8). Although the histology of the metastasis may suggest the primary site of the tumor, not infrequently the cutaneous metastasis may be anaplastic or poorly differentiated and can be designated only as carcinoma, sarcoma, or undifferentiated malignant neoplasm.

PATHOGENESIS AND ETIOLOGY

A tumor may disseminate into the skin through lymphatics. In such cases, cutaneous metastases tend to appear later in the course of the disease and to affect the skin overlying the area of primary tumor. Other neoplasms, such as carcinoma of the kidney and lung, usually spread to the skin hematogenously, to sites distant from the primary tumor.[7, 8] When some malignancies such as carcinoma of the breast and prostate and melanoma metastasize to skin, they have an affinity for epidermal involvement (i.e., epidermotropism), the pathogenesis of which is not well understood.

In general, the location of a cutaneous metastasis is related to the site of the primary neoplasm. Thus, head and neck cutaneous metastases are often associated with

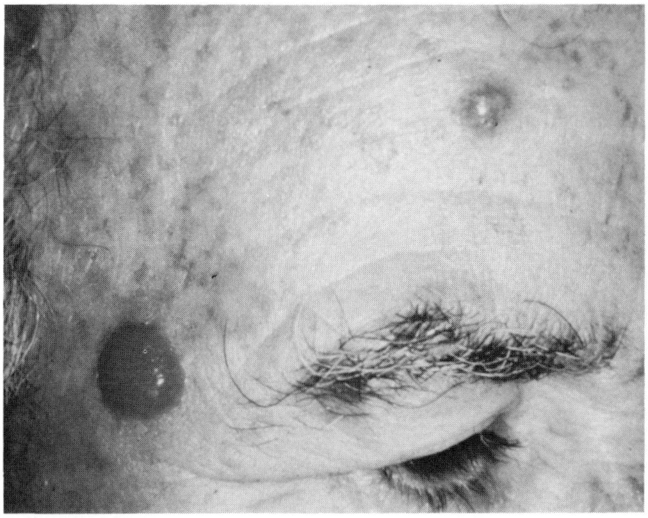

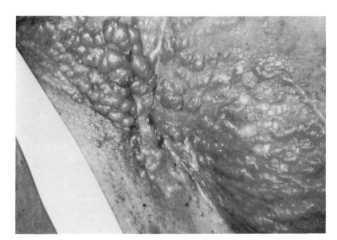

FIGURE 161-2. Nodules of metastatic large cell carcinoma of the lung.

FIGURE 161-4. Indurated pebbly plaque of metastatic melanoma in inguinal fold.

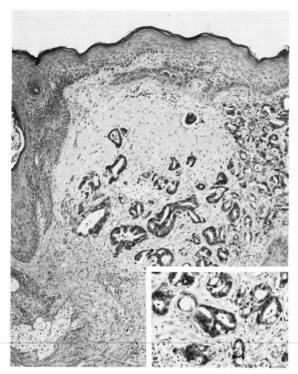

FIGURE 161–5. Metastatic esophageal adenocarcinoma in the scalp. *Inset*, Higher-magnification view of glandular structures.

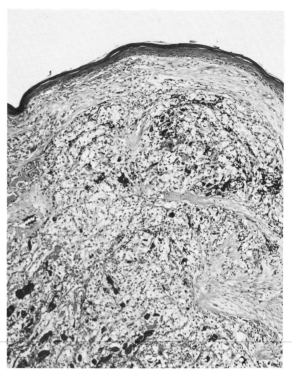

FIGURE 161–7. Metastatic renal cell carcinoma to the neck.

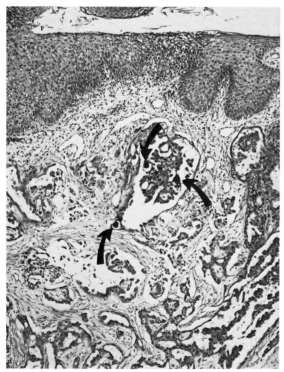

FIGURE 161–6. Metastatic ovarian serous papillary adenocarcinoma in the umbilicus. Note the psammoma bodies (*arrows*).

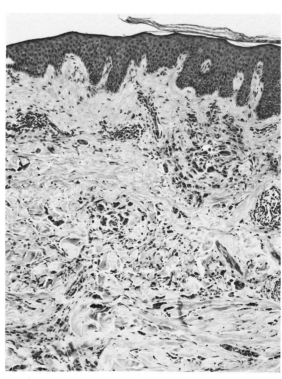

FIGURE 161–8. Metastatic breast carcinoma to the chest wall.

squamous cell carcinoma of the oral cavity or nasopharynx. Chest cutaneous metastases are most frequently associated with breast cancer in women and lung cancer in men. Gastrointestinal neoplasms usually metastasize to the anterior abdominal wall, while pelvic tumors tend to spread to the perineal region. Intra-abdominal malignancies, such as from the stomach, colon, and pancreas, will at times metastasize to the skin of the umbilicus, resulting in the so-called Sister Mary Joseph's nodule. Melanomas and neoplasms associated with vascular invasion, such as renal cell carcinoma, thyroid follicular carcinoma, and choriocarcinoma, show less tendency toward regional localization.

DIAGNOSIS AND DIFFERENTIAL DIAGNOSIS

Clinically, the differential diagnosis of neoplasms metastatic to skin is quite varied and is listed in Table 161–2.

In addition to routine histopathology, special histochemical stains such as periodic acid–Schiff with and without diastase, mucicarmine, Fontana-Masson, and reticulum stains can be helpful in establishing the type of cutaneous metastasis. In recent years, the addition of immunohistochemical markers has provided an important adjunct in evaluating cell types. For example, malignant neural tumors rarely metastasize to skin; therefore, the presence of an infiltrate positive for S-100 protein and/or HMB-45 antigen is likely to indicate metastatic melanoma. Carcinomas are cytokeratin positive, and a variety of keratin monoclonal antibodies can help differentiate between glandular and squamous epithelium. Carcinoembryonic antigen and epithelial membrane antigen are useful for identifying glandular carcinoma and Paget's disease. Some stains are more specific, such as prostate-specific antigen and calcitonin for medullary thyroid carcinoma.

Electron microscopy is another tool for identifying the nature of the cutaneous metastasis. It is best performed

TABLE 161–2. Differential Diagnosis of Neoplasms Metastatic to Skin

Epidermoid/pilar cyst
Lipoma
Neurofibroma
Adnexal tumor
Fibroepithelial polyp
Pyogenic granuloma
Kaposi's sarcoma
Lymphoma
Morphea
Cicatricial alopecia

TABLE 161–3. Treatment of Neoplasms Metastatic to Skin

Surgical excision
Chemotherapy
   Localized
   Isolated limb perfusion
Radiation therapy
Palliation

on properly processed fresh tissue rather than on formalin-fixed, paraffin embedded tissue. Identification of cellular markers such as desmosomes (carcinoma), melanosomes (melanoma), intracytoplasmic mucin (adenocarcinoma), or membrane-bound neurosecretory granules (Merkel cell carcinoma, oat cell carcinoma, carcinoid tumors) may aid in establishing the primary site of malignancy.

TREATMENT

The presence of cutaneous metastases in a patient with internal malignancy is usually a poor prognostic sign because it tends to represent widespread systemic disease. A team approach to treatment employing surgery, chemotherapy, and radiation therapy is needed. The treatment of a specific cutaneous metastasis often depends on whether the lesion interferes with normal function of the body, is disfiguring, or is a source of great pain, frequent bleeding, or possibly secondary infection. Consideration of its contribution to total tumor load must also be considered. Some of the treatment options for cutaneous metastases are listed in Table 161–3.[9]

References

1. Reingold IM. Cutaneous metastases from internal carcinoma. Cancer 1966;19:162–168.
2. Spencer PS, Helm TN. Skin metastases in cancer patients. Cutis 1987;39:119–121.
3. Lookingbill DP, Spangler N, Helm KF. Cutaneous metastases in patients with metastatic carcinoma: A retrospective study of 4020 patients. J Am Acad Dermatol 1993;29:228–236.
4. Brownstein MH, Helwig EB. Metastatic tumors of the skin. Cancer 1972;29:1298–1307.
5. Boring CC, Squires TS, Tong T. Cancer statistics, 1993. CA 1993;43:7–26.
6. Gupta TD, Brasfield R. Metastatic melanoma. Cancer 1984; 17:1323–1339.
7. Brownstein MH, Helwig EB. Spread of tumors to the skin. Arch Dermatol 1973;107:80–86.
8. McKee PH. Cutaneous metastases. J Cutan Pathol 1985;12: 239–250.
9. Healey PM, Malott K, Chalet MD. Cancers metastatic to the skin. In: Friedman RJ, Rigel DS, Kopf AW, et al, eds. Cancer of the Skin. Philadelphia: WB Saunders Co., 1991:347–363.

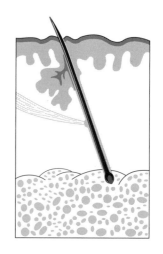

What Diseases of the Skin Are Malformations or Are Predominantly Inherited?

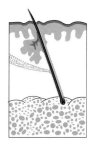

chapter 162

The Ichthyoses: Disorders of Cornification

MARY L. WILLIAMS and PHILIP E. LE BOIT

The disorders of cornification constitute a diverse group characterized by focal or generalized scaling or hyperkeratosis. When generalized, these have been called *ichthyosis*, a term from the Greek root *ichthys* for "fish," to describe a similarity of appearance of the human scaling skin disorders to fish scales. Although widely employed, the term has outlived its usefulness and should be abandoned. In the first place, the term is pejorative. Patients burdened by the onus of a disfiguring skin condition should not bear the additional insult of a derogatory name. There is precedent for changing a disease name to avoid unwanted connotations (e.g., mongolism to Down's syndrome). Second, the term is inaccurate. Some forms show no resemblance to fish scales.[1] The term also does not bear any relationship to disease pathogenesis; that is, the scaling disorder does not present an atavistic reversion to an aquatic ancestor.

These scaling disorders have also been referred to as keratinization disorders. This term may have merit if it is used in its broadest sense to denote all of the processes involved in epidermal terminal differentiation. However, if used narrowly to focus on the formation of keratin filaments per se, other major contributors to stratum corneum function, and in particular, to the lamellar body secretory system, are overlooked. In addition, some true disorders of keratinization are primarily blistering, rather than scaling, disorders (e.g., epidermolysis bullosa simplex arising from mutations in the keratin 5 or 14 genes). Thus the term *keratinization disorders* invites nosologic confusion.

Cornification can be applied broadly to denote all of the processes involved in the formation and maintenance of the stratum corneum. These processes include profilaggrin proteolysis and keratin filament assembly, formation of the cornified envelope, apoptosis and organellar dissolution, and the formation of the lamellar membrane units by means of the lamellar body secretory system. Theoretically, defects involving any of these components could alter stratum corneum function and result in hyperkeratosis. The primary function of the stratum corneum is to provide a barrier to systemic water loss, without which terrestrial life is not possible. The barrier is formed through the secretion of lamellar bodies, an organelle that contains lipid precursors and certain lysosomal-type enzymes, into the extracellular space at the junction of the last granular and first cornified cell layers, and the reorganization of lamellar body membranes to form repeating arrays of membrane bilayers, termed *basic lamellar membrane unit structures*.[2] A secondary function of stratum corneum is to desquamate (i.e., to shed) old, outer corneocytes one by one in an invisible manner and to replace these with newly formed cornified cells (with their surrounding lamellar membrane units) in the inner stratum corneum. It is apparent that abnormalities in both functions of stratum corneum (i.e., barrier function and desquamation) underlie scaling disorders.[3]

Disorders in which desquamation is abnormal without an alteration in the kinetics of epidermal cell replacement (i.e., retention hyperkeratosis) include recessive X-linked ichthyosis (RXLI) and ichthyosis vulgaris. In RXLI, which is caused by deficiency of the enzyme steroid sulfatase, the following pathogenic sequence can be constructed: alteration in the lipid composition of the lamellar membranes through increased cholesterol sulfate and decreased cholesterol content impairs the ultimate breakup of the membrane bilayers and/or the dissolution of corneodesmosomes. Intact desmosomal connections are normally present between corneocytes in the inner layers of stratum corneum, but by mid stratum corneum, only remnants of corneodesmosomes persist. Proteolysis of corneodesmosomes accounts for the shedding of squames from plantar stratum corneum[4] and is likely to be essential for desquamation elsewhere. The proteases involved in corneodesmosomal dissolution may be among the hydrolases residing in lamellar bodies and secreted into the intercellular domain along with the probarrier lipids. Cholesterol sulfate may normally act as an inhibitor of these proteases. The graded hydrolysis of cholesterol sulfate to cholesterol through the action of steroid sulfatase during the outward movement of corneocytes and their membranes would release the protease from inhibition and permit desmosomal degradation. Ultrastructurally, failure to degrade corneodesmosomes in an orderly manner appears to be a common denominator in a wide variety of disorders of cornification.[3]

The notion that disturbance of barrier function may underlie the hyperproliferative disorders of cornification, in which scaling is due to the flooding of the cornified cell compartment by excessive numbers of incompletely cornified cells, derives from experimental work in which it has been demonstrated that either acute or chronic disruption of the permeability barrier results in increased epidermal DNA synthesis.[5] Restoration of a barrier, as for example by covering the skin surface with an occlusive membrane, prevents the increased epidermal DNA synthesis in the acute models (i.e., when a defective barrier is produced by solvent extraction of stratum corneum lipids or removal of the stratum corneum through tape stripping) and normalizes epidermal DNA synthesis in the chronic model of essential fatty acid deficiency. Impaired barrier function is a common feature in a number of disorders of cornification.[6] Hence it is entirely possible that barrier dysfunction may drive the hyperproliferation associated with a number of the disorders. For example, epidermal hyperplasia in disorders in which lamellar bodies are abnormal (e.g., nonbullous congenital ichthyosiform erythroderma, neutral lipid storage disease) may be driven by barrier insufficiency. Similarly, the marked change in phenotype noted in a number of a congenital ichthyoses (i.e., from collodion baby to exfoliative erythroderma in congenital ichthyosiform erythroderma (CIE), or from blistering to hyperkeratosis in bullous ichthyosis) may be driven by the acute requirement for a competent barrier ("xeric stress") presented to the infant at birth.[7] However, it is also possible that some hyperproliferative epidermal disorders may be primary, owing to abnormalities in the regulation of epidermal growth, as evidenced by the hyperkeratotic phenotype in transgenic mice that overexpress the cytokine transforming growth factor$-\alpha$.[8]

ACQUIRED DISORDERS OF CORNIFICATION

Acquired Ichthyoses

Most genetically determined disorders of cornification have their onset of disease in infancy or early childhood, except for the adult form of Refsum's disease, in which the onset may be delayed until the second or third decade. Later onset of a scaling disorder usually indicates an acquired condition and should initiate a search for the cause (Table 162–1). Drugs associated with generalized scaling include several hypocholesterolemic agents, par-

TABLE 162-1. Causes of Acquired Ichthyosis

Drug induced
  Hypocholesterolemic agents
    Nicotinic acid
    Triparanol
    Diazocholesterol
  Other
    Clofazamine
    Cimetidine
    Kava ingestion
Metabolic/Nutritional
  Thyroid dysfunction (especially hypothyroidism)
  Renal failure
  Malabsorption syndromes
  Kwashiorkor
  Zinc deficiency
  Essential fatty acid deficiency
Malignancy
  Carcinoma (especially bronchogenic)
  Lymphoma (especially Hodgkin's and cutaneous T-cell)
Immune Disorders
  Human immunodeficiency virus infection
  Human T-cell lymphotropic virus type II infection
  Collagen vascular disease (especially systemic lupus erythematosus)
Other
  Sarcoidosis
  Radiotherapy

ticularly nicotinic acid, triparanol, and diazacholesterol,[9] as well as clofazamine,[10] and cimetidine.[11] Metabolic causes to be considered include thyroid dysfunction (particularly hypothyroidism), renal failure, malabsorption syndromes, and zinc deficiency. An underlying malignancy, particularly bronchogenic carcinoma and lymphoma, including Hodgkin's disease and cutaneous T-cell lymphoma, should be considered.[12] Sarcoidosis can be excluded by skin biopsy. Acquired ichthyosis is seen frequently in human immunodeficiency virus (HIV) infection[13] and may be a sign of human T-cell lymphotropic virus type II (HTLV-II) infection with profound helper T-cell depletion. Other causes of acquired ichthyosis include collagen vascular disease,[14] particularly systemic lupus erythematosus, radiation therapy, and chronic kava (an intoxicating beverage of the South Pacific) ingestion.[15]

Pityriasis Rotunda

Pityriasis rotunda is considered by most authors to be a localized form of acquired ichthyosis occurring predominantly in South African blacks and Japanese, although it has been reported in other ethnic groups, including West Indian and American blacks.[16-18] The disorder is clinically distinctive and is characterized by sharply circumscribed, strictly round, scaly patches, which may be slightly hyperpigmented but lack erythema or infiltration. Lesions are usually multiple, but countable, and vary in size from 0.5 to more than 25 cm. Most cases are reported in adults 20 to 45 years of age, but children and the elderly may also be affected.

The histopathologic findings in pityriasis rotunda include lamellar and compact hyperkeratosis with a diminished, but tenuously granular layer and sometimes slight epidermal atrophy. Despite the clinical similarity to dermatophytosis, fungal scrapings and cultures are negative and the disorder is resistant to most therapies, including antifungal agents. Pityriasis rotunda has been frequently linked to underlying disease, especially tuberculosis, malnutrition, malignant tumors, and hepatic disease.[18] In South African blacks, it has been particularly linked to hepatocellular carcinoma, and in Japanese women, to uterine and ovarian disease, as well as tuberculosis.[16] In whites, the disorder may not herald underlying disease and may be a familial trait.[19]

GENETICALLY TRANSMITTED, GENERALIZED DISORDERS OF CORNIFICATION: MAJOR FORMS

Ichthyosis Vulgaris

Clinical Description

Ichthyosis vulgaris is a relatively common autosomal dominant trait with an estimated incidence range between 1:250 and 1:6000.[20, 21] Difficulty in determining its true incidence derives from its relatively mild clinical spectrum, which merges with that of dry skin. Ichthyosis vulgaris commonly occurs in association with atopic dermatitis. Delineation of the dry skin of atopic dermatitis from the scaling of ichthyosis vulgaris may not be possible on clinical grounds alone, and ultrastructural demonstration of abnormal keratohyaline granules is required for a definitive diagnosis.[22] When ultrastructural criteria are used, ichthyosis vulgaris has been found to occur in approximately 4% of patients with atopic dermatitis.

Scaling is not usually evident at birth but appears during infancy and early childhood. Onset after 5 years of age is uncommon[23]; therefore, the appearance of an ichthyosis vulgaris–like pattern of scaling in the adult should suggest an acquired ichthyosis and lead to a search for the cause.

In ichthyosis vulgaris, scales are fine and light colored. Scaling is most prominent on the extremities, particularly the lower legs. The flexures are always spared. Involvement of the palms and soles is characteristic. Generally, involvement is mild and manifested by increased skin markings, but in some instances a true keratoderma (diffuse palmoplantar hyperkeratosis) is present. The trunk is usually only mildly involved. Scaling on the face, when present, is limited to the lateral margins. Erythroderma is absent.

Pathology

The most notable histopathologic feature in ichthyosis vulgaris is hyperkeratosis occurring above a thinned or absent granular layer. This is an unusual occurrence, since nearly all conditions that produce hyperkeratosis do so in conjunction with a thickened granular layer (Fig. 162–1). The hyperkeratosis of ichthyosis vulgaris is lamellar or compact and often plugs the orifices of hair follicles, especially when keratosis pilaris is present. The

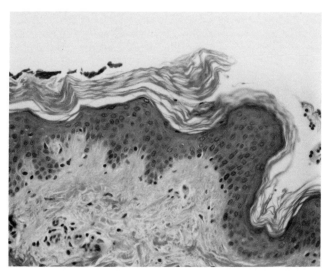

FIGURE 162–1. Ichthyosis vulgaris is characterized by lamellar hyperkeratosis above an epidermis that has a thinned granular layer. Similar changes are seen in some specimens from patients with acquired ichthyosis.

epidermis is sometimes slightly thinned, and its rete ridge pattern is somewhat muted. Ultrastructural examination demonstrates that the few keratohyaline granules that can be found are smaller than normal and have a crumbly or spongy appearance.

Pathogenesis and Etiology

The genetic cause of ichthyosis vulgaris has not been defined. The major protein of the keratohyaline granule, profilaggrin, and its proteolytic cleavage product, filaggrin, are decreased in involved epidermis; similar abnormalities are evident in cultured keratinocytes.[24] Therefore, a defect in the regulation of profilaggrin gene expression has been postulated.[24] Labeling indices are normal; thus ichthyosis vulgaris is a retention hyperkeratosis.[6] Filaggrin is generated by proteolysis of profilaggrin during cornification and is postulated to provide a scaffold around which keratin filaments organize to form the keratin fibrillar network within cornified cells. Keratinization proceeds normally in ichthyosis vulgaris, however, suggesting that either filaggrin is not essential to this process or that the small residual quantities in ichthyosis vulgaris suffice.[25] In outer stratum corneum, filaggrin is hydrolyzed to amino acids, which are postulated to act osmotically, drawing water into the corneocytes and thereby hydrating the stratum corneum.[26] By imbibing water, corneocytes swell, exerting mechanical forces against the weakened intercellular connections of outer corneocytes, thus promoting desquamation. In ichthyosis vulgaris, this process is impaired, leading to stratum corneum retention. Abnormal persistence of desmosomes into outer stratum corneum layers may also contribute to the hyperkeratosis in this disorder.[27]

Diagnosis and Differential Diagnosis

The scales in RXLI tend to be darker than in ichthyosis vulgaris; and while antecubital and popliteal fossae are spared in both disorders, in RXLI the neck flexure usually is not. However, palms and soles are typically spared. Despite these differential features, the phenotypes of RXLI and ichthyosis vulgaris may overlap. Therefore, when a certain diagnosis is required (e.g., for purposes of genetic counseling), a biochemical diagnosis of steroid sulfatase deficiency should be obtained to confirm or exclude RXLI.

Mildly affected patients with nonbullous CIE can be distinguished by their uniform flexural and facial involvement as well as often by a subtle erythroderma. Patients with ichthyosis vulgaris, however, usually have atopic dermatitis, and active dermatitis may produce flexural lichenification and even a mild erythroderma. Resolution of the dermatitis through appropriate therapy will usually permit the correct diagnosis to be appreciated. Similarly, the flexural lichenification of atopic dermatitis in the patient with ichthyosis vulgaris may also closely resemble the flexural ridging of bullous ichthyosis. In the latter instance, a skin biopsy specimen will demonstrate epidermolytic hyperkeratosis.

The onset of ichthyosis after childhood is likely to represent an acquired, rather than genetic, disorder of cornification. Search for the underlying cause in these patients is indicated.

Finally, scaling in some of the ichthyosiform "syndromes" may be mild and suggest ichthyosis vulgaris (e.g., trichothiodystrophy and Refsum's disease).

Treatment

Although a relatively mild form of ichthyosis, ichthyosis vulgaris can be difficult to treat effectively because of the coexistent atopic diathesis in most patients. Most keratolytic agents are irritating to some degree, and irritancy is not well tolerated by atopic patients and may flare their dermatitis. Mild keratolytics, such as 10% urea creams or 5% to 10% lactic acid in hydrophilic ointment (Aqua Gycolic or Lac Hydrin), may be tolerated if the dermatitis is not active. Many patients will prefer simple emollient therapy. The relatively mild extent of disease usually does not warrant treatment with systemic retinoids.

Recessive X-Linked Ichthyosis

Clinical Description

RXLI is a relatively common genetic trait (estimated incidence: 1:2000 to 1:6000 males) that affects males only and is characterized by a nonerythrodermic, generalized hyperkeratosis of mild to moderate severity. Typically, the cutaneous disorder is not evident at birth and first manifests as a pronounced peeling or desquamation at 1 or 3 weeks of age.[28] Thereafter, the characteristic pattern of a "dirty" brown scaling develops on the extremities and, to a lesser degree, on the trunk (Fig. 162–2). During childhood, the scalp is often involved with a crusted hyperkeratosis and involvement of the periauricular region and neck flexure is typical. In adults, the

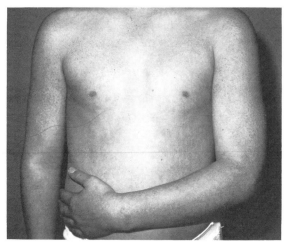

FIGURE 162–2. Recessive X-linked ichthyosis. Note dark color of scales, truncal involvement, and sparing of antecubital fossae.

scalp is usually not clinically involved, but involvement of neck and axilla may persist. Typically, the popliteal and antecubital fossae are spared, as are palms and soles. Marked seasonal fluctuations in disease severity, with improvement in warm weather, are characteristic, but the disorder does not remit with age.

RXLI is due to deficiency of the enzyme, steroid sulfatase. Extracutaneous manifestations of the enzyme deficiency are recognized and include corneal opacities, placental sulfatase deficiency syndrome, elevated serum steroid sulfate levels, cryptorchidism, and, perhaps, testicular cancer.[29] Asymptomatic opacities of Descemet's membrane are evident on slit-lamp examination of some patients; but a negative eye examination does not exclude the diagnosis at any age, nor is the eye examination reliable for identifying female carriers.[30] The placental sulfatase deficiency syndrome represents the prenatal manifestation of this genetic trait and is characterized by very low maternal urinary estriol levels in the presence of fetal and placental well-being (in most other settings, low urinary estrogen levels in late pregnancy signify serious fetal or placental disease). An increased incidence of failure of labor to initiate or progress may be associated with the placental sulfatase deficiency syndrome. Undescended testes are found in approximately 20% of patients with RXLI.[31] Testicular cancer unrelated to testicular maldescent has also been reported in several patients with RXLI.[29] Hence, genital examination is an important part of the evaluation and follow up of all patients with RXLI. In addition to these systemic signs of steroid sulfatase deficiency, a variety of abnormalities affecting other organ systems are described in association with RXLI, owing to deletional mutations affecting neighboring genes ("contiguous gene syndromes"). A variety of RXLI and contiguous gene phenotypes have been described,[32] including obesity, hypogonadism, and mental retardation (Rud's syndrome); Kallman's syndrome (anosmia and hypogonadotrophic hypogonadism); short stature and chondrodysplasia punctata; mirror movements; and ocular albinism.

Pathology

The epidermis in RXLI shows slight hyperplasia with a normal, thickened, or slightly thinned granular layer. Compact and lamellar hyperkeratosis is present and can plug adnexal orifices.

Pathogenesis and Etiology

RXLI is due to deficiency of the microsomal enzyme steroid sulfatase, which is required to desulfate cholesterol sulfate and the entire series of sulfated steroid hormones that occur in parallel to their nonsulfated, active counterparts.[33] The steroid sulfatase gene is located at the tip of the short arm of the X chromosome in a region that escapes X-inactivation. Hence, normal females have approximately twice the amount of active steroid sulfatase enzyme as do normal males. Steroid sulfatase activity in carrier females is similar to that of normal males, and activity in RXLI males is absent. The mutation usually arises by gene deletion, and the frequent associated deletion of neighboring genes accounts for the phenomenon of contiguous gene syndromes.

RXLI is a retention hyperkeratosis with normal epidermal proliferation rates but stratum corneum retention. Both enzyme and its substrate, cholesterol sulfate, are localized to the intercellular membranes in stratum corneum.[34] As corneocytes and their membranes move outward toward the surface, the enzyme hydrolyzes cholesterol sulfate to cholesterol. In some manner this promotes dyshesion of corneocytes, perhaps by permitting corneodesmosome proteolysis.[3]

Diagnosis and Differential Diagnosis

RXLI should be considered in all males with a generalized, nonerythrodermic disorder of cornification. The diagnosis can be established either by direct enzymatic assay in skin, leukocytes, or cultured fibroblasts or by measurement of elevated stratum corneum or plasma cholesterol sulfate levels.[35] The latter can also be inferred by altered mobility of the β (low-density) lipoprotein fraction on serum lipoprotein electrophoresis.[36] At least some flexural sparing, particularly of the antecubital or popliteal fossae is the rule in RXLI, while patients mildly affected with CIE show no flexural sparing. Clinical criteria to distinguish RXLI from ichthyosis vulgaris are not invariably reliable but include a darker scale pattern, sparing of palms and soles, involvement of the neck flexure, and greater truncal involvement in RXLI. In males with multisystemic disease and a scaling disorder, the possibility of RXLI and a contiguous gene syndrome should be considered. In some instances the genomic deletions are large enough to be visualized by chromosomal banding studies.

Treatment

The disorder responds well to topical therapies, including the α-hydroxy acids (e.g., Lac-Hydrin) or propylene glycol (60% in water) overnight under occlusion. Systemic retinoid therapy is rarely indicated. In most patients exposure to a warm, humid climate is beneficial.

Lamellar Ichthyosis and Nonbullous Congenital Ichthyosiform Erythroderma

Clinical Description

The autosomal recessive group of primary disorders of cornification (i.e., disease primarily limited to the skin) are characterized clinically by congenital onset, usually as a collodion baby, and later by a generalized ("head to toe"), uniform involvement of the skin surface with hyperkeratosis and erythroderma. All flexures are involved, as is the face. Palmoplantar involvement parallels the severity of involvement elsewhere on the body surface. Facial involvement is characteristic and in severely affected patients results in ectropion as well as underdevelopment of soft tissue portions of the nose and ear.

A wide range of clinical phenotypes is recognized within this group.[37-39] A uniformly severe phenotype, designated classic lamellar ichthyosis, is characterized by very large, dark, plate-like scales and marked facial involvement with ectropion (Fig. 162–3).[39] Erythroderma is present in this phenotype, but it is much less striking at first inspection than the dense scaling. In contrast, the clinical spectrum of nonbullous CIE is broad and includes both patients with intense erythroderma and marked ectropion as well as patients with a very mild clinical phenotype.[39] Recognition of the severely affected patient with CIE is not difficult (Fig. 162–4). Erythroderma is the most striking clinical feature (Fig. 162–5). Scaling is uniform and generalized. As in other ichthyoses, scales on the lower legs may be large, dark, and plate-like; however, elsewhere, scales tend to be smaller, finer, and lighter. As in classic lamellar ichthyosis, facial involvement may result in severe ectropion as well as underdevelopment of soft tissue structures. In more mildly affected patients, erythroderma may be very subtle and ectropion absent. Here the clinical clues to the correct diagnosis include generalized involvement without flexural sparing and facial tautness. History of con-

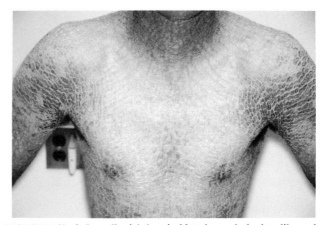

FIGURE 162–3. Lamellar ichthyosis. Note large, dark plate-like scales with mild underlying erythroderma.

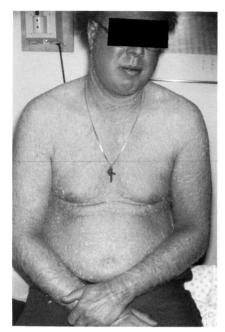

FIGURE 162-4. Nonbullous congenital ichthyosiform erythroderma. Note generalized erythroderma and diffuse, fine white scaling.

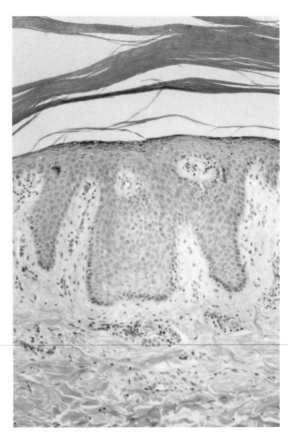

FIGURE 162-6. Lamellar ichthyosis is characterized by more marked hyperkeratosis than ichthyosis vulgaris, along with psoriasiform epidermal hyperplasia.

genital onset as a collodion baby may also suggest a diagnosis of CIE.

The skin of the "collodion" (collodion is a sticky substance that hardens in the air and has been used to treat wounds and coat photographic film) baby at birth is thickened, taut, shiny, and inelastic, thus resembling a dried film of flexible collodion. The collodion baby is not a disease entity but represents a clinical phenotype that may have a variety of underlying causes, most commonly lamellar ichthyosis and CIE. In the collodion baby, ectropion and eclabion are usually present. There is an increased incidence of premature births. In addition to the complications associated with prematurity, collodion babies are at risk for several complications arising from their abnormal skin, including skin infection and septicemia, hypernatremic dehydration, and temperature instability.

Pathology

Lamellar ichthyosis demonstrates more striking hyperkeratosis than does any other disorder of cornification except for harlequin ichthyosis. The granular layer is continuously present, and the epidermis often shows psoriasiform hyperplasia with broad rete ridges (Fig. 162-6). In nonbullous CIE there tends to be less marked hyperkeratosis, and even parakeratosis above a focally diminished granular layer can be present in biopsy specimens. Sometimes a few neutrophils can be present in the parakeratotic foci, simulating psoriasis.

Pathogenesis and Etiology

The underlying cause of neither lamellar ichthyosis nor CIE has been defined. Although the accumulation of n-alkanes in CIE scale was originally reported to be a distinguishing biochemical feature, n-alkanes in scales have since been found to be environmental contaminants, and hence unrelated to the underlying defect.[40] The labeling index (percentage of basal cells taking up

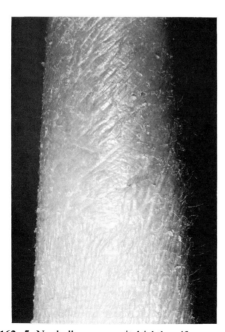

FIGURE 162-5. Nonbullous congenital ichthyosiform erythroderma. Note intense erythroderma with taut, white scales.

radiolabeled thymidine, indicating DNA replication) of CIE is increased, while in lamellar ichthyosis it is normal or nearly so[41]; hence, CIE is a hyperproliferative disorder while lamellar ichthyosis is primarily a retention hyperkeratosis. The hyperproliferation in CIE may be secondary to a defect involving lamellar body formation and/or secretion and resulting in impaired barrier function. Ultrastructurally, lamellar bodies are abnormal, often lacking a normal complement of internal membranes.[42] Many are not secreted into the intercellular space at the stratum corneum–stratum granulosum interface but are retained as lipid droplets and membrane remnants within corneocytes. Others are secreted, but their contents fail to form the normal lamellar unit structures (a repeating pattern of electron-dense and electron-lucent lamellar sheets) within the stratum corneum intercellular domain. Instead, disorganized membrane arrays are formed that provide a poor barrier to water loss.[43]

The collodion baby phenotype may represent a retention hyperkeratosis. In CIE this phenotype may derive from deficiency of lamellar body–derived proteases required to degrade corneodesmosomes.[42] A barrier is not required in the aqueous environment in utero, hence the stimulus for hyperproliferation producing the exfoliative erythrodermic phenotype does not develop until after birth.[7]

Diagnosis and Differential Diagnosis

The severely affected child or adult with either the classic lamellar ichthyosis or CIE phenotypes presents an unmistakable clinical picture, while the patient who is more mildly affected with CIE may require a diagnosis by exclusion. Flexural involvement should be present for the diagnosis, and a subtle erythroderma or facial tautness is usually demonstrable. History of a congenital onset as a collodion baby is also helpful. A dominantly inherited form of lamellar ichthyosis has been described by Traupe and coworkers.[44] The clinical phenotype is that of generalized, nonerythrodermic hyperkeratosis with pronounced palmoplantar involvement. Ultrastructurally, a prominent transforming zone between the granular and cornified cell layers is noted.[45] Onset as a collodion baby[46] and presence of a severe, mutilating palmoplantar keratoderma[47] has been noted in other kindreds with dominant pedigrees. RXLI and bullous ichthyosis can be excluded by biochemical testing and skin biopsy, respectively. One of the ichthyosis-associated multisystem disorders should be considered in patients with signs or symptoms referable to other organ systems. A peripheral blood smear to exclude neutral lipid storage disease should be obtained in all patients with CIE of Mediterranean or Middle Eastern descent. Hair studies may be needed to exclude Netherton's syndrome or trichothiodystrophy.

A definitive diagnosis in a collodion baby may not be possible until the mature clinical pattern has evolved. Some collodion babies will resolve to normal skin or a very mild ichthyosis phenotype.[48] This pattern, termed *self-resolving collodion baby* or *lamellar exfoliation of the newborn*, also appears to be inherited as an autosomal recessive trait. The collodion baby phenotype has also been reported on occasion in trichothiodystrophy, ichthyosis follicularis, Sjögren-Larsson, and Netherton's syndromes, as well as neonatal Gaucher's disease and the Neu-Laxova syndrome. Another congenital onset pattern is that of pronounced peeling or desquamation. RXLI and Sjögren-Larsson syndrome typically present in this manner, as does X-linked hypohidrotic ectodermal dysplasia.[49]

Treatment

Treatment is aimed at maintaining supple skin as well as improvement in appearance. Topical keratolytic agents, such as α-hydroxy acids and salicylic acid, are beneficial but often require highly motivated patients, owing to the need for daily total-body applications. In addition, the stinging and irritancy from topical keratolytics are not well tolerated by young children who lack motivation to improve their appearance. For these children, aggressive topical therapy is usually not indicated. Systemic absorption of topical medications is to be expected because the stratum corneum, although thickened, does not provide an effective barrier. Infants and young children are also at increased risk for systemic toxicity due to a higher surface area to volume ratio, as well as immaturity of detoxification and excretory mechanisms. Systemic salicylism from topical salicylic acid preparations is well recognized, and elevated blood urea nitrogen from topical urea preparations has occurred. Organic acidosis is a theoretical risk in infants treated with topical lactic or glycolic acids. More severely affected patients are candidates for treatment with oral retinoids; however, careful consideration of long-term risks is mandatory, particularly bone toxicity (i.e., premature epiphyseal closure in children) and teratogenicity in women of childbearing age. Optimal management may require relatively high doses (e.g., isotretinoin, 1–2 mg/kg per day; etretinate, 1 mg/kg per day), increasing the risk of dose-dependent side effects. Moreover, the disease can be expected to recur when treatment is interrupted.

Collodion babies should be kept in a humidified environment to minimize the formation of deep fissures as the membrane is shed. Serum electrolytes should be closely monitored, because of the high risk for hypernatremic dehydration caused by the loss of free water across the skin. These infants are also at high risk for septicemia. Clinical signs of systemic infection, which are notoriously difficult to assess in neonates, may be further obscured in the collodion baby who is experiencing temperature instability due to excessive evaporative water losses. Systemic antibiotic therapy should be initiated at the earliest sign of infection and should be directed against *Staphylococcus aureus*, in addition to the usual nursery pathogens. Physicians should avoid undue pessimism in counseling new parents of a collodion baby because resolution to normal or early normal skin may occur in some kindreds. If a severe CIE or lamellar ichthyosis phenotype develops, the need for family support in adjusting to a child with potentially severe cosmetic impairment cannot be overemphasized. Support from other parents of affected children can be very helpful and may be arranged through the lay organization FIRST (Foundation for Ichthyosis and Related Skin Types, PO Box 20921, Raleigh, NC 27619-0921). Development of a healthy self-image in the child begins with a good parent–child adjustment in infancy. The anticipated normalcy of the child in all other respects should be emphasized. The hyperkeratosis may result in impaired sweating and heat prostration. Patients can be taught to anticipate times of heat stress and to externally cool off by dousing with cool water. When these precautions are used, these individuals should enjoy a full range of activities.

Families at risk for lamellar ichthyosis or CIE may be offered prenatal diagnosis. This is achieved by fetoscopy and fetal skin biopsy at about 22 weeks' gestation. Skin ultrastructure demonstrates premature and excessive keratinization in affected infants. Experience has been relatively limited; therefore, parents should be counseled of the possibility of false-negative results (missed diagnosis) as well as the risk of fetal loss from the procedure (approximately 5%).[50]

Bullous Ichthyosis (Epidermolytic Hyperkeratosis)

Clinical Description

Bullous ichthyosis is a rare autosomal dominant trait characterized in the neonate with widespread blistering and denuded skin, and thereafter by a generalized ichthyosiform erythroderma. At least half of cases occur sporadically and must be assumed to represent new mutations. Other names for the disorder (e.g., bullous CIE and epidermolytic hyperkeratosis) are in common use but may led to confusion either with other disorders of cornification (e.g., nonbullous CIE) or with entities sharing the same histopathology. Eponyms have also been employed to separate out two disorders of differing severity: the ichthyosiform erythroderma of Brocq and a milder nonerythrodermic form known as ichthyosa bullosa of Siemens.[31] Sahn and associates[51] have reported a kindred expressing an annular, polycyclic phenotype in which pruritic, annular hyperkeratotic plaques slowly enlarge and then resolve. In other kindreds, lesions are restricted to distal extremities.[52] A wide spectrum of disease severity is encountered in this disorder, with most of the variability between, rather than within, kindreds.[53] It is hoped that further analysis of the mutations in keratins 1 and 10, which are now recognized to underlie the disorder, will elucidate the basis for this phenotypic diversity. Indeed, several groups have recently reported that mutations in keratin 2e underlie the milder, Siemens variant.

At birth, widespread denuded skin is present, precipitated by the trauma of passage through the birth canal (Fig. 162–7). Hyperkeratosis may not be appreciated initially. Mechanically induced blistering is uncommon after the neonatal period; later on, blisters are usually focal and induced by secondary infection. Hyperkeratosis is usually generalized and in some patients includes the palm and soles (Fig. 162–8). Flexures are characteristically involved with a peculiar ridging or exaggerated

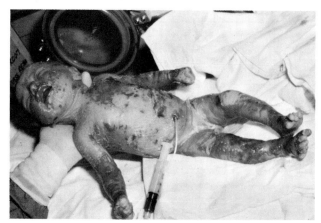

FIGURE 162–7. Bullous ichthyosis (epidermolytic hyperkeratosis) in a neonate. Note widespread areas of denuded skin.

lichenification pattern. Scales in these areas often become macerated and secondarily colonized by bacteria, producing a foul odor. Another distinctive clinical feature is the tendency for stratum corneum to be shed in full-thickness sheets, often leaving a red, tender base (the Mauserung phenomenon).[31] The face is involved, but ectropion does not develop. In some patients the involvement is predominantly focal and limited to extensor and flexure surfaces of elbows and knees and palms and soles. Erythroderma is prominent in some patients and minimal or absent in others in the Siemens variant.

Pathology

The epidermal reaction pattern, epidermolytic hyperkeratosis affects nearly the entire integument in bullous ichthyosis. Epidermal reaction patterns are sets of mor-

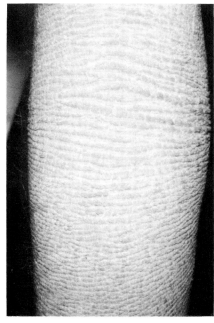

FIGURE 162–8. Bullous ichthyosis. Note characteristic flexural ridging.

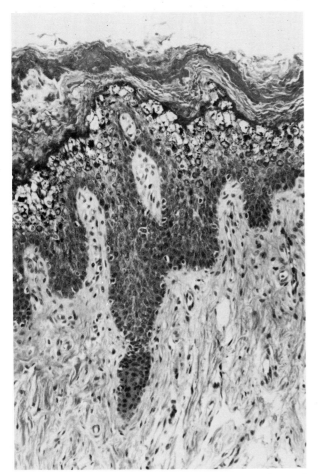

FIGURE 162-9. Epidermolytic hyperkeratosis features reticular alteration of the superficial spinous and granular layers along with hyperkeratosis. Note coarse keratohyaline and trichohyaline granules in the spinous and granular zones in hematoxylin and eosin–stained sections.

phologic features common to several different clinical conditions. Epidermolytic hyperkeratosis can be seen in solitary acanthomas, in epidermal nevi, in hyperkeratosis of the palms and soles, in an annular eruption (annular epidermolytic ichthyosis),[51] and as an incidental microscopic finding affecting only a rete ridge or two. It is characterized by reticular alteration of the epidermis, produced by intracytoplasmic vacuolization of the spinous and granular layers (Fig. 162–9). This is coupled with the occurrence of enlarged keratohyaline and trichohyaline–like granules in the upper half of the epidermis. There is hyperkeratosis and slight papillated epidermal hyperplasia. Blistering in congenital bullous ichthyosis occurs by coalescence of intracytoplasmic vacuoles.

Pathogenesis and Etiology

Bullous ichthyosis is due to mutations either of the keratin 1 gene on chromosome 12 or of the keratin 10 gene on chromosome 17.[54] Keratins 1 and 10 are expressed as a pair in differentiating, suprabasilar keratinocytes. These mutations presumably affect their ability to form a normal cytoskeleton, resulting in the abnormally aggregated tonofilaments that characterize the diagnostic

ultrastructure of this disorder. The previous demonstration that mutations in keratins 5 and 14, the pair normally expressed in basal epidermis, underlie epidermolysis bullosa simplex[55] supports the link between disruption of the keratin filament cytoskeletal network and intraepidermal blistering. In bullous ichthyosis, hyperkeratosis does not develop until after birth. This phenotypic shift at birth may be consequent to the requirement for a competent barrier with extrauterine life.[7] Disruption of the cytoskeletal network may impair lamellar body secretion, leading to increased water loss. Epidermal hyperplasia would result, with consequent expression of the hyperproliferative keratins K6 and K16. Expression of these alternate keratins could account for amelioration of the blistering phenotype after the neonatal period. Recently, several groups have demonstrated that mutations in the keratin 2e gene on chromosome 12 underlie the milder clinical and histopathologic variant (Siemens type).[55a]

Diagnosis and Differential Diagnosis

All other causes of widespread blistering in the neonate must be excluded.[56] Electron microscopy may be required to establish the diagnosis during the neonatal period, if light microscopy supports an intraepidermal blistering disease, but the characteristic features of epidermolytic hyperkeratosis are not seen. In older patients, the diagnosis is suggested by a history of blistering in infancy, as well as by the characteristic clinical features, especially flexural ridging. In mildly affected patients the condition may be mistaken for ichthyosis vulgaris, with flexural lichenification due to concomitant atopic dermatitis. However, in these instances the skin biopsy will be diagnostic of epidermolytic hyperkeratosis. The histopathology of epidermolytic hyperkeratosis is seen in a variety of clinical settings, including some epidermal nevi (Fig. 162–10) and isolated palmoplantar keratoderma (Vörner type). Palmoplantar hyperkeratosis with this histopathology represents a distinct genetic entity; that is, generalized bullous ichthyosis does not occur in these kindreds. In contrast, it is likely that epidermal nevi that exhibit epidermolytic hyperkeratosis represent somatic mutations for the bullous ichthyosis gene(s), since some offspring of parents with such epidermal nevi have exhibited generalized bullous ichthyosis.[31] Indeed, mosaicism for keratin gene mutations has been recently demonstrated in keratinocytes from epidermolytic epidermal nevi and adjacent normal skin.[56a] Ichthyosis hystrix type Curth-Macklin is a rare dominantly inherited disorder of cornification that bears some clinical resemblance to bullous ichthyosis, particularly in the ridged pattern of hyperkeratotic scales, but differs clinically by the absence of blistering.[57] There is also a marked variability in the phenotypic spectrum within these kindreds, with some family members expressing only acral hyperkeratoses or palmoplantar keratoderma and others exhibiting a generalized hyperkeratosis.[57, 58] Histologically, there is perinuclear pallor in granular cells, without acantholysis, and a marked prominence of binucleate keratinocytes. Ultrastructurally, keratin filaments form dense, perinuclear shells.

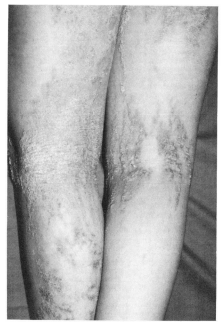

FIGURE 162–10. Extensive bilateral epidermal nevus with histopathology of epidermolytic hyperkeratosis. This form has been termed *ichthyosis hystrix.*

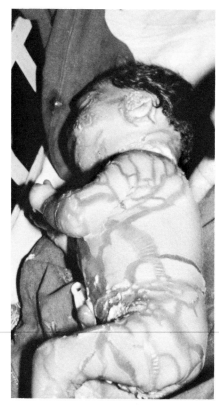

FIGURE 162–11. Harlequin ichthyosis in neonate. Note massive plate-like scales with deep fissures in between.

Treatment

The neonate with bullous ichthyosis should be handled gently to minimize mechanical trauma and watched carefully for signs of sepsis and fluid and electrolyte imbalance. Management of the mature, hyperkeratotic phenotype is complicated by the tendency of scales to be shed as full-thickness stratum corneum, leaving a pink, tender base. For this reason, many patients do not tolerate the irritancy of topical keratolytics. Synthetic retinoids may produce a similar, "therapeutic paradox," that is, desquamation to a tender, dysfunctional base.[59] Antibacterial soaps and topical and/or systemic antibiotics may be required to manage the problems of offensive body odor and secondary infections.

Harlequin Ichthyosis

Clinical Description

The infant at birth presents a grotesque appearance because of the massive, plate-like scales that distort facial features and restrict breathing and feeding (Fig. 162–11). Severe ectropion and eclabion are present, and hands may be deformed by mitten-like skin encasements, although normal bone structures can be demonstrated radiographically. Many of these infants are stillborn, and others do not survive the neonatal period. Previously termed the *harlequin fetus* to denote the fatal outcome, several reports of long-term survivors in recent years indicate that this grim prognosis is not invariably realized.[60, 61] Whether these survivors can be attributed to early institution of retinoid therapy or to generally improved care of the sick neonate and/or to a milder dis-

ease expression is unclear. The later phenotype of survivors is dramatically different from their neonatal picture. The thick scales are replaced by a severe, exfoliative erythroderma, similar to the transition of the collodion baby to CIE phenotype. Like CIE, harlequin ichthyosis is also inherited as an autosomal recessive trait, but the segregation of this very severe phenotype within kindreds implies that it is a distinct genetic trait.[62]

Pathology

Harlequin ichthyosis is produced by massive lamellar and compact hyperkeratosis. Concentric rings of keratin that plug follicular orifices and are interspersed throughout the cornified layer are conspicuous (Fig. 162–12). Some specimens have shown papillated epidermal hyperplasia with perinuclear vacuoles and a diminished granular layer, while in others the granular layer has been intact. Lipid-containing inclusions are often present on ultrastructural examination.

Pathogenesis and Etiology

The underlying cause of harlequin ichthyosis has not been defined, but ultrastructural studies point to a severe defect in lamellar body formation.[63] Virtually no normal lamellar bodies are seen; instead, cells are distended by numerous vesicular structures that are not secreted into the stratum corneum. As in CIE, absence of lamellar body secretory contents in utero would lead to a failure to degrade corneodesmosomes and a retention hyperker-

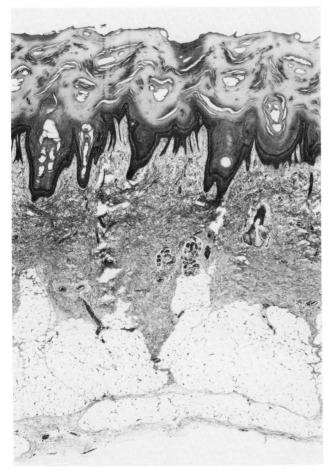

FIGURE 162–12. In harlequin ichthyosis there is massive hyperkeratosis that distends adnexal orifices, accompanied by thinning of adnexal epithelial walls.

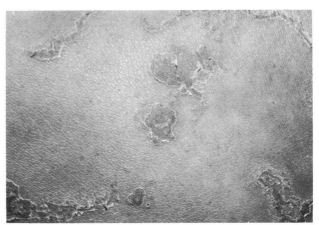

FIGURE 162–13. Netherton's syndrome with ichthyosis linearis circumflexa. Note characteristic double-edged scale.

MULTISYSTEM DISORDERS WITH GENERALIZED SCALING

Netherton's Syndrome

Clinical Description

Netherton's syndrome is a rare, autosomal recessive trait characterized by the triad of ichthyosis, structural defects of the hair shaft, and atopic diathesis. The features of each component of the triad are distinctive. *Ichthyosis linearis circumflexa* is the term adopted by Comel to describe a pattern of bizarre, migratory, polycyclic scaling with a characteristic double-edged scale (Fig. 162–13). This pattern, although pathognomonic of Netherton's syndrome, is an inconstant feature. Early on, the more typical pattern is of a psoriasiform erythroderma, with a prominent, seborrheic-like scaling of the scalp and face (Fig. 162–14).[65] Generalized erythema is

atosis,[7] while after birth the requirement for a competent barrier would result in a hyperproliferative state.

Treatment

Treatment of the neonate with harlequin ichthyosis is similar to that of the collodion baby.[64] In addition, retinoids may facilitate loosing and shedding of the abnormal scales; etretinate (1 mg/kg per day) has been used.[60, 61] Mental development in long-term survivors appears to be normal; however, growth retardation is present and may be secondary to the high caloric requirements of the hyperproliferative epidermis. Provision of adequate calories to maintain growth is an important goal in these children.

Diagnosis and Differential Diagnosis

The facial features and digits of the neonate with restrictive dermopathy are also distorted by inelastic skin, but hyperkeratotic plates are not seen. Some infants with the Neu-Laxova syndrome have had a harlequin ichthyosis phenotype.

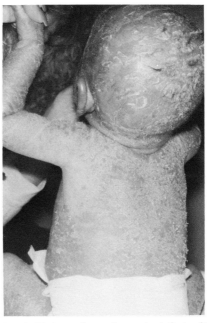

FIGURE 162–14. Netherton's syndrome in infant with exfoliative erythroderma and extensive scalp dermatitis.

noted at birth, followed by peeling or hyperkeratosis. Pruritus, flexural erythema, and lichenification are often present but may be a manifestation of underlying atopic diathesis. The hair shaft defect diagnostic of Netherton's syndrome is trichorrhexis invaginata, a "ball and socket intussusception" of the distal into the proximal hair shaft (Fig. 162–15). Other hair shaft defects may also be present, including pili torti and trichorrhexis nodosa. The atopic diathesis is manifested in approximately two thirds of patients by atopic dermatitis, allergic rhinitis, and/or an elevated serum IgE level.[66] Anaphylactic or angioedema reactions to foods, particularly nuts, are frequently reported. Other inconstant features of the syndrome include recurrent infections, aminoaciduria, neurologic deficits, and mental retardation. Growth retardation is noted in approximately 20% of patients.[66] It has been appreciated that infants with Netherton's syndrome may present with a Leiner's disease-like phenotype, with erythroderma, diarrhea, and failure to thrive.[67] The basis for the severe gastrointestinal symptoms is unclear, but jejunal villus atrophy can be demonstrated in some. Hypernatremic dehydration may also develop in erythrodermic infants.[68] Definitive diagnosis may be difficult during infancy because of a paucity of hair. Hairs for analysis should be collected from regions with abnormal or short hairs; eyebrows, eyelashes, and body hairs may also demonstrate the defect.

Pathology

Biopsy specimens of ichthyosis linearis circumflexa have shown a spongiotic, psoriasiform dermatitis. The characteristic scale is largely parakeratotic.

Pathogenesis and Etiology

The underlying defect in Netherton's syndrome is not known.

Diagnosis and Differential Diagnosis

Leiner's disease has been applied to the syndrome of erythroderma, diarrhea, and failure to thrive in infancy.

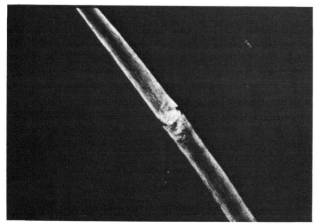

FIGURE 162–15. Hair in Netherton's syndrome demonstrating trichorrhexis invaginata shown in polarized light.

Although previously attributed to a deficiency of the C5 component of complement, it is now apparent that this phenotype may have many causes, including atopic dermatitis and immunodeficiency syndromes, as well as Netherton's syndrome.[69] Omenn's syndrome is an autosomal recessive form of combined T- and B-cell immunodeficiency with diffuse erythema and hyperkeratosis, alopecia, recurrent infections, and failure to thrive.[70, 71] It shares many common features with the graft-versus-host disease that arises in infants with severe combined immunodeficiency syndrome following intrauterine maternal-fetal transfusions, including eosinophilia and lymphocytosis and hepatosplenomegaly, and is associated with alopecia and extensive dermatitis. However, in Omenn's syndrome, chimerism cannot be demonstrated. Deal and colleagues[72] have described an autosomal recessive trait in inbred Pakistani and Arab kindreds with Fanconi's syndrome, flexion deformities, and failure to thrive that is associated with generalized ichthyosis.

Sjögren-Larsson Syndrome

Clinical Description

Sjögren-Larsson syndrome is an autosomal recessive trait due to deficiency of the enzyme fatty alcohol oxidoreductase.[73] The syndrome is characterized by ichthyosis, spastic diplegia or quadriplegia, mental retardation, and speech defects.[74] A generalized, "dandruff-like" hyperkeratosis is evident at birth, but a collodion baby phenotype is not observed. The ichthyosis is usually of moderate severity and tends to spare the face and palms and soles. Accentuation of flexures, forming a ridged, hyperkeratotic pattern, and accentuation of skin markings on the lower abdomen are typical. As in other disorders of cornification, the scales on the lower legs tend to form a lamellar pattern. Erythema is usually mild or absent, and pruritus is common. Hair and nails are normal. Neurologic signs, weakness, spasticity, and mental retardation are usually evident by 3 years of age. The retardation is nonprogressive, but motor function may deteriorate with age. Ocular abnormalities include blepharitis, conjunctivitis, corneal erosions and opacities, photophobia, and retinal "glistening dots."[75] The latter finding, although pathognomonic of Sjögren-Larsson syndrome, may not be present in young children.

Sjögren-Larsson syndrome was first reported within an inbred population of Northern Sweden, but confirmed cases have been found in many ethnic groups; hence the diagnosis should be considered in all patients with generalized hyperkeratosis and central nervous system dysfunction. The diagnosis can be initially confirmed by histochemical assay for alcohol dehydrogenase in epidermis on skin biopsy[76] and definitively established by enzyme assay in cultured fibroblasts or leukocytes.[73] Carriers can be detected by intermediate enzyme activity levels in cultured fibroblasts.[77] Prenatal diagnosis by enzyme assay in chorionic villus cells or amniocytes is possible.[77a]

Pathology

Ichthyotic skin of the Sjögren-Larsson syndrome shows papillated epidermal hyperplasia and either basket-weave orthokeratosis or hyperkeratosis, with the latter sometimes affecting follicular orifices.[78]

Pathogenesis and Etiology

Sjögren-Larsson syndrome is due to deficiency of the fatty aldehyde dehydrogenase component of the fatty alcohol: nicotinamide adenine dinucleotide–oxidoreductase enzyme complex.[73] Histochemical demonstration of deficient alcohol dehydrogenase activity in epidermis strongly suggests that the enzyme deficiency is directly related to the abnormal cornification.[76] However, the metabolic link remains to be determined, since fatty alcohols are not recognized constituents of stratum corneum lipids. Ultrastructurally, abnormal membrane remnants are found within corneocytes.[79] These may derived from unsecreted lamellar bodies, some of which are also abnormal in structure or may represent other retained membrane structures during incomplete cornification.

Treatment

Dietary restriction of long-chain fatty acids through the provision of fat in the form of medium-chain triglycerides has been associated with a marked improvement in ichthyosiform dermatosis in a few patients, as well as some improvement in neurologic status.[80, 81] In other patients, however, there has been no clinical response to dietary treatment.

Neutral Lipid Storage Disease (Chanarin-Dorfman Syndrome)

Clinical Description

Neutral lipid storage disease (Chanarin-Dorfman syndrome) is an autosomal recessive trait; most cases are in persons of Middle Eastern or Mediterranean descent.[82, 83] Skin involvement is generalized with a mild erythroderma and fine white scaling pattern. Lichenification over the dorsa of the hands and extensor surfaces is a common clinical feature. The onset is at or soon after birth. Generalized hyperkeratosis is usually the most striking clinical feature, but the underlying defect (intracellular triglyceride storage) is expressed in virtually all cells, and abnormalities of other organ systems can be elucidated on careful examination. Myopathy, with weakness and elevated levels of (creatine phosphokinase) muscle enzymes, cataracts, neurosensory deafness, and hepatomegaly are the most frequently observed abnormalities. Mild to moderate mental retardation and growth retardation are present in some patients. All patients exhibit prominent lipid vacuoles in circulating leukocytes (Fig. 162–16). The peripheral blood smear is diagnostic, but it must be recognized that automated methods of differential counting do not detect this abnormality. Heterozygotes are asymptomatic but can be

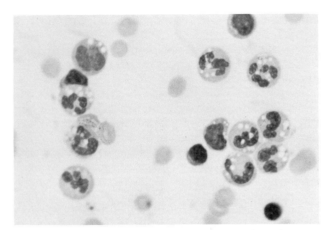

FIGURE 162–16. Peripheral blood smear from patient with neutral lipid storage disease. Note vacuoles in monocytes and polymorphonuclear leukocytes.

detected by the presence of vacuoles in some circulating eosinophils.[83]

Pathology

There is epidermal hyperplasia accompanied by hyperkeratosis, sometimes with foci of parakeratosis in affected skin. Lipid droplets are present in cells of both the basilar and granular layers and can render the cytoplasm of some of these keratinocytes foamy.

Pathogenesis and Etiology

The metabolic defect underlying neutral lipid storage disease is an inability to degrade triacylglycerides that are synthesized within the cell.[84, 85] In contrast, triglycerides imported into the cell in the form of serum lipoproteins are degraded normally though the action of the lysosomal enzyme acid lipase (deficient in Wolman's disease); and serum triglyceride levels are normal due to normal activity of the extracellularly active enzyme lipoprotein lipase. Presumably, the function of another cytosolic lipase is deficient in neutral lipid storage disease, but the precise enzymatic defect has not been defined. In skin, lipid vacuoles are evident in the basal layer, as well as acrosyringia of sweat glands and many dermal cells, including fibrocytes. Ultrastructurally, lamellar bodies are abnormal, showing vacuolization and disruption of the normal laminations.[86] These alterations result in abnormal stratum corneum intercellular lamellae, which, in turn, result in increased transepidermal water loss and stimulus for epidermal hyperplasia.

Differential Diagnosis

A peripheral blood smear should be examined in all patients with a nonbullous CIE phenotype if they come from the Middle East or Mediterranean basin or if they show signs of a multisystem disease. In Wolman's disease (cholesterol ester storage disease), lipid vacuoles are found only in lymphocytes, while in neutral lipid storage disease the vacuoles are in monocytes, polymorphonuclear leukocytes, and eosinophils, and not in lymphocytes.

Trichothiodystrophy

Trichothiodystrophy (i.e., sulfur-deficient brittle hair) is the common feature of a bewildering number of syndromes,[87, 88] most of which are inherited in an autosomal recessive pattern. Eponyms and acronyms associated with trichothiodystrophy include Marinesco-Sjögren syndrome, Tay syndrome, Pollitt syndrome, Sabinas syndrome, BIDS (brittle hair, intellectual impairment, decreased fertility, short stature), IBIDS (ichthyosis, plus BIDS), PIBIDS (photosensitivity plus IBIDS), and SIBIDS (osteosclerosis plus IBIDS).[87, 89, 90] The tendency for uniformity of phenotype within pedigrees has favored genetic heterogeneity as the explanation for this clinical diversity and has implied that the sulfur-deficient hair phenotype is a nonspecific finding. On the other hand, the substantial overlap of clinical phenotypes between subsets of patients has favored pleiotropism of one or a few genes. Even more puzzling has been the demonstration that fibroblasts from some clinically photosensitive and even some nonphotosensitive patients belong to the xeroderma pigmentosum (XP) complementation group D, yet these patients lack the XP phenotype of dispigmentation and predilection for skin cancer.[91] Bootsma and Hoeijmakers[91] have proposed a reconciling theory, namely, that mutations in one or more genes involved in the unwinding of DNA, which regulate both gene transcription and DNA repair, may underlie trichothiodystrophy as well as some forms of XP and Cockayne's syndrome.

Generalized hyperkeratosis of varying degrees of severity is a common but inconstant feature in the trichotiodystrophy syndromes. Onset as a collodion baby is documented in several instances, followed by a generalized hyperkeratosis, including palmoplantar involvement. Erythroderma is usually not a striking feature. Other patients have later onset of an exaggerated dry skin, often with truncal scaling. Pruritus and an eczematous dermatitis are often noted. Trichothiodystrophy should be excluded by hair mount and analysis of hair sulfur content in all children with scaling skin and brittle hair.

KID (Keratitis/Ichthyosis/Deafness) Syndrome

Clinical Description

The acronym KID syndrome denotes the triad of progressive corneal inflammatory disease (*keratitis*), a distinctive and unusual ichthyosiform erythroderma (*ichthyosis*), and a congenital, usually profound neurosensory *deafness*.[92, 93] Two eponyms, Burns' syndrome and Sentor's syndrome, have also been applied to this trait to honor the authors who described the first case and first recognized the syndrome, respectively. Vertical transmission in two kindreds is consistent with autosomal dominant inheritance,[94, 95] with most cases representing new mutations. Wilson and coworkers[96] have

suggested that there is also a more severe, autosomal recessive form with progressive hepatic disease, growth failure, and mental retardation (Desmons-Britten syndrome).

The cutaneous phenotype is distinctive. In contrast to most other disorders of cornification, accentuated scaling is not seen. Instead there is a generalized hyperkeratosis, producing a striking ridging or lichenification over acral surfaces, with markedly hyperkeratotic perioral plaques, often impairing an aged or leonine appearance. An underlying erythroderma is often appreciated. Palms and soles exhibit a distinctive, dense, rugose keratoderma that has been likened to the grained pattern of leather. At birth the skin is thickened, rough, and red or covered with a vernix-like material. Alopecia is often noted at birth; hair may subsequently grow, only to be later lost through a progressive alopecia.[94] Eyebrows and eyelashes are sparse, and nails are often thickened and dystrophic. Teeth may be carious, and oral leukoplakia may be present. Impaired sweating and heat intolerance are reported in many patients, presumably due to sweat duct obstruction rather than gland hypoplasia. Approximately half of patients suffer from recurrent skin infections, both bacterial and fungal, but studies of immune function have been for the most part unrevealing. Cutaneous and mucocutaneous squamous cell carcinomas have been reported in as many as 15% of patients.[97] These malignancies often occur early, in the second or third decades, and may be multiple.

The keratitis usually begins in infancy with purulent blepharitis or keratoconjunctivitis with photophobia and progresses with corneal opacities and ulcerations, neovascularization, and pannus formation. In contrast, the deafness is congenital and nonprogressive. Other extracutaneous defects include neuromuscular signs of tight heel cords and talipes equinovarus. Postnatal growth retardation occurs in about 30% of patients, but mental retardation is uncommon and may be indicative of the autosomal recessive form.[96]

Pathology

There is epidermal hyperplasia with hyperkeratosis and a normal or thickened granular layer. Vacuoles are sometimes apparent in keratinocytes of the granular layer. Excessive accumulation of glycogen within small nerves and hair erector muscles can also occur.

Pathogenesis and Etiology

The underlying defect is unknown. A cochleosaccular abnormality of the inner ear is described, consistent with an embryonic developmental defect. Similar inner ear abnormalities are reported in Refsum's disease, which is another multisystemic disorder with ichthyosis and deafness. Peroxisomal studies in one patient were normal.[96]

Diagnosis and Differential Diagnosis

The clinical picture of KID syndrome is usually distinctive and presents little problem in the diagnosis. In some patients corneal disease may not develop until the adult years[98]; hence absence of this feature does not exclude the diagnosis. Reports of a KID-like phenotype without deafness[99] suggests that deafness, too, may not be an invariable feature.[96]

Treatment

Treatment with systemic retinoids should be undertaken with caution, since worsening of the keratitis is reported[100] and many patients do not respond.[93] An anecdotal account of improvement in skin and eye changes, as well as decreased incidence of new skin malignancies, in a patient treated with long-term oral ketoconazole is reported.[101] Careful follow-up of adolescents and young adults with KID syndrome for early diagnosis of malignancy is indicated.

Refsum's Disease (Phytanic Acid Storage Disease)

Refsum's disease (adult type) is a rare, autosomal recessive trait due to deficiency of the peroxisomal enzyme phytanic acid α-hydroxylase, required to degrade phytanic acid, a branched-chain fatty acid.[102] Phytanic acid derives from phytol, a major component of chlorophyll, and is concentrated in the fat of herbivores. Disease symptoms, due to the accumulation of branched-chain fatty acids, are often delayed until the second or third decade. Night blindness due to retinitis pigmentosa is usually the presenting sign.[103] Unfortunately, diagnosis is often delayed until the fourth or fifth decades. The neurologic signs are episodic and include cerebellar ataxia and peripheral and cranial polyneuropathy. Bony anomalies of the hands and feet (bilateral shortening of metacarpals and phalanges), lenticular opacities, and hyperkeratosis are also seen in most patients. The scaling disorder is usually not the presenting feature and ranges in severity from mild palmoplantar hyperkeratosis to severe truncal scaling. The epidermis is hyperproliferative, and phytanic acid accumulates in all acylated epidermal lipids.[104] Elevated serum phytanic acid levels confirm the diagnosis. Dietary restriction of products containing chlorophyll and animal fat improves the symptoms, including neurologic signs and the scaling disorder,[105] although ocular disease may not improve.[103] In acutely ill patients, plasmaphoresis may be indicated.

Conradi-Hünermann and CHILD Syndromes (Chondrodysplasia Punctata Syndromes with Scaling Skin)

Chondrodysplasia punctata is a clinical term for calcified stippling of the epiphyses. Although it is a transient radiographic abnormality during infancy and childhood, it may be seen in many diverse clinical settings, several of which share the common feature of peroxisomal deficiency. Ichthyosis is a clinical feature of three partial or global peroxisomal deficiency syndromes with chondrodysplasia punctata: rhizomelic chondrodysplasia

punctata, the Conradi-Hünermann syndrome, and the CHILD syndrome.[106]

Rhizomelic chondrodysplasia punctata is a rare, autosomal recessive trait characterized by severe short-limbed dwarfism, mental retardation, and death in infancy. Ichthyosis is said to occur in one third of patients but is poorly described in the literature. Biochemically, these patients exhibit a partial deficiency of peroxisomal function, with impaired synthesis of ether lipids (plasmalogen deficiency) and accumulation of branched chain fatty acids (phytanic acid).

Conradi-Hünermann syndrome is an X-dominant, male lethal trait, characterized by an ichthyosiform erythroderma patterned along the lines of Blashko, in association with focal cataracts and asymmetric limb reduction defects.[107] Bands of ichthyosiform erythroderma alternating with normal skin are noted at birth. These resolve, usually during the first year, and are replaced by bands of follicular atrophoderma (Fig. 162–17). In the scalp, these are represented by spiraling bands of alopecia. Postinflammatory pigmentary changes may also be present. Limb reduction defects are often localized to limbs with the greatest skin involvement. Cataracts are focal and often asymptomatic.

Daughters of affected women have a 50% chance of inheriting the trait, and, like their mothers, will express the disease in a focal, patterned manner. In contrast, only sons inheriting the normal maternal X chromosome survive fetal life, and, hence, all male offspring are normal. Happle[108] has proposed that the focal expression of the disease in females with this and several other X-dominant traits (e.g., carriers of hypohidrotic ectodermal dysplasia, incontinentia pigmenti) is due to "functional mosaicism" within the affected tissues, because in fe-

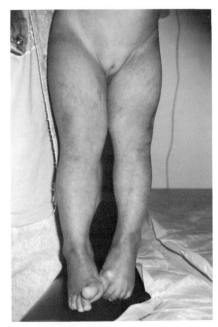

FIGURE 162–17. Conradi-Hünermann syndrome after resolution of the scaling disorders. Note bands of postinflammatory hyperpigmentation and limb asymmetry.

males, only one X chromosome is active within cells. Random inactivation of one X chromosome during early fetal development (lyonization) accounts for the distribution of disease along morphogenic lines. The severity of disease varies greatly from patient to patient, presumably reflecting the extent to which the mutant X chromosome is the active X chromosome in the affected tissues.

Deficiency of the peroxisomal enzyme dihydroxyacetone phosphate acyltransferase, which is required for the synthesis of ether lipids, has been demonstrated in cultured fibroblasts from several patients with Conradi-Hünermann syndrome, although the peroxisomal phenotype in this disorder has not been completely characterized. Emami and colleagues[109] have demonstrated in a mouse homologue of this disease (the Bare patches mouse) that the peroxisomal defect can only be demonstrated in affected skin during the time the disease is active. Loss of a nonviable cell population and overgrowth by neighboring normal cells could account for this progression, although developmentally regulated expression of the mutant gene is also possible.

CHILD syndrome is an acronym for *c*ongenital *h*emidysplasia with *i*chthyosiform erythroderma and *l*imb *d*efects.[110] The most striking feature of this rare syndrome is the limitation of defects to one half of the body. In the typical case there are severe limb reduction defects and organ hypoplasias ipsilateral to an ichthyosiform erythroderma that affects is only one side of the body and spares the face. A number of organ systems are affected by hypoplasia, including the cardiac, pulmonary, renal, and endocrine systems. Involvement is usually right sided, presumably owing to the lethality of left-sided organ hypoplasias. It has been suggested that CHILD and Conradi-Hünermann syndromes may be allelic traits that differ primarily in the timing of the mutational event (or X-inactivation), in view of the commonality of clinical features (ichthyosis, limb reduction defects, chondrodysplasia punctata), inheritance pattern (X-dominant, male lethal), and peroxisomal phenotype (decreased catalase and dihydroxyacetone phosphate acyltransferase activities).[106, 109] Also, like CHILD syndrome, Conradi-Hünermann syndrome is often predominantly unilateral; and conversely, patients with CHILD syndrome may have some contralateral skin involvement. The ichthyosiform erythroderma of CHILD syndrome may similarly resolve over time, although flexures usually remain involved (ptychotropism).[111]

The relationship between peroxisomal deficiency and scaling dermatosis is unclear. Infantile Refsum's disease is a global peroxisomal deficiency syndrome characterized by the onset in infancy of retinitis pigmentosa, deafness, hepatomegaly, facial dysmorphism, and growth and mental retardation. Despite increased serum phytanic acid levels, skin changes have not been described in this disorder, nor in the other global peroxisome deficiency syndrome Zellweger's syndrome. In rhizomelic chondrodysplasia punctata, phytanic acid oxidation is impaired but in CHILD syndrome it is not.[106] Moreover, the phytanic acid oxidation defect in rhizomelic chondrodysplasia punctata is distinct from both adult and infantile Refsum's diseases by complementation analysis.[112]

Gaucher's Disease (Glucocerebrosidase Deficiency)

Gaucher's disease is a lysosomal storage disease due to deficiency of the enzyme β-glucocerebrosidase. Several clinical subtypes are recognized arising from different allelic mutations: type I—the common, chronic adult, non-neuropathic form; type II—the rapidly progressive, acute neuropathic, infantile onset form; and type III—the subacute neuropathic, slowly progressive and late childhood onset form.[113] Recently it has been appreciated that a subgroup of patients with type II is characterized by congenital onset and a fulminant course resulting in neonatal death. At birth, most have exhibited a collodion baby phenotype.[114, 115] A similar phenotype is observed in transgenic mice homozygous for a mutation disrupting the active site of the glucocerebrosidase gene.[116] In epidermis, glucocerebrosidase is a lamellar body enzyme. After secretion within the intercellular domains of stratum corneum, glucocerebrosidase cleaves glucosylceramide to free ceramide, which is one of the major lipid components of the stratum corneum membranes. This hydrolysis of glucosylceramide appears to be required for the final step in the formation of the lamellar membranes of stratum corneum and hence for formation of a functional permeability barrier. Ichthyosis is not described in the other forms of Gaucher's disease, probably because in these less severe forms there is sufficient residual enzyme activity in epidermis.[114, 116] Type II Gaucher's disease should be considered in neonates with collodion membranes or a restrictive dermopathy phenotype (see later)[114] when there is evidence of other organ system involvement, particularly hepatosplenomegaly, hydrops fetalis, neurologic signs, and or apnea.

Neu-Laxova Syndrome

The Neu-Laxova syndrome is a rare, autosomal recessive trait of multiple congenital anomalies and death in utero or during the neonatal period. A severe, generalized hyperkeratosis, often with marked eclabion and ectropion, is present in all patients. In addition to the severe disorder of cornification, the most constant features are severe intrauterine growth retardation, severe microcephaly with central nervous system hypoplasia; abnormal facies with a slanted forehead, flattened nose, and deformed ears; generalized edema; and limb deformities, often with joint contractures.[117] Curry and colleagues[118] have noted the marked heterogeneity of phenotype and proposed a classification, based primarily on the severity of the skeletal manifestations. Some have had a harlequin ichthyosis phenotype. Fatty infiltration in epidermis, dermis, and subcutis, as well as liver and adrenal glands in some patients, suggests an inborn error of lipid metabolism.[117] The association in one instance of this phenotype with glucocerebrosidase deficiency implies that in at least some patients the Neu-Laxova syndrome is a form of neonatal Gaucher's disease.

Restrictive Dermopathy

Restrictive dermopathy is a rare, autosomal recessive trait with fetal akinesia deformation sequence (i.e., joint contractures, intrauterine growth retardation, polyhydramnios, and pulmonary hypoplasia) due to rigid tense skin.[119] Patients are born prematurely and usually die of restrictive pulmonary disease within the perinatal period, although survival to 4 months of age is reported.[120] Marked skin inflexibility may be responsible for most of the phenotypic features, including widened sutures and enlarged fontanelle, fixed facial expression with a small pinched nose, ectropion, and microstomia with the mouth held open in an "O" position. However, skeletal anomalies in some patients, with hypoplastic bones and deficient ossification centers, as well as natal teeth and retinal hyperpigmentation suggest that not all features can be attributed to the skin defect. Scalp hair is often normally present, but eyebrows, eyelashes, and body hair absent. Nails may be long, discolored, and hypoplastic. Traumatic erosions, with a cleft at the dermoepidermal junction, or spontaneous full-thickness lacerations of the skin over joints are described; healing is delayed.

The basis for the marked skin rigidity is unclear.[119] The epidermis often appears hyperplastic, with hyperkeratosis and focal parakeratosis. Diffuse scaling is described, but the hyperkeratosis is insufficient to account for the skin rigidity. Epidermal appendages are immature and often rudimentary. Elastic fibers are absent at the light microscopic level and are present but extremely small at the ultrastructural level. Paradoxically, this feature would be expected to produce skin laxity. Although the dermis is thin, there is a condensed, fibrotic pattern in the collagen, with loss of the rete ridges. It is possible that these collagen abnormalities account for skin rigidity.

Ichthyosis Follicularis

The IFAP syndrome (ichthyosis follicularis with alopecia and photophobia) is a rare trait characterized by generalized hyperkeratosis with extensive spiny follicular hyperkeratoses and congenital noncicatricial alopecia.[121, 122] Marked photophobia is a striking clinical sign. Numerous ophthalmologic abnormalities are described and include corneal opacities, erosions, and keratitis that may progress to neovascularization. Some patients develop psoriasiform plaques on acral surfaces; others have nail dystrophy. Onset at birth with a mild collodion baby phenotype is described.[122] Systemic signs are highly variable and include growth retardation, mental retardation, seizures, recurrent skin and respiratory tract infections, vertebral defects, renal anomalies, and hernias.[121-123] Skin histopathology demonstrates follicular hyperkeratosis with absent or atopic sebaceous glands; eccrine glands are normal.[121] Both X-linked recessive and autosomal dominant inheritance patterns have been proposed. Similar follicular prominence may be seen in KID syndrome. Distinguishing features are deafness and a distinctive, leathery palmoplantar hyperkeratosis in KID syndrome. Keratosis follicularis spinulosa decalvans, an X-linked trait with reduced expression in females,[124] can be distinguished by the progressive development of cicatricial alopecia, follicular keratotic spines on the dorsal fingers, and, in some patients, palmoplantar keratoderma.[125] Although photophobia may be present, generalized hyperkeratosis and the other systemic signs of IFAP syndrome are not.

Zunich-Kaye Syndrome

The Zunich-Kaye syndrome is also known by the acronym CHIME syndrome, for coloboma, heart defects, ichthyosiform dermatosis, mental retardation, and ear anomalies.[126, 127] The disorder appears to be inherited as an autosomal recessive trait. The disorder of cornification is quite distinctive and is characterized by migratory, figurative, erythematous, and hyperkeratotic plaques of varying size, most pronounced over the anterior torso and proximal limbs, with intervening, normal skin.[126] On the face, a distinctive pattern of lamellar ridged, vertically oriented scales on an erythematous base is seen. The skin disorder is not evident at birth but usually appears within the first weeks of life. Palms and soles are hyperkeratotic. Hair is sparse and fine but without structural defects. All patients have exhibited retinal colobomas and severe mental retardation. Congenital heart defects include tetralogy of Fallot, transposition of the great vessels, and peripheral pulmonic stenosis.

Schwachman's Syndrome

Schwachman's syndrome is an autosomal recessive trait characterized by exocrine pancreatic insufficiency, growth retardation, skeletal defects, neutropenia, recurrent infections, and impaired neutrophil chemotaxis. Ichthyosiform or eczematous changes occur in as many as two thirds of patients.[128] Skin involvement appears to be quite variable. Skin changes are not noted at birth, but scaling usually begins in early infancy and may improve later in childhood. Some patients have a marked ichthyosiform erythroderma, particularly on the extremities, with diffuse white scaling without erythroderma elsewhere,[129] while others exhibit xerosis, follicular hyperkeratosis, and eczematous dermatitis.[130] The extent to which nutritional deficiencies, particularly zinc and essential fatty acid deficiency, may underlie these skin changes has not been examined in all cases. The delayed onset of the skin disease and fluctuating disease severity are consistent with a nutritional component.

Cardio-Facio-Cutaneous Syndrome

The cardio-facio-cutaneous (CFC) syndrome is a rare syndrome of multiple anomalies and mental retardation.[131] All patients have typical faces: a high forehead with bitemporal constriction, down slanting palpebral fissures, a depressed nasal bridge and posteriorly rotated ears. Most have cardiac anomalies. Growth retardation, splenomegaly, and hernias are also frequently noted. The cutaneous signs are quite variable and in most reports poorly described. Scalp hair is usually sparse, is curly, and is variably described as thin, brittle, woolly, or friable. Hair shafts exhibit variable diameter and irregular twists.[132] Eyebrows and eyelashes are usually sparse. Skin changes are also quite variable and include ichthyotic changes, especially over extensor surfaces, follicular hyperkeratosis, eczematous patches, and occasionally, palmoplantar hyperkeratosis. Skin on the dorsa of the hands may be thick or redundant, as a residum of fetal lymphedema. Nails and teeth may be dysplastic. Hemangiomas and café-au-lait spots are also reported. All cases have been sporadic. The underlying defect is unknown, but increased plasma levels of medium-chain free fatty acids have been noted in two patients, suggesting an underlying defect in mitochondrial lipid metabolism.[133]

Rud's Syndrome

Rud's syndrome is the triad of ichthyosis, hypogonadism, mental retardation, and seizures. It has been suggested that this is a heterogeneous group of disorders with at least three subsets: (1) an X-linked recessive form with steroid sulfatase deficiency (i.e., RXLI and a contiguous gene syndrome); (2) an X-linked recessive form without steroid sulfatase deficiency; and (3) an autosomal recessive form. Given the genetic heterogeneity, the eponym no longer serves any purpose.

OTHER DISORDERS OF CORNIFICATION

Erythrokeratodermia Variabilis

Clinical Description

Erythrokeratodermia variabilis is a rare autosomal dominant trait characterized by fixed hyperkeratotic plaques and a changing configurate erythroderma.[134] The onset is usually at birth, or within the first few months, but may be delayed until late childhood or early adulthood. The hyperkeratotic plaques are most frequently distributed on the face and extensor surfaces of the extremities. They are often dark and densely hyperkeratotic. In some patients the surrounding skin is normal, while others have a diffuse, leathery hyperkeratosis. The number and extent of plaques is usually progressive until puberty and stable thereafter. Resolution at menopause has been reported. There is often a dense palmoplantar keratoderma. The most striking clinical feature is the variable erythrodermic component in which geographic patterns of erythema induced by exposure to cold, heat, or wind or emotional stress are observed to shift and change within minutes, hours, or days.

The underlying cause is unknown. No difference in cutaneous reactivity to vasoconstrictors or vasodilators has been demonstrated. In a large Dutch kindred, close linkage to the Rh blood group system on chromosome 1p has been demonstrated.[135] Scaling is due to retention hyperkeratosis, since epidermal kinetics are normal. The disorder has responded well in several anecdotal reports to oral retinoids.[136]

Pathology

There is slightly papillated epidermal hyperplasia with hyperkeratosis. Acantholytic parakeratotic cells resembling the grains of Darier's disease are sometimes present in the lower part of the cornified layer.

Diagnosis and Differential Diagnosis

A number of somewhat similar phenotypes have been reported in the literature, but whether these represent distinct entities is unclear.[134] Genodermatoses en cocardes initially described by Degos is a dominantly inherited trait characterized by annular erythematous plaques forming a polycentric or target-like appearance. Unlike erythrokeratodermia variabilis, in this disorder the erythema is associated with the hyperkeratotic lesions and both resolve and recur together. Familial annular erythema can be excluded by the absence of hyperkeratotic lesions.

Erythrokeratolysis hiemalis is a distinctive, dominantly inherited trait described in kindreds originating in the Oudtshoorn district of South Africa.[137] Lesions occur in cyclical attacks, often provoked by cold weather or local bacterial infection, and are characterized by symmetrically distributed erythematous patches that peel from the center outward. Lesions predominate on the palms and soles but may occur elsewhere on the body. The histopathology is distinctive and demonstrates epidermal hyperplasia accompanied by vacuolization and necrosis of a portion of the upper spinous layer, giving rise to parakeratosis. There is expansion of the basal zone of the epidermis. These changes are most pronounced at the advancing edge of lesions and diminish centrally. This disorder may be the same as genodermatosis en cocardes of Degos. In erythrokeratodermia progressiva symmetrica, erythema occurs in association with fixed, hyperkeratotic plaques. The occurrence of phenotypes resembling both erythrokeratodermia variabilis and erythrokeratodermia progressiva symmetrica within the same kindred suggests these disorders may be genetically related.[138] Other focal disorders of cornification may be considered in the differential diagnosis. In pityriasis rotunda, which is an acquired focal disorder of cornification, erythroderma is absent. The Zunich-Kaye syndrome is characterized by focal migratory hyperkeratotic plaques with or without erythema and perioral hyperkeratosis forming a characteristic, lamellar pattern. Associated defects, including deafness, seizures, and mental retardation, point to a multisystemic disease. Hereditary lactate dehydrogenase M-subunit deficiency is an autosomal recessive trait with myoglobinuria and easy fatigability.[139] Skin lesions are described as the childhood onset of migratory, circinate erythematous patches over acral surfaces, palms, and soles, as well as follicular hyperkeratoses. The plaques peel in an inward direction, with flares in the spring and summer and resolution in the winter. The histopathology demonstrates parakeratosis, acanthosis, and pale, swollen spinous and granular cells. The lactate dehydrogenase isozyme in epidermis and muscle is composed of four M-subunits, leading to virtual absence of lactate dehydrogenase activity in skin and hair follicles.[137] Serum lactate dehydrogenase levels may be normal, however. Annually recurring acroerythema may be the same entity.[140] Giroux and Barbeau[141] described a large French-Canadian kindred with a dominantly inherited trait of focal erythematous plaques that tend to resolve during summer and in middle adult years with progressive neurologic disease occurring after age 40.

Erythrokeratodermia Progressiva Symmetrica

Clinical Description

The original description of this autosomal dominant trait is credited to Gottron. The disorder is characterized by psoriasiform plaques that are distributed in a strikingly symmetrical manner, predominantly over the head, extremities (including palms and soles), and buttocks (Fig. 162–18).[141] The trunk is usually relatively spared. The onset is not congenital but usually occurs in the first year of life. Lesions are progressive throughout childhood and may be static thereafter or even partially resolve. The disorder is resistant to topical therapies but responds well to oral retinoids.[141, 142]

Pathology

The histopathologic features of erythrokeratodermia progressiva symmetrica appear to be variable. There is often slight epidermal hyperplasia, with both compact

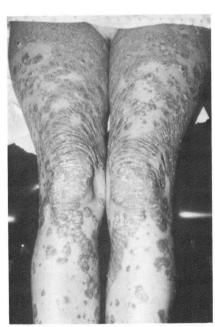

FIGURE 162–18. Erythrokeratodermia progressiva symmetrica. Note well-circumscribed psoriasiform plaques in a strikingly symmetrical distribution.

hyperkeratosis and parakeratosis, which sometimes has a globular quality. Follicular plugging can be present. In some specimens, there are perinuclear vacuoles in cells of the granular layer.[143, 144]

Diagnosis and Differential Diagnosis

Erythrokeratodermia progressiva symmetrica differs from psoriasis clinically by the striking failure to respond to topical therapies and histologically by the absence of Munro's abscesses. It is likely that many patients considered under the rubric of familial pityriasis rubra pilaris may represent erythrokeratodermia progressiva symmetrica. Erythrokeratodermia variabilis differs by the occurrence of changing, evanescent annular erythemas bearing no resemblance to the keratotic plaques.

Peeling Skin Syndrome

The peeling skin syndrome is a rare autosomal recessive trait characterized by cycles of spontaneous desquamation of full-thickness stratum corneum sheets.[145, 146] There is generalized hyperkeratosis, with an underlying erythroderma and diffuse palmoplantar hyperkeratosis, often accompanied by significant pruritus. Hairs may be easily plucked. The disorder may present at or soon after birth as generalized erythema. The peeling regions demonstrate psoriasiform acanthosis with parakeratosis and a split at the stratum granulosum–stratum corneum interface, whereas nonlesional skin demonstrates hyperorthokeratosis.[145] No consistent biochemical changes have been associated with the syndrome. Patients with a nonerythrodermic form in which the split occurs higher, within the stratum corneum, are reported.[147]

Darier's Disease

Clinical Description

Darier's disease (Darier-White disease, keratosis follicularis) is an autosomal dominant trait with an estimated incidence of 1:50,000 to 1:100,000. Many cases are sporadic and presumably represent new mutations.[148] Approximately 75% of patients have the onset of their disease in the first or second decades, but delayed onset until the fifth or later decades is not infrequent. The disorder appears to be fully penetrant, with a wide range of expressivity both within and between kindreds.[148, 149] Keratotic papules in a seborrheic distribution are present in more than 90% of patients (Fig. 162–19). Involvement of flexures, particularly axillae, groins, and inframammary folds, is seen in 80% of patients. In most patients, flexural involvement is mild, but some form extensive, macerated papillomatous plaques (Fig. 162–20). Virtually all patients have hand involvement, which includes nail dystrophy, palmar pits, and acrokeratoses. Hand involvement may be the initial site of involvement in childhood. Nail changes are highly characteristic and include short, broad nails, with longitudinal white and red streaks, nail fragility with V-shaped notches at the

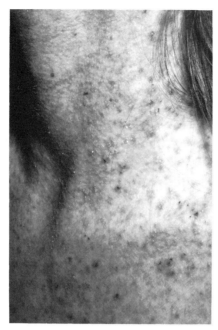

FIGURE 162–19. Darier's disease. Note inflammatory, keratotic papules on neck and chest.

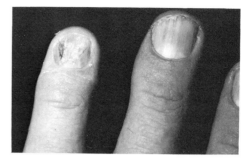

FIGURE 162–21. Nails in Darier's disease. Note severe nail dystrophy in index finger, while adjacent nail exhibits red and white vertical bands and distal notching.

free edge, longitudinal ridges, and subungual hyperkeratoses (Fig. 162–21).[148] Hemorrhagic macules due to trauma are found in some kindreds.[150] Oral manifestations are present in 15% to 50% of patients and include white papules on the hard palate and cobblestoning on the buccal mucosa and gingival margins. Other mucosal epithelia may be involved, including rectal mucosa, hypopharynx, and larynx.

The disease can be triggered by ultraviolet light B exposure,[151] and many patients note onset or flares of the disease after sun exposure. Heat and sweating may also trigger disease. Lithium therapy has been associated with severe flares in several instances.[148, 152] Bullous Darier's disease is a rare variant.[148] A cornifying variant with widespread keratotic plaques has also been described. Hormonal dependency with improvement on estrogen therapy has been observed in some patients,[153] but many

women do not observe changes in disease activity in relation to estrogen status.

Patients are at increased risk for widespread herpes simplex infections (eczema herpeticum), and one fourth of patients suffer from recurrent bacterial skin infections. Immunologic defects have been sought to account for this predisposition, but many patents show no immune deficiency; and in those in whom immune defects are reported, no consistent pattern of immune alterations has emerged.[154] It seems likely that immune abnormalities may be the consequence, rather than cause, of the extensive skin disease. Salivary stones with ductal obstruction are an unusual complication of the disease, but sialadenitis with intermittent salivary gland swelling may occur in one fourth of patients. Bone cysts have been reported in a few patients, but this appears to be a rare manifestation of the disease.[155] Mental deficiency has been noted in some kindreds, as have other neuropsychiatric disorders.[148, 156] However, whether these complaints are part of the disease syndrome or are secondary to the severe social isolation and disability that the skin disease may impose is unclear.[148] A high incidence of suicide ideation has been noted.[157]

Pathology

Darier's disease is characterized by focal acantholytic dyskeratosis occurring in small foci that become confluent (Fig. 162–22). In focal acantholytic dyskeratosis, suprabasal clefts lie beneath columns of acantholytic and dyskeratotic cells. The corps ronds of Darier's disease are simply acantholytic, dyskeratotic cells with prominent perinuclear vacuoles, and grains are their parakeratotic counterparts. The name "keratosis follicularis" is a misnomer because there is no consistent relationship of these foci to follicular epithelium. The epidermis of affected areas may be markedly hyperplastic. Focal acantholytic dyskeratosis is also evident in affected nail bed epithelium.

Pathogenesis and Etiology

The underlying defect in Darier's disease has not been defined. Cultured keratinocytes become acantholytic, indicating that the genetic defect is resident within the epidermis. Moreover, the observation that keratinocytes of Darier's disease secrete a substance that induces

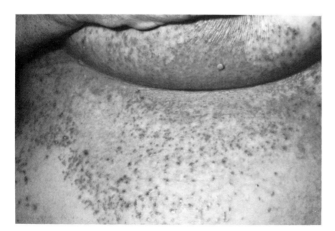

FIGURE 162–20. Darier's disease. Note inflammatory plaque in inframammary fold with keratotic papules at the periphery.

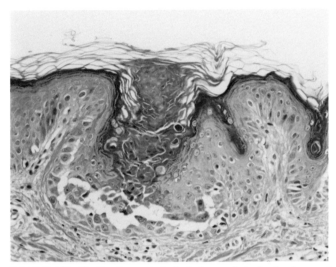

FIGURE 162-22. Focal acantholytic dyskeratosis is the fundamental pathologic alteration in Darier's disease. There are suprabasilar clefts above which are acantholytic and dyskeratotic cells.

acantholysis in normal keratinocytes has suggested that abnormal epidermal proteolytic activity may underlie the disease pathogenesis.[158] However, whether such proteases are the site of the primary defect or represent a later step in disease pathogenesis is unclear.

Diagnosis and Differential Diagnosis

The combination of the clinical picture and histopathology are distinctive and usually present little diagnostic difficulty. Patients with disease localized to a segmental pattern following Blashko's lines are reported[159] and presumably represent a somatic mutation for the Darier's disease gene. Such patients may be at risk for affected offspring with the generalized disease if the mutation affects the germ plasm; however, no such instances of familial transmission have been reported. Acrokeratosis verruciformis of Hopf is an unrelated autosomal dominant trait. Although the acral keratoses are similar to those of Darier's disease, they do not show the Darier's histopathology.[160] The intertriginous lesions of Hailey-Hailey disease may resemble the verrucous papillomatous plaques of Darier's disease, but the other cutaneous, nail, and mucosal signs of Darier's disease are not present. Other disorders with the histopathology of Darier's disease (e.g., Grover's disease, warty dyskeratomas) are sufficiently different clinically to present little confusion. Familial dyskeratotic comedones is an autosomal dominant trait with widespread comedonal lesions predominantly on extremities that show the histopathology of Darier's disease.[161] Other cutaneous signs of Darier's disease are absent.

Treatment

Once established the disease tends to persist and gradually extend. The cutaneous lesions respond well to oral retinoids (e.g., etretinate, 0.5 mg/kg per day). To avoid long-term toxicities, patients should receive the lowest dose that will suppress their disease. Intermittent therapy may suffice for some patients. Macerated, intertriginous lesions respond poorly to retinoids. Here, antibacterial soaps and oral antibiotics may be needed. Sun protection should be encouraged in all patients.

Hailey-Hailey Disease

Hailey-Hailey disease (benign familial pemphigus) is an autosomal dominant trait in which flexural involvement with moist vegetative plaques or scaly patches with vesiculopustules is the characteristic clinical sign. The disorder typically has onset in the second to fourth decade and may gradually improve with age. These lesions are similar to the flexural lesions of Darier's disease, but in Hailey-Hailey disease distinct keratotic papules are not seen. In some patients, extraflexural sites are involved, with scaly, often circinate plaques on trunk, extremities, scalp, and face. Papular plaques bearing a resemblance to genital warts may be an occasional presentation.[162] Unlike Darier's disease, palmar keratoses are not seen, oral involvement is rare, and nail changes are limited to longitudinal white streaks without fragility.[163] Despite limited clinical overlap, the preponderance of evidence suggests that Hailey-Hailey and Darier's disease are distinct genetic disorders. The histopathology is also distinctive and demonstrates suprabasilar acantholysis that may also affect the spinous layer. In contrast to Darier's disease, dyskeratotic acantholytic cells are uncommon. The epidermis is hyperplastic with slender elongated dermal papillae lined by a intact basal layer that projects into the suprabasal cleft. These structures have been likened to intestinal villi. Hyperkeratosis and parakeratosis are commonly found (Fig. 162-23). Ultrastructural examination indicates that the microvilli of lesional keratinocytes are initially affected and that subsequently desmosomes are engulfed by keratinocytes.

Lesions are provoked by a variety of traumatic stimuli. Treatment with topical steroids and antibiotics is often beneficial. Rarely, surgical treatment by excision and grafting, CO_2 laser, and dermabrasion are indicated for resistant plaques.[164] The underlying defect in cellular adhesion has not been defined, although this seems to be an inherent abnormality of Hailey-Hailey keratinocytes, since they dissociate (acantholysis) in cell culture.[154] As in Darier's disease, an increased role for epidermal protease activity has been proposed, but whether this is the initiating event is unclear.

Porokeratosis

Clinical Description

The porokeratoses are a group of disorders having in common a distinctive histopathologic structure—the cornoid lamella. At least four clinical forms can be delineated: (1) porokeratoses of Mibelli (including linear porokeratosis); (2) porokeratosis plantaris, palmaris et disseminata; (3) punctate porokeratosis of palms and soles; and (4) disseminated superficial actinic porokeratosis. Most of these are inherited as autosomal dominant traits. The occurrence of more than one form within the same

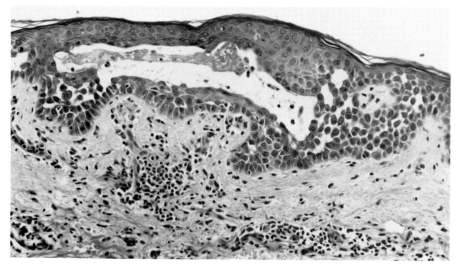

FIGURE 162-23. The histopathologic features of Hailey-Hailey disease include suprabasilar clefts with diffuse acantholysis of the roof of the blister.

kindred or patient suggests that they may be expressions of the same or closely related genetic traits.[165, 166]

Porokeratosis of Mibelli is an autosomal dominant trait characterized by one or more well-demarcated erythematous, hyperkeratotic plaques outlined by a thickened, keratotic border often several millimeters in height (Fig. 162-24). A furrow is evident running along the keratotic ridge. The inner portion of the lesion is less keratotic and may even be atrophic. Lesions are single or few in number and may occur anywhere, including mucous membranes. The initial lesion may be small (<1 cm) and slowly expands to exceed 10 cm in size. Most lesions have their onset in the first decade. In several instances, malignant degeneration to squamous cell carcinoma has been observed. Some patients have multiple lesions that are oriented in a linear or nevoid pattern. Although some authorities recognize linear porokeratosis as a distinct subtype, Mibelli also observed this morphology in his original report. Linear porokeratosis has been observed in monozygotic twins; a mutation affecting a clone of cells distributed along morphogenic lines is proposed. Another linear variant is the porokeratotic eccrine ostial and dermal duct nevus.[167] Here, hyperkeratotic papules are grouped in a linear or nevoid array or coalesce to form plaques. Histopathologically, distention and plugging of eccrine ducts by coronoid lamella-like parakeratotic plugs are seen.

Porokeratosis palmaris et plantaris disseminata is a rare autosomal dominant form that differs from the Mibelli form in the multiplicity of lesions.[168] Lesions too numerous to count develop over both sun-shielded and sun-exposed regions of the neck, trunk, and extremities. Face and scalp are usually spared, and mucous membranes may be involved.[169] The onset is usually in the second or third decade, often beginning with hyperkeratotic papules on the palms and soles. Like disseminated superficial actinic porokeratosis, lesions on glabrous skin are small (<1 cm), have a fine keratotic border, and may be pruritic. Malignant degeneration is reported.

Disseminated superficial actinic porokeratosis was first delineated by Chernosky and Freeman.[170] The condition is common in whites and is more frequent in women. It has its onset in the third and fourth decades as multiple (usually more than 50), small erythematous or atrophic patches with a fine keratotic border, limited to the sun-exposed portions of the extremities.[171] Pruritus may be exacerbated during the summer, when the lesions may become more erythematous and keratotic. They begin as keratotic, often folliculocentric, papules and slowly enlarge. Malignant degeneration is rarely observed. In addition to ultraviolet light, psoralens plus ultraviolet light A (PUVA) therapy may induce these lesions. Immunosuppression has also been associated with their appearance.[172]

Pathology

Cornoid lamellation is the hallmark of the porokeratoses. In this reaction pattern, narrow, sometimes slanting columns of parakeratotic cells are produced by an epidermis in which there are perinuclear vacuoles and individually dyskeratotic cells. Coronoid lamellae define the outer borders of lesions of porokeratosis (Fig. 162-25). The centers of lesions of porokeratosis of Mibelli commonly show psoriasiform epidermal hyperplasia, and those of actinic porokeratosis are frequently the sites of epidermal atrophy, sometimes accompanied by lichenoid lymphocytic infiltrates.

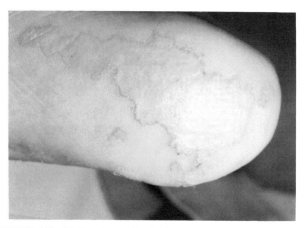

FIGURE 162-24. Porokeratosis of Mibelli on plantar skin. Note keratotic border with furrow.

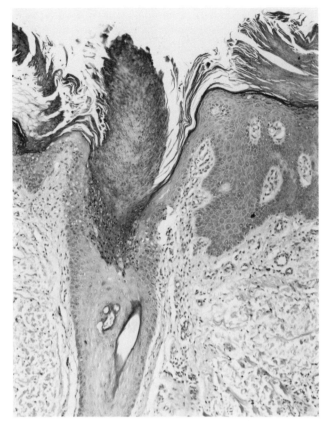

FIGURE 162–25. The cornoid lamella, a vertical or slanting column of parakeratosis, is the hallmark of all of the forms of porokeratosis. In porokeratosis of Mibelli, shown here, the epidermis within the area bounded by cornoid lamellation often shows psoriasiform hyperplasia.

Pathogenesis and Etiology

The lesions of porokeratosis were postulated by Reed and Leone[173] to represent proliferations of an abnormal clone of keratinocytes, perhaps stimulated by actinic damage. A genetic factor that predisposes to their induction could account for the dominant inheritance pattern in most forms of porokeratosis. Immunosuppression has also been linked to the formation of both disseminated superficial actinic and Mibelli types of porokeratotis.[172] Rarely, porokeratosis occurs as a reaction to a drug. Keratinocytes from porokeratotic lesions are frequently aneuploid,[174] supporting the concept of an abnormal clone and underscoring the premalignant nature of porokeratosis. Mibelli originally proposed the derivation of porokeratosis from intraepidermal eccrine ductal cells. However, this theory has fallen into disfavor, because eccrine units are rarely observed in association with porokeratotic lesions. Cytochemical studies have again suggested that porokeratotic lesions may derive from epidermal cells with lumen-forming ability,[175] although lumina are not present histopathologically in any of the forms of porokeratosis.

Treatment

Because of the risk of malignant degeneration, as well as the tendency to enlarge over time, treatment of porokeratosis of Mibelli is usually indicated. Topical 5-fluor-

ouracil or ablation by surgery, dermabrasion, or CO_2 laser may be used. Recurrences are common. Patients with porokeratosis disseminata may benefit from oral retinoids. A number of therapies have been proposed for disseminated superficial actinic porokeratosis, including topical retinoids, cryosurgery, and topical 5-fluorouracil, as well as retinoids plus PUVA. Systemic retinoids are reported to both improve and exacerbate disseminated superficial actinic porokeratosis.[176]

PALMOPLANTAR KERATODERMAS

The palmoplantar keratodermas (PPKs) encompass numerous entities. The initial approach to the patient should focus on determining if the condition is part of a more generalized disorder of cornification (e.g., pityriasis rubra pilaris, psoriasis) or if it is predominantly localized to the palms and soles and whether it is acquired or genetically determined. The differential diagnosis of the genetic forms requires determination of the inheritance pattern and clinical evaluation of the pattern of involvement: focal versus diffuse, extension onto dorsal surfaces (transgrediens) or distant sites, and potential for constriction (pseudoainhum). As in the inherited generalized disorders of cornification (the ichthyoses), PPKs may also be part of a symptom-complex. Case reports of PPKs in association with other organ system abnormalities abound; many of these may represent unique or "private" mutations.[177]

Acquired Palmoplantar Keratoderma

An acquired PPK should be considered in the patient with adult onset of disease and no known familial predisposition. Like acquired ichthyoses, it demands evaluation for an underlying cause. Calluses are a common form of focal acquired PPK that represent a response to chronic frictional injury. The focal hyperkeratosis is due to underlying epidermal hyperplasia and incomplete differentiation.[178] Removal of the hyperkeratosis by keratolytics or manual paring relieves the discomfort; however, the callus will recur unless the underlying stimulus is relieved. Diffuse palmoplantar hyperkeratosis may similarly develop on palms or soles in response to chronic mechanical trauma. These hyperkeratoses are usually functional (i.e., protective from further mechanical injury). Painful callosities sometimes develop in women after menopause (keratoderma climacterium) or bilateral oophorectomy, occasionally in association with hyperhidrosis. Improvement following topical or systemic estrogen replacement therapy suggests the disorder may have a hormonal basis.[179] A psoriasiform pattern of palmoplantar erythema and hyperkeratosis has been associated in a few instances with eccrine syringofibroadenomatosis.[180] Onset is usually after age 40, and a portion of the lesions may have a distinctive "tapioca pudding" appearance.

Like acquired ichthyosis, adult onset of palmoplantar hyperkeratosis may signify an underlying malignancy.[181] An unusual pattern of hyperkeratosis characterized by a rugose or honeycombed morphology ("tripe palms") has been associated with a variety of internal malignancies,[182] as well as bullous pemphigoid.[183] Acanthosis nigricans is also present in some patients, and "tripe palms" may represent a palmar manifestation of this disorder. Cutaneous T-cell lymphoma may also present as an acquired PPK; here the skin biopsy will reveal the correct diagnosis.[184] Punctate palmar keratoses are also associated in some surveys with an increased risk of bladder and lung cancer; these lesions, however, are quite common in the population.[185] The Howel-Evans syndrome is the association of diffuse PPK with esophageal cancer and is inherited as an autosomal dominant trait.[186] The earliest sign of the disease is diffuse follicular hyperkeratosis. Additional cutaneous signs include axillary follicular cysts, thinning of lateral eyebrows, and perhaps marked solar elastosis. The PPK may not develop until adulthood but usually precedes the development of esophageal carcinoma by one or two decades. Esophageal dysplasia precedes the development of overt carcinoma. Close follow-up with annual esophagoscopy is recommended.[186, 187] Unfortunately, retinoid therapy does not appear to prevent progression of the esophageal disease.[188]

Inherited Palmoplantar Keratodermas: Diffuse Forms

Unna and Vörner Forms of PPK

The autosomal dominantly inherited form of diffuse PPK without transgrediens has been designated by two eponyms, the Unna-Thost form and the Vörner form, to denote histopathologic differences: the Unna-Thost form demonstrates orthohyperkeratosis, while the Vörner form shows epidermolytic hyperkeratosis. It has been suggested that the Vörner form is the most common.[189] Features of epidermolytic hyperkeratosis may be focal and relatively subtle and may be easily overlooked. Indeed, re-examination of members of the kindred originally described by Thost has demonstrated the histopathology of epidermolytic hyperkeratosis;[190] hence this portion of the eponym should be discarded. Nielsen[191] has documented the occurrence of the Unna form in northern Sweden, hence it seems appropriate to continue to distinguish these two forms. Clinically, both forms are identical, with a sharply marginated, diffuse palmoplantar hyperkeratosis. A very dense keratoderma results in a yellow, waxy appearance, often rimmed with erythema. The onset is usually in infancy, but delay until childhood may occur. The initial involvement may be focal, over pressure points, only later becoming diffuse. Knuckle pads and occasionally hyperkeratotic patches on elbows and knees may occur, but spill over to the dorsal surfaces (transgrediens) is absent. Blistering is uncommon, even in the Vörner form, and may signify secondary dermatophytosis.[191] Hyperhidrosis is usually present. Mechanical debridement in conjunction with topical keratolytic therapy is the main line of therapy. Some patients may require oral retinoid therapy to maintain mechanical function. However, the long-term risks of retinoid treatment

must be considered in these patients who will require lifelong therapy. Also some patients with the Vörner type do not tolerate retinoid therapy, because of the tendency to desquamate to a tender, insufficiently keratinized base.[59] Low serum biotin levels with improvement on oral biotin supplements has been reported in one kindred.[192]

Recently, mutations in the keratin 9 gene have been described in the Vörner form.[193] Keratin 9 is a keratin species normally expressed only on palms and soles and is a likely candidate for the genetic defect. It should be noted in genetic counseling that patients with the Vörner type of PPK are not at risk for offspring with the generalized disease (bullous ichthyosis).

Mutilating Forms of PPK

The mutilating keratoderma of Vohwinkel is inherited as an autosomal dominant trait and is characterized by infantile onset of keratoderma often with a diffuse, honeycombed pattern. Star-shaped hyperkeratoses typically develop over the dorsa of the digits, elbows, and knees. The keratoderma is severely disabling and typically leads to the development of fibrous constrictions of the digits (pseudoainhum) and autoamputation. Retinoid therapy may prevent progression of the disease.[194] Associated abnormalities in some patients include deafness, cicatricial alopecia, reticulate hyperpigmentation, corneal dystrophy, lipomatosis, and osteoporosis.

Olmsted's syndrome is the association of massive, mutilating keratoderma with severe nail dystrophy and periorificial sharply marginated, hyperkeratotic plaques.[195] Similar verrucous plaques may be present in flexures, and linear or star-shaped fish hyperkeratotic streaks have been described in some patients. Alopecia, follicular hyperkeratoses, and oral leukokeratoses are additional dermatologic signs. Psychomotor delay, short stature, and hypermobile joints have been described in some patients. Autosomal dominant inheritance has been proposed.

Mutilating keratoderma has also been described in kindreds with an autosomal recessive inheritance pattern. Pujol and associates[196] reported mutilating keratoderma in association with a generalized ichthyosiform dermatosis (fine white scales over entire body since birth) and keratotic papules forming symmetrical, linear cords. Another recessive phenotype with hearing loss, cicatricial alopecia, and perianal hyperkeratoses is also described.

Scleroatrophic Forms of Palmoplantar Keratoderma

Huriez syndrome is an autosomal dominant trait with a diffuse, often relatively mild keratoderma in association with scleroatrophy and sclerodactyly.[197] The keratoderma has its onset in infancy or childhood, with the progressive development of scleroatrophy on the dorsa of the hands. Although sclerodactyly is the most striking feature, Raynaud's phenomenon does not occur. Nails may be abnormal with aplasia, ridging, or clubbing. Squamous cell carcinomas may develop on the atrophic skin in the third or fourth decades. PPK sclerodactyly, and scleroatrophy are also seen in the autosomal domi-

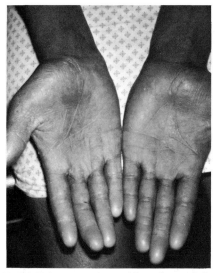

FIGURE 162–26. Palmar atrophy and hyperkeratosis in patient with dyskeratosis congenita.

nant, Kindler-Weary syndrome, in association with acral blistering, generalized poikiloderma, and reticulate hyperpigmentation. PPK with scleroatrophy is seen in most patients with dyskeratosis congenita (Zinsser-Engmann-Cole syndrome) (Fig. 162–26).[198] Reticulate hyperpigmentation with poikiloderma, particularly on the neck, upper chest, and arms, nail dystrophy and oral leukokeratosis are the most constant features of this X-linked recessive syndrome. Other signs include epiphora due to epithelia hyperplasia of the lacrimal duct, hyperhidrosis, alopecia, mechanically induced blisters, hepatosplenomegaly, dental caries, and mild mental and growth retardation. Skin changes are progressive and may not have their onset until mild childhood. Dyspigmentation and nail dystrophy are usually the presenting signs. Approximately 50% of patients develop Fanconi's anemia. An increased incidence of spontaneous and blastogen-induced chromosomal fragility has been noted in some patients.[199] Squamous cell carcinomas, arising from areas of leukoplakia or skin atrophy, as well as esophageal carcinoma, lymphoma, and hematologic malignancies, occur in high incidence. Females may be affected, but whether autosomal forms also occur is controversial.[200, 201] The X-linked recessive form has been mapped to Xq28.[202]

PPK with Transgrediens

Mal de Meleda is a severe, autosomal recessive form of PPK with transgrediens originally described among inbred inhabitants of the Yugoslavian island of Meleda (Mljet), although a similar phenotype is reported from other ethnic groups.[203] The onset is at birth or shortly thereafter with erythema and hyperkeratosis of palms and soles spreading to the dorsa of the hands and feet in a stocking-and-glove pattern or forming focal, circumscribed hyperkeratotic plaques, often in association with plaques on elbows, knees, or angles of the mouth. Nails are dystrophic, and pseudoainhum may develop. Other

associated abnormalities include scrotal tongue, brady-dactyly and syndactyly, and palmar hair. Kindreds exhibiting a dominantly inherited PPK with transgrediens (Greither's syndrome) are also reported.[204]

Papillon-Lefèvre syndrome is an autosomal recessive trait of diffuse PPK with transgrediens and focal keratotic plaques on elbows and knees, in association with severe periodontopathy, leading to premature loss of both primary and secondary teeth. The keratoderma has its onset in the first 3 years of life.[205] Fragile nails, alopecia, and eyelid cysts may be additional dermatologic features. Calcification of the falx cerebri occurs in some patients. The cause of the periodontitis is unknown, but some patients exhibit abnormalities of T- and/or B-cell function, impaired leukocyte chemotaxis, or intracellular killing. Recurrent skin infections occur in one fifth of patients, but systemic infections are rarely associated. Periodontitis and premature loss of teeth are reported in some heterozygotes. Treatment with oral retinoids may assist in the preservation of teeth[206] and may either reduce[207] or increase the risk of pyogenic infections in patients with immune defects.[208]

Ectodermal dysplasias with PPK can be distinguished because teeth themselves are abnormal in these syndromes (enamel dysplasia, adontia, hypodontia), whereas in Papillon-Lefèvre syndrome no abnormalities in tooth structure are evident. Acrodynia (mercury intoxication) may produce palmoplantar erythema and desquamation and premature eruption of teeth with enamel defects, in association with muscle pain, tachycardia, and psychic disturbance.[205]

Diffuse PPK and Multisystemic Disease

Kindreds are described with PPK and progressive sensorineural deafness.[209] The keratoderma is often focal and has its onset in later childhood than most other PPK. The association of PPK and deafness also occurs in pachyonychia congenita, Papillon-Lefèvre syndrome, Olmsted's syndrome, Clouston's syndrome, and the Vohwinkel form of PPK. A syndrome of PPK, deafness, and leukonychia has also been reported.[210] Clouston's syndrome (hidrotic ectodermal dysplasia) is an autosomal dominant trait with generalized alopecia, diffuse PPK, nail dystrophy, and dental dysplasia. PPK may be seen in epidermolysis bullosa simplex of both the Dowling-Meara and Koebner types.[211] Protonotarios and associates[212] have described four kindreds from the Greek island of Naxos with diffuse PPK in association with right ventricular cardiomyopathy (arrhythmogenic right ventricular dysplasia) and sudden death. Diffuse or punctate PPK is a feature of the Naegeli-Franceschetti-Jadassohn syndrome, an autosomal dominant trait with reticulate hyperpigmentation that fades after infancy, hypohidrosis, and severe enamel defects leading to early loss of dentition.[213] Absence of dermatoglyphics and nail dystrophy, including malalignment of the great toenails, are also features. Speckled hyperpigmentation in association with punctate palmoplantar keratoses and acral blistering may be a distinct autosomal dominant trait.[214] Two kindreds are reported with PPK and spastic paraplegia; in one, autosomal dominant inheritance was proposed,[177] while the other kindred also exhibited mental retardation and an X-linked inheritance pattern.[215] PPK and Charcot-Marie-Tooth disease have also been associated.[216] PPK has been reported in association with a wide variety of other abnormalities in a single patient or kindred, and many of these may represent so-called private mutations unique to that kindred.[177]

Inherited Palmoplantar Keratoderma: Focal Forms

Striate PPK is characterized by linear bands of hyperkeratosis that follow the midline of one or more digits, often continuing across the palm in a linear fashion.[217] Plantar involvement may be nummular and centered over pressure points. The trait is inherited in an autosomal dominant manner and may not be expressed until late childhood or adulthood, when it is precipitated by mechanical stress. Painful hereditary callosities are also inherited as an autosomal dominant trait in which focal hyperkeratosis of one to several centimeters in diameter develops on palms and soles over pressure points.[218] Palmoplantar hyperkeratosis is the most constant feature of the autosomal dominant pachyonychia congenita (Jadassohn-Lewandowsky syndrome).[219] Focal keratosis over pressure points develops with weight bearing, often accompanied by blistering and hyperhidrosis (Fig. 162–27). Other common features include nail dystrophy with subungual hyperkeratosis, oral leukokeratosis, and follicular hyperkeratoses.

Small or punctate hyperkeratoses are also inherited as a dominant trait, but in most instances they occur sporadically and may be environmentally included. An increased incidence of atopy has been noted.[220] Two variants are recognized: punctate keratoses of the palms and soles and keratotic pits of the palmar creases. Both are quite common, occurring in 11% and 3% of dermatology patients, and both forms are more common in men and blacks.[221] Punctate keratoses are 1- to 3-mm hyperkeratotic papules distributed over palms and soles. Lesions on the soles may be larger and symptomatic over pressure points and may be single or multiple. Keratotic pits of the palmar creases are discrete depressions in linear arrays. They can be painful and may require surgical intervention. Punctate keratoses are associated in some series with an increased incidence of smoking, as well as

with bladder and lung cancer;[185] both genetic and environmental factors may be involved in their formation. An association between punctate palmoplantar keratoses and gastrointestinal malignancy has also been reported. The differential diagnosis of punctate keratoses of the palms and soles is extensive and includes acquired causes (e.g., warts, arsenical keratoses, syphilis, and yaws) and other genetic traits (e.g., Darier's disease, basal cell nevus syndrome, and Cowden's disease). Punctate keratoses with fine "music box" spines may show the full histopathology of porokeratosis (coronoid lamella) or may only show a mound of parakeratosis. Like other punctate keratoses, punctate porokeratotic keratoderma has an adult onset and is usually sporadic; but familial cases are reported.[222] These keratoses respond to topical 5-fluorouracil therapy.[223]

In tyrosinemia type II (Richner-Hanhart syndrome) focal keratoses may develop over pressure points on the palms and soles. Dendritic corneal ulcerations and mental retardation are the other major clinical signs of this autosomal recessive disorder, which is caused by deficiency of the hepatic enzyme tyrosine aminotransferase. Serum tyrosine levels are markedly elevated, and normalization of tyrosine levels by dietary restriction may prevent full expression of the disease.[224]

References

1. Ackerman AB. Classification of ichthyoses. J Am Acad Dermatol 1985; 6:1047–1048.
2. Elias PM, Menon GK. Structural and lipid biochemical correlates of the epidermal permeability barrier. Adv Lipid Res 1991; 24:1–26.
3. Williams ML. Lipids in normal and pathological desquamation. Adv Lipid Res 1991;24:211–262.
4. Egelrud T, Hofer P-A, Lundström A. Proteolytic degradation of desmosomes in plantar stratum corneum leads to cell dissociation in vitro. Acta Derm Venereol 1988;68:93–97.
5. Proksch E, Feingold KR, Mao-Quiang M, Elias PM. Barrier function regulates epidermal DNA-synthesis. J Clin Invest 1991; 87:1668–1673.
6. Frost P, van Scott EJ. Ichthyosiform dermatoses: Classification based on anatomic and biometric observations. Arch Dermatol 1966;94:113–126.
7. Williams ML, Elias PM. From basket weave to barrier: Unifying concepts for the pathogenesis of the disorders of cornification. Arch Dermatol 1993;129:626–629.
8. Dominey AM, Wang XJ, King LE Jr, et al. Targeted overexpression of transforming growth factor alpha in the epidermis of transgenic mice elicits hyperplasia, hyperkeratosis, and spontaneous, squamous papillomas (abstract). Cell Growth Diff 1993; (12):1071–1082.
9. Williams ML, Feingold KR, Grubauer G, Elias PM. Ichthyosis induced by cholesterol-lowering drugs: Implications for epidermal cholesterol homeostasis. Arch Dermatol 1987;123: 1535–1538.
10. Carver CV. Clofazimine-induced ichthyosis and its treatment. Cutis 1982;29:341–343.
11. Greist MC, Epinette WW. Cimetidine-induced xerosis and asteatotic dermatitis. Arch Dermatol 1982;118:253–254.
12. Cooper MF, Wilson PD, Hartop PJ, et al. Acquired ichthyosis and impaired dermal lipogenesis in Hodgkin's disease. Br J Dermatol 1980;102:689–693.
13. Kaplan MH, Sadick NS, McNutt NS, et al. Acquired ichthyosis may be a marker of concomitant infection with HIV-1 and HTLV-II in intravenous drug users and occurs after profound helper T-cell depletion. J Am Acad Dermatol 1993;29:701–708.
14. Humbert P, Agache P. Acquired ichthyosis: A new cutaneous marker of autoimmunity. Arch Dermatol 1991;127:263–264.

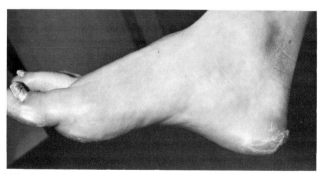

FIGURE 162–27. Pachyonychia congenita. Note focal hyperkeratotic plaques over pressure points and marked subungual hyperkeratosis.

15. Ruze P. Kava-induced dermopathy: A niacin deficiency: Lancet 1990;335:1442-1445.
16. Rubin MG, Mathes B. Pityrasis rotunda: Two cases in black Americans. J Am Acad Dermatol 1986;14:74-78.
17. Berkowitz I, Hodkinson JH, Kew MC, et al. Pityriasis rotunda as a cutaneous marker of hepatocellular carcinoma: A comparison with its prevalence in other diseases. Br J Dermatol 1989; 120:545-549.
18. Griffin LJ, Massa MC. Acquired ichthyosis and pityriasis rotunda. Clin Dermatol 1993;11:27-32.
19. Lodi A, Betti R, Chiarelli G, et al. Familial pityriasis rotunda. Int J Dermatol 1990;29:483-485.
20. Ziprkowski I, Feinstein A. A survey of ichthyosis vulgaris in Israel. Br J Dermatol 1972;86:1-7.
21. Well RS, Kerr CB. Clinical features of autosomal dominant and sex-linked ichthyosis in an English population. Br Med J 1966;1:947-950.
22. Fartasch M, Haneke E, Anton-Lemprecht I. Ultrastructural study of the occurrence of autosomal dominant ichthyosis vulgaris in atopic eczema. Arch Dermatol Res 1987;279:270-272.
23. Kuikkanen K. Ichthyosis vulgaris. Acta Derm Venereol 1969; 49(Suppl 62):1-71.
24. Fleckman P, Holbrook KA, Dale BA, et al. Keratinocytes cultured from subjects with ichthyosis vulgaris are phenotypically abnormal. J Invest Dermatol 1987;88:640-645.
25. Manabe M, Sanchez M, Sun T-T, et al. Interaction of filaggrin with keratin filaments during advanced stages of normal human epidermal differentiation and in ichthyosis vulgaris. Differentiation 1991;48:43-50.
26. Scott IR, Richards S, Harding G, et al. Does establishment of stratum corneum proteins yield functionally active molecules? Ann NY Acad Sci 1988;548:125-136.
27. Elsayed-Ali H, Barton S, Marks R. Stereological studies of desmosomes in ichthyosis vulgaris. Br J Dermatol 1992;126:24-28.
28. Hoyer H, Lykkesfeldt G, Ibsen HH, Bandrup F. Ichthyosis of steroid sulphatase deficiency: Clinical study of 76 cases. Dermatologica 1986;172:184-190.
29. Lykkesfeldt G, Bennett P, Lykkesfeldt AE. Testis cancer: Ichthyosis constitutes a significant risk factor. Cancer 1991;67:730-734.
30. Okano M, Kitano Y, Yoshikawa K, et al. X-linked ichthyosis and ichthyosis vulgaris: Comparison of their clinical features based on biochemical analysis. Br J Dermatol 1988;119:777-783.
31. Traupe H. The Ichthyoses: A Guide to Clinical Diagnosis, Genetic Counseling, and Therapy. Berlin: Springer-Verlag, 1989.
32. Schnur RE, Trask BJ, van den Engh G, et al. An Xp22 microdeletion associated with ocular albinism and ichthyosis: Approximation of breakpoints and estimation of deletion size by using cloned DNA probes and flow cytometry. Am J Hum Genet 1989;45:706-720.
33. Shapiro LJ. Steroid sulfatase deficiency and the genetics of the short arm of the human X chromosome. Adv Human Genet 1985;14:331-381.
34. Elias PM, Williams ML, Maloney MB, et al. Stratum corneum lipids in disorders of cornification: II. Steroid sulfatase and cholesterol sulfate in normal desquamation and the pathogenesis of recessive X-linked ichthyosis. J Clin Invest 1984;74:1414-1421.
35. Shackleton CHL, Reid S. Diagnosis of recessive X-linked ichthyosis: Quantitative HPLC/mass spectrometric analysis of plasma for cholesterol sulfate. Clin Chem 1989;35:1906.
36. Epstein EH Jr, Krauss RM, Shackleton CHL. X-linked ichthyosis: Increased blood cholesterol sulfate and electrophonetic mobility of low-density lipprotein. Science 1981;214:659-660.
37. Bernhardt M, Baden HP. Report of a family with an unusual expression of recessive ichthyosis: Review of 42 cases. Arch Dermatol 1986;122:428-433.
38. Arnold M-L, Anton-Lamprecht L, Albrecht-Nebe H. Congenital ichthyosis with hypogonadism and growth retardation—a new syndrome with peculiar ultrastructural features. Arch Dermatol Res 1992;284:198-208.
39. Williams ML, Elias PM. Heterogeneity in autosomal recessive ichthyosis: Clinical and biochemical differentiation of lamellar ichthyosis and nonbullous congenital ichthyosiform erythroderma. Arch Dermatol 1985;121:477-488.
40. Williams ML, Vogel JS, Ghadially R, et al. Exogenous origin of n-alkanes in pathological scale. Arch Dermatol 1992;128: 1065-1071.
41. Hazell M, Marks R. Clinical, histologic and cell kinetic discriminants between lamellar ichthyosis and nonbullous congenital ichthyosiform erythroderma. Arch Dermatol 1985;121:489-493.
42. Menon GK, Ghadially RG, Williams ML, Elias PM. Lamellar bodies as delivery sources of hydrolytic enzymes: Implications for normal and abnormal desquamation. Br J Dermatol 1992;126: 337-345.
43. Ghadially RG, Williams ML, Hou SYE, Elias PM. Membrane structural abnormalities in the stratum corneum of the autosomal recessive ichthyoses. J Invest Dermatol 1992;99:755-763.
44. Traupe H, Kolde G, Happle R. Autosomal dominant lamellar ichthyosis: A new skin disorder. Clin Genet 1984;25:101-105.
45. Kolde G, Happle R, Traupe H. Autosomal dominant lamellar ichthyosis: Ultrastructural characteristics of a new type of congenital ichthyosis. Arch Dermatol Res 1985;278:1-5.
46. Rossmann-Ringdahl I, Anton-Lamprecht I, Swanbeck G. A mother and two children with nonbullous congenital ichthyosiform erythroderma. Arch Dermatol 1986;122:559-564.
47. Camisa C, Rossana C. Variant of keratoderma hereditaria mutilans (Vohwinkel's syndrome): Treatment with orally administered isotretinoin. Arch Dermatol 1984;120:1323-1328.
48. Frenk E, de Techtermann F. Self-healing collodion baby: Evidence for autosomal recessive inheritance. Pediatr Dermatol 1992;9:95-97.
49. The Executive and Scientific Advisory Boards of the National Foundation for Ectodermal Dysplasias. Scaling skin in the neonate: A clue to the early diagnosis of X-linked hypohidrotic ectodermal dysplasia (Christ-Siemens-Touraine syndrome). J Pediatr 1989;114:600-602.
50. Perry TB, Holbrook KA, Hoff MS, et al. Prenatal diagnosis of congenital non-bullous ichthyosiform erythroderma (lamellar ichthyosis). Prenatal Diagn 1987;7:145-155.
51. Sahn EE, Weimer CE Jr, Garen PD. Annular epidermolytic ichthyosis: A unique phenotype. J Am Acad Dermatol 1992;27: 348-355.
52. Mills CM, Marks R. Acral epidermolytic hyperkeratosis. Br J Dermatol 1993;128:342-347.
53. McGrath JM, Cerio R, Wilson-Jones E. The phenotypic heterogeneity of bullous ichthyosis—a case report of three family members. Clin Exp Dermatol 1991;16:25-27.
54. Syder AJ, Yu, QC, Paller AS, et al. Genetic mutations in the K1 and K10 genes of patients with epidermolytic hyperkeratosis: Correlation between location and disease severity. J Clin Invest 1994;93:1533-1542.
55. Epstein E. Molecular genetics of epidermolysis bullosa. Science 1992;256:799-804.
55a. Rothnagel JA, Traupe H, Wojcik S, et al. Mutations in the rod domain of keratin 2e in patients with ichthyosis bullosa of Siemens. In press.
56. Frieden I. Blisters and pustules in the newborn. Curr Probl Pediatr 1989;19:551.
56a. Paller AS, Syder AJ, Chan Y-M, et al. Genetic and clinical mosaicism in a type of epidermal nevus. N Engl J Med, in press.
57. Ollendorff-Curth H, Allen FH Jr, Schnyder UW, et al. Follow-up of a family group suffering from ichthyosis hystrix type Curth-Macklin. Hummangenetik 1972;17:37-48.
58. Niemi K-M, Virtanen I, Kanerva L, et al. Altered keratin expression in ichthyosis hystrix Curth-Macklin: A light and electron microscopic study. Arch Dermatol Res 1990;282:227-233.
59. Fritsch P, Hönigsmann H, Jaschke E. Epidermolytic palmoplantar keratoderma. Br J Dermatol 1978;99:561-568.
60. Roberts LJ. Long-term survival of a harlequin fetus. J Am Acad Dermatol 1989;21:335-339.
61. Rogers M, Scarf C. Harlequin baby treated with etretinate. Pediatr Dermatol 1989;6:261-267.
62. Unamuno P, Pierola JM, Fernandez E, et al. Harlequin foetus in four siblings. Br J Dermatol 1987;11:569-572.
63. Milner ME, O'Guin WM, Holbrook KA, et al. Abnormal lamellar granules in harlequin ichthyosis. J Invest Dermatol 1992;99:824-829.
64. de Merchant K, Hartwick E, Lee P, et al. Nursing a special patient: The infant with congenital ichthyosis—harlequin syndrome. Neotatal Network 1991;9:27-33.
65. Krafchik BR. Netherton syndrome. Pediatr Dermatol 1992; 9:157-160.
66. Greene SL, Muller SA. Netherton's syndrome: Report of a case

and review of the literature. J Am Acad Dermatol 1985;13: 329–337.

67. Pradeaux L, Olives JP, Bonafe JL, et al. Manifestations digestives et nutritionnelles du syndrome de Netherton. Arch Fr Pediatr 1991;48:95–98.

68. Jones SK, Thomason LM, Surbrugg SK, et al. Neonatal hypernatraemia in two siblings with Netherton's syndrome. Br J Dermatol 1986;116:741–743.

69. Shield JPH, Judge MR, Reardon W, et al. Lethal congenital erythroderma: A newly recognised genetic disorder. Clin Genet 1992;41:273–277.

70. Pupo RA, Tyring SK, Raimer SS, et al. Omenn's syndrome and related combined immunodeficiency syndromes: Diagnostic considerations in infants with persistent erythroderma and failure to thrive. J Am Acad Dermatol 1991;25:442–446.

71. Llorente CP, Amoros JI, de Frutos FJO, et al. Cutaneous lesions in severe combined immunodeficiency: Two case reports and a review of the literature. Pediatr Dermatol 1991;8:314–321.

72. Deal JE, Barratt TM, Dillon MJ. Fanconi syndrome, ichthyosis, dysmorphism, jaundice and diarrhoea—a new syndrome. Pediatr Nephrol 1990;4:308–313.

73. Rizzo WB, Dammann AL, Craft DA, et al. Sjögren-Larsson syndrome: Inherited defect in the fatty alcohol cycle. J Pediatr 1989;115:228–234.

74. Liden S, Jagell S. The Sjögren-Larsson syndrome. Int J Dermatol 1984;23:247–253.

75. Jagell S, Polland W, Sandgren O. Specific changes in the fundus typical for the Sjögren-Larsson syndrome: An ophthalmological study of 35 patients. Acta Ophthalmol 1980;58:321–330.

76. Judge MR, Lake BD, Smith VV, et al. Depletion of alcohol (hexanol) dehydrogenase activity in the epidermis and jejunal mucosa in Sjögren-Larsson syndrome. J Invest Dermatol 1990;95:632–634.

77. Kelson TL, Craft DA, Rizzo WB. Carrier detection for Sjögren-Larsson syndrome. J Inherited Metab Dis 1992;15:105–111.

77a. Rizzo WB, Craft DA, Kelson TL, et al. Prenatal diagnosis of Sjögren-Larsson syndrome using enzymatic methods. Prenatal Diag 1994;14:577–581.

78. Hofer PA, Jagell S. Sjögren-Larsson syndrome: A dermato-histopathological study. J Cutan Pathol 1982;9:360–376.

79. Ito M, Oguro K, Sato Y. Ultrastructural study of the skin in Sjögren-Larsson syndrome. Arch Dermatol Res 1991;283: 141–148.

80. Hooft C, Kriekemans J, van Acker K, et al. Sjögren-Larsson syndrome with oxidative enteropathy: Influence of medium-chain triglycerides on the symptomatology. Helv Paediatr Acta 1967;5:447–458.

81. Guilleminault C, Harpey JP, Lafourcade J. Sjögren-Larsson syndrome: Report of two cases in twins. Neurology 1973;23: 367–373.

82. Chanarin I, Patel A, Slavin G, et al. Neutral-lipid storage disease: A new disorder of lipid metabolism. Br Med J 1975;1:553–555.

83. Williams ML, Koch TK, O'Donnell JJ, et al. Ichthyosis and neutral lipid storage disease. Am J Med Genet 1985;20:711–726.

84. Williams ML, Coleman RA, Placzek D, et al. Neutral lipid storage disease: Evidence for a functional defect in phospholipid-linked triacylglycerol metabolism. Biochem Biophys Acta 1991;1096:162–169.

85. Salvayre R, Negre A, Radom J, et al. Independence of triacylglycerol-containing compartments in cultured fibroblasts from Wolman disease and multisystemic lipid storage myopathy. FEBS Lett 1989;250:35–39.

86. Elias PM, Williams ML. Neutral lipid storage disease with ichthyosis: Defective lamellar body contents and intracellular dispersion. Arch Dermatol 1985;121:1000–1008.

87. Itin PH, Pittelkow MR. Trichothiodystrophy: Review of sulfur-deficient brittle hair syndromes and association with the ectodermal dysplasias. J Am Acad Dermatol 1990;22:705–717.

88. Price VH. Trichothiodystrophy: Update. Pediatr Dermatol 1992;9:369–370.

89. Hersh JH, Klein LR, Joyce MR, et al. Trichothiodystrophy and associated anomalies: A variant of SIBIDS or new symptom complex? Pediatr Dermatol 1993;10:117–122.

90. McCuaig C, Marcoux D, Rasmussen JE, et al. Trichothiodystrophy associated with photosensitivity, gonadal failure, and striking osteosclerosis. J Am Acad Dermatol 1993;28:820–826.

91. Bootsma D, Hoeijmakers JHJ. Engagement with transcription. Nature 1993;363:114–188.

92. Harms M, Gilardi S, Levy PM, et al. KID syndrome (keratitis, ichthyosis, and deafness) and chronic mucocutaneous candidiasis: Case report and review of the literature. Pediatr Dermatol 1984;2:1–7.

93. Langer K, Konrad K, Wolff K. Keratitis, ichthyosis and deafness (KID) syndrome: Report of three cases and a review of the literature. Br J Dermatol 1990;122:689–697.

94. Nazzaro V, Blanchet-Bardon C, Lorette G, et al. Familial occurrence of KID (keratitis, ichthyosis, deafness) syndrome. J Am Acad Dermatol 1990;23:385–388.

95. Grob JJ, Breton A, Bonafe JL, et al. Keratitis, ichthyosis, and deafness (KID) syndrome. Arch Dermatol 1987;123:777–782.

96. Wilson GN, Squires RH Jr, Weinberg AG. Keratitis, hepatitis, ichthyosis, and deafness: Report and review of KID syndrome. Am J Med Genet 1991;40:255–259.

97. Morris MR, Namon A, Shaw GY, et al. The keratitis, ichthyosis, and deafness syndrome. Otolaryngol Head Neck Surg 1991; 104:526–528.

98. McGrae JD. Keratitis, ichthyosis, and deafness (KID) syndrome with adult onset of keratitis component. Int J Dermatol 1990;29:145–146.

99. Judge MR, Misch K, Wright P, et al. Palmoplantar and periorificial keratoderma with corneal epithelial dysplasia: A new syndrome. Br J Dermatol 1991;125:186–188.

100. Hazen PG, Carney JM, Langston RHS, et al. Corneal effect of isotretinoin: Possible exacerbation of corneal neovascularization in a patient with the keratitis, ichthyosis, deafness ("KID") syndrome. J Am Acad Dermatol 1986;14:141–142.

101. Hazen PG, Walker AE, Stewart JJ, et al. Keratitis, ichthyosis, and deafness (KID) syndrome: Management with chronic oral ketoconazole therapy. Int J Dermatol 1992;31:58–59.

102. Steiner D. Refsum disease. In: Scriver CR, Beaudet AL, Sly WS, Vale D, eds. The Metabolic Basis of Inherited Disease. New York: McGraw-Hill, 1989:1533–1550.

103. Clardige KG, Gibberd RB, Sidey MC. Refsum disease: The presentation and ophthalmic aspects of Refsum disease in a series of 23 patients. Eye 1992;6:371–375.

104. Dykes PJ, Marks R, Davies MG, et al. Epidermal metabolism in heredopathia atactica polyneuritiformis (Refsum's disease). J Invest Dermatol 1978;70:126–129.

105. Masters-Thomas A, Bailes J, Billimoria JD, et al. Heredopathia atactica polyneuritiformis (Refsum's disease). J Hum Nutr 1980;34:245–250.

106. Emami S., Rizzo WB, Hanley KP, et al. Peroxisomal abnormality in fibroblasts from involved skin of CHILD syndrome. Arch Dermatol 1992;128:1213–1222.

107. Happle R. X-Linked dominant chondrodysplasia punctata: Review of literature and report of a case. Hum Genet 1979; 53:65–73.

108. Happle R. Lyonization and the lines of Blaschko. Hum Genet 1985;70:200–206.

109. Emami S, Hanley KP, Esterly NB, et al. X-linked dominant ichthyosis with peroxisomal deficiency: An ultrastructural and ultracytochemical study of the Conradi-Hünermann syndrome and its murine homologue, the bare patches mouse. Arch Dermatol 1994;130:325–336.

110. Happle R, Koch H, Lenz W. The CHILD syndrome: Congenital hemidysplasia with ichthyosiform erythroderma and limb defects. Eur J Pediatr 1980;134:27–33.

111. Happle R. Ptychotropism as a cutaneous feature of the CHILD syndrome. J Am Acad Dermatol 1990;23:763–766.

112. Poll-The BT, Skjeldal OH, Stokke O, et al. Phytanic acid alpha-oxidation and complementation analysis of classical Refsum and peroxisomal disorders. Hum Genet 1989;81:175–181.

113. Martin BM, Sidransky E, Ginns EI. Gaucher's disease: Advances and challenges. Adv Pediatr 1989;36:277–306.

114. Sidransky E, Sherer DM, Ginns EI. Gaucher disease in the neonate: A distinct Gaucher phenotype is analogous to a mouse model created by targeted disruption of the glucocerebrosidase gene. Pediatr Res 1992;32:494–498.

115. Lui K, Commens C, Choong R, et al. Collodion babies with Gaucher's disease. Arch Dis Child 1988;63:854–856.

116. Holleran WM, Ginns EI, Menon GK, et al. Epidermal consequences of glucocerebrosidase deficiency: Permeability barriers

alteration and basis for skin lesions in type 2 Gaucher disease. J Clin Invest 1994;93:1756–1764.

117. Tolmie JL, Mirtimer G, Doyle D, et al. The Neu-Laxova syndrome in female sibs: Clinical and pathological features with prenatal diagnosis in the second sib. Am J Med Genet 1987;27:175–182.

118. Curry CJ. Letter to the editor: Further comments on the Neu-Laxova syndrome. Am J Med Genet 1982;13:442–444.

119. Welsh KM, Smoller BR, Holbrook KA, et al. Restrictive dermopathy: Report of two affected siblings and a review of the literature. Arch Dermatol 1992;128:228–231.

120. Verloes A, Mulliez N, Gonzales M, et al. Restrictive dermopathy, a lethal form of arthrogryposis multiplex with skin and bone dysplasias: Three new cases and review of the literature. Am J Med Genet 1992;43:539–547.

121. Eramo LR, Esterly NB, Zierserl EJ, et al. Ichthyosis follicularis with alopecia and photophobia. Arch Dermatol 1985;121:1167–1174.

122. Hamm H, Meinecke P, Traupe H. Further delineation of the ichthyosis follicularis, atrichia, and photophobia syndrome. Eur J Pediatr 1991;150:627–629.

123. Martino F, D'Eufemia P, Pergola MS, et al. Child with manifestations of dermotrichic syndrome and ichthyosis follicularis-alopecia-photophobia (IFAP) syndrome. Am J Med Genet 1992;44:233–236.

124. van Osch LDM, Oranje AP, Keukens FM, et al. Keratosis follicularis spinulosa decalvans: A family study of seven male cases and six female carriers. J Med Genet 1992;29:36–40.

125. Rand R, Baden HP. Keratosis follicularis spinulosa decalvans: Report of two cases and literature review. Arch Dermatol 1983;119:22–26.

126. Zunich J, Esterly NB, Holbrook KA, Kaye CI. Congenital migratory ichthyosiform dermatosis with neurologic and ophthalmologic abnormalities. Arch Dermatol 1985;121:1149–1156.

127. Zunich J, Esterly NB, Holbrook KA, Kaye CI. Autosomal recessive transmission of neuroectodermal syndrome. Arch Dermatol 1988;124:1188–1189.

128. Aggett PJ, Cavanaugh HPC, Matthew DJ, et al. Schwachman's syndrome: A review of 21 cases. Arch Dis Child 1980;55:331–347.

129. Goeteyn M, Oranje AP, Vuzevski VD, et al. Ichthyosis, exocrine pancreatic insufficiency, impaired neutrophil chemotaxis, growth retardation, and metaphyseal dysplasia (Schwachman syndrome): Report of a case with extensive skin lesions (clinical, histological, and ultrastructural findings). Arch Dermatol 1991;127:225–230.

130. Mortureaux P, Taieb A, Bazeille J-ES, et al. Schwachman syndrome: A case report. Pediatr Dermatol 1992;9:57–61.

131. Reynolds JF, Neri G, Herrmann JP, et al. New multiple congenital anomalies/mental retardation syndrome with cardio-facio-cutaneous involvement—the CFC syndrome. Am J Med Genet 1986;25:413–427.

132. Piérard GE, Soyeur-Broux M, Estrada JA, et al. Cutaneous presentation of the cardio-facio-cutaneous syndrome. J Am Acad Dermatol 1990;22:920–922.

133. Graham JM Jr, Reynolds JF, Kelley RI, et al. Cardio-facio-cutaneous (CFC) syndrome: Studies of peroxisomal and fatty acid metabolism. Proceedings of the Greenwood Genetics Center, 1988 Smith Workshop.

134. Cram DL. Erythrokeratoderma variabilis and variable carcinate erythrokeratodermas. Arch Dermatol 1970;101:68–73.

135. van der Schroeff JG, van Leeuwen-Cornelisse I, van Haeringen A, et al. Further evidence for localization of the gene of erythrokeratodermia variabilis. Hum Genet 1988;80:97–98.

136. Rappaport IP, Goldes JA, Goltz RW. Erythrokeratodermia variabilis treated with isotretinoin: A clinical, histologic, and ultrastructural study. Arch Dermatol 1986;122:441–445.

137. Findlay GH, Morrison JGL. Erythrokeratolysis hiemalis—keratolytic winter erythema or "Oudtshoorn Skin." Br J Dermatol 1978;98:491–495.

138. Macfarlane AW, Chapman SJ, Verbov JL. Is erythrokeratodermia one disorder? A clinical and ultrastructural study of two siblings. Br J Dermatol 1991;124:487–491.

139. Takayasu S, Fujiwara S, Waki T. Hereditary lactate dehydrogenase M-subunit deficiency: Lactate dehydrogenase activity in skin lesions and in hair follicles. J Am Acad Dermatol 1991;24:339–342.

140. Nazzari G, Crovato F. Annually recurring acroerythema and hereditary lactate dehydrogenase M-subunit deficiency. J Am Acad Dermatol 1992;27:262–263.

141. Giroux J-M, Barbeau A, Erythrokeratodermia with ataxia. Arch Dermatol 1972;106:183–188.

142. Ruiz-Maldanado R, Tamayo L, del Castillo V, et al. Erythrokeratodermia progressiva symmetrica: Report of 10 cases. Dermatologica 1982;164:133–141.

143. Nazzaro V, Blanchet-Bardon C. Progressive symmetric erythrokeratodermia: Histological and ultrastructural study of patient before and after treatment with etretinate. Arch Dermatol 1986;122:434–440.

144. Niemi K-M, Kanerva L. Histologic and ultrastructural study of a family with erythrokeratodermia progressiva symmetrica. J Cutan Pathol 1993;20:242–249.

145. Levy SB, Goldsmith LA. The peeling skin syndrome. J Am Acad Dermatol 1982;7:606–613.

146. Mevorah B, Frenk E, Saurat JH, et al. Peeling skin syndrome: A clinical, ultrastructural and biochemical study. Br J Dermatol 1987;116:117–125.

147. Silverman AK, Ellis CN, Beals TF, et al. Continual skin peeling syndrome: An electron microscopic study. Arch Dermatol 1986;122:71–75.

148. Burge SM, Wilkinson JD. Darier-White disease: A review of the clinical features in 163 patients. J Am Acad Dermatol 1992;27:40–50.

149. Beck AL Jr, Finocchio AF, White JP. Darier's disease: A kindred with a large number of cases. Br J Dermatol 1977;97:335–339.

150. Foresman PL, Goldsmith LA, Ginn L, et al. Hemorrhagic Darier's disease. 1993;129:511–512.

151. Baba T, Yaoita H. UV radiation and keratosis follicularis. Arch Dermatol 1984;120:1484–1487.

152. Milton GP, Peck GL, Fu J-JL. Exacerbation of Darier's disease by lithium carbonate (correspondence). J Am Acad Dermatol 1990;23:926–928.

153. Espy PD, Stone S, Jolly HW Jr. Hormonal dependency in Darier's disease. Cutis 1976;17:315–320.

154. Patrizi A, Ricci G, Neri I, et al. Imunological parameters in Darier's disease. Dermatologica 1989;178:138–140.

155. Crisp AJ, Payne CMER, Adams J, et al. The prevalence of bone cysts in Darier's disease: A survey of 31 cases. Clin Exp Dermatol 1984;9:78–83.

156. Svendsen IB, Albrectsen B. The prevalence of dyskeratosis follicularis (Darier's disease) in Denmark: An investigation of the heredity in 22 families. Acta Derm Venereol 1950;39:256–269.

157. Denicoff KD, Lehman ZA, Rubinow DR, et al. Suicidal ideation in Darier's disease. J Am Acad Dermatol 1990;22:196–198.

158. Burge SM, Cederholm-Williams SA, Garrod DR, et al. Cell adhesion in Hailey-Hailey disease and Darier's disease: Immunocytological and explant-tissue-culture studies. Br J Dermatol 1991;125:426–435.

159. Starink TM, Woerdeman MJ. Unilateral systematized keratosis follicularis: A variant of Darier's disease or an epidermal naevus (acantholytic dyskeratotic epidermal naevus)? Br J Dermatol 1981;105:207–214.

160. Panja RK. Acrokeratosis verruciformis (Hopf)—a clinical entity? Br J Dermatol 1977;96:643–652.

161. Hall JR, Holder W, Knox JM, et al. Familial dyskeratotic comedones: A report of three cases and review of the literature. J Am Acad Dermatol 1987;17:808–814.

162. Langenburg AL, Berger TG, Cardenelli M, et al. Genital benign chronic pemphigus (Hailey-Hailey disease) presenting as condylomas. J Am Acad Dermatol 1992;26:951–955.

163. Burge SM. Hailey-Hailey disease: The clinical features, response to treatment and prognosis. Br J Dermatol 1992;126:275–282.

164. Kirtschig G, Gieler U, Happle R. Treatment of Hailey-Hailey disease by dermabrasion. J Am Acad Dermatol 1993;38:784–786.

165. Commens CA, Shumack SP. Linear porokeratosis in two families with disseminated superficial actinic porokeratosis. Pediatr Dermatol 1987;4:209–214.

166. Dover JS, Phillips TJ, Burns DA, et al. Disseminated superficial actinic porokeratosis: Coexistence with other porokeratotic variants. Arch Dermatol 1986;122:887–889.

167. Aloi FG, Pippione M. Porokeratotic eccrine ostial and dermal duct nevus. Arch Dermatol 1986;122:892–895.

168. Guss SB, Osbourn RA, Lutzner MA. Porokeratosis plantaris, palmaris, et disseminata: A third type of porokeratosis. Arch Dermatol 1971;104:366–373.
169. Patrizi A, Passarini B, Minghetti G, et al. Porokeratosis palmaris et plantaris disseminata: An unusual clinical presentation. J Am Acad Dermatol 1989;21:415–418.
170. Chernosky ME, Freeman RG. Disseminated superficial actinic porokeratosis (DSAP). Arch Dermatol 1967;96:611–624.
171. Shumack SP, Commens CA. Disseminated superficial actinic porokeratosis: A clinical study. J Am Acad Dermatol 1989; 20:1015–1022.
172. Neumann RA, Knobler RM, Metze D, et al. Disseminated superficial porokeratosis and immunosuppression. Br J Dermatol 1988;119:375–380.
173. Reed RJ, Leone P, Porokeratosis—a mutant clonal keratosis of the epidermis. Arch Dermatol 1970;101:340–347.
174. Beers B, Jaszcz W, Sheetz K, et al. Porokeratosis palmaris et plantaris disseminata. Arch Dermatol 1992;128:236–239.
175. Ma AS-P, Bell DJ, Dinneen AM. Aberrant proliferation of lumen-forming cells in stratified epithelium of porokeratosis skin. J Invest Dermatol 1990;95:388–392.
176. Knobler RM, Neumann RA. Exacerbation of porokeratosis during etretinate therapy. Acta Derm Venereol 1990;70:319.
177. Powell FC, Venencie PY, Gordon H, et al. Keratoderma and spastic paralysis. Br J Dermatol 1983;109:589–596.
178. Thomas SE, Dykes PJ, Marks R, et al. Plantar hyperkeratosis: A study of callosities and normal plantar skin. J Invest Dermatol 1985;85:394–397.
179. Zultak M, Bedeaux C, Blanc D, et al. Keratoderma climacterium treatment with topical estrogen (letter). Dermatologica 1988; 176:151–152.
180. Lui H, Stewart WD, English JC, et al. Eccrine syringofibroadenomatosis: A clinical and histologic study and review of the literature. J Am Acad Dermatol 1992;267:805–813.
181. Khanna SK, Agnone FA, Leibowitz AI, et al. Nonfamilial diffuse palmoplantar keratoderma associated with bronchial carcinoma. J Am Acad Dermatol 1993;28:295–297.
182. Cohen PR, Kurzrock R. Malignancy-associated tripe palms. J Am Acad Dermatol 1992;27:271–272.
183. Razack EMA, Premalatha S, Rao NR, et al. Acanthosis palmaris in a patient with bullous pemphigoid. J Am Acad Dermatol 1987;16:217–219.
184. Aram H, Zeidenbaum M. Palmoplantar hyperkeratosis in mycosis fungoides. J Am Acad Dermatol 1985;13:897–899.
185. Cuzick J, Babiker A, De Stavola BL, et al. Palmar keratoses in family members of individuals with bladder cancer. J Clin Epidemiol 1990;43:1421–1426.
186. O'Mahony MY, Hellier M, Huddy P, et al. Familial tylosis and carcinoma of the oesophagus. J R Soc Med 1984;77:514–517.
187. Ashworth MT, Nash JRG, Ellis A, et al. Abnormalities of differentiation and maturation in the oesophageal squamous epithelium of patients with tylosis: Morphological features. Histopathology 1991;19:303–310.
188. Marger RS, Marger D. Carcinoma of the esophagus and tylosis: A lethal genetic combination. Cancer 1993;72:17–19.
189. Hamm H, Happle R, Butterfass T, et al. Epidermolytic palmoplantar keratoderma of Vörner: Is it the most frequent type of hereditary paloplantar keratoderma? Dermatologica 1988; 177:138–145.
190. Küster W, Becker A. Indication for the identity of palmoplantar keratoderma type Unna-Thost with type Vörner: Thost's family revisited 110 years later. Acta Derm Venereol 1992;72:120–122.
191. Gamborg Nielsen P. Hereditary palmoplantar keratoderma in the northernmost county of Sweden. Acta Derm Venereol 1985; 65:224–229.
192. Menni S, Saleh F, Piccinno R, et al. Palmoplantar keratoderma of Unna-Thost: Response to biotin in one family. Clin Exp Dermatol 1992;17:337–338.
193. Reis A, Hennies HC, Langbein L, et al. Keratin 9 gene mutations in epidermolytic palmoplantar keratoderma (EPPK). Nature Genet 1994;6:174–179.
194. Rivers JK, Duke EE, Justus DW. Etretinate: Management of keratoma hereditaria mutilans in four family members. J Am Aad Dermatol 1985;13:43–49.
195. Atherton DJ Sutton C, Jones BM. Mutilating palmoplantar keratoderma with periorificial keratotic plaques (Olmsted's syndrome). Br J Dermatol 1990;122:245–252.
196. Pujol RM, Moreno A, Alomar A, et al. Congenital ichthyosiform dermatosis with linear keratotic flexural papules and sclerosing palmoplantar keratoderma. Arch Dermatol 1989;125:103–106.
197. Patrizi A, Di Lernia V, Patrone P. Palmoplantar keratoderma with sclerodactyly (Huriez syndrome). J Am Acad Dermatol 1992;26:855–857.
198. Davidson HR, Connor JM. Dyskeratosis congenita. J Med Genet 1988;25:843–846.
199. Schneider A, Mayer U, Gebhart E, et al. Blastogen-induced fragility may differentiate pancytopenia congenital dyskeratosis from Fanconi anaemia. Eur J Pediatr 1988;148:37–39.
200. Pai GS, Morgan S, Whetsel C. Etiologic heretogeneity in dyskeratosis congenita. Am J Med Genet 1989;32:63–66.
201. Drachtman RA, Alter BP. Dyskeratosis congenita: Clinical and genetic heterogeneity: Report of a new case and review of the literature. Am J Pediatr Hematol Oncol 1992;297–304.
202. Connor JM, Gatherer D, Gray FC, et al. Assignment of the gene for dyskeratosis congenita to Xq28. Hum Genet 1989;72: 348–351.
203. Kastl I, Anton-Lamprecht I, Gamborg Nielsen P. Hereditary palmoplantar keratosis of the Gamborg Neilsen type. Arch Dermatol Res 1990;282:363–370.
204. Sybert VP, Dale BA, Holbrook KA. Palmar-plantar keratoderma: A clinical, ultrastructural, and biochemical study. J Am Acad Dermatol 1988;18:75–86.
205. Haneke E. The Papillon-Lefèvre syndrome: Keratosis palmoplantaris with periodontopathy: Report of a case and review of the cases in the literature. Hum Genet 1979;51:1–35.
206. Gelmetti C, Nazzaro V, Cerri D, et al. Long-term preservation of permanent teeth in a patient with Papillon-Lefèvre syndrome treated with etretinate. Pediatr Dermtaol 1989;6:222–225.
207. Bergman R, Friedman-Birnbaum R. Papillon-Lefèvre syndrome: A study of the long-term clinical course of recurrent pyogenic infections and the effects of etretinate treatment. Br J Dermatol 1988;119:731–736.
208. Tosti A, Manuzzi P, Bardazzi F, et al. Is etretinate dangerous in Papillon-Lefèvre syndrome? Dermatologica 1988;176:148–150.
209. Sharland M, Bleach NR, Goberdhan PD, et al. Autosomal dominant palmoplantar hyperkeratosis and sensorineural deafness in three generations. J Med Genet 1992;29:50–52.
210. Crosby EF, Vidurrizaga RH. Knuckle pads, leukonychia, deafness, and keratosis palmoplantaris: Report of a family. Johns Hopkins Med J 1976;139:90–92.
211. Haber RM, Ramsay CA, Boxall LBH. Epidermolysis bullosa simplex with keratoderma of the palms and soles. J Am Acad Dermatol 1985;12:1040–1044.
212. Protonotarios N, Tsatsopoulou A, Patsourakos P, et al. Cardiac abnormalities in familial palmoplantar keratosis. Br Heart J 1986;56:321–326.
213. Itin PH, Lautenschlager S, Meyer R, et al. Natural history of the Naegeli-Franceschetti-Jadassohn synrome and further delineation of its clinical manifestation. J Am Acad Dermatol 1993;28: 942–950.
214. Boss JM, Matthews CNA, Peachey RDG, et al. Speckled hyperpigmentation, palmoplantar punctate keratoses and childhood blistering: A clinical triad, with variable associations: A report of two families. Br J Dermatol 1981;105:579–585.
215. Fitzsimmons JS, Fitzsimmons EM, McLachlan JI, et al. Four brothers with mental retardation, spastic paraplegia and palmoplantar hyperkeratosis: A new syndrome? Clin Genet 1983; 23:329–335.
216. Rabbiosi G, Borroni G, Pinelli P, et al. Palmoplantar keratoderma and Charcot-Marie-Tooth disease. Arch Dermatol 1980; 116:789–790.
217. Ortega M, Quintana J, Camacho F. Keratosis palmoplantar striata (Brunauer-Fuhs type). Acta Derm Venereol. 1982;63: 273–275.
218. Baden HP, Bronstein BR, Rand RE. Hereditary callosities with blisters. J Am Acad Dermatol 1984;11:409–415.
219. Kansky A, Basta-Juzbasic, Videnic N, et al. Pachyonychia con-

genita (Jadassohn-Lewandowsky syndrome)—evaluation of symptoms in 36 patients. Arch Dermatol Res 1993;285:36–37.

220. Anderson WA, Elam MD, Lambert WC. Keratosis punctata and atopy: Report of 31 cases with a prospective study of prevalence. Arch Dermatol 1984;120:884–890.

221. Rustad OJ, Vance JC. Punctate keratoses of the palms and soles and keratotic pits of the palmar creases. J Am Acad Dermatol 1990;22:468–476.

222. Lestringant GG, Berge T. Porokeratosis punctata palmaris et plantaris: A new entity? Arch Dermatol 1989;125:816–819.

223. Osman Y, Daly TJ, Don PC. Spiny keratoderma of the palms and soles. J Am Acad Dermatol 1992;26:879–881.

224. Goldsmith LA. Tyrosinemia II: A large North Carolina kindred. Arch Intern Med 1985;145:1697–1700.

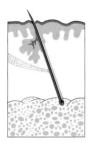

Congenital Alopecias and Disorders of Melanosome Transfer to Hair Follicles

JACK L. ARBISER

DEFINITION

Congenital alopecias represent a heterogeneous group of rare genetic and developmental disorders. Hair development requires the close coordination of multiple cell types of ectodermal and mesodermal origin, and thus hair development is susceptible to multiple forms of genetic insults. At present, the genetic and developmental basis of few of these disorders is understood, and even in the case where a defective gene has been isolated, the pathophysiology of these disorders is not well understood. Recent advances in reverse genetics, transgenic mice, mice created through homologous recombination, and naturally occurring strains of mice will help in the elucidation of these disorders in the future. Because there are few trends in the genetic alopecias, they will be classified into metabolic and developmental disorders, and a description of the salient features will be given.

METABOLIC DISORDERS

Vitamin D–Resistant Rickets

Vitamin D–resistant rickets, also known as vitamin D–dependent rickets type 2, is a rare autosomal recessive disorder characterized by a defective receptor to vitamin D.[1-4] The patient is thus insensitive to physiologic levels of calcitriol (1,25-dihydroxyvitamin D). Clinically, these patients are noted to have non-scarring alopecia, rachitic bones, mild hypocalcemia and hypophosphatasia, high levels of alkaline phosphatase, generalized aminoaciduria, and secondary hyperparathyroidism. Scalp hair is noted to fall out between the ages of 2 and 4 months.[5, 6] Therapy for this disorder includes pharmacologic doses of vitamin D and calcium supplementation, in an attempt to overcome the defective response to vitamin D. The response is variable. Abnormalities of the hair shaft have not been noted, and the alopecia usually spares the eyelashes. Despite correction of laboratory values and skeletal changes by therapy, the alopecia is not affected by vitamin D.[5, 6] This disorder is distinct from the X-linked recessive hypophosphatemic rickets, of which alopecia is not a prominent feature.

Scalp biopsy from a patient with this condition revealed a normal number and normal light microscopic appearance of follicles.[5] Vitamin D likely plays an important but not well understood role in hair development, perhaps by influencing calcium binding proteins.[7]

Menkes' Kinky Hair Syndrome

Menkes' kinky hair syndrome is a rare X-linked deficiency of copper metabolism. This defect results in increased intracellular copper metabolism in certain tissues, and decreased copper metabolism in other tissues. The deficiency of copper in certain tissues results in decreased activity of copper dependent enzymes, such as tyrosinase, dopamine hydroxylase, cytochrome oxidase, and lysyl oxidase.[8] Diminished activity of these enzymes leads to some of the clinical stigmata of Menkes' syndrome, such as hypopigmentation of hair (Fig. 163–1). The hair is twisted on its longitudinal axis, as in pili

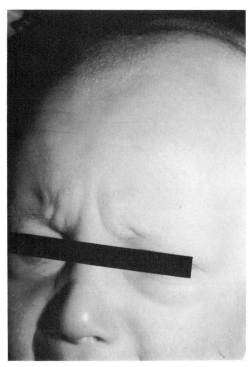

FIGURE 163-1. Sparse, lusterless, lightly pigmented hair in an infant with Menkes' kinky hair syndrome. The hair is extremely short, caused by breakage at defective areas in the hair shaft.

torti.[9] Other clinical findings include mental retardation, degeneration of large vessel elastin, and metaphyseal abnormalities. No clinical treatment is effective in ameliorating the course of the disease.[9] Prenatal diagnosis is available through copper measurements of fetal cells.[10] Female carriers may have hypopigmentation following Blaschko's lines.[11]

Mouse homologues of this disorder exist as the mottled mouse.[12] Recently, the human and mouse genes have been cloned, and the gene has been found to be a copper transporting ATPase gene with homology to bacterial metal transporters.[8, 13-15] The gene is expressed in most tissues, but not in liver.[8] The gene product is very widely distributed, so gene therapy will likely not be effective for this disorder, but understanding the function of the Menkes gene may lead to effective therapy.

Disorders of Amino Acid Metabolism

Argininosuccinic aciduria is a deficiency of the urea cycle enzyme argininosuccinate lyase, which converts argininosuccinate to arginine. Clinical features of this disorder include mental retardation, hepatomegaly, dry and brittle hair with red fluorescence, trichorrhexis nodosa, monilethrix, and epilepsy.[16] Clinical improvement has been noted by dietary supplementation with arginine. On polarizing microscopy, alternating light and dark bands are observed. Amino acid analysis of affected hair is essentially normal, but the polarized microscopic appearance can be reversed by placing these patients on a diet with low protein and with arginine supplementa-

tion.[17] Serum levels of arginine are normal, but citrulline levels are elevated.[18]

Homocystinuria, a deficiency of cystathionine beta synthase, is characterized by diluted hair pigmentation, ectopia lentis, marfanoid habitus, osteoporosis, and thrombotic tendency.[19] A subset of patients respond to pyridoxine therapy.[19, 20] Homocysteine has been shown to be a growth factor for vascular smooth muscle.[21]

SYNDROMES OF PREMATURE AGING

Several syndromes of premature aging have been noted, and the defect in all of these disorders remains obscure. Hutchinson-Gilford progeria syndrome is an autosomal recessive disorder with an incidence of 1 in 8 million births.[22] Clinically, this disorder is characterized by onset during the first year of life, in contrast to Werner's syndrome, which is first noted toward the end of the first decade.[23] Dermatologic findings in these disorders include alopecia and prominent scalp veins, loss of subcutaneous fat, dystrophic nails, scleredematous skin and yellowish discoloration of the skin, as well as hyperlipidemia (Fig. 163-2).[22-24] Alopecia develops at the age of a few months, and is progressive.[21] Alopecia is prominent in Werner's syndrome, but at a later age.

MARIE-UNNA HYPOTRICHOSIS

Marie-Unna hypotrichosis is an autosomal dominant disorder characterized by sparse hair at birth, with hair growth in early childhood. The hair at this period has an unusual texture, and has been described as "horse-tail" like.[25] Eyelashes, eyebrows, and pubic and axillary hair are sparse. Alopecia is noted to worsen at puberty, most notably at the vertex and scalp. Grossly, the hair appears flat and twisted. Electron microscopy reveals fractures of cortex and medullary cells.[26] No other ectodermal structures appear to be affected. Histologically, atrophy and

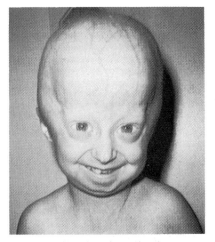

FIGURE 163-2. Progeria. Alopecia, subcutaneous atrophy, prominent scalp veins, and bird-like appearance. (From Fleischmajer R, Nedwich A: Progeria [Hutchinson-Gilford]. Arch Dermatol 107:253, 1973. Copyright © 1973, American Medical Association.)

follicular plugging is observed, with irregularities in the shape of the internal root sheath.[26]

CONGENITAL TRIANGULAR ALOPECIA

Congenital triangular alopecia is an uncommon developmental defect characterized by decreased hair mass, but not decreased hair number, on an isolated portion of the temporal scalp, and is unilateral in 80% of cases.[27] This defect may appear several years after birth.[27] Scalp biopsy of these areas reveals increased numbers of vellus hair follicles and decreased terminal hairs.[28] This defect is permanent, but may be treated with scalp reduction.[29] Inasmuch as medical treatment is ineffective in this condition, it must be differentiated from alopecia areata, and differentiation on clinical grounds alone may be difficult.

TRICHORHINOPHALANGEAL SYNDROME

Trichorhinophalangeal syndrome is a rare syndrome characterized by alopecia and brittle hair, associated with a bulbous nose, mandibular hypoplasia, and cone-shaped epiphyses of the digits.[30] This disorder is associated with an interstitial deletion of chromosome 8q24 and is subdivided into three divisions, based on clinical findings.[30, 31] All three forms are characterized by fine, sparse hair, which is present from birth. No diagnostic abnormalities of the hair shaft are noted. Trichorhinophalangeal syndrome type II is also known as Langer-Giedion syndrome, and differs from type I in that it has multiple cartilaginous exostoses of long bones, ribs, and vertebrae. Type III is characterized by shortening of metatarsals, metacarpals, and phalanges. The differential diagnosis of trichorhinophalangeal syndrome includes anhidrotic ectodermal dysplasia, Larsen's syndrome, oral-facial-digital syndrome, and Coffin-Siris syndrome.[30, 31]

ANHIDROTIC ECTODERMAL DYSPLASIA (CHRIST-SIEMENS-TOURAINE SYNDROME)

Anhidrotic ectodermal dysplasia is an X-linked recessive disorder characterized by hypotrichosis, absence of sweat glands, and hypodontia in affected males.[32, 33] The earliest presentation may be extensive exfoliation of the skin as a newborn.[32, 33] Female carriers may show tooth malformations and slight abnormalities of breasts and sweat glands.[10] Other clinical features include short stature, saddle-nose, periocular hyperpigmentation, and decreased mucous glands of the respiratory tract (Figs. 163–3 and 163–4). Patients may have frequent respiratory infections, and care must be taken to avoid hyperthermia.[32, 33] Linkage studies have narrowed the X-linked anhidrotic ectodermal dysplasia gene to Xq12-q13.1.[34] This disorder may occur in females as a consequence of a balanced X autosomal translocation and nonrandom X chromosome inactivation.[34] The presence of these balanced translocations may be very important in the eventual cloning of this gene, inasmuch as some of these translocations may interrupt the gene

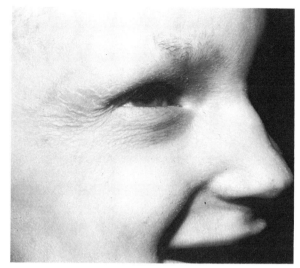

FIGURE 163–3. Fine wrinkling and hyperpigmentation around the eyes of a boy with anhidrotic ectodermal dysplasia.

itself.[32] Prenatal diagnosis is now available for this disease through linkage analysis performed on DNA obtained through fetoscopy.[35] The mouse tabby gene, which is also an X-linked trait, may be the mouse homologue of the gene.[32]

HIDROTIC ECTODERMAL DYSPLASIA (CLOUSTON'S SYNDROME)

Hidrotic ectodermal dysplasia is an autosomal dominant disorder that differs from anhidrotic ectodermal dysplasia in that sebaceous and eccrine function appear normal, but patients have nail dystrophy, hyperpigmentation of skin overlying joints, mental retardation, and alopecia. Analysis of hair from these patients has shown

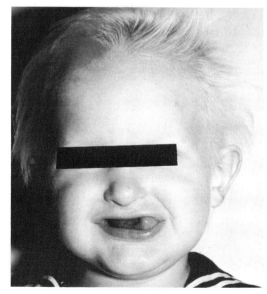

FIGURE 163–4. Typical facies of a boy with anhidrotic ectodermal dysplasia showing the depressed nasal bridge and prominent forehead, chin, and ears. Note light-colored, fly-away hair and absence of teeth.

reduced birefringence with polarized light, and a disorganized fibrillar structure.[36, 37]

ALOPECIA CONGENITA

Alopecia congenita is probably a heterogeneous group of disorders characterized by alopecia present at birth and no other abnormalities.[38] Because of the likely heterogeneity of this disorder, there is no clear pattern of inheritance. Several studies have looked for abnormalities in patients with these disorders.[39] No consistent abnormalities have been found, with some patients having only vellus hairs, and others having terminal hairs. Three patterns have been described, including ones with rudimentary hair and normal-appearing pilosebaceous units, hair present with abnormal pilosebaceous units, and absence of hair bulbs in the presence of sebaceous glands.[40]

CARTILAGE-HAIR HYPOPLASIA

Cartilage-hair hypoplasia is an extremely rare autosomal recessive disorder characterized by short limbs, fine skin, sparse, thin body hair, hyperextensible joints, and defective T helper cell function.[41-44] Hair in this disorder has an abnormally small diameter and decreased central pigmentation.[41] The immunodeficiency in this disorder is clinically manifested with multiple verrucae, anergy to skin antigens, and decreased response to phytohemagglutinin. Mild noncyclic neutropenia, especially of granulocytes, has been noted, as well as delayed skin graft rejection.[41] Natural killer cell function has been noted to be normal.[42] Patients with this disorder have been noted to have recurrent cutaneous infections with staphylococcus and bronchitis, and lethal varicella infection has been noted in these patients. This disorder is found in increased frequency in patients of old Amish or Finnish descent.[44]

KERATOSIS PILARIS ATROPHICANS

Keratosis pilaris atrophicans describes a heterogeneous group of disorders of uncertain genetic transmission that are characterized by the triad of follicular hyperkeratosis, inflammation, and atrophy.[45] These disorders include keratosis pilaris atrophicans faciei (ulerythema ophryogenes), atrophoderma vermiculatum, and keratosis follicularis spinulosa decalvans. These disorders are characterized by follicular inflammation and scarring. Early pathologic changes include compact hyperkeratosis of the infundibulum and isthmus.[46] Hair loss begins in early childhood, progresses to scarring alopecia at puberty, and may also involve eyebrows, trunk, and the extensor surfaces of the arms. This disorder may be associated with atopy, palmoplantar hyperkeratosis, and punctate corneal lesions. Retinoid, keratolytic, and topical corticosteroid therapy has been generally unsuccessful in treatment of these disorders.[45]

INCONTINENTIA PIGMENTI

Incontinentia pigmenti, or Bloch-Sulzberger disease, is an X-linked dominant disorder of neuroectoderm.[47, 48] Clinically, it is characterized by four stages. The first, or vesiculobullous stage, appears within the first 3 weeks of life. The second, or verrucous stage, appears as linear verrucous lesions, which may follow Blaschko's lines (Fig. 163–5). The third stage appears as pigmented lines and whorls, primarily on the trunk, and is usually not present after puberty. The fourth stage of incontinentia pigmenti is the atrophic stage, characterized by atrophy especially on the legs. Eccrine glands and hair are absent in these atrophic areas.[10] Other clinical findings include segmental alopecia, nail dystrophy, dental anomalies, especially conical and pegged teeth, ocular neovascularization, and seizures. The central nervous system is affected in approximately 30% of all patients.[47] Genetic mapping has linked this disorder to two distinct loci on the X chromosome, at Xp11.21, and Xq28. Males with this

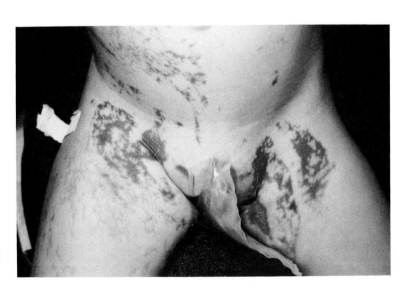

FIGURE 163–5. Extensive tan and dark brown reticulated hyperpigmented lesions on the torso and thighs of a girl with incontinentia pigmenti.

disorder have often been found to have a karyotype of 47 XXY.[48] Mouse homologues of this disorder exist, including the tattered mouse and the striated mouse, which may be useful in elucidating the pathophysiology of this disorder.[48]

CONRADI-HUNERMANN SYNDROME

Conradi-Hunermann syndrome is an X-linked dominant disorder of intracellular organelles known as peroxisomes.[49] Clinically, this disorder is manifested by punctate calcifications in cartilaginous areas, such as the epiphyses, larynx, and trachea.[49-51] These calcifications are transient, but are associated with assymetrical shortening of long bones.

Cutaneous findings of Conradi-Hunermann syndrome include follicular plugging, keratinocyte calcification, cicatricial alopecia, and follicular atrophoderma. An erythroderma is often present at birth, and adherent thick yellow scale is present.[49-51] Sectorial cataracts are present in the majority of patients.[10] The mouse mutant bare patches appear to be the murine homologue of Conradi-Hunermann syndrome.[52]

NETHERTON'S SYNDROME

Netherton's syndrome is a disorder of uncertain genetic transmission characterized by hair shaft defects, especially trichorrhexis invaginata, atopy, and ichthyosis (Fig. 163–6). This disorder has also been called ichthyosis linearis circumflexa. The differential diagnosis includes lamellar ichthyosis, Leiner's disease, and acrodermatitis enteropathica.[53] These patients have recurrent bacterial infections of the skin and otitis, with organisms including *Staphylococcus aureus, Pseudomonas*, and streptococcal species. A patient studied by Greene and

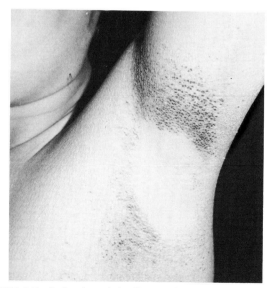

FIGURE 163–6. Sparing of the flexures is noted in this boy with X-linked ichthyosis. Clinically this disorder can be confused with ichthyosis vulgaris.

Muller was noted to have subnormal intelligence and decreased neutrophil phagocytic ability.[53] Hair defects noted in Netherton's syndrome include pili torti, monilethrix, and trichorrhexis nodosa. Aminoaciduria may be seen in these patients, but it may be secondary to long-term corticosteroid use. Multiple attempts at therapy have been tried, but with little success. These attempts include topical corticosteroids, antibiotics, keratolytics, emollients, systemic retinoids, and psoralens plus ultraviolet A. Systemic retinoids were noted to cause worsening of erythroderma.[53]

LOOSE ANAGEN HAIR SYNDROME

Loose anagen hair syndrome is a disorder characterized by the easy removal of anagen hairs from the scalp during a hair pull.[55] Clinically, this is manifested as the painless loss of clumps of hair. Histologically, this disorder is characterized by distortion of the hair bulb and poor adhesion of the outer root sheath to the vitreous layer. Plucked hairs do not stain with cinnamaldehyde, which preferentially stains inner-root sheath proteins. Examination of plucked hairs by scanning electron microscopy reveals absence of the cuticle and root sheaths, as well as ridging and grooving of the shaft. Incomplete keratinization was noted in the inner root sheath and cuticle. This disorder often appears in lighter colored hair and tends to improve with age. Inheritance may be autosomal dominant.[55]

MONILETHRIX

Monilethrix is an uncommon disorder of hair characterized by periodic constrictions that lead to hair shaft breakage and alopecia (Figs. 163–7 and 163–8). Children are born with normal-appearing hair, which is lost within the first 4 months of life. Multiple attempts to treat this disorder have been made, including depilation with thallium salts, radiation therapy, and intralesional corticosteroids, but therapy is largely unsuccessful. Hair has been noted to improve during pregnancy. Systemic steroids have been noted to improve monilethrix in one case, but side effects make this modality impractical. Keratosis pilaris has been noted in a few cases of monilethrix.[56]

TRICHOTHIODYSTROPHY

Trichothiodystrophy is a rare and heterogeneous disorder with the primary feature of brittle hair shafts (Fig. 163–9). The hair protein has been found to contain an abnormally low sulfur content. Detailed microscopic examination reveals a deficient cuticle. Other associated clinical features include photosensitivity, mental retardation, ichthyosis, nail dystrophy, dental anomalies, and decreased fertility (Fig. 163–10).[57, 58] Recently fibroblasts from a subset of these patients have been found to be deficient in repair of DNA damage due to ultraviolet light, and mutations in the ERCC-2 gene have been

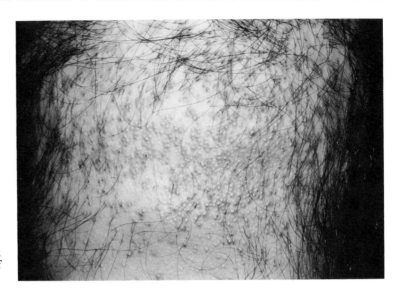

FIGURE 163–7. Posterior scalp of a patient with monilethrix showing sparse hair and hyperkeratotic papules. (Courtesy of Benjamin K. Fisher, MD, Toronto, Ontario.)

found in some of these patients. The ERCC-2 gene is also mutated in xeroderma pigmentosum D patients.[59] The reason behind the differences in clinical phenotypes between these two disorders with a mutation in the same gene is unknown, although it may be secondary to modification of phenotype by other genes. Other DNA repair genes have been implicated in trichothiodystrophy as well.[60]

DISORDERS OF MELANIN TRANSFER: GRISCELLI'S SYNDROME AND CHÉDIAK-HIGASHI SYNDROME

Griscelli's syndrome is a rare autosomal recessive disorder that has been observed in Saudi Arabia. These patients usually present at 3 to 4 months of age with silver-tinged hair, neurologic abnormalities, and recurrent pyogenic infections.[61] Leukocytes are normal in number upon initial presentation, but pancytopenia is a major cause of mortality after age 1. Lymphohistiocytic infiltration of liver, spleen, skin, and central nervous system are commonly observed, with prominent erythrophagocytosis.[61]

Characteristic cutaneous findings include clumping of melanin within hair shafts and little transfer of melanin from melanocytes to keratinocytes. Electron microscopy reveals melanocytes containing stage 3 and 4 melanosomes, and keratinocytes that lack melanosomes.[61, 62]

Immunologically, patients may have normal levels of immunoglobulins, but decreased T cell response to mitogens. Chemotherapy with methotrexate, cytoxan, vincristine, VP-16, and steroids may be effective for ameliorating progression of this disorder, but bone marrow transplantation is the only effective therapy.[61, 63]

The differential diagnosis of this disorder includes Chédiak-Higashi disorder, a recessive disorder of melanocytes and granulocytes that is characterized by defects in natural killer cells. Patients with Chédiak-Higashi syndrome do not have the prominent histiocytosis of Griscelli's syndrome, and in general, have a more indolent clinical course, with death in the teenage years. Recently, cyclosporine has been found to be useful in maintaining remissions in this disease.[63]

Chédiak-Higashi syndrome is a rare autosomal recessive disorder whose pathogenesis is not well understood. The basic defect appears to be in the lysosome and melanosome. The defect in the melanosome prevents transfer of melanosomes to keratinocytes, and the hair shaft reveals clumped melanin granules, which are diagnostic of this disorder. The failure in melanosome transfer results in pale blond hair, sometimes with a metallic sheen, and pale skin.[64] Numerous other tissue types have demonstrated abnormalities, including granulocytes, fibroblasts, and renal epithelial cells.[64] Natural killer lymphocyte activity is deficient in this disorder.

Clinically, children with Chédiak-Higashi syndrome have recurrent bacterial infections, especially with *Staph-*

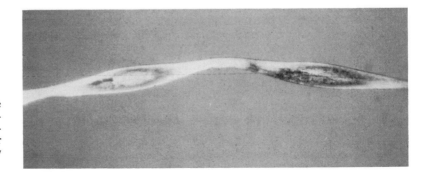

FIGURE 163–8. Monilethrix (beaded hair, nodose hair). Variable hair shaft thickness and node-like deformities occur. (Courtesy of Joseph McGuire, M.D.; reprinted from Hurwitz S: Hair disorders. In: Schachner LA, Hansen RC (eds). Pediatric Dermatology. New York: Churchill-Livingstone, 1988.)

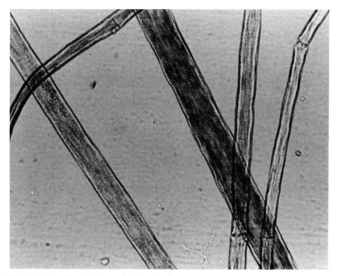

FIGURE 163-9. Several hair shafts show the clean breaks (trichoschisis) characteristic of hairs from patients with trichothiodystrophy.

ylococcus aureus. After the first decade of life, patients develop into an accelerated phase, characterized by lymphocytic infiltrates, pancytopenia, and hepatosplenomegaly. This accelerated phase is lethal unless treated with bone marrow transplantation. Death in the accelerated phase is usually secondary to hemorrhage or infection.[66]

Many animal models of this disease exist, notably the beige mouse and the Aleutian mink.[67] Neutrophils from the beige mouse have been demonstrated to have de-

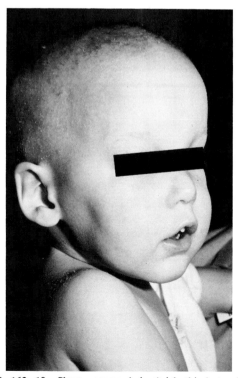

FIGURE 163-10. Short, sparse hair (trichothiodystrophy) and ichthyosiform scales over the entire skin surface in a patient with Tay syndrome.

creased protease activity, which may account for the increased rate of infection in this disorder.[68]

RECENT DISCOVERIES FROM THE WORLD OF MICE

Advances in reverse genetics, transgenic mice, and targeted deletions of known genes have led to the discovery of genes that affect hair patterns and coloration. The mouse genome contains numerous endogenous retroviral sequences, which insert into genes, or excise themselves from existing genes, permitting expression of new genes that affect mouse hair.

The mouse hairless mutant is a strain of mice born with hair that develops total alopecia after 1 month of age. The lack of hair makes these mice attractive models for skin carcinogenesis. This mutation has been found to be a result of a retroviral insertion, and cloning the flanking sequences of the retrovirus has led to the isolation of the mouse hairless gene.[69] The hairless gene has been found to be expressed in hair follicles and the brain, and may be a zinc finger transcription factor.[69]

Elegant studies have led to the characterization of the agouti gene of mice. The agouti gene is a dominant gene, and when expressed in mice, leads to yellow hairs in mice.[70] The agouti gene product regulates the ration of eumelanin and pheomelanin produced by follicular melanocytes.[70, 71] Expression of the dominant agouti gene also leads to susceptibility to various tumors, obesity, and non–insulin dependent diabetes. Multiple alleles of the agouti gene have been characterized, and the agouti gene was originally isolated due to its proximity to an endogenous retrovirus.[70] Multiple factors influence expression of the agouti gene, such as relationship to nearby retroviruses, methylation of DNA, and altered transcripts of the gene.[71] Perhaps a human syndrome characterized by blond hair, obesity, and non–insulin dependent diabetes will be the human analogue of the agouti syndrome.

Waved 1 and waved 2 are two spontaneously appearing mutations characterized by waviness of whiskers and fur, with bending and kinking of hairs.[72, 73] Hair follicles in these mice have been noted to be misaligned. Creation of mice that lacked the transforming growth factor alpha (TGF-α) gene led to mice that have the waved phenotype, and crossing these mutant mice with waved 1 mice did not lead to correction of the defect, implying that the waved 1 mice were mutant in the TGF-α gene.[72, 73] The waved 2 mice have been found to have a mutation in the epidermal growth factor receptor gene (EGFR), which is also the receptor for TGF-α.[74] TGF-α transcripts have been found in the inner root sheath, whereas the EGFR transcripts are found along the outer root sheath, from the bulb to the epidermis.[74] This close geographic juxtaposition implies that the interaction of TGF-α with its receptor EGFR is crucial for the development of normal hair.

Expression of exogenous genes in the skin can have profound effects on hair in mice. Using the promoter of keratin 5, a mutant adenovirus E1a oncoprotein, which binds to the product of the retinoblastoma gene product, resulted in hairs with an absent inner root sheath, and crooked hairs. Again, the disruption of normal signaling apparatus in the vicinity of the hair shaft leads to disturbances in hair growth.[75] It is likely that some of the genetic defects seen in alopecia will involve these signaling pathways.

References

1. Takeda E, Kuroda Y, Saijo T, et al. la-hydroxyvitamin D₃ treatment of three patients with 1,25-dihydroxyvitamin D receptor defect rickets and alopecia. Pediatrics 1987;80:97–101.
2. Eli C, Liberman UA, Rosen JF, et al. A cellular defect in hereditary vitamin-D dependent rickets type II: Defective nuclear uptake of 1,25-dihydroxyvitamin D in cultured skin fibroblasts. N Engl J Med 1981;304:1588–1591.
3. Brooks MH, Bell NH, Love L, et al. Vitamin D dependent rickets type II. Resistance of target organs to 1,25-dihydroxyvitamin D. N Engl J Med 1978;298:996–999.
4. Feldman D, Chen T, Cone C, et al. Vitamin D resistant rickets with alopecia: Cultured skin fibroblasts exhibit defective cytoplasmic receptors and unresponsiveness to 1,25(OH)2D3. J Clin Endocrinol Metab 1982;55:1020–1022.
5. Hochberg Z, Gilhar A, Haim S, et al. Calcitriol-resistant rickets with alopecia. Arch Dermatol 1985;121:646–647.
6. Takeda E, Kuroda Y, Saijo T, et al. la-hydroxyvitamin D₃ treatment of three patients with 1,25-dihydroxyvitamin D–receptor defect rickets and alopecia. Pediatrics 1987;80:97–101.
7. Saurat JH, Didierjean L, Pavlovitch JH, et al. Skin calcium binding protein is localized in the cytoplasm of the basal layer of the epidermis. J Invest Dermatol 1981;76:221–223.
8. Levinson B, Vulpe C, Elder B, et al. The mottled gene is the mouse homologue of the Menkes disease gene. Nature Genet 1994; 6:369–373.
9. Menkes JH. Kinky hair disease: Twenty five years later. Brain Dev 1988;10:77–79.
10. Bolognia JL, Orlow SJ, Glick SA. Lines of Blaschko. J Am Acad Dermatol 1994;31:157–190.
11. Horn N. Copper incorporation studies on cultured cells for prenatal diagnosis of Menkes disease. Lancet 1976;1:1156–1158.
12. Mercer JF, Grimes A, Ambrosini L, et al. Mutations in the murine homologue of the Menkes gene in dappled and blotchy mice. Nature Genet 1994;6:374–378.
13. Vulpe C, Levinson B, Whitney S, et al. Isolation of a candidate gene for Menkes disease and evidence that it encodes a copper transporting ATPase. Nature Genet 1993;3:7–13.
14. Mercer JF, Livingston J, Hall P, et al. Isolation of a partial candidate gene for Menkes disease by positional cloning. Nature Genet 1993;3:20–25.
15. Chelly J, Tumer Z, Tonnesen T, et al. Isolation of a candidate gene for Menkes disease that encodes a potential heavy metal binding protein. Nature Genet 1993;3:14–19.
16. Chernosky ME, Owens P. Trichorrhexis nodosa. Clinical and investigative studies. Arch Dermatol 1966;94:577–585.
17. Baden HP, Baden LA, Shih VE, Kolodny EH. Dietary management reverses grooving and abnormal polarization of hair shafts in argininosuccinase deficiency. Am J Med Genet 1991;40:211–213.
18. Baden HP, Hooker PA. Advances in genetics in dermatology. In: Harris H, Hirschhorn K, eds. Advances in Human Genetics 12. New York: Plenum Press, 1982:89–188.
19. Collins FS, Summer GK, Schwartz RP, Parke JC Jr. Neonatal argininosuccinic aciduria—survival after early diagnosis and dietary management. J Pediat 1980;96:429–431.
20. McKusick VA. Mendelian Inheritance in Man; 6th edition, Baltimore: Johns Hopkins Press, 1983.
21. Tsai JC, Perrella MA, Yoshizumi M, et al. Promotion of vascular smooth muscle cell growth by homocysteine: A link to atherosclerosis. Proc Natl Acad Sci USA 1994;91:6369–6373.
22. DeBusk FL. The Hutchinson-Gilford progeria syndrome. J Pediatr 1972;80:697–724.
23. Erdem N, Gunes AT, Avci O, Osma E. A case of Hutchinson-Gilford progeria syndrome mimicking scleredema in early infancy. Dermatology 1994;188:318–321.
24. Bauer EA, Uitto J, Tan EM, Holbrook KA. Werner's syndrome. Evidence for preferential regional expression of a generalized mesenchymal cell defect. Arch Dermatol 1988;124:90–101.
25. Muller SA. Alopecia: Syndromes of genetic significance. J Invest Dermatol 1973;60:475–492.
26. Stevanovic DV. Hereditary hypotrichosis congenita: Marie-Unna type. Br J Dermatol 1970;83:331–337.
27. Kubba R, Rook A. Congenital triangular alopecia. Br J Dermatol 1976;95:657–659.
28. Trakimas C, Sperling LC, Skelton HG, et al. Clinical and histologic findings in temporal triangular alopecia. J Am Acad Dermatol 1994;31:205–209.
29. Tosti A. Congenital triangular alopecia. Report of fourteen cases. J Am Acad Dermatol 1987;16:991–993.
30. Carrington PR, Chen H, Altick JA. Trichorhinophalangeal syndrome, type 1. J Am Acad Dermatol 1994;31:331–336.
31. Ludecke HJ, Johnson C, Wagner MJ, et al. Molecular definition of the shortest region of deletion overlap in the Langer-Giedion syndrome. Am J Human Genet 1991;49:1197–1206.
32. Zonana J. Hypohidrotic ectodermal dysplasia: Molecular genetic research and its clinical applications. Semin Dermatol 1993; 12:241–246.
33. Reed WB, Lopez DA, Landing BH. Clinical spectrum of anhidrotic ectodermal dysplasia. Arch Dermatol 1970;102:134–143.
34. Thomas NS, Chelly J, Zonana J, et al. Characterization of molecular DNA rearrangements within the Xq12-q13.1 region, in three patients with X-linked hypohidrotic ectodermal dysplasia. Hum Mol Genet 1993;2:1679–1685.
35. Zonana J. Schinzel A, Upadhyaya M, et al. Prenatal diagnosis of X-linked hypohydrotic ectodermal dysplasia by linkage analysis. Am J Med Genet 1990;35:132–135.
36. Rajagopalan KV, Tay CH. Hidrotic ectodermal dysplasia: Study of a large Chinese pedigree. Arch Dermatol 1977;113:481–484.
37. Gold RJ, Scriver CR. Properties of hair keratin in an autosomal dominant form of ectodermal dysplasia. Am J Human Genet 1972;24:549–561.
38. Gillespie JB. Congenital and familial alopecia totalis. Am J Dis Child 1937;53:132–136.
39. Baden HP, Kubilus J. Analysis of hair from alopecia congenita. J Am Acad Dermatol 1980;3:623–626.
40. Porter PS. Genetic disorders of hair growth. J Invest Dermatol 1973;60:493–502.
41. Lux SE, Johnston RB, August CS, et al. Chronic neutropenia and abnormal cellular immunity in cartilage hair hypoplasia. N Engl J Med 1970;282:231–236.
42. Pierce GF, Brovall C, Schacter BZ, Polmar SH. Impaired culture generated cytotoxicity with preservation of spontaneous natural killer-cell activity in cartilage-hair hypoplasia. J Clin Invest 1983;71:1737–1742.
43. Brennan TE, Pearson RW. Abnormal elastic tissue in cartilage-hair hypoplasia. Arch Dermatol 1988;124:1411–1414.
44. McKusick VA, Eldridge R, Hostetler JA, et al. Dwarfism in the Amish II. Cartilage-hair hypoplasia. Bull Johns Hopkins Hosp 1965;116:285–326.
45. Rand R, Baden HP. Keratosis follicularis spinulosa decalvans. Arch Dermatol 1983;119:22–26.
46. Baden HP, Byers HR. Clinical findings, cutaneous pathology, and response to therapy in 21 patients with keratosis pilaris atrophicans. Arch Dermatol 1994;130:469–475.
47. Landy SJ, Donnai D. Incontinentia pigmenti. J Med Genet 1993;30:53–59.
48. Gorski JL, Burright EN. The molecular genetics of incontinentia pigmenti. Semin Dermatol 1993;12:255–265.
49. Happle R. X-linked dominant chondrodysplasia punctata: Review of literature and report of a case. Hum Genet 1979;53:65–73.
50. Kalter DC, Atherton DJ, Clayton PX. X-linked dominant Conradi-Hunermann syndrome presenting as congenital erythroderma. J Am Acad Dermatol 1989;21:248–256.
51. Edidin DV, Esterly NB, Bamzai AK, et al. Chondrodysplasia punctata: Conradi-Hunermann syndrome. Arch Dermatol 1977; 113:1431–1434.
52. Emani S, Hanley KP, Esterly NB, et al. X-linked dominant icthyosis with peroxisomal deficiency: An ultrastructural and ultracytochemical study of the Conradi-Hunermann syndrome and its murine homologue, the bare patches mouse. Arch Dermatol 1994;130:325–337.

53. Greene SL, Muller SA. Netherton's syndrome. Report of a case and review of the literature. J Am Acad Dermatol 1985; 13:329–337.
54. Baden HP, Kevdar JC, Magro CM. Loose anagen hair as a cause of hereditary hair loss in children. Arch Dermatol 1992;128: 1349–1353.
55. Solomon IL, Green OC. Monilethrix: Occurrence in seven generations, with one case that responded to endocrine therapy. N Engl J Med 1963;24:1279–1282.
56. Carnabuci GJ, Rosenberg PE. Monilethrix and keratosis pilaris. Arch Dermatol 1967;96:564–567.
57. Price VH, Odom RB, Ward WH, Jones FT. Trichothiodystrophy: Sulfur-deficient brittle hair as a marker for a neuroectodermal symptom complex. Arch Dermatol 1980;116:1374–1384.
58. Sarasin A, Blanchet-Bardon C, Renault G, et al. Prenatal diagnosis in a subset of trichothiodystrophy patients defective in DNA repair. Br J Dermatol 1992;127:485–491.
59. Johnson RT, Squires S. The XPD complementation group. Insights into xeroderma pigmentosum, Cockayne's syndrome, and trichothiodystrophy. Mutat Res 1992;273:97–118.
60. Stefanini M, Vermeulen W, Weeda G, et al. A new nucleotide-excision repair gene associated with the disorder trichothiodystrophy. Am J Hum Genet 1993;53:817–821.
61. Schneider LC, Berman RS, Shea CR, et al. Bone marrow transplantation for the syndrome of pigmentary dilution and lymphohistiocytosis. J Clin Immunol 1990;10:146–153.
62. Hurvitz H, Gillis R, Klaus S, et al. A kindred with Griscelli disease: Spectrum of neurological involvement. Eur J Pediatr 1993; 152:402–405.
63. Stephan JL, Donadieu J, Ledeist F, et al. Treatment of familial hemophagocytic lymphohistiocytosis with antithymocyte globulins, steroids, and cyclosporine A. Blood 1993;82:2319–2323.
64. Paller AS. Genetic immunodeficiency diseases. In: Fitzpatrick TB, Eisen AZ, Wolff K, et al., eds. Dermatology in General Medicine. New York: McGraw-Hill, 1987:1950–1961.
65. Oliver JM. Impaired microtubule function correctable by cyclic GMP and cholinergic agonists in the Chediak-Higashi syndrome. Am J Pathol 1976;85:395–416.
66. Brak Y, Nir E. Chediak-Higashi syndrome: Am J Pediat Hematol Oncol 1987;9:42–55.
67. Windhorst DB, Padgett G. The Chediak-Higashi syndrome and the homologous trait in animals. J Invest Dermatol 1973;60:529–537.
68. Takeuchi KH, Swank RT. Inhibitors of elastase and cathepsin G in Chediak-Higashi (beige) neutrophils. J Biol Chem 1989;264: 7431–7436.
69. Cachon-Gonzalez MB, Fenner S, Coffin JM, et al. Structure and expression of the hairless gene of mice. Proc Natl Acad Sci USA 1994;91:7717–7721.
70. Bultman SJ, Michaud EJ, Woychik RP. Molecular characterization of the mouse agouti locus. Cell 1992;71:1195–1204.
71. Michaud EJ, van Vugt MJ, Sweet HO, et al. Differential expression of a new dominant agouti allele is correlated with methylation state and is influenced by parental lineage. Genes Dev 1994;8: 1463–1472.
72. Luetteke NC, Qiu TH, Peiffer RL, et al. TGFa deficiency results in hair follicle and eye abnormalities in targeted and waved-1 mice. Cell 1993;73:263–278.
73. Mann GB, Fowler KJ, Gabriel A, et al. Mice with a null mutation of the TGF-α gene have abnormal skin architecture, wavy hair, and curly whiskers and often develop corneal inflammation. Cell 1993;73:249–261.
74. Luetteke NC, Phillips HK, Qiu TH, et al. The mouse waved-2 phenotype results from a point mutation in the EGF receptor tyrosine kinase. Genes Dev 1994;8:399–413.
75. Missero C, Serra C, Stenn K, Dotto GP. Skin-specific expression of a truncated E1A oncoprotein binding to p105-Rb leads to abnormal hair follicle maturation without increased epidermal proliferation. J Cell Biol 1993;121:1109–1120.

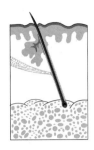

chapter 164

The Ectodermal Dysplasias

J. TIMOTHY WRIGHT and JO-DAVID FINE

DEFINITION

The ectodermal dysplasias are an extensive and diverse group of hereditary conditions that, from a pathogenetic perspective, include all conditions having a developmental defect that embryologically affects the ectoderm.[1] Although there is no consensus on the nosology of ectodermal dysplasias or agreement on which conditions should be included under this general heading, there are considered to be over 120 conditions classifiable as ectodermal dysplasias.[1, 2] Disorders classically described as ectodermal dysplasias clearly present clinical features in tissues of both ectodermal and nonectodermal origin. The term *ectodermal dysplasia* was originally proposed to describe a group of conditions having hypotrichosis, hypodontia, onychodysplasia, and anhidrosis. *Hypohidrosis* is considered a more accurate term than *anhidrosis* because affected individuals have decreased sweating but do not show a complete absence of sweat glands.[3] More recent definitions have included any one of these cardinal features plus at least one additional sign of ectodermal involvement.[1] It is generally agreed that ectodermal dysplasias include conditions that appear to be a primary ectodermal defect. Several of the ectodermal dysplasias and their most prominent clinical features are presented in Table 164–1. Since most ectodermal defects have not as yet been characterized at the molecular level, the diagnosis and delineation of ectodermal dysplasias remain principally clinical.

CLINICAL DESCRIPTION

Although structures of ectodermal origin are most frequently involved in ectodermal dysplasias, a variety of nonectodermal structures may also be involved.[4] This is not surprising given the complex ectodermal-mesenchymal interactions involved in tissue induction, histogenesis, and morphogenesis during embryologic development. Structures including the limbs, bones, palate, neurologic tissue, internal organs, and reproductive structures may be affected (Table 164–2). Hair is the most frequently altered tissue, with 90% of patients with ectodermal dysplasia showing changes in hair distribution, structure, quality, or composition (Fig. 164–1).[1] Often the hair will be twisted (pili torti) and small in diameter, have longitudinal grooves, and have an irregular cross-sectional shape and abnormal pattern of cuticulae (Fig. 164–2). The other most common features in ectodermal dysplasia involve the skin (85%), teeth (80%), nails (75%), face (72%), psychomotor growth and development (61%), eyes (60%), limbs (48%), and hearing (24%).[1]

The skin of persons with ectodermal dysplasia is most commonly hyperplastic but may also be aplastic. Palmar-plantar hyperkeratosis and generalized ichthyosiform erythroderma are common. Increased or decreased pigmentation may also occur, depending on the tissue site and type of ectodermal dysplasia present. Abnormal sweat gland structure and/or function and altered dermatoglyphics are also common in the ectodermal dysplasia.[4]

DIAGNOSIS

The ectodermal dysplasias are inherited as autosomal dominant and recessive and X-linked dominant and recessive mendelian traits.[1, 5] Individuals with ectodermal dysplasia often have no prior family history, making determination of the mode of inheritance impossible in the absence of precise DNA probes. Furthermore, in many patients the disease is difficult to diagnose or subclassify due to its diverse and highly variable clinical

TABLE 164-1. Characteristics of Select Ectodermal Dysplasias

Condition	Mode of Inheritance	Hair	Teeth	Nails	Sweat	Skin	Other Features
Hypohidrotic ectodermal dysplasia (Christ-Siemens-Touraine syndrome)	XR	Hypotrichosis; hypochromic, dry, scant eyebrows and lashes	Hypodontia, peg-shaped incisors, delayed eruption	Generally normal	Hypohidrosis; may have hyperthermia	Dry, decreased sebaceous glands, increased pigmented areas	Photophobia, decreased lacrimal function, hypoplastic maxilla
Hidrotic ectodermal dysplasia (Clouston's syndrome)	AD	Hypotrichosis; hypochromic, fine, dry, scant eyebrows	Occasional hypodontia, spaced dentition	Dystrophic, discolored, paronychia	Normal	Dry, palmoplantar hyperkeratosis	Cataract, thickened skull bones
Ectrodactyly-ectodermal dysplasia-clefting syndrome (EEC syndrome)	AD	Hypotrichosis; fine, dry, scant eyebrows and lashes	Hypodontia, peg-shaped incisors, microdontia	Dysplastic, thin, brittle, striated, pits	Rarely hypohidrosis without hyperthermia	Dry, eczematous areas, palmoplantar hyperkeratosis	Cleft lip/palate, syndactyly, ectrodactyly
Hypohidrotic ectodermal dysplasia and cleft lip/palate (Rapp-Hodgkin syndrome)	AD? XD?	Coarse, wiry, pili torti, sparse on scalp and eyebrows	Hypodontia, enamel hypoplasia, peg-shaped incisors	Dysplastic, narrow, diminished	Hypohidrosis, decreased sweat glands	Dry, coarse, thickened knee/elbow extensor surface	Cleft lip/palate, hypoplastic maxilla
Incontinentia pigmenti (Bloch-Sulzberger syndrome)	XD? AD?	Thin; alopecia	Hypodontia, peg-shaped teeth, delayed eruption	Dystrophic	Normal	Neonatal vesicular eruption, whorled hyperpigmentation	Cataract, atrophy of optic nerve, cleft lip/palate (rare)
Palmar-plantar hyperkeratosis/periodontal destruction (Papillon-Lefévre syndrome)	AR	Occasionally thin	Premature tooth loss, periodontal degeneration	Occasionally dystrophic	Palmoplantar hyperhidrosis	Palmoplantar hyperkeratosis	Liver dysfunction (rare), dura mater calcification

Mode of Inheritance: XR, X-linked recessive; XD, X-linked dominant; AD, autosomal dominant; AR, autosomal recessive; notations followed by ? are still uncertain (most probable inheritance pattern listed first).

Data from Freire-Maia N, Pinheiro M. Ectodermal Dysplasias: A Clinical and Genetic Study. New York: Alan R Liss, 1984.

TABLE 164-2. Tissues Involved in Ectodermal Dysplasias

Tissue	Clinical and Structural Characteristics
Hair	Sparse or absent, may be of small diameter, abnormal cross-sectional shape, longitudinal fissures, hypopigmentation, dystrophic bulb, abnormal slant
Teeth	Absent or reduced in number, peg-shaped, hypoplastic enamel, large pulp chambers (taurodontism), periodontal degeneration
Nails	Absent, thin, brittle, hyperconvex, conical, narrow, broad, thickened, hypopigmented, hyperpigmented, slow growing
Sweat glands	Regional absence, hypoplastic ducts and pores, functional alteration (decreased/increased sweat production)
Bones and limbs	Craniofacial deformities, cleft palate, syndactyly, ectrodactyly (split hands and feet), polydactyly, micromelia, generalized osteoporosis, osteosclerosis
Special senses	Microphthalmia, cataract formation, photophobia, frequent conjunctivitis, congenital deafness, conductive hearing loss
Glands	Decreased lacrimation, supernumerary nipples, mammary gland hypoplasia, decreased numbers of sebaceous and mucous glands, decreased saliva
Internal organs	Abnormal liver and kidney function, congenital heart disease
Reproductive organs	Hypospadias, hypogonadism, cryptorchidism, amenorrhea
Neurologic system	Mental retardation, hypotonia, seizures

Data from Holbrook KA. Structural abnormalities of the epidermally derived appendages in skin from patients with ectodermal dysplasia: Insight into developmental errors. In: Salinas CF, Opitz JM, Paul NW, eds. Recent Advances in Ectodermal Dysplasias. New York; Alan R Liss, 1988.

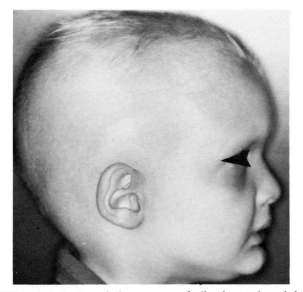

FIGURE 164-1. Alopecia is a common finding in ectodermal dysplasia.

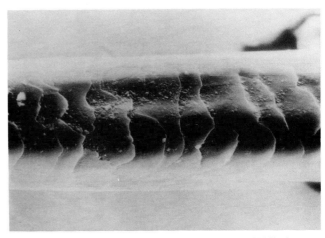

FIGURE 164-2. Scanning electron microscopy ($\times 2000$) shows an abnormal hair shaft morphology in ectodermal dysplasia. (From Wright JT. Hair ultrastructure in X-linked ectodermal dysplasia. Birth Defects 1988;24(2):281–283.)

features. Careful analysis of the family history and evaluation of all at-risk individuals for subtle clinical features is, therefore, essential in obtaining an accurate diagnosis. Localization of the gene for X-linked recessive hypohidrotic ectodermal dysplasia to the Xq13.1 region now provides an accurate method for the diagnosis of cases both prenatally and postnatally in this specific type of ectodermal dysplasia.[6] Further application of molecular biological techniques to the study of ectodermal dysplasia will lead to additional means for diagnosis and subclassification in the near future.

Clinical delineation of inheritance in females with ectodermal dysplasia can be especially challenging since they may have an autosomal type or an X-linked form or, alternatively, represent an X-linked carrier. Delineation of the mode of inheritance is especially important in these cases to determine future recurrence risks. Female carriers of X-linked recessive ectodermal dysplasia frequently (60%–80%) show characteristics of ectodermal dysplasia due to lyonization.[7-10] Female cells express only one of their X chromosomes, with the other being inactivated and forming the cellular bar body. Females expressing a high percentage of X chromosomes having the X-linked ectodermal dysplasia gene are more likely to have clinical features of the syndrome. Careful examination of carrier females shows that dental involvement (i.e., missing, small, or cone-shaped teeth) are present in about 70% of cases (Fig. 164–3) in addition to features such as hypotrichosis and hypohidrosis.[7-9]

TREATMENT

Appropriate management of patients with ectodermal dysplasia often requires a team approach, owing to the diverse spectrum of involvement.[11] Clearly, the nature of required treatments and interventions may be as varied as the disorders. Unfortunately, all interventions are preventive or palliative. Genetic evaluation and counseling should be provided to all families with ectodermal dys-

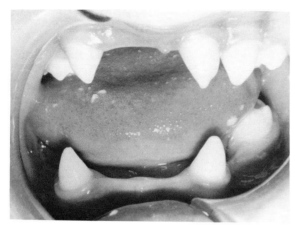

FIGURE 164–3. Severe abnormalities of the teeth are found in many patients with ectodermal dysplasia.

plasia. Individuals with severe hyperthermia may need to curtail activities causing exertion that could raise the body core temperature. Hyperthermia can be an acute problem for severely affected individuals living in warm climates. Febrile seizures and even death have been reported in patients with ectodermal dysplasia having significant hypohidrosis and secondary hyperthermia.[12]

Dermatologic therapy is rendered primarily in response to the xerosis, which may be striking in some patients. Individuals with severe hypotrichosis and hypodontia will benefit from hair and dental prostheses. These interventions are often best initiated before school age, thereby facilitating optimal socialization and peer interaction. Even very young children with severe hypodontia (Fig. 164–3) may be managed with conventional removable dental prostheses.[8] Severe hypodontia secondary to ectodermal dysplasia may also be treated using endosseous implants that serve as a foundation for fixed dental prostheses.[13] Implant therapy is now being performed in young teenage patients with ectodermal dysplasia and provides the advantage of having teeth that are fixed in the mouth as opposed to removable dentures. The placement of an endosseous implant–supported dental prosthesis requires a relatively sophisticated surgical procedure. It is costly, and the long range survival of the implant remains uncertain.

References

1. Freire-Maia N, Pinheiro M. Ectodermal Dysplasias: A Clinical and Genetic Study. New York: Alan R Liss, 1984:251.
2. Freire-Maia N, Pinheiro M. Ectodermal dysplasia: Some recollections and a classification. In: Salinas CF, Opitz JM, Paul NW, eds. Recent Advances in Ectodermal Dysplasias. New York: Alan R Liss, 1988:3–14.
3. Flesher Z: Hereditary ectodermal dysplasia: Report of a case with experimental study. Arch Dermatol Syph 1944;49:410–414.
4. Holbrook KA. Structural abnormalities of the epidermally derived appendages in skin from patients with ectodermal dysplasia: Insight into developmental errors. In: Salinas CF, Opitz JM, Paul NW, eds. Recent Advances in Ectodermal Dysplasias. New York: Alan R Liss, 1988:15–44.
5. Airenne P: X-linked hypohidrotic ectodermal dysplasia in Finland. Proc Finn Dent Soc 1981;77(Suppl 1):1–107.
6. Zonana J, Jones M, Browne D, et al: High-resolution mapping of the X-linked hypohidrotic ectodermal dysplasia (EDA) locus. Am J Hum Genet 1992;51:1036–1046.
7. Nakata M, Koshiba H, Eto K, et al: A genetic study of anodontia in X-linked hypohidrotic ectodermal dysplasia. Am J Hum Genet 1980;32:908–919.
8. Wright JT, Finley WH: X-linked recessive hypohidrotic ectodermal dysplasia: Manifestations and management. J Ala Med Sci 1986;23:84–87.
9. Pinheiro M, Freire-Maia N: Christ-Siemens-Touraine syndrome: A clinical and genetic analysis of a large Brazilian kindred: III. Carrier detection. Am J Med Genet 1979;4:129–134.
10. Larsen WG: The Lyon hypothesis. Arch Dermatol 1968;97: 342–343.
11. Farrington FH. The team approach to the management of ectodermal dysplasias. In: Salinas CF, Opitz JM, Paul NW, eds. Recent Advances in Ectodermal Dysplasias, New York: Alan R Liss, 1988:237–242.
12. Ramchander V, Jankey N, Ramkissoon BA, et al: Anhidrotic ectodermal dysplasia in an infant presenting with pyrexia of unknown origin. Clin Pediatr 1978;17:51–54.
13. Guckes AD, Brahim JS, McCarthy GR, et al: Using endosseous dental implants for patients with ectodermal dysplasia. J Am Dent Assoc 1991;122:59–62.

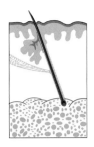

chapter 165

Incontinentia Pigmenti

JACKSON MACHADO-PINTO and LOREN E. GOLITZ

DEFINITION

Incontinentia pigmenti, also called Bloch-Sulzberger syndrome or Bloch-Siemens syndrome, is an X-linked, dominantly inherited disorder that affects, almost exclusively, females.[1-3] The incontinence of pigment from which its name derives is the result of inflammation.

CLINICAL DESCRIPTION

The natural history of incontinentia pigmenti is characterized by progression through three successive stages. In the first stage, a vesiculobullous eruption is present at birth or appears within 2 weeks in 90% of the patients. The vesicles are frequently in a linear arrangement, and the extremities are predominantly affected (Fig. 165–1). Eosinophilia of up to 50% in the peripheral blood is usual.[4]

The vesiculobullous stage is followed by a verrucous stage at 2 to 6 weeks of age. Rarely the vesicular stage of incontinentia pigmenti occurs in utero and patients can be born with verrucous lesions. Linear verrucous and papillomatous lesions develop in previous vesicular areas (Fig. 165–2).

In the third stage, the verrucous lesions give way to bizarre, whorled brown to slate-gray macular pigmentation that is most prominent on the trunk (Fig. 165–3).[3] This pigmentation gradually fades after 16 weeks of age. Occasionally, residual hypopigmentation remains for variable periods of time in the previously hyperpigmented areas.[5]

In up to 33% of the patients there may be patchy cicatricial alopecia resembling pseudopelade of Brocq. The nails may be small and dystrophic or show transverse striations or spooning.[1-3]

Although constitutional signs are absent,[6] associated extracutaneous anomalies are relatively common.[7] Partial anodontia and/or conical teeth are the typical dental defects. Convulsive disorders occur in 13% of patients,[1]

and mental retardation and/or spastic paresis may also be present.[3] Ocular abnormalities include cataracts, papillitis, congenital retinal folds, and optical atrophy.[3]

Incontinentia pigmenti may be associated with an increased frequency of childhood neoplasms. Retinoblastoma, Wilms' tumor, acute myelocytic leukemia, paratesticular rhabdomyosarcoma, and rhabdoid tumor of the kidney have been reported.[8]

PATHOLOGY

Histologically, the vesicular lesions are characterized by eosinophilic spongiosis, which is a distinct but nonspecific reaction pattern that consists of intercellular edema and focal exocytosis of eosinophils into the epidermis (Fig. 165–4). The areas showing eosinophilic spongiosis are often surrounded by isolated or clustered dyskeratotic cells. In the dermis there is a patchy infiltrate of mononuclear cells and many eosinophils.[9]

The verrucous lesions of the second stage show hyperkeratosis, papillomatosis, acanthosis, and scattered dyskeratotic cells within the epidermis (Fig. 165–5). There is often hydropic degeneration of the basement membrane zone. The dermis contains an infiltrate of lymphocytes and eosinophils. There may be exocytosis of some eosinophils into the epidermis. Dermal melanophages are present.[9]

The pigmented whorls of the third stage display an accumulation of melanophages in the superficial dermis, at times accompanied by epidermal atrophy and hydropic change in the basal layer.[9]

PATHOGENESIS AND ETIOLOGY

Incontinentia pigmenti is believed to represent an X-linked, dominantly inherited disease that is lethal for the hemizygous male.[1, 2] The relative infrequency of normal male siblings and the increased spontaneous abor-

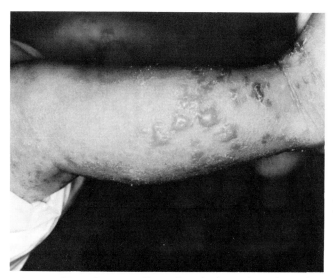

FIGURE 165–1. First stage of incontinentia pigmenti showing vesicular lesions in linear arrangement.

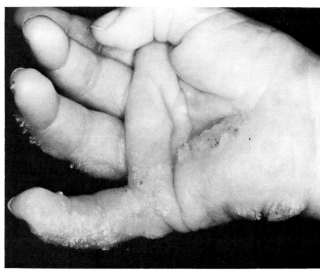

FIGURE 165–2. Second stage of incontinentia pigmenti showing linear verrucous lesions on the palm.

tion rate in affected females is consistent with this hypothesis.[10] The occurrence of rare cases in males has not been adequately explained thus far. They could represent somatic mutations,[1] a coexistence of Klinefelter's syndrome (XXY),[11] or a half-chromatid mutation.[12] Investigation of palm prints in incontinentia pigmenti revealed partial sweat gland aplasia in five of eight patients, which led Rott to classify incontinentia pigmenti as a form of X-linked anhidrotic ectodermal dysplasia.[13]

A constant feature of incontinentia pigmenti is the presence of blood eosinophilia in the vesiculobullous phase. It has been proposed that basophils in early lesions of incontinentia pigmenti may play a role in the attraction of eosinophils through the release of eosinophil chemotactic factor.[14] Keratinocyte-derived leukotriene B$_4$ may play a role in the accumulation of eosinophils within the epidermis in the vesiculobullous stage of the disease.[15] There is evidence of altered immunologic reactivity manifested by neutrophil and lymphocytic dysfunction.[16, 17]

DIAGNOSIS AND DIFFERENTIAL DIAGNOSIS

The combination of linear bullae followed by linear warty lesions in a newborn female infant is considered pathognomonic for incontinentia pigmenti.[4] The differential diagnosis includes those diseases that may clinically present with a vesiculobullous eruption at birth or shortly after, such as neonatal herpes simplex, infantile acropustulosis,[18] epidermolysis bullosa (see Chapter 78),[4] and neonatal herpes gestationis.[19] Rarely, blisters may occur in infants born of mothers with herpes gestationis. However, they disappear spontaneously after a few weeks

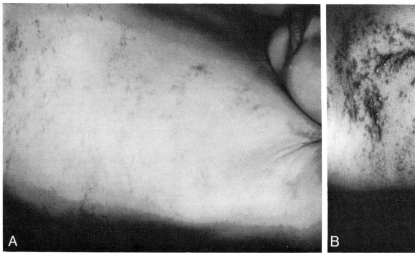

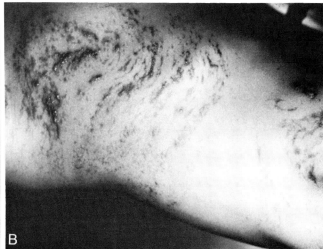

FIGURE 165–3. *A* and *B*, Third stage of incontinentia pigmenti showing bizarre pigmentation on the trunk. (*B*, courtesy of Richard B. Odom, M.D.)

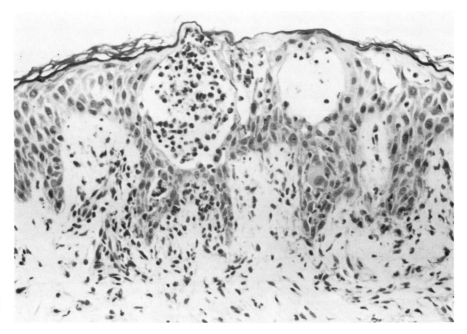

FIGURE 165–4. First stage of incontinentia pigmenti showing spongiotic vesicles and eosinophilic spongiosis (×160).

leaving no residual pigmentation.[19] Diseases that manifest with splashed pigmentation in older infants, such as the Franceschetti-Jadassohn syndrome (chromatophore nevus of Naegeli) and postinflammatory hyperpigmentation from atopic eczema or other causes, should also be considered in the differential diagnosis of incontinentia pigmenti in its third stage.[6] The differential diagnosis of the rare cases resulting in hypopigmentation includes nevus achromicans of Ito.

The disease processes listed in the differential diagnosis lack the triphasic evolution of incontinentia pigmenti

and do not display the same associated abnormalities, if any. Some disappear after a few days leaving no hyperpigmentation; others show hyperpigmentation without the preceding inflammatory changes. The hyperpigmentation does not show the characteristic whorled pattern seen in incontinentia pigmenti.

Histologically, the differential diagnosis of incontinentia pigmenti includes diseases that may show eosinophilic spongiosis, including acute arthropod reactions, infantile acropustulosis, transient neonatal pustular melanosis, and erythema toxicum neonatorum (Table

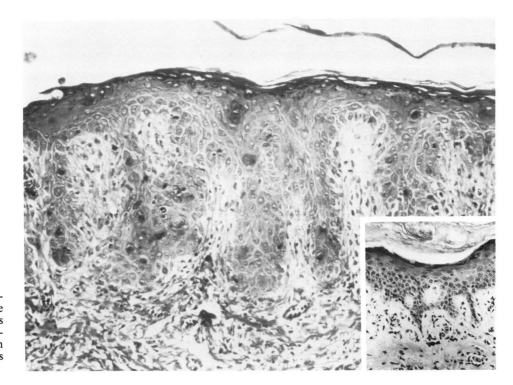

FIGURE 165–5. Second stage of incontinentia pigmenti showing single and clustered dyskeratotic cells (×100). *Inset,* Third stage of incontinentia pigmenti showing melanin pigment in dermal macrophages (×100).

TABLE 165-1. Histologic Differential Diagnosis of Incontinentia Pigmenti

Bullous pemphigoid
Pemphigus vulgaris/foliaceus
Arthropod bite reaction/scabies
Herpes gestationis
Dermatitis herpetiformis
Acute dermatitis
Milker's nodule

165–1). Infantile acropustulosis and transient neonatal pustular melanosis show a predominance of neutrophils within the epidermis, but eosinophils are also common. Erythema toxicum neonatorum shows eosinophils and spongiosis, but there is a tendency for the spongiosis to occur around follicular orifices. The presence of dyskeratotic cells in association with eosinophilic spongiosis in incontinentia pigmenti may help to differentiate it from these other conditions. Although pemphigus vulgaris (see Chapter 74), bullous pemphigoid (see Chapter 75), halogenoderma,[9] granulocytic spongiotic papulovesiculosis,[20] and lichen planus pemphigoides[21] may show eosinophilic spongiosis, they are extremely rare in the neonatal period. They also display clinical, histopathologic, or immunofluorescence features that distinguish them from incontinentia pigmenti. Changes identical to those of the second stage of incontinentia pigmenti can be found in rare epidermal nevi.[22]

TREATMENT

No treatment is necessary except for control of secondary infection of the vesiculobullous lesions. Systemic therapy with corticosteroids or sulfapyridine has not been successful.[4] Skilled dental intervention can minimize cosmetic disability related to the dental abnormalities. Neurologic and ophthalmologic consultation is advisable. Genetic counseling should be offered to all families with incontinentia pigmenti.

References

1. Carney RG. Incontinentia pigmenti: A world statistical analysis. Arch Dermatol 1976;112:535–542.
2. Wiklund DA, Weston WL. Incontinentia pigmenti: A four-generation study. Arch Dermatol 1980;116:701–703.
3. Kang S, Sober AJ. Disturbances of melanin pigmentation. In: Moschella SA, Hurley HJ, eds. Dermatology, 3rd ed, vol II. Philadelphia: WB Saunders Co., 1992:1456–1457.
4. Bleehen SS, Ebling FJG, Champion RH. Disorders of Skin Colour. In: Champion RH, Burton JL, Ebling FGJ, eds. Rook/Wilkinson/Ebling Textbook of Dermatology, 5th ed, vol III. London: Blackwell Scientific Publications, 1992:1580–1582.
5. Alper JC. The Genodermatoses and their Significance in Pediatric Dermatology. Dermatol Clin 1986;4:45.
6. Arnold HC, Odom RB, James WD. Some genodermatoses. In: Arnold HC, Odom RB, James WD, eds. Andrews' Diseases of the Skin, 8th ed. Philadelphia: WB Saunders Co., 1990:637–639.
7. Peltonen L. Incontinentia pigmenti in four generations. Dermatologica 1986;172:201–204.
8. Roberts WM, Jenkins JJ, Moorhead EL II, et al. Incontinentia pigmenti, a chromosomal instability syndrome, is associated with childhood malignancy. Cancer 1988;62:2370–2372.
9. Lever WF, Schaumburg-Lever G. Congenital diseases (Genodermatoses). In: Lever WF, Schaumburg-Lever G. Histopathology of the Skin, 7th ed. Philadelphia: JB Lippincott, 1990:93–95.
10. Person JR. Incontinentia pigmenti: A failure of immune tolerance? J Am Acad Dermatol 1985;1:120–123.
11. Prendiville JS, Gorski JL, Stein CK, et al. Incontinentia pigmenti in a male with Klinefelter's syndrome. J Am Acad Dermatol 1989;20:937–940.
12. Lenz W. Half-chromatid mutations may explain incontinentia pigmenti in males. Am J Hum Genet 1975;27:690–691.
13. Rott HD. Partial sweat gland aplasia in incontinentia pigmenti (Bloch-Sulzberger): Implications for nosologic classification. Clin Genet 1984;26:36–38.
14. Schmalstieg FC, Jorizzo JL, Tschen J, et al. Basophils in incontinentia pigmenti. J Am Acad Dermatol 1984;10:362–364.
15. Takematsu H, Terui T, Torinoki W, et al. Incontinentia pigmenti: Eosinophilic chemotactic activity of the crusted scales in the vesiculobullous stage. Br J Dermatol 1986;115:61–66.
16. Jessen RT, Epps DEV, Goodwin JS, et al. Incontinentia pigmenti. Arch Dermatol 1978;114:1182–1186.
17. Menni S, Piccinno R, Biolchini A, et al. Immunologic investigations in eight patients with incontinentia pigmenti. Pediatr Dermatol 1990;7:275–277.
18. Vignon-Pennamen MD, Wallach D. Infantile acropustulosis. Arch Dermatol 1986;122:1155–1160.
19. Chorzelski TP, Jablonska S, Beutner EH, et al. Herpes gestationis with identical lesions in the newborn. Arch Dermatol 1976;112:1129–1131.
20. Sayami S, Tagami H. Granulocytic spongiotic papulovesiculosis: A new entity? Br J Dermatol 1984;110:504–506.
21. Sobel S, Miller R, Shatin R. Lichen planus pemphigoides: Immunofluorescence findings. Arch Dermatol 1976;112:1280–1283.
22. Fletcher V, Williams ML, Lane AT. Histologic changes resembling the verrucous phase of incontinentia pigmenti within epidermal nevi: Report of two cases. Pediatr Dermatol 1985;3:69–74.

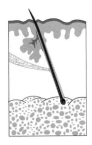

chapter 166

Neurofibromatosis, Tuberous Sclerosis, and Other Neurocutaneous Disorders

NEIL S. GOLDBERG and RANDALL K. ROENIGK

Neurocutaneous syndromes are disorders in which cutaneous and neurologic abnormalities are prominent and may share a common embryology. Most are genetically determined developmental disorders. A partial inventory of neurocutaneous disorders is listed in Table 166–1. Neurofibromatosis and tuberous sclerosis are discussed in detail in this chapter, and Proteus and Leopard syndromes are briefly described as well.

Neurofibromatosis Type 1

DEFINITION

The term *neurofibromatosis* implies neurofibromatosis type 1 (NF1), which formerly was known as as von Recklinghausen's disease, classic neurofibromatosis, or peripheral neurofibromatosis. NF is no longer considered a single disease. Unqualified NF1 is a multisystem disorder characterized by café-au-lait macules, neurofibromas, Lisch nodules, optic gliomas, bony dysplasias, intertriginous freckling, and autosomal dominant inheritance.

The incidence of NF1 is approximately 1 in 3500. There is no gender or racial preference, and 50% of cases appear to be spontaneous mutations.[1]

CLINICAL DESCRIPTION

Cutaneous Features

Neurofibromas

There are three types of neurofibromas: cutaneous, subcutaneous, and plexiform. The cutaneous type are pink, rubbery tumors that can be pedunculated or sessile, can number from just a few to over 1000 (Fig. 166–1), and vary in size from a few millimeters to more than 1 meter (average, 0.5 to 1.0 cm). Although all sites can be affected, the glans penis is rarely involved. Neurofibromas of the female areola and nipple are virtually pathognomonic for NF1 (Fig. 166–2). The lesions herniate easily through the dermis with gentle pressure, a finding called buttonholing. Subcutaneous neurofibromas may be firm, feeling like a pencil eraser. Cutaneous and subcutaneous neurofibromas appear initially in childhood, increase in number during puberty and pregnancy, and continue to appear at a slower rate throughout adulthood.

Plexiform neurofibromas are congenital and nearly pathognomonic for NF1. They are similar to a combination of cutaneous and subcutaneous types and feel like a "bag of worms." They can be large but may be subtle at birth when the only sign of a plexiform neurofibroma may be a hair whorl or patch of hyperpigmentation.

TABLE 166-1. Neurocutaneous Syndromes

Neurofibromatosis	Lentiginosis-deafness-cardiomyopathy (leopard syndrome)
Tuberous sclerosis	Biotin-responsive multiple carboxylase deficiency
Incontinenti pigmenti	Klippel-Trenauney-Weber syndrome
Hypomelanosis of Ito	Neurocutaneous lipomatosis
Neurocutaneous melanosis	Phenylketonuria
Albinism	Homocystinuria
Waardenberg's syndrome	Argininosuccinic aciduria
Albright's syndrome	Fabry's disease
Linear sebaceous nevus syndrome	Menkes' kinky hair syndrome
Epidermal nevus syndrome	Citrullinemia
Proteus syndrome	Refsum's syndrome
Basal cell nevus syndrome	Fucosidosis
Focal dermal hypoplasia	Chédiak-Higashi syndrome
Sjögren-Larsson syndrome	von Hippel–Lindau disease
Neuroichthyosis	Xeroderma pigmentosum
Sturge-Weber syndrome	Cockayne's syndrome
Ataxia-telangiectasia	Poikiloderma congenitale
Cutaneomeningospinal angiomatosis (Cobb syndrome)	Progeria
Hereditary-hemorrhagic telangiectasia (Osler-Weber-Rendu)	Familial dysautonomia

Café-au-Lait Macules

The café-au-lait spot is a homogeneous tan-brown macule with smooth, sharp borders (Fig. 166–3). It can vary in size from a few millimeters to many centimeters (average, 1–3 cm). Café-au-lait macules are found everywhere except the scalp, eyebrows, palms, and soles. They are congenital but may not be visible for the first few months of life.

Intertriginous Freckling

Intertriginous freckling, or Crowe's sign, consists of small 1- to 3-mm in diameter tan-brown macules. Freckling may be universal in NF1, but it is considered diagnostic of NF1 only when it is present in the axilla or groin. It is in these locations only that they can be reliably and consistently distinguished from solar freckles,

which in contrast fade when sun exposure diminishes. Freckles are not miniature café-au-lait macules. The number of café-au-lait macules is fixed at birth, while freckles appear later in childhood and continue to appear through adulthood, especially in areas of friction such as the waistband.

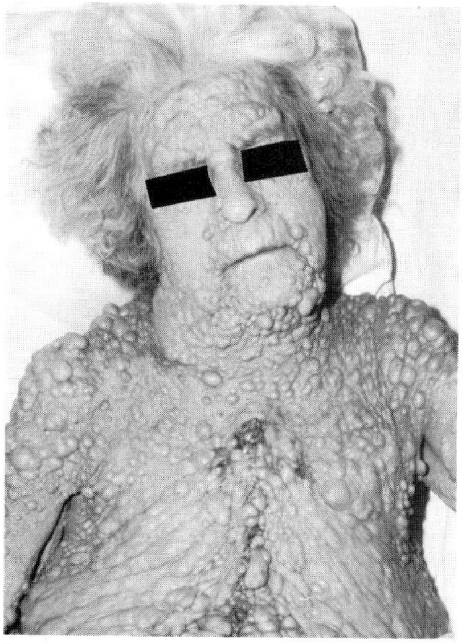

Extracutaneous Features

Central Nervous System and Eye

The most common manifestation of NF1 is Lisch nodules. These are melanocytic hamartomas of the iris. They look like three-dimensional translucent brown spots. They do not interfere with vision and require a slit lamp to visualize in most cases. Lisch nodules appear in childhood. In one study, only 5% of children less than 3 years old had Lisch nodules, but that went up rapidly to 42% of 3- to 4-year-olds and then to 55% of 5- to 6-year-olds.[2] Lisch nodules are rarely seen in patients who do not have NF1.[3, 4]

FIGURE 166–1. Neurofibromatosis type 1. Elderly woman with an uncountable number of cutaneous neurofibromas.

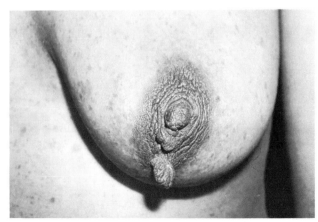

FIGURE 166–2. Close-up of areola revealing neurofibromas. Presence of neurofibromas in this location is very characteristic of neurofibromatosis type 1.

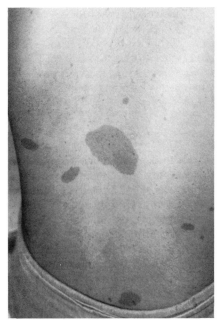

FIGURE 166-3. Typical café-au-lait macules in a young girl with neurofibromatosis type 1.

Optic gliomas are the prototypical central nervous system (CNS) lesions of NF1. Although present in approximately 15% of patients with NF1, 80% of those may be asymptomatic.[5] They appear in childhood, but most are not progressive.

Orthopedic Features

Two lesions of the bone are considered specific for NF1: sphenoid wing dysplasia and pseudarthrosis of the tibia. Although only 0.5% of patients with NF1 have pseudarthrosis, which presents as congenital bowing of the tibia, half of all cases of congenital pseudarthrosis are due to NF1.[6, 7] The osseous lesions are not due to neurofibromas, and their etiology is unknown. Vertebral scalloping, macrocephaly, short stature, and scoliosis (all types) are all frequently seen but are not diagnostic.

Course and Complications

NF1 is a progressive disease. It worsens with age; limited disease early in life is no guarantee of mild disease later.[8] NF1 can also be viewed as a familial cancer-prone syndrome. The lifetime risk for cancer in NF1 patients is approximately 5% above the lifetime risk of the general population.[8] The prototypical adult NF1-specific cancer is neurofibrosarcoma. It can develop within plexiform neurofibroma or within large nerves. It is seldom associated with typical cutaneous or subcutaneous neurofibromas. Pheochromocytomas, malignant melanoma, and embryonal tumors such as Wilms' tumor and rhabdomyosarcoma are also more common in NF1. Children have an increased risk for other cancers such as leukemia. The association of juvenile xanthogranuloma, NF1,

and juvenile chronic myelogenous type leukemia is well documented.[9]

Cosmetic disfigurement is a complication of NF1. For as many as one third of patients with NF1, cutaneous neurofibromas represent their major concern (see the section on surgical management). Craniofacial and spinal plexiform neurofibromas can be associated with profound morbidity and even mortality. Craniofacial plexiform neurofibromas affect as many as 5% of patients with NF1 and can cause facial disfigurement, proptosis, visual changes, and respiratory compromise. A localized area of hyperpigmentation or hypertrichosis overlying the midline on the back could be a plexiform neurofibroma of the spinal cord and should be evaluated. Other nonspecific complications include chronic pruritus, hypertension, constipation, and headaches (Table 166–2).[3] Two thirds of patients with NF1 have mild disease; of the remaining third, one half have severe but correctable problems and one half have persistent, severe difficulties.[10]

TABLE 166-2. Five Categories of Complications

Psychosocial Burden
Mental retardation
School performance problems
Emotional and behavioral disturbances

Developing in Childhood and Causing Lifelong Morbidity
Plexiform neurofibromas (head and neck)
Scoliosis (severe)
Pseudarthrosis
Delayed development or abnormal puberty

"Treatable" Complications that can Develop at any Age
Seizures
Spinal neurofibromas
Visceral neurofibromas
Endocrine tumors
Renal artery stenosis and other vascular lesions
Aqueductal stenosis

CNS and Malignant Tumors
Optic gliomas
Other CNS tumors: astrocytomas, neurilemmomas, meningiomas, schwannomas
Rhabdomyosarcoma
Neurofibrosarcoma

Complications with Minimal Effect on Life-style
Pruritus
Macrocephaly
Short stature
Headaches
Constipation
Hypertension

Data from Huson SM, Compston DAS, Harper PS. A genetic study of von Recklinghausen neurofibromatosis in South Wales: II. Guidelines for genetic counseling. J Med Genet 1989;26:712–721.

PATHOLOGY

Although pedunculated cutaneous neurofibromas commonly occur sporadically, plexiform neurofibromas are almost exclusively seen in patients with neurofibromatosis.

Café-au-lait macules are produced by basilar hyperpigmentation of the epidermis. Giant melanosomes are visible in basilar keratinocytes by routine microscopy, and their detection does not require the complex method of dopa incubation of fresh epidermis.[11]

PATHOGENESIS AND ETIOLOGY

The precise cause of NF1 is unknown. The NF1 gene is a huge gene on the long arm of chromosome 17 near the centromere.[12] Its size presents a large target for spontaneous mutations.[13] The gene is evolutionarily conserved and expressed ubiquitously. The gene product, called neurofibromin, appears to function as a guanosine triphosphatase activating protein (GTPase activating protein [GAP]), converting the oncogene *ras* from its active (guanosine triphosphate [GTP]) to inactive form (guanosine diphosphate [GDP]).[14] The oncogene *ras* is highly conserved though at evolution and controls basic cellular functions such as growth, development and differentiation. A defective GAP, as in patients with NF1, results in the uncontrolled growth of some tissues and the NF1 phenotype. Neurofibromin acts as a tumor suppressor. Many different mutations of the NF1 gene have been described, but no correlation between mutations and phenotype has been documented. Even in the same family, with presumably identical genetic mutations, there is tremendous variability of phenotypic expression.

DIAGNOSIS AND DIFFERENTIAL DIAGNOSIS

Diagnostic Criteria

The advent of sophisticated neuroimaging and diagnostic criteria have made the diagnosis of NF1 much more straightforward. Seven clinically useful criteria were described at a National Institutes of Health–sponsored consensus conference in 1987,[15] were updated in 1990,[16] and are listed in Table 166-3. Two criteria are required for a definitive diagnosis, one for a presumptive diagnosis. The criterion for café-au-lait macules is remarkably similar to the original contribution of Crowe and Schull.[17] The size (1.5 cm) was chosen so café-au-lait macules could be reliably and consistently distinguished from solar freckles. Since café-au-lait macules are present at birth or soon after, they are the most important clinical criterion for identifying NF1 in children. Patients with NF1 may have fewer than six café-au-lait macules, but anyone with six or more requires at least a presumptive diagnosis of NF1 or another form of neurofibromatosis.

In a study of children younger than 6 years old at risk for NF1, 94% (150 of 160) were successfully classified.[18] Café-au-lait macules were almost always the first feature

TABLE 166-3. Criteria for Neurofibromatosis Type I

Two of seven criteria are required for a definitive diagnosis:
1. Six or more café-au-lait macules over 5 mm in greatest diameter in prepubertal individuals and over 15 mm in greatest diameter postpubertal individuals.
2. Freckling in the axillary or inguinal regions.
3. Two or more neurofibromas of any type or one plexiform neurofibroma.
4. Two or more Lisch nodules.
5. Optic glioma.
6. A distinctive osseous lesion such as sphenoid wing dysplasia or thinning of the long bone cortex with or without pseudarthrosis.
7. First-degree relative with neurofibromatosis type 1 by these criteria.

Reproduced with permission, from Mulvihill JJ (moderator). Neurofibromatosis 1 (Recklinghausen's disease) and neurofibromatosis 2 (bilateral acoustic neurofibromatosis): An update. Ann Intern Med 1990;113:39-52.

to appear, followed by freckles and Lisch nodules, and finally neurofibromas. Thus the absence of these later features in a young child does not rule out NF1.

If a child of an NF1 parent reaches the age of 5 and has neither café-au-lait macules nor Lisch nodules, it is unlikely that he has inherited the gene for NF1. It becomes progressively less likely each year that other features do not develop. Because nearly all adults with NF1 have Lisch nodules, their absence virtually excludes a diagnosis of NF1. In parents or adult family members at risk for NF1 because of an affected child, parent, or sibling, the absence of café-au-lait macules, neurofibromas, and Lisch nodules virtually excludes the possibility of NF1.

The discovery of the NF1 gene has not had as much impact on diagnosis as might have been expected.[19, 20] Linkage analysis can only be used for diagnosis when several affected family members can be studied and when useful markers are available. Linkage analysis can be used to diagnose NF1 prenatally or perinatally in presymptomatic individuals.

Suggested Evaluation

The history and physical examination should concentrate on the skin and CNS. Head circumference, height, blood pressure, and screening for scoliosis are especially important. Ophthalmologic examination to identify Lisch nodules is required. Testing for learning disabilities is suggested. Routine laboratory tests are useless.

Guidelines from the National Institutes of Health consensus conference state that routine computed tomography (CT) and magnetic resonance imaging (MRI) screening of patients with NF1 is not likely to be any value[16]; however, MRI can help confirm the diagnosis of NF1 and rule out a presumptive diagnosis in an at-risk individual. In a disease with so many potential CNS problems, a baseline evaluation with MRI is valuable; however, the frequency with which it should be repeated is unknown. MRI has replaced CT scan as the study of choice for diagnosis and management of NF1.[21] Lesions known as "bright spots" that are not known to be associated with any clinical signs are invisible on CT but occur in the majority of NF1 patients studied with MRI.[21] Optic gliomas are also better visualized with MRI.[21]

DIFFERENTIAL DIAGNOSIS

Other disorders that can be confused with NF1 (Table 166–4) include McCune-Albright syndrome (polyostotic fibrous dysplasia, irregular skin pigmentation, and sexual precocity); Watson syndrome (café-au-lait macules, dull intelligence, and pulmonary stenosis); and Proteus syndrome (Fig. 166–4). Proteus syndrome includes mesodermal malformations, hemihypertrophy, scoliosis, cerebriform masses of palms and soles, and subcutaneous masses that can be mistaken for neurofibromas.[22] Review of the original documentation on Joseph Merrick, the Elephant Man, suggests that he was afflicted with Proteus syndrome and not neurofibromatosis. Noonan's syndrome has also been confused with NF1 but is probably a distinct genetic disorder on a separate chromosome.[23]

The clinical heterogeneity of NF1 is one of its salient features. Even in the same family there will be wide variability of expression. Monozygotic twins demonstrate that there is genetic control of the type of NF1 lesions, but there is no genetic control over their location and number.[24]

Neurofibromatosis type 2 (NF2) is the only other type of NF having its own universally accepted criteria (Tables 166–5 and 166–6).[15, 16] The gene for NF2 is distinct from NF1 and is on chromosome 22. Formerly known as central neurofibromatosis, NF2 is characterized by bilateral acoustic neuromas. The characteristic

TABLE 166–4. Differential Diagnosis of Neurofibromatosis Type 1
McCune-Albright syndrome
Watson syndrome
Noonan's syndrome
Proteus syndrome

cutaneous features include neurofibromas and schwannomas but not café-au-lait macules or freckling.

Among the other types of neurofibromatosis, the most useful are segmental neurofibromatosis (NF5) and neurofibromatosis with only café-au-lait macules (NF6). In NF5 the stigmata are confined to only a part of the body. Unfortunately, no strict definition for NF5 exists and reported cases of localized, true segmental and bilateral disease are comingled.[25] NF5 may be the result of postzygotic mutation, chimerism, or mosaicism. Transmission of the NF1 gene cannot be predicted in all cases of NF5, and future systemic involvement beyond the involved segment cannot be ruled out.[25] NF6 should be considered in patients who present with six or more café-au-lait macules and no other features of neurofibromatosis. It is currently thought that perhaps café-au-lait macules can be transmitted as an independent trait in the absence of other classic NF1 stigmata.[25a]

TREATMENT

There is no cure for NF1. Ultimately, knowledge of the genetic mechanism of NF1 may lead to specific therapy. Management is based on genetic counseling and moni-

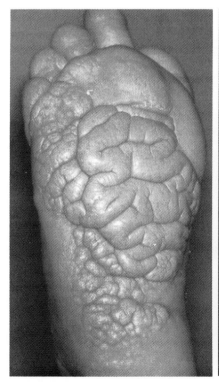
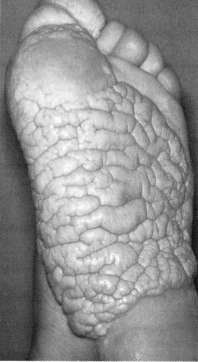

FIGURE 166–4. Characteristic cerebriform masses involve the plantar surfaces and are a variety of the subcutaneous masses that can be mistaken for neurofibromas in Proteus syndrome. (From Samlaska CP, Levin SW, James WD, Benson PM, et al. Proteus syndrome. Arch Dermatol 1989;125:1109–1114. Copyright 1989, American Medical Association.)

**TABLE 166-5. Criteria for
Neurofibromatosis Type 2**

1. Bilateral eighth nerve masses seen with appropriate imaging techniques

or

2. A first-degree relative with neurofibromatosis type 2

and

either:

unilateral eighth nerve mass

or

two of the following: neurofibromas, meningioma, glioma, schwannoma, or juvenile posterior subcapsular lenticular opacity

Reproduced with permission, from Mulvihill JJ (moderator). Neurofibromatosis 1 (Recklinghausen's disease) and neurofibromatosis 2 (bilateral acoustic neurofibromatosis): An update. Ann Intern Med 1990;113:39-52.

**TABLE 166-6. Types of
Neurofibromatosis[24]**

NF1	Classic or peripheral
NF2	Central or acoustic
NF3	Mixed
NF4	Variant
NF5	Segmental
NF6	Café-au-lait only
NF7	Late-onset
NF8	Not otherwise specified

From Bauer M, Lubs H, Lubs ML. Variable expressivity of NF1 in identical twins. Neurofibromatosis 1988;1:323-329.

toring for and treatment of complications. Identification of children at risk is important because early intervention in children with learning disabilities due to neurofibromatosis is extremely valuable.

There are now over 100 regional neurofibromatosis centers for evaluation and management of affected patients and their families. For all subjects with NF1 routine age-specific cancer screening examinations are indicated. The development of focal neurologic complaints, especially referred pain, or a history of a rapidly enlarging mass, suggests neurofibrosarcoma in a patient with NF1.

Surgical Management

The surgical treatment of cutaneous neurofibromas depends on the number and size of the tumors and the patient's motivation. For patients with hundreds of tumors and substantial functional problems, management is different from that of a patient with a small number of tumors in a limited area. Optimally, a patient with NF1 will be treated on a regular basis to minimize each procedure.

Traditionally, surgical excision has been the treatment of choice and is often the most reasonable.[26] Neurofibromas are mid- to deep dermal and subcutaneous tumors that are easily identified clinically and surgically. Excision usually results in few recurrences; however, new neurofibromas may develop in adjacent tissue. The excision is carried down to the subcutaneous tissue, and the wound is closed in a layered fashion. If one attempts to remove dozens of smaller lesions in one session, punch excisions may be performed and the wounds either allowed to heal by secondary intention or by suturing. A mild sedative for patients having a large number of cutaneous neurofibromas treated is sometimes helpful.

Another method to treat cutaneous neurofibromas is electrosurgery, principally electrosection with the loop.[27] Since many neurofibromas are exophytic, one may take a forceps, pull up the lesion, and with the loop or a straight-tipped electrosurgical apparatus simply shave-excise the lesions to an appropriate depth. This is a quick and simple method and obtains immediate hemostasis. The wounds may not require suturing, and sometimes over 100 tumors can be removed in one session. An alternative for facial neurofibromas is dermabrasion,[28] but recurrence from the deeper portion of the lesions should be anticipated.

The CO_2 laser has been used to treat over 100 tumors in one session lasting approximately 1 hour (Fig. 166-5). Local anesthetic is required while sedation is optional. Using approximately 10 W of energy, the CO_2 laser beam (10,600 nm) is focused so the epidermis, dermis, and underlying neurofibroma are vaporized precisely, much like an excision. The neurofibroma can be expressed through the dermal excision by manual pressure to ex-

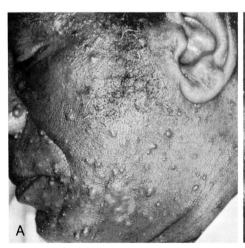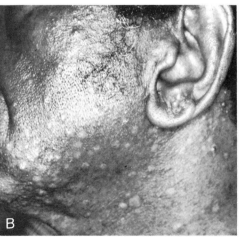

FIGURE 166-5. *A*, Dozens of small cutaneous neurofibromas on the cheek and neck before treatment with the CO_2 laser. *B*, Four months after surgery the wounds have healed with slight pigmentation and without recurrence of the tumors at this point. (*A* and *B* courtesy of Mayo Foundation.)

pose the tumor. Then the base of the entire lesion is vaporized to avoid recurrence. The CO_2 laser is normally used for smaller neurofibromas, and the defect can be either allowed to heal by secondary intention or closed with a small suture or staple. There is no advantage over excision in using the CO_2 laser for larger lesions. The neodymium:yttrium-aluminum-garnet (Nd:YAG) laser (1064 nm) causes much deeper coagulation (4 mm) but does not cause complete tissue death. This laser may be helpful in debulking large tumors. In all cases, procedures are usually repeated over the patient's lifetime.

Treatment of plexiform neurofibromas is beyond the scope of dermatologic surgery.[30] Even a biopsy of suspected plexiform lesion is fraught with danger and should be performed only by experienced surgeons.

Café-au-lait macules are a cosmetic problem for some patients. They may be treated with excision or dermabrasion. Because recurrence of these café-au-lait macules is at least 50%, lasers are available that may be preferable for treating these benign pigmented lesions. Lasers and wavelengths to consider are the flashlamp pumped-dye (510 nm), the Q-switched ruby (694 nm), the Q-switched frequency doubled YAG (1,064, 532 nm), the argon pumped tunable dye (argon, 488 and 514 nm; dye, 577– 630 nm), and the copper vapor (511 and 578 nm). Although the wavelengths of these lasers vary, all are partially absorbed by melanin. Since melanin in café-au-lait spots is normally at the dermoepidermal junction and superficial papillary dermis, laser photoablation may result in dispersal of the pigment and induction of resorption of melanin without substantially damaging adjacent normal collagen and appendages. Selective photothermolysis may occur because pulsed-dye, YAG, and Q-switched ruby lasers provide a high-powered emission in a very brief pulse. Laser treatment can be performed without anesthetic in most cases. Expense of the equipment and frequent recurrence are major limitations.

Tuberous Sclerosis

DEFINITION

Tuberous sclerosis, or Bourneville's disease, is an autosomal dominant disorder characterized by seizures, mental retardation, and a variety of skin lesions such as "ash leaf" macules, facial angiofibromas, ungual fibromas, and shagreen patches. It can affect almost every organ but the most frequently involved are brain, eye, skin, kidneys, heart, and lung. Although originally named after the characteristic brain lesion, the cortical tuber, the disease is more properly referred to as tuberous sclerosis complex (TSC) to emphasize the multiplicity of tissues involved. *Epiloia* is an obsolete term that emphasized epilepsy and retardation (anoia).

There is no sex, race, or geographic predilection among subjects with TSC. The phenotype varies from family to family and even within families. The increasing prevalence and incidence in published studies over the past 30 years is mostly due to reporting increased numbers of less severely affected cases, with a higher prevalence in younger persons.[31–36] The decreased prevalence in older persons is probably due to diminished life expectancy in TSC.[31, 32] A British study documented the overall prevalence as 1 in 27,000, but as 1 in 12,000 in those younger than 10 years of age, and concluded that the birth incidence could be as high as 1 in 10,000.[32]

CLINICAL DESCRIPTION

Cutaneous Features

Ninety-six percent of patients with TSC and their affected relatives have one or more of the five typical skin signs, of which maybe three are pathognomonic.[37] In order of decreasing frequency they are

1. Hypomelanotic macules
2. Multiple facial angiofibromas
3. Periungual fibromas
4. Shagreen patches
5. Fibrous plaques

The skin manifestations as a group are thus the most common in TSC and are important for diagnosis.

Hypomelanotic Macules

The hypomelanotic or "ash leaf" macule is found in 90% of affected individuals.[37] Most patients with TSC will have more than four white spots.[38] The macules are often present at birth but may not be recognized until the skin has been exposed to ultraviolet light.[37] The hypopigmented macules are off-white, not snow-white like those of vitiligo. There are three types of spots[39]:

1. Polygonal (like a thumbprint), 0.5 to 2.0 cm and the most frequent
2. Lance-ovate (ash leaf), 1.0 to 12 cm and highly characteristic but not the most common (Fig. 166–6)

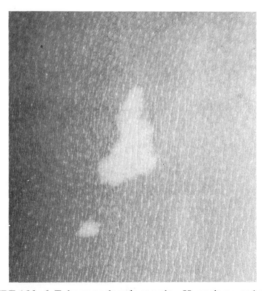

FIGURE 166–6. Tuberous sclerosis complex. Hypopigmented macule with typical "ash leaf" appearance in a young child.

3. Confetti-like, 1 to 3 mm, and rare but more specific and composed of an abundance of tiny white macules

The hypomelanotic lesions are like a reverse image of café-au-lait macules with the same sharp borders. Identification with Wood's light examination may show from one to hundreds of hypopigmented but not depigmented lesions. Although common, hypomelanotic macules are not specific: 0.8% of neonates normally have white spots; the prevalence is 0.4% for white children and 2.4% for black children.[40] The hypomelanotic macules may be confused clinically with vitiligo, but the shape, random distribution, presence at birth, and histology help distinguish them. They also have to be differentiated from nevus anemicus, nevus depigmentosus, piebaldism, and Vogt-Koyanagi-Harada syndrome (Table 166–7). Electron microscopy reveals that melanosomes are reduced in number, diameter, and melanization.

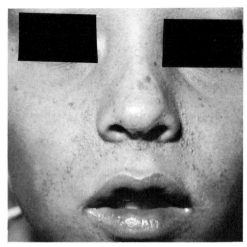

FIGURE 166–7. Tuberous sclerosis complex. Typical facial angiofibromas in a young boy.

Multiple Facial Angiofibromas

Most patients have at least one of three different connective tissue hamartomas: (1) facial angiofibromas, (2) ungual fibromas, and (3) shagreen patches. When present in the typical bilateral and symmetrical distribution, multiple facial angiofibromas are pathognomonic for TSC.[37] Originally called adenoma sebaceum, the confusion was due to the presence of abundant, normal sebaceous glands in the areas where angiofibromas are most common. When every patient with tuberous sclerosis had to have angiofibromas (Vogt's triad: seizures, mental retardation and angiofibromas) to make the diagnosis,[41] the prevalence of angiofibromas was 100%. Today it is well recognized that fewer than half (47%) of patients with TSC have angiofibromas.[37]

Angiofibromas are found over the cheeks, nasolabial folds, and chin; they cross the midline over the nasal bridge and chin. They are rarely seen on the upper lip (Fig. 166–7). The distribution is usually symmetrical, but one side may be predominant. Angiofibromas first appear as small red spots at age 3 or 4 and are usually present by age 5.[37] They seldom appear after puberty and only very rarely in infancy.[42] They can be recognized clinically; biopsy is rarely required. There are no consistent differences in histology between the angiofibromas of TSC and sporadic angiofibromas or fibrous papules.

Periungual Fibromas

The periungual or subungual fibroma is pathognomonic of TSC.[43] It does not develop until the second decade and is present in 20% of patients with TSC.[37] It continues to grow slowly after puberty and can present as

a longitudinal groove in the nail plate. The toes are affected more often than the fingers, and females are afflicted more often than males.

Shagreen Patch

From the French *peau de chagrin*, which means "skin with the appearance of untanned leather," the shagreen patch presents as a skin-colored or yellow-brown plaque and can resemble the skin of an orange. It is located on the dorsal surface, especially on the lumbosacral area, and is rare on the abdomen or chest. Most often this lesion appears after puberty, but it may be seen earlier. Shagreen patches are found in 19% of all patients with TSC but are not diagnostic by themselves.[37] They have been reported in patients who do not appear to have TSC.[45]

Fibrous Plaques

Most fibrous plaques are skin-colored to yellow-brown, smooth elevations of the skin of the forehead and scalp with a rubbery consistency (Fig. 166–8). They can occur with or precede angiofibromas. The plaques usually present in the first 2 to 3 years of life but may be present at birth and then grow very slowly after that. They are hamartomas that histologically resemble angiofibromas. They are probably pathognomonic for TSC,[37] but their frequency is unknown.

Other Cutaneous Findings

Other skin signs that are of no known diagnostic value include café-au-lait macules, skin tags, and nevi.

Extracutaneous Features

The most common extracutaneous organs affected by TSC are the CNS, eyes, kidneys, heart, and lung. Symptoms in all of these organs depend on the size, number, and location of lesions.

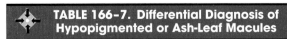

TABLE 166–7. Differential Diagnosis of Hypopigmented or Ash-Leaf Macules

Vitiligo
Nevus depigmentosus
Nevus anemicus
Piebaldism
Vogt-Koyanagi-Harada syndrome

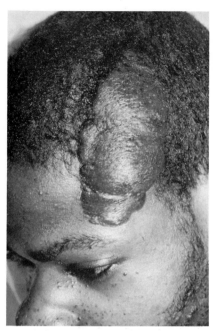

FIGURE 166-8. Tuberous sclerosis complex. Fibrous plaque of the forehead of a severely retarded young man with seizures.

Central Nervous System

There are two nontumorous features—seizures and mental retardation—and three characteristic tumors—cortical tubers, subependymal nodules, and subependymal giant cell tumors.

Seizures. Seizures are the most common presenting feature in TSC.[37] They are second only to skin findings as a whole in the overall frequency of occurrence. They most often begin early in life. Since asymptomatic children rarely present for evaluation for TSC, the number of seizure-free children is small.

Mental Retardation. In a study from the Mayo Clinic, 47% of patients with TSC suffered from mental retardation and 47% were of normal intelligence (the remainder were not known).[37] Of course, as more asymptomatic patients with TSC are found, the fraction of mentally retarded individuals will decrease.

There is a definite correlation with the occurrence of seizures early in life and mental retardation. Among those with seizures, the later in life they begin, and less frequent they occur, the smaller the chance that the patient will be mentally retarded.[45] There is also a correlation with the size and number of tubers: the more numerous and larger the tubers, the more chance there is of mental retardation.[38] There are, however, patients with tubers who never have seizures and are mentally normal. The few reported cases of mental retardation without seizures are not well documented.[38]

Cortical Tubers, Subependymal Nodules, and Giant Cell Tumors. The disease is named after these firm tumors. Tubers are hamartomatous proliferations of glial and neuronal tissues and can give rise to gliomas. There may be as many as 40 lesions per patient, and the distribution is random but symmetrical. The size varies from a few millimeters to a few centimeters.

Subependymal nodules are firm, pea-sized and larger excrescences on the ventricular wall. They resemble solidified wax drippings or "candle gutterings" and can calcify early in life. They are similar in their composition to cortical tubers and can also give rise to gliomas, which are often termed *giant cell subependymomas* because of the multinucleated astrocytes that are their hallmark. When they grow slowly and are asymptomatic, they are called *subependymal nodules*; when they grow excessively and obstruct CSF circulation, they are called *tumors*.

Eye

Retinal hamartomas, called retinal gliomas or phakomas, are found in one eye in at least 50% of patients with TSC.[46] They are pathognomonic for TSC when they are typical in appearance, multiple, and far from the optic disk. They are asymptomatic and require no treatment.

Kidneys

Two renal lesions are seen in TSC: cysts and angiomyolipomas; both can be single, multiple, unilateral, or bilateral. Renal cysts, found in 18%, are more common in children,[47] and cause few problems unless they are numerous or large.[38] Angiomyolipomas, seen in 45%,[48] are hamartomas made of adipose tissue, smooth muscle, and connective tissue and are more common in adults.[47] Although common, they are an infrequent cause of clinical problems. Considered pathognomonic when multiple, they are benign and require treatment only if symptomatic. There is also an increased incidence of renal cell carcinoma in patients with TSC.[49]

Heart

Even though the rhabdomyoma (another hamartoma) is the most common cardiac tumor of infancy, it is still considered unusual. This is probably because most are asymptomatic. In one study in which all infants with TSC were studied by echocardiography, rhabdomyomas were seen in 43%.[37] They cause symptoms by obstructing blood flow, causing arrhythmias, and impairing contractility.[37] Intrauterine cardiac failure may be the cause of hydrops fetalis,[50] stillbirth, or neonatal death.[51] The tumors can be seen with MRI and CT as well as echocardiography. Surgery is required if the lesions are symptomatic.

Lung

The two manifestations of TSC that involve the lung are cystic disease and lymphangiomyomatosis, a condition in which smooth muscle proliferates in the walls of pulmonary lymphatic vessels. Both almost always involve women and are found in less than 1% of patients with TSC.[37] The fibrosis of the lung gives the radiographic appearance of "honeycomb lungs."

Course and Complications

The prognosis of TSC depends on what organs are involved and to what degree these organs are compromised. In a study of the causes of death in 49 patients with TSC, almost half were found to have died of brain abnormalities: 10 from tumors and 13 from complications of severe mental retardation.[49] Renal involvement was the second most common cause of death and the most frequent cause of mortality in those older than 30 years of age. All of the deaths associated with renal compromise were in patients older than 10 years old. Of 11 renal deaths, 2 were from renal cell carcinoma, 2 were from bleeding angiomyolipomas, and 7 were from renal failure.

PATHOLOGY

The adenoma sebaceum of TSC is indistinguishable pathologically from the sporadic angiofibroma, which is discussed in Chapter 146. Periungual fibromas are similar histopathologically to acquired digital fibrokeratomas and appear to arise in the dermis of the proximal nail fold.[52] The shagreen patch is a form of connective tissue nevus.[53]

PATHOGENESIS AND ETIOLOGY

It is well established that TSC is an autosomal dominant disorder with variable expression.[37] Since up to 68% of cases may be spontaneous, the diagnosis of TSC will be made more often without than with a family history, and the issue of nonpenetrance is important. Older reports of "bona fide skipped generations" are very rare and controversial; they are not reliable because methods were inadequate to delineate occult disease.[38] In one study of 26 apparently normal, unaffected relatives of patients with TSC, 4 were found to be affected after imaging studies of the CNS.[54] There are also many reported cases of multiple affected siblings from apparently normal parents. This implies that gonadal mosaicism may occur in some cases.[55, 56]

The molecular genetic approach used so successfully in NF1 has not worked as well for TSC. Although there is tremendous intrafamilial variability in TSC, there is even more interfamilial variability; this implies that a portion of the variability may be genetically determined. The gene for TSC has been "linked" to portions of chromosome 9 (called *candidate gene TSC1*) and 16 (TSC2). There appears to be no phenotypic difference between cases linked to 9 and those linked to 16. Recently, candidate gene TSC2 was identified when it was found to contain five TSC-specific deletions. The gene appears to be highly conserved through vertebrate evolution, and the transcript is widely expressed. The gene protein product is called *TUBERIN* and is homologous to GAP3. TUBERIN appears to act as a tumor suppressor in much the same way that the NF1 gene product behaved.[57a] There are no unique groupings of patients and families that correspond to any specific mutations.

It is possible that TSC may be caused by mutations of more than one gene. Since many complex proteins are made up of more than one polypeptide chain, each of which is encoded by a separate gene, these complex proteins may be rendered dysfunctional through mutations in more than one gene. If TSC can be thought of as a disease in which the CNS lesions are the result of problems with migration, alignment, and proliferation of neural tissue, then many different proteins may act in concert to direct these functions. Mutations of any one of these proteins can be imagined to be responsible for the TSC phenotype. Another possibility is that TSC may be caused by mutations in either a gene encoding a ligand or a gene encoding its receptor. Although genetic heterogeneity is not a difficult concept to understand, it imposes considerable problems in analyzing genetic data[47] and makes use of these data for diagnosis impossible at this time.

DIAGNOSIS AND DIFFERENTIAL DIAGNOSIS

The clinical criteria developed by Gomez[58] were revised in 1992[59] and have evolved to reflect better understanding of variability of TSC (Table 166–8). Like NF1, there are no markers or blood tests to confirm a clinical diagnosis. The criteria have now been ranked in order of significance to distinguish between common but nonspecific features such as hypomelanotic macules and apparently pathognomonic features such as facial angiofibromas.

A cortical tuber or any of the six hamartomas listed under primary criteria are dependable diagnostic features by themselves. Multiple lesions are considered to be more reliable evidence than single ones, and histologic confirmation is better than visual or radiologic identification. Because some features are age related, their usefulness is limited for diagnosis of the young. Several specific features such as facial angiofibromas and ungual fibromas are simply not present at birth. Since it is not possible to have different criteria for different ages, there is a need to periodically reassess children at risk for TSC as they get older, just as in NF1.

Common lesions are more significant if associated with ones that are more specific for TSC. While some patients may defy classification, the criteria are structured so that a patient classified as having definitive TSC is virtually assured of having the disease. On the other hand, it may be very difficult to confirm the diagnosis in minimally affected cases.

Criteria are divided into primary, secondary, and tertiary levels. Diagnoses are also divided into three levels: definite, probable, and suspect. One feature from the primary category is required for an unquestionable, definitive diagnosis of TSC. A definite diagnosis can also be made with two secondary or one secondary and two tertiary features.[59]

The suggested evaluation for TSC includes a total-body cutaneous examination with a Wood's light and an ophthalmologic examination to look for retinal hamartomas. Echocardiography is suggested for all infants but is not helpful in adults.[60] An electroencephalogram is not

TABLE 166-8. Diagnostic Criteria* for Tuberous Sclerosis

Primary Features

Facial angiofibromas[†]
Multiple ungual fibromas[†]
Cortical tuber[‡]
Subependymal nodule or giant cell astrocytoma[‡]
Multiple calcified subependymal nodules protruding into the ventrical[§]
Multiple retinal astrocytomas[†]

Secondary Features

Affected first-degree relative
Cardiac rhabdomyoma[†§]
Other retinal hamartoma or achromic patch[†]
Cerebral tubers[§]
Noncalcified subependymal nodules[§]
Shagreen patch[†]
Forehead plaque[†]
Pulmonary lymphangiomyomatosis[‡]
Renal cysts[‡]

Tertiary Features

Hypomelanotic macules[†]
"Confetti" skin lesions[†]
Renal cysts[§]
Randomly distributed enamel pits in deciduous and/or permanent teeth
Hamartomatous rectal polyps[‡]
Bone cysts[§]
Pulmonary lymphangiomyomatosis[§]
Cerebral white matter "migration tracts" or heterotopias[§]
Gingival fibromas[†]
Hamartoma of other organs[‡]
Infantile spasms

*Definite: either one primary feature, two secondary features, or one secondary plus two tertiary features; Probable: either one secondary plus one tertiary feature or three tertiary features; and Suspect: either one secondary feature or two tertiary features.
[†]Histologic confirmation is not required *if* the lesions are clinically obvious.
[‡]Histologically confirmed.
[§]Radiographic evidence.
Data from Roach ES, Smith M, Huttenlocher P, et al. Report of the Diagnostic Criteria Committee of the National Tuberous Sclerosis Association. J Child Neurol 1992;7:221–224.

useful for diagnosis, but it is very helpful for management of seizures.

Although the calcified subependymal nodule is one of the most characteristic radiologic findings in TSC, and CT is superior to MRI in identifying these nodules (the head CT is abnormal in 89%),[37] MRI has emerged to be the test of choice for the diagnosis of TSC.[21, 61] Although the MRI is not as sensitive in locating calcifications, it can still identify subependymal nodules.[21, 62] The MRI, in fact, is frequently abnormal at birth[63] and is more sensitive than CT in the identification of cortical tubers.[62] The CT is still preferred by some[64] because even though it is less sensitive than MRI it is more specific and it is less expensive and more available. Since the advent of CT and MRI, conventional skull radiographs are no longer used to look for intracerebral calcifications.

A skeletal survey and renal ultrasound examination are not helpful for diagnosis.[34, 60] Radiographs may demonstrate cystic lesions of the metatarsals and metacarpals as well as osteomatous thickening of the skull, pelvis, and long bones.

For suspected asymptomatic carriers, the use of neuroimaging after a skin and eye examination is controversial;[60] but most clinicians suggest neuroimaging is useful if interpreted by a radiologist familiar with TSC. Because of the increased sensitivity, MRI is probably the test of choice in this setting.[21, 65]

There is no way to consistently diagnose TSC prenatally. Cardiac rhabdomyomas have been described as early as 22 to 24 weeks' gestation with fetal echocardiography[66] and cortical tubers and subependymal nodules have been visualized at 33 weeks' gestation using MRI.[67]

TREATMENT

Management of TSC consists of monitoring for and treatment of complications. Seventy percent of deaths in one study were potentially treatable or preventable.[49] Deaths from brain tumors can be reduced by monitoring with serial brain scans. MRI is preferable to CT in this regard since there is less radiation. Early surgical intervention for problem tumors and continued improvement of surgical techniques may reduce mortality further.[47] Seizures need to be aggressively controlled.[47] Radiographs for women of child-bearing age are useful to look for honeycomb lungs, and serial renal function studies are required because of the frequency of renal complications in adults with TSC.[49]

Genetic counseling is extremely important for families of persons with TSC. Since it is an autosomal dominant disorder with suspected complete penetrance, 50% of children of an affected parent are at risk. For families with an affected child in whom no evidence of TSC can be detected in either parent there is still a finite risk for transmission to future children. Since gonadal mosaicism and nonpenetrance can never be completely ruled out, the risk for having future children with TSC is probably 2% to 5%,[33] rather than the 1 in 10,000 risk that would be expected if the event were unrelated.

In many neurologically normal patients with TSC, the presenting complaint is unresponsive "acne" as the facial angiofibromas increase in size. Management of these lesions can substantially improve the quality of life. Surgical excision of facial angiofibromas can be performed, but this is limited to small areas of perinasal skin or particularly troublesome individual tumors in other sites. It is preferable to perform this procedure in stages for patients with multiple tumors, and punch excisions with suture closure can be utilized. Up to 15 lesions per session can be treated at 3- to 6-month intervals.

An alternate procedure is dermabrasion. However, the deeper half of the angiofibroma may remain after superficial dermabrasion. Dermabrasion may be an effective one-stage procedure but can result in atypical hypertrophic scarring. The scarring may be related to the technique, to the nature of the angiofibromas, or to the young age (preteen and early teen years) at which the dermabrasion may be performed. A reasonable compromise may be excision of larger tumors at a young age followed by superficial dermabrasion when the patient is older.

Facial angiofibromas can also be treated with various lasers. CO_2 laser ablation has been used successfully,[68-70] but the argon and other continuous-wave lasers are surprisingly effective in this condition, too.[71] The continuous-wave argon laser targets hemoglobin (chromophore) but causes significant tissue destruction beyond this target. The fibrosis and tissue shrinkage that follows treatment limits the usefulness of the argon laser in port-wine stains but is especially beneficial when treating individual angiofibromas. For lesions with a prominent vascular component, either the flashlamp pumped tunable dye, argon pumped tunable dye, copper vapor, or krypton lasers may be effective. Anesthesia may be required for some patients.

Surgical treatment of periungual fibromas may be indicated if the tumors are painful or disfiguring. These tumors usually arise under the proximal or lateral nail folds. Partial or complete nail avulsion may be required in some cases.[72] An electrosurgical instrument of CO_2 laser may be helpful to treat the base of the fibroma. When the fibroma occurs underneath the proximal nail fold, one must be careful to avoid damaging the extensor tendon attachment to the distal phalanx. The nail fold and matrix are no more than 1 to 2 mm away from this attachment. Thermal damage from electrosurgery may damage the adjacent normal tendon and restrict digital movement. The more precise CO_2 laser is preferable in this case. The procedures can be performed with local anesthesia after digital block with plain lidocaine. Lesions occasionally recur, but more often new lesions develop years later.

The shagreen patch, or collagenoma, seldom needs treatment since it is frequently asymptomatic, occurs on covered skin, and poses little cosmetic deformity. Excision, dermabrasion, and CO_2 or ND:YAG laser ablation might be considered under exceptional circumstances.

Proteus Syndrome

Proteus syndrome is a congenital hamartomatous condition that can involve any structure of the body. There are only about 50 reported cases to date.[73] It is named after the Greek god Proteus, whose name means "the polymorphous." The major manifestations are macrodactyly, regional gigantism, hemihypertrophy, a variety of subcutaneous masses, epidermal nevi, skull anomalies and other exostoses, scoliosis, hemangiomas, and cerebriform thickening of the palms and soles (see Fig. 166–4).[22, 73]

Proteus syndrome is often mistaken for other more common disorders, especially NF1. The "Elephant Man" may even have had Proteus syndrome.[74] It may be the result of a dominant lethal gene surviving by mosaicism.[75]

Leopard Syndrome

"Leopard" is an acronym for *l*entigines, *e*lectrocardiographic abnormalities, *o*cular hypertelorism, *p*ulmonary stenosis, *a*bnormal genitalia, *r*etarded growth, and *d*eafness. It is also known as lentiginosis-deafness-cardiomyopathy syndrome. The lentigines are present at birth and increase in number, size, and darkness with age. The cardiac disease requires the most medical attention.

References

1. Stumpf DA, Alksne JF, Annegers JF, et al. Neurofibromatosis. Arch Neurol 1987;45:575–578.
2. Lubs M-L, Bauer MS, Formas ME, Djokic B. Lisch nodules in neurofibromatosis type 1. N Engl J Med 1991;324:1264–1266.
3. Huson SM, Compston DAS, Harper PS. A genetic study of von Recklinghausen neurofibromatosis in South Wales: II. Guidelines for genetic counseling. J Med Genet 1989;26:712–721.
4. Charles SJ, Moore AT, Yates JRW, Ferguson-Smith MA. Lisch nodules in neurofibromatosis 2. Arch Ophthalmol 1989;107:1571–1572.
5. Listernick R, Charrow J, Greenwald MJ, Esterly NB. Optic gliomas in children with NF1. J Pediatr 1989;114:788–792.
6. McElhannon HM Jr. Congenital pseudarthrosis of the tibia. South Med J 1975;68:824–827.
7. Riccardi VM. Von Recklinghausen neurofibromatosis. N Engl J Med 1981;305:1617–1627.
8. Riccardi VM. Neurofibromatosis: Phenotype, Natural History, and Pathogenesis, 2nd ed. Baltimore: Johns Hopkins University Press. 1992:213–223; 280–316.
9. Cooper PH, Frierson HF, Kayne AL, Sabio H. Association of juvenile xanthogranuloma with juvenile myeloid leukemia. Arch Dermatol 1984;120:371–375.
10. Goldberg NS. Neurofibromatosis (von Recklinghausen's disease). In: Demis DJ, ed. Clinical Dermatology, 20th revision, vol 4, unit 24-2. Philadelphia: JB Lippincott, 1993.
11. Slater C, Hayes M, Saxe N, et al. Macromelanosomes in the early diagnosis of neurofibromatosis. Am J Dermatopathol 1986;8:284–289.
12. Wallace MR, Marchuk DA, Andersen LB, et al. Type 1 neurofibromatosis gene: Identification of a large transcript disrupted in three NF1 patients. Science 1990;249:181–186.
13. Goldberg NS, Collins FS. The hunt for the neurofibromatosis gene. Arch Dermatol 1991;127:1705–1707.
14. Xu G, O'Connell P, Viskochill D, et al. The NF type 1 gene encodes a protein related to GAP. Cell 1990;62:599–608.
15. Neurofibromatosis Conference Statement. Arch Neurol 1988;45:575–578.
16. Mulvihill JJ (moderator). Neurofibromatosis 1 (Recklinghausen's disease) and neurofibromatosis 2 (bilateral acoustic neurofibromatosis): An update. Ann Intern Med 1990;113:39–52.
17. Crowe FW, Schull WJ. Diagnostic importance of café-au-lait spot in neurofibromatosis. Arch Dermatol 1953;91:758–766.
18. Obringer AC, Meadows AT, Zackai EH. The diagnosis of NF1 in the child under the age of 6 years. Am J Dis Child 1989;143:717–719.
19. Hoffman KJ, Boehm CD. Familial neurofibromatosis type 1: Clinical experience with DNA testing. J Pediatr 1992;120:394–398.
20. Upadhyaya M, Fryer A, MacMilan J, Broadhead W, Hudson SM, Harper PS. Prenatal diagnosis and presymptomatic detection of neurofibromatosis type 1. J Med Genet 1992;29:180–183.
21. Truhan AP, Filipek PA. Magnetic resonance imaging: Its role in the neuroradiologic evaluation of neurofibromatosis, tuberous sclerosis, and Sturge-Weber syndrome. Arch Dermatol 1993;129:219–226.
22. Samlaska CP, Levin SW, James WD, Benson PM, Walker JC, Perlik PC. Proteus syndrome. Arch Dermatol 1989;125:1109–1114.

23. Sharland M, Taylor R, Patton MA, Jeffrey S. Absence of linkage of Noonan syndrome to the neurofibromatosis type 1 locus. J Med Genet 1992;29:188–190.
24. Bauer M, Lubs H, Lubs ML. Variable expressivity of NF1 in identical twins. Neurofibromatosis 1988;1:323–329.
25. Goldberg NS. What is segmental neurofibromatosis? J Am Acad Dermatol 1992;26:638–641.
25a. Arnsmeier AL, Riccardi VM, Paller AS. Familial multiple cafe au lait spots. Arch Dermatol 1994;130:1425–1426.
26. Bromley GS, Sherman JE, Goulian D. Neurofibromatosis: Distribution of lesions and surgical treatment. Ann Plast Surg 1982;8:272–276.
27. Roberts AH, Crockett DJ. An operation for the treatment of cutaneous neurofibromatosis. Br J Plast Surg 1987;38:292–293.
28. Hanke CW, Conner AC, Reed JC. Treatment of multiple facial neurofibromas with dermabrasion. J Dermatol Surg Oncol 1987;12:631–637.
29. Roenigk RK, Ratz JL. CO_2 laser treatment of cutaneous neurofibromas. J Dermatol Surg Oncol 1987;13:187–190.
30. Krueger W, Weisberger E, Bullantyne AJ, Goepfert H: Plexiform neurofibroma of the head and neck. Am J Surg 1979;138:517–520.
31. Hunt A, Lindenbaum RH, Tuberous sclerosis: A new estimate of prevalence within the Oxford region. J Med Genet 1984;21:272–277.
32. Sampson JR, Scahill SJ, Stephenson JBP, et al. Genetic aspects of tuberous sclerosis in the west of Scotland. J Med Genet 1989;26:28–31.
33. Osborne JP. Diagnosis of tuberous sclerosis. Arch Dis Child 1988;63:1423–1425.
34. Webb DW, Thomas RD, Osborne JP. Echocardiography and genetic counseling in tuberous sclerosis. J Med Genet 1992;29:487–489.
35. Weiderholt WC, Gomez MR, Kurland LT. Incidence and prevalence of tuberous sclerosis in Rochester, Minnesota, 1950 through 1982. Neurology 1985;35:600–602.
36. Zaremba J. Tuberous sclerosis: A clinical and genetic investigation. J Ment Defic Res 1968;12:63–80.
37. Gomez MR. Tuberous sclerosis. In: Gomez MR, ed. Neurocutaneous Diseases, A Practical Approach. Boston: Butterworths, 1987:30–52.
38. Gomez MR. Phenotypes of the tuberous sclerosis complex with a revision of the diagnostic criteria. Ann NY Acad Sci 1991;615:1–7.
39. Fitzpatrick TB. History and significance and white macules, earliest visible sign of tuberous sclerosis. Ann NY Acad Sci 1991;615:26–35.
40. Alper JC, Holmes LB. The incidence and significance of birthmarks in a cohort of 4,641 newborns. J Pediatr Dermatol 1983;1:58–68.
41. Vogt H. Zur Diagnostik der tuberosen Sklerose. Z Erforsch Behandl Jugendl Schwachsinns 1908;2:1–12.
42. Lagos JC, Gomez MR. Tuberous sclerosis: Reappraisal of a clinical entity. Mayo Clin Proc 1967;42:26–49.
43. Rogers RS. Dermatologic manifestations. In: Gomez MR, ed. Tuberous Sclerosis, 2nd ed. New York: Raven Press, 1988:111–132.
44. Rocha G, Winkleman, RK. Causes of death in patients with tuberous sclerosis. Arch Dermatol 1962;85:722–729.
45. Gomez MR. Neurologic and psychiatric features. In Gomez MR, ed. Tuberous Sclerosis, 2nd ed. New York: Raven Press, 1988:21–36.
46. Robertson DM. Ophthalmic findings. In: Gomez MR, ed. Tuberous Sclerosis, 2nd ed. New York: Raven Press, 1988:89–109.
47. Stefansson K. Tuberous sclerosis. Mayo Clin Proc 1991;66:868–871.
48. Stilwell TJ, Gomez MR, Kelalis PP. Renal lesions in tuberous sclerosis. J Urol 1987;138:477–481.
49. Shepherd CW, Gomez MR, Lie JT, Crowson CS. Mayo Clin Proc 1991;66:792–796.
50. Ostor AG, Fortune DW. Tuberous sclerosis initially seen as hydrops fetalis. Arch Pathol Lab Med 1978;102:34–39.
51. Sharp D, Robertson DM. Tuberous sclerosis in an infant of 28 weeks gestational age. Can J Neurol Sci 1983;10:59–62.
52. Kint A, Baran R. Histopathologic study of Koenen tumors: Are they different from acquired digital fibrokeratoma? J Am Acad Dermatol 1988;18:369–372.
53. Nickel WR, Reed WB. Tuberous sclerosis (review of cutaneous lesions). Arch Dermatol 1962;85:209–226.
54. Cassidy SB, Pagon RA, Pepin M, et al. Family studies in tuberous sclerosis: Evaluation of apparently unaffected parents. JAMA 1983;249:1302–1304.
55. Wilson J, Carter C. Genetics of tuberous sclerosis. Lancet 1978;1:340.
56. Michel JM, Diggle JH, Brice J, et al. Two half-siblings with tuberous sclerosis, polycystic kidneys, and hypertension. Dev Med Child Neurol 1983;25:239–244.
57. Haines JL, Short MP, Kwiatkowski DJ, et al. Localization of one gene for tuberous sclerosis within 9q32-9q34 and further evidence for heterogeneity. Am J Hum Genet 1991;49:764–772.
57a. European chromosome 16 tuberous sclerosis consortium. Cell 1993;75:1305–1315.
58. Gomez MR. Criteria for diagnosis. In: Gomez MR, ed. Tuberous Sclerosis, 2nd ed. New York: Raven Press, 1988:9–20.
59. Roach ES, Smith M, Huttenlocher P, et al. Report of the diagnostic criteria committee of the National Tuberous Sclerosis Association. J Child Neurol 1992;7:221–224.
60. Fryer AE, Chalmers AH, Osborne JP. The value of investigation for genetic counseling in tuberous sclerosis. J Med Genet 1990;27:217–223.
61. Nixon JR, Houser OW, Gomez MR, Okazaki H. Cerebral tuberous sclerosis MR imaging. Radiology 1989;170:869–873.
62. Roach ES, Williams DP, Laster DW. Magnetic resonance imaging in tuberous sclerosis. Arch Neurol 1987;44:301–303.
63. Altman NR, Purser RK, Post MJD. Tuberous sclerosis: Characteristics at CT and MR imaging. Radiology 1988;167:527–532.
64. Roach ES, Kerr J, Mendelsohn D, Laster DW, Raeside C. Diagnosis of symptomatic and asymptomatic gene carriers of tuberous sclerosis by CCT and MRI. Ann NY Acad Sci 1991;615:112–122.
65. Terwey B, Doose H. Tuberous sclerosis: Magnetic resonance imaging of the brain. Neuropediatrics 1987;18:67–69.
66. Crawford DC, Garrett C, Tynan M, Neville BG, Allan LD. Cardiac rhabdomyomata as a marker for the antenatal detection of tuberous sclerosis. J Med Genet 1983;20:303–312.
67. Mirlesse V, Wener H, Jacquemard F, et al. Magnetic resonance imaging in antenatal diagnosis of tuberous sclerosis. Lancet 1992;340:1163.
68. Spenier CW, Achauer BM, Vanderkam VM. Treatment of extensive adenoma sebaceum with a carbon dioxide laser. Ann Plast Surg 1988;20:586–589.
69. Weston J, Apfelberg DB, Maser MR et al. Carbon dioxide laser-abrasion treatment of adenoma sebaceum in tuberous sclerosis. Ann Plast Surg 1985;15:132–137.
70. Wheeland RG, Bailin PL, Kantor GR, et al. Treatment of adenoma sebaceum with carbon dioxide laser vaporization. J Dermatol Surg Oncol 1985;11:861–864.
71. Janniger CK, Goldberg DJ. Angiofibromas in tuberous sclerosis: Comparison of treatment by carbon dioxide and argon laser. J Dermatol Surg Oncol 1990;16:317–320.
72. Baran R, Haneke E. Management of neoplasms in the nail. In: Roenigk RK, Roenigk HH Jr, eds. Surgical Dermatology: Advances in Current Practice. St. Louis: CV Mosby, 1993:219–234.
73. Vaughn RY, Selinger AD, Howell CG, et al. Proteus syndrome: Diagnosis and surgical management. J Pediatr Surg 1993;28:5–10.
74. Cohen MM. Further diagnostic thoughts about the elephant man. Am J Med Genet 1988;29:777–782.
75. Lacombe D, Taieb A, Vergnes P, et al. Proteus syndrome in 7 patients: Clinical and genetic considerations. Genet Couns 1991;2:93–101.

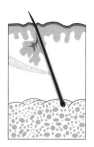
Basal Cell Nevus Syndrome

ERVIN EPSTEIN, JR.

DEFINITION

The basal cell nevus syndrome (BCNS) (nevoid basal cell carcinoma syndrome, Gorlin's syndrome, Gorlin-Golitz syndrome) is a rare inherited disorder characterized by one or more of a large number of abnormalities, most commonly cutaneous basal cell carcinomas, pits of the palms and soles, cysts of the jaws, and ectopic calcification of cranial membranes.

CLINICAL DESCRIPTION

Although patients with BCNS probably were described at least a century ago, the initial clear definition of the salient manifestations was published but 3 decades ago,[1, 2] and still unknown is the true incidence of some less common manifestations or even whether some abnormalities are truly due to a gene defect common to the BCNS as opposed to being present fortuitously in one or two patients with BCNS. The most comprehensive review of clinical manifestations is that of Gorlin,[3] and the most complete survey of abnormalities in a defined population of patients with BCNS is that of Evans and coworkers.[4] Although ascertainment bias may be difficult to avoid, one estimate of the prevalence of BCNS is 1 in 55,600,[4] and in one registry of hereditary tumors the number of families with BCNS was but 4 of 90, this being fewer than the number of families with any of the other studied heritable cancers: retinoblastoma, familial adenomatous polyposis, von Hippel-Lindau disease, and multiple endocrine neoplasia type II.[5]

Basal cell carcinomas are the hallmark of the syndrome, and patients may have several dozen or hundreds (Fig. 167–1). They typically begin around puberty, but the initial lesion may develop only in adulthood, and new tumors usually continue to appear even in later years. As is true of sporadic basal cell carcinomas, the tumors occur more commonly on sun-exposed areas and are fewer in black patients with BCNS. However, a greater percentage of basal cell carcinomas occur on the trunk in patients with BCNS than in patients with sporadic basal cell carcinomas (approximately 1:3 vs. 1:10), and the same study found no clear correlation between numbers of basal cell carcinomas and amount of (patient-reported) sun exposure.[6] Many of the basal cell carcinomas have an appearance no different from that of sporadic basal cell carcinomas, and their biologic behavior is similar: they metastasize only very rarely[7] and are occasionally locally aggressive, especially around the eyes and ears. Other lesions, especially on the trunk, may be more nonspecific, appearing as tiny nontranslucent papules that the unwary may misdiagnose as "tags" or nevi.

The second cutaneous abnormality characteristic of BCNS is the presence of pits of the palms and soles (Fig. 167–2). These are 1 to 3 mm in diameter, asymptomatic, ice pick-like defects in the stratum corneum. Occasionally they are red or, in manual workers, made more prominent by their accumulation of dirt.

The third commonly reported skin abnormality is the presence of superficial milia and of deeper cysts, the latter of which may be at unusual sites (e.g., the acra).

Jaw cysts (odontogenic keratocysts) are often the presenting sign of BCNS, beginning typically at the end of the first decade but sometimes developing initially much later.[8] These are usually asymptomatic but may present as jaw pain and swelling and may cause dysfunction, such as by causing loss of teeth or by eroding into a sinus.[9, 10] Usually more than one cyst is present. Radiolucencies in other bones are also common (e.g., at the fingers[11]), and sclerotic lesions of bones may be confused with metastatic disease.[12]

Another typical feature is calcification of the dural membranes separating the lobes of the brain, particularly

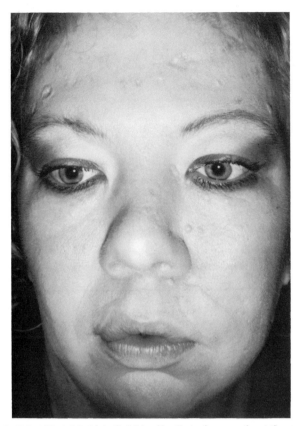

FIGURE 167–1. Multiple facial basal cell carcinomas about the nose, left inner canthus, forehead, and cheeks of this 32-year-old woman who has the typical "facies" of a patient with basal cell nevus syndrome. She has frontal bossing and ocular hypertelorism. (Courtesy of June K. Robinson, M.D.)

ably occur more often in patients with BCNS than in the general population, the more common tumors are medulloblastomas. These occur typically at age 2, considerably earlier than the age of development in patients with sporadic tumors. Although their exact incidence is unknown because they may cause death before other BCNS abnormalities are seen, an incidence of 3% to 5% is often quoted, and one study found that 1% to 2% of patients with medulloblastoma have BCNS.[14]

Ovarian fibromas also occur commonly. They do not inhibit fertility; they often calcify and so present on radiographic examination of the abdomen and pelvis with an unusual appearance that may be confused with calcified uterine leiomyomas; and they can become symptomatic if they twist on their pedicle, a complication requiring prompt surgical intervention to prevent destruction of the ovary. Although more commonly developing after adolescence, they have been reported rarely in young children.[15]

Cysts of the mesentery (lymphomesenteric cysts) may be large enough to be apparent on abdominal palpation. Calcification of the cyst walls can cause a balloon-like appearance on radiographic examinations.

Cardiac fibromas have been reported in young children with BCNS,[16, 17] as have fetal rhabdomyomas.[18]

of the falx cerebri. Like basal cell carcinomas, these calcifications develop earlier in life and in a higher percentage of patients with BCNS than in unaffected individuals.

The third type of skeletal abnormalities are "developmental" (i.e., abnormalities of bony outline). Bifid ribs and changes in skull shape are common. Also occasionally reported are marfanoid habitus (including tall stature, pectus carinatum or excavatum, long limbs), scoliosis, and shortened fourth metacarpals. Skull abnormalities that are usually considered characteristic of BCNS are a large head with bulging ("bossing") of the frontal and temporal bones, which gives the eyes a sunken appearance, and a protruding jaw. In one study, however, it was concluded that in families with BCNS only the probands (who, presumably, were affected more severely) and not other affected individuals have a frontal-occipital head circumference greater than that of a normal population of the same height.[13] Hence, many patients with BCNS have a "typical facies" but many lack any easily recognizable facial pattern. Other reported defects include cleft lip and palate in perhaps 5% of patients.[4]

Brain tumors are probably the most common fatal "complication" of BCNS. Although meningiomas prob-

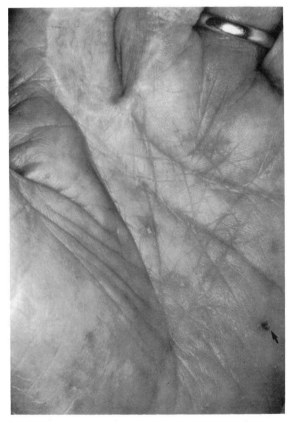

FIGURE 167–2. Palmar pits are individually located either in palmar creases or independent of them. Pits may be 1 to 4 mm in diameter with a violaceous base. The largest pit is marked with an arrow. (Courtesy of June K. Robinson, M.D.)

PATHOLOGY

The range of basal cell carcinomas seen in patients with BCNS is the same as that found in patients with sporadic basal cell carcinomas, as described in Chapter 141.[19] In patients with BCNS who have hundreds of small basal cell carcinomas, the neoplasms are often of the infundibulocystic type (Fig. 167–3) or "nevoid follicular" type.[20] This newly recognized pattern of basal cell carcinoma is believed to arise from vellus follicles. These well-circumscribed neoplasms are located in the superficial dermis and feature small cornifying cysts in the centers of club-like protrusions of cytologically bland basaloid cells. Infundibulocystic basal cell carcinomas were interpreted as trichoepitheliomas in some early reports of BCNS.

The palmar and plantar pits found in patients with BCNS are formed by dells in the normally hyperkeratotic surface of those sites, beneath which there is crowding of basaloid cells at the bases of rete ridges.[21] Rarely, fully developed basal cell carcinomas emanate from these foci.

Although most cutaneous cysts in patients with BCNS are simply infundibular or epidermoid follicular cysts, others are analogous to the odontogenic keratocysts of the jaw that are part of the syndrome.[22] These cysts are lined by squamous epithelium with a festooned inner layer that resembles the cuticular one found in steatocystoma.

PATHOGENESIS AND ETIOLOGY

BCNS is inherited as an autosomal dominant trait, although perhaps 50% to 60% of patients appear to represent new mutations and the fathers of such persons with sporadic cases tend to be older than the average father.[23] No obvious candidate gene has been proposed whose mutations might cause the multitude of phenotypic abnormalities, and the syndrome is possibly caused by the deletion of a region of DNA so large that it contains several genes, more than one of which causes the various abnormalities. Alternatively, the disrupted gene might be pleotropic; that is, it exerts a number of different actions. At this time it seems nearly certain that one function of the gene(s) is to act as a tumor suppressor gene, and it has been suggested for at least a decade[24] that the BCNS fits well with the Knudson model of two-hit carcinogenesis —that two mutations within a single cell are necessary to permit transformation of a cell from the normal to the tumorous state. It seems likely that sporadic basal cell carcinomas develop after ultraviolet irradiation causes mutations in both copies of a tumor suppressor gene whereas those in BCNS develop after such irradiation inactivates the single normal copy of such a gene, the first defect being inherited. After the validation of these hypotheses for inherited and sporadic retinoblastomas, several groups turned to investigation of the molecular genetics of BCNS. Thus far, these investigations have localized the site of the mutations in several dozen BCNS kindreds to a small region of the long arm of chromosome 9 (9q23.3-q34.1) and have indicated that in both sporadic and BCNS-associated basal cell carcinomas a large position of this arm of chromosome 9 is lost, resulting in certain loss of at least one allele of the region harboring the BCNS mutation. Of further interest is the localization of the gene whose mutation causes familial multiple keratoacanthomas to the same region of chromosome 9.[25] Thus one gene or a family of related genes (of previously unknown identity) on chromosome 9q appear to be of fundamental importance in epidermal carcinogenesis, and it is likely that its identity will soon be known.

The function of this gene must still be a matter of speculation. Although basal cell carcinomas in patients with BCNS, as in those with sporadic cases, do not appear to develop strictly as a function of sun exposure,[6, 26] their preponderance in sun-exposed regions and their greatly diminished incidence in patients of African descent suggest that ultraviolet mutagenesis is of at least some importance and that the normal function of the BCNS gene may be in repair of DNA damage. Further clinical evidence implicating faulty DNA repair is the increased sensitivity to x-ray carcinogenesis. There are multiple reports of patients developing numerous basal cell carcinomas in the areas of therapeutic irradiation of medulloblastomas and doing so in a period far shorter

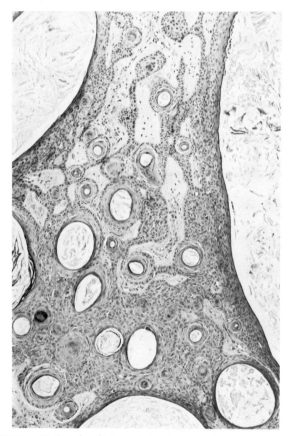

FIGURE 167–3. Infundibulocystic basal cell carcinoma is commonly found incidentally in patients with basal cell nevus syndrome. The pattern seen here is characteristic and shows cords of basaloid and squamous keratinocytes interspersed with small bulbous foci that form keratinizing cysts.

than that expected for x-ray induction of cancers in non–BCNS patients (e.g., 2 years instead of 2 decades). In addition, there is one report of multiple basal cell carcinomas of the hands developing 2 decades after superficial x-irradiation of atopic dermatitis of the hands,[27] and I have seen several members of one kindred with BCNS who developed basal cell carcinomas of the feet several decades after repeated exposure to fluoroscopy irradiation while working in the family shoe store.

Despite these clinical observations, most investigators have found that cells cultured from patients with BCNS unlike, for instance, those from patients with xeroderma pigmentosum have minimal to no detectable abnormal sensitivity to ultraviolet or x-irradiation. One exception is a study in which ultraviolet B light (instead of the otherwise uniformly used shorter wave ultraviolet C light) was used.[28]

DIAGNOSIS AND DIFFERENTIAL DIAGNOSIS

In most instances, the combination of several basal cell carcinomas at a young age, jaw cysts, and palmoplantar pits allows for a ready diagnosis. However, since no single pathognomonic abnormality occurs solely in patients with BCNS and not in otherwise normal individuals, since abnormalities develop in some persons only well into adult life, and since extensive clinical data on the age at onset of different manifestations (studied by different diagnostic interventions) are not available, diagnosis is often uncertain, especially if no family members have more typical abnormalities. In an effort to codify the diagnosis for less typical patients,[4] it was suggested that diagnosis requires two major or one major plus two minor criteria, the major being multiple basal cell carcinomas by 30 years old, odontogenic keratocyst or polystotic bone cyst, three or more palmar or plantar pits, early (by 20 years old) falx calcification, and family history of BCNS. The minor criteria include large skull, cardiac or ovarian fibroma, medulloblastoma, lymphomesenteric cysts, skeletal anomaly, or congenital abnormality such as cleft lip or palate, and polydactyly. In one series of 84 patients, by age 20, 73% had developed a basal cell carcinoma and 82% had developed a jaw cyst, the corresponding numbers at 40 years of age each being 91%. Similarly, in one large family, all patients eventually diagnosed as having BCNS had developed one or more abnormalities (basal cell carcinomas, jaw cysts, or palmar or plantar pits) by age 18 and two or more by age 25.[29]

Differential diagnosis from the point of view of the dermatologist, includes only (1) those patients who develop multiple basal cell carcinomas but have no other phenotypic abnormalities of the BCNS, their underlying defect (if any) being unknown but possibly related to BCNS, and (2) patients with arsenic-induced skin cancers. The latter can be differentiated by their usual development of more squamous cell carcinomas than basal cell carcinomas, by their pigmentary abnormalities, and by the presence on their palms and soles of elevated keratoses rather than depressed pits.

TABLE 167–1. Treatment of Basal Cell Nevus Syndrome
Treatment of Patients with Basal Cell Nevus Syndrome
1. Regular follow-up with complete cutaneous examination for early detection of lesions
2. Sun protection
3. Genetic counseling
4. Dental examinations with surgical treatment of jaw cysts
5. Topical 5-fluorouracil to reduce formation of new lesions
6. Systemic etretinate to prevent new tumor formation may be effective for short periods (1 mg/kg)
Treatment of Individual Lesions of Basal Cell Carcinoma
1. Excisional surgery
2. Electrodesiccation and curettage
3. Cryotherapy
4. Mohs' micrographic surgery

5. Emerging methods
   a. Photodynamic therapy with hematoporphyrin derivative and 630-nm light
   b. Immunotherapy

6. Radiation therapy is contraindicated

TREATMENT

The primary treatment of basal cell carcinomas is the same as that of sporadic basal cell carcinomas—physical destruction (Table 167–1). Differences are those of selection of methods of destruction. Thus, although basal cell carcinomas of the perioral and periauricular areas and of the scalp pose greater threats and therefore require more aggressive management (e.g., by excision), the smaller papules on other areas can be treated for example by cryotherapy without biopsy since their large numbers and generally nonaggressive nature make more vigorous approaches much less attractive. Topical 5-fluorouracil and/or retinoic acid have been reported to reduce the numbers of basal cell carcinomas[30] as has photodynamic therapy. In addition, there is fairly impressive evidence that oral retinoids can retard or stop the development of basal cell carcinomas.[31, 32] Unfortunately, side effects from the dose required for therapeutic efficacy frequently preclude their prolonged use. Of utmost importance is a high frequency of examinations and of treatment of basal cell carcinomas when the tumors are small, and visits as often as monthly may be necessary.

The treatment of jaw keratocysts, like that of visceral tumors and cysts, is surgical. Whether such treatment should be conservative or aggressive is a matter of dispute, but recurrences of keratocysts in patients with BCNS, like those that occur sporadically, are quite common.[33, 34]

References

1. Howell JB, Caro MR. Basal cell nevus: Its relationship to multiple cutaneous cancers and associated anomalies of development. Arch Dermatol 1959;79:67–80.

2. Gorlin RJ, Goltz RW. Multiple nevoid basal cell epithelioma, jaw cysts, and bifid ribs: A syndrome. N Engl J Med 1960;262: 908–912.
3. Gorlin RJ. Nevoid basal cell carcinoma syndrome. Medicine 1987;66:98–113.
4. Evans DGR, Ladusans EJ, Rimmer S, et al. Complications of the naevoid basal cell carcinoma syndrome: Results of a population based study. J Med Genet 1993;30:460–464.
5. Littler M, Harper PS. A regional register for inherited cancers. Br J Med 1989;298:1689–1691.
6. Goldstein AM, Bale SJ, Peck GL, DiGiovanna JJ. Sun exposure and basal cell carcinomas in the nevoid basal cell carcinoma syndrome. J Am Acad Dermatol 1993;29:34–41.
7. Winkler PA, Guyuron B. Multiple metastases from basal cell naevus syndrome. Br J Plastic Surg 1987;40:528–531.
8. Rayner CR, Towers JF, Wilson JSP. What is Gorlin's syndrome? The diagnosis and management of the basal cell naevus syndrome, based on a study of thirty-seven patients. Br J Plast Surg 1976;30:62–67.
9. Friedlander AH, Herbosa EG, Peoples JR. Ocular hypertelorism, facial basal cell carcinomas, and multiple odontogenic keratocysts of the jaws. J Am Dent Assoc 1988;116:887–889.
10. Mustaciuolo VW, Brahney CP, Aria AA. Recurrent keratocysts in basal cell nevus syndrome: Review of the literature and report of a case. J Oral Maxillofac Surg 1989;47:870–873.
11. Dunnick NR, Head GL, Peck GL, Yoder FW. Nevoid basal cell carcinoma syndrome: Radiographic manifestations including cyst-like lesions of the phalanges. Radiology 1978;127:331–334.
12. Yee KC, Tan CY, Bhatt KB, Davies AM. Case report: Sclerotic bone lesions in Gorlin's syndrome. Br J Radiol 1993;66:77–80.
13. Bale SJ, Amos CI, Parry DM, Bale AE. Relationship between head circumference and height in normal adults and in the nevoid basal cell carcinoma syndrome and neurofibromatosis type I. Am J Med Genet 1991;40:206–210.
14. Evans DGR, Farndon PA, Burnell LD, et al. The incidence of Gorlin syndrome in 173 consecutive cases of medulloblastoma. Br J Cancer 1991;64:959–961.
15. Johnson AD, Hebert AA, Esterly NB. Nevoid basal cell carcinoma syndrome: Bilateral ovarian fibromas in a 3½-year-old girl. J Am Acad Dermatol 1986;14:371–374.
16. Cotton JL, Kavey R-EW, Palmier CE, Tunnessen WW Jr. Cardiac tumors and the nevoid basal cell carcinoma syndrome. Pediatrics 1991;87:725–727.
17. Herman TE, Siegel MJ, McAlister WH. Cardiac tumor in Gorlin syndrome. Pediatr Radiol 1991;21:234–235.
18. DiSanto S, Abt AB, Boal DK, Krummel TM. Fetal rhabdomyoma and nevoid basal cell carcinoma syndrome. Pediatr Pathol 1992;12:441–447.
19. Lindberg H, Jepsen FL. The nevoid basal cell carcinoma syndrome: Histopathology of the basal cell tumors. J Cutan Pathol 1983;10:68–73.
20. Walsh N, Ackerman AB. Infundibulocystic basal cell carcinoma: A newly described variant. Mod Pathol 1990;3:599–608.
21. Howell JB, Mehregan AH. Pursuit of the pits in the nevoid basal cell carcinoma syndrome. Arch Dermatol 1970;102:586–597.
22. Barr RJ, Headley JL, Jensen JL, Howell JB. Cutaneous keratocysts of the nevoid basal cell carcinoma syndrome. J Am Acad Dermatol 1986;14:572–576.
23. Jones KL, Smith DW, Harvey MS, et al. Older paternal age and fresh gene mutation: Data on additional disorders. J Pediatrics 1975;86:84–88.
24. Howell JB. Nevoid basal cell carcinoma syndrome: Profile of genetic and environmental factors in oncogenesis. J Am Acad Dermatol 1984;11:98–104.
25. Goudie DR, Yuille MAR, Leversha MA, et al. Multiple self-healing squamous epitheliomata (ESSI) mapped to chromosome 9q22-q31 in families with common ancestry. Nature Genet 1993;3: 165–169.
26. Vitasa BC, Taylor HR, Strickland PT, et al. Association of nonmelanoma skin cancer and actinic keratosis with cumulative solar ultraviolet exposure in Maryland watermen. Cancer 1990;65:2811–2817.
27. Golitz LE, Norris DA, Leukens CA Jr, Charles DM. Nevoid basal cell carcinoma syndrome: Multiple basal cell carcinomas of the palms after radiation therapy. Arch Dermatol 1980;116: 1159–1163.
28. Applegate LA, Goldberg LH, Ley RD, Ananthaswamy HN. Hypersensitivity of skin fibroblasts from basal cell nevus syndrome patients to killing by ultraviolet B but not by ultraviolet C radiation. Cancer Res 1990;50:637–641.
29. Bare JW, Lebo RV, Epstein EH Jr. Loss of heterozygosity at chromosome 1q22 in basal cell carcinomas and exclusion of the basal cell nevus syndrome gene from this site. Cancer Res 1992;52:1494–1498.
30. Strange PR, Lang PG. Long-term management of basal cell nevus syndrome with topical tretinoin and 5-fluorouracil. J Am Acad Dermatol 1992;27:842–845.
31. Hodak E, Ginzburg A, David M, Sandbank M. Etretinate treatment of the nevoid basal cell carcinoma syndrome. Int J Dermatol 1987;26:606–609.
32. Peck GL, DiGiovanna JJ, Sarnoff DS, et al. Treatment and prevention of basal cell carcinoma with oral isotretinoin. J Am Acad Dermatol 1988;19:176–185.
33. Forssell K, Forssell H, Kahnberg K-E. Recurrence of keratocysts: A long-term follow-up study. Int J Oral Maxillofac Surg 1988;17:25–28.
34. Peled M, Kohn Y, Laufer D. Conservative approach to unerupted teeth within cystic lesions in Gorlin's syndrome. Am J Orthodont Dentofac Orthop 1991;99:294–297.

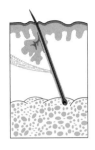

chapter 168

Xeroderma Pigmentosum

JAMES E. CLEAVER and JOHN EPSTEIN

DEFINITION

Xeroderma pigmentosum and the related diseases Cockayne syndrome and trichothiodystrophy are rare genetic diseases inherited as autosomal recessive traits,[1] with an incidence of about 1 per million in Europe and the United States[2, 3] and a higher incidence in Japan[4] and the Middle East.[3]

CLINICAL DESCRIPTION

Xeroderma pigmentosum is characterized by an inordinate susceptibility to develop photodamage and sun-induced skin cancers due, apparently, to ultraviolet (UV) radiation. The skin is normal at birth, and changes are usually first noted between 6 months and 3 years of age but occasionally later.[2, 3, 5] Initial skin changes consist of freckling and dryness of sun-exposed skin (Fig. 168–1). With progression, telangiectasia, angiomas, then depigmented atrophic macules, crusts, ulcers, warty growths, actinic keratoses, and at times vesiculobullous lesions occur. The skin develops the poikilodermatous appearance of chronic, severe actinic damage, leading to skin cancers of all types, especially squamous cell carcinoma and melanoma.[3-5]

Cutaneous Changes

Basal cell carcinomas and squamous cell carcinomas, which are primarily sun induced, are the most common cancers in the general population[6, 7] and in patients with xeroderma pigmentosum.[3] In patients with xeroderma pigmentosum, these malignancies occur at a much higher rate and a much earlier age.[3, 8] Keratoacanthomas, angiomas, and fibrosarcomas also occur in patients with xeroderma pigmentosum.

Malignant melanoma is the third most common skin cancer in patients with xeroderma pigmentosum, as it is in the general U.S. population,[9] but it involves the face, head, and neck significantly less often than do basal cell carcinoma and squamous cell carcinoma.[5, 9, 10] Thus, as with the general population, the role of the sun and the mechanism of its effect on melanoma formation is certainly not as clear as it is for the nonmelanoma skin cancers, even in patients with xeroderma pigmentosum. A 10- to 20-fold increase in internal malignancies over age-matched controls has been reported.[8]

Ocular Changes

Sunlight-induced changes appear primarily on the eyelids, the conjunctivae, and the cornea.[3] Photophobia may be one of the earliest symptoms of the disease. Blepharospasm and conjunctivitis without infection are common. Macular pigmentation, symblepharon, telangiectasia, pinguecula, and pterygium formation of the conjunctivae occur. Corneal vascularization, clouding, keratitis, and ulcers may be seen, with the subsequent development of corneal opacities. The eyelids show the same changes as the adjacent skin. Atrophy of the eyelids, loss of lashes, ectropion, and entropion have also been noted. Squamous cell carcinoma, basal cell carcinoma, and melanomas of the ocular tissues and limbus are almost exclusive to these sun-exposed structures.[3]

Neurologic Abnormalities

Neurologic changes can be important associated symptoms in xeroderma pigmentosum involving up to 18% of patients (Table 168–1).[3]

Oral Changes

Severe atrophy and cancers of the oral structures also appear to be due to sun exposure. In the oral cavity, the

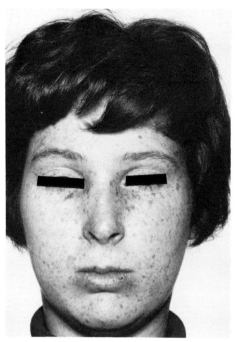

FIGURE 168-1. Freckling and atrophy are typical of the facies of xeroderma pigmentosum.

tip of the tongue may show telangiectasias and other changes, including squamous cell carcinoma.[8]

Photosensitivity

Abnormal acute responses to sun exposure may often be the earliest skin abnormality in patients with xeroderma pigmentosum. These include exaggerated sunburn reaction, delayed appearance of and/or the peak of erythema, excessive persistence of the erythema, telangiectasia and pigmentation persisting for several months, and light and electron microscopic evidence of chronic sun damage following a single UV exposure.[3, 5, 11-14] The clinical action spectrum appears to fall primarily in the UVB range (290–320 nm). Cripps and Ramsay,[11] using a monochromatic source, demonstrated that a patient with xeroderma pigmentosum was most sensitive to 293-nm radiation but responded with erythema into the UVA range up to 340 nm. The minimal erythema dose to UVB radiation is usually normal in patients with xeroderma pigmentosum, and certainly some patients tan without an acute photosensitivity reaction.[13] Some evidence also exists for impaired immune function.[15, 16] Xeroderma pigmentosum cells show a much reduced level of catalase activity, unlike DNA repair-deficient trichothiodystrophy cells, which have normal catalase activity.[17]

Clinical Disease and Complementation Groups

The preceding clinical discussion considered xeroderma pigmentosum generally as a single entity. Cock-

ayne syndrome is a related disease of skin sensitivity to sunlight with other developmental and neurologic abnormalities, but sunlight-induced skin cancers are not more frequent in this disease (see Table 168–1). A small number of patients with both xeroderma pigmentosum and Cockayne syndrome or with both xeroderma pigmentosum and trichothiodystrophy have been reported, suggesting that a single complex xeroderma pigmentosum/ Cockayne syndrome/trichothiodystrophy disease entity should be considered.[18] With the use of complementation (cell hybridization) techniques, the three diseases have been shown to have genetic heterogeneity at the molecular level. Seven groups of xeroderma pigmentosum (A–G) have been classified as showing reduced DNA repair synthesis.[1] An eighth type, named the xeroderma pigmentosum variant, with a postreplication repair defect has also been described (see Table

TABLE 168-1. Clinical Hallmarks of Xeroderma Pigmentosum and Cockayne Syndrome

Clinical Feature	Xeroderma Pigmentosum	Cockayne Syndrome
Solar sensitivity	+	+
Actinic skin changes (especially basal cell and squamous cell carcinoma, melanoma)	+	−
Skin cancers	+	−
Eye abnormalities		
Optic atrophy	−	+
Conjunctivitis	+	−
Cataracts	−	+
Lid atrophy and neoplasia	+	−
Corneal ulcers and scarring	+	−
Pigmentary retinopathy/ degeneration	−	+
Other*		
Mental retardation	+	+
Seizures	+	−
Sensorineural hearing loss	+	+
Microcephaly	+	+
Hyporeflexia	+[†]	−
Poor linear growth	+	+
Cachetic dwarfism	−	+
Skeletal dysplasia	−	+
Large ears, beak nose, long extremities	−	+
Brain abnormalities (shown by imaging)		
Cortical atrophy	+	+
Cerebella atrophy	−	+
Olivopontocerebellar atrophy	+	−
Demyelination	−	+
Basal ganglia calcifications	−	+
Peripheral nerve abnormalities (shown by biopsy)		
Patchy or generalized demyelination	−	+
Neuronal degeneration	+	−
Axon dropout	+	−

*In xeroderma pigmentosum, the neurologic changes are mainly confined to groups A, B, D, and G and can be variable.
†Progressive.
Modified from Greenhaw GA, Hebert A, Duke-Woodside ME, et al. Xeroderma pigmentosum and Cockayne syndrome: Overlapping clinical and biochemical phenotypes. Am J Hum Genet 1992;50: 677–689. University of Chicago, publisher.

168–1).[19–21] Two groups (A, B) with Cockayne syndrome alone[22] and several with various forms of trichothiodystrophy are also known. The two known families in xeroderma pigmentosum group B also exhibit clinical symptoms of Cockayne syndrome, and occasional patients in xeroderma pigmentosum group D show additional symptoms of Cockayne syndrome or trichothiodystrophy.[18] A new complementation group for repair has been identified for a patient with trichothiodystrophy.[23]

Course and Prognosis

In the largest review of patients with xeroderma pigmentosum, only 5% were older than 45 years of age.[3] The average age of death at that time (1975) was 30 years younger than that of the general U.S. population.[24] The cause of death, when recorded, was most commonly cancer and less commonly infection or various other complications. A few patients have a normal life span.

PATHOLOGY

The neoplasms that arise in the skin of patients with xeroderma pigmentosum are indistinguishable from their sporadic counterparts. Malignant melanomas, on occasion, arise in contiguity with solar lentigines in patients with xeroderma pigmentosum, which has led to speculation that the lentigines are precursors of melanoma.

The non-neoplastic skin of patients with xeroderma pigmentosum shows the changes that would be seen in chronic severe solar aging, namely, elastosis of the dermis, telangiectases, solar lentigines, basilar hypopigmentation and hyperpigmentation, and melanophages. Scattered keratinocyte nuclei are typical even in the absence of clinically evident lesions, and small foci of compact hyperkeratosis are common.

PATHOGENESIS AND ETIOLOGY

Xeroderma pigmentosum is due to a genetic defect in the biochemical pathways by which damage caused by sunlight (UVB) to DNA is processed to eliminate its carcinogenic potential. The UVB portion of the solar spectrum is undoubtedly the major factor in skin cancer.[6, 7] Action spectra for squamous carcinoma indicate that DNA is the target molecule; the absorption spectrum of DNA correlates well with lethality, mutation induction, and photoproduct formation. The energy absorbed by DNA produces molecular changes, of which the most important are the dimerized photoproducts between adjacent pyrimidines.[25]

The two major photoproducts induced are the cyclobutane pyrimidine dimer and, at about one fourth the frequency, the pyrimidine-pyrimidone (6-4) photoproduct. The ratio of thymine–cytosine cyclobutane dimers to thymine–thymine dimers increases significantly with increasing wavelength in the UVB region. In conjunction with (6-4) photoproducts, which are preferentially induced at thymine–cytosine dipyrimidines, cytosine dimeric lesions may play a major role in UVB (solar) mutagenesis. The (6-4) photoproduct can further undergo a UVB-dependent conversion to its valence photoisomer, the Dewar pyrimidinone.

These photoproducts are repaired by nucleotide excision repair, which replaces them with newly synthesized patches. Several hierarchical levels of regulation set priorities for the repair of various photoproducts and sites in DNA. In the genome overall, (6-4) photoproducts are excised much more rapidly than cyclobutane dimers; 50% of (6-4) photoproducts can be excised in 2 to 6 hours, whereas cyclobutane dimers require 12 to 24 hours.[26] Actively transcribed genes are more rapidly repaired.[27, 28] Within the actively expressed genes, the transcribed strands are repaired faster than the untranscribed strands.[29] The mechanisms underlying these processes can be understood with reference to the various genes involved in the seven excision-defective xeroderma pigmentosum and two Cockayne syndrome complementation groups.

The existence of multiple complementation groups indicates that the initial step of excision involves cooperative action between multiple proteins that bind to damaged sites and to each other to unwind and modify the sites before endonuclease cleavage; the proteins are then displaced by helicases and polymerases. Most of the genes represented by these xeroderma pigmentosum complementation groups have now been cloned and chromosome locations have been identified (Table 168–2), and their functions during excision have been inferred from their DNA sequence and from functions of similar genes in other organisms, especially yeast (see Table 168–2). One repair gene, ERCCI, is not yet associated with any known disease. Several genes, notably those for xeroderma pigmentosum groups B, D, and G, and Cockayne syndrome group B, code for components of transcription factors, the protein complexes that bind to promoter regions and control gene transcription.[30–33]

To a first approximation, repair can be envisaged to operate by the following sequence of events. Photoproducts are highlighted in the genome by the binding of the xeroderma pigmentosum group A and group E gene products. These are photoproduct-specific DNA-binding proteins that have greater affinity for (6-4) photoproducts than for dimers and may bind more readily in the open chromatin of transcriptionally active genes than in untranscribed chromatin.[34–37] Repair is then directed to damaged sites in active genes by the components of transcription factor TFIIH, some of which have helicase function and may serve to partially unwind DNA during transcription and briefly reverse the direction of the transcription apparatus when it stops at damaged sites.[33] Untranscribed regions of the genome are rendered accessible by the functions of the xeroderma pigmentosum group C gene.[38] The damaged regions of the genome are then excised in a 29- to 30-nucleotide piece[39] by a two-protein complex of ERCCI and XPF, which, by analogy with their yeast (Saccharomyces cerevisiae) homologues, Rad 10 and Rad 1, respectively, may form a single-strand–specific nuclease.[40] After excision, the single-

TABLE 168-2. Xeroderma Pigmentosum, Cockayne Syndrome, and Other Repair Genes

Gene	Chromosome Location	Coding Size	Repair Synthesis (%)	Function
XPA	9q34.1	273 aa	2–5	Binding protein *
XPB	2q21	782 aa	3–7	Transcription factor[†]
XPC	3	823 aa	10–20	Inactive gene repair
XPD	19q13.2	760 aa	25–50	Transcription factor[†]
XPE	11	140/41 kd	40–50	2 subunit (120 kd, 40 kd) binding protein*
XPF	16p13		18	Nuclease[‡]
XPG	13q32-33	1330 aa	<2	Transcription factor
XPV			100	Replication factor
ERCCI	19q13.2	297 aa	0	Nuclease[‡]
CSA			100	Coupling factor[§]
CSB	10q21.1	1493 aa	100	Coupling factor[§]
TTDA[‖]			15	

*DNA-binding proteins with higher binding coefficients for (6–4) photoproducts than for dimers.

[†]Components of TFIIH basal transcription factor.

[‡]Xeroderma pigmentosum group F and ERCCI may, like their homologues in *S. cerevisiae* (Rad 1 and Rad 10), form a complex that has single-strand–specific nuclease activity.

[§]These factors are believed to couple transcription apparatus to excision repair and regulate pyrimidine dimer excision exclusively in transcribed genes.

[‖]Two cases of repair deficiency in trichothiodystrophy that complement each other and all excision-defective XP groups are now known. These are designated as the repair genes *TTDA* and *TTDB*.

strand group is protected by single-strand–specific binding protein, also known as RFA, and filled in by polymerase α or δ and proliferating cell nuclear antigen,[41] and the final gap is sealed by DNA ligase.

There may be at least two routes to the complex clinical symptoms of xeroderma pigmentosum, Cockayne syndrome, and trichothiodystrophy. Much of the reduced genomic repair deficiency that includes transcriptionally active regions, such as that seen in xeroderma pigmentosum group A and most group D patients, may result in neuronal decline because of oxidative damage generated but unrepaired in brain and neuronal tissue.[42] The absence of central nervous system symptoms in xeroderma pigmentosum group C, which retains repair of transcribed genes, would be consistent with this idea. Developmental disorders of bone, central nervous system, and retina, such as those seen in Cockayne syndrome and xeroderma pigmentosum group B and occasionally group D, may result from mutations in regions of the proteins that are involved in their dual function of controlling transcription as well as repair.[33] These transcription factors may have pleiotropic effects on many genes in developing tissues, especially neuronal tissues, which require transcription of a larger fraction of the whole suite of human genes than most other tissues. Answers to these questions may now be within reach with the new technique of gene replacement and the use of transgenic animals.

DIAGNOSIS AND DIFFERENTIAL DIAGNOSIS

The primary diagnosis of xeroderma pigmentosum, Cockayne syndrome, or trichothiodystrophy is based on the clinical presentation of the patient (see Table 168–1). Some cases of extensive sun exposure in fair-skinned individuals can mimic xeroderma pigmentosum, and some patients who are sun sensitive but do not fall easily into these categories have been identified.[43, 44] At higher latitudes, very mild cases of xeroderma pigmentosum, especially group E, may blend sufficiently into the general population to be regarded as asymptomatic.

Once a clinical diagnosis has been made, it can be confirmed by laboratory studies. Methods that are particularly useful are (1) determination of UV sensitivity, which would confirm xeroderma pigmentosum groups A through G and Cockayne syndrome groups A and B[45]; (2) determination of deficiencies in DNA repair by unscheduled DNA synthesis or other methods, which will identify xeroderma pigmentosum groups A through G; and (3) determination of the retarded recovery of RNA synthesis after UV irradiation in cultures with normal DNA repair, which will identify Cockayne syndrome groups A and B.[22] The xeroderma pigmentosum variant remains a difficult group for which to make a positive diagnosis, because many laboratory studies do not distinguish variants from normal cells.[21] Eventually, when the spectrum of mutations in xeroderma pigmentosum genes is known, a DNA diagnostic procedure should become available. When families have been confirmed as being at risk for xeroderma pigmentosum, Cockayne syndrome, or trichothiodystrophy, prenatal diagnosis is feasible and has been attempted by several routes. In one systematic study, xeroderma pigmentosum or Cockayne syndrome in the extant child was confirmed in laboratory studies and prenatal studies were carried out for a total of 12 pregnancies in 10 families.[46] In every case, a diagnosis was made within the time necessary for families to plan the pregnancy outcome. Positive diagnoses were made in two pregnancies, not significantly different from expected. (Currently, patient diagnosis is being developed by Dr. David Busch, Armed Forces Institute of Pathology, Washington, DC, and prenatal diagnosis is offered by Dr. James E. Cleaver, University of California, San Francisco.)

TREATMENT

The best therapy is prevention of UV-induced mutation—avoiding exposure to the sun by means of clothing or potent sunscreens and even avoiding exposure during the day before damage occurs[47]—but most patients with xeroderma pigmentosum have already been damaged before precautions could be taken. However, protection is advisable at all stages. Cancers should be removed as soon as possible. Dermabrasion, dermatome shaving, excision and grafting, and topical application of 5-fluorouracil have been used to remove damaged skin with variable success.

A pharmacologic approach to cancer prevention by using retinoids[48] has been applied to xeroderma pigmentosum.[49] 13-*cis*-Retinoic acid was effective in reducing cancer formation, but its toxicity precluded continued use[49]; the development of less toxic derivatives would be worthwhile.

The current treatment regimen is based on improving DNA repair with a small phage T4 endonuclease, endoV, that is encapsulated into liposomes (T4N5).[50, 51] This preparation increases DNA repair synthesis after UV irradiation by 30% in normal human fibroblasts and by 80% in XP12BE cells.[52, 53] It also significantly increases survival of irradiated cells in culture. In mice, T4N5 liposome preparation applied topically reduced UV-induced skin cancers[54] and prevented the suppression of delayed hypersensitivity and contact hypersensitivity induced by UV.[55] This preparation is now being examined for its potential beneficial effects on the skin of patients with xeroderma pigmentosum.

References

1. Cleaver JE, Kraemer KH. Xeroderma pigmentosum. In: Scriver CR, Beaudet AL, Sly WS, eds. The Metabolic Basis of Inherited Disease, vol 2. New York: McGraw-Hill, 1989:2949–2971.
2. Kraemer KH. Hereditary diseases with increased sensitivity to cellular injury. In: Fitzpatrick TB, Eisen AZ, Wolff K, et al., eds. Dermatology in General Medicine. New York: McGraw-Hill. In press.
3. Kraemer KH, Lee MM, Scotto J. Xeroderma pigmentosum: Cutaneous, ocular, and neurologic abnormalities in 830 published cases. Arch Dermatol 1987;123:241–250.
4. Takebe H, Nishigori C, Satoh Y. Genetics and skin cancer of xeroderma pigmentosum in Japan. Jpn J Cancer Res 1987; 78:1135–1143.
5. Epstein JH. Xeroderma pigmentosum and UVL carcinogenesis. In: Fitzpatrick TB, Pathak MA, Harber LC, et al., eds. Sunlight and Man: Normal and Abnormal Photobiological Responses. Tokyo: University of Tokyo Press, 1974:299–315.
6. Urbach F, Epstein JH, Forbes PD. Ultraviolet carcinogenesis: Experimental, global, and genetic aspects. In: Fitzpatrick TB, Pathak MA, Harber LC, et al., eds. Sunlight and Man: Normal and Abnormal Photobiological Responses. Tokyo: University of Tokyo Press, 1974:259–283.
7. Urbach F, ed. The Biologic Effects of Ultraviolet Radiation, with Emphasis on the Skin. Oxford: Pergamon Press, 1969:3–21.
8. Kraemer KH, Lee MM, Scotto J. DNA repair protects against cutaneous and internal neoplasia: Evidence from xeroderma pigmentosum. Carcinogenesis 1984;5:511–514.
9. Kraemer KH, Lee MM, Andrews AD, et al. The role of sunlight and DNA repair in melanoma and nonmelanoma skin cancer: The xeroderma pigmentosum paradigm. J Invest Dermatol. In press.
10. Surveillance, Epidemiology, and End Results: Incidence and Mortality Data, 1973–77. National Cancer Institute Monograph, vol 57. Bethesda, MD: National Institutes of Health, 1981.
11. Cripps DJ, Ramsay CA, Ruch DM. Xeroderma pigmentosum: Abnormal monochromatic action spectrum and autoradiographic studies. J Invest Dermatol 1971;56:281–286.
12. Robbins JH, Kraemer KH, Lutzner MA, et al. Xeroderma pigmentosum: An inherited disease with sun sensitivity, multiple cutaneous neoplasms, and abnormal DNA repair. Ann Intern Med 1974;80:221–248.
13. Ramsay CA, Giannelli F. The erythemal action spectrum and deoxyribonucleic acid synthesis in xeroderma pigmentosum. Br J Dermatol 1975;92:49–56.
14. Ichihashi M, Fujiwara Y. Clinical and photobiological characteristics of Japanese xeroderma pigmentosum variant. Br J Dermatol 1981;105:1–12.
15. Morison WL, Bucana C, Hashem N, et al. Impaired immune function in patients with xeroderma pigmentosum. Cancer Res 1985;45:3929–3931.
16. Norris PG, Limb GA, Hamblin AS, et al. Immune function, mutant frequency, and cancer risk in the DNA repair defective genodermatoses xeroderma pigmentosum, Cockayne's syndrome, and trichothiodystrophy. J Invest Dermatol 1990;94:94–100.
17. Vuillaume M, Daya-Grosjean L, Vincens P, et al. Striking differences in cellular catalase activity between two DNA repair-deficient diseases: Xeroderma pigmentosum and trichothiodystrophy. Carcinogenesis 1992;13:321–328.
18. Wood RD. DNA repair. Seven genes for three diseases (news). Nature 1991;350:190.
19. Burk PG, Lutzner MA, Clarke DD, et al. Ultraviolet-stimulated thymidine incorporation in xeroderma pigmentosum lymphocytes. J Lab Clin Med 1971;77:759–767.
20. Cleaver JE, Greene AE, Coriell LL, et al. Xeroderma pigmentosum variants. Cytogenet Cell Genet 1981;31:188–192.
21. Hessel A, Siegle RJ, Mitchell DL, et al. Xeroderma pigmentosum variant with multisystem involvement. Arch Dermatol 1992; 128:1233–1237.
22. Lehmann AR. Three complementation groups in Cockayne syndrome. Mutat Res 1982;106:347–356.
23. Stefanini M, Vermeulen W, Weeda G, et al. A new nucleotide-excision-repair gene associated with the disorder trichothiodystrophy. Am J Hum Genet 1993;53:817–821.
24. Vital Statistics of the United States, 1975: Life Tables, Hyattsville, MD: U.S. Department of Health, Education, and Welfare, 1977.
25. Cleaver JE, Mitchell DL. Ultraviolet radiation carcinogenesis. In: Holland JF, Frei E III, Bast RC Jr, et al., eds. Cancer Medicine. London: Lea & Febiger, 1993:245–255.
26. Cleaver JE, Cortes F, Lutze LH, et al. Unique DNA repair properties of a xeroderma pigmentosum revertant. Mol Cell Biol 1987; 7:3353–3357.
27. Bohr VA. Gene specific DNA repair. Carcinogenesis 1991;12: 1983–1992.
28. Terleth C, van de Putte P, Brouwer J. New insights in DNA repair: Preferential repair of transcriptionally active DNA. Mutagenesis 1991;6:103–111.
29. Mellon I, Bohr VA, Smith CA, et al. Preferential DNA repair of an active gene in human cells. Proc Natl Acad Sci USA 1986; 83:8878–8882.
30. Park E, Guzder SN, Koken MH, et al. RAD25 (SSL2), the yeast homolog of the human xeroderma pigmentosum group B DNA repair gene, is essential for viability. Proc Natl Acad Sci USA 1992;89:11416–11420.
31. Gulyas KD, Donahue TF. SSL2, a suppressor of a stem-loop mutation in the HIS4 leader encodes the yeast homolog of human ERCC-3. Cell 1992;69:1031–1042.
32. Schaeffer L, Roy R, Humbert S, et al. DNA repair helicase: A component of BTF2 (TFIIH) basic transcription factor. Science 1993;260:58–63.
33. Bootsma D, Hoeijmakers JH. DNA repair: Engagement with transcription (news; comment). Nature 1993;363:114–115.
34. Robins P, Jones CJ, Biggerstaff M, et al. Complementation of DNA repair in xeroderma pigmentosum group A cell extracts

by a protein with affinity for damaged DNA. EMBO J 1991; 10:3913–3921.

35. McLenigan M, Levine AS, Protic M. Differential expression of pyrimidine dimer-binding proteins in normal and UV light-treated vertebrate cells. Photochem Photobiol 1993;57:655–662.

36. Abramic M, Levine AS, Protic M. Purification of an ultraviolet-inducible, damage-specific DNA-binding protein from primate cells. J Biol Chem 1991;266:22493–22500.

37. Takao M, Abramic M, Moos M Jr, et al. A 127 kDa component of a UV-damaged DNA-binding complex, which is defective in some xeroderma pigmentosum group E patients, is homologous to a slime mold protein. Nucl Acids Res 1993;21:4111–4118.

38. Legerski R, Peterson C. Expression cloning of a human DNA repair gene involved in xeroderma pigmentosum group C. Nature 1992;360:610.

39. Huang JC, Svoboda DL, Reardon JT, et al. Human nucleotide excision nuclease removes thymine dimers from DNA by incising the 22nd phosphodiester bond 5′ and the 6th phosphodiester bond 3′ to the photodimer. Proc Natl Acad Sci USA 1992; 89:3664–3668.

40. Tomkinson AE, Bardwell AJ, Bardwell L, et al. Yeast DNA repair and recombination proteins Rad1 and Rad10 constitute a single-stranded-DNA endonuclease. Nature 1993;362:860–862.

41. Shivji KK, Kenny MK, Wood RD. Proliferating cell nuclear antigen is required for DNA excision repair. Cell 1992;69:367–374.

42. Satoh MS, Jones CJ, Wood RD, et al. DNA excision-repair defect of xeroderma pigmentosum prevents removal of a class of oxygen free radical-induced base lesions. Proc Natl Acad Sci USA 1993;90:6335–6339.

43. Greenhaw GA, Hebert A, Duke-Woodside ME, et al. Xeroderma pigmentosum and Cockayne syndrome: Overlapping clinical and biochemical phenotypes. Am J Hum Genet 1992;50:677–689.

44. Cleaver JE, Thomas GH. Clinical syndromes associated with DNA repair deficiency and enhanced sun sensitivity (editorial). Arch Dermatol 1993;129:348–350.

45. Cleaver JE, Thomas GH. Rapid diagnosis of sensitivity to ultraviolet light in fibroblasts from dermatologic disorders, with particular reference to xeroderma pigmentosum. J Invest Dermatol 1988; 90:467–471.

46. Cleaver JE, Volpe J, Charles WC, et al. Prenatal diagnosis of xeroderma pigmentosum and Cockayne syndrome. Prenat Diagn, in press.

47. Davis BE, Koh HK, Rohrer TE, et al. Sunlight avoidance and cancer prevention in xeroderma pigmentosum. Arch Dermatol 1994;130:806–808.

48. Bertram JS, Kolonel LN, Meyskens FL Jr. Rationale and strategies for chemoprevention of cancer in humans. Cancer Res 1987;47: 3012–3031.

49. Kraemer KH, DiGiovanna JJ, Moshell AN, et al. Prevention of skin cancer in xeroderma pigmentosum with the use of oral isotretinoin. N Engl J Med 1988;318:1633–1637.

50. Yarosh DB. Topical application of liposomes. J Photochem Photobiol 1990;6:445–449.

51. Ceccoli J, Rosales N, Tsimis J, et al. Encapsulation of the UV-DNA repair enzyme T4 endonuclease V in liposomes and delivery to human cells. J Invest Dermatol 1989;93:190–194.

52. Kibitel JT, Yee V, Yarosh DB. Enhancement of ultraviolet-DNA repair in denV gene transfectants and T4 endonuclease V-liposome recipients. J Photochem Photobiol 1991;54:753–760.

53. Yarosh DB, Kibitel JT, Green LA, et al. Enhanced unscheduled DNA synthesis in UV-irradiated human skin explants treated with T4N5 liposomes. J Invest Dermatol 1991;97:147–150.

54. Yarosh D, Alas LG, Yee V, et al. Pyrimidine dimer removal enhanced by DNA repair liposomes reduces the incidence of UV skin cancer in mice. Cancer Res 1992;52:4227–4231.

55. Kripke ML, Cox PA, Alas LG, et al. Pyrimidine dimers in DNA initiate systemic immunosuppression in UV-irradiated mice. Proc Natl Acad Sci USA 1992;89:7516–7520.

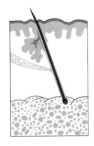

chapter 169

The Porphyrias

MAUREEN B. POH-FITZPATRICK

DEFINITION

Porphyrias are a group of inherited or acquired disorders that result from partial deficiency in activities of the enzymes of the heme biosynthetic pathway. Each porphyria is associated with a specific defective enzyme (Table 169–1), the reduced activity of which results in accumulation of intermediaries or by-products of the pathway in a characteristic pattern.

CLINICAL DESCRIPTION

Although accurate epidemiologic statistics for the prevalence of porphyrias are not available on a worldwide basis, these disorders occur sufficiently commonly to ensure that individuals with porphyria will eventually present to virtually every practicing dermatologist.

Porphyric syndromes share many clinical and pathophysiologic similarities, but they also have many differences. Thus, although some aspects of porphyrias can be discussed in common and some differences can be summarized in tables, many aspects related to only one or a subset of the group are covered in a separate section of this chapter devoted to each syndrome.

Porphyrias are divisible into hepatic or erythropoietic types according to the site in which the heme synthetic defect is predominantly expressed (Table 169–2). Porphyrias can also be divided into those manifesting either cutaneous photosensitivity or neurovisceral symptomatology or both (Table 169–3). Among porphyrias with photocutaneous manifestations, division is possible between those exhibiting immediate or delayed phototoxicity (Table 169–4). Porphyrin-sensitized immediate phototoxicity occurs during or shortly after sunlight exposure and is typified by stinging or burning pain fol-

lowed by erythema, edema, and purpura. Immediate phototoxicity is induced by protoporphyrin, a hydrophobic molecule. Delayed porphyrin-sensitized photocutaneous lesions are induced by the more hydrophilic porphyrins and are indistinguishable among the several forms of porphyrias in which hydrophilic porphyrins accumulate: mechanical fragility, subepidermal blistering with subsequent milia formation and scarring, scarring alopecia, hypertrichosis, pigmentary changes, sclerodermoid lesions that may become calcified, and photoonycholysis.

Classification by inheritance pattern is given in Table 169–5.

The major determinant of porphyrin accumulation patterns, and of the resultant clinical syndromes, is the perturbation of heme biosynthesis created by a particular enzymatic defect. Knowledge of the operation and regulation of this pathway is the key to understanding the biochemical and clinical abnormalities that define each porphyria.

THE HEME BIOSYNTHETIC PATHWAY

The heme biosynthetic pathway is shown in Figure 169–1. Reduced activity of any of its enzymes results in accumulation of its substrates. Large amounts of accumulated substrates escape conversion into pathway intermediaries and enter the blood circulation, either unchanged or as oxidized byproducts of the pathway. The early pathway intermediaries aminolevulinic acid (ALA), porphobilinogen (PBG), and hydroxymethylbilane are molecules termed *porphyrin precursors*. Several subsequent intermediaries in the pathway are cyclic tetrapyrrole molecules termed *porphyrinogens*. Porphyrinogens have eight side chains that may bear carboxyl groups ranging in number from eight (uroporphyrinogen) to two (protoporphyrinogen). Oxidation of porphyrinogens results in formation of porphyrins of similar carboxyl number. This can occur spontaneously, after which the

This work was supported by research grant 5RO1 AR18549 from the National Institute for Arthritis, Musculoskeletal and Skin Diseases.

TABLE 169-1. Enzyme Defects Associated with Porphyrias

Defect	Affected Enzyme
Aminolevulinic acid dehydratase porphyria	Aminolevulinic acid dehydratase (porphobilinogen synthase)
Acute intermittent porphyria	Porphobilinogen deaminase (formerly uroporphyrinogen I synthase)
Congenital erythropoietic porphyria	Uroporphyrinogen III synthase (formerly uroporphyrinogen cosynthase)
Porphyria cutanea tarda	Uroporphyrinogen decarboxylase
Hepatoerythropoietic porphyria	Uroporphyrinogen decarboxalase
Hereditary coproporphyria	Coproporphyrinogen oxidase
Variegate porphyria	Protoporphyrinogen oxidase
Erythropoietic protoporphyria	Ferrochelatase (heme synthase)

TABLE 169-3. Major Manifestations of Porphyrias

Cutaneous
Porphyria cutanea tarda
Erythropoietic protoporphyria
Congenital erythropoietic porphyria
Variegate porphyria—variable
Hereditary coproporphyria—30%

Neurovisceral
Acute intermittent porphyria
Aminolevulinic acid dehydratase porphyria
Hereditary coproporphyria
Variegate porphyria—variable

porphyrins cannot be metabolized further and become byproducts that accumulate in tissues, enter the circulation, and are excreted. The last porphyrinogen in the pathway (protoporphyrinogen) is enzymatically converted to the only intermediary that is a true porphyrin (protoporphyrin).

Porphyrins are red-brown crystalline pigments that are photoactive and cause photosensitivity; porphyrinogens and the porphyrin precursors are colorless and not photoactive. Porphyrins and precursors vary greatly in water solubility; molecules with greater hydrophilicity occur earlier in the pathway. Progressive decarboxylation reduces water solubility. The most hydrophilic compounds (ALA, PBG, and the 8-carboxylic porphyrins) are excreted almost entirely into the urine. The 4-carboxyl coproporphyrins have intermediate solubility properties; these compounds are found in feces as well as urine. The 2-carboxyl protoporphyrin is hydrophobic and is cleared from circulation by hepatobiliary mechanisms and excreted in feces. Physicochemical properties of porphyrins and precursors affect their tissue distribution and the signs and symptoms they may cause.

Two "dead end" branches in the pathway become important when one of two enzymes that normally facili-

tate catalysis along the primary pathway has reduced activity. This first occurs at the point of conversion of hydroxymethylbilane to uroporphyrinogen. To form the isomer III uroporphyrinogen, enzymatic action is required. With deficient activity of uroporphyinogen III synthase, hydroxymethylbilane spontaneously cyclizes to the isomer I uroporphyrinogen.[1] Coproporphyrinogen I is not further metabolized toward heme. The second branch point is at conversion of the 5-carboxylic porphyrinogen to coproporphyrinogen by uroporphyrinogen decarboxylase. With defective uroporphyrinogen decarboxylase activity, 5-carboxylic porphyrinogen undergoes dehydrogenation and decarboxylation catalyzed by coproporphyrinogen oxidase, to form dehydroisocoproporphyrinogen, which eventuates in isocoproporphyrin. Isocoproporphyrin has no physiologic use; it accumulates and is excreted, predominantly in feces.[2]

Accumulation of porphyrins and porphyrin precursors leads to an array of signs and symptoms that typify each clinical syndrome. Characteristic patterns of these metabolites in blood, urine, and feces distinguish porphyrias biochemically and are the usual means of confirming clinical diagnostic suspicions in the laboratory (see Table 169–9).

Although heme biosynthesis proceeds through the same metabolic steps catalyzed by the same sequence of enzymes in erythropoietic and hepatic cells, mechanisms

TABLE 169-2. Major Tissue Source of Excess Porphyrins

Erythropoietic
Protoporphyria (EPP)
Congenital erythropoietic porphyria (CEP)

Hepatic
Acute intermittent porphyria (AIP)
ALA dehydratase porphyria (ALADP)
Porphyria cutanea tarda (PCT)
Variegate porphyria (VP)
Hereditary coproporphyria (HCP)

TABLE 169-4. Phototoxicity Patterns in Porphyrias

Immediate (erythema, edema, pain, purpura)
Erythropoietic protoporphyria

Delayed (fragility, blistering, scarring)
Porphyria cutanea tarda
Hepatoerythropoietic porphyria
Congenital erythropoietic porphyria
Variegate porphyria
Hereditary coproporphyria

TABLE 169-5. Inheritance Patterns of Porphyrias

Autosomal Dominant

Acute intermittent porphyria
Variegate porphyria
Hereditary coproporphyria
Porphyria cutanea tarda
Erythropoietic protoporphyria (some families)

Autosomal Recessive

Congenital erythropoietic porphyria
Aminolevulinic acid dehydratase porphyria
Erythropoietic protoporphyria (some families)

TABLE 169-6. Treatment of Erythropoietic Protoporphyria

Photosensitivity

Physical sunscreens
Beta-carotene
Hypertransfusion

Hepatobiliary Complications

Cholecystectomy, cholelithectomy
Oral adsorbents (cholestyramine, charcoal)
Vitamin E
Bile acids
Iron
Exchange transfusion
Liver transplantation

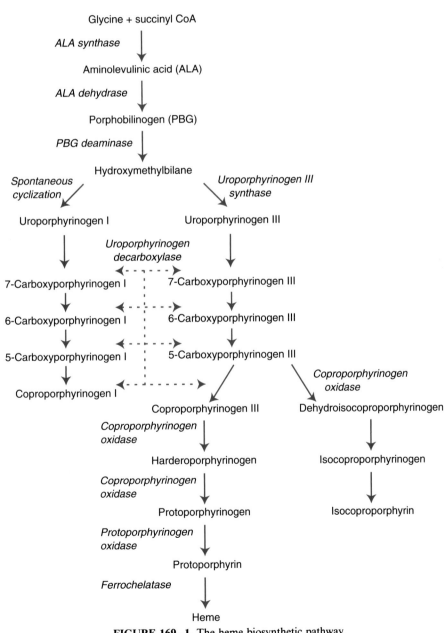

FIGURE 169-1. The heme biosynthetic pathway.

regulating its function in the two cell lines differ in several respects. Details of the complex control mechanisms of heme biosynthesis are beyond the scope of this chapter but can be found elsewhere.[1]

PHOTOCHEMISTRY AND PHOTOBIOLOGY OF PORPHYRINS AND PORPHYRIAS

The electronic configuration of porphyrin molecules permits their absorption of light radiation, with major absorption peaks in the visible violet spectral range (400–410 nm). Long ultraviolet and longer visible light wavelengths can also photoexcite porphyrin molecules, but less strongly. The absorbed energy creates electronically excited-state molecules that can emit light energy (fluorescence), react directly with other biomolecules, or transfer excitation energy to oxygen, creating highly reactive oxygen species. Porphyrin-sensitized toxic-oxygen–dependent events of biologic importance include peroxidation of cell membrane lipids,[3] cross-linking of cell membrane and intracellular proteins,[4-6] inhibition of cell membrane–associated, cytosolic and mitochondrial enzymes,[7-10] loss of membrane integrity and function,[5-7, 9-11] and disruption of intracellular organelles.[12-16] The different kinds of cutaneous lesions that typify various porphyrias apparently result from cascades of events that differ qualitatively or quantitatively (or both) depending on the physiocochemical properties of the porphyrin sensitizers.[9] Events such as disruption of endothelial cell membranes,[14] complement activation,[17] mast cell degranulation with release of inflammatory mediators and proteases,[14, 16] neutrophil recruitment,[14, 17] lysosomal disruption with release of hydrolases and other enzymes,[12, 18] actions of released hydrolases and proteases on structural proteins such as elements of the basement membrane zone or on functional proteins such as enzymes, and perhaps others yet to be elucidated, appear to play interconnected roles in the evolution of the various clinical lesions. Expanded discussions of this complex and still largely speculative topic are available.[19-22]

THE ERYTHROPOIETIC PORPHYRIAS

Congenital Erythropoietic Porphyria

Congenital erythropoietic porphyria (CEP) is an autosomal recessive disorder in which defective activity of uroporphyrinogen III synthase leads to accumulation of the isomer I series of porphyrins (uroporphyrin I to coproporphyrin I) in erythroid cells. These porphyrins are released into plasma by hemolysis or diffusion; are deposited in tissues, bones, and teeth; and are excreted in urine and feces. The diagnosis is often manifested in the neonatal period by pink staining of diapers by porphyrin pigment in urine. Adult-onset cases have also been observed.[23, 24]

CEP is typified by marked cutaneous photosensitivity of the delayed type (Fig. 169–2). Urine, bones, and teeth are stained red-brown. Hemolytic anemia with spleno-

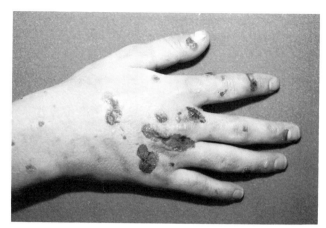

FIGURE 169–2. Hand of a 13-year-old boy with congenital erythropoietic porphyria showing typical lesions of delayed-type porphyric photosensitivity. Blistering, crusted erosions, milia, and photoonycholysis of the thumbnail are evident.

megaly is common; bony fragility has been observed.[25] Some patients are far less severely affected than others.[26]

Laboratory diagnosis is based on demonstration of increased levels of the isomer I porphyrins in blood and urine. In some patients, a large proportion of the abnormally elevated erythrocyte porphyrin content may be zinc protoporphyrin.[26] Assay of the activity of uroporphyrinogen III synthase is the most specific diagnostic test but is a research procedure and is not generally available. The differential diagnosis includes disorders that may present in childhood with porphyrinuria and bullous cutaneous photosensitivity: hepatoerythropoietic porphyria, childhood-onset porphyria cutanea tarda, or rare cases of homozygous inheritance of hepatic porphyrias typically transmitted as autosomal dominant traits. CEP is often distinguishable by its porphyrin biochemical profile in blood, urine, and feces, but in some cases evaluation at a research center that can determine isomer composition of excess porphyrins or assay the activity of uroporphyrinogen III synthase may be required. Rarely, other blistering disorders may simulate CEP, but CEP can be readily excluded by demonstration of normal porphyrin levels in erythrocytes, plasma, and urine.

Treatment of the cutaneous photosensitivity begins with sunlight avoidance; topical sunscreens are not useful unless formulated to block long ultraviolet and visible light wavelengths. Oral beta-carotene for photoprotection typically offers only limited benefit; guidelines for its use are given in the following section on erythropoietic protoporphyria. Circulating porphyrin levels can be lowered by inhibiting erythropoiesis: hypertransfusion regimens[25, 27] and chemically induced bone marrow suppression[28] have been effective in reducing clinical and biochemical disease expression. Splenectomy may decrease the rate of erythrocyte destruction but is not invariably associated with lasting biochemical or clinical benefit. The risks of therapies must be carefully weighed against the severity of the disorder in each individual case.

Erythropoietic Protoporphyria

Typically presenting in childhood as immediate phototoxicity with stinging, burning, erythema, and edema of skin developing within minutes to an hour or so of sunlight exposure, followed by a painful purpura, erythropoietic protoporphyria (EPP) occurs far more frequently than CEP. Vesiculation or hypertrichosis is infrequent. Exposed skin, especially of the dorsum of the hands and occasionally of the face, may become thickened, waxy, leathery, or hyperkeratotic (Fig. 169–3). Facial skin may bear scattered shallow elliptical or linear scars and linear perioral furrowing. Anemia, if present, is typically mild. There is an increased incidence of cholelithiasis at unusually early ages in both males and females. Life-threatening hepatic dysfunction may develop at any age.

A recent study of ferrochelatase activity in several families with EPP suggests that inheritance of more than one gene mutation encoding this enzyme defect may be necessary for disease expression in some families.[29]

Laboratory diagnosis is based on demonstration of increased protoporphyrin in erythrocytes, plasma, and feces, all of which are normal in cases of solar urticaria, the major differential diagnosis for EPP. Urinary porphyrins are normal in EPP unless hepatic failure occurs, producing coproporphyrinuria.

Immediate porphyrin-induced phototoxicity produces acute cutaneous signs and symptoms. Biopsy specimens from the acute wheal-like lesions of EPP demonstrate sparse perivascular and interstitial neutrophilic infiltrates that can invite confusion with solar urticaria. Specimens of long-standing lesions of EPP examined by light microscopy most often reflect effects of chronic damage: markedly thickened papillary dermal capillary walls and an amorphous, hyaline material deposited perivascularly and scattered throughout the dermis.[30, 31] Similar abnormalities, although typically of lesser severity around dermal vessels and more prominent at the dermoepidermal junction, are found in chronically damaged skin in the delayed-type photosensitivity porphyrias, of which porphyria cutanea tarda is the most common.[30, 32]

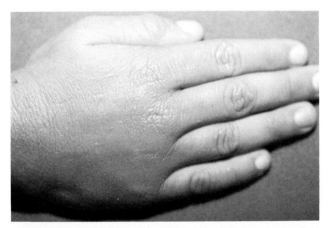

FIGURE 169–3. Hand of a boy with erythropoietic protoporphyria showing chronic changes of thickened skin with accentuated skin markings over the knuckles. A few small scars are present.

Treatment of EPP (see Table 169–6) begins with avoidance of sun exposure. Solar tolerance may be reduced by prior exposure, with dramatically lowered thresholds on days following those during which enough sunlight has been encountered to produce mild tingling.[33] Topical sunscreens must block long ultraviolet and visible light wavelengths to be effective. Preparations containing titanium dioxide or zinc oxide offer the protection of physical barriers; those with agents absorbing well into the ultraviolet A spectrum afford some benefit. Many individuals with EPP can increase their solar tolerance with oral beta-carotene in amounts sufficient to produce carotenodermia.[34] Typical adult doses are 120 to 180 mg per day, increasing to 300 mg per day if efficacy is inadequate at lower doses. Children's doses range from 30 to 120 mg per day. For very young children, the beta-carotene capsules can be opened and the beadlets inside mixed with applesauce or chocolate syrup to facilitate swallowing. Solar tolerance increases slowly; 3 to 4 weeks of treatment may be necessary to reach full benefit. In many latitudes, treatment is needed only in spring and summer months.

Hypertransfusion has been used to ameliorate photosensitivity by reducing endogeneous erythropoiesis, thus reducing porphyrin production.[35] As in CEP, the potential benefits of hypertransfusion must be weighed against the risks of allergic reactions, iron loading, and blood-born infectious diseases.

The dire prognosis of protoporphyrin-induced hepatic dysfunction warrants vigorous medical intervention. Oral cholestyramine resin[36–38] has been used to sequester protoporphyrin in the enteric tract, thus protecting the liver from the toxic effects of its enterohepatic recirculation. Vitamin E has been given concomitantly in the hope of regulating hyperactive porphyrin synthesis. Administration of iron has been followed by clinical improvement in a few cases[37, 39] but has been linked to exacerbation of photosensitivity in others.[40] Infusion of heme analogues, agents apparently effective in "acute attack" porphyrias by reducing hepatic heme synthesis by negative feedback repression of the rate-limiting enzyme ALA synthase, may affect erythropoietic heme synthesis as well[41, 42] but is not suited to long-term treatment. Hypertransfusion or exchange transfusion[37, 43] to reduce new porphyrin formation in the marrow may alleviate protoporphyrin hepatotoxicity; in this potentially fatal context, benefits of reducing the porphyrin load on the liver outweigh the several risks. Administration of cholic acid[38] or chenodeoxycholic acid,[44] in the hope of increasing biliary secretion of protoporphyrin, thus reducing its toxic effects on the liver, yielded mixed results suggesting that further study is needed to clarify the effects of bile acids in this context. Liver transplantation is indicated as a last resort.[45]

Cholecystectomy does not present any more risk for those with EPP than for nonporphyric individuals with gallstones. A potential problem at surgery in patients with EPP was observed after liver transplantation: exposure of skin and intra-abdominal organs to intense operating theater illumination caused porphyrin-sensitized damage with adverse postoperative sequelae.[45] It is probable that patients with EPP with liver failure, who typically have very high circulating prophyrin levels compared with those with gallstones but relatively intact liver function, are at far greater risk of this complication.

THE HEPATIC PORPHYRIAS

Porphyria Cutanea Tarda

Porphyria cutanea tarda (PCT) is the only porphyria with both familial and acquired forms. Heterozygous inheritance of a gene mutation encoding partial deficiency of the activity of the enzyme uroporphyrinogen decarboxylase results in a disorder that presents typically in adults but occasionally in children. Childhood PCT is usually of the familial type. Homozygous inheritance of mutant genes results in a PCT-like disorder in childhood termed *hepatoerythropoietic porphyria* (HEP). Children with HEP can be differentiated from those with heterozygous PCT by demonstration of increased levels of zinc photoporphyrin in erythrocytes of those with HEP but not PCT. Measurement of residual erythrocyte uroporphyrinogen decarboxylase activity also permits differentiation: heterozygous inheritance of a mutant allele results in residual activity of approximately 50% of normal controls, while inheritance of two mutations yields residual activities in the range of 5% to 30%.[46-48]

Clinical signs of PCT and HEP include darkening of the urine and cutaneous photosensitivity of the delayed type, most often manifested by blistering, milia, scarring, and hypertrichosis of sun-exposed skin (Figs. 169–4 and 169–5). Other cutaneous signs (pigmentary changes, sclerodermoid lesions, dystrophic calcification, alopecia,

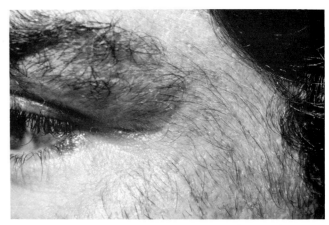

FIGURE 169–5. Facial hypertrichosis in a case of porphyria cutanea tarda. (From Poh-Fitzpatrick MB. The porphyrias. Dermatol Clin 1987;5:55–61.)

photoonycholysis) are variably present; occasionally sclerodermoid changes occur alone. PCT (and HEP) is confirmed in the laboratory by demonstration of the excess porphyrin by-products resulting from the enzyme defect: chiefly uroporphyrin and heptacarboxylic porphyrins in urine and plasma or serum and isocoproporphyrin in feces.[49] In most familial cases of PCT, deficient activity of uroporphyrinogen decarboxylase can be detected in erythrocytes as well as in liver cells, whereas in acquired or sporadic cases the erythrocyte enzyme activity is normal.[50] In some families, PCT occurs with normal erythrocyte enzyme activity.[51]

In sporadic or acquired PCT, and in many familial cases, disease expression requires exposure to additional factors or circumstances: ethanol intake, estrogenic hormone therapies, certain aromatic hydrocarbon hepatotoxins, causes of increased iron stores, or dialysis treatment of chronic renal disease.[52] Serologic evidence of exposure to hepatitis B[53] or C[54] viruses or human immunodeficiency virus[55] is increasingly recognized. Increased incidences of abnormal glucose tolerance and antinuclear antibody tests and of hepatocellular carcinoma are linked to PCT.[52]

In PCT (and in all other porphyrias manifesting delayed-type phototoxicity) bullae form subepidermally and are characterized by "festooning," or upward protrusion of dermal papillae into the blister cavity and little or no dermal inflammatory infiltrate (Fig. 169–6).[32, 56] Sinuous, segmented eosinophilic structures termed *caterpillar bodies,* representing basement membrane material surrounded by degenerating keratinocytes, are seen in the roofs of vesicles in all of the bullous forms of porphyria, including porphyria-like blistering eruptions caused by drugs.[57] Ultrastructural examination of the dermal capillaries and dermoepidermal junction in all porphyrias with photocutaneous manifestations reveals replicated vascular and epidermal basement membranes, suggesting multiple incidents of repair of photodamaged vascular and dermoepidermal junctional elements.[30-32] Deposition of mucopolysaccharides, immunoglobulins, and complement can be demonstrated in these regions.[30] Replication of basal laminae at the dermoepidermal

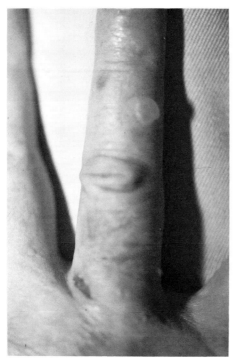

FIGURE 169–4. Hand of a patient with porphyria cutanea tarda showing typical lesions of delayed-type porphyric photosensitivity: bullae, erosions, milia, scarring.

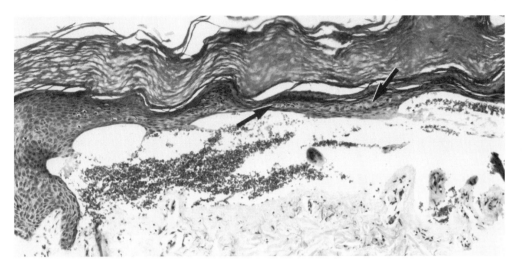

FIGURE 169-6. A cell-poor subepidermal vesicle with festooning of dermal papillae and a "caterpillar body" *(arrows)* in its roof exemplifies the histopathologic findings in porphyric blisters, whether caused by porphyria cutanea tarda or pseudoporphyria due to a drug. The caterpillar body is a strand of basement membrane surrounded by degenerating keratinocytes that give it a segmented appearance.

junction is more prominent in those porphyrias in which blistering and cutaneous fragility are typical, but it also can be seen in skin of individuals exhibiting the immediate-type phototoxicity reaction.[19, 30] Immunohistochemical studies demonstrate that the plane of separation in bullae due to porphyria is in the lamina lucida.[58] Diverse light and electron microscopic investigations of acute and chronic porphyrin-induced cutaneous lesions carried out to gain insight into the pathophysiology have been extensively reviewed elsewhere.[19-21]

Therapeutic interventions can lead to biochemical and clinical remission of PCT (Table 169-7) but have not been successful in HEP. Avoidance of exogenous agents known to exacerbate the disease should be advised. If there are no contraindications, serial phlebotomy or low-dose chloroquine regimens or a combination of the two are the most frequently used therapies. The success of serial phlebotomy protocols appears related to removal of excess hepatic iron stores, which can be monitored by progressive diminution of serum ferritin levels.[59] After ferritin levels reach the lower limit of the normal reference range, levels of circulating and excreted porphyrins continue to decline and cutaneous vasiculation and fragility continue to improve without additional bloodletting.[60] In practice, this can be accomplished by removal of approximately 500 mL of whole blood at weekly or biweekly intervals, while monitoring the hemoglobin level to limit symptoms of iatrogenic anemia; in my

patients I maintain a hemoglobin level above 11 g/dL by judicious spacing of phlebotomy intervals as the ferritin level diminishes. In some patients, serum and urinary porphyrin levels eventually normalize; in others, mildly abnormal levels are maintained for prolonged periods without clinical signs or symptoms. Emergence from remission is signaled by a progressive rise in serum ferritin levels accompanied by slowly rising porphyrin levels. Reinstitution of phlebotomy can reverse this trend before the patient becomes symptomatic; therefore, long-term monitoring of both ferritin and serum or urinary porphyrin levels is recommended.

Oral chloroquine[61] or hydroxychloroquine[62] regimens offer another approach suitable for patients in whom phlebotomy may be contraindicated or technically difficult. Given in low doses, these agents appear to facilitate liberation of porphyrins accumulated in hepatocytes, which are then excreted, accompanied by an increase in urinary iron excretion. Over several months to a year or more such treatments can induce clinical and biochemical remissions. Higher doses are not generally recommended initially because symptomatic hepatotoxicity is produced. Doses of 125 mg twice weekly of chloroquine or 100 mg thrice weekly of hydroxychloroquine appear to be appropriate levels for initiation of treatment. Liver function tests are recommended before treatment and at biweekly intervals thereafter. Glucose-6-phosphate dehydrogenase testing before treatment and interval ophthalmologic evaluations are recommended. It may be possible to increase dosage levels after an initial period without precipitating symptomatic hepatotoxicity.[62] Protocols combining phlebotomy and chloroquine have also been advocated.[63]

Therapies less often used include metabolic alkalinization,[64] iron chelation,[65] plasmapheresis,[66] plasma exchange,[67] oral adsorbents,[68, 69] and vitamin E.[70] Some of these are particularly applicable if venesection or antimalarial agents are relatively or absolutely contraindicated, as in individuals with preexisting anemia or poor renal function. Use of erythropoietin to stimulate erythropoiesis, thereby mobilizing iron stores and providing support for therapeutic phlebotomy, has been used to

TABLE 169-7. Treatment of Porphyria Cutanea Tarda

Physical sunscreens
Phlebotomy
Chloroquine, hydroxychloroquine
Metabolic alkalinization
Iron chelation
Plasmapheresis
Plasma exchange
Oral adsorbents (cholestyramine, charcoal)
Vitamin E
Erythropoietin

TABLE 169-8. Differential Diagnosis of Porphyria Cutanea Tarda

Variegate porphyria
Congenital erythropoietic porphyria
Hereditary coproporphyria
Hepatoerythropoietic porphyria
   (homozygous or compound heterozygous porphyria
   cutanea tarda)
"Pseudoporphyria" due to drugs, tanning beds,
   hemodialysis
Epidermolysis bullosa acquisita
Bullous lupus erythematosus

treat PCT associated with chronic renal failure with hemodialysis.[71]

The differential diagnosis of PCT and HEP (Table 169-8) includes all of the other porphyrias that may present with similar skin lesions (CEP, variegate porphyria, hereditary coproporphyria), all being distinguishable by their different porphyrin laboratory profiles (Table 169-9). A wide array of drugs,[72] exposure to tanning beds,[73] and maintenance hemodialysis treatment[74] are linked to occurrence of photocutaneous bullae that are clinically and histologically similar to those of PCT. Such occurrences have been termed *pseudoporphyria*. Absence of abnormal porphyrin laboratory profiles allows differentiation of these from true PCT. Epidermolysis bullosa acquisita and bullous lupus erythematosus, which may also resemble PCT clinically, are similarly differentiated.

Acute Intermittent Porphyria

Acute intermittent porphyria (AIP) is not manifested by cutaneous photosensitivity but by a wide array of episodic or chronic neurologic dysfunctions that may affect peripheral, autonomic, or central nervous systems. These neurovisceral symptoms occur most often after puberty, vary in frequency and severity, and can be precipitated by many drugs, infections, carbohydrate restriction, or endogenous or exogenous hormonal fluctuations. Similar attacks of potentially life-threatening severity and also characterize aminolevulinic acid dehydratase porphyria, variegate porphyria, and hereditary coproporphyria.

During such episodes, urinary ALA and PBG are excreted copiously in all of the "acute attack" porphyrias and typically remain abnormal even in quiescent periods in AIP. AIP can be confirmed by demonstration of deficient activity of erythrocyte PBG deaminase at about 50% of normal values.

Treatment of AIP (and of the other acute attack porphyrias) is primarily preventive: patients must avoid drugs and factors that induce heme biosynthesis. Once an attack has begun, intensive care may be required. Oral or intravenous loading with glucose may repress the induced heme biosynthetic pathway, as may intravenously administered heme analogues.[1, 75]

Aminolevulinic Acid Dehydratase Porphyria

Aminolevulinic acid dehydratase porphyria (ALADP) is extremely rare; no photosensitivity has been reported. Urinary levels of ALA are markedly increased in the absence of PBG elevations due to profoundly decreased activity of ALA dehydratase.[76]

Hereditary Coproporphyria

Photosensitivity resembling that of PCT occurs in about 30% of cases of hereditary coproporphyria (HCP).[77] Neurovisceral problems are more frequently manifested. Many heterozygotes remain biochemically and clinically silent. As in AIP and variegate porphyria, onset of symptoms in heterozygotes is rare until after puberty. Although laboratory diagnosis of HCP is based on demonstration of increased excretion of coproporphyrin III in both urine and feces as a result of deficient activity of coproporphyrinogen oxidase,[78] levels of ALA and PBG in urine become elevated during "attack" episodes. The differential diagnosis for cases with cutaneous photosensitivity and porphyrinuria includes PCT, variegate porphyria, and late-onset CEP. Neurovisceral symptoms in association with abnormal porphyrin levels bring AIP, variegate porphyria, ALADP, and heavy metal (par-

TABLE 169-9. Key Porphyrin Laboratory Abnormalities

Type of Porphyria	Red Blood Cells	Plasma	Urine	Feces
Aminolevulinic acid dehydratase porphyria	ZnProto		ALA > PBG, Copro III	
Acute intermittent porphyria			ALA, PGB, Uro	
Congenital erythropoietic porphyria	ZnProto, Uro	Uro	Uro I > Copro I	
Porphyria cutanea tarda		Uro > 7-COOH	Uro > 7-COOH	Copro Isocoproporphyrin
Hepatoerythropoietic porphyria	ZnProto	Uro > 7-COOH	Uro > 7-COOH	Copro Isocoproporphyrin
Hereditary coproporphyria		Copro	Copro III, ALA, PBG*	Copro II
Variegate porphyria		+	Copro > Uro / ALA, PBG*	Proto ≥ Copro X-porphyrins
Erythropoietic protoporphyria	Proto	Proto		Proto >> Copro

*May be positive only during active symptoms or acute attack episodes
ALA, aminolevulinic acid; PBG, porphobilinogen; ZnProto, zinc protoporphyrin; Copro, coproprophrin; Uro, uroporphyrin; Proto, protoporphyrin; +, porphyrin present, type not specified.

ticularly lead) poisoning into consideration. A complete porphyrin laboratory profile and blood metal assays usually allow differentiation. The same factors that induce AIP and treatments that may be beneficial in AIP apply to HCP.

Variegate Porphyria

Individuals with variegate porphyria (VP) may exhibit either cutaneous or systemic manifestations or both and can be shown to have approximately 50% reduction in protoporphyrinogen oxidase activity.[79]

The diagnostic porphyrin profile includes elevated levels of both protoporphyrin and coproporphyrin in feces, with protoporphyrin usually in greater proportion. Abnormal porphyrinuria is variably present, with coproporphyrin generally in excess of uroporphyrin when observed. Plasma or serum porphyrin levels are elevated when the disease is active and exhibit a distinctive fluorescence emission spectrum peak that is diagnostic.[80]

The differential diagnosis and approaches to treatment are as noted for the other "acute attack" porphyrias. In the absence of neurovisceral symptoms, misdiagnosis of individuals with VP as having PCT is not uncommon. Several treatments effective in PCT (phlebotomy, chloroquine) are not beneficial and are inappropriate in VP.

References

1. Kappas A, Sassa S, Galbraith RA, et al. The porphyrias. In: Stanbury JB, Wyngaarden JB, Fredrickson DS, eds. The Metabolic Basis of Inherited Disease. New York: McGraw-Hill International Book Co., 1989:1305–1365.
2. Elder GH. Differentiation of porphyria cutanea tarda symptomatica from other types of porphyria by measurement of isocoproporphyrin in faeces. J Clin Pathol 1975;28:601–607.
3. Goldstein BD, Harber LC. Erythropoietic protoporphyria: Lipid peroxidation and red cell membrane damage associated with photohemolysis. J Clin Invest 1972;51:892–901.
4. deGoeij AFPM, van Strallen RJC, van Steveninck J. Photodynamic modification of proteins in human red blood cell membranes induced by protoporphyrin. Clin Chim Acta 1976;71:485–494.
5. Girotti AW. Photodynamic action of protoporphyrin IX on human erythrocytes: Cross-linking of membrane proteins. Biochem Biophys Res Commun 1976;72:1367–1374.
6. Kohn K, Kessel D. On the mode of cytotoxic action of photoactivated porphyrins. Biochem Pharmacol 1979;28:2465–2470.
7. Girotti AW. Bilirubin-sensitized photoinactivation of enzymes in the isolated membrane of the human erythrocyte. Photochem Photobiol 1976;24:525–532.
8. Sandberg S, Glette J, Hope AG, et al. Porphyrin-induced photodamage to isolated human neutrophils. Photochem Photobiol 1981;34:471–475.
9. Sandberg S, Romslo I. Porphyrin-induced photodamage at the cellular and the subcellular level as related to the solubility of the porphyrin. Clin Chim Acta 1981;109:193–201.
10. Dubbelmann TMAR, De Goeij AFPM, van Steveninck J. Photodynamic effects of protoporphyrin on human erythrocytes: Nature of the cross-linking of membrane proteins. Biochim Biophys Acta 1978;511:141–151.
11. Wakulchik SD, Shiltz JR, Bickers DR. Photolysis of protoporphyrin treated human fibroblasts in vitro: Studies on the mechanism. J Lab Clin Med 1980;96:158–167.
12. Allison AC, Mazgnus IA, Young MR. Role of lysosomes and of cell membranes in photosensitization. Nature 1966;209:874–878.
13. Fritsch P, Gschnait F, Honigsmann H, et al. Protective action of beta-carotene against lethal photosensitization of fibroblasts in vitro. Br J Dermatol 1976;94:263–271.
14. Gschnait F, Wolff K, Konrad K. Erythropoietic protoporphyria: Submicroscopic events during the acute photosensitivity flare. Br J Dermatol 1975;92:545–557.
15. Slater TF, Riley PA. Photosensitization and lysosomal damage. Nature 1966;209:151–154.
16. Lim HW, Wasserman SI, Gigli I. Differential effects of protoporphyrin and uroporphyrin on murine mast cells. J Invest Dermatol 1987;88:281–286.
17. Lim HW, Poh-Fitzpatrick MB, Gigli I. Activation of the complement system and generation of chemotactic activity in vivo in patients with porphyrias. J Clin Invest 1984;74:1961–1965.
18. Schothorst AA, Suurmond D, Ploem J. In vitro studies on protoporphyrin uptake and photosensitivity of normal skin fibroblasts and fibroblasts from patients with erythropoietic protoporphyria. J Invest Dermatol 1977;69:551–557.
19. Wolff K, Honigsmann H, Rauschmeier W, et al. Microscopic and fine structural aspects of porphyrias. Acta Derm Venereol 1982;(Suppl 100):17–28.
20. Poh-Fitzpatrick MB. Pathogenesis and treatment of photocutaneous manifestations of the porphyrias. Semin Liver Dis 1982;2:164–176.
21. Lim HW. Pathophysiology of cutaneous lesions in porphyrias. Semin Hematol 1989;26:114–119.
22. Poh-Fitzpatrick MB. Molecular and cellular mechanisms of porphyrin photosensitization. Photodermatology 1986;3:148–157.
23. Deybach JC, de Verneuil H, Phung N, et al. Congenital erythropoietic porphyria (Gunther's disease): Enzymatic studies on two cases of late onset. J Lab Clin Med. 1981;97:551–558.
24. Horiguchi Y, Horio T, Yamamoto M, et al. Late onset erythropoietic porphyria. Br J Dermatol 1989;121:255–262.
25. Piomelli S, Poh-Fitzpatrick MB, Seaman C, et al. Complete suppression of the symptoms of congenital erythropoietic porphyria by long-term treatment with high-level transfusions. N Engl J Med 1986;314:1029–1031.
26. Warner CA, Poh-Fitzpatrick MB, Zaider E, et al. Congenital erythropoietic porphyria: A mild variant with low uroporphyrinogen I levels due to a missense mutation (A66V) encoding residual uroporphyrinogen III synthase activity. Arch Dermatol 1992;128:1243–1248.
27. Haining RC, Cowger ML, Labbe RF, et al. Erythropoietic porphyria: II. The effects of induced polycythemia. Blood 1970;36:297–309.
28. Guarini L, Poh-Fitzpatrick MB, Carriero D, et al: Congenital erythropoietic porphyria (CEP): Suppression of erythropoiesis by treatment with hydroxyurea (HU). Blood 1992;80(Suppl 1):285a.
29. Norris PG, Nunn AV, Hawk JLM, et al. Genetic heterogeneity in erythropoietic protoporphyria: A study of the enzymatic defect in nine affected families. J Invest Dermatol 1990;95:260–263.
30. Epstein JH, Tuffanelli DL, Epstein WL. Cutaneous changes in the porphyrias: A microscopic study. Arch Dermatol 1973;107:689–698.
31. Ryan EA, Madill GT. Electron microscopy of the skin in erythropoietic protoporphyria. Br J Dermatol 1968;80:561–570.
32. Kint A, Geerts ML. Histochemical and electron microscopical study of the bulla from porphyria cutanea tarda. Arch Dermatol Forsch 1973;246:355–364.
33. Poh-Fitzpatrick MB. The "priming phenomenon" for acute phototoxicity in erythropoietic protoporphyria. J Am Acad Dermatol 1989;21:311.
34. Mathews-Roth MM, Pathak MA, Fitzpatrick TB, et al. Beta-carotene as an oral photoprotective agent in erythropoietic protoporphyria. JAMA 1974;228:1004–1008.
35. Dobozy A, Csato M, Siklosi C, et al. Transfusion therapy for erythropoietic protoporphyria. Br J Dermatol 1983;109:571–576.
36. Bloomer JR. Pathogenesis and therapy of liver disease in erythropoietic protoporphyria. Yale J Biol Med 1979;52:39–48.
37. Conley CL, Chisholm JJ. Recovery from hepatic decompensation in protoporphyria. Johns Hopkins Med J 1979;145:237–240.
38. McCullough AJ, Barron D, Mullen KD, et al. Fecal protoporphyrin excretion in erythropoietic protoporphyria: Effect of cholestyramine and bile acid feeding. Gastroenterology 1988;94:177–181.
39. Gordeuk VR, Brittenham GM, Hawkins CW, et al. Iron therapy for hepatic dysfunction in erythropoietic protoporphyria. Ann Intern Med 1986;105:27–31.

40. Milligan A, Graham-Brown RAC, Sarkany I, et al. Erythropoietic protoporphyria exacerbated by oral iron therapy. Br J Dermatol 1988;119:63–66.
41. Watson CJ, Bossenmeier I, Cardinal R, et al. Repression by hematin of porphyrin biosynthesis in red cell precursors in congenital erythropoietic porphyria. Proc Natl Acad Sci USA 1974;71:278–282.
42. Bloomer JR, Pierach CA. Effect of hematin administration to patients with protoporphyria and liver disease. Hepatology 1982;2:817–821.
43. van Wijk HJ, van Hattum J, Baart de la Faille H, et al. Blood exchange and transfusion therapy for acute cholestasis in protoporphyria. Dig Dis Sci 1988;33:1621–1625.
44. van Hattum J, Baart de la Faille H, van den Berg WO, et al. Chenodeoxycholic acid therapy in erythrohepatic protoporphyria. J Hepatol 1986;3:407–412.
45. Bloomer JR, Weimer MK, Bossenmeier IC, et al. Liver transplantation in a patient with protoporphyria. Gastroenterology 1989;97:188–194.
46. Elder GH, Smith SG, Herrero C, et al. Hepatoerythropoietic porphyria: A new uroporphyrinogen decarboxylase defect or homozygous porphyria cutanea tarda? Lancet 1981;1:916–919.
47. Lim HW, Poh-Fitzpatrick MB. Hepatoerythropoietic porphyria: A variant of childhood-onset porphyria cutanea tarda: Porphyrin profiles and enzymatic studies of two cases in a family. J Am Acad Dermatol 1984;11:1103–1111.
48. Toback AC, Sassa S, Poh-Fitzpatrick MB, et al. Hepatoerythropoietic porphyria: Clinical, biochemical and enzymatic studies in a three-generation family lineage. N Engl J Med 1987;316:645–650.
49. Elder GH. Differentiation of porphyria cutanea tarda symptomatica from other types of porphyria by measurement of isocoproporphyrin in feces. J Clin Pathol 1975;28:601–607.
50. Elder GH, Sheppard DM, Enriquez de Salamanca R, et al. Identification of two types of porphyria cutanea tarda by measurement of erythrocyte uroporphyrinogen decarboxylase. Clin Sci 1980;58:477–484.
51. Held JL, Sassa S, Kappas A, et al. Erythrocyte uroporphyrinogen decarboxylase activity in porphyria cutanea tarda: A study of 40 consecutive patients. J Invest Dermatol 1989;93:332–334.
52. Grossman ME, Poh-Fitzpatrick MB. Porphyria cutanea tarda: Diagnosis and management. Med Clin North Am 1980;64:807–827.
53. Rocchi E, Gibertini P, Casanelli M, et al. Hepatitis B virus infection in porphyria cutanea tarda. Liver 1986;6:153–157.
54. LaCour JP, Bodokh I, Castanet J, et al. Porphyria cutanea tarda and antibodies to hepatitis C. Br J Dermatol 1993;128:121–123.
55. Conlan MG, Hoots WK. Porphyria cutanea in association with human immunodeficiency virus infection in a hemophiliac. J Am Acad Dermatol 1992;26:857–859.
56. Feldaker M, Montgomery H, Brunsting LA. Histopathology of porphyria cutanea tarda. Arch Dermatol 1955;24:131–137.
57. Egbert BM, LeBoit PE, McCalmont T, et al. Caterpillar bodies: Distinctive, basement-membrane containing structures in blisters of porphyria. Am J Dermatopathol 1993;15:199–202.
58. Pardo RJ, Penneys NS. Location of basement membrane type IV collagen beneath subepidermal bullous disorders. J Cutan Pathol 1990;17:336–341.
59. Rocchi E, Gibertini P, Cassanelli M, et al. Serum ferritin in the assessment of liver iron overload and iron removal therapy in porphyria cutanea tarda. J Lab Clin Med 1986;107:36–42.
60. Ratnaike S, Blake D, Campbell D, et al. Plasma ferritin levels as a guide to the treatment of porphyria cutanea tarda by venesection. Australas J Dermatol 1988;39:3–7.
61. Taljaard JJF, Shanley BC, Stewart-Wynne EG, et al. Studies on low dose chloroquine therapy in symptomatic porphyria. Br J Dermatol 1972;87:261–269.
62. Malkinson FD, Lovitt L. Hydroxychloroquine treatment of porphyria cutanea tarda. Arch Dermatol 1980;116:1147–1150.
63. Swanbeck G, Wennersten G. Treatment of porphyria cutanea tarda with chloroquine and phlebotomy. Br J Dermatol 1977;97:77–82.
64. Weigand SE, Monckton Copeman PW, Perry H. Metabolic alkalinization in porphyria cutanea tarda. Arch Dermatol 1969;100:544–549.
65. Praga M, Enriquez de Salamanca R, Andres A, et al. Treatment of hemodialysis-related porphyria cutanea tarda with deferoxamine. N Engl J Med 1987;316:547–548.
66. Miyauchi S, Shiraishi S, Miki Y. Small volume plasmapheresis in the management of porphyria cutanea tarda. Arch Dermatol 1983;119:752–755.
67. Disler P, Day R, Burman N, et al. Treatment of hemodialysis-related porphyria cutanea tarda with plasma exchange. Am J Med 1982;72:989–993.
68. Stathers GM. Porphyrin-binding effect of cholestyramine: Results of in vitro and in vivo studies. Lancet 1966;2:780–783.
69. Pimstone NR, Gandhi SN, Mukerji SK. Therapeutic efficacy of oral charcoal in congenital erythropoietic porphyria. N Engl J Med 1987;316:390–393.
70. Ayers S, Mihan R. Porphyria cutanea tarda: Response to vitamin E. Cutis 1978;22:50–52.
71. Anderson KE, Goeger DE, Carson RW, et al. Erythropoietin for the treatment of porphyria cutanea tarda in a patient on long-term hemodialysis. N Engl J Med 1990;322:315–317.
72. Poh-Fitzpatrick MB. Porphyria, pseudoporphyria, pseudopseudoporphyria . . . ? Arch Dermatol 1986;122:403–404.
73. Farr PM, Marks JM, Diffey BL, et al. Skin fragility and blistering due to use of sunbeds. Br Med J 1988;196:1708–1709.
74. Gilchrest B, Rowe JW, Mihm MC. Bullous dermatosis of hemodialysis. Ann Intern Med 1975;83:480–483.
75. Disler PB, Moore MR. The acute attack of porphyria. Clin Dermatol 1985;3:103–111.
76. Doss M, von Tiepermann R, Schneider J, et al. New type of hepatic porphyria with porphobilinogen synthase defect and intermittent acute manifestations. Klin Wochenschr 1979;57:1123–1127.
77. Goldberg A, Rimington C, Lochhead AC. Hereditary coproporphyria. Lancet 1917;1:632–636.
78. Elder GH, Evans GO, Thomas N, et al. The primary enzyme defect in hereditary coproporphyria. Lancet 1976;2:1217–1219.
79. Mustajoki P. Variegate porphyria: Twelve years experience in Finland. Q J Med 1980;49:191–203.
80. Poh-Fitzpatrick MB. A plasma porphyrin fluorescence marker for variegate porphyria. Arch Dermatol 1980;116:543–547.

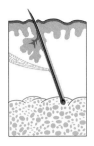

chapter 170

Acrodermatitis Enteropathica

JEFFREY C. DRALUCK and DARRYL M. BRONSON

DEFINITION

Acrodermatitis enteropathica is a rare autosomal recessive disorder characterized by acral and periorificial dermatitis, alopecia, and diarrhea. The disease results from an inability to absorb sufficient amounts of zinc from the diet.

CLINICAL DESCRIPTION

Acrodermatitis enteropathica was first recognized by Brandt[1] in 1936 and named by Danbolt and Closs[2] in 1942. In 1974, Moynahan[3] demonstrated that acrodermatitis enteropathica was an inherited disease of zinc deficiency. Hereditary acrodermatitis enteropathica has been found worldwide with no apparent predilection for race or sex.

The disease is usually not present at birth but typically develops either after weaning from breast milk or during the first few weeks or months of life. The clinical syndrome of acrodermatitis enteropathica is characterized by dermatologic, gastrointestinal, and psychological abnormalities.

Affected individuals develop a symmetrical acral (extensor surfaces of the major joints, fingers, and toes) and periorificial (mouth, nose, eyes, ears, and perineum) vesiculobullous dermatitis that becomes crusted and psoriasiform (Fig. 170–1). Involvement of the digits is manifested by an erythematous dermatitis, paronychial tissue swelling, and nail dystrophy. Perlèche is a common early sign. The tongue and buccal mucosa may either develop superficial aphthous-like lesions or be secondarily infected with *Candida albicans*. Alopecia results when the scalp is involved. In addition, conjunctivitis, blepharitis, and photophobia may be present.

The gastrointestinal disturbance is primarily diarrhea

with irregular exacerbations and remissions. Abdominal pain and foul-smelling stools may be present intermittently or totally absent. Psychological symptoms include mental depression, irritability, and loss of appetite.

Acrodermatitis enteropathica is generally regarded as a disease of infancy and childhood. Before the use of either diiodohydroxyquin or zinc therapy, few affected children survived to adulthood.[4, 5] Of those who survive without therapy, most have milder forms of the disease, often without severe diarrhea.

In several cases, there has been complete remission of the disease at puberty. Absorption of zinc in three adult patients with the disease was shown by Weismann and colleagues to be in the low normal range, in contrast to children with the disease, in whom absorption of zinc is greatly diminished.

PATHOLOGY

Histopathologically, the psoriasiform plaques of acrodermatitis enteropathica are characterized by diffuse parakeratosis and psoriasiform epidermal hyperplasia with characteristic large pale keratinocytes in the upper spinous layers and dyskeratotic cells (Fig. 170–2). In some instances, a subcorneal vesicle is present above the large pale keratinocytes. Four other deficiency diseases, namely, pellagra, necrolytic migratory erythema, neonatal citrullinemia, and maple syrup urine disease, share with acrodermatitis enteropathica the presence of large pale keratinocytes in the superficial epidermis. These diseases also have many clinical features in common.[7]

PATHOGENESIS AND ETIOLOGY

In 1973, Moynahan and Barnes discovered a low plasma zinc level in a patient with a lactose-intolerant

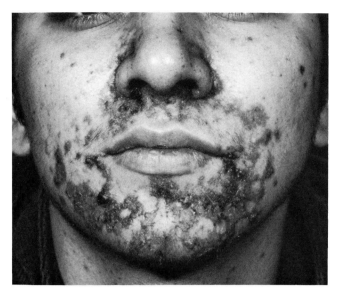

FIGURE 170-1. Acrodermatitis enteropathica. Perioral and facial lesions. (Courtesy of Richard B. Odom, M.D.)

variant of acrodermatitis enteropathica. Supplementation with small amounts of zinc produced a dramatic response.[8] Several other workers have confirmed the observation that acrodermatitis enteropathica is a disorder of deficient zinc absorption from the gastrointestinal tract.[9, 10] The specific defect, however, has not yet been elucidated. A deficient or functionally defective specific intestinal transport protein or zinc binding ligand has been postulated to explain the genetic defect.[11]

Acrodermatitis enteropathica has been reported to flare with pregnancy.[6, 12] The exacerbation of the underlying genetic disease may be explained by an increased demand for zinc by the fetus. However, it is known that serum zinc levels decrease early in pregnancy in normal individuals and return to near-normal levels 8 weeks post partum.[13] Similarly, decreased zinc levels are observed in nonpregnant subjects during the administration of oral contraceptives.[14] It is therefore conceivable that the change in zinc levels observed during pregnancy is primarily due to hormonal effects, rather than from an increased demand by the fetus.[6] Both factors may, however, be operative.

Acquired forms of acrodermatitis enteropathica may occur in patients with a variety of gastrointestinal diseases causing either malabsorption or abnormal excretion of zinc (i.e., as a complication of Crohn's disease), as a consequence of surgery (i.e., in patients who have had small intestine bypass procedures), or secondary to nutritional factors (i.e., in alcoholics with poor nutrition or in patients receiving total parenteral nutrition if the hyperalimentation does not contain zinc). Premature infants are also at risk because the full complement of neonatal zinc is not received until late in the third trimester. When the zinc level in patients with any of these conditions becomes too low, the cutaneous and intestinal manifestations of acrodermatitis enteropathica may develop.

DIAGNOSIS AND DIFFERENTIAL DIAGNOSIS

The clinical constellation of acrodermatitis enteropathica comprises a symmetrical acral and periorificial vesiculobullous dermatitis, alopecia, bouts of diarrhea, and personality changes, including depression, listlessness, and anorexia. Laboratory verification of deficient plasma or serum zinc levels and the rapid and complete response to an increased oral zinc load confirm the diagnosis.

The clinical differential diagnosis is shown in Table 170-1.

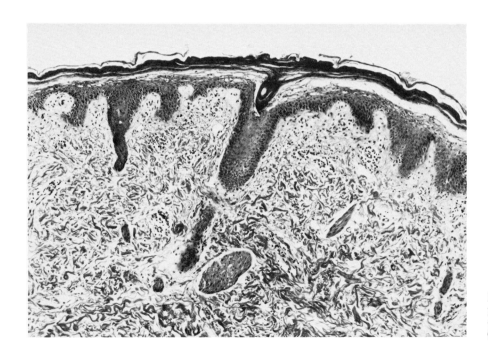

FIGURE 170-2. Acrodermatitis enteropathica. The keratinocytes in the upper part of the epidermis display characteristic pallor (hematoxylin-eosin).

TABLE 170-1. Differential Diagnosis of Acrodermatitis Enteropathica

Severe candidiasis
Pustular psoriasis
Epidermolysis bullosa
Hepatoerythropoietic porphyria
Other deficiency diseases, including necrolytic migratory erythema, pellagra, neonatal citrullinemia, and maple syrup urine disease
Acquired types: association with malabsorption disorders, secondary to nutritional factors, or as a consequence of surgery

TREATMENT

In 1953, Dillaha and colleagues reported successful treatment of acrodermatitis enteropathica with orally administered diiodohydroxyquin (Diodoquin).[15] Oral diiodohydroxyquin was the mainstay of therapy until 1973, when Moynahan and Barnes discovered that acrodermatitis enteropathica was a disease of zinc deficiency that could be remedied with oral zinc sulfate. To date, the mechanism of action of diiodohydroxyquin remains unknown,[10] although some investigators have suggested that diiodohydroxyquin is a source of zinc.[16]

The clinical findings of acrodermatitis enteropathica are now rapidly and dramatically reversed by dietary supplementation with zinc sulfate in a daily dose of 1 to 2 mg/kg in children or 220 mg three times daily in adults. Supplemental zinc should probably be maintained indefinitely and be monitored twice a year, particularly in women of childbearing age who either may become pregnant or want to take oral contraceptives.

References

1. Brandt T. Dermatitis in children with disturbances of the general condition and the absorption of food elements. Acta Dermatol Venereol 1936;17:513–546.
2. Danbolt N, Closs K. Akrodermatitis enteropathica. Acta Dermatol Venereol 1942;23:127–169.
3. Moynahan EJ. Acrodermatitis enteropathica: A lethal inherited human zinc-deficiency disorder. Lancet 1974;2:399–400.
4. Piper EL. Acrodermatitis enteropathica in an adult. Arch Dermatol 1957;76:221–224.
5. Olholm-Larsen P. Untreated acrodermatitis enteropathica in adults. Dermatologica 1978;156:155–166.
6. Weismann K, Hoe S, Knudsen L, et al. Zinc absorption in patients suffering from acrodermatitis enteropathica and in normal adults assessed by whole-body counting technique. Br J Dermatol 1979;101:573–579.
7. Ackerman AB. Acrodermatitis enteropathica. In: Histologic Diagnosis of Inflammatory Skin Diseases, p 512. Philadelphia: Lea & Febiger, 1978.
8. Moynahan EJ, Barnes PM. Zinc deficiency and a synthetic diet for lactose intolerance. Lancet 1973;1:676–677.
9. Lombeck T, Schnippering HG, Ritzl F, et al. Absorption of zinc in acrodermatitis enteropathica. Lancet 1975;1:855.
10. Neldner KH, Hambridge KM. Zinc therapy of acrodermatitis enteropathica. N Engl J Med 1975;292:879–882.
11. Evans GW, Johnson PE. Zinc binding factor in acrodermatitis enteropathica. Lancet 1976;2:1310.
12. Bronson DM, Barsky R, Barsky S. Acrodermatitis enteropathica. J Am Acad Dermatol 1983;9:140–144.
13. Johnson NC. Study of copper and zinc metabolism during pregnancy. Proc Soc Exp Biol Med 1961;108:518–519.
14. Halstead JA, Smith JC Jr. Plasma-zinc in health and disease. Lancet 1970;1:322–324.
15. Dillaha CJ, Lorincz AL, Aavik OR. Acrodermatitis enteropathica: Review of the literature and report of a case successfully treated with Diodoquin. JAMA 1953;152:509–512.
16. Robertson AF, Soto J. Treatment of acrodermatitis enteropathica with zinc sulfate. Pediatrics 1975;55:738.

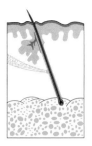

chapter 171

Inherited Enzyme Diseases

Gaucher's Disease

Adelaide A. Hebert and Hope Northrup

All of the inherited disorders of glucosylceramide catabolism are collectively known as Gaucher's disease. Each of the three subtypes of Gaucher's disease is inherited as an autosomal recessive trait. The gene for glucocerebrosidase has been cloned and mapped to chromosome 1q21.[1] In both type 1 and type 2 disease, point mutations have been described.

The three types of Gaucher's disease are related biochemically in that all accumulate the lipid glucosylceramide and all types are deficient in lysosomal glucocerebrosidase (also called acid β-glucosidase). Each subtype represents a grouping of similar phenotypes rather than a single genotype that may or may not be representative of different mutations.

Type 1 (nonneuronopathic) encompasses 99% of the cases of Gaucher's disease evaluated. This form has a chronic time course and manifests with hepatosplenomegaly, thrombocytopenia, anemia, bleeding diathesis, and bone disease. Although the severity and onset of symptoms may vary widely, type 1 disease is distinguished by the lack of neuropathology. This disorder may become manifest at any age and is panethnic, but it occurs more frequently in individuals of Eastern European (Ashkenazi) Jews. This group tends to have less severe disease than the general population, with more severe disease being evident in affected blacks.[1] Genotypes 1226G/1226G tend to have a milder clinical course overall. Those Gaucher's patients with genotypes 1226G/84GG and 1226/1448C often have more severe clinical manifestations.[2]

Type 2 Gaucher's disease (acute neuronopathic) is clinically a stereotypic, rapidly progressive neurovisceral storage disease that is usually fatal within the first 2 years of life. Hepatosplenomegaly is common to this as well as all subtypes of this disorder.

Type 3 (subacute neuronopathic) varies in severity but is usually less rapidly progressive than types 1 or 2. Afflicted children develop ataxia, myoclonus, seizures, and dementia. The degree of hepatosplenomegaly and skeletal involvement is variable, but death occurs in early childhood. All ethnic groups may be affected, but this form of Gaucher's disease is rare. In Northern Sweden, a genetic isolate of type 3 cases has been identified and named Norrbottnian Gaucher's disease. The subtypes of Gaucher's disease are summarized in Table 171–1.

Patients with Gaucher's disease are deficient in glucocerebrosidase, which is a specialized lysosomal acid β-glucosidase.[1] The glucosylceramide accumulates primarily in the lysosomes of the reticuloendothelial cells. Any patient with unexplained splenomegaly should have Gaucher's disease considered in the differential diagnosis. If the serum tartrate noninhibitable acid phosphatase is elevated and if Gaucher's cells are present in the bone marrow, Gaucher's disease is likely. The diagnosis can be confirmed by assay of glucocerebrosidase in white cells or fibroblasts. These assays demonstrate deficiency of glucocerebrosidase activity in patients with Gaucher's disease. The use of 4-methylumbelliferyl-β-D-glucopyranoside substrate provides the most convenient assay of the enzymatic activity.[1] Prenatal diagnosis of Gaucher's disease is possible using either amniocytes or chorionic villi. It is not yet possible to identify Gaucher's disease carriers by current assays.

The skin in adult patients with Gaucher's disease may have an abnormal diffuse yellow-brown skin pigmentation. This may be most evident on the face and legs.[3–5]

TABLE 171-1. Subtypes of Gaucher's Disease

Type 1: Nonneuronopathic Chronic	Type 2: Acute Neuronopathic	Type 3: Subacute Neuronopathic
Clinical Characteristics		
1. Heterogeneous presentation 2. Marked differences in age of symptoms (from birth to 80 years) 3. Marked differences in rate of progression of signs and symptoms 4. Marked differences in number of organ systems involved and rate of progression in organ systems 5. No neurologic involvement 6. Common signs: hepatosplenomegaly; osseous lesions: osteopenia, lytic lesions, osteonecrosis, failed remolding 7. Rare signs: pulmonary infiltration, pulmonary hypertension, cyanosis, clubbing, renal involvement, cirrhosis and liver failure, pericarditis	1. Stereotypic presentation 2. Onset of clinical signs at 3 months 3. Death before 2 years 4. Common signs: hepatosplenomegaly, hypertonic posture, strabismus, trismus, brain stem signs, seizures	1. Heterogeneous presentation 2. Variable age of onset of systemic signs; variable progression 3. Onset of neurologic signs in childhood or adolescence 4. Common signs: hepatosplenomegaly; osseous lesions: osteopenia, lytic lesions, osteonecrosis, failed remolding; slowly progressive dementia; myoclonus; supranuclear ophthalmoplegia
Pathology		
1. Gaucher's cells and variable degree of fibrosis in all organs 2. Perivascular Gaucher's cells in brain 3. Storage in reticuloendothelial cells causing eccentric nucleus and expanded fibrillar cytoplasm	1. Gaucher's cells in all organs, including both perivascular and parenchyma of brain 2. Areas of mild gliosis, cell death, neuronophagia, especially occipital cortex	1. Gaucher's cells in all organs but without marked changes in brain
Biochemistry		
1. Deficiency of glucocerebrosidase 2. Accumulation of glucosylceramide in all organs except brain 3. Cross-reactive material (CRM) to normal enzyme present	1. Deficiency of glucocerebrosidase 2. Accumulation of glucosylceramide in all tissues, including brain 3. CRM present, but altered	1. Deficiency of glucocerebrosidase 2. Accumulation of glucosylceramide in all tissues, including brain, but to a lesser extent than in type 2 3. CRM present, but altered
Genetics		
1. Autosomal recessive inheritance 2. Incidence among Ashkenazim: 1/600–1/2500 3. Incidence among general population: rare 4. Suspect many allelic mutations different from types 2, 3	1. Autosomal recessive inheritance 2. Incidence: rare 3. No ethnic predilection 4. Suspect allelic mutations different from types 1, 3	1. Autosomal recessive inheritance 2. Incidence: rare 3. Panethnic with large Norrbottnian subgroup 4. Suspect allelic mutations, different from types 1, 2

From Barranger JA, Ginns EI: Glycosylceramide lipidoses: Gaucher disease. In: Scriver CR, Beaudet AL, Sly WS, Volle D, eds. The Metabolic Basis of Inherited Disease, 6th edition. New York: McGraw-Hill, 1988:1679.

Gaucher's cells are not found in the skin, but afflicted patients may have increased deposition of hemosiderin and melanin is present in increased amounts in the basal layer of the epidermis.[1]

THERAPY

Enzyme replacement therapy that is macrophage targeted has been developed and tested in patients with Gaucher's disease.[6, 7] This macrophage-targeted human placental glucocerebrosidase (alglucerase) is administered intravenously and has resulted in objective clinical improvement in patients with type 1 Gaucher's disease. The use of alglucerase is superior to other symptomatic therapies, as primary treatment with glucocerebrosidase focuses on removal of the lipid metabolite that causes the pathology.[7–9] The benefits of enzyme-replacement therapy with alglucerase may be due to direct clearance of glucocerebrosidase from the plasma,[10] the targeting of mannose to macrophages,[6] or the interaction with high-affinity mannose receptors.[8]

Hartnup's Disorder

Hope Northrup and Adelaide A. Hebert

Hartnup's disorder is an impairment of neutral amino acid transport that involves the kidneys, the intestine, or both. The diagnosis is based on biochemical rather than clinical abnormalities. Affected individuals show a characteristic urinary pattern of monoaminomonocarboxylic amino acids (alanine, serine, threonine, valine, leucine, isoleucine, phenylalanine, tyrosine, tryptophan, and histidine) and monoaminodicarboxylic amides (glutamine and asparagine), which are excreted in amounts 5 to 20 times normal. Blood amino acids are either low or normal in amount in these patients. Hartnup's disorder is an autosomal recessive trait.[11]

The Hartnup family (after whom the disorder is named) was first brought to attention in 1951 when E. Hartnup was admitted to the Middlesex Hospital, London, England, with mild cerebellar ataxia and a red, scaly rash on the exposed areas of his body. He was thought to have pellagra because his sister, P. Hartnup, had been treated in 1937 with identical symptoms for pellagra. A distinctive pattern of urinary amino acids was noted in the boy. P. Hartnup, the sister, had a recurrence of ataxia and was found to have the same laboratory findings as her brother. The parents were first cousins. The parents and the other six children in the family were tested, with two of the other children showing gross hyperaminoaciduria in the same pattern as E. Hartnup and P. Hartnup. The skin and neurologic problems gradually disappeared in E. Hartnup and P. Hartnup but later occurred briefly in the younger siblings.[12]

The most frequent clinical abnormality seen in Hartnup's patients is an unusual "pellagra-like" skin rash. Affected individuals can have onset from as early as 10 days[13] to as late as 13 years.[14] The rash appears on uncovered areas of the body after sunlight exposure. Histopathologic examination shows changes similar to those in pellagra, acrodermatitis enteropathica, and other conditions in which there are deficiencies of amino acids.[15] Other clinical manifestations that are sometimes seen are primarily neurologic and include ataxia, mental retardation, increased muscle tone, and increased deep tendon reflexes. Ataxia is the most commonly reported neurologic symptom, and it is intermittent in nature. Somatic abnormalities occasionally seen in some Hartnup's patients that are thought to be related to the disease include atrophic glossitis and small stature.

Hartnup's disorder has a widespread distribution with no ethnic predilection. Wherever urine amino acid screening has been performed, cases have been detected. Males and females are equally affected, with consanguinity between parents noted in many families. Initially, general screening of urine amino acids searching for the disorder was performed in institutions for the mentally retarded. Only a handful of cases were diagnosed, leading investigators to believe that mental retardation was a common feature of Hartnup's disorder and that it was a very rare condition. Routine newborn screening has now been conducted in many countries, revealing that Hartnup's disorder is one of the most common amino acid disorders. The composite newborn screening frequency is 1 in 24,000. The great majority of individuals identified prospectively never have any clinical abnormalities associated with Hartnup's disorder. Some investigators even question whether Hartnup's disorder should be considered a disease.[11] The hypothesis of Scriver and colleagues[16] seems to be the most reasonable yet advanced to explain the clinical observations in Hartnup's disorder. These investigators propose that liability to disease in Hartnup's disorder is determined by one or more polygenic factors, the most prominent being plasma amino acid value (low plasma amino acid values in the presence of stress such as diarrhea will result in illness). According to this theory, Hartnup's disease is a multifactorial condition.

THERAPY

Owing to the similarities to pellagra, nicotinic acid and nicotinamide have been utilized as therapies in patients with signs suggesting a deficiency of this vitamin. Amounts from 50 to 300 mg per day given orally have been tried. The rash, ataxia, and psychotic behavior have been reported responsive[14, 17, 18]; however, neither the hyperaminoaciduria nor the intestinal transport defect responds to this therapy.[11,19,20]. In one patient with severe problems (growth failure, developmental delay, chronic diarrhea, hyperactivity, episodic ataxia, and weakness) who was unresponsive to nicotinamide and a protein-enriched diet, tryptophan ethyl ester was successfully utilized to circumvent the intestinal transport defect. The patient had resolution of chronic diarrhea, a significant increase in weight (26%) and height, and an improvement in his gait on an oral dose of 20 mg/kg of tryptophan ethyl ester.[21]

References

1. Barranger JA, Ginns EI. Glucosylceramide lipidoses: Gaucher disease. In: Scriver CR, Beaudet AL, Sly WS, Volle D, eds. The Metabolic Basis of Inherited Disease, 6th edition. New York: McGraw-Hill, 1988:1677–1698.
2. Zimran A, Kay A, Gelbart T, et al. Gaucher disease: Clinical,

laboratory, radiologic and genetic features of 53 patients. Medicine 1992;71:337–353.

3. Thannhauser SJ. Lipidoses, Diseases of Intracellular Lipid Metabolism. New York: Grune & Stratton, 1958.
4. Bloom TF, Groen J, Postma C. Gaucher's disease. Q J Med 1936;5:517.
5. Goldblatt J, Beighton P. Cutaneous manifestations of Gaucher disease. Br J Dermatol 1984;III:331.
6. Barton NW, Brady RO, Dambrosia JM, et al. Replacement therapy for inherited enzyme deficiency: Macrophage-targeted glucocerebrosidase for Gaucher's disease. N Engl J Med 1991; 324:1464–1470.
7. Whittington R. Alglucerase: A review. Drugs 1992;44:73–81.
8. Figueroa ML, Rosenbloom BE, Kay AC, et al. A less costly regimen of alglucerase to treat Gaucher's disease. New Engl J Med 1992;327:1632–1636.
9. Barton NW, Brady RO, Dambrosia JM. Treatment of Gaucher's disease. New Engl J Med 1993;328:1564–1565.
10. Sidransky E, Martin B, Ginns EI. Treatment of Gaucher's disease. New Engl J Med 1993;328:1566.
11. Levy HL. Hartnup's disorder. In: Scriver CR, Beaudet AL, Sly WS, Valle D, eds. The Metabolic Basis of Inherited Disease, 6th edition, vol. 2. New York: McGraw-Hill, 1988:2515–2527.
12. Baron DN, Dent CE, Harris H, et al. Hereditary pellagra-like skin rash with temporary cerebellar ataxia. Constant renal aminoaciduria and other bizarre biochemical features. Lancet 1956;2:421.
13. Somasundaram O, Papakumari M. Hartnup's disease. A report on two siblings. Indian Pediatr 1973;10:455.
14. Oyanagi K, Takagi M, Kitabatake M, Nakao T. Hartnup's disease. Tohoku J Exp Med 1967;91:383.
15. Weedon D. The Skin. New York: Churchill Livingstone, 1992:528.
16. Scriver CR, Mahon B, Levy HL, et al. The Hartnup's phenotype: Mendelian transport disorder, multifactorial disease. Am J Hum Genet 1987;40:401.
17. Halvarsen K, Halvorsen S. Hartnup's disease. Pediatrics 1963; 31:29.
18. Hersov LA. A case of childhood pellagra with psychosis. J Ment Sci 1955;101:878.
19. Seakins JWT, Ersser RS. Effects of amino acid loads on a healthy infant with the biochemical features of Hartnup's disease. Arch Dis Child 1967;42:682.
20. Wong PWK, Lambert AM, Pillai PM, Jones PM. Observations on nicotinic acid therapy in Hartnup's disease. Arch Dis Child 1967;42:642.
21. Jonas AJ, Butler IJ. Circumvention of defective neutral amino acid transport in Hartnup's disease using tryptophan ethyl ester. J Clin Invest 1989;84:200–204.

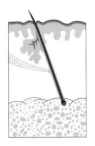

chapter 172

Inherited Elastic Tissue Malformations

KENNETH H. NELDNER

Pseudoxanthoma Elasticum

DEFINITION

Pseudoxanthoma elasticum is an inherited disorder of connective tissue in which the elastic fibers of the skin, retinae, and cardiovascular system become slowly calcified, leaving a canonical spectrum of pathologic events in each of these three organ systems. Both autosomal recessive and autosomal dominant inheritance patterns occur in affected kindreds, with approximately 90% showing an autosomal recessive pattern.[1, 2]

CLINICAL DESCRIPTION

The estimated prevalence of pseudoxanthoma elasticum in the population is 1 in 100,000, although it may be more common due to undiagnosed cases.[1-3] It occurs in all races with an approximate 2 to 1 female predominance. The average age at onset of skin lesions is 13 years; there is a tight clustering of new cases in the 10- to 15-year age group and a broad age range of 2 years to 50 years.[1] Accurate survival data are lacking, although overall longevity is believed to be close to the average survival of the general population. There have been several large studies.[1, 4-7]

Cutaneous Manifestations

There are two major diagnostic features: (1) characteristic yellow-orange, cobblestone, Moroccan leather, plucked chicken skin, linear papules that coalesce to form larger plaques; and (2) a unique localization to flexural sites—predominantly lateral neck (Fig. 172-1), antecubital fossae, axillae (Fig. 172-2), groins and popliteal spaces—with almost perfect symmetry. The initial diagnostic manifestation of pseudoxanthoma elasticum is almost always lateral neck skin lesions. Gradual centripetal extension beyond the primary flexural neck lesions may occur but at greatly varying rates among affected individuals.[1]

Ocular Manifestations

Calcification of the elastic fibers in Bruch's membrane layer of the retina allows for cracking, fissuring, or crazing of this layer, producing angioid streaks most commonly appearing several years after the first skin lesions (Fig. 172-3). Angioid streaks are a hallmark of pseudoxanthoma elasticum and eventuate in nearly 100% of patients, but they are also seen in a diverse group of at least 15 or 16 other conditions unrelated to pseudoxanthoma elasticum[1, 8, 9] and are therefore highly suggestive of pseudoxanthoma elasticum but not pathognomonic.

A mottled, peau d'orange pigmentation of the retina is more often present at the time of onset of the skin lesions and is also highly suggestive of early retinopathy of pseudoxanthoma elasticum. Pseudoxanthoma elasticum retinopathy initially exhibits great clinical heterogeneity, but its severity increases with time. Retinal hemorrhages are the most feared complication and occur with increasing frequency in the fifth decade. By the seventh decade, about 90% of persons with pseudoxanthoma elasticum will have experienced at least one retinal hemorrhage and will have varying degrees of loss of central vision. Patients with pseudoxanthoma elasticum are frequently told by well-meaning physicians that they will eventually "go blind." It is of paramount importance in counseling

1770

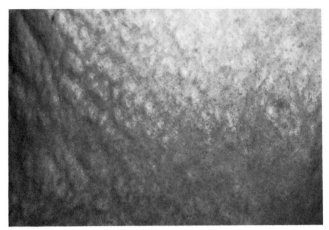

FIGURE 172-1. Typical lesions of pseudoxanthoma elasticum on the lateral neck.

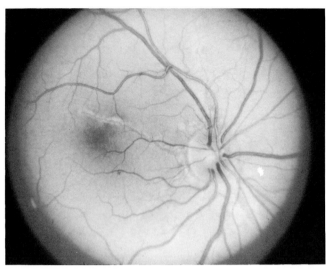

FIGURE 172-3. Pseudoxanthoma elasticum. Retinal photo showing angioid streaks. The most troublesome one is passing through the macula.

patients of any age to stress that pseudoxanthoma elasticum never causes total blindness. Peripheral vision is always preserved so that patients will always be able to get around without assistance, although they may have varying degrees of difficulty with reading and other activities if their condition progresses.

Cardiovascular Manifestations

The cardiovascular manifestations of pseudoxanthoma elasticum are the last to develop—or be recognized clinically. The first sign is often symptomatic calcification of the elastic media and intima of arteries. Early ischemic changes causing intermittent claudication can be detected by noninvasive ankle/brachial blood pressures using Doppler methods.

As in ordinary non-pseudoxanthoma elasticum arteriosclerosis, the gamut of hypertension, myocardial infarction, and stroke occurs in pseudoxanthoma elasticum but with surprisingly little, if any, increased frequency in the pseudoxanthoma elasticum population.[1]

Mitral valve prolapse is common in pseudoxanthoma elasticum,[10] as well as in other connective tissue diseases; it also occurs in normal individuals with no apparent cardiovascular disease. Mitral valve prolapse is seldom symptomatic and is thought to be of no consequence unless accompanied by a murmur of mitral valve insufficiency.

The most significant vascular complication, often occurring in younger patients (second to fourth decade of life), is gastrointestinal (primarily gastric) hemorrhage, which may come without warning and be severe enough to warrant hospitalization, blood transfusion, and occasionally surgery with a partial gastrectomy. Approximately 10% of the patients experience a gastrointestinal hemorrhage some time in their lives; usually this occurs as a single episode, but up to seven or eight over a span of years have been reported. Direct surgical visualization of the bleeding stomach usually shows only diffuse oozing of blood rather than a focal bleeding point.[1, 11]

PATHOLOGY

There are essentially three known pathophysiologic events in pseudoxanthoma elasticum: (1) mineralization of elastic fibers; (2) increased concentrations of glycosaminoglycans and polyanions in the affected dermis[12-14]; and (3) an increase in elastic fibers in the dermis.[15, 16] Before their mineralization the elastic fibers appear normal on light and electron microscopic examination.[1] Some minor amino acid alterations have been reported, but these vary from study to study and may depend on the experimental method used.[1, 17, 18]

The principal finding in the lesional skin of patients with pseudoxanthoma elasticum is an accumulation of fragmented elastic fibers in the mid and deep reticular dermis. The fibers are visible in sections stained with hematoxylin and eosin if they are impregnated with calcium; the more calcified the fibers are, the more baso-

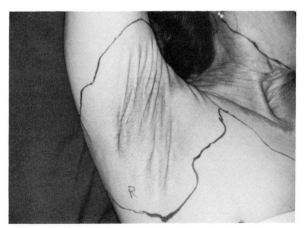

FIGURE 172-2. Pseudoxanthoma elasticum. Late, severe involvement of the lateral neck and axillae showing the skinfolds that may develop in the axillae.

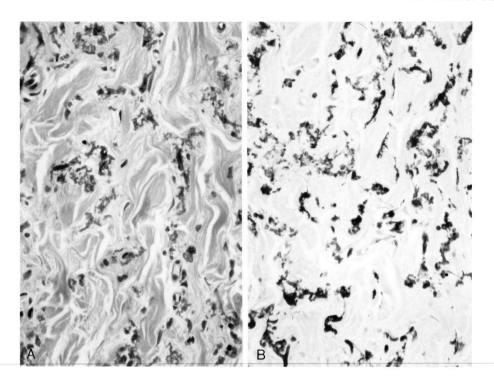

FIGURE 172-4. Pseudoxanthoma elasticum. Skin biopsy specimen showing fragmented calcified elastic fibers in the mid and deep dermis. The fibers are purple in hematoxylin and eosin-stained sections *(A),* and black with a von Kossa stain for calcium *(B).*

philic they appear. Special stains for elastic tissue (Fig. 172-4) and calcium can be used to confirm the diagnosis if needed. An "unwinding" of collagen fibers to produce so-called flower figures has also been reported.[19, 20]

The skin lesions are the direct result of fragmentation of the calcified elastic fibers and the resulting loss of elasticity, although the increased concentration of glycosaminoglycans and an increase in total elastic content no doubt also contribute to the clinical appearance of the skin lesions. Calcification of the elastic laminae of visceral blood vessels accounts for many of the hemorrhagic complications seen in patients with pseudoxanthoma elasticum.

PATHOGENESIS AND ETIOLOGY

The basic reasons for elastic fiber calcification in pseudoxanthoma elasticum are unknown. Theories have implicated the known increase in glycosaminoglycans because normal bone mineralization requires sulfated polyanions,[21] which inhibit the transformation of amorphous calcium carbonate to apatite. An abnormal protease that in some way renders the elastic fiber susceptible to calcification has been proposed.[22] Others[23, 24] have found the dermal elastic fibers in pseudoxanthoma elasticum to be more resistant to pancreatic elastase digestion than normal non–pseudoxanthoma elasticum elastic fibers.

An early classification of pseudoxanthoma elasticum into four separate phenotypes (two autosomal dominant and two autosomal recessive) with 55% of the patients showing autosomal dominant inheritance[7] conflicts with more recent studies.[1] The current consensus is that approximately 90% of the patients fall into the autosomal recessive category and that genetic subtypes cannot be based on phenotypic or biochemical differences because none have thus far been detected.[1] The gradual progression of the disorder with time eventually places all patients into a similar phenotype, albeit with great clinical variation. Autosomal dominant and autosomal recessive patients have no apparent clinical phenotypic differences. A new classification takes into account some of the unusual minimal expressions seen in otherwise unaffected family members.[25]

Molecular abnormalities in elastic fiber structure or function have been briefly studied by Uitto,[26] who has looked for abnormalities in the elastin gene on chromosome 7 (7q11.2); thus far, however, this area of chromosome 7 appears normal in pseudoxanthoma elasticum. Searches for other candidate genes have not thus far been successful.[27]

DIAGNOSIS AND DIFFERENTIAL DIAGNOSIS

The initial diagnosis of pseudoxanthoma elasticum is based largely on the presence of clinically and histologically characteristic skin lesions in flexural areas. Angioid streaks alone, while highly suggestive of pseudoxanthoma elasticum in an affected family, as previously stated, are not unique to pseudoxanthoma elasticum and usually appear a few years after the onset of skin lesions.[1] The cardiovascular manifestations (except gastrointestinal hemorrhage) generally appear still later, commonly in the fourth decade of life or later. Again, there is great clinical heterogeneity among all aspects of pseudoxanthoma elasticum.

The diagnosis may be more complicated in cases in which typical elastic fiber alterations occur in the scars of a patient with a family history but no other discernible signs of pseudoxanthoma elasticum.[28] Likewise, sparse or questionable angioid streaks have rarely been observed in patients without clinically detectable skin lesions or with minute histologic foci of pseudoxanthoma elasticum in skin lesions that are not discernible clinically. These incomplete expressions or formes frustes are difficult to categorize. They may represent minimal expressions in a heterozygote carrier of the pseudoxanthoma elasticum gene or may be early stages of the classic syndrome that will be more fully expressed in future years. As the next decade clarifies the genetic basis for pseudoxanthoma elasticum and brings an increased medical awareness of the disorder, pseudoxanthoma elasticum will probably be proven to be far more common than currently recognized.

The differential diagnosis of pseudoxanthoma elasticum is brief. Despite the namesake, cutaneous xanthomas have little or no clinical resemblance to pseudoxanthoma elasticum. Severe actinic damage to the lateral neck skin does bear a superficial resemblance to pseudoxanthoma elasticum, but the sharply marginated photodistribution places it in a different category and, if any doubt remains, the histopathology is distinct for each condition.

Several nonheritable conditions mimic pseudoxanthoma elasticum. Patients receiving long-term penicillamine therapy occasionally develop skin lesions that clinically resemble pseudoxanthoma elasticum, though seldom in flexural locations, but have no histologic resemblance to pseudoxanthoma elasticum.[29]

There is an interesting group of acquired forms of "localized acquired cutaneous pseudoxanthoma elasticum" with skin lesions that are clinically and histologically similar to classic hereditary pseudoxanthoma elasticum but are not in typical flexural sites and, with rare questionable exceptions, are not accompanied by retinal and cardiovascular involvement.[30] One form can be precipitated by repeated rubbing of calcium salts into damp skin[31, 32]; another form has been described predominantly in black obese, multiparous, hypertensive women with pseudoxanthoma elasticum–like skin lesions confined to the chest and abdomen.[33] The hypertension appears to be of non–pseudoxanthoma elasticum origin. Angioid streaks rarely develop, but occasionally a patient has streaks, which raises the possibility of true hereditary pseudoxanthoma elasticum. This form has also been called periumbilical perforating pseudoxanthoma elasticum or perforating calcific elastosis; however, the lesions occur anywhere on the chest or abdomen and the associated perforating lesions are not similar to the elastosis perforans serpiginosa–type annular perforating lesions associated with hereditary pseudoxanthoma elasticum. There is confusion in the literature about the nosologic position of periumbilical pseudoxanthoma elasticum. The more inclusive name of localized acquired cutaneous pseudoxanthoma elasticum, which encompasses all the nonheritable forms of the disorder, is preferred.[30]

Overlap syndromes with pseudoxanthoma elasticum have been described, the most common being Marfan's and Ehlers-Danlos syndromes.[4] Very rare associations with Paget's disease of bone, tumoral calcinosis, and congenital hyperphosphatasia have also been reported.[34]

TREATMENT

Despite the incurable nature of pseudoxanthoma elasticum (or any other heritable disorder), there are numerous measures that can be recommended to alter the course of the disease and prevent or minimize risk factors (Table 172–1). Knowledge of the natural course, complications, genetics, and potential aggravating factors is essential for the consultant. In general, the earlier in life prophylactic measures are instituted, the more effective they will be.

A summary of treatment recommendations follows:

1. Begin moderate dietary calcium restriction (600 to 800 mg per day) as early in life as possible.[35] This is of proven value in the childhood or adolescent years, and prudence suggests that moderate lifelong calcium restriction is of value in slowing the natural course of pseudoxanthoma elasticum.[1]

2. Care should be taken to avoid head trauma and very heavy lifting and straining, which are known to precipitate retinal hemorrhages. As a general measure, adolescents should avoid weightlifting and head-contact sports (e.g., boxing, football, soccer) and concentrate on noncontact sports (e.g., swimming, track).

3. Elevated serum lipids aggravate the long-term course of pseudoxanthoma elasticum.[1] If levels are elevated, they should be controlled through diet and exercise if possible and by drugs if necessary.

4. Intermittent claudication is often the earliest sign of vascular calcification. If it is present, a lifelong maintenance of normal weight and a regular exercise program are highly recommended to stimulate the development of collateral circulation. Pentoxifylline (Trental) has been helpful in some individuals but should be used with caution in those patients with previous, threatened, or actual gastric or retinal hemorrhages.

5. Retinal hemorrhages are often preceded by subretinal net (membrane) formation, which can often be detected by the patient with an Amsler grid and confirmed by intravenous fluorescein angiography. Laser therapy for retinal hemorrhages is of questionable value and is thought by some to stimulate new areas of neovascularization, which may foster more hemorrhages in the future.[36] Supplements of vitamins A, C, E, and zinc are

◀ TABLE 172–1. Treatment of Pseudoxanthoma Elasticum
Maintenance of a low calcium diet
Avoidance of head-contact sports
Control of serum lipids
Exercise and weight control
Use of an Amsler grid
Limitation of the number of pregnancies
Control of hypertension
Avoidance of tobacco
Awareness of possible gastrointestinal hemorrhage
Avoidance of aspirin and nonsteroidal anti-inflammatory drugs
Use of antibiotics before surgery if mitral valve prolapse with a murmur is present
Genetic counseling

recommended by some ophthalmologists to reduce the risk of retinal hemorrhages. Interferon alfa-2a has been used experimentally in the treatment of retinal hemorrhages in patients with pseudoxanthoma elasticum but needs confirmation before it can be recommended with confidence.[37]

6. Pregnancy and childbirth are well tolerated,[38] but multiple pregnancies tend to aggravate the course of the disorder.[1]

7. Hypertension aggravates the cardiovascular complications and should be controlled with diet and exercise if possible and by drugs if necessary.

8. Tobacco use in any form aggravates pseudoxanthoma elasticum.

9. Acute severe gastrointestinal hemorrhage may occur with little or no warning; therefore, careful watch for melena or any gastrointestinal upset is important. Aspirin and the nonsteroidal anti-inflammatory drugs should be avoided except for occasional use. These drugs and pentoxifylline should be assiduously avoided if there are any symptoms of gastrointestinal upset or threatened retinal hemorrhage.

10. Mitral valve prolapse is common in pseudoxanthoma elasticum (and many other conditions) but is of no consequence unless accompanied by a murmur of mitral valve insufficiency. If a murmur is present, antibiotics are recommended before dental or other surgical procedures are performed.

11. Genetic counseling is essential for all patients.

Ehlers-Danlos Syndrome

In 1901 and 1908, respectively, Ehlers,[39] a Copenhagen dermatologist, and Danlos,[40] a Paris dermatologist, independently reported patients with thin, hyperelastic skin, frequent cutaneous hemorrhages, loose jointedness, and cutaneous pseudotumors. By 1949, the eponym Ehlers-Danlos syndrome was well established and an autosomal dominant inheritance pattern recognized. By 1967, a much greater clinical heterogeneous nature of the syndrome was beginning to be reported and three clinical types were recognized. McKusick, in 1972, described seven types. There are now 9 (and possibly 10) types delineated, and all three major inheritance patterns—autosomal dominant, autosomal recessive, and X-linked—have been observed. The reader interested in Ehlers-Danlos syndrome is referred to several extensive studies.[41-43]

CLINICAL DESCRIPTION

Except for one of the types (type V), the skin is light in color, thin, smooth with a velvety feel, and extremely hyperelastic such that when pulled it rapidly retracts when released (Fig. 172–5).[41] (The circus "rubber man" or "human pretzel" has Ehlers-Danlos syndrome.)

Cutaneous fragility (dermatorrhexis) is markedly in-

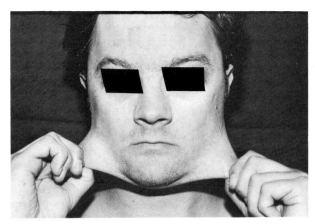

FIGURE 172–5. Hyperelastic skin of the face of a patient with Ehlers-Danlos syndrome.

creased and is particularly troublesome over bony pressure points (knees, elbows, forehead, shins) where mild trauma causes gaping "fish mouth" wounds that are difficult to close because the skin does not hold sutures well. Healing is slow, leaving a thin, shiny, cigarette paper–like scar. Such lacerations are common during childhood when minor trauma is common. After multiple traumatic episodes with scarring and cutaneous hemorrhages, soft, heaped-up pseudotumors develop (Fig. 172–6). In time, small buckshot-sized spheroids develop within the pseudotumors. Elastosis perforans serpiginosa and piezogenic papules on the lateral heel margins occur in some patients.

Another feature of Ehlers-Danlos syndrome skin is easy bruisability and hemorrhage believed due to the poor connective tissue support of the vasculature and direct involvement of the vessel wall. Gingival bleeding after brushing is a common experience, as is excessive hemorrhage after surgical procedures.[44] Life-threatening cerebral and coronary aneurysms may occur, especially in type IV.[45, 46]

The other major characteristic of Ehlers-Danlos syndrome is hyperextensibility of the joints with marked laxity of the joint capsules, ligaments, and tendons (Figs. 172–7 and 172–8). This may range from moderate to the unbelievable. Except for type IV, the most severely

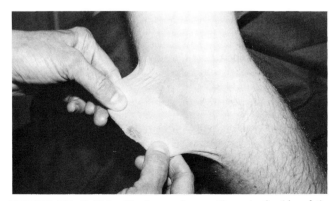

FIGURE 172–6. Ehlers-Danlos syndrome. Hyperelastic skin of the elbow with a pseudotumor on the elbow.

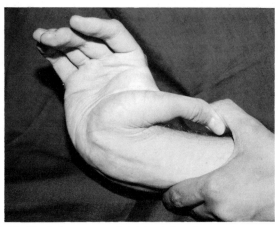

FIGURE 172-7. Hyperextensible joints of the fingers of a patient with Ehlers-Danlos syndrome.

affected individuals can perform such feats as placing their ankles behind their necks or placing their head between their knees—while bending backward! These traits are usually apparent when the child begins to walk. Additional joint and bone complications include pes planus, joint dislocations, spinal deformity, joint effusions, osteoarthritis, talipes, and congenital hip dislocation.

Hernias of all types are common. Pregnancy is often complicated by premature rupture of the membranes and premature delivery with severe postpartum hemorrhage in all types, but especially in type IV.[47] Ocular complications include blue sclerae, strabismus, redundant eyelids, retinal detachment, retinal hemorrhages, and rupture of the globe.

The prevalence of Ehlers-Danlos syndrome is not well established. Estimates range from 1:156,000[48] to a much higher frequency,[49] based on the assumption that many mild expressions of the disorder go undiagnosed. There is no known racial, ethnic, or geographic predisposition.

PATHOLOGY AND PATHOGENESIS

For practical purposes, skin biopsy does not play a role in the diagnosis of Ehlers-Danlos syndrome, since observations of such features as dermal thinning and decreased diameter of collagen bundles by routine light microscopy and distorted arrangement of fibrils on ultrastructural examination have been contradictory. Studies of the extracellular matrix in the various types of Ehlers-Danlos syndrome have been comprehensively summarized.[41, 50] The possibility of a single basic genetic defect is unlikely and remains unknown. There are probably multiple genetic defects to account for the clinical heterogeneity seen in this disorder.

In brief, Ehlers-Danlos syndrome types I, II, and III have a loose, disorderly arrangement of apparently normal collagen fibers but lack a specific known biochemical defect. Approximately 90% of all cases fall into one of these three types and differ only in degrees of severity. Type IV has a known deficiency of collagen type III. As a result, tissues rich in collagen type III (e.g., skin, blood vessels, internal organs) are more severely affected while collagen type III poor structures (e.g., bone, cartilage) are less affected. Ehlers-Danlos syndrome types I, II, and III are the most common types with severe vascular complications.[51]

Type V has only been reported in nine patients and is probably inherited in an X-linked pattern.[52] Most symptoms and signs are relatively mild. There is no known biochemical marker for this type.

In type VI (ocular-scoliotic type) patients have a deficiency of hydroxylysine owing to a basic deficiency of lysyl hydroxylase.[41, 53, 54] This type is apparent in neonates who have severe muscular hypotonia and kyphoscoliosis. Retinal detachment with hemorrhage and rupture of the globe may occur early in life.

Type VII is characterized by especially severe laxity of the ligaments and joint capsules, which allows for enormous joint hypermobility and recurrent subluxations. Congenital hip dislocation is present in nearly all patients. Two defects in collagen cross-linking have been found, one in α_1 (I) chains[55] (type VII A) and the other in α_2 (I) chains (type VII B). Another variant (type VII C) with dermatosparaxis has been proposed.

In type VIII there are mild skin and joint changes but a dramatic loss of primary and secondary teeth much earlier than normal, secondary to a gingivitis and an absorptive periodontosis.[56, 57]

Type IX (occipital horn syndrome) is very rare (reported in about 13 patients) and is characterized by relatively sparse skin and joint manifestations.[58] Diverticula of the urinary bladder have been described.[59] A defect in copper transport has been discovered, suggesting that this type should no longer be classified with Ehlers-Danlos syndrome. Serum ceruloplasmin and copper levels are low and fibroblast copper concentration is high, all of which impair normal lysyl oxidase production and activity.[60]

Type X (found in four of six members of one family) has moderate skin and joint manifestations and a distinguishing feature of plasma and cellular fibronectin dysfunction and a platelet aggregation defect.[61]

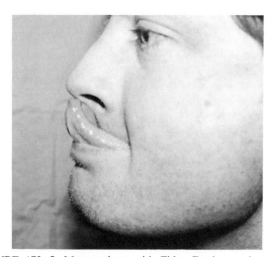

FIGURE 172-8. Most patients with Ehlers-Danlos syndrome can touch their nose with the tip of their tongue (a positive Gorlin sign).

TABLE 172–2. Ehlers-Danlos Syndrome

Type	Skin Signs			Joint Laxity	Complications	Inheritance	Primary Defect
	Elasticity	Fragility	Bruising				
I (gravis)	(+++)	(+++)	(++)	(+++)	Bowel, aorta rupture	AD	Unknown
II (mitis)	(++)	(++)	(+)	(++)	Few complications (often undiagnosed)	AD	Unknown
III (hypermobile)	(+)	(+)	(+)	(+++)	Arthritis muscle pain	AD	Unknown
IV	(−)	(+++)	(+++)	(+)	Aneurysms with rupture; severe obstetric hemorrhage; pneumothorax	AD	Type III collagen deficiency
V	(+++)	(+)	(+)	(+)	Same as I, II, and III but less severe	Probably XL	
VI	(+++)	(++)	(++)	(+++)	Muscle hypotonia; kyphoscoliosis; osteoporosis; eye globe rupture	AR	Lysyl hydroxylase deficiency in most cases
VII	(++)	(+)	(+)	(++++)	Severe ligament and joint laxity; congenital hip arthritis	AD	Missing N-telopeptid of α_1 (I) or α_2 (I) chains of collagen type I (three possible subtypes)
VIII	(+)	(++)	(++)	(++)	Periodontal disease with early loss of teeth	AD	Unknown
IX	(+/−)	(+)	(−)	(+)	Skin more lax than hyperelastic; "occipital horns"; osteoporosis; bladder; diverticulae	XL	Lysyl oxidase deficiency with abnormal copper homeostasis
X	(+)	(+)	(+)	(++)	Petechiae	?	?Fibronectin defect

TABLE 172-3. Differential Diagnosis of Ehlers-Danlos Syndrome
Disorders with Joint Laxity
Marfan's syndrome
Marfanoid hypermobility syndrome
Larsen's syndrome
Osteogenesis imperfecta
Stickler's hereditary arthrophthalmopathy syndrome
Pseudoachondroplasia
Morquio's syndrome
Fragile X syndrome
Trisomy-8 mosaic syndrome
Disorders with Hyperelastic Skin
Noonan's syndrome
Cutis laxa
De Barsy's syndrome
Gerodermia osteodysplastica hereditaria
Menkes' kinky hair disease
Wrinkly skin syndrome
Syndrome with Mitral Valve Prolapse Abnormalities Similar to Ehlers-Danlos Syndrome
Familial mitral valve prolapse
Annuloaortic ectasia
Marfan's syndrome
Syndromes with Vascular Fragility and Hemorrhagic Complications Similar to Type IV
Hemophilia
von Willebrand's disease
Scurvy
Dysfibrinogenemia
Factor XIII deficiency
Marfan's syndrome (arterial rupture)

The recognized types of Ehlers-Danlos syndrome are summarized in Table 172-2.

The great clinical, biochemical, and genetic heterogeneity of the syndrome has created a haven for splitters. As new minor variants are described, claims are being made for even more types of Ehlers-Danlos syndrome, including progeroid[62, 63] and familial hypermobile[64] forms and forms that overlap with other entities.[41, 65]

DIAGNOSIS AND DIFFERENTIAL DIAGNOSIS

The diagnosis of all types is based initially on the clinical findings of hyperelastic skin and joint laxity even though these findings are minimal in some of the rare types (IV, VII, IX, and X). Types I, II, and III have the most severe skin and joint involvement and comprise about 90% of all cases. Types IV, VI, VII, and IX have biochemical abnormalities (see section on pathology) that must be identified to correctly diagnose the type.

Accurate diagnosis of type IV is important because of potential life-threatening hemorrhagic complications. Absence of collagen type III is required for the diagnosis. Type VI may have a deficiency of lysyl hydroxylase and hydroxylysine (type VI A) or rarely may have normal lysyl hydroxylase activity (type VI B). Types IV and VII can be diagnosed prenatally.[66]

There are other heritable syndromes that may have features of hyperelastic skin or joint hyperextensibility similar to those of Ehlers-Danlos syndrome; however, they are seldom combined as in Ehlers-Danlos syndrome. Some of the disorders to be considered in the differential diagnoses of Ehlers-Danlos syndrome are summarized in Table 172-3.

TREATMENT

Treatment is largely symptomatic, although various specific prophylactic measures are now possible. Genetic counseling is of vital importance and should obviously be given before the reproductive years.

Some of the more important prophylactic and therapeutic measures include the following:

1. Physical therapy and exercise programs for those with the most severe skin, muscle, and joint involvement (especially those with types I, II, and III).

2. Protective garments should be worn over bony prominences to pad fragile skin and reduce tears. Extra suturing precautions are required to close torn and ragged wounds (especially in those with types I, II, and III).

3. Vigorous contact sports should be avoided in patients with any type of Ehlers-Danlos syndrome.

4. Counseling is of particular importance in persons with type IV Ehlers-Danlos syndrome because of increased risks for sudden arterial hemorrhages and bowel perforation. Such patients should wear medical-alert bracelets.

5. Patients with type VI with severe kyphoscoliosis may require early surgical bracing of the spine. They should also carry cards or wear bracelets describing possible rupture of the ocular globe.

6. In type VII, frequent joint subluxations may be prevented by wearing appropriate braces or supports over the most susceptible joints.

7. The platelet aggregation defect in type X has thus far not responded to attempts at correction with human fibronectin. Future refinements in this area may be more successful.

8. Those patients with mitral valve prolapse and a murmur of mitral valve regurgitation should take antibiotics before surgery and dental procedures.

9. Antirheumatic drugs are indicated for articular pain.

10. Vitamins and minerals (vitamins C and A, plus zinc and iron) taken to promote collagen and elastin synthesis have had questionable results but at least in moderate doses will do no harm.

Acrokeratoelastoidosis

DEFINITION

Acrokeratoelastoidosis is a condition in which small hyperkeratotic papules occur on the hands or feet with disrupted elastic tissue in the underlying dermis.

CLINICAL DESCRIPTION

The papules of acrokeratoelastoidosis are small (2 to 4 mm) and shiny. They tend to occur on the dorsal hands, usually over the knuckles and often in groups. The lateral margins of the palms and soles may also be involved. They most commonly appear during childhood or adolescence and usually remain throughout life.[67]

PATHOLOGY

Microscopic examination shows slight hyperkeratosis, with a gently delled epidermal surface. The disorder is histologically not a true proliferative "elastoidosis" but rather an "elastorrhexis." Elastic tissue stains are needed to show that fibers in the reticular dermis are fragmented and diminished in number, although some thicker and tortuous fibers may be interspersed.

PATHOGENESIS AND ETIOLOGY

Other than showing an autosomal dominant inheritance pattern, no other cause is known. The fact that cases occur in childhood tends to rule out excessive sun exposure or heavy use of the hands.

DIAGNOSIS AND DIFFERENTIAL DIAGNOSIS

The diagnosis is based on the clinical appearance, early onset, hereditary predisposition, and the histologic finding of decreased and fragmented elastic fibers in the reticular dermis.

Two conditions resemble acrokeratoelastoidosis clinically:

1. Focal acral hyperkeratosis differs only in that the dermis has a normal histologic appearance (i.e., without elastorrhexis). A positive family history is variable. The onset is usually early (second to third decade). The hands and/or feet may be involved.

2. Keratoelastoidosis marginalis[70] (also called degenerative collagenous plaques of the hands by Burks[71]) causes clinically similar lesions on the margins of the hands of older persons who have had excessive sun exposure and hard use of their hands over many years. Histopathologic examination can distinguish this condition from acrokeratoelastoidosis, in that the superficial dermis in keratoelastoidosis marginalis shows thick, vertically and diagonally arranged collagen bundles with interspersed elastotic material.

TREATMENT

Essentially no treatment is needed. Shave excision or electrodesiccation may be tried but may leave scars.

References

1. Neldner KH. Pseudoxanthoma elasticum. Clin Dermatol 1988; 6:1–159.
2. Katagiri K, Fujiwara S, Shinkai H, et al. Heterogeneity of clinical features of pseudoxanthoma elasticum. J Dermatol 1991; 18:211–217.
3. Berlyne GM, Bulmer HG, Platt R. The genetics of pseudoxanthoma elasticum. Q J Med 1961;30:201–212.
4. McKusick VA. Heritable Disorders of Connective Tissue, 5th edition. Beighton P, ed. St. Louis: Mosby–Year Book, 1993.
5. Goodman RM, Smith EW, Paton D, et al. Pseudoxanthoma elasticum: A clinical and histopathological study. Medicine 1963; 42:297–334.
6. Eddy DD, Farber EM. Pseudoxanthoma elasticum: Internal manifestations: A report of cases and a statistical review of the literature. Arch Dermatol 1962;86:729–740.
7. Pope FM. Two types of autosomal recessive pseudoxanthoma elasticum. Arch Dermatol 1974;110:209–212.
8. Paton D. The Relation of Angioid Streaks to Systemic Disease. Springfield, IL: Charles C Thomas, 1972.
9. Connor PJ, Juergens JL, Perry HO, et al. Pseudoxanthoma elasticum and angioid streaks: A review of 106 cases. Am J Med 1961;30:537–543.
10. Lebwohl MG, Distefano D, Prioleau PG, et al. Pseudoxanthoma elasticum and mitral valve prolapse. N Engl J Med 1982; 307:228–231.
11. Yamamura H, Hiraide A, Tabuse H, et al. A report of pseudoxanthoma elasticum with upper gastrointestinal hemorrhage. Nippon Ceba Gakkai Zasshi 1991;92:1027–1030.
12. Smith JG Jr, Davidson EA, Taylor RW. Cutaneous acid mucopolysaccharides in pseudoxanthoma elasticum. J Invest Dermatol 1964;43:429–430.
13. Longas MO, Wisch P, Lebwohl M, et al. Glycosaminoglycans of skin and urine in pseudoxanthoma elasticum: Evidence for chondroitin-6-sulfate alteration. Clin Chim Acta 1986;55:227–236.
14. Martinez-Hernandez A, Huffer WE. Pseudoxanthoma elasticum: Dermal polyanions and the mineralization of elastic fibers. Lab Invest 1974;31:181–186.
15. Smith JG Jr, Davidson EA, Clark RD. Dermal elastin in actinic elastosis and pseudoxanthoma elasticum. Nature 1962;195: 716–717.
16. Uitto J, Paul JL, Brockley K, et al. Elastic fibers in human skin: Quantitation of elastic fibers by computerized digital image analyses and determination of elastin by radioimmunoassay of desmosine. Lab Invest 1983;49:499–505.
17. Schwartz E, Cruickshank FA, Lebwohl M. Determination of desmosines in elastin-related skin disorders by isocratic high performance liquid chromatography. Exp Mol Pathol 1990;52:63–68.
18. Pasquali-Ronchetti I, Volpin D, Baccarani-Contri M, et al. Pseudoxanthoma elasticum: Biochemical and ultrastructural studies. Dermatologica 1981;163:307–325.
19. Danielsen L. Morphological changes in pseudoxanthoma elasticum and senile skin. Acta Derm Venereol 1979(Suppl 83);1–79.
20. Danielsen L. Morphologic changes in pseudoxanthoma elasticum and senile skin. Int J Dermatol 1982;21:604–605.
21. Blumenthal NC, Posner AS, Silverman LD, et al. Effect of proteoglycans on in vitro hydroxyapatite formation. Calcif Tissue Int 1979;27:75–82.
22. Gordon SC, Hinkle LL, Shaw E. Cysteine protease characteristics of the proteoglycanase activity from normal and pseudoxanthoma elasticum fibroblasts. J Lab Clin Med 1983;102:400–410.
23. Schwartz E, Cruickshank FA, Lebwohl MG. Elastase-like protease

and elastolytic activities expressed in cultured dermal fibroblasts from lesions in skin of patients with pseudoxanthoma elasticum, actinic elastosis and cutis laxa. Clin Chim Acta 1988;176: 219–224.

24. Schwartz E, Thieberg M, Cruickshank FA, et al. Elastase digestion of normal and pseudoxanthoma elasticum lesional skin elastins. Exp Mol Pathol 1991;55:190–195.
25. Lebwohl MG, Neldner KH, Pope FM, et al. Classification of pseudoxanthoma elasticum. In press.
26. Uitto J. Biochemistry of the elastic fibers in normal connective tissues and its alterations in diseases. J Invest Dermatol 1979;72:1–10.
27. Christiano AM, Lebwohl MG, Boyd CD, et al. Workshop on pseudoxanthoma elasticum. Molecular Biology and Pathology of the Elastic Fibers. Jefferson Medical College, Philadelphia, PA, June 10, 1992. J Invest Dermatol 1992;99:660–663.
28. Lebwohl MG, Phelps RG, Yannuzzi L, et al. Diagnosis of pseudoxanthoma elasticum by scar biopsy in patients without characteristic skin lesions. N Engl J Med 1987;317:347–350.
29. Meyrick Thomas RH, Kirby JDT. Elastosis perforans serpiginosa and pseudoxanthoma elasticum-like skin change due to D-penicillamine. Clin Exp Dermatol 1985;10:386–391.
30. Neldner KH, Martinez-Hernandez A. Localized acquired cutaneous pseudoxanthoma elasticum. J Am Acad Dermatol 1979;1: 523–530.
31. Christensen OB. An exogenous variety of pseudoxanthoma elasticum in old farmers. Acta Derm Venereol 1978;58:319–321.
32. Otkjaer-Nielsen A, Christensen OB, Hentzer B, et al. Saltpeter-induced dermal changes electron microscopically indistinguishable from pseudoxanthoma elasticum. Acta Derm Venereol 1978;58:323–327.
33. Hicks J, Carpenter CL, Reed RJ. Periumbilical perforating pseudoxanthoma elasticum. Arch Dermatol 1979;115:300–303.
34. Najjar SS, Farah FS, Kurban AK, et al. Tumoral calcinosis and pseudoxanthoma elasticum. J Pediatr 1968;72:243–247.
35. Renie WA, Pyeritz RE, Combs J, et al. Pseudoxanthoma elasticum: High calcium intake in early life correlates with severity. Am J Med Genet 1984;19:235–244.
36. Singerman LJ, Hatem G. Laser treatment of choroidal neovascular membranes in angioid streaks. Retina 1981;1:75–83.
37. Fung WE. Interferon-α 2a for treatment of age-related macular degeneration. Am J Ophthalmol 1991;112:349–350.
38. Berde C, Willis DC, Sandberg EC. Pregnancy in women with pseudoxanthoma elasticum. Obstet Gynecol Surv 1983;35: 279–284.
39. Ehlers E. Cutis Laxa, Neigung zu haemorrhagien in der haut, Lockerung mehrerer Artikulationen. Dermatol Z 1901;8:173–174.
40. Danlos HA. Un cas de cutis laxa avec tumeurs par contusion chronique des coudes et des genouz (xanthoma juvénile pseudo-diabétique de MM, Hallopeau et Macé de Lépinay). Bull Soc Fr Dermatol Syphiligr 1908;19:70–72.
41. Steimmann B, Royce PM, Superti-Furga A. The Ehlers-Danlos syndrome. In: Royce PM, Steinman B, eds. Connective Tissue and Its Heritable Disorders: Molecular, Genetic and Medical Aspects. New York: Wiley–Liss, 1993;351–407.
42. Byers PH, Holbrook KA. Ehlers-Danlos syndrome. In: Emery AEH, Rimoin DL, eds. Principles and Practice of Medical Genetics, 2nd ed. Edinburgh: Churchill Livingstone, 1990; 1065–1081.
43. Gorlin RJ, Cohen MM, Levin LS. Ehlers-Danlos syndrome. In: Syndromes of the Head and Neck, 3rd ed. New York: Oxford University Press, 1990:429–441.
44. Welbury RR. Ehlers-Danlos syndrome: Historical review, report of two cases in one family and treatment needs. ASDC Tour Dentistry Children 1989;56:220–224.
45. Erickson UH, Aunsholt NA, Neilsen TT. Enormous right coronary arterial aneurysm in a patient with type IV Ehlers-Danlos syndrome. Int J Cardiol 1992;35:259–261.
46. Ruby ST, Kramer J, Cassidy SB, Tsipouras P. Internal carotid artery aneurysm: A vascular manifestation of type IV Ehlers-Danlos syndrome. Conn Med 1989;53:142–144.
47. Pope FM, Nicholls AC. Pregnancy and Ehlers-Danlos syndrome type IV. Lancet 1983;1:249–250.

48. Breighton P. The Ehlers-Danlos Syndrome. London: William Heinemann Medical Books, 1970.
49. Holzberg M, Hewan-Lowe KO, Olansky AJ. The Ehlers-Danlos syndrome: Recognition, characterization, and importance of a milder variant of the classic form. J Am Acad Dermatol 1988;19:656–666.
50. Pope FM, Daw SC, Narcisi P, et al. Prenatal diagnosis and prevention of inherited abnormalities of collagen. J Inherit Metab Dis 1989;53:142–144.
51. Sparkman RS. Ehlers-Danlos syndrome type IV: Dramatic, deceptive, and deadly. Am J Surg 1984;147:703–704.
52. Beighton P, Curtis D. X-linked Ehlers-Danlos syndrome type V: The next generation. Clin Genet 1985;27:472–478.
53. Krane SM, Pinnell SR, Erbe RW. Lysyl-protocollagen hydroxylase deficiency in fibroblasts from siblings with hydroxylysine deficiency in fibroblasts from siblings with hydroxylysine-deficiency collagen. Proc Natl Acad Sci USA 1972;69:2899–2903.
54. Hautala T, Byers MG, Eddy RL, et al. Cloning of human lysyl hydroxylase: Complete cDNA-derived amino acid sequence and assignment of the gene (PLOD) to chromosome 1p36.2-p36.3. Genomics 1992;13:62–69.
55. Beighton P, de Paepe A, Danks D, et al. International nosology of heritable disorders of connective tissue, Berlin, 1986. Am J Med Genet 1988;29:581–594.
56. Satoris DJ, Luzzatti L, Weaver DD, et al. Type IX Ehlers-Danlos syndrome: A new variant with pathognomonic radiographic features. Radiology 1984;152:665–670.
57. Biesecker LG, Erickson RP, Glover TW, et al. Molecular and cytologic studies of Ehlers-Danlos syndrome type VIII. Am J Med Genet 1991;41:284–288.
58. Hoffman GS, Filie JD, Schumacher HR Jr, et al. Intractable vasculitis, resorptive osteolysis, and immunity to type I collagen in type VIII Ehlers-Danlos syndrome. Arthritis Rheum 1991;34: 1466–1475.
59. Rabin JM, Hirschfield L, Baldlani GH. Type IX Ehlers-Danlos syndrome: Bladder diverticula with transitional cell carcinoma. Urology 1991;36:563–566.
60. Peltonen L, Kuivaniemi H, Palotie A, et al. Alterations in copper and collagen metabolism in the Menkes syndrome and a new subtype of the Ehlers-Danlos syndrome. Biochemistry 1983;22:6156–6163.
61. Arneson MA, Hammerschmidt DE, Furcht LT, et al. A new form of Ehlers-Danlos syndrome: fibronectin corrects defective platelet function. JAMA 1980;244:144–147.
62. Hernández A, Aguirre-Negrete MG, Gonzáles-Flores S, et al. Ehlers-Danlos features with progeroid facies and mild mental retardation. Clin Genet 1986;30:456–461.
63. Kresse H, Rosthøj S, Quentin E, et al. Glycosaminolglycan-free small proteoglycan core protein is secreted by fibroblasts from a patient with a syndrome resembling progeroid. Am J Hum Genet 1987;41:436–453.
64. Beighton PH, Horan FT. Dominant inheritance in familial generalised articular hypermobility. J Bone Joint Surg [Br] 1970;52:145–147.
65. Hartsfield JK Jr, Lousseff BG. Phenotypic overlap of Ehlers-Danlos syndrome types IV and VIII. Am J Med Genet 1990;37:465–470.
66. Cohn DH, Byers PH. Clinical screening for collagen defects in connective tissue diseases. Clin Perinatol 1990;17:793–809.
67. Highet AS, Rook A, Anderson JR. Acrokeratoelastoidosis. Br J Dermatol 1982;106:337–344.
68. Costa OG. Acrokeratoelastoidosis. Arch Dermatol 1954;170: 228–231.
69. Korc A, Hansen R, Lynch P. Acrokeratoelastoidis of Costa in North America. J Am Acad Dermatol 1985;12:832–836.
70. Koscard E. Keratoelastoidosis marginalis of the hands. Dermatologica 1954;131:169–175.
71. Burks JW, Wise LJ, Clark WH. Degenerative collagenous plaques of the hands. Arch Dermatol 1960;82:362–366.
72. Dowd PM, Harman RPM, Black MM, Focal acral hyperkeratosis. Br J Dermatol 1983;109:97–103.

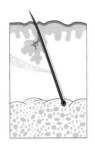

chapter 173

Focal Dermal Hypoplasia and Aplasia Cutis Congenita

ILONA J. FRIEDEN

Focal Dermal Hypoplasia

DEFINITION

Focal dermal hypoplasia (Goltz syndrome; Goltz-Gorlin syndrome) is an X-linked recessive disorder characterized by ectodermal and mesodermal abnormalities. Since its initial description in 1962, over 200 cases have been described, most of them in females.[1-5] The skin, bones, and teeth are the most common sites of involvement, but multiple other organ systems can be affected.

CLINICAL DESCRIPTION

Several diverse skin lesions have been noted, primarily in linear patterns corresponding to the lines of Blashko. These include pink or reddish-brown atrophic-appearing macules in a cribriform pattern (Fig. 173-1); poikiloderma; scar-like areas; soft, yellow-brown fat "herniation", macular hyper- and hypopigmentation, and papillomatous areas, particularly around mucous membranes and periorificial areas. At birth, areas of aplasia cutis may be noted. An inflammatory or desquamative phase, and even blistering or crusting may be present, occasionally preceding the development of other skin findings.[2, 6] Other less common cutaneous manifestations include hyper- and hypohidrosis, lichenoid follicular papules, urtication or intense erythema upon stroking the skin, radial folds around the mouth, and keratototic lesions of the palms and soles.[2] The hair may be brittle, sparse,

contain areas of localized poliosis, and may be totally missing with areas of scarring noted. The nails may also be absent, poorly developed, dystrophic, spooned, grooved, or hypopigmented. In addition to the diverse array of skin lesions, the severity of skin and systemic manifestations may vary considerably; in mild cases, only faint reddish-brown linear atrophic areas may be present, making diagnosis elusive, until a more severely affected offspring is born.[7]

Skeletal abnormalities are very common, especially syndactyly, often of the third and fourth fingers or of the second and third toes. Other reported skeletal abnormalities include short stature; hemiatrophy; microcephaly; complete hypoplasia, absence, or fusion of digits; camptodactyly; clinodactyly; kyphosis; scoliosis; fusion of vertebrae; rib anomalies; and multiple giant cell tumors of the bone.[2, 8] The radiologic finding of osteopathia striata, multiple lines extending from the epiphysis into the diaphysis, which may be present in a number of other congenital disorders, is relatively common in focal dermal hypoplasia, and may be helpful in cases with an uncertain diagnosis.[9, 10]

Oral and dental abnormalities are also relatively common, occurring in approximately one half of affected patients.[11] These include missing teeth, enamel defects, irregular spacing, malocclusion, notching of incisors, extra teeth, mandibular hypoplasia, prognathism, papillomatous lip and gingival lesions, and in rare instances, cleft lip and palate.[12] Papillomatous lesions of the hypopharynx and larynx have also been reported.[13]

Eye abnormalities, including (rarely) anophthalmia; aniridia; increased intercanthal distance; strabismus; nystagmus; colobomas of the iris, choroid, retina, or optic nerve; heterochromia; blue sclera; and clouding of

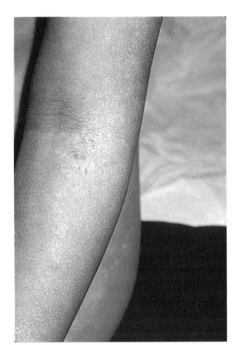

FIGURE 173–1. Linear atrophic lesion on the arm of a patient with Goltz syndrome.

PATHOLOGY

The histopathologic findings of focal dermal hypoplasia depend on the type of skin lesion on which a biopsy is performed.[15] Areas of aplasia cutis congenita demonstrate absence of appendages and a thinner than normal dermis, either covered by an epidermis or devoid of one. The atrophic areas, whether irregular in shape or linear, have clusters of adipocytes that are abnormally situated in the mid or upper reticular dermis or in the papillary dermis. These collections are not in continuity with the subcutaneous fat, indicating that they are malformations rather than herniations as some authors have proposed.[2, 16] The papillary dermis in atrophic areas is often thickened, with increased number of small vessels, and the appearance of atrophy results from diminished reticular dermal colagen fibers. The periorificial papillomas have narrow stalks, rugose surfaces, and epidermal hyperplasia with hyper- or parakeratosis. Lipomatous lesions appear to be the result of progressive enlargement of the fatty deposits found in atrophic defects, with large nodules of lipocytes that elevate the cutaneous surface.[16] In very mild cases, where only atrophic linear lesions are present, the characteristic changes with fat high in the dermis may not be seen; multiple biopsies may be necessary to adequately document the diagnosis.[7]

PATHOGENESIS AND ETIOLOGY

Focal dermal hypoplasia is generally believed to be an X-linked recessive disorder that is usually lethal in hemizygous males, but despite this, 12% of reported cases are in males (unlike incontinentia pigmenti, where only 3% of reported cases are males). Some reports have linked

the cornea or vitreous, have been reported. The wide variety of other described manifestations include facial asymmetry, mental deficiency (which is relatively uncommon), renal and ureteral anomalies, hernias, rectal prolapse, omphalocele, and cardiac anomalies (Table 173–1).[14]

TABLE 173-1. Systemic Defects Associated with Focal Dermal Hypoplasia

System	Defects	Percentage of Patients Affected
Skin	Area of symmetric linearity of aplasia, poikiloderma	>50
	Hypopigmentation of hyperpigmentation, telangiectasias	>50
	Localized herniation of subcutaneous adipose tissue	>50
	Aplasia cutis congenita	10–50
	Multiple papillomas of mucous membranes, esophageal, periorificial, or intertriginous areas	>50
	Hypertrichosis, cicatricial alopecia, sparsity of hair	<10
Skeleton	Short stature; microcephaly; asymmetry of skull, trunk, and extremities; cleft hand	<10
	Hypoplastic and/or absent digits	10–50
	Polydactyly, syndactyly, cleft symphysis, osteopathia striata of long bones, vertebral abnormalities, scoliosis, rib anomalies	
Dental	Enamel defects, early caries, oligodontias, malformed teeth, unerupted teeth, malplaced teeth	
Eyes	Anophthalmia	10–50
	Microphthalmia, pupil and iris abnormalities, optic atrophy	
Soft tissue	Largeness, asymmetry, anteversion of ears	10–50
	Hearing deficit, neurodevelopmental abnormalities, mental deficiency, cleft palate and lip, transverse facial cleft rarely, hernia, omphalocele, congenital heart disease, renal ectopia, unilateral agenesis or hydronephrosis of kidneys, bifid ureter and renal pelvis	

From Suskan E, Kurkcuoglu N, Uluoglu O. Focal dermal hypoplasia (Goltz syndrome) with horseshoe kidney abnormality. Pediatr Dermatol 1990;7:283–286. Reprinted by permission of Blackwell Scientific Publications, Inc.

focal dermal hypoplasia to Xp22.31, but a definite assignment has not been made.[17] Two pedigrees with father-to-daughter inheritance have led to the alternative hypothesis of an autosomal dominant sex-limited form of inheritance, but one of these father-daughter pedigrees has recently been studied, and a pattern of nonrandom (skewed) X-inactivation consistent with X-linked inheritance, and paternal X chromosome mosaicism has been demonstrated, confirming the X-linked nature of this disease.[18] The wide latitude in severity of manifestations in the condition is likely due to the relative number of mutant X chromosomes that remain active.[19] Opitz has argued that the diverse abnormalities noted may be in part due to the effects of the abnormal gene on the developing apical ectodermal ridges, causing a wide variety of secondary abnormalities.[20] The pathogenesis of the abnormally positioned clusters of adipocytes in focal dermal hypoplasia has been controversial. A defect in dermal connective tissue that results in herniation of subcutaneous lipocytes seems less likely than does the proposition that developmental defect leads to the differential of perivascular primitive mesenchymal cells to lipocytes in abnormally superficial locations. Many of the varied clinical appearances of the cutaneous lesions in focal dermal hypoplasia can be explained by progressive enlargement of the collections of lipocytes over time.[16]

DIAGNOSIS AND DIFFERENTIAL DIAGNOSIS

Diagnosis is made based on the clinical findings, correlated with the skin histopathology of affected skin. Long-bone films looking for osteopathia striata may be helpful in some cases. Eye examinations searching for abnormalities should be performed in all affected individuals. The major conditions in differential diagnosis include incontinentia pigmenti, the epidermal nevus syndrome, linear porokeratosis, and the ectodermal dysplasia–ectrodactyly–clefting syndrome (EEC) (Table 173–2).[21] The first two conditions can usually be distinguished readily by histopathologic findings. The EEC syndrome can have skin changes, primarily dermatitis, but does not show the linear and whorled skin or papillomatous lesions found in focal dermal hypoplasia. Mul-

tiple biopsies of affected skin, careful evaluation of other family members, and radiographs searching for osteopathia striata may be helpful in cases with diagnostic uncertainty.

TREATMENT

There is no specific treatment of focal dermal hypoplasia. Papillomatous lesions may be excised if they become cosmetically or functionally bothersome. Orthopedic surgery may help some limb abnormalities. All affected individuals should have dental and ophthalmologic evaluations, and be carefully monitored for musculoskeletal, genitourinary, and developmental problems. Other family members should be examined for abnormalities. Genetic counseling should be given to the affected individual and family. Even in the absence of a precise genetic marker, prenatal diagnosis may be helpful in identifying a female infant at greater risk by using ultrasound to search for severe skeletal anomalies.

Aplasia Cutis Congenita

DEFINITION

Aplasia cutis congenita is characterized by localized area(s) of absent skin at birth. This clinical finding is caused by a heterogeneous group of diseases including autosomal dominant and recessive genetic disorders, chromosomal abnormalities, teratogens, intrauterine infections, and intrauterine vascular accidents. Moreover, many cases are of unknown etiology and are unassociated with any other discernible abnormalities. In addition to the term *aplasia cutis congenita*, many cases are also described as *congenital localized absence of skin*; the two descriptions are essentially synonymous.

Cordon first described aplasia cutis congenita in 1767.[22] Since this description, more than 500 cases of ACC have been reported. The condition is uncommon, but not rare, has a worldwide distribution, and affects both sexes equally. Several extensive reviews of aplasia cutis congenita and proposals for classification have been published.[23-29]

CLINICAL DESCRIPTION

The clinical findings of aplasia cutis congenita depend at least in part on the cause and location of the defect (Table 173–3). The condition is by definition present at birth, but small lesions may occasionally be overlooked during the newborn period, particularly in an infant with thick hair. Lesions may also appear as scars, rather than skin defects, presumably due to in utero healing.

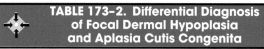

TABLE 173–2. Differential Diagnosis of Focal Dermal Hypoplasia and Aplasia Cutis Congenita

Focal Dermal Hypoplasia

Incontinentia pigmenti
Epidermal nevus syndrome
Linear porokeratosis
EEC syndrome (ectodermal dysplasia–ectrodactyly–clefting syndrome)

Aplasia Cutis Congenita

Obstetric trauma/erosions from scalp electrodes
Neonatal blistering diseases (see Chapter 82)

TABLE 173-3. Classification of Aplasia Cutis Congenita

Category	Body Area Affected	Associated Abnormalities	Inheritance
Group 1: scalp ACC without multiple anomalies	Scalp, usually vertex	Cleft lip and palate; tracheoesophageal fistula; double cervix and uterus; patent ductus arteriosus; omphalocele; polycystic kidney; mental retardation; cutis marmorata telangiectatica congenita	Autosomal dominant or sporadic
Group 2: scalp ACC with associated limb abnormalities	Midline scalp	Limb reduction abnormalities; 2–3 syndactyly; clubfoot; nail absence or dystrophy; skin tags on toes; persistent cutis marmorata; encephalocele; woolly hair; hemangioma; heart disease; cryptorchidism; postaxial polydactyly (1 family)	Autosomal dominant
Group 3: Scalp ACC with associated epidermal and organoid nevi	Scalp, may be asymmetric	Corneal opacities; scleral dermoids; eyelid colobomas; psychomotor retardation; seizures	Sporadic
Group 4: ACC overlying embryologic malformations	Abdomen, lumbar skin, scalp; any site	Meningomyeloceles; spinal dysraphia; cranial stenosis; congenital midline porencephaly; leptomeningeal angiomatosis; ectopia of ear; omphalocele; gastroschisis	Depends on underlying condition
Group 5: ACC with associated fetus papyraceus or placental infarcts	Multiple, symmetric areas, often stellate or linear, on scalp, chest, flanks, axillae, and extremities	Single umbilical artery; developmental delay; spastic paralysis; nail dystrophy; clubbed hands and feet; amniotic bands	Sporadic
Group 6: ACC associated with EB:			
Blistering, usually localized, without multiple congenital anomalies	Extremities	Blistering of skin and/or mucous membranes; absent or deformed nails; metatarsus varus; congenital absence of kidney (seen in cases of recessive, dystrophic EB; dominant, dystrophic EB; and EB simplex)	Depends on EB type: may be autosomal dominant or recessive
Widespread skin fragility with congenital anomalies	Large areas on extremities and torso	Pyloric or duodenal atresia; abnormal ears and nose; ureteral stenosis; renal abnormalities; arthrogryposis; amniotic bands; nail dystrophy	Autosomal recessive
Group 7: ACC localized to extremities without blistering	Pretibial areas; dorsal aspects of hands and feet; extensor areas of wrists	None	Autosomal dominant or recessive
Group 8: ACC caused by specific teratogens	Scalp (with methimazole); any area (with varicella and herpes simplex infections)	Imperforate anus (methimazole); signs of intrauterine infection with varicella and herpes simplex infections	Not inherited
Group 9: ACC associated with malformation syndromes	Scalp; any location	Trisomy 13; 4p—syndrome; many ectodermal dysplasias; Johanson-Blizzard syndrome; focal dermal hypoplasia; amniotic band disruption complex; XY gonadal dysgenesis	Varies, depending on specific syndrome

From Freiden, IJ. Aplasia Cutis Congenita: A clinical review and proposal for classification. J Am Acad Dermatol 1986;14:646–660.
ACC, aplasia cutis congenita; EB, epidermolysis bullosa.

Scalp Aplasia Cutis Congenita

The scalp is the most common site of involvement, occurring in approximately 80% of cases. The size of the defect varies from a few millimeters to as large as 100 cm.[2] Larger defects are often deeper and may extend to the dura or meninges. Seventy to seventy-five per cent of scalp lesions are solitary; 20% are double, and 8% are triple.[23] The lesions may have a variable appearance, with a raw friable surface, crusted, blister-like with a thin or thick membrane covering the defect (Fig. 173–2), or with a mature atrophic scar at the time of birth. The lesions of aplasia cutis of the scalp found in contiguity with organoid nevi are usually round and sharply demarcated, with a thin membranous covering.[24, 29, 30] Atrophic skin and areas of permanent alopecia are occasionally found in contiguity within the scalp.

Although the majority of cases of aplasia cutis congenita of the scalp have no associated abnormalities, multiple abnormalities have been described, including cleft lip and palate, tracheoesophageal fistula, double cervix and uterus, patent ductus arteriosus, coarctation of the aorta, cutis marmorata telangiectatica congenita, arteriovenous fistula, and intestinal lymphangiectasia.[22, 31–35] Scalp aplasia cutis congenita has been reported after maternal ingestion of methimazole, an antithyroid drug.[36] Aplasia cutis congenita of the scalp without associated abnormalities can be inherited as an autosomal dominant condition.

Many cases of the Adams-Oliver syndrome, the association of scalp aplasia cutis congenita with terminal transverse defects of the limbs, have been described.[37–41] The condition is usually an autosomal dominant one, with variable expressivity, even within the same family, but a few cases suggesting autosomal recessive inheritance have been reported.[42] The clinical phenotype consists of mild to severe defects of the scalp and/or underlying bone, and limb defects, including syndactyly, proximal and middle phalangeal reductions, ectrodactyly, and actual distal limb absence. Other associated abnormalities include cutis marmorata telangiectatica congenita, simple pinna, supernumerary nipples, congenital heart defects, woolly hair, and dilated scalp veins. The variable expressivity of this can make the diagnosis difficult, particularly if a good family history is not taken.[39]

Aplasia cutis congenita may be found overlying a diverse group of embryologic malformations including tethered spinal cord, meningomyelocele, midline porencephaly, and arteriovenous malformations. Several cases of a distinctive form of aplasia cutis congenita in association with in utero loss of a twin or triplet fetus or placental infarcts have been reported.[43] Most cases have symmetrical linear and stellate defects on the trunk and extremities, but midline scalp lesions are also fairly common (Fig. 173–3).

Several forms of epidermolysis bullosa (EB) have been reported in association with aplasia cutis congenita. So-called Bart's syndrome, with localized areas of aplasia cutis congenita on the legs without extensive or persistent blistering, is usually due to dominant dystrophic EB.[44, 45] Similar findings have been noted in recessive dystrophic EB, junctional EB, as well as at least one case of EB simplex. A well-defined syndrome of aplasia cutis congenita associated with EB, pyloric atresia, and deformed ears, and limb contractures is due to a severe form of junctional EB.[46]

Several cases of aplasia cutis congenita due to intrauterine infection with herpesvirus infection have been reported. Hutto and colleagues have emphasized the presence of scalp aplasia cutis congenita in cases of intrauterine herpes simplex infection.[47] Other findings of this intrauterine infection include microcephaly, chorioretinitis, and skin vesicles or scarring. In utero varicella infection has caused aplasia cutis congenita of the neck, shoulder, and leg, and can also cause in utero scarring.[48]

Many genetic and chromosomal abnormalities as well as syndromes of malformation without definite genetic basis have associated areas of aplasia cutis congenita. These include trisomy 13, the 4p-syndrome, the oculocerebrocutaneous (Delleman) syndrome, Johanson-Blizzard syndrome, and several forms of ectodermal dysplasia including focal dermal hypoplasia, and so-called ectodermal dysplasia of the face.[24]

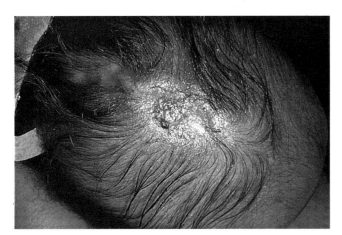

FIGURE 173–2. Aplasia cutis congenita: large scalp defect without other abnormalities.

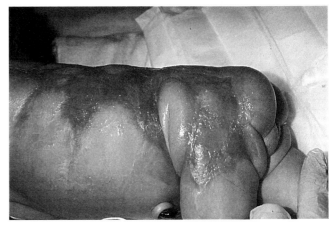

FIGURE 173–3. Aplasia cutis congenita of the torso due to intrauterine death of twin fetus.

PATHOLOGY

Affected skin in aplasia cutis congenita shows a range of findings from complete absence of the epidermis and dermis, with a thin or thick band of scar in their place, either covered by a re-epithelialized epidermis or bare of one. As in other scars, there is diminished elastic tissue. In some cases the subcutis can be absent, either partially or entirely. Appendages are characteristically absent or rudimentary. Occasionally heterotrophic brain tissue is present in scalp lesions clinically indistinguishable from aplasia cutis congenita.[49, 50]

PATHOGENESIS AND ETIOLOGY

Aplasia cutis congenita is a heterogeneous condition, with a number of different causes. Intrauterine vascular disruption may play a role in several forms of aplasia cutis congenita, the most obvious being those cases with the in utero death of a twin or placental infarctions. The association of dilated and tortuous scalp veins and cutis marmorata telangiectatica congenita with the Adams-Oliver syndrome has led some authors to postulate a genetically mediated tendency for vascular compromise affecting "watershed" areas such as the cranial vertex and limbs.[39] Stephan and associates noted that isolated scalp aplasia cutis congenita usually overlies the scalp hair whorl, an area of maximum tensile forces during rapid brain growth, and postulated that a tension-induced disruption of the overlying skin occurs between 10 and 18 weeks of gestation.[37]

DIAGNOSIS AND DIFFERENTIAL DIAGNOSIS
(see Table 173–2)

The diagnosis of aplasia cutis congenita is primarily a clinical one, and skin biopsies are often purposefully avoided, particularly on the scalp, because of the concern about underlying bony defects and potential exposure of connections to the central nervous system. Viral cultures may be helpful in excluding infectious causes of scalp ACC. Biopsy should be undertaken only after assuring that bony defects are not present, because such lesions may extend to the dura of the brain. Imaging studies, particularly magnetic resonance imaging and computed tomography, can be helpful in evaluating the underlying scalp and brain.[32, 51] A retrospective diagnosis of aplasia cutis congenita is occasionally made in older children or adults when a well-circumscribed scar, said to be present from birth or early infancy, is noted on the scalp. Skin biopsy for electron microscopy or immunofluorescent mapping may be helpful in cases where EB, infection, or other causes are suspected (Table 173–3).

Many cases of aplasia cutis congenita have been mistaken for obstetrical trauma including erosions and/or ulcerations from fetal scalp electrodes,[52] but fetal scalp electrodes almost invariably result in small superficial erosions, rather than deep ulcerations. Lesions of aplasia cutis congenita that are covered with a thin epidermal membrane and fluid in the underlying defect may have a

TABLE 173–4. Differential Diagnosis for Aplasia Cutis Congenita
Obstetrical trauma
Blisters in the newborn
Congenital alopecia

blister-like appearance, leading to confusion with other causes of blisters in the newborn period.[53] Areas of congenital alopecia, without absence of skin, may be confused with aplasia cutis congenita, but do not show characteristic scarring on skin biopsy (Table 173–4).

All infants with aplasia cutis congenita should have a complete gestational history, family history, and physical examination with special attention to the extremities, and a search for other abnormalities particularly the hair, teeth, nails, other areas of skin, was well as the eyes and central nervous system. Chromosomal analysis should be considered in those patients where more than one anomaly is present. The placenta, if available, should be closely examined. When possible, family members of patients with scalp aplasia cutis or those with lesions on the extremities suggesting EB should be examined by a dermatologist. Brain ultrasound imaging can be used in young infants to exclude major structural abnormalities of the central nervous system. Magnetic resonance imaging should be performed if neurologic signs and symptoms are present, or plastic surgical repair of a large scalp defect is planned during infancy.

TREATMENT

Virtually all lesions of aplasia cutis congenita will heal with resultant scarring, but the extent of scarring and need for medical and/or surgical intervention are directly related to the size and extent of lesions. Most small lesions of aplasia cutis congenita heal by secondary intention without significant complications, although keloidal scarring has been reported. Such lesions can be managed either with observation alone or with topical antibiotic ointments and sterile dressings.[28, 54] Larger lesions, especially those more than 3 to 4 cm in diameter, are more susceptible to secondary infection and hemorrhage and may require skin grafting.[55] If the dura is exposed, full-thickness skin flaps may help diminish the risk of eschar formation and subsequent infection or hemorrhage.[54] Bone grafting is occasionally necessary.[56]

If a familial form of aplasia cutis congenita is suspected or established, the family should receive genetic counseling. Fetal skin biopsy may aid in prenatal diagnosis of EB; elevated maternal serum or amniotic fluid alpha-fetoprotein has also been reported in this setting.[57]

References

1. Goltz RW, Peterson WC, Gorlin RJ, et al. Focal dermal hypoplasia. Arch Dermatol 1962;86:708–717.
2. Goltz RW, Henderson RR, Hitch JM, et al. Focal dermal hypoplasia syndrome: A review of the literature and report of two cases. Arch Dermatol 1970;101:1–11.

3. Goltz RW. Focal dermal hypoplasia. Pediatr Dermatol 1990; 7:313–314.
4. Gorlin RJ, Meskin LH, Peterson WC, et al. Focal dermal hypoplasia syndrome. Acta Dermato-Venereologica 1963;43:421–440.
5. Hall EH, Terezhalmy GT. Focal dermal hypoplasia syndrome. J Am Acad Dermatol 1983;9:443–451.
6. Mann M, Weintraub R, Hashimoto K. Focal dermal hypoplasia with an initial inflammatory phase. Pediatr Dermatol 1990; 7:278–282.
7. Pujol RM, Casanova JM, Perex M, et al. Focal dermal hypoplasia (Goltz syndrome): Report of two cases with minor cutaneous and extracutaneous manifestations. Pediatr Dermatol 1992; 9:112–116.
8. Sezer G, David R, Revach M, et al. Goltz syndrome with multiple giant-cell tumor-like lesions in bones. Ann Intern Med 1974; 80:714–717.
9. Howell JB, Reynolds J. Osteopathia striata. Hosp Derm Soc 1974;60:178–182.
10. Knockaery D, Dequeker J. Osteopathia striata and focal dermal hyopolasia. Skeletal Radiol 1979;4:223–227.
11. Greer RO, Reissner M. Focal dermal hypoplasia. J Periodontal 1989;6:330–335.
12. Valerius NH. A case of focal dermal hypoplasia syndrome (Goltz) with bilateral cheilo-gnatho-palatoschisis. Acta Paediat Scand 1974;63:287–288.
13. Holzman RS. Airway involvement and anesthetic management in Goltz's syndrome. J Clin Anesth 1991;3:422–425.
14. Suskan E, Kurkcuoglu N, Uluoglu O. Focal dermal hypoplasia (Goltz syndrome) with horseshoe kidney abnormality. Pediatr Dermatol 1990;7:283–286.
15. Ishii N, Baba N, Kanaizuka I, et al. Histopathological study of focal dermal hypoplasia (Goltz syndrome). Clin Exper Dermatol 1992;17:24–26.
16. Howell JB, Freeman RG. Cutaneous defects of focal dermal hypoplasia: An ectomesodermal dysplasia syndrome. J Cutan Pathol 1989;16:237–258.
17. Naritomi K, Izumikawa Y, Nagataki S, et al. Combined Goltz and Aicardi syndromes in a terminal Xp deletion: are they a contiguous gene syndrome? Am J Med 1992;43:839–843.
18. Gorski JL. Father-to-daughter transmission of focal dermal hypoplasia associated with nonrandom X-inactivation: Support for X-linked inheritance and paternal X chromosome mosaicism. Am J Med Genet 1991;40:332–337.
19. Wechsler MA, Papa CM, Haberman F, et al. Variable expression in focal dermal hypoplasia. Am J Dis Child 1988;142:297–300.
20. Opitz, JM. Pathogenetic analysis of certain developmental and genetic ectodermal defects. Birth Defects Original Article Series 1988;24:75–102.
21. Rodini ESO, Nardi A, Guion-Almeida ML, et al. Ectodermal dysplasia, ectrodactyly, clefting, anophthalmia/microphthalmia, and genitourinary anomalies: Nosology of Goltz-Gorlin syndrome versus EEC syndrome. Am J Med Genet 1992;42:276–280.
22. Cordon M: Extrait d'une lettre au sujet de trois enfants de la meme nes avec partie des extremites denuee de peau. J Med Chir Pharmacie 1967;26:556–557.
23. Demmel U: Clinical aspects of congenital skin defects: I. Congenital skin defects on the head of the newborn; II. Congenital skin defects on the trunk and extremities of the newborn; III. Causal and formal genesis of congenital skin defects of the newborn. Eur J Pediatr 1975;121:21–50.
24. Frieden IJ: Aplasia cutis congenita: A clinical review and proposal for classification. J Am Acad Dermatol 1986;14:646–660.
25. Sybert VP: Aplasia cutis congenita: A report of 12 new families and review of the literature. Pediatr Dermatol 1985;3:1–14.
26. Prigent F: Aplasies cutanees congenitales. Ann Dermatol Venereol 1983;110:933–939.
27. Kuster W, Traupe H: Klinik und genetik angeborener hautdefekte. Hautarzt 1988;39:553–563.
28. Blunt K, Quan V, Carr D, et al. Aplasia cutis congenita: A clinical review and associated defects. Neonatal Nework 1992;11:17–27.
29. Frieden I. Golabi M: Aplasia cutis congenita and the epidermal nevus syndrome: A previously unrecognized associaton. Clin Res 1985;33:130.
30. Lantis S, Leyden J, Thew M, Heaton C: Nevus sebaceous of Jadassohn: Part of a new neurocutaneous syndrome? Arch Dermatol 1968;98:117–123.
31. Dallapiccola B, Giannotti A, Marino B, et al. Familial aplasia cutis congenita and coarction of the aorta. Am J Med Genet 1992; 43:762–763.
32. Singman R, Asaikar S, Hotson G, et al. Aplasia cutis congenita and arteriovenous fistula. Arch Neurol 1990;47:1255–1258.
33. Bronspeigel N, Zelnick N, Rabinowitz H, et al. Aplasia cutis congenita and intestinal lymphangiectasia: An unusual associaton. Am J Dis Child 1985;139:509–513.
34. Castle D, Isaacs H, Ramsay M, et al. Hereditary motor and sensory neuropathy type I, associated with aplasia cutis congenita: Possible X-linked inheritance. Clin Genet 1992;41:108–110.
35. Paltzik RL, Aiello AM. Aplasia cutis congenita associated with valvular heart disease. Cutis 1985;36:57–58.
36. Milham S Jr, Elledge W: Maternal methimazole and congenital defects in children. Teratology 1972;5:125.
37. Stephan MJ, Smith DW, Ponzi JW, Alden ER: Origin of scalp vertex aplasia cutis. J Pediatr 1982;101:850–853.
38. Shapiro SD, Escobedo MK: Terminal transverse defects with aplasia cutis congenita (Adams-Oliver syndrome). Birth Defects 1985;21:135–142.
39. Whitley CB, Gorlin RJ. Adams-Oliver syndrome revisited. Am J Med Genet 1991;40:319–326.
40. Arand AG, Ball WS, Crone KR. Congenital scalp defects: Adams-Oliver syndrome. Pediatr Neurosurg 1991;92:203–207.
41. Bork K, Pfeifle J. Multifocal aplasia cutis congenita, distal limb hemimelia, and cutis marmorata telangiectatica in a patient with Adams-Oliver syndrome. Br J Dermatol 1992;127:160–163.
42. Koiffman CP, Wajntal A, Hayke BJ, Catrol RM: Congenital skull defects with distal limb anomalies (Adams-Oliver syndrome—MuKusick 10030): Further suggestion of autosomal recessive inheritance. Am J Med Genet 1988;29:263–268.
43. Mannino FL, Jones KL, Benirschke K: Congenital skin defects and fetus papyraceus. J Pediatr 1977;91:559–564.
44. Bart BJ, Gorlin RJ, Anderson VE, Lyncy FW: Congenital localized absence of skin and associated sbnormalities resembling epidermolysis bullosa: A new syndrome. Arch Dermatol 1966;93:296–304.
45. Butler DF, Berger TG, James WD, et al: Bart's syndrome: Microscopic, ultrastructural, and immunofluorescent mapping features. Pediatr Dermatol 1985;3:113–118.
46. Achiron R, Hamiel-Pinchas O, Engelberg S, et al. Aplasia cutis congenita associated with eipdermolysis bullosa and pyloric atresia: The diagnostic role of prenatal ultrasonography. Prenatal Diagnosis 1992;12:765–771.
47. Hutto C, Arvin A, Jacobs R, et al: Intrauterine herpes simplex infections. J Pediatr 1987;110:97–101.
48. Bailie FB: Aplasia cutis congenita of neck and shoulder requiring a skin graft: A case report. Br J Plast Surg 1983;36:72–74.
49. Commens C, Rogers M, Kan A. Heterotropic brain tissue presenting as bald cysts with a collar of hypertrophic hair. Arch Dermatol 1989;125:1253–1256.
50. Orkin M, Fischer I: Heterotropic brain tissue (heterotopic neural rest). Arch Dermatol 1966;94:699–708.
51. Baldwin HE, Berck CM, Lynfield YL. Subcutaneous nodules of the scalp: Preoperative management. J Am Acad Dermatol 1991;25:819–830.
52. Brown ZA, Jung AL. Stenchever MA. Aplasia cutis congenita and the fetal scalp electrode. Am J Obstet Gynecol 1977;129:351–352.
53. Frieden IJ. Blisters and pustules in the newborn. Curr Probl Ped 1989;9:551–614.
54. Abbott R, Cutting CB, Wisoff JH, et al. Aplasia cutis congenita of the scalp: Issues in its management. Pediatr Neurosurg 1991; 92:182–184.
55. Vinocur CD, Weintraub WH, Wilensky RJ, et al: Surgical management of aplasia cutis congenita. Arch Surg 1976;111:1160–1164.
56. Argenta LC, Dingman RO: Total reconstruction of aplasia cutis congenita involving scalp, skull, and dura. Plast Reconstr Surg 1986;77:650–653.
57. Cowton JAL, Beattie TJ, Gibson AAM, et al: Epidermolysis bullosa in association with aplasia cutis congenita and pyloric atresia. Am J Med Genet 1982;11:319–328.

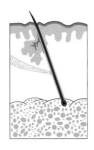

chapter 174

Nevoid Conditions of Epidermis, Dermis, and Subcutaneous Tissue

MAUREEN ROGERS, GAYLE FISCHER, and
PETER HOGAN

In its broadest and original sense, the term *nevus* refers to abnormalities of either structure (malformations) or cellular composition (hamartomas and choristomas) of the skin. These conditions are usually congenital, but sometimes their appearance is delayed into childhood or even young adult life. Nevoid conditions of the skin can be classified according to the malformed tissue or cell of origin (Table 174–1). Cutis verticis gyrata is also discussed in this chapter. Knuckle pads, although sometimes considered with connective tissue nevi, are covered in Chapter 102 on fibromatoses. Developmental cysts and sinuses are discussed in Chapter 143.

Epidermal Nevi

DEFINITION

Epidermal nevi are inborn, stable abnormalities of the epidermis and often also of the papillary dermis. The term *epidermal nevus syndrome* refers to the association of epidermal nevi with abnormalities in other organ systems. It is now clear that this is not a single malformation syndrome but a heterogeneous group of disorders.

CLINICAL FEATURES

Epidermal nevi of the keratinocytic type come in an array of sizes and shapes, ranging from trivial lesions of a few centimeters to catastrophic ones covering much of the trunk, limbs, and head that disfigure a child and can be associated with important extracutaneous abnormalities. There is no racial predilection for epidermal nevi, and, except in the setting of the CHILD (congenital *he*midysplasia, *i*chthyosiform erythroderma, and *l*imb *de*fects) syndrome, they occur equally in males and females. They may involve any area of skin and even extend into the oral cavity. They may be congenital or appear in the first months or years of life or, rarely, later; almost all nevi on the head and neck have been present at birth. Epidermal nevi may enlarge in proportion to the patient's growth or extend far beyond their original distribution. Extension may continue for many months or even several years. Such extension is rare with nevi on the head and neck and with those present at birth, whatever their location.[2]

These nevi show a variety of patterns of keratinization, discussed in detail in the section on pathology. Most of these cannot be distinguished clinically from one another, with a few exceptions. Those in which keratinization is nearly normal but the skin surface is papillated (sometimes called keratinocytic nevi or nevus verrucosus) occur mainly on the trunk and limbs. They vary in color from black through brown to pale gray; most are darker than the surrounding skin, but some are considerably lighter. They may be flat and subtle or very raised and warty. Single or multiple plaques or lines are seen, often arranged in a streaky, swirled, or segmental distribution (Figs. 174–1 and 174–2). Another variant consists of a line of individual small papillomas resembling seborrheic keratoses (Fig. 174–3). Neoplasms rarely develop in epidermal nevi, usually in adult life. Squamous

TABLE 174-1. Nevoid Conditions of the Skin

Nevoid conditions of the epidermis and appendages
  Epidermal nevus, keratinocytic type
  Sebaceous nevus
  Follicular nevus—nevus comedonicus
  Sweat gland nevus (see Chapter 145)
    Apocrine
    Eccrine
  Becker's nevus (see Chapter 132)
  Vascular nevi and malformations (see Chapter 146)
Melanocytic nevi

Dermal and subcutaneous nevi
  Collagen and elastic tissue nevi—cutaneous collagenoma
  Elastic tissue nevus—Buschke-Ollendorff syndrome (nevus
    anelasticus), papular elastorrhexis
  Fat nevi
    Nevus lipomatosus
    Encephalocraniocutaneous lipomatosis
      Congenital lipoma
      Congenital lipomatosis
  Muscular nevi
    Congenital smooth muscle hamartoma
    Congenital rhabdomyomatous mesenchymal
      hamartoma

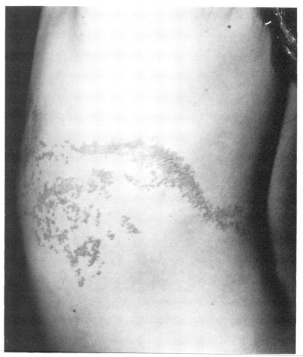

FIGURE 174-2. Epidermal nevus on the trunk.

cell carcinoma, basal cell carcinoma, Bowen's disease, trichoepithelioma, and keratoacanthoma have all been reported to arise in epidermal nevi.[9-12] Conceivably, the nevus in some of these reports may have been a nevus sebaceus, as neoplasms commonly complicated these lesions.

Inflammatory epidermal nevus appears as a linear array of pink to red papules, usually on the lower limb and/or adjacent buttock and hip area, clinically resembling psoriasis or eczematous dermatitis.[2] While inflammatory epidermal nevus has distinct histopathologic features that differ from those of psoriasis, other epidermal nevi with histopathologic features indistinguishable from those of authentic psoriasis (designated *nevoid psoriasis*) may indicate mosaicism for a gene responsible for psoriasis.[13] Nevi of this type often have whitish or micaceous scale, just as do lesions of psoriasis. It is important to note also that psoriasis may spread to an epidermal nevus as a Koebner phenomenon.

PATHOLOGY

In the most common form of epidermal nevus, known as nevus verrucosus, the epidermis is papillated and there is compact hyperkeratosis (Fig. 174-4). This form of epidermal nevus is sometimes mistaken for a seborrheic keratosis, from which it differs by having only rare horn pseudocysts and by papillary dermal fibrosis, which results in the characteristic rigidity of the papillations evident on palpation.

Aberrant keratinization is evident in many of the other forms of epidermal nevus. Epidermolytic hyperkeratosis, which is the histopathologic hallmark of a condition usually considered to be a form of ichthyosis—namely bullous congenital ichthyosiform erythroderma—can occur also in circumscribed forms of epidermal nevus. In

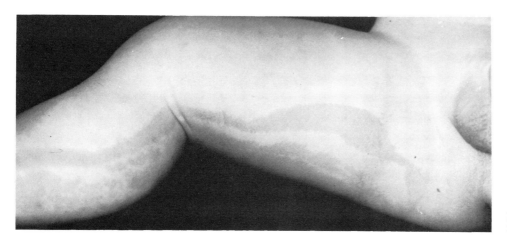

FIGURE 174-1. Epidermal nevus following the lines of Blaschko.

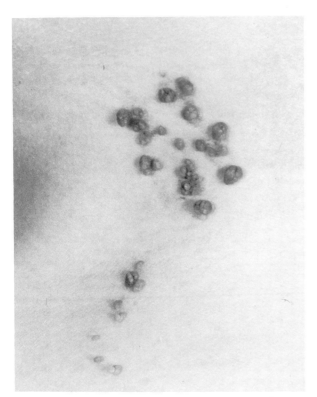

FIGURE 174–3. Epidermal nevus comprising multiple small papillomas.

epidermolytic hyperkeratosis, there is vacuolization throughout the suprabasilar epidermis, with coarse keratohyaline and trichohyaline granules, hyperkeratosis, and sometimes parakeratosis. Other abnormalities of keratinocytic maturation that can be present in epidermal nevi include focal acantholytic dyskeratosis (as occurs in Darier's disease), suprabasilar acantholysis without dyskeratosis (the pattern evident in Hailey-Hailey disease), cornoid lamellation (the hallmark of porokeratosis), and dyskeratosis with hyperkeratosis and infiltrates of eosinophils (as seen in the inflammatory stages of incontinentia pigmenti). All of these findings may reflect mosaicism for genes that would ordinarily produce the corresponding diseases in a widespread distribution.

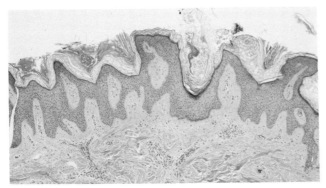

FIGURE 174–4. The epidermis is papillated, hyperkeratotic, and thickened, and the papillary dermis is fibrotic in this verrucous epidermal nevus.

There is a distinctive pattern of cornification seen along with sparse lymphocytic infiltrates in inflammatory epidermal nevus, which is different from that seen in linear or nevoid psoriasis, with which it is often confused. Short stubby columns of parakeratosis, wider than cornoid lamellae, and devoid of the neutrophils found in nevoid psoriasis are the hallmark of this condition. The columns are often situated at the highest points along an undulating epidermal surface.

PATHOGENESIS AND ETIOLOGY

Epidermal nevi arise from the embryonic ectoderm, which gives rise to keratinocytes and also to the cells of epithelial appendages. The mesoderm may also be affected, as the papillary dermis in nevus verrucosus is also abnormal and therapies that do not ablate it are often unsuccessful. Some authors regard epidermal nevi as overlapping with nevus sebaceus, nevus comedonicus, and other cutaneous malformations. Indeed, it was originally believed that these nevi represented variants of a single condition and that the epidermal nevus syndrome was a single condition with great clinical variability.[1, 2] However, Happle[3, 4] proposed that each type of epidermal nevus represents the cutaneous manifestation of a different mosaic phenotype. In favor of the mosaic hypothesis is the fact that most epidermal nevi follow the lines of Blaschko, which do not correspond to any known neural or vascular structures but probably represent the migration tracks of clones of genetically identical cells. Happle pointed out that there are therefore potentially many different "epidermal nevus syndromes" manifested by a spectrum of abnormalities from an epidermal nevus alone to extensive multiorgan involvement. Happle also identifies what he believes are four well-defined epidermal nevus syndromes.[4] The CHILD syndrome, limited to female patients, is an example of functional X chromosome mosaicism explained by the Lyon effect of partial X inactivation. The Proteus syndrome, the nevus sebaceus syndrome, and the nevus comedonicus syndrome, which occur equally in both sexes, are examples of lethal autosomal mutations surviving by mosaicism; the cells carrying the mutation can survive only in close proximity to normal cells. In contrast, the epidermolytic hyperkeratotic type of epidermal nevus is an example of mosaicism involving a nonlethal autosomal dominant mutation; when gonadal mosaicism occurs, the defect may occur in the subsequent generation as a generalized bullous ichthyosis.[5] Epidermal nevi that demonstrate the histologic features of Darier's disease, Hailey-Hailey disease, and porokeratosis probably represent mosaic forms of these conditions.[6, 7] While the vast majority of cases of epidermal nevi are sporadic, rare reports of familial cases occurring in a pattern suggesting an autosomal dominant inheritance[8] indicate that not all of these lesions can be explained on the basis of mosaicism.

There are probably many epidermal nevus syndromes, each representing a particular mosaic phenotype.[4] Most reported associations have been ocular, neurologic, and skeletal, as would be expected because all of these structures, and the epidermis and its epithelial appendages, arise from the embryonic ectoderm; however, a wide variety of other abnormalities are encountered.[1, 2, 20] In general, nevi of the head and neck are associated with ocular and neurologic abnormalities[21] and those on the trunk and limbs with skeletal anomalies. Several entities are well defined. There is a subgroup of patients with nevi of the sebaceous type (see below) on the head and neck who demonstrate ipsilateral hemimegalencephaly and gyral malformations, mental retardation, seizures, and contralateral hemiparesis.[22] In the Proteus syndrome, a folded type of epidermal and dermal nevus is associated with hemihypertrophy, partial gigantism of hands and feet, and a variety of vascular and connective tissue hamartomas.[4, 23] In the CHILD syndrome, an ichthyosiform verrucous epidermal nevus occurs in association with ipsilateral skeletal hypoplasia.[24] Significant developmental abnormalities occur in about 1.7% of all neonates,[25] and some of the other abnormalities occurring in patients with epidermal nevi are certainly fortuitous and not components of any syndrome. However, it seems likely that many of them represent other manifestations of the effect of the genetic event that produced this cutaneous lesion.[6]

Individuals with epidermal nevi have a somewhat increased risk of developing systemic neoplasms, particularly of the urogenital tract, usually at a young age.[1, 20, 26]

DIAGNOSIS AND DIFFERENTIAL DIAGNOSIS

The diagnosis of epidermal nevus is often made clinically. Biopsy is useful to confirm the diagnosis and to detect the specific pathologic change in the affected area. In the case of nevi showing changes of porokeratosis, biopsy is essential because of the risk of carcinoma arising in such lesions.

Verrucous epidermal nevi are sometimes confused with seborrheic keratoses, from which they can generally be distinguished by history and by the presence of small ostia corresponding to the opening of the keratotic tunnels seen histologically as pseudocysts, and with nevus sebaceus, which in its fully developed form is yellow rather than brown.

TREATMENT

Therapy of epidermal nevi is difficult (Table 174–2). Recurrence is almost invariable following cryotherapy, diathermy or dermabrasion. Excision is appropriate for small lesions and narrow linear lesions and for cosmetically troublesome or irritating areas of some widespread nevi. Argon and carbon dioxide lasers have been used,[27-29] sometimes with good result, but again recurrence may occur and there is a risk of hypertrophic scarring; the argon laser is best suited to the softer papillomatous lesions, being ineffective in the harder and more verrucous types.[28] Topical retinoic acid may temporarily flatten very thick areas. There are some reports of the use of oral retinoids in very disfiguring warty lesions,[30] but improvement depends on continued use of

TABLE 174-2. Treatment of Nevoid Conditions of Epidermis, Dermis, and Subcutaneous Tissue

Epidermal Nevi
Electrosurgery
Cryosurgery
Dermabrasion
Argon or CO_2 laser

Sebaceous Nevi, Becker's Nevus
Excision with primary closure or reconstruction with grafting or flaps. Tissue expansion may assist in providing tissue for reconstruction
Laser—use of the Q switch, ruby, YAG, or alexandrite lasers may decrease or eliminate the molecular segmentation of Becker's nevus

these potentially dangerous agents. Despite their benefit in acne, they have not proved effective in nevus comedonicus; a 12% solution of ammonium lactate has been helpful in some cases of this condition[17, 31] and long-term erythromycin in another.[32]

All patients with epidermal nevi should have a detailed physical examination at the time of appearance of their nevus and regular follow-up for several years. It is important to point out, however, that the majority of patients with epidermal nevi have no other important abnormalities.

Nevus Sebaceus

DEFINITION

Nevus sebaceus (of Jadassohn) is a circumscribed abnormality of the skin that includes many of the findings of a verrucous epidermal nevus but also is accompanied by malformations of the dermis, including most prominently abnormal positioning and hypertrophy of sebaceous epithelium. Mesenchymal elements can also be abnormal; hence the name *organoid nevus.*

CLINICAL FEATURES

Nevus sebaceus occurs almost always on the scalp and face, areas rich in sebaceous glands. They are characteristically yellow or occasionally pink in color and are present at birth as fairly flat, hairless plaques, with a smooth waxy surface, linear or oval in shape. They have a tendency to become raised and warty and are often irritable at puberty (Fig. 174–5). Rarely they are significantly raised from birth. The development of a variety of benign and malignant secondary neoplasms in nevus

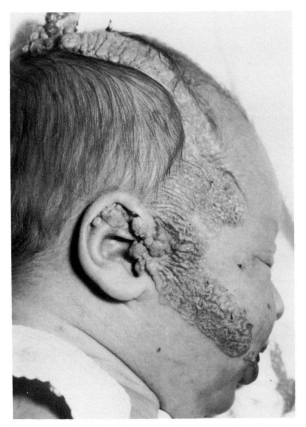

FIGURE 174-5. Extensive nevus sebaceus on face and scalp.

sebaceus is much more common than in epidermal nevi of the keratinocytic type.[14, 15] Benign tumors include trichoblastoma (a benign neoplasm with differentiation toward hair germ), syringocystadenoma papilliferum, nodular hidradenoma, apocrine cystadenoma, tumor of the follicular infundibulum, tricholemmoma, leiomyoma, and keratoacanthoma. Malignant neoplasms include basal cell, squamous cell, sebaceous, and apocrine carcinoma. Most of these occur in adult life, but keratoacanthomas have been reported in childhood.[2, 16] Most of the lesions assumed to be basal cell carcinomas arising in nevus sebaceus are probably trichoblastomas.

PATHOLOGY

The flat alopecic plaques that characterize nevus sebaceus in infants and young children feature diminished numbers of follicular units, and those that are present are often malformed, with abnormally superficial, sometimes bifid, and often misoriented follicular bulbs and broad, misshapen papillae. The epidermal surface is initially flattish and becomes papillated with age.

During puberty, sebaceous lobules enlarge and the epidermis becomes verrucous and hyperkeratotic. Instead of inserting into the sides of follicles, sebaceous glands are abnormally connected to the epidermis itself (Fig. 174-6). Apocrine glands, which are not usually present aside from the axillae, groin, and a few on the breast and

eyelids, are seen in almost half of examples of nevus sebaceus.

Neoplasms complicating nevus sebaceus can resemble their sporadic counterparts, or show unique features that do not correspond to those of any well-described adnexal neoplasm.

PATHOGENESIS AND ETIOLOGY

Many of the same etiologic considerations discussed in the section on epidermal nevi also apply to nevus sebaceus. The occurrence of dermal neoplasms such as leiomyomas indicates that the abnormality is not limited to structures of mesodermal derivation. The enlargement of sebaceous lobules during puberty is presumably due to androgenic stimulation.

DIFFERENTIAL DIAGNOSIS

The differential diagnosis of nevus sebaceus is essentially the same as that of epidermal nevi. Neoplasms arising in nevus sebaceus are best distinguished histologically.

TREATMENT

Many of the therapies attempted for epidermal nevi have also been tried on patients with nevus sebaceus (see Table 174-2). Superficial ablation cannot remove the abnormal dermis, which can spawn some of the neoplasms that arise in this condition. Therefore, complete

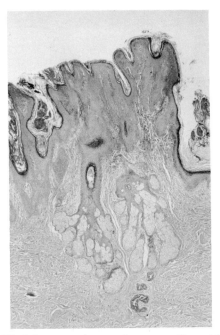

FIGURE 174-6. In nevus sebaceus, there are malformed follicles and sebaceous lobules attached directly to the undersurface of the epidermis, which shows changes similar to those seen in a verrucous epidermal nevus.

excision with conservative margins is the best approach when feasible.

Nevus Comedonicus

The typical nevus comedonicus is composed of dilated follicular openings filled with comedo-like keratin plugs.[17] Groups of these structures occur in a linear or swirled configuration sometimes covering large areas of face, trunk, or limbs. Occasionally, lesions extend from hair-bearing skin onto areas, such as glans penis and palms and soles, that do not usually contain pilosebaceous follicles. Sometimes the plugs are extruded to produce a cribriform appearance. Particularly after puberty, inflamed acne-like cysts and deep scars can develop within the lesion. Mixed entities occur with verrucous change of the epidermis between the comedones.[18] Various secondary tumors, particularly of sweat gland and hair follicle origin, and also basal cell carcinoma have been reported in nevus comedonicus.[19] Nevus comedonicus may be associated with skeletal defects, cerebral anomalies, and cataracts.[4] Histopathologic examination shows bulbous, dilated follicular infundibula that contain laminated keratin. Some lesions in which the cornified contents were columns of parakeratotic cells have been termed *porokeratotic eccrine ostial and dermal duct nevus.* The attached follicular units are often atrophic.

The differential diagnosis of nevus comedonicus includes folliculitis, cribiform atrophy, keratosis pilaris atrophicans, and related conditions; and familial dyskeratotic comedones, an autosomal dominant condition in which focal acantholytic dyskeratosis occurs in the walls of plugged follicles.[19a]

Dermal and Subcutaneous Nevi

CUTANEOUS COLLAGENOMA

Collagenomas are uncommon connective tissue nevi composed of dense dermal collagen, often with a reduction in elastic fibers. Occasionally they occur as solitary lesions,[33] but most commonly they present as multiple asymptomatic, firm, flesh-colored dermal nodules symmetrically distributed on the upper trunk and arms.[33, 34] They vary in size from a few millimeters to several centimeters. They may be slightly elevated, flat, or indented producing a peau d'orange appearance. The usual time of onset is in adolescence. The condition may occur as an autosomal dominant trait—*familial cutaneous collagenoma*—in which it may be associated with other (in particular, cardiac) abnormalities.[35, 36] An identical

clinical picture can occur sporadically and is termed *eruptive collagenoma.*[33] Collagenomas occur in several syndromes, including Proteus syndrome,[37] Down syndrome,[38] and tuberous sclerosis. In tuberous sclerosis, the collagenoma presents as the "shagreen patch," a firm dermal plaque with a pebbly surface, usually in the lumbosacral area.

The dermis is thickened in cutaneous collagenomas, and collagen bundles are haphazard in their orientations. Stains for elastic tissue show either diminished fibers or wide separation of them. The epidermis is usually flat but sometimes is slightly papillated. Collagenomas resemble many other dermal nodules such as leiomyomas and neurilemmomas, and their diagnosis is usually made on biopsy. Excision is curative but may not be practical in patients with many lesions.

ELASTIC TISSUE NEVUS AND THE BUSCHKE-OLLENDORFF SYNDROME

Elastic tissue nevi are dermal papules within which there are increased numbers of elastic fibers. They can occur as solitary or multiple lesions. In the dominantly inherited Buschke-Ollendorff syndrome,[39, 40] multiple connective tissue nevi, usually of the elastic tissue type, but occasionally collagenomas, are associated with osteopoikilosis, or focal thickening of the long bones. The nevi have the apppearance of yellow or flesh-colored papules, nodules, plaques, or streaks. The lesions may be firm and elevated or very subtle and are usually few in number and found symmetrically placed on the trunk. The disseminated papular form—dermatofibrosis lenticularis disseminata—is less common. The skin lesions usually appear before puberty, but the onset may be delayed to adult life. The bone abnormality—osteopoikilosis—is evident as a radiologic change appearing in childhood and consists of multiple circumscribed opacities at the ends of the long bones, in the pelvis, and in the bones of the hands and feet. Like the skin changes, it persists through life. Occasionally, patients have either skin or bone changes alone.

NEVUS ANELASTICUS

In this condition, small grouped papules, which may be yellow or flesh colored, occur on the trunk.[41, 42] Lesions may be so numerous that they produce a diffuse fine wrinkling of the skin. They are found to consist of a focal absence of elastic tissue. Differentiation from middermal elastolysis or from anetoderma can be difficult.

PAPULAR ELASTORRHEXIS

In this recently described entity, small white nonfollicular papules are found in a symmetrical distribution on the trunk. The onset is in the second decade. They demonstrate homogenization of collagen as well as decreased elastin and may represent a variant of nevus anelasticus.[43]

NEVOID CONDITIONS OF ADIPOSE TISSUE — SUPERFICIAL LIPOMATOUS NEVUS

This rare hamartoma, also termed *nevus lipomatosus superficialis,* consists of soft, clustered yellow to skin-colored nodules caused by the abnormal presence of adipose tissue within the dermis.[44] It is usually present at birth or occurs in the early years of life, but later appearance has been reported.[44] The lesions are typically found on the lower trunk, pelvic girdle area, or the thighs but may occur elsewhere. They may follow Blaschko's lines, producing a linear configuration. The clinical appearance is variable.[44-46] The nodules may be sessile or pedunculated and either smooth or verrucous (Fig. 174–7). They may be small, producing a peau d'orange appearance, or large and cerebriform. Occasionally hair or comedones occur in the lesions, and leukodermic and café-au-lait macules have also been described in the area.[45] The lesions usually remain static after their appearance but occasionally have been noted to grow slowly. They are usually asymptomatic, but ulceration from trauma may occur.[45] A solitary form has been described that has the appearance of a papule, skin tag, or nodule. This type is likely to be of later onset and may occur on unusual sites such as the ear or scalp. It is of insidious onset and slow growing.[44] Some investigators do not consider these lesions to be authentic examples of nevus lipomatosus but instead to be acrochordons or skin tags with lipocytes — that is, pedunculated lipofibromas.[44a]

The diagnosis is often made clinically. While the clinical appearance of congenital lesions is nearly pathognomonic, solitary small lesions arising in adult life can resemble ordinary skin tags, from which they differ by having broader bases. Nevus lipomatosus can be removed by shave excision.[46] Histopathologic examination of the resultant specimen shows clusters of adipocytes situated within the dermis, with some even surrounding vessels of the superficial vascular plexus.

ENCEPHALOCRANIOCUTANEOUS LIPOMATOSIS

In this rare sporadic neurocutaneous syndrome, multiple connective tissue nevi, predominantly lipomatous, are associated with neurologic, skeletal, and ocular abnormalities.[47, 48] The cutaneous lesions comprise multiple

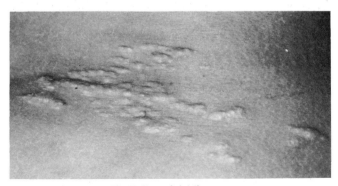

FIGURE 174–7. Superficial lipomatous nevus.

yellow to skin-colored papules and nodules. Telangiectasia may be a feature. The nevi occur in a linear distribution on the head and neck, and there is alopecia when they occur in hair-bearing skin. Lipomas occur in the brain and meninges, and other structural intracranial abnormalities are found ipsilateral to the cutaneous lesions. Neurologic features of the syndrome include developmental delay and infantile-onset seizures, and choristomas are the most common ocular feature. Happle[49] has suggested that this syndrome could be another example of mosaicism involving a lethal autosomal mutation.

CONGENITAL LIPOMA

This very rare nevus, which is usually found on the vulva, is present at birth as a soft, smooth, skin-colored pedunculated nodule.[50] It is easily excised.

CONGENITAL LIPOMATOSIS

In this rare condition, there are excess lipocytes throughout the subcutis and adjacent muscle. This produces the clinical appearance of large lipomatous masses, usually on the upper trunk.[51] There may be an underlying abnormality of ribs and pleura. The condition can be differentiated from diffuse lipomatous hypertrophy producing a generalized skin folding, the so-called Michelin tire baby.[52]

MUSCULAR NEVI

Congenital Smooth Muscle Hamartoma

Smooth muscle hamartomas are uncommon lesions that may be congenital or arise in childhoood or adolescence.[53-56] The typical appearance is of a slightly hyperpigmented plaque or patch, usually located on the trunk, buttocks, or proximal limbs. It is usually solitary but may be quite extensive. Perifollicular papules may be present, and hypertrichosis is a usual feature. The lesion may become raised on firm stroking as a result of the contraction of large arrector pili muscles (pseudo–Darier's sign). The condition is not associated with any systemic abnormalities or malformations. Occasionally the smooth muscle hamartoma is diffuse, with a generalized hypertrichosis and folding of the skin, producing the "Michelin tire baby" appearance[57, 58]; in this situation, other malformations and chromosomal abnormalities have been reported.[57,58] On biopsy, smooth muscle hamartomas are seen to consist of interlacing bundles of mature smooth muscle similar to those seen in leiomyomas. The epidermis is often slightly hyperplastic and hyperpigmented.

Congenital Rhabdomyomatous Mesenchymal Hamartoma

This recently reported dermal and subcutaneous hamartoma presents at birth as a solitary, soft, smooth polypoid lesion. It occurs most commonly on the chin and is composed of disorganized skeletal muscle and adipose tissue.[59, 60] The skeletal muscle elements of this lesion contract and relax with feeding of the infant.

Cutis Verticis Gyrata

The term *cutis verticis gyrata* refers to a hypertrophy and folding of the scalp skin as a result of its overgrowth in relation to the underlying skull. It can occur as an isolated or primary form of unknown etiology[61, 62] or in association with other disorders, including primary pachydermoperiostosis,[61, 62] acromegaly,[63] hypothyroidism,[62] secondary syphilis,[61] tuberous sclerosis,[64] and Apert's syndrome.[64] Occasionally, cutis verticis gyrata–like scalp changes can occur with severe inflammation (e.g., dissecting cellulitis),[61] with congenital melanocytic nevi,[65] or as a result of chronic rotational traction.[66]

In the primary form, scalp changes usually begin around the onset of puberty and progress over a 5- to 10-year period, but onset in the neonatal period has been recorded.[67] The scalp acquires a cerebriform appearance with a convoluted pattern of ridges and furrows. The changes are usually symmetrical and are most prominent on the occipital region. Most patients are male and exhibit severe mental retardation, which may be accompanied by epilepsy and features of cerebral palsy; the condition has been associated with the fragile X syndrome.[68] In pachydermoperiostosis, the scalp changes are identical to those in primary cutis verticis gyrata; the condition is distinguished by the presence of thick folded facial skin, spade-like hands and feet, finger clubbing, cylindrical thickening of the distal arms and legs, sebaceous gland hyperplasia, and hyperhidrosis of the palms and soles.

Cutis verticis gyrata due to acromegaly, hypothyroidism, secondary syphilis, tuberous sclerosis, and Apert's syndrome can be distinguished by the usually minor nature of the scalp changes, the associated clinical features, and appropriate laboratory investigations. If the scalp hypertrophy is due to a congenital melanocytic nevus, the area is well defined and usually pigmented and hypertrichotic; occasionally the pigmentation is slight, leading to diagnostic difficulty. In the absence of other predisposing conditions, a history of severe scalp inflammation or trauma should be sought. Apart from managing any underlying condition that is amenable to therapy, the only treatment for the condition is surgical excision of the redundant skin.[62]

References

1. Solomon LM, Esterly NB. Epidermal and other organoid nevi. Curr Probl Pediatr 1975;6:1–56.
2. Rogers M, McCrossin I, Commens C. Epidermal nevi and the epidermal nevus syndrome. J Am Acad Dermatol 1989; 20:476–488.
3. Happle R. Lethal genes surviving by mosaicism: A possible explanation for sporadic birth defects involving the skin. J Am Acad Dermatol 1987;16:899–906.
4. Happle R. How many epidermal nevus syndromes exist? J Am Acad Dermatol 1991;25:550–556.
5. Nazzaro V, Ermacora E, Santucci B, et al. Epidermolytic hyperkeratosis: Generalized form in children from parents with systematized linear form. Br J Dermatol 1990;122:417–422.
6. Rogers M. Epidermal nevi and the epidermal nevus syndromes: A review of 233 cases. Pediatr Dermatol 1992;9:342–344.
7. Munro CS, Cox NH. An acantholytic dyskeratotic epidermal nevus with other features of Darier's disease on the same side of the body. Br J Dermatol 1992;127:168–171.
8. Meschia JF, Junkins E, Hofman KJ. Familial systematized epidermal nevus syndrome. Am J Med Genet 1992;44:664–667.
9. Braunstein BL, Mackel SE, Cooper PH. Keratoacanthoma arising in a linear epidermal nevus. Arch Dermatol 1982;118:362–363.
10. Cramer SF, Mandel MA, Hauler R, et al. Squamous cell carcinoma arising in a linear epidermal nevus. Arch Dermatol 1981; 117:222–224.
11. Horn MS, Sausker WF, Pierson DL. Basal cell epithelioma arising in a linear epidermal nevus. Arch Dermatol 1981;117:247.
12. Wilkinson SM, Tan CY, Smith AG. Keratoacanthoma arising within organoid naevi. Clin Exp Dermatol 1991;16:58–60.
13. Atherton DJ, Kahana M, Russell-Jones R. Naevoid psoriasis. Br J Dermatol 1989;120:837–841.
14. Fergin PE, Chu AC, Macdonald DM. Basal cell carcinoma complicating naevus sebaceus. Clin Exp Dermatol 1981;6:111–115.
15. Wilson Jones E, Heyl T. Naevus sebaceus. A report of 140 cases with special regard to the development of secondary malignant tumours. Br J Dermatol 1970;82:99–117.
16. Buescher L, DeSpain JD, Diaz-Arias AA, et al. Keratoacanthoma arising in an organoid nevus during childhood: Case report and literature review. Pediatr Dermatol 1991;8:117–119.
17. Cestari TF, Rubim M, Valentini BC. Nevus comedonicus: Case report and brief review of the literature. Pediatr Dermatol 1991;8:300–305.
18. Kim SC, Kang WH. Nevus comedonicus associated with epidermal nevus. J Am Acad Dermatol 1989;21:1085–1088.
19. Dudley K, Barr W, Armin A, et al. Nevus comedonicus in association with widespread follicular tumors. J Am Acad Dermatol 1986;15:1123–1127.
19a. Price M, Russell Jones R. Familial dyskeratotic comedones. Clin Exp Dermatol 1985;10:147–53
20. Eichler C, Flowers F, Ross J. Epidermal nevus syndrome: Case report and review of clinical manifestations. Pediatr Dermatol 1989;6:316–320.
21. Grebe TA, Rimsza ME, Richter SF, et al. Further delineation of the epidermal nevus syndrome: Two new cases with new findings and literature review. Am J Med Genet 1993;47:24–30.
22. Pavone L, Curatolo P, Rizzo R, et al. Epidermal nevus syndrome: A neurologic variant with hemimegalencephaly, gyral malformation, mental retardation, seizures and facial hemihypertrophy. Neurology 1991;41:266–271.
23. Nazzaro V, Cambiaghi S, Montagnani A, et al. Proteus syndrome. J Am Acad Dermatol 1991;25:377–383.
24. Hebert A, Esterly NB, Holbrook KA, et al. The CHILD syndrome. Arch Dermatol 1987;123:503–509.
25. Marden PM, Smith DW, McDonald MI. Congenital anomalies in the newborn infant, including minor variations. J Pediatr 1964;64:357–371.
26. Rongioletti F, Rebora A. Epidermal nevus with transitional cell carcinomas of the urinary tract. J Am Acad Dermatol 1991; 25:856–858.
27. Ratz JL, Bailin PL, Wheeland RG. Carbon dioxide laser treatment of epidermal nevi. J Dermatol Surg Oncol 1986;12: 567–570.
28. Hohenleutner U, Landthaler M. Laser therapy of verrucous epidermal naevi. Clin Exp Dermatol 1993;18:124–127.
29. Ashinoff R. Linear nevus sebaceus of Jadassohn treated with the carbon dioxide laser. Pediatr Dermatol 1993;10:189–191.
30. Happle R, Kastru W, Macher E. Systemic retinoid therapy of systematized verrucous epidermal nevus. Dermatologica 1977; 155:200–205.
31. Milton GP, DiGiovanni JJ, Peck GL. Treatment of nevus comedonicus with ammonium lactate lotion. J Am Acad Dermatol 1989;20:324–328.
32. Glover MT, Ridley CM, Leigh IM. Extensive comedo naevus:

Benefit from long-term erythromycin. Br J Dermatol 1991; 125(Suppl. 38):57–58.

33. Uitto J, Santa Cruz DJ, Eisen AZ. Connective tissue nevi of the skin. J Am Acad Dermatol 1980;3;441–461.

34. Berberian BB, Wood C. Asymptomatic nodules on the back and abdomen: Connective tissue nevi, collagenoma type. Arch Dermatol 1987;123:811–812.

35. Henderson RR, Wheeler CE, Abele DC. Familial cutaneous collagenoma: Report of cases. Arch Dermatol 1968;98:23–27.

36. Hegedus SI, Schorr WF. Familial cutaneous collagenoma. Cutis 1972;10:283–288.

37. Hornstein L, Bove KE, Towbin RB. Linear nevi, hemihypertrophy, connective tissue hamartomas and unusual neoplasms in children. J Pediatr 1987;110:404–408.

38. Kopec AV, Levine N. Generalised connective tissue nevi and ichthyosis in Down's syndrome. Arch Dermatol 1979;115: 623–624.

39. Verbov J, Graham R. Buschke-Ollendorff syndrome: Disseminated dermatofibrosis with osteopoikilosis. Clin Exp Dermatol 1986;11:17–26.

40. Thieberg MD, Stone MS, Siegfried EC. Buschke-Ollendorff syndrome. Pediatr Dermatol 1993;10:86–87.

41. Crivelatto E. Disseminated nevus anelasticus. Int J Dermatol 1986;25:171–173.

42. Starrico R, Mehregan AH. Nevus elasticus and nevus elasticus vascularis. Arch Dermatol 1961;84:943–947.

43. Sears JK, Stone MS, Argenyi Z. Papular elastorrhexis; a variant of connective tissue nevus. Case reports and review of the literature. J Am Acad Dermatol 1988;19(Part 2):409–414.

44. Wilson Jones E, Marks R, Pongsehirun D. Naevus superficialis lipomatosis. Br J Dermatol 1975;93:121–133.

44a. Mehregan A, Tavafoghi V, Gjandchi A. Nevus lipomatosus superficialis cutaneus Hoffmann Zurhelle. J Cutan Pathol 1975; 2:307–13.

45. Dotz W, Prioleau PG. Nevus lipomatosus cutaneus superficialis. Arch Dermatol 1984;120:376–379.

46. Eyre SP, Hebert AA, Rapini RP. Rubbery zosteriform nodules on the back. Arch Dermatol 1992;128:1395–1400.

47. Sanchez NP, Rhodes AR, Mandell F, et al. Encephalocraniocutaneous lipomatosis: A new neurocutaneous syndrome. Br J Dermatol 1981;104:89–96.

48. Grimalt R, Ermacora E, Mistura L, et al. Encephalocraniocutaneous lipomatosis: Case report and review of the literature. Pediatr Dermatol 1993;10:164–168.

49. Happle R, Steijlen PM. Enzephalokraniokutane lipomatose. Ein nichterblicher mosaikphanotyp. Hautarzt 1993;43:19–22.

50. Fukamizu H, Matsumoto K, Inoue K, et al. Large vulvar lipoma. Arch Dermatol 1982;118:447.

51. Lachman RS, Finkelstein J, Mehringer CM, et al. Congenital aggressive lipomatosis. Skel Radiol 1983;9:248–254.

52. Ross CM. Generalised folded skin with an underlying lipomatous nevus, "the Michelin tyre baby." Arch Dermatol 1969;100: 320–323.

53. Berger TG, Levin MW. Congenital smooth muscle hamartoma. J Am Acad Dermatol 1984;11:709–712.

54. Goldman MP, Kaplan RP, Heng MC. Congenital smooth muscle hamartoma. Int J Dermatol 1987;26:448–452.

55. Gange EJ, Su WPD. Congenital smooth muscle hamartoma of the skin. Pediatr Dermatol 1993;10:1021–1023.

56. Johnson MD, Jacobs AH. Congenital smooth muscle hamartoma: A report of six cases and a review of the literature. Arch Dermatol 1989;125:820–822.

57. Glover MT, Malone M, Atherton DJ. Michelin tyre baby syndrome resulting from diffuse smooth muscle hamartoma. Pediatr Dermatol 1989;6:329–331.

58. Schnur RE, Herzberg AJ, Spinner N, et al. Variability in the Michelin tyre baby syndrome. A child with multiple anomalies, smooth muscle hamartoma and familial paracentric inversion of chromosome 7q. J Am Acad Dermatol 1993;28(Part 2):364–370.

59. Mills AE. Rhabdomyomatous mesenchymal hamartoma of skin. Am J Dermatopathol 1989;11:58–63.

60. Ashfaq R, Timmons CF. Rhabdomyomatous mesenchymal hamartoma of skin. Pediatr Pathol 1992;12:731.

61. Polan S, Butterworth T. Cutis verticis gyrata: A report with review of seven new cases. Am J Ment Def 1953;57:613–631.

62. Garden JM, Robinson JK. Essential primary cutis verticis gyrata. Arch Dermatol 1984;120:1480–1483.

63. Abu-Jamra F, Dimick DF. Cutis verticis gyrata. Am J Surg 1966;111:274–277.

64. Palo J, Iivanainen M, Blomqvist K, et al. Aetiological aspects of the cutis verticis gyrata and mental retardation syndrome. J Ment Defic Res 1970;14:33–43.

65. Orkin M, Frichot BC, Zelickson AS. Cerebriform intradermal nevus. A cause of cutis verticis gyrata. Arch Dermatol 1974; 110:575–582.

66. Khare AK, Singh G. Acquired cutis verticis gyrata due to rotational traction. Br J Dermatol 1984;110:125–126.

67. Hseih H, Fisher DE, Bronson DM, et al. Cutis verticis gyrata in a neonate. Pediatr Dermatol 1983;1:153–156.

68. Schepsis C, Palazzo R, Ragusa RM, et al. Association of cutis verticis gyrata with fragile X syndrome and fragility of chromosome 12. Lancet 1989;2:279.

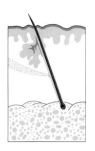

chapter 175

Genodermatoses

JAMES E. SLIGH, JR., and MOISE L. LEVY

Recent developments in the technology of molecular genetics have generated many important advances in the field of inherited disorders of the skin. As many of the genes responsible for these conditions are cloned and characterized, and targeted therapies evolve, there will be new hope for the patients and families suffering with them. Recent understanding of the molecular basis of these diseases has produced new methods for laboratory diagnosis[1] as well as expanded the window of diagnostic possibility to help families make informed decisions during the prenatal period.[2] The next technological step to conquer will be the effective use of somatic gene therapy to correct the gene defects in genodermatoses.

This chapter summarizes the features of certain genodermatoses not covered elsewhere in this text. Included in Tables 175–1 to 175–3 are genodermatoses associated with malignancy, vascular syndromes, and genodermatoses associated with chromosomal instability.

TABLE 175-1. Genodermatoses with Potential for Malignancy

Disease	Inheritance	Cutaneous Findings	Other Manifestations
Basal cell nevus syndrome (Gorlin's syndrome)[3-7]	Autosomal dominant	Basal cell carcinomas erupt as 1-mm to 1-cm papules on the face, trunk, and arms (Fig. 175–1). Shallow (2- to 3-mm) pits of the palms and soles are specific for the disease. Microscopic basal cell carcinomas may also be found incidentally in the walls of some of these pits.	Prognathism, cysts of the mandible and maxilla, and other dental abnormalities, bifid ribs or other skeletal anomalies, intracranial calcification, ovarian fibromas, medulloblastomas, mental retardation, ophthalmologic abnormalities.
Cowden's disease (multiple hamartoma syndrome)[8-10]	Autosomal dominant	Yellowish tan verrucous or papillomatous papules especially on the face and extremities (trichilemmomas). Multiple 1- to 3-mm oral mucosa papillomas may have cobblestone appearance (Fig. 175–2). Palmoplantar keratoses and acral keratoses.	36% of female patients will develop breast carcinoma. Thyroid disease and tumors are frequent. Hamartomatous polyps may involve entire GI tract, but most common in colon. Skeletal abnormalities, adenoid facies, high-arched palate. Genitourinary tract cysts.
Dyskeratosis congenita (Zinsser-Cole-Engmann syndrome)[11-13]	X-linked recessive or autosomal dominant	Reticular pigmentation of the head, neck, and trunk begins in the first decade and progresses to atrophy and telangiectasia. Progressive nail dystrophy and leukoplakia of mucous membranes are also early manifestations of the disease (Fig. 175–3). Other changes include palmoplantar hyperkeratosis and hyperhidrosis.	Bone marrow involvement often manifests with thrombocytopenia or pancytopenia. Hypoplastic marrow and decreased cellular immunity predispose to severe infection. Skeletal and neurologic involvement are common. Leukoplakia may progress to squamous cell carcinoma.

TABLE 175-1. Genodermatoses with Potential for Malignancy (*Continued*)

Disease	Inheritance	Cutaneous Findings	Other Manifestations
Gardner's syndrome[14-18]	Autosomal dominant	Epidermal cysts may be present at birth. Osteomas, most commonly on the face and head. Desmoid tumors occur frequently, especially in females, at sites of incisions or spontaneously. Fibromas.	Adenomatous polyps in the colon > small intestine. Risk of developing carcinomatous changes in gastrointestinal polyps is 100% as early as 9 years of age. Dental anomalies. Thyroid cancer. Retroperitoneal fibrosis. Specific ocular fundus pigmentation. Total colectomy is recommended.
Peutz-Jeghers syndrome[19,20]	Autosomal dominant	Periorificial and acral pigmentation. Melanoplakia most common on lips, buccal mucosa, digits, palms, and soles, and is usually present by age 2. Pigmented macules are brown or black (Fig. 175-4).	Hamartomatous polyps found in jejunum > ileum > stomach > duodenum > colon. Polyps also found in airways and genitourinary tract. Risk for developing malignancy is unknown. Gonadal tumors, cervical and breast cancer.

GI, gastrointestinal.

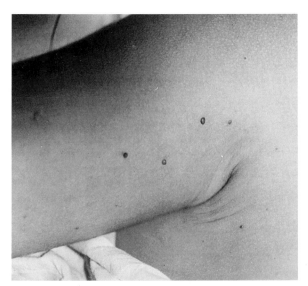

FIGURE 175-1. Multiple hyperpigmented papules representative of basal cell nevi on the arm and chest of a 10 year old with the basal cell nevus syndrome.

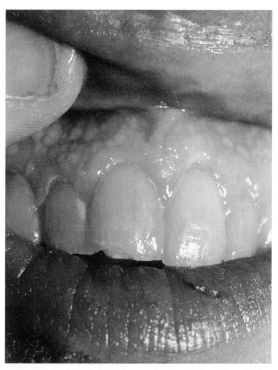

FIGURE 175-2. Multiple soft papules involving the gingiva of a patient diagnosed with Cowden's syndrome. (Courtesy of Adelaide Hebert, M.D.)

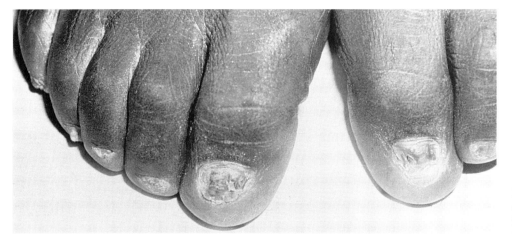

FIGURE 175-3. Onychodystrophy affecting most nails in a girl with dyskeratosis congenita. (Courtesy of N. Prose, M.D.)

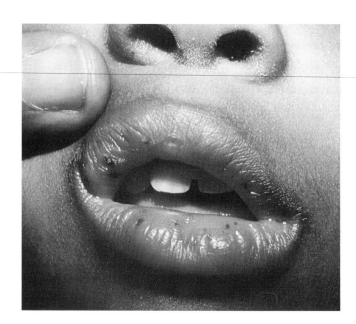

FIGURE 175-4. Multiple hyperpigmented macules distributed over the lips of a child typical of Peutz-Jeghers syndrome. (Courtesy of Adelaide Hebert, M.D.)

TABLE 175-2. Vascular Syndromes

Disease	Inheritance	Cutaneous Findings	Other Manifestations
Bannayan syndrome[21-26]	Autosomal dominant	Arteriovenous malformations, lipomas, and lymphatic-venous malformations. Pigmented macules on the penis.	Growth and mental retardation, macrocephaly, intracranial tumors, macrodactyly, increased size at birth. Hashimoto's thyroiditis also reported.
Blue rubber bleb nevus syndrome[27,28]	Autosomal dominant	1- to 50-mm blue to purplish red sac-like venous malformations distributed over the upper extremities and trunk. Blue macules.	Vascular malformations found on any mucosal surface. Gastrointestinal lesions cause intestinal bleeding, iron deficiency. Visceral venous malformations.
Cobb's syndrome[29]	Sporadic	Nevus flammeus and angiokeratomas. These lesions appear over the trunk in a dermatomal distribution.	Vascular malformations in the spinal cord at the level of the dermatomal lesions. Renal tumors, kyphoscoliosis.
Cutis marmorata telangiectatica congenita[30-33]	Autosomal dominant or sporadic	Deep red reticular mottling of skin from telangiectasias involving extremities > trunk > face (Fig. 175-5). Lesions may fade or thrombose.	Limb asymmetry on the affected side. Macrocephaly. Mental retardation.
Gorham's syndrome[34-36]	Sporadic	Venous malformations that may or may not overlie affected bone. Lymphatic malformations.	Massive replacement of bone with fibrous tissue.
Klippel-Trenaunay syndrome and Parkes Weber syndrome[37-39]	Sporadic	Nevus flammeus and venous varicosities that are present at birth. Hypertrophy of soft tissue and bone (Fig. 175-6). Patients may have angiokeratomas, venous malformations, and lymphatic malformations. Lower extremity is involved more than the upper extremity. Distribution of lesions is usually unilateral.	There is often a compensatory scoliosis when a lower extremity is involved and hypertrophic. Arteriovenous shunts, hemorrhage, epidural vascular malformations can result in hemiplegia secondary to spinal cord paralysis.
Maffucci's syndrome[40-42]	Sporadic	Multiple lymphatic-venous malformations and endochondromas. The vascular lesions may be present at birth, and approximately 80% of the lesions will develop before puberty.	Defects in bone ossification result in easy fractures, short stature, different lengths in the long bones. Predisposed to malignancy, especially chondrosarcoma.
Rendu-Osler-Weber syndrome (hereditary hemorrhagic telangiectasia)[43,44]	Autosomal dominant	Punctate telangiectasias of the skin most common on the face, tongue, lips, nasal mucosa, hands, arms, and fingertips (Fig. 175-7). Often presents as recurrent epistaxis in childhood.	Telangiectasias of the gastrointestinal and genitourinary tract which can be a source of bleeding. Upper GI bleeding is more common than lower. Increased liver function tests, pulmonary arteriovenous fistulae.
Riley-Smith syndrome[45]	Autosomal dominant	Multiple lymphatic-venous malformations and pseudo-papillomas.	Macrocephaly. Growth is normal and there are no associated neurologic manifestations.
Sturge-Weber syndrome[46]	Sporadic (most), autosomal dominant, or autosomal recessive	Capillary malformations of the leptomeninges with an ipsilateral nevus flammeus usually in the distribution of first division of the trigeminal nerve (Fig. 175-8). Up to 20% have facial involvement bilaterally.	Mental retardation, contralateral hemiplegia or hemiparesis, seizures usually beginning in the first year, intracranial calcification, visceral capillary malformations, ocular involvement, glaucoma if V_2 involved.
Von Hippel-Lindau syndrome[47-50]	Autosomal dominant	Port-wine stains, café-au-lait macules. Dermal capillary malformations have a predilection for the head and neck region.	Vascular malformations in the cerebellum and brain stem. Retina also commonly affected (Fig. 175-9). Cystic neoplasms or angiomatous lesions in the kidneys, liver, and pancreas. Tumors in head are a risk for hemorrhage. Pheochromotomas.
Wyburn-Mason syndrome[51-54]	Sporadic	Facial nevus flammeus contiguous with arteriovenous malformations of the optic nerve and retina, enlarged facial veins.	Cirsoid aneurysm of the midbrain and of the optic nerve, nystagmus, retardation, seizures, ataxia (Fig. 175-10).

GI, gastrointestinal.

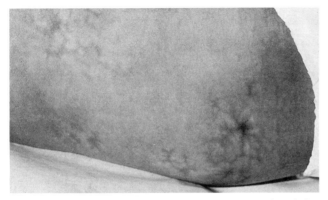

FIGURE 175–5. Telangiectatic erythema over the leg of an infant with cutis marmorata telangiectatica congenita.

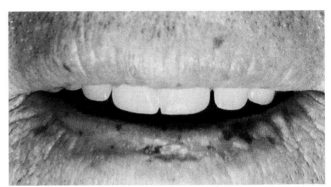

FIGURE 175–7. Multiple telangiectasias involving the lips of a patient with hereditary hemorrhagic telangiectasia.

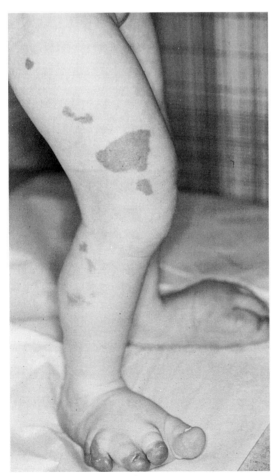

FIGURE 175–6. Capillary and venous malformation with limb hypertrophy typical of the Klippel-Trenaunay syndrome.

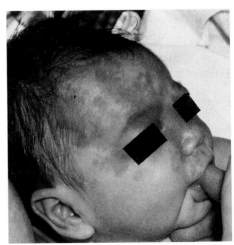

FIGURE 175–8. A capillary malformation involving the first and second branches of the trigeminal nerve in a child with Sturge-Weber syndrome.

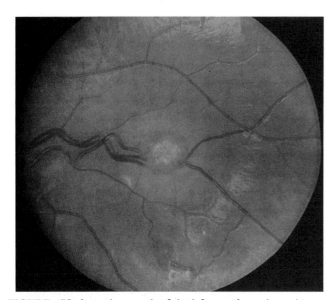

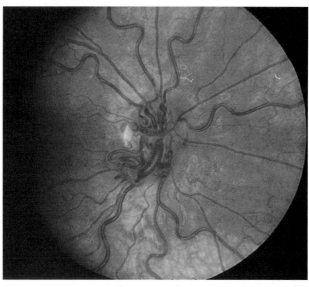

FIGURE 175-9. A photograph of the left eye of a patient with von Hippel–Lindau syndrome. Illustrated are endophytic and exophytic vascular malformations acting as an acquired shunt. There is marked engorgement of the feeding arteriole and hypersaturation of the draining venule. Small areas of lipoproteinaceous exudate are present as well. (Courtesy of R. A. Lewis, M.D.)

FIGURE 175-10. A photograph of the fundus of the right eye of a patient with Wyburn-Mason syndrome. There is marked enlargement of the vasculature of both the right optic disk and adjacent retina. Abnormal arborization and arteriolization of the venous blood and absence of a normal capillary bed are features typical of a congenital arteriovenous malformation. Similar vascular malformations over the pterygopalatine area, orbit, right cerebral hemisphere, eyelids, and forehead were present on the same side. (Courtesy of R. A. Lewis, M.D.)

TABLE 175-3. Genodermatoses Associated with Chromosomal Instability

Disease	Inheritance	Cutaneous Findings	Other Manifestations	Etiology	Laboratory Evaluations
Ataxia-telangiectasia (Louis-Bar syndrome)[55-58]	Autosomal recessive	Cutaneous telangiectasias primarily in sun-exposed areas, atrophy, mottled patches of hypopigmentation and hyperpigmentation, premature hair graying, decreased subcutaneous fat.	Fusiform dilatations of bulbar conjunctival capillaries, cerebellar ataxia, recurrent sinopulmonary infections, increased incidence of lymphoproliferative neoplasia at a young age, abnormal thymic development, cellular and humoral immune system defects, diabetes (Fig. 175-11).	Profound sensitivity to x-ray or gamma irradiation.	Lymphopenia. Balanced translocation between chromosomes 7 and 14. Increased alpha-fetoprotein, increased CEA, chromosomal instability to radiation including amniotic fluid cells.
Bloom's syndrome[59-63]	Autosomal recessive	Telangiectatic erythema in a butterfly distribution over the face, photosensitivity, café-au-lait macules.	Growth and mental retardation, characteristic narrow and pointed facies, immune abnormalities, and increased bacterial infections. Predisposition to malignancy, especially leukemia, testicular atrophy and infertility in males.	DNA ligase I deficiency. Increase in sister chromatid exchange. Spontaneous chromosomal breaks.	Cultured cells (including amniotic fluid cells) show increased sister chromatid exchange (visualized with bromodeoxyuridine labeling) and the formation of quadraradial figures, decreased serum levels of IgA and IgM, reduced number of CD4+ T cells, and impaired mitogen response.
Cockayne's syndrome[64-66]	Autosomal recessive	Early actinic damage, highly prone to developing cutaneous malignancy, premature aging, loss of subcutaneous fat, photosensitivity that heals with scarring and patches of atrophy and hypopigmentation.	Very short stature, deafness, mental retardation, retinal atrophy, type II lipoproteinemia, intracranial calcification, large ears and nose with sunken eyes. Long upper and lower limbs in comparison to body size. Demyelination in peripheral nerves and central nervous system. Cryptorchidism.	Profound sensitivity to ultraviolet radiation. Impaired repair of UV damage in genes being actively transcribed.	Cultured cells (including amniotic fluid cells) show decreased colony-forming ability after UV irradiation, delayed DNA synthesis (S phase) in the cells following irradiation. Delayed nerve conduction velocities. Osteoporosis and intracranial calcification radiographically.
Fanconi's anemia[67-70]	Autosomal recessive	Both hyperpigmentation and hypopigmentation, petechiae.	Aplastic anemia, kidney and spleen hypoplasia, thumb and radius bony abnormalities. Progressive growth failure. High incidence of leukemia.	Chromosomal instability and increased sensitivity to DNA cross-linking agents.	Prenatal diagnosis by quantitation of chromosomal breakage in cultured amniotic fluid cells. Cells are sensitive to agents such as mitomycin C or diepoxybutane.

Progeria[71-73]	Autosomal recessive	External signs of aging, wrinkled skin with prominence of the superficial veins, alopecia (eyelashes and eyebrows may be lost as well), subcutaneous fat atrophy, areas of scleroderma and irregular pigmentation. Midfacial cyanosis and scleroderma may be present at birth.	Die of "old age" in the first two decades of life. Arteriosclerosis, failure to thrive, cessation of growth. Delayed or incomplete tooth development. No sexual development. Osteoporosis. Open anterior fontanelles Glyphic nose.	Unknown	Increased levels of urinary hyaluronic acid. Radiologic findings include thin cranial bones with open sutures and fontanelles. Osteoporosis. Broad metaphyses and thin cortex of long bones.
Rothmund-Thomson syndrome[74-77]	Autosomal recessive	Macular erythema in a photodistribution leading to poikiloderma most extensive in but not limited to sun-exposed skin. Absent or sparse thin hair on head and body, dystrophic nails, hyperkeratotic lesions on thick skin areas (palmoplantar, elbows, and knees) (Figs. 175-12 and 175-13).	Normal life expectancy. Underdeveloped secondary sexual characteristics. Short stature, dysmorphic facial features, malformation of teeth, cataracts, bone defects (Fig. 175-14). May develop osteosarcoma.	Unknown	Aminoaciduria may be present. Multiple abnormal chromosome patterns including trisomy 8 may be found in skin fibroblasts.
Xeroderma pigmentosum[78-81]	Autosomal recessive	Increased photosensitivity and predisposition for development of cutaneous malignancy as early as age 3. Irregular freckling, dry skin, hypopigmentation, hyperpigmentation, telangiectasias, and atrophy in childhood (Fig. 175-15).	May have associated ocular or neurologic abnormalities. Ocular: telangiectasias of the conjunctivae, keratitis, corneal clouding. Neurologic: ataxia, impaired hearing, progressive mental retardation.	Defective DNA repair mechanism. DNA damage accumulates from inability to properly conduct excision repair of UV-damaged DNA such as thymine dimers. Defective genes form many different complementation groups.	Decreased proliferation rate and survival of cultured cells following exposure to UV light. Decreased rate of excision of UV-induced pyrimidine dimers in cultured cells (including amniotic fluid cells)
Werner's syndrome[82-84]	Autosomal recessive	Premature graying and thinning of hair, subcutaneous fat atrophy, acral scleroderma, sparse body hair, hyperkeratosis of the palms and soles.	Early growth arrest, with low body weight. Flat feet, high-pitched or hoarse voice, irregular tooth arrangement. Early bilateral cataracts, poor development of secondary sexual characteristics, survival into the fifth decade and death often associated with atherosclerosis. May have mild senile dementia.	Chromosomal instability. Accelerated aging, reduced in vitro life span of cultured fibroblasts.	Diabetes mellitus or glucose intolerance is frequently present. Increased levels of urinary hyaluronic acid. Reduced life span of fibroblasts cultured in vitro.

CEA, carcinoembryonic antigen; UV, ultraviolet.

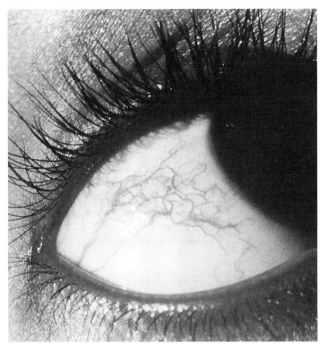

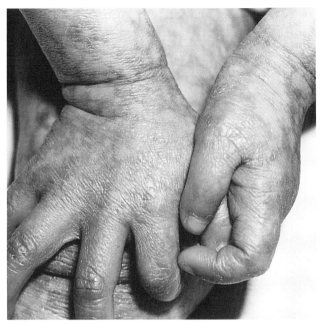

FIGURE 175–13. Poikiloderma and senile appearing skin over the hands of a child with the Rothmund-Thomson syndrome.

FIGURE 175–11. Bulbar telangiectasias in a child with ataxia-telangiectasia.

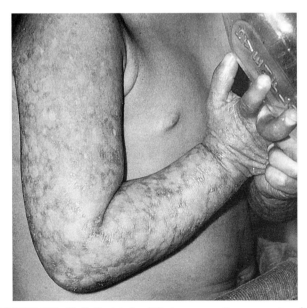

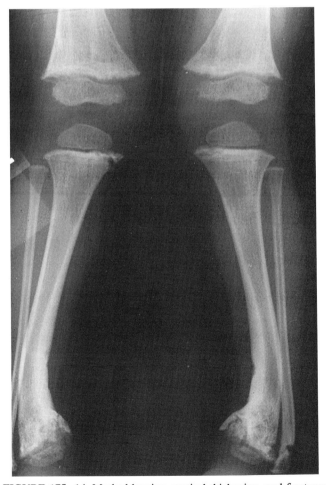

FIGURE 175–12. Reticulated poikiloderma over the upper extremity of a child with the Rothmund-Thomson syndrome.

FIGURE 175–14. Marked bowing, cortical thickening, and fractures involving the right and left tibia of a 4 year old with Rothmund-Thomson syndrome. Also present is a fracture of the left fibula.

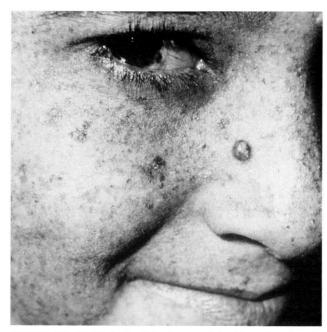

FIGURE 175–15. Marked actinic changes of the skin and conjunctiva in a young girl with xeroderma pigmentosum. A solitary squamous cell carcinoma is present over the nose.

References

1. Levy ML, Magee W. Postnatal testing for unusual genodermatoses. Dermatol Clinics 1994;12:93–97.
2. Sybert VP, Holbrook KA, Levy ML. Prenatal diagnosis of severe dermatologic diseases. Adv Dermatol 1992;7:179–209.
3. Farndon PA, Del Mastro RG, Evans DGR, et al. Location of gene for Gorlin syndrome. Lancet 1992;339:581–582.
4. Gailani MR, Bale SJ, Leffell DJ, et al. Developmental defects in Gorlin syndrome related to a putative tumor suppressor gene on chromosome 9. Cell 1992;69:111–117.
5. Gorlin RJ. Nevoid basal-cell carcinoma syndrome. Medicine 1987;66:98–113.
6. Chenevix-Trench G, Wicking C, Berkman J, et al. Further localization of the gene for nevoid basal cell carcinoma syndrome (NBCCS) in 15 Australian families: Linkage and loss of heterozygosity. Am J Hum Genet 1993;53:760–767.
7. See also Chapter 167 in this book.
8. Weary PE, Gorlin RJ, Gentry WC, et al. Multiple hamartoma syndrome (Cowden's disease). Arch Dermatol 1972;106:682–690.
9. Starink TM, Van Der Veen JPW, Arwert F, et al. The Cowden Syndrome: A clinical and genetic study in 21 patients. Clin Genet 1986;29:222–233.
10. Barax CN, Lebwohl M, Phelps RG. Multiple hamartoma syndrome. J Am Acad Dermatol 1987;17:342–346.
11. Drachtman RA, Alter BP. Dyskeratosis congenita: Clinical and genetic heterogeneity. Am J Pediatr Hematol Oncol 1992; 297–304.
12. Conner JM, Gatherer D, Gray FC, et al. Assignment of the gene for dyskeratosis congenita to Xq28. Hum Genet 1986;72: 348–351.
13. Davidson HR, Conner JM. Dyskeratosis congenita. J Med Genet 1988;25:843–846.
14. Nakamura Y, Lathrop M, Leppert M, et al. Localization of the genetic defect in familial adenomatous polyposis within a small region of chromosome 5. Am J Hum Genet 1988;43:638–644.
15. Bodmer WF, Bailey CJ, Bodmer J, et al. Localisation of the gene for familial adenomatous polyposis on chromosome 5. Nature 1987;328:614–616.
16. Leppert M, Dobbs M, Scambler P, et al. The gene for familial polyposis coli maps to the long arm of chromosome 5. Science 1987;238:1411–1413.
17. Weary PE, Linthicum A, Cawley EP, et al. Gardner's syndrome: A family group study and review. Arch Dermatol 1964;90:20–30.
18. Traboulsi EI, Krush AJ, Gardner EJ, et al. Prevalence and importance of pigmented ocular fundus lesions in Gardner's syndrome. N Engl J Med 1987;316:661–667.
19. Giardiello FM, Welsh SB, Hamilton SR, et al. Increased risk of cancer in the Peutz-Jeghers syndrome. N Engl J Med 1987;316:1511–1514.
20. Spigelman AD, Murday V, Philips RK. Cancer and the Peutz-Jeghers syndrome. Gut 1989;30:1588–1590.
21. Bannayan GA. Lipomatosis, angiomatosis, and macrocephaly. A previously undescribed congenital syndrome. Arch Pathol 1971;92:1–5.
22. Zonana J, Rimoin DL, Davis DC. Macrocephaly with multiple lipomas and hemangiomas. J Pediatr 1976;89:600–603.
23. Ruvalcaba RHA, Myhre S, Smith DW. Sotos syndrome with intestinal polyposis and pigmentary changes of the genitalia. Clin Genet 1980;18:413–416.
24. Higgenbottom MC, Schultz P. The Bannayan syndrome: An autosomal dominant disorder consisting of macrocephaly, lipomas, hemangiomas, and risk for intracranial tumors. Pediatrics 1982;69:632–634.
25. Saul RA, Stevenson RE, Bley R. Mental retardation in the Bannayan syndrome. Pediatrics 1982;69:642–644.
26. Gorlin RJ, Cohen MM, Condon LM, et al. Bannayan-Riley-Ruvalcaba syndrome. Am J Med Genet 1992:44:307–314.
27. Oranje AP. Blue rubber bleb nevus syndrome. Pediatr Dermatol 1986;3:304–310.
28. Moodley M, Ramdial P. Blue rubber bleb nevus syndrome: A case report and review of the literature. Pediatrics 1993;92:160–162.
29. Jessen RT, Thompson S, Smith EB. Cobb syndrome. Arch Dermatol 1977;113:1587–1590.
30. Powel ST, Su WPD. Cutis marmorata telangiectatica congenita. Report of nine cases and review of the literature. Cutis 1984;34:305–312.
31. Rogers M, Poyzer KG. Cutis marmorata telangiectatica congenita. Arch Dermatol 1982;118:895–899.
32. Cohen PR, Zalar GL. Cutis marmorata telangiectatica congenita: Clinicopathologic characteristics and differential diagnosis. Cutis 1988;42:518–522.
33. Picascia DD, Esterly NB. Cutis marmorata telangiectatica congenita: Report of 22 cases. J Am Acad Dermatol 1989;20:1098–1104.
34. Frost JF, Caplan RM. Cutaneous hemangiomas and disappearing bones. Arch Dermatol 1965;92:501–508.
35. Gorham LW, Stout AP. Massive osteolysis (acute spontaneous absorption of bone, phantom bone, disappearing bone). Its relation to hemangiomatosis. J Bone Joint Surg 1955;37A:985–1004.
36. Choma ND, Biscotti, CV, Bauer TW, et al. Gorham's syndrome: A case report and review of the literature. Am J Med 1987;83:1151–1156.
37. Baskerville PA, Ackroyd JS, Browse NL. The Klippel-Trenaunay syndrome: Clinical, radiological, and haemodynamic features and management. Br J Surg 1985;72:232–236.
38. Gloviczki P, Hollier LH, Telander RL, et al. Surgical implications of Klippel-Trenaunay syndrome. Ann Surg 1983;197:353–362.
39. Servelle M. Klippel and Trenaunay's syndrome. Ann Surg 1985;201:365–373.
40. Lewis RJ, Ketcham AS. Maffucci's syndrome: Functional and neoplastic significance. J Bone Joint Surg 1973;55A:1465–1479.
41. Kaplan RP, Wang JT, Amron DM, et al. Maffucci's syndrome: Two case reports with a literature review. J Am Acad Dermatol 1993;29:894–899.
42. Collins PS, Han W, Williams LR, et al. Maffucci's syndrome (hemangiomatosis osteolytica): A report of four cases. J Vasc Surg 1992;16:364–371.
43. Reilly PJ, Nostrant TT. Clinical manifestations of hereditary hemorrhagic telangiectasia. Am J Gastroenterol 1984;79:363–367.
44. McCue CM, Hartenberg M, Nance WE. Pulmonary arteriovenous malformations related to Redu-Osler-Weber syndrome. Am J Med Genet 1984;19:19–27.
45. Riley HD, Smith WR. Macrocephaly, pseudopapilledema, and multiple hemangiomata. Pediatrics 1960;26:293–300.
46. Enjolras O, Riche, MC, Merland JJ. Facial port-wine stains and Sturge-Weber syndrome. Pediatrics 1985;76:48–51.
47. Melmon KL, Rosen SW. Lindau's disease. Am J Med 1964;36:595–617.

48. Kounis NG, Karapanou E, Dimopulos P, et al. The von Hippel–Lindau syndrome: Report of a case and review of the literature. Br J Clin Pract 1989;43:37–41.
49. Neumann HP, Wiestler OD. Clustering of features of von Hippel–Lindau syndrome: Evidence for a complex genetic locus. Lancet 1991;337:1052–1054.
50. Seizinger BR. Toward the isolation of the primary genetic defect in von Hippel–Lindau disease. Ann N Y Acad Sci 1991;615:332–337.
51. Wyburn-Mason R. Arteriovenous aneurysm of the midbrain and retina, facial naevi and mental changes. Brain 1943;66:163–203.
52. Theron J, Newton TH, Hoyt WF. Unilateral retinocephalic vascular malformations. Neuroradiology 1974;7:185–196.
53. Hopen G, Smith JL, Hoff JT, et al. The Wyburn-Mason syndrome. J Clin Neuro Ophthalmol 1983;3:53–62.
54. Patel U, Gupta SC. The Wyburn-Mason syndrome: A case report and review of the literature. Neuroradiology 1990;31:544–546.
55. Cohen LE, Tanner DJ, Schaefer HG, et al. Common and uncommon cutaneous findings with ataxia-telangiectasia. J Am Acad Dermatol 1984;10:431–438.
56. Gatti RA, Bodor E. Vinters HV, et al. Ataxia-telangiectasia: An interdisciplinary approach to pathogenesis. Medicine 1991;70:99–117.
57. Llerena JC, Murer-Orlando M. Bloom syndrome and ataxia-telangiectasia. Semin Hematol 1991;28:95–103.
58. Smith LS, Conerly SL. Ataxia-telangiectasia or Louis-Bar syndrome. J Am Acad Dermatol 1985;12:681–696.
59. Lambert WC, Lambert MW. Diseases associated with DNA and chromosomal instability. In: Alper JC, ed. Genetic Disorders of the Skin. St. Louis: Mosby-Yearbook, 1991:320.
60. Bloom D. The syndrome of congenital telangiectatic erythema and stunted growth. J Pediatr 1966;68:103–113.
61. Giannelli F, Benson PF, Pawsey SA, et al. Ultraviolet light sensitivity and delayed DNA-chain maturation in Bloom's syndrome fibroblasts. Nature 1977;265:466–469.
62. Chan JYH, Becker FF, German J, et al. Altered DNA ligase I activity in Bloom's syndrome cells. Nature 1987;325:357–359.
63. Willis AE, Lindahl T. DNA ligase I deficiency in Bloom's syndrome. Nature 1987;325:355–357.
64. Cockayne EA. Dwarfism with retinal atrophy and deafness. Arch Dis Child 1936;11:1–8.
65. Nance MA, Berry Sa. Cockayne's syndrome; review of 140 cases. Am J Med Genet 1992;42:68–84.
66. Venema J, Mullenders LHF, Natarajan AT, et al. The genetic defect in Cockayne syndrome is associated with a defect in repair of UV-induced DNA damage in transcriptionally active DNA. Proc Natl Acad Sci USA 1990;87:4707–4711.
67. Fanconi G. Familial constitutional panmyelocytopathy, Fanconi's anemia (F.A.) Semin Hematol 1967;4:233–249.
68. Schroeder TM, Tilgen D, Kruger J, et al. Formal genetics of Fanconi's anemia. Hum Genet 1976;32:257–288.
69. Gordon-Smith EC, Rutherford TR. Fanconi anemia: Constitutional aplastic anemia. Semin Hematol 1991;28:104–112.
70. Auerbach AD. Diagnosis of diseases of DNA synthesis and repair that affect the skin using cultured amniotic fluid cells. Semin Dermatol 1984;3:172–184.
71. DeBusk FL. The Hutchinson-Gilford Progeria syndrome. J Pediatr 1972;80:697–724.
72. Parkash H, Sidhu SS, Raghavan R, et al. Hutchinson-Gilford progeria:Familial occurrence. Am J Med Genet 1990;36:431–433.
73. Badame AJ. Progeria. Arch Dermatol 1989;125:540–544.
74. Vennos EM, Collins M, James WD. Rothmund-Thomson syndrome: Review of the world literature. J Am Acad Dermatol 1992;27:750–762.
75. Drouin CA, Mongrain E, Sassesville D, et al. Rothmund-Thomson syndrome with osteosarcoma. J Am Acad Dermatol 1993;28:301–305.
76. Ying KL, Oizumi J, Curry CJR. Rothmund-Thomson syndrome associated with trisomy 8 mosaicism. J Med Genet 1990;27:258–260.
77. Der Kaloustian VM, McGill JJ, Vekemans M, et al. Clonal lines of aneuploid cells in Rothmund-Thomson syndrome. Am J Med Genet 1990;37:336–339.
78. Tanaka K, Wood RD. Xeroderma pigmentosum and nucleotide excision repair of DNA. Trends Biochem Sci 1994;19:83–86.
79. Kraemer KH, Lee MM, Scotto J. Xeroderma pigmentosum: Cutaneous, ocular, and neurologic abnormalities in 830 published cases. Arch Dermatol 1987;123:241–250.
80. Robbins JH, Kraemer KH, Lutzner MA, et al. Xeroderma pigmentosum: an inherited disease with sun sensitivity, multiple cutaneous neoplasms and abnormal DNA repair. Ann Intern Med 1974;80:221–248.
81. See also Chapter 167 of this book.
82. Murata K, Nakashima H. Werner's syndrome: Twenty-four cases with a review of the Japanese medical literature. J Am Geriatr Soc 1982;30:303–308.
83. Epstein CJ, Martin GM, Schultz AL, et al. Werner's syndrome: A review of its symptomatology, natural history, pathologic features, genetics and relationship to the natural aging process. Medicine 1966;45:177–221.
84. Gebhart E, Bauer R, Raub U, et al. Spontaneous and induced chromosomal instability in Werner syndrome. Hum Genet 1988;80:135–139.

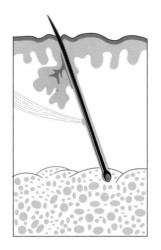

What Are the Disorders of Deposition and Cellular Secretion?

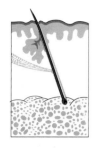

chapter 176

Xanthomas

FRANK PARKER

DEFINITION

Xanthomas, which are localized infiltrates of lipid containing foamy macrophages in either the dermis or tendons, are important clinical clues to underlying systemic disturbances in lipoprotein metabolism that subsequently lead to the development of two life-threatening conditions: atherosclerotic cardiovascular disease and pancreatitis. Patients with certain lipoprotein abnormalities are at risk for the development of premature coronary and peripheral atherosclerosis, while hypertriglyceridemia may cause acute pancreatitis. The lipids that accumulate in xanthomas and in the intima of blood vessels are derived from lipids carried in lipoproteins (1) when the lipoproteins are found in high plasma concentrations or (2) when the lipoprotein levels are normal but their biochemical structure is altered. The lipoproteins then readily cross the endothelium of the vasculature, where they are engulfed by macrophages.[1-3]

CLINICAL DESCRIPTION

Xanthomas usually appear in one of four general forms, occurring either in the skin or in tendons or tendon sheaths: tendinous, planar, tuberous, and eruptive.[3, 4] Although the form of the xanthomas the clinician observes is not solely diagnostic of the specific underlying lipoprotein disturbance, it does serve to alert the physician to a dyslipoproteinemia due to either a primary metabolic aberration or to other diverse conditions, such as diabetes, thyroid disease, pancreatitis, and renal disease, not to mention life-threatening atherosclerosis.

Tendinous xanthomas arise in tendons, ligaments, and fascia and are noted initially as deeply situated, smooth, firm nodules of various sizes covered by normal-appearing, freely movable skin. Some are easily visible, but smaller lesions are detected only on palpation with back-and-forth movement of the tendon. Tendinous xanth-

omas occur most frequently in extensor tendons of the hands (Fig. 176–1), knees, elbows, and Achilles tendons.

The finding of tendinous xanthomas almost always indicates an underlying disturbance in cholesterol and in low-density and intermediate-density lipoprotein metabolism. Coronary atherosclerosis is also a frequent finding. Rarely, tendinous xanthomas are found in the presence of normal plasma cholesterol, as in the case of the syndrome of cerebrotendinous xanthomatosis due to the accumulation of cholesterol and in several cases where plant sterols (B-sitosterol, campesterol and stigmasterol) abnormally accumulate in the blood due to increased absorption through the gut.

Planar xanthomas appear as yellow, soft, and either macular or slightly elevated smooth-surfaced plaques. The most common planar xanthoma is xanthelasma palpebrarum, which occurs on the eyelids (Fig. 176–2). Although such xanthomas suggest the presence of underlying hypercholesterolemia, when these are seen in patients younger than 40 to 50 years of age only about half will have plasma lipid elevations. The incidence of associated hypercholesterolemia and premature coronary atherosclerosis is greater when xanthelasma develops in young persons. A frequent accompanying clinical finding in patients with tendinous xanthomas, xanthelasmas, and hypercholesterolemia is corneal arcus, consisting of whitish yellow infiltrates of cholesterol, triglyceride, and phospholipid in the peripheral corneal limbus.

A second type of planar xanthoma has been termed *xanthoma striatum palmare* and appears as flat, yellow to orange, linear lesions in the creases of the palms and fingers. Conditions causing elevated plasma cholesterol and triglycerides (increases in very-low-density and intermediate-density lipoproteins) are usually associated with this form of xanthomas. Their presence always suggests an underlying problem in lipoprotein metabolism.

A third form of planar xanthomatosis is extensive, yellow-orange infiltrative, soft plaques that diffusely involve the face, neck, and even upper portions of the

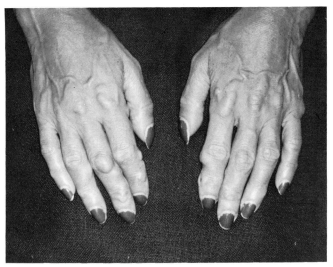

FIGURE 176-1. The hands are a common site for tendinous xanthomas.

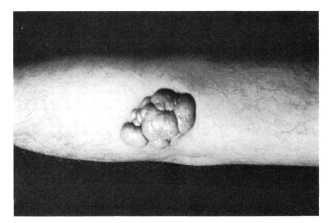

FIGURE 176-3. Tuberous xanthomas are frequently found on the skin over the dorsal aspects of joints.

trunk and arms observed in association with paraproteinemias or various causes of cholestatic liver disease. Increases in blood cholesterol levels are usually reported, although normal blood lipid levels are occasionally found in patients with some paraproteinemias with diffuse planar xanthomatosis.

Other variants of planar xanthomas are *intertriginous xanthomas*, appearing as flat to slightly raised, yellow plaques with a corrugated surface seen within and adjacent to finger webs, axillae, buttocks, and antecubital and popliteal fossae. Such lesions occur in conjunction with hypercholesterolemia.

Tuberous xanthomas appear as yellow to red papules that evolve into larger firm nodules, usually over exten-

sor surfaces of the body (elbows, knees, buttocks) as well as the palms (Fig. 176-3). Such xanthomas indicate a systemic alteration in lipid metabolism when cholesterol and/or triglyceride amounts are increased. Typically, increases in intermediate-density lipoproteins (as occurs in type III, dysbetalipoproteinemia) lead to tuberous xanthomas, but they can also occur with increases in low-density lipoproteins as well (familial hypercholesterolemia).

Eruptive xanthomas are characterized by small, yellow, cutaneous papules, 1 to 4 mm in diameter, with an erythematous halo around the base (Fig. 176-4). They erupt suddenly in crops over the extensor surfaces of the arms, legs, and buttocks. These forms of xanthomas develop almost exclusively in the presence of lactescent, hyperlipemic plasma due to elevated serum levels of triglycerides when they are carried by large light-scattering lipoproteins (i.e., chylomicrons, very-low-density lipoproteins, and intermediate-density lipoproteins). Commonly, the hypertriglyceridemia causes not only eruptive xanthoma but also lipemia retinalis (retinal vessels and the fundus appear pale pink to yellow) and acute pancreatitis.

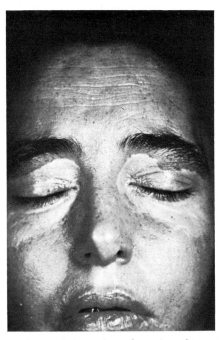

FIGURE 176-2. Xanthelasma have formed confluent plaques surrounding the eyes of this patient.

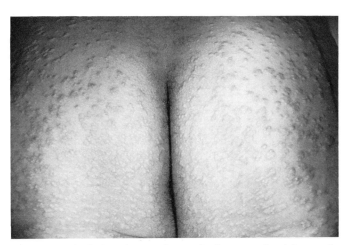

FIGURE 176-4. Eruptive xanthomas begin as small, pink to red papules that later become yellow as the lesions accumulate foamy macrophages.

PATHOLOGY

The various forms of cutaneous xanthomas due to altered lipid metabolism have in common the accumulation of macrophages with foamy cytoplasm but differ in respect to their location and the degree of fibrosis that accompanies them. The nature of the lipid within foam cells is not ascertainable with conventional histologic techniques. Frozen sections can be stained with oil red O, Sudan black, or other stains to demonstrate lipid, and polarized light demonstrates cholesterol crystals.

In tendinous xanthomas the dense fibrous tissue of a tendon is expanded by foamy macrophages and giant cells. Planar xanthomas vary in the density of dermal infiltration by foam cells. Xanthelasma shows clusters of foamy macrophages and Touton giant cells in the dermis. Touton giant cells are distinguished by a wreath-like arrangement of nuclei, with a center of eosinophilic cytoplasm and a foamy periphery (Fig. 176–5). Most other forms of planar xanthoma have sparse infiltration by foam cells. Tuberous xanthomas feature large masses of mononuclear foamy macrophages in the dermis. Fibrosis supervenes in older lesions. Eruptive xanthomas begin with a deposition of eosinophilic material between collagen bundles and dermal infiltrates of mononuclear cells. Macrophages gradually become lipidized, and eventually form nodular masses of foam cells in the

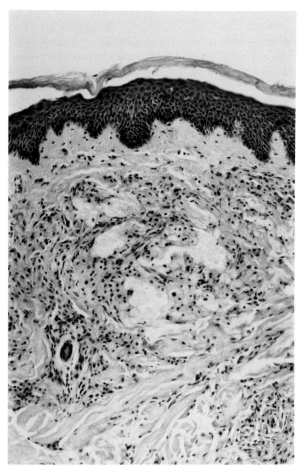

FIGURE 176–6. In eruptive xanthoma, lipid accumulates so rapidly in the dermis that some of it escapes phagocytosis by macrophages. Neutrophils are sometimes present in early lesions. Note the foamy macrophages, which are not found in papules of granuloma annulare.

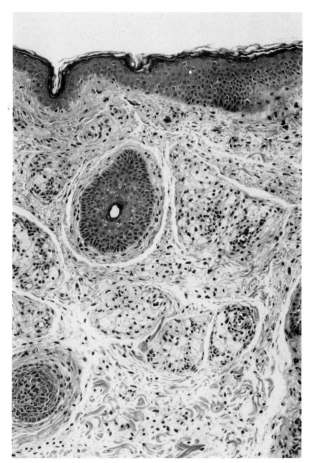

FIGURE 176–5. Xanthelasma feature masses of foamy macrophages sometimes accompanied by Touton giant cells.

dermis. The deposition of lipid appears to be so rapid that it is present not only within macrophages but extracellularly (Fig. 176–6). A few neutrophils and interstitial mucin are often present as well.[5]

PATHOGENESIS

Lipoproteins and Their Metabolism

Plasma lipoproteins are spherular particles composed of lipids (cholesterol, cholesterol esters, triglycerides, and phospholipids) and specific polypeptides called apoproteins. Lipoproteins have a hydrophobic core of nonpolar triglycerides and cholesterol esters surrounded by a hydrophilic surface lipid monolayer of free cholesterol, phospholipids, and the apoproteins. This stable configuration facilitates solubilization of the lipids, allowing them to be transported to appropriate tissues in the body. The lipid–protein combinations impart distinctive chemical, physical, and immunologic properties, which allow for segregating lipoproteins into five major groups on the basis of both ultracentrifugation and electrophoresis. Each group, therefore, has two designations depending on their density or ability to float in various salt densities or their movement in an electrical field on paper or agarose gel electrophoresis. These groups are (1) chylomicrons; (2) very-low-density lipoproteins (VLDLs) or pre-β-lipoproteins; (3) intermediate-density lipoproteins (IDLs) or broad-β lipoproteins; (4) low-density lipoproteins (LDLs) or β-lipoproteins; and (5) high-density lipoproteins (HDLs) or α-lipoproteins.

This grouping of lipoproteins on the basis of ultracentrifugation and electrophoresis depends on the type and amount of apoproteins as well as on the kinds of lipids carried by each group. The various lipoproteins actually represent a spectrum of complexes containing varying concentrations of apoproteins, triglycerides, and cholesterol. Apoproteins and cholesterol are dense while triglycerides are light, less dense, and readily float in the watery milieu of the plasma. Thus those lipoproteins that contain large amounts of cholesterol and apoprotein (HDL and LDL) are small, compact, and dense lipoproteins that do not float readily in ultracentrifuge, while those lipoproteins rich in triglyceride and relatively apoprotein sparse float rapidly in the ultracentrifuge and are of large size (chylomicrons, VLDC, and IDL). These latter lipoproteins are large enough (25–500 nm) to scatter transmitted light and therefore cause plasma lactescence.

Apoproteins are polypeptides that are characterized by their amino acid composition and immunologic characteristics. At least 12 apoproteins have been recognized and are named according to the lipoprotein group on which they are found in greatest abundance. Thus apoproteins AI through III are found predominantly in HDL, apoprotein B-100 is predominantly found on LDL; apoprotein CI through CIII are found on chylomicrons and VLDL; and E2, E3, and E4 apoproteins are distributed on chylomicrons, VLDL, and IDL.

Apoproteins play an important role in lipoprotein metabolism and hyperlipoproteinemia. The apoproteins provide the means to emulsify and solubilize lipids, playing a crucial role in the structure of lipoproteins. Other crucial functions include (1) certain apoproteins serve as cofactors for enzymes involved in lipoprotein metabolism (e.g., apoprotein CII); and (2) apoproteins are specific ligands for high-affinity cellular receptors (apoproteins B-200 and E2 and E3).

Metabolism of Plasma Lipoproteins

There are two sources from which circulating plasma lipoproteins are formed: (1) exogenous dietary fat incorporated into lipoproteins formed in the intestines and (2) endogenously synthesized fats of hepatic origin. Thus, two general metabolic lipoprotein cascades that are interrelated are constantly at work (Fig. 176–7).

Exogenous Lipoprotein Transport. Triglyceride-rich chylomicrons are formed in the intestinal mucosa from ingested animal and vegetable fats—triglycerides and cholesterol. Apoproteins CI, CII, CIII, and E2 through E4 are transferred to the large triglyceride-rich chylomicrons from HDL in the circulation. An enzyme found in capillary endothelium, lipoprotein lipase (LPL), hydro-

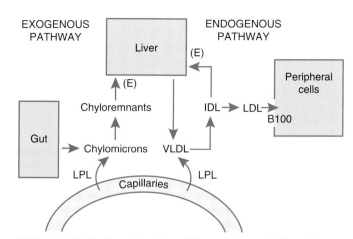

FIGURE 176–7. General outline of lipoprotein metabolism. Exogenous pathway: chylomicrons originate in the intestine and are converted to chyloremnants. Endogenous pathway: very-low-density lipoproteins (VLDL) are formed in the liver and are converted to intermediate-density lipoproteins (IDL) and low-density lipoproteins (LDL). Lipoprotein lipase (LPL) plays a crucial role in converting chylomicrons to remnants and VLDL to IDL. Apoproteins E (E) and B (B) are important in mediating the binding and catabolism of the lipoproteins to cell surface receptors, which include LDL, IDL, and remnants.

lyzes the triglycerides in the core of chylomicrons, converting them to cholesterol-rich chylomicron remnants that are rapidly removed by the liver E2 through E4 receptor binding of the E2 through E4 apoproteins on the chylomicron remnants. LPL is activated by apoprotein CII on the chylomicron surface.

Endogenous Lipoprotein Transport. VLDL are synthesized in the liver to transport triglycerides to peripheral tissues where their fatty acids are used as an energy source. These triglycerides incorporated into VLDL in the liver are continuously synthesized from plasma fatty acids and glycerol (obtained from the catabolism of carbohydrates). Indeed, ingestion of glucose, carbohydrates, and alcohol stimulates endogenous synthesis of VLDL since these substances are metabolized to glycerol in the liver. Cholersterol incorporated into the VLDL is synthesized in the liver from mevalonic acid. The rate-limiting step in cholesterogenesis, 3-hydroxy-3-methylglutaryl-coenzyme A (HMG-CoA) to mevalonic acid catalyzed by HMG-CoA reductase, controls the amount of endogenous cholesterol synthesis in the liver and peripheral cells. The enzymatic step is under negative feedback control so that the more cholesterol present (in the liver or peripheral cells), such as might be ingested in the diet, the less endogenous cholesterol synthesis.

Apoproteins B-100 is combined with triglycerides and cholesterol synthesized in the liver to form nascent VLDL. When VLDL is secreted into the circulation apoproteins CI through CIII, E2 through E4 and A are added to VLDL by transfer from circulating HDL. Like chylomicrons, VLDL triglycerides are hydrolyzed by LPL in capillary endothelium, the enzyme again depending on apoprotein CII as a cofactor activating the enzyme that hydrolyzes triglycerides in the VLDL to convert them to remnant lipoproteins or IDL (IDL contain less amounts of triglycerides and more cholesterol than VLDL). Thus, LPL, in the presence of CII apoprotein on the surface of chylomicrons and VLDL converts these two lipoproteins to "remnant" lipoproteins since their triglycerides are hydrolyzed from their cores. Lack of LPL activity results therefore in the accumulation of both chylomicrons and VLDL. LPL activity varies under a number of conditions. Insulin and thyroid hormones are required for appropriate activity, and estrogens and corticosteroids impair LPL hydrolytic reactions.

Some of the remnant or IDL, formed after the hydrolysis of triglycerides from the VLDL, are cleared from the plasma by the liver, and this catabolism of IDL depends on specific apoprotein E receptors in the liver. Most of the IDL escape hepatic uptake and remain in the circulation where more triglycerides and all apoproteins except B-100 are removed, leaving cholesterol-rich apoprotein B-100 containing LDL. LDL are metabolized after binding to specific cellular receptors in the liver and peripheral tissue that recognize apoprotein B-100 carried by the LDL. These LDL receptors serve as biochemical magnets attracting the LDL particles to attach to cell surfaces. Binding of LDL to cell receptors leads to cellular internalization and degradation of the LDL, which provides intracellular cholesterol for use within the cell. Internalization of cholesterol from the LDL also inhibits endogenous cellular cholesterol synthesis by repression of the activity of cellular HMG-CoA reductase (negative feedback control) and at the same time decreases the B-100 receptors synthesized by the cell.

The factors controlling the concentration of LDL in the circulation (and hence serum cholesterol because LDL carry significant quantities of cholesterol in the plasma) depend on three things: (1) synthesis of VLDL and their subsequent conversion to LDL (recall that cholesterogenesis in the liver partially controls the formation of VLDL); (2) catabolism of LDL by liver and peripheral cells, which depends on the binding of apoprotein B-100 on LDL by B-100 receptors; and (3) excretion of cholesterol from the body by oxidation to bile salts that are excreted into the gut, where they are used to solubilize and absorb dietary fats. Some of the bile acids are reabsorbed from the ileum and returned to the liver for reuse (the so-called enterohepatic pathway), but small amounts are lost in the feces. Thyroid hormones modulate the rate of cholesterol oxidation to bile salts so hyperthyroidism causes decreased serum cholesterol levels by accelerating the oxidation to bile salts and loss of salts in the stool, while hypothyroidism retards this process, resulting in hypercholesterolemia.

Reverse Cholesterol Transport System. HDL not only serve as a source of various apoproteins that they transfer to and from various lipoproteins, but they also function as a vehicle for transport of cholesterol from peripheral cells back to the liver. HDL bind to special receptors on peripheral cell membranes, whereby free cholesterol is released by peripheral cells to be taken up by HDL, which contains an enzyme, lecithin-cholesterol acyltransferase, and apoprotein AI, a cofactor for the enzyme. The enzyme and apoprotein AI add fatty acid to free cholesterol in the HDL, resulting in cholesterol esters, which are then transferred to LDL, chylomicron

remnants, and chylomicrons, which are eventually returned to the liver and out in the bile—a reverse cholesterol transport system from the cells in the body to excretion in the bile. This process appears to be antiatherogenic because it leads to elimination of excess cholesterol from the body.

Lipoproteins Atherogenicity and Propensity to Form Xanthomas

Certain lipoproteins are atherogenic, including LDL, VLDL, IDL, and possibly chylomicron remnants, while HDL appears to protect against atherogenesis.[6]

In general, chylomicrons and VLDL when found in high concentrations predispose to eruptive xanthomas; elevated levels of LDL are associated with tendinous and planar xanthomas (xanthelasma and intertriginous xanthomas); while IDL, when increased, can cause tuberous xanthomas and xanthoma striatim palmare.

Disorders of Lipoprotein Metabolism

Abnormal accumulation of lipoprotein in the plasma results from (1) excessive production, (2) defective removal or decreased catabolism, or (3) a combination of both mechanisms. Defective removal of lipoprotein has been shown to be due to several processes, including enzyme deficiencies, defective formation of certain apoproteins that serve as ligands for cellular receptors, and deficiencies in cellular receptors. Thus, changes in plasma lipids and lipoproteins are often secondary to apoprotein and receptor disturbances.

These metabolic aberrations in lipoprotein metabolism may be seen either as a primary manifestation of specific genetic disorders (primary hyperlipoproteinemia)[7] or as an associated phenomenon secondary to specific underlying disease (e.g., diabetes, hypothyroidism, pancreatitis)—so-called secondary hyperlipoproteinemia.

Differentiation between primary and secondary hyperlipoproteinemias may be difficult because of similar symptomatology, abnormal laboratory tests, and lipoprotein alterations, but this differentiation is the cornerstone of successful diagnosis and therapy.

Primary Hyperlipoproteinemias

Primary hyperlipoproteinemias can be divided into familial conditions, in which genetic predisposition is associated with the presence of the lipoprotein disorder in family members in readily recognized genetic inheritance patterns, and the sporadic, in which neither genetic nor secondary factors play a role.[7]

The familial hyperlipoproteinemias can be understood on the metabolic basis of these monogenic conditions, which can be divided into three general categories:

1. Triglyceride-rich lipoprotein removal defects. Lack of LPL normal activity results in defects of removal of chylomicrons and VLDL. The enzyme, LPL may be

recessively genetically deficient or there may be an autosomal recessive deficiency of apoprotein CII—the LPL activator. The lack of apoprotein CII on chylomicrons and VLDL results in the inability of LPL to recognize these lipoproteins so they are not cleared from the circulation even though LPL activity is normal. This is a striking example of the crucial importance that apoproteins play in lipoprotein metabolism where an apoprotein defect leads to widespread lipid alterations. When chylomicrons and VLDL accumulate in the circulation (whether due to lack of LPL or apoprotein CII), the *hyperlipemic syndrome* results. These large lipoproteins scatter light, causing lipemia or lactescent plasma along with lipemia retinalis, abdominal pain, hepatosplenomegaly, pancreatitis, and eruptive xanthomas.

2. *Excessive triglyceride-rich lipoprotein production.* Endogenous familial hypertriglyceridemia is a common monogenic dominantly inherited condition that results primarily from accelerated hepatic production of VLDL especially after ingestion of carbohydrates and alcohol. Many patients are obese (obesity increases VLDL production), and some display glucose intolerance and mild decreases in LPL activity (decreasing clearance of VLDL). The elevation of VLDL results in the hyperlipemic syndrome with eruptive xanthomas as well as xanthomas striatum palmaris. Cardiovascular disease is common.

3. *Familial dysbetalipoproteinemia* or *broad beta disease* is a condition defined by high concentrations of chylomicron remnants and IDL that lead to tuberous and eruptive xanthomas, accelerated coronary and peripheral atherosclerosis, and lipemic plasma.[6] The underlying genetic defect is the synthesis of an abnormal form of apoprotein E—a form that does not bind normally to apoprotein E chylomicron remnant or IDL apoprotein E receptors in the liver. This production of abnormal apoprotein E causes alterations in the stereo configuration of the apoprotein E ligands on the surface of IDL and chyloremnants so that apoprotein E receptors do not recognize these lipoproteins and they are not taken up by the liver in the normal manner and thus accumulate in the circulation. IDL and chyloremnants cause a single broad band extending from the prebeta to the beta lipoproteins on electrophoretic separation. Hence the name broad beta disease.

Familial hypercholesterolemia is the second monogenetic defect in lipoprotein catabolism in which plasma LDL accumulate because of the autosomally dominantly inherited deficiency in removal—in this case due to a lack of the formation of high-affinity apolipoprotein B-100 LDL receptors in the liver and peripheral tissue. Those heterozygotes for familial hypercholesterolemia have one normal and one abnormal gene for LDL receptors. Their cells produce only half the normal number of LDL apolipoprotein B-100 receptors, and as a result LDL is removed from the plasma at only two-thirds the normal rate. There is also overproduction of LDL because the lack of uptake of LDL cholesterol into the liver results in no negative feedback on cholesterol genesis and thus endogenous cholesterol synthesis accelerates (i.e., less external cholesterol gets into cells) so there is no

"braking effect" on cholesterogenesis. This results in hyperbetalipoproteinemia of twofold to threefold over normal from the time of birth, with symptoms developing in the third to sixth decades when tendinous and tuberous xanthomas, xanthelasmas, arcus senilis, and premature atherosclerotic cardiovascular disease develop. In rare subjects who are homozygous for the disease and inherit two mutant genes at the LDL locus, few or no functional LDL receptors are present so LDL is removed from the circulation at only one third of the normal rate. Overproduction of LDL is even greater, resulting in a sixfold to eightfold elevation in plasma LDL. In such patients, symptomatic coronary atherosclerosis develops before the age of 20, with plasma cholesterol values exceeding 800 mg/dL, and cutaneous and tendinous xanthomas evolve in the first few years of life. Occasionally, intertriginous xanthomas are seen evolving in the finger webs, axillae, buttocks, and antecubital and popliteal fossae.

The third dominant inherited condition that leads to a lipoprotein removal defect is a newly described genetic abnormality termed *familial defective apoprotein B-100* in which there is an amino acid substitution in the apoprotein B-100 impairing the ability of the LDL receptor to recognize and bind LDL. This results in lack of normal clearing of LDL and phenotypic changes similar to those patients with familial hypercholesterolemia.

Thus defects in the structure of apoprotein E or B-100 or the LDL receptor disrupts metabolic pathways in lipoprotein metabolism and leads to elevation of specific types of lipoproteins. These hyperlipoproteinemias also clearly make the point that basic defects in protein (apoprotein) and receptor formation lead to lipid abnormalities and widespread, often fatal consequences.

Secondary Hyperlipoproteinemias

Serum lipoprotein abnormalities occur in association with a number of underlying diseases that occasionally cause xanthomatosis. These diseases can induce symptoms, lipoprotein changes, and xanthomas that mimic the primary lipoproteinemias. For this reason, secondary diseases must be looked for in evaluating patients with xanthomatosis. The following outlines the lipoprotein abnormalities and etiologies of these changes in certain secondary conditions:

1. *Diabetes mellitus.* The lack of adequate LPL activity in the absence of insulin leads to the "hyperlipemia syndrome" with elevations in chylomicrons and VLDL. Eruptive xanthomas, lipemic sera, lipemia retinalis, and pancreatitis occur.

2. *Pancreatitis.* Hyperlipidemia due to increases in levels of VLDL and chylomicrons are associated with the "hyperlipemic syndrome" in pancreatitis in two ways. The lipemia can be primary, preceding and serving as the cause of pancreatitis (high chylomicron and VLDL levels cause hemorrhagic pancreatitis) or the lipemia can be secondary to an initial episode of pancreatitis (destruction of the pancreas can cause insulin deficiency with LPL insufficiency).

3. *Drugs causing or accentuating hyperlipoproteinemia.* Estrogens and corticosteroids decrease LPL activity

and occasionally cause elevations in chylomicrons and VLDL, with resulting hyperlipemic syndrome and eruptive xanthomas. 13-*cis*-Retinoic acid (Accutane) and etretinate cause increases in VLDL with occasional eruptive xanthomas and pancreatitis.

4. *Hypothyroidism.* Two mechanisms altering lipoprotein metabolism explain a wide range of lipoprotein patterns seen in hypothyroidism. First, myxedema is associated with increases in LDL and hypercholesterolemia owing to the crucial role thyroid hormones play in oxidizing hepatic cholesterol to bile salts (there is decreased conversion when thyroid hormones are low). Second, thyroid hormones are needed for LPL activity, and in myxedema LPL activity is decreased, impairing chylomicron and VLDL clearance. Thus one can see xanthelasma or eruptive xanthomas depending on the lipoproteins found in increased amounts.

5. *Cholestatic liver disease.* Hypercholesterolemia is seen in patients with obstructive liver disease in which an abnormal cholesterol-rich lipoprotein, "lipoprotein X," accumulates. Lipoprotein X, secreted by the liver in the presence of cholestasis, has an unusual structure consisting of apoprotein C and albumin. This lipoprotein has a β-lipoprotein mobility and it carries large amounts of free cholesterol and phospholipids. Congenital malformations of the biliary tract, failure of bile canaliculi to develop in the newborn, and biliary cirrhosis in adults are major causes of cholestatic syndromes that lead to extensive palmar xanthomas, tuberous xanthomas, and xanthelasmas. Pruritus and jaundice are also seen in these patients.

6. *Dysgammaglobulinemia and paraproteinemia.* Diseases with paraproteinemia such as multiple myeloma, Waldenström's macroglobulinemia, cryoglobulinemia, and, occasionally, lymphomas may be associated with elevations in chylomicrons, VLDL, and LDL levels. These lipoproteinemias are believed to be caused by binding of various lipoproteins by the abnormal circulating paraproteins, with resulting diminished clearance of lipoproteins. Extensive planar xanthomas are seen as golden yellow plaques over the head, neck, and trunk. In some patients, with xanthomatosis and dysgammaglobulinemia, no serum lipoprotein abnormalities are seen.

Normolipidemic Xanthomatosis

Xanthomas can arise in the absence of elevated blood lipids (or at least in the absence of hypercholesterolemia or hypertriglyceridemia) or lipoproteins. Indeed, xanthelasmas commonly occur without associated lipoprotein elevations. At least three general mechanisms can be identified in playing a role in the evolution of xanthomatous infiltrates.

1. Alterations in lipoprotein content or structure in which normal amounts of lipoproteins are found but there is an accumulation of unusual lipids within the lipoproteins that predispose to their accumulations in skin and other tissues. Examples are *cerebrotendinous xanthomatosis* in which cholestanol accumulates in lipoproteins and tissues due to an autosomal recessive defi-

ciency in oxidation of cholesterol to bile salts and *phytosterolemia* in which plant sterols are excessively absorbed from the gastrointestinal tract and accumulate in LDL, causing xanthelasmas, tendinous and cutaneous xanthomas, and atherosclerosis. There are also examples of patients with normal plasma cholesterol where alterations in apoprotein content lead to xanthomatosis and atherosclerosis.

2. Lymphoproliferative changes in the skin with secondary accumulation of lipids in macrophages. This may be the mechanism of the formation of widespread planar xanthomas in patients with paraproteinemias and normal lipoprotein levels.

3. Local tissue abnormalities such as inflammatory reactions in the skin increase vascular permeability to otherwise normal levels of lipoproteins in the circulation. This reaction, termed dystrophic xanthomatosis, can be seen in patients with atopic dermatitis, epidermolysis bullosa, and mycosis fungoides.

DIAGNOSIS AND DIFFERENTIAL DIAGNOSIS

Finding xanthomas mandates a careful history and physical examination, with attention directed to the familial incidence of xanthomas or premature atherosclerotic disease, as well as to lipemia retinalis, arcus senilis, hepatosplenomegaly, and abdominal pain. Biopsy may be necessary to rule out other conditions.

Quantitative measurement of fasting plasma cholesterol and triglyceride levels is the initial step in dealing with patients with xanthomas. If these levels are elevated, then lipoprotein measurements are performed.

If lipoprotein levels are elevated, every effort must be made to determine if the alterations are a primary genetic defect or due to a secondary underlying disease such as diabetes or thyroid disease (which are treated directly).

Patients with normocholesterolemic xanthomas may require special studies on apoprotein content and a search for unusual lipids (i.e., cholestanol, phytosterols).

Differential Diagnosis (Table 176–1)

Tendinous xanthomas are nearly pathognomonic clinically when multiple lesions are present. Giant cell tumor of tendon sheath or pigmented villonodular tenosynovitis also causes nodular expansion of tendons, but the lesions are usually solitary.

TABLE 176-1. Differential Diagnosis of Xanthomas
Tendinous xanthoma
Giant cell tumor of the tendon sheath
Planar xanthoma
Sebaceous hyperplasia
Syringoma
Milia

The different forms of planar xanthomas elicit somewhat different differential diagnoses. Xanthelasmas are pathognomonic when multiple small plaques are present on the eyelids, but early, small lesions can be confused with sebaceous hyperplasia, syringoma, or milia. Necrobiotic xanthogranuloma can produce yellow plaques on the eyelids, but the lesions are bulky and far fewer. Diffuse or generalized planar xanthomas do not have the flexural distribution seen in xanthoma disseminatum, which is unrelated to hyperlipidemia, but both can feature yellow plaques. Early lesions of xanthoma disseminatum are orange rather than yellow.

Tuberous xanthomas can be confused with nodular lesions of erythema elevatum diutinum and with rheumatoid nodules because all of these occur over the dorsal surfaces of joints. Tuberous xanthomas on the elbows can be accompanied by lesions on the buttocks, which do not occur in the other conditions. Tuberous xanthomas tend to be softer than rheumatoid nodules or nodules of erythema elevatum diutinum. The histopathology of these conditions is distinctive.

Eruptive xanthomas can be confused clinically and histologically with generalized granuloma annulare. Incipient lesions of eruptive xanthoma can be painful, and contiguous lesions sometimes fuse to form tuberoeruptive xanthomas, occurrences that do not happen in granuloma annulare. Although infiltrates of macrophages and mucin are common to both conditions histologically, foamy macrophages and interstitial lipid do not occur in granuloma annulare. Both juvenile xanthogranuloma and its adult counterpart can present with yellow papules. The so-called micronodular form usually occurs in children, in whom eruptive xanthomas are rare, while the macrondular form in adults features only a few lesions.

TREATMENT

The choice of treatment to resolve xanthomas (and, it is hoped, atheromatous infiltrates) depends on the underlying lipoprotein abnormality.[8] An understanding of where the metabolic processes that regulate normal plasma levels of each lipoprotein group go wrong provides a rational understanding of how therapy can normalize the hyperlipoproteinemia.

If a secondary condition is responsible for the hyperlipoproteinemia, the condition should be specifically treated (e.g., insulin for diabetes, thyroid replacement for hypothyroidism), but if no secondary disease is found, then two major approaches to therapy are available for treating primary hyperlipoproteinemias: (1) diet and (2) antihyperlipidemic drugs.

Diet

Dietary manipulation alone is often effective in lowering lipoproteins in most primary hyperlipoproteinemias except in familial hypercholesterolemia. There are four general ways by which alterations in the diet are helpful:

1. Decrease in total caloric intake to reduce weight. This decreases VLDL, IDL, and LDL synthesis so that improvement is seen in endogenous familial hypertriglyceridemia (VLDL), broad beta disease (IDL), and familial hypercholesterolemia (LDL).

2. Change in distribution of triglyceride and cholesterol intake. Restricting dietary triglyceride decreases production of chylomicrons, and this is useful in treating hyperchylomicronemic conditions (lack of LPL or apoprotein CII deficiency). Restricting cholesterol intake can decrease LDL by 10% to 15%.

3. Alter carbohydrate intake. Since carbohydrates, glucose, and alcohol stimulate the endogenous cascade of the lipoprotein metabolic cycle (VLDL, IDL, LDL), restriction of these dietary ingredients help in treating endogenous familial hypertriglyceridemia and broad beta disease.

4. Altering the type of triglycerides in the diet. Saturated fats (triglycerides) increase plasma cholesterol and LDL by decreasing the LDL receptors in the liver. Polyunsaturated fats, on the other hand, tend to lower LDL by interfering with cholesterol absorption in the gut and preventing bile salt reabsorption in the ileum. Omega-3 polyunsaturated fats also seem to have antithrombotic effects that are of benefit in preventing atherosclerotic thrombotic events. The intake of large quantities of fiber (oat bran, pectin, psyllium) also seem to decrease cholesterol and LDL.

Antilipid Pharmacologic Agents

When dietary restrictions, alterations, and weight reduction are ineffective a number of drugs may be added to the regimen. Details of drug therapy are not the purpose of this review, but three types of drugs affect lipoprotein metabolism:

1. Drugs altering cholesterol and bile salt absorption. These anion exchange resins, cholestyramine and colestipol, sequester cholesterol and bile salts in the intestine, enhancing their excretion in the feces and thereby decrease LDL. They are therefore useful in treating familial hypercholesterolemia and apoprotein B-100 deficiency.

2. Drugs altering lipoprotein synthesis and catabolism, including nicotinic acid, clofibrate, gemfibrozil, dextrothyroxine, probucol, and nicotinic acid. Clofibrate, gemfibrozil, and probucol decrease the synthesis of VLDL in the liver and secondarily the level of IDL and LDL (which are primarily derived from VLDL), and therefore these medications are useful in treating the hyperlipoproteinemic conditions in the endogenous cascade of lipoprotein metabolism. Dextrothyroxine lowers LDL by accelerating oxidation of liver cholesterol to bile acids with subsequent loss in the stool.

3. Drugs altering endogenous cholesterol synthesis such as lovastatin, which penetrates cells where it inhibits HMG-CoA reductase so that hepatic intracellular cho-

lesterol synthesis is blocked. Lovastatin also stimulates the production of LDL receptors in the liver and has thus proven to be extremely effective in patients with familial hypercholesterolemia who lack LDL receptors.

PROGNOSIS

Diet and drugs have had considerable success in clearing eruptive xanthomas. Tuberous xanthomas, found in broad beta disease, resolve with weight reduction, diet (restricted carbohydrates), and drug therapy. Tendinous and tuberous xanthomas and xanthelasma seen in familial hypercholesterolemia, although difficult to resolve, have been reported to regress with strict dietary restriction of cholesterol and a combination of drugs, especially lovastatin and cholestyramine.

References

1. Parker F, Odland GF. Ultrastructural and lipid biochemical comparisons of human eruptive tuberous and planar xanthomas. Isr J Med Sci 1973;9:395.
2. Parker F. Hyperlipoproteinemia and xanthomatosis. In: Callen JF, ed. Cutaneous Aspects of Internal Disease. Louisville, KY: Year Book Medical Publishers, 1980.
3. Parker F. Xanthomas and hyperlipidemias. J Am Acad Dermatol 1985;13:1.
4. Fleischmajer R. Cutaneous and tendon xanthomas. Dermatologica 1964;128:113.
5. Cooper PH. Eruptive xanthoma: A microscopic simulant of granuloma annulare. J Cutan Pathol 1986;13:207–215.
6. Scanu AM, Lann RM, Berg K. Lipoprotein (a) and atherosclerosis. Ann Intern Med 1991;115:209–218.
7. Mahley RW, Weisgreiber KH, Innerarity TL, Rail ST. Genetic defects in lipoprotein metabolism. JAMA 1991;265:78–83.
8. Blum CB, Levy RI. Current therapy for hypercholesterolemia. JAMA 1987;261:3582–3587.

chapter 177

Amyloidosis

KEN HASHIMOTO

Amyloid is a filamentous substance of uniform diameter (6 to 10 nm) with fibrils that are straight and neither branch nor anastomose (Fig. 177-1).[1] Varying amounts of amorphous materials are embedded on these filaments. Amyloid stains metachromatically with basic aniline dyes, such as crystal violet, and orthochromatically with dyes used to stain cotton, such as Congo red and Dylon. Pinkish red stains of Congo red or Dylon should exhibit greenish birefringence under polarized light. Thioflavin-T binds amyloid and exhibits fluorescence under an appropriate filter combination. These tinctorial characteristics of amyloid filaments are related to their β-pleated antiparallel sheet configuration. Chemically, amyloids are diverse; keratin, immunoglobulins, insulin, thyrocalcitonin, and other substances are known to be amyloidogenic and each amyloid produced from these building materials satisfies the criteria mentioned earlier.

There are many subtypes of amyloidoses (Table 177-1). However, only a dozen or so produce skin lesions. Amyloidoses are classified mainly according to their chemical origins. Other considerations include whether the condition is systemic or localized and isolated or familial and its etiologic factors and clinical appearance.

Systemic Amyloidosis

In this category of amyloidoses, skin involvement accompanies more serious systemic disease. Nevertheless, in amyloidosis derived from altered light chains (AL amyloidosis), for example, skin signs may precede the systemic symptoms.

SYSTEMIC AL AMYLOIDOSIS

Clinical Description

Systemic AL amyloidosis can be associated with multiple myeloma or other gammopathies. Those patients with myeloma are designated as having myeloma-associated amyloidosis, and those without gammopathy, who are more numerous, have primary systemic amyloidosis. Some cases seem to begin without an immunocyte dyscrasia, which develops later, or a dyscrasia is discovered after repeated examinations with more sensitive methods.

Cutaneous lesions may occur in 30% to 40% of cases.[2] Clinical findings[2-4] in AL amyloidosis are most often (1) macroglossia with or without hardening of oral mucous

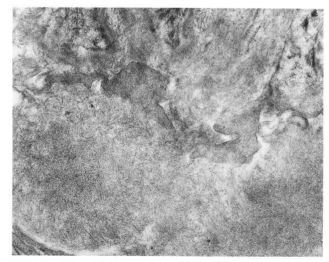

FIGURE 177-1. Lichen amyloidosus. Amyloid filaments are rigid, straight, nonbranching, and nonanastomosing. The filaments are randomly arranged (×4500).

**TABLE 177-1. Chemical Origin
of Various Amyloids**

Precursor	Type of Amyloid
Systemic Amyloidosis	
Immunoglobulin light chains	Monoclonal gammopathy- and myeloma-associated amyloidosis (AL)
Serum amyloid AA protein	Reactive systemic (secondary) amyloidosis (AA)
Prealbumin	Familial and senile forms of systemic amyloidosis
β_2-Microglobulin	Amyloidosis associated with long-term hemodialysis
Organ-Limited Amyloidoses	
Procalcitonin	Amyloid in medullary carcinoma of thyroid
Cystatin C	Icelandic familial cerebrovascular amyloidosis
β-Protein	In Alzheimer's disease, Down syndrome, senile dementia
Atrial natriuretic peptide	Isolated atrial amyloid
Islet amyloid polypeptide (IAPP)	In islets of Langerhans in type 2 diabetes
Insulin	Iatrogenic amyloid
Keratin proteins	Skin-limited amyloidoses

membrane, (2) periorbital waxy papules and plaques with ecchymosis, and (3) pinch hemorrhages (Fig. 177–2). Less commonly, amyloid deposition becomes more generalized and causes purpuric or ecchymotic lesions on folded areas such as the retroauricular and nasolabial folds, neck, umbilicus, and anogenital area. Waxy, shiny, and frequently semi-translucent papulonodules may also be found in flexural areas. Massive amyloid deposition can result in leonine facies, condyloma lata–like growths in the genital skin, and xanthomatous lesions in other sites. Postpurpuric hemosiderin pigmentation and jaundice due to hepatic involvement may occur. Perivascular deposition of amyloid may produce cord-like blood vessel thickening. Diffuse dermal infiltration can cause induration, and when the fragile amyloid in the lesion is split it may produce hemorrhagic bulla. Alopecia and nail dystrophy can occur. AL amyloidosis is primarily a systemic disease. Typically, elderly patients begin to complain of fatigue and weight loss. Carpal tunnel syndrome is common.

Pathology

The primary sites of amyloid deposition in the skin in systemic AL amyloidosis are around small vessels, sweat glands, and lipocytes (so-called amyloid rings). Thus, even a biopsy specimen of clinically normal skin can reveal amyloid. In more advanced lesions, amyloid is found diffusely in the dermis and subcutis. The papillary dermis can also be involved. Masses of amyloid are often fissured, forming small islands. Despite the fact that amyloid is foreign to the skin, inflammatory cells are absent or few. No plasma cells are present either within the lesion or at its periphery. Purpuric lesions show ex-

travasation of erythrocyte from venules whose walls are weakened by infiltration by amyloid.

Pathogenesis and Etiology

Whether or not the foci of plasma cell proliferation are found in the bone marrow, the amyloid substance is derived from monoclonal expansion of plasma cells. These cells produce either λ or κ light chain of immunoglobulin, which may be fragmented by lysosomal enzymes after repeated phagocytosis by macrophages to produce amyloid light-chain proteins.[5] The final AL amyloid is conjugated with neutral polysaccharides and therefore is often periodic acid–Schiff (PAS) positive and diastase resistant. This synthetic step may take place in the liver; skin deposition seems to be secondary to the production of AL protein at another site because there are insufficient plasma cells or macrophages in lesional skin. Amyloid filaments of all types have affinity to amyloid P component, a nonfibrillary glycoprotein. Normal elastic fiber microfibrils (elastofibril or fibrillin) have the

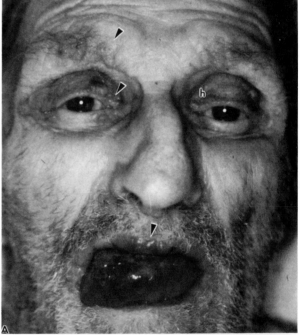

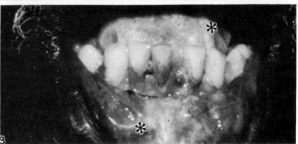

FIGURE 177-2. AL amyloidosis. *A,* Waxy papulonodular eruptions tend to form plaques on eyebrows, eyelids, and upper lip (*arrowheads*). An enlarged tongue (macroglossia) is hemorrhagic and so are the upper eyelids (h). In *B,* an enlarged and hardened tongue and lower lip show impressions of teeth (*asterisks*).

amyloid P component. Elastic fibers are often embedded in amyloid, probably because of this affinity. Blood vessels and eccrine glands, the sites of predilection for cutaneous amyloid deposition, are surrounded by elastic fibers.

Diagnosis and Differential Diagnosis

Diagnosis is possible if the patient exhibits macroglossia, periorbital ecchymotic papulonodules, and pinch hemorrhage. Tumefactive lesions should be differentiated from nodular amyloidosis and hyalinosis cutis et mucosae. However, nodular amyloidosis may be a variant of AL amyloid. Histologic and immunohistochemical differentiation between the amyloid deposited in the AL type and that deposited in the nodular type is impossible. Hyalinosis cutis et mucosae or lipoid proteinosis is usually inherited as an autosomal recessive trait, although it may occur as an isolated case. Beady nodules along palpebral borders and around the nostrils, if present, are helpful in the differential diagnosis. Colloid milium of the face features amber-colored, semitranslucent papulonodules that can form plaques, often with hemorrhage. Only biopsy and laboratory studies can separate this condition from AL amyloidosis (Table 177–2). Detection of Bence Jones protein in urine and monoclonal light chain in serum or urine with immunoelectrophoresis is essential for the differential diagnosis.

Treatment

There is no effective therapy for AL amyloidosis. Chemotherapy for multiple myeloma with melphalan-prednisone[6] or colchicine (1 to 2 mg per day),[7] which is effective for secondary amyloidosis due to familial Mediterranean fever, has been used with variable results. Amyloid is insoluble; and once deposited in the tissue, it is difficult to remove with ordinary tissue proteases. Temporary relief of gastrointestinal symptoms may be obtained with systemic antibodies, but no change is seen in the skin lesions.

SYSTEMIC AA AMYLOIDOSIS

Clinical Description

Systemic AA amyloidosis is also referred to as secondary systemic amyloidosis because there are preceding chronic inflammatory diseases such as rheumatoid arthritis and familial Mediterranean fever or chronic infectious diseases such as osteomyelitis, bronchiectasis, and lepromatous leprosy. Amyloids associated with familial Mediterranean fever and Muckle-Wells syndrome are of the AA type. Skin lesions are rare, but the subcutaneous fat of the lower abdomen or rectal mucosa contains AA amyloid.[8] Predilection sites of AA amyloid deposition are parenchymatous organs such as kidney (nephrosis, uremia), liver (speckle or wax liver), and spleen (sago or lardaceous spleen).

Pathology

As in AL amyloidosis, amyloid deposition in AA amyloidosis is seen surrounding blood vessels, lipocytes (amyloid rings), and eccrine glands. As more amyloid accumulates in the skin, it can be found diffusely in the dermis.

Pathogenesis

AA amyloid is not immunoglobulin but is instead derived from the amino-terminal portion of serum amyloid A (SAA)–related protein. SAA is an α-globulin and apparently present in normal sera in association with high-density lipoproteins, but its cleavage into AA amyloid may be stimulated in chronic inflammation or infections.[9]

TABLE 177–2. Differential Diagnosis of Amyloid, Colloid, and Hyalin

Type of Disorder	Amyloid Stains*	Congo Red After KMnO$_4$	Lipid	Keratin	Amyloid Ultrastructure†	Site of Skin Deposition
Amyloids						
Primary systemic	+++	+++	–	–	+++	Diffuse dermal perivascular
Secondary systemic	+++	–	–	–	+++	Subcutaneous fat
Skin-limited						
Lichenoid-macular	+++	+++	–	+++	+++	Papillary dermis
Poikiloderma-like	+++	+++	–	++		
Nodular	+++	+++	–	–	+++	Dermis
Familial	+++	+++	–	–	+++	Papillary dermis
Colloid milium	+	+	–	–	+++	Papillary dermis
Hyalinosis cutis et mucosae	±	±	±	–	–	Dermis
Hyalin in porphyrias	+	+	±	–	–	Vascular in papillary dermis

*Amyloid stains include alkaline Congo red, Dylon, crystal violet metachromasia, periodic acid–Schiff after diastase, and P-component.
†Six- to 10-nm straight, nonbranching filaments.
Modified from Hashimoto K. Cutaneous amyloidoses. In: Demis DJ, ed. Clinical Dermatology, 19th revision, vol. 2, unit 12–21. Philadelphia: JB Lippincott, 1992:1–13.

Diagnosis and Differential Diagnosis

Aspiration needle biopsy of the subcutaneous fat tissue of the lower abdomen is more sensitive than rectal biopsy.[10] AA amyloid in tissue sections becomes alkaline Congo red negative after it is treated with potassium permanganate.[11] This oxidation method is useful to differentiate AA amyloid from AL or keratin amyloids, which are alkaline Congo red positive after permanganate treatment.

Treatment

Correction of an underlying disease may not alleviate secondary AA amyloidosis, because once deposited in the tissue, amyloid is difficult to remove. However, colchicine is significantly effective for AA amyloidosis secondary to familial Mediterranean fever.[7]

FAMILIAL AMYLOIDOTIC POLYNEUROPATHY

Clinical Description

Familial amyloidotic polyneuropathy is a relatively new discovery in the long history of amyloidosis. In this autosomal dominant disease the site of primary amyloid deposition is in peripheral nerves. Clinical symptoms may simulate muscular dystrophy, multiple sclerosis, leprosy, or syringomyelia. Skin lesions consist of multiple atrophic scars and poorly healed ulcers of limbs, particularly at pressure points. Petechiae develop after gentle stroking of the skin.[12] There are Portuguese, Japanese, and Swedish groups of patients.[13-17] Japanese patients have long been isolated as lepers.[14, 15]

Pathology

In addition to the peripheral nerves, kidney, pancreas, and testes may be involved. Unlike other systemic amyloidoses, the liver and spleen are spared. In the skin, blood vessels, arrector pili muscles, and elastic fibers are infiltrated with amyloid.[13, 16] Dermal blood vessels and cutaneous nerves are not involved in the Swedish type.[17]

Pathogenesis

Prealbumin has been believed to produce this type of amyloid, which is designated as AFP.[18]

Diagnosis and Differential Diagnosis

Leprosy with neural involvement has a similar clinical appearance with trophic ulcers, atrophic scars, deformities of joints, and contractures of limbs. Amyloid and acid-fast stains of biopsy specimens and a lepromin skin test will facilitate the differential diagnosis.

MUCKLE-WELLS SYNDROME

Clinical Description

Widely spread geographical (urticarial) skin lesions, limb pain, fever, and nephropathy (predominantly amyloidal) occur in "aguey bouts."[19] As periodical attacks with these symptoms advance, progressive deafness begins. The trait is dominantly inherited with variable penetrance.

Pathology

There is elevated polyclonal serum α-globulin. Tissue-deposited amyloid is the permanganate-sensitive AA type.[4, 11, 20] Skin lesions have not carefully been examined in this rare disease.

FAMILIAL MEDITERRANEAN FEVER

Clinical Description

As sporadic attacks of fever are repeated, amyloidosis develops with clinical evidence of peritonitis, pleuritis, and synovitis. Skin lesions may develop in the form of erysipelas-like erythema of legs and feet and of Henoch-Schönlein purpura.[20, 21] Inheritance is autosomal recessive.

Pathology

Parenchymatous organs such as spleen (lardaceous spleen), kidneys, adrenals, and pulmonary alveolar septa are involved. Hepatic sinusoids are spared. The amyloid is the permanganate-sensitive AA type. Skin lesions have not been studied.

β_2-MICROGLOBULIN AMYLOID

In addition to carpal tunnel tissue, synovia, and bone, β_2-microglobulin amyloid may deposit in the skin as groups of small shiny lichenoid papules on the arms and trunk in a patient who has undergone long-term hemodialysis.[22]

Skin-Limited Keratin Amyloidoses

In this large group of amyloidoses, only skin involvement occurs and amyloid is largely derived from keratin. As degenerating keratinocytes drop off into the dermis, they are enveloped by basement membrane components that become a part of amyloid.[22-27]

IDIOPATHIC KERATIN AMYLOIDOSES

Clinical Description

Lichen amyloidosus, macular amyloidosis, and biphasic amyloidosis (a combination of both) are related and most often affect dark-skinned races such as Asians, Latinos, and those of Middle Eastern extraction. Typically, lichen amyloidosus affects the extensor surfaces of the extremities, such as the shins (Fig. 177–3A; see color plate) and outer arms. Lesions on the upper back are relatively common. The condition is more frequent in males, occurring most often between 50 and 60 years of age.[28] Small pruritic papules become larger and confluent as the patient constantly scratches because of intense pruritus. Well-developed lesions are hyperpigmented, lichenified, and hyperkeratotic. Papules and small nodules similar to prurigo nodularis are strewn over a grater-like rough skin surface. Excoriations and hemorrhagic crusts are common.

Macular amyloidosis is more common in women. Frequent sites are areas subject to friction such as the upper back, neck, shin (Fig. 177–4), thigh, and buttocks. In contrast to the lichenoid variety, pruritus is not usually noted. Typically, a middle-aged woman seeks medical attention when neck lesions creep up to the face and cannot be concealed with high-necked clothing. Macular lesions consist of hyperpigmentation with a characteristically rippled pattern (i.e., parallel waves of hyperpigmentation). Constant friction with nylon brush or towel may cause macular amyloidosis (i.e., friction or irritant amyloidosis).[29]

Biphasic amyloidosis[29] shows both lichenoid and macular amyloidoses in the same location (Fig. 177–3B) or at separate sites. Lichenoid lesions are pruritic. The peak incidence of the biphasic type is between 50 and 60 years of age.

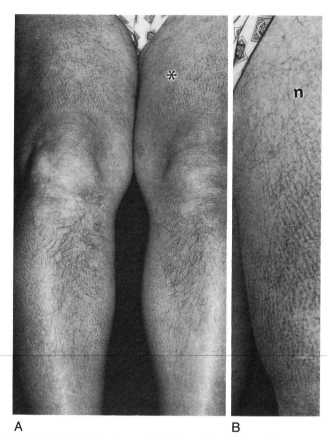

A   B

FIGURE 177–4. Macular amyloidosis. *A*, Shins and anterior thighs of this woman show rippled pattern of hyperpigmentation. Area designated by *asterisk* is shown enlarged in *B*.

Pathology

The epidermis is acanthotic and hyperkeratotic in lichenoid lesions. There may be eosinophilic cytoid bodies in the epidermis, which are rich in disulfide bonds and are Congo red positive (Fig. 177–5).[31] Amyloid in Congo red–stained sections turns greenish when viewed under polarized light. Thus, amyloid or a precursor is already present in the epidermis, albeit in scant quantities. Amyloid deposition principally expands dermal papillae and presses rete ridges into thin septa (Fig. 177–6; see color plate). Amyloid globules can be scattered in the upper reticular dermis, but perivascular deposition as seen in systemic amyloidoses is not prominent. In macular amyloidosis, the lesional epidermis is often atrophic and the amount of amyloid deposition may be very small; repeated alkaline Congo red stain is often required to demonstrate it. In routinely processed tissue, Congo red or Dylon stains may be weak and crystal violet or toluidine blue stain can be negative. Considering that all of the special stains for amyloid are nonspecific, electron microscopic demonstration of amyloid filaments should re-

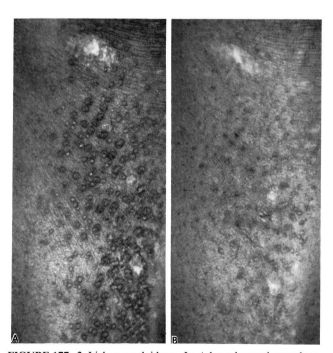

FIGURE 177–3. Lichen amyloidosus. In *A*, hyperkeratotic papulonodules become confluent in lower part of this picture. In *B*, after the treatment with mercaptoethanol-urea solution,[36] most papules have subsided but hyperpigmentation remains; this is the picture of biphasic amyloidosis. (See color plate.)

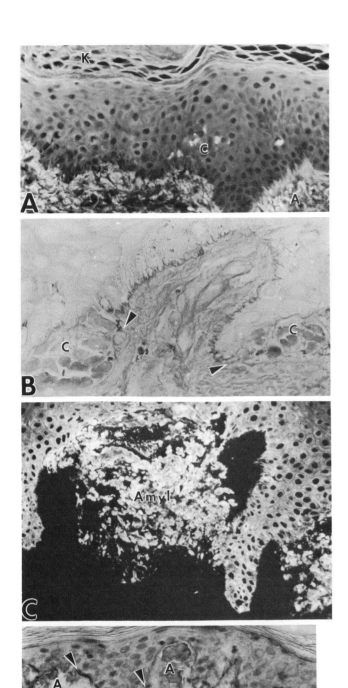

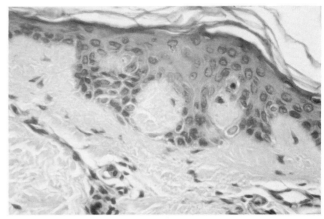

FIGURE 177–6. Lichen amyloidosus. Pink globular materials accumulated in dilated papillary dermis. An apoptotic basal cell with a pyknotic nucleus is seen in acanthotic epidermis (hematoxylin-eosin, ×130). (See color plate.)

FIGURE 177–5. *A*, DACM stain for disulfide bonds in lichen amyloidosus lesion. Several cytoid bodies (c) in the lower epidermis, hyperkeratotic basket-weave keratin (K), and amyloid (A) in the upper dermis are fluorescent (i.e., disulfide positive). *B*, PAS stain with diastase predigestion demonstrates cytoid bodies (c) in a cluster at the dermoepidermal junction, where the basement membrane (*arrowheads*) is disrupted. *C*, Antikeratin antibody–labeled amyloid (Amyl) as well as epidermal keratin. *D*, Laminin immunoperoxidase stain. Basement membrane is disrupted (*arrowheads*) where amyloid (A) is deposited, presumably because degenerated keratinocytes dropping down from the epidermis have caused the breakage. (*A, C,* and *D,* ×200; *B,* ×320.)

main as the gold standard in amyloid diagnosis in general. If an immunostain for keratin (see Fig. 177–5*C*) is also negative, electron microscopy can be performed for definitive analysis; however, for practical purposes the demonstration of eosinophilic globules and melanophages in the papillary dermis of a patient with a characteristic clinical picture generally suffices.

Pathogenesis and Etiology

Trauma, insect bites, mild chronic infection, and other injurious factors may be involved in the initial damage to the epidermal keratinocytes. The predilection sites for lichen amyloidosus (e.g., the shins) are such trauma-prone locations. However, pruritic conditions such as atopic dermatitis and prurigo nodularis do not lead to keratin-derived amyloidosis. Racial and hereditary background is therefore important.

Cytoid bodies as are seen in the lesional epidermis of idiopathic keratin amyloidoses are present in the epidermis and papillary dermis of lichen planus and discoid lupus erythematosus. However, they do not become amyloid, perhaps because they are degraded or removed[22] by an intense T-cell infiltrate.

No matter what the cause of keratinocyte damage might be, the first step in keratinocyte-derived amyloidosis appears to be apoptosis (i.e., nuclear pyknosis and fragmentation followed by cytoplasmic disruption). Tonofilaments become thicker and bundled into a wavy mass that occupies the whole cytoplasm; this is called filamentous degeneration[23] and can be seen on light microscopy as cytoid bodies or hyaline bodies. Amyloid keratin contains proteins with disulfide bonds[31] that are rich in upper epidermal keratinocytes. However, the most commonly found keratin species in lichenoid, macular, and biphasic amyloidoses are basal layer keratins—numbers 5 (58 kd), 10 (56.5 kd), and 14 (50 kd); it is presumed that in these conditions the major source of amyloid is the lower epidermal keratinocytes. During filamentous degeneration and after dropping into the dermis there must be certain modifications, and sulfhy-dryl linkages, rich in lower epidermal keratinocytes, may be reduced to disulfide bonds. Components of the dermoepidermal junction such as hemidesmosomes, lamina densa (laminin, type IV collagen) (see Fig. 177–5B and D), PAS-positive diastase-resistant neutral mucopolysaccharides, and anchoring fibrils (type VII collagen) can be demonstrated on electron microscopy (see Fig. 177–1)[32] as well as immunohistochemically.[26, 27]

All types of amyloid have affinity to amyloid P-component,[33] and keratin amyloid is no exception. Elastic fiber microfibrils have amyloid P-component. Thus, the oxytalan and elaunin fibers of the papillary dermis, the elastic fibers of arrector muscles, and the periappendageal elastic fibers may be the sites of deposition of keratin-derived amyloid.[34] In fact, the initial deposition of amyloid in the papillary dermis may be due not only to its proximity to the epidermis but also to its network of fine elastic fibers. In established lesions, keratin epitopes can be demonstrated even in the reticular dermis. Raw keratins, such as derived from ruptured epidermal cysts, elicit a vigorous foreign-body reaction in the dermis. In contrast, amyloid keratins stay there quietly.

Diagnosis and Differential Diagnosis

Atopic dermatitis with prurigo nodularis should be differentiated from lichen amyloidosus. For macular amyloidosis, the differential diagnosis is often poikilodermas of various etiologies (Civatte type, mycosis fungoides, dermatomyosis, scleroderma), postinflammatory hyperpigmentation, erythema dyschromicum perstans, dyskeratosis congenita, and, if on the face, melasma (Table 177–3).

Today, most pathology laboratories perform immunostains. It is more specific and easier to use antikeratin antibodies than to use conventional amyloid stains. There are many polyclonal antikeratin antibodies such as Dako's whole keratin antibodies that react with keratins 5, 10, and 14 and are tolerant of formalin fixation. The staining of the epidermis serves as an internal control

---

TABLE 177–3. Differential Diagnosis of Primary Cutaneous Amyloidosis

Macular Amyloidosis

Atopic dermatitis
Poikiloderma of Civatte
Poikilodermatomyositis
Postinflammatory hyperpigmentation
Dyskeratosis congenita
Melasma

Lichen Amyloidosus

Prurigo nodularis
Pretibial myxedema
Lichen nitidus
Lichen simplex chronicus
Hypertrophic lichen planus

TABLE 177–4. Treatment of Primary Cutaneous Amyloidosis

Etretinate
Topical dimethyl sulfoxide
Topical retinoic acid (0.05%)
Topical mercaptoethanol-urea solution
High-potency topical or intralesional corticosteroids

(see Fig. 177–5C). There is no other disease that gives diffuse keratin staining of the upper dermis, and therefore this method is diagnostic.

Treatment

Etretinate therapy for 10 to 20 weeks has been shown to be effective in some cases of lichen amyloidosus.[35, 36] Topical dimethyl sulfoxide (50%), retinoic acid (0.05%), fluorinated corticosteroids, and mercaptoethanol-urea solution[37] (Fig. 177–3B) give some relief (Table 177–4). Dermabrasion removes the source of amyloid keratin and is reportedly very effective with long-term remission.[38]

ACTINIC AMYLOIDOSIS

Both ultraviolet A and B light cause keratinocyte degeneration. Chronic exposure to actinic rays produces a large number of damaged keratinocytes in which filamentous degeneration of tonofilaments occurs (Fig. 177–7).[23] These keratinocytes are observed as cytoid bodies on light microscopy and eventually drop into the dermis to form keratin amyloid. The most common example is the keratin amyloid found in actinic keratosis.[26, 39] The colloid substance in juvenile colloid milium is actually keratin amyloid[41] in spite of its clinical resemblance to colloid milium of the adult face. Concha amyloidosis[41] is limited to the auricular concha or helix of the ear, where actinic radiation often causes lesions of discoid lupus erythematosus. Clinically, there are cobblestone-like, aggregated, waxy or pearly papules and nodules that may form a plaque. Mild pruritus may be present. Chronic psoralens and ultraviolet A light therapy frequently produces keratin amyloid in the upper dermis.[42] No clinical symptoms are elicited.

OTHER KERATIN AMYLOIDOSES

Familial primary cutaneous amyloidosis is seen with or without Sipple's syndrome (medullary thyroid carcinoma) with manifestations of macular and lichenoid amyloidoses.[45, 46]

Anosacral amyloidosis occurs in the perianal and sacral region of the older individual with radiating streaks of hyperkeratotic skin.[47]

Vitiliginous amyloidosis consists of small or large, continuous or mottled deposition (amyloidosis cutis

Amyloidogenesis By Filamentous Degeneration

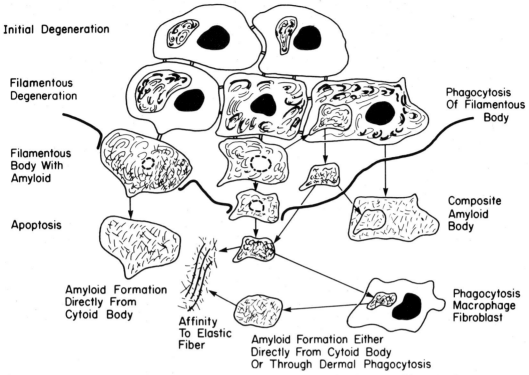

FIGURE 177-7. Schematic presentation of filamentous degeneration. (From Hashimoto K. Cutaneous amyloidoses. In: Demis DJ, ed. Clinical Dermatology, 19th revision, vol. 2, unit 12-21. Philadelphia: JB Lippincott, 1992:1-13.)

dyschromica).[48] In South America this type composes 10% of skin-limited amyloidoses.[49]

EPITHELIOMA KERATIN AMYLOIDOSIS

Epithelial tumors derived from the epidermis contain keratin species (numbers 5, 10, 14, and 15), which become amyloid in lichenoid, macular, and biphasic amyloidoses. Basal cell carcinoma, Bowen's disease, and seborrheic keratosis are commonly laden with stromal and sometimes parenchymal amyloid.[18, 26] Neoplastic cells undergo apoptosis and accumulate in the stroma, where they become keratin amyloid.

Clinically, there are no special signs or symptoms to distinguish those amyloid-positive epithelial tumors from ordinary ones in which no amyloid is deposited.

Histologically, unusually eosinophilic globules in the stroma raise suspicion of amyloid formation. Amyloid of epithelial tumors shares all ultrastructural and immunohistochemical characteristics of idiopathic keratin amyloid.

INSULIN AMYLOIDOSIS

Amyloid filaments can be produced from insulin, for example, in pancreatic islet amyloid polypeptide (IAPP) of non–insulin-dependent (type 2) diabetes mellitus and amyloid in insulinoma.[50, 51] Repeated injection of porcine insulin on the same site can produce insulin amyloid in the skin.[52]

NODULAR AMYLOIDOSIS

Clinical Description

Nodular or tumefactive amyloidosis was described by Gottron in 1950 under the name of amyloidosis cutis nodularis atrophicans diabetica.[53] Single or multiple lesions can occur anywhere, but the face, scalp, and leg are common sites (Fig. 177-8). Middle-aged women are most often affected with this relatively rare amyloidosis.[28] Individual lesions are waxy, yellowish tumor-like nodules or atrophic plaques. Some nodules are semitransparent and appear like bulla, while others are covered with telangiectases or hemorrhagic skin (see Fig. 177-8). Nodular amyloidosis may be associated with Sjögren's syndrome.[54, 55] Such cases can have SSA/Ro or SSA/La antibodies and may exhibit photosensitivity, including subacute cutaneous lupus erythematosus, which shares SSA/Ro or SSB/La antibodies with Sjögren's syndrome.[56]

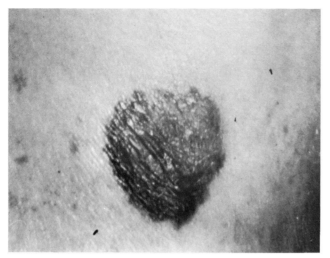

FIGURE 177-8. Nodular amyloidosis. A lesion on the lower leg shows an atrophic surface with hemorrhage.

Pathology

There is massive infiltration of the entire dermis and often the subcutis by amyloid. Perivascular and periappendageal deposition may be particularly heavy (Fig. 177-9). Immunoglobulin κ or λ light chains or both are demonstrable in this amyloid.[57, 58] Epitopes of keratins, type IV collagen, and laminin are absent,[26] suggesting that this amyloid is of immunoglobulin origin. Some lesions contain plasma cells,[59] which produce immunoglobulin locally.

Pathogenesis

Immunoglobulin light chains are demonstrated in all cutaneous amyloidoses. These are not essential compo-

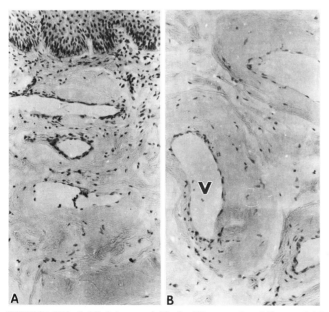

FIGURE 177-9. Nodular amyloidosis. Glassy eosinophilic amyloid occupies the entire dermis, particularly perivascular areas (V) (*A*, ×75; *B*, ×150).

nents in keratin amyloidoses, and elution with various buffers can remove them.[60] Tight meshworks of amyloid filaments, regardless of their chemical origins, trap immunoglobulins. However, in some cases of nodular amyloidosis λ chain cannot be eluted while other immunoglobulin chains (κ, α, γ, μ) can be removed.[57] The purified amyloid fibril protein was identified as having a λ light component.[58] It is not known if all cases of nodular amyloidosis eventually become systemic AL amyloidosis with multiple myeloma, and nodular amyloidosis may simply be a forme fruste of AL amyloidosis. Sjögren's syndrome is not associated with systemic AL amyloidosis.

Diagnosis and Differential Diagnosis

The clinical differential diagnosis includes cutaneous lymphoma, pseudolymphoma, sarcoidosis, Sweet's syndrome, colloid milium, and hyalinosis cutis et mucosae. Nodular lesions of AL amyloidosis are usually a part of more generalized cutaneous manifestations.

Treatments

Small numbers of nodular amyloidosis lesions are best treated by surgical removal. Intralesional corticosteroid injections, if repeated, reduce the size of the nodule.

References

1. Glenner GG. Amyloid deposits and amyloidosis. The β-fibrilloses. N Engl J Med 1980;302:1283-1293.
2. Rubinow A, Cohen AS. Skin involvement in generalized amyloidosis: A study of clinically involved and uninvolved skin in 50 patients with primary and secondary amyloidosis. Ann Intern Med 1978;88:781-785.
3. Brownstein MH, Helwig EB. The cutaneous amyloidoses: II. Systemic forms. Arch Dermatol 1970;102:20-28.
4. Breathnach SM. Amyloid and amyloidosis. J Am Acad Dermatol 1988;18:1-16.
5. Glenner GG, Ein D, Eanes ED, et al. Creation of "amyloid" fibrils from Bence Jones proteins in vitro. Science 1971;174:712-714.
6. Kyle RA, Greipp PR. Primary systemic amyloidosis: Comparison of melphalan and prednisone versus placebo. Blood 1978; 52:818-827.
7. Zemer D, Pras M, Sohar E, et al. Colchicine in the prevention and treatment of the amyloidosis of familial Mediterranean fever. N Engl J Med 1986;314:1001-1005.
8. Wright JR, Calkins E, Ozdemir AL. Clinical implications of differentiating the common forms of generalized amyloidosis: A reexamination of an old idea. In: Glenner GG, Costa PP, Freitas F, eds. Amyloid and Amyloidosis. Amsterdam: Excerpta Medica, 1980:17-24.
9. Benditt EP, Eriksen N. Amyloid protein SAA is associated with high density lipoprotein from normal serum. Proc Natl Acad Sci USA 1977;74:4025-4028.
10. Orfila C, Giraud P, Modesto A, et al. Abdominal fat tissue aspirate in human amyloidosis: Light, electron, and immunofluorescence studies. Hum Pathol 1986;17:366-369.
11. Wright JR, Calkins E, Humphrey RL. Potassium permanganate reaction in amyloidosis. Lab Invest 1977;36:274-281.
12. Rubinow A, Cohen AS. Skin involvement in familial amyloidotic polyneuropathy. Neurology 1981;31:1341-1345.
13. Andrade C. A peculiar form of peripheral neuropathy: Familiar atypical generalized amyloidosis with special involvement of the peripheral nerves. Brain 1952;75:408-427.

14. Araki S, Kurihara T, Tawara S, et al: Familial amyloidotic polyneuropathy in Japanese: Clinical, pathophysiological, biochemical, and therapeutic studies. In: Glenner GG, Costa PP, Freitas F, eds. Amyloid and Amyloidosis. Amsterdam: Excerpta Medica, 1980; 65–77.

15. Kito S, Itoga E, Ito Y, et al. Clinical and biochemical studies of the Ogawa village type hereditary amyloidosis with DMSO therapy. In: Glenner GG, Costa PP, Freitas F, eds. Amyloid and Amyloidosis. Amsterdam: Excerpta Medica, 1980;153–165.

16. Shiraham T, Cohen AS, Ribinow A, et al. Ultrastructure of skin biopsies from patients with heredofamilial amyloid polyneuropathy. In: Glenner GG, Costa P, Freitas F, eds. Amyloid and Amyloidosis. Amsterdam: Excerpta Medica, 1980;132–138.

17. Cohen AS, Rubinow A, Ginter D, et al. Preliminary report on a recently discovered family of Swedish origin with heredofamilial amyloid polyneuropathy. In: Glenner GG, Costa P, Freitas F, eds. Amyloid and Amyloidosis. Amsterdam: Excerpta Medica, 1980; 78–85.

18. Glenner GG. A retrospective and prospective overview of the investigations on amyloid and amyloidosis: The β-fibrilloses. In: Glenner GG, Costa PP, Freitas F, eds. Amyloid and Amyloidosis. Amsterdam: Excerpta Medica, 1980;3–13.

19. Muckle TJ. The Muckle-Wells syndrome. Br J Dermatol 1979;100:87–92.

20. Sohar E, Gafni J, Pras M, et al. Familial Mediterranean fever: A survey of 470 cases and a review of the literature. Am J Med 1967;43:227–253.

21. Sato KC, Kumakiri M, Koizumi H, et al. Lichenoid skin lesions as a sign of β_2-microglobulin-induced amyloidosis in a long-term haemodialysis patient. Br J Dermatol 1993;128:686–689.

22. Hashimoto K. Editorial: Progress on cutaneous amyloidoses. J Invest Dermatol 1984;82:1–3.

23. Kumakiri M, Hashimoto K. Histogenesis of primary localized cutaneous amyloidosis: Sequential change of epidermal keratinocytes to amyloid via filamentous degeneration. J Invest Dermatol 1979;73:150–162.

24. Kobayashi H, Hashimoto K. Amyloidogenesis in organ-limited cutaneous amyloidosis: An antigenic identity between epidermal keratin and skin amyloid. J Invest Dermatol 1983;80:66–72.

25. Eto H, Hashimoto K, Fukaya T, et al. Differential staining of cytoid bodies and skin-limited amyloids with monoclonal anti-keratin antibodies. Am J Pathol 1984;116:473–481.

26. Hashimoto K, Ito K, Taniguchi Y, et al. Keratin in cutaneous amyloidoses. In: Parrish LC, Crissey JT, eds. Clinics in Dermatology, Cutaneous Amyloidoses, vol. 8, No. 2. New York: Elsevier 1990:55–65.

27. Horiguchi Y, Fine J-D, Leigh IM. Lamina densa malformation involved in histogenesis of primary localized cutaneous amyloidosis. J Invest Dermatol 1992;99:12–18.

28. Wang W-J. Clinical features of cutaneous amyloidoses. In: Wong C-K, Breathnach SM, guest eds. Clinics in Dermatology, Cutaneous Amyloidosis, vol. 8, No. 2. New York: Elsevier 1990:13–19.

29. Hashimoto K, Ito M, Kumakiri M, et al. Nylon brush amyloidosis. Arch Dermatol 1987;123:633–637.

30. Brownstein MH, Hashimoto K, Greenwald G. Biphasic amyloidosis link between macular and lichenoid forms. Br J Dermatol 1973;88:25–29.

31. Mukai H, Kanzaki T, Nishiyama S. Sulfhydryl and disulfide stainings in amyloids of skin-limited and systemic amyloidosis. J Invest Dermatol 1984;82:4–8.

32. Kumakiri M, Hashimoto K, Tsukinaga I, et al. Presence of basal lamina-like substance with anchoring fibrils within the amyloid deposits of primary localized cutaneous amyloidosis. J Invest Dermatol 1983;81:153–157.

33. Pepys MB, Baltz ML, de Beer FC, et al. Biology of serum amyloid P component. Ann NY Acad Sci 1982;389:286–298.

34. Breathnach SM. The cutaneous amyloidoses: Pathogenesis and therapy. Arch Dermatol 1985;121:470–475.

35. Helander I, Hopsu-Havu VK. Treatment of lichen amyloidosus by etretinate. Clin Exp Dermatol 1986;11:574–577.

36. Aram H. Failure of etretinate (Ro 10-9359) in lichen amyloidosus. Int J Dermatol 1986;25:206.

37. Hashimoto K. Cutaneous Amyloidoses. In: Demis DJ, ed. Clinical Dermatology, 19th revision, vol. 2, unit 12–21. Philadelphia: JB Lippincott, 1992:1–13.

38. Wong C-K, Phil D, Li W-M. Dermabrasion for lichen amyloidosus. Arch Dermatol 1982;118:302–304.

39. Hashimoto K, King LE Jr. Secondary localized cutaneous amyloidosis associated with actinic keratosis. J Invest Dermatol 1973; 61:293–299.

40. Hashimoto K, Nakayama H, Chimenti S, et al. Juvenile colloid milium: Immunohistochemical and ultrastructural studies. J Cutan Pathol 1989;16:164–174.

41. Hicks BC, Weber PJ, Hashimoto K, et al. Primary cutaneous amyloidosis of the autricular concha. J Am Acad Dermatol 1988;18:19–25.

42. Hashimoto K, Kumakiri M. Colloid-amyloid bodies in PUVA-treated human psoriatic patients. J Invest Dermatol 1979; 72:70–80.

43. Nagao S, Iijima S. Light and electron microscopic study of Riehl's melanosis: Possible mode of its pigmentary incontinence. J Cutan Pathol 1974;1:165–175.

44. Masu S, Sato A, Seiji M. Electron microscopic studies on Civatte body in Riehl's melanosis. Tohoku J Exp Med 1980;131:177–196.

45. Kousseff BG, Espinoza C, Zamore GA. Sipple syndrome with lichen amyloidosis as a paracrinopathy: Pleiotropy, heterogeneity, or a contiguous gene? J Am Acad Dermatol 1991;25:651–657.

46. Vasily DB, Bhatia SG, Uhlin SR. Familial primary cutaneous amyloidosis: Clinical, genetic and immunofluorescent studies. Arch Dermatol 1978;114:1173–1176.

47. Yanagihara M. Ano-sacral cutaneous amyloidosis. Jpn J Dermatol 1981;91:463–471.

48. Morishima T. A clinical variety of primary localized cutaneous amyloidosis characterized by dyschromia (amyloidosis cutis dyschromica). J Dermatol 1970;80:43–52.

49. Ollague W, Ollague J, Ferretti H. Epidemiology of primary cutaneous amyloidoses in South America. In: Clinics in Dermatology, Cutaneous Amyloidoses, vol. 8, No. 2. New York: Elsevier 1990; 25–35.

50. Glenner GG, Eanes ED, Bladen HA. β-pleated sheet fibrils: A comparison of native amyloid with synthetic protein fibrils. J Histochem Cytochem 1974;22:1141–1158.

51. Westermark P, Wernstedt C, Wilander E, et al. Amyloid fibrils in human insulinoma and islets of Langerhans of the diabetic cat are derived from a neuropeptide-like protein also present in normal islet cells. Proc Natl Acad Sci USA 1987;84:3881–3885.

52. Dische FE, Wernstedt C, Westermark GT, et al. Insulin as an amyloid-fibril protein at sites of repeated insulin injections in a diabetic patient. Diabetologia 1988;31:158–161.

53. Gottron HA. Amyloidosis cutis nodularis atrophicans diabetica. Dtsch Med Wochenschr 1950;75:19–24.

54. Haneda S, Hamamatsu T. Cutaneous amyloidosis associated with Sjögren's syndrome. Hifu Rinsho 1979;21:81.

55. Yamazaki S, Iwakura N, Furuya T. A case of nodular amyloidosis associated with Sjögren's syndrome. Hifu Rinsho 1979;21:87.

56. Lee LA. Neonatal lupus erythematosus. J Invest Dermatol 1993;100:9S–13S.

57. Ito K, Hashimoto K, Kambe N, et al. Roles of immunoglobulins in amyloidogenesis in cutaneous nodular amyloidosis. J Invest Dermatol 1987;89:415–418.

58. Kitajima Y, Hirata H, Kagawa Y, et al. Partial amino acid sequence of an amyloid fibril protein from nodular primary cutaneous amyloidosis showing homology to λ immunoglobulin light chain of variable subgroup III (A λ III). J Invest Dermatol 1990;95:301–303.

59. Masuda C, Mohri S, Nakahima H. Histopathological and immunohistochemical study of amyloidosis cutis nodularis: Comparison with systemic amyloidosis. Br J Dermatol 1988;119–33–43.

60. MacDonald DM, Black MM, Ramnarain N. Immunofluoresence studies in primary localized cutaneous amyloidosis. Br J Dermatol 1977;96:635–641.

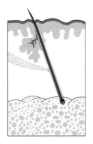

chapter 178

Cutaneous Ossification and Calcification

KALMAN L. WATSKY

DEFINITION

New bone formation or calcium deposition in the skin may be present in a variety of clinical settings, both inherited and acquired (Table 178–1).[1,2] Osteoma cutis, formation of new bone in the skin, may be primary or secondary. Primary cutaneous ossification frequently occurs in Albright's hereditary osteodystrophy and as idiopathic osteoma cutis. In secondary cases of cutaneous ossification, bone formation occurs within a preexisting lesion, usually a tumor. Calcinosis cutis is the deposition of calcium in the skin and subcutaneous tissues. Four principal forms of calcinosis cutis are recognized: metastatic calcinosis, dystrophic calcinosis, idiopathic calcinosis, and subepidermal calcified nodule.[2]

CLINICAL PRESENTATION

Cutaneous Ossification

Primary osteoma cutis occurs in the absence of any preexisting cutaneous lesion. There are both generalized and localized forms. The latter may present as (1) a single large plaque noted at birth, or during the first 2 years of life; (2) an isolated nodule in an older child or adult; or (3) multiple papules on the face (primarily seen in women).[1-4] Levels of calcium and phosphorus in the serum of patients in all of these groups are normal.[1] Multiple facial osteomas typically occur in young women with a long history of acne vulgaris; however, the occurrence of these lesions in patients with no history of acne, or in anatomic sites where acne does not usually occur, suggests that acne vulgaris does not always play an etiologic role in this condition.[5] The tetracycline double-labeling technique has been used to evaluate a patient with

multiple miliary osteomas and showed a high rate of remodeling and mineralization.

In generalized osteoma cutis, multiple stone-hard lesions of varying sizes are present in widespread locations. Although rarely idiopathic,[7] the underlying cause is most typically Albright's hereditary osteodystrophy.[8] Osteoma cutis may be present at birth, or arise later in life, and may affect any site. Patients with Albright's hereditary osteodystrophy and osteoma cutis may develop hypocalcemia secondary to pseudohypoparathyroidism, although they may be normocalcemic at presentation.[9] Albright's hereditary osteodystrophy is also characterized by pseudohypoparathyroidism (in which patients have normal serum calcium values), as well as short stature, characteristic facies (rounded with a flattened nose), and numerous skeletal abnormalities, the most significant being shortening of some of the metacarpal bones. Bone formation in Albright's hereditary osteodystrophy may also be seen in subcutaneous tissue, along fascial planes, and in periarticular regions.[8]

Secondary or metaplastic osteoma cutis is a more common condition. An analysis of 425 cases of osteoma cutis by workers at the Armed Forces Institute of Pathology showed that 86% of cases were secondary and the remainder primary.[4] Cutaneous neoplasms are the most important group of disorders demonstrating secondary ossification, especially pilomatricomas, in which bone formation is seen in 14% to 20% of cases.[2] Occasionally ossification can occur in other tumors—for example, chondroid syringoma, basal cell carcinoma, pilar cysts, and nevi.[3, 4] Rarely, metaplastic ossification may be seen in scars or in inflammatory processes of the skin such as morphea, scleroderma, dermatomyositis, and myositis ossificans progressiva.[1, 4] Some cases of osteoma cutis resist classification, such as the form associated with unilateral linear basal cell nevus and unilateral anodontia.[10]

TABLE 178-1. Differential Diagnosis and Evaluation of Cutaneous Ossification and Calcification

Condition	Clinical Examples	Calcium/Phosphorus
Osteoma Cutis		
Primary osteoma cutis		
Localized	Isolated nodule, multiple papules	Normal
Generalized	Albright's hereditary osteodystrophy	Normal, hypocalcemia
Secondary osteoma cutis		
Neoplasms	Pilomatricoma, others	Normal
Inflammatory processes	Morphea, myositis ossificans progressiva	Normal
Calcinosis Cutis		
Metastatic calcification	Renal failure patients with firm nodules around large joints, white papules/plaques, calciphylaxis	Hypercalcemia/hyperphosphatemia
Dystrophic calcification		
Universalis	Dermatomyositis	Normal
Circumscripta	Scleroderma, subcutaneous fat necrosis of the newborn	Normal
Neoplasms	Pilomatricoma, others	Normal
Other	Local infiltration, traumatic implantation	Normal
Idiopathic calcification		
Tumoral calcinosis	Subcutaneous masses	Hyperphosphatemia
Scrotal calcinosis	Nodules on scrotum	Normal
Cutaneous calculi	Fascial or mucosal nodules	Normal

Cutaneous Calcification

Metastatic calcification develops in the setting of hypercalcemia or hyperphosphatemia. The former may result from (1) primary hyperparathyroidism, (2) excessive intake of vitamin D, (3) excessive intake of milk and alkali, or (4) extensive destruction of bone.[1, 2] Hyperphosphatemia is primarily seen in the setting of chronic renal failure.[11] Metastatic calcification in subcutaneous tissues presents as firm or fluctuant nodules often around large joints. Cutaneous metastatic calcinosis is rare and appears as firm, white papules or symmetrical nodular plaques. These lesions may occur in a linear array, and occasionally a granular, white substance may be expressed from them.[1,2,11] An unusual patient with secondary hyperparathyroidism as a result of chronic renal failure developed epidermal and follicular calcification in lesions of toxic epidermal necrolysis.[12] The media of arteries and arterioles are especially prone to metastatic calcification and may lead to vascular occlusion and cutaneous ulceration and necrosis, particularly on the lower extremities. The term *calciphylaxis* has been used to describe such instances of widespread cutaneous and systemic calcification and has been noted especially in patients with the acquired immunodeficiency syndrome (AIDS) and renal failure[1, 13] (Figs. 178-1 and 178-2). Patients with end-stage renal failure may also develop calcifying panniculitis as part of systemic calciphylaxis.[14] A familial form of tumoral calcinosis, often associated with hyperphosphatemia, has also been reported.[1, 15]

In dystrophic cutaneous calcification, the calcium is deposited in previously damaged tissue, the values for serum calcium and phosphorus are normal, and there is no internal involvement.[1, 2] Dystrophic calcification is not uncommonly seen in connective tissue diseases. In dermatomyositis, calcinosis cutis is seen more often in children than in adults and presents in one of three ways: (1) small subcutaneous papules and plaques, (2) large tumorous deposits in the intermuscular fascial planes that appear "popcorn-like" on plain x-ray and can limit motion, and (3) widespread exoskeleton (calcinosis universalis). Spontaneous resolution may be associated with hypercalcemia.[1, 2, 16] Smaller deposits of calcium in areas of sclerosis (calcinosis circumscripta) are more typical in patients with systemic scleroderma (especially in the CREST syndrome [calcinosis cutis, Raynaud's phenomenon, esophageal dysfunction, sclerodactyly, and telangiectasia]) and may rarely be seen in widespread morphea. These deposits favor a periarticular location, especially the fingers, although intra-articular, paraspinous, and intervertebral calcifications have been observed in adults.[1,2,16] Calcinosis cutis is unusual in lupus erythematosus and is seen primarily in patients with long-standing systemic disease and predominantly involves the buttocks and extremities. This calcification is not associated with panniculitis and may be asymptomatic despite significant roentgenographic changes.[17] Dystrophic calcinosis cutis is also seen in subcutaneous fat necrosis of the

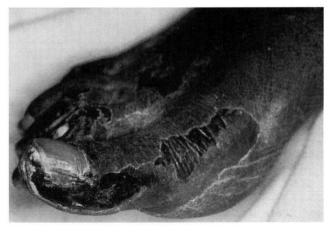

FIGURE 178-1. An HIV-positive patient with renal failure and a high calcium-phosphorus product unresponsive to parathyroidectomy developed gangrene of the distal extremities.

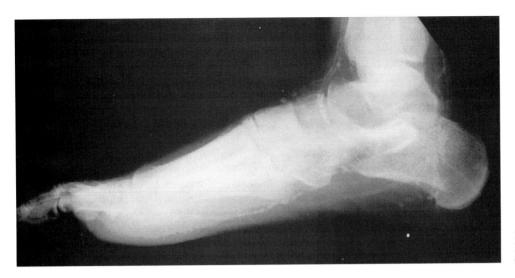

FIGURE 178–2. Same patient as in Figure 178–1. Plain x-rays revealed calcific arteries.

newborn, a self-healing disorder characterized by firm nodules and plaques on the cheeks, buttocks, and proximal extremities. Occasionally the nodules extrude their contents; symptomatic hypercalcemia as a result of spontaneous resolution of these lesions has rarely been reported.[18] Calcification of the auricular cartilage presents as an inflexible ear and is usually secondary to local injury, although numerous systemic conditions have also been associated with this finding.[19, 20] Dystrophic calcinosis cutis has also been reported in the subcutaneous nodules of Ehlers-Danlos syndrome.[2]

Numerous benign and malignant cutaneous neoplasms may also be a focus for calcification. Pilomatricoma features calcification of anucleate keratinocytes (ghost or shadow cells), hence the name *calcifying epithelioma of Malherbe.* Secondary ossification can occur in pilomatricoma as well. Many other neoplasms, including basal cell carcinomas and melanomas, may also undergo calcification. Local infiltration of tissues by intravenously administered calcium salts[21] or as a result of traumatic implantation of calcium salts (e.g., during electroencephalography)[22] may lead to dystrophic calcinosis cutis. In neonates, calcified nodules can occur after numerous heel sticks[23] and cephalhematomas acquired during delivery may also calcify.

In idiopathic calcinosis cutis, no underlying cutaneous disease may be identified, although clinically these lesions closely resemble those seen in dystrophic calcinosis cutis. Tumoral calcinosis, which consists of numerous large subcutaneous calcified masses sometimes in association with papular and nodular calcinosis cutis, is considered a special manifestation of idiopathic calcinosis cutis. The disease is typically familial and associated with hyperphosphatemia.[2, 15] A subcategory of idiopathic calcinosis cutis is idiopathic calcinosis of the scrotum, in which numerous asymptomatic nodules arise on the scrotal skin, enlarge with the passage of time, and occasionally extrude their calcified contents. Despite past questions as to whether such lesions represented calcification of an underlying cyst, an extensive investigation using immunohistochemical techniques showed no evidence for keratin and concluded that these lesions were indeed idiopathic.[24, 25] The subepidermal calcified nodule, also known as cutaneous calculus, is usually a single, verrucous nodule on the face of a child. However, there may be multiple lesions, which may arise at any time between birth and adult life.[26] A similar lesion has been identified in oral mucosa and appears to be analogous.[27]

PATHOLOGY

The pathologic appearance of cutaneous ossification is that of spicules of bone of varying size within the dermis, or in the subcutaneous tissue. Osteocytes, cement lines, and haversian canals are seen along with osteoblasts.[2] The x-ray appearance is that of true bone.[1] In calcinosis cutis, deposits of calcium stain deep blue with hematox-

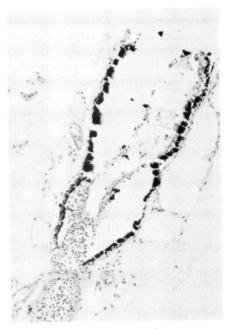

FIGURE 178–3. Calcification in the wall of a subcutaneous vessel in a patient with calciphylaxis (von Kossa stain).

TABLE 178-2. Treatment of Cutaneous Ossification and Calcification

Osteoma Cutis	Calcinosis Cutis
Tretinoin	Aluminum hydroxide
Etidronate disodium	Warfarin
Surgery	Intralesional adrenal steroids
	Etidronate disodium
	Surgery

ylin-eosin and black with the von Kossa stain. Typically, the calcium occurs as large deposits when located in the subcutaneous tissues and as granules and smaller deposits in the dermis. Deposits of calcium in vessels, as can be seen in calciphylaxis, are most pronounced in the internal elastic membrane of arteries or arterioles (Fig. 178–3).[2] The x-ray appearance is that of radiodense deposits.[1] Evaluation of calcium and phosphorus metabolism should be an essential part of the work-up of patients with either cutaneous ossification or calcification.[1,2]

TREATMENT

A variety of treatments have been attempted for osteoma cutis and cutaneous calcification (Table 178–2). Treatment of primary osteoma cutis presenting as multiple miliary osteomas with etidronate disodium did not lead to objective improvement.[5] In another patient with post-acne osteoma cutis, treatment with 0.05% tretinoin cream led to the transepidermal elimination of some osteomas.[6] Surgical therapies have also been successful.[6] Surgical excision is an effective treatment for cutaneous neoplasms that demonstrate secondary ossification.

Treatment of the underlying condition may lead to improvement in metastatic calcification. Several treatments have been reported to be effective in dystrophic cutaneous calcification, including aluminum hydroxide, low-dose warfarin, intralesional adrenal steroids, and etidronate disodium.[28-31] Surgical treatment of subcutaneous calcifications of polymyositis or dermatomyositis has also been reported.[32] Surgical excision is also an effective therapy for localized calcinosis cutis and for neoplasms with secondary calcification.

References

1. Orlow SJ, Watsky KL, Bolognia JL. Skin and bones II. J Am Acad Dermatol 1991;25:447–462.
2. Lever WF, Schaumburg-Lever G. Histopathology of the Skin, 6th edition. Philadelphia: JB Lipincott, 1983:420–422, 660–663.
3. Burgdorf W, Nasemann T. Cutaneous osteomas: A clinical and histopathologic review. Arch Dermatol Res 1977;260:121–135.
4. Roth SI, Stowell RE, Helwig EB. Cutaneous ossification: Report of 120 cases and review of the literature. Arch Pathol 1963;76:44–54.
5. Goldminz D, Greenberg RD. Multiple miliary osteoma cutis. J Am Acad Dermatol 1991;24:878–881.
6. Moritz DL, Elewski B. Pigmented postacne osteoma cutis in a patient treated with minocycline: Report and review of the literature. J Am Acad Dermatol 1991;24:851–853.
7. O'Donnell TF, Geller SA. Primary osteoma cutis. Arch Dermatol 1971;104:325–326.
8. Eyre WG, Reed WB. Albright's hereditary osteodystrophy with cutaneous bone formation. Arch Dermatol 1971;104:635–642.
9. Prendiville JS, Lucky AW, Mallory SB, et al. Osteoma cutis as a presenting sign of pseudo-hypoparathyroidism. Pediatr Dermatol 1992;9:11–18.
10. Aloi FG, Tomasini CF, Isaia G, et al. Unilateral linear basal cell nevus associated with diffuse osteoma cutis, unilateral anodontia, and abnormal bone mineralization. J Am Acad Dermatol 1989;20:973–978.
11. Katz AI, Hampers CL, Merrill JP. Secondary hyper-parathyroidism and renal osteodystrophy in chronic renal failure. Medicine 1969;48:333–374.
12. Solomon AR, Lomite SL, Headington JT. Epidermal and follicular calciphylaxis. J Cutan Pathol 1988;15:282–285.
13. Cockerell CJ, Dolan ET. Widespread cutaneous and systemic calcification, calciphylaxis, in patients with the acquired immune deficiency syndrome and renal disease. J Am Acad Dermatol 1992;26:559–562.
14. Lowry LR, Tschen JA, Wolf JE, Yen A. Calcifying panniculitis and systemic calciphylaxis in an end-stage renal patient. Cutis 1993;51:245–247.
15. Pursley TV, Prince MJ, Chausmer AB, et al. Cutaneous manifestation of tumoral calcinosis. Arch Dermatol 1979;115:1100–1102.
16. Wheeler CE, Curtis AC, Cawley EP, et al. Soft tissue calcification, with special reference to its occurrence in the "collagen diseases." Ann Intern Med 1952;36:1050–1075.
17. Rothe MJ, Grant-Kels JM, Rothfield NF. Extensive calcinosis cutis with systemic lupus erythematosus. Arch Dermatol 1990;126:1060–1063.
18. Thomsen RJ. Subcutaneous fat necrosis of the newborn and idiopathic hypercalcemia. Arch Dermatol 1980;116:1155–1158.
19. Larson PL, Weinstock MA, Welch RH. Calcification of the auricular cartilage. Cutis 1992;50:55–57.
20. Gordon DL. Calcification of auricular cartilage. Arch Intern Med 1964;113:23–27.
21. Goldminz D, Barnhill R, McGuire J, Stenn KS. Calcinosis cutis following extravasation of calcium chloride. Arch Dermatol 1988;124:922–925.
22. Lee FA, Gwinn JL. Roentgen patterns of extravasation of calcium gluconate in the tissue of the neonate. J Pediatr 1975;86:598–601.
23. Leung A. Calcification following heel sticks. J Pediatr 1985;106:168.
24. Song DH, Lee H, Kang WH. Idiopathic calcinosis of the scrotum: Histopathologic observations of fifty-one nodules. J Am Acad Dermatol 1988;19:1095–1101.
25. Wright S, Navsana IH, Leigh IM. Idiopathic scrotal calcinosis is idiopathic. J Am Acad Dermatol 1991;24:727–730.
26. Tezuka T. Cutaneous calculus: Its pathogenesis. Dermatologica 1980;161:191–199.
27. El-Mofty SK, Santa Cruz D. Mucosal calcified nodule: The oral counterpart of the subepidermal calcified nodule. Oral Surg Oral Med Oral Pathol 1992;73:472–475.
28. Wang W-J, Lo W-L, Wong C-K. Calcinosis cutis in juvenile dermatomyositis: Remarkable response to aluminum hydroxide therapy. Arch Dermatol 1988;124:1721–1722.
29. Berger RG, Featherstone GL, Raasch RH, et al. Treatment of calcinosis universalis with low dose warfarin. Am J Med 1987;83:72–76.
30. Hazen PG, Walker AE, Carney JF, Stewart JJ. Cutaneous calcinosis of scleroderma. Successful treatment with intralesional adrenal steroids. Arch Dermatol 1982;18:366–367.
31. Rabens SF, Bethune JE. Disodium etidronate therapy for dystrophic cutaneous calcification. Arch Dermatol 1975;111:357–361.
32. Shearin JC, Pickrell K. Surgical treatment of subcutaneous calcifications of polymyositis or dermatomyositis. Ann Plast Surg 1980;5:381–385.

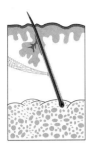

chapter 179

The Cutaneous Mucinoses

ALFREDO REBORA and FRANCO RONGIOLETTI

The cutaneous mucinoses are a heterogeneous group of disorders in which mucin accumulates in the skin either diffusely or focally. Mucin is a jelly-like amorphous mixture of glycosaminoglycans (GAGS) — mainly hyaluronic acid and dermatan sulfate bound to small amounts of chondroitin sulfate and heparin sulfate. All types of GAGS can be demonstrated in tissue sections by the Alcian-blue stain at pH 2.5 or the colloidal iron stain. Inasmuch as the causes of these conditions are unknown, mucinoses can be divided into those in which mucin deposition results in clinically distinctive lesions (Table 179–1) and diseases in which mucin deposition is an epiphenomenon (Table 179–2).[1, 2] Differential diagnosis of these conditions is detailed in Table 179–3, and treatment strategies are listed in Table 179–4.

DERMAL MUCINOSES WITH DISTINCTIVE FEATURES

Lichen Myxedematosus

Definition

Lichen myxedematosus is a localized or generalized papular eruption due to dermal deposition of mucin without thyroid disease.

Clinical Description

Lichen myxedematosus has three forms — a localized type affecting a single site, a disseminated type involving more than one site, and a generalized type, termed scleromyxedema or the Gottron-Arndt syndrome, affecting large portions of the skin or even the whole body.

Lichen myxedematosus is most commonly seen in patients 30 to 50 years old and affects both sexes equally. It features multiple, waxy, flat-topped papules that remain isolated (Fig. 179–1) or coalesce into plaques.[3] Linear and annular, nodular, urticarial, or cyst-like lesions may also be seen. In scleromyxedema, a sclerodermatous induration affects the mouth and fingers.[4] Vertical furrows on the glabella give some patients a leonine appearance. The elbows, forearms, upper trunk, and neck are also involved. The scalp and mucosae are usually spared.

A serum paraprotein is present in most cases of lichen myxedematosus. It is usually a 7S-IgG with lambda light chains. Unpredictably, a small number of patients with lichen myxedematosus develop myeloma or Waldenström's macroglobulinemia. Other laboratory tests are usually normal in localized or disseminated lichen myxedematosus. Two patients with lichen myxedematosus and human immunodeficiency virus infection have been reported. Scleromyxedema has a number of internal manifestations including neurologic, cardiovascular, renal, and rheumatologic disorders as well as necrotizing myopathy, dermatomyositis, esophageal aperistalsis, and laryngeal involvement. Most patients, though, have no visceral involvement.

The localized and disseminated types of lichen myxedematosus may clear spontaneously. The prognosis of the generalized form, scleromyxedema, is worse. It is often progressive. Death may result from pneumonia, thrombosis, or, rarely, from internal organ involvement.

Pathology

All forms of lichen myxedematosus show increased amounts of mucin in the mid- and upper reticular dermis, and varying degrees of fibroplasia. The proliferation of fibroblasts and collagen bundles is most marked in scleromyxedema, where they are arranged haphazardly in the dermis (Fig. 179–2). In late lesions of scleromyxedema, a whorled pattern may be evident. In all of

TABLE 179-1. Cutaneous Mucinoses with Distinctive Features (with Clinicopathologic Evidence and Specificity)

A. Dermal
   1. Lichen myxedematosus
   2. Acral persistent papular mucinosis
   3. Reticular erythematous mucinosis
   4. Scleredema
   5. Dysthyroidotic mucinoses
      a. Localized (pretibial) myxedema
      b. Generalized myxedema
      c. Papular mucinosis associated with thyroid disease
   6. Papular and nodular mucinosis associated with lupus erythematosus
   7. Self-healing juvenile cutaneous mucinosis
   8. Cutaneous mucinosis of infancy
   9. Cutaneous toxic mucinoses
      a. Papular mucinosis of the toxic oil syndrome
      b. Papular mucinosis of the eosinophilia-myalgia syndrome
  10. Neuropathia mucinosa cutanea
  11. Cutaneous focal mucinosis
  12. Mucous cyst
      a. Digital
      b. Of the oral mucosa
  13. Miscellaneous mucinoses
B. Follicular
   1. Pinkus' follicular mucinosis
   2. Urticaria-like follicular mucinosis

From Rongioletti F, Rebora A: Les mucinoses cutanees. Ann Dermatol Venereol 1993;120:75-87.

the forms of lichen myxedematosus, elastic fibers are fragmented and diminished and there are perivascular infiltrates of lymphocytes. Mucin may fill the walls of myocardial vessels, and the interstitium of kidney, pancreas, adrenals, and nerves.

Pathogenesis and Etiology

The etiology of lichen myxedematosus is unknown. As in many other dermal mucinoses, fibroblasts are the presumed source of GAGS. Whether the cutaneous changes of lichen myxedematosus are induced by paraproteinemia is not known. Lichen myxedematosus serum, even after paraprotein elution, incites fibroblast proliferation.

Diagnosis and Differential Diagnosis

Histopathology and the presence of a monoclonal gammopathy help distinguish lichen myxedematosus from several papular eruptions that have a similar appearance such as granuloma annulare, lichen amyloidosus, lichen planus and other lichenoid eruptions, and eruptive collagenoma. Scleromyxedema can be distinguished from systemic scleroderma and scleredema in which papules do not occur.

Treatment

No therapy is curative. Intralesional hyaluronidase and steroids have been disappointing. Electron-beam and radiotherapy, extracorporeal photochemistherapy,

PUVA, retinoids, dermabrasion, plasmapheresis, melphalan, cyclophosphamide, methotrexate, local steroids, and dimethyl sulfoxide have been useful.[4, 5] Potentially toxic drugs should be limited to patients who are disfigured, disabled, or very ill.

Acral Persistent Papular Mucinosis

Acral persistent papular mucinosis affects mostly women with multiple, symmetrical, ivory or flesh colored, 2- to 5-mm wide papules. They are located on the back of the hands and wrists and can persist for over a decade.

Mucin deposits that are large, focal, and well circumscribed are present in the upper dermis, sparing a subepidermal zone. Only rarely is the number of fibroblasts increased.[6]

It is not clear if acral persistent papular mucinosis is a variant of lichen myxedematosus or a distinct entity.[7] Topical steroids and hyaluronidase have proved useless.

TABLE 179-2. Disorders Associated with Histologic Deposition of Mucin

A. Epithelial Mucinosis
   1. Mycosis fungoides
   2. Spongiotic dermatitis
   3. Basal cell carcinoma
   4. Warts
   5. Keratoacanthoma
   6. Squamous cell carcinoma
B. Dermal Mucinosis
   1. Lupus erythematosus
   2. Dermatomyositis
   3. Scleroderma
   4. Degos' disease
   5. Granuloma annulare
   6. Pachydermoperiostosis
   7. UV radiation and PUVA
   8. Hypertrophic scar
   9. Actinic elastosis
  10. Hereditary progressive mucinous histiocytosis
  11. Epithelial tumors (basal cell carcinoma, eccrine tumors)
  12. Mesenchymal tumors (fibroma, malignant fibrous histiocytoma, myxosarcoma, lipoma, liposarcoma)
  13. Neural tumors (neurofibroma, neurilemoma, neuromyxoma)
C. Follicular Mucinosis
   1. Lymphoma
   2. Pseudolymphoma
   3. Cutaneous leukemia
   4. Spongiotic dermatitis
   5. Lupus erythematosus
   6. Hypertrophic lichen planus
   7. Insect bites
   8. Angiolymphoid hyperplasia with eosinophilia
   9. Hodgkin's disease
  10. Lichen striatus
  11. Sarcoidosis
  12. Photo-induced eruptions
  13. Familial reticuloendotheliosis

UV, ultraviolet; PUVA, psoralen plus ultraviolet A.
From Rongioletti F, Rebora A: The new cutaneous mucinoses. A review with an up-to-date classification of cutaneous mucinoses. J Am Acad Dermatol 1991;24:265-70.

TABLE 179-3. Differential Diagnosis of Cutaneous Mucinoses

Localized or Disseminated Types of Lichen Myxedematosus

Granuloma annulare
Lichen amyloidosus
Lichen planus
Lichenoid eruptions
Eruptive collagenoma

Generalized Lichen Myxedematosus (Scleromyxedema)

Systemic scleroderma
Scleredema

Reticular Erythematous Mucinosis

Lupus erythematosus
Jessner's lymphocytic infiltrate
Seborrheic dermatitis

Scleredema

Systemic scleroderma
Scleromyxedema
Generalized myxedema
Sclerema neonatorum
Trichinosis
Dermatomyositis
Edema of cardiac or renal origin

Localized (Pretibial) Myxedema

Lichen simplex chronicus
Lymphedema
Elephantiasis
Hypertrophic lichen planus

Generalized Myxedema

Edema of cardiac or renal origin
Scleredema
Scleromyxedema
Acute diffuse scleroderma

Follicular Mucinosis

Follicular mucinosis associated with cutaneous T-cell
  lymphoma
Lichen planus
Keratosis pilaris
Pityriasis rubra pilaris
Secondary syphilis
Alopecia mucinosa
Other non-scarring alopecias

 TABLE 179-4. Treatment of Cutaneous Mucinoses

Lichen Myxedematosus

Intralesional hyaluronidase
Local, intralesional, and systemic corticosteroids
Retinoids
Electron-beam and radiotherapy
Dermabrasion
Plasmapheresis
Melphalan
Cyclophosphamide
Methotrexate
Local dimethylsulfoxide
PUVA

Reticular Erythematous Mucinosis

Antimalarials

Scleredema

"Wait and see" (possible spontaneous clearing)
Cyclophospamide (?)
Systemic corticosteroids (?)
Electron beam therapy (?)

Pretibial Myxedema

"Wait and see" (possible spontaneous clearing)
Occlusive or intralesional corticosteroids
Plasmapheresis (?)
Gradient pneumatic compression (?)

Generalized Myxedema

Early thyroid replacement

Follicular Mucinosis

"Wait and see" (possible spontaneous clearing)
Topical, intralesional, and systemic corticosteroids
X-rays
Dapsone
Antimalarials
Psoralens plus ultraviolet A
Interferon alfa-2b

Clinical Description

Plaque-like cutaneous mucinosis and REM are most likely different aspects of the same rare syndrome.[8, 9] REM occurs most often in middle-aged women, although men and children are not spared.

Reddish macules and papules merge into reticulate annular or plaque-like, slightly pruritic lesions in the midback or chest (Fig. 179–3), at times spreading to the abdomen. Sun exposure worsens the eruption, but it has even been beneficial.[10] Phototesting may reproduce REM lesions. Usually, REM is not associated with systemic diseases and altered laboratory tests. However, hypothyroidism, discoid lupus erythematosus (LE), breast and colon carcinoma, diabetes, myxedema, Hashimoto's thyroiditis, and thrombocytopenia have been reported.[11]

Reticular Erythematous Mucinosis (Plaque-like Cutaneous Mucinosis, REM Syndrome, Midline Mucinosis)

Definition

Reticular erythematous mucinosis (REM) is a persistent photoaggravated erythematous reticular or plaque-like eruption in the midline of the back or chest.

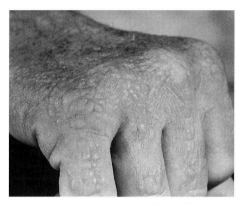

FIGURE 179-1. Lichen myxedematosus. Typical lesions consisting of waxy, 4- to 5-mm wide, lichenoid papules, isolated or coalescing into plaques on the upper limbs. (From Rongioletti F, Rebora A: Les mucinoses cutanees. Ann Dermatol Venereol 1993;120:75-87.)

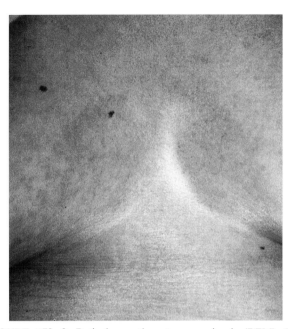

FIGURE 179-3. Reticular erythematous mucinosis (REM). Erythematous macules and papules coalesce into a reticulate or plaque-like lesion in the middle of the chest. (Courtesy of Richard Odom, M.D.)

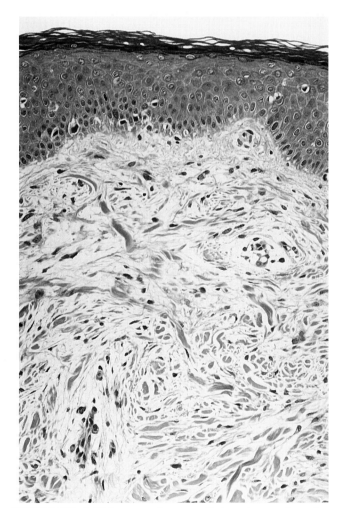

FIGURE 179-2. Lichen myxedematosus features increased numbers of haphazardly arranged spindled cells in the dermis, with delicate, similarly oriented collagen bundles separated by mucin.

Oral contraceptives, menses, and pregnancy may promote or exacerbate REM.[10] REM may clear spontaneously even after 15 years.[10]

Pathology

There are small amounts of mucin interstitially in the upper dermis, along with a perivascular and, at times, perifollicular T-cell infiltrate.[12] Usually, direct immunofluorescence is negative, but granular deposits of IgM, IgA, and C3 have been very rarely seen at the dermoepidermal junction.

Pathogenesis and Etiology

Sunlight may be a causal or promoting factor. Tubuloreticular inclusions have been detected in endothelial cells and pericytes in lesional skin.[12] Although these inclusions occur in viral infections, they can also be produced by high levels of interferon and are found in endothelial cells in lupus erythematosus. The relationship to lupus erythematosus is to be elucidated.

Diagnosis and Differential Diagnosis

Lupus erythematosus shows involvement of the epidermis histologically and IgG and C3 deposits at the dermoepidermal junction. An unusual form of lupus erythematosus known as tumid lupus erythematosus can be impossible to distinguish microscopically from REM, but clinically presents as scattered smooth-topped papules. Jessner's lymphocytic infiltration usually lacks mucin deposits. Seborrheic dermatitis is a scaling disorder and involves the scalp and face.

Treatment

Antimalarials are usually effective in clearing the lesions of REM in 2 to 4 weeks.

Scleredema

Definition

This disorder is a symmetrical diffuse induration of the upper part of the body due to thickening of the dermis and deposition of mucin.

Clinical Description

There are three types of scleredema, although a simpler division into patients with and without diabetes has been suggested.[13] The first type affects mostly middle-aged females, but also children. It is preceded by fever, malaise, and infection, usually streptococcal, of upper and lower respiratory tract. The skin of the cervicofacial region, then of the trunk and proximal upper limbs, suddenly hardens. The face is expressionless, and opening the mouth and swallowing are difficult because of involvement of the tongue and pharynx. This type usually resolves in a few months.

The second type shares the same clinical features, but has a subtle onset without preceding illness and persists for years.

The third type occurs mainly in obese middle-aged males with insulin-dependent diabetes (scleredema diabeticorum). The onset is subtle and the disorder persistent. Erythema and induration of the back are common, irrespective of whether hyperglycemia is corrected.

Serositis, dysarthria and dysphagia, myositis, ocular and cardiac abnormalities, parotiditis, monoclonal gammopathy, and myeloma may occur in all forms. There may be also hyperparathyroidism, rheumatoid arthritis, Sjögren's syndrome, and malignant insulinoma.[14] Scleredema causes little morbidity besides the limitation of movement. Type I may clear in 1 to 2 years, whereas the other types last longer. Type III scleredema is occasionally fatal.

Pathology

The principal alteration in scleredema is thickening of the dermis, with mucin deposition between collagen bundles. At times, the mucin deposition can be so slight that multiple biopsies or stains of unfixed frozen sections are needed to detect it.[15] There is a sparse perivascular lymphocytic infiltrate with mast cells. Direct immunofluorescence is usually negative, but IgG and C3 have been found at the dermoepidermal junction. Mucin also accumulates in skeletal muscle and in the heart.[16]

Pathogenesis and Etiology

Streptococcal hypersensitivity, injury to lymphatics, paraproteinemia, and diabetes may play a role. Fibroblasts cultured from lesional skin show enhanced collagen production.

Diagnosis and Differential Diagnosis

The early edematous stages of systemic scleroderma may be confused with scleredema. However, Raynaud's phenomenon and acrosclerosis occur in scleroderma. Scleromyxedema differs in that it causes papules rather than diffuse dermal induration. Myxedema, sclerema neonatorum, trichinosis, dermatomyositis, and edema of cardiac or renal origin can be easily differentiated.

Treatment

There is no specific treatment. Systemic and intralesional steroids and intralesional hyaluronidase, methotrexate, ultraviolet rays, antibiotics, and penicillamine have not been helpful. Cyclophosphamide and electron-beam therapy have been of benefit.[17]

Dysthyroidotic Mucinosis Associated with Altered Thyroid Function

Localized (Pretibial) Myxedema

Definition. Localized or pretibial myxedema is a cutaneous induration of the shins due to mucin deposition, associated with hyperthyroidism or occurring after thyroidectomy.

Clinical Description. Localized myxedema is one of the signs of Graves' disease (0.4% to 5%) along with goiter, exophthalmos, thyroid acropathy, and high blood levels of long-acting thyroid-stimulating hormone.[18] Rarely, it occurs in Hashimoto's thyroiditis without thyrotoxicosis, in hypothyroidism following treatment of Graves' disease, and even in euthyroid patients.[19]

Localized myxedema develops as erythematous to skin-colored, sometimes purple-brown or yellowish, waxy, indurated, peau d'orange nodules or plaques. Usually, they are located on the anterolateral aspect of the legs (Fig. 179–4) or feet. Localized myxedema may also

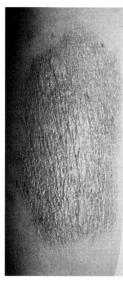

FIGURE 179–4. Localized (pretibial) myxedema. Indurated plaque on the pretibial region.

present as a diffuse non-pitting edema on the shins or feet evolving into elephantiasis. More rarely, localized myxedema affects face, shoulders, upper limbs, and lower abdomen.[20] Large plaques are often painful and pruritic. Hypertrichosis and hyperhidrosis are confined to pretibial myxedematous skin.

Usually, localized myxedema morbidity is little, but entrapment of peroneal nerves by mucinous connective tissue may cause foot drop or faulty dorsiflexion.

Pathology. Large quantities of mucin are stored in the reticular dermis, causing collagen bundles to separate and the dermis to thicken (Fig. 179–5). A grenz zone of normal collagen is also observed. There is a perivascular and periadnexal lymphocytic infiltrate with mast cells and large stellate fibroblasts. Elastic fibers are reduced. The epidermis is often papillated, hyperplastic, and hyperkeratotic.

Pathogenesis and Etiology. A serum factor (unrelated to long-acting thyroid stimulating hormone) could incite fibroblasts to produce mucin. An insulin-like growth factor,[21] traumas, and a lymphatic obstruction due to mucin may play a role.[22]

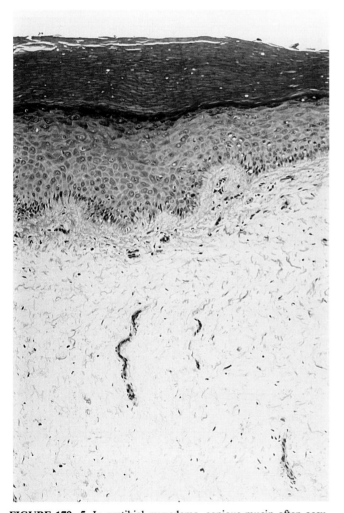

FIGURE 179–5. In pretibial myxedema, copious mucin often accumulates in the reticular dermis. In this case, only a few strands of residual collagen fibers are visible. Note the epidermal hyperplasia and hyperkeratosis, common features in pretibial myxedema.

Diagnosis and Differential Diagnosis. Lichen simplex chronicus, lymphedema, elephantiasis, and hypertrophic lichen planus lack mucin deposition and are generally not seen in the setting of thyroid disease.

Treatment. Steroids administered under occlusive dressings or delivered by intralesional injection may help. Usually, skin grafting is followed by relapses. Plasmapheresis and gradient pneumatic compression[23] have been of benefit. Therapy of hyperthyroidism does not improve the cutaneous lesions and, often, localized myxedema develops after it. Localized myxedema may also clear spontaneously.

Generalized Myxedema

Definition. Generalized myxedema is a manifestation of severe hypothyroidism in which mucin is stored in the dermis leading to induration of the skin.[18]

Clinical Description. Hypothyroidism may be congenital (cretinism), juvenile, or adult onset. Congenital hypothyroidism affects 1 of 5000 neonates and may cause a distinctive syndrome of dwarfism, mental retardation, and systemic and cutaneous symptoms. Somnolence, constipation, feeding problems, poor muscle tone, persistence of jaundice, and respiratory problems all suggest the diagnosis. More than 33% of infants have no symptoms.

Periorbital tissues, the tongue, lips, hands, and genitals are puffy. The skin is dry, cold, and pale. Nails and hair are dry and brittle, and there can be patch alopecia. Presence of a clavicular pad is diagnostic.

Juvenile hypothyroidism develops in a previously euthyroid child. Features are short stature, abnormal physical and mental development, retardation of sexual maturity, and poor performance at school. Hypertrichosis may develop on the shoulders and upper back.

Adult hypothyroidism is the most common form. It can be seen in women 40 to 60 years old as the result of an autoimmune disease, ordinarily Hashimoto's thyroiditis, or of therapy of Graves' disease, or, more rarely, of pituitary or hypothalamic failure.

The initial symptoms are subtle, including mental and physical sluggishness, weight gain, constipation, leg cramps, loss of appetite, and cold intolerance.[24] The face has a dull expression. Eyelids, lips, tongue, and hands are puffy, the nose is broad, the speech hoarse and slurred. The skin is pale, cool, waxy, and dry for the absence of sweating with ichthyosis or eczema craquelé. Hair and nails are dry and brittle. A diffuse non-scarring alopecia is common. Purpura on the limbs, blue teleangiectatic fingertips, delayed wound healing, and xanthomas are present.[25] Cardiomegaly, megacolon or bowel obstruction, psychiatric symptoms, serositis, carpal tunnel syndrome, and seventh nerve paralysis may be associated.

Pathology. Mucin deposits, mainly perivascular and perifollicular, splay collagen bundles and may spread to fat and nerves. Fibroblasts are not increased. Elastic fibers are reduced. Psychiatric symptoms are caused by mucin deposits in the brain.

Pathogenesis and Etiology. Generalized myxedema is produced by quantitative or functional deficiency of thyroxin. Impaired degradation, rather than an increased synthesis of GAGS, has been suggested.

Diagnosis and Differential Diagnosis. The diagnosis is made clinically. Low levels of T3 and T4 confirm the diagnosis. The thyroid-stimulating hormone level is high in primary hypothyroidism and low in secondary hypothyroidism, in which myxedema does not occur.

Treatment. Early treatment is crucial for proper mental development of neonates with hypothyroidism. T4 and thyroid-stimulating hormone levels should be measured 3 to 6 days after birth and treatment begun before the fourth month. Usually, symptoms subside with thyroxin treatment and recur if it is stopped.[26] Even areas of hair loss regrow with treatment. If untreated, patients can die as a result of "myxedema coma."

Papular Mucinosis Associated with Thyroid Disease

Papular mucinosis resembling multiple focal cutaneous mucinosis and differing from generalized or localized myxedema has been associated with Hashimoto's thyroiditis.[27] Correction of thyroxin levels cured this condition in a hypothyroidal myxedematous patient.[28]

Papular and Nodular Mucinosis in Lupus Erythematosus

Papular and nodular mucinosis (PNM) occurs in 1.5% of lupus erythematosus cases as symptomless skin-colored, at times reddish, 0.5- to 2-cm wide papules and nodules rarely merging into plaques.[29, 30] They are better seen with tangential light (Fig. 179–6). Central depression and pigmentation may be additional features. The back and V of the neck are mostly involved. Only in three cases did PNM begin or worsen after sun exposure.[29]

PNM antedates lupus erythematosus or begins with it. The course may be related to disease activity. Usually, patients with lupus erythematosus who develop PNM have systemic disease, with renal (50%) and articular (40%) involvement. Twenty percent of patients have discoid lupus erythematosus only.

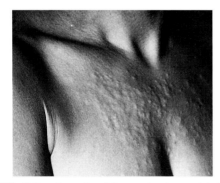

FIGURE 179–6. Papular and nodular mucinosis associated with lupus erythematosus. Flesh-colored, sometimes erythematous, papular and nodular lesions giving a "lumpy" appearance to the skin of the chest.

Mucin abounds in the upper and mid-dermis. The epidermal changes of lupus erythematosus can be absent or subtle, but a lupus band may be seen on direct immunofluorescence.[29]

Only a few patients respond to antimalarials, the remainder requiring systemic steroids. In at least two cases, PNM did not clear at all in spite of the good response of other symptoms of lupus erythematosus.[29]

Self-Healing Juvenile Cutaneous Mucinosis

Self-healing juvenile cutaneous mucinosis develops acutely in children as asymptomatic papules in linear, infiltrated, non-tender, slightly pruritic erythematous plaques. They give a corrugated appearance to the skin. The face, neck, scalp, trunk, and thighs are affected. Deep nodules are present on the face and, along with arthritis, on knees, elbows, and fingers.[31]

Mucin is stored in the upper reticular dermis with a mild increase of fibroblasts and mast cells and a perivascular infiltrate in the papillary dermis. Mucin with the staining properties of sialomucin can be found in the periarticular nodules.

Self-healing juvenile cutaneous mucinosis clears spontaneously, but arthralgia occasionally recurs.[32]

Cutaneous Mucinosis of Infancy

In cutaneous mucinosis of infancy, 1- to 2-mm wide, opalescent papules are grouped on the elbows. Isolated or linear papules affect upper arms and the back of hands.[33] Onset is early (fourth month) or even congenital.[34]

Mucin is so superficial as to look as "enclosed by epidermal cells." Fibroblasts do not proliferate, and a perivascular round cell infiltrate may be seen in the papillary dermis.

Cutaneous mucinosis of infancy has no spontaneous resolution. Topical steroids and tretinoin were ineffective in one patient.

Cutaneous Toxic Mucinoses

Though unrelated epidemiologically, toxic oil syndrome and L-tryptophan-associated eosinophilia-myalgia syndrome share some clinical features among which are mucinous papules.[35]

Papular Mucinosis in Toxic Oil Syndrome

Toxic oil syndrome results from the ingestion of adulterated rapeseed oil. The pathogenetic mechanism is still obscure.

The onset of this condition is acute with fever, a pruritic eruption, peripheral eosinophilia, and an often fatal interstitial pneumopathy. Three to 4 months after onset, symptomless, white or yellow, non-confluent, 1- to 5-mm wide papules develop on the limbs.[36] Lesions clear spontaneously or are followed by sclerodermoid changes.

Papular Mucinosis in Eosinophilia-Myalgia Syndrome

Eosinophilia-myalgia syndrome is a systemic illness related to a contaminant of L-tryptophan-containing products.

A severe generalized myalgia with blood eosinophilia, constitutional symptoms, and scleroderma marks the disease. Papular mucinosis may develop 1 to 5 months after the onset of the illness. White or skin-colored, 1- to 3-mm wide, itching papules affect limbs and, less often, shoulders, abdomen, and scalp. Mucin gathers in the upper and mid-dermis. Fibroblasts are increased.[37] Papules subside slowly after L-tryptophan discontinuation.

Neuropathia Mucinosa Cutanea

A young man had livedo on his legs and hyperesthesia. Hypertrophic (onion-like) intradermal nerves were encased by mucin.[38]

Cutaneous Focal Mucinosis

The lesion is a symptomless, skin-colored papule or nodule, less than 1 cm wide, on the face, trunk, or limbs of adults.[39] Only rarely has cutaneous focal mucinosis been linked to a thyroid disorder without myxedema, and with REM and scleromyxedema.[40]

Mucin is dispersed through the upper and middermis. Fibroblasts may be either increased or reduced. Elastic fibers are absent.[41] Cleft-like spaces, but no cysts, are seen.

Cutaneous focal mucinosis may be an angiomyxoma or the result of a "muciparous" reaction of the connective tissue to nonspecific stimuli.

Lesions of cutaneous focal mucinosis can be surgically excised. Relapses are uncommon.

Mucous Cysts

Mucous Digital Cyst (Myxoid Cyst, Synovial Cyst, Myxoid Pseudocyst)

Mucous digital cyst occurs at any age, mostly in women, as a raised, cystic nodule, almost translucent, seldom wider than 2 cm. Usually, it is located on the fingers (rarely the toes) at the nail base. Clear viscous material comes out, but older cysts may be solid. Mucous digital cyst may become verrucous and black colored after internal bleeding. The adjacent nail may show a longitudinal furrow and a Heberden's (osteophytic) nodule. Early mucous digital cyst may disclose dermal mucin-filled cleft-like spaces, but a large nonencapsulated cyst is typical.

Mucous digital cyst is neither a cyst nor a tumor, but the result of connective tissue degeneration. Trauma is a promoting factor.

Excision, incision and drainage, aspiration of the content, and intralesional injections of triamcinolone or sclerosant agents are used, but relapses are frequent.[42]

Any associated osteophytic nodule should be removed because it would promote relapses.

Mucous Cyst of the Oral Mucosa (Mucocele)

Mucoceles are single, symptomless, dome-shaped, translucent, blue-whitish cysts that contain a clear, viscous fluid. They are usually located on the inner surface of the lower lip or on the floor of the mouth. Most are smaller than 1 cm in diameter, and wax and wane over several months. Rarely, multiple mucoceles arise in the superficial labial epithelium and can resemble a blistering disease. Mucoceles result either from a ruptured mucous salivary gland duct or from retention of mucus due to obstruction of a duct.

In early mucoceles, small mucin-filled spaces are surrounded by or intermixed with edematous, acutely inflamed granulation tissue. In older lesions, large cystic spaces develop. Rarely, a true cyst develops that is lined by columnar epithelium. Mucoceles contain sialomucin—mucin produced by epithelial cells rather than fibroblasts, and that contains nonsulfated GAGS. Unlike connective tissue–derived mucin, sialomucin stains well with periodic acid–Schiff following digestion with diastase. It is also Alcian-blue positive and colloidal iron positive, like connective tissue–derived mucin.

Mucoceles can be excised or treated with cryotherapy. They may even disappear spontaneously.[43]

Miscellaneous Mucinoses

Other mucinoses, possibly variants of the aforementioned ones, are *atypical tuberous myxedema, cutaneous focal mucinosis with spontaneous healing*, and some not well-defined papular and nodular mucinoses.

In atypical tuberous myxedema, large mucinous nodules occur on the limbs. Only their size distinguishes atypical tuberous myxedema from lichen myxedematosus.[44] Atypical tuberous myxedema has been incorrectly used also to mean lichen myexedematosus, scleromyxedema, and other euthyreotic mucinoses.

Papules resembling cutaneous focal mucinosis in a patient with diabetes mellitus and no thyroid abnormality spontaneously cleared after biopsy.[45]

DISTINCTIVE FOLLICULAR MUCINOSES

Mucin accumulates in follicular epithelium in two distinctive clinical conditions—alopecia mucinosa and urticaria-like follicular mucinosis. Otherwise, follicular mucinosis is a histologic epiphenomenon most often seen in cutaneous T-cell lymphomas and other skin disorders (see Table 179–2). Alopecia and follicular mucinosis are discussed in detail in Chapter 135.

Urticaria-like follicular mucinosis occurs in middle-aged men. Urticarial pruritic papules or plaques recur on the head and neck on an erythematous "seborrheic" background and fade, leaving a red macule that persists for a few weeks. Hairy regions may be involved, but neither follicular plugging nor alopecia occur. Urticaria-like follicular mucinosis waxes and wanes irregularly over 2 months to 15 years. There are no associated systemic diseases.[46] Sunlight has controversial effects, but it helped in at least 2 cases.[47]

As in Pinkus' follicular mucinosis, mucin-filled cystic spaces occupy hair follicles, close to the "bulge." In the upper dermis, lymphocytes and eosinophils are seen around blood vessels and hair follicles. Direct immunofluorescence showed vascular C3 deposits in only one patient.[47] The prognosis is good. Antimalarials were helpful in two patients.

References

1. Rongioletti F, Rebora A. The new cutaneous mucinoses. A review with an up-to-date classification of cutaneous mucinoses. J Am Acad Dermatol 1991;24:265–270.
2. Rongioletti F, Rebora A. Les mucinoses cutanees. Venereol 1993;120:75–87.
3. Farmer ER, Hambrick GW Jr, Shulman LE. Papular mucinosis. A clinicopathologic study of four patients. Arch Dermatol 1982;118:9–13.
4. Koeppel MG, Advilinac, Terrier G, et al. Electron beam therapy in Arndt-Gottron's scleromyxedema. Br J Dermatol 1993;129:733–735.
5. Bonnetblanc JM, Bedane C. Regression of scleromyxedema with topical betamethasone and dimethylsulfoxide: A 30 month follow-up. Arch Dermatol 1991;127:1733–1734.
6. Rongioletti F, Rebora A, Crovato F. Acral persistent papular mucinosis: A new entity? Arch Dermatol 1986;122:1237–1239.
7. Rebora A, Rongioletti F. Acral persistent papular mucinosis and lichen myxedematosus. Dermatology 1992;185:81.
8. Perry HO, Kierland RR, Montgomery H. Plaque-like form of cutaneous mucinosis. Arch Dermatol 1960;82:980–985.
9. Steigleder GK, Gartmann H, Linker V. REM syndrome: Reticular erythematous mucinosis (round-cell erythematosis), a new entity? Br J Dermatol 1974;91:191–199.
10. Quimby SR, Perry HO. Plaque-like cutaneous mucinosis; its relationship to reticular erythematous mucinosis. J Am Acad Dermatol 1982;6:856–861.
11. Braddock SW, Davis CS, Davis RB. Reticular erythematous mucinosis and thrombocytopenic purpura: Report of a case and review of the world literature, including plaque-like cutaneous mucinosis. J Am Acad Dermatol 1988;19:859–868.
12. Chavaz P, Polla L, Saurat JH. Paramyxovirus-like inclusions and lymphocyte type in the REM syndrome. Br J Dermatol 1982;106:741–743.
13. Venencie PY, Powell FC, Su WPD, et al. Scleredema: A review of thirty-three cases. J Am Acad Dermatol 1984;11:128–134.
14. Matsunaga J, Hara M, Tagami H. Scleredema of Buschke associated with malignant insulinoma. Br J Dermatol 1992;126:527–528.
15. Cole HG, Winkelman RK. Acid mucopolysaccharide staining in scleredema. J Cutan Pathol 1990;17:211–213.
16. Black MM. Mucinosis. In: Champion RH, Burton JL, Ebling FJG, eds. Textbook of Dermatology, 5th edition, vol. IV. Oxford: Blackwell, 1992:2325–2333.
17. Angeli-Besson C, Koeppel MC, Jacquet P, et al. Electron-beam therapy in scleredema adultorum with associated monoclonal hyperaminoglobulinemia. Br J Dermatol 1994;130:396–397.
18. Heymann WR. Cutaneous manifestations of thyroid disease. J Am Acad Dermatol 1992;26:885–902.
19. Srebnik A, Ophyr J, Brenner S. Euthyroid pretibial myxedema. Int J Dermatol 1992;32:431–432.
20. Noppakun N, Bancheun K, Chandraprasert S. Unusual locations of localized myxedema in Graves' disease. Arch Dermatol 1986;122:85–90.
21. Kriss JP. Pathogenesis and treatment of pretibial myxedema. Endocrinol Metab Clin North Am 1987;16:409–415.
22. Bull RH, Coburn PR, Mortimer PS. Pretibial myxedema: A manifestation of lymphoedema? Lancet 1993;341:403–404.
23. Schleicher SM, Milstein HJ. Treatment of pretibial mucinotisuiter gradient pneumatic compression. Arch Dermatol 1994;130:842–844.
24. Levy EG. Thyroid disease in the elderly. Med Clin North Am 1991;75:151–167.
25. Signore RJ, von Weiss J. Alopecia of myxedema: Clinical response to levothyroxine sodium. J Am Acad Dermatol 1991;25:902–904.
26. Diven DG, Gwinup G, Newton RC. The thyroid. Dermatol Clin 1989;7:547–557.
27. Shuppli R, Forrer J. Eine ungewohnliche Form von bullloser Mucinose der Haut bei Hashimoto-Thyreoiditis. Dermatologica 1981;162:307–312.
28. Jakubovic HR, Salama SSS, Rosenthal D. Multiple cutaneous focal mucinosis with hypothyroidism. Ann Int Med 1982;96:56–58.
29. Rongioletti F, Parodi A, Rebora A. Papular and nodular mucinosis as a sign of lupus erythematosus. Dermatologica 1990;180:221–223.
30. Kobayashi T, Shimuizu H, Shimizu S, et al. Plaque-like cutaneous lupus mucinosis. Arch Dermatol 1993;128:383–384.
31. Bonerandi JJ, Andrac L, Follana J, et al. Mucinose cutanee juvenile spontanement resolutive: Etude anatomo-clinique et ultrastructurale. Ann Dermatol Venereol 1980;107:51–57.
32. Pucevich MV, Latour DL, Bale GR, et al. Self-healing juvenile cutaneous mucinosis. J Am Acad Dermatol 1984;11:327–332.
33. Lum D. Cutaneous mucinosis of infancy. Arch Dermatol 1980;116:198–200.
34. McGrae JD. Cutaneous mucinosis of infancy: A congenital and linear variant. Arch Dermatol 1983;119:272–273.
35. Rongioletti F, Rebora A. Cutaneous toxic mucinoses. J Am Acad Dermatol 1992;26:789–790.
36. Fonseca E, Contreras F. Cutaneous mucinosis in the toxic oil syndrome. J Am Acad Dermatol 1987;16:139–140.
37. Valicenti JMK, Fleming MG, Pearson RW, et al. Papular mucinosis in L-tryptophan-induced eosinophilia-myalgia syndrome. J Am Acad Dermatol 1991;25:54–58.
38. Vakilzadeh F. Neuropathia mucinosa cutanea. Hautarzt 1988;40:167–168.
39. Johnson WC, Helwig EB. Cutaneous focal mucinosis: A clinicopathological and histochemical study. Arch Dermatol 1966;93:13–20.
40. Rongioletti F, Amantea A, Balus L, et al. Cutaneous focal mucinosis associated with reticular erythematous mucinosis and scleromyxedema. J Am Acad Dermatol 1991;24:656–657.
41. Wiek M, Schmoeckel C. Cutaneous focal mucinosis. A histopathological and immunohistochemical analysis of 11 cases. J Cutan Pathol 1994;21:446–452.
42. Audebert C. Treatment of mucoid cyst of fingers and toes by injection of sclerosant. Dermatol Clin 1987;7:179–188.
43. Lattanand A, Johnson WC, Graham JH. Mucous cyst (mucocele). Arch Dermatol 1970;101:673–678.
44. Suter L, Vakilzadeh F, Macher E. Atypical tuberous myxedema Jadassohn-Dosseker. Dermatologica 1980;161:265–269.
45. Suhonen R, Niemi KM. Cutaneous focal mucinosis with spontaneous healing. J Cutan Pathol 1983;10:334–339.
46. Enjolras O, Guillemette J, Hewitt J. Dermatose ortiee avec mucinose folliculaire. Ann Dermatol Venereol 1980;107:491–495.
47. Crovato F, Nazzari G, Nunzi E, et al. Urticaria-like follicular mucinosis. Dermatologica 1985;170:133–135.

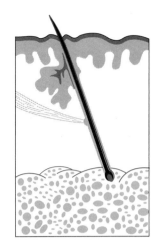

What Are the Dermatologic Manifestations of Internal Disease? What Are the Dermatologic Disorders Commonly Found in Pediatrics?

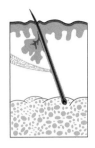

chapter 180

Paraneoplastic Syndromes

DAVID I. McLEAN and HARVEY LUI

DEFINITION

What constitutes a true paraneoplastic syndrome? There are two essential criteria: (1) the dermatosis must develop only after the genesis of the malignant tumor, and (2) the dermatosis and the malignant tumor should follow a parallel course.[1] The second criterion means that removal of the cancer results in resolution of the dermatosis, while tumor recurrence can cause relapse of the dermatosis. Clearly, the paraneoplastic dermatosis cannot occur in the absence of the cancer, if the term *paraneoplastic* is to be retained.

Paraneoplastic conditions must have a proven association of the cutaneous eruption with a tumor. This is not difficult where both the dermatosis and the cancer are rare. It becomes a major problem, however, where the dermatosis is very common, such as the seborrheic keratoses of the sign of Leser-Trélat, and the presumed association is with a wide spectrum of common neoplasms. In this situation, the literature is replete with anecdotal reports of dubious significance. Case-controlled studies are needed, but few are available. Much that appears in the literature should be questioned.

This discussion of paraneoplastic syndromes includes only those dermatoses that are caused by, and are located at a distance from, the tumor. Preexisting conditions that can be associated with cancer, such as arsenical keratoses, or the sebaceous neoplasms found in patients with the Muir-Torre syndrome, are therefore not included. In addition, although cutaneous infiltrates produced by the tumor cells themselves or by substances synthesized by the tumor (e.g., amyloid, melanin) can be definite skin signs of internal cancer, they are not generally considered to be true paraneoplastic conditions.

NECROLYTIC MIGRATORY ERYTHEMA

Necrolytic migratory erythema, also known as the glucagonoma syndrome, is a prototypical paraneoplastic syndrome in which a unique specific cutaneous alteration is produced by a distant tumor. This dermatosis is a marker for a glucagon-producing tumor of the pancreas.[2-5] Necrolytic migratory erythema is manifested by erythema, vesicles, pustules, bullae, and erosions that typically involve the face and the intertriginous areas, particularly the groin (Fig. 180–1). Necrolytic migratory erythema is often initially mistaken for an intertriginous candidal infection. The eruption can also involve the shins, ankles, and feet, as well as the fingertips. The vesicles are often very superficial, tend to become confluent, and rupture easily. Brownish-red papules are often scattered over much of the skin surface.[6, 7] Peripheral expansion of the lesions results in an arcuate or gyrate morphology. Associated abnormalities include glossitis, stomatitis, dystrophic nails, alopecia, weight loss, anemia, and diabetes.[8]

Most patients with necrolytic migratory erythema have a pancreatic islet cell tumor of the glucagon-producing type resulting in high serum glucagon levels and mild diabetes mellitus. Resection of the tumor clears the eruption, sometimes within 48 hours.[4, 7, 9] The cutaneous eruption is most likely due to excess catabolism of amino acids as a result of enhanced hepatic uptake.

Rarely, the dermatitis can occur in patients without cancer but with hepatic cirrhosis and hyperglucagonemia,[10] pancreatitis,[11] or celiac sprue.[12] Pathologic examination shows psoriasiform epidermal hyperplasia with pallor, ballooning, and necrosis of the upper spinous layer of the epidermis. This pattern is identical to that

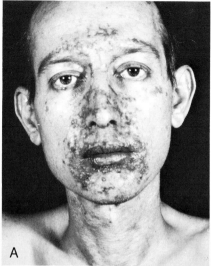
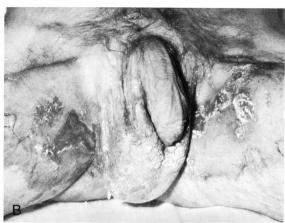

FIGURE 180-1. *A,* Patient with necrolytic migratory erythema and a glucagon-secreting pancreatic carcinoma. *B,* Same patient as in *A,* showing typical groin erosions. (*A* courtesy of Department of Dermatology, Massachusetts General Hospital.)

seen in a variety of deficiency diseases such as acrodermatitis enteropathica and pellagra and reflects a common pathophysiology, namely the toxic effects of amino acid deficiency on keratinocytes. While the diagnosis can be suspected on biopsy, confirmation may require serum glucagon levels. Localization of the tumor, which is usually in the tail of the pancreas, requires computed tomography, arteriography, or both.

HYPERTRICHOSIS LANUGINOSA ACQUISITA

In hypertrichosis lanuginosa acquisita, there is excessive growth of lanugo (vellus) hairs. These long, soft, downy hairs initially cover the face and ears (Fig. 180-2), but eventually all hair-bearing skin may be involved. Associated abnormalities include glossitis, which is often painful, and red papules occurring extensively on the tongue.[13] Fully expressed hypertrichosis lanuginosa acquisita is usually secondary to malignant tumors, but excessive lanugo hair growth also can be caused by anorexia nervosa or drugs such as steroids, phenytoin, diazoxide, streptomycin, penicillamine, and minoxidil.[14]

Hypertrichosis lanuginosa acquisita secondary to malignancy is usually abrupt in its onset and is rapidly progressive. Neoplasms reported in association with hypertrichosis lanuginosa acquisita include tumors of colon,[13, 15-17] rectum,[15, 18, 19] bladder,[20] lung,[14, 21, 22] pancreas,[23] gallbladder,[24] uterus,[25] and breast,[26] and lymphoma.[25,27]

SWEET'S SYNDROME

Sweet's syndrome (see also Chapter 38), or "acute febrile neutrophilic dermatosis,"[28] consists of tender, red plaques and nodules that can appear anywhere on the skin surface but occur most commonly on the face and extremities (Fig. 180-3; see color plate). Individual lesions may appear edematous and translucent. Vesicles or vesicopustules may cover the surface of the plaques, which tend to expand peripherally with central clearing.

When ulceration occurs, lesions resemble those of pyoderma gangrenosum.[29-31] Pyrexia and neutrophilia are common,[32] and there can be an associated arthritis, conjunctivitis, or episcleritis.[33]

Sweet's syndrome as a paraneoplastic condition is most commonly associated with leukemia, particularly acute myelocytic leukemia,[34, 35] although other leukemias or lymphomas have been reported.[36-45] Solid tumors, which are much less commonly associated, include adenocarcinoma, embryonal testicular carcinoma, ovarian carcinoma, gastric carcinoma, and adenocarcinoma of the prostate and rectum.[46-51] Pyoderma gangrenosum and Sweet's syndrome can also be produced in patients treated with leukocyte colony stimulation factor.[52] Cancer-associated Sweet's syndrome is often character-

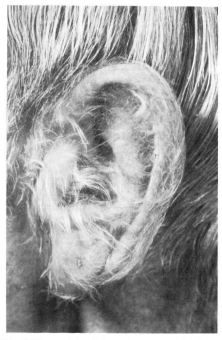

FIGURE 180-2. Hypertrichosis lanuginosa acquisita in a patient with lung cancer.

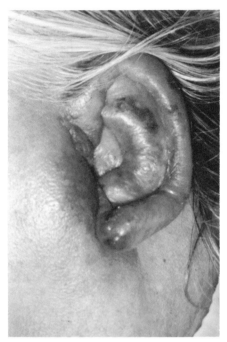

FIGURE 180-3. Patient with acute myelogenous leukemia and Sweet's syndrome. (See color plate.)

ized by anemia, absence of fever, and lack of neutrophilia.[53]

SUBCUTANEOUS FAT NECROSIS

Paraneoplastic subcutaneous fat necrosis is found in association with acinar cell adenocarcinoma of the pancreas (see also Chapter 71). Non-paraneoplastic subcutaneous fat necrosis is clinically similar and can occur with pancreatitis[54] and pancreatic pseudocyst,[55] presumably secondary to elevation of lipase, amylase, or trypsin. Both are frequently associated with polyarthralgia, which can affect most of the joints of the body, with ankle involvement being particularly common. The polyarthralgia is probably the result of fat necrosis of the periarticular soft tissue. Osteolytic bone lesions can occur secondary to intraosseous fat necrosis.[56] There is frequently a concomitant fever and eosinophilia.[57-59]

The skin lesions of subcutaneous fat necrosis may or may not be painful. Lesions occur most commonly on the legs, buttocks, and trunk and can present as either fluctuant, violaceous nodules, or ulcers that heal with scarring.

ERYTHEMA GYRATUM REPENS

Erythema gyratum repens is a cutaneous eruption consisting of concentric, raised, erythematous bands migrating in waves over the body surface and resulting in a wood-grain pattern (Fig. 180-4; see color plate).[60] These bands move quickly—up to 1 cm per day.[60] This eruption is almost pathognomonic for the presence of an internal malignant neoplasm. The erythematous bands can be flat or raised, and they are frequently surmounted by a fine marginal desquamation.

Almost all cases of erythema gyratum repens are paraneoplastic and are most commonly associated with carcinoma of the breast,[60-62] lung,[63-68] bladder,[69] prostate,[69] cervix,[70, 71] stomach, and esophagus, and with multiple myeloma.[72,73] All cases of erythema gyratum repens must be thoroughly investigated for an internal malignancy (see also Chapter 38).

PRURITUS

Paraneoplastic pruritus can occur in patients whose skin appears normal or xerotic. It is usually generalized and, unlike benign pruritus, often is paroxysmal and has a "burning" quality.[74]

Paraneoplastic pruritus is most commonly associated with leukemia and lymphoma, where it is usually a late symptom. Indeed, pruritus is one of the most common cutaneous manifestations of leukemia, probably exceeded only by purpura. The pruritus of leukemia is usually less severe than that associated with lymphoma and is more often generalized.[75, 76] The severity of the pruritus tends to parallel the course of the disease in both leukemia and lymphoma.[77] Severe and paroxysmal pruritus associated with bathing is a rather specific marker for polycythemia rubra vera, being present in half of patients.[78]

Pruritus associated with solid tumors is most commonly secondary to cancers of the pancreas and stomach,[76] and the appearance of severe pruritus after treatment of the primary tumor may herald a tumor recurrence.[79]

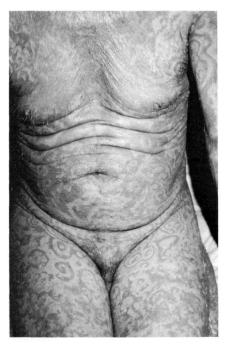

FIGURE 180-4. Erythema gyratum repens secondary to internal cancer. (See color plate.) (Courtesy of D. Lookingbill, M.D., Hershey, PA.)

Renal and hepatic involvement by primary or metastatic cancer can also produce pruritus secondary to the accumulation of pruritogenic metabolites in the skin.

MULTIPLE ERUPTIVE SEBORRHEIC KERATOSES

Multiple eruptive seborrheic keratoses, also known as the sign of Leser-Trélat, have been mentioned in association with many internal malignancies, including tumors of the stomach,[80, 81] breast,[82-84] prostate,[85] lung,[86] and colon[87-89]; malignant melanoma[90]; as well as lymphoma,[91-94] primary lymphoma of the brain,[95] and mycosis fungoides.[96] This condition has also been mentioned in association with hyperkeratosis of the palms and soles[80] and acanthosis nigricans.[97]

Evidence to support the presumed relationship of seborrheic keratoses to malignant disease is meager,[98] although there are many anecdotal reports. Most of the cancers so described are common. Seborrheic keratoses are ubiquitous in the elderly, who are also at greatest risk for developing cancer. To prove an uncommon causal relationship between a common cancer and a common skin sign is difficult.

Pseudoeruptive seborrheic keratoses can occur secondary to any inflammatory skin eoeruption.[99-101] Inflammatory dermatoses often tend to center around preexisting skin papillomas and seborrheic keratoses, making them suddenly appear to "erupt." It is common to see an increase in the prominence of seborrheic keratoses in patients with generalized dermatitis from any cause. The sign of Leser-Trélat may or may not be a true paraneoplastic entity.

COLLAGEN-VASCULAR DISEASE

Dermatomyositis in adults can be a marker for internal neoplasia, and the development of the dermatomyositis can predate the diagnosis of the cancer. Bronchogenic carcinoma is the most common associated tumor, with breast, ovary, cervix, and gastrointestinal tumors also reported in many patients.[102]

The association of cancer with adult dermatomyositis is real. In one series, approximately 37% of the 650 patients with dermatomyositis but not polymyositis had an underlying malignancy.[102] Other large series have found that roughly a quarter of patients with dermatomyositis had malignancies.[103, 104] In contrast, polymyositis is less strongly associated with cancer than dermatomyositis. In 153 patients with polymyositis-dermatomyositis, there was a malignant tumor in 8.5%, and in 19.2% of men over the age of 50 years.[105] More recent studies combining polymyositis patients with those with dermatomyositis show a similarly tenuous relationship with cancer.[106, 107] From this evidence, it would appear that adults with dermatomyositis, but perhaps not with polymyositis, should be investigated thoroughly for evidence of an associated malignant tumor.[108-111]

Systemic lupus erythematosus (SLE) is only rarely associated with malignant neoplasia. However, there are clearly recognized associations between SLE and thymoma[112-116] and lymphoma.[117-119]

PARANEOPLASTIC ACROKERATOSIS OF BAZEX

Paraneoplastic acrokeratosis of Bazex is a symmetrical dermatosis that most commonly affects the digits, nails, feet, ears, and nose with an erythematous to violaceous, scaling eruption that, except for a bluer hue, resembles psoriasis.[120] There is gradual progression of the eruption to include involvement of the cheeks, elbows, knees, and central trunk. Bullae and acanthosis nigricans can also be present. Nail changes include subungual hyperkeratosis, onychomadesis (shedding), flaky white surface changes to the nail plate, and periungual fissuring and suppuration.[121-123]

Bazex's syndrome is almost always associated with cancer, usually of the upper respiratory system, which includes cancer of the tongue, pharynx, esophagus, and lung. The eruption frequently predates evidence of the cancer.[120, 124]

ERYTHRODERMA

Erythroderma is a diffuse and generalized erythema and scaling of the entire skin surface that is usually not associated with malignancy (see Chapter 31). However, cancer-associated erythroderma is well documented and occurs mainly in association with hematologic malignancies, particularly T-cell leukemia and lymphoma, where there is direct infiltration of the skin by the malignant cells.[125, 126] True paraneoplastic erythroderma (i.e., not associated with direct tumor cell infiltration) occurs in association with solid tumors of lung, liver, prostate, thyroid, colon, pancreas, and stomach.[125] In these cases, erythroderma is usually a late sign.[126]

ACQUIRED ICHTHYOSIS

Paraneoplastic ichthyosis is a true hyperkeratosis and can be differentiated clinically and histologically from simple dry skin (xerosis) (Fig. 180-5). While the ichthyosis usually occurs as a late manifestation of a lymphoma, it may precede the diagnosis by several years.[127] In addition to lymphomas (Hodgkin's, non-Hodgkin's, and mycosis fungoides), and myeloma, acquired ichthyosis has been associated with cancer of the breast, cervix, and lung; Kaposi's sarcoma; leiomyosarcoma; and rhabdomyosarcoma.[128-133]

ACANTHOSIS NIGRICANS

Acanthosis nigricans can be of benign or malignant causation.[134] Benign acanthosis nigricans can be idiopathic, or secondary to obesity; to endocrinopathies such as diabetes, polycystic ovary disease (Stein-Leventhal

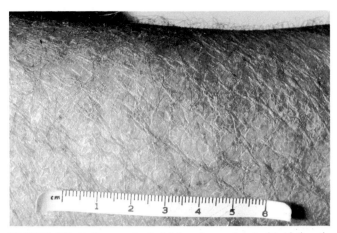

FIGURE 180–5. Paraneoplastic ichthyosis associated with histiocytic lymphoma. A distinct erythema is evident within the fissures.

syndrome), Addison's disease, pituitary tumors, or pinealoma; or to drugs such as nicotinic acid, glucocorticoids, and diethylstilbestrol.

Clinically, acanthosis nigricans is manifested as a gray-brown, symmetrical, velvety thickening of the skin with increased skinfold markings. The most common sites of involvement are the axilla, base of the neck, groin, and antecubital fossa. However, there can be generalized skin involvement including the mucous membranes. Pruritus is also a feature of acanthosis nigricans. Unlike the benign form, malignant acanthosis nigricans is usually of sudden onset, is rapidly progressive, and is often pruritic. Diffuse keratoderma involving the palms and soles is also common in the malignant form. Otherwise, acanthosis nigricans is clinically indistinguishable from benign acanthosis nigricans. The appearance of acanthosis nigricans can precede other evidence of the internal malignant disease. There may be an association with eruptive seborrheic keratoses.

Malignant acanthosis nigricans is usually due to an intra-abdominal tumor, with gastric adenocarcinoma being the most common.[135, 136] Acanthosis nigricans has also been described in association with a plethora of other malignant diseases, including carcinoma of the gallbladder,[137] liver,[138] and lung[139, 140]; Hodgkin's lymphoma[141]; and mycosis fungoides.[142–144]

Both benign and malignant acanthosis nigricans have similar histologic findings. The velvety texture of the condition is due to papillomatosis, and its color is in large part the result of hyperkeratosis.

HERPES GESTATIONIS

Herpes gestationis has been described in association with both hydatiform moles[145, 146] and germ cell tumors.[147]

PEMPHIGUS

Paraneoplastic pemphigus (see also Chapter 74) is a recently characterized distinct eruption with well-charac-

terized clinicopathologic features.[148] Morphologically the lesions can show features of both pemphigus and erythema multiforme, while histologically there is dyskeratosis of keratinocytes and basal layer vacuolization in addition to suprabasal acantholysis.[149] There is a well-defined association between both pemphigus vulgaris and pemphigus foliaceus and thymoma, with or without clinical myasthenia gravis.[150–154] Pemphigus vulgaris has also been associated with lymphoma, especially Hodgkin's disease,[155–157] and Kaposi's sarcoma.[158, 159] The relationship of pemphigus vulgaris to solid tumors is less well defined. Most reports are isolated cases that suggest, but do not prove, a causal relationship. It is possible that many of the earlier cases represented paraneoplastic pemphigus as described above.

BULLOUS PEMPHIGOID

Most cases of bullous pemphigoid temporally associated with cancer are age, rather than cancer related.[160, 161] There are rare reports that suggest that bullous pemphigoid can occur as a true paraneoplastic condition.[162, 163]

THROMBOPHLEBITIS

The association of peripheral thrombophlebitis (phlebothrombosis) with gastric carcinoma was first noted by Trousseau in the nineteenth century. Other cancers include tumors of pancreas, prostate, lung, liver, bowel, gallbladder, and ovary, as well as lymphoma and leukemia. The sometimes "migratory" nature of the thrombophlebitis probably relates to a generalized hypercoagulable state (Fig. 180–6).

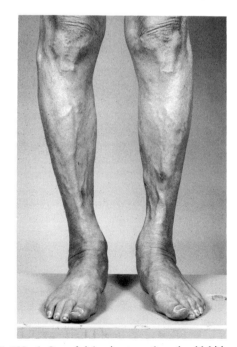

FIGURE 180–6. Superficial migratory thrombophlebitis of the left pretibial skin in a patient with pancreatic carcinoma.

Mondor's disease, usually benign but sometimes associated with breast cancer,[164, 165] is thrombophlebitis of the anterior chest wall presenting as a tender or nontender cord.

Patients younger than 50 years with deep venous thrombosis appear to have a very significant risk of occult cancer (relative risk, 19.0).[166] Paraneoplastic deep venous thrombosis is often associated with low hemoglobin and an eosinophilia.[167]

FLUSHING

Acquired pronounced flushing, usually of the central face and upper trunk, can be a manifestation of carcinoid tumors—the carcinoid syndrome.[168] These cancers can arise from bronchus, stomach, pancreas, and thyroid, or from teratomas. Tumors metastatic from the small bowel are the most likely to produce flushing, although flushing can also be produced from gastric tumors. Gastric tumor flushing typically occurs immediately after food intake. Carcinoid of the bronchus can be associated with a particularly prolonged flushing and with periorbital edema. Wheezing, diarrhea, and abdominal pain are also features of the carcinoid syndrome.[169]

The flushing of carcinoid syndrome can become gyrate as it fades. After many episodes, telangiectasia, chronic diffuse erythema, and cutaneous sclerosis can develop. A pellagra-like dermatosis, secondary to tryptophan diversion from niacin to serotonin production, can also occur in conjunction with carcinoid tumors.

Although the diarrhea seen in carcinoid appears to be secondary to serotonin release, the flushing of carcinoid syndrome appears to be secondary to the release of other vasoactive substances, such as substance P, from the tumor.[170] A somatostatin analogue (octreotide) can block at least some of the flushing.[171, 172]

Vasoactive substances causing flushing can also be released in patients with extensive localized, or systemic mastocytosis, and in patients with pheochromocytoma.

XANTHOMAS

Plane xanthomas are the most common paraneoplastic xanthomas, and the cancer association is usually with multiple myeloma.[173-176] Xanthomas have also been associated with other hematopoietic malignancies, including lymphocytic, myelocytic, and myelomonocytic leukemia; leukemic lymphocytic reticuloendotheliosis; diffuse histiocytic lymphoma; and cutaneous T-cell lymphoma.[177-183] Juvenile xanthogranuloma can be associated with juvenile chronic myeloid leukemia.[184]

Although most patients with paraneoplastic xanthomas are hyperlipoproteinemic, they may be normolipemic.[185] Purpura within xanthomas can be a feature of diffuse plane xanthomas associated with malignant disease.[186] Hemorrhagic bullae have been present in a normolipemic patient with xanthoma disseminatum and multiple myeloma.[187]

TELANGIECTASIA

Localized, grouped telangiectatic vessels on the anterior chest wall can be a marker for an underlying primary breast carcinoma.[188] When that is the case, an indurated, warm, subcutaneous plaque can be located immediately beneath the telangiectatic area. Telangiectatic vessels can also be the first evidence of dermal or subcutaneous metastases of breast cancer, as well as other malignant tumors. Progressive telangiectases have also been associated with distant carcinoid tumors (see Flushing), and with adenocarcinoma of the hepatic bile duct.[189]

PURPURA

Purpura from paraneoplastic causes can occur by a wide variety of mechanisms, including thrombocytopenia, consumption coagulopathy, hyper- or dysglobulinemia, vascular fragility, and vasculitis.

Lymphoma, most commonly Hodgkin's disease, is the most common cause of immune thrombocytopenic purpura (ITP) associated with malignant disease, and the ITP may precede other evidence of the lymphoma. Purpura can also result from disseminated intravascular coagulation (DIC). Paraneoplastic DIC is most commonly associated with acute lymphocytic or myelomonocytic leukemia, including T-cell acute lymphocytic leukemia.[190] While clinically significant DIC is relatively uncommon, many cancer patients have biochemical evidence of the process. Thrombotic thrombocytopenic purpura, when associated with cancer, is usually a late manifestation.

Purpura can also be associated with the hyperglobulinemia, such as that seen in association with multiple myeloma or lymphoma. Acral purpura, often associated with Raynaud's phenomenon, can be secondary to the presence of cryoglobulins. Purpura, usually palpable, can also be associated with vasculitis, or septicemia, which in turn can be associated with cancer.[191]

CUTANEOUS ISCHEMIA

Evidence of compromised peripheral circulation, such as Raynaud's phenomenon or frank gangrene, can be a marker for many malignant neoplasms.

Anecdotal accounts of peripheral ischemia have been associated with many malignant neoplasms, including carcinoma of the pancreas, stomach, small bowel, ovary, and kidney; polycythemia rubra vera; myeloma; lymphoma; and leukemia.[192-197] There is often an associated hyperviscosity secondary to hyperglobulinemia, including cryoglobulinemia, or to an increased number of circulating cells, causing sludging.

CONCLUSION

Paraneoplastic syndromes tell us something profound about the skin, and about the cancer. The tumor is producing a biologically active product that causes a distinctive skin reaction. The skin, in turn, reacts in a unique way to that tumor product, resulting in a distinctive cutaneous eruption. These skin eruptions also allow us to diagnose cancers at an earlier and, hopefully, more treatable stage. Paraneoplastic syndromes are important to us both as clinicians and as scientists.

References

1. McLean D. Cutaneous paraneoplastic syndromes. Arch Dermatol 1986;122:765-767.
2. McGavran MH, Under RH, Recant L, et al. A glucagon-secreting alpha-cell carcinoma of the pancreas. N Engl J Med 1966;274:1408-1413.
3. Wilkinson DS. Necrolytic migratory erythema with carcinoma of the pancreas. Trans St. John's Dermatol Soc 1973;59:244-250.
4. Mallinson CN, Bloom SR, Warin AP, et al. A glucagonoma syndrome. Lancet 1974;2:1-5.
5. Montenegro-Rodas F, Samaan NA. Glucagonoma tumors and syndrome. Curr Probl Cancer 1981;6:3-54.
6. Church RE, Crane WAJ. A cutaneous syndrome associated with islet-cell carcinoma of the pancreas. Br J Dermatol 1967;79:284-286.
7. Sweet RD. A dermatosis specifically associated with a tumour of pancreatic alpha cells. Br J Dermatol 1974;90:301-308.
8. Shupack JL, Berczeller PH, Stevens DM. The glucagonoma syndrome. J Dermatol Surg Oncol 1978;4:242-247.
9. Kahan RS, Perez-Figaredo RA, Neimanis A. Necrolytic migratory erythema. Arch Dermatol 1977;113:792-797.
10. Doyle J, Schroeter A, Rogers R. Hyperglucagonaemia and necrolytic migratory erythema in cirrhosis—possible pseudoglucagonoma syndrome. Br J Dermatol 1979;100:581-587.
11. Thivolet J. Necrolytic migratory erythema without glucagonoma. Arch Dermatol 1981;117:4.
12. Goodenberger D, Lawley T, Strober W, et al. Necrolytic migratory erythema without glucagonoma: Report of two cases. Arch Dermatol 1979;115:1429-1423.
13. Hegedus SI, Schorr WF. Acquired hypertrichosis lanuginosa and malignancy. Arch Dermatol 1972;106:84-88.
14. Knowling MA, Meakin JW, Hradsky NS, Pringle JF. Hypertrichosis lanuginosa acquisita associated with adenocarcinoma of the lung. Can Med Assoc J 1982;126:1308-1310.
15. van der Lugt L, Dudok de Wit C. Hypertrichosis lanuginosa acquisita. Dermatologica 1973;146:46-54.
16. Dyall-Smith D, Varigos G, Thomas R. Hypertrichosis lanuginosa acquisita and adenocarcinoma of the colon. Australas J Dermatol 1987;28:1-6.
17. Davies RA, Newman DM, Phillips MJ, et al. Acquired hypertrichosis lanuginosa as a sign of internal malignant disease. Can Med Assoc J 1978;118:1090-1096.
18. Fretzin DF. Malignant down. Arch Dermatol 1967;95:294-297.
19. Hensley GT, Glynn KP. Hypertrichosis lanuginosa as a sign of internal malignancy. Cancer 1969;24:1051-1056.
20. Lyell A, Whittle CH. Hypertrichosis lanuginosa, acquired type. Proc Roy Soc Med 1951;44:576-577.
21. Potter B, Fretzin DF. Hypertrichosis lanuginosa and anaplastic carcinoma. Arch Dermatol 1966;94:801-802.
22. Ikeya T, Izumi A, Suzuki M. Acquired hypertrichosis lanuginosa. Dermatologica 1978;156:274-282.
23. McLean DI, MacAulay JC. Hypertrichosis lanuginosa acquisita associated with pancreatic carcinoma. Br J Dermatol 1977;96:313-316.
24. Herzberg JJ, Potjan K., Gebauer D. Hypertrichose lanugineuse acquise. Ann Dermatol Symp (Paris) 1969;96:129-134.
25. Samson MK, Buroker TR, Henderson MD, et al. Acquired hypertrichosis lanuginosa. Cancer 1975;36:1519-1521.
26. Wadskow S, Bro-Jorgensen A, Sondergaard J. Acquired hypertrichosis lanuginosa. Arch Dermatol 1976;112:1442-1444.
27. Jemec GBE. Hypertrichosis lanuginosa acquisita. Arch Dermatol 1986;122(7):805-808.
28. Sweet RD. An acute febrile neutrophilic dermatosis. Br J Dermatol 1964;76:349-356.
29. Goldin D, Wilkinson DS. Pyoderma gangrenosum with chronic myeloid leukemia. Proc Roy Soc Med 1974;67:1239-1240.
30. Sheps M, Shapero H, Ramsay C. Bullous pyoderma gangrenosum and acute leukemia. Arch Dermatol 1978;114:1842-1843.
31. Burton JL. Sweet's syndrome, pyoderma gangrenosum and acute leukemia. Br J Dermatol 1980;102:239.
32. Cohen PR, Kurzrock R. Sweet's syndrome and malignancy. Am J Med 1987;82:1220-1226.
33. Krauser RE, Schumacher HR. The arthritis of Sweet's syndrome. Arthritis Rheum 1975;18:35-41.
34. Klock JC, Oken RL. Febrile neutrophilic dermatosis in acute myelogenous leukemia. Cancer 1976;37:922-927.
35. Goodfellow A, Calvert H. Sweet's syndrome and acute myeloid leukemia. Lancet 1979;2:478-479.
36. Spector JI, Zimbler H, Levine R, et al. Sweet's syndrome. JAMA 1980;244:1131-1132.
37. Meulders Q, Allal A, Egggers S, Ferrant A. Sweet's syndrome and myelodysplastic syndrome in a patient with metastatic breast carcinoma. Am J Med 1986;86:138-139.
38. Krilov LR, Jacobson M, Shende A. Acute febrile neutrophilic dermatosis (Sweet's syndrome). Pediatr Infect Dis J 1987; 6:77-79.
39. Tuncer AM. Acute lymphoblastic leukemia and Sweet's syndrome. Acta Haematol 1988;80:224.
40. Visani G, Patrizi A, Colombini R, et al. Sweet's syndrome and chronic lymphocytic leukemia associated with scirrhous breast cancer. Haematologica 1990;75:173-175.
41. Gisser SE. Acute febrile neutrophilic dermatosis (Sweet's syndrome) in a patient with hairy cell leukemia. Am J Dermatopathol 1983;5:283-288.
42. Apted JH. Sweet's syndrome (acute febrile neutrophilic dermatosis) associated with multiple myeloma. Australas J Dermatol 1984;25:15-17.
43. Berth-Jones J, Hutchinson PE. Sweet's syndrome and malignancy. Br J Dermatol 1989;121:123-127.
44. Krolikowski FJ, Reuter K, Shultis EW. Acute febrile neutrophilic dermatosis (Sweet's syndrome) associated with lymphoma. Hum Pathol 1985;16:520-522.
45. Vestey JP, Judge M. Sweet's syndrome and non-Hodgkin's lymphoma: The first report of this association. Acta Derm Venereol 1985;65:564-566.
46. Greer KE, Pruitt JL, Bishop GF. Acute febrile neutrophilic dermatosis (Sweet's syndrome). Arch Dermatol 1975;111: 1461-1463.
47. Shapiro L, Baraf CS, Richheimer LL. Sweet's syndrome (acute febrile neutrophilic dermatosis). Arch Dermatol 1971;103:81-84.
48. Nguyen KQ, Hurst CG, Pierson DL, Rodman OG. Sweet's syndrome and ovarian carcinoma. Cutis 1983;32:152-154.
49. Uchida H, Ikari Y, Hashizume S, et al. A case of Sweet's syndrome with early gastric cancer. Dermatologica 1990; 181:224-227.
50. Dyall-Smith D, Billson V. Sweet's syndrome associated with adenocarcinoma of the prostate. Australas J Dermatol 1988; 29:25-27.
51. Mali-Gerrits MG, Rampen FH. Acute febrile neutrophilic dermatosis (Sweet's syndrome) and adenocarcinoma of the rectum. Clin Exp Dermatol 1988;13:105-106.
52. Johnson ML, Grimwood RE. Leukocyte colony stimulating factors: A review of associated neutrophilic dermatoses and vasculitides. Arch Dermatol 1994;130:77-81.
53. Cohen PR, Kurzrock R. Sweet's syndrome and cancer. Clin Dermatol 1993;11:149-157.
54. Hughes PSH, Apisarnthanarax P, Mullins JF. Subcutaneous fat necrosis associated with pancreatic disease. Arch Dermatol 1975;111:506-510.
55. Zimmermann I, Urbaniak M, Karwowski A. Coexistence of arthritis, subcutaneous fat necrosis, and pseudocyst of pancreas. Rheumatol Int 1986;6:45-48.
56. Radin DR, Colletti PM, Forrester DM, Tang WW. Pancreatic acinar cell carcinoma with subcutaneous and intraosseous fat necrosis. Radiology 1986;158:67-68.
57. Belsky H, Cornell NW. Disseminated focal fat necrosis following radical pancreatico-duodenectomy for acinous carcinoma of head of pancreas. Ann Surg 1966;141:556-562.
58. MacMohon HE, Brown PA, Shen EM. Acinar cell carcinoma of

the pancreas with subcutaneous fat necrosis. Gastroenterology 1965;49:555–559.

59. Mullin GT, Caperton EM, Crespin SR, Williams RC. Arthritis and skin lesions resembling erythema nodosum in pancreatic disease. Ann Intern Med 1968;68:75–87.

60. Gammel JA. Erythema gyratum repens. Arch Dermatol Syph 1952;66:494–505.

61. Purdy MJ. Erythema gyratum repens. Arch Dermatol 1959;80:590–591.

62. Jacobs R, Eng AM, Solomon LM. Carcinoma of the breast, pemphigus vulgaris and gyrate erythema. Int J Dermatol 1978;17:221–224.

63. Schneeweiss J. Erythema gyratum repens. Proc Roy Soc. Med 1959;52:367–368.

64. Gold SC. Erythema gyratum repens. Proc Roy Soc Med 1959;52:367–368.

65. Solomon H. Erythema gyratum repens. Arch Dermatol 1969;100:639.

66. Olsen TG, Milroy SK, Jones-Olsen S. Erythema gyratum repens with associated squamous cell carcinoma of the lung. Cutis 1984;34(4):351–352.

67. Graham-Brown RA. Bullous pemphigoid with figurate erythema associated with carcinoma of the bronchus. Br J Dermatol 117(3):385–388.

68. Appell ML, Ward WQ, Tyring SK. Erythema gyratum repens. Cancer 1988;62(3):548–550.

69. Thomson J, Stankler L. Erythema gyratum repens. Br J Dermatol 1970;82:406–411.

70. Duperrat B, Guilaine J, Demay C. Erythema gyratum en rapport avec un carcinome cervical metastatique. Bull Soc Franc Derm Syph l961;68:20–21.

71. van Dijk E. Erythema gyratum repens. Dermatologica 1961;123:301–310.

72. Barriere H, Litoux P, Bureau B, et al. Erythema gyratum repens de gammel et ichtyose acquise associes a un cancer de l'oesophage. Ann Dermatol Venereol 1978;105:319–321.

73. Thivolet MM, Gallois P, Perrot H. Une Dermatose paraneoplasique meconnue: L'erythema giratum repens. Rev Lyonnaise de Med 1970;19:789–795.

74. Cormia FE, Domonkos AN. Cutaneous reactions to internal malignancy. Med Clin North Am 1965;49(Suppl. 3):655–680.

75. Wiener K. Skin Manifestations of Internal Disorders. London: H. Kimpton, 1947.

76. Newbold PCH. Skin markers of malignancy. Arch Dermatol 1970;102:680–692.

77. Feiner AS, Mahmood T, Wallner SF. Prognostic importance of pruritus in Hodgkin's disease. JAMA 1978;240:2738–2740.

78. Wasserman LR. The treatment of polycythemia vera. Semin Hematol 1976;13:57–78.

79. Shoenfeld Y, Weiberger A, Ben-Bassat M, Pinkhas J. Generalized pruritus in metastatic adenocarcinoma of the stomach. Dermatologica 1977;155:122–124.

80. Millard LG, Gould DJ. Hyperkeratosis of the palms and soles associated with internal malignancy and elevated levels of immunoreactive human growth hormone. Clin Exp Dermatol 1976;1:363–368.

81. Kameya S, Noda A, Isobe E, Watanabe T. The sign of Leser-Trélat associated with carcinoma of the stomach. Am J Gastroenterol 1988;83:664–666.

82. Lynch HT, Fusaro RM, Pester JA, Lynch JF. Leser-Trélat sign in mother and daughter with breast cancer. J Med Genet 1982;19:2218–221.

83. Friedman-Birnbaum R, Haim S. Seborrheic keratosis and papillomatosis: Markers of breast adenocarcinoma. Cutis 1983;32:161–162.

84. Venencie PY, Perry HO. Sign of Leser-Trélat: Report of two cases and review of the literature. J Am Acad Dermatol 1984;10:83–88.

85. Gitlin MC, Pirozzi DJ. The sign of Leser-Trélat. Arch Dermatol 1975;111:792.

86. Doll CD, McCagh MF, Welton WA. Sign of Leser-Trélat. JAMA 1977;238:236–237.

87. Walter JA, Lewis JG, Robinson TWE. Eruptive basal cell papillomata with carcinoma of the caecum. Proc Roy Soc Med 1972;65:595–596.

88. Kovary PM, Vakilzadeh F, Macher E, et al. Monoclonal gammopathy in scleredema. Arch Dermatol 1981;117:536–539.

89. Heng MC, Soo-Hoo K, Levin S, Petresek D. Linear seborrheic keratoses associated with underlying malignancy. J Am Acad Dermatol 1988;18:1316–1321.

90. Fanti PA, Metri M, Patrizi A. The sign of Leser-Trélat associated with malignant melanoma. Cutis 1989;44:39–41.

91. Safai B, Grant JM, Good RA. Cutaneous manifestation of internal malignancies (II). The sign of Leser-Trélat. Int Soc Trop Dermatol 1978;17:494–495.

92. Halevy S, Halevy J, Feuerman EJ. The sign of Leser-Trélat in association with lymphocytic lymphoma. Dermatologica 1980;161:183–186.

93. Wagner RF, Wagner KD. Malignant neoplasms and the Leser-Trélat sign. Arch Dermatol 1981;117:598–599.

94. Dantzig PI. Sign of Leser-Trélat. Arch Dermatol 1973;108:700–701.

95. Kaplan DL, Jegasothy B. The sign of Leser-Trélat associated with primary lymphoma of the brain. Cutis 1984;34:164–165.

96. Toonstra J, Ramselaar CG, Van der Putte SC. Leser-Trélat sign in mycosis fungoides. Dermatologica 1985;171:247–249.

97. Ballin DB. Acanthosis nigricans. Arch Dermatol 1955; 71:746–747.

98. Rampen HJ, Schwengle LE. The sign of Leser-Trélat, does it exist? J Am Acad Dermatol 1989;21:50–55.

99. Berman A, Winkelmann RK. Seborrheic keratosis. Arch Dermatol 1982;118:615–618.

100. Brown FC. Sign of Leser-Trélat. Arch Dermatol 1974;110:129.

101. Bruckner N, Katz RA, Hood AF. Pemphigus foliaceus resembling eruptive seborrheic keratoses. Arch Dermatol 1980;116:815–816.

102. Andreev VC. Skin manifestations in visceral cancer. In: Mali H, Nijmegen, eds. Current Problems in Dermatology. Basel: S Karger, 1978.

103. Bonnetblanc JM, Bernard P, Fayol J. Dermatomyositis and malignancy. Dermatologica 1990;180(4):212–6.

104. Callen JP, Hyla JF, Bole GG, Kay DR. The relationship of dermatomyositis and polymyositis to internal malignancy. Arch Dermatol 1980;116:295–298.

105. Bohan A, Peter JB, Bowman RL, Pearson CM. A computer assisted analysis of 153 patients with polymyositis and dermatomyositis. Medicine 1977;56:255–286.

106. Manchul LA, Jin A, Pritchard KI, et al. The frequency of malignant neoplasms in patients with polymyositis-dermatomyositis. A controlled study. Arch Intern Med 1985;145(10):1835–1839.

107. Lakhanpal S, Bunch TW, Ilstrup DM, Melton LJ. Polymyositis dermatomyositis and malignant lesions: Does an association exist? Mayo Clin Proc 1986;61(8):645–653.

108. Callen JP. The value of malignancy evaluation in patients with dermatomyositis. J Am Acad Dermatol 1982;6:253–259.

109. Richardson JB, Callen JP. Dermatomyositis and malignancy. Med Clin North Am 1989;73(5):1211–1220.

110. Basset-Sequin N, Roujeau JC, Gherardi R, et al. Prognostic factors and predictive signs of malignancy in adult dermatomyositis. Arch Dermatol 1990;126(5):633–637.

111. Cox NH, Lawrence CM, Langtry JA, Ive FA. Dermatomyositis. Disease associations and an evaluation of screen investigations for malignancy. Arch Dermatol 1990;126(1):61–65.

112. Singh BN. Thymoma presenting with polyserositis and the lupus erythematosus syndrome. Aust Ann Med 1969;18:55–58.

113. Larsson O. Thymoma and systemic lupus erythematosus in the same patient. Lancet 1963;2:665–666.

114. Kough RH, Barnes WT. Thymoma associated with erythroid aplasia, bullous skin eruption and the lupus erythematosus cell phenomenon. Ann Intern Med 1964;61:308–315.

115. Takigawa M, Hayakawa M. Thymoma with systemic lupus erythematosus, red blood cell aplasia, and herpes virus infection. Arch Dermatol 1974;110:99–102.

116. Beutner EH, Chorzelski TP, Hale WL, Hausmanowa-Petrusewicz I. Autoimmunity in concurrent myasthenia gravis and pemphigus erythematosus. JAMA 1968;203:845–849.

117. Green JA, Dawson AA, Walker W. Systemic lupus erythematosus and lymphoma. Lancet 1973;2:753–756.

118. Fournie GJ, Conte JJ, Delsol G, et al. Systemic lupus erythematosus and malignant histiocytosis. Lancet 1978;2:1305–1306.

119. Wyburn-Mason R. SLE and lymphoma. Lancet 1979;1:156.

120. Jacobsen F, Abildtrup N, Laursen S, et al. Acrokeratosis paraneoplastica (Bazex syndrome). Arch Dermatol 1984;120:502–504.

121. Bazex A, Griffiths A. Acrokeratosis paraneoplastica—a new cutaneous marker of malignancy. Br J Dermatol 1980;102:301–306.

122. Baran R. Paraneoplastic acrokeratosis of Bazex. Arch Dermatol 1977;113:1613.

123. Bazex A, Dupre A, Christol B, Cantala P. Paraneoplastic acrokeratosis. Fourteenth International Congress of Dermatology. Excerpta Medica, 1972;248:53–54.

124. Richard M, Giroux JM. Acrokeratosis paraneoplastica (Bazex syndrome). J Am Acad Dermatol 1987;16:178–183.

125. Nicolis GD, Helwig EB. Exfoliative dermatitis. Arch Dermatol 1973;108:788–797.

126. Abrahams I, McCarthy JT, Sanders SL. 101 cases of exfoliative dermatitis. Arch Dermatol 1963;87:96–101.

127. Stevanovic DV. Hodgkin's disease of the skin. Arch Dermatol 1960;82:96–99.

128. Krakowski A, Brenner S, Covo J, et al. Acquired ichthyosis in Kaposi's sarcoma. Dermatologica 1973;147:348–351.

129. Majekodunmi AE, Femi-Pearse D. Ichthyosis: Early manifestations of intestinal leiomyosarcoma. Br Med J 1974;3:734.

130. Flint GL, Flam M, Soter NA. Acquired ichthyosis. Arch Dermatol 1975;111:1446–1447.

131. Young, Steinman HK. Acquired ichthyosis in a patient with acquired immunodeficiency syndrome and Kaposi's sarcoma. J Am Acad Dermatol 1987;16:395–396.

132. Bechtel MA, Callen JP. Disseminated Kaposi's sarcoma in a patient with acquired ichthyosis. J Surg Oncol 1984;26:22–26.

133. Grattan CE, Williams DM, Raafat F, Manna V. Acquired ichthyosis in a child with rhabdomyosarcoma. Pediatr Dermatol 1988;5:167–169.

134. Brown J, Winkelmann RK. Acanthosis nigricans: A study of 90 cases. Medicine 1968;47:33–51.

135. Curth HO. Significance of acanthosis nigricans. Arch Dermatol 1952;66:80–100.

136. Rigel DS, Jacobs MI. Malignant acanthosis nigricans: A review. J Dermatol Surg Oncol 1980;6:923–927.

137. Arora A, Choudhuri G, Tandon RK. Acanthosis nigricans associated with adenocarcinoma of the gallbladder. Am J Gastroenterol 1985;80:896–897.

138. Muramatsu T, Matsumoto H, Yamashina Y, et al. Pemphigus foliaceus associated with acanthosis nigricans–like lesions and hepatocellular carcinoma. Int J Dermatol 1989;28:462–463.

139. Horiuchi Y, Katsuoka K, Yoshimura H, et al. Acanthosis nigricans and Leser-Trélat sign associated with squamous cell carcinoma and adenocarcinoma of the lung. Int J Dermatol 1986;25:459–460.

140. Menzies DG, Choo-Kang J, Buxton PK, Campbell IW. Acanthosis nigricans associated with alveolar cell carcinoma. Thorax 1988;43:414–415.

141. Janier M, Blanchet-Bardon C, Bonvalet D, et al. Malignant acanthosis nigricans associated with non-Hodgkin's lymphoma. Dermatologica 1988;176:133–137.

142. Willemze R, Scheffer E, Van Vloten WA. Mycosis fungoides simulating acanthosis nigricans. Am J Dermatopathol 1985;7:367–371.

143. Neill SM, Monk BE, du Vivier A. Mycosis fungoides associated with acanthosis nigricans. J Roy Soc Med 1985;78:79–81.

144. Schweitzer WJ, Goldin HM, Bronson DM, Brody PE. Acanthosis nigricans associated with mycosis fungoides. J Am Acad Dermatol 1988;19:951–953.

145. Dupont C. Herpes gestationis with hydatidiform mole. Trans St. John's Hosp Derm Soc 1974;60:103.

146. Tillman WG. Herpes gestationis with hydatidiform mole and chorion epithelioma. Br Med J 1950;1:1471.

147. Halkier-Sorensen L, Beck HI, Sogaard H. Herpes gestationis in association with neoplasma malignum generalisata. Acta Derm Venereol Suppl (Stockh) 1985;120:96–100.

148. Mehregan D, Oursler J, Leiferman K, et al. Paraneoplastic pemphigus: A subset of patients with pemphigus and neoplasia. J Cutan Pathol 1993;10:203–210.

149. Horn T, Anhalt G. Histologic features of paraneoplastic pemphigus. Arch Dermatol 1992;128:1091–1095.

150. Peck SM, Osserman KE, Weiner LB, et al. Studies in bullous disease. N Engl J Med 1968;279:951–958.

151. Stillman MA, Baer RL. Pemphigus and thymoma. Acta Derm Venereol (Stockh) 1972;52:393–397.

152. Vetters JM, Saikia NK, Wood J, Simpson JA. Pemphigus vulgaris and myasthenia gravis. Br J Dermatol 1973;88:437–441.

153. Safai B, Gupta S, Good RA. Pemphigus vulgaris associated with a syndrome of immunodeficiency and thymoma: A case report. Clin Exp Dermatol 1978;3:129–134.

154. Imamura S, Takigawa M, Ikai K, et al. Pemphigus foliaceus, myasthenia gravis, thymoma and red cell aplasia. Clin Exp Dermatol 1978;3:285–291.

155. Naysmith A, Hancock BW. Hodgkin's disease and pemphigus. Br J Dermatol 1976;94:695–696.

156. Sood VD, Pasricha JS. Pemphigus and Hodgkin's disease. Br J Dermatol 1974;90:575–578.

157. Saikia NK. Extraction of pemphigus antibodies from a lymphoid neoplasm and its possible relationship to pemphigus vulgaris. Br J Dermatol 1972;86:411–414.

158. Pisanty S, Garfunkel A. Kaposi's sarcoma. J Oral Med 1970;25:89–92.

159. Rosenmann E. Kaposi's disease in a patient with pemphigus vulgaris. Isr J Med Sci 1966;2:269–274.

160. Stone SP, Schroeder AL. Bullous pemphigoid and associated malignant neoplasms. Arch Dermatol 1975;111:991–994.

161. Lindelöf B, Islam N, Eklund G, Arfors L. Pemphigoid and cancer. Arch Dermatol 1990;126:66–68.

162. Rook AJ. A pemphigoid eruption associated with carcinoma of the bronchus. Trans St. John's Hosp Derm Soc 1968;54:152–154.

163. Goodnough LT, Muir A. Bullous pemphigoid as a manifestation of chronic lymphocytic leukemia. Arch Intern Med 1980;140:1526–1527.

164. Vieta JO, Heymann AD. Mondor's disease. N Y State J Med 1977;77:120–121.

165. Miller DR, Cesario TC, Slater LM. Mondor's disease associated with metastatic axillary nodes. Cancer 1985;56:903–904.

166. Goldberg RJ, Seneff M, Gore JM, et al. Occult malignant neoplasm in patients with deep venous thrombosis. Arch Intern Med 1987;147:251–253.

167. Aderka D, Brown A, Zelikovski A, Pinkhas J. Idiopathic deep vein thrombosis in an apparently healthy patient as a premonitory sign of occult cancer. Cancer 1986;57:1846–1849.

168. Thorn GW, Adams RD, Braunwald E, et al. Harrison's Principles of Internal Medicine, 8th edition. New York: McGraw-Hill, 1977.

169. Aldrich LB, Moattari AR, Vinik AI. Distinguishing features of idiopathic flushing and carcinoid syndrome. Arch Intern Med 1988;148(12):2614–2618.

170. Vinik AI, Gonin J, England BG, et al. Plasma substance P in neuroendocrine tumors and idiopathic flushing. J Clin Endocrinol Metab 1990;70:1702–1709.

171. Balks HJ, Conlon JM, Creutzfeldt W, Stockmann F. Effect of a long-acting somatostatin analogue (octreotide) on circulating tachykinins and the pentastrin-induced carcinoid flush. Eur J Clin Pharmacol 1989;36:133–137.

172. Oberg K, Norheim I, Theodorsson E, et al. The effects of octreotide on basal and stimulated hormone levels in patients with carcinoid syndrome. J Clin Endocrinol Metab 1989;68:796–800.

173. Marien KJC, Smeenk G. Plane xanthomata associated with multiple myeloma and hyperlipoproteinemia. Br J Dermatol 1975;93:407–415.

174. Moschella SL. Plane xanthomatosis associated with myelomatosis. Arch Dermatol 1970;101:683–687.

175. Wilson DE, Flowers CM, Hershgold EJ, Eaton RP. Multiple myeloma, cryoglobulinemia and xanthomatosis. Am J Med 1975;59:721–729.

176. Roberts-Thomson PJ, Venables GS, Onitriri AC, Lewis B. Polymeric IgA myeloma, hyperlipidaemia and xanthomatosis: A further case and review. Postgrad Med J 1975;51:44–51.

177. Lynch PJ, Winkelmann RK. Generalized plane xanthoma and systemic disease. Arch Dermatol 1966;93:639–646.

178. Haqqani MT, Hunter RD. Normolipemic plane xanthoma and histiocytic lymphoma. Arch Dermatol 1976;112:1470–1471.

179. Mays JA, Neerhout RC, Bagby GC, Koler RD. Juvenile chronic granulocytic leukemia. Am J Dis Children 1980;134:654–658.

180. O'Donnell J, Tansey P, Chunt P, et al. Acute myelomonocytic

leukemia presenting as a xanthomatous skin eruption. J Clin Pathol 1982;35:1200–1203.

181. Statham B, Fairris G, Cotterill J. Atypical eruptive histiocytosis—a marker of underlying malignancy? Br J Dermatol 1982;110:103–105.

182. McCadden ME, Glick AD, King LE Jr. Mycosis fungoides associated with dystrophic xanthomatosis. Arch Dermatol 1987;123:91–94.

183. Vail JT Jr, Adler KR, Rotherberg J. Cutaneous xanthomas associated with chronic myelomonocytic leukemia. Arch Dermatol 1985;121:1318–1320.

184. Cooper PH, Frierson HF, Kayne AL, Sabio H. Association of juvenile xanthogranuloma with juvenile myeloid leukemia. Arch Dermatol 1984;120:371–375.

185. Feingold KR, Castro GR, Ishikawa Y, et al. Cutaneous xanthoma in association with paraproteinemia in the absence of hyperlipidemia. J Clin Invest 1989;83:796–802.

186. Weber G, Pilgrim M. Contribution to the knowledge of normolipaemic plane xanthomatosis. Br J Dermatol 1974;90:465–469.

187. Maize JC, Ahmed AR, Provost TT. Xanthoma disseminatum and multiple myeloma. Arch Dermatol 1974;110:758–761.

188. Weber FP. Bilateral thoracic zosteroid spreading marginate telangiectasia—probably a variety of "carcinoma erysipelatodes" (C. Rasch)—associated with unilateral mammary carcinoma, and better termed "carcinoma telangiectaticum." Br J Dermatol 1933;45:418–423.

189. Rosenbaum FF, Santer DG, Claudon DB. Essential telangiectasia, pulmonic and tricuspid stenosis, and neoplastic liver disease: A possible new clinical syndrome. J Lab Clin Med 1953;42:941–942.

190. French AJ, Lilleyman JS. Bleeding tendency of T-cell lymphoblastic leukemia. Lancet 1979;2:469–470.

191. Selly WB, Zolin WD. Disseminate intradermal bacterial colonization presenting as palpable purpura in lymphoblastic leukemia. J Am Acad Dermatol 1983;8:714–717.

192. Hawley PR, Johnston AW, Rankin JT. Association between digital ischaemia and malignant disease. Br Med J 1967;3:208–212.

193. Palmer HM. Digital vascular disease and malignant disease. Br J Dermatol 1974;91:476–477.

194. Palmer HM, Vedi KK. Digital ischaemia and malignant disease. Practitioner 1974;213:819–822.

195. Brown GE, Giffin HZ. Peripheral arterial disease in polycythemia vera. Arch Intern Med 1930;46:705–717.

196. Fagrell B, Mellstedt H. Polycythemia vera as a cause of ischemic digital necrosis. Acta Chir Scand 1978;144:129–132.

197. Narita H, Ogata K, Kikuchi I, Inoue S. A case of cryoglobulinemic gangrene in myeloma with fatal outcome despite successful skin grafting. Dermatologica 1980;160:125–130.

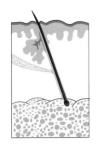

chapter 181

Hirsutism and Its Related Endocrine Disorders

ARTHUR C. HUNTLEY

DEFINITION

Hirsutism is the abnormal growth of terminal hair in androgen-sensitive areas such as the moustache and beard regions (Fig. 181–1). The presence of terminal hair in these regions is not necessarily abnormal for some women and the determination of whether a patient has hirsutism must take into consideration the normal hair pattern for the genetic makeup of the individual.

Excess hair may also be present in *hypertrichosis*, in which uniformly long smooth, silky hair is distributed over the entire body rather than just the androgen-sensitive areas. Hypertrichosis is a common occurrence when the patient is on certain medication (cyclosporin, minoxidil), in association with certain malignancies, and accompanying metabolic disorders in hypothyroidism, anorexia nervosa, and starvation.

In hirsutism, a woman has terminal hair in the characteristic male distribution of androgen-responsive areas, including the moustache and beard regions, the pubic escutcheon, the back, chest, and thighs. The upper lip, chin, lower abdomen, and thighs are the most sensitive areas to evaluate.[1] Hirsutism is usually described according to the density of terminal hair in these target areas. A scoring system that allows for an objective evaluation is useful for diagnosis and measuring the success of therapy.

CLINICAL PRESENTATION

Polycystic Ovarian Syndrome

In the majority of hirsute women, *polycystic ovarian syndrome,* a group of related disorders that culminate in the development of chronic anovulation, hyperadrenogenism, relative insulin resistance, and acanthosis nigricans, is considered. The anovulation is usually perimenarchal in onset. When the hirsutism occurs together with menstrual disturbances and results in long-lasting amenorrhea, Stein-Leventhal syndrome should be considered. Further signs of virilization such as hypertrophy of the clitoris or husky voice are rare. Obesity is common. Enlarged cystic ovaries are decisive for diagnosis.

Laboratory evaluation indicates a high serum luteinizing hormone (LH) level and normal or low follicle-stimulating hormone (FSH) concentrations (i.e., increased ratio of LH to FSH). Testosterone concentrations in polycystic ovarian syndrome patients are usually mildly elevated (not greater than 200 ng/dl).[2]

Ovarian Tumors

Neoplasms of the ovary may be responsible for excess ovarian androgen production either by direct secretion of testosterone or by stimulation of adjacent ovarian stroma and thecal tissue to secrete this hormone. Multiple tumor types have been noted for androgen production, including tumors of the granulosa theca cell and Sertoli-Leydig cell, hilar and lipoidal cell tumors, and gonadoblastomas. Serum free testosterone levels may be only slightly elevated but are generally above 200 ng/dl. Patients who present with virilization (acne and hirsutism) should be evaluated for one of these tumors. Transvaginal ultrasonography can usually give a satisfactory image of the ovaries. In the presence of an adnexal mass, a laparoscopy seems warranted.

Cushing's Disease and Syndrome

Cushing's disease and syndrome are conditions of hypercortisolism, which may be accompanied by hirsutism.

1853

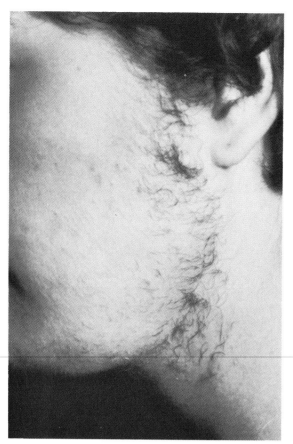

FIGURE 181-1. Hirsutism of the face in a patient with hyperandrogenemia. (From Bergfeld WF. Hair disorders. In: Moschella SL, Hurley HJ, eds. Dermatology, 3rd edition. Philadelphia: WB Saunders Co., 1992:1553.)

In Cushing's disease the secretion is due to excess pituitary adrenocorticotropic hormone (ACTH) secretion. In Cushing's syndrome, the hypercortisolism is pituitary independent. The clinical diagnosis is usually made on the presence of common physical signs such as moon facies and buffalo hump, and the hirsutism is a secondary consideration. The traditional tests are a 24-hour urinary cortisol (normal levels less than 100 ng/24 hours) or low-dose dexamethasone suppression testing. The corticotropin-releasing hormone is an alternative evaluation that may be performed on ambulatory patients. There is some evidence that the initial test of choice may become overnight high-dose dexamethasone followed by plasma ACTH measurements by radioimmunoassay.[4] Diagnosis is still best established by using 24-hour urine free cortisol. If cortisol is elevated, plasma ACTH is measured.

Hyperprolactinemia

Some patients with elevated prolactin from pituitary tumors also develop hirsutism. The mechanisms of hypercortisolism is not understood in these patients. When patients present with hirsutism and inappropriate lactation, serum prolactin evaluation is warranted.

Congenital Adrenal Hyperplasia

Congenital adrenal hyperplasia occurs when there is a partial blockage of the synthesis of cortisol. This form of adrenal hyperandrogenism results from excess corticotropin levels and thus increased androgen secretion. Several enzymes are associated with this syndrome. The genes encoding each of the steroid biosynthetic enzymes have now been cloned, and the mutations in these genes that cause the various forms of congenital adrenal hyperplasia are being determined.[5] These enzyme deficiencies usually manifest early in life, with the patient developing ambiguous genitalia. However a subset of these deficiencies is considered to be late-onset or attenuated, in which the clinical manifestations are hirsutism or anovulation.

The measurement of baseline steroid levels in hirsute patients may not be helpful in differentiating among the causes of increased androgen production. A substantial proportion of women with hirsutism have mild defects in adrenal steroidogenesis, revealed by an ACTH stimulation test, that are indicative of late-onset (non-classic) congenital adrenal hyperplasia.[6]

The most common enzyme causing adrenal hyperplasia is 21-hydroxylase deficiency. The diagnosis is usually made by demonstration of an increased concentration of 17-hydroxyprogesterone, the substrate for the deficient enzyme.

11β-hydroxylase deficiency is a much less common condition, present in approximately 0.8% of hirsute women. The usual screening test is measurement of 17-hydroxyprogesterone. Levels below 200 ng/dl are usually normal, whereas 800 ng/dl are usually associated with the enzyme deficiency. Levels between 200 and 800 ng/dl warrant further testing with ACTH-stimulation testing. Diagnosis is made by measuring 11 deoxycortisol after adrenal stimulation.[7]

Adrenal Neoplasms

Adenoma and carcinoma of the adrenal gland may cause very high dehydroepiandrosterone sulfase (DHEA-S) or testosterone levels. Evaluation usually includes computed tomography and magnetic resonance imaging.

Idiopathic Hirsutism (?Peripheral Increased Androgen Metabolism)

Many patients have hirsutism in the face of normal adrenal and ovarian function, including normal levels of bound and free serum testosterone. This subset of patients has been hypothesized to have an increased metabolism of testosterone within the target tissue.[8] This condition is supposedly characterized by increased 5 α-reductase activity resulting in increased conversion of testosterone to dihydrotestosterone. Tests have not substantiated this theory because dihydrotestosterone metabolites such as androsterone sulfate can be measured and they are normal.[9] It is important to note that there still is a subset of women with hirsutism of undetermined cause.

PATHOLOGY

Other than an increased number of terminal hairs, there is no specific histopathologic finding to establish the diagnosis of hirsutism.

PATHOGENESIS AND ETIOLOGY

In women, there are three sources of circulating androgens: ovarian, adrenal, and peripheral tissue conversion of precursors. The ovaries and adrenal glands produce testosterone, androstenedione, and dehydroepiandrosterone (DHEA). The adrenal cortex also produces DHEA-S. Of these compounds, testosterone is the physiologically active compound. Normal daily production of testosterone in women is 0.2 to 0.3 mg, with approximately one third coming from ovarian production and the remainder coming from ovarian and adrenal precursors metabolized to testosterone by peripheral tissue. Ovarian and perhaps adrenal testosterone production are normally regulated by the pituitary via LH.

Androstenedione, DHEA, and DHEA-S, although designated as weak androgens, are best thought of as androgen precursors because they can be converted to testosterone in peripheral tissues. Androstenedione is a weak androgen secreted about equally by adrenal and ovarian tissue. DHEA-S is also a relatively weak androgen, but this one is produced almost exclusively by the adrenal glands (about 20 mg/day). Both DHEA and DHEA-S secretion by the adrenal glands are thought to be episodic in synchrony with secretion of cortisol.[10] This production appears to be gonadotropin independent and ACTH responsive.

Peripheral conversion of androgen precursors appears to be the major source of circulating androgen. When human skin is incubated with DHEA, androstenedione and testosterone are formed,[11] as well as DHEA-S, Δ^5-androstene-3β, 17β-diol, and Δ^4-androstenedione.[12] In general, serum testosterone reflects ovarian androgen production more than adrenal, and DHEA-S is used as an indicator of adrenal androgen production.

The precursor compound for androgens and for other steroids is cholesterol. The conversion of cholesterol into an array of compounds including cortisone is dependent on a number of enzymes, including 3β-OL dehydrogenase, 17-hydroxylase, 21-hydroxylase, and 11-hydroxylase. The absence or deficiency of any of these enzymes can result in a shunting of this biosynthetic pathway to the production of androgens, resulting in a virilizing syndrome and hirsutism. (see Chapter 133)

DIAGNOSIS AND DIFFERENTIAL DIAGNOSIS

The baseline examination utilizing a scale to indicate the extent of the hirsutism can be used for future evaluation of treatment efficacy. Examination is performed to rule out a number of conditions such as Cushing's syndrome, prolactinoma, gonadal dysgenesis, and exogenous hormone. The presence of virilization as demonstrated by concurrent acne, deepening of the voice,

TABLE 181–1. Differential Diagnosis of Hirsutism
Hypertrichosis Secondary to
Medications (cyclosporine, minoxidil) Malignancies Metabolic disorders (porphyria, hypothyroidism, mucopolysaccharidosis, anorexia nervosa, starvation) Congenital generalized
Androgenic Hirsutism in Women
Polycystic ovarian syndrome Ovarian tumors Cushing's disease and syndrome Acromegaly Hyperprolactinemia Congenital adrenal hyperplasia: (21-hydroxylase deficiency, 11ß-hydroxylase deficiency) Adrenal neoplasms Medications (androgens, anabolic steroids, diazoxide, phenytoin (Dilantin), danazol, progesterone)
Idiopathic Hirsutism

amenorrhea, increased muscle mass, and clitoral hypertrophy may indicate the presence of severe androgen excess and warrants an exhaustive investigation for serious disease, such as an androgen-secreting tumor. (Table 181–1).[13]

Although it has long been the rule that patients who have normal menses do not need a hormonal evaluation, a study of 129 women presenting with the chief complaint of hirsutism reported that half of the 40% with regular menstrual cycles had elevated levels of one or more androgens.[14] It is therefore suggested that a screening work-up be done on all patients with hirsutism. This should include a serum free testosterone, LH, FSH, DHEA, and DHEA-S, 17α-hydroxyprogesterone, and an ultrasound examination (for polycystic ovaries).

For patients with virilism, the investigation involves imaging, selective venous sampling, or laparotomy.

TREATMENT OF HIRSUTISM

General Considerations

Before initiating therapy for patients with hirsutism, there should be an accurate identification of any underlying abnormalities in androgen production or metabolism. It is important to rule out the presence of a malignancy, especially in patients with more virilization. History should be taken to insure that the hirsutism is not due to medications such as androgens, anabolic steroids, danazol, and progestational compounds.

Medical treatment usually manages to decrease the rate of hair growth but may not eliminate the need for physical removal of undesired hair.[15] Areas of the body that appear to respond to medical therapy include the hair on the face, chest, abdomen, and upper thighs. In

TABLE 181–2. Treatment of Hirsutism
Elevated Levels of 17α-hydroxyprogesterone and Dehydroepiandrosterone Sulfate
Glucocorticoid suppression
Idiopathic Hirsutism
Anti-androgens: estrogen-dominant oral contraceptive Spironolactone Synthetic progestins: medroxyprogesterone acetate and megestrol Dexamethasone Gonadotropin-releasing hormone agonist Ketoconazole Cyproterone acetate Flutamide

contrast, hair around the nipples, on the arms, back, and lower legs responds less well. The medical therapy used in the treatment of hirsutism is not used during pregnancy.

In the presence of elevated levels of 17 α-hydroxyprogesterone and DHEA-S, the presumptive diagnosis is adrenal source of androgens. The treatment of choice is then glucocorticoid suppression (Table 181–2).

When there is hirsutism in the setting of normal menses and normal serum testosterone and DHEA-S, the diagnosis is usually considered to be idiopathic hirsutism, or perhaps a disorder of peripheral androgen metabolism such as increased peripheral conversion of testosterone to dihydrotestosterone. The antiandrogens are usually the drug of choice.

The anti-androgens are usually effective and are first-line agents for most causes of hirsutism. The combination of spironolactone and oral contraceptive is excellent for treating this condition.[16] Oral contraceptives serve to prevent a contraindicated pregnancy as well as to control dysfunctional bleeding caused by the spironolactone. Patients with adrenal hyperplasia are usually treated with either dexamethasone or anti-androgens. Spironolactone may also be given in combination with dexamethasone.

Specific Agents

Oral Contraceptives

The most commonly used agents for the treatment of hirsutism, oral contraceptives suppress the secretion of LH, increase sex hormone–binding globulin concentrations, and decrease testosterone and DHEA-S concentrations. Oral contraceptives are effective for lowering androgens from both ovarian and adrenal sources. In addition, with increased levels of sex hormone–binding globulin, there is less free (active) testosterone. Recommended oral contraceptives for this treatment are estrogen dominant and contain progestin with minimal androgenic activity, such as ethynodiol diacetate. Side effects include increasing plasma lipids. Oral contracep-

tives that contain norgestrel appear to be less effective than those with norethindrone or ethynodiol diacetate.[17] Once the hirsutism has been treated, changing to bimonthly treatment may be effective in maintaining the remission.[18]

Synthetic Progestins

Synthetic progestins alone may be used to treat hirsutism. Both medroxyprogesterone acetate and megestrol are weak anti-androgens and suppress gonadotropin secretion and testosterone production. Administration is continuous at 20 to 40 mg per day orally or 150 mg intramuscularly every 6 weeks to 3 months. Reported side effects include disorders of thrombosis, hepatic dysfunction, depression, and water retention or weight gain.

Dexamethasone

Dexamethasone is often successful in treatment of hirsutism of ovarian or adrenal origin. It can be given orally in doses as low as 0.25 mg every other day. Doses higher than 0.5 mg daily have the potential risk of suppressing the adrenal-pituitary axis. Dexamethasone may be the agent of choice in treatment of congenital adrenal hyperplasia. In these cases, dosages up to 1.0 mg daily may be needed to suppress corticotropin secretion.

Gonadotropin-releasing Hormone Agonists

These drugs work by desensitization of gonadotropin-releasing hormone receptors on the gonadotropes, resulting in decreased gonadotropin secretion. Side effects resulting from hyperestrogenemia include irregular menstrual bleeding, endometrial atrophy, hot flushes, vaginal dryness, and osteoporosis. These agents appear to have demonstrated efficacy in polycystic ovarian disease.

Ketoconazole

As an oral antifungal drug, ketoconazole is well known for feminizing side effects in men. This agent inhibits cytochrome P-450–dependent enzymes involved in adrenal and gonadal steroid synthesis. It may be useful in a number of instances including polycystic ovarian disease, adrenal adenoma or carcinoma, Cushing's disease, and idiopathic hirsutism. The anti-androgen doses range from 400 to 1200 mg per day. Side effects include a rare hepatotoxicity, hair loss, nausea, fatigue, headaches, and vaginal bleeding. It should be reserved for patients with hyperandrogenism unresponsive to other medical therapy.[19]

Spironolactone

This is a potassium-sparing diuretic that has anti-androgen side effects. It acts by inhibiting 5 α-reductase activity and interfering with binding of dihydrotestosterone to its receptor. Testosterone synthesis is also inhibited by spironolactone. It is administered in dosages from 50 to 200 mg per day. Larger doses appear to be more efficacious. Side effects include abnormal menstrual bleeding and breast tenderness.

Cyproterone Acetate

This anti-androgen compound is not available in the United States but is widely used in Europe for the treatment of hirsutism. It is a synthetic progestin that works as a competitive inhibitor of testosterone and dihydrotestosterone to androgen receptors, and also inhibits gonadotropin secretion. Because it induces hepatic enzymes, it increases the metabolic clearance of testosterone. It is administered in a dosage of 50 to 200 mg per day on days 5 to 14 of the menstrual cycle or as a monthly 300-mg intramuscular injection. Side effects include weight gain, abnormal menstrual bleeding, fatigue, nausea, and headache.

Flutamide

Although not yet available in the United States, this nonsteroidal anti-androgen appears to act solely through the blockade of the androgen receptor. It is often administered in conjunction with oral contraceptives to inhibit gonadotropin rise (and to prevent pregnancy). Recommended dosages are 250 mg twice daily. Side effects include the deterioration of menstrual function and dry skin. Favorable effects may be noted within 3 months of therapy.[20]

References

1. Derksen J, Moolenaar AJ, Van Seters AP, Kock DF. Semiquantitative assessment of hirsutism in Dutch women. Br J Dermatol 1993;128(3):259–263.
2. Kessel B, Liu J. Clinical and laboratory evaluation of hirsutism. Clin Obstet Gynecol 1991;34:805–816.
3. Chang RJ, Nakamura RM, Judd HJ, Kaplan SA. Insulin resistance in nonobese patients with polycystic ovarian disease. J Clin Endocrinol Metab 1983;57:356.
4. Kaye TB, Crapo L. The Cushing syndrome: An update on diagnostic tests [see comments]. Ann Intern Med 1990;112(6):434–444.
5. Miller WL. Congenital adrenal hyperplasias. Endocrinol Metab Clin North Am 1991;20(4):721–749.
6. Siegel SF, Finegold DN, Lanes R, Lee PA. ACTH stimulation tests and plasma dehydroepiandrosterone sulfate levels in women with hirsutism [see comments]. N Engl J Med 1990;323(13):849–854.
7. Azziz R, Boots LR, Parker CR Jr, et al. 11 beta-hydroxylase deficiency in hyperandrogenism. Fertil Steril 1991;55(4):733–741.
8. Kettel LM. Management of hirsutism. West J Med 1992;156:648–649.
9. Zwicker H, Rittmaster RS. Androsterone sulfate: Physiology and clinical significance in hirsute women. J Clin Endocrinol Metab 1993;76:112–116.
10. Rosenfeld RS, Rosenberg BJ, Fukushima DK, et al. 24-hour secretory pattern of dehydroisoandrosterone and dehydroisoandrosterone sulfate. J Clin Endocrinol Metab 1975;40:850–855.
11. Cameron ERD, Baillie AH, Mailne JA, Thompson J. Transformation in vitro of (7α-³H)-dehydroepiandrosterone to (³H)-testosterone by skin from men. J Endocrinol 1966;35:xix–xx.
12. Gallegos AJ, Berliner DL. Transformation and conjugation of dehydroepiandrosterone by human skin. J Clin Endocrinol Metab 1967;27:1214–1218.
13. Barth JH. Hirsute women: Should they be investigated? J Clin Pathol 1992;45:188–192.
14. Mehta A, Matwijiw I. Taylor P, et al. Should androgen levels be measured in hirsute women with normal menstrual cycles? Int J Fertil 1992;37:354–357.
15. Schriock EA, Schriock ED. Treatment of hirsutism. Clin Obstet Gynecol 1991;14:852–863.
16. Pittaway DE, Maxon WS, Wentz AC. Spironolactone in combination drug therapy for unresponsive hirsutism. Fertil Steril 1985;43:878–882.
17. Pang S. Relevance of biological properties of progestogens of oral contraceptives in the treatment of androgen excess symptoms. J Clin Endocrinol Metab 1990;71:5.
18. Porcile A, Gallardo E. Oral contraceptives containing disogestrel in the maintenance of the remission of hirsutism: Monthly versus bimonthly treatment. Contraception 1991;44:533–540.
19. Weber MM, Luppa P, Engelhardt D. Inhibition of human adrenal androgen secretion by ketoconazole. Klin Wochenschr 1989;67:707.
20. Marcondes JAM, Wajchenberg BL, Minnani SL, et al. Treatment of hirsutism in women with flutamide. Fertil Steril 1992;57:543–547.

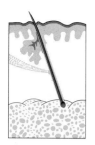

chapter 182

Inherited Abnormalities of Amino Acid Metabolism

ELIZABETH F. SHERERTZ

Skin lesions are often a critical clinical feature of some inborn errors of metabolism. The cutaneous manifestations may be so characteristic of a specific disorder that the dermatologist may have important diagnostic input when consulting on a pediatric patient with developmental delay or neurologic symptoms.

This chapter focuses on those inborn errors of amino acid metabolism with prominent cutaneous features, and that may be treated with appropriate nutritional intervention (Table 182–1). Some defects of amino acid metabolism are covered elsewhere in this text: for example, albinism (Chapter 131). Other inborn errors of metabolism, such as zinc deficiency (Chapter 170), Menkes' disease (Chapter 163), and glycogen storage disease, (Chapter 171) are covered elsewhere in the text.

PHENYLKETONURIA

Clinical Description

Phenylketonuria (PKU) is an autosomal recessive disorder (incidence about one in 12,000) associated with an eczematous dermatitis in about 30% of affected children, even without a family history of atopy.[1-3] Urine screening of newborns for PKU is routine in the United States and elsewhere. The eczema is typically flexural involvement of the extremities. There is also dilution of pigment in skin and hair, due to decreased melanin synthesis (Fig. 182–1).[4] Sclerodermatous changes may occur in the first year of life, beginning in the buttock and thigh areas, and then advancing to involve the trunk and proximal extremities, eventuating in contractures.[5, 6] The induration involves the muscles, subcutaneous tissue, and dermis.

Each of these skin abnormalities in PKU can be prevented or improved with dietary phenylalanine restriction. However, excessive phenylalanine restriction, leading to deficiency of this essential amino acid, has been associated with oral lesions and a generalized eczematous reaction.[7]

Pathogenesis and Etiology

PKU is caused by a deficiency of the enzyme phenylalanine hydroxylase, which catalyzes the conversion of phenylalanine to tyrosine. Accumulation of phenylalanine and metabolites are associated with "mousy" body odor, developmental delay, and mental retardation.

Diagnosis and Differential Diagnosis

Although a urine screening test is commonly used, the diagnosis of PKU is most reliably made from measurement of plasma phenylalanine (>20 mg/ml). Elevation may be most marked after a protein meal. The clinical differential diagnosis includes atopic dermatitis with coincidental neurologic abnormalities and childhood scleroderma.

Treatment

Treatment of infants with a low-phenylalanine diet will improve skin changes and prevent mental retardation.[8]

TABLE 182–1. Dermatologic Signs of Disorders of Amino Acid Metabolism

Disease	Metabolic Defect	Major Clinical Features	Dermatologic Signs	Effect of Treatment on Skin Involvement
Phenylketonuria (PKU)	Phenylalanine hydroxylase deficiency	Developmental delay Mental retardation	Flexural eczema Scleroderma-like changes • proximal • childhood onset Pigment dilution	Dietary phenylalanine restriction improves skin; skin may darken with diet
Tyrosinemia, type II (Richner-Hanhart syndrome)	Hepatic tyrosine aminotransferase deficiency	Photophobia Corneal scarring Developmental delay Mental retardation	Hyperkeratosis • hands and feet • painful, focal Leukokeratosis of tongue	Dietary phenylalanine and tyrosine restriction improves skin
Albinism Oculocutaneous • classic • other (see Chapter 131)	Absence of tyrosinase Tyrosinase positive	Decreased pigment Decreased visual acuity, photophobia	Decreased pigmentation of skin, hair, eyes	No repigmentation (photoprotection is essential)
Prolidase deficiency	Reduced activity of prolidase	Mental retardation Splenomegaly Recurrent infections	Skin ulcers • legs	Manganese supplementation (prolidase cofactor) may help
Argininosuccinic aciduria	Deficiency of argininosuccinate lyase		Trichorrhexis nodosa Dry, brittle hair	Hair may improve spontaneously with age
Multiple biotin-dependent carboxylase deficiency	Holocarboxylase Synthetase deficiency (early onset) Biotinidase deficiency (later onset)	Seizures, ataxia Failure to thrive Hypotonia Keratoconjunctivitis Metabolic acidosis	Seborrheic-like dermatitis Refractory candida intertrigo Pigment dilution Diffuse alopecia	Biotin treatment improves skin
Homocystinuria	Cystathionine synthase deficiency (pyridoxine-dependent)	Lens dislocation Other eye abnormalities Osteoporosis—spine Developmental delay Vascular occlusion	Pigment dilution Brittle hair Malar flushing Livedo reticularis	Methionine-restricted diet and pyridoxine supplementation may improve skin
Hartnup disease	Defective intestinal transport of tryptophan	Occasional ataxia Retardation	Pellagra-like rash Photosensitivity	Oral nicotinamide improves skin
Maple syrup urine disease	Branched-chain amino acids accumulate	Hypoglycemia seizures, acidosis Growth retardation Urine odor	Exfoliative erythroderma associated with inadequate dietary intake of branched-chain amino acids	Skin improves with less restriction of diet
Alkaptonuria	Homogentisic acid oxidase deficiency	Dark urine Discoloration and degeneration of cartilage	Dark cerumen Cutaneous ochronosis	

TYROSINEMIA II (RICHNER-HANHART SYNDROME)

Clinical Description

Tyrosinemia has autosomal recessive inheritance, and a biochemical carrier state has not been identified. Painful dendritic corneal ulcers with neovascularization may occur in the first year of life. Mild mental retardation may be a feature. Skin lesions in tyrosinemia II occur early in life, as do ophthalmologic symptoms of lacrimation, pain, and photophobia. The skin lesions begin as blisters or crusts and evolve into painful localized hyperkeratoses of the hands and feet, particularly on the tips of digits (Fig. 182–2). There may be hyperhidrosis.[9, 10] Leukokeratosis of the tongue may occur.

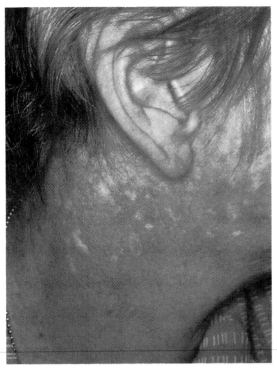

FIGURE 182-1. Fair skin and an ill-defined poorly circumscribed eczematous eruption in a patient with phenylketonuria.

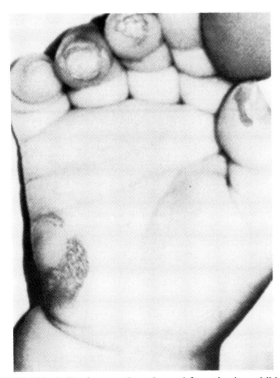

FIGURE 182-2. Erosions on the palm and fingertips in a child with tyrosinemia II (Richner-Hanhart syndrome). From Goldsmith LA. Tyrosinemia II. Lessons in molecular pathophysiology. Pediatr Dermatol (1983;1:25–34. Reprinted by permission of Blackwell Scientific Publications, Inc.)

Pathology

The hyperkeratotic palmar and plantar lesions have an inflammatory stage that is, in some families, characterized by epidermolytic hyperkeratosis. In fully developed lesions there is compact hyperkeratosis punctuated by vertical columns of parakeratotic cells situated above dells in the epidermal surface. Multinucleated keratinocytes are evident in the superficial spinous zone, and ultrastructural examination shows aggregated tonofilaments as well as needle-shaped inclusions.

Pathogenesis and Etiology

There is a deficiency of hepatic tyrosine aminotransferase, which is the rate-limiting enzyme of tyrosine catabolism. This results in tyrosinemia and in elevated urinary tyrosine metabolites, both of which can be measured to establish the diagnosis. A tyrosine load test can also be done.[10] Tissue damage may be due to intracellular crystallization of tyrosine, leading to lysosomal release of proteolytic enzymes and subsequent inflammation.

Diagnosis and Differential Diagnosis

The diagnosis of tyrosinemia is confirmed by increased plasma or urinary levels of tyrosine. Clinically, the palmar-plantar blistering may be initially confused with epidermolysis bullosa. Progression to hyperkeratotic lesions may raise the diagnosis of epidermolytic hyperkeratosis. The concomitant ocular symptoms and signs should raise suspicion of tyrosinemia in an infant with painful palmar-plantar hyperkeratosis.

Treatment

A low-tyrosine, low-phenylalanine diet may rapidly resolve clinical symptoms and signs, and is the treatment of choice. Oral retinoids have also been demonstrated to improve skin lesions, but without any effect on plasma tyrosine levels.[12] Skin lesions do not respond to conventional keratolytic therapy.

ARGININOSUCCINIC ACIDURIA

Clinical Description

Argininosuccinic aciduria has autosomal recessive inheritance, and major features of hepatomegaly, seizures, and mental retardation are due to hyperammonemia. Changes of trichorrhexis nodosa and brittle hair have been reported in about half of patients with argininosuccinic aciduria.[13] The hair changes do not correlate with the argininosuccinic acid levels. Polarized microscopy of hair demonstrates no uniform cortical or medullary structure, and fluorescent microscopy of acridine orange-stained hair shows red rather than typical green fluorescence.[14, 15] Nails may also be involved, but the skin in general is normal.

Pathogenesis and Etiology

The essential urea cycle enzyme, argininosuccinate lyase, is deficient in argininosuccinic aciduria. This results in an increase in blood ammonia, citrullinemia, and large amounts of argininosuccinate excreted in the urine. The mechanism for the hair defect is not known, although cystine content of the hair was low in one patient.[16]

Diagnosis and Differential Diagnosis

The diagnosis of argininosuccinic aciduria is made with the finding of increased plasma and urinary argininosuccinic acid. A screen for urinary amino acids is helpful in this regard. The diagnosis should be considered in a child with unusually dry, brittle, uncombable hair, or hair that is "not growing" (due to breakage). The differential diagnosis includes tinea capitis, trichotillomania, and exogenous trauma due to styling or hair care.

Treatment

Increased amounts of arginine in the diet may improve hair.[17] Dialysis, low-protein diet, and supplementation of sodium benzoate and sodium phenylacetate to activate alternate nitrogen excretion pathways can influence the morbidity of this and other urea cycle enzyme disorders.[18]

ALKAPTONURIA

Clinical Description

Alkaptonuria is rare (1 in 250,000) and has an autosomal recessive inheritance. Connective tissue discoloration and degeneration occurs in the third or fourth decade, leading to ochronotic arthropathy, which particularly involves the spine and larger joints. The skin signs of alkaptonuria are delayed in onset, and the diagnosis is usually made because of family history or diaper discoloration. Dark ear cerumen and greenish blue pigmentation of the axillae may occur in childhood. Darkening of ear cartilage and punctate pigmentation of sweat glands in skin overlying cartilage (ears, nose) does not occur until adulthood.[19]

Pathogenesis and Etiology

The catabolic enzyme homogentisic acid oxidase is deficient, which prevents breakdown of an intermediate product of phenylalanine and tyrosine metabolism. Homogentisic acid is excreted in the urine, often turning it dark. Homogentisic acid also accumulates in connective tissues, where it inhibits collagen cross-linking.

The discoloration is due to oxidation of homogentisic acid, leading to ochronotic pigment.

Diagnosis and Differential Diagnosis

The diagnosis of alkaptonuria is made by the demonstration of homogentisic acid in the urine by its reducing ability. The presence of homogentisic acid in the urine can interfere with some urine tests and lead to a mistaken diagnosis of glycosuria or diabetes. Alternatively, specific enzymatic assay or gas chromatography can be done. For dark urine, the differential diagnosis includes porphyrias, hepatobiliary disease, and hemoglobinuria. For the cutaneous pigmentation, exogenous ochronosis can be differentiated by absence of joint or urinary findings. Other causes of hyperpigmentation could be considered, such as Addison's disease, hemochromatosis, argyria, or pellagra, but may usually be differentiated clinically by lack of cartilaginous involvement.

Treatment

Supportive therapy for the arthropathy is indicated, but there is no effective treatment for the disease progression.

INBORN ERRORS OF BIOTIN DEFICIENCY (MULTIPLE BIOTIN-DEPENDENT CARBOXYLASE DEFICIENCY)

Biotin serves as an essential cofactor for metabolism of organic acids derived from the branched-chain amino acids. There are two heritable types of biotin deficiency: a neonatal form due to holocarboxylase synthetase deficiency, and an autosomal recessive later-onset form due to a deficiency of biotinidase.[20, 21] Biotinidase helps to recycle biotin from carboxylases. Cutaneous signs may be heralding features, and include a bright red, scaling eruption most pronounced in intertriginous areas, and patchy to total alopecia. Biotin administration improves skin lesions and alopecia.

Other clinical findings are metabolic acidosis, developmental failure to thrive, hypotonia, and seizures.

HOMOCYSTINURIA

Skin changes affect about 50% of patients with this autosomal recessive disorder, and are light-colored skin hair, with a livedo reticularis vascular pattern on the extremities. Homocystinuria is due to a deficiency of the pyridoxine-dependent cystathionine synthase, which converts homocysteine to cystathionine. Major clinical features are lens dislocation, osteoporosis, and tendency toward thromboembolic disease. Methionine restriction and pyridoxine supplementation can be helpful in some cases.[22]

HARTNUP DISEASE

Hartnup disease has impaired transport of neutral amino acids, such as tryptophan, in the intestine and renal tubule, which results in reduced synthesis of nicotinamide. Occasional patients with Hartnup disease may have intermittent clinical features similar to pellagra: photosensitive desquamating eruption, whose histopathology also resembles that of pellagra, and neuropsychiatric symptoms.[23]

PROLIDASE DEFICIENCY

Prolidase is an enzyme that lyses carboxy-terminal imidodipeptides. In the autosomal recessive prolidase deficiency, childhood onset of recurrent, refractory skin ulcerations may occur. Some reports describe an amyloid-like substance in the walls of vessels in ulcerated skin.[24] Low intelligence, infections, and dysmorphic features may also occur. Dietary administration of proline and manganese (a cofactor) may help wound healing in this setting.[25]

References

1. Knox WE. Incidence and inheritance. In: Lyman FI, eds. Phenylketonuria. Springfield, IL: Thomas, 1963:49–50.
2. Bickel H. The effects of a phenylalanine-free and phenylalanine-poor diet in phenylpyruria oligophrenia. Exp Med Surg 1954; 12:114–117.
3. Fleischer TL, Zeligman I. Cutaneous findings in phenylketonuria. Arch Dermatol 1960;81:898–903.
4. Tourian A, Sidbury SB. Phenylketonuria and hyperphenylalaninemia. In: Stanbury JB, Wyngaarden JB, Frederickson DS, et al., eds. The Metabolic Basis of Inherited Disease. New York: McGraw-Hill, 1983:270–286.
5. Jablonska S, Stachow A. Scleroderma-like lesions in phenylketonuria. In: Jablonska S, ed. Scleroderma and Pseudoscleroderma, 2nd edition. New York: Academic Press, 1976:489–498.
6. Guillet GY, Dore N, Hehmstre JP, Battin J. Pseudoscleroderma and phenylketonuria. Int J Dermatol 1983;22:422–426.
7. Rouse BM. Phenylalanine deficiency syndrome. J Pediatr 1966;69:246–249.
8. Scriver CR, Kaufman S, Woo SLC. The hyperphenylalaninemias. In: Scriver DR, Beaudet AL, Sly WS, Valle D, eds. The Metabolic Basis of Inherited Disease, 6th edition. New York: McGraw-Hill, 1989:495–546.
9. Goldsmith LA, Kang E, Bienfang DC, et al. Tyrosinemia with plantar and palmar keratosis and keratitis. J Pediatr 1973;83: 798–805.
10. Goldsmith LA, Laberge C. Tyrosinemia and related disorders. In: Scriver CR, Beaudet AL, Sly WS, Valle D, eds. The Metabolic Basis of Inherited Disease, 6th edition. New York: McGraw-Hill, 1989:547–562.
11. Shimizu N, Ito M, Ito K, et al. Richner-Hanhart's syndrome. Electron microscopy of the skin lesion. Arch Dermatol 1990; 126:1342–1346.
12. Hunziker N, Brun R, Jeanneret JP. Richner Hanhart syndrome (RHS)—tyrosinemia type II and oral aromatic retinoid (Ro 10-9359), report of two cases. In: Orfanos CE, Braun-Falco O, Farber EM, et al., eds. Retinoids: Advances in Basic Research and Therapy. New York: Springer-Verlag, 1982:453.
13. Irons M, Levy HL: Metabolic syndromes with dermatologic manifestations. Clin Rev Allergy 1986;4:101–124.
14. Coryell ME, et al. A familial study of a human enzyme defect, argininosuccinic aciduria. Biochem Biophys Res Commun 1962; 14:307.
15. Levin B, et al. Argininosuccinic aciduria. An inborn error of amino acid metabolism. Arch Dis Child 1961;36:622.
16. Potter JL, Timmons GD, Silvidi AA. Argininosuccinic aciduria: The hair abnormality revisited. Am J Dis Child 1980;134: 1095–1096.
17. Hartlage RL, et al. Argininosuccinic aciduria: Perinatal diagnosis and early dietary management. J Pediatr 1974;85:86.
18. Batshaw ML, Brusilau S, Waber L, et al. Treatment of inborn errors of urea synthesis: Activation of alternative pathways of waste nitrogen synthesis and excretion. N Engl J Med 1982;306: 1387–1392.
19. Le Du BN: Alcaptonuria. In: Scriver CR, Beaudet AL, Sly WS, Valle D, eds. The Metabolic Basis of Inherited Disease, 6th edition. New York: McGraw-Hill, 1989:775–790.
20. Nyhan WL. Inborn errors of biotin metabolism. Arch Dermatol 1987;123:1696–1698.
21. Wolf B, Grier RE, Allen RJ, et al. Phenotypic variation in biotinidase deficiency. J Pediatr 1983;103:233–237.
22. Mudd SH, Levy HL, Skovby F: Disorders of transsulfuration. In: Scrivner DR, Beaudet AL, Sly WS, Valle D (eds). The Metabolic Basis of Inherited Disease, 6th edition. New York: McGraw-Hill, 1989:698–729.
23. Wilaken B, Yu JS, Brown DA. Natural history of Hartnup disease. Arch Dis Child 1977;52:38–40.
24. Pierard GE, Cornil F, Lapiere CM. Pathogenesis of ulcerations in deficiency of prolidase. The role of angiopathy and of deposits of amyloid. Am J Dermatopathol 1984;6:491–497.
25. Der Kaloustian VM, Freij BJ, Kurban AK. Prolidase deficiency: An inborn error of metabolism with major dermatological manifestations. Dermatologica 1982;164:293–304.

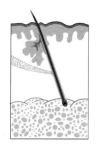

chapter 183

Dermatologic Manifestations of Internal Disease

JOSEPH L. JORIZZO and JEFFREY P. CALLEN

A detailed review of all dermatologic signs of internal disease is beyond the scope of this chapter. Many of the topics in this discussion are reviewed in detail elsewhere in this text. Tables are heavily utilized in this chapter to present an overview of data relevant to these topics. A systems approach is used.

CUTANEOUS RHEUMATOLOGY

Topics traditionally included as cutaneous rheumatology are as follows: lupus erythematosus (Chapter 24), dermatomyositis (Chapter 25), scleroderma, Raynaud's phenomenon and related conditions (Chapters 62 and 98), vasculitides (Chapters 57 to 59 and 67), and miscellaneous disorders, usually including: rheumatoid arthritis (Chapter 47), pyoderma gangrenosum (Chapter 39), psoriatic arthritis (Chapter 27), Behçet's disease (Chapter 40), Sweet's syndrome (Chapter 38), bowel bypass/bowel-associated dermatosis-arthritis syndrome (Chapter 44), Reiter's syndrome (Chapter 28), Kawasaki disease (Chapter 184), and relapsing polychondritis (Chapter 56).

Cutaneous conditions reported in patients with rheumatoid arthritis are summarized in Table 183–1[1, 2] (Figs. 183–1 and 183–2). Dermatologists should be particularly careful to couple laboratory evaluation with a conscientious complete cutaneous examination including examination of all mucosal surfaces, nails and nail folds, hair, and the entire cutaneous surface in this group of patients. Because clinical criteria are published for the diagnosis of many of these disorders, dermatologists should be familiar with the criteria and should incorporate them into a focused thorough history including relevant negatives. It is very helpful to think in terms of

clinicopathologic basis and pathogenesis of lesions. For example, in patients with systemic lupus erythematosus, photodistributed lesions with an interface histopathology (e.g., discoid lesions, subacute lesions, and poikilodermatous lesions) have different implications and are treated differently than vessel-based lesions such as lesions of small or larger vessel vasculitis.

Sjögren's syndrome describes the occurrence of keratoconjunctivitis sicca and xerostomia in association with an autoimmune disorder. The skin can be frequently involved in either primary Sjögren's syndrome or secondary Sjögren's syndrome (Table 183–2) (Figs. 183–3 and 183–4; see color plate).

CUTANEOUS REACTION PATTERNS WITH PROMINENT SYSTEMIC MANIFESTATIONS

A number of classic mucocutaneous conditions have many internal disease associations. These dermatologic conditions have been thoroughly reviewed elsewhere in this textbook including: urticaria (Chapter 41), erythema multiforme (Chapter 22), erythema nodosum (Chapter 68), generalized pruritus (Chapter 8), erythroderma (Chapter 31), and purpura (Chapter 26).

An excellent partial differential diagnosis of purpura has been published by Piette and is reproduced in Table 183–3.[3] (See also Figs. 183–5 to 183–10 and Fig. 183–9 color plate). It is impractical and certainly not cost effective to approach the patient with a cutaneous reaction pattern with the idea of excluding all associations with every laboratory evaluation described for that association. A guiding principle would be to utilize a careful and complete history and physical examination, often con-

1863

TABLE 183-1. Some Dermatologic Conditions Reported in Patients with Rheumatoid Arthritis

Palisading Granulomas

Rheumatoid nodules (Fig. 183-1)
Superficial ulcerating rheumatoid necrobiosis
Rheumatoid papules

Vasculitis

Mild — Bywater's lesions
Moderate — Necrotizing venulitis
Severe — Larger vessel vasculitis

Pyoderma Gangrenosum

Evanescent Erythema of Still's Disease

Bullous Diseases

Bullous pemphigoid
Pemphigus
Dermatitis herpetiformis
Epidermolysis bullosa acquisita

Miscellaneous Lesions

Palmar erythema
Nail fold capillary dilatation
Atrophic skin over bony prominences
Patchy hyperpigmentation
Red lunulae
Pigmented purpuric eruption
Amyloidosis

Cutaneous Lesions Due to Rheumatologic Therapy

Naproxen	Pseudoporphyria (Fig. 183-2)
Penicillamine	Pemphigus
	Lichenoid drug eruption
	Elastosis perforans serpiginosa
Gold	Lichenoid drug eruption

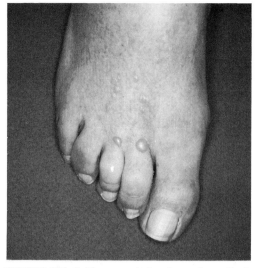

FIGURE 183-2. Naproxen-induced pseudoporphyria.

TABLE 183-2. Mucocutaneous Changes Associated with Sjögren's Syndrome

Primary Sjögren's Syndrome

Defining characteristics
  Keratoconjunctivitis sicca
  Diminished salivary gland flow
  Abnormal salivary gland biopsy
  Positive autoantibody test
Skin conditions associated with Sjögren's syndrome
  Vasculitis (Fig. 183-3)
  Annular erythema
  Subacute cutaneous lupus erythematosus (Fig. 183-4)

Diseases Associated with Secondary Sjögren's Syndrome

Lupus erythematosus
  Subacute cutaneous lupus erythematosus
Rheumatoid arthritis
Scleroderma
Exclusions:
  Sarcoidosis
  Lymphoma
  Graft-versus-host disease
  Human immunodeficiency disease

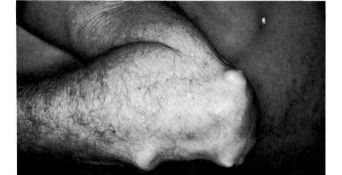

FIGURE 183-1. Rheumatoid nodule.

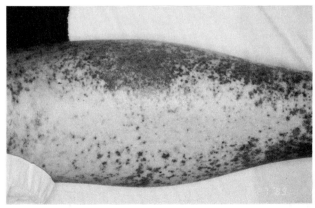

FIGURE 183-3. Small vessel vasculitis in Sjögren's syndrome. (See color plate.)

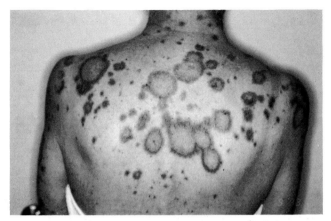

FIGURE 183–4. Subacute cutaneous lupus erythematosus in a patient with Sjögren's syndrome. (See color plate.)

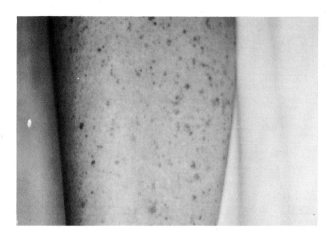

FIGURE 183–5. Thrombocytopenia.

TABLE 183–3. Partial Differential Diagnosis for Purpura

Petechiae (nonpalpable) (Fig. 183–5)	Palpable Purpura (Fig. 183–8)
Hemostatically relevant thrombocytopenia (<50,000/mm³)	Classical type
Idiopathic thrombocytopenic purpura	Small vessel leukocytoclastic vasculitis syndromes
Thrombotic thrombocytopenic purpura (some cases)	Idiopathic
DIC	Post-infectious
Drug-related thrombocytopenia	Drug induced
Peripheral destruction: quinidine, quinine	IgA predominant (includes most Henoch-Schönlein
Marrow: idiosyncratic or dose-related	purpura)
Marrow infiltration, fibrosis, or failure	Mixed cryoglobulinemia
Abnormal platelet function	Associated with lupus, rheumatoid arthritis, Sjögren's
Congenital or hereditary platelet function defects	Small vessel lesions of Wegener's, Churg-Strauss,
Acquired platelet function defects (e.g., aspirin, renal or	lymphomatoid granulomatosis
hepatic insufficiency, monoclonal gammopathy)	PLEVA syndrome
Thrombocytosis in myeloproliferative diseases	Erythema multiforme (some variants)
(>1,000,000/mm³)	Target lesions
Elevated intravascular pressure (Valsalva maneuver–like	Erythema multiforme
etiologies)	Retiform or livedoid purpura
Chronic pigmented purpura (occasionally palpable, due to	Bland occlusion syndromes (retiform morphology without
inflammation) (Fig. 183–6)	early erythema)
	Ecthyma gangrenosum
	Monoclonal cryoglobulinemia, cryofibrinogenemia
Ecchymotic (Fig. 183-7)	DIC and purpura fulminans (some forms) (Fig. 183-9)
	Protein C deficiency
Procoagulant defect (often localized to sites of minor	Coumadin necrosis
trauma)	Heparin necrosis
Hemophilia	Cholesterol emboli
Anticoagulants	Oxalate crystal occlusion
Disseminated intravascular coagulation	Antiphospholipid antibody syndrome (Fig. 183-10)
Vitamin K deficiency	Atrophie blanche and livedoid vasculitis (some forms)
Hepatic insufficiency with poor procoagulant synthesis	Cutaneous calciphylaxis
Poor dermal support of vessels (usually localized to sites of	"Hybrid" lesions (both retiform morphology and prominent
minor trauma)	early erythema)
Corticosteroid therapy, topical or systemic	IgA-predominant small vessel
Scurvy	leukocytoclastic vasculitis (some)
Systemic amyloidosis (light-chain related)	Syndromes of small and medium vessel leukocytoclastic
Ehlers-Danlos syndrome, primarily Types I, IV, VI, VIII, and X	vasculitis, such as rheumatic vasculitis, polyarteritis,
Pseudoxanthoma elasticum	Wegener's, etc. (occasionally)
Other	Some early lesions of coumadin or heparin necrosis
Benign hypergammaglobulinemic purpura of	demonstrate erythema, but this tends to be at the margin
Waldenström (due to mild vessel inflammation; usually	of large, confluent areas of necrosis
causes macular hemorrhage, but can produce	
palpable purpura)	

PLEVA, pityriasis lichenoides et varioliformis acuta; DIC, disseminated intravascular coagulation.
From Piette WW. Purpura. In: Callen JP, Jorizzo JL, et al., eds. Dermatological Signs of Internal Disease, 2nd edition. Philadelphia: WB Saunders, 1995:87–95.

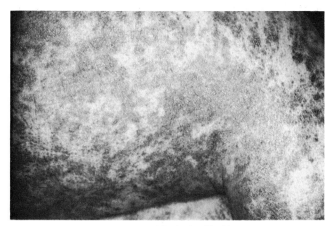

FIGURE 183-6. Capillaritis.

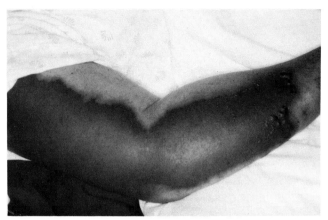

FIGURE 183-9. Disseminated intravascular coagulation. (See color plate.)

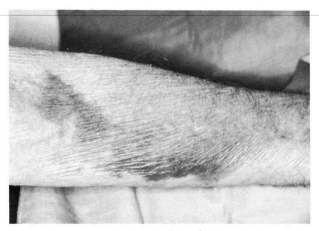

FIGURE 183-7. Ecchymotic purpura.

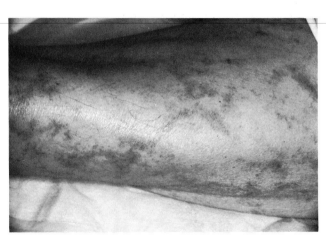

FIGURE 183-10. Antiphospholipid antibody syndrome with livedo reticularis.

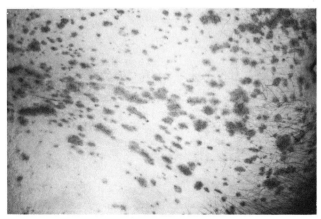

FIGURE 183-8. Palpable purpura.

ducted by a primary care physician in conjunction with the dermatologist, and screening laboratory tests. Abnormalities can then be pursued thoroughly but in a stepwise conscientious manner.

CUTANEOUS HEMATOLOGY AND ONCOLOGY

Disorders of interest to dermatologists and to hematologists/oncologists are also well covered in the following chapters of this textbook: skin signs of internal malignancy (Chapter 183), metastatic disease (Chapter 161), leukemia/lymphoma (Chapters 159 and 160), dysproteinemias (Chapter 182), histiocytosis (Chapters 154 and 155), vascular neoplasms (Chapter 146), cutaneous T-

TABLE 183-4. Criteria Used to Associate Dermatoses and Neoplasia

Concurrent onset
Parallel course
Uniform neoplasm (site of cell type)
Statistical association
Genetic association

From Callen JP. Skin signs of internal malignancy. In: Callen JP, Jorizzo JL, et al., eds. Dermatological Signs of Internal Disease, 2nd edition. Philadelphia: WB Saunders Co., 1995:111–121.

cell lymphoma (Chapter 158), pigmented lesions (Chapter 150), and cutaneous reactions to chemotherapeutic agents (Chapter 44).

Skin signs of internal malignancy are summarized in Tables 183–4 and 183–5. Table 183–4 summarizes Curth's criteria for the associations of dermatoses and neoplasia, and Table 183–5 represents the application of these criteria to specific claimed associations (Figs. 183–11 to 183–20; see color plate for Figs. 183–16 and 183–19).[4] The use of Curth's criteria is important to establish whether a given criteria is a chance occurrence or truly a malignancy-associated event.

TABLE 183-5. Paraneoplastic Disorders

Disorders that Fit Curth's Criteria

Acanthosis nigricans and possibly the sign of Leser-Trélat (Fig. 183–11)
Bazex's syndrome
Carcinoid syndrome
Erythema gyratum repens (Fig. 183–12)
Hypertrichosis lanuginosa (Fig. 183–13)
Ectopic ACTH syndrome
Glucagonoma syndrome (Fig. 183–14)
Neutrophilic dermatoses (Fig. 183–15)
Paget's disease (Fig. 183–16)
Paraneoplastic pemphigus (Fig. 183–17)

Disorders Associated Statistically with Cancer

Acrochordon
Bowen's disease (Fig. 183–18)
Dermatomyositis (Figs. 183–19 and 183–20)
Extramammary Paget's disease
Exfoliative dermatitis
Mycosis fungoides
Palmar keratoses
Pruritus
Porphyria cutanea tarda
Pityriasis rotunda

Dermatoses Possibly Associated with Cancer

Arsenical keratoses
Erythema annulare centrifugum
Acquired ichthyosis
Multicentric reticulohistiocytosis
Necrobiotic xanthogranuloma
Classical pyoderma gangrenosum
Polymyositis
Tripe palms
Vasculitis
Vitiligo

ACTH, adrenocorticotropic hormone. From Callen JP. Skin signs of internal malignancy. In: Callen JP, Jorizzo JL, et al., eds. Dermatological Signs of Internal Disease, 2nd edition. Philadelphia: WB Saunders Co., 1995:111–121.

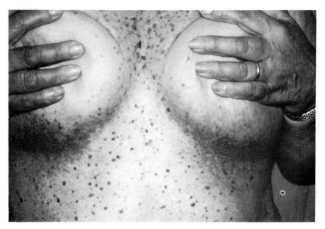

FIGURE 183–11. Acanthosis nigricans.

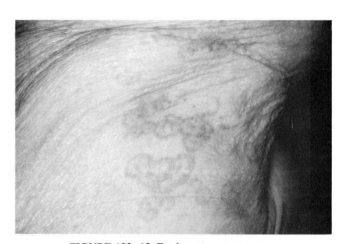

FIGURE 183–12. Erythema gyratum repens.

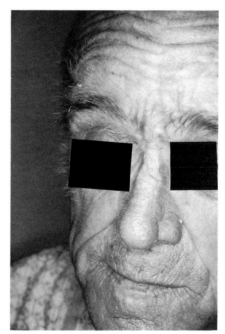

FIGURE 183–13. Hypertrichosis lanuginosa.

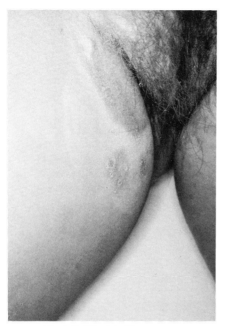

FIGURE 183-14. Glucagonoma.

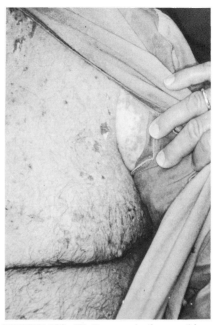

FIGURE 183-17. Paraneoplastic pemphigus.

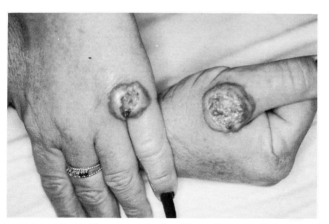

FIGURE 183-15. Sweet's syndrome. (From Callen JP. Skin signs of internal malignancy. In: Callen JP, Jorizzo JL, et al., eds. Dermatological Signs of Internal Disease, 2nd edition. Philadelphia, WB Saunders Co., 1995:111-121.)

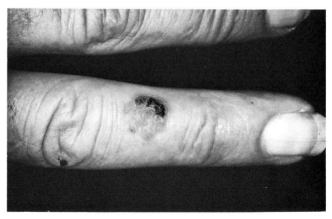

FIGURE 183-18. Bowen's disease.

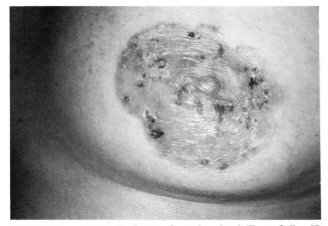

FIGURE 183-16. Paget's disease. (See color plate.) (From Callen JP. Skin signs of internal malignancy. In: Callen JP, Jorizzo JL, et al., eds. Dermatological Signs of Internal Disease, 2nd edition. Philadelphia: WB Saunders Co., 1995:111-121.)

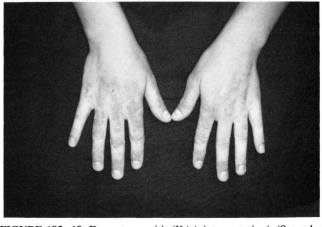

FIGURE 183-19. Dermatomyositis (KAA interpretation). (See color plate.)

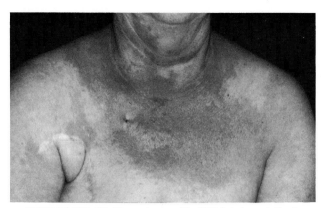

FIGURE 183–20. Dermatomyositis (ICAA interpretation).

CUTANEOUS ENDOCRINOLOGY AND METABOLIC DISEASE

Endocrine disease, particularly diabetes mellitus, is an area where cutaneous manifestations may be important clues to diagnosis. Patients with endocrine disease are especially susceptible to various associated mucocutaneous disorders. Areas of cutaneous endocrinology and metabolic disease discussed elsewhere in this textbook include diabetes mellitus (Chapters 46 and 47, but not specifically discussed), thyroid disease (not specifically discussed), lipids (Chapter 176), androgen-related disorders (Chapter 133), adrenal disease (not specifically discussed), porphyria (Chapter 169), and amino acid metabolism (Chapter 182).

Diabetes mellitus is a very common medical disease with sequelae that affect almost every organ system. The skin is definitely no exception. Necrobiosis lipoidica diabeticorum is discussed elsewhere (Chapter 47). Table 183–6 summarizes cutaneous manifestations of diabetes mellitus (Figs. 183–21 to 183–29, see color plate for Fig. 183–22). Several recent reviews have been published on this topic.[5-7]

Thyroid disease is also associated with considerable cutaneous changes. Current reviews highlight these dermatologic manifestations and associations.[8, 9] Tables 183–7 and 183–8 summarize dermatologic manifesta-

TABLE 183–6. Selected Dermatologic Associations of Diabetes Mellitus

Dermatosis	Clinical Description	Modifying Factors
Rubeosis	Chronic flushed appearance to face, neck, and even extremities	Improved by good diabetic control. Flares with vasodilators.
Diabetic dermopathy	Hyperpigmented patches—primarily on the lower legs.	Precipitated by trauma.
Diabetic bullae (Fig. 183–21)	Tense bullae primarily on the lower extremities. Multiple variants may exist.	Uncertain role of trauma.
Necrobiosis lipoidica diabeticorum (Fig. 183–22)	Well circumscribed, yellow-brown patches often on lower extremities with pronounced epidermal atrophy with raised red border. Ulceration is common.	Intralesional corticosteroids, aspirin, dipyridamole and pentoxifylline may be beneficial. Uncertain role of trauma in induction of lesions.
Disseminated granuloma annulare (Fig. 183–23)	Although several studies suggest an association, current opinion and several other studies argue against a true association.	—
Cutaneous perforating diseases (Fig. 183–24)	Diabetic patients undergoing renal dialysis may develop one of 3 types of these clinicopathologically distinctive papular lesions as often as 5%–10% of the time.	Excoriation may induce lesions.
Vitiligo	Idiopathic macular eruption with absence of melanocytes from these lesions.	May be associated with anti-insulin antibodies in some patients.
Scleredema adultorum of Buschke	Dramatic induration of the skin of the neck and upper back occurs due to the glycosaminoglycan deposition. Waxy induration of the extremities may effect joint mobility.	—
Acanthosis nigricans (Fig. 183–25)	Velvety epidermal thickening with hyperpigmentation primarily in the axillary, inguinal, and neck folds.	Pathogenesis may be related to insulin-like epidermal growth factor-like effects.
Lipodystrophy	A number of variants of generalized and partial lipodystrophies can occur in association with diabetes mellitus.	Congenital and acquired, familial and sporadic variants occur. (Localized lipodystrophy may also occur at insulin injection sites)
Acral erythema	An acral erysipelas-like erythema has been described in elderly diabetics.	Due to small vessel vasculopathy.
Acral dry gangrene	Acral gangrene usually of the feet occurs with increased incidence in elderly patients with diabetes mellitus	Due to larger and small vessel vascular disease.
Leg ulcers	Chronic, therapy-resistant ulcers on the lower legs.	Multifactorial.

Continued

TABLE 183-6. Selected Dermatologic Associations of Diabetes Mellitus (*Continued*)

Dermatosis	Clinical Description	Modifying Factors
Cutaneous infectious with dermatophytes, yeast, and bacteria	Examples: Candidiasis of all locations, dermatophytosis, erythrasma, tinea versicolor, impetigo, mucor.	IMaceration, occlusion, antibiotics.
Neurotropic ulcers (Fig. 183-26)	Deep refractory skin ulcers at sites of pressure	Sensory neuropathy reduces ability to escape injury from chronic trauma.
Eruptive xanthomas (Fig. 183-27)	Yellow-red papules with a sudden onset in a generalized distribution.	High triglyceride levels that can occur with poor diabetic control leads to these lesions.
Yellow skin (Fig. 183-28)	Diffuse yellowish hue to the skin.	Elevated serum carotene produces this.
Hemodermatosis (Fig. 183-29)	Bronzing of skin due to melanin— "bronze diabetes"	Excess iron stores, cirrhosis, heart failure.

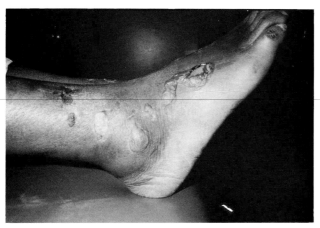

FIGURE 183-21. Bullous diabeticorum.

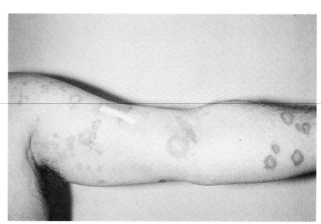

FIGURE 183-23. Granuloma annulare.

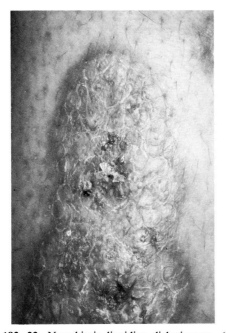

FIGURE 183-22. Necrobiosis lipoidica diabeticorum. (See color plate.)

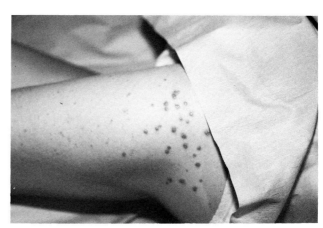

FIGURE 183-24. Kyrle's disease.

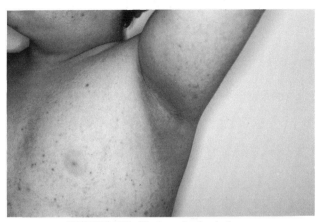

FIGURE 183–25. Acanthosis nigricans.

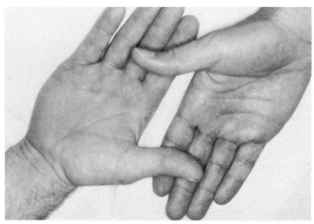

FIGURE 183–28. Carotenemia.

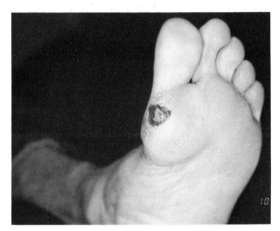

FIGURE 183–26. Neurotropic ulcer.

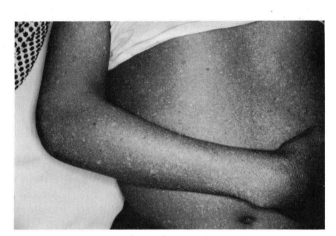

FIGURE 183–29. Hemochromatosis.

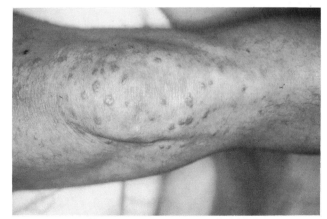

FIGURE 183–27. Eruptive xanthomas.

TABLE 183–7. Dermatologic Manifestations of Hyperthyroidism

Skin	Fine, velvety, or smooth
	Warm and moist (increased sweating); rarely dry
	Hyperpigmentation (localized or generalized)
	Vitiligo (see Fig. 183–30)
	Urticaria, dermatographism
	Pretibial myxedema and thyroid acropachy (see Fig. 183–31)
Hair	Fine, thin
	Alopecia (diffuse and mild; rarely severe)
	Alopecia areata
Nails	Onycholysis
	Koilonychia
	Clubbing with thyroid acropachy

From Rosen T, Kleman GA. Thyroid and the skin. In: Callen JP, Jorizzo JL, et al., eds. Dermatological Signs of Internal Disease, 2nd edition. Philadelphia: WB Saunders Co., 1995:189–195.

TABLE 183-8. Dermatologic Manifestations of Hypothyroidism

Skin	Dry, rough or coarse; cold and pale; puffy, boggy or edematous (myxedema)
	Yellow discoloration as a result of carotemia
	Ichthyosis and palmoplantar hyperkeratosis
	Easy bruising (capillary fragility)
	Eruptive bruising (capillary fragility)
	Eruptive and tuberous xanthomas (rare)
Hair	Dull, coarse, and brittle
	Slow growth (increase in telogen or resting hairs)
	Alopecia (lateral third of eyebrows, rarely diffuse)
Nails	Thin, brittle, striated
	Slow growth
	Onycholysis (rare)

From Rosen T, Kleman GA. Thyroid and the skin. In: Callen JP, Jorizzo JL, et al., eds. Dermatological Signs of Internal Disease, 2nd edition. Philadelphia: WB Saunders Co., 1995:189–195.

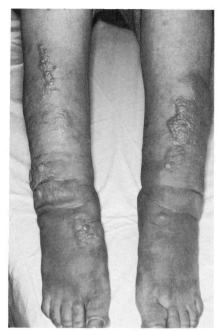

FIGURE 183-31. Pretibial myxedema.

tions of hyperthyroidism and hypothyroidism, respectively[10] (Figs. 183–30 and 183–31).

Adrenal disease can classically be manifested as excessive glucocorticoid activity (Cushing's syndrome) or as insufficient glucocorticoid activity (Addison's disease). Features of these syndromes are outlined in Tables 183–9 and 183–10, respectively, and in a recent review.[11]

Nutritional deficiencies remain a primary social, political, moral, ethical, and economic issue in impoverished areas of the world. Chapter 182 and several recent references highlight this area.[12, 13] Table 183–11 is a summary of selected dermatologic aspects of nutritional deficiency (Figs. 183–32 and 183–33).

CUTANEOUS GASTROENTEROLOGY

Cutaneous aspects of gastroenterology are discussed in detail elsewhere in this textbook, particularly cutaneous diseases associated with gastrointestinal abnormalities (not discussed in one specific chapter), cutaneous hepatology (not discussed in one specific chapter), and cutaneous aspects of pancreatic disease (Chapters 71 and 180). Table 183–12 is a list of selected cutaneous associ-

TABLE 183-9. Cushing's Syndrome—Some Dermatologic Features

Altered Subcutaneous Fat Distribution

Rounded facies
Fullness of cheeks (moon facies)
Dorsal cervical vertebral fat deposits (buffalo hump)
Pelvic girdle fat deposition
Reduced fat in the arms and legs

Skin Atrophy

Global atrophy with epidermal and dermal components affected
Striae on abdominal flanks, arms, and thighs
Cutaneous fragility and slowly healing ulcers
Purpura (reduced connective tissue support)

Cutaneous Infections

Pityriasis versicolor
Dermatophytosis
Candidiasis

Appendageal Effects

Steroid acne
Hirsuitism

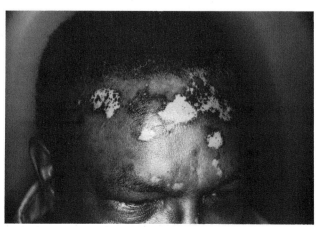

FIGURE 183-30. Vitiligo.

TABLE 183–10. Addison's Disease—Some Dermatologic Manifestations

Hyperpigmentation (MSH-like effects)
    Sun-exposed skin
    Sites of trauma
    Axillae, perineum, nipples
    Palmar creases
    Nevi
    Mucous membranes
    Hair
    Nails
Loss of ambisexual hair in postpubescent females
Fibrosis and calcification of cartilage of the ear (rare)
Increased loss of salt in sweat
Vitiligo (association in some patients)
Chronic mucocutaneous candidiasis (association in some
    patients)

MSH, melanocyte-stimulating hormone.

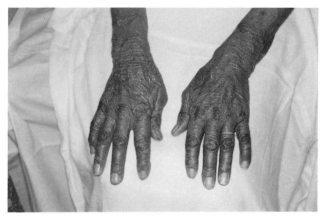

FIGURE 183–32. Pellagra.

TABLE 183–11. Dermatologic Manifestations of Nutritional Disorders

Nutritional Deficiency	Dermatologic Manifestations
Protein	Scaling of skin, hyper- and hypopigmentation, cutaneous ulcers, hyperkeratosis, petechial hemorrhage in "flaky paint" pattern. "Flag sign" of hair. Nails become thin and soft.
Essential fatty acid	Dry scaly skin, diffuse alopecia, resembles acrodermatitis enteropathica, periorificial dermatitis.
Vitamin A	Follicular hyperkeratosis, night blindness, xerophthalmia, keratomalacia, keratinizing metaplasia of mucous membranes, slow wound healing.
Vitamin B_1 (thiamine)	Orogenital dermatitis.
Vitamin B_2 (riboflavin)	Inflammation of lips, flattened lingual papillae, seborrheic-like dermatitis, and genital dermatitis. "Oro-oculo-genital syndrome."
Vitamin B_6 (pyridoxine)	Periorificial and seborrheic-like dermatitis, angular stomatitis, glossitis.
Vitamin B_{12} (cobalamin)	Brown reticular hyperpigmentation on the finger pulps. Brown mottling on nape of neck, axillae, lateral abdominal area, and hands and feet.
Niacin (Fig. 183–32)	Pellagra (dermatitis, diarrhea, dementia, and when untreated—death). Photodistributed brownish-red scaly dermatitis. "Cassal's necklace." Sebaceous gland prominence—"goose skin." Oro-oculo-genital syndrome.
Biotin	Alopecia and periorificial dermatitis.
Pantothenic acid	"Burning feet syndrome."
Folic acid	Similar to those of vitamin B_{12}.
Vitamin C (ascorbic acid) (Fig. 183–33)	Follicular hyperkeratosis ("cork screw hair"), perifollicular hemorrhage, petechiae, gum hemorrhage, peripheral edema, delayed wound healing, sicca syndrome.
Vitamin D	Rickets, alopecia, bone and cartilage abnormalities.
Vitamin E (tocopherol)	Seborrheic dermatitis-like eruption.
Vitamin K	Purpura to frank hemorrhage.
Zinc	Acrodermatitis enteropathica—dry, scaly plaques to vesiculobullous, pustular, erosive lesions acral and periorificial distribution. Candidal colonization, Beau's lines, and trichonodosis are common.
Copper	Menkes' kinky-hair syndrome (pili torti) and depigmentation of hair and skin. Defective elastin formation with dilated dermal blood vessels.
Iron	Koilonychia ("spoon nails"), angular stomatitis, glossitis with flattening of lingual papillae. Generalized pruritus.
Selenium	Loss of pigmentation of hair and skin. Curling of hair, Terry's nails (white nail bed).

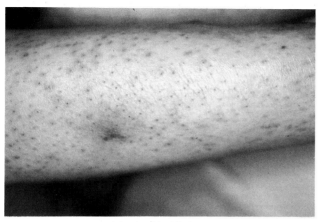

FIGURE 183-33. Scurvy.

ations of Crohn's disease and ulcerative colitis.[14] Table 183-13 lists dermatologic conditions associated with gastrointestinal hemorrhage[15] (Figs. 183-34 to 183-38). Cutaneous hepatology has been the subject of recent reviews.[16, 17] Table 183-14 is a list of selected dermatologic aspects of liver disease (Figs. 183-39 and 183-40).

TABLE 183-12. Some Cutaneous Associations of Crohn's Disease and Ulcerative Colitis

Erythemas (including annular erythemas)
Urticaria
Erythema nodosum
Necrotizing venulitis
Larger vessel necrotizing vasculitis
Pustular vasculitis
Pyoderma gangrenosum (Fig. 183-34)
Oral lesions
    Specific granulomas (Crohn's disease only)
    Aphthosis
    Angular cheilitis
    Pyostomatitis vegetans
Metastatic Crohn's disease
Finger clubbing
Acquired acrodermatitis enteropathica (zinc deficiency)
Striae
Epidermolysis bullosa acquisita
Psoriasis
Exfoliative erythroderma
Vitiligo
Lichen nitidus
Lichen planus

From Sherertz EF, Jorizzo JL. Skin lesions associated with gastrointestinal disease. In: Yamada T, Alpers DH, Owyang, C, et al., eds. Textbook of Gastroenterology. Philadelphia: JB Lippincott, 1991: Chapter 44.

TABLE 183-13. Gastrointestinal Hemorrhage and the Skin

Disorder	Cutaneous Findings	Gastrointestinal Features	Other Pertinent Findings	Treatment and Comments
Hereditary hemorrhagic telangiectasia (Osler-Weber-Rendu disease)	Macular mat-like telangiectasia with facial, mucosal, or acral distribution (Figs. 183-35 and 183-36)	Recurrent hemorrhage in the upper gastrointestinal (UGI) tract	Epistaxis, often as a presenting manifestation, and arteriovenous malformations (pulmonary, central nervous system, hepatic)	Treatment consists of blood replacement and (?) estrogens; lasers may be useful Autosomal dominant Surgical resection of lesions
Blue rubber bleb nevus syndrome	Large subcutaneous blue cavernous hemangiomas, purple-black rubbery compressible angiomas, and irregular blue-black papules and macules	Gastrointestinal (GI) vascular malformations	Vascular malformations may occur elsewhere	Autosomal dominant or sporadic
Pseudoxanthoma elasticum	Yellow papules on intertriginous surfaces, redundant lax skin (Fig. 183-37). "Plucked chicken" skin.	UGI hemorrhage; occasional lower GI hemorrhage	Angioid streaks on the retina, hypertension, premature atherosclerosis, and vascular calcification; caused by calcification and fragmentation of elastic fibers	No known treatment; replace blood loss; four heritable types: two autosomal dominant, two autosomal recessive
Ehlers-Danlos syndrome, type IV (ecchymotic type)	Translucent, hyperextensible, and fragile skin; marked bruisability	UGI hemorrhage secondary to arterial rupture or intestinal perforation	Minimal joint hyperextensibility	Autosomal dominant; deficiency of synthesis of type III collagen
Gardner's syndrome	Epidermal cysts, lipomas, and desmoid tumors	Lower GI hemorrhage and adenomatous colonic polyps; adenocarcinoma is a late symptom	Osteomas and mandibular cysts	Autosomal dominant; total colectomy
Peutz-Jeghers syndrome	Melanotic macules on mucosal surfaces or occasionally acral skin	Hamartomatous polyps throughout GI tract, intussusception, or hemorrhage	Possible increase in frequency of breast cancer and ovarian cancer; GI cancer is rare but does occur	Autosomal dominant; remove symptomatic areas of the bowel

TABLE 183-13. Gastrointestinal Hemorrhage and the Skin (*Continued*)

Disorder	Cutaneous Findings	Gastrointestinal Features	Other Pertinent Findings	Treatment and Comments
Cowden's syndrome (multiple hamartoma syndrome)	Facial or periorificial papules (tricholemmomas), mucosal papules in a cobblestone pattern, and acral hyperkeratotic papules (Fig. 183-38)	Hamartomatous polyps in the small and large intestines	Fibrocystic disease of the breast, thyroid tumors, and breast carcinoma (often bilateral)	Autosomal dominant; remove polyps, if symptomatic; mastectomy
Muir-Torre syndrome	Sebaceous neoplasia and multiple keratoacanthomas	Multiple malignancies of the GI tract causing occult blood loss	Malignancies also reported to occur in the larynx and the genitourinary tract; also lymphomas	Autosomal dominant; remove symptomatic areas of the bowel
Cronkhite-Canada syndrome	Circumscribed areas of lentiginous hypermelanosis, alopecia, and generalized nail thinning	Adenomatous GI polyps and diarrhea; abdominal pain	Weight loss	Malignant degeneration is unusual
Vasculitis	Palpable purpura, livedo reticularis nodules, and ulcers	Ulcerations from vascular inflammation in <10% of patients with cutaneous vasculitis; may be more common in patients with IgA circulating immune complexes	Arthritis and nephritis	Corticosteroids or immunosuppressives or both
Malignant atrophic papulosis (Degos' disease)	Early signs include pale red papules with central necrosis, then later, atrophic, white (ivory) scars	Similar lesions on the GI mucosa; hemorrhage may result in death	Central nervous system disease, pleuritis, and pericarditis	Skin biopsy: wedge-shaped ischemic necrosis with dermal mucin
Scurvy	Perifollicular purpura	Collagen degeneration in the vessel walls; mild GI blood loss results in anemia	Conjunctival hemorrhage and gingivitis with easy bleeding	Vitamin C replacement
Kaposi's sarcoma (including classic Kaposi's and acquired immunodeficiency syndrome (AIDS))	Purpuric macules, papules, and nodules	Lesions on the GI mucosa result in bleeding	In AIDS, typical associated problems; possible lymphomas in classic Kaposi's sarcoma	In classic Kaposi's sarcoma chemotherapy may be helpful
Inflammatory bowel disease				
Ulcerative colitis	Erythema nodosum, pyoderma gangrenosum and vasculitis	Uniform and continuous mucosal inflammation with neutrophils resulting in ulceration, hemorrhage, and hyperemia; submucosa and small intestine are spared; rectum is usually involved (>95%); toxic megacolon may develop	Aphthous ulcerations, arthritis, and chronic blood loss; malignant degeneration as a late consequence	Sulfonamides (especially azulfidine) or corticosteroids; total colectomy
Crohn's disease (regional enteritis or granulomatous colitis)	Erythema nodosum, pyoderma gangrenosum, vasculitis, and perirectal fistulae	Chronic inflammation extending through all layers of the intestinal wall with or without granuloma formation; cobblestoning of the colonic mucosa; skip areas are very common, but rectal involvement is <50%	Aphthous ulcerations, arthritis, and chronic blood loss	Azulfidine, metronidazole, corticosteroids or adreno-corticotropic hormone and immunosuppressives (azathioprine or possibly cyclosporine); avoid surgery!

From Callen JP, Fabré VC. Cutaneous manifestations of systemic disease. In: Moschella SL, Hurley HJ, eds. Dermatology. Philadelphia: WB Saunders Co., 1992:1682-1718.

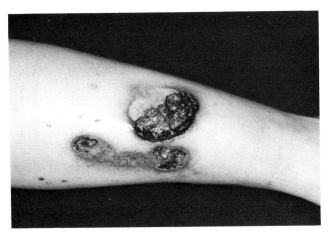

FIGURE 183–34. Pyoderma gangrenosum.

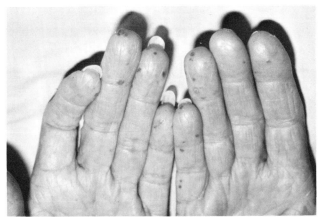

FIGURE 183–36. Hereditary hemorrhagic telangiectasia.

CUTANEOUS INFECTIOUS DISEASE

Cutaneous infectious disease is a vast collection of topics that are of central importance to the interface between dermatology and internal medicine and are discussed elsewhere in this text. The following topics are traditional and are covered in this textbook as described: viral diseases (Chapters 121 to 125), fungal diseases (Chapters 117 to 120), bacterial diseases (Chapters 105 to 107), sexually transmitted diseases (Chapter 108), protozoan diseases (Chapter 127), and rickettsial diseases (Chapter 109).

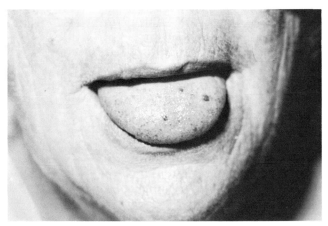

FIGURE 183–35. Hereditary hemorrhagic telangiectasia.

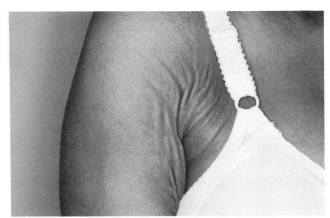

FIGURE 183–37. Pseudoxanthoma elasticum.

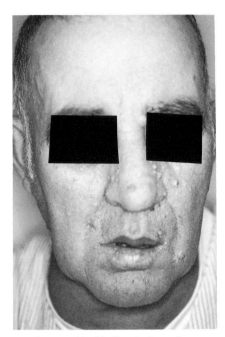

FIGURE 183-38. Cowden's syndrome.

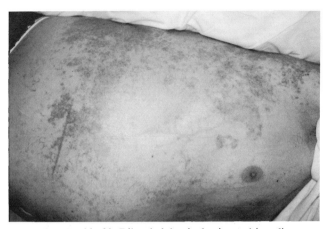

FIGURE 183-39. Dilated abdominal veins and jaundice.

TABLE 183-14. Dermatologic Aspects of Liver Disease

Liver Disease	Dermatologic Associations
Cirrhosis	Spider angiomas and other telangiectasias Palmar erythema Dilated abdominal wall veins (Fig. 183-39) Terry's nails (white nail bed) Muehrcke's nails (transverse white bands) Sparse axillary pubic and pectoral hair Gynecomastia Pruritus Jaundice (Fig. 183-39)
Primary biliary cirrhosis	Jaundice Hyperpigmentation Xanthomas—eruptive, xanthelasma, planar xanthomas Pruritus (Fig. 183-40)
Hemochromatosis ("bronze diabetes")	Hyperpigmentation—generalized
Wilson's disease	Kayser-Fleischer ring—(golden brown or greenish) brown circle of pigment in Descemet's membrane at the periphery of the cornea Blue lunulae
Viral hepatitis	Small vessel necrotizing vasculitis Polyarteritis nodosa Gianotti-Crosti syndrome (papular acrodermatitis of childhood) Essential mixed cryoglobulinemia Urticaria Erythema multiforme Erythema nodosum Erythema cyanosis Raynaud's phenomenon

OTHER SYSTEMIC DISEASES WITH CUTANEOUS MANIFESTATIONS

Sarcoidosis is a multisystem disease with major cutaneous manifestations. This topic is well covered elsewhere in this textbook (Chapter 45). Cardiovascular diseases and the skin are not specifically discussed elsewhere in this text. Table 183-15 is a review of cardiopulmonary and dermatologic abnormalities that are features of multisystem disorders (Figs. 183-41 to 183-46, see color plate for Fig. 183-45). Table 183-16 is a summary of cutaneous findings that occur in cardiac disorders.[18] Pulmonary disorders are listed in Table 183-17 (Figs. 183-47 and 183-48).

Text continued on page 1882

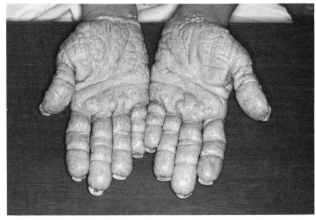

FIGURE 183-40. Primary biliary cirrhosis.

TABLE 183-15. Cardiac Abnormalities in Multisystem Disorders with Prominent Cutaneous Features

Disease	Cardiac Manifestation	Cutaneous Features	Comments
Primary systemic amyloidosis	Congestive heart failure, conduction disturbances, cardiomegaly	Pinch purpura, waxy skin (Fig. 183-41)	Proteinuria, associated with myeloma
Behçet's disease	Pericarditis	Oral and genital aphthae, pathergy, pustular vasculitis (Fig. 183-42)	Eye involvement (hypopyon), CNS disease, colitis
Carcinoid syndrome	Endocardial plaque—tricuspid insufficiency conduction defects, pulmonic stenosis, right-sided heart failure, asthmatic attacks	Flushing, sclerodermoid changes	Serotonin-producing tumor of the intestine, usually metastatic to liver at the onset of symptoms
Cutis laxa	Aortic dilatation and rupture, pulmonary artery stenosis, cor pulmonale	Marked looseness of the skin	Variable inheritance patterns
Dermatomyositis	Non-specific ECG changes, conduction defects, pericarditis (rare), congestive heart failure	Gottron's papules, heliotrope rash, poikiloderma, photosensitive eruption	Cardiac involvement is a poor prognostic sign
Malignant atrophic papulosis (Degos' disease)	Pericarditis, pericardial effusion	Ivory scars, infarcts of the skin	Unknown cause, often rapidly fatal
Diabetes mellitus	Coronary artery disease		
Ehlers-Danlos syndrome	Aortic, pulmonary artery dilatation, mitral, tricuspid valve prolapse, arterial rupture	Hyperelasticity of the skin, "cigarette paper" scars, ecchymoses	Cardiac disease is limited to types I, III, and IV
Exfoliative erythroderma	High-output cardiac failure	Exfoliative dermatitis	Various causes include eczemas, psoriasis, lymphoma, drugs, etc.
Fabry's disease	Mitral valve prolapse, conduction defects, cardiomyopathy, congestive heart failure, myocardial infarction, CVAs	Angiokeratoma corporis diffusum	X-linked recessive inheritance deficiency of alpha-galactosidase A; lipiduria leads to end-stage renal disease
Hemochromatosis	Congestive heart failure, supraventricular arrhythmias	Generalized bronze hyperpigmentation	Diabetes mellitus, cirrhosis
Hypereosinophilic syndrome			
Kawasaki disease (mucocutaneous lymph node syndrome)	Coronary arteritis, coronary artery aneurysms, myocardial infarction	Glossitis, cheilitis, acral erythema, edema and desquamation (Fig. 183-43) Polymorphous exanthem, conjunctival injection (uveitis)	High fever, lymphadenopathy; treatment wtih immune globulin is very helpful
Neonatal lupus erythematosus	Congenital heart block (most often complete)	Transient LE rash (often nonscarring) (Fig. 183-44)	Rash and cardiac disease rarely occur in the same patient; a pacemaker may become necessary
Systemic lupus erythematosus	Verrucous endocarditis (Libman-Sacks) (most often of the mitral valve), pericarditis, coronary arteritis	Malar erythema (butterfly rash), photosensitivity, DLE, SCLE skin lesions	Anticardiolipin antibody may be more common in LE patients with mitral regurgitation and/or valvular vegetations
Lipid disorders—hyperlipoproteinemias	Coronary artery disease	Tuberous xanthomas, tendon xanthoma, planar xanthoma (xanthelasma) Xanthelasma, juvenile arcus senilis Planar xanthomas, tuberous xanthomas	Type IIA—increased LDL, cholesterol, normal triglyceride. Type IIB—increased LDL and VLDL, cholesterol, mild increased triglyerides Type III—defect results in increased cholesterol and triglycerides
LEOPARD syndrome	ECG abnormalities (unspecified)	Multiple lentigines	L = lentigines, E = ECG abnormality, O = ocular hypertelorism, A = abnormalities of the genitalia, R = retardation of growth, D = deafness

TABLE 183-15. Cardiac Abnormalities in Multisystem Disorders with Prominent Cutaneous Features (*Continued*)

Disease	Cardiac Manifestation	Cutaneous Features	Comments
Multicentric reticulohistiocytosis	Pericarditis, congestive heart failure, coronary artery disease, cardiomegaly	Erythematous to violaceous nodules on the face and hands, mucosal nodules may occur	Synovium is affected also
Myxomas (Carney's syndrome, NAME and LAMB syndromes)	Atrial myxoma	Cutaneous myxoma, lentigines	Carney's syndrome includes growths of the adrenal, pituitary, and testes
Neurofibromatosis	Hypertension due to pheochromocytoma	Café-au-lait spots, neurofibromas, axillary freckling	
Pseudoxanthoma elasticum	Early-onset atherosclerotic vascular disease; aortic aneurysm	Yellow papules on intertriginous skin; loss of elasticity, redundant skin	Angioid streaks on ophthalmoscopy
Relapsing polychondritis	Aortic insufficiency, dissecting aortic aneurysms	Beefy, red, floppy ears (Fig. 183–45)	Joint involvement, tracheal collapse
Rheumatic fever	Pancarditis in acute phase; late manifestations include mitral and/or aortic valve disease	Erythema marginatum, subcutaneous nodules	Rare in the U.S. Follows pharyngitis due to group A β-hemolytic streptococcus Polyarthritis, chorea, fever
Sarcoidosis	Conduction defects, congestive heart failure	Papules, nodules, plaques, lesions in scars, etc.	Pulmonary disease, lymphadenopathy Presence of cardiac involvement is associated with poor prognosis
Scleroderma	Conduction defects, cor pulmonale, pericarditis, visceral Raynaud's phenomenon	Sclerosis (acral and/or central), telangiectasis, calcinosis	Raynaud's phenomenon, pulmonary fibrosis, esophageal dysmotility Cardiac disease associated with poor prognosis
Tuberous sclerosis	Cardiac rhabdomyomas	Adenoma sebaceum, periungual and subungual fibromas, ash-leaf macule; shagreen patch	Renal hamartomas, CNS tumors, mental retardation, seizures
Vasculitis	Coronary artery vasculitis	Palpable purpura, nodules, livedo reticularis, ulcerations	Arthritis, GI colic or bleeding Cardiac involvement is rare
Werner's syndrome	Premature atherosclerosis, coronary artery disease	Premature graying, alopecia, sclerodermoid changes, loss of subcutaneous fat, ankle ulcerations	Bird-like facies, high-pitched voice, inherited as an autosomal recessive Myocardial infarction is usually responsible for death by 5th decade

Adapted from Callen JP. Cardiovascular diseases and the skin. In: Callen JP, Jorizzo JL, et al., eds. Dermatological Signs of Internal Disease, 2nd edition. Philadelphia: WB Saunders Co., 1995:301–306.

CNS, central nervous system; ECG, electrocardiogram; CVA, cerebrovascular accident; LE, lupus erythematosus; DLE, drug-induced lupus erythematosus; SCLE, subacute cutaneous lupus erythematosus; LDL, low-density lipoproteins; VLDL, very low density lipoprotein; NAME, nevi, atrial myxomas, myxomas, ephelides; LAMB, lentigenes, atrial myxoma, mucocutaneous myxoma, blue nevi; GI, gastrointestinal.

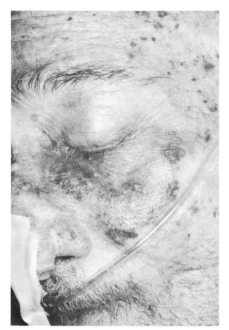

FIGURE 183–41. Amyloidosis.

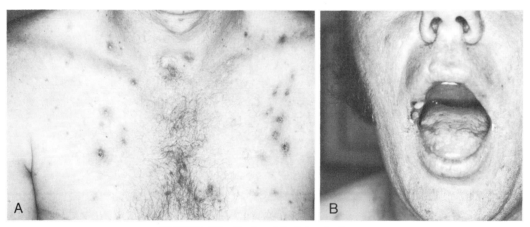

FIGURE 183–42. *A* and *B*, Behçet's disease.

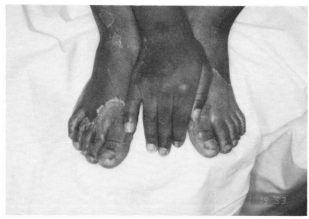

FIGURE 183–43. Kawasaki disease.

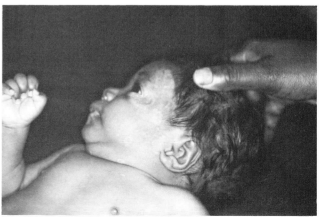

FIGURE 183–44. Neonatal lupus erythematosus.

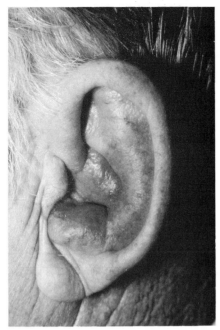

FIGURE 183–45. Relapsing polychondritis. (See color plate.)

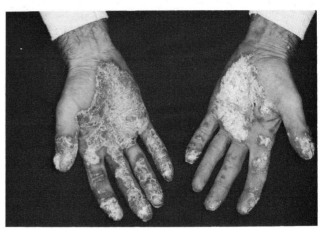

FIGURE 183–46. Reiter's disease.

TABLE 183–16. Cutaneous Findings Observed in Association with Primary Cardiac Abnormalities

Cardiac Disorder	Cutaneous Changes
Coronary artery disease	Xanthomas, skin changes of diabetes, changes of premature aging, ? presence of an earlobe crease
Hypertension:	
Pheochromocytoma	Neurofibromatosis, café-au-lait spots
Renovascular	Features of scleroderma
Cholesterol emboli	Palpable purpura, livedo reticularis, ulcerations
Often follows an invasive procedure such as catheterization or angiography	
Bacterial endocarditis	Osler's nodes, Janeway's lesions, petechiae, purpuric pustules, splinter hemorrhages
Left atrial myxoma	Changes of syndromes with myxomata
	Embolic phenomena as in cholesterol emboli
Drug therapy for cardiac diseases:	
Amiodarone	Photosensitivity, resultant slate blue-gray pigmentation
β blockers	Flare of psoriasis
Minoxidil	Hypertrichosis
Quinidine	Petechiae (thrombocytopenia), photosensitivity
Procainamide HCl	Drug-induced lupus erythematosus (LE)
Thiazide diuretics	Photosensitivity, drug-induced subacute cutaneous LE

From Callen JP. Cardiovascular diseases and the skin. In: Callen JP, Jorizzo JL, et al., eds. Dermatological Signs of Internal Disease, 2nd edition. Philadelphia: WB Saunders Co., 1995:301–306.

TABLE 183–17. Pulmonary Disease and the Skin

Disorder	Cutaneous Findings	Pulmonary Disease	Other Features	Treatment and Comments
Sarcoidosis	Papules, nodules, plaques Lupus pernio (Figs. 183–47 and 183–48) Erythema nodosum (EN)	Pulmonary fibrosis, granulomas, Bilateral hilar lymphadenopathy (BHL), upper respiratory disease	Bone cysts, hypercalcemia, arthritis, uveitis	Hydroxychloroquine for cutaneous lesions Combination of EN, BHL, arthritis known as Löfgren's syndrome — a self-limited benign variant of sarcoidosis Corticosteroids for scarring lesions and progressive pulmonary involvement
Tuberculosis	Lupus vulgaris Scrofuloderma	Cavitating infiltrates Unilateral hilar lymphadenopathy	Fever, debilitation	Isoniazid, rifampicin
Mycoplasma pneumonia	Erythema multiforme or Stevens-Johnson syndrome	Pneumonitis — "walking pneumonia"		Erythromycin
Varicella pneumonia	Typical lesions	Pneumonitis	More common in adults, pregnancy	Can result in death, acyclovir may be effective
Human immunodeficiency virus infection	Kaposi's sarcoma, opportunistic infections	*Pneumocystis carinii* pneumonitis	Opportunistic infections, diarrhea	Pentamidine, zovirudine
Lymphomatoid granulomatosis	Nodules or plaques or papules Facial location is common	Angiocentric, angiodestructive infiltrate of atypical lymphocytes	Lymphoma may develop	Immunosuppressive therapy
Wegener's granulomatosis	Vasculitic lesions, cutaneous granulomas	Cavitary pulmonary nodules Pulmonary vasculitis	Glomerulonephritis (may be rapidly progressive) Upper respiratory tract inflammation Sinusitis, iritis, mononeuritis multiplex, pericarditis, arthritis, mucosal ulceration	Anti-neutrophil cytoplastic antibody may aid in diagnosis Corticosteroids, cyclophosphamide
Dermatomyositis	Gottron's papules, heliotrope, photosensitivity, poikiloderma	Pulmonary fibrosis, aspiration pneumonia, hypoventilation	Proximal symmetric muscle weakness	Corticosteroids, immunosuppression
Scleroderma	Sclerosis, telangiectasia, calcinosis, Raynaud's phenomenon	Pulmonary fibrosis, cor pulmonale, visceral Raynaud's phenomenon Late — lung cancer	Esophageal dysmotility, arthritis	D-penicillamine
Blastomycosis	Verrucous, ulcerating lesions, pustules at the periphery	Patchy fibrotic infiltrate; chest radiograph may be normal.	Testicular involvement	Amphotericin-B, ? ketoconazole Skin lesions represent dissemination
Hereditary hemorrhagic telangiectasia	Mucosal and acral telangiectatic mats	Pulmonary A-V malformation	Epistaxis, recurrent GI bleeding, A-V malformation in other organs	None known to be effective

Cutaneous aspects of renal disease are discussed in various chapters, but are not considered as a group elsewhere in this textbook. Table 183–18 is an overview of cutaneous changes that are particularly prevalent in patients with renal disease[19] (Figs. 183–49 to 183–54). Table 183–19 is taken from material in a recent review.[19] The skin is commonly affected in patients with renal disease. Changes occur from at least four possible avenues: (1) those changes seen that occur with uremia; (2) those changes due to multisystem disorder; (3) changes related to dialysis; and (4) changes due to the presence of a transplanted kidney and the therapy used to prevent rejection.

Pruritus is a feature of uremia, but in addition it occurs

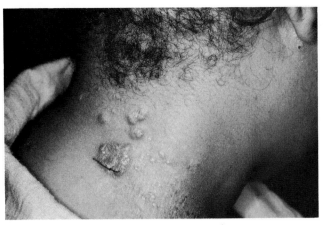

FIGURE 183–47. Sarcoidosis.

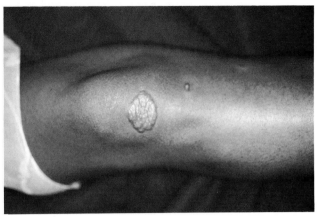

FIGURE 183–48. Sarcoidosis.

TABLE 183-18. Renal Disease and the Skin

Disorder	Cutaneous Findings	Renal Abnormality	Other Findings	Treatment	Comment
Cutaneous changes of ESRD	1. Pale color, sallowness 2. Xerosis, if severe ichthyosis 3. Pruritus—may be severe 4. Metastatic calcinosis 5. Uremic frost 6. Gangrene	ESRD of various causes	1. Anemia of chronic disease 2. — 3. ? Increased tissue mast cell numbers 4. Calcium × phosphorus >60 5. Severe uremia 6. Calcification of vessel walls	1. Recombinant erythropoietin 2. Emollients 3. Ultraviolet light 4. Antacids that bind phosphate 5. Dialysis or transplant 6. Vascular surgery	3. May be due to 2° hyperpara-thyroidism 4. Abnormal calcium metabolism
Multisystem Disorders Systemic lupus erythematosus	Malar erythema, cutaneous LE lesions, photosensitivity, alopecia, Raynaud's phenomenon, vasculitis	Glomerulone-phritis—focal, membranous or diffuse proliferative	Arthritis, CNS disease, cytopenia, multiple antibodies (anti-nDNA, anti-Sm), hypocomple-mentemia	Dependent on the severity of the renal lesion	
Scleroderma	Raynaud's phenomenon, calcinosis, sclerosis, telangiectasia	Malignant hypertension, rapidly progressive renal impairment	Esophageal dysmotility, pulmonary fibrosis	Angiotensin converting enzyme inhibitors	
Polyarteritis nodosa	Livedo reticularis, palpable purpura, nodules	Glomerulone-phritis, renal artery aneurysms, hypertension	Arthritis, myositis, fever, pleuritis, pericarditis, mononeuritis multiplex, abdominal pain, GI bleeding	Corticosteroids, cyclophos-phamide	Rule out hepatitis B infection, vasculitis of the medium and small arteries
Neurofibroma-tosis	Café-au-lait spots, neurofibromas	Hypertension (malignant), pheochromo-cytoma	Seizures, CNS tumors, peripheral nerve tumors	Removal	Evaluate other family members, and other endocrine organs
Tuberous sclerosis	Adenoma sebaceum, ash-leaf macule, shagreen patch, periungual fibroma (Figs. 183–49 and 183–50)	Renal hamartoma (angiomyoli-poma)	CNS tumors, mental retardation, cardiac rhabdomyoma, seizures	Surgical removal	Autosomal dominant

Continued

TABLE 183-18. Renal Disease and the Skin (*Continued*)

Disorder	Cutaneous Findings	Renal Abnormality	Other Findings	Treatment	Comment
Fabry's disease	Angiokeratoma corporis diffusum (Fig. 183-51)	Accumulation of ceramide trihexoside (glycosphingo-lipid) in the glomerulus with proteinuria and renal failure	Mitral valve prolapse, conduction defects, congestive heart failure, myocardial infarction, CVAs, painful crises in childhood	Renal transplantation	Deficiency of alpha-galactosidase A, X-linked recessive
Nail-patella syndrome	Hypoplasia of nails and patella	Progressive renal failure, proteinuria	Skeletal abnormalities, in particular the iliac crest	None known	
Sarcoidosis	Papules, nodules, plaques	Calcium stones	Lymphadenop-athy, uveitis, pulmonary fibrosis	Corticosteroids are helpful in hypercalcemia	
1° systemic amyloidosis	Pinch purpura	Proteinuria	Congestive heart failure, paraprotein, myeloma	None known	
Cutaneous changes related to dialysis	Pruritis	ESRD	None	Ultraviolet light	
	Splinter hemorrhages	ESRD	None	None	
	Bullous dermatosis of hemodialysis	ESRD	None	Sunscreens	Rule out porphyria
	Kyrle's disease	ESRD	Diabetes mellitus	? Topical tretinoin	
Cutaneous changes in transplant patients	Infections Fungal Viral—atypical herpes simplex (Fig. 183-52), multiple warts Norwegian scabies Bacterial Cushing's syndrome	ESRD			Due to immunosup-pression
		ESRD		Reduce corticosteroid dosage	Due to corticosteroid use
	Cancer Squamous cell carcinoma (Figs. 183-53 and 183-54) Anogenital carcinoma Kaposi's sarcoma	ESRD		Reduce immunosup-pressive dosage	Due to immunosup-pression

ESRD, end-stage renal disease; LE, lupus erythematosus; GI, gastrointestinal; CNS, central nervous system; CVA, cerebrovascular accident.

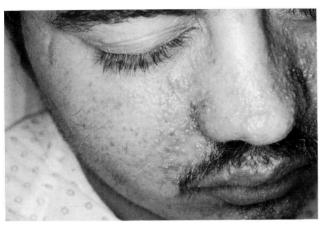

FIGURE 183–49. Tuberous sclerosis.

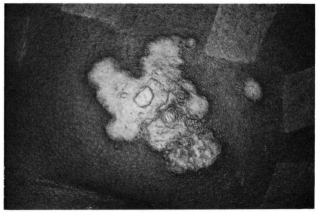

FIGURE 183–52. Atypical herpes simplex virus in transplant patient.

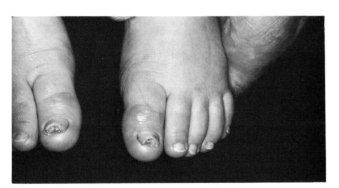

FIGURE 183–50. Tuberous sclerosis.

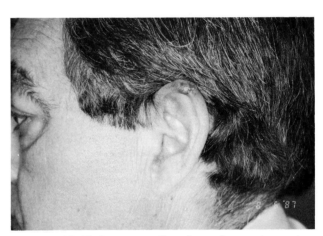

FIGURE 183–53. Squamous cell carcinoma in transplant patient.

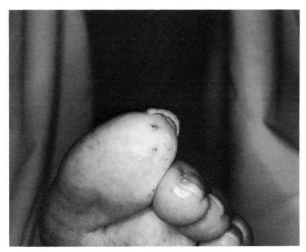

FIGURE 183–51. Fabry's disease.

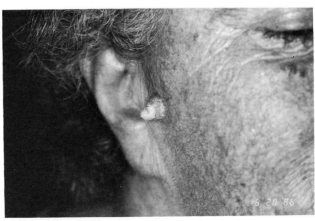

FIGURE 183–54. Squamous cell carcinoma in transplant patient.

TABLE 183-19. Dermatologic Conditions Particularly Prevalent in Patients on Renal Dialysis

Uremic pruritus
Bullous disease of dialysis ("pseudo" porphyria)
Perforating diseases
　Kyrle's disease
　Reactive perforating folliculitis
　Reactive perforating collagenosis
Contact dermatitis
Acroangiodermatitis ("pseudo" Kaposi's sarcoma)
Staphylococcus aureus carriage with folliculitis, furunculosis, etc.
"Dialysis acne" (from testosterone-like medications to stimulate hematopoiesis)

Data from Jorizzo JL, Sheretz EF. Cutaneous changes in renal disorders. In: Fitzpatrick TB, Eisen AZ, Wolff K, eds. Dermatology in General Medicine. New York: McGraw Hill, 1993: Chapter 165.

TABLE 183-20. Life-Threatening Systemic Disorders with Prominent Cutaneous Features

Infectious Diseases

Erysipelas
Cellulitis
Necrotizing fasciitis
Ecthyma gangrenosum
Meningococcemia
Rocky Mountain spotted fever

HIV-Associated Disorders

Kaposi's sarcoma
Cryptococcosis
Histoplasmosis
Tuberculosis (scrofuloderma)
Bacillary angiomatosis
Varicella-zoster virus infection
Cytomegalovirus infection
Herpes simplex virus infection

Collagen Vascular Disease

Systemic lupus erythematosus
Dermatomyositis
Relapsing polychondritis
Behçet's disease

Vascular Diseases

Angioedema—hereditary or allergic
Kawasaki disease
Vasculitis
Cholesterol emboli
Degos' disease

Malignancies with Rapid Evolution

Mycosis fungoides (d'emblé form)
Lymphoma/leukemia (HTLV-1 associated)
Melanoma (nodular)
Histiocytosis X (Letterer-Siwe)
Cutaneous metastases

Miscellaneous

Systemic mastocytosis
Graft-versus-host disease

HIV, human immunodeficiency virus.
From Kerdel FA. Life-threatening disorders. In: Callen JP, Jorizzo JL, et al., eds. Dermatological Signs of Internal Disease, 2nd edition. Philadelphia: WB Saunders Co., 1995:397–402.

in nonuremic patients on hemodialysis. It is still unclear why patients with chronic renal failure on dialysis have pruritus. The pruritus may be localized or generalized, it is usually worse during dialysis, but may occur around the clock. Patients with abnormal calcium-phosphorus metabolism seem to be more often affected by pruritus. Thus one postulate holds that secondary hyperparathyroidism is at least indirectly related to the pruritus. Furthermore, some patients with pruritus have improved when parathyroidectomy is performed. Most patients respond at least partially to soporific antipruritic agents. Many patients also respond to sub-erythemogenic doses of ultraviolet B phototherapy.

Patients with renal transplantation are given the immunosuppressive agents cyclosporine, azathioprine and/or corticosteroids in order to prevent rejection. The combination of these drugs predisposes the patient to two major problems, infection and malignancy.

In addition, many unique dermatoses and variations in clinical presentation of common dermatoses are seen in patients who have acquired immune suppression as occurs from infection with the human immunodeficiency virus, with malignancy, and with drug-induced immunosuppression following organ or tissue transplantation. The issues are discussed well elsewhere in this textbook (Chapter 125).

Psychocutaneous diseases play a significant role in the practice of medical dermatology. These entities are reviewed in Chapter 89. Neurocutaneous disorders are the subject of Chapter 148.

Pregnancy is an important physiologic state that is associated with its own specific dermatoses and with modification of other dermatoses. Chapter 37 reviews these issues. Mast cell disease is the subject of Chapter 41. Internal disease can produce profound effects on the nails (Chapter 136), hair (Chapters 133 to 135), and mucous membranes (Chapters 138 and 139). Leg ulcers are also potential dermatologic clues to underlying disease and are discussed elsewhere in this book (Chapter 65).

Dermatology is too often viewed as a specialty dealing with outpatients who do not have life-threatening disease. In reality, a number of dermatologic patients do have life-threatening dermatoses.[20] Table 183–20 is a summary of selected life-threatening systemic disorders with prominent cutaneous features. Table 183–21 is a summary of cutaneous conditions with potentially life-threatening systemic complications.[20]

The use of systemic drugs for skin disease has been the subject of recent reviews.[21, 22] Table 183–22 is a summary of some important dermatoses selectively requiring systemic medications with some element of risk.[23]

TABLE 183-21. Cutaneous Conditions with Potential Life-Threatening Systemic Complications

Sclerema neonatorum
Mechanobullous diseases
Hemangiomas
Staphylococcal scalded skin syndrome (see Chapter 106)
Erythema multiforme/Stevens-Johnson Syndrome (see Chapter 22)
Toxic epidermal necrolysis
Pustular psoriasis
Impetigo herpetiform (see Chapter 79)
Pemphigus (see Chapter 74)
Spider bites

From Kerdel FA. Life-threatening disorders. In: Callen JP, Jorizzo JL, et al., eds. Dermatological Signs of Internal Disease, 2nd edition. Philadelphia: WB Saunders Co., 1995:397–402.

TABLE 183-22. Some Important Dermatoses Selectively Requiring Systemic Medications *with an Element of Risk

Psoriasis

Cyclosporine
Methotrexate
PUVA
Retinoids

Acne Vulgaris

Retinoids

Vasculitis

Azathioprine
Corticosteroids
Dapsone

Lupus Erythematosus

Antimalarials
Corticosteroids
Cyclosporine
Dapsone
Retinoids

Pyoderma Gangrenosum

Corticosteroids
Cyclosporine
Dapsone

Pemphigus Vulgaris

Azathioprine
Corticosteroids
Cyclosporine

Bullous Pemphigoid

Corticosteroids
Cyclosporine
Dapsone

TABLE 183-22. Some Important Dermatoses Selectively Requiring Systemic Medications *with an Element of Risk (Continued)

Dermatitis Herpetiformis

Dapsone

Mycosis Fungoides

Methotrexate
PUVA

Disorders of Keratinization

Retinoids

Atopic Dermatitis, Severe

Azathioprine
Corticosteroids
Cyclosporine
PUVA

*Note: The drugs listed under each heading are those on which this chapter focuses and are not an exhaustive list of therapeutic options. The listing of drugs is alphabetic and does not imply a therapeutic sequence.
PUVA, psoralens with ultraviolet A light therapy.
From Wolverton SE. Systemic therapy for cutaneous disease. In: Callen JP, Jorizzo JL, et al., eds. Dermatological Signs of Internal Disease, 2nd edition. Philadelphia: WB Saunders Co., 1995:417–420.

References

1. Jorizzo JL, Daniels JC. Dermatologic conditions reported in patients with rheumatoid arthritis. J Am Acad Dermatol 1983;8:439–453.
2. Smith ML, Jorizzo JL, Semble E, et al. Rheumatoid papules: Lesions showing features of vasculitis and palisading granuloma. J Am Acad Dermatol 1989;20:348–352.
3. Piette WW. Purpura. In: Callen JP, Jorizzo JL, et al., eds. Dermatological Signs of Internal Disease, 2nd edition. Philadelphia: WB Saunders Co., 1995:87–95.
4. Callen JP. Skin signs of internal malignancy. In: Callen JP, Jorizzo JL, et al., eds. Dermatological Signs of Internal Disease, 2nd edition. Philadelphia: WB Saunders Co., 1995:111–121.
5. Huntley AC. The cutaneous manifestations of diabetes mellitus. Dermatol Clin 1992;7:531–546.
6. Lovitt MH, Dover JS. Necrobiosis lipoidica. J Am Acad Dermatol 1991;25:735–748.
7. Sibbald RG, Schachter RK. The skin and diabetes mellitus. Int J Dermatol 1984;23:567–584.
8. Diven DG, Gwinup G, Newton RC: The thyroid. Dermatol Clin 1989;7:547–558.
9. Heyman WR. Cutaneous manifestations of thyroid disease. J Am Acad Dermatol 1992;26:885–902.
10. Rosen T, Kleman GA. Thyroid and the skin. In: Callen JP, Jorizzo JL, et al., eds. Dermatological Signs of Internal Disease, 2nd edition. Philadelphia: WB Saunders Co., 1995:189–195.
11. Feingold KR, Elias PM. Endocrine-skin interactions. J Am Acad Dermatol 1988;19:1–20.
12. Miller SJ. Nutritional deficiency and the skin. J Am Acad Dermatol 1989;21:1–30.
13. Delahoussaye AR, Jorizzo JL. Cutaneous manifestations of nutritional disorders. Dermatol Clin 1989;7:559–570.
14. Shererz EF, Jorizzo JL. Skin lesions associated with gastrointestinal disease. In: Yamada T, Alpers DH, Owyang C, et al., eds. Textbook of Gastroenterology. Philadelphia: JB Lippincott, 1991: Chapter 44.

15. Callen JP, Fabre VC. Cutaneous manifestations of systemic disease. In: Moschella SL, Hurley HJ, eds. Dermatology, 3rd edition. Philadelphia: WB Saunders Co., 1992: Chapter 66.
16. Sarkany I. The skin-liver connection. Clin Exp Dermatol 1988; 13:151–159.
17. Greer KE. Cutaneous hepatology. In: Callen JP, Jorizzo JL, et al., eds. Dermatologic Signs of Internal Disease, 2nd edition. Philadelphia: WB Saunders Co., 1995:233–239.
18. Callen JP. Cardiovascular diseases and the skin. In: Callen JP, Jorizzo JL, et al., eds. Dermatological Signs of Internal Disease, 2nd edition. Philadelphia: WB Saunders Co., 1995:301–306.
19. Jorizzo JL, Sheretz EF. Cutaneous changes in renal disorders. In: Fitzpatrick TB, et al., eds. Dermatology in General Medicine. New York: McGraw Hill, 1993: Chapter 165.
20. Kerdel FA. Life-threatening disorders. In: Callen JP, Jorizzo JL, et al., eds. Dermatological Signs of Internal Disease, 2nd edition. Philadelphia: WB Saunders Co., 1995:397–402.
21. Wolverton SE, Wilkin JK, eds. Systemic Drugs for Skin Diseases. Philadelphia: WB Saunders Co., 1991.
22. Wolverton SE. Monitoring for adverse effects from systemic drugs used in dermatology. J Am Acad Dermatol 1992;26:661–669.
23. Wolverton SE. Systemic therapy for cutaneous disease. In: Callen JP, Jorizzo JL, et al., eds. Dermatological Signs of Internal Disease, 2nd edition. Philadelphia: WB Saunders Co., 1995:417–420.

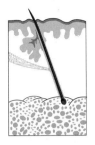

chapter 184

Pediatric Dermatology

BERNARD A. COHEN

The anatomy and physiology of the skin in children is both quantitatively and qualitatively different from that of adults. As a result, the practitioner must learn to recognize distinctive patterns of skin disease in children and pediatric variations of disorders that occur at all ages. Safe and effective medical management requires a understanding of the basic principles of growth and development in childhood and the special sensitivities of the parents and family.

NORMAL DEVELOPMENT[1, 2]

The average newborn weighs 3.5 kg (7.5 pounds) and is 50 cm (20 inches) long. After a brief period of weight loss, full-term infants regain their birth weight usually by 10 days of age. Growth proceeds at a rapid clip, with weight doubling at 5 months and tripling at 1 year of age. The average infant grows 25 to 30 cm (10 to 12 inches) during the first year and develops a marked increase in subcutaneous fat, which peaks at about 9 months of age. During the second year the rate of growth decelerates, with weight increasing about 5 pounds per year and height about 2.5 inches per year until the pubertal growth spurt. Appetite decreases, fat begins to decrease, and a leaner, more muscular toddler emerges.

The head circumference, which is 34 to 35 cm at birth, reaches 47 cm at 1 year, two thirds of the size at maturity. By the end of the second year, the brain reaches 80% of the adult size. The first teeth erupt between 5 and 9 months of age, and a rough estimate of age in months can be calculated by adding 6 to the number of teeth present.

The first year is a period of rapid development of gross motor, fine motor, language, and social skills. Although premature infants are often developmentally delayed, most catch up to their full-term counterparts by 2 years of age. Sensory and social deprivation especially during the neonatal period may interfere with normal development, particularly in children who develop severe medi-

cal complications of prematurity. Difficulties with parent-infant bonding resulting from a prolonged nursery admission also increase the risk of child abuse, which often presents with dermatologic clues.[3]

NORMAL NEWBORN SKIN

The skin of the neonate differs from that of the adult in several ways. In the full-term child, the skin is thinner, less hairy, has decreased eccrine gland activity, and fewer functional melanocytes.[4] Differences are magnified in the preterm infant, where the epidermis is about half the thickness of the full-term infant and adult. Additionally, there is a marked decrease in melanocytes, dermal collagen, and elastic fibers, and there is total anhidrosis. Consequently, newborns are poorly equipped to handle thermal stress and the effects of sunlight exposure. They have increased transepidermal water loss, and increased transcutaneous penetration of toxic substances and medications that are deliberately or inadvertently applied to the skin surface. They are more likely to develop blisters or erosions in response to heat, chemical irritants, mechanical trauma, and inflammatory dermatoses.

BARRIER PROPERTIES AND THE USE OF TOPICAL AGENTS

The barrier properties of the skin reside primarily in the stratum corneum.[5-8] Although keratinization begins at 24 weeks' gestation, it is not complete until close to term. In full-term infants transepidermal water loss and absorption of topical agents are similar to those of older children and adults. However, epidermal maturation is delayed by several days in infants born at 36 weeks and by at least several weeks in children born before 32 weeks. Epidermal maturation and subsequent barrier function may be further delayed by epidermal injury resulting from mechanical, thermal, and chemical

1889

trauma, infection, hyperemia, and ischemia. Finally, in any infant or child, the high surface area–to–volume ratio exaggerates the risk of transcutaneous absorption of topical agents.

Percutaneous absorption of toxic substances in normal preterm infants and term infants with disruption of the epidermal barrier has been well documented.[5-9] Aniline dyes used to mark diapers have caused methemoglobinemia. Topical steroids can produce local atrophy, systemic effects, and adrenal suppression. Accidental exposure to pentachlorophenol in nursery linens has been associated with poisoning, and topical application of povidine iodine has resulted in elevated plasma iodine levels and thyroid dysfunction (Fig. 184–1). Isopropyl alcohol, ethyl and methyl alcohol, chlorhexidine, and other substances are readily absorbed and may produce toxic reactions.

In general the use of topical agents in newborns should be restricted to those agents that are safe when administered systemically. Antiseptic agents and topical antibiotics should be used with caution and applied only to small areas of skin, particularly during the first few weeks of life in premature infants under 30 weeks' gestation.

SKIN CARE IN THE NEWBORN

At birth the skin is covered with a greasy, white material with a pH of 6.7 to 7.4. Although the function of this vernix caseosa is unknown, it may have lubricating and antibacterial properties. Beneath the vernix, the skin has a pH of 5.5 to 6.0. Overwashing, particularly with harsh soaps, may result in irritation, alkaline pH, and a decrease in normal barrier function. Consequently, bathing should only be done gently with tepid tap water. The use of mild soaps should be restricted to the umbilicus, diaper area, neck, axillae, and other areas where bacteria are most numerous.

According to a recent survey of neonatologists, there is no consensus on routine skin care in the nursery.[10] A majority of infants receive a bath within the first day of life. The same is true of almost half the tiny premature babies admitted to intensive care nurseries. In many nurseries, babies are subsequently bathed daily.

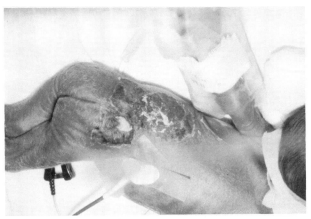

FIGURE 184–1. Betadine burn in nursery.

Injury to the skin can be reduced by judicious placement and removal of tape, monitor electrodes, and adhesives. The use of topical cleansing agents and adhesive removers should be kept to a minimum. When lubrication is necessary, small amounts of petrolatum or other bland, fragrance-free preparations can be applied.

Methods of preventing skin breakdown in healthy premature infants and sick full-term babies vary around the country and include regular repositioning and cushioning with lambs' wool and water beds. A recent study documented that a water-in-oil emollient (Eucerin cream) was effective in decreasing the incidence of dermatitis in premature infants of 29 to 36 weeks' gestation without increasing cutaneous bacteria.[11] A subsequent study with a preservative-free petrolatum wool wax ester ointment (Aquaphor) applied twice daily for 2 weeks to premature infants younger than 33 weeks' gestation gave similar results.[12] Moreover, bacterial colonization and the incidence of neonatal sepsis was lower in the treated group. Once skin breakdown has occurred, topical antibiotics and antifungals can be used with caution, and occlusive as well as semi-occlusive dressings may be helpful. Close monitoring for the development of cellulitis and sepsis includes daily dressing changes and surveillance cultures as indicated by clinical findings.

THERMOREGULATION IN NEWBORNS

Cold stress is a major risk for the newborn, particularly the tiny premature infant. Decreased thickness of the skin results in increased heat loss from radiation and conduction. Minimal subcutaneous fat in the premature neonate decreases the infant's ability to respond to cooling. A recent survey of skin care practices in the nation's intensive care nurseries indicated that use of a plastic wrap covering forming a mini-isolette was the most popular method for reducing heat and insensible water loss while children were kept under radiant warmers. Semipermeable polyurethane membranes have also been used successfully. Once the infant is in an isolette, humidified air is used almost universally.

In some premature infants and in full-term babies, hyperthermia may be a problem particularly when phototherapy or insulated clothing is used. Although sweat glands are anatomically complete at 28 weeks' gestation, they may not be fully functional until 2 to 4 weeks after birth. Apnea, poor feeding, and temperature instability associated with miliaria crystallina may be early signs of heat stress.

In addition to increased thermal stress, phototherapy may be associated with the development of phototoxic reactions and the bronze baby syndrome.[13] Bilirubin absorbs maximally in the blue wavelengths of light between 420 nm and 470 nm. Phototherapy, using blue fluorescent light bulbs, converts toxic unconjugated bilirubin into water soluble unconjugated isomers which are readily excreted by the liver and the kidneys without the need for conjugation. Coincidental exposure to photosensitizers such as sulfonamides and methylene blue may result in a severe phototoxic reaction. Moreover, infants with a significant component of conjugated bilirubin may develop a grayish brown pigmentation. Although pigmentation may last for months, the clinical significance of the bronze baby syndrome is unclear. Infants with conjugated hyperbilirubinemia are likely to have a serious underlying medical problem such as newborn sepsis and should be thoroughly investigated.

SUN PROTECTION

The melanoma epidemic, the risk of developing non-melanoma skin cancer, and "age" related changes in the skin have been closely linked to the effects of cumulative ultraviolet light exposure. It has been estimated that three quarters of lifetime sun exposure occurs in the first two decades of life.[14] Consequently, the practicing dermatologist must train pediatricians and parents about aggressive and early solar protection.

Although the use of sunscreens in children under 6 months of age is not routinely recommended, these children are not ambulatory and can be readily protected by physical barriers (e.g., clothing, umbrella, stroller covers).[15] However, regular use of sunscreens, particularly in light-complected individuals, should begin as soon as children walk at 9 to 12 months of age. Hypoallergenic, water-resistant products with an SPF of 15 to 30 are well tolerated by most children and should be applied at least 15 to 30 minutes before going outdoors. Although products with SPFs greater than 30 are more effective at preventing histologic changes associated with ultraviolet light exposure, it is not clear if this is clinically important. Moreover, the risk of contact allergic and irritant reactions may increase with increasing concentrations of the active ingredients.

Although some physicians have voiced concern about decreased levels of active vitamin D_3 as a result of aggressive sunscreen use in children, recent studies suggest that this is not a significant clinical problem.

Counseling regarding safe sun should also include tips on the use of clothing, hats, and sunglasses as a physical barrier and avoidance of midday sun exposure. Discussions with teenagers should also emphasize the dangers of artificial sun tanning devices. Unfortunately, children who have not been trained to protect their skin early in life are unlikely to change their behavior as adolescents.[16]

EVALUATION OF THE SKIN IN INFANTS AND CHILDREN

Although skin lesions in infants and young children are often benign and transient, some may herald the onset of life-threatening dermatoses, whereas others provide clues to underlying systemic disorders.

Initially, the clinician must obtain a detailed history of the onset and course of lesions, associated medical problems, topical and systemic medications, and evidence of pruritus. A review of neonatal records and photographs from parents will help to establish the presence of congenital malformations and nevoid anomalies. Maternal records may reveal intrauterine exposure to infectious, toxic, or pharmacologic agents. The family history may suggest a hereditary or infectious disorder, and the clinician may need to interview and examine family members for similar problems.

Examination of the skin must include the hair, nails, teeth, mucous membranes, and genitals. The dermatologist may need assistance for turning the sick infant in an isolette in the intensive care nursery. In the full-term nursery or outpatient office, care must be taken to avoid cold stress by exposing only a small portion of the body surface at any time.

Several excellent pediatric dermatology texts and atlases are available for a more detailed evaluation of the skin in infants and children.[17-19] The following discussion will focus on disorders that occur primarily in infants and young children or where the expression of skin lesions varies considerably from the adult presentation.

CHILD ABUSE

Cutaneous findings often provide the first clues of child abuse and neglect, and early recognition of these clues by the dermatologist may be life-saving (see Chapter 95). Over 2,500,000 cases occur annually in the United States, and over 1200 have a fatal outcome. Although neglect accounts for over half of the cases, over 40% are associated with physical or sexual abuse.[3, 20, 21]

Physical findings that should raise the clinical suspicion include the presence of bruises, crusts, abrasions, and the imprint of the object that caused the injury in unusual locations such as the mid back, buttocks, genitals, upper arms, ears, and feet (Figs. 184-2 and 184-3). The presence of old bruises and scars supports a suspicion of chronic and recurrent injury. Cigarette burns and hot water dip (Figs. 184-4 and 184-5) injuries should be considered abuse until proven otherwise.

A vague history that is not compatible with the cutaneous findings and a history that varies with different caretakers or the same caretaker at different times is typical of physical abuse. Other red flags include a delay in presentation for care of injuries, inappropriate parental concern, abnormal parent-child interactions in the office, and a history of repeated visits to the emergency room or physician's office for accidents, fractures, and/or ingestions.

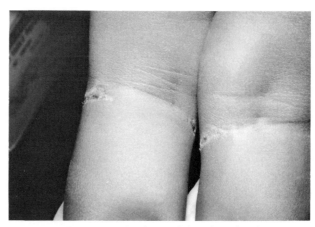

FIGURE 184-2. Ligature injury (rope burn).

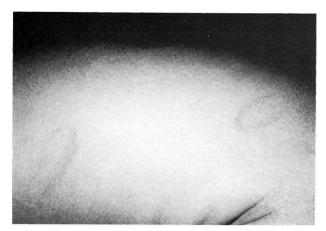

FIGURE 184-3. Lamp loop lesions.

The careful, sensitive, nonjudgmental clinician may uncover other parental and child risk factors for abuse. Parents who were themselves abused as children, who have limited coping skills or family support, who have alcohol, drug, or psychiatric problems, who are unemployed, or who are in their adolescent years seem to be most prone to abuse their own children. Children under 3 years of age who were born prematurely, who have chronic medical disorders or congenital anomalies, or who are under foster care are at greatest risk.

The diagnosis of neglect and sexual abuse can pose a more difficult challenge. Poor hygiene and growth, missed health maintenance visits, delayed vaccinations, and a delay in presentation for skin disease (infected insect bites, chronic tinea capitis or corporis, untreated chronic eczema, chronic diaper dermatitis) may be the result of neglect. Except in the case of acute rape and sodomy, physical findings in sexual abuse may be subtle. The presence of anogenital trauma or urethritis or vaginitis and positive cultures for gonorrhea or a darkfield examination consistent with syphilis is diagnostic. However, other infections associated with sexual activity in adults including genital warts, molluscum contagiosum, and herpes simplex are usually acquired in a non-abuse setting.

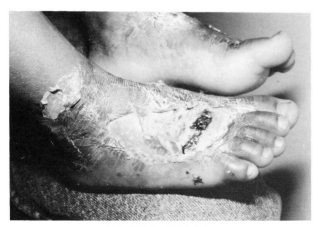

FIGURE 184-4. Dip injury.

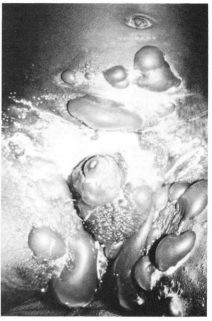

FIGURE 184-5. Hot water injury.

Before 1980 there were fewer than 20 cases of anogenital warts reported in children, and the majority were known or suspected to have been acquired from sexual abuse.[22] During the last decade there has been an explosion in pediatric case reports that has followed the epidemic of condyloma in young sexually active adults. Moreover, several large series of carefully investigated children have demonstrated that the majority of pediatric infections are acquired by an innocent nonvenereal route. Although the clinician must raise the issue of sexual exposure in any child who presents with anogenital warts, other sources, particularly perinatal contact with maternal condyloma, should be considered. Unfortunately, maternal lesions may be subclinical and regress spontaneously before the diagnosis is made. Indirect contact with maternal and paternal human papilloma virus may occur during bathing, diaper changes, and toileting in infants and toddlers. Finally, the specificity of human papilloma virus types for well-defined clinical lesions has been undermined by the recovery of human papilloma virus associated with nonvenereal warts from anogenital lesions in children and adults.

Whenever physical or sexual abuse is suspected, the child deserves a careful cutaneous and medical examination. Historical data from emergency room, nursery, and primary care records must be reviewed. All abused children should be reported to the appropriate authorities and released only to caretakers who can assure their safety.

NEONATAL DERMATOSES (Fig. 184-6)[23]

Transient Vascular Phenomena

During the first few weeks of life, cold stress may be associated with a number of transient vascular phenom-

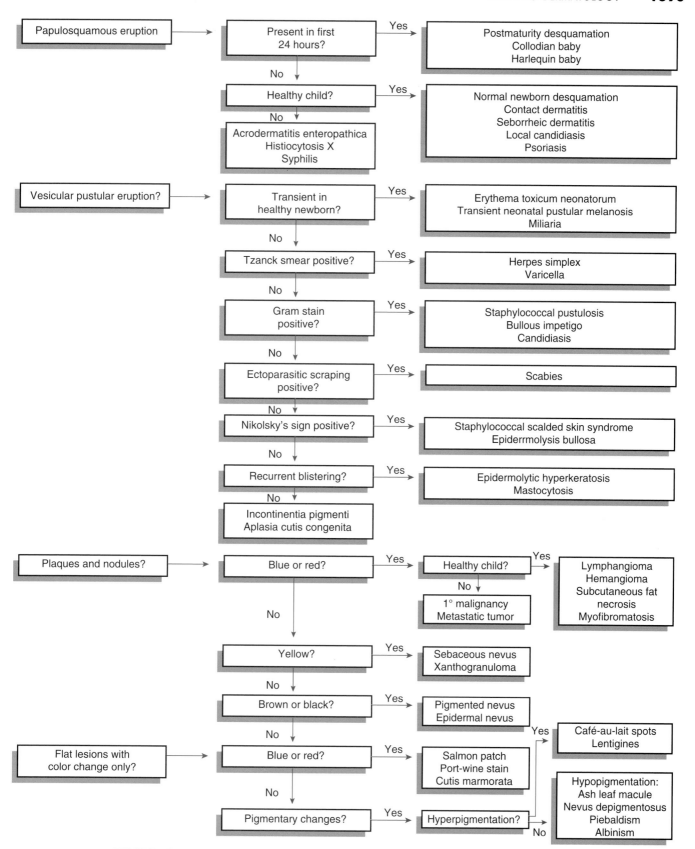

FIGURE 184-6. Algorithm for evaluation of neonatal rashes. (From A Colour Atlas of Pediatric Dermatology by B. A. Cohen, Mosby – Year Book an imprint of Times Mirror International Publishers Ltd. London, UK, 1883.)

ena. Acrocyanosis, in which the hands and feet become variably and symmetrically blue, disappears quickly when the child is bundled or warmed. Central cyanosis of the lips or face may be a marker for underlying cardiac or pulmonary disease. Cutis marmorata or livedo reticularis also develops with cold exposure. Diffuse marbling or mottling appears on the trunk and extremities for seconds to minutes intermittently up to 1 month of age. If cutis marmorata persists beyond the neonatal period, associated disorders including Down syndrome, trisomy 18, hypothyroidism, and Cornelia de Lange's syndrome should be considered. Congenital phlebectasia (cutis marmorata telangiectatica congenita) may mimic persistent cutis marmorata. Although this permanent vascular anomaly may be generalized, lesions are usually localized to a small part of the skin surface. Infants with congenital phlebectasia deserve a careful medical evaluation for other mesodermal and neuroectodermal anomalies.

The harlequin color change is noted when the infant is placed in the lateral decubitus position. The dependent half of the body turns deep red in contrast to the pale upper half. The color reverses when the infant is rocked from side to side. Although this phenomenon may develop in up to 10% of infants, the color change usually lasts for under a minute. Recurrences are common during the first month of life. The cause is unknown, and it has not been associated with serious underlying disease.

Minor Anomalies

Minor congenital anomalies, such as skin tags of the auricle, epicanthal folds, simian creases, and café-au-lait spots, are of little or no physiologic consequence and occur in up to half of newborns. Nearly 10% of newborns have three or more minor anomalies, many of which are inherited in a multifactorial familial pattern. Although the risk of an associated syndrome with multiple major anomalies is low, the presence of multiple minor anomalies should prompt a thorough pediatric evaluation to exclude occult major defects, such as structural congenital heart disease, congenital cataracts, cleft palate, and choanal atresia.

When anomalies involve two or more structures in the skin, a hereditary ectodermal dysplasia should be considered.[24] This is a heterogeneous group of disorders commonly associated with systemic findings. Distinctive cutaneous defects may suggest specific genodermatoses that may also be confirmed by evaluating other family members.[25, 26] For example, careful skin examinations of mothers of infants with neonatal seizures may reveal reticulated linear scarring associated with burned-out incontinentia pigmenti. In tuberous sclerosis, asymptomatic adults may show evidence of mild disease expression with subtle facial angiofibromas and/or hypopigmented macules and café-au-lait spots.

The purpose of genetic counseling is to prevent births of children with life-threatening disorders. In most cases this means identifying heterozygotes from high-risk populations or parents who have already had an affected child. Universal neonatal screening for a number of inborn errors of metabolism, such as phenylketonuria and

congenital hypothyroidism, are routinely performed in the United States. Early diagnosis of these disorders allows for immediate intervention at birth and prevention of serious complications. None of the genodermatoses has been sufficiently characterized to allow for cost-effective routine screening.

In families where previous children have been affected with genodermatoses, associated systemic anomalies may be detected with standard prenatal diagnostic techniques. Ultrasonography has been performed routinely since the 1970s to assess gestational age, multiple fetuses, and placental localization. It can also be used to evaluate fetal central nervous system malformations; craniofacial defects; skeletal anomalies; renal, cardiac, and gastrointestinal disease; and fetal tumors. The progression of cutaneous anomalies such as lymphangiomas and arteriovenous malformations can be followed by ultrasound before delivery. Fetal cells obtained from amniocentesis can be evaluated for chromosomal aberrations, sex-linked disorders, and inherited metabolic disorders. Fetal cells can also be subjected to DNA probes as these markers become available for genodermatoses in the near future. Amniocentesis can be safely performed at 15–16 weeks' gestation with less than a 0.5% risk of fetal loss. However, studies that require culturing of fetal cells may not yield results until well into the second trimester.

In families at high risk for bearing a child with a serious genetic disorder, fetal tissue can be obtained by chorionic villus sampling at 8 to 11 weeks' gestation for DNA marker studies and biochemical analysis. Although this allows for earlier diagnosis of an affected baby, the risk of fetal loss ranges between 1% and 2%.

At this time, fetal skin biopsy diagnosis can be obtained for histologic examination, electron microscopy, and biochemical and histologic markers. Detection of some variants of epidermolysis bullosa, harlequin fetus, and lamellar ichthyosis has been possible using this technique. However, fetoscopy cannot usually be performed until well into the second trimester, and the risk of fetal loss may approach 5%. Moreover, the detection of ultrastructural and/or biochemical aberrations may be delayed by normal variations in the development of these markers in the fetus.

Benign Pustular Dermatoses

Several innocent pustular eruptions that occur commonly in neonates must be distinguished from potentially serious infections.

Erythema toxicum neonatorum develops in up to 70% of healthy full-term infants typically on the second or third day of life. Erythematous macules and papules evolve over hours into 2- to 3-mm yellow papules and pustules on a broad urticarial base, giving a "flea-bitten" appearance (Fig. 184–7). Although any part of the skin surface may be involved, lesions tend to cluster on the trunk, face and proximal extremities. Cultures of material obtained from pustules are sterile, and smears usually reveal sheets of neutrophils and eosinophils. Although biopsy is not needed for diagnosis, specimens taken to rule out other vesiculopustular conditions show

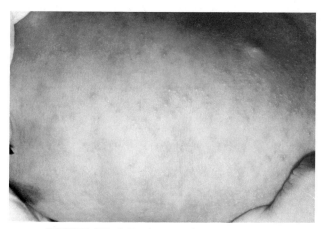

FIGURE 184–7. Erythema toxicum neonatorum.

that erythema toxicum neonatorum is a pustular folliculitis in which neutrophils and eosinophils predominate.

Transient neonatal pustular melanosis commonly develops in utero or during the first day of life.[27] Macules or pustules on the sacrum or buttock may be the only cutaneous finding (Fig. 184–8). However, pustules can spread over much of the skin surface. Pustules tend to aggregate on the chin, neck, upper chest, sacrum, abdomen, and thighs. Lesions typically arise on a noninflammatory base, and over a period of several days develop a central crust, then dry, leaving a collarette of scale, and finally heal with postinflammatory hyperpigmentation that resolves over 4 to 6 weeks. The pustules are subcorneal collections of neutrophils with few eosinophils. Pigment in basal keratinocytes, rather than an accumulation of melanophages accounts for the hyperpigmentation of resolving macules.[28] Unlike erythema toxicum neonatorum, scrapings from pustules of transient neonatal pustular melanosis show mostly neutrophils. This dermatosis occurs in only 4% of newborns, primarily in black males.

Both erythema toxicum neonatorum and transient neonatal pustular necrosis must be distinguished from *staphylococcal pustulosis* (see Chapter 82). Pustules in staphylococcal infection tend to be relatively large compared with the surrounding erythema. They often cluster in the diaper area, around the umbilical stump, or intertriginous areas. Gram's stain of purulent exudate reveals gram-positive cocci, and cultures are positive for *Staphylococcus aureus*. Prompt local care with compresses and topical antibiotics may result in rapid clearing. Widespread lesions require oral antibiotics. If the infant is febrile or appears ill in any way, a thorough evaluation for possible sepsis, hospital admission, and parenteral antibiotics are usually warranted. These benign pustular dermatoses should also be distinguished from candidiasis (see Chapter 119) and herpes simplex (see Chapter 121). In many infants, candidiasis presents as white plaques of thrush on the tongue, gingivae, and buccal mucosa. In disseminated cutaneous candidiasis, 3- to 4-mm pustules on a red base involve the entire skin surface.[29] Within 5 to 7 days the pustules dry and go on to desquamate. In healthy full-term infants this infection is usually self limited. However, in premature infants the risk of candidal septicemia is high, and specimens should be cultured and patients treated with parenteral amphotericin. Gram's stain or potassium hydroxide preparation of pus reveals yeast forms and pseudohyphae. Herpes simplex can be excluded by performing a Tzanck smear. However, suspicious lesions should also be sent for viral culture, which may demonstrate positive findings as early as 12 to 24 hours later. Only 50% of newborns with disseminated herpes simplex develop cutaneous lesions, and even clinically trivial primary cutaneous lesions may result in life-threatening disseminated disease (Fig. 184–9).

Scabies may also develop in the first several weeks of life and is often confused with viral and bacterial infections (Fig. 184–10; see Chapter 128). In newborns scabies follows exposure to infested hospital staff, family members, or day care workers. Affected infants usually present with nonspecific symptoms such as poor eating, increased fussiness, and poor weight gain. Large numbers of hockey stick–shaped burrows are often noted on the palms and soles in addition to the trunk and scalp. However, as in older individuals, the development of a hypersensitivity reaction to the *Sarcoptes scabei* mite may result in a widespread eczematous eruption that obscures the primary lesions. The excellent safety profile of 5% permethrin cream (Elimite cream) makes this product the treatment of choice in a pediatric setting.

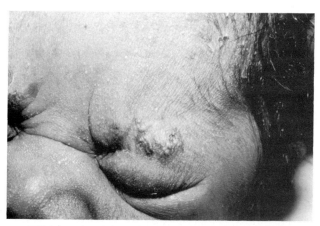

FIGURE 184–8. Transient neonatal pustular melanosis.

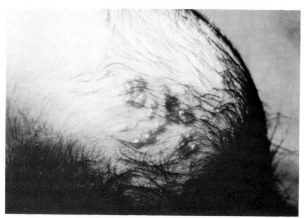

FIGURE 184–9. Herpes simplex.

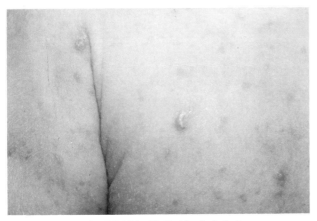

FIGURE 184-10. Scabies in infant.

Acropustulosis of infancy is a chronic, relapsing, pruritic eruption characterized by the presence of sterile vesicles and pustules on the palms and soles (Fig. 184-11).[30, 31] However, lesions may spread to the scalp, trunk, buttocks, and extremities. Onset may occur during the first several months of life and episodes typically last from 1 to 3 weeks, with intervening remissions of 1 to 3 weeks. During flares, infants are usually fussy and the pruritus is severe. Disease-free intervals tend to increase until the eruption resolves between 18 months and 3 years of age. Histopathology shows subcorneal pustules containing predominantly neutrophils. The presence of intense pruritus particularly on the palms and soles often suggests the diagnosis of scabies, which can only be excluded by repeated negative ectoparasite scrapings. Although infants may respond quickly to oral dapsone, short courses of medium- or high-potency topical steroids to small areas can be used effectively and safely.

In *miliaria* 2- to 3-mm vesicles (miliaria crystallina) and inflammatory papules and pustules (miliaria rubra) appear in both term and preterm infants usually after the first 1 to 2 weeks of life in response to thermal stress (see Chapter 93).[32] Lesions erupt in crops on the skin creases, scalp, face, and trunk. Cooling and loosening of clothing results in rapid resolution of lesions.

Neonatal acne develops in at least 20% of newborns at

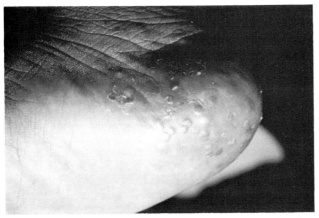

FIGURE 184-11. Acropustulosis of infancy.

birth or within the first few weeks of life (see Chapter 49).[33] Closed comedones predominate on the face. However, extensive eruptions over the trunk and occasionally the extremities may also include inflammatory papules and pustules. Lesions resolve without treatment within 1 to 3 months. The risk of severe acne in adolescence does not seem to be increased in these children.

Scaly Dermatoses

At 7 to 10 days of life physiologic desquamation peaks, with large sheets of scale peeling from the extremities, leaving normal skin beneath. Deep cracking and fissuring of the skin the first day of life should alert the practitioner to the risk of postmaturity syndrome. In these infants peeling may be noted in the delivery room. Other cutaneous markers include decreased subcutaneous fat and meconium staining. These children require close monitoring during the first few days of life for increased risk of temperature instability, hypoglycemia, hypocalcemia, poor feeding, and sepsis.

Ichthyosis refers to a heterogeneous group of genodermatoses some of which present in the newborn period (see Chapter 162).[34, 35] In the newborn, the first clues of disease include generalized scaling and erythema typical of an erythroderma (congenital ichthyosiform erythroderma) or a thick cellophane-like collodion membrane (lamellar ichthyosis). In the erythrodermic infant bacterial infections, such as staphylococcal and streptococcal disease, disseminated candidiasis, and rare toxic epidermal necrolysis can be excluded by the absence of blisters or pustules, a Nikolsky sign, or positive scrapings and cultures. Affected children may develop a chronic erythroderma or thick generalized plate-like scales associated with ectropion and eclabium. Although both of these autosomal recessive variants are associated with a thickened stratum corneum, the ineffective cutaneous barrier results in increased heat and transcutaneous water loss and an increased risk of infection. A third variant of congenital ichthyosis presents in the newborn with widespread blistering (bullous congenital ichthyosiform erythroderma or epidermolytic hyperkeratosis) and may be confused with epidermolysis bullosa or other primary bullous diseases. Over the first few months of life, distinctive scaling increases particularly in the flexures as the blistering subsides. Epidermolytic hyperkeratosis is inherited in an autosomal dominant pattern.

Diaper dermatitis includes a number of acute and chronic disorders that present with rash primarily or initially in the diaper area (see Chapter 11). In its most common form, it represents an irritant contact dermatitis resulting from repeated exposure to urine and feces under occlusion.[36-38] Although ammonia from urine was first thought to play a leading role in the development of irritant dermatitis, recent studies suggest that feces is the principal culprit. Once the epidermal barrier is disrupted, the skin may become sensitive to mild irritants such as soap, detergents, and various topical agents.

Irritant reactions are usually confined to the convex surfaces of the diaper area including the scrotum, labia majora, anterior thighs, suprapubic area, and buttocks.

The inguinal creases are usually spared. When secondary infection with candidal, staphylococcal, or streptococcal organisms occurs, the creases become involved. Treatment consists of gentle, regular cleaning of the diaper area with plain water and mild soap, avoidance of additional irritants, and the use of barrier pastes such as zinc oxide. Painful, fiery red patches will respond to brief courses of low-potency topical steroids, and secondary infection should be treated with topical antibiotics or antifungals when indicated. The addition of oral antibiotics may trigger diarrhea and further insult to the perianal skin. Prolonged use of topical steroids should be avoided because of the risk of atrophy.

Persistent or recurrent diaper dermatitis may be the first sign of infantile psoriasis.[39] Bright red scaly patches and plaques may spread over the trunk and to other creases. A skin biopsy may be necessary to distinguish psoriasis from seborrhic and contact dermatitis. In seborrheic dermatitis, lesions may disseminate to the scalp, intertriginous areas, and trunk. The eruption is dramatic, but topical steroid responsive, self-limited, and asymptomatic. Most cases of seborrheic dermatitis resolve during the first year of life. Infantile seborrheic dermatitis can be differentiated from atopic dermatitis, which invariably spares the warm, moist, protected diaper area. Unprotected areas including the face and extensor surfaces of the arms and legs are most severely affected. Eczema does not usually involve the groin until children are toilet trained.

The rare child who develops chronic diaper dermatitis and growth failure deserves a careful evaluation for an underlying medical disorder. Recalcitrant diaper dermatitis and candidiasis may be a marker for hereditary and acquired immunodeficiency. An erosive diaper dermatitis with lesions disseminated to the face and skin creases should alert the clinician to the possibility of a nutritional deficiency associated with cystic fibrosis, acrodermatitis enteropathica, urea enzyme cycle defects, or biotinidase deficiency. Diets lacking in zinc, biotin, or essential fatty acids or amino acids will result in similar rash. In histiocytosis X an erosive diaper rash is accompanied by similar patches on other body creases and the scalp. Patches often develop a hemorrhagic component, and mucous membranes may also be involved. Lymphadenopathy and hepatosplenomegaly may also be prominent, and skin biopsies show characteristic histiocytic infiltrates.

Vesiculobullous Eruptions

Blistering eruptions in the newborn may present a confusing clinical picture. Once common bacterial, viral, and fungal infections have been excluded, only a limited number of disorders remain.

Several conditions, which do not commonly blister, may present with vesiculation in infancy because of decreased efficacy of intraepidermal attachments and dermal-epidermal adhesion. In rare cases of bullous mastocytosis, recurrent blistering may be so severe that fluid and electrolyte balance is disrupted and the risk of infection is high (see Chapter 152).[40] More commonly, children with solitary mastocytomas or urticaria pigmentosa occasionally develop localized areas of blistering that are often mistaken for bullous impetigo. In both settings blistering decreases with increasing age.

Localized or widespread blistering on a noninflammatory base especially over bony prominences and areas of mechanical trauma should suggest the diagnosis of epidermolysis bullosa (see Chapter 73). These disorders can be characterized by histopathologic and clinical findings, inheritance patterns, and biochemical and molecular markers.[41, 42] Epidermolytic hyperkeratosis and pachyonychia congenita are both commonly associated with blistering in infants and should be considered in the differential diagnosis of epidermolysis bullosa.[43, 44] Unlike epidermolysis bullosa, a Nikolsky sign is absent in both disorders and characteristic clinical findings develop within the first 1 to 3 months of life. In epidermolytic hyperkeratosis the histopathology is diagnostic and will exclude epidermolysis bullosa. The most common types of pachyonychia congenita are autosomal dominant, and a family history may confirm the diagnosis.

Localized or widespread linear blistering on an urticarial base in an infant girl is suggestive of incontinentia pigmenti (see Chapter 165).[45] In many cases the course is mild and lesions are limited to the skin. Subsequent swirling hyperpigmentation may resolve in childhood, leaving barely detectable reticulated scars. When this X-linked dominant disorder, which is lethal in males, is suspected, a careful examination of the mother is required to detect the subtle residual scarring.

Lumps and Bumps

Although cutaneous malignancies are rare, two forms of panniculitis cause self-limited disease regularly in otherwise healthy infants.

In subcutaneous fat necrosis of the newborn, red or hemorrhagic nodules and plaques up to 3 cm in diameter appear most commonly on areas exposed to trauma and cold stress, such as the cheeks, back, buttocks, arms, and thighs during the first few days of life.[46, 47] Although the cause is unknown, complicated deliveries, hypothermia, perinatal asphyxia, and maternal diabetes predispose to the development of fat necrosis. In most cases the general health of the child is unaffected. However, recalcitrant life-threatening hypercalcemia has been rarely reported. Skin biopsies characteristically demonstrate fat necrosis, foreign body giant cells, and residual lipocytes with needle-shaped clefts in a radial arrangement. Most lesions resolve without scarring in 1 to 2 months. However, some nodules become fluctuant, ulcerate, and heal with atrophy.

Cold panniculitis appears as red indurated nodules and plaques on the cheeks of infants exposed to cold weather (see Chapter 70).[48] It also occurs as a complication of sucking on cold teething rings and popsicles. Lesions may develop within 1 to 3 days of exposure and resolve within 1 month. The lack of fever and other systemic symptoms helps to distinguish cold panniculitis from facial or buccal cellulitis. The high saturation of fatty acids in the fat of young infants compared with older

TABLE 184-1. Histologic Diagnosis of 775 Superficial Lumps Excised in Children

Type	Number
Epidermal inclusion cysts	459 (59%)
Congenital malformations (pilomatrixoma, lymphangioma, brachial cleft cyst)	117 (15%)
Benign neoplasms (neural tumors, lipoma, adnexal tumors)	56 (7%)
Benign lesions of undetermined origin (xanthomas, xanthogranulomas, fibromatosis, fibromas)	50 (6%)
Self-limiting processes (granuloma annulare, urticaria pigmentosa, insect bite reaction)	47 (6%)
Malignant tumors	11 (1.4%)
Miscellaneous	35 (4%)

Reproduced by permission of PEDIATRICS, Vol. 72, page 147, copyright 1983.

children and adults may explain the propensity for the fat to solidify at low temperatures, resulting in panniculitis.

Slowly growing nodules in the newborn may be associated with hamartomatous nevi or cysts, which account for the majority of tumors excised by surgeons in young children. (Table 184–1).[49, 50] Milia are a common, self-limited developmental anomaly that involves the face, trunk, and occasionally the extremities in many infants. Milia and epidermal inclusion cysts also occur after trauma as evidenced by the heel-stick nodules (Fig. 184–12) that appear on the feet of nursery intensive care unit graduates at 4 to 6 months of life. The lesions usually calcify and then regress within several years.

Rarely, cutaneous metastases provide the first clue of malignancy in the newborn or infant. The rapid growth of a congenital plaque or nodule may be an early finding in congenital leukemia, adrenal carcinoma, rhabdomyosarcoma, Wilms' tumor, or neuroblastoma. The presence of cutaneous neuroblastoma with multi-organ involvement but without bony involvement is typical of an unusual self-limited variant of neuroblastoma. Skin biopsies enable both diagnosis and staging.

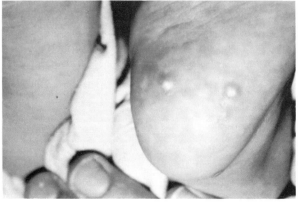

FIGURE 184–12. Hell-stick nodules.

Pediatric Surgery

Between 2 years of age and adolescence, children are at greatest risk of developing prominent scarring. Results are also site dependent. Head and neck wounds heal best, whereas widening of scars occurs more commonly on the trunk and extremities.[51] Hypertrophic scars and keloids arise most frequently on the ears, upper lip, upper central trunk, and mid abdomen especially in children with a genetic predisposition. Pediatric developmental factors should also be considered when planning elective surgery. For instance, excision of a nevus in the diaper should be postponed until after toilet training to reduce the risk of wound infection. Tissue expanders are not well tolerated in infants and toddlers; however, school-age children may cooperate with complicated preoperative and postoperative wound care.

Dermatologists should also take advantage of new approaches to outpatient sedation and topical anesthesia to help with minor surgical procedures in the pediatric patient. Intranasal midazolam provides brief sedation with rapid onset and rapid recovery and little risk of respiratory suppression. Oral chloral hydrate, intramuscular meperidine, promethazine, and chlorpromazine, and oral midazolam can be used when longer sedation is required. Many hospitals have anesthesiologists who will work with clinicians in designing safe, effective outpatient sedation. EMLA (eutectic mixture of lidocaine and prilocaine) cream can be used alone or in combination with sedation before minor procedures such as curettage of molluscum, skin biopsies (before injection of local anesthesia), and laser surgery.[52] For best results, parents apply the cream under plastic wrap occlusion 90 to 120 minutes before coming to the office.

KAWASAKI DISEASE

Kawasaki disease is a disease of uncertain etiology that occurs primarily in infants and young children. This disease was first reported in 1967 as the mucocutaneous lymph node syndrome and subsequently named after the physician who first described it. The diagnosis of Kawasaki disease is made when a patient fulfills five of six clinical criteria, which include: fever for at least 5 days, desquamation of the palms and soles, conjunctivitis, strawberry tongue or other oral mucous membrane involvement, polymorphous exanthemous eruption, and lymph node enlargement. A perineal eruption occurring early in the disease has also been described. Treatment involves a combination of aspirin and intravenous gammaglobulin to prevent the most serious sequela of coronary aneurysm.

References

1. Illingsworth RS. The Development of the Infant and Young Child, Abnormal and Normal, 7th edition. New York: Churchill Livingstone, 1983.
2. Levine M, Carey W, Crocker A, Gross R. Developmental-Behavioral Pediatrics. Philadelphia: WB Saunders Co., 1983.
3. Carrasco M, Davis HW. Child abuse and neglect. In Davis HW, Zitelli BJ, eds. Atlas of Pediatric Physical Diagnosis, 2nd edition. Singapore: Wolfe, 1992:6.1–6.28.

4. Maibach HI, Boisitis EK. Neonatal Skin Structure and Function. New York: Marcel Dekker, 1982.
5. Nachman RL, Esterly NB. Increased skin permeability in preterm infants. J Pediatr 1971;79:628–632.
6. Fanaroff AA, Wald M, Gruber HS, Klaus MH. Insensible water loss in low birth weight infants. Pediatrics 1972;50:236.
7. Barker N, Hadroft J, Rutter N. Skin permeability in the newborn. J Invest Dermatol 1987;88:409.
8. Hammarlund K, Sedin G. Transepidermal water loss in newborn infants. Acta Pediatr Scand 1979;68:795.
9. West DP, Worober S, Solomon LM. Pharmacology and toxicology of infant skin. J Invest Dermatol 1981;76:147.
10. Personal communication (unpublished abstract from a national survey, Johns Hopkins), 1992.
11. Lane AT, Drost SS. Effects of repeated application of emollient cream to premature neonates' skin. Pediatrics 1993;92:415–419.
12. Nopper AJ, Horii K, Sookdeo-Drost S, et al. Topical ointment therapy reduces the risk of nosocomial infection in premature infants. Poster presentation. 1994; Society for Pediatric Dermatology, Hilton Head, South Carolina.
13. Onishe S, Itah S, Isobe K, et al. Mechanism of development of bronze baby syndrome in neonates treated with phototherapy. Pediatrics 1082;69:273.
14. Stern RS, Weinstein MC, Baker SG. Risk reduction for nonmelanoma skin cancer with childhood sunscreen use. Arch Dermatol 1986;122:537–545.
15. Morelli JG, Weston WL. What sunscreen should I use for my 3-month baby? (Letter) Pediatrics 1993;9:882.
16. Banks BA, Silverman RA, Schwartz RH, Tunnessen WW. Attitudes of teenagers toward sun exposure and sunscreen use. Pediatrics 1992;89:40–42.
17. Schachner LA, Hansen RC. Pediatric Dermatology. Boston: Churchill Livingston, 1988.
18. Weston W. Practical Pediatric Dermatology. Boston: Little, Brown, 1985.
19. Cohen BA. Atlas of Pediatric Dermatology. London: Wolfe, 1993.
20. Helfer RE, Kempe RS, eds. The Battered Child, 4th edition. Chicago: University of Chicago Press, 1987.
21. Krugman RD, ed. Child abuse and neglect. Pediatr Ann 1992; 21:471–511.
22. Cohen BA, Honig P, Androphy E. Anogenital warts in children, clinical and virologic evaluation for sexual abuse. Arch Dermatol 1990;126:1575–1580.
23. Hurwitz S. Skin lesions in the first year of life. Contemporary Pediatrics 1993;10:110–128.
24. Friere-Maia N, Pinheiro M. Ectodermal Dysplasias. A Clinical and Genetic Study. New York: Alan R. Liss, 1984.
25. Milunsky A. Genetic Disorders and the Fetus: Diagnosis, Prevention and Treatment, 2nd edition. New York: Plenum, 1986.
26. Alper JC. Genetic Disorders of the Skin. St. Louis: Mosby Yearbook, 1991.
27. Ramamurthy RS, Reveri M, Esterly NB, et al. Transient neonatal pustular melanosis. J Pediatr 1976;88:831–835.
28. Whitley R, Arvin A, Priber C, et al. Predictors of morbidity and mortality in neonates in herpes simplex infection. N Eng J Med 1991;324:450–454.
29. Chapel TA, Gagliardi C, Nicholas W. Congenital cutaneous candidiasis. J Am Acad Dermatol 1982;6:926–928.
30. Jarratt M, Ramsdell W. Infantile acropustulosis. Arch Dermatol 1979;115:834–836.
31. Kahn G, Rywlin AM. Acropustulosis of infancy. Arch Dermatol 1979;115:831–834.
32. Holzle E, Kligman AM. The pathogenesis of miliaria rubra: Role of the resident microflora. Br J Dermatol 1978;99:117–137.
33. Ginkis FL, Hall WK, Tolman MM. Acne neonatorum. Arch Dermatol 1952;66:717–721.
34. Rand RE, Baden HP. The ichthyoses—a review. J Am Acad Dermatol 1983;8:285–305.
35. Williams ML. The ichthyoses—pathogenesis and prenatal diagnosis: A review of recent advances. 1983;1:1–24.
36. Stein H. Incidence of diaper rash when using cloth and disposable diapers. J Pediatr 1982;101:723.
37. Berg RW, Buckingham KW, Stewart RL. Etiologic features in diaper dermatitis: The role of urine. Pediatr Dermatol 1986;3:102.
38. Lane AT, Rehder PA, Helin K. Evaluation of diapers containing absorbent gelling material with conventional disposable diapers in newborn infants. Am J Dis Child 1990;144:315.
39. Neville EA, Finn OA. Psoriasiform napkin dermatitis—a followup study. Br J Dermatol 1975;92:279–285.
40. Caplan RM. The natural course of urticaria pigmentosa. Arch Dermatol 1983;87:146–157.
41. Pessar A, Verdicchio JF, Caldwell D. Epidermolysis bullosa. The pediatric dermatologic management and therapeutic update. Arch Dermatol 1988;3:99.
42. Fine JD. Editorial: Changing clinical and laboratory concept in inherited epidermolysis bullosa (editorial). Arch Dermatol 1988;124:523–526.
43. Schonfeld PH. The pachyonychia congenita syndrome. Acta Derm Venereol (Stockh) 1980;60:45–49.
44. Soderquist NA, Reed WB. Pachyonychia congenita with epidermal cysts and other congenital dyskeratoses. Arch Dermatol 1968; 97:31–33.
45. Cohen BA. Incontinentia pigmenti. Neurol Clin North Am 1987; 5:361.
46. Thomsen RJ. Subcutaneous fat necrosis of the newborn and idiopathic hypercalcemia. A report of a case. Arch Dermatol 1980;116:1155.
47. Norwood-Galloway A, Lebwohl M, Phelp RG, et al. Subcutaneous fat necrosis of the newborn with hypercalcemia. J Am Acad Dermatol 1987;16:435–439.
48. Rotman H. Cold panniculitis in children. Arch Dermatol 1966;94:720–724.
49. Knight PJ, Reiner CB. Superficial lumps in children, what, when, and why? Pediatrics 1983;72:147–153.
50. Sell EJ, Alansen RC, Struck-Pierce S. Calcified nodules in the heel. A complication of neonatal intensive care. J Pediatr 1980;96:473.
51. Peacock EE. Surgery of scars. In Serafin P, Georgiade NG, eds. Pediatric Plastic Surgery. St Louis: Mosby, 1988, 126–127.
52. de Waard-van der Spek FB, Oranje AP, Lillieborg S, Stolz E. Treatment of molluscum contagiosum using lidocaine/prilocaine cream (EMLA) for analgesia. J Am Acad Dermatol.

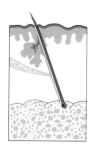

Index

Note: Page numbers in *italics* refer to illustrations; page numbers followed by t indicate tables. Plate numbers refer to color plates in the front of the book.

A

AA3 antigen, in dermoepidermal junction, 624
  in epidermolysis bullosa, 642t
Abrasions, from marine environment, 797–798, *798*, 798t
Abscess(es), dental, and sinus tract to skin, vs. acne, 469
  cutaneous drainage of, 1337
  in actinomycosis, 1007–1008, *1008*
  in psoriasis, of nails, 1297
  Munro's, 109
  Pautrier's, 109
  resident flora in, 926–927
Acantholysis, blisters in, 95, *95*, *96*, 96t
  definition of, 105
  in Hailey-Hailey disease, 1701, *1702*
  in squamous cell carcinoma, 1385, *1386*
Acantholytic dermatosis, transient, 341–343, *342*, 342t, *343*, 343t
Acantholytic dyskeratosis, focal, 107
  in Darier's disease, 1700, *1701*
Acanthoma, large cell, vs. stucco keratosis, 1447
  pale cell, *1442*, 1442–1443, *1443*, 1443t
  pilar sheath, 1465
Acanthoma fissuratum, 773t, 773–774, 774t
Acanthosis, 105
Acanthosis nigricans, oral lesions in, 1325
  paraneoplastic, 1846–1847, *1867*, 1867t
  with diabetes, 1869t, *1871*
Accessory nerve, spinal, anatomy of, *118*, 119
Accutane. See *Isotretinoin (Accutane)*.
Acetic acid, and wound healing, 566t
Acetowhite warts, 1102, 1117
Aciduria, and alopecia, 1713
  argininosuccinic, 1859t, 1860–1861
Acinetobacter species, in interdigital infection, 928, 929
  in normal cutaneous flora, 926
Acitretin. See also *Retinoids*.
  for lichen planus, 239t
  for lupus erythematosus, discoid, 276
  for psoriasis, 309–310, 315
  for skin carcinoma, 1429–1431
Acne, and folliculitis, 463, 941, 946
  and scarring, papular, vs. anetoderma, 911t
    surgery for, *473*, 473–479
  clinical findings in, 461–464, *462–464*
  definition of, 461
  diagnosis of, 468–470, *469*, 469t
  drug reactions in, 423, 464, *464*

Acne (*Continued*)
  in neonate, 715t, 719, 1896
  infundibular cysts with, 1450, *1451*
  pathogenesis of, 465–468, 466t, 468t
  pathology of, 464–465
  treatment of, 470t–472t, 470–473
Acne agminata, 468, 987
Acne conglobata, 463
Acne fulminans, 463, *463*
Acne keloidalis nuchae, 470
  and alopecia, *1282*, 1282–1283, *1283*
Acne mechanica, 772–773, 773t, 852, 853
Acne rosacea, 485–496. See also *Rosacea*.
Acne varioliformis, 468–469
Acquired immunodeficiency syndrome, 1137–1155. See also *Human immunodeficiency virus infection*.
Acral arteriovenous hemangioma, 1507t, 1511, *1512*
Acral lentiginous melanoma, clinical findings in, 1580, *1580*, Plate 11
  pathology of, 1583, *1584*
Acral sites, definition of, 105
Acroangiodermatitis, 1507t, 1507–1508, *1508*
Acrocephalosyndactyly, with acne, 464
Acrocyanosis, 829, 830
Acrodermatitis, Epstein-Barr virus infection and, 1082, 1133, *1134*, Plate 9
Acrodermatitis chronica atrophicans, in Lyme borreliosis, 967, 968, 969t
  vs. anetoderma, 911t
Acrodermatitis continua, of Hallopeau, 298
Acrodermatitis enteropathica, 1763–1765, *1764*, 1765t, 1873t
Acrodynia, tooth abnormalities with, 1324t
Acrokeratoelastoidosis, 1778
Acrokeratosis of Bazex, paraneoplastic, 1846
Acrokeratosis verruciformis, of Hopf, vs. stucco keratosis, 1447
Acropustulosis, of infancy, 189, *190*, 716t, 719–720, *720*, 1896, *1896*
Acrosyringium, anatomy of, 36, *40*
  embryology of, 5
Acrotrichium, 30
Actinia equina stings, 790
Actinic amyloidosis, 1824, *1825*
Actinic cheilitis, 1380
Actinic granuloma, 442
  vs. granuloma annulare, 441, 441t
Actinic keratosis, 1378–1380. See also *Keratosis, actinic*.
Actinic porokeratosis, 1701–1703

Actinic prurigo, *761*, 761t, 761–762, 762t
  vs. polymorphic light eruption, 760t, 761t
Actinic reticuloid syndrome, 763, 768–770, *769*, 769t, 770t, Plate 5
Actinic vasculopathy, 735
Actinodendron plumosom stings, 790
Actinomycetoma, 1069–1070, 1071t
Actinomycin D (dactinomycin), and folliculitis, 429–430
Actinomycosis, 1007–1009, *1008*, 1008t, *1009*
Acyclovir, for Epstein-Barr virus infection, 1084
  for herpes simplex infection, 1077–1078, *1078*
    genital, 1347
    in dermabrasion, for acne scars, 478
    in erythema multiforme, 252t, 253
    in neonate, 718
    with human immunodeficiency virus infection, 1139–1140
  for lymphomatoid papulosis, 1637
  for varicella-zoster infection, 1081, *1081*, 1131
    in immunosuppressed patient, 1156, 1157
    with human immunodeficiency virus infection, 1140, 1141
Adams-Oliver syndrome, 1784, 1785
Adamson fringes, 29, *30*
Adapin (doxepin), for neurotic excoriations, 784
  for urticaria, 402
Addison's disease, 1872, 1873t
Adenocarcinoma, digital papillary, 1481, *1482*
  in Paget's disease, extramammary, *1487*, 1487–1488, *1488*, 1488t
    mammary, 1488–1489, *1489*
  of pancreas, subcutaneous fat necrosis with, 1845
  of sweat glands, 1480–1481
  of umbilicus, metastatic, 1674, *1676*
Adenoma, digital papillary, 1481–1482
  sebaceous, 1472, *1472*
    vs. acne, 469
Adenylate cyclase, in DNA photodamage, 1369
Adhesion molecules, in alopecia areata, 1271
  in inflammatory response, 146–151
Adhesives, cyanoacrylate, and burn injury, 846
Adipocytes, embryology of, 5
Adiposus dolorosa, 1526

Adnexa. See also specific structures, e.g., *Eccrine glands.*
  epithelial cysts of, surgery for, 1456–1461, 1458t, *1459–1462*
    with nonsquamous lining, 1454–1456, *1456–1458*
    with squamous lining, 1450–1454, 1451t, *1451–1456*
  epithelial structures of, definition of, 107
Adrenal gland, cortical hyperfunction of, and hirsutism, 1853–1854
  disorders of, cutaneous signs of, 1872, 1872t, 1873t
  topical corticosteroids and, 164, 166
Adrenergic drugs, for urticaria, 402
Adrenergic urticaria, 393–394
Advancement flaps, after skin cancer excision, 1409–1411, *1409–1411*
Aeromonas hydrophila infection, 943, 946, 947
AF1 monoclonal antibody, in dermoepidermal junction, 625–626
  in epidermolysis bullosa, 642t
AF2 monoclonal antibody, in dermoepidermal junction, 625–626
  in epidermolysis bullosa, 642t
Afipia felis infection, 1023–1024
African trypanosomiasis, *1174*, 1174–1175
Aging, and physical abuse, 843
  and wound healing, 566
  of skin, ultraviolet light and, 732–746. See also *Photoaging.*
  premature, 1713, *1713*, 1803t
Agminated lesions, definition of, 105
Agouti gene, and hair color, in mice, 1718
AIDS, 1137–1155. See also *Human immunodeficiency virus infection.*
Ainhum, vs. Dupuytren's disease, 908
Albendazole, for cysticercosis, 1187–1188
  for enterobiasis, 1184
  for gnathostomiasis, 1184
  for hookworm infestation, 1183
  for larva migrans, cutaneous, 1182
  for strongyloidiasis, 1183
Albinism, ocular, 1223, 1223t
  oculocutaneous, 1219–1223, 1220t, 1221t, *1222*
Albopapuloid lesions, in Pasini epidermolysis bullosa, 640
Albright's hereditary osteodystrophy, 1828, 1829t
Alcohol, and flushing, 534t
  ethyl, and wound healing, 566t
  isopropyl, in antiseptic solutions, 129, 129t
Aleppo evil, 1163
Alexandrite laser, in tattoo removal, 455t, 458
Algae, and skin infection, 1072
Alkaptonuria, 1859t, 1861
Alkyl mercury compounds, and burn injury, 844t
Allergy, and contact dermatitis, 167–173. See also *Contact dermatitis.*
  to cnidarian stings, 787–788
  to tattoo dyes, 453, 455
  with photosensitization, 726–730, *729*, 729t–731t
  and urticaria, 394–395, 400–401
Allografts, for leg ulcers, 569t, 569–570, *570*
Allylamines, for dermatophytosis, 1052–1054, 1053t, 1054t
Alopecia, androgenetic, 1250–1257
  clinical findings in, 1250–1252, *1251, 1252*
  definition of, 1250
  diagnosis of, *1255*, 1255–1256
  diffuse, 1275, *1276*

Alopecia (*Continued*)
  pathogenesis of, 1254–1255
  pathology of, 1252–1253, *1253*
  treatment of, 1256t, 1256–1257
  vs. alopecia areata, 1272t
  chemotherapy and, 426–427
  congenital disorders and, 1712–1717, *1713–1718*
  diffuse, 1274–1278
    clinical findings in, *1274*, 1274–1275
    definition of, 1274
    etiology of, 1275–1277, *1276*, 1277t
    pathology of, 1275
    treatment of, 1276–1277
  evaluation of, punch biopsy in, 124
  genetic abnormalities and, in mice, 1718–1719
  hair replacement surgery for, mini-micrografts in, *1260*, 1260–1261, *1261, 1263*
    punch grafting in, *1258*, 1258–1260, *1259*
  in anhidrotic ectodermal dysplasia, 1714, *1714*
  in Conradi-Hünermann syndrome, 1716
  in keratosis pilaris atrophicans, 504, *504*, 1715
  in loose anagen hair syndrome, 1716
  in lupus erythematosus, discoid, 260, *261*
    systemic, 263
  in Marie-Unna hypotrichosis, 1713–1714
  in monilethrix, 1716, *1717*
  in Netherton's syndrome, 1716, *1716*
  in progeria, 1713, *1713*
  in psoriasis, 301
  in syphilis, 951, *951*
  in trichorhinophalangeal syndrome, 1714
  in trichotillomania, 780t, 781t, *782*, 782–783
  involutional, 1275
  scalp lifting for, 1263–1265, *1264*
  scalp reduction for, *1262*, 1262–1263, *1263*
  scarring, definition of, 1280
    pediatric, *1292*, 1292t, 1292–1293, 1293t
    primary, classification of, 1280, 1281t
      lymphocyte-associated, 1285t, 1285–1290, 1286t, *1286–1288*, 1288t–1290t, *1290*
      pustulofollicular, 1281t–1284t, 1281–1285, *1281–1285*
    secondary, 1291, 1291t, *1292*
  sports-related, 851
  temporoparieto-occipital flap surgery for, *1265*, 1265–1266
  tick bites and, 816
  tinea capitis and, 1045, *1045, 1046*, 1285, *1285*
  triangular, congenital, 1714
  with ichthyosis linearis circumflexa, 1693, *1693*
Alopecia areata, 1269–1274
  clinical findings in, 1269–1270, *1270*
  definition of, 1269
  diagnosis of, 1271, 1272t
  pathogenesis of, 1270–1271
  pathology of, 1270, *1270*
  treatment of, 1271–1274, 1273t
Alopecia congenita, 1715
Alopecia mucinosa, 1289–1290, *1290*, 1290t
  in T-cell lymphoma, 1641
Alpha chains, in dermal extracellular collagen, 859, *860*
Alpha$_1$-antitrypsin deficiency, and panniculitis, *605*, 605–607, *606*, 606t, 607t
Alpha-6-beta-4 integrin, 621

Alpha-tocopherol, deficiency of, cutaneous signs of, 1873t
  for pityriasis rubra pilaris, 334–335
Alprazolam, for neurotic excoriations, 784
Altomeris io caterpillar, and dermatitis, 809, *809*
Aluminum chloride, in hemostasis, 133
Aluminum chloride hexahydrate, for hyperhidrosis, 1316, 1316t
Amalgam, dental, and oral mucosal pigmentation, 1323
Amebiasis, 1172–1173, *1173*
American trypanosomiasis, *1173*, 1173–1174
Amikacin, for nocardiosis, 1007, 1008t
Amino acids, in Hartnup's disorder, 1768
  metabolism of, disorders of, 1858–1862, 1859t, *1860*
  and alopecia, 1713
Aminolevulinic acid, in porphyria, 1753, *1755*, 1760, 1760t
β-Aminoproprionitrile, for hypertrophic scars, 903
Amiodarone, and hyperpigmentation, 1237
  and phototoxicity, 726, *729*, Plate 4
Amitriptyline, for pudendal neuralgia, 1355
Ammonia, in urine, and diaper dermatitis, 184–187, *185*, 185t, 186t, Plate 1
Ammonium, quaternary, and wound healing, 566t
Amoxicillin, and serum sickness–like reaction, 418
  for chancroid, 976
  for Lyme borreliosis, 969, 969t
Amphophilic lesions, definition of, 105
Amphotericin B, for blastomycosis, 1067, 1067t
  for coccidioidomycosis, 1064, 1064t
  for cryptococcosis, 1061, 1061t
  for histoplasmosis, 1065–1066, 1066t
  for opportunistic fungal infection, 1072
  for sporotrichosis, 1063, 1063t
Ampicillin, and rash, in cytomegalovirus infection, 1084
  for *Haemophilus influenzae* infection, 946
Amputation, dermatitis after, 774t, 774–775, 775t
Amputation neuroma, 1537, *1538*, 1541t, 1542t
Amylase, in pancreatic panniculitis, 610, 611
Amyloidosis, 1818–1826
  actinic, 1824, *1825*
  insulin, 1825
  keratin, 1824–1825
  idiopathic, *1822*, 1822–1824, *1823*, 1824t, Plate 14
  lichen, *86, 1818, 1822*, 1822–1824, *1823*, 1824t, Plate 14
  nodular, 1825–1826, *1826*
  oral lesions in, 1328
  systemic, cardiac features of, cutaneous signs with, 1878t, *1880*
    renal disease in, cutaneous signs with, 1884t
  secondary, 1820–1821
  with altered light chains, 1818–1820, *1819*
  types of, 1818, 1819t
  vs. scleroderma, 888t
Amyloidotic polyneuropathy, familial, 1821
Anafranil, for trichotillomania, 783
Anagen, in hair growth, 30, *31*, 105, 1247, 1248
  loose hair in, 1716
  vs. alopecia areata, 1272t

Anaphylaxis, chemotherapy and, 428
   in drug reactions, 415–416
Anaplasia, definition of, 105, *105*
Anchoring fibrils, dermal, 863–864, *864*
   in epidermolysis bullosa, 867–869, *868, 869*
Anchoring filament–associated basement
   membrane components, in
   dermoepidermal junction, 625–626
Anchoring filament–associated proteins, in
   dermoepidermal junction, 623–624
Ancylostoma infestation, 1183
   and cutaneous larva migrans, 1181, 1181t
Androgens, and hirsutism, 1853–1857, *1854,*
   1855t, 1856t
   and sebaceous gland activity, in acne, 465
   for urticaria, 403
   in alopecia, 1250–1257. See also *Alopecia, androgenetic.*
   in hair follicle growth, 1248t, 1248–1249, *1249*
Androstenedione, in hair follicle growth,
   1249, *1249*
   in hirsutism, 1855
Androsterone sulfate, in hirsutism, 1854
Anemia, aplastic, antimalarial drugs and, 275
   Fanconi's, 1802t
   in epidermolysis bullosa, 643
Anemone larvae, and seabather's eruption,
   792–793, 1186, 1187t
Anemone stings, 789–790, *790*
Anesthesia, 130t, 130–131
   for adnexal epithelial cyst removal, 1460
   for dermabrasion, for acne scars, 476–477
   for electrosurgery, for rhinophyma,
   493–494
   for liposuction, 1532, 1533
      for hyperhidrosis, 1316
   in pediatric surgery, 1898
Anetoderma, 910–912, *911,* 911t
   atrophy in, *100*
   dermal elastic fibers in, 875
   in human immunodeficiency virus
   infection, 1145
Aneurysms, capillary, thrombosed, 1509
   in Behçet's disease, 386–387
   punch hair grafting and, 1259
Angina bullosa hemorrhagica, 1333
Angioblastoma, 1507t, *1510,* 1510–1511, *1511*
Angiodermatitis, acral, 1507t, 1507–1508, *1508*
Angioedema, chemotherapy and, 428
   clinical findings in, *395,* 395–396
   definition of, 392, *393*
   diagnosis of, 399–400, *401*
   in drug reactions, 415–416
Angioendotheliomatosis, reactive, 1507t,
   1508–1509
Angiofibroma, facial, in tuberous sclerosis,
   1736, *1736,* 1739–1740
Angiogenesis, 1492–1495, 1493t, 1495t
   in wound healing, *564,* 565
Angiogenin, 1493t, 1494
Angioid streaks, in pseudoxanthoma
   elasticum, 1770, *1771*
Angioimmunoblastic lymphadenopathy, 1666
Angiokeratoma, 1507t, *1514,* 1514–1515
   genital, 1352, *1352*
Angiokeratoma corporis diffusum, cardiac
   disorders with, 1878t
   renal disease with, 1884t, *1885*
Angioleiomyoma, 1522, 1523, *1523*
Angiolipoma, 1526–1527, *1527*
Angiolymphoid hyperplasia, with
   eosinophilia, 1507t, 1511–1513, *1512*

Angioma, spider, 1509
   tufted, acquired, 1507t, *1510,* 1510–1511, *1511*
Angioma serpiginosum, 1509
   of Hutchinson, vs. pigmented purpura, 293
Angiomatosis, bacillary, 1023–1028
   clinical findings in, 1025, *1025, 1026,*
   Plate 8
   diagnosis of, 1027, 1027t
   epidemiology of, 1024–1025
   historical aspects of, 1023–1024
   pathology of, *1026,* 1026–1027
   treatment of, 1028
   cutaneomeningospinal, 1506
Angiomyolipoma, renal, in tuberous
   sclerosis, 1737
Angiosarcoma, *1516,* 1516–1518, *1517*
   and lymphedema, 554, 556, 1516
Angiotrophic lymphoma, 1664, 1666
Angiotropin, 1493t, 1494
Anhidrotic ectodermal dysplasia, 1714, *1714,*
   1721, 1722t, 1723t
Animal bites, bacterial infection of, 943, 947
Annular sarcoidosis, *87*
Anonychia, 1301
Anthelix, chondrodermatitis nodularis of,
   507, *508,* 510, *510*
Anthralin, for alopecia areata, 1271, 1273t,
   1274
   for psoriasis, 305t, 306
      with phototherapy, 313
Anthrax, 1030–1032, *1031,* 1031t, 1032t
Antiandrogens, for alopecia, 1256
Anti-angiogenic factors, 1495, 1495t
Antianxiety drugs, for neurotic excoriations,
   784
Anti–basement membrane autoantibodies,
   and dermatosis, in pregnancy, 370
   in epidermolysis bullosa, 642, 642t
Antibiotics. See also specific drugs, e.g.,
   Penicillin.
   adverse reactions to, in human
   immunodeficiency virus infection,
   1145
   and hyperpigmentation, 1237
   for acne, 466–468, 470–472, 471t
   for anthrax, 1031–1032, 1032t
   for bacterial skin infections, uncommon,
   946t, 946–947
   for bowel-associated dermatosis-arthritis
   syndrome, 376, 376t
   for cellulitis, 925, 925t
   for erysipelas, 925, 925t
   for impetigo, 920–921, 921t
   for plague, 1034, 1034t
   for staphylococcal infection, 922–923,
   923t
   for streptococcal infection, 923t
   for tularemia, 1035
   hypersensitivity to, 416–417
      in Epstein-Barr virus infection, 1082
   in wound healing, 566, 566t, 568
   skin reactions to, 416–417
Antibodies. See also *Autoantibodies.*
   anthyroid, in granuloma annulare, 441
   antinuclear, in scleroderma, 885
      stratified epithelium-specific, ulcerative
      stomatitis with, chronic, 1333
   antiphospholipid, 456t, 545t, 547–550
      with livedo reticularis, 1865t, *1866*
   monoclonal, fibril-specific, in
      dermoepidermal junction, 625–626
      in epidermolysis bullosa, 642t
Anticoagulants. See also specific drugs, e.g.,
   Heparin.
   and skin necrosis, *419,* 419–420

Anticoagulants (*Continued*)
   for Köhlmeier-Degos syndrome, 546t, 552
   use of, biopsy after, 121–122
Anticonvulsants, for pudendal neuralgia,
   1355–1356
Antidepressants, for neurotic excoriations, 784
   for pudendal neuralgia, 1355
   for trichotillomania, 783
Antigen-presenting cells, in allergic contact
   dermatitis, 167–173, *169, 170,* 171t
   in inflammatory response, 142
Antigens, bullous pemphigoid, 619–620,
   620, 667–668
   cicatricial pemphigoid, 620–621
   processing of, in allergic contact dermatitis,
   169, 169–171, *170,* 170t
Antihistamines, for mastocytosis, 1607, 1607t
   for urticaria, 401–402
Anti-inflammatory drugs. See also
   Corticosteroids and specific drugs, e.g.,
   Aspirin.
   nonsteroidal, for systemic lupus
   erythematosus, 277
      in psoriasis, 301
Antimalarial drugs, and pigmentation
   disorders, 422, 1237
   for discoid lupus erythematosus, 275t,
   275–276
   for morphea, 898, 899t
   for sarcoidosis, 437
Anti-neutrophil cytoplasmic autoantibodies,
   in arteritis, 524–526
Antinuclear antibodies, in scleroderma, 885
   stratified epithelium-specific, ulcerative
   stomatitis with, 1333
Antioxidants, in epidermis, 52–53
   in facial skin care, 80–81
Antiperspirants, for hyperhidrosis, 1315–1316
Antiphospholipid syndrome, 545t, 546t,
   547–550
   with livedo reticularis, 1865t, *1866*
Antisepsis, 128–129, 129t
Antiseptics, in wound healing, 566, 566t
Antithyroid antibodies, in granuloma
   annulare, 441
α_1-Antitrypsin deficiency, and panniculitis,
   605, 605–607, *606,* 606t, 607t
Antivenin, for black widow spider bites, 813
Anus, in lymphogranuloma venereum, 980
   warts of, child abuse and, 1892
Aorta, coarctation of, hemangioma with,
   1498
Apert's syndrome, with acne, 464
Aphthosis, complex, vs. Behçet's disease, 389t
Aphthous stomatitis, in Behçet's disease, 385, *386*
   in human immunodeficiency virus
   infection, 1148, 1337t
   recurrent, 1330–1331
Aplasia cutis congenita, 1782t, 1782–1785,
   1783t, *1784,* 1785t
   vs. blistering disorders, 717t
Aplastic anemia, antimalarial drugs and, 275
Apocrine glands. See also *Sweat glands.*
   anatomy of, 32–34, *34, 35*
   carcinoma of, 1486–1487
   embryology of, 5
   hidradenitis of, 481–483, *482,* 482t, *483*
   hidradenoma papilliferum of, 1486, *1486,*
   1486t
   hydrocystoma of, 1455–1456, *1457*
   in Paget's disease, extramammary, 1487
      mammary, 1488–1489
   rare tumors of, 1476, 1477t
   syringocystadenoma papilliferum of, 1484t,
   1485, 1485–1486, 1486t

Aponeurotic system, muscular, superficial, 114
Apoproteins, in xanthoma, 1812–1813
Apoptosis, definition of, 105, *106*
Apresoline, and lupus erythematosus, 266
Aquagenic urticaria, 395, 400
Aquatic skin disorders, 787–802
    abrasions in, 797–798, *798*, 798t
    cnidarian stings and, 787–791, 788t, *789, 790*, 791t
    contact dermatitis in, 795–797
    envenomation in, 798–802, 801t
    in seabather's eruption, 791–793, *792*, 793t, 794t, 1186–1187, *1187*, 1187t
    in swimmer's itch, *793*, 793–795, 794t, 795t, 1186, 1187t
    lacerations in, 797–798, *798*, 798t
Arachidonic acid, in mastocytosis, 1605
Arachnid bites, 805t, 811–813, *811–813*, 815–816, *816*
    and Lyme borreliosis, 965–966, 970
    and rickettsial infection, 1011, 1012, 1016, 1019
    and tularemia, 944, *944*, 1035
Aralen. See *Chloroquine.*
Areola, sebaceous glands of, 30, *32*
Argininosuccinic aciduria, 1859t, 1860–1861
    and alopecia, 1713
Aromatase, in androgenetic alopecia, 1254–1255
    in hair follicle growth, 1249, *1249*
Arotinoids, for psoriasis, 309
Arsenic, and pigmentation disorders, 421–422
    and skin cancer, vs. basal cell nevus syndrome, 1745
Arsobal, for trypanosomiasis, 1175
Arteries. See also *Blood vessels.*
    digital, in Raynaud's phenomenon, 538
    disease of, and leg ulcers, 561, *561*, 562t
    in skin, structure of, 21
    of face, anatomy of, *112*, 115
Arterioles, in skin, 21
Arteriovenous fistula, punch hair grafting and, 1259
Arteriovenous hemangioma, acral, 1507t, 1511, *1512*
Arteriovenous malformations, 1496t, 1503–1504, 1506
Arteritis, giant cell, 515–517, *516*, 516t
    infrared radiation and, 825
    of multiple vessels. See *Polyarteritis.*
Arthritis, in Behçet's disease, 386
    in Lyme borreliosis, 966–967, 969t
    in polychondritis, relapsing, 513
    in Reiter's syndrome, 322–325, 325t
    psoriatic, 301–302
    pyoderma gangrenosum with, 380, 380t
    rheumatoid, cutaneous signs of, 1863, *1864*, 1864t
        in mixed connective tissue disease, 268
        subcutaneous nodules in, 444–447, *445, 446*, 446t
        with bowel-associated dermatosis, 375–376, 376t
        vs. Behçet's disease, 389t
Arthroconidia, in dermatophytosis, 1050
Arthropod bites, 804–807, 811–817. See also specific types, e.g., *Tick bites.*
    reaction to, vs. Wells' syndrome, 362
Ascorbic acid (vitamin C), deficiency of, 1873t, *1874*
    cutaneous signs of, 1873t, *1874*
    gastrointestinal hemorrhage in, 1875t
    in wound healing, 567
    in facial skin care, 80
Ash leaf macules, in tuberous sclerosis, *1735*, 1735–1736

Ashy dermatosis, 1238
Asparaginase, allergy to, 428
Aspergillosis, 1071, 1072
    in immunosuppressed patient, 1157
    in neonate, 714, 715t
    with human immunodeficiency virus infection, 1142
Asphalt, and burn injury, 846
Aspirin, and Reye's syndrome, 1079, 1081
    as anticoagulant, biopsy after, 121–122
    for antiphospholipid syndrome, 546t, 550
    for flushing, 535
    for Köhlmeier-Degos syndrome, 546t
    for livedo vasculopathy, 545, 546t
    for mastocytosis, 1607
Astemizole, for urticaria, 402
Astringents, in facial cleansing, 80
Atabrine (quinacrine), and pigmentation disorders, 422
    for discoid lupus erythematosus, 275, 275t
Ataxia, with telangiectasia, 1802t, *1804*
Atheroembolism, cutaneous, 545t, 546t, 546–547, *547*, 1881t
Atherosclerosis, with xanthoma, 1809, 1813
Athletes, skin disorders in, 849–853. See also *Sports.*
Athlete's foot (tinea pedis), 851, 928–929, 1044t, 1045–1047, *1046, 1047*
Atopic dermatitis, 195–202
    clinical findings in, 195–196, *196*
    differential diagnosis of, 199–200, 200t
    epidemiology of, 195
    light-exacerbated, vs. actinic reticuloid syndrome, 770, 770t
    of hand, 188, 190, 191
    pathogenesis of, *198*, 198–199
    pathology of, 197–198
    treatment of, 200t, 200–202, 1887t
    vs. seborrheic dermatitis, 216
    with human immunodeficiency virus infection, 1146
Atopic eczema, heat therapy for, 826
Atopy, definition of, 105
Atrium, myxoma of, cutaneous signs with, 1879t, 1881t
Atrophic papulosis, malignant, 545t, 546t, 551–552
    and gastrointestinal hemorrhage, 1875t
    cardiac disorders with, 1878t
Atrophie blanche, livedo vasculopathy and, 543, *544*
Atrophoderma of Pasini and Pierini, 895, 897, 898
    vs. anetoderma, 911t
Atrophoderma vermiculatum, 504
Atrophy, cutaneous, assessment of, *100*, 100–101, *101*, 101t
Atypia, definition of, 105, *105*
Auchmeromyia luteola infestation, 820
Aurelia aurita stings, 788, *789*
Auricular muscles, anatomy of, 114
Auricular nerve, greater, anatomy of, *118*, 119
Auriculotemporal nerve, anatomy of, 117
Auriculotemporal syndrome, hyperhidrosis in, 1313–1314
Auspitz sign, in plaque psoriasis, 296
Australian box jellyfish stings, 787–789, *790*, 791t
Autoantibodies, anti–basement membrane, and dermatosis, in pregnancy, 370
    in epidermolysis bullosa, 642, 642t
    anti-neutrophil cytoplasmic, in arteritis, 524–526
    in Sweet's syndrome, 374
    in systemic lupus erythematosus, 273, 273t

Autoimmunity, and dermatitis, in pregnancy, 370
    and pruritus, 155t
    cicatricial pemphigoid antigen in, 620–621
    in vitiligo, 1211–1212
    psoralen–ultraviolet radiation therapy and, in treatment of psoriasis, 315
Autonomic nervous system, in skin, 23–25, *25*
    in sweat gland function, 1308
Avascular necrosis, of bone, in systemic lupus erythematosus, 265
Axilla, hidradenitis suppurativa of, 481–483, *482*, 482t, *483*
    odor in, bacterial flora and, 927–928
    trichomycosis of, 927, *928*
Axons, anatomy of, 1536–1537
Azathioprine, for actinic reticuloid syndrome, 770t
    for Behçet's disease, 390, 390t
    for lupus erythematosus, discoid, 276
        systemic, 277–278
    for pemphigoid, bullous, 670, 671
        cicatricial, 677
    for pemphigus, paraneoplastic, 661, 661t
    for pemphigus foliaceus, 658, 658t
    for pemphigus vulgaris, 654t, 655
    for polymyositis, 288t, 289
    for psoriasis, 311–312
    for Reiter's syndrome, 325, 325t
Azelaic acid, for melasma, 1236
Azidothymidine (zidovudine), adverse reactions to, in human immunodeficiency virus infection, 1145
Azulfidine (sulfasalazine), for discoid lupus erythematosus, 276
    for urticaria, 402–403

B

B cells. See *Lymphocytes.*
Bacillary angiomatosis, 1023–1028. See also *Angiomatosis, bacillary.*
Bacille Calmette-Guérin, immunization with, in human immunodeficiency virus infection, 1142
    in prevention of leprosy, 1003
Bacillus anthracis infection, 1030–1032, *1031*, 1031t, 1032t
Bacitracin, and wound healing, 566t
Bacterial infection. See also specific organisms, e.g., *Streptococcus pyogenes.*
    and erythema nodosum, 593, 594t
    and leg ulcers, 562t
    by normal cutaneous flora, 926–929, *927, 928*
    in toxic epidermal necrolysis, 706, 710t
    in wound healing, 565–566, 566t
    of animal bite wounds, 943, 947
    of genitalia, 1343–1344
    of insect bite wounds, 943–944, *944*, 947
    oral, 1335, 1336t, 1337t
    vaginal, diagnosis of, 1343, 1343t
    with human immunodeficiency virus infection, 1138, *1138*
Bactrim. See *Trimethoprim, with sulfamethoxazole.*
Baghdad sore, 1163
Baker-Gordon formula, in chemical peel, for photoaging, 742t, *744*, 744–746, 745t, *746*
Balanitis, in Reiter's syndrome, 322, 323t, *324*
Balanoposthitis, diagnosis of, 1342t
Balloon cell, 105
Balloon cell nevi, 1566

Ballooning degeneration, 105
Bannayan-Zonana syndrome, 1506, 1799t
Banner-type transposition flap, after skin
   cancer excision, 1414
Barium, and burn injury, 844t
Barrier function, of epidermis, 46
   against microorganisms, 51–52
   biochemical mechanisms of, 51t, 52–53
   homeostasis in, 48–50, *50*
   in neonate, 1889–1890, *1890*
   two-compartment model of, 50–51, 51t
Bartholin's cyst, 1352
Bartholin's glands, staphylococcal infection
   of, 1343
Bartonellosis, 1024t, 1024–1028, *1026*, 1027t
Basal cell, definition of, 105–106
Basal cell carcinoma, 1387–1391. See also
   Carcinoma.
Basal cell nevus syndrome, 1742–1745,
   1743, 1744, 1745t, 1796t, *1797*
   infundibular cysts in, 1450–1451
Basal layer, in gestation, 3
   structure of, 5–6, *6*
Basaloid cells, definition of, 106
Basement membrane. See also
   Dermoepidermal junction.
   collagen in, 862, *862*
   definition of, 106
   immunoglobulin M antibodies to, and
      dermatosis, in pregnancy, 370
   in tricholemmoma, 1470, *1470*
   keratinocytes in, 59
Basement membrane proteins, in
   dermoepidermal junction,
   hemidesmosomal-associated, 619–621,
   620
   lamina densa–associated, 624–625
Basement membrane zone, linear
   immunoglobulin A deposits in, in
   bullous dermatosis, 698–702, *699–701*,
   700t, 701t
Bazex's acrokeratosis, paraneoplastic, 1846
Bazin's erythema induratum, 985–987, *987*,
   Plate 7
BCNU, for lymphoma, cutaneous T-cell,
   1652
   for lymphomatoid papulosis, 1636t, 1637
Beaded lines, juxtaclavicular, configuration
   of, *87*
Beard, shaving of, and pseudofolliculitis,
   499–502, *500*, 500t
Beau's lines, 1302
Bedbug bites, *805*, 807, 807t
Bee stings, 807t, 807–808, 808t
Behçet's disease, 385–391
   acneiform eruption in, 469
   cardiac features of, cutaneous signs with,
      1878t, *1880*
   clinical findings in, 385–387, *386*
   diagnosis of, 388, 388t, 389t
   neonatal, 716t
   oral lesions in, 1330–1331
   pathogenesis of, 387–388
   pathology of, 387, *387*
   treatment of, 388–391, 390t
   vs. chancroid, 975, 975t
Benadryl (diphenhydramine), for nummular
   dermatitis, 213, 213t
   for pseudoparkinsonian side effects of
      pimozide, 781
Benznidazole, for trypanosomiasis, 1174
Benzophenones, and photoallergy, *729*,
   Plate 5
   in sunscreens, 754
Benzo-porphyrin derivative, in photodynamic
   therapy, for skin carcinoma, 1427

Benzoyl peroxide, and wound healing, 566t
   for acne keloidalis nuchae, 1283, 1283t
Benztropine mesylate, for
   pseudoparkinsonian side effects of
   pimozide, 781
Berloque dermatitis, vs. melasma, 1235
Besnier's prurigo gestationis, 369–370
Beta-blockers, in psoriasis, 301
Beta-carotene, for photosensitivity, in
   erythropoietic protoporphyria, 1757
Betamethasone, after dermabrasion, for acne
   scars, 478
   augmented, 163–164
   for alopecia areata, 1271–1274, 1273t
   for contact dermatitis, 181
   for seborrheic dermatitis, 165
   potency of, 163
Beta$_2$-microglobulin, in amyloidosis, 1821
Bilharziasis (schistosomiasis), 1184–1186,
   1185
   and swimmer's itch, *793*, 793–795, 794t,
      795t
Biliary cirrhosis, primary, and pruritus, 158
   cutaneous signs of, *1877*, 1877t
Biliary tract, disorders of, and
   hyperlipidemia, with xanthoma, 1815
   in prurigo gravidarum, 369
   in Langerhans cell histiocytosis, 1611
Bilobed transposition flap, after skin cancer
   excision, 1415–1416, *1416*
Biopsy, delay of, reasons for, 121–122
   in dermatomyositis, 286
   in graft-versus-host reaction,
      sclerodermoid, 231, *231*
   in polymyositis, 286
   of genitalia, 1343
   of leg ulcer, 563
   of melanoma, 124, 125, 1589–1590, *1590*
   of nevi, melanocytic, 1569–1571, *1570,
      1571*
   shave, for actinic keratosis, 1396
      for skin carcinoma, 1398
   site selection for, 120t, 120–121
   specimen handling in, 122–123
   types of, 121, *123*, 123–128, *125, 126*
Biotin, deficiency of, 1859t, 1861
   and alopecia, diffuse, 1276
   cutaneous signs of, 1873t
   for nail brittleness, 1303
Birbeck granules, in allergic contact
   dermatitis, *170*, 170–171, 171t
   in embryology, 4
   in epidermal structure, *11–13*
   in Langerhans cell histiocytosis, 1612, *1612*
Bird mite bites, *814*, 814–815, *815*
Birthmarks, arteriovenous malformations
   and, 1496t, 1503–1504, 1506
   hemangiomas and, 1496t, 1496–1501,
      1497, 1498, 1500
   lymphatic malformations and, 1496t,
      1504, *1504*, 1505
   nevus simplex and, 1496t, 1502–1503
   port-wine stains as, 1496t, 1501–1502,
      1502
   syndromes associated with, 1505–1506
   venous malformations and, 1496t, 1503,
      1503
Bismuth, and pigmentation disorders, 421
Bite wounds, octopus, 800
Bitemporal scalp lift, 1263, *1264*
Bites, bacterial wound infection after,
   943–944, *944*, 947
   insect, 804–807, *805*, 805t, *806*, 807t
      reaction to, vs. Wells' syndrome, 362
   mite, 813–815, *814, 815*
   spider, 811–813, *811–813*

Bites (*Continued*)
   tick, 805t, 815–816, *816*
      and Lyme borreliosis, 965–966, 970
      and rickettsial infection, 1011, 1012,
         1016, 1019
      and tularemia, 944, *944*, 1035
Bitumen, and burn injury, 844t, 846
Black widow spider bites, 812–813, *813*
Blaschko's lines, in hypomelanosis of Ito,
   1226, 1227, 1227t
   in lichen striatus, 245
Blastomycosis, *1066*, 1066–1067, 1067t,
   1068t
   of lung, cutaneous signs with, 1882t
Bleeding. See *Hemorrhage.*
Bleomycin, and hyperpigmentation, 1237
Blindness, night, in Refsum's disease, 1695
Blisters, 615–721. See also *Bulla(e)* and
   Vesicle(s).
   blood-filled, oral, 1333
   definition of, 106
   friction and, in athletes, 850, 853
   grafting of, for vitiligo, 1216
   in dactylitis, distal, 921
   in neonate, 712, 713t–717t
      infectious, 712–718, 713t–715t
      transient, 715t, 719, *719*
      uncommon, 713t, 716t, 717t, 719–721,
         720
   pressure and, vs. toxic epidermal
      necrolysis, 710t
Bloch-Sulzberger syndrome, 1725–1728. See
   also *Incontinentia pigmenti.*
Blood, clotting of. See *Coagulation.*
   disorders of, and leg ulcers, 562t
   and pruritus, 155t, 158
   cutaneous signs of, 1866–1867
   dapsone and, 702, 702t
   in hypereosinophilic syndrome,
      352–358. See also
      Hypereosinophilic syndrome.
   in Langerhans cell histiocytosis, 1611
   in systemic lupus erythematosus, 272t,
      273–274
   in toxic epidermal necrolysis, 706
   pyoderma gangrenosum with, 380, 380t
   loss of. See *Hemorrhage.*
   lymphoma spread through, cutaneous
      T-cell, 1646–1647, *1647*, 1649, *1650*,
      1650t
   transfusion of, trypanosomiasis prevention
      in, 1174
Blood vessels. See also *Arteries, Capillaries,*
   and *Veins.*
   benign tumors of, 1507t, *1509–1515*,
      1509–1516
   development of, 1492–1495, 1493t, 1495t
   disorders of, cutaneous signs of, 1886t
      in Behçet's disease, 386–387
      in genodermatoses, 1799t, *1800, 1801*
      in neonate, and transient dermatoses,
         1892–1894
   hyperplasia of, 1506–1509, 1507t, *1508*
   in collagen-vascular disease, 1846, 1886t
   in graft-versus-host disease, 228
   in radiation dermatitis, 837, *838*
   in scleroderma, 885–887, *888*
   in skin, 21–23, *24, 25*
   in systemic lupus erythematosus, 263–264
   in thermoregulation, 55
   inflammation of. See *Vasculitis.*
   leaking of, interleukin-2 and, in
      erythroderma, 338
   malformations of, and birthmarks, 1496t,
      1496–1506. See also *Birthmarks.*
   vs. blistering disorders, 716t

Blood vessels (*Continued*)
occlusive disease of, noninflammatory, in
small vessels, 543–552
of dermis, 876–877
of face, anatomy of, *112*, 115
of neck, anatomy of, 119
oral, lesions of, 1325–1326
regrowth of, in wound healing, *564*, 565
sarcoma of, *1516*, 1516–1518, *1517*
trauma to, drug abuse and, 840
Bloom's syndrome, 765, 1366, *1367*, 1802t
Blue nevus, 1568, *1568*, Plate 10
and melanoma, 1580
Blue rubber bleb nevus syndrome, 1505, 1799t
gastrointestinal hemorrhage in, 1874t
Bluefarb-Stewart syndrome, 1507
Blushing, 534
BM-40 protein, in dermoepidermal junction,
625
Boils, vs. acne, 469
Bone, disorders of, in neurofibromatosis, 1731
in Rothmund-Thomson syndrome,
1803t, *1804*
in syphilis, congenital, 960t
retinoids and, 310
formation of, in skin, 1828, 1829t,
1830–1831, 1831t
necrosis of, avascular, in systemic lupus
erythematosus, 265
osteolysis of, in Gorham's syndrome, 1506
Bone marrow, disorders of, in
hypereosinophilic syndrome, 354
transplantation of, and graft-versus-host
disease, 225–226
with allogeneic graft, acute reaction
in, 226–230, *227*, 227t–229t,
228, Plate 1
chronic reaction in, *230*, 230–232,
231
with autologous graft, 232–233
Boots, Unna's, in leg ulcer management, 567
Borrelia burgdorferi, and Jessner's
lymphocytic infiltrate, 345
in Lyme disease, 965–970. See also *Lyme
borreliosis*.
in lymphoid hyperplasia, 1627, 1629
in morphea, 898
Botfly larvae, in furuncular myiasis, 818, *819*
Botryomycosis, 926
Bourneville's disease, 1735–1740. See also
Tuberous sclerosis.
Boutonneuse fever, 1012t, 1016–1017
Bowel. See *Intestine*.
Bowenoid papulosis, 1103, *1104*, 1108, 1352,
1352
Bowen's disease, *1380*, 1380–1381, 1381t,
1868
of vulva, 1353, *1353*
periungual, 1305
Box jellyfish stings, 787–789, *790*, 791t
Boyd's perforating vein, varicosity of, *578*
Brain, tumors of, in basal cell nevus
syndrome, 1743
Brain stem, melanocytes in, in vitiligo, 1211
Breast, cancer of, metastasis of, to skin,
1674, *1675*, *1676*, 1677
Paget's disease of, 1488–1489, *1489*, *1868*,
Plate 15
removal of, angiosarcoma after, and
lymphedema, 554, 556, 1516
silicone implant in, and scleroderma, 887,
888t, 892t, 893–894
Brevibacterium epidermidis infection,
interdigital, 928, 929
Brill-Zinsser disease, 1012t, 1018

Bristleworms, and dermatitis, 796–797
Brocq's pseudopelade, 1285–1287, *1286*,
1286t
Bromhidrosis, 1317
Bromine, and burn injury, 844t
Brown recluse spider bites, *811*, 811–812, *812*
Brucellosis, 1032t, 1032–1033, 1033t
Bruch's membrane, calcification in, in
pseudoxanthoma elasticum, 1770
Brugia malayi infestation, 1179
Bubonic plague, *1033*, 1033–1034, 1034t
Buccal branch, of facial nerve, anatomy of,
113, 116, 116t, 117
Buccal mucosa, biopsy of, 128
vermilion border of, sebaceous glands of,
30–31, 1325
Buccal nerve, anatomy of, 117
Buccinator muscle, anatomy of, 113, *113*
Bulb, of hair follicle, *28*, 28–29
Bulge, definition of, 106
Bulla(e), assessment of, 94–96, *95–97*, 96t
genital, diagnosis of, 1342t
in epidermolysis bullosa, 635–645. See
also *Epidermolysis bullosa*.
in herpes gestationis, 679, *680*
in incontinentia pigmenti, 1725–1728
in lupus erythematosus, systemic, 264, *264*,
269–270, *270*, 274, 278
in lymphoma, T-cell, 1644
in morphea, 896–898
in neonate, 1897
in porphyria cutanea tarda, 1758, *1758*,
1759
in scabies, 1196, *1196*
with diabetes, 1869t, *1870*
Bullous dermatosis, and scarring alopecia,
1290–1291
chronic, neonatal onset of, 716t, 720
diagnosis of, 700–701, *701*, 701t
linear immunoglobulin A, 698–702,
699–701, 700t, 701t
treatment of, 701–702, 702t
Bullous ichthyosis, 1688–1690, *1688–1690*
genetic mutation in, 63, 1689
Bullous impetigo, 921, *921*
in staphylococcal scalded skin syndrome,
935, *935*, 936, *936*
Bullous pemphigoid, 664–671. See also
Pemphigoid, bullous.
Bullous pemphigoid antigens, 15, *19*, 864,
865
in dermoepidermal junction, 619–620,
620, 667–668
Bullous pyoderma gangrenosum, 381, *381*
atypical, 375
Bunostomum phlebotomum infestation, and
cutaneous larva migrans, 1181, 1181t
Bupivacaine, in anesthesia, 130, 130t
Buried sutures, *136*, 136–137
Burkitt's lymphoma, Epstein-Barr virus
infection in, 1082, 1083
Burkitt-type lymphoblastic lymphoma, 1664,
1664
Burning mouth syndrome, 1328
Burns, chemical, 843–847, 844t, 845t, *846*
child abuse and, 1891, *1892*
vs. toxic epidermal necrolysis, 710t
Burow's wedge advancement flap, after skin
cancer excision, 1410
Burrows, assessment of, 101–102, *102*
in scabies, 101, *102*, 1196, *1196*, 1197
in tungiasis, 820–821, *821*
Buschke-Löwenstein condyloma, 1353, 1385
Buschke-Ollendorff syndrome, 1792
Buschke's scleredema, with diabetes, 1869t

Buspirone (BuSpar), for neurotic
excoriations, 784
Busulfan, and hyperpigmentation, 1237
Butterfly larvae, and dermatitis, 809–810
Butterfly sign, in neurotic excoriations, 783,
783
Buttock, gangrene of, perinatal, 715t
Bypass surgery, intestinal, and dermatitis-
arthritis syndrome, 375–376, 376t

C

Cabbage head jellyfish stings, 788
Cachectin (tumor necrosis factor-α), in
angiogenesis, 1493t, 1494
in inflammatory response, 144t, 144–145,
151
in urticaria, 397t, 398
Cadherins, in inflammatory response, 150
in pemphigus foliaceus, 657
Café-au-lait macules, 1563
in neurofibromatosis, 1730, *1731*, 1732,
1735
Calabar swellings, in loiasis, 1180
Calcifying epithelioma, of Malherbe,
1468–1470, *1469*, 1830
Calcinosis, of scrotum, idiopathic, 1352
Calciphylaxis, 1829, *1830*, 1831
Calcipotriol, for psoriasis, 307
Calcitonin gene-related peptide, in Raynaud's
phenomenon, 538–539, 542
Calcitriol, for psoriasis, 307
rickets resistant to, and alopecia, 1712
Calcium, deposition of, in acne scar tissue,
after dermabrasion, 479
in skin, 1828–1831, *1829*, 1829t, *1830*,
1831t
in keratinocyte differentiation, 66
in pseudoxanthoma elasticum, 1770, 1773
with steroid therapy, for lupus
erythematosus, systemic, 277
Calcium channel blockers, for urticaria, 402
Calcium gluconate, for hydrofluoric acid
burn, 847
Calf muscle, pump function of, in venous
ulceration, 560, *560*
Calluses, 1703
Calmette-Guérin bacillus, immunization
with, in human immunodeficiency virus
infection, 1142
in prevention of leprosy, 1003
Cancer. See also specific types, e.g.,
Melanoma.
and erythema nodosum, 593, 594t
and palmoplantar keratoderma, 1703–1704
chemotherapy for, and hyperpigmentation,
1237
cyclosporine and, 311
dermatoses with, 1843–1849. See also
Paraneoplastic dermatosis.
erythema gyratum repens with, 349, 350
genodermatoses and, 1796t, *1797*, 1797t,
1798
heat therapy for, 826
in chondroid syringoma, 1478–1479
infrared radiation and, 824
metastasis of, definition of, 109
to skin, 1674t, 1674–1677, *1675*, *1676*,
1677t
in neonate, 1898
methotrexate and, 309
of mouth, 1329–1330
in acquired immunodeficiency
syndrome, 1337t

Cancer (*Continued*)
    papillomavirus and, 1335
    papillomavirus and, 1100, 1103–1104,
      1110–1111, 1335
    pyoderma gangrenosum with, 381
    radiation dermatitis and, 837, *837*, 838
    testicular, with ichthyosis, X-linked
      recessive, 1684
    ultraviolet-induced, molecular mechanisms
      of, 1369–1374, *1370*, 1370t, *1371,
      1373*
    with dermatomyositis, 285–286
    with Sweet's syndrome, 373
Candidiasis, 1056–1058, *1057*, 1057t, *1058*,
    1058t
    genital, *1057*, 1057t*1345*, 1345–1346
    in diaper dermatitis, 184, *185*, 186, 186t,
      187, 1057t, Plate 1
    in immunosuppressed patient, 1157
    in neonate, 714, 715t
    oral, 1335–1336, 1337t
      in human immunodeficiency virus
        infection, 1148
      vs. lichen planus, 238, 238t
    vaginal, *1345*, 1345–1346
      after antibiotic therapy, for acne, 472
      diagnosis of, 1343, 1343t
    vulvar, and vestibulitis, 1354
    with human immunodeficiency virus
      infection, 1144
Capillaria infestation, and larva migrans,
    1181, 1181t
Capillaries. See also *Blood vessels.*
    dilatation of, in pigmented purpura, 293
    hemangioma of, lobular, 1507t, *1509*,
      1509–1510, *1510*
      oral, 1325–1326
    in Raynaud's phenomenon, 538
    in Rocky Mountain spotted fever, 1013
    in scleroderma, 886–887, *888*
    in skin, 21–23, *24*
    inflammation of, in purpura, with systemic
      disease, 1865t, *1866*
    loops of, in nail folds, 1304
    malformations of, and port-wine stains,
      1496t, 1501–1502, *1502*
    thrombosed aneurysms of, 1509
Carbamazepine, for pudendal neuralgia,
    1355–1356
    hypersensitivity to, 417
Carbocaine, in anesthesia, 130, 130t
Carbolic acid (phenol), and burn injury,
    845t, 846
    in chemical peel, for photoaging, 742t,
      743–746, *744*, 745t, *746*
Carboxylase deficiency, biotin-dependent,
    1859t, 1861
Carboxypeptidase, in urticaria, 398
Carboxyporphyrinogens, in heme
    biosynthesis, in porphyria, 1754, 1754t,
    1755
Carbuncles, staphylococcal infection and, 922
Carcinoid syndrome, and flushing, 1848
    cardiac features of, cutaneous signs with,
      1878t
Carcinoid tumors, vs. scleroderma, 887, 888t
Carcinoma, basal cell, 1381t, *1387–1390*,
    1387–1391
    clinical findings in, *1387*, 1387–1388,
      1388
    cryosurgery for, *1394*, 1397–1398
    curettage for, *1394*, 1396–1397, *1397*
    definition of, 1387
    electrodesiccation for, *1394*, 1396–1397,
      1397

Carcinoma (*Continued*)
    excision of, *1394*, 1398–1400, *1399*
    in basal cell nevus syndrome,
      1742–1745, *1743, 1744*, 1745t,
      1796t
    laser surgery for, 1398
    Mohs micrographic surgery for, 1393t,
      1394, *1394*, 1394t, 1403–1408,
      1404–1406, 1406t
    pathology of, 1388–1391, *1389, 1390*
    pigmented, vs. melanoma, 1586–1587,
      1587, Plate 12
    radiation therapy for, *1394, 1400*,
      1400–1402, 1401t, 1402t, *1403*
    treatment of, 1393, 1393t, 1394, *1394*,
      1394t
    vs. trichoepithelioma, 1466–1468, *1467*
    definition of, 1363
    excision of, reconstructive surgery after,
      1408–1423. See also *Reconstructive
      surgery.*
    in digital papillary adenoma, 1481, *1482*
    in hidradenoma, 1480–1481
    in Paget's disease, extramammary, *1487*,
      1487–1488, *1488*, 1488t
      mammary, 1488–1489, *1489*
    in poroma, 1480
    in xeroderma pigmentosum, 1747, 1803t,
      1805
    interferons for, 1427–1429, *1428*
    Merkel cell, 1391–1393, *1392*, 1392t, 1393t
    of apocrine glands, 1486–1487
    of eccrine glands, microcystic, 1483, *1483,
      1484*
    mucinous, 1484–1485
    of genitalia, 314, 1352–1353, *1353*
    of sweat ducts, syringoid, 1483–1484, 1484t
    photodynamic therapy for, 1423–1427,
      1425, 1426
    pilomatrix, 1471
    retinoids for, 1429–1431
    sebaceous, *1473*, 1473–1474, *1474*
    squamous cell, after renal transplantation,
      1884t, *1885*
      curettage for, 1396–1397, *1397*
      definition of, 1383–1385, *1384*
      development of, in lichen planus, 236,
        1331
      differential diagnosis of, 1381t
      electrodesiccation for, *1394*, 1396–1397,
        1397
      excision of, 1398–1400, *1399*
      in epidermolysis bullosa, dystrophic,
        640, *640*, 645
      in situ (Bowen's disease), *1380*,
        1380–1381, 1381t, *1868*
        of vulva, 1353, *1353*
        periungual, 1305
      laser surgery for, 1398
      Mohs micrographic surgery for,
        1403–1408, *1404, 1405*, 1406t
      of genitalia, psoralen–ultraviolet
        radiation therapy and, 314
      oral, 1329
      pathogenesis of, 1387
      pathology of, 1385–1386, *1386*
      periungual, 1305
      radiation therapy for, 1400–1402,
        1401t, 1402t
      solar keratosis and, 1379
      treatment of, 1393, 1395, *1395*, 1396t
    verrucous, 1385–1386, *1386*
      oral, 1329
    with human immunodeficiency virus
      infection, 1149, *1149*, 1155

Carcinoma (*Continued*)
    with lupus vulgaris, 985, *986*, Plate 7
Cardiac. See *Heart.*
Cardio-facio-cutaneous syndrome,
    1697–1698
Caries, dental, sinus tracts from, to skin, vs.
    acne, 469
Carmustine, for lymphoma, cutaneous T-cell,
    1652
    for lymphomatoid papulosis, 1636t, 1637
Carotenemia, with diabetes, 1870t, *1871*
Carrión's disease, 1024t, 1024–1028, *1026*,
    1027t
Cartilage, inflammation of, in relapsing
    polychondritis, 512–514, *513*, 513t,
    514t
    with dermatitis, nodular, 507–510, *508*,
      509t, *510*
Cartilage link proteins, in inflammatory
    response, 150
Cartilage-hair hypoplasia, 1715
Carukia barnesi stings, 789
Castleman's disease, and pemphigus, 660
Catagen phase, in hair cycle, 30, *31*, 106,
    1248
Cataracts, in atopic dermatitis, 196–197
    psoralen–ultraviolet radiation therapy and,
      315
    radiation exposure and, 837
Caterpillars, and dermatitis, *809*, 809–810,
    810
Catfish stings, 800–801
Cat-scratch disease, clinical findings in,
    1025–1026
    diagnosis of, 1027t, 1027–1028
    epidemiology of, 1024–1025
    historical aspects of, 1023–1024
    pathology of, 1027
    treatment of, 1028
Cautery, for macrocomedones, 471–472
CD44 glycoprotein, in inflammatory
    response, 150
CD4-positive T helper cells, in atopic
    dermatitis, 198, *198*, 199
Cefaclor, and serum sickness–like reaction,
    418
Cefazolin, for staphylococcal infection, 923t
    for streptococcal infection, 923t
Ceftriaxone, for chancroid, 976, 976t
    for Lyme borreliosis, 969t
Celestone. See *Betamethasone.*
Cellulitis, *Aeromonas hydrophila* infection
    and, 943
    gastrointestinal bacterial flora and,
      941–942, 942t
    Haemophilus influenzae infection and,
      939–940
    in Wells' syndrome, 360, *361*, Plate 3
    of scalp, and alopecia, *1281*, 1281–1282,
      1282t
    streptococcal, *924*, 924t, 924–926, 925t
      diagnosis of, 945
Cement, and burn injury, 844t, 846
Central nervous system. See *Nervous system.*
Centroblastic lymphoma, *1662*, 1663–1664
Centrocytic lymphoma, *1662*, 1663
Cephalexin, for cellulitis, of scalp, 1282, 1282t
    for folliculitis decalvans, 1284, 1284t
    for staphylococcal infection, 923t
      with pyoderma, in neonate, 712
    for streptococcal infection, 923t
Cephalic histiocytosis, benign, 1622
Cephalopod bites, 800
Cephalosporium infection, and mycetoma,
    1070, 1071t

Cercaria, in dermatitis, *793*, 793–795, 794t, 795t, 1186, 1187t
  in schistosomiasis, 1185, *1185*
Cerebrum, thrombosis of, in antiphospholipid syndrome, 548
  in Sneddon's syndrome, 548
Cervical branches, of facial nerve, anatomy of, *113*, 116, 116t, 117, 119
Cervical nerves, transverse, anatomy of, *118*, 119
Cervical plexus, anatomy of, *118*, 119
Cervix uteri, mucopurulent inflammation of, 1344
C1-esterase inhibitor, in angioedema, *395*, 395–396, 400
Cestode larva infestation, 1187–1188
Chagas' disease, *1173*, 1173–1174
Chanarin-Dorfman syndrome, *1693*, 1693–1694
Chancres, in syphilis, 949, *950*, 953
  tuberculous, 984
Chancroid, 973–976, *974*, 975t, 976t
  vs. syphilis, 956
Chédiak-Higashi syndrome, 1221t, 1222, 1717–1718
Cheilitis, actinic, 1380
  retinoids and, 310
Cheilitis glandularis, 1329
Cheilitis granulomatosa, 1327
Chemical burns, 843–847, 844t, 845t, *846*
Chemical exposure, and cutaneous T-cell lymphoma, 1648
  and scleroderma, 891–894, 892t, *893*
Chemical peel, for acne scars, 474
  for photoaging, 741–746, *742*, 742t, 743t, *744–746*, 745t, 746t
  patient selection for, 742t, 742–743
Chemical stimuli, and pruritus, 155t, 157
Chemokines, in inflammatory response, 143–144, 151
Chemosurgery, 1403–1408. See also *Mohs micrographic surgery.*
Chemotherapy, allergic reactions to, 428
  and acral erythema, 428, *428*, Plate 3
  and actinic keratosis, 429
  and alopecia, 426–427
  and eccrine disorders, 428–429, *429*, Plate 3
  and hyperpigmentation, 1237
  and lichen planus–like reaction, 430
  and lymphocyte increase, skin reaction in, 429
  and melanocytic nevi, benign, 430
  and nail dystrophies, 427
  and pigmentary changes, 427
  and Raynaud's phenomenon, 429
  dactinomycin in, and folliculitis, 429–430
  drugs in, and contact dermatitis, 430
  for Kaposi's sarcoma, 1154
  for leukemia, 1672–1673
  for melanoma, 1594
  local skin reactions to, 428
  mithramycin in, flushing reaction to, 430
  sclerotic reactions to, 429
  skin reactions to, 426–430, 427t, *428, 429*, Plate 3
  with radiation therapy, and skin reactions, 427–428
  for skin carcinoma, 1402
Cherry hemangioma, 1507t, 1515
Cheyletiella mite bites, 813, *814*
Chickenpox, 1078–1081. See also *Varicella-zoster infection.*
Chiclero's ulcer, 1163
Chigger bites, 815, *815*
  and typhus, 1018, *1019*

Chilblains, 829–830
  homelessness and, 841
  in systemic lupus erythematosus, 263
Child. See also *Infant* and *Neonate.*
  abuse of, physical, 841–842, *843, 1891*, 1891–1892, *1892*
    sexual, 842–843, 1892
  acne in, 463
  alopecia in, scarring, *1292*, 1292t, 1292–1293, 1293t
  Epstein-Barr virus infection in, 1082
  genital warts in, 1106
  histiocytoma in, eruptive, generalized, 1622
    indeterminant cell, 1620
  histiocytosis in, cephalic, benign, 1622
    classification of, 1620, 1621t
    Langerhans cell, 1610
    malignant, 1623–1624
  ichthyosis in. See *Ichthyosis.*
  laryngeal papillomatosis in, 1106
  lipoblastoma in, 1529–1530
  lymphohistiocytosis, hemophagocytic, 1623
  morphea in, pansclerotic, 896, 898
  mucinosis in, cutaneous, self-healing, 1838
  nevus lipomatosus superficialis in, 1526
  panniculitis in, cold exposure and, 609–610
  rhabdomyosarcoma in, *1525*, 1525–1526
  skin evaluation in, 1891
  sunscreen use by, 756t, 756–757, 1891
  surgery in, 1898
  syphilis in, congenital, 957t, 959, *960*, 960t
  toxic shock syndrome in, 932
  xanthogranuloma in, 1620–1622, *1621, 1622*, 1622t
  xanthoma disseminatum in, 1623
CHILD syndrome, 1696
  epidermal nevi in, 1787, 1789, 1790
CHIME syndrome, 1697
Chironex fleckeri stings, 787–789, *790*, 791t
Chitin, modified, anti-angiogenic effect of, 1495
Chlamydia trachomatis infection, and lymphogranuloma venereum, 976t, 979–981, *980*
  and urethritis, 1344
Chloracne, 463–464
Chlorambucil, for pemphigus vulgaris, 654t, 655
  with prednisone, for cutaneous T-cell lymphoma, 1653
Chloramphenicol, for granuloma inguinale, 979
  for Rocky Mountain spotted fever, 1015, 1016t
  for tularemia, 947, 1035
Chlorhexidine, and wound healing, 566t
  for candidiasis, oral, 1336
  in antiseptic solutions, 129, 129t
Chlorins, in photodynamic therapy, for skin carcinoma, 1427
Chloroma, with granulocytic leukemia, 1672
Chloroquine, and pigmentation disorders, 422
  for discoid lupus erythematosus, 275t, 275–276
  for morphea, 898
  for porphyria cutanea tarda, 1759
Chlorpromazine, and hyperpigmentation, 1237
Cholecystectomy, in protoporphyria, 1757–1758
Cholestasis, and hyperlipidemia, with xanthoma, 1815
  and pruritus, 155t, 158
  in prurigo gravidarum, 369

Cholesterol embolism, 545t, 546t, 546–547, *547*, 1881t
Cholesterolosis, extracellular, 528–530, *529*, 530t
Cholinergic urticaria, 392–394, 400
Chondritis, in relapsing polychondritis, 512–514, *513*, 513t, 514t
Chondrodermatitis nodularis, 507–510, *508*, 509t, *510*
Chondrodysplasia punctata, with scaling skin, *1695*, 1695–1696, 1716
Chondroid syringoma, *1477*, 1478–1479, *1479*
Chondroitin 6-sulfate proteoglycan, in dermoepidermal junction, 625
  in epidermolysis bullosa, 642t
Choriocarcinoma, with herpes gestationis, 683
Chorion proteins, glycine in, 62, 63
Christ-Siemens-Touraine syndrome, 1714, *1714*, 1722t
Chromic acid, and burn injury, 844t
Chromoblastomycosis, 1067–1069, *1069*, 1069t
Chrysaora quinquecirrha stings, 788
Chrysarobin, for psoriasis, 306
Chrysops flies, as vectors of loiasis, 1180
Churg-Strauss syndrome, 522–527, *523, 526*, 526t
  vs. hypereosinophilic syndrome, 356
Chymase, in urticaria, 397t, 398
Cicatricial pemphigoid. See also *Pemphigoid.*
Cicatricial pemphigoid antigen, 620–621
Cigarette smoking, in protease inhibitor deficiency panniculitis, 605, 607
Cimetidine, for androgenetic alopecia, 1257
Cimex lectularius, 805
Cinnamates, in sunscreens, 754
Ciprofloxacin, for chancroid, 976, 976t
  for *Pseudomonas* infection, 946
Cirrhosis, biliary, primary, and pruritus, 158
  cutaneous signs of, *1877*, 1877t
  methotrexate and, 308
Civatte bodies, definition of, 106, *106*
  in lichen planus, 237
Civatte's poikiloderma, vs. melasma, 1235
C-kit proto-oncogene, in inflammatory response, 145
Clarithromycin, for leprosy, 1001
Clark's nevus, 1571–1574, *1572, 1573*, Plates 10 and 11
  vs. melanoma, 1588
Clavulanate, for chancroid, 976
Clear cell hidradenoma, *1477*, 1480–1481, *1481*, 1481t
Cleft, definition of, 106
  of lip, with ectodermal dysplasia, 1722t
  of palate, with ectodermal dysplasia, 1722t
  sternal, hemangioma with, 1498
Climacteric, flushing in, 534, 535
Clindamycin, for actinomycosis, 1008t, 1009
  for bowel-associated dermatosis-arthritis syndrome, 376, 376t
  for staphylococcal infection, 922–923, 923t
  for streptococcal infection, 923t
Clobetasol, 163–164
  for Behçet's disease, 389, 390t
  for lichen sclerosus, genital, 1351
  for lupus erythematosus, subacute cutaneous, 278
Clofazimine, and hyperpigmentation, 1237
  for leprosy, 1001, 1001t, 1002
Clofibrate, for hyperlipidemia, with xanthoma, 1816
Clomipramine, for trichotillomania, 783
Clonidine, for flushing, climacteric, 535

Clostridial infection, and cellulitis, 941–942
Clothing, as barrier to ultraviolet radiation, 755
Clotrimazole, for candidiasis, 1058, 1058t
    oral, 1336
Clotting. See *Coagulation.*
Clouston's syndrome, 1714–1715, 1722t
Clubbing, of nail plate, 1298t, 1301
Clutton's joint, in congenital syphilis, 960t
Cnidarian stings, 787–791, 788t, *789, 790,* 791t
Coagulation, disorders of, in Kasabach-Merritt syndrome, 1498
    in livedo reticularis, 544, *544,* 545
    screening for, before biopsy, 121
    in electrosurgery, for rosacea, 489, 489t, 491, *491–493*
    in surgery, 131–134, *132*
    in wound healing, 564, *564*
    intravascular, disseminated, and purpura, 1848, 1865t, *1866,* Plate 15
Coagulation factor VIII, in Raynaud's phenomenon, 539
Coarctation, of aorta, hemangioma with, 1498
Cobalamin deficiency, 1873t
Cobb's syndrome, 1506, 1799t
Cocaine, abuse of, 839–841, *840*
Coccidioidomycosis, 1063–1064, 1064t, 1068t
Cochliomyia hominivorax larvae, in furuncular myiasis, 819
Cockayne's syndrome, 765, 1802t
    clinical findings in, 1747–1749, 1748t
    DNA repair system in, 1366, 1367, 1748–1751, 1750t
Cockayne-Touraine epidermolysis bullosa, 640
Coelenterata stings, 787–791, 788t, *789, 790,* 791t
Cogentin, for pseudoparkinsonian side effects of pimozide, 781
Colchicine, for amyloidosis, 1820
    for Behçet's disease, 390, 390t
    for erythema elevatum diutinum, 530
    for erythema nodosum, 594
    for scleroderma, 889
    for Sweet's syndrome, 375, 375t
    for urticaria, 402
    for venulitis, cutaneous, 588
Cold, exposure to, 826, 826t
    and acrocyanosis, 829, 830
    and cryoglobulinemia, 833
    and erythema, 832–833
    and erythrocyanosis, 829–831
    and frostbite, *826,* 826–828, 841, 849, 852
    and immersion foot, 777, 828
    and livedo reticularis, 831–832, *832,* 832t
    and panniculitis, 609–610, 1897–1898
    and perniosis, 829–830, 841
    and Raynaud's phenomenon, 537–539
    and urticaria, *393,* 394, 400
    in neonate, 1890, 1892–1894, 1897–1898
    sports-related, 849, 852
Cold creams, in facial cleansing, 79
Colitis, ulcerative, cutaneous signs of, 1872–1874, 1874t, 1875t, *1876*
    pyoderma gangrenosum with, 379, 382, 383
Collagen, degeneration of, definition of, 107
    in acne scar treatment, 474
    in dermal extracellular matrix, biology of, 858–861, *860, 861*

Collagen *(Continued)*
    genetic heterogeneity of, 859t, 861–865, *862–865*
    in dermal structure, 17, *22*
    in dermoepidermal junction, 14, 16, *19, 20, 22,* 624, 625
    in Ehlers-Danlos syndrome, 865–866, *866,* 1775
    in epidermolysis bullosa, 642t, 643–644, 867–869, *867–869*
        dystrophic, 627–628
    in epidermolysis bullosa acquisita, 686, 687, *687,* 688t
    in granuloma annulare, 441
    in keloids, 869–871, 901, *901,* 902
    in scleroderma, 882, 885–886, *886.* See also *Scleroderma.*
    lamellar, definition of, 108
Collagenase inhibitors, anti-angiogenic effect of, 1495, 1495t
Collagenoma, cutaneous, 1792
Collagenosis, perforating, reactive, 407, *408,* 409, *410,* 410t
Collagen-vascular disease, cutaneous signs of, 1886t
    paraneoplastic, 1846
Collarette, of epithelium, definition of, 106, *106*
Collodion, in Gaucher's disease, 1696
    in ichthyosis, lamellar, *1685, 1686,* 1686–1688
Colloid bodies, definition of, 106, *106*
    in lichen planus, 237
Colloid dressings, for psoriasis, 306
Colloid milium, diagnosis of, *94*
    vs. amyloidosis, 1820, 1820t
Colon. See *Intestine.*
Colony-stimulating factors, in inflammatory response, 145, 145t
Combes' solution, in chemical peel, for photoaging, 742t, 743, *744, 745*
Combs, hot, and scarring alopecia, 1285–1286
Comedones, cautery for, 471–472
    definition of, 106
    diagnosis of, *93*
    in acne, 462, 466
Complement, deficiency of, and systemic lupus erythematosus, 267–268, 268t
    in bullous pemphigoid, 668
    in venulitis, 586–588
Complement fixation testing, in lymphogranuloma venereum, 980
Computed tomography, of skin carcinoma, 1400, *1400*
Condyloma. See also *Papillomavirus infection* and *Verrucae.*
    of Buschke and Lowenstein, 1353, 1385
Condylomata lata, in syphilis, 951, 952, *952,* 954
    vs. papillomavirus infection, 1102, *1103*
Cone shells, envenomation by, 799–800
Congo floor maggot infestation, 820
Conjunctiva, inflammation of, in psoriasis, 301
    in Reiter's syndrome, 322
    lesions of, in epidermolysis bullosa acquisita, *687*
    in pemphigoid, cicatricial, 674, *675*
Connective tissue, diseases of, and Raynaud's phenomenon, 537–541, 540t
    in dermal extracellular matrix, 857–876. See also *Dermis, extracellular matrix of.*
    mixed disease of, 268
    nevi of, vs. anetoderma, 911t

Conradi-Hünermann syndrome, *1695,* 1695–1696
    alopecia with, 1716
Contact dermatitis, allergic, 167–173
    corticosteroids and, topical, 166
    immune response in, antigen processing in, 171–173, 172t
        antigen-presenting cells in, *169,* 169–171, *170,* 171t
        B cells in, 167–168
        T cells in, 167–169, *168, 169*
    papules in, *92*
    poison ivy and, *87*
    vesicles in, *95,* 96t
    vs. actinic reticuloid syndrome, 770, 770t
    vs. polymorphic light eruption, 760t
    vs. syphilis, 956
    with atopic dermatitis, 199
    chemotherapeutic agents and, 430
    genital, 1350
    irritant, of diaper region, 184, *185,* 186, Plate 1
    marine life and, 795–797
    occupational, 173–181
        diagnosis of, 180, 180t
        epidemiology of, 174–175, *175–177*
        morphology of, 175–179, *178*
        pathology of, *179,* 179–180, *180*
        treatment of, 180t, 180–181, 181t
    sports-related, 850, 853
    with venous ulcer, of leg, 558, *559*
Contact urticaria, 395, 400
Contraceptives, and diffuse alopecia, 1275
    for androgenetic alopecia, 1257
    for hirsutism, 1856
Contracture, Dupuytren's, 908–909, *909*
Copper, deficiency of, cutaneous signs of, 1873t
    in water, and hair discoloration, 849–850, 852–853
    metabolism of, in Ehlers-Danlos syndrome, 866
        in Menkes' kinky hair syndrome, 1712–1713, *1713*
    Wilson's disease of, cutaneous signs of, 1877t
Coproporphyria, hereditary, 1760t, 1760–1761
Coproporphyrinogen, in heme biosynthesis, in porphyria, 1754, 1754t, *1755*
Coral cuts, 798, *798,* 798t
Coral stings, 791
Cords, assessment of, 101, 102, *102*
    of cells, definition of, 106
Cordylobia anthropophaga larvae, in furuncular myiasis, 819
Corn emperor moth, larva of, and dermatitis, 809, *809*
Cornea, conical, in atopic dermatitis, 197
    disorders of, in xeroderma pigmentosum, 1747
    inflammation of, rosacea and, 485–486
        with ichthyosis and deafness, 1694–1695
    pustular dermatosis of, 327–329, *328, 329,* 329t
        vs. pustular psoriasis, 298–299
Corneocytes, in stratum corneum, 47–48
Corner sutures, 137, *137*
Cornification, disorders of, 1681–1706. See also *Ichthyosis.*
    acquired, 1682t, 1682–1683
    in Darier's disease, 1699–1701, *1700, 1701*
    in erythrokeratodermia, 1698–1699, *1699*

Cornification (*Continued*)
  in Hailey-Hailey disease, 1701, *1702*
  in palmoplantar keratoderma,
    1703–1706, *1705, 1706*
  in peeling skin syndrome, 1699
  in porokeratosis, 1701–1703, *1702, 1703*
Cornified envelope, synthesis of, 11, 47, *47*
Cornified layer, barrier function of, 46
  against electric current, 53
  against microorganisms, 51–52
  biochemical mechanisms of, 51t, 52–53
  homeostasis in, 48–50, *50*
  two-compartment model of, 50–51, 51t
  basket weave, definition of, 106
  disorders of, 1681–1706. See also
    Ichthyosis.
  formation of, *47,* 47–48
  in dry skin, 76
  in epidermal structure, 6, *16*
  in gestation, 3
  keratinocyte differentiation in, 66–67
  structure of, 48
Cornoid lamella, definition of, 106
Coronary arteries, disorders of, cutaneous
    signs with, 1878t, 1879t, 1881t
Corrugator supercilii muscle, anatomy of,
    114
Corticosteroids, abuse of, by athletes, 852
  anabolic, and acne, 463, *464,* 852
  and hyperlipidemia, with xanthoma,
    1814–1815
  and perioral dermatitis, 497, *498*
  and wound healing impairment, 567
  anti-angiogenic effect of, 1495, 1495t
  endogenous, and striae, in adolescent
    athletes, 851
  for acantholytic dermatosis, 343, 343t
  for acne keloidalis nuchae, 1283, 1283t
  for alopecia areata, 1271–1274, 1273t
  for atopic dermatitis, 201
  for Behçet's disease, 389, 390, 390t
  for bowel-associated dermatosis-arthritis
    syndrome, 376, 376t
  for brown recluse spider bites, 812
  for bullous pemphigoid, 670t, 670–671
  for cellulitis, of scalp, 1282, 1282t
  for chondrodermatitis nodularis, 509
  for Churg-Strauss syndrome, *526,* 527
  for dermatomyositis, 288t, 288–289
  for epidermolysis bullosa acquisita,
    688–689
  for Epstein-Barr virus infection, 1083–1084
  for erosive pustular dermatosis, of scalp,
    1284, 1284t
  for erythema nodosum, 594
  for erythroderma, 339, 339t
  for hemangioma, of infancy, 1500–1501
  for herpes gestationis, 683
  for herpes simplex infection, in erythema
    multiforme, 254
  for hidradenitis suppurativa, 481
  for hypereosinophilic syndrome, 357, *357*
  for hypertrophic scars, 903, 904
  for Jessner's lymphocytic infiltrate, 346
  for keloids, 903, 904
  for Langerhans cell histiocytosis, 1614
  for lichen planopilaris, 1288, 1288t
  for lichen planus, 238–239, 239t
  for lupus erythematosus, discoid, 274–275
    with scarring alopecia, 1289, 1289t
    subacute cutaneous, 278
    systemic, 277–278
  for lupus panniculitis, 276
  for nail disorders, 1300, 1302
  for nummular dermatitis, 213, 213t
  for pemphigoid, cicatricial, 677, 677t

Corticosteroids (*Continued*)
  for pemphigus, oral, 1332
    paraneoplastic, 661, 661t
  for pemphigus foliaceus, 658, 658t
  for pemphigus vulgaris, 654, 654t
  for photoallergy, 730
  for polyarteritis, microscopic, *526,* 527
  for polyarteritis nodosa, 520
  for polychondritis, relapsing, 514, 514t
  for polymyositis, 288t, 288–289
  for pruritic urticarial papules and plaques
    of pregnancy, 367–368
  for psoriasis, 305t, 305–306, 1300
  for pyoderma gangrenosum, 383t, 383–384
  for reversal reactions, in leprosy,
    1002–1003
  for sarcoidosis, 436–437
  for scarring, after laser ablation, of warts,
    1116
  for scleroderma, 889
    chemically induced, 891, 893
  for seborrheic dermatitis, 217, 217t
  for Sweet's syndrome, 375, 375t
  for temporal arteritis, 517
  for toxic shock syndrome, 933
  for urticaria, 402
  for vitiligo, 1214
  for vulvar disorders, 1357, *1357*
  for Wegener's granulomatosis, *526,* 527
  for Wells' syndrome, 362–363
  in diaper dermatitis, 186, 186t
  in toxic epidermal necrolysis, 709–710
  injection of, and atrophy, vs. anetoderma,
    911t
  receptors of, in keratinocyte differentiation,
    70
  systemic, for psoriasis, 312
  topical, 160–166
    indications for, 164t, 164–165
    mechanism of action of, 160
    potency of, 160–163, 162t, *163*
    side effects of, 164–166, 165t
    superpotent, 163–164
    withdrawal of, and panniculitis, 608–609,
      609t
Cortisol, excess secretion of, and hirsutism,
    1853–1854
Corymbiform lesions, 106
Corynebacterium infection, in pitted
    keratolysis, 928
Corynebacterium minutissimum infection,
    and erythrasma, 927, *927,* Plate 6
    genital, 1343–1344
    interdigital, 928
Corynebacterium species, and axillary odor,
    927–928
  in normal cutaneous flora, 926
Cosmetics, and acne, 464, *464*
Cotrimoxazole, for head louse infestation,
    1193
Cotton, intravenous injection of, in drug
    abusers, 839
Coumarins, and skin necrosis, 419, *419,*
    545t, 546t, 550
Cowden's disease, 1470, *1470,* 1796t, *1797*
  gastrointestinal hemorrhage in, 1875t,
    1877
  oral lesions in, 1326
Cowhage spicules, and pruritus, 155–156
Cowpox, 1096t, 1096–1097
Coxiella burnetii infection, 1012t, 1019
Coxsackievirus infection, and oral lesions,
    1335t
  and rash, 1124t, 1125t, 1131–1132, *1132*
CREST syndrome, 882
Critical line of Ayber, 29, *29*

Crockett's perforating veins, varicosity of, *578*
Crohn's disease, cutaneous signs of,
    1872–1874, 1874t, 1875t, *1876*
  genital ulceration in, vs. chancroid, 975,
    975t
  oral lesions in, 1334
  pyoderma gangrenosum with, 379–380,
    383
Cronkhite-Canada syndrome, 1875t
Crosti's disease, 1664
Crowe's sign, in neurofibromatosis, 1730
Crusts, assessment of, 97–98, *98*
  in acne, 462, *462*
  in dermatitis herpetiformis, 691, *692*
  in impetigo, *97,* 920, *921*
  in staphylococcal scalded skin syndrome,
    935, *935*
  in varicella-zoster infection, 1079, *1080*
Cryoanesthesia, for dermabrasion, for acne
    scars, 476–477
Cryoglobulinemia, 833
  in vasculitis, *523,* 524, 525, 526t
Cryotherapy, for actinic keratosis, 1395,
    1397–1398
  for basal cell carcinoma, 1393t, 1394,
    1394, 1397–1398
  for hypertrophic scars, 903
  for Kaposi's sarcoma, 1154
  for keloids, 903
  for melanoacanthoma, 1448
  for pale cell acanthoma, 1443
  for pseudofolliculitis barbae, 501–502
  for seborrheic keratosis, 1446
  for stucco keratosis, 1447
  for warts, 1113
    genital, 1349
Cryptococcosis, 1060–1061, *1061,* 1061t,
    1068t
  oral lesions in, 1335
  with human immunodeficiency virus
    infection, *1141,* 1141–1142
Ctenocephalides canis bites, *806*
Culicoides grahami midge, as vector of
    streptocerciasis, 1179
Curettage, for pathologic study, 127
  of carcinoma, basal cell, before excision,
    1400
    with electrodesiccation, *1394,*
      1396–1397, *1397*
    before Mohs micrographic surgery,
      1403, *1404*
Curth-Macklin ichthyosis hystrix, 1689
Cushing's disease, and hirsutism, 1853–1854
Cushing's syndrome, and hirsutism,
    1853–1854
  cutaneous signs of, 1872, 1872t
  topical corticosteroids and, 164, 166
Cuterebra larvae, in furuncular myiasis,
    818–819
Cuticle, of hair follicle, 28, *28,* 1246
  of nail fold, anatomy of, 36, *40*
    embryology of, 5
Cutis laxa, 913–915, *914,* 915t
  cardiac disorders with, 1878t
  dermal elastic fibers in, 875, *875,* 913–915
  thermal radiation and, 825
  vs. anetoderma, 911t, 912
  X-linked, 866, 913
Cutis marmorata, 831
  in neonate, 1894
Cutis marmorata telangiectatica congenita,
    1503, 1799t
Cutis rhomboidalis nuchae, 733, *733*
Cutis verticis gyrata, 1794
Cyanea capillata stings, 788–789
Cyanoacrylate adhesives, and burn injury, 846

Cyclobutane, in DNA photodamage, 1365, *1365*, 1366
  in xeroderma pigmentosum, 1749
Cyclophosphamide, allergy to, 428
  and hyperpigmentation, 1237
  for Churg-Strauss syndrome, *526*, 527
  for lupus erythematosus, systemic, 277–278
  for pemphigoid, cicatricial, 677
  for pemphigus, paraneoplastic, 661, 661t
  for pemphigus foliaceus, 658, 658t
  for pemphigus vulgaris, 654t, 654–655
  for polyarteritis, microscopic, *526*, 527
  for polyarteritis nodosa, 520
  for Wegener's granulomatosis, *526*, 527
Cyclosporine, for actinic reticuloid syndrome, 770t
  for alopecia areata, 1273t
  for atopic dermatitis, 202
  for Behçet's disease, 390t, 390–391
  for epidermolysis bullosa acquisita, 689
  for erythroderma, 339, 339t
  for lichen planus, 239, 239t
  for pemphigus, paraneoplastic, 661, 661t
  for pityriasis rubra pilaris, 335
  for psoriasis, 310–311
  for pustulosis, palmoplantar, 192
  for pyoderma gangrenosum, 383t, 384
  for urticaria, 403
  with marrow transplantation, and graft-versus-host disease, 225, 232–233
Cylindroma, 1476–1477, *1477, 1478*
Cyproheptadine, for urticaria, 402
Cyproterone acetate, for hirsutism, 1857
  with ethinyl estradiol, for acne, 471
Cyst(s), adnexal epithelial, surgery for, 1456–1461, 1458t, *1459–1462*
  with nonsquamous lining, 1454–1456, *1456–1458*
  with squamous lining, 1450–1454, 1451t, *1451–1456*
  Bartholin's, 1352
  definition of, 106
  epidermal inclusion, 1450–1451, 1451t, *1451–1454*
    in amputee dermatitis, 774, 775
  genital, diagnosis of, 1343t
  in basal cell nevus syndrome, 1742–1745
  in hidradenitis suppurativa, 481, 482, *482*
  in steatocystoma multiplex, 1454–1455, *1456, 1457*
  miliary, 1451–1452, *1455*
    after chemical peel, 746
  colloid, diagnosis of, *94*
    vs. acne, 469
  mucous, 1839
    periungual, 1299t, 1305
  of lung, in tuberous sclerosis, 1737
  renal, in tuberous sclerosis, 1737
  trichilemmal, 1452–1453, *1455*
    proliferating, 1453–1454, *1456*
  vellus hair, eruptive, 1451, *1454*
Cystathionine synthase deficiency, 1859t, 1861
  and alopecia, 1713
Cysticercosis, 1187–1188
Cytochrome P450, in dermatophytosis, 1053
Cytokines, in collagen gene expression, 865
  in epidermal barrier function, 52
  in inflammatory response, 143t–145t, 143–146, 151
  in keratinocyte activation, 67–68
Cytomegalovirus, in herpes simplex infection, 1139
  infection by, 1084–1086, *1085*, 1086t
    oral lesions in, 1335t

Cytophagic histiocytic panniculitis, *612*, 612–613
Cytosine, in DNA photodamage, *1365*, 1366
Cytoxan. See *Cyclophosphamide.*

D

Dabska tumor, 1516, 1517
Dactinomycin, and folliculitis, 429–430
Dactylitis, blistering, 922
Danazol, for urticaria, 403
Dandy-Walker malformation, hemangioma with, 1498
Dapsone, for acropustulosis, in infant, 720
  for alopecia areata, 1273t
  for Behçet's disease, 390, 390t
  for bowel-associated dermatosis-arthritis syndrome, 376, 376t
  for brown recluse spider bites, 812
  for bullous dermatosis, linear IgA, 701, 702, 702t
  for bullous pemphigoid, 670
  for cellulitis, of scalp, 1282, 1282t
  for dermatitis herpetiformis, 694–695
  for erythema elevatum diutinum, 530
  for granuloma annulare, 441–442
  for leprosy, 1000–1002, 1001t
  for lupus erythematosus, discoid, 276
    systemic, bullous, 278
  for mycetoma, 1070
  for pemphigoid, cicatricial, 677
  for pyoderma gangrenosum, 383, 383t
  for subcorneal pustular dermatosis, 329
  for Sweet's syndrome, 375, 375t
  for urticaria, 402
Darier's disease, 1300, 1699–1701, *1700, 1701*
  oral lesions in, 1325
  vs. acantholytic dermatosis, 341
  vs. seborrheic dermatitis, 217
Darier's sign, in mastocytosis, 1602, *1603*, 1606
Darkfield examination, for syphilis, 954–955, *955*
Daunorubicin, and hyperpigmentation, 1237
Deafness, with keratitis and ichthyosis, 1694–1695
  with palmoplantar keratoderma, 1705
  with piebaldism, 1225
Debridement, for leg ulcers, 568
Decubitus ulcer, assessment of, *100*
Deerfly fever (tularemia), 943–944, *944*, 1034–1035, 1035t
Degos' disease, 545t, 546t, 551–552
  and gastrointestinal hemorrhage, 1875t
  cardiac disorders with, 1878t
Degos' genodermatoses en cocardes, 1698
Dehydroepiandrosterone, in androgenetic alopecia, 1255, 1256
  in hair follicle growth, 1249, *1249*
  in hirsutism, 1855
Delhi boil, 1163
Delleman syndrome, 1784
Demodex folliculorum infestation, in rosacea, 486, *486*, 487
  vs. acne, 469
Dendrocytes, dermal, 877–878
Dennie-Morgan fold, in atopic dermatitis, 196
Dental. See *Teeth.*
Deoxyribonucleic acid. See *DNA.*
Depigmentation, for vitiligo, 1215
Deposits, in skin, definition of, 107
Depressor anguli oris muscle, anatomy of, 112, *113*

Depressor labii inferioris muscle, anatomy of, 112, *113*
Depressor septi muscle, anatomy of, *113*, 114
Dercum's disease, 1526
Dermabrasion, for acne scars, *473*, 474–479
  for angiofibromas, in tuberous sclerosis, 1736, *1736*, 1739–1740
  for photoaging, 741
Dermacentor andersoni tick, *816*
Dermacentor ticks, as vectors of Rocky Mountain spotted fever, 1011
Dermal hyperplasia, focal, tooth abnormalities with, 1324t
Dermal hypoplasia, focal, 1780–1782, *1781*, 1781t, *1782t*
Dermanyssus gallinae bites, 814, *814*
Dermatitis, acral. See *Acrodermatitis.*
  arthritis with, bowel-associated, 375–376, 376t
    vs. Behçet's disease, 389t
  atopic, 195–202. See also *Atopic dermatitis.*
  autoimmune, in pregnancy, 370
  berloque, vs. melasma, 1235
  caterpillars and, *809*, 809–810, *810*
  cercarial, *793*, 793–795, 794t, 795t, 1186, 1187t
  contact, 167–181. See also *Contact dermatitis.*
  definition of, 107
  diaper, 184–187, *185*, 185t, 186t, 1896–1897, Plate 1
    candidiasis and, 1057t
    in adults, 776, 777
  exfoliative, drug-induced, 420
    vs. toxic epidermal necrolysis, 710t
    with erythroderma, 197, 336, 338
    cardiac disorders in, 1878t
  factitial, 780t, 781t, 784–785, *785*
  in amputees, 774t, 774–775, 775t
  in Lyme borreliosis, 967, 968, 969t
  in pityriasis lichenoides, 256–258, *257*, 258t
  inflammatory response in, 141–151. See also *Inflammatory response.*
  interface, 108
  lichenoid, 235–241. See also specific disorders, e.g., *Lichen planus.*
  moths and, 810–811
  nummular, 211–213, *212*, 212t, 213t. See also *Nummular dermatitis.*
  of feet, 188–193, 191t, 192t, 197
  of hands, 188–189, 188–193, 191t, 192t, 197
  papular, Spangler's, in pregnancy, 370
  perioral, 497–498, *498*, 498t
    vs. acne, 469
  photosensitivity, in actinic reticuloid syndrome, 763, 768–770, *769*, 769t, 770t, Plate 5
  radiation and, 836–838, *837, 838*
  rheumatoid neutrophilic, 376–377
  seborrheic, 214–217. See also *Seborrheic dermatitis.*
  spongiotic, in pityriasis rosea, 218–220. See also *Pityriasis rosea.*
  ultraviolet light exposure and, in human immunodeficiency virus infection, 1146, *1146*
  vs. sensitive skin, 78
Dermatitis herpetiformis, 691–696, *692, 693*, 694t, 695t
  biopsy of, site for, 120, 120t
  clinical findings in, 691–692, *692*
  definition of, 691
  differential diagnosis of, 694, 694t
  oral lesions in, 1333

Dermatitis herpetiformis (*Continued*)
  pathogenesis of, 694
  pathology of, 692–694, *693*
  treatment of, 694–696, 695t
  vs. bullous dermatosis, linear IgA, 698,
    700–701, 701t
  vs. subcorneal pustular dermatosis, 329
Dermatobia hominis larvae, in furuncular
  myiasis, 818, *819*
Dermatofibroma, 1552–1555, *1553*, 1553t,
  1554, 1555t
  nodules in, *95*, 95t
Dermatofibrosarcoma protuberans, 1553t,
  1555t, *1555–1557*, 1555–1558
Dermatographism, in urticaria, *393*, 400
Dermatoheliosis, 735
Dermatomyositis, *1868, 1869*, Plate 15
  cancer with, 285–286, 1846
  cardiac disorders with, 1878t
  clinical findings in, in adults, *284*, 284–285
    in children, 285
  diagnosis of, 283, 286–287, 287t
  epidemiology of, 283
  pathogenesis of, 287–288
  pathology of, 286, *286*
  photosensitivity in, 766
  pulmonary disease in, cutaneous signs
    with, 1882t
  treatment of, 288t, 288–289
Dermatophytosis, 1043–1054
  and scarring alopecia, 1285, *1285*
  configuration of, *87*
  diagnosis of, 1051–1052, 1052t
  genital, 1345
  pathogenesis of, 1050–1051
  pathology of, 1049–1050, *1050*
  treatment of, 1052–1054, 1053t, 1054t
  types of, 1043–1049, 1044t, *1044–1049*
  with human immunodeficiency virus
    infection, 1143–1144
Dermatosis papulosa nigra, 1441–1442,
  1442, 1442t
Dermis, blood vessels of, 876–877
  collagen in, in scleroderma, 882, 885–886,
    886. See also *Scleroderma*.
  dendrocytes in, 877–878
  disorders of, 882–915. See also specific
    disorders, e.g., *Keloids*.
  elastic fibers of. See *Elastic fibers*.
  embryology of, 5
  extracellular matrix of, 857–858, 859t
    collagen fibers in, biology of, 858–861,
      860, 861
    disorders of, in Ehlers-Danlos
      syndrome, 865–866, *866*
      genetic heterogeneity of, 859t,
        861–865, *862–865*
    glycosaminoglycans in, 857–858, 859t,
      876
    proteoglycans in, 857–858, 859t, 876
  fibrillin in, 857, 859t, *870, 871, 872*,
    873–874
  hypoplasia of, focal, 1780–1782, *1781*,
    1781t, 1782t
    vs. anetoderma, 911t
  junction of, with epidermis, 617–628. See
    also *Dermoepidermal junction*.
  layers of, 857, *858*
  lymphatic system of, 877
  macrophages in, 878
  mast cells in, 877
  structure of, 3, *4*, 16–21, *22, 23*, 857–878
Dermoepidermal junction, 13–16, *19–22*,
  617–628
  anatomy of, *618*, 618–619

Dermoepidermal junction (*Continued*)
  basal epidermal keratins in, 621
  basement membrane proteins in,
    hemidesmosomal-associated, 619–621,
    620
    lamina densa–associated, 624–625
  development of, 626
  embryology of, 3
  functions of, 617–618
  in epidermolysis bullosa, 628, 635, 636t,
    638–639, *639*
    dystrophic, 627–628
    kalinin genes in, 628, 642t, 644
  in epidermolysis bullosa simplex, 626–627,
    627
  lamina lucida in, 15, *19, 22*, 618, 618–619
    proteinaceous components of, 621–624
  structure of, 13–16, *19–22*
Desipramine, for neurotic excoriations, 784
Desmogleins, in epidermal structure, *9*
  in inflammatory response, 150
  in pemphigus foliaceus, 657
Desmons-Britten syndrome, 1694
Desmoplakins, in epidermal structure, *9*
Desmoplasia, definition of, 107
Desmoplastic melanoma, clinical findings in,
  1580
  pathology of, 1585, *1585*
Desmoplastic nevi, 1566
Desmoplastic trichoepithelioma, 1468, *1468*
Desmosomes, in dry skin, 76, *77*
  in epidermal structure, 6, *9–11*
Dexamethasone, for hirsutism, 1856
Dextrothyroxine, for hyperlipidemia, with
  xanthoma, 1816
DFMO, for trypanosomiasis, 1175
Diabetes mellitus, cardiac disorders with,
  1878t
  dermatoses associated with, 1869, 1869t,
    1870, 1870t, *1871*, Plate 15
  granuloma annulare with, 441
  hyperlipidemia with, and xanthoma, 1814,
    1870t, *1871*
  necrobiosis lipoidica with, 446t, *447*,
    447–448, *448*, Plate 4
  perforating dermatosis with, 408, *408*,
    1869t, *1870*
  vs. scleroderma, 888t
Diadema antillarum, and skin wounds, 799
Dialysis, cutaneous changes with, 1884t,
  1886t
Dianette, for acne, 471
Diaper dermatitis, 184–187, *185*, 185t, 186t,
  1896–1897, Plate 1
  candidiasis and, 1057t
  in adults, 776, *777*
Dibenzoylmethanes, in sunscreens, 754
Dicloxacillin, for folliculitis decalvans, 1284,
  1284t
  for staphylococcal infection, 923t
    with pyoderma, in neonate, 712
  for streptococcal infection, 923t
  with skin grafting, composite, after cancer
    excision, 1423
Diet, and sweating, 1313
  as aid to management, of dermatitis
    herpetiformis, 694–696
    of toxic epidermal necrolysis, 706, 710t
    of xanthoma, 1816
  deficiencies of, and alopecia, diffuse,
    1275–1276, 1277t
    and diaper dermatitis, 1897
    and wound healing impairment, 567
    cutaneous signs of, 1872, *1873*, 1873t,
      1874

Diethylcarbamazine, for filariasis, 1179
  for loiasis, 1180
  for toxocariasis, 1183
  in onchocerciasis, 1177, 1178
Diffuse idiopathic skeletal hyperostosis,
  retinoids and, 310
Diflorasone diacetate, 163–164
Digitate dermatosis, 222
Digitation, definition of, 107, *107*
Digits, blistering infection of, 922, *922*
  deformities of, in epidermolysis bullosa,
    dystrophic, 641, *641*, 645
    in trichorhinophalangeal syndrome, 1714
    with acne, 464
    with ectodermal dysplasia, 1722t
  fibroma of, 1305
  infection between, 928–929
  ischemia of, in Raynaud's phenomenon,
    537–542, 540t, 541t
  mucous cyst of, 1839
  nails of. See *Nail(s)*.
  papillary adenoma of, 1481, *1482*
  trauma to, sports and, 850, 853
Dihematoporphirin ether, in photodynamic
  therapy, for skin carcinoma, 1426–1427
Dihydrotestosterone, and sebaceous gland
  activity, in acne, 465
  in genital development, 1340
  in hair follicle growth, 1249, *1249*
  in hirsutism, 1854
Diiodohydroxyquin, for acrodermatitis
  enteropathica, 1765
Diloxanide, for amebiasis, 1173
Diltiazem, for perniosis, 829
Diodoquin, for acrodermatitis enteropathica,
  1765
Diphenhydramine, for nummular dermatitis,
  213, 213t
  for pseudoparkinsonian side effects of
    pimozide, 781
Diphtheria A toxin–interleukin 2 gene
  fusion product, for cutaneous T-cell
  lymphoma, 1653
Diprosone. See *Betamethasone*.
Dipyridamole, for Köhlmeier-Degos
  syndrome, 546t
  for livedo vasculopathy, 545, 546t
Dirofilariasis, 1181
Discoid dermatitis, 211–213. See also
  Nummular dermatitis.
Discoid lupus erythematosus. See *Lupus
  erythematosus, discoid*.
Disodium cromoglycate, for mastocytosis,
  1607
Disseminated intravascular coagulation, and
  purpura, 1848, 1865t, *1866*, Plate 15
DNA, in Bloom's syndrome, 765
  in Cockayne's syndrome, 765
  in xeroderma pigmentosum, 765,
    1748–1751, 1750t
  of papillomaviruses, 1108–1109
  photodamage to, 737–738, 1364–1366,
    1365
    and enzyme activation, 1369
    and mutagenesis, 1367, *1368*
    repair of, 1366t, 1366–1367
  synthesis of, in epidermal barrier function,
    49–50, *50*
Dodd's perforating veins, varicosity of, *578*
Domestic violence, 841–843, *843*
Donovanosis (granuloma inguinale), 976t,
  977, 977–979
  vs. chancroid, 975, 975t
  vs. syphilis, 956
DOPA, in melanocytes, 13, *1204*, 1206–1207

Doppler ultrasonography, in diagnosis of leg ulcers, 563
Doucas-Kapetanakis purpura, 291–292
Dowling-Meara epidermolysis bullosa, 637–638, 642, 643
   genetic mutation in, 9, 61–62, 626–627, *627*
   with palmoplantar keratoderma, 1705
Doxepin, for neurotic excoriations, 784
   for urticaria, 402
Doxorubicin, and hyperpigmentation, 1237
   extravasation of, 428
Doxycycline, for acne, 471, 471t
   for acne keloidalis nuchae, 1283, 1283t
   for bacillary angiomatosis, 1028
   for cellulitis, of scalp, 1282, 1282t
   for folliculitis decalvans, 1284, 1284t
   for granuloma inguinale, 976t
   for Lyme borreliosis, 969, 969t
   for lymphogranuloma venereum, 976t, 981
   for *Mycobacterium marinum* infection, 990
   for Rocky Mountain spotted fever, 1015, 1016t
   for rosacea, 488
   for syphilis, 957t
   for typhus, 1017
Dracunculosis, 1180–1181
Drechslera infection, in immunosuppressed patient, 1157
Dressings, for leg ulcers, 568, 568t
Drithocreme (anthralin), for alopecia areata, 1271, 1273t, 1274
   for psoriasis, 305t, 306
   with phototherapy, 313
Drug abuse, and skin infection, 839–840
   and skin trauma, 839–841, *840*
Drug reactions, 412–423
   and acne, 423, 463, *464*
   and alopecia, diffuse, 1277, 1277t
   and erythema multiforme, 251
   and erythema nodosum, 593, 594t
   and erythermalgia, 533, 534, 534t
   and exacerbation of skin disease, 423
   and flushing, 534t–535t
   and linear IgA bullous dermatosis, 700
   and lupus erythematosus–like syndrome, 266–267, 267t, 423
   and pemphigus, 422–423
   and photosensitivity, 420
      vs. actinic reticuloid syndrome, 770, 770t
   and phototoxicity, 726–730, 727t–729t, 731t
   and pigmentation disorders, 420–422, *421*
   and skin necrosis, *419*, 419–420, 545t, 546t, 550
   and toxic epidermal necrolysis, 704, 707–710, 708t, 710t
   definition of, 412
   diagnosis of, *413*, 413t, 413–414
   epidemiology of, 412–413, 413t
   exanthematous, *413, 414*, 414–415
   exfoliative dermatitis in, 420
   fixed eruptions in, 420–421, *421*
      vs. chancroid, 975, 975t
   hypersensitivity syndrome in, 416–417
   in human immunodeficiency virus infection, 423, 1145
   lichenoid, 423
      vs. lichen planus, 238, 238t
   pustular, 422
   serum sickness in, 417–418
   serum sickness–like, 418
   to chemotherapeutic agents, 426–430, 427t, *428, 429*, Plate 3
   to vancomycin, in red man syndrome, 420

Drug reactions (*Continued*)
   urticarial, *413*, 415–416
   vasculitis in, 418–419
   vs. syphilis, 956, 957
Drysol, in hemostasis, 133
Dum-Dum fever, 1163
Dupuytren's disease, 908–909, *909*
Duranest, in anesthesia, 130, 130t
Dust mite infestation, in atopic dermatitis, 199
Dysbetalipoproteinemia, and xanthoma, 1814
Dyschondroplasia, in Maffucci's syndrome, 1506
Dysgammaglobulinemia, and hyperlipidemia, with xanthoma, 1815
Dyshidrotic eczema, 188, *189*, 190, 191
Dyskeratosis, acantholytic, focal, definition of, 107
   definition of, 107
   in Darier's disease, 1700, *1701*
   intraepithelial, hereditary benign, oral lesions in, 1325
Dyskeratosis congenita, 1705, *1705*, 1796t, *1798*
   oral lesions in, 1329
Dysplasia, definition of, 107

E

Ear, chondrodermatitis nodularis of, 507–510, *508*, 509t, *510*
   in keratitis/ichthyosis/deafness syndrome, 1694–1695
   in Langerhans cell histiocytosis, 1611
   in vitiligo, 1211
   inflammation of, external, in swimmers, 851, 853
      Pseudomonas aeruginosa infection and, 940, *941*, Plate 6
   muscles of, anatomy of, 114
   polychondritis of, relapsing, 512–513, *513*
Eating, and flushing, 534t
Ecchymosis, in purpura, with systemic disease, 1865t, *1866*
Eccrine glands. See also *Sweat glands.*
   adenoma of, digital papillary, 1481–1482
   anatomy of, 34–36, *36–40*, 1308–1309, *1309*
   carcinoma of, microcystic, 1483, *1483, 1484*
      mucinous, 1484–1485
      syringoid, 1483–1484, 1484t
   cylindroma of, 1476–1477, *1477, 1478*
   disorders of, chemotherapy and, 428–429, *429*, Plate 3
   embryology of, 5
   hidradenoma of, clear cell, *1477*, 1480–1481, *1481*, 1481t
   hydrocystoma of, 1456–1457, *1458*
   hypersecretion by, 1307–1308, 1311–1317, 1312t, *1313–1315*, 1316t
   in thermoregulation, 55–56
   physiology of, 1307–1310, *1310*
   poroma of, *1477*, 1479–1480, *1480*, 1480t
   spiradenoma of, *1477, 1482*, 1482–1483, 1483t
   syringoma of, 1477–1479, *1477–1479*, 1478t
Echinoderms, and skin wounds, 798–799
Echovirus infection, and rash, 1124t, 1125t, 1131–1132, *1132*
Ecthyma, 921, *922*
Ecthyma gangrenosum, 945, *945*
   in neonate, 713

Ectodermal dysplasia, 1721–1724
   anhidrotic, 1714, *1714*, 1722t
   clinical findings in, 1721, 1722t, *1723*, 1723t
   definition of, 1721
   diagnosis of, 1721–1723, *1724*
   hidrotic, 1714–1715, 1722t
   tooth abnormalities with, 1324t
   treatment of, 1723–1724
   with palmoplantar keratoderma, 1705
Ectrodactyly, with ectodermal dysplasia, and cleft lip and palate, 1722t
Eczema, atopic, heat therapy for, 826
   dyshidrotic, 188, *189*, 190, 191
   in actinic reticuloid syndrome, 768, 769, *769*, 769t, Plate 5
   in amputee dermatitis, 774, 775
   vs. plaque psoriasis, 297
   with human immunodeficiency virus infection, 1145–1146
   with venous ulcer, of leg, 558
Eczematid-like purpura, of Doucas and Kapetanakis, 291–292
Edema, in erythema multiforme, 247–248, *248*
   lymphatic, 554–557, *555*, 555t, 556t
      in filariasis, 1179
      with angiosarcoma, 554, 556, 1516
   of amputation stump, 774
   with venous ulcer, of leg, 558
Edwardsiella lineata larvae, and seabather's eruption, 792–793, 1186, 1187t
Eflornithine, for trypanosomiasis, 1175
Ehlers-Danlos syndrome, *1774*, 1774–1777, *1775*, 1776t, 1777t
   cardiac disorders in, 1878t
   collagen abnormalities in, 865–866, *866*
   gastrointestinal hemorrhage in, 1874t
Ehrlichia infection, 816, 1012t, 1019
Eicosanoids, in urticaria, 398
Eicosapentaenoic acid, dietary, for psoriasis, 312
Elasmobranch fish, and skin injury, 797
Elastic fibers, in acrokeratoelastoidosis, 1778
   in anetoderma, 910–912, *911*, 911t
   in cutis laxa, 875, *875*, 913–915
   in dermal structure, 17, *23*, 870–873, 871–874
   in Ehlers-Danlos syndrome, *1774*, 1774–1777, *1775*, 1776t, 1777t
   in pseudoxanthoma elasticum, *874*, 874–875, 1770–1774, *1771, 1772*, 1773t
Elastic tissue nevus, 1792
Elastin, in dermal extracellular matrix, 857, 859t, *870–873*, 871–874
Elastolysis, vs. anetoderma, 911t, 912
Elastolytic giant cell granuloma, 441, 441t, 442
Elastorrhexis, papular, 1792
Elastosis, definition of, 107
   solar, 734–735, *735*, 875–876, *876*, Plate 5
   thermal, 825
Elastosis perforans serpiginosa, 407–410, *408, 409*, 410t
Elaunin fibers, in dermal structure, 17
Elderly, physical abuse of, 843
   wound healing in, 566
Electrical current, low-voltage, skin resistance to, 53
Electrical stimulation, in leg ulcer management, 570
Electrocoagulation, for rosacea, 489, 489t, 491, *491–493*
   in surgery, *132*, 132–133

Electrodesiccation, for rosacea, 489t, 489–491, *490*
  with curettage, for basal cell carcinoma, 1396–1397, *1397*
Electrofulguration, for rosacea, 489t, 489–491
Electrosurgery, for hypertrophic scars, 905
  for keloids, 905
  for neurofibromatosis, 1734
  for rosacea, 489t, 489–493, *490–493*
    in rhinophyma, *493*, 493–496, *495*
  for warts, 1113
Elephantiasis, in filariasis, 1179
Elimite (permethrin), for louse infestation, 1192, 1194–1195
  for scabies, 1198
Elliptical biopsy, technique of, 127
Embolism, in hypereosinophilic syndrome, 353, 355, 357–358
  of atheromatous plaques, 545t, 546t, 546–547, *547*, 1881t
Emetine hydrochloride, for amebiasis, 1173
Emollients, for dry skin, 77
  in facial skin care, 80
Emotional dysfunction, with atopic dermatitis, 197
Emphysema, with cutis laxa, 913
Employment, antigen exposure in, and contact dermatitis, 173–181. See also *Contact dermatitis.*
  chemical exposure in, and burns, 843–847, 844t, 845t
  and lymphoma, 1648
Enamel, hypoplasia of, in epidermolysis bullosa, junctional, 639
Encephalocraniocutaneous lipomatosis, 1793
Endocarditis, bacterial, cutaneous signs of, 1881t
  with hypereosinophilic syndrome, 353, 355
Endocrine neoplasia, multiple, oral lesions in, 1327
Endophytic structure, definition of, 107
Endothelial cell growth factors, 1493t, 1494
Endothelial cells, leukocyte adhesion to, in inflammatory response, 149–151
Endothelin-1, in Raynaud's phenomenon, 539
Energy, increased expenditure of, in toxic epidermal necrolysis, 706, 710t
Entactin, in dermoepidermal junction, 15, 16, 625
Entamoeba histolytica infection, 1172–1173, *1173*
Enterobiasis, 1183–1184
Enteropathy, gluten-sensitive, with dermatitis herpetiformis, 691, 694–696
Enterovirus infection, and rash, 1124t, 1125t, 1131–1132, *1132*
Enzyme-linked immunosorbent assay, in Lyme borreliosis, 968–969
Eosinophilia, angiolymphoid hyperplasia with, 1507t, 1511–1513, *1512*
  in atopic dermatitis, 198
  in hypereosinophilic syndrome, 352–358. See also *Hypereosinophilic syndrome.*
Eosinophilia-myalgia syndrome, in scleroderma, chemically induced, 891, 892, 892t, *893*
  papular mucinosis in, 1839
Eosinophilic fasciitis, in morphea, 897, 898
  vs. scleroderma, 887, 888t
Eosinophilic folliculitis, in human immunodeficiency virus infection, 1144, *1144*
  pustular, in neonate, 717t, 720–721
Eosinophilic granuloma, in Langerhans cell histiocytosis, 1610–1611, 1613

Eosinophilic ulcer, of oral mucosa, 1333–1334
Eosinophils, in incontinentia pigmenti, 1725, 1726, *1727*
  in Wells' syndrome, 360, 361, *361*, Plate 3
Ephedrine, for urticaria, 402
Ephelides (freckles), 1561
  in neurofibromatosis, 1730
  in xeroderma pigmentosum, 1747, *1748*
Epidermal growth factor, in keratinocyte activation, 67
Epidermal inclusion cysts, 1450–1451, 1451t, *1451–1454*
  in amputee dermatitis, 774, 775
Epidermal nevi, 1787–1790, *1788*, 1788t, *1789*, 1790t
  differential diagnosis of, 1441, 1442t
  vs. lichen striatus, 245–246
  vs. stucco keratosis, 1447
Epidermis, barrier function of, 46
  against microorganisms, 51–52
  biochemical mechanisms of, 51t, 52–53
  homeostasis in, 48–50, *50*
  two-compartment model of, 50–51, 51t
  differentiation of, 46–47, *47*
  hyperplasia of, definition of, 107
  junction of, with dermis, 13–16, *19–22*, 617–628. See also *Dermoepidermal junction.*
  lamellar bodies in, *47*, 48, *49*
  necrolysis of, toxic, 247–254, 704–710. See also *Erythema multiforme* and *Toxic epidermal necrolysis.*
  protective function of, against electric current, low-voltage, 53
    against ultraviolet radiation, 53
  structure of, 3, *4*, 5–6, *6–16*
  suture of, simple interrupted, *134*, 134–135
Epidermodysplasia verruciformis, *1105*, 1105–1106
Epidermolysis bullosa, 635–645
  and alopecia, scarring, 1291
  classification of, 635–636, 636t
  clinical findings in, 636–641, *637, 639–641*
  definition of, 635
  diagnosis of, 644, 644t
  dystrophic, 635, 636t, 639–641, *640, 641*, 867–869, *867–869*
  epidemiology of, 636
  genetic mutations in, 9, 61–62, 626–628, *627*
  in neonate, 1897
  junctional, 635, 636t, 638–639, *639*
    kalinin genes in, 628, 642t, 644
    oral lesions in, 1332
  pathogenesis of, 643–644
  pathology of, 641–643, *642*, 642t, *643*
  prognosis of, 645
  tooth abnormalities with, 639, 1324t
  treatment of, 644–645, 645t
  with aplasia cutis congenita, 1784
  with palmoplantar keratoderma, 1705
Epidermolysis bullosa acquisita, 685–689
  clinical findings in, 685, *686*
  definition of, 685
  diagnosis of, 687–688, *688*, 688t, *689*
  pathogenesis of, 686–687, *687, 688*
  pathology of, 685–686, *686*
  treatment of, 688–689
  vs. bullous pemphigoid, 669–670
Epidermolytic hyperkeratosis, 1688–1690, *1688–1690*
  genetic mutation in, 63, 1689
Epidermophyton flocculosum infection, 1043, 1044t, 1046–1048, 1051

Epidermopoiesis, 107
Epidermotropism, 107
Epilation, for pseudofolliculitis barbae, 500–501
Epiligrin, in epidermolysis bullosa, 642t, 644
Epinephrine, for urticaria, 402
  in anesthesia, 130–131
  for liposuction, for hyperhidrosis, 1316
Epithelioid cells, definition of, 107
Epithelioid hemangioendothelioma, 1516, 1517
Epithelioid hemangioma, 1507t, 1511–1513, *1512*
Epithelioid tubercle, definition of, 107
Epithelioma, calcifying, of Malherbe, 1468–1470, *1469*, 1830
  definition of, 107
  of hair follicles, 1466–1468, *1467, 1468*
  sebaceous, 1472–1473
Epithelioma keratin amyloidosis, 1825
Epithelium, adnexal, cysts of, surgery for, 1456–1461, 1458t, *1459–1462*
  with nonsquamous lining, 1454–1456, *1456–1458*
  with squamous lining, 1450–1454, 1451t, *1451–1456*
  structures of, definition of, 107
  collarette of, definition of, 106, *106*
  focal hyperplasia of, papillomavirus infection and, 1103, *1103*, 1335
Epithelium-specific antinuclear antibody, stratified, ulcerative stomatitis with, 1333
Eponychium, embryology of, 5
Epoprostenol, for Raynaud's phenomenon, 541–542
Epstein-Barr virus infection, 1082–1084, *1083*, 1083t
  and oral lesions, 1148, 1335t
  and rash, 1124t, 1125t, 1132–1134, *1134*, Plate 9
  in Rosai-Dorfman disease, 1618
Epulis, in pregnancy, 1325–1326
Equestrian panniculitis, 829
Erosions, assessment of, 98–99, *100*
  in dermatitis herpetiformis, 691, *692*
  in pemphigus vulgaris, 651, *652*
  in pustular dermatosis, of scalp, and alopecia, *1284*, 1284t, 1284–1285
  with blisters and pustules, in neonate, 712, 714t, 716t, 720
Eruption, polymorphic, definition of, 109
  light and, 758–761, *759, 760*, 760t, 761t
    vs. Jessner's lymphocytic infiltrate, 346
Eruptive histiocytoma, 1662
Eruptive xanthoma, 1810, *1810*, 1811, 1816
Erysipelas, 923, 923–925, 925t
Erysipelothrix rhusiopathiae infection, 943, 946, 947
Erythema, acral, chemotherapy and, 428, *428*, Plate 3
  with diabetes, 1869t
  cold exposure and, 832–833
  in chemical peel, for photoaging, 743, 744, 746
  in coccidioidomycosis, 1063
  in dermatomyositis, *284*, 284–285, Plate 2
  in diaper dermatitis, 184, *185*
  in granuloma annulare, 439
  in graft-versus-host disease, 226, *227*, 227t, Plate 1
  in impetigo, 920, *920, 921*
  in lichen planopilaris, 1287, *1287*
  in lupus. See *Lupus erythematosus.*
  in rosacea, 485, 487t, 487–488
  in sclerosing panniculitis, 603, *604*

Erythema (*Continued*)
in serum sickness, 417
in sunburn, 736
necrolytic migratory, 1843–1844, *1844,
1868*
psoralen–ultraviolet radiation therapy and,
in treatment of psoriasis, 314
toxic, of pregnancy, 367
with reticular mucinosis, 1834t,
1834–1836, *1835*
Erythema ab igne, *824,* 824–825
Erythema annulare centrifugum, 348–349,
349, 349t, Plate 2
Erythema chronicum migrans, in Lyme
borreliosis, 966, *966,* 968, 969t, Plate 6
Erythema dyschromicum perstans, 241, 1238
Erythema elevatum diutinum, 528–530,
529, 530t
Erythema gyratum repens, *349,* 349t,
349–350, 1845, *1845,* Plate 14
paraneoplastic, *1867*
Erythema induratum, of Bazin, 985–987,
987, 988t, Plate 7
Erythema infectiosum, 1124t, 1125t, *1128,*
1128–1129, Plate 8
Erythema marginatum rheumaticum, 349t,
350, 350–351
Erythema multiforme, 247–254
clinical findings in, 247–249, *248, 249*
definition of, 247
diagnosis of, 248, 251–252
mycoplasmal infection and, 251, 1882t
oral lesions in, 1333
vs. lichen planus, 238, 238t
pathogenesis of, 250–251
pathology of, 249–250, *250*
treatment of, 252t, 252–254
vs. polymorphic light eruption, 758–760,
760, 761t
vs. toxic epidermal necrolysis, 704, 710t
vs. toxic shock syndrome, 933, 934t
Erythema nodosum, 591–594, *592, 593,* 593t
in sarcoidosis, 434–435
subcuticular inflammation in, *94*
vs. nodular vasculitis, 595–596, 597t
Erythema nodosum leprosum, 585, 998, 1002
Erythema toxicum neonatorum, 715t, 718,
1893, 1894–1895, *1895*
Erythermalgia, 533–534, 534t
Erythrasma, 927, *927,* Plate 6
genital, 1343–1344
Erythrocyanosis, 829–831
Erythroderma, 336–339, *337,* 338t, 339t,
Plate 2
clinical findings in, 336–338, *337,* 338t
diagnosis of, 338, 338t
drug-induced, 420
exfoliative, 336, 338
cardiac disorders in, 1878t
in atopic dermatitis, 197
in ichthyosis, lamellar, 1685, *1685, 1686*
in lymphoma, T-cell, 1640, *1640,* 1641,
1642, 1655
in pityriasis rubra pilaris, 331, *332,* 332t,
Plate 2
paraneoplastic, 1846
pathogenesis of, 337
pathology of, 337
treatment of, 339, 339t
Erythrodermic psoriasis, *86,* 295t, 300, Plate
1. See also *Psoriasis.*
Erythrokeratoderma, vs. atopic dermatitis,
200
Erythrokeratodermia progressiva symmetrica,
1699, *1699*

Erythrokeratodermia variabilis, 1698–1699
Erythrokeratolysis hiemalis, 1698
Erythromelalgia, 533–534, 534t
Erythromycin, and wound healing, 566t
for acne, 471, 471t
for acne keloidalis nuchae, 1283, 1283t
for actinomycosis, 1008t, 1009
for bacillary angiomatosis, 1028
for bowel-associated dermatosis-arthritis
syndrome, 376, 376t
for bullous pemphigoid, 670
for chancroid, 976, 976t
for erythrasma, genital, 1344
for folliculitis decalvans, 1284, 1284t
for granuloma inguinale, 976t, 979
for Lyme borreliosis, 969, 969t
for lymphogranuloma venereum, 976t,
981
for staphylococcal infection, 923t
for streptococcal infection, 923t
Erythroplakia, oral, 1328–1329
Erythroplasia of Queyrat, 1380
Erythropoietic porphyria, 1753, 1754t, *1756,*
1756–1758, *1757,* 1760t
tooth abnormalities with, 1324t
vs. blistering disorders, in neonate, 717t
Erythropoietic protoporphyria, 1755t, *1757,*
1757–1758, 1760t
Eschar, 97, *98,* 107
Esophagus, cancer of, and palmoplantar
keratoderma, 1704
metastasis of, to skin, 1674, *1676*
strictures of, in epidermolysis bullosa, 643,
645
Espundia, 1163
Estradiol, for androgenetic alopecia, 1257
with cyproterone acetate, for acne, 471
Estrogens, and hyperlipidemia, with
xanthoma, 1814–1815
and lupus erythematosus, 271
for androgenetic alopecia, 1257
for hirsutism, 1856
in genital development, 1341
Ethambutol, for tuberculosis, 989
Ethinyl estradiol, for alopecia, androgenetic,
1257
with cyproterone acetate, for acne, 471
Ethionamide, for leprosy, 1001
Ethyl alcohol, and wound healing, 566t
Ethylene oxide, and burn injury, 844t
Etidocaine, in anesthesia, 130, 130t
Etoposide, for Langerhans cell histiocytosis,
1614
for lymphoma, cutaneous T-cell, 1654
Etretinate. See also *Retinoids.*
and hyperlipidemia, with xanthoma,
1815
for Darier's disease, 1701
for erythroderma, 339, 339t
for ichthyosis, harlequin, 1691
lamellar, 1687
for lichen planus, 239t
for pityriasis rubra pilaris, 334, 335
for psoriasis, 309–310, 315
for skin carcinoma, 1429–1431
Eumelanins, *1204,* 1207
Eumycetoma, 1069–1070, 1071t
Eutrombicula alfreddugesi bites, 815, *815*
Exanthem, viral, 1123–1134. See also *Viral
infection.*
Exanthem subitum, in herpesvirus-6
infection, 1087, 1087t, 1124t, 1125t,
1129–1130, *1130*
Exanthematous drug eruption, *413, 414,*
414–415

Exanthematous pustulosis, acute generalized,
vs. toxic epidermal necrolysis, 710t
drug-induced, 422
Excisional biopsy, technique of, 127
Excoriations, assessment of, *100*
in acne, 463
neurotic, 780t, 781t, *783,* 783–784
pruritus and, 154
Exercise. See also *Sports.*
and urticaria, 392
Exfoliative dermatitis, drug-induced, 420
vs. toxic epidermal necrolysis, 710t
with erythroderma, 197, 336, 338
cardiac disorders in, 1878t
Exoendophytosis, definition of, 107
Exophiala werneckii infection, and tinea
nigra, 1037–1038, *1038,* 1038t
Exophytosis, definition of, 107
Exostoses, of jaws, 1328, *1328*
subungual, 1301
Eye(s), disorders of, with dermal hypoplasia,
focal, 1780–1781, 1781t
in albinism, 1219–1223, 1220t, 1221t,
1222, 1223t
in atopic dermatitis, 196–197
in Behçet's disease, 386, 388t
in erythema multiforme, 249, 252t,
253–254
in hypereosinophilic syndrome, 354
in leprosy, 998
in Lyme borreliosis, 967
in neurofibromatosis, 1730–1731
in onchocerciasis, 1178
in pemphigoid, cicatricial, 674, *675*
in polychondritis, relapsing, 513
in pseudoxanthoma elasticum, 1770–1771,
1771, 1773–1774
in psoriasis, 301
in Reiter's syndrome, 322
in rosacea, 485–486
in Sturge-Weber syndrome, 1505
in Sweet's syndrome, 373
in toxic epidermal necrolysis, 710t
in tuberous sclerosis, 1737
in varicella-zoster infection, *1079,* 1080
with human immunodeficiency virus
infection, 1141
in vitiligo, 1210
in von Hippel–Lindau syndrome, 1799t,
1801
in Wyburn-Mason syndrome, 1799t, *1801*
in xeroderma pigmentosum, 1747, 1748t,
1803t, *1805*
toxicity to, antimalarial drugs and, 275–276
retinoids and, 310
Eyeglass frames, and acanthoma fissuratum,
773t, 773–774, 774t
Eyelid(s), carcinoma of, radiation therapy
for, 1400, *1400,* 1402
sebaceous, *1473,* 1473–1474, *1474*
Dennie-Morgan fold in, in atopic
dermatitis, 196
meibomian glands of, 31
muscles of, anatomy of, *113,* 114
psoriasis of, 301
xanthoma of, 1809, *1810,* 1816

F

Fabry's disease, angiokeratoma in, 1514–1515
cardiac disorders in, 1878t
renal disease in, cutaneous signs with,
1884t, *1885*
Face, anatomy of, blood supply in, *112,* 115
lymphatic system in, 115, *116*

Face (*Continued*)
    muscles in, 112–114, *113*
    sensory nerves in, 112, *112*
    skin tension lines in, 114–115
    topographic, 111–112, *112*
    hemiatrophy of, in morphea, 896, 897
    skin care of, normal, 79–81, *80*
Facial artery, anatomy of, *112*, 115
Facial nerve, anatomy of, 113, *113*, 116t, 116–117
    branches of, in neck, *118*, 119
Factitial dermatitis, 780t, 781t, 784–785, *785*
Famciclovir, for varicella-zoster infection, 1081
Fanconi's anemia, 1802t
Farmer's neck, 733, *733*
Fascicles, definition of, 107
Fasciitis, eosinophilic, in morphea, 897, 898
    vs. scleroderma, 887, 888t
    necrotizing, 942, 942t, 945–946
        genital, 1344
    palmar, 908–909, *909*
Fat. See also *Lipids.*
    in nevus lipomatosus superficialis, 1526
    subcutaneous, blood supply of, 28
        embryology of, 5
        hypertrophy of, liposuction for, *1531*, 1531–1534
        in skin grafting, after cancer excision, 1421, *1422*
        inflammation of. See *Panniculitis.*
        insulating function of, 46
        necrosis of, paraneoplastic, 1845
        of newborn, in sclerema, 599–600, *600*, 600t
        necrosis of, *600*, 600–602, *601*, 601t, 1845, 1897
        structure of, 3, *4*, 28
        tumors of, 1526–1530, *1527–1529*
        liposuction for, *1530*, 1530–1531
Fatigue, chronic, Epstein-Barr virus infection in, 1082
Fatty acid deficiencies, and alopecia, diffuse, 1276
    cutaneous signs of, 1873t
Fatty alcohol oxidoreductase deficiency, in Sjögren-Larsson syndrome, 1692, 1693
Favre-Racouchot disease, 733, *734*
Favus, 1045, *1046*
    and scarring alopecia, 1285, *1285*
Feet. See *Foot.*
Ferguson-Smith keratoacanthoma, 1382
Ferric subsulfate, in hemostasis, 133
Ferritin, in porphyria cutanea tarda, 1759
Fetus. See also *Pregnancy.*
    angiogenesis in, 1492
    harlequin, 1690
    herpes simplex virus transmission to, 714, 715t
    loss of, antiphospholipid syndrome and, 549–550
    skin development in, 3–5
    syphilis transmission to, 957t, 958, 959, *960*, 960t
    teratogenicity to, retinoids and, 310
    varicella transmission to, 715t, 718
Fibrel, in acne scar treatment, 474
Fibrillar tissue, definition of, 107
Fibrillin, in dermal extracellular matrix, 857, 859t, *870*, 871, *872*, 873–874
Fibrils, anchoring, collagen in, 863–864, *864*
    in epidermolysis bullosa, 867–869, *868, 869*
Fibrinolysis, in livedo vasculopathy, 544
Fibroblast growth factors, in angiogenesis, 1493t, 1493–1494

Fibroblasts, in radiation dermatitis, 837, *838*
Fibrohistiocytoma, 1552–1555, *1553*, 1553t, *1554*, 1555t
Fibrokeratoma, digital, acquired, 1305
Fibroma, of nerve sheath, 1540–1544, 1541t, 1542t, *1543*
    oral, 1326, *1326*
    ovarian, in basal cell nevus syndrome, 1743
    periungual, 1301
        in tuberous sclerosis, 1736, 1740
    subungual, 1301
Fibromatosis, palmar, 908–909, *909*
Fibronectin, in dermal extracellular matrix, 858, 859t
    in dermal structure, 18–21
    in dermoepidermal junction, 16, 624
Fibroplasia, in wound healing, *564*, 565
Fibrosarcoma, of nerve sheath, 1546, *1546*
Fibrosis, collagen gene defect in, *869*, 869–871
    definition of, 107
Fibrotic tracts, definition of, 107
Fibrous plaques, in tuberous sclerosis, 1736, *1737*
Fibrous tracts, definition of, 107
Fibrous tumors, in dermatofibroma, 1552–1555, *1553*, 1553t, *1554*, 1555t
    in dermatofibrosarcoma protuberans, 1553t, 1555t, *1555–1557*, 1555–1558
Fibroxanthoma, atypical, 1553t, 1555t, *1558*, 1558–1559
Filaggrin, in epidermal differentiation, 9–11, 47
    in epidermal structure, 6, *15, 16*
    in ichthyosis vulgaris, 1683
    in keratinocyte differentiation, in granular layer, 64–65, *65*
Filariasis, *1174*, 1179
Finasteride, for alopecia, androgenetic, 1257
Fingernails. See *Nail(s).*
Fingers. See also *Digits.*
    contracture of, in Dupuytren's disease, 908–909, *909*
    in scleroderma, 882, *883*, 887–889
    deformities of, in epidermolysis bullosa, 641, *641*, 645
Fire ant stings, 807t, 808t, 808–809, *809*
Fire coral stings, 791
Fish oils, for psoriasis, 312
Fish skin, toxins in, and dermatitis, 797
Fish tank granuloma, 989t, 990, *990*, Plate 7
Fissures, assessment of, 99–100
Fistula, arteriovenous, punch hair grafting and, 1259
    odontogenic-cutaneous, 1337
Fitzpatrick classification, of skin photosensitivity, 739t, 739–740, 742–744, 746
Flame figures, in Wells' syndrome, 361, *361*, Plate 3
Flap surgery, after skin cancer excision, 1408–1417
    advancement, 1409–1411, *1409–1411*
    rotation, 1411–1413, *1412, 1413*
    selection of technique in, 1416–1417
    terminology of, 1408–1409
    transposition, 1413–1416, *1414–1416*
    temporoparietal-occipital, for alopecia, *1265*, 1265–1266
Fleas, as vectors, of typhus, 1018
    bites of, 804, 805t, *806*, 807, 807t
    in tungiasis, 820–821, *821*
Flies, as vectors, of loiasis, 1180
    of onchocerciasis, 1177
    bites of, 805, 805t, 807t

Flies (*Continued*)
    larvae of, in furuncular myiasis, 818–820, *819*
    in wound myiasis, 820, *820*
Flolan, for Raynaud's phenomenon, 541–542
Flow cytometry, in T-cell lymphoma, 1649–1650, *1650*
Fluconazole, for candidiasis, 1058t, 1346
    for coccidioidomycosis, 1064
    for cryptococcosis, 1061, 1061t
    for pityriasis versicolor, 1040t, 1040–1041
    for *Pityrosporum* folliculitis, 1040t, 1041
Flucytosine, for chromoblastomycosis, 1069
    for cryptococcosis, 1061, 1061t
Fludarabine monophosphate, for T-cell lymphoma, 1653
Fluocinolone, for contact dermatitis, 181
Fluocinonide, for lichen planus, 239, 239t
Fluorescent antibody testing, for herpes simplex virus infection, 123
    for syphilis, 955, 956t
Fluorethyl, in cryoanesthesia, for dermabrasion of acne scars, 476–477
Fluoroquinolones, for Rocky Mountain spotted fever, 1015, 1016t
5-Fluorouracil, for actinic keratosis, 1395
    for papillomavirus infection, genital, 1349
Fluoxetine, for trichotillomania, 783
Flushing, 534–535, 535t, 536t
    mithramycin and, 430
    paraneoplastic, 1848
Flutamide, for androgenetic alopecia, 1257
    for hirsutism, 1857
Flutists, acne mechanica in, 772
Fly. See *Flies.*
Folic acid deficiency, cutaneous signs of, 1873t
Follicles. See *Hair follicles.*
Food, allergy to, in atopic dermatitis, 199, 201
Foot, cellulitis of, vs. gout, 924
    dermatitis of, 188–193, 191t, 192t, 197
    in epidermolysis bullosa, 637, *637*, 641, *641*
    sole of, keratoderma of, 1703–1706, *1706*
    porokeratosis of, 1701–1703, *1702*
    psoriasis of, pustular, 298
    tinea of, 851, 928–929, 1044t, 1045–1047, *1046, 1047*
    trench, 776–777, 777t, 828
Football players, acne mechanica in, 772
Fordyce's angiokeratoma, 1514, *1514*
Fordyce's spots, 30–31, 1325
Foreign body granuloma, 452–454, 454t
    in drug abusers, 839
Forest yaws, 1163
Formalin, in biopsy, 122
Formication, 780–781
Foscarnet, adverse reactions to, in human immunodeficiency virus infection, 1145
    for cytomegalovirus infection, 1086
    for herpes simplex infection, 1078
    for herpesvirus-6 infection, 1088, 1130
    for varicella-zoster infection, 1081
    with human immunodeficiency virus infection, 1141
Fournier's gangrene, 942, 946–947, 1344
Fragrances, in skin care products, sensitivity to, 79
Framboesia, 962
Francisella tularensis infection, 943–944, *944*, 947, 1034–1035, 1035t
Freckles, 1561
    in neurofibromatosis, 1730
    in xeroderma pigmentosum, 1747, *1748*
Free radicals, and facial skin damage, 52–53, 80–81
Freon, in cryoanesthesia, for dermabrasion of acne scars, 476–477

Frey's syndrome, hyperhidrosis in, 1313–1314
Friction, and acanthoma fissuratum, 773t, 773–774, 774t
  and acne, 464
  and acne mechanica, 772–773, 773t, 852, 853
  and amputee dermatitis, 774t, 774–775, 775t
  and athlete's nodules, 775t, 775–776, 776t, 851
  and calluses, 1703
  and sports injuries, 850–851, 853
Frontal bone, anatomy of, 111
Frontoparietal scalp lift, 1263, *1264*
Frostbite, *826*, 826–828
  homelessness and, 841
  sports-related, 849, 852
Fulguration, in electrosurgery, for rosacea, 489t, 489–491
Fungal infection. See also specific infections, e.g., *Candidiasis.*
  and erythema nodosum, 593, 594t
  biopsy of, 122
  dermatophytic, 1043–1054. See also *Dermatophytosis.*
  in atopic dermatitis, 197
  in immunosuppressed patient, 1157
  interdigital, 929
  of genitalia, *1345*, 1345–1346
  oral, 1335–1336, 1337t
  superficial, 1037–1041, 1038t, *1038–1040*, 1040t
Furuncles, staphylococcal infection and, 922
Furuncular myiasis, 818–820, *819*
Fusarium infection, 1072
  in immunosuppressed patient, 1157

G

GADD 153, in DNA repair, after photodamage, 737–738
Gallbladder, removal of, in protoporphyria, 1757–1758
Gambian sleeping sickness, 1174–1175
Gamma globulin, for dermatomyositis, 288t, 289
  for polymyositis, 288t, 289
Gamma-delta T-cell lymphoma, 1642, 1645
Ganciclovir, for cytomegalovirus infection, 1085–1086
  for herpesvirus-6 infection, 1088, 1130
Gangrene, acral, with diabetes, 1869t
  Fournier's, 942, 946–947, 1344
  in systemic lupus erythematosus, 264
  in trench foot, 777
  of buttock, perinatal, 715t
  paraneoplastic, 1848
Gardner's syndrome, 1797t
  gastrointestinal hemorrhage in, 1874t
  infundibular cysts with, 1450–1451
  oral abnormalities in, 1324t
Gastritis, in syphilis, 952
Gastrocnemius muscle, pump function of, in venous ulceration, 560, *560*
Gastroenteritis, *Aeromonas hydrophila* infection and, 943
Gastrointestinal tract, bacterial flora of, and cellulitis, 941–942, 942t
  cancer of, metastasis of, to skin, 1674, *1676*
  disorders of, and dermatitis-arthritis syndrome, 375–376, 376t, 389t
    cutaneous signs of, 1872–1874, 1874t, 1875t, *1876, 1877*

Gastrointestinal tract (*Continued*)
    in acrodermatitis enteropathica, 1763–1765, *1764*, 1765t, 1873t
    in Behçet's disease, 387, 389t
    in blue rubber bleb syndrome, 1505
    in epidermolysis bullosa, junctional, 639, 643, 645
    in hypereosinophilic syndrome, 354
    in mastocytosis, 1604
    in scleroderma, 884
    in toxic epidermal necrolysis, 705–706
  hemorrhage in, in pseudoxanthoma elasticum, 1771, 1774
  inflammatory disease of, pyoderma gangrenosum with, 379–380, 382, 383
Gaucher's disease, 1696, 1766–1767, 1767t
Gelfoam, in hemostasis, 133
Gemfibrozil, for hyperlipidemia, with xanthoma, 1816
Genes, and life-threatening disorders, parental counseling on, 1894
  collagen, and dermal structure, 859t, 861–865, *862–865*
    in Ehlers-Danlos syndrome, 866
    in epidermolysis bullosa, 627–628, 686, 687, 867–869, *869*
  disorders of. See also specific disorders, e.g., *Conradi-Hünermann syndrome.*
    and dermatosis, 1796
      chromosomal instability in, 1802t, 1803t, *1804, 1805*
      in vascular syndromes, 1799t, *1800, 1801*
      with malignant potential, 1796t, *1797*, 1797t, *1798*
  DNA repair system in, 1366–1367, *1368*
  elastin, 872–873, *873*
    in albinism, 1219–1223, 1220t, 1221t, *1222*, 1223t
    in carcinogenesis, 1363
      ultraviolet-induced, 1369–1374, *1370*, 1370t, *1371, 1373*
    in cutis laxa, 913–914
    in dermal hypoplasia, focal, 1781–1782
    in epidermolysis bullosa, 635–636, 636t
    in granuloma annulare, 441
    in hypomelanosis of Ito, 1226–1227
    in ichthyosis, bullous, 1689
    in keratin formation, 9
      defects of, and epidermolysis bullosa simplex, 61–62, 626–627, *627*
      in epithelial development, 60–61, *61*
      in keratinocyte differentiation, 62–63
    in melanocyte system, 1205, 1207
    in pemphigus vulgaris, 653–654
    in piebaldism, *1224*, 1224–1225
    in pseudoxanthoma elasticum, 1772
    in psoriasis, 303
    in Waardenburg's syndrome, 1225
  kalinin, in epidermolysis bullosa, junctional, 628, 642t, 644
  tumor-suppressing, mutations of, in skin cancer, *1370*, 1371–1374, *1373*
Genistein, anti-angiogenic effect of, 1495, 1495t
Genitalia, anatomy of, 1340–1341, *1341*
  aphthae of, in Behçet's disease, 385
  bacterial infection of, 1343–1344
  chancroid of, 973–976, *974*, 975t, 976t
  contact dermatitis of, 1350
  disorders of, classification of, 1340, 1341t
    diagnosis of, 1341–1343, 1342t, 1343t
    with systemic disease, 1352
  embryology of, 1340
  fungal infection of, *1057*, 1057t, *1345*, 1345–1346

Genitalia (*Continued*)
    granuloma of, 976t, *977*, 977–979
    herpes simplex infection of, 1074–1075, 1346–1347. See also *Herpes simplex infection.*
    in leprosy, 999
    in Reiter's syndrome, 322, 323t, 324
    injury to, in child abuse, 1892
    intertrigo of, 1350
    lentigines of, mucosal, 1563
    lichen planus of, 1350–1351
    lichen sclerosus of, *1351*, 1351–1352
    lichen simplex chronicus of, 1350
    louse infestation of, *1193*, 1193–1195, *1194*, 1194t, 1195t
    lymphogranuloma venereum of, 976t, 979–981, *980*
    molluscum contagiosum of, 1346
    necrotizing fasciitis of, 1344
    pain in, 1353–1356, *1354, 1355*, Plate 9
    papillomavirus infection of, 1102t, 1102–1104, *1102–1104*, 1106, 1347–1349, *1348*
    pemphigoid of, cicatricial, 674–675
    piedra of, white, 1345
    psoriasis of, 300–301, 1350
    trichomoniasis of, 1176–1177, 1343t
    tumors of, *1352*, 1352–1353, *1353*
    varicella-zoster infection of, 1347
Genitoanorectal syndrome, in lymphogranuloma venereum, 980
Genodermatoses, 1796–1805. See also *Genes.*
Genodermatoses en cocardes, 1698
Gentamicin, and wound healing, 566t
  for tularemia, 947
Gentian violet, in prevention of trypanosomiasis, 1174
Geographic tongue, 1327, *1327*
German measles (rubella), 1124t, 1125t, 1127–1128
  oral lesions in, 1335t
Germinal centers, definition of, 107
Gestation. See *Fetus* and *Pregnancy.*
Giacomini's vein, anatomy of, *577*
Gianotti-Crosti syndrome, 1082, *1083*
  rash in, 1124t, 1125t, 1133–1134, *1134*, Plate 9
Giant cell arteritis, 515–517, *516*, 516t
  infrared radiation and, 825
Giant cell granuloma, elastolytic, 441, 441t, 442
Giant cell tumors, in tuberous sclerosis, 1737
Giant cells, definition of, 107–108
  in xanthogranuloma, 1621, *1621, 1622*
  in xanthoma, 1809, 1811, *1811*
Gingiva, hyperplasia of, 1328
  in acquired immunodeficiency syndrome, 1337t
  in Kaposi's sarcoma, 1151, *1152*
  leukemic infiltration of, 1671
Gingivostomatitis, in herpes simplex infection, 1335, 1335t
Glioma, nasal, *1547*, 1547–1549, 1548t
  optic, in neurofibromatosis, 1731
  retinal, in tuberous sclerosis, 1737
Glogau classification, of photoaging, 742, 742t
Glomangioma, 1513, *1513*
Glomeruloid hemangioma, 1516
Glomerulonephritis, after impetigo, 921
  in toxic epidermal necrolysis, 706
Glomus bodies, in dermal blood vessels, 23, *25*
Glomus tumors, 1507t, *1513*, 1513–1514, *1514*
  of nail bed, 1301
Glossina flies, as vectors of trypanosomiasis, 1174

Glossitis, benign migratory, 1327, *1327*

Glucagonoma, and necrolytic migratory erythema, 1843–1844, *1844, 1868*

Glucantine, for leishmaniasis, 1169

Glucocerebrosidase, in Gaucher's disease, 1696, 1766, 1767, 1767t

Glucosylceramide, in Gaucher's disease, 1766, 1767t

Glue, and burn injury, 846

Gluteal cleft, frictional injury in, sports-related, 851

Gluten-sensitive enteropathy, with dermatitis herpetiformis, 691, 694–696

Glycams, in inflammatory response, 150

Glycerol, for dry skin, 77

Glyceryl para-aminobenzoic acid, in sunscreens, 754

Glycine, in keratinocyte differentiation, 62–63

Glycolic acid, in chemical peel, for photoaging, 742t, 743, 743t

Glycoproteins, CD44, in inflammatory response, 150
  in dermoepidermal junction, 15–16

Glycosaminoglycans, in dermal structure, 18
  in extracellular matrix, 857–858, 859t, 876

Gnathostoma infestation, 1184
  and cutaneous larva migrans, 1181, 1181t

Goeckerman regimen, in phototherapy, for psoriasis, 306, 313

Gold, analogues of, anti-angiogenic effect of, 1495, 1495t
  and pigmentation disorders, 422, 1237

Gold salts, for pemphigus foliaceus, 658, 658t
  for pemphigus vulgaris, 654t, 655

Goltz's syndrome, 1780–1782, *1781*, 1781t, 1782t
  vs. anetoderma, 911t

Gonadotropin-releasing hormone, agonists of, for hirsutism, 1856

Gonococcal infection, skin lesions in, *944*, 944–945

Gorham's syndrome, 1506, 1799t

Gorlin's sign, in Ehlers-Danlos syndrome, *1775*

Gorlin's syndrome (basal cell nevus syndrome), 1742–1745, *1743, 1744*, 1745t, 1796t, *1797*
  infundibular cysts in, 1450–1451

Gottron's papules, in dermatomyositis, 284, *284*, 286

Gougerot-Blum lichenoid purpura, 291–293, *292*

Gout, vs. cellulitis, 924

Grafting, after skin carcinoma excision, composite, 1421–1423, *1424*
  full-thickness, 1420–1421, *1421–1423*
  split-thickness, 1417–1420, *1417–1420*
  for acne scars, 474
  for keloids, 904
  for leg ulcers, 568–570, *569*, 569t, *570*
  for vitiligo, 1215–1216
  immunosuppression with, 1155–1157. See also *Immunosuppression.*
  of hair, mini-micrograft technique in, *1260*, 1260–1261, *1261, 1263*
    punch technique in, *1258*, 1258–1260, *1259*
  of kidney, cutaneous changes with, 1884t, *1885*, 1886

Graft-versus-host disease, 225–233
  and toxic epidermal necrolysis, 708
  oral lesions in, 1334
  vs. scleroderma, 888t

Graft-versus-host disease (*Continued*)
  with marrow transplantation, 225–226
    allogeneic, acute reaction in, 226–230, *227*, 227t–229t, *228*, Plate 1
      chronic reaction in, *230*, 230–232, *231*
    autologous, 232–233

Granular cell tumor, of nerve sheath, 1541t, 1545–1546, *1546*

Granular layer, in epidermal structure, 6, *14, 15*
  in gestation, 3
  keratinocytes in, 63–66, *65*

Granular lymphocytic leukemia, cutaneous manifestations of, 1670

Granulation tissue, definition of, 108
  in wound healing, *564, 565*

Granulocyte colony-stimulating factor, in inflammatory response, 145

Granulocyte/macrophage colony-stimulating factor, in inflammatory response, 145

Granuloma, actinic, 442
  vs. granuloma annulare, 441, 441t
  dermal, 878
  eosinophilic, in Langerhans cell histiocytosis, 1610–1611, 1613
  foreign bodies and, 452–454
    in drug abusers, 839
  in alopecia, scarring, 1291, 1291t
  in cheilitis, 1327
  in diaper dermatitis, 184, 186
  in lymphoma, T-cell, 1641, 1644
    with slack skin, 1666
  in rosacea, 485, 487t
  in Wells' syndrome, 360, *361*, Plate 3
  Miescher's radial, in erythema nodosum, 592, *593*
  Mycobacterium marinum infection and, 989t, 990, *990*, Plate 7
  pyogenic, 1507t, *1509*, 1509–1510, *1510*
    oral, 1325–1326
  reticulohistiocytic, 1616
  with inflammation, 433–459. See also specific disorders, e.g., *Sarcoidosis.*
  with slack skin, 1641, 1644, 1666
  vs. anetoderma, 911t

Granuloma annulare, 438–442, *439, 440*, 441t, 442t
  arcuate dermal erythema in, 439
  diagnosis of, 441, 441t
  generalized, 438, *439*
  in human immunodeficiency virus infection, 1145
  linear, 439
  localized, 438, *439*
  pathogenesis of, 440–441
  pathology of, 439–440, *440*
  perforating, 438–439
  subcutaneous, 438
  treatment of, 441–442, 442t
  with diabetes, 1869t, *1870*

Granuloma faciale, 530–532, *531*, 531t

Granuloma fissuratum, 773t, 773–774, 774t

Granuloma inguinale, 976t, *977*, 977–979
  vs. chancroid, 975, 975t
  vs. syphilis, 956

Granulomatosis, lymphomatoid, 1667
  pulmonary disease in, cutaneous signs with, 1882t
  Wegener's, 522–527, *523, 525, 526*, 526t
    oral lesions in, 1334
    pulmonary disease in, cutaneous signs with, 1882t
    vs. polychondritis, relapsing, 513

Granulomatous inflammation, definition of, 108

Graves' disease, with herpes gestationis, 680

Greither's syndrome, 1705

Griscelli's syndrome, 1717

Griseofulvin, for dermatophytosis, 1054

Grocers' itch, 814–815

Ground substance, in dermal structure, 17–18

Grover's disease, 341–343, *342*, 342t, *343*, 343t

Growth factors, in angiogenesis, 1493t, 1493–1494
  in collagen gene expression, 865
  in elastin gene expression, 873
  in hair development, in mice, 1718
  in keloids, 869–871, 902
  in leg ulcer management, 570
  in melanoma, 1586

Growth regulation, in photoaged skin, 738

Growth retardation, with atopic dermatitis, 197

Grysbowski keratoacanthoma, 1382

Guanosine triphosphate, binding of, in *ras* gene mutations, 1371, *1371*

Gummas, in syphilis, 953

Gums. See *Gingiva.*

Guttate hypomelanosis, idiopathic, 1228, 1228t

Guttate psoriasis, *87*, 295t, 299, *299*. See also *Psoriasis.*

H

Haarscheibe, 25

Haemophilus ducreyi infection, and chancroid, 973–976, *974*, 975t, 976t

Haemophilus influenzae infection, 939–940, 946

Hailey-Hailey disease, 1701, *1702*
  vs. acantholytic dermatosis, 341

Hair, anatomy of, 1245–1250, *1246*, 1246t, 1248t, *1249*
  brittle, in trichothiodystrophy, 1694
  discoloration of, in swimmers, 849–850, 852–853
  excessive growth of, in hirsutism, 1853–1857, *1854*, 1855t, 1856t
    in hypertrichosis lanuginosa acquisita, 1844, *1844*
    topical corticosteroids and, 166
  genetic abnormalities of, in mice, 1718–1719
  growth of, biochemistry of, 1248t, 1248–1249, *1249*
    phases of, 1247–1248
  hypoplasia of, with cartilage hypoplasia, 1715
  in ectodermal dysplasia, 1721, 1722t, *1723*, 1723t
  loss of. See *Alopecia.*
  racial differences in, 41
  removal of, from operative site, 129

Hair follicle disks, 25

Hair follicles, anatomy of, 28–30, *28–31*, 1245–1247, *1246*
  autonomic effects on, 23–25, *25*
  center cell lymphoma of, *1662*, 1663–1664
  cysts of, infundibular, 1450–1451, 1451t, *1451–1454*
    surgery for, 1456–1461, 1458t, *1459–1462*
  trichilemmal, 1452–1453, *1455*
    proliferating, 1453–1454, *1456*
  degeneration syndrome of, 1286, *1286*

Hair follicles (*Continued*)
  embryology of, 4–5
  growth of, biochemistry of, 1248t, 1248–1249, *1249*
  hyperkeratosis of, with ichthyosis, 1697
  in granuloma faciale, 530, *531*
  in keratosis pilaris, 503–504, *504*
  in lichen spinulosus, *505*, 505–506, 506t
  inflammation of, 461–506
    and scarring alopecia, in folliculitis decalvans, *1283*, 1283–1284, 1284t
    bacterial infection and, 922
    dactinomycin and, 429–430
    dermatophytic, pathology of, 1050
    eosinophilic, in human immunodeficiency virus infection, 1144, *1144*
      pustular, in neonate, 717t, 720–721
    gram-negative, 463, 941, 946
    in acne, 461–479. See also *Acne*.
    Malassezia furfur infection and, 1038t, 1040t, 1041
    pruritic, in pregnancy, 370
    Pseudomonas aeruginosa infection and, 940–941, *941*
    sports-related, 851–853
  keratosis of, scarring, *1292*, 1292t, 1292–1293
  leiomyoma of, 1522–1523, *1523*
  lichen planus of, 236, 237, 239
    and scarring alopecia, *1287*, 1287–1288, 1288t
  lymphoid, definition of, 109
  lymphoma of, *88*
  melanin transfer disorders of, 1717–1718
  melanocytes in, 1205
  mucinosis of, 1833t, 1839–1840
    and scarring alopecia, 1289–1290, *1290*, 1290t
    definition of, 107
    in lymphoma, T-cell, 1641, 1644
  occlusion of, in hidradenitis suppurativa, 481–483, *482*, 482t, *483*
  papules of, 90, 91t, *93*
  pilar sheath acanthoma in, 1465
  pilomatricoma of, 1468–1470, *1469*, 1830
  pilomatrix carcinoma of, 1471
  pustules in, 96, *97*
  racial differences in, 41
  sebaceous, 31
  structure of, 3, *4*
  trichoepithelioma of, 1466–1468, *1467, 1468*
    desmoplastic, 1468, *1468*
  trichofolliculoma of, *93*, 1466, *1466*
  tricholemmoma of, 1470, *1470*
  tumors of, 1464–1474
  vellus, eruptive cysts of, 1451, *1454*
  Winer's dilated pore of, 1464–1465
Hair replacement surgery, mini-micrografts in, *1260*, 1260–1261, *1261, 1263*
  punch grafting in, *1258*, 1258–1260, *1259*
Hairy cell leukemia, cutaneous manifestations of, 1670
  vs. Langerhans cell histiocytosis, 1613
Hairy leukoplakia, oral, Epstein-Barr virus and, 1083, *1083*, 1084, 1148
  in acquired immunodeficiency syndrome, 1336–1337
Hairy tongue, 1327–1328
Hallopeau's acrodermatitis continua, 298
Hallopeau-Siemens epidermolysis bullosa, *640*, 640–642, *641*, 645, *867*, 867–869, *868*

Halo nevus, 1566–1567
  vs. melanoma, 1588
Halobetasol propionate, 163–164
Hamartoma. See also *Nevus (nevi)*.
  definition of, 108
  multiple, in Cowden's disease, 1796t, *1797*
  of muscle, 1793–1794
Hamilton classification, of androgenetic alopecia, 1250, *1251*
Hand, contracture of, in Dupuytren's disease, 908–909, *909*
  dermatitis of, 188–193, 191t, 192t
    atopic, 197
    pathology of, 190
  palm of, fasciitis of, 908–909, *909*
    in epidermolysis bullosa, 641, *641*
    keratoderma of, 1703–1706, *1705*
    petechiae of, sports and, 850–851, 853
    pitting of, in basal cell nevus syndrome, 1742, *1743*
    porokeratosis of, 1701–1703
    psoriasis of, pustular, 298
  pustulosis of, *189*, 189–192, *190*
  skin care of, normal, *81*, 81–82
  tinea of, 1046–1047, *1047*, 1052t
Hand-foot-and-mouth disease, 1132, *1132*, 1335t
Hand-Schüller-Christian disease, 1610
Hansen's disease, 993–1003. See also *Leprosy*.
Harlequin color change, in neonate, *1893*, 1894
Harlequin ichthyosis, 66, *1690*, 1690–1691, *1691*
Hartnup disease, 1768, 1859t, 1862
Haxthausen's disease, 609
Heaf test, for tuberculosis, 987
Hearing, loss of, with keratitis and ichthyosis, 1694–1695
  with palmoplantar keratoderma, 1705
  with piebaldism, 1225
Heart, congenital block of, lupus erythematosus and, 265–266, 278
  disorders of, cutaneous signs with, 1877, 1878t, 1879t, *1880, 1881*, 1881t, Plate 15
    in cardio-facio-cutaneous syndrome, 1697–1698
    in Lyme borreliosis, 967, 969t
    in pseudoxanthoma elasticum, 1771, 1773, 1774, 1879t
    in scleroderma, 884, 1879t
    in tuberous sclerosis, 1228, 1737, 1879t
    with androgenetic alopecia, 1252
    with hypereosinophilic syndrome, 353, 355
Heat, and urticaria, 392–394, 400
  in infrared radiation, 823
    and erythema ab igne, *824*, 824–825
    cutaneous effects of, 823–824
  in therapy, for atopic eczema, 826
    for infectious disease, 826
    for psoriasis, 825
    for skin cancer, 826
  preservation of, skin in, 53–56
    in neonate, 1890
Heck's disease, 1103, *1103*, 1335
Heel, petechiae of, sports and, 850, 853
Heliotrope, in dermatomyositis, 284, *284*, Plate 2
Helix, chondrodermatitis nodularis of, 507, *508*, 509–510, *510*
Hemangioendothelioma, epithelioid, 1516, 1517
  kaposiform, 1499

Hemangioendothelioma (*Continued*)
  retiform, 1516
  spindle cell, 1516, 1517
Hemangioma, arteriovenous, acral, 1507t, 1511, *1512*
  capillary, lobular, 1507t, *1509*, 1509–1510, *1510*
  cherry, 1507t, 1515
  epithelioid, 1507t, 1511–1513, *1512*
  glomeruloid, 1516
  hemosiderotic, 1507t, *1515*, 1515–1516
  in neonate, vs. blistering disorders, 716t
  microvenular, 1516
  multinucleate cell, 1516
  of infancy, 1496t, 1496–1501, *1497, 1498, 1500*
  oral, 1325–1326
  sclerosing, 1552–1555, *1553*, 1553t, *1554*, 1555t
  sinusoidal, 1516
Hemangiomatosis, neonatal, diffuse, 1498
Hematoma, after liposuction, 1532
  scalp reduction and, 1262
  subungual, 1298t, 1300
Hematoporphyrin derivate, in photodynamic therapy, for skin carcinoma, 1424, 1426–1427
Heme, biosynthesis of, in porphyria, 1753–1756, *1755*, 1755t
Hemiatrophy, facial, in morphea, 896, 897
Hemidesmosomes, in dermoepidermal junction, 14–15, *19–22*, 618, 618–619
  basement membrane proteins associated with, 619–621, *620*
  in keratinocyte attachment, to basement membrane, 59
Hemochromatosis, cardiac disorders with, 1878t
  with diabetes, 1870t, *1871*
Hemophagocytic lymphohistiocytosis, 1623
Hemorrhage, after dermabrasion, for acne scars, 479
  control of, in surgery, 131–134, *132*
  from varicose veins, 575
  gastrointestinal, cutaneous signs of, 1874, 1874t, 1875t, *1876*
    in pseudoxanthoma elasticum, 1771, 1774
  in amyloidosis, 1819, *1819*
  punctate, in pityriasis rosea, 219
  splinter, of nails, 1298t, 1300
Hemorrhagic telangiectasia, hereditary, 1799t, *1800*, 1882t
  and gastrointestinal hemorrhage, 1874t, *1876*
Hemosiderotic hemangioma, 1507t, *1515*, 1515–1516
Hemostasis, in surgery, 131–134, *132*
Hendersonula toruloidea infection, vs. tinea pedis, 1046
Henle's layer, in hair follicle, 28, *28*, 29, *30*
Henoch-Schönlein purpura, *523*, 524, 525, 526t, 585, 586
Heparan sulfate proteoglycan, in dermoepidermal junction, 624–625
Heparin, and skin necrosis, 419–420
  anti-angiogenic effect of, 1495
  for coumarin-induced skin necrosis, 546t, 550
  for livedo vasculopathy, 546t
  in urticaria, 397, 397t
  use of, biopsy after, 121–122
Hepatitis, in syphilis, 952
  viral, cutaneous signs of, 1877t
Hepatitis B virus infection, in Gianotti-Crosti syndrome, 1133, 1134

Hepatoerythropoietic porphyria, 1758, 1760, 1760t
Herald patch, in pityriasis rosea, 218–220, 219t
Herlitz epidermolysis bullosa, 638–639, *639*, 642
Hermansky-Pudlak syndrome, 1221t, 1222
Heroin, abuse of, 839, 840
Herpangina, oral lesions in, 1335t
Herpes gestationis, 679–684, *680, 681*, 683t
    and neonatal blistering eruption, 720
    paraneoplastic, 1847
    vs. bullous pemphigoid, 669
Herpes simplex infection, 1074–1078, 1077t, *1078*
    after renal transplantation, 1884t, *1885*
    and erythema multiforme, 250–254, 252t
    clinical findings in, 1074–1076, *1075, 1076*
    definition of, 1074
    diagnosis of, 1076–1077, *1077*, 1077t
        biopsy in, 123
    epidemiology of, 1074
    genital, 1074–1075, *1075, 1076, 1346*, 1346–1347
    in dermabrasion, for acne scars, management of, 478
    in immunosuppressed patient, 1156
    in neonate, 714–718, 715t, 1075, *1893*, 1895, *1895*
    lesions of, configuration of, *87*
    oral lesions in, 1074–1076, *1075*, 1077t, 1335, 1335t
    pathology of, 1076, *1077*
    sports-related, 851, 853, 1075
    treatment of, 1077–1078, *1078*
    vs. chancroid, 975, 975t
    vs. syphilis, 955
    with human immunodeficiency virus infection, *1139*, 1139–1140
Herpes zoster, 1078–1081. See also *Varicella-zoster infection.*
Herpesvirus infection, 1074–1088
    and aplasia cutis congenita, 1783t, 1784
    and dermatitis, vs. Behçet's disease, 389t
    in atopic dermatitis, 197, 201
Herpesvirus-6 infection, 1086–1088, 1087t
    and roseola, 1124t, 1125t, 1129–1130, *1130*
    in Rosai-Dorfman disease, 1618
Herpetiform dermatitis, 691–696. See also *Dermatitis herpetiformis.*
Herpetiform lesions, definition of, 108
12-HETE, for psoriasis, 312
Hexachlorophene, and wound healing, 566t
    in antiseptic solutions, 129, 129t
Hibernoma, 1529
Hibiclens (chlorhexidine), and wound healing, 566t
    for candidiasis, oral, 1336
    in antiseptic solutions, 129, 129t
Hidradenitis suppurativa, 481–483, *482, 483*, 483t
Hidradenocarcinoma, 1480–1481
Hidradenoma, clear cell, *1477*, 1480–1481, *1481*, 1481t
Hidradenoma papilliferum, 1486, *1486*, 1486t
Higoumenakis' sign, in syphilis, congenital, 960t
Hippel-Lindau syndrome, 1799t, *1801*
Hirschsprung's disease, with hypopigmentation, 1225, 1225t
Hirsutism, clinical findings in, 1853–1854
    definition of, 1853, *1854*
    diagnosis of, 1855, 1855t
    pathogenesis of, 1855
    treatment of, 1855–1857, 1856t

Histamine, and pruritus, 158
    in mastocytosis, 1605, 1607, 1607t
    in sunburn, 736
    in urticaria, 397, 397t
        solar, 762, 763
Histiocytic panniculitis, cytophagic, *612*, 612–613
Histiocytoma, eruptive, 1622
    indeterminant cell, 1620
Histiocytoma cutis, 1552–1555, *1553*, 1553t, *1554*, 1555t
Histiocytosis, cephalic, benign, 1622
    hemophagocytic, 1623
    Langerhans cell, 1610–1614, *1611, 1612*, 1613t, 1614t, Plate 13
        malignant, 1624
        oral abnormalities with, 1324t
        vs. seborrheic dermatitis, 216
    malignant, 1623–1624
    of reticular structures, congenital, self-healing, 716t, 1610
    multicentric, 1616–1617, *1617*, 1617t
        cardiac disorders in, cutaneous signs with, 1879t
    sinus, 1617–1619, *1618*, 1619t
        with lymphadenopathy, vs. Langerhans cell histiocytosis, 1613
Histocompatibility complex, major. See *Major histocompatibility complex.*
Histoplasmosis, 1064–1066, 1065t, 1066t, 1068t
    with human immunodeficiency virus infection, 1142
HIV infection, 1137–1155. See also *Human immunodeficiency virus infection.*
Hives, 392–403. See also *Urticaria.*
Hodgkin's lymphoma, and hyperhidrosis, 1312
    vs. lymphomatoid papulosis, 1632, *1633*, 1634, 1635t, 1637
Homelessness, skin trauma associated with, 841
Homocystinuria, 1859t, 1861
    and alopecia, 1713
Homogentisic acid oxidase deficiency, in alkaptonuria, 1859t, 1861
Homomenthyl salicylate, in sunscreens, 754
Hookworm infestation, 1143
Hopf's acrokeratosis verruciformis, vs. stucco keratosis, 1447
Horner's syndrome, hyperhidrosis in, 1313, 1314
Hornet stings, 807–808, 808t
Horns, cutaneous, 98, *99*
Horse riding, and perniosis, 829
Horton's disease (temporal arteritis), 515–517, *516*, 516t
    infrared radiation and, 825
Hot flashes, 534, 535
Hot tub folliculitis, 851, 853, 940–941, *941*
Howel-Evans syndrome, 1704
H-plasty, after skin cancer excision, 1410, *1410*
Human immunodeficiency virus infection, 1137–1155
    anetoderma in, 1145
    bacterial infection with, 1138, *1138*
    clinical findings in, 1137–1138
    cryptococcosis in, 1060, 1061, *1061*
    cytomegalovirus infection in, 1084–1086, 1086t
    drug reactions in, 423, 1145
    eczema with, 1145–1146
    Epstein-Barr virus infection with, 1083, *1083*, 1084

Human immunodeficiency virus infection *(Continued)*
    folliculitis in, eosinophilic, 1144, *1144*
    fungal infection with, superficial, 1143–1144
        systemic, *1141*, 1141–1142
    granuloma annulare in, 1145
    herpes simplex infection with, *1139*, 1139–1140
    herpesvirus-6 infection with, 1086, 1088
    histoplasmosis with, 1065
    insect bite reactions in, 1144–1145
    Kaposi's sarcoma in, 1149–1155. See also *Kaposi's sarcoma.*
    leishmaniasis with, 1143
    life-threatening disorders with, cutaneous signs of, 1886t
    lymphoma with, 1155
    melanoma with, 1149
    molluscum contagiosum with, 1138–1139, *1139*
    mycobacterial infection with, 991, 1142
    oral lesions in, 1148, 1336–1337, 1337t
    papular mucinosis in, 1145
    photosensitivity in, *1146*, 1146–1147
    pityriasis rubra pilaris with, 331, 333, 335, 1148
    psoriasis with, *1147*, 1147–1148
    psoriatic arthritis with, 302
    pulmonary disease in, cutaneous signs with, 1882t
    rash in, 1124t, 1125t, 1130, *1130*, Plate 8
    Reiter's syndrome with, 1148
    salivary gland disease in, 1148–1149
    scabies with, 1143, *1143*
    seborrheic dermatitis with, 214, 216, 1146, 1147, *1147*
    skin carcinoma with, 1149, *1149*, 1155
    strongyloidiasis with, 1143
    syphilis with, 959–961
    toxic epidermal necrolysis in, 708–709
    varicella-zoster infection with, *1140*, 1140–1141
    vasculitis in, 1149
Human leukocyte antigens, in Behçet's disease, 387–388
    in dermatitis herpetiformis, 691–694
    in herpes gestationis, 682
    in lupus erythematosus, 271
    in pemphigus foliaceus, 657–658
    in pemphigus vulgaris, 653–654
    in psoriasis, 302–304
    in Reiter's syndrome, 323
Human papillomavirus infection, 1100–1117. See also *Papillomavirus infection.*
Human T-lymphocyte virus infection, in adult T-cell lymphoma/leukemia, 1667–1668
Humectants, for dry skin, 77
Hunter's perforating veins, varicosity of, *578*
Huriez syndrome, 1704
Hutchinson-Gilford progeria syndrome, 1713
Hutchinson's angioma serpiginosum, vs. pigmented purpura, 293
Hutchinson's sign, in acral lentiginous melanoma, 1580, *1580*, Plate 11
Hutchinson's teeth, in congenital syphilis, 960, 960t
Huxley's layer, in hair follicle, *28*, 28–29, *30*
Hyalinosis, vs. amyloidosis, 1820, 1820t
Hyalohyphomycosis, 1072
Hydatidiform mole, with herpes gestationis, 683
Hydralazine, and lupus erythematosus, 266

Hydroa vacciniforme, *763*, 763–764
  vs. polymorphic light eruption, 760t
Hydrocolloid dressings, for psoriasis, 306
Hydrocortisone, for atopic dermatitis, 201
  for seborrheic dermatitis, 217, 217t
  topical, 160, 162–163
Hydrocystomas, 1455–1456, *1457, 1458*
Hydrofluoric acid, and burn injury, 845t,
  846–847
Hydrogen peroxide, and wound healing, 566t
Hydroid stings, 790–791, 794t
Hydroquinone, for melasma, 1236
α-Hydroxy acids, in chemical peel, for
  photoaging, 742t, 743, 743t
Hydroxychloroquine, and pigmentation
  disorders, 422
  for dermatomyositis, 288
  for lichen planus, 239–240
  for lupus erythematosus, discoid, 275t,
    275–276
  for morphea, 898
  for pemphigus foliaceus, 658, 658t
  for porphyria cutanea tarda, 1759
  for venulitis, cutaneous, 588
Hydroxylase deficiency, and adrenal
  hyperplasia, with hirsutism, 1854
Hydroxylysine deficiency, in Ehlers-Danlos
  syndrome, 1775, 1776t, 1777
Hydroxymethylbilane, in heme biosynthesis,
  in porphyria, 1753, 1754, *1755*
17-Hydroxyprogesterone, in adrenal
  hyperplasia, with hirsutism, 1854
Hydroxysteroid dehydrogenase, in hair
  follicle growth, 1249, *1249*
Hydroxyurea, for hypereosinophilic
  syndrome, 357, *357*
  for psoriasis, 310
Hydroxyzine, for nummular dermatitis, 213,
  213t
  for urticaria, 402
Hydrozoa stings, 790–791, 794t
Hylesia moth, and dermatitis, 810–811
Hymenopteran stings, 807t, 807–808, 808t
Hyperadrenocorticism, and hirsutism,
  1853–1854
  cutaneous signs of, 1872, 1872t
  topical corticosteroids and, 164, 166
Hypercalcemia, and skin calcification, *1829*,
  1829t, 1829–1831, *1830*, 1831t
Hypercholesterolemia, and xanthoma, 1814,
  1816–1817
Hyperchromasia, definition of, 108
Hypercortisolism, and hirsutism, 1853–1854
Hypereosinophilic syndrome, 352–358
  clinical findings in, 352–354, 353t
  diagnosis of, 355–356, 356t
  pathogenesis of, 354–355
  pathology of, 354
  treatment of, 356–358, *357*
Hyperextensibility, of joints, in Ehlers-Danlos
  syndrome, 866, *866*, 1774–1775, *1775*,
  1777, 1777t
Hypergranulosis, definition of, *107*, 108
Hyperhidrosis, clinical findings in, 1311
  definition of, 1311
  differential diagnosis of, 1312t,
    1312–1314, *1313*
  pathogenesis of, 1307–1308, 1311–1312
  tooth abnormalities with, 1324t
  treatment of, *1314*, 1314–1317, *1315*,
    1316t
Hyperimmunoglobulin E syndrome, 717t, 721
Hyperkeratosis. See also *Keratosis.*
  definition of, 108
  epidermolytic, 1688–1690, *1688–1690*

Hyperkeratosis (*Continued*)
  genetic mutation in, 63, 1689
  in dermatitis, of palms, 188–191
  in epidermal nevi, 1788–1789, *1789*
  in erythrokeratodermia variabilis, 1698
  in ichthyosis follicularis, 1697
  in peeling skin syndrome, 1699
  in tyrosinemia, 1859, 1859t, *1860*
  palmoplantar, 1703–1706, *1705, 1706,*
    1722t
  subungual, 1298t, 1300–1301
Hyperlipidemia, and coronary artery disease,
  cutaneous signs with, 1878t
  and xanthoma, 1813–1817
  retinoids and, 310, 1815
Hyperostosis, diffuse idiopathic, retinoids
  and, 310
Hyperphosphatemia, and skin calcification,
  1829, 1829t
Hyperpigmentation, 1233–1240, 1234t
  acne and, 462
  chemically induced, 1234t, 1236–1238,
    1237
  in erythema dyschromicum perstans, 1238
  in fixed drug eruption, 420–421, *421*
  in melasma, 1233–1236, *1234, 1235,*
    1235t, 1236t
  in Mongolian spot, 1240
  in nevus of Ito, 1239–1240
  in nevus of Ota, 1239–1240
  postinflammatory, 89t, *91*, 1238–1239
    in pityriasis rosea, 219
  with epidermolysis bullosa, 638
Hyperplasia, definition of, 108
  epidermal, definition of, 107
Hyperprolactinemia, and hirsutism, 1854
Hypersensitivity, and serum sickness,
  417–418
  in drug reactions, 415–417
Hypertension, cutaneous signs of, 1879t,
  1881t
  venous, and leg ulceration, 560, *560*
Hyperthermia, in neonate, 1890
Hyperthyroidism, and alopecia, diffuse, 1275
  with herpes gestationis, 680
Hypertrichosis, topical corticosteroids and,
  166
  vs. hirsutism, 1853, 1855t
Hypertrichosis lanuginosa, 1844, *1844, 1867*
Hypertrophy, definition of, 108
Hyphae, in dermatophytosis, 1049, *1050*
Hypochondriacal psychosis, and delusions of
  parasitosis, 780t, 780–782, 781t
Hypoderma larvae, in furuncular myiasis, 819
Hypodermitis sclerodermaformis (sclerosing
  panniculitis), 603–605, *604*, 605t
  with venous ulcer, of leg, 558–559, *559*
Hypoesthesia, scalp reduction and, 1262
Hypohidrosis, in ectodermal dysplasia, 1714,
  1714, 1721, 1722t, 1723t
Hypomelanosis, guttate, idiopathic, 1228,
  1228t
  in tuberous sclerosis, *1735*, 1735–1736
  of Ito, 1226–1227, *1227*, 1227t
Hyponychium, anatomy of, 40, *40*
Hypopigmentation, 1219–1230
  after lichen striatus, 244, *245*
  in albinism, 1219–1223, 1220t, 1221t,
    1222, 1223t
  in hypomelanosis, idiopathic guttate, 1228,
    1228t
  of Ito, 1226–1227, *1227*, 1227t
  in nevus depigmentosus, 1225–1227, 1226t
  in piebaldism, 1223–1225, *1224*, 1224t,
    1225t

Hypopigmentation (*Continued*)
  in tuberous sclerosis, 1226t, 1226–1228,
    1228t
  in Waardenburg's syndrome, 1225, 1225t
  infection and, 1229–1230
  inflammatory disorders and, 1228–1229,
    1229
Hypoplasia, definition of, 108
Hypopyon, in subcorneal pustular
  dermatosis, 327, *328*
Hypothalamus, in thermoregulation, 54
Hypothyroidism, and alopecia, diffuse, 1275
  and cutaneous mucinosis, 1834t, *1836*,
    1836–1838, *1837*
  and hyperlipidemia, with xanthoma, 1815
  in hypersensitivity syndrome,
    drug-induced, 417
Hypotrichosis, Marie-Unna, 1713–1714

I

Ichthyocrinotoxism, 797
Ichthyosis, 1681–1706. See also *Cornification.*
  acquired, 1682, 1682t
  bullous, 63, 1688–1690, *1688–1690*
  harlequin, 66, *1690*, 1690–1691, *1691*
  in cardio-facio-cutaneous syndrome, 1698
  in Gaucher's disease, 1696
  in neonate, 1896
  in pityriasis rotunda, 1682–1683
  in restrictive dermopathy, 1697
  in Rud's syndrome, 1698
  in Schwachman's syndrome, 1697
  in Sjögren-Larsson syndrome, 1692–1693
  in Zunich-Kaye syndrome, 1697
  lamellar, *1685*, 1685–1688, *1686*
  paraneoplastic, 1846, *1847*
  scale in, 98, *99*
  with chondrodysplasia punctata,
    1695–1696
  with keratitis and deafness, 1694–1695
  X-linked recessive, 1681–1682, *1684*,
    1684–1685
Ichthyosis follicularis, 1697
Ichthyosis hystrix, 1689, *1690*
Ichthyosis linearis circumflexa, alopecia with,
  1693, *1693*
  in Netherton's syndrome, 1691, *1691*, 1692
Ichthyosis vulgaris, *1683*, 1683–1684
  in atopic dermatitis, 196
Iloprost, for Raynaud's phenomenon, 541
Imipramine, for pudendal neuralgia, 1355
Immersion foot, 777–778, 778t, 828
Immune globulin, for toxic shock syndrome,
  933–935
  for varicella-zoster infection, 1081
Immune system, complement deficiency in,
  and systemic lupus erythematosus,
  267–268, 268t
  in allergic contact dermatitis, 167–173,
    168t, *168–170*, 171t, 172t
  in atopic dermatitis, 198, 198–199
  in erythema multiforme, 251
  in graft-versus-host disease, 225–233. See
    also *Graft-versus-host disease.*
  in granuloma annulare, 440–441
  in inflammatory response, 141–143
    adhesion molecules in, 146–150
    cytokines in, 143t–145t, 143–146, 151
  in leprosy, 995t, 996–997
  in papillomavirus infection, 1109
  in photoaging, 739
  in pityriasis rosea, 220
  in scleroderma, 884–885

Immune system (*Continued*)
in sunburn, 737
in systemic lupus erythematosus, 272t, 272–273, 273t
in toxic epidermal necrolysis, 706
in vitiligo, 1211–1212
Langerhans cells in, epidermal, 53
photosuppression of, in tumor development, 1367–1369, *1369*
skin in, 40–41
vasculitides mediated by, 524, 525, 526t
Immunoblastic lymphoma, B-cell, 1664
Immunocytoma, 1663
Immunodeficiency, acquired, 1137–1155. See also *Human immunodeficiency virus infection.*
cytomegalovirus infection in, 1084–1086, 1086t
in neonate, diaper dermatitis in, 1897
papillomavirus infection in, 1105
vs. atopic dermatitis, 199–200, 200t
Immunofluorescent testing, in lupus erythematosus, 270–271
in Lyme borreliosis, 968–969
in lymphogranuloma venereum, 980
in Rocky Mountain spotted fever, 1014–1015, *1015*
Immunoglobulin A, in dermatitis herpetiformis, 693, 694
in erythema elevatum diutinum, 529
in pemphigus foliaceus, 658
in subcorneal pustular dermatosis, 327–329
linear deposition of, and oral lesions, 1333
in bullous dermatosis, 698–702, *699–701*, 700t, 701t
Immunoglobulin E, excess of, and vesicular eruption, in neonates, 717t, 721
Immunoglobulin E–mediated hypersensitivity, in drug reactions, 415–416
Immunoglobulin G, in bullous pemphigoid, 666, *667*, 668
in epidermolysis bullosa acquisita, 686–688, 688t
in herpes gestationis, 681–682
in pemphigus, paraneoplastic, 660–661, *661*
in pemphigus foliaceus, 656
in pemphigus vulgaris, 651, 653, *653*
Immunoglobulin light chains, in amyloidosis, 1818–1820, 1826
Immunoglobulin M, in anti–basement membrane autoantibody dermatosis, in pregnancy, 370
in linear dermatosis, in pregnancy, 370
Immunoglobulins, as adhesion molecules, in inflammatory response, 148–149, 151
in pemphigoid, cicatricial, 675, 676, *676*
in venulitis, cutaneous, 586–588
Immunoperoxidase testing, for herpes simplex virus infection, 123
Immunosuppression, and cancer, 1155
and fungal infection, 1157
and herpes simplex infection, 1156
and papillomavirus infection, 1155–1156
and *Pseudomonas* infection, 1157
and varicella-zoster infection, 1156–1157
for graft-versus-host disease, 232
for keloids, 903
in lymphoma, cutaneous T-cell, 1647
ultraviolet light and, in tumor development, 1367–1369, *1369*
Immunotherapy, for graft-versus-host disease, 230
for melanoma, 1593–1595

Impetiginization, definition of, 108
Impetigo, *920*, 920–921, *921*, 921t
bullous, in staphylococcal scalded skin syndrome, 935, *935*, 936, *936*
crusts in, *97*, 920, *921*
sports-related, 851
vs. subcorneal pustular dermatosis, 329
Impetigo herpetiformis, in pregnancy, *368*, 368–369
Imuran. See *Azathioprine.*
In situ neoplasms, definition of, 108, *108*
Incisional biopsy, technique of, 127
Inclusion cysts, epidermal, 1450–1451, 1451t, *1451–1454*
in amputee dermatitis, 774, 775
Incontinentia pigmenti, 1722t, 1725–1728
alopecia with, *1715*, 1715–1716
clinical findings in, 1725, *1726*
definition of, 1725
diagnosis of, 1726–1728, 1728t
in neonate, 1897
pathogenesis of, 1725–1726
pathology of, 1725, *1727*
tooth abnormalities with, 1324t
treatment of, 1728
Indomethacin, for erythema nodosum, 594
for venulitis, cutaneous, 588
Infant. See also *Neonate.*
acne in, 463
acropustulosis in, 189, 190, 716t, 719–720, *720*, 1896, *1896*
birthmarks in, 1496t, 1496–1506. See also *Birthmarks.*
cornification disorders in, 1683–1698. See also *Cornification* and *Ichthyosis.*
Epstein-Barr virus infection in, 1082
lupus erythematosus in, 265–266, *267*
treatment of, 278
mucinosis in, cutaneous, 1838
seborrheic dermatitis in, 214–217, *215*, 216t, 217t
skin evaluation in, 1891
Infiltrate, definition of, 108
mixed inflammatory cell, definition of, 109
Inflammatio cutis racemosa (livedo reticularis), 831–832, *832*, 832t
in systemic lupus erythematosus, 263
with antiphospholipid antibody syndrome, 1865t, *1866*
Inflammatory cell infiltrate, mixed, definition of, 109
Inflammatory response, adhesion molecules in, 146–151
cytokines in, 143t–145t, 143–146, 151
immune system in, 141–143
in wound healing, *564*, 564–565
leukocyte–endothelial cell adhesion in, sequential step model of, 150–151
neovascularization in, 1493
pathways of, 141–151
Infraorbital nerve, anatomy of, 117
Infrared radiation, and erythema ab igne, *824*, 824–825
cutaneous effects of, 823–824
heat transmission in, 823
Infratrochlear nerve, anatomy of, 117
Infundibular cysts, 1450–1451, 1451t, *1451–1454*
in amputee dermatitis, 774, 775
Infundibulum, of hair follicle, 28, *28*, 30
Ingram technique, in phototherapy, for psoriasis, 313
Inguinal syndrome, in lymphogranuloma venereum, 979, *980*

Injection injury, drug abuse and, 839–840, *840*
Ink, in tattoos, 452–459. See also *Tattoos.*
Insects. See also specific types, e.g., *Fleas.*
as disease vectors, 804, 805t
bites of, 804–807, *805*, 805t, *806*, 807t
bacterial infection of, 943–944, *944*, 947
hypersensitivity to, in human immunodeficiency virus infection, 1144–1145
reaction to, vs. Wells' syndrome, 362
Insulin, in amyloidosis, 1825
Integrins, $\alpha 6\beta 4$, 621
in inflammatory response, 146–148
in keratinocyte attachment, to basement membrane, 59
in keratinocyte differentiation, 62
Intensity theory, of pruritus, 155, 156
Interface dermatitis, 108
Interferons, anti-angiogenic effect of, 1495, 1495t
for Behçet's disease, 390t, 390–391
for hemangioma, of infancy, 1501
for hypertrophic scars, 903
for Kaposi's sarcoma, 1154–1155
for keloids, 903
for lymphoma, cutaneous T-cell, 1654
for lymphomatoid papulosis, 1637
for papillomavirus infection, genital, 1349
for skin carcinoma, 1427–1429, *1428*
in atopic dermatitis, 198–199, 202
Interleukin 2 gene–diphtheria A toxin fusion product, for lymphoma, cutaneous T-cell, 1653
Interleukins, and pemphigus vulgaris, acute, 422–423
for erythroderma, and vascular leak syndrome, 338
in angiogenesis, 1493t, 1495
in atopic dermatitis, *198*, 198–199
in chemotherapy regimens, skin reaction to, 429
in elastin gene expression, 873
in epidermal barrier function, 52
in inflammatory response, 143–145, 143t–145t, 151
in keratinocyte activation, 67–68
in Wells' syndrome, 361
Intertrigo, 776–777, 777t
genital, 1350
Intestine, Crohn's disease, genital ulceration in, vs. chancroid, 975, 975t
Crohn's disease of, oral lesions with, 1334
disorders of, dermatosis-arthritis syndrome with, 375–376, 376t
vs. Behçet's disease, 389t
in Hartnup's disorder, 1768
in linear IgA bullous dermatosis, 700
gluten-sensitive disorder of, with dermatitis herpetiformis, 691, 694–696
large, enlargement of, with hypopigmentation, 1225, 1225t
ulcerative inflammation of, cutaneous signs of, 1872–1874, 1874t, 1875t, *1876*
pyoderma gangrenosum with, 379, 382, 383
Intraepithelial dyskeratosis, hereditary benign, oral lesions in, 1325
Intraepithelial neoplasia, genital, 1340, 1341t, *1352*, 1352–1353
Intravascular coagulation, disseminated, and purpura, 1848, 1865t, *1866*, Plate 15
Involucrin, in keratinocyte differentiation, in granular layer, 63–64

Iodine, in antiseptic solutions, 129, 129t
　with povidone, and wound healing, 566t
　toxicity of, in neonate, 1890, *1890*
Iodophors, in antiseptic solutions, 129, 129t
Iodoquinol, for amebiasis, 1173
Iontophoresis, for hyperhidrosis, *1314*, 1314–1315, *1315*
Iris, Lisch nodules in, in neurofibromatosis, 1730
Iron, deficiency of, and alopecia, diffuse, 1276
　cutaneous signs of, 1873t
　for protoporphyria, erythropoietic, 1757
　in porphyria cutanea tarda, 1759–1760
Iron oxide, in sunscreens, 754
Irritant contact dermatitis. See also *Contact dermatitis.*
　acne treatment and, 472
　occupational, 173–181
　of diaper region, 184, *185*, 186, Plate 1
Irukandji syndrome, 789
Ischemia, cutaneous, paraneoplastic, 1848
　digital, in Raynaud's phenomenon, 537–542, 540t, 541t
Island flaps, after skin cancer excision, 1411, *1411*
Islet cell tumors, and necrolytic migratory erythema, 1843
Isoflavonoids, anti-angiogenic effect of, 1495, 1495t
Isoniazid, for tuberculosis, 989
Isopropyl alcohol, in antiseptic solutions, 129, 129t
Isotretinoin (Accutane). See also *Retinoids.*
　and hyperlipidemia, with xanthoma, 1815
　for acantholytic dermatosis, 343, 343t
　for acne, 468, 470–473, *472*, 472t
　for cellulitis, of scalp, 1282, 1282t
　for ichthyosis, lamellar, 1687
　for lichen planus, 239, 239t
　for lupus erythematosus, discoid, 276
　for lymphomatoid papulosis, 1637
　for photoaging, 741
　for pityriasis rubra pilaris, 334
　for skin carcinoma, 1429–1431
Isthmus, of hair follicle, 28, *28*, 30, *31*
Itching, 154–158. See also *Pruritus.*
Ito's hypomelanosis, 1226–1227, *1227*, 1227t
Ito's nevus, 1239–1240, 1568
Itraconazole, for aspergillosis, 1072
　for blastomycosis, 1067, 1067t
　for candidiasis, 1058t
　for chromoblastomycosis, 1069
　for coccidioidomycosis, 1064
　for dermatophytosis, 1054
　for histoplasmosis, 1065–1066, 1066t
　for pityriasis versicolor, 1040, 1040t
　for *Pityrosporum* folliculitis, 1040t, 1041
Ivermectin, for cutaneous larva migrans, 1182
　for filariasis, 1179
　for loiasis, 1180
　for onchocerciasis, 1178
　for strongyloidiasis, 1183
Ixodid tick bites, 815–816, *816*
　and Lyme borreliosis, 965–966, 970

J

Jadassohn-Lewandowsky syndrome (pachyonychia congenita), oral lesions in, 1325
　palmoplantar keratoderma in, 1706, *1706*
　tooth abnormalities with, 1324t
Jadassohn-Pellizari anetoderma, 910
Jarisch-Herxheimer reaction, 958

Jaws, abscess of, in actinomycosis, 1007, *1008*
　anatomy of, 111–112
　cysts of, in basal cell nevus syndrome, 1742, 1745
　tori of, 1328, *1328*
Jejunoileal bypass surgery, and dermatitis-arthritis syndrome, 375–376, 376t
Jellyfish, larvae of, and seabather's eruption, 792–793, 1186, *1187*, 1187t
　stings of, 787–789, 788t, *789, 790*, 791t
Jessner's lymphocytic infiltrate, 344–346, *345*, 346t
Jessner's solution, in chemical peel, for photoaging, 742t, 743, 744, *744, 745*
Job's syndrome, 717t, 721
Jock itch (tinea cruris), 851, *1048*, 1048–1049, 1052t
Joggers, injuries in, 851, 853
Johanson-Blizzard syndrome, 1783t, 1784
Joints, in alkaptonuria, 1861
　in Ehlers-Danlos syndrome, 866, *866*, 1774–1775, *1775*, 1777, 1777t
　inflammation of. See *Arthritis.*
　pain in, in systemic lupus erythematosus, 265
Jugular vein, anatomy of, 119
Juri flap, for alopecia, *1265*, 1265–1266

K

Kala-azar, 1163–1165
Kalinin, in dermoepidermal junction, 623–624
　in epidermolysis bullosa, 642t, 644
　junctional, 628, 642t, 644
Kallin syndrome, 638
Kallman's syndrome, 1684
Kaposiform hemangioendothelioma, 1499
Kaposi's sarcoma, 1149–1155
　and gastrointestinal hemorrhage, 1875t
　clinical findings in, *1151*, 1151–1153, *1152*
　differential diagnosis of, 1153–1155, 1154t
　epidemiology of, 1149–1151, 1150t, 1151t
　herpesvirus-6 infection in, 1088
　oral lesions in, 1151, 1152, *1152*, 1329
　pathogenesis of, 1153
　pathology of, 1153
　vs. acroangiodermatitis, 1507, 1508, *1508*
　vs. angiosarcoma, 1517
　vs. hemosiderotic hemangioma, 1515–1516
　vs. melanoma, 1587, *1587*, Plate 12
Kasabach-Merritt syndrome, 1498, 1499
Katayama fever, 1186
Kawasaki disease, 1898
　cardiac disorders in, cutaneous signs with, 1878t, *1880*
　rash in, 1124t, 1125t
　vs. toxic shock syndrome, 933, 934t
Keloids, 900–905
　clinical findings in, 900, *901*
　collagen gene defect in, *869*, 869–871
　definition of, 900
　diagnosis of, 902
　in morphea, 896, 897
　pathogenesis of, 901–902
　pathology of, 900, 901, *901*
　treatment of, 902–905, *904, 905*
Kenalog. See *Triamcinolone.*
Keratin(s), as basal cell–specific markers, 60–61, *61*
　basal epidermal, 621
　function of, 7
　gene expression of, 9
　in epidermal differentiation, 47

Keratin(s) (*Continued*)
　in epidermal nevi, 1787–1789
　in epidermolysis bullosa, 626–627, *627*
　in hair, 1246–1247
　in ichthyosis, bullous, 1689
　in infundibular cysts, 1450, *1452, 1543*
　in trichilemmal cysts, 1453, 1454, *1456*
　in Vörner palmoplantar keratoderma, 1704
　pairing of, 7–9
Keratin amyloidosis, 1824–1825
　idiopathic, *1818, 1822*, 1822–1824, *1823*, 1824t, Plate 14
Keratinocytes, 58–70
　activated, 67–68
　cytokines derived from, 145t, 145–146
　differentiation of, in granular layer, 63–66, *65*
　initiation of, 62–63
　nuclear receptors in, 68–70, *69*
　in alopecia areata, 1270, *1270*
　in basal layer, as stem cells, 58–59, *60*
　attachment of, to basement membrane, 59
　in production of basement membrane components, 59
　phenotypes of, 60–61, *61*
　in cornified envelope, 11
　in epidermal structure, 5–9, *8, 10, 14–16*
　in epidermolysis bullosa, 641–643, *642*
　in grafting, for leg ulcers, 569
　in herpes simplex infection, 1076, *1077*
　in immune system, 41
　in melanoacanthoma, 1448, *1448*
　in pigmentation system, *1204*, 1205–1206, *1206*
　in tricholemmoma, 1470, *1470*
　in verruca vulgaris, 1106–1110, *1107, 1108*
Keratitis, rosacea and, 485–486
　with ichthyosis and deafness, 1694–1695
Keratoacanthoma, 1381t, 1381–1383, *1382*
　retinoids for, 1430
Keratoconus, in atopic dermatitis, 197
Keratocysts, of jaw, in basal cell nevus syndrome, 1742, 1745
Keratoderma, in erythroderma, 336
　palmoplantar, 1703–1706, *1705, 1706*
Keratoderma blennorhagicum, in Reiter's syndrome, 322, *323*, 323t
Keratoelastoidosis, 1778
Keratohyalin, in epidermal differentiation, 47, *47*
Keratohyalin granules, in epidermal structure, 6, *14, 15*
　in keratinocyte differentiation, 65
Keratolysis, pitted, 928, *928*
Keratosis. See also *Hyperkeratosis.*
　actinic, 1378–1380, *1379*, 1381t
　assessment of, 98
　chemotherapy and, 429
　retinoids for, 1430
　treatment of, 1395–1396, *1396*
　cryosurgery in, 1395, 1397–1398
　with cornoid lamella, 1701–1703, *1702, 1703*
　assessment of, 97, 98, *98–100*
　follicular, scarring, *1292*, 1292t, 1292–1293
　seborrheic, *92, 93, 1444*, 1444–1446, *1445*, 1445t
　in rosacea, electrodesiccation of, *490*, 490–491
　multiple eruptive, paraneoplastic, 1846
　vs. dermatosis papulosa nigra, 1441
　stucco, 1446–1447, 1447t

Keratosis follicularis (Darier's disease), 1699–1701, *1700, 1701*
  oral lesions in, 1325
  vs. acantholytic dermatosis, 341
  vs. seborrheic dermatitis, 217
Keratosis follicularis spinulosa decalvans, 504, *504*
Keratosis lichenoides chronica, 241
Keratosis pilaris, 503–504
Keratosis pilaris atrophicans, 504, *504*, 1715
Kerion, and scarring alopecia, 1285
Ketoconazole, for blastomycosis, 1067, 1067t
  for candidiasis, 1058, 1058t
    genital, 1346
  for chromoblastomycosis, 1069
  for coccidioidomycosis, 1064
  for dermatophytosis, 1054
  for hirsutism, 1856
  for histoplasmosis, 1065–1066, 1066t
  for pityriasis versicolor, 1040t, 1041
  for *Pityrosporum* folliculitis, 1040t, 1041
  for seborrheic dermatitis, 165, 215, 217, 217t
Ketron-Goodman pagetoid reticulosis, 1641
KF-1 antigen, in dermoepidermal junction, 625
  in epidermolysis bullosa, 642t
KID syndrome, oral abnormalities in, 1324t
Kidney(s), cancer of, metastasis of, to skin, 1674–1675, *1676*
  cyclosporine toxicity to, 311
  disorders of, cutaneous signs with, 1882–1886, 1883t, 1884t, *1885*, 1886t
    in Hartnup's disorder, 1768
    in hypereosinophilic syndrome, 354
    in leprosy, 999
    in polyarteritis nodosa, 519
    in scleroderma, 884, 886
    in syphilis, 952
    in systemic lupus erythematosus, 265, 272t
    in toxic epidermal necrolysis, 706
    in tuberous sclerosis, 1737
  failure of, perforating dermatosis with, 408, *409*
  inflammation of, after impetigo, 921
Kimura's disease, vs. angiolymphoid hyperplasia with eosinophilia, 1513
Kindler-Weary syndrome, 1704–1705
Kinky hair syndrome, Menkes', 866, 1712–1713, *1713*
Klein-Waardenburg syndrome, 1225, 1225t
Klippel-Trenaunay syndrome, 1504–1505, 1799t, *1800*
Knee, synovitis of, in congenital syphilis, 960t
Knuckles, injury to, sports-related, 853
Koebner epidermolysis bullosa, 637, 643
  genetic mutation in, 9, 61–62
  with palmoplantar keratoderma, 1705
Koebner phenomenon, in acquired perforating dermatosis, 408, *409*
  in plaque psoriasis, 296
Köhlmeier-Degos syndrome, 545t, 546t, 551–552
  and gastrointestinal hemorrhage, 1875t
  cardiac disorders with, 1878t
Koilonychia, 1298t, 1301
Koplik's spots, in measles, 1125t, 1126, 1127
Krause end-bulbs, 28
Kveim-Siltzbach test, for sarcoidosis, 436
Kwashiorkor, and alopecia, diffuse, 1276
Kwell (lindane), for louse infestation, 1192, 1194–1195
  for scabies, 1198
    with human immunodeficiency virus infection, 1143, *1143*

Kyphoscoliosis, in Ehlers-Danlos syndrome, 1775
Kyrle's disease, *408*, 408–411, *409*, 410t
  with diabetes, *1870*

L

Labial artery, inferior, anatomy of, 115
Lacerations, from marine environment, 97–798, *798*, 798t
Lacrimal glands, in Sjögren's syndrome, 268, 1863, 1864t
Lacrimal nerve, anatomy of, 117
Lactate dehydrogenase M-subunit deficiency, 1698–1699
Lactic acid, skin sensitivity to, 79
Lamella, cornoid, definition of, 106
Lamellar bodies, epidermal, 6, *47*, 48, *49*
  in keratinocyte differentiation, 65–66
Lamellar collagen, definition of, 108
Lamellar ichthyosis, *1685*, 1685–1688, *1686*
Lamina densa, in dermoepidermal junction, 16, *19*, 22, 618–619
  in epidermolysis bullosa, 642, *643*
Lamina lucida, immunoglobulin A deposition in, and bullous dermatosis, 698, 701, *701*
  in dermoepidermal junction, 15, *19*, 22, *618*, 618–619
  proteinaceous components of, 621–624
  in epidermolysis bullosa, 642, *642*
Laminated orthokeratosis, definition of, 108
Laminins, in dermoepidermal junction, 14–16, *19*, 621–623
Langer-Giedion syndrome, 1714
Langerhans cell histiocytosis, 1610–1614, *1611, 1612*, 1613t, 1614t, Plate 13
  malignant, 1624
  oral abnormalities with, 1324t
  vs. seborrheic dermatitis, 216
Langerhans cells, depletion of, in sunburn, 737
  in allergic contact dermatitis, *169*, 169–173, *170*, 171t
  in atopic dermatitis, *198*, 199
  in embryology, 3–4
  in epidermal structure, 6, *11–13*
  in graft-versus-host disease, 227–228
  in immune system, 40, 53
  in photosuppression, 1368
  in inflammatory response, 142
Langerhans granules (Birbeck granules), in allergic contact dermatitis, *170*, 170–171, 171t
  in embryology, 4
  in epidermal structure, *11–13*
  in histiocytosis, 1612, *1612*
Lanugo hairs, in embryology, 4
  in hypertrichosis, paraneoplastic, 1844, *1844*, *1867*
Large cell acanthoma, vs. stucco keratosis, 1447
Large intestine. See *Intestine.*
Larva migrans, cutaneous, 85, *87*, 1181t, 1181–1182, *1182*
  visceral, in toxocariasis, 1183
Larynx, in epidermolysis bullosa, 639, 645
  papillomatosis of, juvenile, 1106
Laser surgery, for acne scars, 474
  for angiofibromas, in tuberous sclerosis, 1740
  for hemangioma, of infancy, 1499–1500, *1500*
  for hyperpigmentation, postinflammatory, 1239

Laser surgery (*Continued*)
  for hyperpigmented nevi, 1240
  for hypertrophic scars, 904–905
  for Kaposi's sarcoma, 1154
  for keloids, 904–905, *905*
  for melanocytic nevi, 1569t
  for melasma, 1236
  for neurofibromatosis, *1734*, 1734–1735
  for photoaging, 741
  for port-wine stain, 1502, *1502*
  for rosacea, 489
  for skin carcinoma, 1398
  for warts, 1114–1117, 1115t, 1116t
    genital, 1349
  in tattoo removal, 454t–456t, 454–459, *456, 457*
  indications for, 1115, 1115t
Lathyrogenic agents, for hypertrophic scars, 903
  for keloids, 903
Laugier-Hunziker syndrome, oral pigmentation in, 1324–1325
LDA-1, in dermoepidermal junction, 625
Lead, and pigmentation disorders, 422
Leg, amputation of, dermatitis after, 774t, 774–775, 775t
  ulcers of, 558–571. See also *Ulcer(s), of leg.*
Leiner's disease, 214
  vs. Netherton's syndrome, 1692
Leiomyoma, 1522–1523, *1523*
Leiomyosarcoma, 1523–1524, *1524*
Leishmaniasis, 1163–1170
  clinical findings in, 1163–1165, 1164t, *1165*
  definition of, 1163
  diagnosis of, 1167–1169, *1168*, 1168t
  pathogenesis of, 1167, *1167*
  pathology of, 1165–1167, *1166*
  treatment of, 1169–1170, 1170t
  with human immunodeficiency virus infection, 1143
Lennert's lymphoma, 1667
Lens, cataracts of, in atopic dermatitis, 196–197
  radiation exposure and, 837
  damage to, psoralen–ultraviolet radiation therapy and, 315
Lentigines, 89t, *90*, 1561–1563, *1562*, 1562t, Plate 9
  chemical peel for, 743, 746t
  psoralen–ultraviolet radiation therapy and, in treatment of psoriasis, 314
  solar, vs. stucco keratosis, 1447
Lentiginous melanoma, acral, clinical findings in, 1580, *1580*, Plate 11
  pathology of, 1583, *1584*
Lentigo maligna melanoma, clinical findings in, 1579, *1579*, Plate 11
  pathology of, 1582–1583, *1583*
LEOPARD syndrome, 1740, 1878t
Lepidopterism, 810–811
Lepromin skin test, 994, 995t, 1000
Leprosy, 993–1003
  borderline, 995t, 997, 999
  clinical findings in, 994–999, 995t, *996, 997*, Plate 7
  complications of, 997–998
  definition of, 993
  diagnosis of, 1000, 1000t
  epidemiology of, 993–994
  erythema nodosum in, 585, 998, 1002
  indeterminate, 997, 999
  lepromatous, 994–997, 995t, *996, 997*, 999, *999*, Plate 7
  pathogenesis of, 999–1000
  pathology of, 999, *999*, Plate 7
  prevention of, 1003

Leprosy (*Continued*)
   treatment of, 1000–1003, 1001t
   tuberculoid, 994, 995t, *996*, 999, Plate 7
Leptospirosis, vs. toxic shock syndrome, 933, 934t
Leser-Trélat syndrome, paraneoplastic, 1846
   seborrheic keratosis in, 1444
Letterer-Siwe disease, 1610, 1611, 1613
   vs. atopic dermatitis, 200
   vs. seborrheic dermatitis, 216
Leukemia, and pruritus, 1845
   chemotherapy for, skin reaction to, 429
   cutaneous manifestations of, 1670–1673, *1671*, 1673t
   hairy cell, vs. Langerhans cell histiocytosis, 1613
   monocytic, 1623–1624, *1671*, 1671–1672
   oral lesions in, 1330
   Sweet's syndrome with, 1844–1845, *1845*, Plate 14
   vasculitis with, cutaneous, 584
   vs. hypereosinophilic syndrome, 354
   with T-cell lymphoma, in adult, 1666–1668
      treatment of, 1656
Leukeran (chlorambucil), for pemphigus vulgaris, 654t, 655
   with prednisone, for cutaneous T-cell lymphoma, 1653
Leukocyte antigens. See *Human leukocyte antigens.*
Leukocytes, adhesion of, to endothelial cells, 149–151
   elevated level of, in hypereosinophilic syndrome, 352, 354–355
   polymorphonuclear, in plaque psoriasis, 297
Leukocytoclasis, definition of, 108, *108*
   in vasculitis, 584–589, 585t, *585–587*, 586t, 588t
Leukoderma, in piebaldism, 1223, *1224*
Leukokeratosis, oral, in pachyonychia congenita, 1325
Leukonychia, 1303, *1303*
Leukonychia trichophytica, 1048, *1048*
Leukoplakia, definition of, 108
   oral, 1328–1329
      vs. lichen planus, 238, 238t
   oral hairy, Epstein-Barr virus and, 1083, *1083*, 1084, 1148
      in acquired immunodeficiency syndrome, 1336–1337
Leukotriene B$_4$, for psoriasis, 312
Leukotrienes, in mastocytosis, 1605
   in urticaria, 398
Levator anguli oris muscle, anatomy of, 113, *113*
Levator labii superioris muscles, anatomy of, 113, *113*
Lewandowsky's rosacea, 485, 487t, 987
Lice, as vectors of typhus, 1017
   infestation by, 1190–1195, 1191t
      of body, 1190–1191, 1192t
      of scalp, 1191–1193, 1192t
      pubic, *1193*, 1193–1195, *1194*, 1194t, 1195t
Lichen amyloidosus, 86, *1818, 1822*, 1822–1824, *1823*, 1824t, Plate 14
Lichen aureus, 291–293
Lichen myxedematosus, 1832–1833, 1834t, *1835*
Lichen nitidus, *240*, 240–241
   papules in, *92*
Lichen planopilaris, 236, 237, 239
   and scarring alopecia, *1287*, 1287–1288, 1288t

Lichen planus, 235–240, *236, 237*, 238t, 239t,
   clinical findings in, 235–236, *236*, Plate 1
   diagnosis of, 86, *87*, 238, 238t
   epidemiology of, 236
   erosive, vs. Behçet's disease, 389t
   genital, 1350–1351
   malignant transformation in, 236
   natural history of, 236
   of nails, 1302
   oral, 238, 238t, 1331, *1331*
   papules in, *92, 93*
   pathogenesis of, 238
   pathology of, 237, *237*
   treatment of, 238–240, 239t
   vs. erythema dyschromicum perstans, 1238
   vs. plaque psoriasis, 297
   vs. syphilis, 957
Lichen planus–like reaction, to chemotherapy, 430
Lichen sclerosus, genital, *1351*, 1351–1352
   vs. scleroderma, 888t
Lichen sclerosus et atrophicus, 895, *896*, 897, 898
   atrophy in, *100*
   discoloration in, 104, *104*
   in Lyme borreliosis, 967–968
   vs. anetoderma, 911t
   vs. vitiligo, 1214
Lichen scrofulosorum, 985, 986, 988t
Lichen simplex chronicus, 205–206, *206*, 206t
   genital, 1350
   plaques in, *93*
   scale in, *98*
Lichen spinulosus, *505*, 505–506, 506t
   papules in, *93*
Lichen striatus, 244–246, *245*, 246t
Lichenification, definition of, 108–109
   with erythroderma, 336, *337*, Plate 2
Lichenoid drug eruptions, 423
   vs. lichen planus, 238, 238t
Lichenoid graft-versus-host reaction, after marrow transplantation, 230, 231
Lichenoid lesions, definition of, 109
Lichenoid purpura, of Gougerot and Blum, 291–293, *292*
Lidocaine, for Behçet's disease, 390, 390t
   in anesthesia, 130t, 130–131
      for dermabrasion, for acne scars, 476
      for genital biopsy, 1343
      for liposuction, for hyperhidrosis, 1316
Light, exposure to. See *Photo-* entries and *Ultraviolet light.*
   spectrum of, 751, 1364, *1364*
Light chains, in amyloidosis, 1818–1820, 1826
Limbs, hypertrophy of, in Klippel-Trenaunay syndrome, 1505
Lindane, for louse infestation, 1192, 1194–1195
   for scabies, 1198
      with human immunodeficiency virus infection, *1143*
Lindsay's half and half nail, 1301
Linear immunoglobulin A disease, 698–702, *699–701*, 700t, 701t
   oral lesions in, 1333
Linear immunoglobulin M dermatosis, in pregnancy, 370
Linuche unguiculata larvae, and seabather's eruption, 792–793, 1186, 1187t
Lionfish stings, 801–802
Lion's mane jellyfish stings, 788–789
Lip, cleft, with ectodermal dysplasia, 1722t
   Fordyce's spots on, 30–31, 1325
   inflammation of, actinic, 1380

Lip (*Continued*)
   retinoids and, 310
   granulomatous, 1327
   with salivary gland involvement, 1329
   melanotic macules of, 1323–1324
   solar keratosis of, 1380
Lipase, in pancreatic panniculitis, 610, 611
Lipid storage disease, neutral, *1693*, 1693–1694
Lipids, elevated blood level of, and coronary artery diesase, cutaneous signs with, 1878t
   retinoids and, 310, 1815
   in epidermal barrier function, 48–51
   in sebum, in acne, 465–466, 466t
   in stratum corneum, in keratinocyte differentiation, 67
   in xanthoma, 1809, *1811*, 1811–1817, *1812*
Lipoatrophy, *100*, 101, *101*
Lipoblastoma, 1529–1530
Lipodermatosclerosis, 603–605, *604*, 605t
   with venous ulcer, of leg, 558–559, *559*
Lipodystrophy, atrophy in, *100*, 101, *101*
   with diabetes, 1869t
Lipoid proteinosis, oral abnormalities with, 1324t
Lipoma, 1526–1527, *1527*
   blood vessels in, 1526–1527, *1527*
   congenital, 1793
   liposuction for, *1530*, 1530–1531
   pleomorphic, 1528–1529, *1529*
   spindle cell, 1528
Lipomatosis, encephalocraniocutaneous, 1793
Lipomatous nevi, superficial, 1526, 1793, *1793*
Liposarcoma, 1530, *1531*
Liposomes, in treatment of leishmaniasis, 1170
Liposuction, for fat hypertrophy, *1531*, 1531–1534
   for hidradenitis suppurativa, 482–483, *483*
   for hyperhidrosis, 1316–1317
   for lipoma, *1530*, 1530–1531
Lisch nodules, in neurofibromatosis, 1730
Listeriosis, in neonate, 712–713
Livedo reticularis, 831–832, *832*, 832t
   in systemic lupus erythematosus, 263
   with antiphospholipid antibody syndrome, 1865t, *1866*
Livedo vasculopathy, 543–545, *544*, 545t, 546t
Livedoid lesions, in polyarteritis nodosa, 520, 520t, 521
Liver, disorders of, as contraindication to cyclosporine treatment, 311
   cholestatic, and hyperlipidemia, with xanthoma, 1815
      and pruritus, 155t, 158
   in prurigo gravidarum, 369
   cutaneous signs of, 1874, *1877*, 1877t
   in porphyria, *1758*, 1758–1761, *1759*, 1759t, 1760t
   in protoporphyria, erythropoietic, 1757–1758
   toxicity to, methotrexate and, 308–309
   psoralen–ultraviolet radiation therapy and, 315
   retinoids and, 310
Lobular panniculitis, definition of, 109
Loiasis, 1180
Loricrin, in keratinocyte differentiation, 64
Lotrisone, for vulvar disorders, *1357*
Louis-Bar syndrome, 1802t, *1804*
Louse. See *Lice.*
Lovastatin, for hyperlipidemia, with xanthoma, 1816–1817
Loxosceles reclusa bites, *811*, 811–812, *812*

Lucio's phenomenon, 998, 1003
Ludwig classification, of androgenetic
    alopecia, 1250, *1252*
Lung(s), cancer of, metastasis of, to skin,
    1674, *1675*, 1677
  disorders of, cutaneous signs with, 1877,
    1882t, *1883*
  in actinomycosis, 1008
  in Churg-Strauss syndrome, 523, 527
  in Langerhans cell histiocytosis, 1611
  in lymphoma, cutaneous T-cell, 1656
  in sarcoidosis, 435
  in scleroderma, 884, 886
  in tuberous sclerosis, 1737
  in tularemia, 1035
  in Wegener's granulomatosis, 523, 527
Lunula, anatomy of, 36–40, *40*
  disorders of, 1298t, 1301
Lupus erythematosus, 260–278
  and livedo reticularis, *832*
  discoid, and scarring alopecia, *1288*,
    1288–1289, 1289t
    biopsy of, site for, 120t
    clinical findings in, 260, *261*
    diagnosis of, 272, 272t
    oral lesions in, 1332–1333
    pathogenesis of, 271–272
    pathology of, 268–271, *269*, 269t
    treatment of, 274t, 274–276, 275t
    vs. Jessner's lymphocytic infiltrate,
      345–346
  drug-induced, 266–267, 267t, 423
  mucinosis in, 1838, *1838*
  neonatal, 265–266, *267*
    erosions in, 716t, 720
    heart block in, cutaneous signs with,
      1878t, *1880*
    treatment of, 278
  photosensitivity in, 766
  subacute cutaneous, 265, *266*, 274
    treatment of, 278
  systemic, biopsy of, site for, 120t
    cardiac disorders in, cutaneous signs
      with, 1878t
    clinical findings in, 261–265, 262t,
      262–264
    complement deficiency and, 267–268,
      268t
    diagnosis of, 272t, 272–274, 273t
    oral lesions in, 1332
    overlap syndromes with, 268
    pathogenesis of, 271–272
    pathology of, 268–271, 269t, *270*
    photodermatitis in, 84–85, *86*, Plate 1
    renal disease in, cutaneous signs with,
      1883t
    treatment of, 274t, 276–278, 277t
    with malignancy, 1846
  treatment of, 1887t
  types of, 260, 261t
  vasculitis in, 524, 526t
  vs. lichen planus, 238, 238t
  vs. polymorphic light eruption, 760t
  vs. vitiligo, 1213
Lupus panniculitis, clinical findings in, 261,
    262
  pathology of, 269, *270*
  treatment of, 276
Lupus pernio, 434
Lupus vulgaris, 985, *986*, 988, *988*, 988t,
    Plate 7
Lyme borreliosis, 965–970, *966*, 969t, Plate 6
  clinical findings in, *966*, 966–968, Plate 6
  definition of, 965
  diagnosis of, 968–969, 969t

Lyme borreliosis (*Continued*)
  biopsy in, 122–123
  epidemiology of, 965–966
  pathogenesis of, 968
  pathology of, 968
  treatment of, 969t, 969–970
Lymph nodes, in melanoma, 1589, 1592,
    1592
  Kawasaki disease of, 1898
    cardiac disorders in, cutaneous signs
      with, 1878t, *1880*
    rash in, 1124t, 1125t
    vs. toxic shock syndrome, 933, 934t
Lymphadenopathy, angioimmunoblastic,
    1666
  in erythroderma, 336–337
  with sinus histiocytosis, 1617–1619, *1618*,
    1619t
  vs. Langerhans cell histiocytosis, 1613
Lymphadenosis benigna cutis, in Lyme
    borreliosis, 967, 968, 969t
Lymphangiomyomatosis, of lung, in
    tuberous sclerosis, 1737
Lymphatic system, angiosarcoma of, 1516
  in Kaposi's sarcoma, 1152
  in skin, 23
  malformations of, 1496t, 1504, *1504*
  of dermis, 877
  of face, anatomy of, 115, *116*
  of neck, 119
Lymphedema, 554–557, *555*, 555t, 556t
  in filariasis, 1179
  with angiosarcoma, 554, 556, 1516
Lymphoblastic lymphoma, Burkitt-type,
    1664, *1664*
Lymphocyte toxicity assay, in cutaneous
    drug reaction, 414
Lymphocytes, B, in allergic contact
    dermatitis, 167–168
  in inflammatory response, 142
  in Jessner's lymphocytic infiltrate, 344
  in lupus erythematosus, 272
  in lymphoid hyperplasia, 1626–1629
  in lymphoma, 1660–1665. See also
    Lymphoma.
  proliferations of, and pemphigus, 660
  in alopecia areata, 1270, *1270*
  in leprosy, 995t, 996
  in lichen planus, 237, *237*
  in scarring alopecia, 1285t, 1285–1290,
    1286t, *1286–1288*, 1288t–1290t, *1290*
  in venulitis, cutaneous, 588
  increase of, chemotherapy-induced, 429
  T, helper, in atopic dermatitis, *198*,
    198–199
    in allergic contact dermatitis, 167–169,
      168, 169
    in immune system, 40–41
    in inflammatory response, 142
    in Jessner's lymphocytic infiltrate,
      344–345
    in leukemia, adult, cutaneous
      manifestations of, 1670
    in lupus erythematosus, 272
    in lymphoid hyperplasia, 1626–1629
    in lymphoma, 1639–1656. See also
      Lymphoma.
    in photoaged skin, 739
    in scleroderma, 885
    in toxic shock syndrome, 932–933
Lymphocytic infiltrate, Jessner's, 344–346,
    345, 346t
Lymphocytic leukemia, cutaneous
    manifestations of, 1670, *1671*, 1672
Lymphocytic lymphoma, 1663

Lymphocytoma, cutaneous, photosensitivity
    in, 766
  diagnosis of, *94*
Lymphoepithelioid lymphoma, 1667
Lymphogranuloma venereum, 976t,
    979–981, *980*
  vs. chancroid, 975, 975t
  vs. syphilis, 956–957
Lymphogranulomatosis X, 1666
Lymphohistiocytosis, hemophagocytic, 1623
Lymphoid follicles, definition of, 109
Lymphoid hyperplasia, cutaneous,
    1626–1629, *1627*, 1628t, 1629t
Lymphoma, and pemphigus, *659*, 660
  angiotropic, 1664, 1666
  classification of, 1660, 1661t
  cutaneous, B-cell, 1660–1665
    clinical findings in, 1662, *1662*
    definition of, 1660–1662, *1661*
    pathology of, *1662*, 1662–1665, *1664*,
      1665t
    prognosis of, 1662, *1663*
    semimalignant, 1665, 1665t
    treatment of, 1665
  diagnosis of, 1665t, 1667
  etiology of, 1667
  T-cell, 1639–1656
    clinical findings in, 1639–1642,
      1640–1642
    definition of, 1639
    diagnosis of, 1648–1649
    non–mycosis fungoides, 1665–1667,
      1666
    pathogenesis of, 1645t, 1645–1648,
      1647, 1647t
    pathology of, *1642–1644*, 1642–1645
    prognosis of, 1650–1651
    staging of, 1649–1650, *1650*, 1650t
    treatment of, 1651t, 1651–1654
      by stage of disease, 1651, 1651t,
        1654–1656
    vs. actinic reticuloid syndrome, 770,
      770t
  Epstein-Barr virus infection in, 1082, 1083
  follicular, *88*
  follicular center cell, *1662*, 1663–1664
  follicular mucinosis with, 1289–1290
  histiocytic, 1623–1624
    and panniculitis, 612–613
  Hodgkin's, and hyperhidrosis, 1312
    vs. lymphomatoid papulosis, 1632, *1633*,
      1634, 1635t, 1637
  immunoblastic, 1664
  in immunosuppressed patient, 1155
  Ki-1–positive, 1666
    vs. lymphomatoid papulosis,
      1634–1637, 1635t
  lymphocytic, 1663
  lymphoepithelioid, 1667
  oral lesions in, 1329
  papulosis with, lymphomatoid, 1631–1632
  subcuticular, *94*
  with human immunodeficiency virus
    infection, 1155
  with leukemia, adult T-cell, 1666–1668
Lymphomatoid granulomatosis, 1667
  pulmonary disease in, cutaneous signs
    with, 1882t
Lymphomatoid papulosis, *92*, 1631–1637
  clinical findings in, 1631–1632, *1632*
  definition of, 1631
  diagnosis of, 1634–1637, 1635t
  pathogenesis of, 1633–1634
  pathology of, 1632, *1633, 1634*
  treatment of, 1636t, 1637

Lymphomatoid papulosis (*Continued*)
  vs. pityriasis lichenoides, 257–258, 1634, 1635t
Lymphomesenteric cysts, in basal cell nevus syndrome, 1743
Lymphonodular pharyngitis, 1335t
Lymphoproliferative disorders, and xanthomatosis, 1815
  pyoderma gangrenosum with, 380, 380t
Lymphotoxin, in inflammatory response, 144–145
Lyngbya majuscula, and dermatitis, 795–796
Lysosomal storage disorders, in Gaucher's disease, 1696
Lysyl hydroxylase, in Ehlers-Danlos syndrome, 866, 1775, 1776t, 1777

M

Macrocomedones, cautery for, 471–472
Macroglossia, in amyloidosis, 1328
Macrophage colony-stimulating factor, in inflammatory response, 145
Macrophages, dermal, 878
  in leprosy, 995t, 996–997
  in wound healing, 564, 564–565
  in xanthoma, 1809, 1811, *1811*
Macular amyloidosis, *1822*, 1822–1824, 1824t
Macule(s), assessment of, 88–89, 89t, *89–92*
  café-au-lait, 1563
    in neurofibromatosis, 1730, *1731*, 1732, 1735
    genital, diagnosis of, 1342, 1342t
  hypomelanotic, in tuberous sclerosis, *1735*, 1735–1736
  in erythema dyschromicum perstans, 241
  in graft-versus-host disease, 226, *227*, 227t, Plate 1
  in leprosy, 994, *996*, Plate 7
  in leukemia cutis, *1671*
  in Peutz-Jeghers syndrome, 1797t, *1798*
  in syphilis, 950, *950*
  melanotic, oral, 1323–1324
  of nail bed, in psoriasis, 1297
Maculopapular lesions, definition of, 109
Madelung's disease, 1526
Madurella infection, and mycetoma, 1069, 1070, 1071t
Maffucci's syndrome, 1506, 1799t
Maggot infestation, furuncular, 818–820, *819*
  of wounds, 820, *820*
Magnetic resonance imaging, of neurofibromatosis, 1732–1733
Majocchi purpura annularis telangiectodes, 291
Major histocompatibility complex, in allergic contact dermatitis, 168–170
  in herpes gestationis, 682–683
  in inflammatory response, 142
  in marrow transplantation, 226
  in toxic shock syndrome, 932–933
Mal de Meleda, 1705
Malar eminences, rash over, in lupus erythematosus, 262, *262*, 272t
Malaria, drugs used for. See *Antimalarial drugs.*
Malassezia furfur infection, and folliculitis, 1038t, 1040t, 1041
  and pityriasis versicolor, 1038t, *1039*, 1039–1041, *1040*, 1040t
  in acne, 466, 467
Malherbe's calcifying epithelioma, 1468–1470, *1469*, 1830

Malignancy. See also *Cancer* and specific types, e.g., *Sarcoma.*
  definition of, 109
Malnutrition. See *Diet.*
Mandible, abscess of, in actinomycosis, 1007, *1008*
  anatomy of, 111–112
  cysts of, in basal cell nevus syndrome, 1742, 1745
  tori of, 1328, *1328*
Mandibular branch, of facial nerve, anatomy of, *113*, 116, 116t, 117
Mannans, in dermatophytosis, 1051
Man-of-war stings, 787, 789, 791t
Mansonella streptocerca infestation, 1179
Mantoux test, for tuberculosis, 987
Maple syrup urine disease, 1859t
Marasmus, and alopecia, 1276
Marcaine, in anesthesia, 130, 130t
Marfan's syndrome, elastosis perforans serpiginosa with, 407, *408*
  fibrillin in, 873–874
Marie-Unna hypotrichosis, 1713–1714
Marine life, and skin disorders, 787–802.
  See also *Aquatic skin disorders.*
Marinesco-Sjögren syndrome, 1694
Marrow, disorders of, in hypereosinophilic syndrome, 354
  transplantation of, and graft-versus-host disease, 225–226
    with allogeneic graft, acute reaction in, 226–230, *227*, 227t–229t, *228*, Plate 1
    chronic reaction in, *230*, 230–232, *231*
    with autologous graft, 232–233
Marzola scalp lift, 1263, *1264*
Mast cells, dermal, 877
  in bullous pemphigoid, 668
  in immune dysfunction, *198*
  in urticaria, 396–399, 397t, 398t
  in venulitis, cutaneous, 588
Mastectomy, angiosarcoma after, and lymphedema, 554, 556
Mastocytoma, 1602–1603, *1603*, 1606t
Mastocytosis, 1602–1607
  clinical findings in, 1602–1604, *1603, 1604*, Plate 12
  cutaneous, 88
    in neonate, 716t
  definition of, 1602
  diagnosis of, 1605–1606, 1606t
  pathogenesis of, 1604–1605
  pathology of, 1604, *1605*, Plate 13
  treatment of, 1606–1607, 1607t
Mastoid process, anatomy of, 112
Matrical zone, of follicular bulb, 29, *29*
Mattress suture, vertical, *135*, 135–136
Maturation, of cells, definition of, 109
Maxilla, abscess of, in actinomycosis, 1007, *1008*
  anatomy of, 111
  cysts of, in basal cell nevus syndrome, 1742, 1745
  tori of, 1328
Max-Joseph spaces, in lichen planus, 237
Mazzotti reaction, in onchocerciasis, 1177, 1178
Measles, 1124t, 1125t, 1126–1127, *1127*, Plate 8
  German (rubella), 1124t, 1125t, 1127–1128
  oral lesions in, 1335t
Mebendazole, for enterobiasis, 1184
  for gnathostomiasis, 1184
  for hookworm infestation, 1183

Mebendazole (*Continued*)
  for strongyloidiasis, 1183
  for toxocariasis, 1183
  for trichinosis, 1180
Mechlorethamine, for erythroderma, 339, 339t
  for lymphoma, cutaneous T-cell, 1651–1652
  for lymphomatoid papulosis, 1636t, 1637
Mediterranean fever, familial, and amyloidosis, 1820, 1821
Mediterranean spotted fever, 1012t, 1016–1017
Medroxyprogesterone, anti-angiogenic effect of, 1495
  for hirsutism, 1856
Medulla, of hair, anatomy of, 1247
Megacolon, congenital, with hypopigmentation, 1225, 1225t
Megalopyge opercularis caterpillar, and dermatitis, 809–810, *810*
Megestrol, for hirsutism, 1856
Meglumine antimoniate, for leishmaniasis, 1169
Meibomian glands, 31
Meischer's granuloma, 441, 441t, 442
Meissner corpuscles, 27, *27*
Mel B, for trypanosomiasis, 1175
Melanin, in lesion pigmentation, 103–104
  in skin pigmentation, 11–13, *17, 18*
  protective function of, against ultraviolet radiation, 53
  transfer of, to hair follicles, disorders of, 1717–1718
Melanoacanthoma, *1447*, 1447–1448, *1448*, 1448t
  oral, 1324
Melanoblasts, 1203–1205, *1204*
Melanocytes. See also *Pigmentation.*
  biology of, *1206*, 1206–1207
  embryology of, 1203–1205, *1204*
  histology of, 1205–1206
  in freckles, 1561
  in lentigines, 1561–1563, *1562*, 1562t, Plate 9
  in nevi, 1561–1574. See also *Nevus (nevi), melanocytic.*
  loss of, in vitiligo, 1210–1216. See also *Vitiligo.*
Melanogenesis, ultraviolet light and, 752
Melanoma, 1576–1595
  clinical findings in, 1577–1581, *1578–1581*, Plates 11 and 12
  definition of, 1576
  diagnosis of, 1586–1588, *1587*, 1588t, 1595, Plate 12
  epidemiology of, 1576–1577, *1577*
  genital, 1353
  host response to, 1586
  in situ, 108, *108*
  in xeroderma pigmentosum, 1747
  malignant, oral, 1329–1330
  management of, 1588–1595
    biopsy in, 124, 125, 1589–1590, *1590*
    immunotherapy in, 1593–1595
    in metastatic disease, 1594–1595
    staging in, 1589t, 1590–1591
    surgery in, 1591–1594, *1592*
  metastatic, epidermotropic, diagnosis of, *94*
    management of, 1594–1595
    to skin, 1674
  Mohs micrographic surgery for, 1407–1408, 1592–1593
  p53 tumor suppressor gene mutations in, 1374

Melanoma (*Continued*)
  pathogenesis of, 1586
  pathology of, 1581t, 1581–1586, *1582–1585*
  reporting of, 1588, 1589t
  vs. Langerhans cell histiocytosis, 1613
  vs. melanoacanthoma, 1448
  with human immunodeficiency virus infection, 1149
  with longitudinal melanonychia, 1303–1304
Melanonychia, longitudinal, 1303–1304
Melanophages, definition of, 109
Melanosis, pustular, in neonate, 715t, 718, *719, 1893*, 1895, *1895*
  Riehl's, vs. melasma, 1235
Melanosomes, 11–13, *17, 18*
Melanotic macules, oral, 1323–1324
Melarsoprol, for trypanosomiasis, 1175
Melasma, 1233–1236, *1234, 1235*, 1235t, 1236t
Membrane-coating (lamellar) granules, in epidermal structure, 6, *47*, 48, *49*
  in keratinocyte differentiation, 65–66
Mendes da Costes epidermolysis bullosa, 638
Meningioma, cutaneous, 1547–1549, 1548t, *1549*
Meningitis, syphilitic, 958–959
Meningocele, rudimentary, 1548t
Meningococcemia, rash in, 1124t, 1125t
  skin lesions in, 944
Meningospinal angiomatosis, 1506
Menkes' kinky hair syndrome, 866, 1712–1713, *1713*
Menopause, flushing in, 534, 535
Menstruation, disorders of, androgenetic alopecia with, 1256
  tampon use in, and toxic shock syndrome, 931–932
Mental nerve, anatomy of, 117
Mental retardation, in tuberous sclerosis, 1737
Mentalis muscle, anatomy of, 112, *113*
Mepivacaine, in anesthesia, 130, 130t
Mercury, and pigmentation disorders, 421, 1237
Merkel cell carcinoma, 1391–1393, *1392*, 1392t, 1393t
Merkel cells, in embryology, 3
Merkel nerve endings, 25
Merosin, in dermoepidermal junction, 622, 623
Mesenchymal hamartoma, rhabdomyomatous, 1793–1794
Mesentery, cysts of, in basal cell nevus syndrome, 1743
Metabolic disorders, and alopecia, 1712–1713, *1713*
  and ichthyosis, 1682, 1682t
  in alkaptonuria, 1859t, 1861
  in argininosuccinic aciduria, 1859t, 1860–1861
  in biotin deficiency, 1859t, 1861
  in Gaucher's disease, 1766–1767, 1767t
  in Hartnup disease, 1768, 1859t, 1862
  in homocystinuria, 1859t, 1861
  in phenylketonuria, 1858, 1859t, *1860*
  in prolidase deficiency, 1859t, 1862
  in tyrosinemia, 1859t, 1859–1860, *1860*
  vs. atopic dermatitis, 199–200, 200t
Metastasis, definition of, 109
  of melanoma, *94*, 1594–1595, 1674
  to skin, 1674t, 1674–1677, *1675, 1676*, 1677t
    in neonate, 1898
Methacholine, in diagnosis, of urticaria, 400

Methotrexate, for acantholytic dermatosis, 343
  for Behçet's disease, 390, 390t
  for dermatomyositis, 289
  for erythroderma, 339, 339t
  for keloids, 903
  for lymphoma, cutaneous T-cell, 1654
  for lymphomatoid papulosis, 1636t, 1637
  for polychondritis, relapsing, 514, 514t
  for polymyositis, 289
  for psoriasis, 307–309, 316
  for Reiter's syndrome, 325, 325t
Methoxypsoralen. See also *Psoralens.*
  with ultraviolet radiation, for lichen planus, 239, 239t
    for psoriasis, 313–315
    for vitiligo, 1214–1215
Methylprednisolone, for bullous pemphigoid, 670
  for Churg-Strauss syndrome, 527
  for dermatomyositis, 288
  for Langerhans cell histiocytosis, 1614
  for polyarteritis, microscopic, 527
  for polymyositis, 288
  for pyoderma gangrenosum, 383t, 384
  for Wegener's granulomatosis, 527
Metronidazole, for amebiasis, 1173
  for bowel-associated dermatosis-arthritis syndrome, 376, 376t
  for dracunculosis, 1181
  for rosacea, 488
  for trichomoniasis, 1177
  for vaginosis, bacterial, 1344
Mibelli's angiokeratoma, 1514, *1514*
Mibelli's porokeratosis, 1701–1703, *1702, 1703*
Microabscesses, in psoriasis, of nails, 1297
  Munro's, 109
  Pautrier's, 109
Micrococcus sedentarius infection, in pitted keratolysis, 928
Micrococcus species, in normal cutaneous flora, 926
β_2-Microglobulin, in amyloidosis, 1821
Micrografting, of hair, *1260*, 1260–1261, *1261, 1263*
Microsporum infection, 1043–1049, 1044t, *1049*
Microvesiculation, definition of, 109
Midges, as vectors of streptocerciasis, 1179
Miescher-Melkersson-Rosenthal syndrome, oral lesions in, 1327
Miescher's radial granulomas, in erythema nodosum, 592, *593*
Milia, 1451–1452, *1455*
  after chemical peel, 746
  colloid, diagnosis of, *94*
    vs. amyloidosis, 1820, 1820t
  vs. acne, 469
Miliaria, in neonate, 715t, 718–719, *1893*, 1896
  vs. polymorphic light eruption, 760t
Miliary tuberculosis, 985, 988, 988t
Milker's nodule, 1097–1098
Millepora alcincornis stings, 791
Milroy's disease, 555–556
Mini-micrografting, of hair, *1260*, 1260–1261, *1261, 1263*
Minocycline, and pigmentation disorders, 422, 1237, *1237*
  anti-angiogenic effect of, 1495
  for acne, 471, 471t
  for acne keloidalis nuchae, 1283, 1283t
  for bowel-associated dermatosis-arthritis syndrome, 376, 376t

Minocycline (*Continued*)
  for cellulitis, of scalp, 1282, 1282t
  for folliculitis decalvans, 1284, 1284t
  for granuloma inguinale, 979
  for leprosy, 1001
  for *Mycobacterium marinum* infection, 990
  for nocardiosis, 1007, 1008t
  for rosacea, 488
Minoxidil, for alopecia, androgenetic, 1256, 1257
  for alopecia areata, 1271, 1273t, 1274
Mite bites, 813–815, *814, 815*
Mite infestation, burrows in, 101, *102*
  demodectic, in rosacea, 486, *486*, 487
    vs. acne, 469
  in atopic dermatitis, 199
  scabietic, *1195–1197*, 1195–1198, 1197t
    in neonate, 715t, 718, *1893*, 1895, *1896*
    vs. chancroid, 975t
    with human immunodeficiency virus infection, 1143, *1143*
Mite larvae, as vectors of typhus, 1018, *1019*
Mithramycin, flushing reaction to, 430
Mitis variant, of epidermolysis bullosa, 641, *641*
Mitral valve, prolapse of, in pseudoxanthoma elasticum, 1771, 1774
Mitsuda reaction, in leprosy, 994
Mixed connective tissue disease, 268
Mixed inflammatory cell infiltrate, definition of, 109
Mohs micrographic surgery, for basal cell carcinoma, 1393t, 1394, *1394*, 1394t, 1403–1408, *1404–1406*, 1406t
  for dermatofibrosarcoma protuberans, 1557–1558
  for incompletely excised tumors, 1407
  for melanoma, 1407–1408, 1592–1593
  for Paget's disease, extramammary, 1488
  for recurrent tumors, 1407
  for sebaceous carcinoma, 1474
  for subclinically spreading tumors, 1406–1407
  historical aspects of, 1403
  indications for, 1405–1406, *1406*, 1406t
  limitations of, 1408
  technique of, 1403–1405, *1404, 1405*
Moisture, and immersion foot, 776–777, 777t, 828
  and intertrigo, 776–777, 777t
  and nail disorders, 1297, 1302–1303
  and papillomavirus infection, 1104–1105
Moisturizers, in skin care, of face, 80–81
  of hands and body, 82
  natural, 76
Molars. See also *Teeth.*
  mulberry, in congenital syphilis, 960t
Mole, hydatidiform, with herpes gestationis, 683
Molluscum contagiosum, *1098*, 1098–1099
  genital, 1346
  papules in, *92, 93*
  with human immunodeficiency virus infection, 1138–1139, *1139*
Mollusks, envenomation by, 799–800
Mondor's disease, paraneoplastic, 1848
Mongolian spot, 1240, 1568
Monilethrix, alopecia in, 1716, *1717*
Moniliform lesions, definition of, 109
Monkeypox, 1096
Monobenzone, in depigmentation, for vitiligo, 1215
Monochloroacetic acid, and burn injury, 845t

Monoclonal antibodies, fibril-specific, in dermoepidermal junction, 625–626
  in epidermolysis bullosa, 642t
Monocytes, in immune dysfunction, *198*, 199
  in wound healing, 564
  plasmacytoid, in Jessner's lymphocytic infiltrate, 345, 346
Monocytic leukemia, 1623–1624, *1671*, 1671–1672
Mononucleosis, cytomegalovirus in, 1084, 1086t
  Epstein-Barr virus in, 1082–1084, 1083t
  oral lesions in, 1335t
  vs. herpesvirus-6 infection, 1087, 1087t
Monsel's solution, in hemostasis, 133
Montenegro test, for leishmaniasis, 1168–1169
Montgomery's tubercles, 30, *32*
Moon jellyfish stings, 788, *789*
Morbilliform drug eruption, 415
Morphea, 895–899
  clinical findings in, 895–897, *896*
  definition of, 895
  differential diagnosis of, 898, 898t
  in Lyme borreliosis, 967–968
  pathogenesis of, 898
  pathology of, *897*, 897–898
  treatment of, 898–899, 899t
Morphine, injection of, and pruritus, 157–158
Mosquito bites, 805, 805t, 807t
Moths, and dermatitis, 810–811
  larvae of, and dermatitis, *809*, 809–810, *810*
Mouth, biopsy of, 128
  black lesions of, 1323–1325, *1324*
  blue lesions of, 1323–1325, *1324*
  burning syndrome of, 1328
  cancer of, 1329–1330, 1335, 1337t
  dental disorders in. See *Teeth.*
  dermatitis around, 497–498, *498*, 498t
    vs. acne, 469
  dryness of, 1328
  in amyloidosis, 1328
  in Cowden's disease, 1326, 1796, *1797*
  in epidermolysis bullosa, junctional, 639
  in erythema multiforme, 249, 252t, 253
  in herpes simplex infection, 1074–1076, *1075*, 1077t, 1335, 1335t
  in human immunodeficiency virus infection, 1148, 1336–1337, 1337t
  in Kaposi's sarcoma, 1151, 1152, *1152*
  in pemphigoid, cicatricial, 674, *675*
  in pemphigus vulgaris, 651, 652, *652*
  in scleroderma, 883, *883*
  in systemic lupus erythematosus, 263
  in xeroderma pigmentosum, 1747–1748
  infections of, bacterial, 1335, 1336t, 1337t
    fungal, 1335–1336, 1336t
    viral, 1334–1335, 1335t, 1337t
  lichen planus in, 238, 238t, 1331, *1331*
  mucocele of, 1839
  mucous membranes of, disorders of, 1323–1337
  muscles of, anatomy of, 112–113, *113*
  pink lesions in, 1326, *1326*
  premalignant lesions of, 1328–1329
  psoriasis of, 300
  red lesions in, 1325–1326
  tongue lesions in. See *Tongue.*
  tori in, 1328, *1328*
  ulcerative disorders of, 1330–1334, *1331*
  white lesions of, 1325
  yellow lesions of, 1325
Mucha-Habermann disease, 256–258, *257*, 258t

Mucinosis, 1832–1840
  acral persistent, papular, 1833
  dysthyroidotic, 1834t, *1836*, 1836–1838, *1837*
  erythematous, reticular, 1834t, 1834–1836, *1835*
  focal, 1839
  follicular, 1833t, 1839–1840
    and scarring alopecia, 1289–1290, *1290*, 1290t
    definition of, 107
    in lymphoma, T-cell, 1641, 1644
  in eosinophilia-myalgia syndrome, 1839
  in human immunodeficiency virus infection, 1145
  in lichen myxedematosus, 1832–1833, 1834t, *1835*
  in lupus erythematosus, 1838, *1838*
  in scleredema, 1834t, 1836
  in toxic oil syndrome, 1838
  in tuberous myxedema, atypical, 1839
  juvenile, self-healing, 1838
  toxic, 1838–1839
  with neuropathy, 1839
Mucinous carcinoma, of eccrine glands, 1484–1485
Muckle-Wells syndrome, 1820, 1821
Mucocele, 1839
  oral, 1326
Mucocutaneous corpuscles, 28
Mucocutaneous lymph node syndrome (Kawasaki disease), 1898
  cardiac disorders in, cutaneous signs with, 1878t, *1880*
  rash in, 1124t, 1125t
  vs. toxic shock syndrome, 933, 934t
Mucoepithelial dysplasia, hereditary, oral lesions in, 1326
Mucormycosis, oral lesions in, 1335
Mucous cysts, 1839
  periungual, 1299t, 1305
Mucous membranes, oral, disorders of, 1323–1337. See also *Mouth.*
Mucuna pruriens, and pruritus, 155–156
Mud wrestling, and folliculitis, 851, 941
Muehrcke's lines, 1301
Muir-Torre syndrome, 1472
  gastrointestinal hemorrhage in, 1875t
Multinucleate cell hemangioma, 1516
Multiple endocrine neoplasia, oral lesions in, 1327
Münchausen syndrome, child as proxy in, 842
Munro's microabscess, 109
Mupirocin, and wound healing, 566t
  for impetigo, 920–921
  for staphylococcal infection, 922, 923t
  for streptococcal infection, 923t
Murine typhus, 1012t, 1018
Muscles, in hypereosinophilic syndrome, 354
  nevi of, 1793–1794
  of calf, pump function of, in venous ulceration, 560, *560*
  of face, 112–114, *113*
  of neck, 118–119
  pain in, in scleroderma, chemically induced, 891, 892, 892t, *893*
    with eosinophilia, and papular mucinosis, 1839
  tumors of, 1522–1526, *1523–1525*, 1526t
Muscular aponeurotic system, superficial, anatomy of, 114
Muscular dystrophy, with epidermolysis bullosa, 638
Musicians, acne mechanica in, 772

Myalgia, with eosinophilia, and papular mucinosis, 1839
  in scleroderma, chemically induced, 891, 892, 892t, *893*
Myasthenia gravis, with epidermolysis bullosa, 638
Mycetoma, 1069–1071, *1070*, 1070t, 1071t
  in nocardiosis, 1006, *1007*
Mycobacterial infection, with human immunodeficiency virus infection, 991, 1142
Mycobacterial infections, tuberculous, 983–991
Mycobacterium avium infection, 989t, 991, 1142
Mycobacterium chelonei infection, 989t, 991
Mycobacterium fortuitum infection, 989t, 991
Mycobacterium kansasii infection, 989t, 990–991, 1142
Mycobacterium leprae infection, 993–1003. See also *Leprosy.*
Mycobacterium marinum infection, 989t, 990, *990*, 1142, Plate 7
Mycobacterium scrofulaceum infection, 991
Mycobacterium ulcerans infection, 989t, 990
Mycoplasma pneumoniae infection, and erythema multiforme, 251, 1882t
Mycosis. See *Fungal infection.*
Mycosis fungoides. See also *Lymphoma, cutaneous T-cell.*
  and hypopigmentation, 1229, *1229*
  atrophy in, *101*
  chemical exposure and, 1648
  clinical findings in, 1639, 1641
  diagnosis of, 1648
  follicular mucinosis with, 1289
  treatment of, 1887t
  vs. lymphomatoid papulosis, 1632, 1634, *1634*
  vs. small plaque parapsoriasis, 222–224
Myelogenous leukemia, cutaneous manifestations of, 1671–1672
Myelosuppression, methotrexate and, 308
Myiasis, furuncular, 818–820, *819*
  of wounds, 820, *820*
Myrmecia, pathology of, 1107, *1107*
Myxedema, and cutaneous mucinosis, 1834t, *1836*, 1836–1838, *1837*
  pretibial, *1872*
    and hyperhidrosis, 1313
    glycosaminoglycans in, 876
  tuberous, atypical, 1839
Myxoid cysts, 1839
  periungual, 1299t, 1305
Myxoid liposarcoma, 1530
Myxoid pseudocyst, 1839
Myxolipomas, 1527
Myxoma, cardiac, cutaneous signs with, 1879t, 1881t
  of nerve sheath, 1541t, *1544*, 1544–1545, *1545*

N

Nadolol, for flushing, 535
Naegeli-Franceschetti-Jadassohn syndrome, 1705
Nafcillin, for staphylococcal infection, 923t
  for streptococcal infection, 923t
Nail(s), anatomy of, 1295, *1296*
  candidiasis of, 1057t
  disorders of, clinical findings in, 1296–1297, *1297*
    in dyskeratosis congenita, 1796t, *1798*

Nail(s) (*Continued*)
in ectodermal dysplasia, 1721, 1722t, 1723t
dystrophy of, chemotherapy and, 427
embryology of, 5
fibromas around, in tuberous sclerosis, 1736, 1740
fungal infection of, *1047*, 1047–1048, *1048*, 1050, 1052t, 1057t
growth of, 1295
in Darier's disease, 1699–1700, *1700*
ingrown, 1299t, 1304–1305
pigmentary disorders of, *1303*, 1303–1304
psoriasis of, 300, 316, 1297, *1300*
Nail bed, anatomy of, 40, *40*, 1295, *1296*
disorders of, 1297–1301, 1298t, 1299t, *1300*
papillary adenoma of, 1481–1482
Nail folds, anatomy of, 36–40, *40*, 1295, *1296*
disorders of, 1299t, 1304–1305
in dermatomyositis, 285
embryology of, 5
Nail plate, anatomy of, 36, *40*, 1295, *1296*
disorders of, 1298t, 1299t, 1301–1303
embryology of, 5
Nail-patella syndrome, renal disease with, 1884t
Nairobi medium, in diagnosis of chancroid, 975
Napkin (diaper) dermatitis, 184–187, *185*, 185t, 186t, 1896–1897, Plate 1
candidiasis and, 1057t
in adults, 776, 777
Naproxen, and pseudoporphyria, *1864*
Nasal nerve, dorsal external, anatomy of, 117
Nasalis muscle, anatomy of, 113, *113*
Nattrassia infection, vs. tinea pedis, 1046
Natural killer cells, in graft-versus-host disease, 227–229
Natural moisturizing factor, 76
Necator americanus infestation, 1183
Neck, anatomy of, blood supply in, 119
lymphatic system in, 119
muscles in, 118–119
nerves in, *118*, 119
topographic, 117–118, *118*
Necrobiosis, rheumatoid, 444, *445*
Necrobiosis lipoidica, 446t, *447*, 447–448, *448*, Plate 4
Necrobiosis lipoidica diabeticorum, 1869t, *1870*, Plate 15
Necrobiotic xanthogranuloma, 446t, 448–450, *449*
Necrolysis, epidermal, toxic, 704–710. See also *Toxic epidermal necrolysis.*
Necrolytic migratory erythema, 1843–1844, *1844*, *1868*
Necrosis, anticoagulant-induced, *419*, 419–420, 545t, 546t, 550
definition of, 109
Necrotizing fasciitis, 942, 942t, 945–946
genital, 1344
Necrotizing sialometaplasia, 1333
Necrotizing vasculitis, 584–589, 585t, *585–587*, 586t, 588t
Neisseria gonorrhoeae infection, skin lesions in, *944*, 944–945
Nematocysts, in cnidarian stings, 788, 791t
Nematode infestations, *1177*, 1177–1184, *1178*, 1181t, *1182*
Neodymium:YAG laser, in tattoo removal, 455t, 458
Neomycin, and wound healing, 566t
Neonate. See also *Child* and *Infant.*
aplasia cutis in, 1782t, 1782–1785, 1783t, *1784*, 1785t

Neonate (*Continued*)
blistering disorders in, 712, 713t–717t
infectious, 712–718, 713t–715t
transient, 715t, 719, *719*
uncommon, 713t, 716t, 717t, 719–721, *720*
congenital skin anomalies in, minor, 1894
cornification disorders in, 1683–1698. See also *Cornification* and *Ichthyosis.*
dermatoses in, evaluation of, *1893*
vascular, transient, 1892–1894
erythema toxicum in, 715t, 718, 1894–1895, *1895*
growth of, 1889
herpes simplex infection in, 714–718, 715t, 1075, 1895, *1895*
lupus erythematosus in, 265–266, *267*, 278, 716t, 720
heart block in, cutaneous signs with, 1878t, *1880*
nodules in, 1898, *1898*
panniculitis in, 1897–1898
pustular disorders in, 712, 713t–717t, *1893*, 1894–1896, *1895*, *1896*
infectious, 712–718, 713t–715t
transient, 715t, 718–719, *719*
uncommon, 713t, 716t, 717t, 719–721, *720*
scaly dermatoses in, 1896–1897
sclerema in, 599–600, *600*, 600t
skin in, barrier function of, 1889–1890, *1890*
care of, 1890
normal, 1889
subcutaneous fat necrosis in, *600*, 600–602, *601*, 601t
syphilis in, 957t, 959, 960t, 1324t
thermoregulation in, 1890–1894
topical drug use in, 1890, *1890*
toxoplasmosis in, 1175, *1175*
vesicobullous eruptions in, 1897
Neoplasms. See *Cancer* and *Tumor(s).*
Neovascularization, inflammation and, 1493
Nephr-. See *Kidney(s).*
Nerve(s). See also *Neur-* entries.
disorders of, in leprosy, 994, 995t, 996, *996*, 998, 1003
in varicella-zoster virus infection, 1078–1081
melanoma of, 1580, 1585
neuroma of, 1537–1539, *1538*, *1539*, 1541t, 1542t
of face, *113*, 116t, 116–117
tumors of, classification of, 1536, 1537t
histogenesis of, 1536–1537
Nerve sheath, fibromas of, 1540–1544, 1541t, 1542t, *1543*
granular cell tumor of, 1541t, 1545–1546, *1546*
malignant tumor of, 1546, *1546*
myxoma of, 1541t, *1544*, 1544–1545, *1545*
schwannoma of, 1539–1540, *1540*, 1541t, 1542t
Nerve tissue, ectopic, tumors of, 1546–1549, *1547*, 1548t, *1549*
Nervous system, ablative surgery of, for hyperhidrosis, 1308
central, in Behçet's disease, 386
in syphilis, 957t, *958*, 958–959
with human immunodeficiency virus infection, 960, 961
in systemic lupus erythematosus, 265, 272t
in tuberous sclerosis, 1737, 1738, 1739t
in hypereosinophilic syndrome, 353–354
in Langerhans cell histiocytosis, 1611

Nervous system (*Continued*)
in Lyme borreliosis, 967
in lymphoma, cutaneous T-cell, 1656
in pruritus, 154–157
in skin, 23–28, *25–27*
in Sturge-Weber syndrome, 1505
in sweat gland function, 1308
in thermoregulation, 54
in xeroderma pigmentosum, 1747, 1748t, 1750
injury to, and hyperhidrosis, 1308
Netherton's syndrome, *1691*, 1691–1692, *1692*
alopecia with, 1716, *1716*
vs. atopic dermatitis, 200
Neu-Laxova syndrome, 1696–1697
Neuralgia, pudendal, *1355*, 1355–1356
Neurilemmoma, 1539–1540, *1540*, 1541t, 1542t
Neuroblastoma, cutaneous, 1547–1549, 1548t, *1549*
Neurocutaneous syndromes, 1729, 1730t
Neuroepithelioma, peripheral, 1547
Neurofibroma, solitary, 1540–1544, 1541t, 1542t, *1543*
vs. anetoderma, 911t
Neurofibromatosis, clinical features of, cutaneous, 1729–1730, *1730*
extracutaneous, 1730–1731
complications of, 1731, 1731t
definition of, 1729
diagnosis of, 1732–1733, 1732t–1734t, *1733*
hypertension in, cutaneous signs with, 1879t
pathogenesis of, 1732
pathology of, 1732
progression of, 1731
renal disease in, cutaneous signs with, 1883t
treatment of, 1733–1735, *1734*
vs. solitary neurofibroma, 1540
Neurofibrosarcoma, 1546, *1546*
Neurolemmoma, 1539–1540, *1540*, 1541t, 1542t
Neuroma, palisaded encapsulated, 1537–1539, *1538*, *1539*, 1541t, 1542t
traumatic, 1537, *1538*, 1541t, 1542t
Neuronopathy, in Gaucher's disease, 1766, 1767t
Neuropathia mucinosa cutanea, 1839
Neuropathy, amyloidotic, familial, 1821
Neuropeptide Y, in perniosis, 829
Neurosarcoma, 1546, *1546*
Neurosyphilis, 957t, *958*, 958–959
with human immunodeficiency virus infection, 960, 961
Neurothekeoma, 1541t, *1544*, 1544–1545, *1545*
Neurotic excoriations, 780t, 781t, *783*, 783–784
Neurotropic ulcer, with diabetes, 1870t, *1871*
Neurotropism, definition of, 109
Neutral lipid storage disease, *1693*, 1693–1694
Neutropenia, cyclic, oral lesions in, 1334
Neutrophilic dermatosis, in bowel-associated dermatosis-arthritis syndrome, 375–376, 376t
in Sweet's syndrome, 372–375, *373*, 373t–375t, Plate 3
rheumatoid, 376–377
Neutrophils, in wound healing, 564
Nevoid lesions, definition of, 109
Nevus (nevi), balloon cell, 1566
basal cell, 1742–1745, *1743*, *1744*, 1745t, 1796t, *1797*
infundibular cysts with, 1450–1451

Nevus (nevi) (*Continued*)
  blue, 1568, *1568*, Plate 10
  blue rubber bleb, 1505, 1799t
    gastrointestinal hemorrhage with, 1874t
  connective tissue, vs. anetoderma, 911t
  dermal, *92*, 1792–1793, *1793*
  desmoplastic, 1566
  differential diagnosis of, 1565–1569,
    1566t, *1566–1568*, Plate 10
  elastic tissue, 1792
  epidermal, 1787–1790, *1788*, 1788t, *1789*,
    1790t
    differential diagnosis of, 1441, 1442t
    vs. lichen striatus, 245–246
    vs. stucco keratosis, 1447
  halo, 1566–1567, 1588
  in albinism, 1220t, 1221t, 1223t
  melanocytic, 1561–1574
    and melanoma, 1580, 1586
    atypical, 1571–1574, *1572, 1573*, 1588,
      Plates 10 and 11
    benign, chemotherapy and, 430
      vs. malignant, 1569
    clinical findings in, 1563–1565, *1564,
      1565*, Plates 9 and 10
    congenital, 1569
    treatment of, 1569t, 1569–1571, *1570,
      1571*
    vs. melanoma, 1587–1588, 1588t
  muscular, 1793–1794
  of Ito, 1239–1240, 1568
  of Ota, 89t, *92*, 1239–1240, 1568
  oral, 1324–1325
  pathogenesis of, 1565
  penetrating, deep, 1568–1569
  persistent, *1567*, 1567–1568
  sebaceous, 1790t, 1790–1792, *1791*
  Spitz, 1566, *1566, 1567*, Plate 10
    multiple, configuration of, *87*
  sponge, white, 1325
  subcutaneous, 1793–1794
Nevus anelasticus, 1792
Nevus araneus, 1509
Nevus comedonicus, 1792
Nevus depigmentosus, 1225–1227, 1226t
Nevus flammeus, 1496t, 1501–1502, *1502*,
  1505, 1506
Nevus lipomatosus superficialis, 1526, 1793,
  1793
Nevus simplex, 1496t, 1502–1503
  vs. port-wine stain, 1501
Nevus spilus, 1567
Newborn. See *Neonate.*
Niacin deficiency (pellagra), cutaneous signs
  of, *1873*, 1873t
  photosensitivity in, 766
  vs. Hartnup's disorder, 1768
Niacinamide, for bullous pemphigoid, 670
  for erythema elevatum diutinum, 530
Nicein, in epidermolysis bullosa, 642t, 644
Nicotinamide, for Hartnup's disorder,
  1768
Nicotine, and stomatitis, 1329
Nicotinic acid, deficiency of, and pellagra,
  photosensitivity with, 766
  for Hartnup's disorder, 1768
Nidogen, in dermoepidermal junction, 15,
  16, 625
Nifedipine, for perniosis, 829
  for Raynaud's phenomenon, 541
    in scleroderma, 887
  for urticaria, 402
Nifurtimox, for trypanosomiasis, 1174
Night blindness, in Refsum's disease, 1695
Nikolsky sign, in pemphigus vulgaris, 652
Nimorazole, for trichomoniasis, 1177

Nipples, frictional injury to, in joggers, 851,
  853
  sebaceous glands of, 30, *32*
Niridazole, for dracunculosis, 1181
Nitrogen mustard, for alopecia areata, 1273t
  for Langerhans cell histiocytosis, 1614
  for lymphoma, cutaneous T-cell,
    1651–1652
Nits, in pediculosis, 1190–1195, 1192t, *1194*
Nix (permethrin), for louse infestation, 1192,
  1194–1195
  for scabies, 1198
Nocardiosis, 1006–1007, *1007*, 1007t, 1008t
  and mycetoma, 1069, 1070, 1071t
Nodular infiltrates, definition of, 109
Nodular melanoma, clinical findings in,
  1579–1580, *1580*, Plate 11
  pathology of, 1583–1584, *1584*
Nodular vasculitis, 594–596, *595, 596*, 597t
Nodule(s), assessment of, 93–94, *94, 95*, 95t
  athlete's, 775t, 775–776, 776t, 851
  dermal, differential diagnosis of, 1464,
    1465t
  genital, diagnosis of, 1342, 1343t
  in acne, 462, *462*
  in amyloidosis, 1819, *1819*, 1822, *1822*,
    1825–1826, *1826*, Plate 14
  in bacillary angiomatosis, 1025, *1025,
    1026*, Plate 8
  in basal cell carcinoma, *1387*, 1387–1389,
    1389
  in chondrodermatitis, 507–510, *508*, 509t,
    510
  in dermatofibroma, 1552, *1553*
  in dermatofibrosarcoma protuberans,
    1555, *1555*, 1556, *1557*
  in erythema elevatum diutinum, 528, *529*
  in erythema induratum, of Bazin, 986,
    987, *987*, Plate 7
  in erythema nodosum, 592, *592*
  in fibroxanthoma, atypical, 1558, *1558*
  in Kaposi's sarcoma, 1151, *1152*
  in leprosy, 994, *996*
  in leukemia cutis, 1670, 1671, *1671*
  in lymphoma, T-cell, *1640*, 1642, *1642*
  in lymphomatoid papulosis, 1631, *1632*
  in mucinosis, in lupus erythematosus,
    1838, *1838*
  in mycetoma, 1069, *1070*
  in necrotizing vasculitides, *523*, 524, *526*
  in neonate, *1893*, 1898, *1898*
  in pale cell acanthoma, 1442, *1442*
  in pancreatic panniculitis, 610, *610*
  in prurigo, *207*, 207–208, 208t
  in rosacea, 485, *486*, Plate 4
  in sporotrichosis, 1062, *1062*
  in squamous cell carcinoma, 1383, *1384*
  in subcutaneous fat necrosis, of newborn,
    600, *600, 601*
  in syphilis, 951, *951*, 953, *953*
  in trichomycosis axillaris, 927, *928*
  Lisch, in neurofibromatosis, 1730
  milker's, 1097–1098
  of ear, differential diagnosis of, 509, 509t
  pseudorheumatoid, 438
  rheumatoid, 444–447, *445, 446*, 446t
    in systemic lupus erythematosus, 264
  subcutaneous, differential diagnosis of,
    1464, 1465t
  subependymal, in tuberous sclerosis, 1737
Nonsteroidal anti-inflammatory drugs, for
  lupus erythematosus, systemic, 277
  in psoriasis, 301
Norethindrone, for alopecia, androgenetic,
  1257
Norpramin, for neurotic excoriations, 784

Nose, carcinoma of, excision of, skin grafting
  after, 1421–1422, *1422–1424*
  glioma of, *1547*, 1547–1549, 1548t
  in leprosy, 998–999
  in trichorhinophalangeal syndrome, 1714
  muscles of, anatomy of, *113*, 113–114
  rosacea of, 485, *486*, Plate 4
  electrosurgery for, *493*, 493–496, *495*
Notalgia paresthetica, 208–209, 209t
Novocain, in anesthesia, 130, 130t
Nuclear matrix acceptor protein, in hair
  follicle growth, 1249
Nuclear receptors, in keratinocyte
  differentiation, 68–70, *69*
Nummular dermatitis, clinical findings in,
  211, *212*
  configuration of, *87*
  diagnosis of, 212, 212t
  of hands and feet, 188, 190, 191
  pathogenesis of, 212
  pathology of, 211
  treatment of, 212–213, 213t
  vs. atopic dermatitis, 199
  with human immunodeficiency virus
    infection, 1146
Nutrition. See *Diet.*
Nystatin, for candidiasis, 1058, 1058t, 1336

O

Obesity, and hidradenitis suppurativa, 482
Obsessive-compulsive disorder, and
  trichotillomania, 782–783
Occipital horn syndrome, 1775, 1776t
Occipital nerve, lesser, anatomy of, *118*, 119
Occipitoparietal scalp lift, 1263, *1264*
Occlusive agents, for dry skin, 77
Occupational exposure, and contact
  dermatitis, 173–181. See also *Contact
  dermatitis.*
  to chemicals, and burns, 843–847, 844t,
    845t
  and lymphoma, 1648
Ochronosis, exogenous, vs. melasma, 1235
Octopus bites, 800
Octyl salicylate, in sunscreens, 754
Oculocerebrocutaneous syndrome, 1784
Oculoglandular syndrome, in
  trypanosomiasis, 1173, *1173*
Odland (lamellar) bodies, in epidermal
  structure, 6, *47*, 48, *49*
  in keratinocyte differentiation, 65–66
Odor, axillary, bacterial flora and, 927–928
  in bromhidrosis, 1317
Ogna epidermolysis bullosa simplex, 638
Oil drop sign, in psoriasis, of nails, 1297
Oil toxicity, and mucinosis, 1838
  and scleroderma, 891, 892t
Olmsted's syndrome, 1704
Omenn's syndrome, vs. Netherton's
  syndrome, 1692
Onchocerciasis, *1177*, 1177–1179, *1178*
Oncogenes, in inflammatory response, 145
  in papillomavirus infection, 1110–1111
  in ultraviolet-induced carcinogenesis,
    1369–1372, *1370*, 1370t, *1371*
Onychodystrophy, chemotherapy and, 427
  in dyskeratosis congenita, 1796t, *1798*
  in psoriasis, 300
Onychogryphosis, 1298t, 1299t, 1301
Onycholysis, 1297–1300, 1298t, 1299t, *1300*
Onychomycosis, candidiasis and, 1057t
  clinical findings in, *1047*, 1047–1048, *1048*
  diagnosis of, 1297
  differential diagnosis of, 1052t
  pathology of, 1050

Onychorrhexis, 1302
Ophthalmic artery, branches of, anatomy of, 115
Opioid drugs, injection of, and pruritus, 157–158
Oral mucosa. See *Mouth.*
Orap, for delusions of parasitosis, 781, 782
Orbicularis oculi muscle, anatomy of, *113,* 114
Orbicularis oris muscle, anatomy of, 113, *113*
Orbit, erythema of, in dermatomyositis, 284, *284,* Plate 2
   hemangioma of, in infant, 1500–1501
   muscles of, anatomy of, *113,* 114
Orf, *1097,* 1097–1098
Organoid nevus, 1790
Oriental sore, 1163
Oriental spotted fever, 1012t, 1016
Ornidyl, for trypanosomiasis, 1175
Ornithonyssus bites, 813–814, *814, 815*
Oroya fever, 1024, 1024t, 1026, 1028
Orthokeratosis, compact, definition of, 106
   definition of, 109
   laminated, definition of, 108
   scale in, *98*
Orthopoxvirus infection, 1093–1096, *1094,* 1094t, 1095t
Osler-Weber-Rendu syndrome, 1799t, *1800,* 1882t
   gastrointestinal hemorrhage in, 1874t, *1876*
Osmidrosis, 1317
Ossification, cutaneous, 1828, 1829t, 1830–1831, 1831t
Osteodystrophy, Albright's hereditary, 1828, 1829t
Osteolysis, in Gorham's syndrome, 1506
Osteoma cutis, 1828, 1829t, 1831, 1831t
Osteonectin, in dermoepidermal junction, 625
Ota's nevus, 89t, *92,* 1239–1240, 1568
Otitis externa, in swimmers, 851, 853
   Pseudomonas aeruginosa infection and, 940, *941,* Plate 6
Ovaries, cancer of, metastasis of, to skin, 1674, *1676*
   fibromas of, in basal cell nevus syndrome, 1743
   polycystic, and hirsutism, 1853
   tumors of, and hirsutism, 1853
Overweight, and hidradenitis suppurativa, 482
Oxacillin, for staphylococcal infection, 923t
   for streptococcal infection, 923t
Oxsoralen. See also *Psoralens.*
   for dermatitis, of hands and feet, 192
Oxybenzone, and photoallergy, *729,* Plate 5
   in sunscreens, 754
Oxygen, in free radicals, and facial skin damage, 52–53, 80–81
   in photodynamic therapy, for skin carcinoma, *1425,* 1426
   in wound healing, 566
Oxytalan fibers, in dermal structure, 17
Oxytetracycline, for acne, 471t
Oysters, *Vibrio vulnificus* contamination of, 942

P

p53 tumor suppressor gene, mutations of, in skin cancer, *1370,* 1371–1374, *1373*
Pachyonychia congenita, oral lesions in, 1325
   palmoplantar keratoderma in, 1706, *1706*
   tooth abnormalities with, 1324t
Pacini corpuscles, 27, *27*
Padimate O, in sunscreens, 754
Pagetoid cells, definition of, 109
Pagetoid pattern, definition of, *108,* 109, *109*

Pagetoid reticulosis, in lymphoma, T-cell, 1641, 1644
Paget's cells, definition of, 109, *109*
Paget's disease, extramammary, 1353, *1487,* 1487–1488, *1488,* 1488t
   mammary, 1488–1489, *1489, 1868,* Plate 15
Pain, genital, diagnosis of, 1342, 1342t
   perineal, 1342t, 1356
   vulvar, 1353–1356, *1354, 1355,* Plate 9
   with erythema, 533–534, 534t
Palate, cleft, with ectodermal dysplasia, 1722t
   erosion of, in Reiter's syndrome, 323, *324*
   papillary hyperplasia of, 1326
Pale cell acanthoma, *1442,* 1442–1443, *1443,* 1443t
Palm. See *Hand.*
Pancreas, cancer of, subcutaneous fat necrosis with, 1845
   disease of, and panniculitis, *610,* 610–611, *611*
   tumors of, and necrolytic migratory erythema, 1843–1844, *1844, 1868*
Pancreatitis, hyperlipidemia with, and xanthoma, 1814
   in toxic epidermal necrolysis, 706
Panniculitis, 591–613
   biopsy of, 124
   cold injury and, 609–610
   cytophagic histiocytic, *612,* 612–613
   equestrian, 829
   in erythema nodosum, 591–594, *592, 593,* 593t
   in neonate, 1897–1898
   in nodular vasculitis, 594–596, *595, 596,* 597t
   lobular, definition of, 109
   lupus, clinical findings in, 261, *262*
      pathology of, 269, *270*
      treatment of, 276
   pancreatic disease and, *610,* 610–611, *611*
   papules in, *92*
   protease inhibitor deficiency and, *605,* 605–607, *606,* 606t, 607t
   sclerosing, 603–605, *604,* 605t
      with venous ulcer, of leg, 558–559, *559*
   steroid withdrawal and, 608–609, 609t
Panniculus. See *Fat, subcutaneous.*
Pansclerotic morphea, of childhood, 896, 898
Pantothenic acid deficiency, cutaneous signs of, 1873t
Papilla, dermal, anatomy of, 1247
Papillary adenoma, digital, 1481–1482
Papillary hyperplasia, of palate, 1326
Papillomas, in yaws, 962, *962*
Papillomatosis, definition of, 109
Papillomavirus infection, 1100–1117. See also *Verrucae.*
   and oral lesions, 1334–1335
   clinical description of, 1101–1104, *1101–1104*
   diagnosis of, 1101, 1102t, 1111
   epidemiology of, 1104–1106, *1105*
   genital, 1102t, 1102–1104, *1102–1104,* 1106, 1347–1349, *1348*
   genotypes of, 1100, 1101t
   immune response to, 1109
   in immunosuppressed patient, 1155–1156
   molecular biology of, 1109–1110
   oncogenes in, 1110–1111
   pathogenesis of, 1108–1109
   pathology of, 1106–1108, *1106–1108*
   treatment of, 1111t, 1111–1114, 1112t
   laser therapy in, 1114–1117, 1115t, 1116t
Papillon-Lefèvre syndrome, 1705, 1722t
   tooth abnormalities with, 1324t, 1722t

Papular elastorrhexis, 1792
Papular mucinosis. See *Mucinosis.*
Papule(s), assessment of, 89–90, 91t, *92, 93*
   bowenoid, 1103, *1104,* 1108, 1352, *1352*
   genital, diagnosis of, 1342, 1343t
   Gottron's, in dermatomyositis, 284, *284,* 286
   in acantholytic dermatosis, transient, 341, *342*
   in acne, 462
   in acne scars, vs. anetoderma, 911t
   in acroangiodermatitis, 1507, *1508*
   in amyloidosis, 1819, *1819,* 1822, *1822,* Plate 14
   in bacillary angiomatosis, 1025, *1025,* Plate 8
   in bartonellosis, 1026, *1026*
   in basal cell nevus syndrome, 1796t, *1797*
   in Behçet's disease, 386
   in Cowden's syndrome, 1796t, *1797*
   in cryptococcosis, with human immunodeficiency virus infection, 1141, *1141*
   in Darier's disease, 1699, *1700*
   in dermatosis papulosa nigra, 1441–1442, *1442,* 1442t
   in elastosis perforans serpiginosa, 407, *408*
   in eruptive xanthoma, 1810, *1810*
   in hemosiderotic hemangioma, 1515, *1515*
   in histiocytosis, sinus, 1617, *1618*
   in Kaposi's sarcoma, 1151, *1151, 1152*
   in Langerhans cell histiocytosis, 1610, *1611*
   in leukemia cutis, 1670, 1671, *1671*
   in lichen myxedematosus, 1832, *1835*
   in lichen nitidus, 240, *240*
   in lichen planopilaris, 1287, *1287*
   in lichen planus, 86, *87*
   in lichen spinulosus, 505, *505*
   in lichen striatus, 244, *245*
   in mastocytosis, cutaneous, *88*
   in melanoacanthoma, 1447, *1447*
   in molluscum contagiosum, 1098, *1098*
   in neonate, evaluation of, *1893*
   in papillomavirus infection, genital, 1348, *1348*
   in perforating collagenosis, reactive, 407, *408*
   in perforating dermatosis, acquired, 408, *408*
   in pityriasis lichenoides, 256, *257*
   in polymorphic light eruption, 758, 759, *759, 760*
   in pseudofolliculitis barbae, 499, *500*
   in rosacea, 485, *486,* Plate 4
   in sarcoidosis, 433–434, *434*
   in sebaceous hyperplasia, 1471, *1471*
   in seborrheic keratosis, 1444, *1444*
   in Spangler's dermatitis, in pregnancy, 370
   in syphilis, *950–952,* 951, 952, 954
   in systemic lupus erythematosus, 264
   penile, pearly, *1348,* 1352
   piezogenic, in runners, 851, 853
   urticarial, pruritic, with plaques, in pregnancy, 365–368, *366,* 367t, 368t
      vs. herpes gestationis, 683
   with necrosis, in tuberculid infection, 985, 986, *986,* Plate 7
Papuloerythroderma, 1667
   in lymphoma, T-cell, 1641, *1642*
Papulonecrotic tuberculid, 985, 986, *986,* 988t, Plate 7
Papulosis, atrophic, malignant, 545t, 546t, 551–552
   and gastrointestinal hemorrhage, 1875t

Papulosis (*Continued*)
    cardiac disorders with, 1878t
    bowenoid, 1103, *1104*, 1108, 1352, *1352*
    lymphomatoid, 1631–1637. See also
        Lymphomatoid papulosis.
Papulosquamous diseases, definition of, 109
Para-aminobenzoic acid, in sunscreens,
    752–754
Paracoccidioidomycosis, oral lesions in, 1335
Paragonimiasis, 1187
Parakeratosis, definition of, 109
    scale in, *98*
Paralysis, tick bites and, 816
Paraneoplastic dermatosis, 1843–1849, *1844,*
    1845, 1847, 1867, 1867t, *1867–1869,*
    Plate 15
    acanthosis nigricans in, 1846–1847, *1867,*
        1867t
    acrokeratosis of Bazex in, 1846
    bullous pemphigoid in, 1847
    collagen-vascular disease in, 1846
    erythema gyratum repens in, 1845, *1845,*
        Plate 14
    erythroderma in, 1846
    flushing in, 1848
    herpes gestationis in, 1847
    hypertrichosis lanuginosa in, *1844, 1844,*
        1867
    ichthyosis in, 1846, *1847*
    ischemia in, 1848
    necrolytic migratory erythema in,
        1843–1844, *1844*
    pemphigus in, 658–661, *659*, 660t, *661,*
        661t, 1847, *1868*
    pruritus in, 1845–1846
    purpura in, 1848
    seborrheic keratosis in, 1846
    subcutaneous fat necrosis in, 1845
    Sweet's syndrome in, 1844–1845, *1845,*
        1868, Plate 14
    telangiectasia in, 1848
    thrombophlebitis in, *1847*, 1847–1848
    xanthomas in, 1848
Parapoxvirus infection, 1093, 1096t,
    1096–1098, *1097*
Paraproteinemia, and hyperlipidemia, with
    xanthoma, 1815
    with necrobiotic xanthogranuloma, 449
Parapsoriasis, 222–224, *223, 224,* 224t
Parasitosis, 1163–1198. See also specific
    infestations, e.g., *Leishmaniasis.*
    and pruritus, 155t
    delusions of, 780t, 780–782, 781t
Parkes Weber syndrome, 1503, 1505, 1799t
Parkinsonism, pimozide side effects
    mimicking, 781
Paromomycin, for amebiasis, 1173
Paronychia, 1299t, 1304
Parotid gland, anatomy of, *113,* 115–116
Parsol 1789, in sunscreens, 754
Parvovirus B19 infection, and erythema
    infectiosum, 1124t, 1125t, *1128,*
    1128–1129, Plate 8
Pasini epidermolysis bullosa, 640
Pasini-Pierini atrophoderma, 895, 897, 898
    vs. anetoderma, 911t
Pasteurella multocida infection, in bite
    wounds, 943, 947
Patch(es), assessment of, 88–89, 89t, *89–92*
    in lymphoma, T-cell, 1639–1640, *1640,*
        1642, 1643, 1648, 1654–1655
    in pityriasis rosea, 218–220, 219t
    in syphilis, *950, 950–951, 951*
    shagreen, in tuberous sclerosis, 1736, 1740
Patella, hypoplasia of, with nail hypoplasia,
    and renal disease, 1884t

Pattern theory, of pruritus, 157
Pautrier's microabscess, 109
Pedicles, in flap reconstruction, after skin
    cancer excision, 1408–1409
Pediculosis capitis, 1191–1193, 1192t
Pediculosis corporis, 1190–1191, 1192t
Pediculosis pubis, *1193*, 1193–1195, *1194,*
    1194t, 1195t
Pediculus humanus corporis, as vector of
    typhus, 1017
Pedunculated skin, definition of, 109
Peeling skin syndrome, 1699
Pellagra, cutaneous signs of, *1873*, 1873t
    photosensitivity in, 766
    vs. Hartnup's disorder, 1768
Pemphigoid, bullous, 664–671
    biopsy of, site for, 120, 120t
    clinical findings in, 664–665, *665*
    definition of, 664
    differential diagnosis of, 668–670, 669t
    paraneoplastic, 1847
    pathogenesis of, 667–668
    pathology of, 665–666, *666, 667*
    psoralen–ultraviolet radiation therapy
        and, in treatment of psoriasis,
        315
    treatment of, 670t, 670–671, 1887t
    vesicles in, 96, *97*
    vs. cicatricial, 669, 676
    vs. linear IgA bullous dermatosis,
        700–701, 701t
    cicatricial, 674–677
      and alopecia, 1291
      clinical findings in, 674–675, *675*
      definition of, 674
      diagnosis of, 676, 676t
      pathogenesis of, 675–676
      pathology of, 675, *676*
      treatment of, 677, 677t
      vs. bullous, 669, 676
      oral lesions in, 1332
      vs. lichen planus, 238, 238t
Pemphigoid antigens, 15, *19*
    bullous, 619–620, *620,* 864, *865*
    cicatricial, 620–621
Pemphigoid gestationis, 679–684. See also
    Herpes gestationis.
Pemphigus, 651–661
    biopsy of, site for, 120, 120t
    drug-induced, 422–423
    in Hailey-Hailey disease, 1701, *1702*
      vs. acantholytic dermatosis, 341
    oral lesions in, 1331–1332
    paraneoplastic, 658–661, *659*, 660t, *661,*
        661t, 1847, *1868*
    vs. toxic epidermal necrolysis, 710t
Pemphigus erythematosus, 264
Pemphigus foliaceus, 655t, 655–658, *656,*
    658t
    immune response in, cadherins in, 150
    vs. subcorneal pustular dermatosis, 329
Pemphigus vegetans, 651, 652
Pemphigus vulgaris, 651–655, *652,* 652t,
    653, 654t
    immune response in, cadherins in, 150
    maternal, and neonatal blistering eruption,
        720
    oral, vs. lichen planus, 238, 238t
    treatment of, 1887t
    vs. Behçet's disease, 389t
D-Penicillamine, anti-angiogenic effect of,
    1495, 1495t
    for morphea, 898
    for scleroderma, 889
Penicillin, for actinomycosis, 1008t, 1009
    for anthrax, 1031

Penicillin (*Continued*)
    for erysipelas, 925
    for Lyme borreliosis, 969, 969t
    for pinta, 963
    for staphylococcal infection, 923t
    for streptococcal infection, 923t
    for syphilis, 957t, 957–958
      endemic, 963
      with human immunodeficiency virus
        infection, 961
    for yaws, 963
    skin reactions to, 416
Penis, balanitis of, in Reiter's syndrome, 322,
    323t, *324*
    Bowen's disease of, 1380
    papules of, pearly, *1348,* 1352
Pentamidine isethionate, for trypanosomiasis,
    1175
Pentostam, for leishmaniasis, 1169
Pentoxifylline, for atheroembolism,
    cutaneous, 546t, 547
    for livedo vasculopathy, 546t
Perforating collagenosis, reactive, 407, *408,*
    409, *410*, 410t
Perforating skin disorders, 407–411,
    408–410, 410t, 411t
    with diabetes, 1869t, *1870*
Perforating veins, varicosity of, 575–576,
    576, 578
Periarteritis. See *Polyarteritis.*
Periderm, 3
Perifolliculitis capitis, *1281*, 1281–1282,
    1282t
Perineum, hidradenitis suppurativa of, 481,
    482
    pain in, 1342t, 1356
Perineurium, tumor invasion by, in
    squamous cell carcinoma, 1385
    Mohs micrographic surgery for,
        1406–1407
Periodontal disease, in acquired
    immunodeficiency syndrome, 1337t
Perioral dermatitis, 497–498, *498,* 498t
    vs. acne, 469
Periostitis, in congenital syphilis, 960t
Permethrin, for louse infestation, 1192,
    1194–1195
    for scabies, 1198
Perniosis (chilblains), 829–830
    homelessness and, 841
    in systemic lupus erythematosus, 263
Pertofrane, for neurotic excoriations, 784
Peruvian wart, 1024t, 1024–1028, *1026,*
    1027t
Petechiae, 89t
    in purpura, with systemic disorders, *1865,*
        1865t, *1866*
    sports and, 850–851, 853
Petroleum jelly, for dry skin, 77
Peutz-Jeghers syndrome, 1797t, *1798*
    gastrointestinal hemorrhage in, 1874t
Phaeoannellomyces werneckii infection, and
    tinea nigra, 1037–1038, *1038,* 1038t
Phaeohyphomycosis, 1072
Phagocytes, in granuloma annulare, 441
Phakomas, in tuberous sclerosis, 1737
Phakomatosis pigmentovascularis, 1505
Pharyngitis, lymphonodular, 1335t
Phenformin, for livedo vasculopathy, 545
Phenobarbital, hypersensitivity to, 417
Phenol, and burn injury, 845t, 846
    in chemical peel, for photoaging, 742t,
        743–746, *744,* 745t, *746*
Phenothiazines, and pigmentation disorders,
    422
Phenylbutazone, for gnathostomiasis, 1184

Phenylketonuria, 1858, 1859t, *1860*
vs. albinism, 1222
Phenytoin, for epidermolysis bullosa, 644–645
for pudendal neuralgia, 1355–1356
hypersensitivity to, 417
Pheomelanins, *1204*, 1207
Phialophora jeanselmi infection, and mycetoma, 1070, 1071t
pHisoHex (hexachlorophene), and wound healing, 566t
in antiseptic solutions, 129, 129t
Phlebectasia, congenital, 1503
Phlebitis, chemotherapy and, 428
cords in, 102, *102*
in Behçet's disease, 386–387
paraneoplastic, *1847*, 1847–1848
Phlebotomus sandflies, as vectors of bartonellosis, 1025
Phlebotomy, for porphyria cutanea tarda, 1759
Phospholipids, antibodies to, syndrome of, 545t, 546t, 547–550
with livedo reticularis, 1865t, *1866*
Phosphonoformic acid. See *Foscarnet*.
Phosphorus, and burn injury, 845t
imbalance of, and calcification of skin, 1829, 1829t
Photoaggravated disorders, 765t, 765–766
Photoaging, 732–746
definition of, 732, 733
differential diagnosis of, 733t, 739
pathogenesis of, 738–739
pathology of, 733–735, *734–736*, Plate 5
prevention of, 739t, 739–740, 740t
treatment of, medical, 740–741, 741t
surgical, 741–746, *742*, 742t, 743t, *744–746*, 745t, 746t
Photoallergy, and urticaria, 394–395, 400–401
clinical findings in, 726–727, 729, 729t, Plate 5
definition of, 726
diagnosis of, 730, 730t
pathogenesis of, 729t, 729–730
pathology of, 727
treatment of, 730, 731t
Photobiology, 725, *726*, 726t, 727t
Photocarcinogenesis, 1367
Photodamage, 732–746
clinical findings in, 733, *733*, 733t, *734*
definition of, 732–733
pathogenesis of, 736–738
pathology of, 734–735, *734–736*, Plate 5
prevention of, 739t, 739–740, 740t
sensitivity to, variations in, 739t, 739–740, 742–744, 746
treatment of, 740
Photodermatitis, in lupus erythematosus, systemic, 84–85, *86*, Plate 1
Photodermatosis, DNA abnormalities and, 765
idiopathic, 758–766, 759t
in actinic prurigo, *761*, 761t, 761–762, 762t
in hydroa vacciniforme, *763*, 763–764
in polymorphic eruption, 758–761, *759*, *760*, 760t, 761t
in solar urticaria, *762*, 762–763
Photodynamic therapy, for skin cancer, 1423–1427, *1425, 1426*
Photoplethysmography, in diagnosis, of leg ulcers, 563
of varicose veins, 579–580

Photosensitivity, in actinic reticuloid syndrome, 763, 768–770, *769*, 769t, 770t, Plate 5
in dermatomyositis, 766
in drug reactions, 420
in human immunodeficiency virus infection, *1146*, 1146–1147
in lupus erythematosus, 263, *263*, 766
in lymphocytoma, cutaneous, 766
in pellagra, 766
in porphyria, 1756, *1756*
in porphyria cutanea tarda, 1758, *1758*
in protoporphyria, erythropoietic, 1755t, 1757, *1757*
in psoriasis, 766
sunscreens for, 755t, 756t, 757
variations in, 739t, 739–740, 742–744, 746
Phototherapy, for alopecia areata, 1273t, 1274
for dermatitis, atopic, 201–202
of hands and feet, 191–193
for graft-versus-host disease, 230
for Langerhans cell histiocytosis, 1614
for lichen planus, 239, 239t
for lymphoma, cutaneous T-cell, 1652, 1654, 1655
for lymphomatoid papulosis, 1636t, 1637
for mastocytosis, 1607
for psoriasis, 305t, 306, 312–315
in combination therapy, 315–316
for urticaria, 403
for vitiligo, 1214–1215
psoralens in. See *Psoralens*.
skin reactions to, effect of chemotherapy on, 427–428
toxicity of, in neonate, 1890–1891
Phototoxicity, and contact dermatitis, occupational, 178
clinical findings in, 726–727, *728*, 728t, *729*, Plate 4
definition of, 726
diagnosis of, 730, 730t
pathogenesis of, 728–729
pathology of, 727
treatment of, 730, 731t
Physalia stings, 787, 789, 791t
Phytanic acid storage disease, 1695
Phytosterolemia, and xanthomatosis, 1815
Piebaldism, 1223–1225, *1224*, 1224t, 1225t
vs. vitiligo, 1213
Piedra, 1038t, 1038–1039
white, genital, 1345
Piedraia hortae infection, 1038–1039
Pigmentation, 11–13, *17, 18*
changes in, chemotherapy and, 427
in chemical peel, for photoaging, 746
with atopic dermatitis, 196
with dermabrasion, for acne scars, 475, 478
deficiency of, 1219–1230
disorders of, acne and, 462
after lichen striatus, 244, *245*
and nail discoloration, *1303*, 1303–1304
chemically induced, 1234t, 1236–1238, *1237*
drug reactions and, 420–422, *421*
genital, diagnosis of, 1342, 1342t
in albinism, 1219–1223, 1220t, 1221t, *1222*, 1223t
in erythema dyschromicum perstans, 1238
in hypomelanosis, idiopathic guttate, 1228, 1228t
of Ito, 1226–1227, *1227*, 1227t
in melanoacanthoma, *1447*, 1447–1448, *1448*, 1448t

Pigmentation (*Continued*)
in melasma, 1233–1236, *1234, 1235*, 1235t, 1236t
in Mongolian spot, 1240
in nevus depigmentosus, 1225–1227, 1226t
in nevus of Ito, 1239–1240
in nevus of Ota, 1239–1240
in Peutz-Jeghers syndrome, 1797t, *1798*
in piebaldism, 1223–1225, *1224*, 1224t, 1225t
in tuberous sclerosis, 1226t, 1226–1228, 1228t
in vitiligo, 1210–1216. See also *Vitiligo*.
in Waardenburg's syndrome, 1225, 1225t
infection and, 1229–1230
inflammatory disorders and, 89t, *91*, 219, 1228–1229, *1229*, 1238–1239
port-wine stain with, 1505
ultraviolet light exposure and, 735
with epidermolysis bullosa, 638
excess of, 1233–1240, 1234t
in purpuric dermatosis, 291–293, *292*, 293t
incontinence of, 1722t, 1725–1728. See also *Incontinentia pigmenti*.
melanocytes in, 1203–1207. See also *Melanocytes*.
of hair, genetic abnormalities and, in mice, 1718
melanin transfer disorders and, 1717–1718
of oral cavity, 1323–1325, *1324*
Pigmentosa reticularis, dermatopathic (livedo reticularis), 831–832, *832*, 832t
in systemic lupus erythematosus, 263
with antiphospholipid antibody syndrome, 1865t, *1866*
Pilar cysts, 1452–1453, *1455*
proliferating, 1453–1454, *1456*
Pilar sheath acanthoma, 1465
Pilomatricoma, 1468–1470, *1469*, 1830
Pilomatrix carcinoma, 1471
Pilosebaceous unit. See also *Hair follicles* and *Sebaceous glands*.
tumors of, 1464–1474
Pimozide, for delusions of parasitosis, 781, 782
Pincer nail, 1301–1302
Pinta, 961–963
Piperazine, for enterobiasis, 1184
Piritrexim, for psoriasis, 308
Pitch, and burn injury, 844t, 846
Pitted keratolysis, 928, *928*
Pitting, of nails, 1303
palmar, in basal cell nevus syndrome, 1742, *1743*
Pityriasis alba, hypopigmentation in, 1229
vs. vitiligo, 1214
Pityriasis lichenoides, 256–258, *257*, 258t
vs. lymphomatoid papulosis, 257–258, 1634, 1635t
Pityriasis rosea, 218–220, *219*, 220t, 221t
diagnosis of, *86*, 220, 220t
vs. psoriasis, guttate, 299
vs. syphilis, 957
Pityriasis rotunda, 1682–1683
Pityriasis rubra pilaris, *98*, 331–335, *332*, 332t, *333*, 334t, Plate 2
with human immunodeficiency virus infection, 1148
Pityriasis versicolor, 1038t, *1039*, 1039–1041, *1040*, 1040t
hypopigmentation in, 1229–1230
Pityrosporum infection, and folliculitis, vs. acne, 469

Pityrosporum orbiculare infection, and folliculitis, 922
Pityrosporum ovale (*Malassezia furfur*) infection, and acne, 466, 467
and folliculitis, 1038t, 1040t, 1041
and seborrheic dermatitis, 215–216
Plague, 943, *1033*, 1033–1034, 1034t
Plakoglobin, in pemphigus vulgaris, 653
Plaque(s), assessment of, 90–91, *93*, 93t
atheromatous, embolism of, 545t, 546t, 546–547, *547*, 1881t
fibrous, in tuberous sclerosis, 1736, *1737*
in Behçet's disease, 386
in blastomycosis, 1066, *1066*
in Darier's disease, 1699, *1700*
in dermatofibrosarcoma protuberans, 1555, *1555*, 1556, *1556*
in erythema elevatum diutinum, 528, *529*
in erythrokeratodermia progressiva symmetrica, 1699, *1699*
in granuloma faciale, 530, *531*
in Kaposi's sarcoma, *1151*, 1152, *1152*
in Langerhans cell histiocytosis, 1610, *1611*
in leukemia cutis, 1670, 1671, *1671*
in lichen planus, 86, *87*
in lupus erythematosus, discoid, with scarring alopecia, 1288, *1288*
in lymphoma, T-cell, 1639–1641, *1640, 1643*, 1643–1645, 1648, 1654–1655
in morphea, 895, *896*, 897
in necrobiotic xanthogranuloma, 449, *449*
in neonate, evaluation of, *1893*
in papillomavirus infection, genital, 1348, *1348*
in parapsoriasis, 222–224, *223, 224*, 224t
in psoriasis, 295t, 295–297, *296, 297*
in sarcoidosis, 434
in sclerosing panniculitis, 603, *604*
in *Staphylococcus aureus* infection, with human immunodeficiency virus infection, 1138, *1138*
in Sweet's syndrome, 372, *373*, Plate 3
in syringocystadenoma papilliferum, 1484t, 1485, 1486
in syringoid sweat duct carcinoma, 1483–1484, 1484t
urticarial, pruritic, with papules, in pregnancy, 365–368, *366*, 367t, 368t
vs. herpes gestationis, 683
Plaque-like cutaneous mucinosis, 1834t, 1834–1836, *1835*
Plaquenil. See *Hydroxychloroquine.*
Plasmacytoid monocytes, in Jessner's lymphocytic infiltrate, 345, 346
Plasmacytoma, extramedullary, 1664
Plasmapheresis, for pemphigus vulgaris, 655
for urticaria, 403
Plasminogen activator, for livedo vasculopathy, 545, 546t
Platelet factor 4, anti-angiogenic effect of, 1495, 1495t
Platelet-activating factor, in Wells' syndrome, 361
Platelet-derived endothelial cell growth factor, 1493t, 1494
Platelets, deficiency of, biopsy in, 121–122
Platysma muscle, anatomy of, 112, *113*
Pleomorphism, definition of, 109
Plethysmography, in diagnosis, of leg ulcers, 563
of varicose veins, 579–580
Pleurisy, in systemic lupus erythematosus, 265
Plexus, vascular, superficial, definition of, 110
Pneumococcal infection, 940
Pneumonia, cutaneous signs of, 1882t

Pneumonic plague, 1034
Pneumonitis, methotrexate and, 309
Podophyllin, for papillomavirus infection, genital, 1349
POEMS syndrome, glomeruloid hemangioma in, 1516
seborrheic keratosis in, 1446
Poikiloderma, in dermatomyositis, 284–286
in lymphoma, T-cell, 1641, 1644, *1644*
in Rothmund-Thomson syndrome, 1803t, *1804*
of Civatte, vs. melasma, 1235
with erythroderma, 336
Poison ivy, and dermatitis, *87*
Pollen, in atopic dermatitis, 199
Pollitt syndrome, 1694
Polyangiitis, microscopic, 522–527, *523, 526*, 526t
systemic, 584
Polyarteritis, microscopic, 522–527, *523, 526*, 526t
Polyarteritis nodosa, 519–521, *520*, 520t
benign cutaneous, 832
diagnosis of, *523*, 526t
renal disease in, cutaneous signs with, 1883t
Polychondritis, relapsing, 512–514, *513*, 513t, 514t
cardiac disorders in, cutaneous signs with, 1879t, *1881*, Plate 15
Polycystic ovarian syndrome, and hirsutism, 1853
Polycythemia rubra vera, and pruritus, 158
Polymorphic eruption, definition of, 109
light-induced, 758–761, *759, 760*, 760t, 761t
Polymorphic light eruption, vs. Jessner's lymphocytic infiltrate, 346
Polymorphonuclear leukocytes, in plaque psoriasis, 297
Polymyalgia rheumatica, infrared radiation and, 825
Polymyositis, diagnosis of, 283, 286–287, 287t
epidemiology of, 283
in adults, clinical findings in, *284*, 284–285
in mixed connective tissue disease, 268
malignancy with, 285–286
paraneoplastic, 1846
pathogenesis of, 287–288
treatment of, 288t, 288–289
Polyneuropathy, amyloidotic, familial, 1821
Polypoid lesion, definition of, 109–110
Polyvinyl chloride toxicity, vs. scleroderma, 887, 888t
Pomades, and acne, 464, *464*
Pompholyx, 188, *189*, 190, 191
Pore, dilated, of Winer, 1464–1465
Porocarcinoma, 1480
Porokeratosis, 1701–1703, *1702, 1703*
Poroma, *1477*, 1479–1480, *1480*, 1480t
Porphobilinogen, in heme biosynthesis, in porphyria, 1753, *1755*
Porphyria, 1753–1761
acute intermittent, 1760, 1760t
aminolevulinic acid dehydratase, 1760, 1760t
classification of, 1753, 1754t, 1755t
clinical findings in, 1753, 1754t
definition of, 1753, 1754t
erythropoietic, 1753, 1754t, *1756*, 1756–1758, *1757*, 1760t
tooth abnormalities with, 1324t
vs. blistering disorders, in neonate, 717t
heme biosynthetic pathway in, 1753–1756, *1755*, 1755t

Porphyria (*Continued*)
in hereditary coproporphyria, 1760t, 1760–1761
photobiology of, 1756
photochemistry of, 1756
variegate, 1760t, 1761
Porphyria cutanea tarda, *1758*, 1758–1760, *1759*, 1759t, 1760t
with human immunodeficiency virus infection, 1146
Portuguese man-of-war stings, 787, 789, 791t
Port-wine stain, 1496t, 1501–1502, *1502*
in Proteus syndrome, 1506
in Sturge-Weber syndrome, 1505
with pigmentation disorders, 1505
Potassium iodide, for erythema nodosum, 594
for sporotrichosis, 1063
for Sweet's syndrome, 375, 375t
Potassium permanganate, for erythroderma, 339t
Povidone, with iodine, and wound healing, 566t
toxicity of, in neonate, 1890, *1890*
Poxvirus infections, 1093–1099, *1094*, 1094t–1096t, *1097, 1098*
Praziquantel, for cysticercosis, 1187
for gnathostomiasis, 1184
for schistosomiasis, 1186
Prednisolone, for hemangioma, of infancy, 1500
Prednisone, for antiphospholipid syndrome, 546t, 550
for Behçet's disease, 390, 390t
for bowel-associated dermatosis-arthritis syndrome, 376, 376t
for brown recluse spider bites, 812
for bullous dermatosis, linear IgA, 702t
for bullous pemphigoid, 670–671
for cellulitis, 925
of scalp, 1282, 1282t
for Churg-Strauss syndrome, *526*, 527
for contact dermatitis, 181
for dermatomyositis, 288t, 288–289
for epidermolysis bullosa acquisita, 688–689
for erosive pustular dermatosis, of scalp, 1284, 1284t
for erythema nodosum, 594
for erythroderma, 339, 339t
for hemangioma, of infancy, 1500
for herpes gestationis, 683
for herpes simplex infection, in erythema multiforme, 254
for hidradenitis suppurativa, 481
for hypereosinophilic syndrome, 357, *357*
for Jessner's lymphocytic infiltrate, 346
for lichen planopilaris, 1288, 1288t
for lichen planus, 239, 239t
for loiasis, 1180
for lupus erythematosus, systemic, 277–278
for nail matrix disorders, 1302
for nummular dermatitis, 213, 213t
for pemphigoid, cicatricial, 677
for pemphigus, paraneoplastic, 661, 661t
for pemphigus foliaceus, 658, 658t
for pemphigus vulgaris, 654, 654t
for photoallergy, 730
for polyarteritis, microscopic, *526*, 527
for polychondritis, relapsing, 514, 514t
for polymyositis, 288t, 288–289
for pruritic urticarial papules and plaques of pregnancy, 368
for pseudofolliculitis barbae, 501
for pyoderma gangrenosum, 383, 383t, 384
for reversal reactions, in leprosy, 1003

Prednisone (*Continued*)
for scleroderma, 889
for Sweet's syndrome, 375, 375t
for temporal arteritis, 517
for trichinosis, 1180
for urticaria, 402
for Wegener's granulomatosis, 526, 527
for Wells' syndrome, 363
with chlorambucil, for lymphoma, cutaneous T-cell, 1653
Pregnancy, acrodermatitis enteropathica in, 1764, 1765
alopecia in, diffuse, 1275
and varicose veins, 576
autoimmune dermatitis in, 370
dermatoses in, 365–370
epulis in, 1325–1326
erythema infectiosum in, 1128, 1129
fetal loss in, antiphospholipid syndrome and, 549–550
herpes gestationis in, 679–684, *680, 681,* 683t
herpes simplex virus infection in, transmission of, to fetus, 714, 715t
immunoglobulin M anti--basement membrane autoantibody dermatosis in, 370
impetigo herpetiformis in, *368,* 368–369
linear immunoglobulin M dermatosis in, 370
Lyme borreliosis in, 969t, 970
methotrexate contraindicated in, 308
pruritus in, 155t
of Besnier, 369–370
with cholestasis, 369
with folliculitis, 370
with urticarial papules and plaques, 365–368, *366,* 367t, 368t
vs. herpes gestationis, 683
psoriasis in, 301, 368, *368*
retinoid teratogenicity in, 310
rubella in, 1127, 1128
Spangler's papular dermatitis in, 370
syphilis in, 957t, 958, 959
toxoplasmosis in, 1175, 1176
varicella infection in, transmission of, to fetus, 715t, 718
Pregnane ring, in topical corticosteroids, 162, *163*
Prepuce, sebaceous glands of, 30
Pressure-induced urticaria, 394, 400
Pretibial lesions, in epidermolysis bullosa, dystrophic, 640
Pretibial myxedema, *1872*
and cutaneous mucinosis, 1834t, *1836,* 1836–1837, *1837*
and hyperhidrosis, 1313
glycosaminoglycans in, 876
Probucol, for hyperlipidemia, with xanthoma, 1816
Procainamide, and lupus erythematosus, 266
Procaine, in anesthesia, 130, 130t
Procerus muscle, anatomy of, *113,* 114
Profilaggrin, 9
in keratinocyte differentiation, in granular layer, 64–65, *65*
Progeria, 1713, *1713,* 1803t
Progesterone, and autoimmune dermatitis, in pregnancy, 370
for androgenetic alopecia, 1257
Progestins, for hirsutism, 1856
Prolactin, blood level of, elevated, and hirsutism, 1854
in androgenetic alopecia, 1256
Prolidase deficiency, 1859t, 1862

Prolyl hydroxylation, in dermal extracellular collagen, 859–861, *861*
Pronestyl, and lupus erythematosus, 266
Propionibacterium acnes, in acne, 465–467
in androgenetic alopecia, 1253
Propionibacterium species, in normal cutaneous flora, 926
Proquazone, for Jessner's lymphocytic infiltrate, 346
Prostaglandins, for Raynaud's phenomenon, 541–542
in urticaria, 398
Protease inhibitor deficiency, and panniculitis, 605, 605–607, *606,* 606t, 607t
Protein C deficiency, in coumarin-induced skin necrosis, 546t, 550
in neonate, vs. blistering disorders, 717t
Protein deficiency, cutaneous signs of, 1873t
Protein kinase C, in DNA photodamage, 1369
Protein S deficiency, in neonate, vs. blistering disorders, 717t
Proteinosis, lipoid, oral abnormalities with, 1324t
Proteoglycans, in dermal extracellular matrix, 857–858, 859t, 876
in dermoepidermal junction, 15–16, *19*
Proteus syndrome, 1506, 1740
vs. neurofibromatosis, 1733, *1733*
Proto-oncogenes, c-*kit,* in inflammatory response, 145
in ultraviolet-induced carcinogenesis, 1370, *1370,* 1370t
Protoporphyria, erythropoietic, 1755t, *1757,* 1757–1758, 1760t
Protoporphyrinogen, in heme biosynthesis, in porphyria, 1753, 1754t, *1755*
Prototheca infection, 1072
Protozoal infestation, 1172–1177, *1173–1176*
and erythema nodosum, 593, 594t
Prozac, for trichotillomania, 783
Prurigo, *207,* 207–208, 208t
actinic, *761,* 761t, 761–762, 762t
vs. polymorphic light eruption, 760t, 761t
Prurigo gravidarum, 369
Prurigo nodularis, *207,* 207–208, 208t
Pruritus, clinical description of, 154, 155t
definition of, 154
genital, diagnosis of, 1342, 1342t
grocers', 814–815
in atopic dermatitis, treatment of, 201
in cutaneous disease, 155t, 158
in dermatomyositis, 285
in lichen simplex chronicus, 205–206
in notalgia paresthetica, 208–209, 209t
in pityriasis rosea, 218, 220
in pregnancy, 365–370. See also *Pregnancy.*
in prurigo. See *Prurigo.*
in swimmers, *793,* 793–795, 794t, 795t, 1186, 1187t
in systemic disease, 155t, 158
localized, 209, 209t
neurology of, 154–157
paraneoplastic, 1845–1846
pathology of, 154
pharmacology of, 157–158
renal disorders and, 1883t, 1883–1886, 1884t
with purpuric dermatosis, pigmented, 291–292
with urticarial papules and plaques, in pregnancy, 365–368, *366,* 367t, 368t
vs. herpes gestationis, 683
Pseudarthrosis, of tibia, in neurofibromatosis, 1731

Pseudoainhum, in palmoplantar keratoderma, 1703, 1704
vs. Dupuytren's disease, 908–909
Pseudoallescheria boydii infection, and mycetoma, 1069, 1070, 1071t
Pseudocysts, in seborrheic keratosis, 1444, *1445*
myxoid, 1839
Pseudofolliculitis barbae, 499–502, *500,* 500t
Pseudoglandular structures, definition of, 110
Pseudo-Kaposi's sarcoma, 1507t, 1507–1508, *1508*
Pseudolymphoma, 1665, 1665t
cutaneous, 1626
Pseudomonas aeruginosa infection, 940–941, *941,* 946, Plate 6
and ecthyma gangrenosum, in neonate, 713
and septicemia, skin lesions with, 945, *945*
in whirlpool folliculitis, 851, 853
interdigital, 929
Pseudomonas infection, in immunosuppressed patient, 1157
Pseudoparkinsonism, pimozide and, 781
Pseudopelade of Brocq, 1285–1287, *1286,* 1286t
Pseudoporphyria, naproxen and, *1864*
Pseudorheumatoid nodules, 438
Pseudosyndactyly, in epidermolysis bullosa, 641, *641,* 645
Pseudoxanthoma elasticum, 1770–1774
cardiac disorders in, cutaneous signs with, 1879t
clinical findings in, 1770–1771, *1771*
definition of, 1770
dermal elastic fibers in, *874,* 874–875
diagnosis of, 1772–1773
gastrointestinal hemorrhage in, 1874t, *1876*
pathogenesis of, 1772
pathology of, 1771–1772, *1772*
treatment of, 1773t, 1773–1774
Psoralens, and phototoxicity, 726, *728*
for dermatitis, atopic, 201–202
of hands and feet, 191–193
with phototherapy, and lentigo, 1563
for alopecia areata, 1273t, 1274
for Langerhans cell histiocytosis, 1614
for lichen planus, 239, 239t
for lymphoma, cutaneous T-cell, 1652, 1654, 1655
for lymphomatoid papulosis, 1636t, 1637
for mastocytosis, 1607
for psoriasis, 313–316
for vitiligo, 1214–1215
Psoriasiform hyperplasia, irregular, definition of, 108
Psoriasiform lesions, definition of, 110
Psoriasis, 295–316
arthritis in, 301–302
definition of, 295
diaper dermatitis in, 1897
differential diagnosis of, 295, 295t
drug reactions in, 423
epidemiology of, 302
erythrodermic, 295t, 300
diagnosis of, *86,* Plate 1
genital, 300–301, 1350
guttate, 295t, 299, *299*
configuration of, *87*
heat therapy for, 825
historical aspects of, 295
inverse, 295t, 299–300
nail lesions in, 300, 316, 1297, *1300*
of feet, *189,* 189–192
of hands, 189, *189, 190*
of scalp, 301

Psoriasis (*Continued*)
oral lesions in, 1325
pathogenesis of, 302–304
photosensitive, 766
plaques in, 295t, 295–297, *296, 297*
pustular, *97,* 295t, 297–299
in impetigo herpetiformis, in pregnancy, 368, *368*
vs. generalized exanthematous pustulosis, drug-induced, 422
treatment of, for nail involvement, 316
outcome of, assessment of, 304, 305t
phototherapy in, 305t, 306, 312–316
systemic, 305t, 307–312, 315–316, 1887t
topical, 305t, 305–307
triggering factors in, 301
vs. lichen planus, 238, 238t
vs. seborrheic dermatitis, 216
vs. syphilis, 957
with human immunodeficiency virus infection, *1147,* 1147–1148
with subcorneal pustular dermatosis, 328
Psychological disorders, and alopecia, diffuse, 1277
and delusions of parasitosis, 780t, 780–782, 781t
and factitial dermatitis, 780t, 781t, 784–785, *785*
and neurotic excoriations, 780t, 781t, *783,* 783–784
and skin disorders, 779–785
general approach to, 779–780
and trichotillomania, 780t, 781t, *782,* 782–783
mistaken attribution of skin disorders to, 785
with atopic dermatitis, 197
Pterygium, dorsal, 1302
ventral, 1298t, 1301
Pubic hair, louse infestation of, *1193,* 1193–1195, *1194,* 1194t, 1195t
Pudendal neuralgia, *1355,* 1355–1356
Pulsed-dye laser, in wart ablation, 1117
Punch biopsy, technique of, 121, *123,* 123–124
Punch elevation, for acne scars, 474
Punch grafting, for acne scars, 474
of hair, *1258,* 1258–1260, *1259*
Purpura, Henoch-Schönlein, *523, 524, 525,* 526t, 585, 586
in lymphoma, T-cell, 1644
in necrotizing vasculitides, *523, 524, 526*
palpable, venulitis and, 584, *585*
paraneoplastic, 1848
pigmented, 291–293, *292,* 293t
systemic disorders and, 1863–1866, *1865,* 1865t, *1866*
Purpurins, in photodynamic therapy, for skin carcinoma, 1427
Puss caterpillar, and dermatitis, 809–810, *810*
Pustule(s), assessment of, 96–97, *97*
genital, diagnosis of, 1342t
in acne, 462
in candidiasis, 1056–1057, *1057*
in drug eruptions, 422
in eosinophilic folliculitis, in neonate, 717t, 720–721
in erosive dermatosis, of scalp, and alopecia, *1284,* 1284t, 1284–1285
in impetigo herpetiformis, 368, *368*
in lymphoma, T-cell, 1644
in melanosis, in neonate, 715t, 718, *719, 1893,* 1895, *1895*
in psoriasis, 295t, 297–299, 304. See also *Psoriasis.*

Pustule(s) (*Continued*)
in rosacea, 485, *486*
in syphilis, 951–952, *952*
neonatal disorders and, 712, 713t–717t, *1893,* 1894–1896, *1895, 1896*
infectious, 712–718, 713t–715t
transient, 715t, 718–719, *719*
uncommon, 713t, 716t, 717t, 719–721, *720*
spongiform, 110
subcorneal, 110, 327–329, *328, 329,* 329t
Pustulofollicular alopecia, scarring, 1281t–1284t, 1281–1285, *1281–1285*
Pustulosis, exanthematic, acute generalized, vs. toxic epidermal necrolysis, 710t
drug-induced, 422
palmoplantar, *189,* 189–192, *190*
Pyoderma, genital, 1343
staphylococcal infection and, in neonate, 712, 715t
Pyoderma faciale, 463, *463*
Pyoderma gangrenosum, 379–384, 380t, *380–382,* 382t, 383t, Plate 3
bullous, atypical, 375
clinical findings in, 379–381, *380,* 380t, *381,* Plate 3
diagnosis of, 382t, 382–383
pathogenesis of, 382
pathology of, 381–382, *382*
treatment of, 383t, 383–384, 1887t
vs. Behçet's disease, 389t
Pyogenic granuloma, 1507t, *1509,* 1509–1510, *1510*
oral, 1325–1326
Pyostomatitis vegetans, 381, *381,* 1334
Pyrantel pamoate, for enterobiasis, 1184
for hookworm infestation, 1183
Pyrazinamide, for tuberculosis, 989
Pyrethroids, for louse infestation, 1192, 1194–1195
Pyridoxine deficiency, cutaneous signs of, 1873t
Pyrimethamine, for toxoplasmosis, 1175
Pyrimidine, in DNA photodamage, *1365,* 1365–1366
in xeroderma pigmentosum, 1749
Pyrvinium pamoate, for enterobiasis, 1184

Q

Q fever, 1012t, 1019
Q-switched laser, in tattoo removal, 453, *453,* 454t–456t, 455–459
Queensland tick typhus, 1012t, 1016
Queyrat's erythroplasia, 1380
Quinacrine, and pigmentation disorders, 422
for discoid lupus erythematosus, 275, 275t

R

Rabbit fever (tularemia), 943–944, *944,* 947, 1034–1035, 1035t
Radiation, infrared, and erythema ab igne, *824,* 824–825
cutaneous effects of, 823–824
heat transmission in, 823
ultraviolet. See *Ultraviolet light.*
Radiation injury, and alopecia, scarring, 1291, *1292*
and ataxia-telangiectasia, 1802t
and cancer, 837, *837,* 838
and dermatitis, 836–838, *837, 838*

Radiation therapy, for hypertrophic scars, 904
for Kaposi's sarcoma, 1154
for keloids, 904
for Langerhans cell histiocytosis, 1614
for lymphoma, cutaneous T-cell, 1651–1656
for melanoma, 1594
for skin carcinoma, *1394, 1400,* 1400–1402, 1401t, 1402t, *1403*
skin reactions in, chemotherapy and, 427–428
with marrow transplantation, and epidermal cell changes, vs. graft-versus-host disease, 229
Radicals, free, and facial skin damage, 52–53, 80–81
Raeder's syndrome, hyperhidrosis in, 1314
Ramsay Hunt syndrome, 1080
Rapeseed oil, contaminated, and toxic oil syndrome, mucinosis with, 1838
scleroderma in, 891, 892t
Rapp-Hodgkin syndrome, 1722t
ras oncogenes, in skin cancer, *1371,* 1371–1372
Rash, in cytomegalovirus infection, 1084
in herpesvirus-6 infection, 1087, 1087t
in rickettsial disease, 1011–1013, 1012t, *1013,* 1016–1018, *1019*
in systemic lupus erythematosus, 262, *262*
viral, 1123–1134. See also *Viral infection.*
Rat mite, tropical, bites of, 813–814, *814*
Raynaud's phenomenon, 537–542, 540t, 541t
chemotherapy and, 429
clinical findings in, 537–538
definition of, 537
diagnosis of, 540t, 540–541
in scleroderma, 882, 884
treatment of, 887–889
in systemic lupus erythematosus, 263
paraneoplastic, 1848
pathogenesis of, 538–539
pathology of, 538
treatment of, 541t, 541–542
Reactive perforating collagenosis, 407, *408,* 409, *410,* 410t
Reagin blood test, for syphilis, 955
Recklinghausen's disease, 1729–1735. See also *Neurofibromatosis.*
Reconstructive surgery, after skin cancer excision, flaps in, advancement, 1409–1411, *1409–1411*
rotation, 1411–1413, *1412, 1413*
terminology of, 1408–1409
transposition, 1413–1416, *1414–1416*
grafting in, composite, 1421–1423, *1424*
full-thickness, 1420–1421, *1421–1423*
split-thickness, 1417–1420, *1417–1420*
Rectum, in granuloma venereum, 980
Red man syndrome, 420
5α-Reductase, in androgenetic alopecia, 1254–1255
in hair follicle growth, 1249, *1249*
Reed-Sternberg cells, vs. lymphomatoid papulosis, 1632, *1633,* 1634, 1635t, 1637
Refsum's disease, 1695
Reiter's syndrome, 322–325, *323,* 323t–325t, *324*
conjunctivitis in, vs. psoriasis, 301
cutaneous signs of, *1881*
vs. Behçet's disease, 389t
vs. pustular psoriasis, 299
with human immunodeficiency virus infection, 1148

Relapsing polychondritis, 512–514, *513*,
513t, 514t
cardiac disorders in, cutaneous signs with,
1879t, *1881*, Plate 15
Renal. See *Kidney(s)*.
Rendu-Osler-Weber syndrome, 1799t, *1800*,
1882t
gastrointestinal hemorrhage in, 1874t, *1876*
Respiratory tract. See also *Lung(s)*.
disorders of, in Churg-Strauss syndrome,
523, 527
in hypereosinophilic syndrome, 354
in toxic epidermal necrolysis, 706
in Wegener's granulomatosis, 523, 527
obstruction of, hemangioma and, in
infancy, 1498
Restrictive dermopathy, 1697
Rete ridges, in lichen nitidus, 240, *240*
in skin structure, 5, *6*
Reticular erythematous mucinosis, 1834t,
1834–1836, *1835*
Reticularis multiplex (livedo reticularis),
831–832, *832*, 832t
in systemic lupus erythematosus, 263
with antiphospholipid antibody syndrome,
1865t, *1866*
Reticulohistiocytoma, of back, 1664
Reticulohistiocytosis, congenital, self-healing,
716t, 1610
multicentric, 1616–1617, *1617*, 1617t
cardiac disorders in, cutaneous signs
with, 1879t
Reticuloid syndrome, actinic, 763, 768–770,
769, 769t, 770t, Plate 5
Reticulosis, pagetoid, in lymphoma, T-cell,
1641, 1644
Retiform hemangioendothelioma, 1516
Retina, disorders of, antimalarial drugs and,
in treatment of lupus erythematosus,
275–276
in pseudoxanthoma elasticum,
1770–1771, *1771*, 1773–1774
in von Hippel–Lindau syndrome, 1799t,
1801
gliomas of, in tuberous sclerosis, 1737
Retin-A. See *Retinoic acid*.
Retinitis pigmentosa, in Refsum's disease,
1695
Retinoic acid (tretinoin), and hyperlipidemia,
with xanthoma, 1815
for acne keloidalis nuchae, 1283, 1283t
for alopecia, androgenetic, 1257
for melasma, 1236
for perforating collagenosis, reactive, 410
for photoaging, 740–741, 741t
for pseudofolliculitis barbae, 501
for skin carcinoma, 1429–1431
receptors of, in keratinocyte differentiation,
69, *69*
Retinoids, and hyperlipidemia, with
xanthoma, 1815
effect of, on wrinkling, 735, *736*
for acantholytic dermatosis, 343, 343t
for acne, 468, 470–473, *472*, 472t
for acne keloidalis nuchae, 1283, 1283t
for alopecia, androgenetic, 1257
for cellulitis, of scalp, 1282, 1282t
for Darier's disease, 1701
for erythroderma, 339, 339t
for ichthyosis, harlequin, 1691
lamellar, 1687
for lichen planus, 239, 239t
for lupus erythematosus, discoid, 276
for lymphomatoid papulosis, 1637
for measles, 1127

Retinoids (*Continued*)
for melasma, 1236
for perforating collagenosis, reactive, 410
for photoaging, 740–741, 741t
for pityriasis rubra pilaris, 334t, 334–335
for pseudofolliculitis barbae, 501
for psoriasis, 309–310, 315
for skin carcinoma, 1429–1431
in facial skin care, 81
Retinyl palmitate, for measles, 1127
in facial skin care, 81
Reversal reactions, in leprosy, 997–998,
1002–1003
Reye's syndrome, 1079, 1081
Rhabdomyoma, 1524–1525
of heart, in tuberous sclerosis, 1228, 1737
cutaneous signs with, 1879t
Rhabdomyomatous mesenchymal
hamartoma, 1793–1794
Rhabdomyosarcoma, *1525*, 1525–1526
Rhagades, in congenital syphilis, 960t
Rheumatic fever, cardiac disorders in,
cutaneous signs with, 1879t
erythema marginatum with, *350*, 350–351
Rheumatoid arthritis, cutaneous signs of,
1863, *1864*, 1864t
in mixed connective tissue disease, 268
Rheumatoid neutrophilic dermatitis, 376–377
Rheumatoid nodules, 444–447, *445, 446*,
446t
in systemic lupus erythematosus, 264
Rhinophyma, 485, *486*, Plate 4
electrosurgery for, *493*, 493–496, *495*
Rhizomelic chondrodysplasia, 1695
Rhodesiense sleeping sickness, 1174–1175
Rhombic transposition flap, after skin cancer
excision, 1414, *1415*
Rhus dermatitis, configuration of, *87*
Rhytidosis, ultraviolet light exposure and,
Plate 5, 733t, 733–735, *734–736*
chemical peel for, 741–746, *742*, 742t,
743t, *744–746*, 745t, 746t
Riboflavin deficiency, cutaneous signs of,
1873t
Richner-Hanhart syndrome, 1859t,
1859–1860, *1860*
palmoplantar keratoderma in, 1706
Rickets, and alopecia, 1712
Rickettsial infection, 1011–1019
and ehrlichiosis, 1012t, 1019
and Mediterranean spotted fever, 1012t,
1016–1017
and Oriental spotted fever, 1012t, 1016
and Q fever, 1012t, 1019
and Queensland tick typhus, 1012t, 1016
and Rocky Mountain spotted fever,
1011–1016. See also *Rocky Mountain
spotted fever*.
and Siberian tick typhus, 1012t, 1016
and South African tick-bite fever, 1012t,
1016, *1016*
and typhus, 1012t, 1017–1019, *1019*
Rickettsialpox, 1017
Ridley-Jopling classification, of leprosy, 994,
995t
Riehls' melanosis, vs. melasma, 1235
Rifampin, for cellulitis, of scalp, 1282, 1282t
for leprosy, 1000–1002, 1001t
for tuberculosis, 989
Riley-Smith syndrome, 1506, 1799t
Risorius muscle, anatomy of, 113, *113*
Ritter disease, 935, *935*
Rochalimaea henselae infection, 1023–1028.
See also *Angiomatosis, bacillary* and
Cat-scratch disease.

Rocky Mountain spotted fever, 1011–1016
clinical findings in, 1011–1013, 1012t, *1013*
diagnosis of, 1014–1015, *1015*, 1015t
pathogenesis of, 1014
pathology of, 1013–1014, *1014*
rash in, 1124t, 1125t
treatment of, 1015–1016, 1016t
vs. toxic shock syndrome, 933, 934t
Rogaine (minoxidil), for alopecia,
androgenetic, 1256, 1257
for alopecia areata, 1271, 1273t, 1274
Romana's sign, in trypanosomiasis, 1173,
1173
Rosacea, 485–496
clinical findings in, 485–486, *486*, Plate 4
definition of, 485
diagnosis of, 487t, 487–488
electrosurgery for, 489t, 489–493, *490–493*
in rhinophyma, *493*, 493–496, *495*
laser surgery for, 489
Lewandowsky's, 485, 487t, 987
medical treatment of, 488t, 488–489
pathogenesis of, 487
pathology of, *486*, 486–487
vs. acne, 469, *469*
with human immunodeficiency virus
infection, 1146–1147
Rosacea fulminans, 463, *463*
Rosai-Dorfman disease, 1617–1619, *1618*,
1619t
vs. Langerhans cell histiocytosis, 1613
Roseola, in herpesvirus-6 infection, 1087,
1087t, 1124t, 1125t, 1129–1130, *1130*
Rotation flaps, after skin cancer excision,
1411–1413, *1412, 1413*
Rothmund-Thomson syndrome, 765, 1803t,
1804
tooth abnormalities with, 1324t
Rowing, frictional injury in, to gluteal cleft,
853
Rubella, 1124t, 1125t, 1127–1128
oral lesions in, 1335t
Rubeola, 1124t, 1125t, 1126–1127, *1127*,
Plate 8
Rubeosis, with diabetes, 1869t
Ruby laser, Q-switched, in tattoo removal,
455t, 457–458
Rud's syndrome, 1684, 1698
Ruffini corpuscles, 27–28
Rugby players, herpes gladiatorum in, 851,
853
Runners, injuries in, 851, 853
Running sutures, 136, *136*

S

Sabinas syndrome, 1694
Sagartia elegans stings, 790
Sailor's neck, 733, *733*
Salicylates. See also *Aspirin*.
and Reye's syndrome, 1079, 1081
in sunscreens, 754
Salivary glands, in Sjögren's syndrome,
cutaneous signs with, 1863, *1864*,
1864t, *1865*, Plate 15
in lupus erythematosus, 266, 268
metaplasia of, necrotizing, 1333
parotid, anatomy of, *113*, 115–116
sicca syndrome of, in human
immunodeficiency virus infection,
1148–1149
Salmon patch, 1496t, 1502–1503
vs. port-wine stain, 1501
Salmonella typhi infection, 945

Sandflies, as vectors, of bartonellosis, 1025
  of leishmaniasis, 1163, 1167, *1167*
Saphenous vein, anatomy of, 576, *577*
Sarcoidosis, 433–437
  and hypopigmentation, 1229, *1229*
  annular, *87*
  cardiac disorders in, cutaneous signs with,
    1879t
  cutaneous signs of, 433–435, *434*, 1882t,
    1883
  definition of, 433
  diagnosis of, 436, 436t
  epidemiology of, 433
  pathogenesis of, 435–436
  pathology of, 435, *435, 436*
  renal disease in, cutaneous signs with, 1884t
  systemic disease in, 435
  treatment of, 436–437, 437t
Sarcoma, in dermatofibrosarcoma
    protuberans, 1553t, 1555t, *1555–1557,*
    1555–1558
  Kaposi's, 1149–1155. See also *Kaposi's
    sarcoma.*
  of fatty tissue, 1530, *1531*
  of muscle, 1523–1526, *1524, 1525*
  of nerve sheath, 1546, *1546*
  with granulocytic leukemia, 1672
Sarcoptes scabiei infestation. See *Scabies.*
Saucerization biopsy, technique of, 124–127,
    126
Scabies, *1195–1197*, 1195–1198, 1197t
  burrows in, 101, *102*, 1196, *1196*, 1197
  in neonate, 715t, 718, *1893, 1895, 1896*
  vs. chancroid, 975t
  with human immunodeficiency virus
    infection, 1143, *1143*
Scalded skin syndrome, staphylococcal, 934t,
    935, 935–937, *936*
  rash in, 1124t, 1125t
  vs. toxic epidermal necrolysis, 707,
    710t
Scales, assessment of, 97, *97–99*, 98
  in ichthyosis, 1681–1706. See also
    Ichthyosis.
  in neonate, 1896–1897
  with chondrodysplasia, *1695*, 1695–1696,
    1716
Scalp, anatomy of, lymphatic system in, 115,
    116
  muscles in, 114
  aplasia cutis congenita of, 1783t, 1784,
    1784, 1785
  cellulitis of, and alopecia, *1281,*
    1281–1282, 1282t
  disorders of, in temporal arteritis, 516, 516t
  in cutis verticis gyrata, 1794
  lifting of, for alopecia, 1263–1265, *1264*
  louse infestation of, 1191–1193, 1192t
  psoriasis of, 301
  pustular dermatosis of, and alopecia, *1284,*
    1284t, 1284–1285
  reduction surgery of, for alopecia, *1262,*
    1262–1263, *1263*
  tinea of, and scarring alopecia, 1285, *1285*
    clinical findings in, 1043–1045, 1044t,
      1045, 1046
    differential diagnosis of, 1052t
    vs. alopecia areata, 1272t
  trichilemmal cysts of, 1453–1454, *1456*
Scapula, scaphoid, in congenital syphilis, 960t
Scarlet fever, rash in, 1124t, 1125t
  vs. toxic shock syndrome, 934t
Scars, after acne, papular, vs. anetoderma,
    911t
  surgery for, *473*, 473–479

Scars (*Continued*)
  after curettage and electrodesiccation, for
    carcinoma, 1396
  after laser ablation, of warts, 1116
  after punch hair grafting, 1260
  definition of, 110
  hypertrophic, 900–905
    clinical findings in, 900, *901*
    definition of, 900
    diagnosis of, 902
    pathogenesis of, 901–902
    pathology of, 900–901
    treatment of, 902–905
  in alopecia, 1280–1293. See also *Alopecia,
    scarring.*
  in hydroa vacciniforme, 763, *764*
  in lupus erythematosus, management of,
    274
  keloid, 900–905. See also *Keloids.*
Schamberg's disease, 291–293, *292*
Schistosomiasis, 1184–1186, *1185*
  and swimmer's itch, *793*, 793–795, 794t,
    795t
Schizophrenia, bromhidrosis in, 1317
Schizotrypanum cruzi infection, *1173,*
    1173–1174
Schwachman's syndrome, 1697
Schwann cells, anatomy of, 1536–1537
Schwannoma, 1539–1540, *1540*, 1541t, 1542t
  malignant, 1546, *1546*
Schweninger-Buzzi anetoderma, 910
SCL-70 antibodies, in scleroderma, 885
Scleredema, 1834t, 1836
  vs. scleroderma, 887, 888t
  with diabetes, 1869t
Sclerema neonatorum, 599–600, *600*, 600t
Scleroatrophy, in palmoplantar keratoderma,
    1704–1705, *1705*
Sclerodactyly, Raynaud's phenomenon in,
    540
Scleroderma, cardiac disorders in, cutaneous
    signs with, 1879t
  chemically induced, 891–894, 892t, *893*
  clinical findings in, 882–884, *883*
  definition of, 882
  diagnosis of, 886–887, 887t, *888*, 888t
  in mixed connective tissue disease, 268
  pathogenesis of, 884–885
  pathology of, 885–886, *886*
  pulmonary disease in, cutaneous signs
    with, 1882t
  Raynaud's phenomenon in, 537, 538, 540
  renal disease in, cutaneous signs with, 1883t
  treatment of, 887–889
Sclerodermoid graft-versus-host reaction,
    after marrow transplantation, *230,*
    230–232, *231*
Scleromyxedema, vs. scleroderma, 887, 888t
Sclerosing hemangioma, 1552–1555, *1553,*
    1553t, *1554*, 1555t
Sclerosing panniculitis, 603–605, *604*, 605t
  with venous ulcer, of leg, 558–559, *559*
Sclerosis, cutaneous, chemotherapy and, 429
  definition of, 110
  systemic. See *Scleroderma.*
Sclerotherapy, for telangiectasia, 574–575,
    575, 580, 580–581
  for varicose veins, 574, *580*, 580–581
  for venous malformations, 1503
Scoliosis, in Ehlers-Danlos syndrome, 1775
Scopulariopsis brevicaulis infection, of nail,
    1047, 1072
Scorpion bites, 817
Scorpion fish stings, 801–802
Scorpion stings, 817

Scrofuloderma, 984–985, 988, 988t
Scrotum, calcinosis of, idiopathic, 1352
Scrub typhus, 1012t, 1018–1019, *1019*
Scurvy, and gastrointestinal hemorrhage,
    1875t
  cutaneous signs of, 1873t, *1874*
Scytalidium infection, vs. tinea pedis, 1046
Sea anemone larvae, and seabather's
    eruption, 792–793
Sea anemone stings, 789–790, *790*
Sea blubber stings, 788–789
Sea cucumbers, and dermatitis, 797
Sea lice, 1186, 1187t
Sea nettle stings, 788
Sea urchins, and skin wounds, 798–799
Sea wasp stings, 787–789, *790*, 791t
Seabather's eruption, 791–793, *792*, 793t,
    794t, 1186–1187, *1187*, 1187t
Seaweed, and dermatitis, 795–796
Sebaceous glands, adenoma of, 1472, *1472*
  anatomy of, 30–32, *32, 33, 1246*
  carcinoma of, *1473*, 1473–1474, *1474*
  embryology of, 4–5
  epithelioma of, 1472–1473
  hyperplasia of, *1471*, 1471–1472
  in acne, 461, *462*, 465–466, 466t. See also
    Acne.
  in steatocystoma multiplex, 1454–1455,
    1456, 1457
  in vermilion border, 30–31, 1325
  secretions of, normal variations in, 75, 76t
Sebaceous nevi, 1790t, 1790–1792, *1791*
Sebaceous trichofolliculoma, 1466
Seborrhea, in perioral dermatitis, 497, 498
Seborrheic dermatitis, 214–217
  clinical findings in, 214–215, *215*
  diagnosis of, 216t, 216–217
  light-exacerbated, vs. actinic reticuloid
    syndrome, 770, 770t
  pathogenesis of, 215–216
  pathology of, 215
  treatment of, 165, 217, 217t
  vs. acne, 469
  vs. atopic dermatitis, 199
  vs. plaque psoriasis, 297
  with human immunodeficiency virus
    infection, 214, 216, 1146, 1147, *1147*
Seborrheic keratosis, *92, 93, 1444,*
    1444–1446, *1445*, 1445t
  in rosacea, electrodesiccation of, *490,*
    490–491
  multiple eruptive, paraneoplastic, 1846
  stucco, 1446–1447, 1447t
  vs. dermatosis papulosa nigra, 1441
Seizures, in tuberous sclerosis, 1737
Selectins, in inflammatory response, 149–151
Selectivity theory, of pruritus, 156–157
Selenium deficiency, cutaneous signs of, 1873t
Selenium oxychloride, and burn injury, 845t
Selenium sulfide, for seborrheic dermatitis,
    217, 217t
Senear-Usher syndrome, 264
Sensory receptors, in skin, *25–27*, 25–28
Septicemia, in plague, 1034
  Pseudomonas aeruginosa infection and,
    skin lesions with, 945, *945*
Septra. See *Trimethoprim, with
    sulfamethoxazole.*
Seroma, after liposuction, 1532
Serositis, in systemic lupus erythematosus, 265
Serum sickness, 417–418
Serum sickness–like reactions, 418
Sessile excrescence, definition of, 110
Sexual abuse, 841–843, 1892
Sézary syndrome, 1640, *1640*

Shagreen patch, in tuberous sclerosis, 1736, 1740
Shave biopsy, technique of, 121, 124–127, *125*
Shave excision, for actinic keratosis, 1396
   for skin carcinoma, 1398
Shaving, and pseudofolliculitis barbae, 499–502, *500*, 500t
Shellfish, *Vibrio vulnificus* contamination of, 942
Shin, saber, in syphilis, congenital, 960t
Shingles, 1078–1081. See also *Varicella-zoster infection.*
Shivering, in thermoregulation, 54
Sialometaplasia, necrotizing, 1333
Sialomucins, in inflammatory response, 150
Siberian tick typhus, 1012t, 1016
Sicca syndrome, in human immunodeficiency virus infection, 1148–1149
Siderophage, definition of, 110
Silicone, implants of, and scleroderma, 887, 888t, 892t, 893–894
   in gel dressings, for hypertrophic scars, 903
      for keloids, 903
Silver, and hyperpigmentation, 1237
Silver nitrate, in hemostasis, 133
Sinequan (doxepin), for neurotic excoriations, 784
   for urticaria, 402
Sinus histiocytosis, 1617–1619, *1618*, 1619t
   with lymphadenopathy, vs. Langerhans cell histiocytosis, 1613
Sinus tracts, definition of, 110
   from dental caries to skin, vs. acne, 469
   in hidradenitis suppurativa, 481, *482*
Sinusoidal hemangioma, 1516
Sjögren-Larsson syndrome, 1692–1693
Sjögren's syndrome, cutaneous signs of, 1863, *1864*, 1864t, *1865*, Plate 15
   in lupus erythematosus, 266, 268
Skin. See also specific structures, e.g., *Hair follicles*, and disorders, e.g., *Lupus erythematosus.*
   blood vessels of, 21–23, *24, 25*
   care of, normal, 75–82, 76t, *77*, 78t, *80, 81*
      of body, 81–82
      of face, 79–81, *80*
      of hands, *81*, 81–82
   disorders of, diagnosis of, chronology in, 102–103, *103*
      clinical, 84–87, 85t, *85–88*
      color in, 88–89, 89t, *89–92*, 103–104, *104*
      lesion configuration in, 104–105, 105t
      lesion consistency in, 104
      terminology in, *105–109*, 105–110
   dryness of, normal, 76, *77, 77*
   embryology of, 3–5, *4*
   in immune system, 40–41
   in temperature regulation, 53–56
   innervation of, 23–28, *25–27*
   lesions of, types of, 88–102. See also specific lesions, e.g., *Papule(s).*
   normal variations in, 75, 76t
   perforating disorders of, 407–411, *408–410*, 410t, 411t, 1869t, *1870*
   pigmentation of, 11–13, *17, 18*
   racial differences in, 41
   sensitivity of, 78–79
   structure of, 3, *4*
   tension lines in, resting, anatomy of, 114–115
Slack skin, granulomatous, vs. anetoderma, 911t

Sleeping sickness, African, *1174*, 1174–1175
Small intestine. See *Intestine.*
Smallpox, 1093–1095, *1094*, 1094t, 1095t
Smoking, in protease inhibitor deficiency panniculitis, 605, 607
Sneddon's syndrome, 548
Soap, in facial cleansing, 79
   in skin care, of hands and body, 81
Soapfish toxin, and dermatitis, 797
Sodium hypochlorite, and wound healing, 566t
Solar elastosis, 734–735, *735*, 875–876, *876*, Plate 5
Solar keratosis, 1378–1380. See also *Keratosis, actinic.*
Solar lentigines, vs. stucco keratosis, 1447
Solar urticaria, idiopathic, *762*, 762–763
   vs. polymorphic light eruption, 760, 760t
Sole. See *Foot.*
Solenopsis stings, 807t, 808t, 808–809, *809*
South African tick-bite fever, 1012t, 1016, *1016*
Southern blot technique, in cutaneous T-cell lymphoma, 1648–1649
Sowda, 1178
Spangler's papular dermatitis, in pregnancy, 370
Spanish toxic oil syndrome, cutaneous mucinosis in, 1838
   scleroderma in, 891, 892t
Sparganosis, 1188
Specificity theory, of pruritus, 156
Spectacle frames, and acanthoma fissuratum, 773t, 773–774, 774t
Sperm, methotrexate toxicity to, 309
Sphenoid wing dysplasia, in neurofibromatosis, 1731
Spider angioma, 1509
Spider bites, 811–813, *811–813*
Spinal accessory nerve, anatomy of, *118*, 119
Spinal cord, in angiomatosis, 1506
   injury to, and hyperhidrosis, 1311–1312
Spindle cell carcinoma, pathology of, 1385, *1386*
Spindle cell hemangioendothelioma, 1516, 1517
Spindle cell lipoma, 1528
Spindle cell nevus, vs. melanoma, 1587
Spindle cells, in nerve sheath myxoma, 1544, *1544*
   in neurofibroma, 1540, *1543*
Spine, scoliosis of, in Ehlers-Danlos syndrome, 1775
Spines, in keratotic lesions, 98, *99*
Spinous layer, 3
Spiradenoma, *1477, 1482*, 1482–1483, 1483t
Spiramycin, for toxoplasmosis, 1175
Spirometra larva, in sparganosis, 1188
Spironolactone, for alopecia, androgenetic, 1257
   for hirsutism, 1856–1857
Spitz nevi, 1566, *1566, 1567*, Plate 10
   multiple, configuration of, *87*
   vs. melanoma, 1587
Spleen, enlargement of, in T-cell lymphoma, 1656
Sponge nevus, white, 1325
Sponges, absorbable, in hemostasis, 133
   and dermatitis, 796
Spongiform pustules, definition of, 110
Spongiosis, blisters in, 95, *95, 96*, 96t
   definition of, 110
   in acantholytic dermatosis, 341–342, *343*
   in contact dermatitis, occupational, 179, *179*

Spongiosis (*Continued*)
   in incontinentia pigmenti, 1725, *1727*
   in pityriasis rosea, 218–220, *219*, 220t, 221t
   papules in, *92*
Spores, in dermatophytosis, 1050
Sporotrichosis, 1061–1063, *1062*, 1063t
   with human immunodeficiency virus infection, 1142
Sports, and acne mechanica, 772–773, 852, 853
   and athlete's foot, 851, 928–929
   and cold injury, 849, 852
   and friction injury, 850–851, 853
      nodules in, 775t, 775–776, 776t, 851
   and infectious skin disease, 851–852
   and skin disorders, 849–853, 850t, 852t
      regional classification of, 850t
   and steroid abuse, 852
   and sun exposure, 849, 852
   and urticaria, 852
   aquatic, and skin disorders, 787–802. See also *Aquatic skin disorders.*
   equipment in, and contact dermatitis, 850, 853
Spotted fever, Mediterranean, 1012t, 1016–1017
   Oriental, 1012t, 1016
   Rocky Mountain, 1011–1016. See also *Rocky Mountain spotted fever.*
Squamous cells, definition of, 110
   in carcinoma. See *Carcinoma.*
Stanazolol, for sclerosing panniculitis, 605
   for urticaria, 403
Staphylococcal infection, 919–923, 925–929
   and carbuncles, 922
   and furuncles, 922
   and pustules, in folliculitis, *97*
      in neonate, *1893*, 1895
   and pyoderma, in neonate, 712, 715t
   and scalded skin syndrome, 934t, *935*, 935–937, *936*
      rash in, 1124t, 1125t
      vs. toxic epidermal necrolysis, 707, 710t
   and toxic shock syndrome, 931–935, 934t
   interdigital, 928, 929
   recurrent, 922–923, 923t
   with human immunodeficiency virus infection, 1138, *1138*
Staphylococcus aureus infection, and abscesses, 926
   and dactylitis, distal blistering, 922
   and ecthyma, 921, *922*
   and folliculitis, 922
   and impetigo, *920*, 920–921, *921*
      genital, and pyoderma, 1343
   in atopic dermatitis, 197, 199, 201
   topical corticosteroids and, 165
   with scabies, 1196, 1197
Staphylococcus epidermidis, in acne, 465–467
Staphylococcus species, in normal cutaneous flora, 926
Starfish, and skin wounds, 798–799
Stasis dermatitis, with venous ulcer, of leg, 558
Steatocystoma multiplex, 1454–1455, *1456, 1457*
Stellate cells, in nerve sheath myxoma, 1544, *1544*
Stem cells, epidermal, 5–6
   follicular, anatomy of, 1247
   keratinocytic, in basal layer, 58–59, *60*
Sternum, clefting of, hemangioma with, 1498
Steroids. See *Corticosteroids.*
Stevens-Johnson syndrome, 247–254. See also *Erythema multiforme.*
   vs. Behçet's disease, 389t

Stevens-Johnson syndrome (*Continued*)
    vs. toxic epidermal necrolysis, 704, 708,
        710t
    vs. toxic shock syndrome, 933, 934t
Stewart-Treves syndrome, 554, 556, 1516
Stibogluconate, for leishmaniasis, 1169
Stingrays, and skin injury, 797, 800
Stings, by insects, 807–809, 808t, *809*
    by marine life, 798–802, 801t
        and contact dermatitis, 795–797
        cnidarian, 787–791, 788t, *789, 790,* 791t
    by scorpions, 817
Stomach. See also *Gastrointestinal tract.*
    hemorrhage in, in pseudoxanthoma
        elasticum, 1771, 1774
    inflammation of, in *Aeromonas hydrophila*
        infection, 943
    in syphilis, 952
Stomatitis, aphthous, in Behçet's disease,
        385, 386
    in human immunodeficiency virus
        infection, 1148, 1337t
    recurrent, 1330–1331
    herpes simplex infection and, 1335, 1335t
    in pemphigus, paraneoplastic, 659, *659*
    in Reiter's syndrome, 323, 323t, *324,* 325
    lichenoid, 1331
    nicotine and, 1329
    pyoderma gangrenosum with, 381, *381*
    ulcerative, chronic, with stratified
        epithelium-specific antinuclear
        antibody, 1333
Stomolophus meleagris stings, 788
Stonefish stings, 801–802
Strands, definition of, 110
Stratum corneum. See *Cornified layer.*
Stratum germinativum (basal layer), in
        gestation, 3
    structure of, 5–6, *6*
Stratum granulosum (granular layer), in
        epidermal structure, 6, *14, 15*
    in gestation, 3
    keratinocytes in, 63–66, *65*
Stratum lucidum, in epidermal structure, 6
Stratum spinosum, in gestation, 3
Streptocerciasis, 1179
Streptococcal infection, 919–926
    and cellulitis, *924,* 924t, 924–926, 925t
        diagnosis of, 945
    and erysipelas, *923,* 923–925, 925t
    and toxic shock–like syndrome, 933,
        934t
    genital, and pyoderma, 1343
Streptococcus pneumoniae infection, 940
Streptococcus pyogenes infection, and
    cellulitis, perianal, 925–926
    and dactylitis, blistering, 922
    and ecthyma, 921
    and impetigo, 920–921
    and psoriasis, 301
    sports-related, 851
Streptomyces infection, and mycetoma, 1069,
    1070, 1071t
Streptomycin, for granuloma inguinale, 979
    for mycetoma, 1070
    for plague, 1034t
    for tularemia, 947, 1035
Striae, in adolescent athletes, 851
Striae atrophica, vs. anetoderma, 911t
Striae distensae, in keloids, 901
Strongyloidiasis, *1182,* 1182–1183, Plate 9
    and larva migrans, cutaneous, 1181, 1181t
    vs. hypereosinophilic syndrome, 356
    with human immunodeficiency virus
        infection, 1143
Stucco keratosis, 1446–1447, 1447t

Sturge-Weber syndrome, 1799t, *1800*
    cutaneous vascular malformations with,
        1505
Subcorneal pustules, 110, 327–329, *328,
        329,* 329t
Subcutaneous fat. See *Fat, subcutaneous.*
    inflammation of. See *Panniculitis.*
Subcuticular running sutures, 136, *136*
Subependymomas, giant cell, in tuberous
        sclerosis, 1737
Substance P, in perniosis, 829
Sucking, intrauterine, and blisters, in
        neonate, 715t, 719, *719*
Sucquet-Hoyer canal, 23, *25*
Suction blisters, grafting of, for vitiligo, 1216
Sulfadiazine, and wound healing, 566t
    for nocardiosis, 1007, 1008t
    for toxoplasmosis, 1175
Sulfamethoxazole. See *Trimethoprim.*
Sulfapyridine, for bullous dermatosis, linear
        IgA, 701–702, 702t
    for bullous pemphigoid, 670
    for dermatitis herpetiformis, 695
Sulfasalazine, for discoid lupus
        erythematosus, 276
    for urticaria, 402–403
Sulfisoxazole, for lymphogranuloma
        venereum, 976t, 981
    for nocardiosis, 1008t
Sulfonamides, for erythema elevatum
        diutinum, 530
    reactions to, in human immunodeficiency
        virus infection, 423, 1145
    in hypersensitivity syndrome, 416–417
Sulzberger-Garbe syndrome, 211
Sunburn, 736–737. See also *Photodamage.*
Sunlight, heat transmission in, 823
    spectrum of, 751, 1364, *1364*
    ultraviolet radiation in. See *Ultraviolet light.*
Sunscreens, 78, 78t, 739, 752–757, 753t,
        755t, 756t
    active ingredients in, 753t, 753–755
    development of, 752
    evaluation of, 752–753
    for children, 756t, 756–757, 1891
    for normal skin, 755t, 755–757
    for photosensitive skin, 755t, 756t, 757
    guidelines for use of, 756t, 757
    in facial skin protection, 81
    in lupus erythematosus, 274
    in melasma, 1236
Supraclavicular nerves, anatomy of, *118,* 119
Supraorbital nerve, anatomy of, 117
Supratrochlear nerve, anatomy of, 117
Suramin, for trypanosomiasis, 1175
Surfer's knots, 775t, 775–776, 776t, 851
Surgery. See also specific indications, e.g.,
        Carcinoma, and techniques, e.g., *Laser
        surgery.*
    alopecia after, diffuse, 1277
    anesthesia in, 130t, 130–131
    antisepsis in, 128–129, 129t
    hemostasis in, 131–134, *132*
    suture techniques in, 134–137, *134–137*
Sutton's disease, 1330
Sutures, in flap reconstruction, 1409
    in skin grafting, split-thickness, 1419,
        1420, *1420*
    techniques of, 134–137, *134–137*
Sweat ducts, carcinoma of, 1483–1484, 1484t
Sweat glands. See also *Apocrine glands* and
        Eccrine glands.
    absence of, with ectodermal dysplasia,
        1714, 1721, 1722t, 1723t
    anatomy of, 32–36, *34–40,* 1308–1309,
        1309

Sweat glands (*Continued*)
    autonomic effects on, 23–25, *25,* 1308
    disorders of, in ectodermal dysplasia, 1721,
        1722t, 1723t
    hypersecretion by, 1307–1308,
        1311–1317. See also *Hyperhidrosis.*
    in thermoregulation, 55–56
    physiology of, 36, 1307–1310, *1310*
Sweet's syndrome, 372–375, *373,* 373t–375t,
        Plate 3
    paraneoplastic, 1844–1845, *1845, 1868,*
        Plate 14
    vs. Behçet's disease, 389t
    vs. rheumatoid neutrophilic dermatitis, 377
Swimmer's itch, *793,* 793–795, 794t, 795t,
        1186, 1187t
Swimming, and hair discoloration, 849–850,
        852–853
    and otitis externa, 851, 853
Swimming pool granuloma, 989t, 990, *990,*
        Plate 7
Sycosis barbae, chronic, 499–502, *500,* 500t
    vs. acne, 469–470
Symblepharon, in epidermolysis bullosa
        acquisita, *687*
    in pemphigoid, cicatricial, 674, *675*
Synovial cysts, 1839
    periungual, 1299t, 1305
Synovitis, in congenital syphilis, 960t
Syphilis, 949–961
    anetoderma after, *911*
    central nervous system in, 957t, *958,*
        958–961
    condylomata lata in, 951, 952, *952,* 954
        vs. papillomavirus infection, 1102, *1103*
    congenital, 957t, 958, 959, *960,* 960t, 1324t
    definition of, 949
    endemic, 961, 963
    epidemiology of, 953
    false-positive test for, in systemic lupus
        erythematosus, 274
    genital lesions in, 1344
    hair loss in, vs. alopecia areata, 1272t
    laboratory tests for, 954–955, *955,* 956t
    latent, 952
    mucocutaneous, late, 952–953, 957, 957t
    pathology of, 953–954, *954*
    primary, clinical findings in, 949–950, *950*
        differential diagnosis of, 955–957, 956t
    secondary, clinical findings in, 950–952,
        950–952
        differential diagnosis of, 956t, 957
        vs. lichen planus, 238, 238t
        vs. psoriasis, guttate, 299
    skin lesions in, 945
    transmission of, 953
    treatment of, 957t, 957–958
    vs. Behçet's disease, 389t
    vs. chancroid, 974–975, 975t
    with human immunodeficiency virus
        infection, 959–961
Syringocystadenoma papilliferum, 1484t,
        1485, 1485–1486, 1486t
Syringoid carcinoma, of sweat ducts,
        1483–1484, 1484t
Syringoma, 1477–1478, *1477–1479,* 1478t
Systematized lesions, definition of, 110
Systemic lupus erythematosus. See *Lupus
        erythematosus.*
Systemic sclerosis. See *Scleroderma.*

T

T cells. See *Lymphocytes.*
T_3 receptors, in keratinocyte differentiation,
        70

Tabes dorsalis, 959

Tache noir, in rickettsial fever, 1016, *1016*
  sports and, 850–851, 853

Tachyphylaxis, topical corticosteroids and, 165

Taenia solium larva, in cysticercosis, 1187–1188

Talon noir, sports and, 850, 853

Tampons, in toxic shock syndrome, 931–932

Tanning, ultraviolet light exposure and, 732, 736–737, 752

Tapeworm larva, in cysticercosis, 1187–1188
  in sparganosis, 1188

Tar, and burn injury, 844t, 846

Tar preparations, for atopic dermatitis, 201
  for psoriasis, 306, 313

Targetoid hemosiderotic hemangioma, 1507t, *1515*, 1515–1516

Tattoos, 452–459
  amalgam, 1323
  clinical appearance of, 452–453
  for vitiligo, 1216
  histology of, 453, *453*
  laser surgery for, 454t–456t, 454–459, *456, 457*

Tay syndrome, 1694

Tedania ignis, and dermatitis, 796

Teeth, abscesses of, cutaneous drainage of, 1337
  caries of, and sinus tract to skin, vs. acne, 469
  disorders of, in dermatologic disease, 1323, 1324t
    in ectodermal dysplasia, 1721–1724, 1722t, 1723t, *1724*
    in epidermolysis bullosa, 639, 1324t
    in syphilis, congenital, 960, 960t
    with dermal hypoplasia, focal, 1780, 1781t
    with palmoplantar hyperkeratosis, 1722t
  extraction of, actinomycotic abscess after, 1007–1008, *1008*

Telangiectasia, 1509
  assessment of, 101, *101, 102*
  ataxia with, 1802t, *1804*
  clinical findings in, 575
  diagnosis of, 578–580, 579t
  hemorrhagic, hereditary, 1799t, *1800*, 1882t
    and gastrointestinal hemorrhage, 1874t, *1876*
  in Bloom's syndrome, 1802t
  in rosacea, 485, 491, *492, 493*
  in scleroderma, 883, 883–884
  paraneoplastic, 1848
  sclerotherapy for, 574–575, *575, 580*, 580–581

Telangiectasia macularis eruptiva perstans, 1603–1604, 1606t

Telemactis rufa stings, 790

Telogen, definition of, 110
  effluvium in, after punch hair grafting, 1259–1260
  and alopecia, diffuse, *1274*, 1274–1278, *1276*, 1277t
  vs. alopecia areata, 1272t
  in hair growth, 30, *31*, 1247, 1248

Temovate. See *Clobetasol.*

Temperature regulation, in toxic epidermal necrolysis, 706
  skin in, 53–56
  in neonate, 1890–1891

Temporal arteritis, 515–517, *516*, 516t
  infrared radiation and, 825

Temporal artery, anatomy of, 115
  superficial, in flap surgery, for alopecia, 1265

Temporal bone, mastoid process of, anatomy of, 112

Temporal branch, of facial nerve, anatomy of, *113*, 116, 116t, 117

Temporoparieto-occipital flap surgery, for alopecia, *1265*, 1265–1266

Tendons, xanthomas in, 1809, *1810*, 1811, 1815

Tension lines, anatomy of, 114–115

Terbinafine, for dermatophytosis, 1054

Terbutaline, for urticaria, 402

Terfenadine, for urticaria, 402

Terry's nail, 1300–1301

Testes, cancer of, with ichthyosis, X-linked recessive, 1684
  disorders of, in leprosy, 999

Testosterone, and sebaceous gland activity, in acne, 465
  in androgenetic alopecia, 1254–1256
  in genital development, 1340
  in hair follicle growth, 1249, *1249*
  in hirsutism, 1853–1855

Tetracycline, for acne, 471, 471t
  for acne keloidalis nuchae, 1283, 1283t
  for actinomycosis, 1008t, 1009
  for anthrax, 1031
  for Behçet's disease, 389, 390t
  for bowel-associated dermatosis-arthritis syndrome, 376, 376t
  for bullous pemphigoid, 670
  for cellulitis, of scalp, 1282, 1282t
  for erythema elevatum diutinum, 530
  for erythrasma, genital, 1344
  for folliculitis decalvans, 1284, 1284t
  for granuloma inguinale, 976t, 979
  for lymphogranuloma venereum, 976t, 981
  for perioral dermatitis, 498
  for plague, 1034t
  for Rocky Mountain spotted fever, 1015, 1016t
  for rosacea, 488
  for syphilis, 957t, 958
  for tularemia, 1035

Textile workers, anthrax in, 1030–1032

Thalidomide, for erythema nodosum leprosum, 1002
  for graft-versus-host disease, 232

Thermoregulation, in toxic epidermal necrolysis, 706
  skin in, 53–56
  in neonate, 1890–1894

Thiabendazole, for dracunculosis, 1181
  for gnathostomiasis, 1184
  for hookworm infestation, 1183
  for larva migrans, cutaneous, 1182
  for strongyloidiasis, 1183
  for toxocariasis, 1183
  for trichinosis, 1180

Thiamine deficiency, cutaneous signs of, 1873t

Thiazide, and phototoxicity, *728*

Thimble jellyfish larvae, and seabather's eruption, 792–793

Thioredoxin, in hair follicle growth, 1249

Thiotepa, and eccrine disorders, 429

Thrombocytopenia, and purpura, *1865*, 1865t

Thromboembolism, in hypereosinophilic syndrome, 353, 355, 357–358

Thrombophlebitis, cords in, 102, *102*
  in Behçet's disease, 386–387
  paraneoplastic, *1847*, 1847–1848

Thrombosis, drug abuse and, 840
  in antiphospholipid syndrome, 548–550
  in capillary aneurysms, 1509
  in coumarin-induced skin necrosis, 546t, 550

Thrombosis (*Continued*)
  in Köhlmeier-Degos syndrome, 551–552
  in livedo vasculopathy, 544, *544*

Thymine, in DNA photodamage, 1365, *1365*, 1366

Thymoma, and pemphigus, 660

Thymopentin, for atopic dermatitis, 202

Thyroid, antibodies to, in granuloma annulare, 441
  disorders of, and alopecia, diffuse, 1275
  dermatoses associated with, 1869–1872, 1871t, *1872*, 1872t
  hyperfunction of, with herpes gestationis, 680
  hypofunction of, and cutaneous mucinosis, 1834t, *1836*, 1836–1838, *1837*
  and hyperlipidemia, with xanthoma, 1815
  in hypersensitivity syndrome, drug-induced, 417

Thyroid hormone receptors, in keratinocyte differentiation, 70

Tibia, pseudarthrosis of, in neurofibromatosis, 1731

Tick bites, 805t, 815–816, *816*
  and Lyme borreliosis, 965–966, 970
  and rickettsial infection, 1011, 1012, 1016, 1019
  and tularemia, 944, *944*, 1035

Ticlopidine, for livedo vasculopathy, 546t

Tin ethyletiopurpurin, in photodynamic therapy, for skin carcinoma, 1427

Tinea. See also *Dermatophytosis.*
  with human immunodeficiency virus infection, 1143–1144

Tinea barbae, 1049, 1052t

Tinea capitis, and scarring alopecia, 1285, *1285*
  clinical findings in, 1043–1045, 1044t, *1045, 1046*
  differential diagnosis of, 1052t
  vs. alopecia areata, 1272t

Tinea corporis, 1043, *1044*, 1044t, 1052t

Tinea cruris (jock itch), 851, *1048*, 1048–1049, 1052t

Tinea facei, 1049, *1049*, 1052t

Tinea imbricata, 1049, 1052t

Tinea manuum, 1046–1047, *1047*, 1052t

Tinea nigra, 1037–1038, *1038*, 1038t

Tinea pedis (athlete's foot), 851, 928–929, 1044t, 1045–1047, *1046, 1047*, 1052t

Tinea unguium, *1047*, 1047–1048, *1048*, 1052t

Tinea versicolor, 1038t, *1039*, 1039–1041, *1040*, 1040t
  hypopigmentation with, 1229–1230
  scale in, *98*
  vs. vitiligo, 1214

Tinidazole, for amebiasis, 1173
  for trichomoniasis, 1177

Tissue plasminogen activator, for livedo vasculopathy, 545, 546t

Titanium dioxide, in sunscreens, 754

Tocopherol, deficiency of, cutaneous signs of, 1873t
  for pityriasis rubra pilaris, 334–335

Toenails. See *Nail(s).*

Toes. See also *Digits.*
  deformities of, in epidermolysis bullosa, dystrophic, 641, *641*, 645
  spaces between, infection of, 928–929
  trauma to, sports and, 850, 853

Tomography, computed, of skin carcinoma, 1400, *1400*

Toners, in facial cleansing, 80

Tongue, disorders of, in temporal arteritis, 516, 516t
geographic, 1327, *1327*
hairy, 1327–1328
hairy leukoplakia of, Epstein-Barr virus and, 1083, *1083*, 1084
in acquired immunodeficiency syndrome, 1336–1337
hypertrophy of, in amyloidosis, 1328
Tooth. See *Teeth*.
Topoisomerase I, antibodies to, in scleroderma, 885
TORCH syndrome, 1084
Tori, of jaws, 1328, *1328*
Touton giant cells, in xanthogranuloma, 1621, *1622*
in xanthoma, 1809, 1811, *1811*
Toxic epidermal necrolysis, 247–254, 704–710. See also *Erythema multiforme*.
clinical findings in, 704–707, *705*, Plate 4
definition of, 704
differential diagnosis of, 709, 710t
etiology of, 707–709, 708t
in neonate, vs. blistering disorders, 716t
pathogenesis of, 709
pathology of, 707, *707*
treatment of, 709–710, 710t
Toxic oil syndrome, mucinosis in, 1838
scleroderma in, 891, 892t
Toxic shock syndrome, 931–935, 934t
Toxocariasis, 1183
Toxoplasmosis, *1175*, 1175–1176, *1176*
Trabecula, definition of, 110
Trachea, disorders of, in epidermolysis bullosa, 639, 645
Trachyonychia, 1303
Transforming growth factors, in angiogenesis, 1493t, 1494
in collagen gene expression, 865
in elastin gene expression, 873
in hair development, in mice, 1718
in keloids, 869–871, 902
Transfusion, trypanosomiasis prevention in, 1174
Transglutaminase K, in keratinocyte differentiation, 66–67
Transgrediens, in palmoplantar keratoderma, 1705
Transplantation. See *Grafting*.
Transposition flaps, after skin cancer excision, 1413–1416, *1414–1416*
selection of technique for, 1416–1417
Trauma, and neuroma, 1537, *1538*, 1541t, 1542t
and pyoderma gangrenosum, 379, *380*
and skin changes, in neonate, 715t, 719
drug abuse and, 839–841, *840*
in child abuse, 841–843, *843*, *1891*, 1891–1892, *1892*
Trematode infestation, 1184–1187, *1185, 1187*, 1187t
Trench foot, 777–778, 778t, 828
Treponema carateum infection, and pinta, 961–963
Treponema pallidum infection, and syphilis, 949–961. See also *Syphilis*.
and yaws, *962*, 962–963
Tretinoin. See *Retinoic acid*.
Triactis producta stings, 790
Triacylglyceride metabolism, in neutral lipid storage disease, 1693
Triamcinolone, for acne keloidalis nuchae, 1283, 1283t
for atopic dermatitis, 201
for Behçet's disease, 390t
for cellulitis, of scalp, 1282, 1282t

Triamcinolone (*Continued*)
for chondrodermatitis nodularis, 509
for cysts, inflamed, 1457
for erosive pustular dermatosis, of scalp, 1284, 1284t
for erythema nodosum, 594
for granuloma annulare, 441
for hidradenitis suppurativa, 481
for hypertrophic scars, 903
for keloids, 903
for lichen planus, 239, 239t
for lupus erythematosus, discoid, 274
with scarring alopecia, 1289, 1289t
for nail matrix disorders, 1302
for nummular dermatitis, 213, 213t
for paronychia, 1304
for pemphigoid, cicatricial, 677
for psoriatic onycholysis, 1300
for pyoderma gangrenosum, 383, 383t
for scarring, after laser ablation, of warts, 1116
injection of, for topical corticosteroid–resistant dermatitis, 165
Trichilemmal cysts, 1452–1453, *1455*
proliferating, 1453–1454, *1456*
Trichinosis, 1180
Trichloroacetic acid, in chemical peel, for acne scars, 474
for photoaging, 742t, 743–744, *744, 745*
Tricho-dento-osseous syndrome, 1324t
Trichoepithelioma, 1466–1468, *1467, 1468*
Trichofolliculoma, *93*, 1466, *1466*
Trichohyalin granules, in hair follicles, 29, *30*
in keratinocyte differentiation, 65
Tricholemmal sheath, definition of, 110
Tricholemmoma, 1470, *1470*
Trichomalacia, definition of, 110
Trichomoniasis, 1176–1177, 1343t
Trichomycosis, axillary, 927, *928*
genital, 1344
Trichophyton infection, clinical findings in, 1043–1049, 1044t, *1044–1049*
with human immunodeficiency virus infection, 1143–1144
Trichorhinophalangeal syndrome, 1714
Trichosporon beigelii infection, and piedra, 1038–1039
genital, 1345
Trichosporon infection, in immunosuppressed patient, 1157
Trichothiodystrophy, 1694, 1716–1717, *1718*, 1747–1750
Trichotillomania, 780t, 781t, *782*, 782–783
vs. alopecia areata, 1272t
Triethylenethiophosphoramide, and eccrine disorders, 429
Trifluridine, for herpes simplex virus infection, 1078
Trigeminal nerve, anatomy of, 112, *112*, 117
Triglycerides, in xanthoma, 1812, 1814, 1816
Triiodothyronine receptors, in keratinocyte differentiation, 70
Trimethoprim, for acne, 471, 471t
with sulfamethoxazole, adverse reactions to, in human immunodeficiency virus infection, 1145
contraindication to, with methotrexate therapy, 308
for bowel-associated dermatosis-arthritis syndrome, 376, 376t
for chancroid, 976
for granuloma inguinale, 976t, 979
for head louse infestation, 1193

Trimethoprim (*Continued*)
for mycetoma, 1070
for nocardiosis, 1007, 1008t
Trimethylpsoralen. See also *Psoralens*.
with ultraviolet radiation, for vitiligo, 1214
Trioxsalen. See also *Psoralens*.
for dermatitis, of hands and feet, 192
Trumpet nail, 1301–1302
Trypanosomiasis, African, *1174*, 1174–1175
American, *1173*, 1173–1174
Tryptase, in urticaria, 397t, 397–398
Tryptophan, and scleroderma, 891–893, 892t, *893*
deficiency of, and pellagra, photosensitivity with, 766
ethyl ester of, for Hartnup's disorder, 1768
Tsetse fly, as vector of trypanosomiasis, 1174
Tuberculid infection, 985–987, *986, 987*, 988t, Plate 7
Tuberculoid leprosy, 994, 995t, *996*, 999, Plate 7
Tuberculosis, cutaneous signs of, 1882t
hematogenous, 985, *986*, Plate 7
of skin, 983–991
definition of, 983
diagnosis of, 987–988, *988*, 988t
in scrofuloderma, 984–985, 988, 988t
inoculation and, 984, 988t
warty, 984, *984*, 988, 988t
orificial, 985, 988, 988t
treatment of, 988–989, 989t
Tuberous myxedema, atypical, 1839
Tuberous sclerosis, 1226t, 1226–1228, 1228t, 1735–1740
cardiac disorders in, cutaneous signs with, 1879t
clinical features of, cutaneous, 1735–1736, *1735–1737*, 1736t
extracutaneous, 1736–1737
course of, 1738
definition of, 1735
diagnosis of, 1738–1739, 1739t
pathogenesis of, 1738
pathology of, 1738
renal disease in, cutaneous signs with, 1883t, *1885*
tooth abnormalities with, 1324t
Tuberous xanthoma, 1810, *1810*, 1811, 1816
Tularemia, 943–944, *944*, 947, 1034–1035, 1035t
Tumor(s). See also *Cancer* and specific neoplasms, e.g., *Fibroma*.
adrenal, and hirsutism, 1854
and bullous pemphigoid, 665
and leg ulcers, 562t
and lymphedema, 554
and pemphigus, 658–661, *659*, 660t, *661*, 661t, 1847, *1868*
vs. toxic epidermal necrolysis, 710t
angiogenesis in, 1492–1493
carcinoid, vs. scleroderma, 887, 888t
dermatoses with, 1843–1849. See also *Paraneoplastic dermatosis*.
epidermal, benign, 1441–1448
fibrous, 1552–1559
glomus, 1507t, *1513*, 1513–1514, *1514*
of nail bed, 1301
in lymphoma, T-cell, 1640–1641, *1641, 1643*, 1643–1644, 1655
in situ, 108, *108*
of apocrine glands, 1476, 1477t, 1485–1489, *1485–1489*, 1486t, 1488t
of eccrine glands, 1476–1485
of fat, 1526–1530, *1527–1529*
liposuction for, *1530*, 1530–1531

Tumor(s) (*Continued*)
  of genitalia, *1352,* 1352–1353, *1353*
    vs. chancroid, 975t
  of hair follicles, 1464–1474
  of muscle, 1522–1526, *1523–1525,* 1526t
  of nerves, 1536–1549
  of pilosebaceous unit, 1464–1474
  of skin, assessment of, 93, *94, 95,* 95t
  oral, in multiple endocrine neoplasia, 1327
  ovarian, and hirsutism, 1853
  ultraviolet radiation and, 735, 1367–1369,
    1368, 1369
  vasculitis with, cutaneous, 584
Tumor necrosis factors, in angiogenesis,
  1493t, 1494
  in inflammatory response, 144t, 144–145,
    151
  in urticaria, 397t, 398
Tumor suppressor genes, mutations of, in
  skin cancer, *1370,* 1371–1374, *1373*
Tungiasis, 820–821, *821*
Tylotic skin, definition of, 110
Typhoid fever, skin lesions in, 945
Typhoidal tularemia, 1035
Typhus, 1012t, 1017–1019, *1019*
  Queensland tick, 1012t, 1016
  Siberian tick, 1012t, 1016
Tyrosinase, in albinism, 1219–1222, 1220t,
  1221t, *1222*
  in melanin synthesis, 13, *1204,* 1206, 1207
Tyrosinemia, type II, 1859t, 1859–1860, *1860*
  palmoplantar keratoderma in, 1706
Tyson's glands, 30
Tzanck test, in herpes simplex infection, 123,
  1076–1077, *1077*

U

Ulcer(s), aphthous, in human
  immunodeficiency virus infection, 1148,
  1337t
  assessment of, 98–99, *100*
  atheroembolism and, 545t, 547
  drug abuse and, 840
  eosinophilic, of oral mucosa, 1333–1334
  genital, diagnosis of, 1342t
  hemangioma and, in infancy, 1498, 1499,
    1500
  in amebiasis, 1172, *1173*
  in Behçet's disease, 385, *386,* 387
  in chancroid, 973–976, *974,* 975t, 976t
  in cryptococcosis, with human
    immunodeficiency virus infection,
    1141, *1141*
  in granuloma inguinale, *977,* 977–978
  in herpes simplex infection, genital, 1346,
    1346, 1347
  in leishmaniasis, 1163, *1164*
  in livedo vasculopathy, 543, *544,* 546t
  in lymphoma, T-cell, 1642, *1642*
  in necrobiosis lipoidica, 447, *447,* Plate 4
  in nodular vasculitis, 595, *595*
  in pyoderma gangrenosum, 379, *380,*
    381–383, *382,* 382t, Plate 3
  in rheumatoid necrobiosis, 444, *445*
  in syphilis, 949, *950,* 952, *952*
  in varicella-zoster infection, with human
    immunodeficiency virus infection,
    1140, *1140*
  in yaws, 962, *962*
  Mycobacterium ulcerans infection and, 990
  of leg, 558–571
    arterial, 561, *561*
    definition of, 558
    diagnosis of, 561–563, 562t

Ulcer(s) (*Continued*)
  incidence of, 558
  management of, 567–571, 568t, *569,*
    569t, *570*
    venous, 558–560, *559, 560*
    wound healing in, 563–567, *564,* 566t,
      567t
  oral, 1330–1334, *1331*
    in systemic lupus erythematosus, 263
  tuberculous, metastatic, 985, *986*
  with blisters and pustules, in neonate, 712,
    714t
  with diabetes, 1869t, 1870t, *1871*
Ulcerative colitis, cutaneous signs of,
  1872–1874, 1874t, 1875t, *1876*
  pyoderma gangrenosum with, 379, 382, 383
Ultrasonography, in diagnosis of leg ulcers,
  563
Ultraviolet light. See also *Photo-* entries.
  and skin drying, 76
  and skin injury, 77–78, 78t
  clothing as barrier to, 755
  exposure to, allergic reaction to, 726–730,
    729, 729t–731t, Plate 5
    and actinic reticuloid syndrome,
      768–770, *769,* 769t, 770t, Plate 5
    and amyloidosis, 1824, *1825*
    and basal cell carcinoma, 1391
    and bullous pemphigoid, 664–665
    and carcinogenesis, DNA damage in,
      1367
      molecular mechanisms of, 1369–1374,
        1370, 1370t, *1371, 1373*
    and DNA damage, 1364–1366, *1365*
      in mutagenesis, 1367, *1368*
      repair of, 1366t, 1366–1367
    and hydroa vacciniforme, *763,* 763–764,
      764
    and immunosuppression, in tumor
      development, 1367–1369, *1369*
    and lentigo, 1563
    and melanoma, 1576–1577, 1578t, 1595
    and melasma, 1235
    and polymorphic eruption, 758–761,
      759, 760, 760t, 761t
      vs. Jessner's lymphocytic infiltrate, 346
    and skin aging, 732–746. See also
      Photoaging.
    and skin cancer, 1363
    and skin damage, 732–746. See also
      Photodamage.
    and urticaria, 394–395, 400–401, *762,*
      762–763
    biologic response to, 725, *726,* 726t, 727t
    in Bloom's syndrome, 765
    in Cockayne's syndrome, 765, 1802t
    in lupus erythematosus, 84–85, *86, 263,*
      263, 271, 274, 766, Plate 1
    in xeroderma pigmentosum, 765,
      1747–1751, *1748,* 1748t, 1750t
    protection against, sunscreens for,
      752–757. See also *Sunscreens.*
    sports-related, 849, 852
    toxic reaction to, 726–730, *728,* 728t,
      729, 730t, 731t, Plate 4
      with drug reaction, 420
    with infrared radiation, 823–824
  in solar spectrum, 751, 1364, *1364*
  in therapy. See *Phototherapy.*
  radiation intensity of, 751
  skin as barrier to, 53
  skin response to, acute, 751–752
    chronic, 752
  windows as barrier to, 755
Umbilicated lesion, definition of, 110

Umbilicus, adenocarcinoma of, metastatic,
  1674, *1676*
Uncein, in dermoepidermal junction, 623
  in epidermolysis bullosa, 642t, 644
Uncinaria infestation, 1183
  and cutaneous larva migrans, 1181, 1181t
Unna's boots, in leg ulcer management, 567
Unna's paste, in chemical peel, for
  photoaging, 742t
Unna-Thost palmoplantar keratoderma, 1704
Urethra, anatomy of, 1341, *1341*
Urethritis, in Reiter's syndrome, 322
  nongonococcal, 1344
Urine, and diaper dermatitis, 184–187, *185,*
  185t, 186t, Plate 1
Uroporphyrinogen, in heme biosynthesis, in
  porphyria, 1753, 1754, 1754t, *1755*
Urticaria, 392–403
  chemotherapy and, 428
  cholinergic, 392–394, 400
  clinical findings in, 392–395
  definition of, 110, 392, *393*
  diagnosis of, 399–400, *401*
  etiology of, 392, 394t, 399
  exercise-induced, 852
  in drug reactions, *413,* 415–416
  in follicular mucinosis, 1839–1840
  in Sweet's syndrome, 374–375
  insect bites and, 804, 805, *806*
  pathogenesis of, 396–399, 397t, 398t
  pathology of, 396
  solar, idiopathic, *762,* 762–763
    vs. polymorphic light eruption, 760, 760t
  treatment of, 400–403, *401*
  venulitis and, 585t, 585–586, *586*
  with papules and plaques, pruritic, in
    pregnancy, 365–368, *366,* 367t,
    368t
    vs. herpes gestationis, 683
Urticaria pigmentosa, 1603, *1603,* 1606t
Urticarial vasculitis, in systemic lupus
  erythematosus, 263–264
Uta, 1163
Uterine cervix, mucopurulent inflammation
  of, 1344

V

Vaccinia infection, 1095, 1095t
Vacuolar alteration, definition of, 110
Vagina, anatomy of, 1341, *1341*
  candidiasis of, 1343, 1343t, *1345,*
    1345–1346
    after antibiotic therapy, for acne, 472
  infection of, diagnosis of, 1343, 1343t
Vaginitis, diagnosis of, 1342t
  nonspecific, 1344
  streptococcal infection and, 1343
Vaginosis, bacterial, 1344
Valley fever, 1063
Vancomycin, and red man syndrome, 420
  for staphylococcal infection, 923t
  for streptococcal infection, 923t
Varicella-zoster infection, 1078–1081,
  1079–1081, 1081t
  and oral lesions, 1335t
  and pneumonia, 1882t
  genital, 1347
  in immunosuppressed patient, 1156–1157
  in neonate, 715t, 718
  lesions of, configuration of, *87*
  rash in, 1124t, 1125t, 1131
  vs. smallpox, 1094, 1094t
  with human immunodeficiency virus
    infection, *1140,* 1140–1141

Varicose veins, 574–581. See also *Veins, varicose.*
Variola infection, 1093–1095, *1094*, 1094t, 1095t
Vascular cell adhesion molecule-1, in inflammatory response, 147, 149
Vascular endothelial cell growth factor, 1493t, 1494
Vascular leak syndrome, interleukin-2 and, in erythroderma, 338
Vascular plexus, superficial, definition of, 110
Vasculitis, 515–532
 and gastrointestinal hemorrhage, 1875t
 and leg ulcers, 562t
 definition of, 110
 drug-induced, 418–419
 immune complex, in granuloma annulare, 440–441
 in human immunodeficiency virus infection, 1149
 in polyarteritis, microscopic, 522–527, *523, 526,* 526t
 in polyarteritis nodosa, 519–521, *520,* 520t
 in Rocky Mountain spotted fever, 1013–1014, *1014*
 in systemic lupus erythematosus, 263–264
 in temporal arteritis, 515–517, *516,* 516t
 leukocytoclastic, 584–589, 585t, *585–587,* 586t, 588t
 nodular, 594–596, *595, 596,* 597t
 of coronary arteries, cutaneous signs with, 1879t
 treatment of, 1887t
Vasculopathy, actinic, 735
 livedo, 543–545, *544,* 545t, 546t
Vegetation, cutaneous, definition of, 110
Veins. See also *Blood vessels.*
 disease of, and leg ulcers, 558–560, *559, 560,* 562t
 fistula to, from artery, punch hair grafting and, 1259
 in thermoregulation, 55
 inflammation of, chemotherapy and, 428
  cords in, 102, *102*
  in Behçet's disease, 386–387
  paraneoplastic, *1847,* 1847–1848
 insufficiency of, clinical findings in, 575
  definition of, 574
 malformations of, 1496t, *1503,* 1503–1506, *1504*
 of face, anatomy of, 115
 varicose, clinical findings in, 575
  definition of, 574
  diagnosis of, 577–580, 578t
  pathogenesis of, 576–577
  pathology of, 575–576, *576–578*
  sclerotherapy for, 574, *580,* 580–581
Vellus hair cysts, eruptive, 1451, *1454*
Vellus hairs, definition of, 110
 in alopecia, androgenetic, 1250, 1252, *1253*
 in hypertrichosis, paraneoplastic, 1844, *1844, 1867*
Venous lakes, 1509
Venules, cutaneous, 21, 23
Venulitis, cutaneous, 584–589, 585t
 clinical findings in, 584–586, *585,* 585t, *586*
 diagnosis of, 588
 laboratory findings in, 586t, 586–587, *587*
 pathogenesis of, 587–588
 treatment of, 588–589
Vermilion border, sebaceous glands of, 30–31, 1325
Vermix caseosa, 5

Verocay bodies, in schwannoma, 1539, *1540*
Verrucae (warts), 1100–1117. See also *Papillomavirus infection.*
 anogenital, child abuse and, 1892
 configuration of, *87*
 contour of, *92*
 electrocoagulation for, 491, *491*
 flat, 1101, *1101,* 1102t, 1107, *1108*
 genital, 1102t, 1102–1104, *1102–1104,* 1106
 periungual, 1299t, 1305
 Peruvian, 1024t, 1024–1028, *1026,* 1027t
 plane, vs. acne, 469
 vs. stucco keratosis, 1447
Verrucous (warty) lesions, definition of, 110
 in carcinoma, 1385–1386, *1386*
  genital, 1353
  oral, 1329
 in incontinentia pigmenti, 1725, *1726*
 in syringocystadenoma papilliferum, 1484t, 1485, *1486*
 in syringoid carcinoma, 1484, 1484t
 in tuberculosis, 984, *984,* 988, 988t
Versican, in dermal extracellular matrix, 876
Vertical mattress suture, *135,* 135–136
Vesicle(s), assessment of, 94–96, *95–97,* 96t
 genital, diagnosis of, 1342t
 in herpes simplex virus infection, 1074–1077, *1075–1077*
 in hydroa vacciniforme, 763, *764*
 in incontinentia pigmenti, 1725, 1726, *1726, 1727,* 1728
 in neonate, 716t, 720, 1897
 in polymorphic light eruption, 758, 759, *759, 760*
 in varicella-zoster virus infection, 1079, 1080, *1080*
 insect bites and, 804, *806*
Vesicopustules, 97
Vesiculobullous disease, and scarring alopecia, 1290–1291
Vestibulitis, vulvar, 1354, *1354,* Plate 9
Vibrio vulnificus infection, 942, 946, 947
Villous lesions, definition of, 110
Vinblastine, for angiolymphoid hyperplasia with eosinophilia, 1513
Vincristine, for hypereosinophilic syndrome, 357
Violinists, acne mechanica in, 772
Viral infection, and erythema nodosum, 593, 594t
 and hepatitis, cutaneous signs of, 1877t
 and lupus erythematosus, 271
 genital, *1346,* 1346–1349, *1348*
 in atopic dermatitis, 197, 201
 in lymphoma, cutaneous T-cell, 1647
 in Rosai-Dorfman disease, 1618
 oral, 1334–1335, 1335t, 1337t
 rash in, enteroviruses and, 1124t, 1125t, 1131–1132, *1132*
  epidemiology of, 1123, 1126t
  Epstein-Barr virus and, 1124t, 1125t, 1132–1134, *1134*
  history in, 1123–1126, 1126t
  human immunodeficiency virus and, 1124t, 1125t, 1130, *1130,* Plate 8
  in erythema infectiosum, 1124t, 1125t, *1128,* 1128–1129, Plate 8
  in Gianotti-Crosti syndrome, 1124t, 1125t, 1133–1134, *1134,* Plate 9
  in measles, 1124t, 1125t, 1126–1127, *1127,* Plate 8
  in roseola, 1124t, 1125t, 1129–1130, *1130*
  in rubella, 1124t, 1125t, 1127–1128

Viral infection (*Continued*)
 pathophysiology of, 1126
 physical examination in, 1124t–1126t, 1126
 varicella and, 1124t, 1125t, 1131
Virilization, and hirsutism, 1855
Vitamin A. See also *Retinoids.*
 deficiency of, cutaneous signs of, 1873t
 in wound healing, 567
Vitamin B$_1$ deficiency, cutaneous signs of, 1873t
Vitamin B$_2$ deficiency, cutaneous signs of, 1873t
Vitamin B$_6$ deficiency, cutaneous signs of, 1873t
Vitamin B$_{12}$ deficiency, cutaneous signs of, 1873t
Vitamin C, deficiency of, cutaneous signs of, 1873t, *1874*
 gastrointestinal hemorrhage in, 1875t
 in wound healing, 567
 in facial skin care, 80
Vitamin D, deficiency of, cutaneous signs of, 1873t
 for psoriasis, 307
 receptors of, in keratinocyte differentiation, 69–70
 rickets resistant to, and alopecia, 1712
 with steroid therapy, for systemic lupus erythematosus, 277
Vitamin E, deficiency of, cutaneous signs of, 1873t
 for pityriasis rubra pilaris, 334–335
 in facial skin care, 80–81
Vitamin K, deficiency of, cutaneous signs of, 1873t
 in wound healing, 567
 in coumarin-induced skin necrosis, 546t, 550
Vitiligo, 104, *104,* 1210–1216, *1211,* 1211t, 1213t, 1214t
 clinical findings in, 1210–1212, *1211,* 1211t
 definition of, 1210
 differential diagnosis of, 1213t, 1213–1214
 macules in, 88, 89t, *90*
 pathogenesis of, 1212–1213
 pathology of, 1212
 treatment of, 1214t, 1214–1216
 with diabetes, 1869t
 with thyroid disease, *1872*
Vohwinkel palmoplantar keratoderma, 1704
von Hippel–Lindau syndrome, 1799t, *1801*
von Recklinghausen's disease, 1729–1735. See also *Neurofibromatosis.*
von Willebrand factor, in Raynaud's phenomenon, 539
von Zumbusch pustular psoriasis, 297–298
 vs. generalized exanthematous pustulosis, drug-induced, 422
Vörner palmoplantar keratoderma, 1704
Vulva, anatomy of, 1341, *1341*
 candidiasis of, *1345,* 1345–1346
 disorders of, topical therapy for, 1356–1357, *1357*
 intraepithelial neoplasia of, classification of, 1340, 1341t
 pain in, 1353–1356, *1354, 1355,* Plate 9
 diagnosis of, 1342, 1342t
 tumors of, 1352–1353, *1353*
 vestibulitis of, 1354, *1354,* Plate 9
Vulvitis, Zoon's, 1354–1355
Vulvovaginitis, diagnosis of, 1342t
 streptococcal infection and, 1343
V-Y plasty, after skin cancer excision, *1411*

W

Waardenburg's syndrome, 1225, 1225t
Warfarin, as anticoagulant, biopsy after, 121–122
   for antiphospholipid syndrome, 546t, 549
Warts, 1100–1117. See also *Papillomavirus infection* and *Verrucae.*
   Peruvian, 1024t, 1024–1028, *1026,* 1027t
Wasp stings, 807t, 807–808, 808t
Water, and urticaria, 395, 400
   copper in, and hair discoloration, 849–850, 852–853
   sunscreen resistance to, 753
Water sports, and skin disorders, 787–802. See also *Aquatic skin disorders.*
Weber-Cockayne epidermolysis bullosa, 637, *637,* 643
   genetic mutation in, 9, 61–62
Webster transposition flap, after skin cancer excision, 1414–1415
Wegener's granulomatosis, 522–527, *523, 525, 526,* 526t
   oral lesions in, 1334
   pulmonary disease in, cutaneous signs with, 1882t
   vs. polychondritis, relapsing, 513
Weibel-Palade bodies, 23
Weight, and hidradenitis suppurativa, 1482
   loss of, alopecia with, diffuse, 1275–1276
Wells' syndrome, 360–363, *361,* 362t, Plate 3
Werner's syndrome, 1713, 1803t
Whirlpool folliculitis, 851, 853, 940–941, *941*
White sponge nevus, 1325
Whitlow, herpetic, 1076, *1076*
Wickham's striae, in lichen planus, 235, *236,* 237, Plate 1
Willebrand factor, in Raynaud's phenomenon, 539
Wilson's disease, cutaneous signs of, 1877t
Windows, ultraviolet radiation blocking by, 755
Winer's dilated pore, 1464–1465
Wohlfahrtia larvae, in furuncular myiasis, 819
Wolman's disease, vs. neutral lipid storage disease, 1693–1694
Woringer-Kolopp disease, 1641, 1644
Workplace, antigen exposure in, and contact dermatitis, 173–181. See also *Contact dermatitis.*
   chemical exposure in, and burns, 843–847, 844t, 845t
   and lymphoma, 1648

Woronoff's ring, in plaque psoriasis, 296
Wounds, care of, after laser ablation of warts, 1116
   healing of, biology of, 563–567, *564,* 566t, 567t
   myiasis of, 820, *820*
WR 6026, for leishmaniasis, 1170
Wrestlers, herpes gladiatorum in, 851, 853, 1075
Wrinkles, ultraviolet light exposure and, 733t, 733–735, *734–736,* Plate 5
   chemical peel for, 741–746, *742,* 742t, 743t, *744–746,* 745t, 746t
Wuchereria bancrofti infestation, *1174,* 1179
Wyburn-Mason syndrome, 1506, 1799t, *1801*

X

Xanthelasma, pathology of, 1811, *1811*
Xanthelasma palpebrarum, 1809, *1810,* 1816
Xanthoerythroderma perstans, 222
Xanthogranuloma, juvenile, 1620–1622, *1621, 1622,* 1622t
   nodules in, *94*
   necrobiotic, 446t, 448–450, *449*
Xanthoma, 1809–1817
   clinical findings in, 1809–1810, *1810*
   definition of, 1809
   diagnosis of, 1815t, 1815–1816
   fibrous, atypical, 1553t, 1555t, *1558,* 1558–1559
   paraneoplastic, 1848
   pathogenesis of, 1811–1815, *1812*
   pathology of, 1811, *1811*
   prognosis of, 1817
   treatment of, 1816–1817
   with diabetes, 1814, 1870t, *1871*
Xanthoma disseminatum, 1623
Xenobiotics, metabolism of, epidermal, 52
Xeroderma pigmentosum, 765, 1747–1751, 1803t, *1805*
   and melanoma, 1576
   carcinoma with, retinoids for, 1430–1431
   clinical findings in, 1747–1749, *1748,* 1748t
   definition of, 1747
   diagnosis of, 1750–1751
   DNA photodamage and, 737, 738
   DNA repair system in, 1364, 1366–1367
   pathogenesis of, 1749–1750, 1750t
   pathology of, 1749
   treatment of, 1751
Xerosis, in atopic dermatitis, 196
   retinoids and, 310

Xerostomia, 1328
Xylocaine. See *Lidocaine.*

Y

Yangtze River fever, 1186
Yaws, *962,* 962–963
   forest, 1163
Yeast infection. See specific organisms, e.g., *Malassezia furfur.*
Yersinia pestis infection, 943, *1033,* 1033–1034, 1034t

Z

Zidovudine, adverse reactions to, 1145
   for Kaposi's sarcoma, 1154–1155
Zinc, deficiency of, and alopecia, diffuse, 1276
   cutaneous signs of, 1873t
   for alopecia areata, 1273t
   malabsorption of, and acrodermatitis enteropathica, 1763–1765
Zinc oxide, in sunscreens, 754
Zinc protoporphyrin, in porphyria, 1760t
Zinc pyrithione, for seborrheic dermatitis, 217, 217t
Zinsser-Engmann-Cole syndrome (dyskeratosis congenita), 1705, *1705,* 1796t, *1798*
   oral lesions in, 1329
Zoonotic infection, and anthrax, 1030–1032, *1031,* 1031t, 1032t
   and brucellosis, 1032t, 1032–1033, 1033t
   and plague, *1033,* 1033–1034, 1034t
   and tularemia, 1034–1035, 1035t
   poxviruses in, 1096t, 1096–1098, *1097*
Zoon's vulvitis, 1354–1355
Zoster, 1078–1081. See also *Varicella-zoster infection.*
Zosteriform lesions, definition of, 110
Z-plasty, after skin cancer excision, *1412,* 1413
Zunich-Kaye syndrome, 1697
Zyderm Collagen, in acne scar treatment, 474
Zygoma, anatomy of, 111
Zygomatic branch, of facial nerve, anatomy of, 113, *113,* 116, 116t, 117
Zygomatic nerve, anatomy of, 117
Zygomaticus muscles, anatomy of, 113, *113*
Zygomycosis, 1072
   in immunosuppressed patient, 1157